The Complete
Directory
for People with
Chronic Illness

2011/12
Tenth Edition

The Complete Directory for People with Chronic Illness

- Condition Descriptions
- Associations
- Publications
- Research Centers
- Support Groups
- Websites

A SEDGWICK PRESS Book

Grey House Publishing

PUBLISHER:	Leslie Mackenzie
EDITOR:	Richard Gottlieb
EDITORIAL DIRECTOR:	Laura Mars
PRODUCTION MANAGER:	Kristen Thatcher
PRODUCTION ASSISTANTS:	Cathy Hughes, Nicole Palumbo, Erica Schneider
MARKETING DIRECTOR:	Jessica Moody

A Sedgwick Press Book
Grey House Publishing, Inc.
4919 Route 22
Amenia, NY 12501
518.789.8700
FAX 518.789.0545
www.greyhouse.com
E-MAIL: books@greyhouse.com

First edition published 1994
Tenth edition published 2011
Printed in Canada
All rights reserved
The complete directory for people with chronic illness – 1994-2011

       1053 p.; 27.5 cm
       Other title: DCI
       ISSN: 1080-7659

1.   Chronic diseases – United States – Directories. 2. Chronic Diseases – Bibliography. 3. Chronic Disease – United States – Directories. 4. Social Support – United States – Directories. 5. Information Services – United States – Directories. 6. Rehabilitation – United States – Directories. I. Title: DCI.

RC108 .C645
616' .0025'73   96-640803

ISBN: 978-1-59237-741-1

Table of Contents

Introduction

Health care professionals estimate that 133 million Americans currently suffer from a chronic illness and, due to the aging of our population, this number will reach 171 million by 2030. This tenth edition of *The Complete Directory for People with Chronic Illness* offers a comprehensive overview of 89 specific chronic illnesses from Addison's to Wilson's Disease. Each chapter includes an easy-to-understand medical description, plus a wide range of condition-specific support services and information resources that deal with the variety of issues concerning those with a chronic illness, as well as those who support the chronic illness community.

> *"...The strength of this source is ... in the information referral portion of each entry: the wide range of resources and organizations presented that can assist with additional information and support ..."*
>
> **American Reference Books Annual, 2010**

"Chronic" comes from the Greek word *chronos* meaning time (Greek god Chronos is often depicted as Father Time). Chronic Illness Alliance defines chronic illness as ... *an illness that is permanent or lasts a long time. It may get slowly worse over time [or] go away. It may cause permanent changes to the body [and] will certainly affect the person's quality of life.* National Center for Health Statistics defines chronic illness as *lasting 3 months or more.*

However you define chronic illness, this new edition provides thousands of ways to deal with the many aspects of chronic disease. It includes associations, state agencies, libraries & resource centers, research centers, magazines, newsletters, audio & video tapes, hot lines, support groups and web sites. In addition to chapters dealing with specific chronic conditions, this edition includes several chapters relevant to the chronic illness community in general, such as wish foundations, death and bereavement groups and medical homes – primary care settings in the community.

The Complete Directory for People with Chronic Illness provides critical information to those dealing for the first time with the stress and crucial need-to-know issues, as well as to those already coping with chronic disease. *How can I connect with others with diabetes? What cancer treatment is best for me? When do I need to protect my 2-year old with a heart condition from normal play? Why is my healthy child angrier than his chronically ill sibling?* You'll find ways to answer these questions and more in the pages of this edition.

In addition to patients and their families, this directory offers sought-after support for hospital and medical center personnel, especially discharge planners, social service workers, and disability coordinators. *The Complete Directory for People with Chronic Illness* is full of resources crucial for people with chronic illness as they transition from diagnosis to home, home to work, and work to community life.

The Complete Directory for People with Chronic Illness provides, in one source, **comprehensive, critical, immediate information** – from national associations to children's books. It is the perfect choice for those who find navigating the Internet overwhelming (we've done it for you), as well as for those who feel comfortable surfing the Net (we provide valuable, specific web sites).

Educational Material
- To access information by specific chronic illness, body system, or disorder category, the cross-referenced *Chronic Illness – Body System* chart in the front of the book makes it easy.
- *Next Steps After Your Diagnosis* is a detailed, 21-page article, with information and support resources in five important categories, listed below, plus critical phone numbers and web sites.
  1. Take the Time you Need
  2. Get the Support you Need
  3. Talk with Your Doctor
  4. Seek out Information
  5. Decide on a Treatment Plan

Arrangement

The 89 chronic condition chapters are arranged alphabetically by name of the disorder. Each chapter begins with a brief description of the illness, written in layman's terms, with probable causes, symptoms and treatment options.

Following each description are disease-specific resources. Chapters contain the following: **National Associations; State Agencies; Libraries & Resource Centers; Magazines, Newsletters, Pamphlets; Research Centers; Books for Adults; Books for Children; Support Groups & Hotlines; Audio & Video Resources; Web Sites.**

This reference work profiles 10,905 listings. Thousands have been verified or updated, with more data points, more web sites, more key executives. Listings include the name of the organization or publication, address, phone, 8,559 fax numbers, 5,626 e-mails, 8,693 web sites, and 8,816 key executives. Brief descriptions and other details are included depending on the type of listing; Associations, for example, may include year founded and yearly dues, while Magazines may include frequency and number of pages.

In addition to the 89 chapters of chronic illnesses, *The Complete Directory for People with Chronic Illness* includes several supplemental chapters in the back of the book designed to provide value to individuals with chronic illness and their families: **General Resources** – information relevant to the general chronic illness community; **Wish Foundations** – organizations devoted to granting wishes of chronically and terminally ill individuals; and **Death & Bereavement** – support services for those who find themselves or a loved one close to death or grieving a loss.

Rounding out this directory are two indexes that allow users additional access to the information: **Entry Name Index** and **Geographic Index**.

The Complete Directory for People with Chronic Illness is also available for subscription on G.O.L.D. – Grey House OnLine Database. Subscribers to G.O.L.D. can access their subscription via the Internet and do customized searches that make finding information quicker and easier. Visit http://gold.greyhouse.com for more information.

CHRONIC ILLNESS — BODY SYSTEM

The following chart lists the chronic illness and its body system(s) or disorder category. Chronic conditions not listed do not fall into a specific system(s). A cross-reference chart follows that lists the information in reverse — body system or disorder categories followed by chronic illnesses.

CHRONIC ILLNESS . . . . **BODY SYSTEM/DISORDER CATEGORY**

Addison's Disease . . . . Endocrine
Aging . . . . Cells & Tissues
AIDS/HIV . . . . Immune, Infectious Disease
Allergies . . . . Immune
Alzheimer's Disease . . . . Nervous
Amyotrophic Lateral Sclerosis . . . . Nervous
Arthritis . . . . Muscular, Skeletal
Asthma . . . . Respiratory
Ataxia . . . . Nervous
Attention Deficit Hyperactivity Disorder . . . . Behavioral, Developmental
Autistic Spectrum Disorders . . . . Behavioral, Developmental
Brain Tumors. . . . . Nervous
Carpal Tunnel Syndrome. . . . . Muscular, Skeletal, Nervous
Celiac Disease . . . . Gastrointestinal
Cerebral Palsy . . . . Nervous, Muscular
Chronic Fatigue Syndrome . . . . Immune
Chronic Pain . . . . Nervous
Cooley's Anemia (Thalassemia) . . . . Blood
Congential Heart Disease . . . . Cardiovascular
Crohn's Disease. . . . . Gastrointestinal
Cystic Fibrosis. . . . . Respiratory, Gastrointestinal
Diabetes Mellitus. . . . . Endocrine
Down Syndrome . . . . Developmental
Eating Disorders (Anorexia Nervosa, Bulimia) . . . . Behavioral
Endometriosis . . . . Reproductive
Fabry Disease . . . . Gastrointestinal
Fibromyalgia Syndrome . . . . Muscular, Skeletal
Gastrointestinal Disorders. Gastrointestinal
Gaucher's Disease. . . . . Gastrointestinal
Growth Disorders . . . . Developmental
Head Injuries . . . . Nervous
Hearing Impairment . . . . Sensory
Heart Disease. . . . . Cardiovascular
Hemophilia . . . . Blood
Hepatitis . . . . Infectious Disease
Hydrocephalus. . . . . Nervous
Hypertension . . . . Cardiovascular
Impotence . . . . Reproductive
Incontinence . . . . Urinary
Infertility . . . . Reproductive
Kidney Disease . . . . Gastrointestinal

CHRONIC ILLNESS . . . . **BODY SYSTEM/DISORDER CATEGORY**

Liver Disease. . . . . Gastrointestinal
Lung Disease. . . . . Respiratory
Lupus Erythematosus . . . . Cells & Tissues
Mental Illness: General . . . . Behavioral
Mental Illness: Depression . . . . Behavioral
Mental Illness: Schizophrenia. . . . . Behavioral
Migraine . . . . Cardiovascular, Nervous
Multiple Sclerosis . . . . Nervous
Muscular Dystrophy . . . . Nervous
Myasthenia Gravis. . . . . Nervous
Neurofibromatosis. . . . . Nervous, Dermatologic
Osteogenesis Imperfecta . . . . Skeletal
Osteoporosis . . . . Skeletal
Paget's Disease . . . . Skeletal
Parkinson Disease . . . . Nervous
Post-Polio Syndrome. . . . . Muscular, Skeletal
Prader Willi Syndrome . . . . Endocrine
Raynaud's Disease. . . . . Cardiovascular
Sarcoidosis . . . . Cells & Tissues, Respiratory
Scleroderma. . . . . Cells & Tissues, Dermatologic
Scoliosis . . . . Skeletal
Seizure Disorders . . . . Nervous
Sexually Transmitted Diseases . . . . Reproductive, Infectious Disease
Sickle Cell Disease . . . . Blood
Sjogren's Syndrome . . . . Cells & Tissues
Skin Disorders. . . . . Dermatologic
Sleep Disorders . . . . Dermatologic
Spina Bifida. . . . . Nervous, Skeletal
Spinal Cord Injuries . . . . Nervous
Stroke. . . . . Nervous
Substance Abuse . . . . Behavioral
Tay Sachs Disease. . . . . Nervous
Thyroid Disease. . . . . Endorcrine
Tick-Borne Disease . . . . Infectious Disease
Tourette Syndrome . . . . Nervous
Tuberculosis . . . . Respiratory, Infectious Disease
Tuberous Sclerosis . . . . Nervous, Dermatologic
Turner Syndrome. . . . . Endocrine
Ulcerative Colitis. . . . . Gastrointestinal
Visual Impairment. . . . . Sensory
War Syndromes . . . . Nervous
Wilson's Disease . . . . Gastrointestinal

BY BODY SYSTEM/DISORDER CATEGORY

Behavioral
Attention Deficit Disorder; Autism; Eating Disorders; Mental Illness; Substance Abuse

Blood
Cooley's Anemia; Hemophilia; Sickle Cell Disease

Cardiovascular
Heart Disease; Hypertension; Migraine; Raynaud's Disease

Cells & Tissues
Aging; Lupus Erythematosus; Scleroderma; Sjogren's Syndrome

Dermatologic
Neurofibromatosis; Scleroderma; Skin Disorders; Tuberous Sclerosis

Developmental
Attention Deficit Disorder; Autism; Down Syndrome; Growth Disorders

Endocrine
Addison's Disease; Diabetes; Turner Syndrome

Gastrointestinal
Celiac Disease; Crohn's Disease; Cystic Fibrosis; Fabry Disease; Gastrointestinal Disorders; Gaucher's Disease; Kidney Disease; Liver Disease; Ulcerative Colitis

Immune
AIDS; Allergies; Chronic Fatigue Syndrome

Infectious Disease
AIDS; Hepatitis; Sexually Transmitted Diseases; Tick-Borne Disease; Tuberculosis

Muscular
Arthritis; Carpal Tunnel Syndrome; Cerebral Palsy; Fibromyalgia Syndrome; Post-Polio Syndrome

Nervous
Agent Orange Related Injuries; Alzheimer's Disease; Amyotrophic Lateral Sclerosis; Ataxia; Brain Tumors; Carpal Tunnel Syndrome; Cerebral Palsy; Charcot-Marie-Tooth Disorder; Chronic Pain; Gulf War Syndrome; Head Injuries; Hydrocephalus; Multiple Sclerosis; Muscular Dystrophy; Myasthenia Gravis; Neurofibromatosis; Parkinson Disease; Seizure Disorders; Spina Bifida; Spinal Cord Injuries; Stroke; Tourette Syndrome; Tuberous Sclerosis

Reproductive
Endometriosis; Impotence; Infertility; Sexually Transmitted Diseases

Respiratory
Asthma; Cystic Fibrosis; Lung Disease; Tuberculosis

Skeletal
Arthritis; Carpal Tunnel Syndrome; Fibromyalgia Syndrome; Osteognesis Imperfecta; Osteoporosis; Paget's Disease; Post-Polio Syndrome; Scoliosis; Spina Bifida

Sensory
Hearing Impairment; Visual Impairment

Urinary
Incontinence

Next Steps After Your Diagnosis: Finding Information and Support

Introduction

Your doctor* gave you a diagnosis that could change your life. This article can help you take the next steps.

Every person is different, of course, and every person's disease or condition will affect them differently. But research shows that after getting a diagnosis, many people have some of the same reactions and needs.

About this Article

Next Steps After Your Diagnosis offers general advice for people with almost any disease or condition. And it has tips to help you learn more about your specific problem and how it can be treated.

The information in this article is presented in a simple way to help you scan the material and read only what you need right now. Organizations, publications, and other resources are included if you would like to know more. The on-line version www.ahrq.gov/consumer/diaginfo.htm has many additional resources and their Internet links.

Five Basic Steps

This article describes five basic steps to help you cope with your diagnosis, make decisions, and get on with your life.

Step 1: Take the time you need.
Do not rush important decisions about your health. In most cases, you will have time to carefully examine your options and decide what is best for you.

Step 2: Get the support you need.
Look for support from family and friends, people who are going through the same thing you are, and those who have "been there." They can help you cope with your situation and make informed decisions.

---

* Your medical care might come from a doctor, nurse, physician assistant, or another kind of clinician or health care practitioner. To keep it simple, in this article we use the term "doctor" to refer to any of these professionals with whom you might interact.

Step 3: Talk with your doctor.

Good communication with your doctor can help you feel more satisfied with the care you receive. Research shows it can even have a positive effect on things such as symptoms and pain. Getting a "second opinion" may help you feel more confident about your care.

Step 4: Seek out information.

When learning about your health problem and its treatment, look for information that is based on a careful review of the latest scientific findings published in medical journals.

Step 5: Decide on a treatment plan.

Work with your doctor to decide on a treatment plan that best meets your needs.

As you take each step, remember this: Research shows that patients who are more involved in their health care tend to get better results and be more satisfied.

Step 1:
Take the time you need.

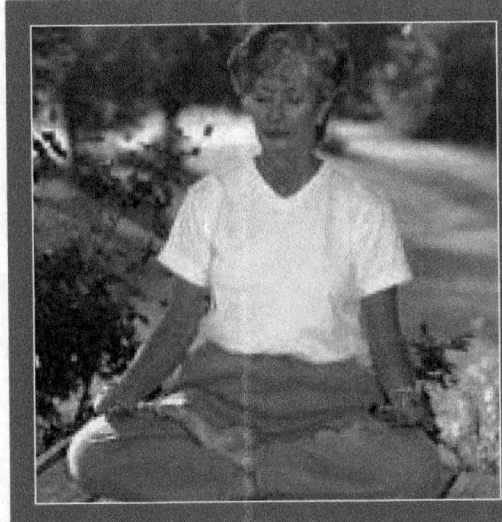

Take time to breathe. Don't panic, and don't feel pressured into making a rush decision.

Alexis, cancer survivor

A diagnosis can change your life in an instant.

Like so many other people in your situation, you might be feeling one or more of the following emotions after getting your diagnosis:

- Afraid
- Alone
- Angry
- Anxious
- Ashamed
- Confused
- Depressed
- Helpless
- In denial
- Numb
- Overwhelmed
- Panicky
- Powerless
- Relieved (that you finally know what's wrong)
- Sad
- Shocked
- Stressed

It is perfectly normal to have these feelings. It is also normal, and very common, to have trouble taking in and understanding information after you receive the news – especially if the diagnosis was a surprise. And it can be even harder to make decisions about treating or managing your disease or condition.

Take time to make your decisions.

No matter how the news of your diagnosis has affected you, do not rush into a decision. In most cases, you do not need to take action right away. Ask your doctor how much time you can safely take.

Taking the time you need to make decisions can help you:

- Feel less anxious and stressed.

- Avoid depression.

- Cope with your condition.

- Feel more in control of your situation.

- Play a key role in decisions about your treatment.

Step 2:
Get the support you need.

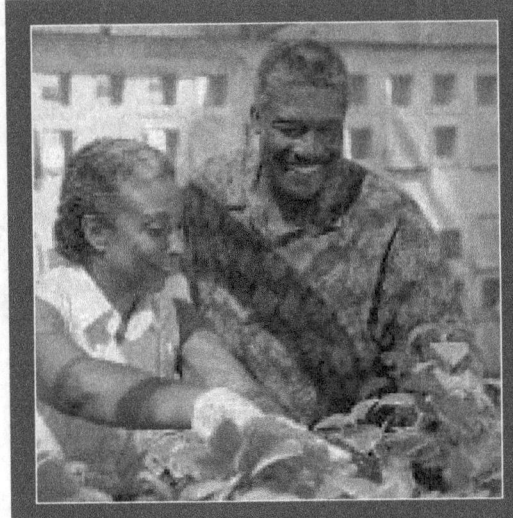

I was shocked when I was diagnosed with diabetes. The extra support I got from my friends and support group really helped me adjust to the new lifestyle I had to adopt.

Richard, person with diabetes

You do not have to go through it alone.

Sometimes the emotional side of illness can be just as hard to deal with as the physical side. You may have fears or concerns. You may feel overwhelmed. No matter what your situation, having other people to turn to will help you know you are not alone.

Here are the kinds of support you might want to seek:

▓ Family and friends.

Talking to family and friends you feel close to can help you cope with your illness or condition. Just knowing that someone is there can be a comfort.

Sometimes it is hard to ask for help. And sometimes your family and friends want to help, but they do not want to intrude, or they do not know how to ask or what to offer. Think about specific ways people can help you. One idea is to ask someone to come with you to a doctor's appointment to help ask questions, take notes, and talk with you afterward.

If you do not have family or friends who can provide support, other people or groups can.

Support or self-help groups.

Support groups are made up of people with the same disease or condition who get together to share information and concerns and to help one another. Support groups may or may not be led by experts. Self-help groups are similar to support groups but usually are led by the participants. The names "support group" and "self-help group" sometimes are used to refer to either kind.

Research on support groups shows that participants feel less anxious, experience less depression, have a better quality of life, and have more success coping with their disease or condition. Similar findings have been reported for self-help groups.

On-line support or self-help groups.

The Internet has support or self-help groups for people whose concerns and situations may be similar to yours. You can also find "message boards," where you can post questions and get answers. These on-line communities can help you connect with people who can give you support and provide information.

But be careful. Not every idea or treatment you come across in these groups will be scientifically proven to be safe and effective. If you read about something interesting and new, check it out with your doctor.

Counselor or therapist.

A good counselor or therapist can help you cope with sadness, depression, and feelings of being overwhelmed. If you think this kind of help might be right for you, ask your doctor or other health care professional to recommend someone in your area.

People like you.

You might want to meet and talk with someone in your own situation. Someone who has "been there" can talk about the real-life outcomes of their treatment choices as well as how they have learned to live with their disease or condition. Some advocacy or support groups can help you make this kind of contact.

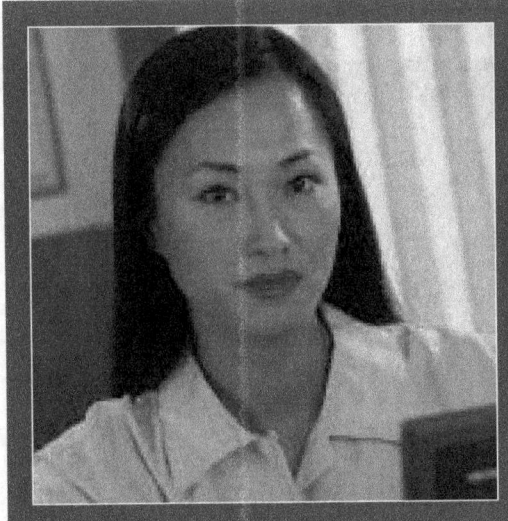

If only I had known what it would be like to live with the after-effects of this type of surgery, I might have chosen a different kind.

Susan, who underwent surgery for a digestive disease

Help is available.

Take advantage of the support that is available to you. See "Where to Find More Information" on page xxx for specific places to find support. An expanded list appears in the on-line version of this article at www.ahrq.gov/consumer/diaginfo.htm.

Step 3:
Talk with your doctor.

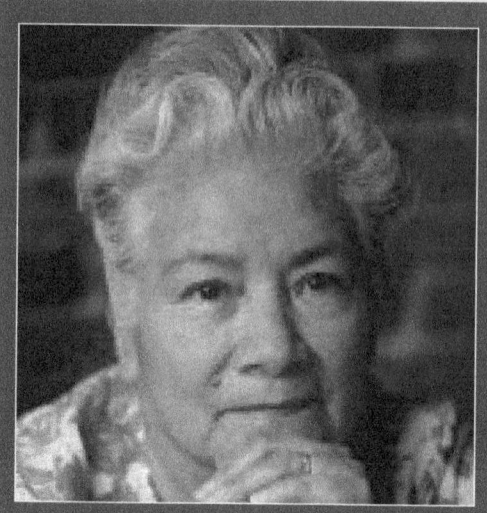

I had trouble under-standing what my doctor was telling me. The words were too technical, and there was too much to absorb. I finally asked her to slow down and keep it simple. That helped a lot.

Dana, person with heart disease

Your doctor is your partner in health care.

You probably have many questions about your disease or condition. The first person to ask is your doctor.

It is fine to seek more information from other sources; in fact, it is important to do so. But consider your doctor your partner in health care—someone who can discuss your situation with you, explain your options, and help you make decisions that are right for you.

It is not always easy to feel comfortable around doctors. But research has shown that good communication with your doctor can actually be good for your health. It can help you to:

• Feel more satisfied with the care you receive.

• Have better outcomes (end results), such as reduced pain and better recovery from symptoms.

Being an active member of your health care team also helps to reduce your chances of medical mistakes, and it helps you get high-quality care.

Of course, good communication is a two-way street. Here are some ways to help make the most of the time you spend with your doctor.

Prepare for your visit.

- Think about what you want to get out of your appointment. Write down all your questions and concerns. Some suggested questions are listed on page xxiii.

- Prepare and bring to your doctor visit a list of all the medicines you take.

- Consider bringing along a trusted relative or friend. This person can help ask questions, take notes, and help you remember and understand everything once you leave the doctor's office.

Give information to your doctor.

- Do not wait to be asked.

- Tell your doctor everything he or she needs to know about your health—even the things that might make you feel embarrassed or uncomfortable.

- Tell your doctor how you are feeling—both physically and emotionally.

- Tell your doctor if you are feeling depressed or overwhelmed.

Get information from your doctor.

- Ask questions about anything that concerns you. Keep asking until you understand the answers. If you do not, your doctor may think you understand everything that is said.

- Ask your doctor to draw pictures if that will help you understand something.

- Take notes.

- Tape record your doctor visit, if that will be helpful to you. But first ask your doctor if this is okay.

- Ask your doctor to recommend resources such as Web sites, booklets, or tapes with more information about your disease or condition.

Also see "Ten Important Questions to Ask Your Doctor After a Diagnosis," on page xxiii.

Do not hesitate to seek a second opinion.

A second opinion is when another doctor examines your medical records and gives his or her views about your condition and how it should be treated. You might want a second opinion to:

- Be clear about what you have.

- Know all of your treatment choices.

- Have another doctor look at your choices with you.

It is not pushy or rude to want a second opinion. Most doctors will understand that you need more information before making important decisions about your health.

Check to see whether your health plan covers a second opinion. In some cases, health plans require second opinions.

Here are some ways to find a doctor for a second opinion:

- Ask your doctor. Request someone who does not work in the same office, because doctors who work together tend to share similar views.

- Contact your health plan or your local hospital, medical society, or medical school.

- Use the Doctor Finder on-line service of the American Medical Association at www.ama-assn.org.

Get information about next steps.

- Get the results of any tests or procedures. Discuss the meaning of these results with your doctor.

- Make sure you understand what will happen if you need surgery.

- Talk with your doctor about which hospital is best for your health care needs.

Finally, if you are not satisfied with your doctor, you can do two things: (1) talk with your doctor and try to work things out, and/or (2) switch doctors, if you are able to. It is very important to feel confident about your care.

To learn more, see "Where to Find More Information" on page xxx. The online version of this article includes additional resources.

Ten Important Questions to Ask Your Doctor After a Diagnosis

These 10 basic questions can help you understand your disease or condition, how it might be treated, and what you need to know and do before making treatment decisions.

1. What is the technical name of my disease or condition, and what does it mean in plain English?

   _____

2. What is my prognosis (outlook for the future)?

   _____

3. How soon do I need to make a decision about treatment?

   _____

4. Will I need any additional tests, and if so what kind and when?

   _____

5. What are my treatment options?

   _____

6. What are the pros and cons of my treatment options?

   _____

7. Is there a clinical trial (research study) that is right for me? (See page xxiv.)

   _____

8. Now that I have this diagnosis, what changes will I need to make in my daily life?

   _____

9. What organizations do you recommend for support and information?

   _____

10. What resources (booklets, Web sites, audiotapes, videos, DVDs, etc.) do you recommend for further information?

    _____

Step 4:
Seek out information.

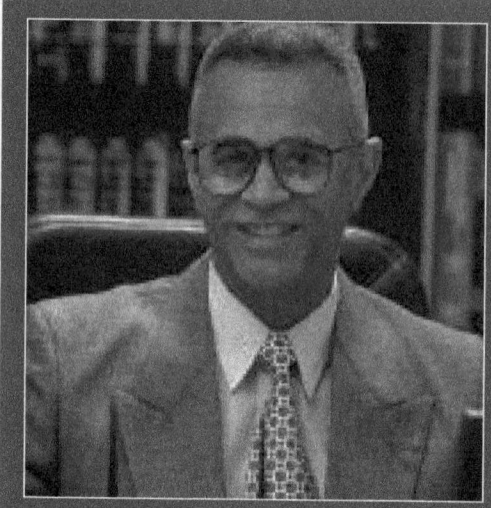

I'm really glad I took the time to research my options. It stopped me from jumping into a treatment that would have been completely wrong for me.

Seth, prostate cancer survivor

Now that you know your treatment options, you can learn which ones are backed up by the best scientific evidence. "Evidence-based" information—that is, information that is based on a careful review of the latest scientific findings in medical journals—can help you make decisions about the best possible treatments for you.

Evidence-based information comes from research on people like you.

Evidence-based information about treatments generally comes from two major types of scientific studies:

- **Clinical trials** are research studies on human volunteers to test new drugs or other treatments. Participants are randomly assigned to different treatment groups. Some get the research treatment, and others get a standard treatment or may be given a placebo (a medicine that has no effect), or no treatment. The results are compared to learn whether the new treatment is safe and effective.

- **Outcomes research** looks at the impact of treatments and other health care on health outcomes (end results) for patients and populations. End results include effects that people care about, such as changes in their quality of life.

Take advantage of the evidence-based information that is available.

Health information is everywhere—in books, newspapers, and magazines, and on the Internet, television, and radio. However, not all information is good information. Your best bets for sources of evidence-based information include the Federal Government, national nonprofit organizations, medical specialty groups, medical schools, and university medical centers.

Some resources are listed below, grouped by type of information. See "Where to Find More Information" on page xxx for additional ideas. The online version of Next Steps After Your Diagnosis lists many more, and includes links to Internet sites.

■ Information.

Information about your disease or condition and its treatment is available from many sources. Here are some of the most reliable:

- **healthfinder®:** www.healthfinder.gov/organizations/OrgListing.asp
  The healthfinder® site—sponsored by the U.S. Department of Health and Human Services—offers carefully selected health information Web sites from government agencies, clearinghouses, nonprofit groups, and universities.

- **Health Information Resource Database:**
  www.health.gov/nhic/#Referrals
  Sponsored by the National Health Information Center, this database includes 1,400 organizations and government offices that provide health information upon request. Information is also available over the telephone at 800-336-4797.

- **MEDLINEplus®:** www.nlm.nih.gov/medlineplus
  MedlinePlus® has extensive information from the National Institutes of Health and other trusted sources on over 650 diseases and conditions. The site includes many additional features.

- **National nonprofit groups** such as the American Heart Association, American Cancer Society, and American Diabetes Association can be valuable sources of reliable information. Many have chapters nationwide. Check your phone book for a local chapter in your community. The Health Information Resource Database (www.health.gov/nhic/#Referrals) can help you find national offices of nonprofit groups.

- **Health or medical libraries** run by government, hospitals, professional groups, and other reliable organizations often welcome consumers. For a list of libraries in your area, go to the MedlinePlus® "Find a Library" page at http://www.nlm.nih.gov/medlineplus/libraries.html.

Current medical research.

You can find the latest medical research in medical journals at your local health or medical library, and in some cases, on the Internet. Here are two major online sources of medical articles:

- **MEDLINE/PubMed®:** http://www.ncbi.nlm.nih.gov/entrez/query.fcgi PubMed® is the National Library of Medicine's database of references to more than 14 million articles published in 4,800 medical and scientific journals. All of the listings have information to help you find the articles at a health or medical library. Many listings also have short summaries of the article (abstracts), and some have links to the full article. The article might be free, or it might require a fee charged by the publisher.

- **PubMed Central:** http://www.pubmedcentral.nih.gov/ PubMed Central is the National Library of Medicine's database of journal articles that are available free of charge to users.

Clinical trials.

Perhaps you wonder whether there is a clinical trial that is right for you. Or you may want to learn about results from previous clinical trials that might be relevant to your situation. Here are two reliable resources:

- **ClinicalTrials.gov:** http://clinicaltrials.gov/ct/g ClinicalTrials.gov provides regularly updated information about federally and privately supported clinical research on people who volunteer to participate. The site has information about a trial's purpose, who may participate, locations, and phone numbers for more details. The site also describes the clinical trial process and includes news about recent clinical trial results.

- **Cochrane Collaboration:** www.cochrane.org The Cochrane Collaboration writes summaries ("reviews") about evidence from clinical trials to help people make informed decisions. You can search and read the review abstracts free of charge at http://www.cochrane.org/

reviews/index.htm. Or you can read plain-English consumer summaries of the reviews at www.informedhealthonline.org.

The full Cochrane reviews are available only by subscription. Check with your local medical or health library (see page xxxii) [link back to library section in on-line version] to see whether you can access the full reviews there.

Outcomes research.

Outcomes research provides research about benefits, risks, and outcomes (end results) of treatments so that patients and their doctors can make better informed decisions. The U.S. Agency for Healthcare Research and Quality (AHRQ) supports improvements in health outcomes through research, and sponsors products that result from research such as:

- **National Guideline Clearinghouse™:** www.guideline.gov
  The National Guideline Clearinghouse™ is a database of evidence-based clinical practice guidelines and related documents. Clinical practice guidelines are documents designed to help doctors and patients make decisions about appropriate health care for specific diseases or conditions. The clearinghouse was originally created by AHRQ in partnership with the American Medical Association and America's Health Insurance Plans.

Steer clear of deceptive ads and information.

While searching for information either on or off the Internet, beware of "miracle" treatments and cures. They can cost you money and your health, especially if you delay or refuse proper treatment. Here are some tip-offs that a product truly is too good to be true:

- Phrases such as "scientific breakthrough," "miraculous cure," "exclusive product," "secret formula," or "ancient ingredient."

- Claims that the product treats a wide range of ailments.

- Use of impressive-sounding medical terms. These often cover up a lack of good science behind the product.

- Case histories from consumers claiming "amazing" results.

- Claims that the product is available from only one source, and for a limited time only.

- Claims of a "money-back guarantee."

- Claims that others are trying to keep the product off the market.

- Ads that fail to list the company's name, address, or other contact information.

To learn more about finding evidence-based information, see "Where to Find More Information," page xxx. The on-line edition of this article has many additional resources.

Step 5:
Decide on a treatment plan.

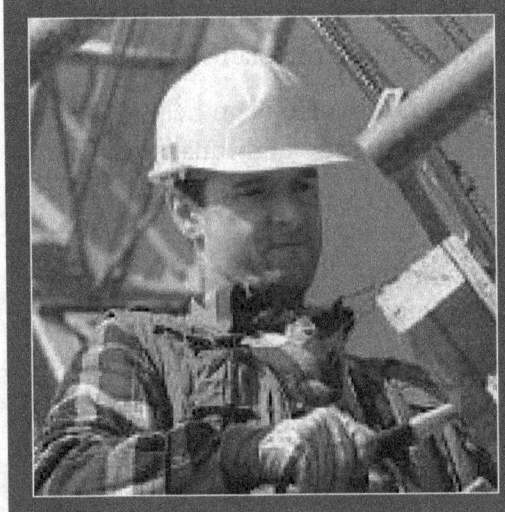

My doctor told me I had done one of the hardest but most important things a patient has to do: Face up to the diagnosis and make decisions. It feels good to be where I am now.

Bob, person with a neurological disorder

At this point, you have learned about your disease or condition and how it can be treated or managed. Your information may have come from the following sources:

- Your doctor.

- Second opinions from one or more other doctors.

- Other people who are or were in the same situation as you.

- Information sources such as Web sites, health or medical libraries, and nonprofit groups.

Work with your doctor to make decisions.

When you are ready to make treatment decisions, you and your doctor can discuss:

- Which treatments have been found to work well, or not work well, for your particular condition.

- The pros and cons of each treatment option.

Make sure that your doctor knows your preferences and feelings about the different treatments – for example, whether you prefer medicine over surgery.

Once you and your doctor decide on one or more treatments that are right for you, you can work together to develop a treatment plan. This plan will include everything that will be done to treat or manage your disease or condition—including what you need to do to make the plan work.

Remember, being an active member of your health care team helps to reduce your chances of medical mistakes, and it helps you get high-quality care.

Take another deep breath.

You have taken important steps to cope with your diagnosis, make decisions, and get on with your life. Remember two things:

- Call on others for support as you need it.

- Make use of evidence-based information for any future health decisions.

Where to Find More Information

Get the support you need.

American Self-Help Group Clearinghouse
http://mentalhelp.net/selfhelp/

National Board for Certified Counselors (NBCC)
3 Terrace Way, Suite D
Greensboro, NC 27403-3660
336-547-0607.
www.nbcc.org

National Institute of Mental Health
Public Information and Communications Branch
6001 Executive Boulevard, Room 8184, MSC 9663
Bethesda, MD 20892-9663
Phone: 866-615-6464 (toll-free)
TTY: 301-443-8431
http://www.nimh.nih.gov/HealthInformation/GettingHelp.cfm

Talk to your doctor.

Be an Active Member of Your Health Care Team. Food and Drug Administration. 2004. http://www.fda.gov/cder/consumerinfo/ active_member.htm. Phone: 888-INFO-FDA (888-463-6332).

Be Informed: Questions to Ask Your Doctor Before You Have Surgery. Agency for Healthcare Quality and Research. 1995. http://www.ahrq.gov/consumer/surgery.htm. Phone: 800-358-9295.

Five Steps to Safer Health Care. Agency for Healthcare Research and Quality. 2003. http://www.ahrq.gov/consumer/5steps.htm. Phone: 800-358-9295.

Getting a Second Opinion Before Surgery. Centers for Medicare & Medicaid Services. 2004. www.medicare.gov/Publications/Pubs/pdf/02173.pdf. Phone: 800-MEDICARE (800-633-4227).

How to Get a Second Opinion. National Women's Health Information Center. 2003. http://www.4woman.gov/pub/secondopinion.htm. Phone: 1-800-994-WOMAN.

Quick Tips – When Planning for Surgery. Agency for Healthcare Research and Quality. 2002. http://www.ahrq.gov/consumer/quicktips/ tipsurgery.htm. Phone: 800-358-9295.

Quick Tips – When Talking with Your Doctor. Agency for Healthcare Research and Quality. 2002. http://www.ahrq.gov/consumer/quicktips/ doctalk.htm. Phone: 800-358-9295.

Talking with Your Doctor: A Guide for Older People. National Institute on Aging. 2002. www.niapublications.org/pubs/talking/index.asp. Phone: 800-222-2225. |

Seek out information.

2005 Toll-Free Numbers for Health Information. National Health Information Center. www.health.gov/nhic/pubs/tollfree.htm. Phone: 800-336-4797.

AARP Health Guide. AARP. 2004. www.aarp.org/health/healthguide. Phone: 888-OUR-AARP (888-687-2277).

HON Code of Conduct (HONcode) for Medical and Health Web Sites Health on the Net Foundation. http://www.hon.ch/HONcode/

How to Evaluate Health Information on the Internet: Questions and Answers. National Cancer Institute. 2003. http://cis.nci.nih.gov/fact/2_10.htm. Phone: 800-4-CANCER (800-422-6237).

How to Find Medical Information. National Institute of Arthritis and Musculoskeletal and Skin Diseases. 2001. http://www.niams.nih.gov/hi/topics/howto/howto.htm. Phone: 877-22-NIAMS (877-226-4267) (toll-free).

JAMA Patient Page: Health Information on the Internet. The Medem Network. http://www.medem.com/medlb/article_detaillb.cfm?article_ID=ZZZLJLLLTMC&sub_cat=603

National Guideline Clearinghouse™. Agency for Healthcare Research and Quality. http://www.guideline.gov/

NOAH: New York Online Access to Health. http://www.noah-health.org/

A User's Guide to Finding and Evaluating Health Information on the Web. Medical Library Association. 2003. http://www.mlanet.org/resources/userguide.html#1

Virtual Treatments Can Be Real-World Deceptions. Federal Trade Commission. 2001. http://www.ftc.gov/bcp/conline/pubs/alerts/mrclalrt.htm

Your Guide to Choosing Quality Health Care. Agency for Healthcare Research and Quality. 2002. http://www.ahrq.gov/consumer/qntool.htm. Phone: 800-358-9295.

AHRQ consumer publications:

20 Tips to Help Prevent Medical Errors—Practical tips and questions to ask. (AHRQ 00-P038)

20 Tips to Help Prevent Medical Errors in Children (AHRQ 02-P034)

Five Steps to Safer Health Care—Shorter version of 20 Tips. (AHRQ 03-M007)

Ways You Can Help Your Family Prevent Medical Errors!—Easy-to-read version, with drawings. (AHRQ 01-0017)

Your Guide to Choosing Quality Health Care—Based on research about the information people want and need when choosing health plans, doctors, treatments, hospitals, and long-term care. (AHRQ 99-012)

Improving Health Care Quality: A Guide for Patients and Their Families—Short version of *Your Guide to Choosing Quality Health Care*. (AHRQ 01-0004)

Quick Checks for Quality—Checklist to use when choosing health plans, doctors, treatments, hospitals, and long-term care. (AHRQ 99-R027)

Quick Tips:
>   *When Getting Medical Tests* (AHRQ 01-0040b)
>   *When Getting a Prescription* (AHRQ 01-0040c)
>   *When Planning for Surgery* (AHRQ 01-0040d)
>   *When Talking with Your Doctor* (AHRQ 01-0040a)

To order AHRQ publications:

For electronic copies of these publications, go to the AHRQ Web site at www.ahrq.gov/consumer

For print copies, contact the AHRQ Publications Clearinghouse at 800-358-9295.

Description

1 Addison's Disease

Addison's disease is a rare disorder that stems from the malfunction of the adrenal glands located on top of the kidneys. In this disease, there is a deficiency of hormones produced by the adrenal cortex, the gland's firm outer layer. Most often, Addison's disease results from destruction of the adrenal gland. This glandular destruction may result from unusual infections, malignant tumors, an autoimmune process or other rare disorders. At least half of all cases of Addison's disease result from patient's developing antibodies against their own adrenal tissue (autoimmune process).

There can be increased water excretion in the urine and lowered blood pressure, which can lead to severe dehydration and other major complications. The symptoms of Addison's disease increase with the progression of the disease. Early signs may include fatigue, loss of appetite, low blood pressure (hypotension), weakness and significant loss from the kidneys of water and minerals. Other symptoms may include darkened scars and skin folds, as well as dark freckles on the head and shoulders. In the later stages, nausea may develop, as well as dizziness, further dehydration, low blood sugar (hypoglycemia) and mental changes including confusion.

Patients who are treated early have an excellent prognosis, but it is imperative that treatment be instituted immediately and vigorously. In order to counteract the hormonal loss, physicians prescribe steroid hormone replacement therapy. Certain doses of hormones need to be increased during times of illness and surgery. Treatment should never be stopped, even for a day, without the advice of a physician. Persons on treatment should wear an alert bracelet to let emergency medical providers know of their diagnosis.

National Agencies & Associations

2 Endocrine Society
8401 Connecticut Avenue   301-941-0200
Chevy Chase, MD 20815   888-363-6274
Fax: 301-941-0259
e-mail: societyservices@endo-society.org
www.endo-society.org
Source of state-of-the-art research and clinical advancements in endocrinology and metabolism. Dedicated to promoting excellence in research education and clinical practice in the field of endocrinology. Prime advocate and integrative force for clinicians.
Kelly E. Mayo, President
Alan D. Rogol, VP Physician in Practice

3 National Adrenal Diseases Foundation
505 Northern Boulevard   516-487-4992
Great Neck, NY 11021   Fax: 516-829-5710
e-mail: nadfmail@aol.com
www.nadf.us
Nonprofit organization dedicated to offer support information and research for individuals having diseases of the adrenal glands. Goals of the organization include assisting patients through informational and educational activities as well as support programs.
Paul Marguli, MD, Medical Director
Melanie G Wong, Executive Director

4 National Institute of Diabetes & Digestive & Kidney Diseases
National Institutes of Health
31 Center Drive   301-496-3583
Bethesda, MD 20892-2560   800-860-8747
Fax: 703-738-4929
e-mail: ndic@info.niddk.nih.gov
www.diabetes.niddk.nih.gov
Conducts and supports research on many of the most serious diseases affecting public health. The Institute supports much of the clinical research on the diseases of internal medicine and related subspecialty fields as well as many basic science disciplines.
Dr. Griffin Rodgers, Acting Director

Support Groups & Hotlines

5 National Health Information Center
PO Box 1133   310-565-4167
Washington, DC 20013   800-336-4797
Fax: 301-984-4256
e-mail: info@nhic.org
www.health.gov/nhic
Offers a nationwide information referral service, produces directories and resource guides.

Magazines

6 Endocrine News
Endocrine Society
8401 Connecticut Avenue   301-941-0200
Chevy Chase, MD 20815   888-363-6274
Fax: 301-941-0259
e-mail: societyservices@endo-society.org
www.endo-society.org
Endocrine News is the source of trends and insights for members of the endocrine community.
Monthly
Kelly E Mayo PhD, President
Scott Hunt, Executive Director

Newsletters

7 Addison News
6142 Territorial
Pleasant Lake, MI 49272   www2.dmci.net/users/hoffmanrj

8 NADF News
National Adrenal Diseases Foundation
505 Northern Boulevard   516-487-4992
Great Neck, NY 11021   Fax: 516-829-5710
e-mail: nadfmail@aol.com
www.nadf.us
Contains information on the latest research, question and answer column by an endocrinologist and helpful hints for those with Addison's Disease.
Quarterly Monthly
Melanie G Wong, Executive Director
Debbie Benish, Editor

Web Sites

9 Healing Well
www.healingwell.com
An online health resource guide to medical news, chat, information and articles, newsgroups and message boards, books, disease-related web sites, medical directories, and more for patients, friends, and family coping with disabling diseases, disorders, or chronic illnesses.

10 Health Finder
www.healthfinder.gov
A government Web site where you will find information and tools to help you and those you care about stay healthy.

11 Health Link USA
www.healthlinkusa.com

Discussion forum for treatments, symptoms and causes of 700 health conditions, diseases and topics.

12   **Helios Health**

www.helioshealth.com

Online resource for your health information. Detailed information about specific health topics, access to expert advice from our Medical Advisory Board, and up-to-date health news.

13   **Hormone Foundation**

www.hormone.org

Educational resource for you, your loved ones, and your health professionals on the prevention, treatment, and cure of hormone-related conditions.

14   **MedicineNet**

www.medicinenet.com

An online resource for consumers providing easy-to-read, authoritative medical and health information.

15   **Medscape**

www.medscape.com

Search engine providing links to websites with information on illnesses, diseases and disorders.

16   **National Adrenal Disease Foundation**

www.medhelp.org

Non-profit organization dedicated to providing support, information and education to individuals having Addison's disease as well as other diseases of the adrenal glands.

17   **WebMD**

www.webmd.com

Information on Addison's disease, including an overview of the disease, symptoms and home treatment.

Description

18 **Aging**

The elderly population in the United States is growing faster than any other segment of the population, and has done so since 1900. It is estimated that this trend will continue at least through the year 2050. In 2004, there were 36.3 million people in the U.S. older than 65. One in eight persons is over 85 years, classified as 'old old.' By 2040, it is anticipated that one person in five will exceed 65 years of age, and the number of people over 85 will increase to four times their number today, representing the aging of the baby boomers.

Aging is not a disease, but part of the normal life cycle, and many seniors retain good health and live independently for long past the traditional age of retirement. In time, however, most will develop one or more chronic conditions; for those over 75 years of age, the most common conditions are hypertension, heart disease, hearing loss, arthritis, and cataracts. By the year 2030, 150 million Americans are expected to have a chronic condition, and 42 million will be limited in their ability to work or live independently. Treating this population will require many medical and nonmedical services, integrated to provide a comprehensive continuum of care. See also *Alzheimer's Disease.*

National Agencies & Associations

19 **American Association of Homes and Services for the Aging**
2519 Connecticut Avenue NW   202-783-2242
Washington, DC 20008-1520   Fax: 202-783-2255
e-mail: info@LeadingAge.org
www.aahsa.org
National association of more than 4 000 nonprofit nursing homes continuing care retirement communities independent living centers and community service providers serving more than 60,000 older Americans each year.
William L Minnix Jr, President and CEO
Katrinka Smith Sloan, COO and SVP Member Services

20 **American Association of Retired Persons**
601 E Street NW
Washington, DC 20049   888-687-2277
e-mail: member@aarp.org
www.aarp.org
AARP is the nation's leading organization for people age 50 and older. It serves their needs and interests through information and education, advocacy and community services provided by a network of local chapters and experienced volunteers.
Barry Rand, CEO
John Wider, President

21 **Commission on Accreditation of Rehabilitation Services**
6951 E Southpoint Road   520-325-1044
Tucson, AZ 85756   888-281-6531
Fax: 520-318-1129
carf.org
CARF reviews and grants accreditation services nationally and internationally at the request of a facility or program. Their standards are rigorous, so those services that meet them are among the best available.
Amanda Birch, Adminstrator of Operations
Brian Boon, Ph.D., President/Chief Executive Officer

22 **Gerontological Society of America**
1220 L Street NW   202-842-1275
Washington, DC 20005   Fax: 202-842-1150
e-mail: geron@geron.org
www.geron.org
Nonprofit professional organization with more than 5000 members in the field of aging. Provides researchers, educators, practitioners and policy makers with opportunities to understand, advance, integrate and use basic and applied research on aging populations.
James Appleby, Executive Director
Linda Krogh Harootyan, Deputy Executive Director

23 **Institute for Life Course and Aging**
222 College Street   416-978-0377
Toronto, Ontario, M5T-3J1   Fax: 416-978-4771
www.aging.utoronto.ca
The Institute is a research center under the auspices of the School of Graduate Studies at the University of Toronto.
Prof Lynn McDonald, Director
Susan Murphy, Administration

24 **International Federation on Aging**
351 Christie Street   416-342-1655
Toronto, Ontario, MG6-3C3   Fax: 416-392-4157
e-mail: jbarratt@ifa-fiv.org
www.ifa-fiv.org

To inform, educate and promote policies and practice to improve the quality of life of older persons around the world.
Dr Jane Barratt, Secretary General
Greg Shaw, Director, International Relations

25 **National Council on Aging**
1901 L Street NW   202-479-1200
Washington, DC 20036   Fax: 202-479-0735
TTY: 202-479-6674
TDD: 202-479-6674
e-mail: info@ncoa.org
www.ncoa.org
The nation's first charitable organization dedicated to promoting the dignity, independence, well-being and contributions of older Americans. NCOA serves as a national voice and powerful advocate on behalf of older Americans.
James P Firman EdD, President/CEO
S. Stuart Spector, Vice President

26 **Problems of the Elderly Committee**
740 15th Street NW   202-662-1000
Washington, DC 20005-1019   Fax: 202-662-1501
e-mail: crimjustice@abanet.org
www.abanet.org/crimjust
This Committee examines the issues that affect the elderly as victims of street crime, identity theft, financial exploitation and other crimes of which they are targets. The committee looks at issues arising from the aging prisons populations and the elders as perpetrators of crime, also.
Stephen N. Zack, President
Benjamin F Overton, Co-Chair

27 **Senior Resource**
4521 Campus Drive   858-793-7901
Irvine, CA 92612   877-793-7901
Fax: 858-792-9080
e-mail: questions@seniorresource.com
www.seniorresource.com
An agency that helps seniors to understand aging and gives different resources consisting of sociologic changes; metabolic changes; positive aging; and physical changes.
Bryan D Hatchell, Chair

28 **US Administration on Aging**
1 Massachusetts Avenue   202-619-0724
Washington, DC 20201   Fax: 202-357-3555
e-mail: aoainfo@aoa.hhs.gov
www.aoa.gov
The Administration on Aging an agency in the US Department of Health and Human Services is one of the nation's largest providers

of home and community-based care for older persons and their caregivers.
Edwin L Walker, Acting Assistant Secretary
Carol Crecy, Director Office of Communications

State Agencies & Associations

Alaska

29 **AARP Alaska State Office**
3601 C Street
Anchorage, AK 99503
866-227-7447
Fax: 907-341-2270
e-mail: ak@aarp.org
www.aarp.org/states/ak
AARP is a nonprofit nonpartisan membership organization for people age 50 and over. AARP is dedicated to enhancing the quality of life as one ages, in addition to facilitating social change and delivering value to members through information and advocacy.
Fred Jenkins, Development Director
George Hieronymus, AARP Alaska State President

Arizona

30 **AARP Arizona: Phoenix Collier Center**
Collier Center
201 E Washington Street
Phoenix, AZ 85004-2428
866-389-5649
Fax: 602-256-2928
e-mail: azaarp@aarp.org
www.aarp.org/states/az
AARP is a nonprofit nonpartisan membership organization for people age 50 and over. AARP is dedicated to enhancing the quality of life as one ages, in addition to facilitating social change and delivering value to members through information and advocacy.
Leonard J Kirschner PhD, Arizona AARP State President
David Mitchell, Arizona AARP State Director

Arkansas

31 **AARP Arkansas State Office: Little Rock**
1701 Centerview Drive
Little Rock, AR 72211
866-544-5379
Fax: 501-227-7710
e-mail: araarp@aarp.org
www.aarp.org/states/ar
AARP is a nonprofit nonpartisan membership organization for people age 50 and over. AARP is dedicated to enhancing the quality of life as one ages, in addition to facilitating social change and delivering value to members through information and advocacy.
Mary Dillard, Arkansas AARP State President
Pat Jones, Arkansas AARP State Media Relations

California

32 **AARP California State Office: Pasadena**
200 S Los Robles Avenue
Pasadena, CA 91101-2422
866-448-3615
Fax: 626-583-8500
e-mail: calosangeles@aarp.org
www.aarp.org/states/ca
AARP is a nonprofit nonpartisan membership organization for people age 50 and over. AARP is dedicated to enhancing the quality of life as one ages, in addition to facilitating social change and delivering value to members through information and advocacy.
Helen Russ, California AARP State President
Thomas A Porter, California AARP State Director

33 **AARP California State Office: Sacramento**
1415 L Street
Sacramento, CA 95814
866-448-3614
Fax: 916-446-2223
e-mail: casacramento@aarp.org
www.aarp.org/states/ca
AARP is a nonprofit nonpartisan membership organization for people age 50 and over. AARP is dedicated to enhancing the qual-

ity of life as one ages, in addition to facilitating social change and delivering value to members through information and advocacy.
Helen Russ, California State AARP President
Thomas A Porter, California State AARP Director

Colorado

34 **AARP Colorado State Office: Denver**
303 E 17th Avenue
Denver, CO 80203-5012
866-554-5376
Fax: 303-764-5999
e-mail: coaarp@aarp.org
www.aarp.org/states/co
AARP is a nonprofit nonpartisan membership organization for people age 50 and over. AARP is dedicated to enhancing the quality of life as one ages, in addition to facilitating social change and delivering value to members through information and advocacy.
Robert Martinez, Colorado AARP State President
Jon Looney, Colorado AARP State Director

Florida

35 **AARP Florida State Office: St. Petersburg**
400 Carillon Parkway
Saint Petersburg, FL 33716
866-595-7678
Fax: 727-369-5191
TTY: 727-561-9544
e-mail: flaarp@aarp.org
www.aarp.org/states/fl
AARP is a nonprofit nonpartisan membership organization for people age 50 and over. AARP is dedicated to enhancing the quality of life as one ages, in addition to facilitating social change and delivering value to members through information and advocacy.
Kathy Marma, Florida AARP State Media Relations
Thomas Thame MD, Florida AARP State Board of Directors

36 **Goodwill Industries-Suncoast**
Goodwill Industries-Suncoast
10596 Gandy Boulevard
St. Petersburg, FL 33702
727-523-1512
888-279-1988
Fax: 727-563-9300
TTY: 727-579-1068
e-mail: chris.ward@goodwill-suncoast.com
www.goodwill-suncoast.org
A nonprofit, community-based organization whose mission is to help people achieve self-sufficiency through the dignity and power of work, serving people who are disadvantaged, disabled or elderly. The mission is accomplished through providing independent living skills, affordable housing, and training and placement in community employment.
R Lee Waits, President/Chief Executive Officer
Charlie Robinson Jr, Chair

Georgia

37 **AARP Georgia: Atlanta**
999 Peachtree Street NE
Atlanta, GA 30309-4421
866-295-7281
Fax: 404-881-6997
e-mail: gaaarp@aarp.org
www.aarp.org/states/ga
AARP is a nonprofit nonpartisan membership organization for people age 50 and over. AARP is dedicated to enhancing the quality of life as one ages, in addition to facilitating social change and delivering value to members through information and advocacy.
Matthew McWilliams, Georgia AARP State Media Relations
Will Phillips, AARP Georgia Associate State Director

Hawaii

38 **AARP Hawaii State Office: Honolulu**
1132 Bishop Street
Honolulu, HI 96813
808-843-1906
866-295-7282
Fax: 808-843-1908
e-mail: oahuaarp@hawaii.rr.com
www.aarp.org/states/hi
AARP is a nonprofit nonpartisan membership organization for people age 50 and over. AARP is dedicated to enhancing the qual-

ity of life as one ages, in addition to facilitating social change and delivering value to members through information and advocacy.
Stuart TK Ho, AARP Hawaii Interim State President
Barbara Kim Stanton, Hawaii AARP State Director

Idaho

39 AARP Idaho State Office: Meridian
3830 E Gentry Way
Meridian, ID 83642
866-295-7284
Fax: 208-288-4424
e-mail: aarpid@aarp.org
www.aarp.org/states/id
AARP is a nonprofit nonpartisan membership organization for people age 50 and over. AARP is dedicated to enhancing the quality of life as one ages, in addition to facilitating social change and delivering value to members through information and advocacy.
Cheryl Tussey, Idaho AARP State Media Relations
Jim Wordelman, AARP Idaho State Director

Illinois

40 AARP Illinois State Office: Chicago
222 N LaSalle Street
Chicago, IL 60601-1033
866-448-3613
Fax: 312-372-2204
e-mail: aarpil@aarp.org
www.aarp.org/states/il
AARP is a nonprofit nonpartisan membership organization for people age 50 and over. AARP is dedicated to enhancing the quality of life as one ages, in addition to facilitating social change and delivering value to members through information and advocacy.
Evelyn Gooden, Illinois AARP State President
Gerardo Cardenas, Illinois AARP State Media Relations

Indiana

41 AARP Indiana State Office: Indianapolis
One N Capitol Avenue
Indianapolis, IN 46204-2025
866-448-3618
Fax: 317-423-2211
e-mail: inaarp@aarp.org
www.aarp.org/states/in
AARP is a nonprofit nonpartisan membership organization for people age 50 and over. AARP is dedicated to enhancing the quality of life as one ages, in addition to facilitating social change and delivering value to members through information and advocacy.
Martin DeAgostino, Indiana AARP State Media Relations
June Lyle, AARP Indiana State Director

Iowa

42 AARP Iowa State Office: Des Moines
600 E Court Avenue
Des Moines, IA 50309
866-554-5378
Fax: 515-244-7767
e-mail: iaaarp@aarp.org
www.aarp.org/states/ia
AARP is a nonprofit nonpartisan membership organization for people age 50 and over. AARP is dedicated to enhancing the quality of life as one ages, in addition to facilitating social change and delivering value to members through information and advocacy.
Ann Black, Iowa AARP State Media Relations
Bruce Koeppl, Iowa AARP State Director

Kansas

43 AARP Kansas State Office: Topeka
555 S Kansas
Topeka, KS 66603
866-448-3619
Fax: 785-232-8259
e-mail: ksaarp@aarp.org
www.aarp.org/states/ks
AARP is a nonprofit nonpartisan membership organization for people age 50 and over. AARP is dedicated to enhancing the quality of life as one ages, in addition to facilitating social change and delivering value to members through information and advocacy.
Mary Tritsch, Kansas AARP State Media Relations
Maren Turner, Kansas AARP State Director

Kentucky

44 AARP Kentucky State Office: Louisville
10401 Linn Station Road
Louisville, KY 40223
866-295-7275
Fax: 502-394-9918
e-mail: kyaarp@aarp.org
www.aarp.org/states/ky
AARP is a nonprofit nonpartisan membership organization for people age 50 and over. AARP is dedicated to enhancing the quality of life as one ages, in addition to facilitating social change and delivering value to members through information and advocacy.
Bill Harned, AARP Kentucky State President
Fred Smith, Executive Council Community Service

Louisiana

45 AARP Louisiana State Office: Baton Rouge
301 Main Street
Baton Rouge, LA 70825
866-448-3620
Fax: 225-387-3400
e-mail: la@aarp.org
www.aarp.org/states/la
AARP is a nonprofit nonpartisan membership organization for people age 50 and over. AARP is dedicated to enhancing the quality of life as one ages, in addition to facilitating social change and delivering value to members through information and advocacy.
Earl A White, AARP Louisiana State President
Julia Kenny, AARP Louisiana State Director

Maine

46 AARP Maine State Office: Portland
1685 Congress Street
Portland, ME 04102
866-554-5380
Fax: 207-775-5727
e-mail: me@aarp.org
www.aarp.org/states/me
AARP is a nonprofit nonpartisan membership organization for people age 50 and over. AARP is dedicated to enhancing the quality of life as one ages, in addition to facilitating social change and delivering value to members through information and advocacy.
Bruce Kinney, Maine AARP State Advocacy Coordinator
Phyllis Cohn, Maine AARP State Media Relations

Massachusetts

47 AARP Massachusetts State Office: Boston
1 Beacon Street
Boston, MA 02108
866-448-3621
Fax: 617-723-4224
e-mail: ma@aarp.org
www.aarp.org/states/ma
AARP is a nonprofit nonpartisan membership organization for people age 50 and over. AARP is dedicated to enhancing the quality of life as one ages, in addition to facilitating social change and delivering value to members through information and advocacy.
Charlie Desmond, AARP Massachusetts State President
Claire Redmond, Executive Council Member

Michigan

48 AARP Michigan State Office: Lansing
309 N Washington Square
Lansing, MI 48933
866-227-7448
Fax: 517-482-2794
TTY: 877-434-7598
e-mail: miaarp@aarp.org
www.aarp.org/states/mi
AARP is a nonprofit nonpartisan membership organization for people age 50 and over. AARP is dedicated to enhancing the quality of life as one ages, in addition to facilitating social change and delivering value to members through information and advocacy.
Steve Gools, AARP Michigan State Director
Stepheni Schlinker, Michigan AARP State Media Relations

Minnesota

49 **AARP Minnesota State Office: Saint Paul**
30 E Seventh Street
Saint Paul, MN 55101   866-554-5381
                                     Fax: 651-221-2636
                                     e-mail: aarpmn@aarp.org
                                     www.aarp.org/states/mn
AARP is a nonprofit nonpartisan membership organization for people age 50 and over. AARP is dedicated to enhancing the quality of life as one ages, in addition to facilitating social change and delivering value to members through information and advocacy.
Michele Kimball, AARP Minnesota State Director
Amy Gromer McDonough, AARP Minnesota State Media Relations

Missouri

50 **AARP Missouri State Office: Kansas City**
700 W 47th Street
Kansas City, MO 64112-1805   866-389-5627
                                     Fax: 816-561-3107
                                     e-mail: moaarp@aarp.org
                                     www.aarp.org/states/mo
AARP is a nonprofit nonpartisan membership organization for people age 50 and over. AARP is dedicated to enhancing the quality of life as one ages, in addition to facilitating social change and delivering value to members through information and advocacy.
John McDonald, AARP Missouri State Director
Anita K Parran, AARP Missouri State Media Relations

Montana

51 **AARP Montana State Office: Helena**
30 W 14th Street
Helena, MT 59601   866-295-7278
                                     Fax: 406-441-2230
                                     e-mail: mtaarp@aarp.org
                                     www.aarp.org/states/mt
AARP is a nonprofit nonpartisan membership organization for people age 50 and over. AARP is dedicated to enhancing the quality of life as one ages, in addition to facilitating social change and delivering value to members through information and advocacy.
Max Logan, AARP Montana Volunteer State President
Bob Bartholomew, AARP Montana State Director

Nebraska

52 **AARP Nebraska State Office: Lincoln**
301 S 13th Street
Lincoln, NE 68508   866-389-5651
                                     Fax: 402-323-6908
                                     e-mail: neaarp@aarp.org
                                     www.aarp.org/states/ne
AARP is a nonprofit nonpartisan membership organization for people age 50 and over. AARP is dedicated to enhancing the quality of life as one ages, in addition to facilitating social change and delivering value to members through information and advocacy.
Sunny Andrews, AARP Nebraska State President
Devorah Lanner, AARP Nebraska State Media Relations

Nevada

53 **AARP Nevada State Office: Las Vegas**
5820 S Eastern Avenue
Las Vegas, NV 89119   866-389-5652
                                     Fax: 702-938-3225
                                     e-mail: nvaarp@aarp.org
                                     www.aarp.org/states/nv
AARP is a nonprofit nonpartisan membership organization for people age 50 and over. AARP is dedicated to enhancing the quality of life as one ages, in addition to facilitating social change and delivering value to members through information and advocacy.
Deborah Moore, AARP Nevada Spokeswoman
Nancy Andersen, AARP Nevada State Volunteer Coordinator

New Hampshire

54 **AARP New Hampshire State Office-Manchester**
900 Elm Street
Manchester, NH 03101   866-542-8168
                                     Fax: 603-629-0066
                                     e-mail: nh@aarp.org
                                     www.aarp.org/states/nh
AARP is a nonprofit nonpartisan membership organization for people age 50 and over. AARP is dedicated to enhancing the quality of life as one ages, in addition to facilitating social change and delivering value to members through information and advocacy.
Kelly Clark, AARP New Hampshire State Director
Jamie Bulen, AARP New Hampshire State Media Relations

New Jersey

55 **AARP New Jersey State Office: Princeton**
101 Rockingham Row
Princeton, NJ 08540   866-542-8165
                                     Fax: 609-987-4634
                                     e-mail: njaarp@aarp.org
                                     www.aarp.org/states/nj
AARP is a nonprofit nonpartisan membership organization for people age 50 and over. AARP is dedicated to enhancing the quality of life as one ages, in addition to facilitating social change and delivering value to members through information and advocacy.
Sy Larson, AARP New Jersey State President
Jane Margesson, AARP New Jersey State Media Relations

New Mexico

56 **AARP New Mexico State Office: Sante Fe**
535 Cerrillos Road
Santa Fe, NM 87501   866-389-5636
                                     Fax: 505-820-2889
                                     e-mail: nmaarp@aarp.org
                                     www.aarp.org/states/nm
AARP is a nonprofit nonpartisan membership organization for people age 50 and over. AARP is dedicated to enhancing the quality of life as one ages, in addition to facilitating social change and delivering value to members through information and advocacy.
Louis Sarabia, AARP New Mexico State President
Stan Cooper, AARP New Mexico State Director

New York

57 **AARP New York State Office: Albany**
1 Commerce Plaza
Albany, NY 12260   866-227-7442
                                     Fax: 518-434-6949
                                     e-mail: nyaarp@aarp.org
                                     www.aarp.org
AARP is a nonprofit nonpartisan membership organization for people age 50 and over. AARP is dedicated to enhancing the quality of life as one ages, in addition to facilitating social change and delivering value to members through information and advocacy.
Marilyn Pinksy, State President

58 **AARP New York State Office: New York City**
780 3rd Avenue
New York, NY 10017   866-227-7442
                                     Fax: 212-644-6390
                                     e-mail: nyaarp@aarp.org
                                     www.aarp.org/states/ny
AARP is a nonprofit nonpartisan membership organization for people age 50 and over. AARP is dedicated to enhancing the quality of life as one ages, in addition to facilitating social change and delivering value to members through information and advocacy.
Lois Aronstein, AARP New York State Director
Madeleine Moore, AARP New York State President

North Carolina

59   AARP North Carolina State Office: Raleigh
1511 Sunday Drive
Raleigh, NC 27607   866-389-5650
                                              Fax: 919-755-9684
                                              TTY: 919-508-0290
                                         e-mail: ncaarp@aarp.org
                                          www.aarp.org/states/nc
AARP is a nonprofit nonpartisan membership organization for
people age 50 and over. AARP is dedicated to enhancing the quality of life as one ages, in addition to facilitating social change and
delivering value to members through information and advocacy.
Diana D Hatch, AARP North Carolina State President
Bob Garner, Communications Director

North Dakota

60   AARP North Dakota State Office: Bismarck
107 W Main Avenue
Bismarck, ND 58501   866-554-5383
                                              Fax: 701-255-2242
                                         e-mail: ndaarp@aarp.org
                                          www.aarp.org/states/nd
AARP is a nonprofit nonpartisan membership organization for
people age 50 and over. AARP is dedicated to enhancing the quality of life as one ages, in addition to facilitating social change and
delivering value to members through information and advocacy.
Betty Keegan, AARP North Dakota State President
Lyle Halvorson, AARP North Dakota State Media Relations

Ohio

61   AARP Ohio State Office: Columbus
17 S High Street
Columbus, OH 43215-3467   866-389-5653
                                              Fax: 614-224-9801
                                         e-mail: ohaarp@aarp.org
                                          www.aarp.org/states/oh
AARP is a nonprofit nonpartisan membership organization for
people age 50 and over. AARP is dedicated to enhancing the quality of life as one ages, in addition to facilitating social change and
delivering value to members through information and advocacy.
Kathy Keller, AARP Ohio State Media Relations
Joanne Limbach, AARP Ohio State President

Oklahoma

62   AARP Oklahoma State Office: Edmond
126 N Bryant Avenue
Edmond, OK 73034   866-295-7277
                                              Fax: 405-844-7772
                                            e-mail: ok@aarp.org
                                          www.aarp.org/states/ok
AARP is a nonprofit nonpartisan membership organization for
people age 50 and over. AARP is dedicated to enhancing the quality of life as one ages, in addition to facilitating social change and
delivering value to members through information and advocacy.
Robert Bristow, AARP Oklahoma State President
Marjorie Lyons, Executive Council Member

Oregon

63   AARP Oregon State Office: Clackamas
9200 SE Sunnybrook Boulevard
Clackamas, OR 97015-5762   866-554-5360
                                              Fax: 503-652-9933
                                         e-mail: oraarp@aarp.org
                                          www.aarp.org/states/or
AARP is a nonprofit nonpartisan membership organization for
people age 50 and over. AARP is dedicated to enhancing the quality of life as one ages, in addition to facilitating social change and
delivering value to members through information and advocacy.
Ray Miao, AARP Oregon State President
Don Bruland, Director

Pennsylvania

64   AARP Pennsylvania State Office: Harrisburg
30 N 3rd Street
Harrisburg, PA 17101   866-389-5654
                                              Fax: 717-236-4078
                                        e-mail: sgardner@aarp.org
                                          www.aarp.org/states/pa
AARP is a nonprofit nonpartisan membership organization for
people age 50 and over. AARP is dedicated to enhancing the quality of life as one ages, in addition to facilitating social change and
delivering value to members through information and advocacy.
J Shane Creamer, AARP Pennsylvania State President
Steve Gardner, AARP Pennsylvania State Media Relations

South Carolina

65   AARP South Carolina Office: Columbia
1201 Main Street
Columbia, SC 29201   866-389-5655
                                              Fax: 803-251-4374
                                         e-mail: scaarp@aarp.org
                                          www.aarp.org/states/sc
AARP is a nonprofit nonpartisan membership organization for
people age 50 and over. AARP is dedicated to enhancing the quality of life as one ages, in addition to facilitating social change and
delivering value to members through information and advocacy.
Charles A Johnson, AARP SC State President
Patrick Cobb, AARP SC State Media Relations

Tennessee

66   AARP Tennessee State Office: Nashville
150 4th Avenue N
Nashville, TN 37219   866-295-7274
                                              Fax: 615-313-8414
                                         e-mail: tnaarp@aarp.org
                                          www.aarp.org/states/tn
AARP is a nonprofit nonpartisan membership organization for
people age 50 and over. AARP is dedicated to enhancing the quality of life as one ages, in addition to facilitating social change and
delivering value to members through information and advocacy.
Margot Seay, AARP Tennessee State President
Rebecca Kelly, AARP Tennessee State Director

Texas

67   AARP Texas State Office: Austin
98 San Jacinto Boulevard
Austin, TX 78701   866-227-7443
                                              Fax: 512-480-9799
                                         e-mail: rayuso@aarp.org
                                          www.aarp.org/states/tx
AARP is a nonprofit nonpartisan membership organization for
people age 50 and over. AARP is dedicated to enhancing the quality of life as one ages, in addition to facilitating social change and
delivering value to members through information and advocacy.
Rafael Ayuso, AARP Texas State Media Relations
Bob Jackson, AARP Texas State Director

Utah

68   AARP Utah State Office: Midvale
6975 Union Park Center
Midvale, UT 84047   866-448-3616
                                              Fax: 801-561-2209
                                         e-mail: utaarp@aarp.org
                                          www.aarp.org/states/ut
AARP is a nonprofit nonpartisan membership organization for
people age 50 and over. AARP is dedicated to enhancing the quality of life as one ages, in addition to facilitating social change and
delivering value to members through information and advocacy.
Pat Gamble Hovey, Volunteer State President of AARP Utah
Ruby Hammel, Executive Council Advocacy Coordinator

Vermont

69   **AARP Vermont State Office: Montpelier**
199 Main Street
Burlington, VT 05401

866-227-7451
Fax: 802-651-9805
e-mail: vtaarp@aarp.org
www.aarp.org/states/vt

AARP is a nonprofit nonpartisan membership organization for people age 50 and over. AARP is dedicated to enhancing the quality of life as one ages, in addition to facilitating social change and delivering value to members through information and advocacy.
Nancy C Lang, AARP Vermont State President
Dave Reville, AARP Vermont State Media Relations

Virginia

70   **AARP Virginia State Office: Richmond**
707 E Main Street
Richmond, VA 23219

866-542-8164
Fax: 804-819-1923
e-mail: vaaarp@aarp.org
www.aarp.org/states/va

AARP is a nonprofit nonpartisan membership organization for people age 50 and over. AARP is dedicated to enhancing the quality of life as one ages, in addition to facilitating social change and delivering value to members through information and advocacy.
Bill Kallio, AARP Virginia State Director
Tony Hylton, AARP Virginia State Media Relations

Washington

71   **AARP Washington State Office: Seattle**
9750 3rd Avenue NE
Seattle, WA 98115

866-227-7457
Fax: 206-517-9350
e-mail: waaarp@aarp.org
www.aarp.org/states/wa

AARP is a nonprofit nonpartisan membership organization for people age 50 and over. AARP is dedicated to enhancing the quality of life as one ages, in addition to facilitating social change and delivering value to members through information and advocacy.
John Barnett, AARP Washington State President
Doug Shadel, AARP Washington State Director

West Virginia

72   **AARP West Virginia Office: Charleston**
300 Summers Street
Charleston, WV 25301

866-227-7458
Fax: 304-344-4633
e-mail: wvaarp@aarp.org
www.aarp.org/states/wv

AARP is a nonprofit nonpartisan membership organization for people age 50 and over. AARP is dedicated to enhancing the quality of life as one ages, in addition to facilitating social change and delivering value to members through information and advocacy.
Ruth Wagner, AARP West Virginia State President
Ginger Thomp McDaniel, AARP West Virginia State Media Relations

Wisconsin

73   **AARP Wisconsin State Office: Madison**
222 W Washington Avenue
Madison, WI 53703

866-448-3611
Fax: 608-251-7612
e-mail: wistate@aarp.org
www.aarp.org/states/wi

AARP is a nonprofit nonpartisan membership organization for people age 50 and over. AARP is dedicated to enhancing the quality of life as one ages, in addition to facilitating social change and delivering value to members through information and advocacy.
Ethel Percy Andrus, Founder
Albert W Majkrzak, AARP Wisconsin State President

Wyoming

74   **AARP Wyoming State Office: Cheyenne**
2020 Carey Avenue
Cheyenne, WY 82009

866-663-3290
e-mail: wy@aarp.org
www.aarp.org/states/wy

AARP is a nonprofit nonpartisan membership organization for people age 50 and over. AARP is dedicated to enhancing the quality of life as one ages, in addition to facilitating social change and delivering value to members through information and advocacy.
Les Engelter, AARP Wyoming State President
Joanne Bowlby, AARP Wyoming State Media Relations

International

75   **AARP Virgin Islands State Office: St Croix**
4093 Diamond Ruby
Christiansted, VI 00820

866-389-5633
Fax: 340-692-2544
e-mail: viaarp@aarp.org
www.aarp.org/states/vi/

AARP is a nonprofit, nonpartisan membership organization for people age 50 and over. AARP is dedicated to enhancing the quality of life as one ages in addition to facilitating social change and delivering value to members through information, advocacy and service.
Hugo Dennis, Jr., AARP Virgin Islands State President

Libraries & Resource Centers

76   **Aging In America/Morningside House Nursing**
1500 Pelham Parkway S
Bronx, NY 10461

877-244-6469
e-mail: access@aiamsh.org
www.aginginamerica.org

Aging in America is a community-based, social service agency. Morningside House is a provider of specialized medical, nursing and rehabilitative services.
Dr William T Smith, President/CEO

Research Centers

77   **Case Western Reserve University: Center on Aging and Health**
10900 Euclid Avenue
Cleveland, OH 44106

216-368-2000
Fax: 216-368-6389
e-mail: info@case.edu
fpb.case.edu/Centers/UCAH

Research organization conducting supporting and facilitating research into the chronically ill aged person.
Diana L Morris, Executive Director
Evelyn Duffy, Associate Director

78   **Center for the Study of Aging**
706 Madison Avenue
Albany, NY 12208-3604

518-465-6927
Fax: 518-462-1339
e-mail: iapaas@aol.com
www.centerforthestudyofaging.org

Not-for-profit educational and research center for social and medical research on aging health exercise lifelong health and fitness and programs to improve the health and quality of life for older men and women.
Sara Harris, Executive Director
Debra Treadgold, President

79   **Columbia University Center for Geriatrics Gerontology**
College of Physicians and Surgeons
630 West 168th Street
New York, NY 10032

212-305-3595
Fax: 212-305-1343
e-mail: psadmissions@columbia.edu
www.cumc.columbia.edu/dept/ps

Clinical research in geriatric/gerontology and long-term care.
Lee Goldman MD, Dean

80 **Creighton University Center for Healthy Aging**
601 N 30th Street   402-280-4561
Omaha, NE 68131   Fax: 402-280-4623
e-mail: caad@creighton.edu
medicine.creighton.edu/CAAD
Focuses on human development, aging and health care for the elderly.
Patricio F Reyes, Director
Haakon Nygaard, Staff

81 **Landon Center on Aging University of Kansas Medical Center**
University of Kansas Medical Center
3901 Rainbow Boulevard   913-588-1203
Kansas City, KS 66160   800-766-3777
Fax: 913-588-1201
e-mail: rnudo@kumc.edu
www2.kumc.edu/coa
Provides support for interdisciplinary research on the issue of age and aging.
Randolph Nudo, Director
Linda Redford, Associate Director

82 **Purdue University: Center for Research on Aging**
Hanley Hall   765-494-9692
W Lafayette, IN 47907-2055   Fax: 765-494-2180
e-mail: calc@purdue.edu
www.purdue.edu/aging
Social science research on aging health and health care delivery.
Kenneth F Ferraro, Director
Margaret Favorite, Assistant Director

83 **Roy M and Phyllis Gough Huffington Center on Aging**
Huffington Center on Aging
Baylor College of Medicine   713-798-5804
Houston, TX 77030   Fax: 713-798-6688
e-mail: Gretchen@bcm.tmc.edu
www.hcoa.org
Internal unit of Baylor College representing research into the biology of aging.
Gretchen Darlington, Director
Adam Antebi, Associate Professor

84 **University of Pennsylvania Institute on Aging**
3615 Chestnut Street   215-898-3163
Philadelphia, PA 19104-2676   Fax: 215-573-5566
e-mail: aging@mail.med.upenn.edu
www.med.upenn.edu/aging
The mission of the IOA is to improve the health of the elderly by increasing the quality and quantity of clinical and basic research as well as educational programs focusing on normal aging and age-related diseases at the UPSM and across the entire Penn campus.
John Q Trojanowski, Acting Director
Steven E Arnold, Associate Director

Support Groups & Hotlines

85 **Aging Support Group**
Consultants for Aging Families
649 Remington Street   970-498-0730
Fort Collins, CO 80524   e-mail: nanceemc@aol.com
www.fortnet.org/CAF
A source of support, guidance, and accurate, thorough information to help manage the needs and preferences of your older family members.
Nancy McCambridge, Director

86 **Children of Aging Parents**
PO Box 167   215-355-6611
Richboro, PA 18954   800-227-7294
Fax: 215-355-6824
e-mail: info@caps4caregivers.org
www.caps4caregivers.org
A nonprofit, charitable organization that assists the nation's nearly 54 million caregivers of the elderly or chronically ill with reliable information, referrals and support, and to heighten public awareness.

87 **National Health Information Center**
PO Box 1133   310-565-4167
Washington, DC 20013-1133   800-336-4797
Fax: 301-984-4256
e-mail: info@nhic.org
www.health.gov/nhic
A health information referral service sponsored by the Office of Disease Prevention and Health Promotion. NHIC puts health professionals and consumers who have health questions in touch with those organizations that are best able to provide answers.

Books

88 **Activities for the Disabled, Elderly and Adults**
Haworth Press
10 Alice Street   607-722-5857
Binghamton, NY 13904-1580   800-429-6784
Fax: 607-722-0012
www.haworthpress.com
Learn how to effectively plan and deliver activities for a growing number of older people with developmental disabilities. It aims to stimulate interest and continued support for recreation program development and implementation among developmental disability and aging service systems.
136 pages Hardcover
ISBN: 1-560240-92-X

89 **Adult Children and Aging Parents**
American Counseling Association
5999 Stevenson Avenue   703-823-9800
Alexandria, VA 22304-3302   800-347-6647
Fax: 703-823-0252
www.counseling.org
Provides effective intervention strategies and suggestions for counselors who work with older persons, individually and with the family. Offers information on many vital topics such as Alzheimer's Disease, retirement, elder abuse and suicide.
216 pages
ISBN: 0-840354-48-7

90 **Aging and Family Therapy**
Haworth Press
10 Alice Street   607-722-5857
Binghamton, NY 13904-1580   800-429-6784
Fax: 607-722-0012
www.haworthpress.com
Here are creative strategies for use in therapy with older adults and their families. This book provides practitioners with information, insight, reference tools, and other sources that will contribute to more effective intervention with the elderly and their families.
244 pages Hardcover
ISBN: 0-866567-78-3

91 **Aging and Our Families**
Human Sciences Press
233 Spring Street   212-620-8000
New York, NY 10013-1522   800-221-9369
Handbook for family caregivers.
132 pages Paperback
ISBN: 0-898854-41-5

92 **Caregivers' Roller Coaster**
Loyola University Press
3441 N Ashland Avenue   773-281-1818
Chicago, IL 60657-1355   800-621-1008
www.loyolapress.com
A simply written self-help guide for caregivers of the frail elderly. Offers support for men and women, not trained professionals, who find themselves caring for aging family members in their own homes. Offers practical advice and information on Alzheimer's, Medicare, insurance and community services for the elderly.
150 pages
ISBN: 0-829407-45-6

93 **Caring for Those You Love: A Guide to Compassionate Care for the Aged**
Bethany Chaffin, author
Horizon Publishers & Distributors, Inc.

191 N 650 East
Bountiful, UT 84010-3628

801-295-9451
Fax: 801-298-1305
e-mail: hpservice09@hotmail.com
horizonpublishersbookstore.com

Includes helpful information on identifying the problems of the aged. It explains the best and most frequently used treatments prescribed for these problems, and tells how family members can help to meet the physical, emotional, and spiritual needs of aging parents and other loved ones.
108 pages
ISBN: 0-882902-70-9
Duane S Crowther, Owner/CEO
Jean D Crowther, Owner/CEO

94   Continuing Care Retirement Community Directory
American Assoc. of Homes & Services for the Aging
901 E Street NW
Washington, DC 20004-2037

800-508-9442
Fax: 301-206-9789

A national consumer's directory of continuing care retirement communities. This directory is a vital tool for individuals searching and evaluating a community for themselves or a loved one.

95   Court-Related Needs of the Elderly and Persons with Disabilities
Commission on the Mentally Disabled
1800 M Street NW
Washington, DC 20036-5802

202-331-2240
www.statejustice.org/

Report of the National Conference, examines the barriers of the judicial system impeding access for the elderly and persons with disabilities.

96   Creative Movements for Older Adults
Human Sciences Press
233 Spring Street
New York, NY 10013-1522

212-620-8000
800-221-9369

Exercises for the elderly.
172 pages Cloth
ISBN: 0-898854-14-8

97   Diagnosis and Treatment of Old Age
S Karger Publishers
26 W Avon Road
Farmington, CT 06085-1162

860-675-7834
800-828-5479
Fax: 860-675-7302
www.karger.ch/company/karger.htm#10

These papers furnish a concise update on the diagnosis and treatment of Alzheimer's disease.
112 pages Hardcover
ISBN: 3-805548-44-3

98   Elder Care
Center For Public Representation
PO Box 260049
Madison, WI 53726-0049

608-251-4008
800-369-0388
Fax: 608-251-1263
www.law.wisc.edu/pal

A compendium of alternatives for providing and financing long-term care. This practical guide provides the most comprehensive and comforting information to help navigate a number of consumer minefields.
224 pages
ISBN: 0-873371-13-5

99   Elderly in Modern Society
Vance Bibliographier
PO Box 229
Monticello, IL 61856-0229

217-762-3831

A bibliography of laws and human rights for the elderly.
15 pages
ISBN: 0-792001-10-9

100   Falling in Old Age
Reing Tideiksaar PhD, author

Springer Publishing Company
11 W 42nd Street
New York, NY 10036

212-431-4370
877-687-7476
Fax: 212-941-7842
e-mail: cs@springerpub.com
www.springerpub.com

This book provides an enormous body of fall-related research that has been organized by the author into easy, digestible information for geriatric health professionals. Extensively updated and revised for its second edition, the book has direct clinical applications and strategies for preventing and managing falls. It also contains new information on the physical, psychological, and social complications of falling.
412 pages Hardcover
ISBN: 0-826152-91-6

101   Family Carebook
CAREsource Program Development
505 Seattle Tower
0eattle, WA 98101-3021

206-625-9080

Guide to aging, the special needs of older adults, and the demands of providing care and support. Experts explain potential conflicts, planning opportunities and strategies for success.
475 pages Paperback
ISBN: 1-878866-12-5

102   Focus on Geriatric Care and Rehabilitation
Aspen Publishers
7201 McKinney Circle
Frederick, MD 21704-8356

301-251-8500
mail: customer.service@aspenpubl.com
www.aspenpub.com

Written for nurses, occupational therapists and administrators in geriatric settings.
Michael Brown, Publisher

103   From Theory to Therapy: The Development of Drugs for Alzheimer's Disease
Alzheimer's Association
225 N Michigan Avenue
Chicago, IL 60611-1696

800-272-3900
Fax: 866-699-1246
TDD: 312-335-8700
e-mail: media@alz.org
www.alz.org

Provides a layman's explanation of how experimental drugs are being developed and tested for Alzheimer's disease, and information about patient participation in clinical drug trials.

104   Geriatric Rehabilitation Preview
RTC on Aging
7601 E Imperial Highway
Downey, CA 90242-4155

310-940-7402
www.usc.edu/dept/gero/RRTConAging

Covers research, training activities, and other issues pertaining to the rehabilitation of elderly persons with disabilities.

105   Health Care of the Aged
Abraham Monk, PhD, author

Haworth Press
10 Alice Street
Binghamton, NY 13904-1580

607-722-5857
800-429-6784
Fax: 607-722-0012
www.haworthpress.com

Focusing on the need for developing new service delivery models for the aged, this book examines fiscal, political, and social criteria influencing this challenge of the 1990s. The aged are caught in the sweeping changes currently occurring in the financing, organizing and delivery of human health care services.
183 pages Hardcover
ISBN: 1-560240-65-5

106   Healthy Aging: Good Investment & Together We Care: Helping Caregivers Find Supp.
National Council on Aging
1901 L Street NW
Washington, DC 20036

202-479-1200
Fax: 202-479-0735
TDD: 202-479-6674
e-mail: info@ncoa.org
www.ncoa.org

Describes seven model programs that could be used in community-based organizations serving older adults.
2 Book Set
James P Firman, EdD, President/CEO

107 **International Health Guide for Senior Citizen Travelers**
Pilot Books
103 Cooper Street   516-422-2225
Babylon, NY 11702-2368   Fax: 516-669-4173
Covers essential pre-departure health planning such as advice on specific health concerns, disease prevention, specific travel problems, medical preparedness and assistance.
70 pages Paperback
ISBN: 0-875761-39-9
Anne Small, President

108 **Living Well in a Nursing Home**
Lynn Dickinson, Xenia Vosen, author
Hunter House Publishing
1515 1/2 Park Street   510-865-5282
Alameda, CA 94501   800-266-5592
     Fax: 510-865-4295
e-mail: ordering@hunterhouse.com
www.hunterhouse.com
This book concentrates on the positive aspects of nursing homes, providing tips, support and reassurance.
256 pages Paperback
ISBN: 0-897934-60-2

109 **Mentally Impaired Elderly**
Ellen D Taira, author
Haworth Press
10 Alice Street   607-722-5857
Binghamton, NY 13904-1580   800-429-6784
     Fax: 607-722-0012
www.haworthpress.com
Provides effective support and sensitive care for the most vulnerable segment of the elderly population, those with mental impairment.
191 171 pages
ISBN: 1-560241-68-1

110 **Mirrored Lives**
Greenwood Publishing Group, Inc/Praeger Publishers
PO Box 6926
Portsmouth, NH 03802-6926   800-225-5800
     Fax: 877-231-6980
e-mail: service@greenwood.com
www.greenwood.com
Discusses geriatric decline connected to nonterminal illness in old age. Koch takes a sensitive but thorough look at the declining years of his father.
240 pages
ISBN: 0-275936-71-6

111 **Nursing Home Information Services**
925 15th Street NW   202-347-8800
Washington, DC 20005-2301
Lists acceptable nursing homes across the nation and provides information about their costs, admission requirements, standards and programs.

112 **Nursing Home and You: Partners in Caring**
American Assn. of Homes & Services for the Aging
901 E Street NW
Washington, DC 20004-2037   800-508-9442
     Fax: 301-206-9789
Offers information to nursing home staff and family members about caring for persons with Alzheimer's Disease.

113 **Older Americans Information Directory**
Grey House Publishing
4919 Route 22   518-789-8700
Amenia, NY 12501   800-562-2139
     Fax: 518-789-0545
e-mail: books@greyhouse.com
www.greyhouse.com
An invaluable resource that offers up-to-date information on the prevalent social, health and financial issues facing older Americans in the 21st century, as well as recreational and educational opportunities to enrich their lives.
1200 pages
ISBN: 1-592375-43-X
Leslie Mackenzie, Publisher

114 **On Your Behalf**
CAREsource Program Development
505 Seattle Tower   206-625-9080
Seattle, WA 98101
This book takes the mystery out of very important sets of legal options. It gives lay people as well as advisors, service providers, and caregivers the information they need to understand their options and the importance of individual choice.
16 pages Books & Video
ISBN: 1-878866-14-1

115 **Physical Activity and the Aging**
Human Kinetic Publishers
PO Box 5076
Champaign, IL 61825-5076   800-747-4457
     Fax: 217-351-1549
www.humankinetics.com
North America's leading scholars examine the effects of aging on motor function, cardiovascular function, balance, the nervous system, changes in activity level, and possible reasons for activity level changes.
208 pages
ISBN: 0-873222-20-2

116 **Planning for Long-Term Care**
National Council on Aging
1901 L Street NW   202-479-1200
Washington, DC 20036   Fax: 202-479-0735
     TDD: 202-479-6674
e-mail: info@ncoa.org
www.ncoa.org
Identify the various long-term care resources within your family and in your community using this thorough and readable guide.
160 pages
James P Firman, EdD, President/CEO

117 **Read Easy**
CAREsource Program Development
505 Seattle Tower   206-625-9080
Seattle, WA 98101
If books, audio tapes and computers can spark the imagination of the young adult and the middle aged, why not seniors as well? All it takes is commitment to make quality library resources and programs accessible and user-friendly to older readers. Read Easy is an invaluable planning and operations guide, explaining senior needs to library professionals and librarianship principles to senior care professionals.
95 pages
ISBN: 1-878866-13-3

118 **Resources for Elders with Disabilities**
Resources for Rehabilitation
22 Bonad Road   781-368-9080
Winchester, MA 01890   Fax: 781-368-9096
e-mail: orders@rfr.org
www.rfr.org
Provides information that enables elders, family members and other caregivers, and service providers to locate appropriate services. Includes information about rehabilitation, laws that affect elders with disabilities, and self-help groups. Published in large print.

ISBN: 0-929718-31-3

119 **Senior Center Self: Assessment & National Accreditation Manual**
National Council on Aging
1901 L Street NW   202-479-1200
Washington, DC 20036   Fax: 202-479-0735
     TDD: 2024796674
e-mail: info@ncoa.org
www.ncoa.org
Based upon compliance with standards (best practices) developed by the National Institutes of Senior Centers. This program was developed under the auspices of NCOA's National Institute of Senior Centers (NISC).
Book & CD Set
James P Firman, EdD, President/CEO

120 **Senior Citizens and the Law**
Center for Public Representation

PO Box 260049
Madison, WI 53726-0049

608-251-4008
800-369-0388
Fax: 608-251-1263

An introduction to legal problems facing the elderly in Wisconsin. This edition discusses legal problems associated with Social Security, Medicare, SSI, guardianship and its alternatives, community-based services, probate, taxes, private health insurance and consumer protection.
176 pages
ISBN: 0-932622-29-1

121 Successful Models of Community Long Term Care Services for the Elderly
Haworth Press
10 Alice Street
Binghamton, NY 13904-1580

607-722-5857
800-429-6784
Fax: 607-722-0012
www.haworthpress.com

Experienced practitioners provide examples of successful community-based long term care service programs for the elderly.
174 pages
ISBN: 0-866569-87-9

122 Unloving Care
Harper Collins Publishers/Basic Books
10 E 53rd Street
New York, NY 10022-5299

212-207-7000
800-242-7737
Fax: 212-207-7203
www.harpercollins.com

A leading public health expert gives his account of the negative aspects of nursing homes.
305 pages
ISBN: 0-465088-81-3

Magazines

123 AARP Magazine
American Association of Retired Persons
601 East Street NW
Washington, DC 20049

202-434-3525
888-687-2277
e-mail: member@aarp.org
www.aarp.org

Celebrity interviews. Features on health and finance. Movie reviews and more. All with an eye toward the topics and issues you care about most.
A Barry Rand, CEO

124 Abstracts in Social Gerontology
National Council on Aging
1901 L Street NW
Washington, DC 20036

202-479-1200
Fax: 202-479-0735
TDD: 202-479-6674
e-mail: info@ncoa.org
www.ncoa.org

Detailed abstracts are provided for recent major journal articles, books, reports and other materials on many facets of aging, including adult education, demography, family relations, institutional care and work attitudes.
Quarterly
James P Firman, EdD, President/CEO

125 Innovations
National Council on Aging
1901 L Street NW
Washington, DC 20036

202-479-1200
Fax: 202-479-0735
TDD: 2024796674
e-mail: info@ncoa.org
www.ncoa.org

Explores significant developments in the field of aging through opinion articles, profiles and research summaries. Features articles on social trends, articles on specific aging programs and information on NCOA's activities. Members are free.
Quarterly
James P Firman, EdD, President/CEO

126 International Journal of Technology and Aging
Human Sciences Press

233 Spring Street
New York, NY 10013-1522

212-620-8000
800-221-9369
Fax: 212-463-0742

Designed to serve health-care professionals, researchers, academicians and industries concerned with the convergence of two recent trends, the dramatic advances in technology and the rapidly growing elderly population.

127 Modern Maturity
AARP
601 E Street NW
Washington, DC 20049-0003

800-424-3410
e-mail: member@aarp.org
www.aarp.org

Offers news and information of concern to those 50 and older. Features articles on current events, health, recreation, housing, family life, legislation and other issues.
6x Year

Newsletters

128 AARP Bulletin
American Association of Retired Persons
601 East Street NW
Washington, DC 20049

888-687-2277
www.aarp.org

Get daily news about the issues that matter to you.
Bill Novelli, AARP CEO

129 Best Practices
American Assoc. of Homes & Services for the Aging
2519 Connecticut Avenue NW
Washington, DC 20008-1520

202-783-2242
Fax: 202-783-2255
e-mail: info@aahsa.org
www.aahsa.org

Keeps nonprofit aging service providers informed of new trends and developments in quality of care for older persons.

130 Bulletin
AARP
601 E Street NW
Washington, DC 20049

800-424-3410
e-mail: member@aarp.org
www.aarp.org

11x Year

131 CAPSule
Children of Aging Parents
PO Box 167
Richboro, PA 18954-0167

215-355-6611
800-227-7294
Fax: 215-355-6824
e-mail: info@caps4caregivers.org
www.caps4caregivers.org

Newsletter devoted to assisting caregivers of the elderly.
12 pages Quarterly
Lenore Sherman, Executive Director
Karen Rosenberg, Director Senior Services

132 Capital Advantage
Capital Advantage Publishing
2731-A Prosperity Avenue
Fairfax, VA 22031

703-289-4670
Fax: 703-289-4678
e-mail: sales@capitaladvantage.com
www.capitaladvantage.com

Publishes articles on all aspects of aging including legislation, innovative programs and services.
Monthly

133 Center for the Study of Aging Newsletter
University of Pennsylvania Center for Aging Study
3615 Chestnut Street
Philadelphia, PA 19104-4205

215-898-3163
Fax: 215-573-8684
e-mail: www.med.upenn.edu/aging
ageweb@mail.med.upenn.edu

News and information concerning the University and Center aging activities, programs and seminars.

134 **Elderly Health Services Letter**
American Business Publishing
3100 Highway 138   732-681-1133
Wall Township, NJ 0771
Information on trends and developments in the expanding field of
health services for the elderly.
Monthly
Robert Jenkins, Publisher

135 **Geriatric Care News**
DRS Geriatric Publishing Company
7435 SE 71st Street   206-232-9689
Mercer Island, WA 98040-5314
Newsletter for the elderly and their families.
Monthly
Denise Schramke, Publisher

136 **Geriatrics**
7500 Old Oak Boulevard   440-243-8100
Cleveland, OH 44130-3343
Articles for physicians and laypersons relating to care of mid-
dle-aged and elderly persons.
Monthly

137 **Gerontology News**
Gerontological Society of America
1030 15th Street NW   202-842-1275
Washington, DC 20005   Fax: 202-842-1150
                                    e-mail: geron@geron.org
                                    www.geron.org
It reports on policy issues, legislative actions, Society events, re-
search results, and recently released major reports on aging. Regu-
lar features include Washington Updates; Research Highlights;
Grants Available; New Resources and Reports; Data Updates; and
Calls for Papers, Nominations, and Manuscripts.
Carol Ann Schutz, Executive Director

138 **Health After 50: Johns Hopkins Medical Letter**
Johns Hopkins Medical Institutions
550 Broadway   410-955-3182
Baltimore, MD 21205-2011   800-829-9170
                                    e-mail: www.medjhu.edu
Health newsletter for people over 50.
10 pages Monthly
ISBN: 1-042188-2 -
Rodney Friedman, Publisher

139 **Lifelong Health and Fitness**
Center for the Study of Aging
706 Madison Avenue   518-465-4927
Albany, NY 12208-3604   Fax: 518-462-1339
                                    e-mail: iapaas@aol.com
                        www.centerforthestudyofaging-albany.org
A quarterly newsletter published by the Center for the Study of
Aging.
8 pages Quarterly
Sara Harris, Executive Director

140 **NCOA Week**
National Council on Aging
1901 L Street NW   202-479-1200
Washington, DC 20036   Fax: 202-479-0735
                                    TDD: 202-479-6674
                                    e-mail: info@ncoa.org
                                    www.ncoa.org
Breaking news of NCOA initiatives, crucial legislative and policy
issues, research studies, developments in work and volunteering
for older adults, benefits for seniors, trends in aging, grant oppor-
tunities, and more. Members only.
Weekly
James P Firman, EdD, President/CEO

141 **Senior Focus**
National Council on Aging
1901 L Street NW   202-479-1200
Washington, DC 20036   Fax: 202-479-0735
                                    TDD: 202-479-6674
                                    e-mail: info@ncoa.org
                                    www.ncoa.org

Timely, objective, and practical information on health and
wellness, lifestyle, and financial issues for seniors and people who
work with them.
Bi-Monthly
James P Firman, EdD, President/CEO

142 **Vital Aging Report**
National Council on Aging
1901 L Street NW   202-479-1200
Baltimore, MD   Fax: 202-479-0735
                                    TDD: 202-479-6674
                                    e-mail: info@ncoa.org
                                    www.ncoa.org
Packed with news about health and financial matters as well as
United Senior's Health Council's innovative programs and re-
search. The USHC is a program of the National Council on the
Aging. Member price $17.50.
Quarterly
James P Firman, EdD, President/CEO

Pamphlets

143 **American Perceptions of Aging in the 21st Century**
National Council on Aging
1901 L Street NW   202-479-1200
Washington, DC 20036   Fax: 202-479-0735
                                    TDD: 2024796674
                                    e-mail: info@ncoa.org
                                    www.ncoa.org
There are many interesting and important findings related to aging
in America as reported by over 3000 respondents. This chartbook
is intended as a handy reference for scholars, the press and advocates.
James P Firman, EdD, President/CEO

144 **Care of the Elderly in America**
Vance Bibliographies
PO Box 229   217-762-3831
Monticello, IL 61856-0229
A bibliography of aged care in America.
11 pages
ISBN: 1-555905-59-5

145 **Exploring Care Options for a Relative with Alzheimer's Disease**
American Assoc. of Homes & Services for the Aging
2519 Connecticut Avenue NW   202-783-2242
Washington, DC 20008-1520   800-508-9442
                                    Fax: 202-783-2255
                                    e-mail: www.aahsa.org
                                    pub@aahsa.org

146 **Medicare Health Plan Choices: Consumer Update**
National Council on Aging
1901 L Street NW   202-479-1200
Washington, DC 20036   Fax: 202-479-0735
                                    TDD: 202-479-6744
                                    e-mail: info@ncoa.org
                                    www.ncoa.org
Annually updated report contains important information about op-
tions that are available to Medicare beneficiaries. Medicare is
changing, Medigap premiums are going up, and many Medicare
HMOs are dropping service to seniors. Pamphlets available in sin-
gle copies or packs of 50.
James P Firman, EdD, President/CEO

147 **Nonprofit Housing and Care Options for Older People**
American Assoc. of Homes & Services for the Aging
901 E Street NW
Washington, DC 20004-2037   800-508-9442
                                    Fax: 301-206-9789
Offers information on continuing care facilities, retirement communities and more for the elderly and relatives caring for Alzheimer's patients.

148 **Time Out!**
Alzheimer's Association

225 N Michigan Avenue
Chicago, IL 60611-1696

800-272-3900
Fax: 866-669-1246
TDD: 312-335-8700
e-mail: media@alz.org
www.alz.org

Details the Association's position supporting a national respite care policy and recommends actions for federal and state policy makers.
1991 14 pages

Audio & Video

149 **Aphasia: Struggling for Understanding**
Filmakers Library
124 E 40th Street
New York, NY 10016-1798

212-808-4980
Fax: 212-808-4983
e-mail: info@filmakers.com
www.filmakers.com

What if your ability to speak or understand speech was taken away without warning, and you struggled to find words that just won't come? This film is about two people faced with the daunting task of learning to speak again,of regaining their humanity. DVD or VHS, Classroom Rental VHS also available for $65. 14 minutes in length.
DVD or VHS
Sue Oscar, Co-President

Web Sites

150 **Alliance for Aging Research**
www.agingresearch.org
Improving the health and independence of Americans as they age. Promotes medical and behavioral research into the aging process.

151 **American Association of Retired Persons**
www.aarp.org
AARP is the nation's leading organization for people age 50 and older. Information and education, advocacy, and community services provided by a network of local chapters and experienced volunteers throughout the country.

152 **American Society on Aging**
www.asaging.org
An association of diverse individuals bound together by a common goal: to support the commitment and enhance the knowledge and skills of those who seek to improve the quality of life of older adults and their families.

153 **Gerontological Society of America**
www.geron.org
Nonprofit professional organization with more than 5000 members in the field of aging. Provides researchers, educators, practitioners and policy makers with opportunities to understand, advance, integrate and use basic and applied research on aging to improve the quality of life as one ages.

154 **Healing Well**
www.healingwell.com
An online health resource guide to medical news, chat, information and articles, newsgroups and message boards, books, disease-related web sites, medical directories, and more for patients, friends, and family coping with disabling diseases, disorders, or chronic illnesses.

155 **Health Finder**
www.healthfinder.gov
Searchable, carefully developed web site offering information on over 1000 topics. Developed by the US Department of Health and Human Services, the site can be used in both English and Spanish.

156 **Healthlink USA**
www.healthlinkusa.com
Health information concerning treatment, cures, prevention, diagnosis, risk factors, research, support groups, email lists, personal stories and much more. Updated regularly.

157 **Helios Health**
www.helioshealth.com
Online resource for your health information. Detailed information about specific health topics, access to expert advice from our Medical Advisory Board, and up-to-date health news.

158 **MedicineNet**
www.medicinenet.com
An online resource for consumers providing easy-to-read, authoritative medical and health information.

159 **Medscape**
www.medscape.com
Medscape offers specialists, primary care physicians, and other health professionals the Web's most robust and integrated medical information and educational tools.

160 **National Council on Aging**
www.ncoa.org
Seniors Corner includes many resources and health related information on older Americans and their caregivers.

161 **National Institute of Aging**
www.nia.nih.gov
Conducts research on aging, behavioral and social research, neuroscience and neuropsychology, geriatrics, and clinical gerontology.

162 **Research Center**
www.resarch.aarp.org
Online center offering information on consumer issues, demographics, independent living and other items of interest to senior citizens.

163 **US Administration on Aging**
www.aoa.gov
An agency in the US Department of Health and Human Services, is one of the nation's largest providers of home and community-based care for older persons and their caregivers.

164 **WebMD**
www.webmd.com
WebMD provides valuable health information, tools for managing your health, and support to those who seek information.

Description

165 # AIDS/HIV

AIDS, Acquired Immune Deficiency Syndrome, is an infectious disorder that suppresses the normal function of the human body's immune system. AIDS is a result of HIV (Human Immunodeficiency Virus) infection, which destroys the body's ability to fight infections. Specifically, the virus infects and later destroys T-cells, which are a part of the body's immune system that responds to invading organisms. This destructive process is slow and silent, which means that HIV can be contracted years before any symptoms appear. When enough T-cells have been destroyed, the body is invaded by organisms that wouldn't ordinarily be able to cause serious disease. An early symptom of HIV infection is usually an increasing number of infections. Weight loss, fever and night sweats are common. Certain cancers, especially lymphoma and Kaposi's sarcoma, also take advantage of the body's lowered resistance.

HIV transmission requires contact with body fluids and is usually spread from an infected person to a noninfected person by unprotected sexual intercourse, or by sharing needles. Mothers can give HIV infection to their children before and during childbirth and while breastfeeding.

Prevention of HIV infection is the best way to stop the AIDS epidemic. Unfortunately, progress on a vaccine has been disappointing, so avoiding contact with the virus is the primary method of prevention. Avoiding the riskier types of sexual intercourse will reduce one's risk, as will the use of a condom duringvaginal and anal sex. Injecting drug users should not share needles. The use of needle exchange programs has decreased the spread of HIV infection. Women with HIV are encouraged to avoid pregnancy. If pregnant, HIV positive women should stay on medicine directed against HIV and should not breast-feed. Today, infants born to HIV women are treated with medication immediately after birth and this has greatly reduced the incidence of vertical transmission of the infection from mother to child. Until anti-HIV drugs became available, infected persons usually had a rapid downhill course. Today, combination drug treatment can offer most infected persons a long period of relatively good health. However, the treatment regimen is often complex and expensive, involving three or four drugs which must be taken several times a day. Since skipping doses encourages growth of virus that is resistant to the drugs, it is very important to take the drugs exactly as directed.

National Agencies & Associations

166 **AIDS Action**
1424 K Street, NW
Washington, DC 20005
202-408-4848
Fax: 202-408-1818
www.aidsaction.org
National organization dedicated to the development analysis cultivation and encouragement of sound policies and programs in response to the HIV epidemic. We do this through the dissemination of information and the building and use of advocacy.
Donna Crews, Director Government Affairs
Mark Ishaug, President, CEO

167 **AIDS Coalition of Cape Breton**
150 Bentinck Street
Sydney, Nova Scotia, B1P-6H1
902-567-1766
Fax: 902-567-1766
e-mail: christineporter@accb.ns.ca
www.accb.ns.ca
Provides support and advocacy services for PLW HIV/AIDS (people living with HIV/AIDS). Services provided deal with social, legal, ethical and spiritual issues.
Christine Porter, Executive Director
Jo-Anne Rolls, PHA Program Coordinator

168 **AIDS Committee of Durham**
22 King Street West
Oshawa, Ontario, L1H-1A3
905-576-1445
877-361-8750
Fax: 905-576-4610
e-mail: info@aidsdurham.com
www.aidsdurham.com
To provide HIV/AIDS related services to the infected or affected and the general community in the region of Durham.
Doug Willoughby, President
Allan Hooey, Vice President

169 **AIDS Committee of London**
#30-186 King Street
London, Ontario, N6A-3C1
519-434-1601
866-920-1601
Fax: 519-434-1843
e-mail: info@aidslondon.com
www.aidslondon.com
Is a community-based, charitable organization providing HIV-related services to people living with and concerned about HIV/AIDS in London and area.
Brian Lester, Executive Director
Elizabeth Lam, Office Manager

170 **AIDS Committee of Ottawa**
251 Bank Street
Ottawa, Ontario, K2P-1X3
613-238-5014
Fax: 613-238-3425
e-mail: connect@aco-cso.ca
www.aco-cso.ca
Works to empower people living with HIV/AIDS and the PLWHA (persons living with HIV/AID) community in Ottawa through promoting the well being and quality of life of those living with, or close affected by HIV/AIDS.
Kathleen Cummings, Executive Director
Kenda Hoffer, Office Administrator

171 **AIDS Committee of Toronto**
399 Church Street
Toronto, Ontario, M5B-2J6
416-340-2437
Fax: 416-340-8224
www.actoronto.org
Delivers responsive, effective, and valued community-based HIV support services and education, prevention, outreach and fundraising programs that promote health, well-being, worth and rights of individuals and communities living with, affected by and at risk for HIV/AIDS, and increase awareness of HIV/AIDS.
James Forbes, Special Event Manager
Hazelle Palmer, Executive Director

172 **AIDS Committee of York Region**
194 Eagle Street E
Newmarket, Ontario, L3Y-1J6
905-953-0248
800-243-7717
Fax: 905-953-1372
e-mail: edacyr@bellnet.ca
www.acyr.org
The AIDS Committee of York Region envisions an informed and compassionate society, which is supportive of people living with HIV/AIDS who are striving to overcome social and service challenges, working with them towards a healthy and empowered lifestyle.
Radha Bhardwaj, Acting Executive Director

173 AIDS Network
600 Williamson Street
Madison, WI 53703
608-252-6540
Fax: 608-252-6559
TTY: 608-441-3542
e-mail: info@aidsnetwork.org
www.aidsnetwork.org
Provides critical AIDS care and prevention services. Sustained in these efforts by the resources expertise and passion of hundreds of volunteers and donors.
Gerry Haney, Vice President
Mary Vasquez, President

174 AIDS New Brunswick
65 Brunswick Street
Fredericton, NB, E3B-1G5
506-459-7518
800-561-4009
Fax: 506-459-5782
e-mail: info@aidsnb.com
www.aidsnb.com
A provincial organization committed to facilitating community-based responses to the issues of HIV/AIDS. The aim is to promote and support the health and well-being of persons living with and affected by HIV/AIDS and to reduce the spread of HIV/AIDS in New Brunswick.
Nick Scott, Executive Director

175 AIDS Niagara
Normandy Resource Center
St. Catharines, Ontario, L2R-3C9
905-984-8684
800-773-9843
Fax: 905-988-1921
e-mail: info@aidsniagara.com
www.aidsniagara.com
AIDS Niagara is dedicated to improving the quality of life for those infected and/or affected by HIV/AIDS.
Steve Byers, Executive Director
Jody Yurchak, Education & Support Coordinator

176 AIDS PEI
375 University Avenue
Charlottetown, PE, C1A-4N4
902-566-2437
Fax: 902-626-3400
www.aidspei.com
To create a supportive environment for Persons Living with AIDS/HIV, to increase public understanding of the impact of HIV/AIDS, and to reduce the incidence of HIV/AIDS in Prince Edward Island.
Tom Hilton, Executive Director
K. Deanna Carroll, Director

177 AIDS Thunder Bay
574 Memorial Avenue
Thunder Bay, Ontario, P7B-3Z2
807-345-1516
800-488-5840
Fax: 807-345-2505
e-mail: info@aidsthunderbay.org
www.aidsthunderbay.org
Provide quality, compassionate support, education and advocacy around HIV and AIDS, and related issues.
Sandra Cruzo, Vice President
Dennis Eeles, President

178 AIDS Treatment Data Network
611 Broadway
New York, NY 10012
212-260-8868
800-734-7104
e-mail: network@atdn.org
www.atdn.org
The Network is a national independent community-based not-for-profit organization that provides treatment access and advocacy, case management, supportive counseling and English and Spanish language information services to men women and children with HIV.

179 AIDS.ORG
P.O. Box 69491
Los Angeles, CA 90069
323-656-6036
www.aids.org
The mission of AIDS.ORG is to help prevent HIV infections and to improve the lives of those affected by HIV and AIDS by providing education and facilitating the free and open exchange of knowledge at any easy-to-find centralized Web site.
Alain Berrebi, Executive Director
Peter Dobson, Director

180 AIDSinfo
PO Box 6303
Rockville, MD 20849-6303
301-519-0459
800-448-0440
Fax: 301-315-2818
TTY: 888-480-3739
e-mail: contactus@aidsinfo.nih.gov
www.aidsinfo.nih.gov
AIDSinfo is a U.S. Department of Health and Human Services (DHHS) project that offers the latest federally approved information on HIV/AIDS clinical research, treatment and prevention, and medical practice guidelines for people living with HIV/AIDS, their families and friends, health care providers, scientists, and researchers.

181 ANKORS: Kootenay & Boundary HIV/AIDS and Hepatitis C Support Services
101 Baker Street
Nelson, BC, V1L-4H1
250-505-5506
800-421-2437
Fax: 250-505-5507
e-mail: information@ankors.bc.ca
www.ankors.bc.ca
ANKORS' mission is to respond to the evolving needs of those living with and affected by HIV/AIDS and Hepatitis C.
Cheryl Dowden, Executive Director
Gary Dalton, Community Care Team

182 Access AIDS Network
111 Elm Street
Sudbury, Ontario, P3C-1T3
705-688-0500
800-465-2437
Fax: 705-688-0423
e-mail: access@cyberbeach.net
www.accessaidsnetwork.com
A non-profit, community-based charitable organization, committed to promoting wellness, education, harm and risk reduction.
Richard Rainville, Executive Director
Christine Coutu, Clerical Intake Worker

183 Alberta Reappraising AIDS Society
Box 61037
Calgary, Alberta, T2N-4S6
403-289-6609
Fax: 403-206-7717
e-mail: aras@aras.ab.ca
www.aras.ab.ca
Promote critical discussion of the HIV/AIDS dogma.
David Crowe, President
Roger Swan, Treasurer

184 American Autoimmune Related Diseases Association
22100 Gratiot Avenue
Eastpointe, MI 48021
586-776-3900
800-598-4668
Fax: 586-776-3903
e-mail: aarda@aarda.org
www.aarda.org
Awareness, education, referrals for patients with any type of autoimmune disease.
Virginia T. Ladd, President/Executive Director

185 American Civil Liberties Union AIDS Project
125 Broad Street
New York, NY 10004
212-549-2500
www.aclu.org/HIVAIDS/HIVAIDSMain.cfm
Offers legislative and employment information public awareness materials and support for persons with HIV/AIDS and their families.
Anthony D Romero, Executive Director
Susan Herman, President

186 American Federation of Teachers HIV/AIDS Education Project
555 New Jersey Avenue NW
Washington, DC 20001-2029
202-879-4400
www.aft.org
A group of education professionals with the main purpose of their work being the education and public awareness of HIV and AIDS.
Randi Weingarten, President

187 American Foundation for AIDS Research
120 Wall Street   212-806-1600
New York, NY 10005-3908   800-342-2437
                                        Fax: 212-806-1601
                                       TTY: 800-243-7889
                            e-mail: kevin.frost@amfar.org
                                           www.amfar.org
Supports research in basic clinical prevention and public policy
and publishes the HIV/AIDS Treatment Directory.
Kevin Robert Frost, CEO
Bradley Jensen, Chief Financial Officer

**188 Asian & Pacific Islander Wellness Center Community HIV/AIDS
Services**
730 Polk Street   415-292-3400
San Francisco, CA 94109   Fax: 415-292-3404
                                       TTY: 415-292-3410
                             e-mail: info@apiwellness.org
                                       www.apiwellness.org
HIV Care Services is the only integrated HIV services program tar-
geting A&PIs in Northern California. Integrates primary care with
psychiatric mental health HIV treatment psychosocial support
and, in response to evolving needs, targeted HIV prevention.
Lance Toma LCSW, Executive Director
Ann Madden, SPHR, Human Resources Administrator

189 Asian and Pacific Island Wellness Center
730 Polk Street   415-292-3400
San Francisco, CA 94109   Fax: 415-292-3404
                                       TTY: 415-292-3410
                             e-mail: info@apiwellness.org
                                       www.apiwellness.org
Our mission is to educate support empower and advocate for Asian
and Pacific Islander communities - particularly A&PIs living with
or at-risk for HIV/AIDS.
Lance Toma LCSW, Executive Director
Ann Madden, SPHR, Human Resources Administrator

190 Better Existence with HIV
1244 W. Thorndale   773-293-4740
Chicago, IL 60660   Fax: 773-293-4750
                                           www.behiv.org
Private not-for-profit AIDS service organization. Only compre-
hensive AIDS service provider in all northern Cook County. Effec-
tively combines direct service and prevention programs.
Eric Nelson, Executive Director
Julie Supple, Director of Programs

191 Black Coalition for AIDS Prevention
20 Victoria Street   416-977-9955
Toronto, Ontario, M5C-2N8   Fax: 416-977-7664
                           e-mail: blackcap@black-cap.com
                                        www.black-cap.com
A volunteer-driven, charitable, not-for-profit, community-based
organization. We work in partnership with organizations and individuals who support in principle and practice our mission, philosophy and activities.
Angela Robertson, Chair
Trevor Grey, Co-Chair

192 British Columbia Persons with AIDS Society
1107 Seymour Street   604-893-2200
Vancouver, BC, V6B-5S8   800-994-2437
                                       Fax: 604-893-2251
                                 e-mail: info@bcpwa.org
                                           www.bcpwa.org
Exists to enable persons living with AIDS and HIV disease to em-
power themselves through mutual support and collective action.
Ross Harvey, Executive Director
Denise Becker, Chair

193 CDC National Prevention Information Network (NPIN)
PO Box 6003   919-361-4892
Rockville, MD 20849-6003   800-458-5231
                                       Fax: 888-282-7681
                                       TTY: 800-243-7012
                                e-mail: info@cdcnpin.org
                                           www.cdcnpin.org
The CDC National Prevention Information Network (NPIN) is the
U.S. reference, referral, and distribution service for information

on HIV/AIDS, sexually transmitted diseases (STD's), and tuberculosis (TB). NPIN produces, collects, catalogs, processes, stocks,
and disseminates materials and information on HIV/AIDS, STD's,
and TB to organizations and people working in those disease fields
in international, national, state, and local settings.

194 Canadian Foundation for AIDS Research
165 University Avenue   416-361-6281
Toronto, Ontario, M5H-3B8   800-563-2873
                                        Fax: 416-361-5736
                                            www.canfar.ca
A national charitable foundation whose goal is to raise awareness
in order to generate funds for research into all aspects of HIV infec-
tion and AIDS.
Christopher Bunting, President
Jenna Kellner, National Programs Manager

195 Central Alberta AIDS Network Society
4611-50th Avenue   403-346-8858
Red Deer Alberta, T4N-3Z9   877-346-8858
                                        Fax: 403-346-2352
                            e-mail: receptionist@cirsonine.ca
                                            www.caans.org
Central Alberta AIDS Network Society is a local charity and a
Turning Point agency that offers support to individuals who are in-
fected or affected by HIV/AIDS and provides prevention and edu-
cation throughout Central Alberta.
Jennifer Vanderschae, Executive Director
Mel Lewis, Health Promotion Coordinator

196 Children Affected by AIDS Foundation
6033 W Century Boulevard   310-258-0850
Los Angeles, CA 90045   Fax: 310-258-0851
                                 e-mail: caaf@caaf4kids.org
                                            www.caaf4kids.org
The mission of the Children Affected by AIDS Foundation
(CAAF) is to make a positive difference in the lives of children in-
fected with HIV and affected by AIDS. CAAF accomplishes this
by helping meet their diverse, special needs, advocating and edu-
cating.
Jayne Harkness, President
Joe Christina, Founder, Vice President

197 Children's AIDS Fund
PO Box 16433   703-433-1560
Washington, DC 20041   866-829-1560
                                        Fax: 800-557-8529
                          e-mail: info@childrensaidsfund.org
                                       www.childrensaidsfund.org
The Children's AIDS Fund works to limit suffering of children and
their families caused by HIV disease by providing care services
resourced referrals and education.
Anita Smith, President

198 Clinical Focus on Primary Immune Deficiency Diseases
Immune Deficiency Foundation
40 W Chesapeake Avenue   410-321-6647
Towson, MD 21204   800-296-4433
                                        Fax: 410-321-9165
                              e-mail: idf@primaryimmune.org
                                       www.primaryimmune.org
Educational monograph is designed specifically for health care
professionals and focuses on topics relevant to primary immune
deficiency diseases.
Marcia Boyle, President & Founder

199 Committee of Ten Thousand
236 Massachusetts Avenue NE   202-543-0988
Washington, DC 20002   800-488-2688
                                        Fax: 202-543-6720
                            e-mail: cott-dc@earthlink.net
                                            www.cott1.org
Represents people with hemophilia who contracted HIV/AIDS and
Hepatitis C from tainted factor concentrates in the 1970s and
1980s. The only national advocacy and support agency for this se-
riously disabled community.
Corey S Dubin, President
Mary Lou Murphy, Co-Vice President

200   Continuum
255 Golden Gate Avenue
San Francisco, CA 94102

415-437-2900
Fax: 415-437-2550
TTY: 415-861-1399
e-mail: anne@continuumhiv.org
web.mac.com/tenderloinhealth

Empower and dignify the lives of underserved people with HIV and AIDS providing innovative health and human services that establish community, and reduce the rate of HIV infection.
Colm Hegarty, Director Development & Public Relations
Chiquita T Tuttle, Interim Executive Director

201   Deaf AIDS Project Family Service Foundation
Family Service Foundation
5301 76th Avenue
Landover Hills, MD 20784

301-459-2121
866-935-4658
Fax: 301-459-0675
TTY: 301-731-2116
e-mail: ssoulier@fsfinc.org
www.deafnonprofit.net/dap

The AIDS Administration established in 1987 as a division of the Maryland Department of Health and Mental Hygiene leads public health initiatives regarding HIV (Human Immunodeficiency Virus), the virus that causes AIDS.

202   Elizabeth Glaser Pediatric AIDS Foundation
1140 Connecticut Avenue NW
Washington, DC 20036

202-296-9165
888-499-4673
Fax: 202-296-9185
e-mail: info@pedaids.org
www.pedaids.org

Creates a future of hope for children and families worldwide by eradicating pediatric AIDS providing care and treatment to people with HIV/AIDS and accelerating the discovery of new treatments for other serious and life-threatening pediatric illnesses.
Charles Lyons, President/CEO

203   Farha Foundation
576, Sainte-Catherine Street E
Montreal, QC, H2L-2E1

514-270-4900
Fax: 514-270-5363
e-mail: farha@farha.qc.ca
www.farha.qc.ca

A fundraising organization, committed to help men, women and children living with HIV/AIDS.

204   Foundation for Children with AIDS
6221 Blue Grass Avenue
Harrisburg, PA 17112-2331

717-489-0206
888-683-8323
Fax: 717-489-0214
e-mail: info@helpchildrenwithaids.org
www.helpchildrenwithaids.org

A national nonprofit organization founded to improve the quality of life for drug-effected and HIV-infected children and their families. The foundation raises funds for family and community-based services for children and their families affected by HIV.
Nick Cassino, President
Robert Maynard, Vice President

205   HIV West Yellowhead Services
Box 2427
Jasper, Alberta, T0E-1E0

780-852-5274
877-291-8811
Fax: 780-852-5273
e-mail: hivdirector@incentre.net
www.hivwestyellowhead.com

Encourage a positive, healthy lifestyle and provide accurate information to the people living and working in the region.

206   HIV/Hepatitis C in Prison (HIP) Committee
California Prison Focus
San Francisco, CA 94103

510-665-1935
e-mail: contact@prisons.org
www.prisons.org/hivin.htm

The HIV/HCV in Prison Committee of California Prison Focus works on behalf of prisoners to fight for consistent access to quality medical care including access to all new HIV and hepatitis C medications, diagnostic testing and combination therapies.
Michelle Foy, Contact
Judy Greenspan, Contact

207   Health Information Network
PO Box 30762
Seattle, WA 98113

206-784-5655
Fax: 206-784-3240
www.healthinfonetwork.org

Offers information public awareness and support for women with HIV/AIDS and the public in general.
Kathi Knowles, Executive Director

208   Health Information Network for Women and AIDS
Positive Women's Network
2817 Rockefeller Avenue
Everett, WA 98201

425-259-9899
888-651-8931
Fax: 425-259-9880
www.pwnetwork.org

A partnership of women living with and affected by HIV/AIDS supports women in making informed choices about HIV/AIDS and health.
Kerri Mallams, Executive Director
Aisa Bennett, President

209   Heart Touch™ Project
3400 Airport Avenue
Santa Monica, CA 90405

310-391-2558
Fax: 310-391-2168
e-mail: executive@hearttouch.org
www.hearttouch.org

Non-profit educational and service organization devoted to the delivery of compassionate and healing touch to home or hospital-bound men women and children.
Jennifer Noguera, Coordinator Children's Program
Patrick Callahan, Executive Director

210   Immune Deficiency Foundation
40 W Chesapeake Avenue
Towson, MD 21204-4841

410-321-6647
800-296-4433
Fax: 410-321-9165
e-mail: idf@primaryimmune.org
www.primaryimmune.org

The only national charitable organization aimed at fighting the primary immune deficiency diseases. The founders included parents of children with primary immune deficiency immunologists who treat immune deficient patients and other individuals with an immune deficiency.
John Seymour, Vice Chair
Marcia Boyle, Chair President & Founder

211   International Council of AIDS Service Organization
65 Wellesley Street E
Toronto Ontario, M4Y-1G7

416-921-0018
Fax: 416-921-9979
e-mail: icaso@icaso.org
www.icaso.org

A global network of non-governmental and community-based organizations.
Kieran Daly, Executive Director
Sara Simon, Project Manager

212   Life Force: Women Fighting AIDS
57 Willoughby Street
Brooklyn, NY 11201-4300

718-797-0937
Fax: 718-797-4011
e-mail: info@lifeforceinc.org
www.lifeforceinc.org

A support network offering prevention education awareness risk reduction workshops and support for woman with HIV/AIDS.
Sayida Self, Program Director
Linney Smith, Executive Director

213   Living Positive
9912-106 Street
Edmonton, Alberta, T5K-1C5

780-488-5768
800-210-9561
Fax: 780-702-8211
www.edmlivingpositive.ca

Dedicated to providing emotional, spiritual and psychological support to all those living with HIV.
Lance Hansen, Director
Deborah Norris, Chairperson

214   Medical Library Association
65 E Wacker Place
Chicago, IL 60601-7246

312-419-9094
Fax: 312-419-8950
e-mail: info@mlahq.org
www.mlahq.org

Non-profit educational organization of more than 1,100 institutions and 3,600 individual members in the health sciences information field, committed to educating health information professionals, supporting health information research and promoting access to information.
Ruth Holst, President
Carla J Funk, Executive Director

215   Multifaith Works
115 16th Avenue   206-324-1520
Seattle, WA 98122   Fax: 206-324-2041
                              e-mail: info@multifaith.org
                              www.multifaith.org
Non-profit non-denominational organization that provides housing and supportive services to people living with AIDS or other life-threatening illness and community education on issues of human diversity.
Arthur Padilla, Executive Director
Randy Lazenby, President

216   NAMES Project Foundation AIDS Memorial Quilt
AIDS Memorial Quilt
204 14th Street NW   404-688-5500
Atlanta, GA 30318-5304   Fax: 404-688-5552
                              e-mail: info@aidsquilt.org
                              www.aidsquilt.org
International non-governmental non-profit organization that is the custodian of the AIDS Memorial Quilt a poignant memorial and powerful tool for use in preventing new HIV infections.
Julie Rhoad, Executive Director
Roddy Williams, Director of Operations

217   National AIDS Fund
1444 K Street NW   202-408-4848
Washington, DC 20005-1511   888-234-AIDS
                              Fax: 202-408-1818
                              www.aidsfund.org
The National AIDS Fund is one of America's largest philanthropic organizations dedicated to eliminating HIV/AIDS as a major health and social problem. The Fund's primary purpose is channeling critical resources to community-based organizations to fight HIV.
Mark Ishaug, President & CEO
Matthew Kessler, Director of Operations

218   National AIDS Treatment Advocacy Project
580 Broadway   212-219-0106
New York, NY 10012   888-26N-ATAP
                              Fax: 212-219-8473
                              e-mail: info@natap.org
                              www.natap.org
Educate by sending out literature e-mail lists and give forums on how to prevent HIV or how to live with it.
Jules Levin, Executive Director

219   National Coalition on Immune System Disorders
1090 Vermont Avenue NW   202-371-8090
Washington, DC 20005-4953   800-438-2996
                              Fax: 202-371-1945
Professional and lay organizations with a primary interest in the immune system and its diseases.
Robert R Humphreys, Executive Director

220   National Hospice & Palliative Care Organization (NHPCO)
1731 King Street   703-837-1500
Alexandria, VA 22314   800-658-8898
                              Fax: 703-837-1233
                              e-mail: nhpcoinfo@nhpco.org
                              www.nhpco.org
The nation's only advocate for terminally ill patients and their families. Founded in 1978, the NHPCO is the only organization devoted to hospice in the United States. Support is included from state hospice organizations, patients, families, communities, provider program members and professional/volunteer members. Represents hospice care interests to Congress, regulatory agencies, courts, voluntary organizations and the public.
Donald Schumacher, PsyD, President/CEO

221   National Minority AIDS Education Training Center
Howard University

1840 7th Street NW   202-865-8146
Washington, DC 20001-3029   Fax: 202-667-1382
                              e-mail: gdowner@howard.edu
                              www.aetcnmc.org/index
Located at Howard University as a HIV/AIDS training and technical resource for providers of minority HIV-infected patients throughout the country. The NMAETC receives 100% of its funding through the MAI Initiative.
Goulda Downe PhD RD, Principal Investigator
David Luckett, Deputy Director

222   National Native American AIDS Prevention Center
720 S Colorado Boulevard   720-382-2244
Denver, CO 80246   Fax: 720-382-2248
                              e-mail: information@nnaapc.org
                              www.nnaapc.org
To address the impact of HIV/AIDS on American Indians Alaska Natives and Native Hawaiians through culturally appropriate advocacy research education and policy development in support of healthy Indigenous people.
Stacey A Bohlen, President
Robert Foley, Executive Director

223   National Prevention Information Network CDC NPIN
PO Box 6003   404-679-3860
Rockville, MD 20849-6003   800-458-5231
                              Fax: 888-282-7681
                              TTY: 888-232-6348
                              e-mail: info@cdcnpin.org
                              www.cdcnpin.org
The CDC National Prevention Information Network (NPIN) is the U.S. reference referral and distribution service for information on HIV/AIDS, sexually transmitted diseases (STDs) and tuberculosis (TB).
Jay Laudato, Executive Director

224   National Prison Project/ACLU AIDS in Prison Project
125 Broad Street
New York, NY 10004   212-549-2900
                              www.aclu.org
National Prison Project seeks to create constitutional conditions of confinement and strengthen prisoners' rights through class action litigation and public education. Our policy priorities include reducing prison overcrowding and improving prisoner medical care.
Susan N Herman, President
Anthony Romero, Executive Director

225   New England AIDS Education and Training Center
23 Miner Street   617-262-5657
Boston, MA 02215-3318   Fax: 617-262-5667
                              e-mail: aidsed@neaetc.org
                              www.neaetc.org
Our goal is to increase the number of health care providers effectively trained to counsel diagnose treat and manage the care of individuals with HIV infection and to assist in the prevention of high risk behavior which may lead to infection.
Donna M Gallagher RNC MS AN, Project Director
Calvin Cohen MD MS, Co-Research Director

226   North Bay Aids Committee
269 Main Street W   705-497-3560
North Bay, Ontario, P1B-2T8   Fax: 705-497-7850
                              e-mail: acnba@efni.com
                              www.aidsnorthbay.com
To assist and support all persons infected or affected by HIV/AIDS and to limit the spread of the virus through education and outreach strategies.
Stacey L Mayhall, Executive Director
Steve Lamb, Support Services Coordinator

227   Ontario HIV Treatment Network
1300 Yonge Street   416-642-6486
Toronto, ON M41X3   877-743-6486
                              Fax: 416-640-4245
                              e-mail: info@ohtn.on.ca
                              www.ohtn.on.ca
To optimize the quality of life of people living with HIV in Ontario and to promote excellence and innovation in treatment, research, education and prevention through a collaborative network of ex-

cellence representing consumers, providers, researchers and other stakeholders.
Evan Collins, President
Sean Rourke, Executive Director

228 Pediatric AIDS Foundation
11150 Santa Monica Boulevard
Los Angeles, CA 90025-3092
310-314-1459
Fax: 310-314-1469
e-mail: info@pedaids.org
www.pedaids.org
A national nonprofit organization confronting medical problems unique to children infected with HIV/AIDS. The foundation funds critically needed pediatric AIDS research and provides help to hospitals that serve the needs of children with HIV/AIDS.
Charles Lyons, President/CEO
Susie Zeegan, Co-Founder

229 Peel HIV/AIDS Network
160 Traders Boulevard E
Mississauga, Ontario, L4Z 3-4K1
905-361-0523
866-896-8700
Fax: 905-361-1004
e-mail: info@phan.ca
www.phan.ca
Committed to serving people living with and affected by HIV/AIDS and to limit the spread of the virus through support education advocacy and volunteerism.
Ketih Wong, Executive Director
Berkha Gupta, Coordinator Volunteer Services

230 Project Inform
1375 Mission Street
San Francisco, CA 94103
415-558-8669
800-822-7422
Fax: 415-558-0684
e-mail: support@projectforum.org
www.projectforum.org/HIVhealth/infoline
HIV Health Infoline has provided HIV treatment and access to care information, free of charge, to people living with HIV, their providers and support networks. Staffed by highly trained volunteers, the Infoline has the personal experiences and outside connections to answer questions about living healthfully with HIV.
Dana Van Gorder, Executive Director
Michael Allerton, President

231 Resources and Services Database Centers for Disease Control
Centers for Disease Control
PO Box 6003
Rockville, MD 20849
877-242-9760
877-242-9760
Fax: 301-562-1050
TTY: 240-514-2780
e-mail: info@hivatwork.org
www.brta-lrta.org
Describes more than 16 000 organizations that provide HIV and AIDS prevention education and social services. These include public health departments community and social service organizations hospitals and clinics.

232 The AIDS Network
140 King Street East
Hamilton, ON, L8N-1B2
905-528-0854
866-563-0563
Fax: 905-528-6311
e-mail: info@aidsnetwork.ca
www.aidsnetwork.ca
Hours of operation: Monday-Friday, 9am-12pm and 1pm-5pm.
Todd Fraleigh, Executive Director
Tony Mark, President

233 Toronto People with AIDS Foundation
200 Gerard Street E
Toronto, Ontario, M5A-2E6
416-506-1400
Fax: 416-506-1404
e-mail: info@pwatoronto.org
www.pwatoronto.org
The Toronto People with AIDS Foundation exists to promote the health and well-being of all people living with HIV/AIDS by providing accessible, direct, and practical support services.
Murray Jose, Executive Director
Suzanne Paddock, Director, Programs & Services

234 UNICEF USA
125 Maiden Lane
New York, NY 10038
212-686-5522
800-486-4233
Fax: 212-779-1679
e-mail: information@unicefusa.org
www.unicefusa.org
Supports child survival protection and development worldwide through education advocacy and fundraising for AIDS and other conditions.
Caryl M Stern, President and CEO
Edward G Lloyd, Executive Vice President and CFO

235 Well Project
112 Krog Street NE
Atlanta, GA 30307
404-474-3152
888-616-9355
e-mail: info@thewellproject.org
www.thewellproject.org
The Well Project is a not for profit corporation and an initiative conceived developed and administered by HIV+ women and those who are affected by this disease. Our Founder Dawn Averitt Bridge was diagnosed with HIV in 1988.
Dawn Averitt Bridge, Founder & Board President
Richard Averitt, COO

236 Women Alive
1566 Burnside Avenue
Los Angeles, CA 90019
323-965-1564
800-554-4876
Fax: 323-965-9886
e-mail: info@women-alive.org
www.women-alive.org
Coalition of, by and for women living with HIV/AIDS. Created ways to help women connect with each other, bring others out of isolation, exchange information about HIV treatments and take charge of their lives.
Carrie Broadus, Executive Director
Alfredia Thomas, President

237 Women's AIDS Network Women and Children's Service Program
Women and Children's Service Program
10 United Nations Plaza
San Francisco, CA 94101
415-864-4376

State Agencies & Associations

Alabama

238 Alabama Department of Public Health
201 Monroe Street
Montgomery, AL 36104-3000
334-206-5364
800-228-0469
Fax: 334-206-2092
www.adph.org/aids
Offers health education and risk education activities including compiling a state community resource directory.
Danna Cargill, Office Manager
Jane B Cheeks, Division Director

Alaska

239 Alaska Department of Health and Social Services: AIDS/STD Program
3601 C Street
Anchorage, AK 99503-0249
907-269-8000
800-478-0084
Fax: 907-562-7802
e-mail: mollie_cross@health.state.ak.us
www.epi.hss.state.ak.us/hivstd
The HIV/STD Program addresses public health issues and activities with the goal of preventing sexually transmitted diseases (STDs) and HIV infection in Alaska as well as their impact on health. AIDS program offers education to providers and organizations.
John Middaug PhD, Chief Dept of Public Health/Epidemiology
Mollie Cross, Prevention Community Planning Group

Arizona

240   Arizona Department of Health Services
150 N 18th Avenue
Phoenix, AZ 85007
60- 5-2 10
800-334-1540
Fax: 602-542-0883
www.azdhs.gov

Provides HIV and AIDS seropositive surveillance case investigation and analysis and AIDS health education and training for the public.
Margery Sheridan, Division Chief
Will Humble, Interim Director

241   Tucson Interfaith HIV/AIDS Network (TIHAN)
1011 N Craycroft Road
Tucson, AZ 85711
520-299-6647
Fax: 520-784-0620
e-mail: friends@tihan.org
www.tihan.org

Serving interfaith communities of Tucson through compassionate care education training and spiritual support so that we can make more people aware of the health crisis which affects all of us. Also provide non-medical in-home help.
Scott Blades, Executive Director
Aimee Graves, President

Arkansas

242   Arkansas Department of Health AIDS Prevention Program
AIDS Prevention Program
4815 West Markham Street
Little Rock, AR 72205
501-661-2000
www.healthyarkansas.com

Provides educational materials such as pamphlets and films conducts HIV and AIDS research and operates a speakers bureau.
Robin Thomas, Regional Director
Paul Halverson, Director

California

243   Aids, Medicine and Miracles
3288 21st Street
San Francisco, CA 94110-2423
415-252-7111
Fax: 415-252-7117
e-mail: amminfo@aidsmedicineandmiracles.org
www.aidsmedicineandmiracles.org

Provides culturally sensitive counseling and education to stop the spread of HIV infection, and to help people face the emotional, psychological and social changes of living with HIV disease.
Gregg Cassin, Chair
Daniel Ramos, Secretary

244   California Collaborative Treatment Group CCTG Data Center
CCTG Data Center
3900 Fifth Avenue
San Diego, CA 92103-1910
619-543-5006
Fax: 619-298-1359
e-mail: rhaubrich@ucsd.edu
www.cctg.ucsd.edu

The CCTG is a multi-center clinical trials organization founded by Dr. Allen McCutchan in 1986. The primary mission of the CCTG is to improve the scientific basis for HIV patient care and HIV prevention. CCTG develops treatment protocols and drug therapies.
Richard Haub MD, Investigator/Professor of Medicine
Allen McCutc MD, Investigator/Professor of Medicine

245   California Department of Health Services Office of Aids
Office of Aids
1501 Capitol Ave.
Sacramento, CA 95814
916-445-4171
800-458-5231
Fax: 916-440-7404
www.dhs.ca.gov/aids

Works to develop strategies and implement programs for education and prevention testing and counseling supportive care and treatment and research to control the spread of HIV infection.
David Maxwell-Jolly, Director

246   Los Angeles County Department of Health Services
AIDS Programs
600 S Commonwealth Avenue
Los Angeles, CA 90005
213-351-8000
800-243-7889
Fax: 213-738-0825
e-mail: aids@ph.lacounty.org
www.lapublichealth.org

Responsible for planning coordinating and implementing county wide HIV/AIDS efforts.
Charles L Henry, Director
Raymond H Johnson, Chief of Staff

247   San Francisco AIDS Foundation (SFAF)
1035 Market Street
San Francisco, CA 94103
415-487-3000
800-367-AIDS
Fax: 415-487-8079
TTY: 415-487-3012
TDD: 415-487-8099
e-mail: info@aidslifecycle.org
www.sfaf.org

SFAF provides confidential array of services-including financial benefits counseling client advocacy housing assistance HIV prevention efforts and needle exchange.
Neil Giuliano, CEO
Barbara Kimport, VP Development

248   San Francisco Area AIDS Education and Training Center
UCSF Box 1365
50 Beale Street
San Francisco, CA 94105-1365
41- 5-7 91
Fax: 41- 5-7 93
e-mail: sfaetc@ucsf.edu
http://www.sfaetc.ucsf.edu/

Helps to improve the care of people living with HIV and AIDS by supporting state-of-the-art clinical consultation education and training for health care professionals and organizations in Sa Francisco San Mateo and Marin counties.
Jacqueline Tulsky, Medical Director
Ronald H Goldschmidt, Director

Colorado

249   CO Center for AIDS Research: University Colorado Health Sciences Center/CFAR
Division of Infectious Diseases
4200 E 9th Avenue
Denver, CO 80262
303-315-7233
Fax: 303-315-8681
e-mail: colorado.cfar@uchsc.edu
www.uchsc.edu/ccfar

Describes forms and patterns of use of complimentary and alternative medicine (CAM) for the treatment of HIV/AIDS.
Edward N Janoff MD, CFAR Director
Kristin Jones, CFAR Administrator

Connecticut

250   Connecticut Department of Health Services AIDS Programs
AIDS Programs
410 Capitol Avenue
Hartford, CT 06134
860-509-8000
800-842-0038
Fax: 860-509-7853
e-mail: webmaster.dph@ct.gov
www.dph.state.ct.us

Operates a speakers bureau provides training workshops seminars and counseling services conducts meetings and offers information and referral services.
Rosa M Biaggi, Director
William Gerrish, Communications

251   Northwestern Connecticut AIDS Project
100 Migeon Avenue
Torrington, CT 06790-0985
860-482-1596
800-381-2437
Fax: 860-482-3606
e-mail: general@nwctaids.org
www.freewebs.com/nwctaidsproject

A nonprofit organization offering support and a variety of services to people with AIDS and their loved ones. Provides education to all segments of the public about AIDS prevention and treatment.
Patricia Lafayette, Executive Director
Demetria McMilliAn, Program Director Client Services

Delaware

252   Delaware Department of Health and Social Services
Division of Public Health, HIV/STD Program
417 Federal Street   302-744-4700
Dover, DE 19901   888-459-2943
                                       Fax: 302-739-6659
                    e-mail: dhssinfo@state.de.us
                www.dhss.delaware.gov/dhss/dph/index.htm
Provides HIV counseling and testing prevention education and
AIDS surveillance and studies.
Jamie Rivera, Director

District of Columbia

253   Washington DC Department of Health HIV/AIDS Administration
HIV/AIDS Administration
899 North Capitol Street NE
Washington, DC 20002   202-442-5955
                                            www.doh.dc.gov
Mission is to reduce the incidence of HIV/AIDS and number of
deaths related to HIV/AIDS in the District of Columbia by the ap-
plication of sound public health practices and initiatives through
HIV disease surveillance tracking, monitoring, and intervention.
Mohammed Akhter, Director

Florida

**254   Body Positive HIV and AIDS Research and Re Southwest Center
for HIV/AIDS**
1144 E McDowell Road   602-307-5330
Phoenix, AZ 85006   Fax: 602-307-5021
                    e-mail: cweiner@phoenixbodypositive.org
                                          http://swhiv.org/
Body Positive is a non-profit organization created by and for people infected and affected by HIV, that provides the community with
the knowledge, resources and collective strength necessary for individuals to live long and well with HIV and to prevent the spread
of the disease.
Carol A Poore MBA, President and CEO
Andy Myers MD, Medical Director

255   Florida Department of Health Bureau of HIV/AIDS
Bureau of HIV/AIDS
4052 Bald Cypress Way   850- 24- 414
Tallahassee, FL 32399-1715   Fax: 850- 48- 457
                    e-mail: DiseaseControl@doh.state.fl.us
                                        www.doh.state.fl.us
Making voluntary HIV testing a routine part of medical care imple-
menting new models for diagnosing HIV infections outside medi-
cal settings preventing new infections by working with persons
diagnosed with HIV and their partners.
Tom Liberti, Bureau Chief
Janell Clemons, Administrative Assistant

256   Positive Voices
8315 NE 22 Avenue   78- 9-5 28
Miami, FL 33147   888-POS-CONN
                                       Fax: 786-623-0701
                    e-mail: email@positiveconnections.org
                              www.positiveconnections.org
The Center for Positive Connections is a non-profit community
based organization that is run for those infected our community.
Our mission is to provide educational emotional holistic and social
support at all individuals living with HIV/AIDS.

257   TBAN
7402 N 56th Street
Tampa, FL 33674-8333   813-769-5180
                              www.queertampa.com/tan.html
TBAN formerly The Tampa AIDS Network (TAN) is a community
organization which provides prevention education emotional and
physical support services and advocacy on behalf of all persons affected by HIV disease.
Vivian Candelaria, Director

Georgia

**258   Georgia Department of Human Resources: Division of Public
Health**
AIDS Section
2 Peachtree Street NW   40- 6-7 27
Atlanta, GA 30303   800-551-2728
                                       Fax: 404-657-3100
                    e-mail: gdphinfo@dhr.ga.us
                                        http://health.state.ga.us
Provides technical support and assistance to the Public Health Districts to prevent STD and HIV infection ensuring the availability of
quality STD/HIV prevention and treatment by improving quality
assurance guidelines and methods by providing appropriate training.
Brenda Fitzgerald, Director

Hawaii

259   Hawaii Department of Health: Communicable Disease Division
AIDS/Sexually Transmitted Diseases Control Branch
1250 Punchbowl St   80- 5-6 44
Honolulu, HI 96813-2317   Fax: 80- 5-6 44
                    e-mail: janice.okubo@doh.hawaii.gov
                              www.hawaii.gov/health/about/admin
Offers research education surveillance and testing components.
AIDS information and guidelines about the placement of infants
children and adolescents who test positive for HIV in nursery or
school settings are also available.
Chiyome Fuki MD, Director
Loretta Fuddy, Deputy Director

Idaho

**260   Idaho Department of Health and Welfare The STD/AIDS
Program**
The STD/AIDS Program
450 W State Street 1st Floor   208-334-6527
Boise, ID 83720-0036   Fax: 208-332-7346
                    e-mail: apsportal@dhw.idaho.gov
                              www.healthandwelfare.idaho.gov
Program receives federal funding to support testing treatment and
prevention services for Idaho's reportable sexually transmitted in-
fections.
Richard Armstrong, Director
Tom Shananan, Public Information Manager

Illinois

261   AIDS Legal Council of Chicago
180 N Michigan Avenue   312-427-8990
Chicago, IL 60601   866-506-3038
                                       Fax: 312-427-8419
                    e-mail: info@aidslegal.com
                                          www.aidslegal.com
Legal advice and services for persons who are HIV positive or have
AIDS and their companions families etc.
Ann Hilton Fisher, Executive Director
Charles Winstersteen, President

262   Chicago Department of Health
333 S State Street   312-747-9884
Chicago, IL 60604   Fax: 312-747-9765
                                       TTY: 312-747-2374
                    e-mail: publichealth@cdph.org
                                       egov.cityofchicago.org
Offers educational services audiovisual materials surveillance of
HIV and AIDS counseling and referrals.
David Kern, Director

**263   Illinois Department of Public Health: Division of Infectious
Diseases**
535 W Jefferson Street   217-782-4977
Springfield, IL 62761   Fax: 217-782-3987
                                       TTY: 800-547-0466
                                          www.idph.state.il.us
Administers the AIDS Drug Assistance Program (ADAP). Cur-
rently nearly 3 300 clients use ADAP services each month access-

ing 10 000 prescriptions. Client approved for ADAP must re-apply on an annual basis in order to continue to receive services.
Damon Arnold, Director
Randy J Dunn, State Superintendent of Education

264 **Test Positive Aware Network (TPAN)**
5537 N Broadway Street   773-989-9400
Chicago, IL 60640-1405   Fax: 773-989-9494
                                    e-mail: tpan@tpan.com
                                    www.tpan.com
Empowers people living with HIV through peer-led programming support services information dissemination and advocacy. Provides services to the broader community to increase HIV knowledge and sensitivity and to reduce the risk of infection.
Bill Farrand, CEO/Dierctor of Client Services
Thomas Hart, President

Kansas

265 **Kansas Department of Health & Environment Epidemiology & Disease Prevention: HIV**
1000 SW Jackson   785-296-1500
Topeka, KS 66612-1274   Fax: 785-368-6368
                                    e-mail: info@kdheks.gov
                                    www.kdheks.gov
Conducts surveillance of HIV/AIDS in Kansas. Conducts Prevention Program with training for counselors and educators partial funding of counseling test sites and distribution of educational materials. Provides medications and primary care.
Kathy Donner, HIV Prevention Director
Jeni Trimble, HIV Surveillance Director

Louisiana

266 **Louisiana Department of Health & Hospitals : Office of Public Health**
Louisiana AIDS Prevention/Surveillance Program
628 N 4th Street   22- 3-2 80
Baton Rouge, LA 70821-0629   Fax: 22- 3-2 80
                                    e-mail: avis.richard-griffin@la.gov
                                    http://www.dhh.louisiana.gov/offices/?id
The HIV/AIDS Program was established in 1985 to provide leadership policy development and technical assistance including HIV/AIDS education prevention and services to parish health units and community based organizations throughout the state.
William Clark, Medical Director
William Hineman, Director/Program Manager II

Maine

267 **Maine Bureau of Health: Division of Disease Control**
HIV/STD Program
286 Water Street   207-287-8016
Augusta, ME 04333   Fax: 207-287-3498
                                    TTY: 800-606-0215
                                    e-mail: chris.zukas-lessard@maine.gov
                                    www.maine.gov/dhhs/boh/index.htm
Provides technical assistance to state agencies and private organizations regarding AIDS education and policy development.
Chris Zukas-Lessard, Deputy Director
Dora Anne Mills, Director

Massachusetts

268 **Massachusetts Department of Health HIV/AIDS Bureau**
HIV/AIDS Bureau
250 Washington Street   617-624-6000
Boston, MA 02108   800-235-2331
                                    Fax: 617-624-5399
                                    TTY: 617-437-1672
                                    www.mass.gov/dph
Assisting in preventing the spread of the HIV epidemic and the development of appropriate cost-effective health and support services which will maintain patients in the least restrictive setting.
Kevin Cranston, Director
John Auerbach, Commissioner Department of Public Health

269 **New England AIDS Education & Training Center (NEHEC)**
23 Miner Street   617-262-5657
Boston, MA 02215-3318   Fax: 617-262-5667
                                    e-mail: aidsed@neaetc.org
                                    www.neaetc.org
The New England HIV Education Consortium (NEHEC), a HRSA minority AIDS initiative program, is a training and education program serving all six states in the New England region. The principal goal of NEHEC is to address the HIV-related training, educational, and support needs of the full, spectrum of providers as they provide state-of-the-art, quality and compassionate care to individuals living with HIV/AIDS.
Donna M Gallagher RNC/MS/ANP, Principal Investigator/Project Director
Barry Sandberg MS/MPA, Assistant Director/Administrator

Michigan

270 **Michigan Department of Community Health HIV/AIDS Prevention & Intervention Secti**
HIV/AIDS Prevention & Intervention Section
109 Michigan Avenue   517-241-5900
Lansing, MI 48913   888-826-6565
                                    Fax: 517-241-5911
                                    www.michigan.gov/mdch
Gives general public and high-risk education grants supporting educational materials programs and a hotline.
Loretta Davis-Satter, Director Division HIV/AIDS-STD
Chris Hanson, Dental Program Coordinator

Minnesota

271 **Minnesota Department of Health: AIDS/STD Prevention Service**
Office of Infectious Diseases
717 Delaware Street SE   612-676-5414
Minneapolis, MN 55440-9272   877-925-4189
                                    Fax: 612-623-5743
                                    e-mail: indepcweb@health.state.mn.us
                                    www.health.state.mn.us
This division is to prevent death and disability from HIV and other sexually transmitted diseases by providing statewide leadership regarding the prevention of transmission and the availability of health and supportive services for infected persons.
Harry Hull, Director

Mississippi

272 **Mississippi Department of Public Health: STD/HIV Prevention Program**
570 E Woodrow Wilson Drive   601-576-7400
Jackson, MS 39216   866-458-4948
                                    Fax: 601-576-7909
                                    www.msdh.state.ms.us
Funds two statewide hotlines one for the general public and one for the gay community. Both offer health education and risk reduction activities of the Program include baseline evaluation of public knowledge about AIDS through surveys.
Joy Sennett, Director Communicable Disease Office

Missouri

273 **Missouri Department of Health: Bureau of AIDS Prevention**
912 Wildwood   573-751-6400
Jefferson City, MO 65102-0570   866-628-9891
                                    Fax: 573-751-6010
                                    e-mail: info@dhss.mo.gov
                                    www.dhss.mo.gov
Human Immunodeficiency Virus (HIV) disease and infection and Acquired Immunodeficiency Syndrome (AIDS) surveillance monitors and analyzes data on the number of people infected with HIV and/or AIDS and identifies and tracks trends in disease incidence.
Margaret T Donnelly, Director
Bret Fischer, Director

Montana

274 **Montana Deptartment of Health And Human Services**
STD & HIV Prevention Program

1400 Broadway
Helena, MT 59620

406-444-4540
800-233-6668
Fax: 406-444-1861
www.dphhs.state.mt.us

This program receives a Federal grant through the Centers for Disease Control to carry out a health education/risk reduction program to detect and prevent the spread of HIV infection through a number of services.
Jane Smilie, Acting Administrator
Anna Whiting Sorrell, Director

Nevada

275 Nevada Department of Human Resources: Health Program Section
4126 Technology Way
Carson City, NV 89706-2009

775-684-4000
Fax: 775-684-4010
e-mail: nvdhr@dhhs.nv.gov
www.dhhs.nv.gov

Provides HIV counseling and testing a speakers bureau information and referrals resource materials including AIDS video recordings and education.
Harold Cook, Administrator
Mike Wilden, Director

New Hampshire

276 New Hampshire Department of Health and Human Services
Division of Public Health Services
129 Pleasant Street
Concord, NH 03301-4604

603-271-4502
800-852-3345
Fax: 603-271-4934
TTY: 800-735-2964
TDD: 8007352964
www.dhhs.state.nh.us

HIV/AIDS Program receives both state and Federal funding pertaining to AIDS education risk reduction testing and surveillance.
Joyce J Welch, Program Coordinator
James Fredyma, Director

New Jersey

277 New Jersey Department of Health: Division of AIDS Prevention & Control
Division of HIV/AIDS Service (DHAS)
Po Box 360
Trenton, NJ 08625-0360

609-292-7837
800-367-6543
www.state.nj.us/health

Serves to coordinate and direct primary HIV activities within the Department networking with other divisions and agencies to provide information and care programs to populations in need.
Laurence E Ganges, Assistant Commissioner
John Fasanella, Director

278 New Jersey Woman AIDS Network
103 Bayard Street
New Brunswick, NJ 08901

732-846-4462
Fax: 732-846-2674
e-mail: office@njwan.org
www.njwan.org

A leader in identifying issues facing women with HIV/AIDS educating service providers advocating for appropriate policies and building a multicultural women and HIV/AIDS movement.
Monique Howard, Executive Director
Patryce Burgess, Wellness Coordinator

New Mexico

279 New Mexico Health Department: Public Health Division
HIV/AIDS/STD Prevention & Services Bureau
1190 S Saint Francis Drive
Santa Fe, NM 87502-4182

505-827-2613
800-545-2437
Fax: 505-827-2530
www.health.state.nm.us

Provides training programs and HIV education to the general public and professionals risk reduction information AIDS school curriculums classroom presentation information and an AIDS hotline.
Don Maestas, Director

New York

280 New York Department of Health, Office of Public Health: AIDS Institute
AIDS Institute
Empire State Plaza
Albany, NY 12237-0001

518-474-9866
Fax: 518-473-8814
e-mail: hivpubs@health.state.ny.us
www.health.state.ny.us

Awards grants and maintains relationships with regional AIDS service groups, crisis intervention, psychosocial counseling and legal, financial and housing assistance. The Institute also offers preventive education, risk reduction education, HIV counseling and testing and patient care.
Wendy V. Gould, Coordinator Educational Materials

North Carolina

281 North Carolina Department of Health & Natural Resources
HIV/STD Prevention & Care
1931 Mail Service Center
Raleigh, NC 27699-1902

919-707-5000
Fax: 919-870-4829
e-mail: hivstdprevention@ncmail.net
www.ncpublichealth.com

Oversee the AIDS surveillance program HIV counseling testing partner notification health education risk reduction and public information efforts in North Carolina.
Rebecca King, Chief
Jeffrey Engel, Director

Ohio

282 Ohio Department of Health: Division of Preventive Medicine
HIV/AIDS Surveillance Division
246 N High Street
Columbus, OH 43215-0118

614-466-1388
800-777-4775
Fax: 614-644-1909
TTY: 800-332-AIDS
e-mail: Surveillance@odh.ohio.gov
www.odh.ohio.gov

Consists of AIDS surveillance seroprevalence programs, health care worker education, health education and risk reduction projects.
Alvin D Jackson MD, Director of Health
Anne Harnish, Assistant Director

Oklahoma

283 Oklahoma Department of Health: AIDS Division
1000 NE 10th
Oklahoma City, OK 73117-1207

405-271-5600
800-522-0203
Fax: 405-271-5149
www.health.state.ok.us

Provides prevention-related services and funding to the network of AIDS service delivery organizations, both public and private in Oklahoma. The Division provides services and training and certification of AIDS educators, surveillance, and seroprevalence staff.
Rocky D McElvany, Interim Commissioner of Health
Ken Feagins, Director

Oregon

284 Oregon Department of Human Resources Health Division HIV Program
Health Division, HIV Program
800 NE Oregon Street
Portland, OR 97232

971-673-1222
800-777-2437
Fax: 971-673-1299
TTY: 971-673-0372
e-mail: health.webmaster@state.or.us
www.oregon.gov/DHS/ph

HIV Program includes training workshops for AIDS trainers curriculum development or revision and an AIDS hotline through Cascade AIDS Project.
Veda Latin, HST Program Manager
Mitch Zahn, HIV Prevention Manager

285   Pennsylvania Department of Health: Bureau of HIV/AIDS
Division of HIV/AIDS
Room 933   717-783-4677
Harrisburg, PA 17108   800-662-6080
Fax: 717-772-6975
e-mail: c-hivepi@state.pa.us
www.dsf.health.state.pa.us

The purpose of the Division of HIV/AIDS is to develop and implement a multi-dimensional coordinated strategy to prevent disease and change high-risk behaviors as well as provide resources and direction for sustaining preventive behavior and avoiding infection.
Janice P Kopelman MSW LSW, Director

286   Philadelphia Department of Public Health: AIDS Program
AIDS Activities Coordinating Office (AACO)
1101 Market Street   215-685-5600
Philadelphia, PA 19107   800-985-AIDS
Fax: 215-685-5293
www.phila.gov/health

Administers federal state and city funded HIV/AIDS programs in Philadelphia through collaborative service contracts with community-based organizations.
Marla Gold MD, Program Coordinator
Nan Feyler, Chief of Staff

287   Rhode Island Department of Health: Division of Disease Prevention & Control
Office of AIDS/HIV
3 Capitol Hill   401-222-5960
Providence, RI 02908   800-381-AIDS
Fax: 401-222-2488
www.health.state.ri.us

Provides health education and risk reduction activities through its AIDS program. Services include professional conferences, providing assistance for in-service programs, presentation of two courses and organization of an AIDS minority program. Also, provides public health services in HIV/AIDS and Viral Hepatitis. The office develops policies, funds community programs and conducts surveillances.
Paul G. Loberti, Chief Administrator
Lucille Minuto, Assistant Administrator

288   South Carolina Department of Health & Environmental Control
Bureau of Preventive Health Services
2600 Bull Street
Columbia, SC 29201   803-898-3432
www.scdhec.net

Provides services to prevent the spread of sexually transmitted diseases (STD's) and HIV infection to reduce associated illness and death and to provide care and support resources for persons with HIV disease.
Jeff Jones MD, Director

289   Tennessee Department of Health: AIDS Program
Cordell Hull Building, 4th Floor
425 Fifth Avenue N   615-741-3111
Nashville, TN 37243   Fax: 615-741-2491
e-mail: tn.health@tn.gov
health.state.tn.us

Provides HIV/STD education and information, as well as collecting monitoring and distributing data. Provides assistance to individuals, and intervention and treatment services.
Laurel Wood, Program Coordinator
Susan Cooper, Commissioner

290   AIDS Outreach Center (AOC)
400 North Beach Street   817-335-1994
Fort Worth, TX 76111   Fax: 817-335-3617
e-mail: info@aoc.org
www.aoc.org

The staff and volunteers of the AIDS Outreach Center (AOC) provide a wide range of social services, outreach activities, testing and counseling, prevention education programs and public policy advocacy for men, women and children living with HIV, and their loved ones.
Allan Gould Jr, Executive Director
Anthony Powell, President

291   Houston Department of Health and Human Services: Bureau of HIV Prevention
8000 N Stadium Drive   713-794-9020
Houston, TX 77054-1823   Fax: 713-798-0830
TTY: 713-794-9092
www.houstontx.gov/health

Coordinates sexually transmitted disease surveillance, seroprevalence, contract tracing partner notification, public information, minority initiatives and health evaluation/risk reduction.
Stephen L Williams, Director

292   Texas Department of Health: Bureau of HIV and STD Prevention
HIV/STD Division
1100 W 49th Street   512-458-7111
Austin, TX 78756-3199   888-963-7111
TTY: 800-735-2989
TDD: 512-458-7708
www.dshs.state.tx.us

Mission is to prevent, treat, and/or control the spread of HIV, STD, and other communicable diseases to protect the health of the citizens of Texas.
David Lakey, Commissioner

293   Utah Department of Health: Bureau of Communicable Disease Control
Division of Epidemiology & Laboratory Services
288 N 1460 W   801-538-6101
Salt Lake City, UT 84114-2105   800-537-1046
Fax: 801-538-9923
e-mail: rrolfs@utah.gov
www.health.utah.gov/cdc

Secures and distributes funds for AIDS prevention services, provides educational programs and counseling to the general public, AIDS service organizations, health workers and groups at risk.
David Patton, Executive Director
Melissa Stevens-Dimo, Manager, Communicable Diseases

294   Vermont Department of Health: Health Surveillance HIV/AIDS/STD/TB Program
108 Cherry Street   802-863-7200
Burlington, VT 05402-0070   800-464-4343
Fax: 802-865-7754
TTY: 802-863-7235
www.healthvermont.gov

Provides health education and risk reduction activities nurses and other professional training, AIDS presentations, educational and media campaigns and counseling and referrals.
Rod Copeland PhD, Director HIV/AIDS Program

295   Virginia Department of Health: Division of HIV, STD, and Pharmacy Services
109 Governor Street   804-786-6267
Richmond, VA 23219   800-533-4148
Fax: 804-786-7528
e-mail: hiv-stdhotline@vdh.virginia.gov.
www.vdh.virginia.gov

Supports local health departments and community-based organizations in the prevention, surveillance and treatment of HIV and

other STD's, including their complications, through provision of education, information, and health care services.
Casey Riley, Director
Craig Parrish, Pharmacist

Washington

296 Northwest AIDS Education and Training Center (AETC)
901 Boren Avenue   20- 5-3 33
Seattle, WA 98104   Fax: 206-221-4945
                              e-mail: leedave@u.washington.edu
                              http://depts.washington.edu/nwaetc/
Located at the University of Washington, offering HIV treatment education, clinical consultation, capacity building and technical assistance to health care professionals and agencies in Washington, Alaska, Montana, Idaho, and Oregon.
Bernadette Lalonde Ph.D, Principal Investigator/Program Director
Laurie Conratt MBA, State Programs Manager

297 Washington Department of Health: Division of HIV/AIDS Prevention Services
HIV Client Services
PO Box 47840   360-236-3434
Olympia, WA 98504-7840   877-376-9316
                                           Fax: 360-236-3400
                              e-mail: brown.mcdonald@doh.wa.gov
                              www.doh.wa.gov/cfh/HIV_AIDS/Prev_Edu
Provides information and referrals to local, state and national resources relating to HIV/AIDS provides informational and educational materials to individuals, agencies and organizations and actively works with print and broadcast media to promote HIV/AIDS awareness.
Paul Brown, HIV Data Manager
Brown McDonald, HIV Prevention Services Manager

West Virginia

298 West Virginia Department of Health & Human Resources
HIV/AIDS & STD Program
State Capitol Complex   304-558-0684
Charleston, WV 25305-3715   800-352-6513
                                           Fax: 304-558-1130
                              e-mail: wvdhhrsecretary@wvdhhr.org
                                           www.wvdhhr.org
Provides the AIDS-related services in 15 public health HIV-counseling and testing centers which offer by appointment confidential or anonymous testing.
Martha Yeage Walker, Secretary

Wisconsin

299 Wisconsin Department of Health and Social Services: Division of Health
HIV/AIDS/Hepatitis Program
1 West Wilson Street   608-266-1865
Madison, WI 53703   800-438-1282
                                           Fax: 608-267-2832
                                           TTY: 888-701-1251
                              e-mail: DHSwebmaster@wisconsin.gov
                                           www.dhs.wisconsin.gov
Coordinates counseling and testing sites activities and services to HIV-infected persons, produces a report that contains information and recommendations for health care workers, emergency medical technicians and food service workers.
Seth Foldy, Administrator and State Health Officer
Thomas Sieger, Deputy Administrator

Wyoming

300 Wyoming Department of Health HIV/AIDS/Hepatitis Program
HIV/AIDS/Hepatitis Program
401 Hathaway Building   307-777-7656
Cheyenne, WY 82002-0001   866-571-0944
                                           Fax: 307-777-7439
                                           wdh.state.wy.us

100 percent federally funded and responsible for the solicitation development and implementation of community AIDS prevention initiatives.
Brent D Sherard, Director and State Health Officer
Ginny Mahoney, Chief of Staff

Foundations

301 National Hemophilia Foundation
116 West 32nd Street   212-328-3700
New York, NY 10001   800-42H-ANDI
                                           Fax: 212-328-3777
                              e-mail: handi@hemophilia.org
                                           www.hemophilia.org
The National Hemophilia Foundation is dedicated to finding better treatments and cures for bleeding and clotting disorders and to preventing the complications of these disorders through education, advocacy and research.
Alan Kinniburgh, PhD, Chief Executive Officer

Libraries & Resource Centers

302 AIDS Library of Philadelphia
1233 Locust Street   215-985-4851
Philadelphia, PA 19107   Fax: 215-985-4492
                              e-mail: library@aidslibrary.org
                                           www.aidslibrary.org
Improving access to health and support services, preventing HIV transmission, and raising the public awareness of HIV/AIDS related issues.

303 National Library of Medicine
8600 Rockville Pike   301-594-5983
Bethesda, MD 20894   888-346-3656
                                           Fax: 301-402-1384
                              e-mail: custserv@nlm.nih.gov
                                           www.nlm.nih.gov/
The National Library of Medicine (NLM), on the campus of the National Institutes of Health in Bethesda, Maryland, is the world's largest medical library. The Library collects materials in all areas of biomedicine and health care, as well as works on biomedical aspects of technology, the humanities, and the physical, life, and social sciences.
Dr Donald Lindberg, Director
Betsy L Humphreys, Deputy Director

Research Centers

304 CDC National Prevention Information Network (NPIN)
PO Box 6003   404-679-3860
Rockville, MD 20849-6003   800-458-5231
                                           Fax: 888-282-7681
                                           TTY: 800-243-7012
                              e-mail: info@cdcnpin.org
                                           www.cdcnpin.org
The CDC National Prevention Information Network (NPIN) is the U.S. reference, referral, and distribution service for information on HIV/AIDS, sexually transmitted diseases (STDs), and tuberculosis (TB). NPIN produces, collects, catalogs, processes, stocks, and disseminates materials and information on HIV/AIDS, STDs, and TB to organizations and people working in those disease fields in international, national, state, and local settings.

Alabama

305 Centers for AIDS Research: University of Alabama at Birmingham
BBRB 256
Birmingham, AL 35294-1150   205-934-4011
                                           www.uabcfar.uab.edu
Provides expertise, resources, and services not otherwise readily obtained through traditional funding mechanisms.
Michael S. Saag, Director
Carol Z Garrison, President

306 General Clinical Research Center: UAB
Room 907 Medical Education Building
Birmingham, AL 35294   205-934-4852
                                    e-mail: ccts@uab.edu
                                         www.ccts.uab.org

AIDS and genetics research.
Burt Nabors, MD, Director
Stuart Frank, Co-Principal Investigator

307 University of Alabama at Birmingham: National Cooperative Drug/AIDS
UAB Center for AIDS Research
BBRB 256
Birmingham, AL 35294-1150   205-934-4011
                                       www.uabcfar.uab.edu

Dr. Richard Whitley, Principal Investigator

California

308 AIDS Clinical Trials Unit CARES Clinic
CARES Clinic
2nd Floor Research Office   916-914-6322
Sacramento, CA 95814   Fax: 916-325-1955
                                  e-mail: actu@ucdavis.edu
                                  www.ucdmc.ucdavis.edu/actu
The ACTU at Davis Medical Center is dedicated to offering the latest in research clinical trials to HIV/AIDS patients throughout Northern Central California.
Nancy L Fitch, Director
Carol Z Garrison, President

309 Adult Research Opportunities
220 Dickinson Street   619-543-8080
San Diego, CA 92103-8208   Fax: 619-543-5066
                                        www.avrctrials.org
A university-based nonprofit clinical trials unit. Conduct's patient-oriented research and educational programs on HIV and other chronic infections. Studies have pioneered the development of treatments that continue to change the course of the HIV epidemic.
Sandy Matson, Administrative Assistant
Colleen Burks, Finance Assistant

310 Center for AIDS Prevention Studies AIDS Research Institute University of C
AIDS Research Institute, University of California
50 Beale Street   415-597-9100
San Francisco, CA 94105   Fax: 415-597-9213
                                  e-mail: CAPS.Web@ucsf.edu
                                         www.caps.ucsf.edu
The mission of the Center for AIDS Prevention Studies is to conduct domestic and international research to prevent the acquisition of HIV and to optimize health outcomes among HIV-infected individuals.
Stephen F Morin, Director
Susan Kegeles, Co-Director

311 Center for Interdisciplinary Research in Immunology and Diseases at UCLA
UCLA School of Medicine
924 Westwood Blvd. #545
Los Angeles, CA 90095   310-825-6373
                                  dgsom.healthsciences.ucla.edu
Research into immunology and blood disorders with special focus on AIDS and HIV infections.
Albert Glover, Director, Academic Affairs

312 Centers for AIDS Research: North-Central California
UC Davis, Division of Infectious Diseases
4150 V Street   916-734-8033
Sacramento, CA 95817   Fax: 916-734-7766
                                  e-mail: nccfar@ucdavis.edu
                                  www.ucdmc.ucdavis.edu/nccfar
Provides expertise resources and services not otherwise readily obtained through more traditional funding mechanisms.
Richard B Pollard, Division Chief
Krystin E Cheung, Director

313 Centers for AIDS Research: USCD Center for AIDS Research
Center for AIDS Research

University of California San Diego   858-534-5545
La Jolla, CA 92093-0716   Fax: 858-822-5840
                                   e-mail: cfar@ucsd.edu
                                         cfar.ucsd.edu
Provides expertise resources and services and services not otherwise readily obtained through traditional funding mechanisms.
Douglas Richman, Director
Kim Schafer, Administrative Director

314 Centers for AIDS Research: University of California, Los Angeles
UCLA AIDS Institute
10940 Wilshire Blvd.   310-794-4419
Los Angeles, CA 90024-1678   Fax: 310-794-3955
                                  e-mail: ebayrd@mednet.ucla.edu
                                      www.uclaaidsinstitute.org
Provides expertise, resources, and services not otherwise readily obtained through traditional funding mechanisms.
Irvin S.Y. Chen, Director
Dr. Thomas Coates, Associate Director

315 City of Hope National Medical Center Drug Discover/AIDS Group
City of Hope
1500 E Duarte Road
Duarte, CA 91010   626-256-4673
                                        www.cityofhope.org
Developmental research into the treatment of AIDS.
Michael A Friedman MD, President, CEO
Virginia A Opipare, Executive Vice President, Chief Opperato

316 Kaiser Foundation Research Institute
2000 Broadway
Oakland, CA 94612   510-891-3400
                                         www.dor.kaiser.org

Joe V Selby MD, MPH, Director

317 Stanford University General Clinical Research Center
GCRC Administration
300 Pasteur Drive   650-723-4000
Stanford, CA 94305-5251   Fax: 650-725-6698
                                  e-mail: gcrcstanford@stanford.edu
                                      www.med.stanford.edu/gcrc
The Stanford General Clinical Research Center (GCRC) is the major clinical research facility for Stanford University School of Medicine. With patient care units in Stanford University Hospital and Lucile Packard Children's Hospital the center plays a crucial role in the school's bench-to-bedside research mission.
David Stevenson, Associate Program Director
Branimir I Sikic, Program Director

318 Stanford University National Cooperative Drug Discovery/AIDS Group
School of Medicine
300 Pasteur Drive
Stanford, CA 94305   650-723-4000
                                        www.med.stanford.edu
Ellen Jo Baron, Director

319 UCLA AIDS Clinical Research Center
1399 S Roxbury Drive   310-557-2273
Los Angeles, CA 90035   Fax: 310-206-3311
                                       www.uclacarecenter.org

Ronald T Mitsuyana, Director
Judith Currier, Associate Director

320 UCSD Antiviral Research Center
220 Dickinson Street   619-543-8080
San Diego, CA 92103-8208   Fax: 619-543-5066
                                        www.avrctrials.org
Develops treatment protocols and drug therapies and recruits research volunteers for AIDS studies and HIV related disorders.
Jack Degnan, Outreach Manager
Michael Giancola, Community Health Program Representative

321 USC Internal Medicine
1520 San Pablo Street
Los Angeles, CA 90033-1034   800-872-2273
                                   Fax: 213-224-6687
                                     www.usc.edu/health/internal
Research into internal medicine with specialties in cardiovascular endocrinology and diabetes gastrointestinal and liver disease geri-

atric medicine hematology infectious diseases nephrology oncology pulmonary and critical care and rheumatology and immunology.
Alexandra Levine, Head

322 University of California San Francisco Center for AIDS Prevention
Center for AIDS Prevention Studies (CAPS)
50 Beale Street   415-597-9100
San Francisco, CA 94105-3411   Fax: 415-597-9213
e-mail: CAPS.web@ucsf.edu
www.caps.ucsf.edu

The mission of the Center for AIDS Prevention Studies is to conduct domestic and international research to prevent the acquisition of HIV and to optimize health outcomes among HIV-infected individuals.
Stephen F Morin, Director
Susan Kegeles, Co-Director

323 University of California: Institute of Health Policy Studies
513 Parnassus Avenue   415-476-9000
San Francisco, CA 94143-410   Fax: 415-476-0705
e-mail: claire.brindis@ucsf.edu
www.ihps.medschool.ucsf.edu

Health policy and AIDS research.
Claire Brindis, Interim Director
Daniel Dohan, Associate Director of Training

Colorado

324 Centers for AIDS Research: University of Colorado Health Sciences Center
Colorado Center for AIDS Research
4200 East 9th Avenue   303-315-7233
Denver, CO 80262   Fax: 303-315-8681
e-mail: colorado.cfar@uchsc.edu
www.uchsc.edu/ccfar

Describes forms and patterns of use of complimentary and alternative medicine (CAM) for the treatment of HIV/AIDS.
Robert T. Schooley, Director

District of Columbia

325 George Washington National Cooperative: Drug Discovery/AIDS Treatment
Department of Pharmacology & Physiology
2300 Eye Street NW   202-994-3541
Washington, DC 20037-2336   Fax: 202-994-2870
e-mail: phmsmc@gwumc.edu
www.gwumc.edu/pharm

Studies and researches natural products and synthetic anti-AIDS agents.
Susan Ceryak, Associate Research Professor
Jian-Zhong Guo, Associate Research Professor

326 Whitman Walker Clinic AIDS/Medical Services Programs
1701 14th Street NW   202-745-7000
Washington, DC 20009-3840   Fax: 202-745-0238
e-mail: info@wwc.org
www.wwc.org

A non-profit community-based health organization serving the Washington D.C. metropolitan region. Established by and for the gay and lesbian community our clinic is comprised of diverse volunteers and staff who provide or facilitate the delivery of high quality comprehensive accessible health care and community services. Especially committed to ending the suffering of all those infected and affected by HIV/AIDS.
Donald Blanchon, CEO
June Crenshaw, Chair

Florida

327 Department of Epidemiology and Health Policy Research: University of Florida
1329 SW 16th Street   352-265-8035
Gainesville, FL 32608   Fax: 352-265-8047
e-mail: rdarbelles.ichp.ufl.edu
www.ehpr.ufl.edu

Studies into child and adolescent health financing and organization of health care delivery systems community health chronic

conditions transition from pediatric to adult health care access to health care for vulnerable populations quality of life and outcomes research.
Irina Olsen, Assistant Director
Cherrie Bell, Program Assistant

328 Tampa Bay Research Institute
10900 Roosevelt Boulevard N   727-576-6675
Saint Petersburg, FL 33716-2308   Fax: 727-577-9862
e-mail: development@tampabayresearch.org
www.tampabayresearch.org

TBRI is the first independent biomedical research organization of its kind in Florida. Our scientists dedicate their lives work to conquering chronic and infectious diseases while gaining a better understanding of the immune system.
Akiko Tanaka, Co-Founder

329 University of South Florida Center for HIV Education and Research
13301 Bruce B Downs Boulevard   813-974-4430
Tampa, FL 33612-3807   866-352-2382
Fax: 813-974-8451
e-mail: Contact@FCAETC.org
www.usfcenter.org

Serves health care professionals throughout Florida by providing education and information on the transmission control treatment and prevention of HIV and AIDS and by conducting related research and community outreach.
Michael Knox PhD, Director
Martha Fried PhD, Associate Director

Georgia

330 AIDS School Health Education Database Centers for Disease Control
Centers for Disease Control
1600 Clifton Road   404-639-3534
Atlanta, GA 30333   800-232-4636
TTY: 888-232-6348
e-mail: cdcinfo@cdc.gov
www.cdc.gov

An information awareness resource produced by the Division of Adolescent and School Health. The database offers descriptions of various educational resources for professionals relevant to the education of children and youth about HIV infection and AIDS.
Thomas Friedman MD, Director
Harold Jaffe, MD, MA, Associate Director of Science

331 Center for AIDS Research: Emory University Rollins School of Public Health
1518 Clifton Road NE   404-727-2924
Atlanta, GA 30322-4201   Fax: 404-727-9853
e-mail: cfar@emory.edu
www.cfar.emory.edu

Provides expertise resources and services not otherwise readily obtained through more traditional funding mechanisms.
James W Curran, Director
Carlos del Rio, Co-Director for Clinical Science

332 Educational Materials Database Centers for Disease Control
Centers for Disease Control
1600 Clifton Road   404-639-3534
Atlanta, GA 30333-4201   800-232-4636
TTY: 888-232-6348
e-mail: info@cdcnpin.org
www.cdc.gov

A collection of bibliographic descriptions about hard-to-find AIDS and HIV information and educational materials.
Thomas Friedman MD, Director
Harold Jaffe, MD, MA, Co-Director for Clinical Science

333 Emory University: National Cooperative Drug Discovery for AIDS Treatment
Emory Healthcare Pediatrics Department
201 Dowman Drive   404-727-6123
Atlanta, GA 30322   Fax: 404-727-5737
www.pediatrics.emory.edu

Barbara J Stoll MD, Professor, Chair
James W Wagner, President

334   Funding Database Centers for Disease Control
Centers for Disease Control
1600 Clifton Road   404-639-3534
Atlanta, GA 30333   800-232-4636
                                                TTY: 888-232-6348
                                            e-mail: cdcinfo@cdc.gov
                                                       www.cdc.gov
A listing of HIV and AIDS related funding opportunities for community-based and HIV and AIDS service organizations.
Thomas Friedman MD, Director
Harold Jaffe, MD, MA, Associate Director of Science

Illinois

335   Clinical Research Center Northwestern Center for Clinical Researc
Northwestern Center for Clinical Research
750 N Lake Shore Drive   312-503-1709
Chicago, IL 60611   e-mail: nucats@northwestern.edu
                                           www.nucats.northwestern.edu
Colleen De Luca, Associate Director, Administration
Philip Greenland, Director

Indiana

336   Purdue University Center for AIDS Research
School of Pharmacy and Pharmaceutical Sciences
575 Stadium Mall Drive   765-494-1361
W Lafayette, IN 47907-2091   Fax: 765-494-7880
                                      e-mail: oss@pharmacy.purdue.edu
                                                www.pharmacy.purdue.edu
Steve Byrn, Department Head
Stanley L Hem, Associate Department Head

Maryland

337   Center for AIDS Research: Johns Hopkins University School of Medicine
733 N. Broadway
Baltimore, MD 21205-2196   410-955-3182
                                     www.hopkinsmedicine.org/aidsresearch
Provides expertise resources and services not otherwise readily obtained through more traditional funding mechanisms.
Ronald R Peterson, ,President, JHH/HS
Edward D Miller, MD, Dean, CEO

338   Johns Hopkins University: Center for Communication Programs
Johns Hopkins Bloomberg School of Public Health
111 Market Place   410-659-6300
Baltimore, MD 21202   Fax: 410-659-6266
                                           e-mail: info@jhuccp.org
                                                     www.jhuccp.org
Health communications family planning and AIDS prevention research.
Susan Krenn, Director
J Douglass Storey, Associate Director of Communican Science

339   University of Maryland Center for Research, Grants & Contracts
Family Studies Depatment
1142 School of Public Health   301-405-3672
College Park, MD 20742   Fax: 301-314-9161
                                           e-mail: fmst@umd.edu
                                               www.hhp.umd.edu/FMST
Dr. R Narker Bausell, Director
Elaine Anderson, Chair

340   University of Maryland Center for Studies Family Studies Depatrment
1142 School of Public Health   301-405-3672
College Park, MD 20742   Fax: 301-314-9161
                                           e-mail: fmsc@umd.edu
                                               www.sph.umd.edu/fmsc
Dr R Narker Bausell, Director
Elaine Anderson, Chair

341   University of Maryland: Medical Biotechnology Center
725 W Lombard Street   410-706-8181
Baltimore, MD 21201-1513   Fax: 410-706-8184
                                      e-mail: lederer@umbi.umd.edu
                                                    www.umbi.umd.edu

Offers research into AIDS and HIV infection including vaccine development.
W Jonathan Lederer, Director
Kadir Aslan, Assistant Professor

Massachusetts

342   Center for AIDS Research: Harvard Medical School, Division of AIDS
The Landmark Buiding
104 Mt. Auburn Street   617-384-9039
Cambridge, MA 02138   Fax: 617-495-8231
                                      e-mail: aids@hms.harvard.edu
                                              aids.med.harvard.edu/cfar.htm
Provides expertise resources and services not otherwise readily obtained through traditional funding mechanisms.
Bruce Walker, Director

343   Center for Blood Research Harvard Medical School/CBR
Harvard Medical School/CBR
200 Longwood Avenue   617-278-3140
Boston, MA 02115   Fax: 617-278-3131
                                  e-mail: kirchhausen@crystal.harvard.edu
                                                     www.idi.harvard.edu
Offers research into blood disorders including multidisciplinary studies on AIDS and hemophilia cancer and diabetes research as well.
Tomas Kirchhausen, Principal Investigator
Fredrick Alt, President/ Director

344   Centers for AIDS Research: University of Massachusetts Medical School
55 Lake Avenue N   508-856-8989
Worcester, MA 01655   e-mail: publicaffairs@umassmed.edu
                                               www.umassmed.edu/cfar
Provides expertise, resources, and services not otherwise readily obtained through traditional funding mechanisms.
Terence R Floyd MD, Dean

345   Dana Farber Cancer Institute National Drug Discovery Group for AIDS Treatment
Dana-Farber Cancer Institute
450 Brookline Avenue   617-632-3000
Boston, MA 02115-5450   800-408-3324
                                                TTY: 617-632-5330
                                                TDD: 617-632-5330
                           e-mail: dana-farbercontactus@dfci.harvard.edu
                                                    www.dana-farber.org
Edward Benz, President and CEO
Janet E Porter, Executive Vice President and COO

346   Developmental Medicine Center Children's Hospital Boston
Children's Hospital Boston
300 Longwood Avenue   617-355-6000
Boston, MA 02115   Fax: 617-730-0633
                                                TTY: 617-730-0152
                                            www.childrenshospital.org
Studies developmental effects of infants at risk and development effects of congenital HIV infection.
James Mandell, CEO
Sandra Fenwick, President, COO

Michigan

347   University of Michigan: National Cooperative Drug/AIDS Group
School of Dentistry
1011 N University Avenue   734-763-6933
Ann Arbor, MI 48109-1078   Fax: 734-763-3453
                                       e-mail: paulk@umich.edu
                                                    www.dent.umich.edu
Focuses on the design of new drugs to fight AIDS.
John C Drach PhD, Director
Paul H Krebsbach, Department Chair

348   Wayne State University Center for Health Research
College of Nursing
Center for Health Research   313-577-4070
Detroit, MI 48202   Fax: 313-577-4571
                                      e-mail: n.artinian@wayne.edu
                                                www.nursing.wayne.edu/CHR

Facilitates interdisciplinary health research across diverse settings where nursing is practiced and healthcare is provided.
Nancy T Artinian, Director
Barbara K Redman, Dean

New York

349 Aaron Diamond AIDS Research Center
455 First Avenue   212-448-5000
New York, NY 10016   Fax: 212-725-1126
e-mail: webinfo@adarc.org
www.adarc.org
Committed to finding solutions to end the AIDS epidemic. In the decade and a half since HIV was identified researchers have learned more about this virus than about any other in history.
David Ho, Director & CEO
Gerald Friedland MD, Chairman

350 Centers for AIDS Research: Albert Einstein College of Medicine
Albert Einstein College of Medicine
Jack and Pearl Resnick Campus   718-430-2000
Bronx, NY 10461   Fax: 718-430-2374
e-mail: cfaradm@aecom.yu.edu
www.aecom.yu.edu/cfar
Provides consultation and support to the medical and research community in the scientific evaluation of CAM therapies.
Allen M Spiegel MD, Dean
Matthew Scharff MD, CFAR Investigator

351 Centers for AIDS Research: Columbia University College of Physicians
Center for AIDS Research
630 W 168th Street   212-305-1296
New York, NY 10032   e-mail: jka8@columbia.edu
www.cumc.columbia.edu
Provides a comprehensive framework for training educational programs and research which addresses health promotion disease prevention symptom management and quality of life for individuals with HIV. The goal of the Center is to create innovative research and service approaches for the prevention and management of HIV. This objective is fulfilled through research program development and program evaluations.
Lee Goldman MD, Executive Vice President
Lee Bollinger, JD, President of the University

352 Centers for AIDS Research: NYU School of Medicine
522 First Avenue   212-263-8527
New York, NY 10016   e-mail: zinszh01@med.nyu.edu
www.hivinfosource.org/hivis/cfar
Provides expertise resources and services not otherwise readily obtained through traditional funding mechanisms.
Derya Unutmaz MD, Director

353 General Clinical Research Center Mount Sinai School of Medicine
Mount Sinai School of Medicine
One Gustave L Levy Place   212-241-6500
New York, NY 10029-6574   Fax: 212-348-5811
e-mail: hugh.sampson@mssm.edu
www.mssm.edu/gcrc
Focuses on AIDS education and prevention.
Dennis S Charney, Executive Vice President
Jane Whitney, Chief Complience Officer

354 HIV Center for Clinical and Behavioral Studies
1051 Riverside Drive   212-543-5969
New York, NY 10032   Fax: 212-543-6003
e-mail: whiteme@pi.cpmc.comlumbia.edu
www.hivcenternyc.org
Interdisciplinary research center that investigates the behavioral causes and consequences of HIV/AIDS. Focusing on the intersections of HIV infection gender and sexuality; treatment strategies for infected populations; and innovative dissemination of scientific findings.
Anke A Ehrhardt, Director
Heino F L Meyer-Bahlbur, Associate Director

355 Institute for Clinical Research Weill Cornell Medical College
Weill Cornell Medical College

1300 York Avenue   212-746-5454
New York, NY 10065   Fax: 212-746-8970
e-mail: cto@med.cornell.edu
www.med.cornell.edu
The mission of the ICR is to support, advance and promote clinical and translational research enterprises at WCMC. As part of Research and Sponsored Programs (RASP) the ICR streamlines the clinical research process and offers a wide range of services, resources and training.
David J Skorton MD, President of the University
Michelle A Lewis, MS, Director (Research and Sponsored Program

356 SUNY at Buffalo National Cooperative Drug Discovery Group for AIDS Treatment
Department of Biochemistry
140 Farber Hall   716-829-2727
Buffalo, NY 14214-3000   Fax: 716-829-2725
e-mail: jluck@buffalo.edu
www.buffalo.edu
Kenneth M Blumenthal, Professor and Chairman
Elizabeth O'Brocta, Assistant to the Chairman

357 Spellman Center for HIV Related Disease The Spellman Center
The Spellman Center
415 W Fifty-First Street
New York, NY 10019   212-459-8130
www.stclaresny.org
David Kaufman, Director

358 State University of New York: SUNY Stony HIV Treatment Development Center
Center for Infectious Diseases
101 Nicolls Road   631-444-4000
Stony Brook, NY 11794-5120   Fax: 631-444-2493
e-mail: rsteigbigel@notes.cc.sunysb.edu
www.stonybrookmedicalcenter.org
Human immunodeficiency virus research.
Joyce Klien, Director
Laura Coppola, Assistant Director

North Carolina

359 Centers for AIDS Research: Univeristy of North Carolina at Chapel Hill
UNC Center For AIDS Research
Lineberger Cancer Center   919-966-8645
Chapel Hill, NC 27599   e-mail: cfar@med.unc.edu
cfar.med.unc.edu
Administrative and shared research support to synergistically enhance and coordinate high quality AIDS research projects.
Ronald Swanstrom, Director
Myron S Cohen, Associate Director

Ohio

360 Centers for AIDS Research: Case Western University
Department of Medicine
Division of Infectious Diseases   216-368-0271
Cleveland, OH 44106-5029   Fax: 216-368-3055
e-mail: mxl6@case.edu
www.clevelandactu.org
Provides administrative and shared research support to enhance and coordinate high quality AIDS research projects.
Michael M Lederman, Co-Director
Jonathan Karn, Associate Director

Pennsylvania

361 Centers for AIDS Research: University of Pennsylvania
Penn Center for AIDS Research
295 John Morgan Building   215-573-7354
Philadelphia, PA 19104-6140   Fax: 215-573-7356
e-mail: oliviere@mail.med.upenn.edu
www.med.upenn.edu
Also the Children's Hospital and the Wistar Institute provides important services and research for high quality projects.
James A Hoxie, Director
Ronald G Collman, Co-Director

362 Temple University Clinical Research Center Office of Clinical Research
Office of Clinical Research
Medical Education and Research Buil
Philadelphia, PA 19140
215-707-7000
Fax: 215-201-2684
e-mail: tusm@temple.edu
www.temple.edu/medicine
CRC Unit provides space to perform clinical research on 4 West of Temple University Hospital. The CRC Unit has the potential for three rooms for inpatient/outpatient studies and an additional room for outpatient studies.
Antonio Giorgio MD, President

363 Thomas Jefferson University: Center for Research in Medical Education
Jefferson Medical College
1020 Walnut Street
Philadelphia, PA 19107
215-955-6000
Fax: 215-923-7583
e-mail: Joseph.Gonnella@jefferson.edu
www.jefferson.edu/jmc

Joseph Gonne MD, Director
Robert L Barchi MD, President

Rhode Island

364 Centers for AIDS Research: Brown University
The Miriam Hospital
CFAR/RISE Building
Providence, RI 02906
401-793-4068
Fax: 401-793-4704
e-mail: vgodleski@lifespan.org
www.lifespan.org/cfar
Provides expertise resources and services not otherwise readily obtained through traditional funding mechanisms.
Charles C J Carpenter, Director
Susan Cu-Uvin, HIV and Women Core Co-Director

South Carolina

365 Medical University of South Carolina Health Services Administration
Medical University of South Carolina
179 Ashley Avenue
Charleston, SC 29425
843-792-2300
Fax: 843-923-27
www.musc.edu
Devoted to public health policy and health care management including AIDS research.
Sara King, Director
Raymond S Greenburg, President

Tennessee

366 Centers for AIDS Research: Vanderbilt University Medical Center
Division of Infectious Disease
1161 21st Avenue S
Nashville, TN 37232-2582
615-322-8972
e-mail: richard.daquila@vanderbilt.edu
www.mc.vanderbilt.edu/cfar
Provides expertise resources and services not otherwise readily obtained through more traditional funding mechanisms.
Richard D' Aquila, Director
G Fatima Lima Ph.D., Associate Director

Texas

367 Centers for AIDS Research: Baylor College of Medicine
Department of Molecular Virology & Microbiology
One Baylor Plaza
Houston, TX 77030
713-798-3006
Fax: 713-798-5019
e-mail: jbutel@bcm.edu
www.bcm.edu/cfar
A research center that is a branch of the Centers for AIDS Research.
Janet S Butel, Director
William T Shearer, Co-Director

Vermont

368 University of Vermont: Office of Health Promotion Research
1 S Prospect Street
Burlington, VT 05401
802-656-4187
Fax: 802-656-8826
e-mail: ohpr@uvm.edu
www.uvm.edu/~ohpr
Research done into public policy and human health including AIDS information and evaluation.
Anne L Dorwaldt, Assistant Director
Rachael Chicoine, AAS, Research Project Assistant

Washington

369 Centers for AIDS Research: University of Washington, Harborview Medical Center
Center For AIDS & STDs
325 Ninth Avenue
Seattle, WA 98104-2499
206-744-4239
Fax: 206-744-3693
e-mail: worthy@u.washington.edu
www.depts.washington.edu/cfas
Provides administrative and shared research support to synergistically enhance and coordinate high quality AIDS research projects. CFARs accomplish this through core facilities that provide expertise resource and services not otherwise readily obtained through more traditional funding mechanisms.
King K Holmes, Director
Mary Fielder, Assistant to the Director

370 HIV Prevention Trials Unit University of Washington/Seattle HPTU Si
University of Washington/Seattle HPTU Site
Cabrini Medical Tower 901 Boren Av
Seattle, WA 98104
206-520-3800
Fax: 206-520-3801
e-mail: hptu@u.washington.edu
www.depts.washington.edu
A worldwide collaborative clinical trials network established by the National Institutes of Health (NIH) to evaluate the safety and efficacy of non-vaccine prevention interventions alone or in combination using HIV incidence as the primary endpoint.
Connie Celum, Principal Investigator

Support Groups & Hotlines

371 AEGIS AIDS Education Global Information System
PO Box 184
San Juan Capistrano, CA 92693
949-495-1952
Fax: 949-443-1755
e-mail: comments@aegis.org
www.aegis.org
A not-for-profit, tax-exempt, educational corpoation that adds more than 3000 documents each month. Reach more than 10 million users annually, including: the US Federal Government, US Educational Institutions, and Nonprofit organizations both here and abroad.
Vanessa Robison, President
Sister Mary Elizabeth, Assistant Operations Director

372 AIDS Alabama
3521 7th Avenue S
Birmingham, AL 35222
205-324-9822
800-592-2437
Fax: 205-324-9311
e-mail: maryanne@aidsalabama.org
www.aidsalabama.org
Devotes its energy and resources statewide to helping people with HIV/AIDS live healthy, independent lives and works to prevent the spread of HIV. It is our goal to provide housing for those with HIV in the Birmingham area, secure and administer grants for care of persons with HIV statewide, and specialize in targeted prevention education programs.
Elaine Cottle, Executive Director

373 AIDS Hotline of Central New York
AIDS Community Resources
627 W Genesee Street
Syracuse, NY 13204
315-475-2430
800-475-2430
Fax: 315-472-6515
e-mail: information@aidscommunityresources.com
www.aidscommunityresources.com

A not-for-profit, community-based organization providing prevention, education and support services to those infected with and affected by HIV/AIDS Serves Cayuga, Herkimer, Jefferson, Lewis, Madison, Oneida, Onondaga, Oswego and St. Lawrences counties in New York State.
Michael Crinnin, Executive Director

374   AIDS Support Group of Cape Cod
428 S Street
Hyannis, MA 02610
508-778-1957
866-990-2437
Fax: 508-778-4501
e-mail: info@asgcc.org
www.asgcc.org

Our mission is to provide services that maintain and enhance the quality of life for persons living with HIV and AIDS on Cape Cod and Martha's Vineyard and to provide health education, prevention and harm reduction outreach via timely and accurate information about HIV/AIDS, STIs and viral hepatitis.
Krystin St. Onge, Interim Director

375   AIDSinfo
US Department of Health and Human Services
PO Box 6303
Rockville, MD 20849-6303
301-315-2816
800-448-0440
Fax: 301-315-2818
TTY: 888-480-3739
e-mail: contactus@aidsinfo.nih.gov
www.aidsinfo.nih.gov

Offers the latest federally approved information on HIV/AIDS clinical research, treatment and prevention, and medical practice guidelines for people living with HIV/AIDS, their families and friends, health care providers, scientists, and researchers.

376   Alaskan Statewide AIDS Helpline
1057 W Fireweed
Anchorage, AK 99503
907-263-2050
800-478-AIDS
Fax: 907-263-2051
www.alaskanaids.org

A key collaborator within the state of Alaska in the provision of supportive services to persons living with HIV/AIDS and their families and in the elimination of the transmission of HIV infection and its stigma.
Trevor Storrs, Executive Director

377   BABES Network-YWCA
1118 Fifth Ave
Seattle, WA 98101
206-720-5566
888-292-1912
Fax: 206-720-5901
e-mail: the_staff@babesnetwork.org
www.babesnetwork.org

A peer-based program, a sisterhood of women facing HIV together. Reduces isolation, promotes self-empowerment, enhances quality of life and serves the needs of women facing HIV and their families through peer support, advocacy, education and outreach
Rhonda Kimm, Advocacy Coordinator
Amelia Vader, Program Manager

378   COMPASS Program
c/o Institute for Urban Family Health
16 East 16th Street
New York, NY 10003
212-924-7744
Fax: 212-691-4610
e-mail: info@institute2000.org
www.institute2000.org/health/rwp.htm

Medical services include HIV testing and specialized HIV medical care for adults in addition to women's health services including gynecology, PAP tests, family planning and birth control methods. Mental health services includes individual, couples, and family counseling and psychiatric evaluations and monitoring.
Neil Calman MD/ABFP/FAAFP, President/Chief Executive Officer
Weston Willett, Chief Information Officer

379   Cascade AIDS Project Hotline
620 SW Fifth Avenue
Portland, OR 97204
503-223-2437
Fax: 503-223-7087
e-mail: info@cascadeaids.org
www.cascadeaids.org

Provides HIV prevention and services information by phone and internet to youth and adults across Orgeon and the Northwest.
Joseph Sedillo, Hotline Coordinator

380   Dunshee House
303-17th Avenue East
Seattle, WA 98112
206-322-2584
Fax: 206-322-1779
e-mail: josh@dunsheehouse.org
www.dunsheehouse.org

A non-profit organization, builds community and cultivates powerful, healthy lives by providing emotional support and personal development services to those affected by HIV/AIDS, the Queer communities, and those who love them.

381   HEAL
Sidney Hillman Family Pracitce
16 E 16th Street
New York, NY 10003-3105
212-924-7744
e-mail: healweb@thorup.com
www.thorup.com/HEAL

The Health Education AIDS Liaison provides alternative and holistic support groups and resources for people with HIV.

382   HIV/AIDS Prevention Program
Centers for Disease Control and Prevention
1600 Clifton Road NE
Atlanta, GA 30333
800-232-4636
TTY: 888-232-6348
e-mail: cdcinfo@cdc.gov
www.cdc.gov/hiv

As a part of its overall public health mission, CDC provides leadership in helping control the HIV/AIDS epidemic by working with community, state, national, and international partners in surveillance, research, and prevention and evaluation activities. CDC's programs also work to improve treatment, care, and support for persons living with HIV/AIDS and to build capacity and infrastructure to address the HIV/AIDS epidemic in the United States and around the world.
Jonathan Mermin, Director

383   Immunization Division Centers for Disease Control
1600 Tullie Circle NE
Atlanta, GA 30329-2303
404-639-1880
800-311-3435
Fax: 404-639-5258
www.cdc.gov

Robert Janssen, Director

384   King County Crisis Clinic
206-461-3222
866-427-4747
Fax: 206-461-8368
TDD: 206-461-3219
e-mail: info@crisisclinic.org
www.crisisclinic.org

A non-profit organization, we offer an array of support services available to everyone in King County, Washington.

385   Minnesota AIDS Project AIDSLine
1400 Park Avenue
Minneapolis, MN 55404
612-373-2437
800-248-2437
TTY: 888-820-2437
e-mail: mapaidsline@mnaidsproject.org
www.mnaidsproject.org

A statewide, toll-free information and referral service that can answer your questions about HIV and connect you to resources that can help
Lorraine Teel, Executive Director

386   National Health Information Center
PO Box 1133
Washington, DC 20013-1133
310-565-4167
800-336-4797
Fax: 301-984-4256
e-mail: info@nhic.org
www.health.gov/nhic

A health information referral service sponsored by the Office of Disease Prevention and Health Promotion. NHIC puts health professionals and consumers who have health questions in touch with those organizations that are best able to provide answers.

387   Project Inform Hotline
1375 Mission Street
San Francisco, CA 94103-2621
415-558-8669
800-822-7422
Fax: 415-558-0684
e-mail: web@projectinform.org
www.projectinform.org

Represents HIV-positive people in the development of treatments and a cure, supports individuals to make informed choices about their HIV health, advocates for quality health care to respond to HIV and related conditions, and promotes medical strategies that prevent new infections.
Dana Van Gorder, Executive Director

388 STI Resource Center Hotline

919-361-8488
800-227-8922
www.ashastd.org

Provides information, materials and referrals to anyone concerned about sexually transmitted infections.
Lynn Barclay, President/CEO
Deborah Arrindell, VP Health Policy

Books

389 ABC of AIDS
Michael W. Adler, author

BMJ Publishing Group
PO Box 281
Annapolis, MD 20701-0281

800-2FO-NBMJ
Fax: 800-2FA-XBMJ
e-mail: bmjpg@pmds.com
ww.bmjpg.com

118 pages Paperback
ISBN: 0-727915-03-7

390 AIDS & HIV Related Diseases

Harper Collins Publishers
10 East 53rd Street
New York, NY 10022

212-207-7000
www.harpercollins.com

An education guide for professionals and the public which covers such topics as: Understanding HIV and its effect on the immune system; HIV transmission; The history of AIDS and HIV; HIV testing; The natural course of an HIV infection; Medical treatment and those who administer them; The people who have AIDS; AIDS education.
1996 246 pages
ISBN: 0-306450-85-2

391 AIDS & Other Manifestations of HIV Infection

Academic Press (Elsevier)
1183 Westline Industrial Drive
St Louis, MO 63146

800-545-2522
Fax: 800-535-9935
e-mail: usbkinfo@elsevier.com
www.elsevier.com

An essential reference resource providing a comprehensive overview of the biological properties of this etiologic viral agent, its clinicopathological manifestations, the epidemiology of its infection, and present and future therapeutic options.
2004-4th Edi 1000 pages
ISBN: 0-127640-51-7
Gary Wormser, Editor

392 AIDS Alert

American Health Consultants
3525 Piedmont Road
Atlanta, GA 30305

404-262-5476
800-688-2421
Fax: 800-284-3291
www.ahcpub.com

The definitive source of AIDS news and advice for health care professionals. Covers up-to-the-minute developments and guidance on the entire spectrum of AIDS challenges, including treatment, education, precaustion, screening, diagnosis and policy.

393 AIDS and HIV Related Diseases
Josh Powell, author

Plenum Publishing Corporation
233 Spring Street
New York, NY 10013

212-620-8000
800-221-9369
Fax: 212-463-0742
e-mail: books@plenum.com

An education guide for professionals and the public which covers such topics as: Understanding HIV and its effect on the immune

system; HIV transmission; The history of AIDS and HIV; HIV testing; The natural course of an HIV infection; Medical treatment and those who administer them; The people who have AIDS; AIDS education.
1996 243 pages
ISBN: 0-306450-85-2

394 AIDS and Persons with Developmental Disabilities

Commission on the Mentally Disabled
1800 M Street NW
Washington, DC 20036

202-331-2240

A discussion of federal and state laws that defines the rights and responsibilities of individuals with disabilities and service providers with respect to HIV infection.

395 AIDS in the Twenty-First Century: Disease and Globalization
Tony Barnett, Alan Whiteside, author

Palgrave Macmillan
175 Fifth Avenue
New York, NY 10010

212-982-3900
800-221-7945
Fax: 212-777-6359
www.palgrave.com

Presents compelling data and research which reveals the shocking social and economic impact of HIV/AIDS on a global scale
432 pages
ISBN: 1-403900-05-0

396 AIDS, Revised Edition
Alan E. Nourse, M.D., author

Franklin Watts c/o Grolier
90 Old Sherman Tpke
Danbury, CT 06816

203-797-3500
800-621-1115
Fax: 203-797-3197
www.grolier.com

This bestselling book has been updated with the latest findings and research into the AIDS epidemic. Includes new statistical information and findings on HIV and AIDS.
144 pages
ISBN: 0-531106-62-4

397 AIDS: A Communication Perspective

Lawrence Erlbaum Associates Publishers
10 Industrial Avenue
Mahwah, NJ 07430-2262

201-236-9500
Fax: 201-236-6396
www.erlbaum.com

ISBN: 0-805809-98-8

398 AIDS: Distinguishing Between Fact and Opinion
Teresa Opheim, author

Greenhaven Press
PO Box 9187
Farmington Hills, MI 48333-9187

800-877-GALE
Fax: 800-414-5043
e-mail: gale.galeord@thomson.com (E-Mail Orders)
www.galegroup.com/greenhaven

For beginning debaters, reports and classroom use this book offers three debates: Can AIDS be spread by casual contact? Should the Food and Drug Administration make AIDS drugs more available? Is AIDS a moral issue?.
36 pages
ISBN: 0-899086-33-0

399 AIDS: How it Works in the Body
Lorna Greenberg, author

Franklin Watts
96 Leonard Street
London EC2A 4XD,
For readers ages 9-12

www.wattspub.co.uk

64 pages School Binding

400 AIDS: Trading Fears for Facts: A Guide for Young People
Karen Hein, Theresa Foy Digernimo, author

Consumer Reports Books
101 Truman Avenue
Yonkers, NY 10703-1057

www.consumerreports.org

Listed for young adult readers.
232 pages Paperback
ISBN: 0-890437-21-1

401 Amfar AIDS Handbook: The Complete Guide to Understanding HIV and AIDS
Darrell Ward, author

W.W. Norton & Company, Inc.
500 Fifth Avenue   212-354-5500
New York, NY 10110   Fax: 212-869-0856
                                           www.norton.com
Gives a greater understanding of HIV/Aids. The causes and effects, what new treatment options are being developed.
360 pages
ISBN: 0-393316-36-X

402 Black Death: AIDS in Africa
Susan Hunter, author

Macmillan
175 Fifth Avenue
New York, NY 10010   646-307-5151
                                        us.macmillian.com
The untold story of AIDS in Africa, home to 80 percent of the 40 million people in the world currently infected with HIV. Brings the staggering statistics to life and paints for the first time a stunning picture of the most important political issue today.
256 pages
ISBN: 1-403967-17-2

403 Children and the AIDS Virus: A Book for Children, Parents, and Teachers
Rosmarie Hausherr, author

Clarion Books
For readers ages 4-8.
48 pages Library Binding
ISBN: 0-899198-34-1

404 Community Service Delivery for Children with HIV Infection and Families
Geneva, Woodruff & Christopher Hanson, author

South Shore Mental Health Center
6 Fort Street   617-847-1950
Quincy, MA 02169   e-mail: contactus@ssmh.org
                                          www.ssmh.org
A manual providing guidelines for developing community-based, family-centered services for children with HIV infection and their families. Describes how services can be planned and delivered using guiding principles and practices of transagency case management.

405 Coping When You or a Friend is HIV-Positive
Pat Kelly, author

Hazelden Publishing & Educational Services
15251 Pleasant Valley Road   651-257-4010
Center City, MN 55012-0176   800-328-9000
                                           Fax: 651-213-4577
         e-mail: customersupport@hazeldon.org
                                    www.hazelden.org
Provides compassionate counsel for teens who have been diagnosed with the virus.
136 pages Paperback
ISBN: 1-568381-77-8

406 Dancing Against the Darkness: A Journey Through America in the Age of AIDS
Steven Petrow, author

Rowman & Littlefield Publishing Group
4501 Forbes Blvd.   717-794-3800
Lanham, MD 20706   800-462-6420
                                           Fax: 717-794-3803
              e-mail: custserv@rowman.com
                              www.lexingtonbooks.com
218 pages Hardcover
ISBN: 0-669243-09-4

407 Everything You Need to Know About AIDS
Katherine White, author

Rosen Publishing Group
29 E 21st Street   212-777-3017
New York, NY 10010   800-237-9932
                                          Fax: 888-436-4643
      e-mail: customerservice@rosenpub.com
                              www.rosenpublishing.com
Without proper information, our teens remain at risk for AIDS. This volume presents balanced information on the disease and on safer sex precautions, in a language that readers can understand.
64 pages Library Binding
ISBN: 0-823933-14-8
Barbara Taylor, Author

408 Everything You Need to Know About Being HIV Positive
Amy Shire, author

Rosen Publishing Group
29 E 21st Street   212-777-3017
New York, NY 10010   800-237-9932
                                          Fax: 888-436-4643
      e-mail: customerservice@rosenpub.com
                              www.rosenpublishing.com
To teens who need to understand thier options are when living with HIV on a day-to-day basis. This book explains the facts about HIV.
Hardcover
ISBN: 0-823926-14-1
Amy Shire, Author

409 Everything You Need to Know When a Parent has AIDS
Barbara Hermie Draimin, author

Rosen Publishing Group
29 E 21st Street   212-777-3017
New York, NY 10010   800-237-9932
                                          Fax: 888-436-4643
      e-mail: customerservice@rosenpub.com
                              www.rosenpublishing.com
More and more teens have a parent who has AIDS. Teens must learn where they can turn for help in dealing with this difficult situation. By presenting stories of teens in the same situation, this book helps readers deal with their anger and grief.
64 pages Library Binding
ISBN: 0-823916-90-1
Barbara Hermie Draimin DSW, Author

410 Global AIDS: Myths and Facts, Tools for Fighting the AIDS Pandemic
Alexander Irwin, Joyce Millen, author

South End Press
7 Brookline Street   718-874-0089
Cambridge, MA 02139-4146   e-mail: info@southendpress.org
                                    www.southendpress.org
10 myths about HIV/AIDS treatment and prevention while calling for an international movement to fight the disease.
296 pages
ISBN: 0-896086-73-9

411 Guide to Living With HIV Infection
John G. Bartlett, Ann K. Finkbeiner, author

John's Hopkins University Press
2715 N Charles Street   410-516-6900
Baltimore, MD 21218-4363   800-537-5487
                                           Fax: 410-516-6968
                                    www.press.jhu.edu
The most complete source of medical, emotional, social, and practical advice available for those infected with HIV and their loved ones. Provides essential information for making decisions about treatment and testing in a world transformed by new research and pharmacotherapy.
1996 408 pages Paperback
ISBN: 0-801884-85-6

412 Invisible People: How the U.S. Has Slept Through the Global AIDS Pandemic
Greg Behrman, author

Free Press Publishing Co.

1010 W CASS St
Tampa, FL 33606-1307
368 pages
ISBN: 0-743257-55-3

813-254-5888

413 Living Well With HIV and AIDS
Allen L Gifford MD, Kate Loring RN, author
Bull Publishing Company
PO Box 1377
Boulder, CO 80306
800-676-2855
Fax: 303-545-6354
www.bullpub.com
Offers the latest information based on the HIV care guidelines from the Department of Health & Human Services and the Center for Disease Control. Disscusses a shift in treatments emphasis to the ways of managing side effects such as lypodystrophy, redistribution of body fat, cardiac risks, and concerns with vulnerability to other ailments called comorbidities
2005 328 pages Papperback
ISBN: 0-923521-86-8

414 Living on the Edge
Michael Kelly, author
HarperCollins Canada Limited/Order Department
1995 Markham Road
Ontario, Canada M1 B 5M8,
800-387-0117
Fax: 800-668-5788
A gritty, honest, biographical account of one young man's experience from the original diagnosis via the development of the illness, how Michael has learned to live with his illness and how it has affected him and all his friends who support him.
160 pages
ISBN: 0-551027-49-5

415 Local AIDS Sercices: The National Directory
US Conference of Mayors
1620 I Street NW
Washington, DC 20006
202-293-7330
Fax: 202-293-2352
e-mail: info@usmayors.org
www.usmayors.org
2,500 organizations that provide various information and services for AIDS coordinates and other health-related professionals.

416 Lynda Madaras Talks to Teens About AIDS
Lynda Madaras, author
Waterfront Books
98 Brookes Avenue
Burlington, VT 05401
802-658-7477
800-639-6063
e-mail: helpkids@waterfrontbooks.com
www.waterfrontbooks.com
An informative book about the HIV virus and AIDS.
128 pages

417 Night Kites
M.E. Kerr, author
HarperCollins Children's Books
1350 Avenue of the Americas
New York, NY 10019
212-261-6500
www.harperchildrens.com
For young adults.
224 pages Paperback
ISBN: 0-064470-35-0

418 No Longer Immune: A Counselor's Guide to AIDS
American Counseling Association
5999 Stevenson Avenue
Alexandria, VA 22304
703-823-9800
800-347-6647
Fax: 703-823-0252
www.counseling.org
Covers a broad range of issues such as working with specific populations, handling pre- and posttesting situations, coping with fear, grief and survivor guilt, preventing caregiver burnout and dealing with countertransference.
295 pages Paperback
ISBN: 1-556200-64-1

419 Parent Education Program-HIV/AIDS: A Challenge to Us All
Pediatric AIDS Foundation

2950 31st Street
Santa Monica, CA 90405-3092
310-314-1459
800-499-4673
Fax: 310-314-1469
e-mail: info@pedcids.org
www.pedaids.org
This parent meeting kit with a guide book and two videos will help any adult set up a parent meeting on the subject of AIDS. This kit provides accurate information to parents about HIV/AIDS, allows parents to voice concerns and fears, gives examples of appropriate answers to your child's questions about HIV/AIDS and replaces fear with knowledge and compassion.

420 Predicting AIDS and Other Epidemics
Christopher Lampton, author
Franklin Watts
96 Leonard Street
London EC2A 4XD,
www.wattspub.co.uk
144 pages S & L Binding

421 Scarlet Letters
AIDS Project Los Angeles
The David Geffen Center
Los Angeles, CA 90005
213-201-1600
www.apla.org
A bilingual (Spanidh/English) journal targeted at HIV prevention providers in the U.S. The Scarlet Letters features opinion pieces and research-based essays by invited HIV/STD prevention experts.
2 year

422 Teen Guide to AIDS Prevention
Alan E. Nourse, author
Franklin Watts
96 Leonard Street
London EC2A 4XD,
www.wattspub.co.uk
For young adult readers.
61 pages S & L Binding

423 We Have AIDS
Elaine Landau, author
Franklin Watts
96 Leonard Street
London EC2A 4XD,
www.wattspub.co.uk
For young adult readers.
S & L Binding

424 What Is AIDS?
Anna Forbes, author
The Rosen Publishing Group
PowerKids Press
New York, NY 10010
212-777-3017
800-237-9932
Fax: 888-436-4643
www.powerkidspress.com
For reader levels ages 4-8.
1st Edition 24 pages Hardcover

425 Women & AIDS
Diane Richardson, author
Methuen
11-12 Buckingham Gate
London SW1E 6LB,
www.methuen.co.uk
The first sourcebook to provide the information women need by identifying the most accurate sources and providing valuable statistical data.
183 pages Paperback
ISBN: 0-416017-51-7

426 Women and AIDS: A Practical Guide for Those Who Help Others
Continuum Publishing Corporation
370 Lexington Avenue
New York, NY 10017-6503
212-532-3650
Tailored to women, this book grapples with attitudes and realities of AIDS.

427 Women and Aids: Coping and Caring
Plenum Publishing Corportation

233 Spring Street
New York, NY 10013-1522

212-620-8000
800-221-9369
Fax: 212-463-0742
e-mail: info@plenum.com

1996 263 pages
ISBN: 0-306452-58-8
Ann O'Leary, Editor

428   You Have HIV: A Day at a Time
Lynn S. Baker, author

W.B. Saunders Company

www.elsevierhealth.com

258 pages paperback
ISBN: 0-721636-06-3

Children's Books

429   AIDS Overview Series
Lucent Books
Thomson Gale
Farmington Hills, MI 48333-9187

800-877-4253
Fax: 800-414-5043
e-mail: gale.customerservice@thomson.com
www.gale.com/lucent

A straightforward account that teaches young adults all about the growing problem of AIDS.
1998 112 pages
ISBN: 1-560061-93-6

430   AIDS Awareness Library
Rosen Publishing Group
29 E 21st Street
New York, NY 10010

800-237-9932
Fax: 888-436-4643
e-mail: customerservice@rosepub.com
www.rosenpublishing.com

1996 24 pages
ISBN: 0-823974-06-1

431   AIDS To the Point: Confronting Youth Issues
Diana L. Hynson, author

Abingdon Press
201 8th Avenue S
Nashville, TN 37202-0801

615-749-6347
800-251-3320
Fax: 615-749-6577
www.abingdonpress.com

A resource that offers a practical means of talking with teens, individually or in a group, about AIDS. This volume offers teaching articles, ready-to-go programs for teens, leader's guides, worship resources, facts and figures, where to go for help and a section exclusively in Spanish. This is a volume in the To The Point: Confronting Youth Issues series of books.
96 pages Paperback
ISBN: 0-687782-20-1

432   AIDS: How it Works in the Body
Franklin Watts Grolier
90 Old Sherman Turnpike
Danbury, CT 06816-0001

203-797-3500
Fax: 203-797-3197
www.grolier.com

Focuses on the physiological effects AIDS has on the body, explains the causes of the disease, how the immune system works to defend the body and how the HIV virus affects the immune system.
64 pages Grades 5-7
ISBN: 0-531200-74-4

433   AIDS: Trading Fears for Facts a Guide for Teens
Consumer Reports Books
9180 La Saint Drive
Fairfield, OH 45014

914-378-2567
Fax: 914-378-2907

Written specifically for teenage readers and filled with illustrations, this book includes the current facts about AIDS, discusses how the virus is transmitted and precautions that should be taken.

434   AIDS: Trading Fears for Facts: A Guide for Young People
Consumer Reports Books

9180 La Saint Drive
Fairfield, OH 45014

914-378-2567
Fax: 914-378-2907
www.consumerreports.com

1993
ISBN: 0-890432-62-4

435   Dancing Against the Darkness: A Journey Through America in the Age of AIDS
Heath Publishing
125 Spring Street
Lexington, MA 02421-7801

617-822-6650

A professional in the field, this author has chosen people across the nation to interview and use as examples for how the AIDS epidemic has struck America and what kind of lives it has affected.
Grades 7-12

436   Everything You Need to Know When a Parent Has AIDS
Barbara Hermie Draimin, DSW, author

Rosen Publishing Group
29 E. 21st Street
New York, NY 10010

212-777-3017
800-237-9932
Fax: 888-436-4643
e-mail: rosenpub@tribeca.ios.com

More and more teens have a parent who has AIDS. Teens must learn where they can turn up for health in dealing with this difficult situation. By presenting stories of teens in the same situation, this book helps readers deal with their anger and grief.

ISBN: 0-823916-90-1

437   Impact of AIDS
Franklin Watts Grolier
90 Old Sherman Turnpike
Danbury, CT 06816-0001

203-797-3500
800-621-1115
Fax: 203-797-3197
www.grolier.com

Examines the effects of the HIV infection and discusses the efforts in finding a cure for AIDS.
64 pages Grades 5-7
ISBN: 0-531172-25-2

438   Night Kites
Harper Collins
55 Avenue Road
Hazelton, Toronto, M5R3L2,

416-975-9334
www.harpercollins.com

This book focuses on two brothers, one of whom is homosexual and how they interact in the face of AIDS and the intolerance of homosexuality among the many people they know.
Grades 8-12

439   Our Immune System
Sara LeBien, author

Immune Deficiency Foundation
40 W Chesapeake Avenue
Towson, MD 21204-4841

410-321-6647
800-296-4433
Fax: 410-321-9165
e-mail: idf@primaryimmune.org
www.primaryimmune.org

This storybook educates children about primary immunodeficiency diseases through delightful, eye-catching illustrations. The characters explain how the immune system works and describe the treatments for pediatric patients. Children will understand their own bodies and be better prepared to deal with their own primary immunodeficiency.
G. Richard Barr, Chairman
Marcia Boyle, Founder, Chairperson

440   Predicting AIDS and Other Epidemics
Franklin Watts Grolier
90 Old Sherman Turnpike
Danbury, CT 06816-0001

203-797-3500
800-621-1115
Fax: 203-797-3197
www.grolier.com

Surveys the efforts of scientists and researchers to predict the spread of epidemic diseases, including AIDS.
128 pages Grades 7-12
ISBN: 0-531107-85-0

441 Problem of AIDS
Franklin Watts Grolier
90 Old Sherman Turnpike   203-797-3500
Danbury, CT 06816-0001   800-621-1115
                                       Fax: 203-797-3197
                                       www.grolier.com
Part of the Let's Talk About series, this book addresses the questions and answers children and young adults have about AIDS.
32 pages Grades 3-5
ISBN: 0-531171-91-4

442 Teen Guide to AIDS Prevention
Franklin Watts Grolier
90 Old Sherman Turnpike   203-797-3500
Danbury, CT 06816-0001   800-621-1115
                                       Fax: 203-797-3197
                                       www.grolier.com
Directly addresses the questions and fears of teenagers by explaining clearly and simply what AIDS is, how it is spread, and the preventive measures young persons should take.
64 pages Grades 9-12
ISBN: 0-531109-66-6

443 We Have AIDS
Franklin Watts Grolier
90 Old Sherman Turnpike   203-797-3500
Danbury, CT 06816-0001   800-621-1115
                                       Fax: 203-797-3197
                                       www.grolier.com
This book goes beyond statistics and facts and focuses on the personal side of the disease. Offers source notes, a bibliography and an index.
128 pages
ISBN: 0-531108-98-8

444 What's a Virus, Anyway? The Kid's Book About AIDS
Waterfront Books
98 Brookes Avenue   802-658-7477
Burlington, VT 05401-3326
A simple introduction to help adults talk with children about the subject of AIDS.
67 pages

Magazines

445 AIDS Alert
American Health Consultants
3525 Piedmont Road   404-262-5476
Atlanta, GA 30305   800-688-2421
                                       Fax: 404-262-5560
                                       www.ahcpub.com
Covers up-to-the-minute developments and guidance on the entire spectrum of AIDS challenges, including treatment, education, precautions, screening, diagnosis and policy.

446 AIDS Clinical Care
New England Journal of Medicine
860 Winter Street   781-893-3800
Waltham, MA 02451-1413   800-843-6356
                                       Fax: 781-893-0413
                                       e-mail: nejcust@mms.org
                                       www.massmed.org
Up to date information specifically targeted at physicians with AIDS patients.
Monthly

447 AIDS: A Year In Review
Lippincott Williams & Wilkins
Po Box 1620   301-223-2300
Hagerstown, MD 21741   800-638-3030
                                       www.lww.com

448 AIDS: International Monthly Journal
Lippincott Williams & Wilkins
Po Box 1620   301-223-2300
Hagerstown, MD 21741   800-638-3030
                                       www.lww.com

449 AIDS: The Disease State Management Resource
American Health Consultants
Po Box 740056   800-688-2421
Atlanta, GA 30374   Fax: 800-284-3291
                                       www.ahcpub.com

450 Critical Path AIDS Project
2062 Lombard Street
Philadelphia, PA 19146-1315   215-545-2212
                                       www.critpath.org
Articles and reprints on experimental treatments and alternative therapies, and a listing of Philadelphia-area resources.
Monthly

451 Institute on Health Care for the Poor and Underserved at Meharry Medical College
Sage Publications
1005 DB Todd Boulevard   615-327-6819
Nashville, TN 37208   800-669-1269
                                       Fax: 615-327-6362
                                       e-mail: vbrennan@mmc.edu
Offers health care and public health policy research focusing on poor and underserved populations.
100pages 4x a year
Dr. Amy Cato, Director
Dr. Virginia Brennan, Editor

452 Journal of Acquired Immune Deficiency Syndrome
Lippincott Williams & Wilkins
Po Box 1620   301-223-2300
Hagerstown, MD 21741-2601   800-638-3030
                                       www.lww.com
An interdisciplinary journal providing a synthesis of AIDS-related information from all relevant clinical and basic sciences.
Monthly
ISBN: 0-894925-5 -
William A Hazeltine, Editor

453 Journal of the Medical Library Association
Medical Library Association
65 E Wacker Place   312-419-9094
Chicago, IL 60601-7246   Fax: 312-419-8950
                                       e-mail: info@mlahq.org
                                       www.mlahq.org
An international, peer-reviewed journal that aims to advance the practice and research knowledgebase of health science librarianship.
Quarterly
Carla J Funk, Executive Director
Elizabeth Lund, Publications Director

454 POZ Magazine
POZ Publishing
462 Seventh Avenue   212-242-2163
New York, NY 10018-7424   Fax: 212-675-8505
                                       e-mail: poz-editor@poz.com
                                       www.poz.com
A magazine for people living with, and affected by, HIV/AIDS.
60 pages BiMonthly
Regan Hofmann, Editor in Chief
Jennifer Morton, Managing Editor

455 Risky Business
San Francisco AIDS Foundation Materials Dept.
333 Valencia Street   415-861-3397
San Francisco, CA 94103-3547
A comic book style magazine providing accurate information about AIDS using humor and real-life situations. Contains stories that stress the importance of knowing how AIDS is transmitted and prevented.

456 Straight Talk: A Magazine for Teens About AIDS
Custom Publishing Division of Rodale Press
33 E Minor Street   610-967-5171
Emmaus, PA 18098-0001
A lively magazine that includes articles about teens with AIDS, teens involved in peer education and teens at risk for getting infected. Good information is presented in an interesting format for young adults.

457 Washington Update
Committee of Ten Thousand
500 Belmont Street
Brockton, MA 02301   508-587-2512
e-mail: cott-dc@earthlink.net
www.cott1.org
Is a primer on government related issues of importance to COTT's constituency. From health care legislation, to regulatory affairs to Administration policy for chronic diseases. A hands-on journal for grass roots health care advocacy in our Nation's capital.
Bi-Monthly
John Rider, Contact

Newsletters

458 AIDS Alert
American Health Consulants
3525 Piedmont Road
Atlanta, GA 30305   404-262-5476
800-688-2421
Fax: 404-262-5560
e-mail: customerservice@ahcpub.com
www.ahcpub.com
Covers up-to-the-minute developments and guidance on the entire spectrum of AIDS challenges, including treatment, education, precautions, screening, diagnosis and policy.
12 year

459 AIDS Link
University of Cincinnati-Medical Center Info.
231 Bethesda Avenue   513-558-5661
Cincinnati, OH 45267-0001   Fax: 513-558-3136
medcenter.uc.edu/
Aimed at healthcare professionals working with HIV/AIDS inflicted patients.
Rebecca Atterrin, Editor

460 AIDS News
Northern California Chapter of the NHF
7700 Edgewater Drive   510-568-6243
Oakland, CA 94621-3023
Provides current information for people who need to cope mentally and physically with the issues of virus infection and transmission. Provides answers to questions about AIDS, ARC, HIV infection and transmission prevention.
BiMonthly

461 AIDS Policy and Law
LRP Publications
747 Dresher Road
Horsham, PA 19044-0980   www.lrp.com
A report on AIDS policy and law developments from the courts, NIH, federal and state AIDS agencies and advocacy organizations.
24 year

462 AIDS Treatment Data Network
611 Broadway   212-260-8868
New York, NY 10012   800-734-7104
Fax: 212-260-8869
www.atdn.org
Information bulletins covering new treatments, clinical trials, and more.

463 AIDS Treatment News
ATN Publications
PO Box 411256
San Francisco, CA 94141-1256   800-873-2812
www.atnonline.org
Reports on the developments in treatments for HIV disease and related infections. Also covers issues relating to research.
BiMonthly

464 AIDS Update
Dallas Gay Alliance
PO Box 190812
Dallas, TX 75219-0812   214-528-4233
Fax: 214-521-6424
e-mail: info@dgla.org
www.divanet.com/dgla/
Includes general information on AIDS issues and treatments.

465 AIDS Weekly Plus
Charles Henderson
Po Box 5528
Atlanta, GA 31107-0528   e-mail: info@hendersonnet.atl.ga.us
All aspects of AIDS epidemic coverage, including research, treatments, vaccine development, political and public policy.
46 year

466 AIDS/STD News Report
CD Publications
8204 Fenton Street   301-588-6380
Silver Spring, MD 0910   800-666-6380
Fax: 301-588-6385
e-mail: info@cdpublications.com
www.cdpublications.com
Formerly AIDS News Alert, provides grant listings from federal, private, and corporate sources; proposal writing tips; updates on successful programs, and the latest news on AIDS/STD federal/state legislation, research, and successful programs.
24 year

467 APICHA News
Asian & Pacific Islander Coalition on HIV/AIDS
400 Broadway   212-334-7940
New York, NY 10013   866-274-2429
Fax: 212-334-7956
e-mail: apicha@apicha.org
www.apicha.org
Provides information on prevention education, client services and advocacy for Asians and Pacific Islanders.
Quarterly
Therese R Rodriguez, CEO

468 APLA Update
AIDS Project Los Angeles
3550 Wilshire Boulevard
Los Angeles, CA 90010   213-201-1600
www.apla.org
Presents news about AIDS and programs of AIDS Project Los Angeles to people affected by the disease.
20 pages

469 BETA
San Francisco AIDS Foundation
995 Market Street 200   415-487-3000
San Francisco, CA 94103   e-mail: feedback@sfaf.org
www.sfaf.org
Medical information.
Quarterly

470 Being Alive
Being Alive People with HIV/AIDS Action Coalition
621 N San Vincente Boulevard   310-289-2551
West Hollywood, CA 90069   Fax: 310-289-9866
e-mail: info@beingalivela.org
www.beingalivela.org
Medical updates, plus information on AIDS advocacy, a calendar of local events and listings of AIDS support groups.

471 Being Alive Newsletter
Being Alive-People with HIV/AIDS Action Coalition
7531 Santa Monica Boulevard   323-874-4322
West Hollywood, CA 90040   Fax: 323-969-8753
e-mail: kevin@beingalivela.org
www.beingalivela.org
A regularly-published source of information and education for our peers living with HIV/AIDS and for the greater community. Standing articles cover timely issues such as HIV/AIDS treatment options, mental health, substance abuse, nutrition, advocacy, community referrals, and a variety of other topics. Additionally, we feature information on Being Alive events alongside other relevant community events.
Quarterly
Kevin Kurth, Executive Director/Editor

472 CORPUS
AIDS Project Los Angeles
The David Geffen Center
Los Angeles, CA 90005   213-201-1600
e-mail: info@apla.org
www.apla.org

A journal that uses art, cultural criticism, poetry, short stories and humor to reveal the challenges of HIV prevention in gay and bisexual communities.
Annually
Craig E Thompson, Executive Director

473   COTT News
Committee on Ten Thousand
500 Belmont Street
Brockton, MA 02301   508-587-2512
                                 www.cott1.org
A range of information, reportage and viewpoints regarding issues and events of importance to grass roots health care advocacy and support.
John Rider, Contact

474   Center for AIDS Prevention Studies
AIDS Research Institute
74 New Montgomery   415-597-9100
San Francisco, CA 94105   Fax: 415-597-9213
                                e-mail: capsweb@psg.ucsf.edu
                                www.caps.ucsf.edu
Local, national, and international interdisciplinary research.

475   Community Health Funding Report
CD Publications
8204 Fenton Street   301-588-6380
Silver Spring, MD 20910-4571   800-666-6380
                                Fax: 301-588-6385
                                e-mail: chf@cdpublications.com
                                www.cdpublications.com
Covers grants for AIDS and sexually transmitted disease related programs from federal and private sources. Includes news on national and local issues affecting AIDS and STD's and case studies of successful fundraising programs. This biweekly newsletter describes changes in funding streams for community based health programs, including AIDS programs. It lists available federal and private grant opportunities, along with Washington News Medicare/Medicaid.
18 pages BiMonthly
Mike Gerecht, Publisher
Amy Bernstein, Editor

476   Cott Washington Update
Committee of Ten Thousand
236 Massachusetts Avenue NE   202-543-0988
Washington, DC 20002-4971   800-488-2688
                                Fax: 202-543-6720
                                www.cott1.org
Offers legislative updates, information on clinical trials, therapies, book reviews, business and politics, a readers forum and resources pertaining to HIV/AIDS.
10 pages Monthly
Corey Dubin, President
Dave Cavenaugh, Government Relations

477   FOCUS
UCSF AIDS Health Project
1930 Market Street
San Francisco, CA 94102   415-476-3902
                                www.ucsf-ahp.org
Reviews the counseling aspects of AIDS; how HIV-related counseling is affected by the medical, epidemiological, and social realities of AIDS, as well as the emotional response to the disease. It is written for mental health and health care providers working on the front lines and is of interest to researchers, policy makers, and program administrators.
10x/year
James W Dilley MD, Executive Director

478   Gay Men's Health Crisis
119 West 24th Street
New York, NY 10011   212-367-1000
                                www.gmhc.org
Not-for-profit, volunteer-supported and community-based organization committed to national leadership in the fight against AIDS.

479   HIV Counselor PERSPECTIVES
UCSF AIDS Health Project

1930 Market Street
San Francisco, CA 94102   415-476-3902
                                www.ucsf-ahp.org
An educational resource for HIV antibody test counselors, prevention case managers, and other health and mental health professionals, particularly those working in brief counseling venues.
4 year
James W Dilley MD, Executive Director

480   HIV Frontline
Center for AIDS Prevention Studies
University of California   415-552-6356
San Francisco, CA 94114   Fax: 415-597-9213
                                e-mail: CAPSweb@psg.ucsf.edu
                                www.caps.ucsf.edu
Monthly newsletter aimed at mental health and healthcare professionals who counsel people living with HIV/AIDS.
Monthly
Dr. Leon McKusick

481   IDF Advocate
Immune Deficiency Foundation
40 W Chesapeake Avenue
Towson, MD 21204   800-296-4433
                                e-mail: idf@primaryimmune.org
                                www.primaryimmune.org
Mailed to patients, family members, physicians, nurses, industry, government and interested individuals.
3x/year
Marcia Boyle, President/Founder

482   Immune Deficiency Foundation Newsletter
Immune Deficiency Foundation
40 W Chesapeake Avenue   410-321-6647
Towson, MD 21204-4841   800-296-4433
                                Fax: 410-321-9165
                                e-mail: idf@primaryimmune.org
                                www.primaryimmune.org
Offers medical updates and technology news on the latest services, products and treatments for persons with immune diseases.
Tamara Brown, Medical Programs Manager

483   In Focus
Project Inform
205 13th Street   415-558-8669
San Francisco, CA 94103-2461   800-822-7422
                                Fax: 415-558-0684
                                e-mail: web@projectinform.org
                                www.projectinform.org
The organizational newsletter of Project Inform.
20+ pages 3x/year
Skip Emerson, Executive Assistant

484   Just Kids
3 Corners
5th Avenue   212-634-4879
New York, NY 10014
Covers medical and social issues faced by HIV-positive children, teens and their parents.
Annual

485   MLA News
Medical Library Association
65 East Wacker Place   312-419-9094
Chicago, IL 60601-7246   Fax: 312-419-8950
                                e-mail: info@mlahq.org
                                www.mlahq.org
Keeps you at the forefront of association matters and the profession as a whole. Regular departments include calendar, continuing education, employment opportunities, international news, Internet resources, personals, professional development, and technology. Columns include consumer health, expert searching, hospital librarianship, leadership and management, and new members. Members only.
Jean P Shipman, President

486   NMAC Update
National Minority AIDS Council

300 I Street NE
Washington, DC 20002-4389

202-544-1076
www.nmac.org

A newsletter reporting on public policy issues and information on subjects in organizational management.
BiMonthly

487   OUTReach
The San Francisco AID Foundation
995 Market Street
San Francisco, CA 94103

415-487-8000
Fax: 415-487-8009
TDD: 415-487-8099
www.sfaf.org

Features concise articles on a wide range of HIV/AIDS topics.

488   PAACNOTES
101 W Grand Avenue
Chicago, IL 60610-4272

312-222-1326
800-243-3059

A news journal of the Physicians Coalition for AIDS Care featuring articles on clinical management, scientific research and a diverse range of legal, ethical and economic issues directly affecting the care of persons with HIV disease.

489   PWA Rag
Prisoners With AIDS Rights Advocacy Group
1626 Wilcox Avenue
Loa Angeles, CA 90028

770-946-9346
e-mail: RAGNEWS@aol.com
www.hometown.aol.com

Contains articles, treatment updates, and resources for prisoners.

490   Positive Living
APLA
3550 Wilshire Boulevard
Los Angeles, CA 90010

213-201-1600
800-922-2438

Monthly

491   Positive Outlook
2655 Swann Avenue
Tampa, FL 33609

813-877-5696

Focuses on local people and issues in West Central Florida.
Quarterly

492   Positive Social Support Newsletter
Lambda Center
4228 Wisconsin Avenue NW
Washington, DC 20016

202-965-8434
877-252-6232
e-mail: contact@lambcenter.com
www.thelambdacenter.com

Sponsored by and for people with HIV.

493   Positive Voice Newsletter
National Association of People with AIDS (NAPWA)
8401 Colesville Road
Silverspring, MD 20910

240-247-0880
866-846-9366
Fax: 240-247-0574
e-mail: info@napwa.org
www.napwa.org

Frank J Oldham Jr, President/CEO
Peter Kronenberg, VP Communications/Editor

494   Positive Woman
PO Box 34372
Washington, DC 20043-4372

202-898-0372

Provides medical information, including alternative and holistic therapies for HIV-positive women.
BiMonthly

495   Positively Aware
Test Positive Aware Network
5537 N Broadway Street
Chicago, IL 60640

773-989-9400
Fax: 773-989-9494
e-mail: tpan@tpan.com
www.tpan.com

An internationally known and respected magazine devoted to HIV treatment, wellness, and optimum quality of life for those living with HIV, as well as those who care for them.
Bi-monthly
Jeff Berry, Publications Director

496   RAP* Time
Rural Center for AIDS/STD Prevention

Indiana University
Bloomington, IN 47405-3085

812-855-7974
800-566-8644
Fax: 812-855-3936
e-mail: aids@indiana.edu
www.indiana.edu/~aids/

Summarizes current research concerning HIV/STD prevention, particularly in rural settings.
William L Yarber HSD, Senior Director

497   STEP Perspective
Seattle Treatment Exchange Project
1123 E John Street
Seattle, WA 98102-5711

206-329-4857
800-869-7837
e-mail: info@stepproject.org
www.thebody.com

Updates on treatments for HIV and related diseases condensed from journals, conferences and databases by the scientific review committee.

498   Seasons
National Native American AIDS Prevention Center
436 14th Street
Oakland, CA 94612-2011

510-444-2051
Fax: 510-444-1593
e-mail: information@nnaape.org
www.nnaapc.org

Features articles and artwork by Native Americans impacted by HIV/AIDS.
Quarterly

499   Treatment Issues
Department of Medical Information
New York, NY 10011-3601

212-337-1950

The gay men's health crisis newsletter of experimental AIDS therapies.
10x Year

500   Up Front Drug Information
5701 Biscayne Boulevard
Miami, FL 33137-2601

305-757-2566

Provides information on drugs and drug referrals.

501   Walk Talk
AIDS Coalition Silicon Valley
Walk For AIDS Silicon Valley
San Jose, CA 95154

408-451-WALK
Fax: 408-248-7423
e-mail: info@walkforaids.org

The AIDS Coalition Silicon Valley Newsletter highlighting Walk for AIDS Silicon Valley fundraising events, issues and articles about HIV/AIDS service providers in the County.

502   Wisconsin AIDS Update
Wisconsin AIDS/HIV Program, Department of Health
PO Box 309
Madison, WI 53701-0309

608-267-5287
e-mail: webmaildph@dhfs.state.wi.us
www.dhfs.state.wi.us

Includes epidemiological and clinical care articles, selections from the most important current abstracts in ATIN and a statewide list of events and resources.
Quarterly

503   World/Mundo
PO Box 11535
Oakland, CA 94611-0535

415-658-6930

Contains letters, advice, events calendar, and information on support groups in Northern California.

Pamphlets

504   AIDS Medicines in Development
Pharmaceutical Research & Manufacturers of America
950 F Street NW
Washington, DC 20004

202-835-3400
Fax: 202-835-3414
www.phrma.org

An annual chart of antivirals, as well as information on diagnostics and vaccines.

505   AIDS and Hemophilia: Protecting Yourself and Others
Hemophilia Council of California: Bay Area Office

7700 Edgewater Drive
Oakland, CA 94621
510-568-7074
Fax: 510-568-2048
e-mail: hccoak@aol.com
Lori Drake, Mental Health Counselor/Health Educator

506   AIDS, the Law & You
AIDS Action Committee
131 Clarendon Street
Boston, MA 02116-5145
617-536-7733
800-424-2634
Fax: 617-437-6445
e-mail: webmaster@aac.org
www.aac.org
Discusses legal protection against AIDS-related discrimination, HIV testing and the law.

507   Americans with Disabilities Act: What it Means for People with AIDS
American Civil Liberties Union AIDS Project
132 W 43rd Street
New York, NY 10036-6503
212-944-9800
www.aclu.org

508   Basics of HIV Disease: Questions and Answers
National Hemophilia Foundation
116 W 32nd Street
New York, NY 10001-3212
888-463-6643
800-424-2634
Fax: 212-328-3777
www.hemophilia.org
This publication contains basic information about hemophilia and HIV disease.
1992 28 pages
Alan Kinniburgh, PhD, CEO

509   Be Smart About HIV
American Red Cross
1616 Fort Myer Drive
Arlington, VA 22209-3100
703-312-8724
Fax: 703-312-8738
www.redcross.org
This brochure offers very simple and informative information on the HIV virus, in both English and Spanish.
1996
Sandra L Mertz, Product Manager

510   Children with AIDS: Guidelines for Parents and Caregivers
AIDS Task Force of Central New York
627 W Genesee Street
Syracuse, NY 13204-2347
315-415-2430
Offers general information on AIDS, diet and feeding, household chores, and coping with the illness.

511   Clinical Focus
Immune Deficiency Foundation
40 W Chesapeake Avenue
Towson, MD 21204-4841
410-321-6647
800-296-4433
Fax: 410-321-9165
e-mail: idf@primaryimmune.org
www.primaryimmune.org
Biannual publication for medical professionals covering current issues and information regarding clinical approaches to primary immune deficiencies.
BiAnnual
Marcia Boyle, Founder/Chair

512   Clinical Focus on Primary Immune Deficiency Diseases
Immune Deficiency Foundation
40 W Chesapeake Avenue
Towson, MD 21204-4841
410-321-6647
800-296-4433
Fax: 410-321-9165
e-mail: idf@primaryimmune.org
www.primaryimmune.org
educational mongraph is designed specifically for health care professionals and focuses on topics relevant to primary immune deficiency diseases.
Marcia Boyle, Founder/Chair

513   Clinical Presentation of the Primary Immunodeficiency Diseases
Immune Deficiency Foundation

40 W Chesapeake Avenue
Towson, MD 21204-4841
410-321-6647
800-296-4433
Fax: 410-321-9165
e-mail: idf@primaryimmune.org
www.primaryimmune.org
A primer for physicians.
Tamara Brown, Medical Programs Manager

514   Clinical Trials: Talking it Over
NIAID, Office of Communications
Building 31
Bethesda, MD 20892-0001
301-496-5717
Educational pamphlet pertaining to clinical trials.

515   Condoms and Sexually Transmitted Diseases, Especially AIDS
Department of Health and Human Services
National Institutes of Health
Bethesda, MD 20892-0001
202-673-7700
Offers information on condoms and how various forms of protection can be used to prevent sexually transmitted diseases, especially HIV/AIDS.

516   Eating Defensively: Food Safety Advice for Persons with AIDS
AIDSinfo
PO Box 6303
Rockville, MD 20849-6303
301-519-0459
800-448-0440
Fax: 301-519-6616
TTY: 888-480-3739
e-mail: ContactUs@aidsinfo.nih.gov
www.aidsinfo.nih.gov
The food safety advice in this brochure is intended to help persons with HIV infection to reduce the risk of food poisoning, thereby avoiding an illness that could worsen their condition or even cause death.
1992

517   HIV Infection and AIDS
NAID Office of Communications
31 Center Drive
Bethesda, MD 20892-0001
301-496-5717
Offers information on transmission, treatment, early symptoms, diagnosis, prevention and research.

518   HIV and AIDS During Pregnancy
March of Dimes
233 Park Avenue South
New York, NY 10003
212-353-8353
Fax: 212-254-3518
e-mail: NY639@marchofdimes.com
www.marchofdimes.com

519   HIV/AIDS in the Workplace
New York Business Group on Health
386 Park Avenue S
New York, NY 10016-8804
212-252-7440
e-mail: nybgh@nybgh.org
www.nybgh.org
Offers information on federal law and state law regarding HIV/AIDS in the workplace, universal risks, health insurance and other business costs.

520   Hope for Children with AIDS
Pediatric AIDS Foundation
2950 31st Street
Santa Monica, CA 90405-3092
310-394-1459
888-499-4673
Fax: 310-394-1469
e-mail: info@pedaids.org
www.pedaids.org
A brochure offering information on the latest research and advances in the area of pediatric AIDS.

521   How to Keep an Infusion Log
Immune Deficiency Foundation
40 W Chesapeake Avenue
Towson, MD 21204
800-296-4433
e-mail: idf@primaryimmune.org
www.primaryimmune.org
This brochure explains the value of keeping an immune globulin infusion log, as well as practical information on how to set up your personal records.
Marci Boyle, President/Founder

522 IDF Guide for Nurses on Immune Globulin Therapy for Primary Immunodeficiency
Immune Deficiency Foundation
40 W Chesapeake Avenue
Towson, MD 21204   800-296-4433
                                    e-mail: idf@primaryimmune.org
                                    www.primaryimmune.org
This guide provides direction for nurses to administer immune globulin replacement therapy in the safest and most effective way. Information includes: clinical uses for immune globulin replacement therapy; product selection and characteristics; infusions, complications and adverse events of IVIG and SCIG; concomitant medications; nursing interventions and responsibilities and helpful references and resources.
Marcia Boyle, President/Founder

523 IDF Patient and Family Handbook
Immune Deficiency Foundation
40 W Chesapeake Avenue
Towson, MD 21204   800-296-4433
                                    e-mail: idf@primaryimmune.org
                                    www.primaryimmune.org
For patients and family members, contains information about the diagnosis and treatment of primary immunodeficiency diseases, the immune system, specific diseases, therapies, general care, health insurance and issues specific to adult, adolescent and pediatric patients.
R Michael Blaese MD, Editor
Jerry A Winkelstein MD, Editor

524 Immune Deficiency Foundation
40 W. Chesapeake Avenue
Towson, MD 21204   800-296-4433
                                    e-mail: idf@primaryimmune.org
                                    www.primaryimmune.org
Your partner for living with primary immune deficiency diseases. This brochure describes the IDF and its activities and services.

525 Infections Linked to AIDS
NAID Office of Communications
31 Center Drive   301-496-5717
Bethesda, MD 20892-0001
Offers information on infections related to HIV/AIDS and referral numbers of where to receive help.

526 Our Immune System
Sara LeBien, author
Immune Deficiency Foundation
40 W Chesapeake Avenue   410-321-6647
Towson, MD 21204-4841   800-296-4433
                                    Fax: 410-321-9165
                                    e-mail: idf@primaryimmune.org
                                    www.primaryimmune.org
This storybook educates children about primary immunodeficiency diseases through delightful, eye-catching illustrations. The characters explain how the immune system works and describe the treatments for pediatric patients. Children will understand their own bodies and be better prepared to deal with their own primary immunodeficiency.

527 Taking the HIV (AIDS) Test: How to Help Yourself
NAID Office of Communications
31 Center Drive   301-496-5717
Bethesda, MD 20892-0001
Offers information on the AIDS test, how it works, how it can help and should it be taken.

528 Teeens, Sexually Transmitted Diseases & HIV/AIDS
4 Brighton Road
West Sussex, RH13 5BA UK,   e-mail: info@avert.org
                                    www.avert.org
Designed for teens, and contains information on what STD's are, how to avoid becoming infected, safer sex, how to spot symptoms of STD's, STD treatment, information about HIV/AIDS, information about testing and treatment, and advice helplines.

529 Testing Positive for HIV
NAID Office of Communications
31 Center Drive   301-496-5717
Bethesda, MD 20892-0001

Information on what a positive HIV test means, how not to spread the disease to others, and various health and dieting tips.

530 Testing for HIV Infection
American Red Cross
1616 Fort Myer Drive   703-312-8724
Arlington, VA 22209-3100   Fax: 703-312-8738
1996
Sandra L Mertz, Product Manager

531 Women, Sex, and HIV
American Red Cross
1616 Fort Myer Drive   703-312-8724
Arlington, VA 22209-3100   Fax: 703-312-8738
1992
Sandra L Mertz, Product Manager

532 Your Job and HIV: Are There Risks?
American Red Cross
1616 Fort Myer Drive   703-312-8724
Arlington, VA 22209-3100   Fax: 703-312-8738
1992
Sandra L Mertz, Product Manager

Audio & Video

533 AIDS Work: Six Healthcare Workers Face the AIDS Crisis
Fanlight Productions
Icarus Films   718-488-8900
Brooklyn, NY 11201   800-876-1710
                                    Fax: 718-488-8642
                                    e-mail: info@fanlight.com
                                    www.fanlight.com
Two physicians and four nurses reflect on several decades of combined experiences in caring for patients with HIV/AIDS. They discuss facing fear, frustration, burnout and grief as they struggle to deliver compassionate care, as well as the rewards of caring for this population. This inspirational program is invaluable for stress management programs, and in preparing students and new workers for the realities they will face.
VHS
ISBN: 1-572952-20-2
Steve Guy, Producer

534 Does Anyone Die of AIDS Anymore?
Louise Hogarth, author
Fanlight Productions
Icarus Films   718-488-8900
Brooklyn, NY 11201   800-876-1710
                                    Fax: 718-488-8642
                                    e-mail: info@fanlight.com
                                    www.fanlight.com
The answer to this disturbing film's title question is a resounding yes! Despite the much-hyped advances in treatment which, for some patients, have transformed HIV from a death sentence to a chronic illness, tens of thousands of people are still dying of AIDS in the United States. And tens of thousands more will die, even in this rich and medically advanced nation, because of ignorance and denial which have resulted in a 'third wave' of HIV infection.
26 Minutes
ISBN: 1-572958-48-0
Nicole Johnson, Publicity Coordinator

535 Roger's Story: For Cori
Howard Shepps, author
Fanlight Productions
Icarus Films   718-488-8900
Brooklyn, NY 11201   800-876-1710
                                    Fax: 718-488-8642
                                    e-mail: info@fanlight.com
                                    www.fanlight.com
Forty-four year-old Roger shares the harrowing story of his 20-year struggle against heroin, and his recent diagnosis with AIDS.
1989 28 Minutes
ISBN: 1-572950-47-1

536 Too Little, Too Late
Micki Dickoff, author

Fanlight Productions
Icarus Films   718-488-8900
Brooklyn, NY 11201   800-876-1710
                                      Fax: 718-488-8642
                                      e-mail: info@fanlight.com
                                      www.fanlight.com
In this moving video, family members of people with AIDS share their pain and frustration, as well as the solace they have derived from having been able to help their loved one to a peaceful death.
1987 49 Minutes
ISBN: 1-572950-27-7

537 Undetectable: The New Face of AIDS
Jay Corcoran, author

Fanlight Productions
Icarus Films   718-488-8900
Brooklyn, NY 11201   800-876-1710
                                      Fax: 718-488-8642
                                      e-mail: info@fanlight.com
                                      www.fanlight.com
This gripping documentary follows six women and men, straight and gay, of different ethnic and cultural backgrounds, over a three-year period as they deal for the first time with hope. Though the new multi-drug therapies for HIV disease offer a possible reprieve from what was once a death sentence, those who are lucky enough to respond to the drugs nonetheless face both a grueling treatment regimen, and the complex physical and psychological challenges of rebuilding their lives.
2001 56 Minutes
ISBN: 1-572958-45-6

Web Sites

538 AIDS United

www.aidsunited.org
To end the AIDS epidemic in the United States. We will achieve this goal through national, regional and local policy/advocacy, strategic grantmaking, and organizational capacity building. With partners throughout the country, we will work to ensure that people living with and affected by HIV/AIDS have access to the prevention and care services they need and deserve.

539 AIDS.ORG

www.aids.org
The mission of AIDS.ORG is to help prevent HIV infections and to improve the lives of those affected by HIV and AIDS by providing education and facilitating the free and open exchange of knowledge at any easy-to-find centralized website.

540 Children Affected by AIDS Foundation

www.caaf.org
The only organization solely devoted to providing social, educational, recreation and other critical support programs to vulnerable children impacted by HIV/AIDS in the U.S. and other countries.

541 Committee of Ten Thousand

www.cott1.org
A grass-roots, peer-led, education, advocacy and support organization for persons with HIV disease. Dedicated to the belief that persons with HIV/AIDS and all chronic diseases can lead productive and healthy lives

542 HIV/Hepatitis C in Prison (HIP) Committee

www.prisons.org/hivin.htm
Fighting for consistent access to quality medical care including access to all new HIV and Hepatitis C medications, diagnostic testing and combination therapies.

543 Healing Well

www.healingwell.com
A social network and support community for patients, caregivers, and families coping with the daily struggles of diseases, disorders and chronic illness.

544 Health Finder

www.healthfinder.gov

Searchable, carefully developed web site offering information on over 1000 topics. Developed by the US Department of Health and Human Services, the site can be used in both English and Spanish.

545 Healthlink USA

www.healthlinkusa.com
Health information concerning treatment, cures, prevention, diagnosis, risk factors, research, support groups, email lists, personal stories and much more. Updated regularly.

546 Helios Health

www.helioshealth.com
Online resource for your health information. Detailed information about specific health topics, access to expert advice from our Medical Advisory Board, and up-to-date health news.

547 Immune Deficiency Foundation

www.primaryimmune.org
The national patient organization dedicated to improving the diagnosis, treatment and quality of life of persons with primary immunodeficiency diseases through advocacy, education and research.

548 MedicineNet

www.medicinenet.com
An online resource for consumers providing easy-to-read, authoritative medical and health information.

549 Medscape

www.medscape.com
Medscape offers specialists, primary care physicians, and other health professionals the Web's most robust and integrated medical information and educational tools.

550 National AIDS Information Clearinghouse

www.cdcnac.org
Provides information and materials for employers on national, state and local resources related to HIV/AIDS in the workplace.

551 National Minotirty AIDS Education Training

www.nmaetc.org
Located at Howard University, as a HIV/AIDS training and technical resource for providers of minority HIV-infected patients throughout the country. THe NMAETC receives 100% of its funding through the MAI Initiative. THe NMAETC in collaboration with ither HRSA funded programs seeks to influence health care professionals who treat minority HIV-infected patients.

552 New England AIDS Education & Training Ctr.

www.neaetc.org
One of eleven regional education centers funded by the Ryan White CARE Act and sponsored regionally by the Office of Community Programs at the University of Massachusetts Medical Center. The AETC Program is administered by Health Resources and Services Administration (HRSA) HIV/AIDS bureau.

553 People with AIDS Health Group

www.Aidsinfonyc.org
PWA is a non-profit buyers club organized to assist people with AIDS in obtaining medications — as well as provide support groups committed to the self-empowerment of people living with AIDS. They offer three programs: Treatment Education and Support, Advocacy and Public Policy, and Early Treatment Access.

554 Project Inform

www.projectinform.org
Represents HIV-positive people in the development of treatments and a cure, supports individuals to make informed choices about their HIV health, advocates for quality health care to respond to HIV and related conditions, and promotes medical strategies that prevent new infections.

555 San Francisco Area AIDS Education Center

www.ucsf.edu/sfaetc
Helps to improve the care of people living with HIV and AIDS by supporting state-of-the-art clinical consultation, education, and training for health care professionals and organizations in Sa Francisco, San Mateo, and Marin counties.

556 Smart & Strong

www.smartstrong.com

A healthcare education company that supports providers and empowers HIV positive patients through publications, seminars and innovative educational programs.

557 WebMD

www.webmd.com

Information on AIDS related diseases, including articles and resources.

Description

558 Allergies

Allergy means altered reactivity. Allergies are usually characterized by a hypersensitivity to substances, such as pollens, pet dander, certain foods, some medications and molds. Such substances (allergens) can trigger an allergic response in susceptible individuals. Symptoms of allergies may present in a wide spectrum ranging from the mild sneezing, runny nose and congestion of hayfever to life-threatening reactions, known as anaphylaxis. Additional allergic reactions include itchy, watery eyes, skin rashes and asthma. More severe symptoms may include a tingling sensation in the mouth, swelling of the tongue and throat, difficulty breathing, hives, vomiting abdominal cramps, diarrhea, drop in blood pressure, loss of consciousness, and cardiovascular collapse leading to death. Allergic symptoms typically appear within minutes to two hours after the person has been exposed to the allergen.

Approximately 35 million people suffer from allergies in the United States. The cause of allergies is unclear, although there may be a genetic link in some people.

Treatment for allergies depends upon the specific substance, beginning with avoidance. Strict avoidance of the allergy-causing food is the only way to avoid a food allergy reaction. There are no medications that cure food allergies. Most people outgrow their food allergies, although peanuts, nuts, fish and shellfish are often considered life-long allergies.

For non-food allergies, medications such as antihistamines and inhaled bronchodilators, as well as allergy shots to reduce the allergic response, may be prescribed by doctors. Epinephrine, also called adrenaline, is the medication of choice for controlling a severe reaction. Individuals at risk of an anaphylactic reaction should have a bracelet or necklace with that information. Those who are allergic to insect stings should carry and use a pre-filled syringe of epinephrine (epipen) for prompt self-treatment.

National Agencies & Associations

559 Allergy & Asthma Network Mothers of Asthmatics
8201 Greensboro Drive
Fairfax, VA 22102
703-641-9595
800-878-4403
Fax: 703-288-5271
e-mail: info@aanma.org
www.breatherville.org
Leading nonprofit membership organization dedicated to eliminating suffering and death due to asthma, allergies and related conditions through education, advocacy, community outreach and research.
Nancy Sander, Founder/President

560 Allergy Asthma Information Association
295 The West Mall
Toronto, Ontario, M9C-4Z4
416-621-4571
800-611-7011
Fax: 416-621-5034
e-mail: admin@aaia.ca
www.aaia.ca

To develop societal awareness of the seriousness of allergic disease, including asthma, and to enable allergic individuals, their families and caregivers, to increase control over allergy symptoms by providing leadership in information, education, advocacy, in partnership with health care professionals, business, industry and government.
Mary Allen, CEO

561 American Academy of Allergy, Asthma & Immunology
555 East Wells Street
Milwaukee, WI 53202-3823
414-272-6071
800-822-2762
Fax: 414-272-6070
e-mail: info@aaaai.org
www.aaaai.org
Strives to serve the public through information on asthma and allergies, as well as referrals to allergists. Also offers pollen and mold statistics from the Committee on Pollen & Molds.
Kay Whalen, Executive Director
Marianne Canter, Director of Communications

562 American Academy of Environmental Medicine
6505 E Central Avenue
Wichita, KS 67206
316-684-5500
Fax: 316-684-5709
e-mail: administrator@aaemonline.org
www.aaem.com
Offers names of Clinical Ecologists and Allergy Specialists in the United States.
Robin Bernhoft, President
James F Coy MD, Secretary

563 American College of Allergy, Asthma & Immunology
85 West Algonquin Road
Arlington Heights, IL 60005
847-427-1200
Fax: 847-427-1294
e-mail: mail@acaai.org
www.acaai.org
This association focuses its attention on research and public awareness of allergies. Distributes informational brochures and pamphlets, offers referrals and counseling services, as well as patient care.
Dana V Wallace MD, President
Richard W Weber, Vice President

564 American Dietetic Association
120 South Riverside Plaza
Chicago, IL 60606-6995
312-899-0040
800-877-1600
Fax: 312-899-1979
e-mail: media@eatright.org
www.eatright.org
Offers information and support to allergy sufferers. Serves the public through the promotion of optimal nutrition, health, and well-being.
Patricia M Babjak, CEO
Judith Rodriguez, President

565 Association of Birth Defect Children Birth Defect Research for Children
800 Celebration Avenue
Celebration, FL 34747
407-566-8304
e-mail: staff@birthdefects.org
www.birthdefects.org
Offers informational packets on childhood asthma and prevention.
Betty Mekdeci, Contact

566 Asthma and Allergy Foundation of America
8201 Corporate Drive
Landover, MD 20785
202-466-7643
800-727-8462
Fax: 202-466-8940
e-mail: info@aafa.org
www.aafa.org
Nonprofit patient organization dedicated to improving the quality of life for people with asthma and allergies and their caregivers, through education, advocacy and research.
William McLin M.Ed., President & CEO
Liana Burns, Programs Assistant

567 Canadian Society of Allergy and Clinical Immunology
774 Echo Drive
Ottawa, Ontario, K1S-5N8
613-730-6272
Fax: 613-730-1116
e-mail: csaci@royalcollege.ca
www.csaci.ca

Is the advancement of the knowledge and practice of allergy, clinical immunology, and asthma for optimal patient care.
Dr Stuart Carr, President
Dr Paul Keith, Vice President

568 Eczema Association for Science and Education
4460 Redwwod Highway   415-499-3474
San Rafael, CA 94903-1953   800-818-7546
e-mail: info@nationaleczema.org
www.nationaleczema.org
Offers resources and information for allergy patients.
Julie Block, President
Diane Dunn, Communications and Program Manager

569 Food Allergy and Anaphylaxis Network
11781 Lee Jackson Highway
Fairfax, VA 22033-3309   800-929-4040
                                         Fax: 703-691-2713
e-mail: faan@foodallergy.org
www.foodallergy.org
Increases public awareness about food allergies and anaphylaxis advances research and provides education, emotional support and coping strategies to patients; serves as the communication link between the food industry, the government and the airline industry.
Anne Munoz-Furlong, Founder
Jennifer Love, Marketing and Media Communications

570 Immune Deficiency Foundation
40 W Chesapeake Avenue   410-321-6647
Towson, MD 21204-4841   800-296-4433
                                         Fax: 410-321-9165
e-mail: idf@primaryimmune.org
www.primaryimmune.org
The national patient organization dedicated to improving the diagnosis treatment and quality of life of persons with primary immunodeficiency diseases through advocacy education and research.
Marcia Boyle, President & Founder
John Seymour PhD LMFT, Vice Chair

571 National Institute of Allergy and Infectious Diseases
NIAID Office of Communications and Public Liason
6610 Rockledge Drive   301-496-5717
Bethesda, MD 20892-6612   866-284-4107
                                         Fax: 301-402-3573
                                         TDD: 800-877-8339
e-mail: clane@niaid.nih.gov
www.niaid.nih.gov
Conducts and supports research on allergies; focused on understanding what happens to the body during the allergic process. Educates patients and health care workers in controlling allergic disease; offers various research centers that conduct and evaluate educational programs focused on methods to control allergic diseases.
Anthony S Fauci, MD, Director

State Agencies & Associations

California

572 Asthma and Allergy Foundation of America: Southern California Chapter
5900 Wilshire Boulevard   323-937-7859
Los Angeles, CA 90036   800-624-0044
                                         Fax: 323-937-7815
e-mail: Breathingmatters@aafa-ca.org
http://www.aafa.org/display.cfm?id=10&su
Dedicated to controlling and curing asthma and allergic diseases through education, a network of support groups, the support of research and specialized training, increasing public awareness and providing medication and treatment to the under served. Program highlights include the Breathmobile, asthma camps and air power games for children.
Michael Ingram, Executive Director

Colorado

573 Mountain-Plains AIDS Education and Training Center (MPAETC)
12631 E 17th Avenue   303-724-0867
Aurora, CO 80045   Fax: 303-724-0875
e-mail: info@mpaetc.org
www.mpaetc.org
One of 12 regional AETCs funded nationwide by a grant from the U.S. Health Resources and Services Administration through the Ryan White Comprehensive AIDS Resources Emergency (CARE) Act. Provides educational programs about HIV infection for healthcare providers.
Beth Mullin Rotach, Director
Lucy Bradley-Springe, Principal Investigator

Florida

574 Asthma and Allergy Foundation of America: Florida Chapter
200 Orangewood Drive   727-738-1146
Dunedin, FL 34698   Fax: 727-736-4484
e-mail: cherylsmall@aafaflorida.org
www.aafa.org
Works to serve its community through programs, advocacy, education, research and national involvement.
John Little, Executive Director

Maryland

575 Asthma and Allergy Foundation of America: Maryland/Greater Washington, DC
17 Warren Road   410-484-2054
Baltimore, MD 21208   800-727-9333
                                         Fax: 410-484-2043
e-mail: aafamd@rcn.com
www.aafa-md.org
Serves the state of Maryland, District of Columbia and Northern Virginia areas. Dedicated to helping asthma and allergy sufferers successfully manage and control their disease through the education, referrals and research. Major activities include accredited child care provider course, school liaison, asthma camp, patient assistance, college scholarships for high school seniors and professional education courses. Breathmobile, Mobile Asthma Clinic, visiting schools in the city of Baltimore.
Susan Sweitzer, Executive Director

Massachusetts

576 Asthma and Allergy Foundation of America: New England Chapter
109 Highland Ave.   781-444-7778
Needham, MA 02494   877-227-8462
                                         Fax: 781-444-7718
                                         TTY: 877-227-8462
e-mail: aafane@aafane.org
www.asthmaandallergies.org
Serves Massachusetts, Rhode Island, Connecticut, Maine, New Hampshire and Vermont. Program highlights include speakers and exhibits, telephone information and referrals, tobacco control program, scholarship essay contest for high school juniors, advocacy for safer environments and training programs for school, daycare and health professionals.
Elaine Erenrich Rosenburg, Executive Director
Sharon Schumack, Health Education Coordinator

Michigan

577 Asthma and Allergy Foundation of America: Michigan Chapter
2075 Walnut Lake Rd   248-406-4254
West Bloomfield, MI 48323-8768   888-444-0333
                                         Fax: 248-757-2102
e-mail: aafamich@sbcglobal.net
www.aafamich.org
Serves the state of Michigan through public forums, work place educational programs, patient advocacy, Asthma Camp and telephone referrals and information.
Kathleen Felice Slonager, Executive Director
Dr. Rola Bokhari-Panza, President

Missouri

578   Asthma and Allergy Foundation of America: St. Louis Chapter
1500 S Big Bend   314-645-2422
St. Louis, MO 63117   Fax: 314-692-2022
e-mail: aafa@aafastl.org
www.aafastl.org
This chapter has provided children who suffer from asthma and allergies with life saving medications, equipment and educational and emotional support. The founders of the St. Louis chapter identified the apparent need in their community to help children effectively manage their asthma through the provision of medical resources, equipment and education.
Patricia Williams, Executive Director

Oregon

579   Asthma and Allergy Foundation of America: Oregon Chapter
14530 SW 144th Avenue   503-524-2232
Tigard, OR 97224-1445   Fax: 208-474-6839
e-mail: hensches@teleport.com
Serving the state of Oregon.
Sandra L Henschel, Executive Director

Pennsylvania

580   Asthma and Allergy Foundation of America: Southern Pennsylvania Chapter
470 Sentry Parkway East   610-397-1540
Blue Bell, NJ 19422   Fax: 856-224-5893
e-mail: aafasepa@verizon.net
http://www.aafa.org/
In the process of establishing a vital, new program that will aid children with chronic asthma. Many parents, some who are without medical insurance, are unaware of the availability of a medical support system that can help their children. The Children at Risk program will enable parents to have their children evaluated and also receive a free one month supply of medication. Parents will also receive information regarding available options for follow up care and prescription coverage.
Marijo Washburn, Executive Director

Texas

581   Asthma and Allergy Foundation of America: North Texas Chapter
3904 Justin Driveÿ   817-297-3132
Ft. Worth, TX 76036   888-932-2232
Fax: 817-297-6564
e-mail: info@aafatexas.org
www.aafatexas.org
Offers many educational programs and services that touch patients, caregivers, physicians and allied health professionals, including: child care provider education programs, school nurse and respiratory therapist education programs, work site allergy education programs, spacer and peak flow meter distribution to those in need, a toll free hotline, prescription assistance information, free educational materials in English and Spanish, an electronic newsletter, professional education, etc.
Laura Steves, Executive Director

Washington

582   Asthma and Allergy Foundation of America: Washington State Chapter
108 S Jackson Street   206-368-2866
Seattle, WA 98104   800-778-2232
Fax: 206-368-2941
e-mail: aafawa@aafawa.org
www.aafawa.org
Program highlights include trainings for health care professionals on asthma and allergy management, working collaboratively with other local and regional agencies to improve the quality of life for those affected by asthma and allergies, organizing health fairs and other public events and providing educational materials and products.
Penny Nelson, Executive Director

Research Centers

583   Columbus Children's Research Institute
700 Children's Drive   614-722-2000
Columbus, OH 43205   800- 79- 840
Fax: 614- 35- 079
e-mail: John.Barnard@NationwideChildrens.org
www.nationwidechildrens.org
Research institute dedicated to enhancing the health of children by engaging in the high quality cutting-edge research according to the highest scientific and ethical standards.
John A Barnard, Research Institute President
Steve Allen MD, CEO

584   Creighton University Allergic Disease Center
601 N 30th Street   402-280-4403
Omaha, NE 68131-0001   Fax: 402-280-4803
e-mail: casalej@creighton.edu
medicine.creighton.edu/allergy/homepage.
Robert G Townley, Investigator
Thomas B Casale, Chief

585   Mayo Clinic and Foundation: Division of Allergic Diseases
Department of Immunology
200 First Street SW   507-284-2511
Rochester, MN 55905   Fax: 507-284-0161
TTY: 507-284-9786
e-mail: lee.theresa@mayo.edu
www.mayoclinic.org
Provides a focus for research into the causes prevention and management of allergic diseases.
John H Noseworthy MD, President
William C Rupp MD, Vice President, CEO

586   National Jewish Center for Immunology
Goodman Building Room 611   303-398-1287
Denver, CO 80206   800-423-8891
Fax: 303-398-1806
www.nationaljewish.org
Basic and clinical research into the causes and treatments of asthmatic disorders.
Tom Gart, Chairman
Michael Salem, President & CEO

587   National Jewish Center for Immunology and Respiratory Medicine
Goodman Buiilding Room 611   303-398-1287
Denver, CO 80206   800-423-8891
Fax: 303-398-1806
www.nationaljewish.org
Basic and clinical research into the causes and treatments of asthmatic disorders.
Tom Gart, Chairman
Michael Salem, President & CEO

588   Research Institute of Palo Alto Medical Foundation
795 El Camino Real
Palo Alto, CA 94301-2302   650-326-8120
www.pamf.org/research
Clinical and general medical sciences research including allergy and immunology disorders.
Harold S Luft, Director
Marcus Krupp, Director Emeritus

589   Scripps Research Institute
10550 N Torrey Pines Road
La Jolla, CA 92037   858-784-1000
www.scripps.edu
Richard A Lerner MD, President
Douglas A Bingham, Executive Vice President and Chief Opera

590   Texas Children's Allergy and Immunology Clinic
Clinical Care Center
6701 Fannin Street   832-824-1000
Houston, TX 77030   800-364-5437
Fax: 832-825-3072
e-mail: pediai@texaschildrenshospital.org
www.texaschildrenshospital.org
Mark A Wallace, President & CEO
Mark W Kline MD, Physician In Chief

591 University of Florida: General Clinical Research Center
University of Florida
1600 SW Archer Road   352-273-5500
Gainesville, FL 32610-0322   888-635-0763
                                          Fax: 352-273-5541
                                  e-mail: thomprd@ufl.edu
                                          www.med.ufl.edu

Studies on allergies and immunology.
Robert Thompson, Program Director

592 University of Kansas Allergy and Immunology Clinic
University of Kansas Medical Center
3901 Rainbow Boulevard   913-588-5000
Kansas City, KS 66160   TTY: 913-588-7963
                                          TDD: 913-588-7963
                                 e-mail: dstechsc@kumc.edu
                                          www.kumc.edu

This service provides complete evaluation of patients with allergic
diseases such as rhinitis and asthma immunological deficiencies
food and drug intolerances and autoimmune dysfunctions.
Barbara F Atkinson MD, Executive Vice Chancellor
Shelley Gebar, RN, MHA, Chief of Staff

**593 University of Michigan Montgomery: John M. Sheldon Allergy
Society**
Alllergy & Clinical Immunology
24 Frank Lloyd Wright Drive   734-232-2154
Ann Arbor, MI 48106-0380   Fax: 734-647-6263
                             e-mail: echoreed@med.umich.edu
                          www.med.umich.edu/sheldonsociety

Travis A Miller, President

594 University of Texas Southwestern Medical Center at Dallas
University of Texas Southwestern Medical Center
5323 Harry Hines Boulevard   214-648-3111
Dallas, TX 75390   Fax: 214-648-9119
                                   www.utsouthwestern.edu

Immunodermatology department researching allergies and immune disorders.
Daniel K Podolsky MD, President

595 Warren Grant Magnuson Clinical Center
National Institute of Health
9000 Rockville Pike   301-496-2563
Bethesda, MD 20892   800-411-1222
                                          Fax: 301-402-2984
                                          TTY: 866-411-1010
                                 e-mail: prpl@mail.cc.nih.gov
                                          www.cc.nih.gov

Established in 1953 as the research hospital of the National Institutes of Health. Designed so that patient care facilities are close to
research laboratories so new findings of basic and clinical scientists can be quickly applied to the treatment of patients. Upon referral by physicians, patients are admitted to NIH clinical studies.
Michael J Klag MD, Chair
David K Henderson MD, Clinical Director

Support Groups & Hotlines

596 ASTHMA Hotline
American Academy of Allergy, Asthma and Immunology
555 E Wells Street   414-272-6071
Milwaukee, WI 53202   800-822-2762
                                          Fax: 414-272-6070
                                          www.aaai.org

Referral line offering information on allergy and asthma treatments, referrals to an allergy/immunology specialist, lay organization or support groups across the country.

597 National Health Information Center
PO Box 1133   310-565-4167
Washington, DC 20013-1133   800-336-4797
                                          Fax: 301-984-4256
                                     e-mail: info@nhic.org
                                          www.health.gov/nhic

A health information referral service sponsored by the Office of
Disease Prevention and Health Promotion. NHIC puts health professionals and consumers who have health questions in touch with
those organizations that are best able to provide answers.

Books

598 Allergies A to Z
Facts on File
132 W 31st Street   212-967-8800
New York, NY 10001   800-322-8755
                                          Fax: 800-678-3633
                                e-mail: custserv@factsonfile.com
                                          www.factsonfile.com

This vital resource for the one in five Americans who suffer from
alleries provides reliable, up-to-date information on every aspect
of this condition.
Paperback

599 Allergy Alerts from Living with Allergies
American Allergy Association
PO Box 7273   650-322-1663
Menlo Park, CA 94026-7273
These alerts cover a wide range of areas from dyes in medications
to medication interactions, food additives like sulfites, spelt, situa-
tions that could trigger asthma, problems with collagen and even
fabric softeners.

600 Allergy Plants that Cause Sneezing and Wheezing
Asthma and Allergy Foundation of America
1233 20th Street NW   202-466-7643
Washington, DC 20036-2330   800-727-8462
                                          Fax: 202-466-8940
                                          www.aafa.org

Destined to be displayed on coffee tables, the spectacular photographs in this book actually show allergy sufferers what causes
their sneezing and wheezing.
64 pages Paperback

601 Complete Book of Children's Allergies
Allergy Central Products
96 Danbury Road   203-438-9580
Ridgefield, CT 06877-4053   800-422-3878
                                          Fax: 203-431-8963
                                          www.allergycontrol.com

Major childhood allergies, recommendations for treatment.
Softcover

602 Cooking for the Allergic Child
Allergy Central Products
96 Danbury Road   203-438-9580
Ridgefield, CT 06877-4053   800-442-3878
                                          Fax: 203-431-8963
                                          www.allergycontrol.com

More than 300 recipes with nutrients analysis.
Softcover

603 Diets to Help Gluten and Wheat Allergy
HarperCollins Canada Limited/Order Department
1995 Markham Road
Scarborough, M1B 5M8,   800-387-0117
                                          Fax: 800-668-5788

This book offers sound and practical advice on gluten allergy
wheat sensitivity and Celiac disease.
96 pages
ISBN: 0-722529-10-4

604 Food Allergy: A Primer for People
Asthma and Allergy Foundation of America
1233 20th Street NW   202-466-7643
Washington, DC 20036-2330   800-727-8462
                                          Fax: 202-466-8940
                                          www.aafa.org

Food allergies demystified.
66 pages Hardcover

**605 Human Exposure Assessment for Airborne Pollutants: Advances
& Opportunity**
National Academies Press
500 5th Street NW   202-334-3313
Washington, DC 20001   888-624-8373
                                          Fax: 202-334-2451
                                e-mail: customer_service@nap.edu
                                          www.nap.edu

Explores the need for strategies to address indoor and outdoor exposures and examines the methods and tools available for finding out where and when significant exposures occur.
344 pages
ISBN: 0-309042-84-0
Sandy Adams, Publishing Operations Director
Dottie Lewis, Publishing Services Director

606 **Indoor Allergens: Assessing & Controlling Adverse Health Effects**
National Academies Press
500 5th Street NW
Washington, DC 20055
202-334-3313
888-624-8373
Fax: 202-334-2793
e-mail: customer_service@nap.edu
www.nap.edu
This comprehensive and practical volume will be important to allergists and other health care providers; public health professionals; specialists in building design, construction, and maintenance; faculty and students in public health; and interested allergy patients.
350 pages
ISBN: 0-309048-31-6
Sandy Adams, Publishing Operations Director
Dottie Lewis, Publishing Services Director

607 **Infant Formulas for Allergic Infants and Dietetic Concerns for Toddlers**
American Allergy Association
PO Box 7273
Menlo Park, CA 94026-7273
650-322-1663
Offers information on reliable food labels, evaluations of infant formulas, FDA labeling requirements under the new law and more.

608 **New Food Labels**
American Allergy Association
PO Box 7273
Menlo Park, CA 94026-7273
650-322-1663
Offers clear-cut and precise information on new label word definitions.

609 **Pollen Times: By State, By Month**
American Allergy Association
PO Box 7273
Menlo Park, CA 94026-7273
650-322-1663
A comprehensive guide offering information on how to plan vacations while avoiding pollen problems.

610 **Traveling with Allergies: Prepare and Avoid Problems**
American Allergy Association
PO Box 7273
Menlo Park, CA 94026-7273
650-322-1663
Prepare for travel, recognize and minimize the risk, sidestep smoke, food allergies, pollen, mold, dander, weather and emergencies.

Children's Books

611 **All About Allergies**
Dutton Children's Books
375 Hudson Street
New York, NY 10014-3658
212-366-2000
Fax: 212-366-2262
www.pengiunputnam.com

1993 64 pages
ISBN: 0-525674-10-1

612 **Allergies**
Franklin Watts Grolier
90 Old Sherman Turnpike
Danbury, CT 06816-0001
203-797-3500
800-621-1115
Fax: 203-797-3197
www.grolier.com
Covers the major types of allergies, including those of the respiratory and gastrointestinal tracts.
112 pages Grades 7-12
ISBN: 0-531125-16-5

613 **Living with Allergies**
Franklin Watts Grolier

90 Old Sherman Turnpike
Danbury, CT 06816-0001
203-797-3500
800-621-1115
Fax: 203-797-3197
www.grolier.com
Shows how people with allergies are able to overcome their handicap to lead full and productive lives.
32 pages Grades 5-7
ISBN: 0-531108-57-0

Magazines

614 **Allergy & Asthma Today**
Allergy and Asthma Network Mothers of Asthmatics
8201 Greensboro Drive
McLean, VA 22102
800-878-4403
e-mail: info@aanma.org
www.aanma.org
The practical, family-friendly magazine for people living with asthma, allergies and other respiratory conditions. Award-winning and medically reviewed, packed with news and real-life inspiration and success stories, the ultimate resource for patients, families and healthcare providers.
40 pages Quarterly
Laurie Ross, Managing Editor

Newsletters

615 **Advice From Your Allergist**
American College of Allergy & Immunology
85 W Algonguin Road
Alrlington Heights, IL 60005
847-359-2800
www.allergy.mcg.edu
Offers information on the effects, triggers and causes of allergies including house dust, pets, hay fever, hives and exercise.

616 **Food Allergy News**
Food Allergy and Anaphylaxis Network
10400 Eaton Place
Fairfax, VA 22030-2208
703-691-3179
800-929-4040
Fax: 703-691-2713
e-mail: faan@foodallergy.org
www.foodallergy.org
Contains allergy free recipes, practical tips such as birthday party, trick-or-treating and travel tips, a dietitian's column, medical information and product information.
12 pages BiMonthly
Anne Munoz-Furlong, Founder

617 **MA Report**
Allergy and Asthma Network/Mothers of Asthmatics
2751 Prosperity Avenue
Fairfax, VA 22031
703-641-9595
800-878-4403
Fax: 703-573-7794
e-mail: editor@aanma.org
www.breatherville.org
Provides up-to-date medical news, emotional support and practical strategies for overcoming asthma and allergies.
8 pages 8x Year
Mary McGowan, Executive Director
Nancy Sander, Editor-in-Chief

Pamphlets

618 **Allergic Diseases**
National Institute of Allergy & Infectious Disease
31 Center Drive
Bethesda, MD 20892-2520
301-496-5717
www.niaid.nih.gov/default.htm
Offers information on allergies, who gets them, diagnosis and treatments for various types of allergic diseases.

619 **Allergies and You**
American Lung Association
1740 Broadway
New York, NY 10019-4315
212-315-8700

Answers basic questions about allergy, particularly as it relates to asthma.

620 Eating Without Packet
American Allergy Association
PO Box 7273
Menlo Park, CA 94026-7273   650-322-1663
Twelve information sheets describing the most common food allergens, specific problems with common foods and supplements, and the facts on milk ingredient labeling, milk allergies, and milk sensitivity. Included in the packet is a 16-page handbook, Understanding Calcium and Osteoporosis.

621 FAAN Flashbacks
Food Allergy and Anaphylaxis Network
10400 Eaton Place   703-691-3179
Fairfax, VA 22030-2208   800-929-4040
                                         Fax: 703-691-2713
                                  e-mail: faan@foodallergy.org
                                         www.foodallergy.org
Series of reprints on specific topics of Food Allergy News. Specific pamphlets offer information on wheat, milk, soy, egg, fish, peanuts, managing food allergy in schools and anaphylaxis.
Anne Munoz-Furlong, Founder

622 Food Allergy and Atopic Dermatitis
Food Allergy and Anaphylaxis Network
10400 Eaton Place   703-691-3179
Fairfax, VA 22030-2208   800-929-4040
                                         Fax: 703-691-2713
                                  e-mail: faan@foodallergy.org
                                         www.foodallergy.org
The purpose of this booklet is to provide tips and other sources of information to help parents raise a child who is afflicted with atopic dermatitis.
12 pages
Anne Munoz-Furlong, Founder

623 Guide to Gluten-Free Diets
American Allergy Association
PO Box 7273
Menlo Park, CA 94026-7273   650-322-1663
Offers information on safe substitutes for baking and cooking. Differentiates celiac disease from wheat allergy. Sources of gluten in diet with warnings on when to check with the manufacturer.

624 Helpful Hints for the Allergic Patient
American Academy of Allergy, Asthma and Immunology
611 E Wells Street   414-272-6071
Milwaukee, WI 53202-3889   800-822-2762
                                         Fax: 414-272-6070
                                         www.aaaai.org
An informational brochure good for someone who has just been diagnosed with allergies.
8 pages

625 Just One Little Bite Can Hurt! Important Facts About Anaphylaxis
Food Allergy and Anaphylaxis Network
10400 Eaton Place   703-691-3179
Fairfax, VA 22030-2208   800-929-4040
                                         Fax: 703-691-2713
                                  e-mail: faan@foodallergy.org
                                         www.foodallergy.org
Offers information on what anaphylaxis is, what the patient should do if they have a reaction and important medical safety tips regarding the illness.
8 pages Booklet
Anne Munoz-Furlong, Founder

626 Nutrition Guide to Food Allergies
Food Allergy and Anaphylaxis Network
10400 Eaton Place   703-691-3179
Fairfax, VA 22030-2208   800-929-4040
                                         Fax: 703-691-2713
                                  e-mail: faan@foodallergy.org
                                         www.foodallergy.org

Offers answers to the most commonly asked questions about food allergies, common allergy causing foods and resources for the patient.
24 pages
Anne Munoz-Furlong, Founder

627 Something in the Air: Airborne Allergens
National Institute of Allergy & Infectious Disease
9000 Rockville Pike   301-496-5717
Bethesda, MD 20892-0001
Offers information on the symptoms to airborne substances, pollen, mold, dust, animal, chemical allergies and treatments for them.

Audio & Video

628 Alexander, the Elephant Who Couldn't Eat Peanuts
Food Allergy and Anaphylaxis Network
11781 Lee Jackson Highway
                                         800-929-4040
                                         Fax: 703-691-2713
                                         www.foodallergy.org
Helps children cope with their own allergies and teach other children about tolerance. Both videos combine colorful animation with interviews of real-life children with food allergies who talk about their experiences.
Jennifer Roeder, Marketing/Media Communications Director

629 Allergic Rhinitis
American Academy of Allergy, Asthma and Immunology
611 E Wells Street   414-272-6071
Milwaukee, WI 53202-3889   800-822-2762
                                         Fax: 414-272-6070
                                         www.aaaai.org
Allergic rhinitis, often called hay fever, affects the quality of life of millions of Americans. This video covers the causes and symptoms of seasonal and chronic allergic rhinitis, as well as environmental controls and treatments.
10-13 minutes

630 Allergic Rhinitis: Nothing to Sneeze At!
Asthma and Allergy Foundation of America
1233 20th Street NW   202-466-7643
Washington, DC 20036-2330   800-727-8462
                                         Fax: 202-466-8940
                                         www.aafa.org
The basics of allergic rhinitis, with a touch of humor. Common allergens, environmental control, skin testing and immunotherapy medications.
Videotape

631 Allergic Skin Reactions
American Academy of Allergy, Asthma and Immunology
611 E Wells Street   414-272-6071
Milwaukee, WI 53202-3889   800-822-2762
                                         Fax: 414-272-6070
                                         www.aaaai.org
In some people, allergy symptoms include itching redness, rashes, or hives. This video describes the symptoms, triggers, and treatment for common skin reactions such as dermatitis, hives and angioedema.
10-13 minutes

632 An Overview of Allergy
American College of Allergy & Immunology
800 E NW Highway   847-359-2800
Palatine, IL 60067-6580
Strengthen relationships with patients by providing them with the essential information they need.

633 Sinusitis and Sinus Surgery
Milner-Fenwick
2125 Greenspring Drive   410-252-1700
Timonium, MD 21093-3100   800-432-8433
                                         Fax: 410-252-6316
                                  e-mail: sales@milnerfenwick.com
                                         www.milner-fenwick.com
Discusses sinusitis symptoms, causes, evaluation and treatments. Animation depicts how sinuses function and how irritants, aller-

gies, colds or structural abnormalities cause sinus blockages. Also explains the role of medical therapy and irrigation in managing acute sinusitis.

14 minutes
Dolores McKee, Advertising Director

Web Sites

634   American College of Allergy, Asthma & Immunology
www.acaai.org
A professional association of more than 5,000 allergists/immunologists and allied health professionals. Promotes excellence in the practice of the subspecialty of allergy and immunology.

635   American Lung Association
www.lungusa.org
The leading organization working to save lives by improving lung health and preventing lung disease through Education, Advocacy and Research.

636   Asthma and Allergy Foundation of America
www.aafa.org
The leading patient organization for people with asthma and allergies, and the oldest asthma and allergy patient group in the world. Dedicated to improving the quality of life for people with asthma and allergic disease through education, advocacy and research.

637   Birth Defect Research for Children
www.birthdefects.org
Provides parents and expectant parents with information about birth defects and support services for their children

638   Food Allergy and Anaphylaxis Network
www.foodallergy.org
To raise public awareness, to provide advocacy and education, and to advance research on behalf of all those affected by food allergies and anaphylaxis.

639   Healing Well
www.healingwell.com
A social network and support community for patients, caregivers, and families coping with the daily struggles of diseases, disorders and chronic illness.

640   Health Finder
www.healthfinder.gov
Government website where individuals can find information and tools to hel you and those you care about stay healthy.

641   Healthlink USA
www.healthlinkusa.com
Health information concerning treatment, cures, prevention, diagnosis, risk factors, research, support groups, email lists, personal stories and much more. Updated regularly.

642   Helios Health
www.helioshealth.com
Online resource for your health information. Detailed information about specific health topics, access to expert advice from our Medical Advisory Board, and up-to-date health news.

643   Immune Deficiency Foundation
www.primaryimmune.org
National patient organization dedicated to improving the diagnosis, treatment and quality of life of persons with primary immunodeficiency diseases through advocacy, education and research.

644   MedicineNet
www.medicinenet.com
An online resource for consumers providing easy-to-read, authoritative medical and health information.

645   Medscape
www.medscape.com
Medscape offers specialists, primary care physicians, and other health professionals the Web's most robust and integrated medical information and educational tools.

646   WebMD
www.webmd.com

Information on allergies, including articles and resources.

Description

647 Alzheimer's Disease

Alzheimer's disease is a degenerative neurologic disease that attacks the brain and impairs memory, thinking faculties and behavior. As the most common form of dementing illness, it afflicts 4 million adults and is twice as common in women as in men. It primarily affects older people.

In spite of diligent research, the cause of Alzheimer's disease is unknown. The disease runs in families in about 15 to 20 percent of cases, although the remainder may have some genetic component. There are multiple symptoms of Alzheimer's disease, the most pronounced being gradual memory loss. Other symptoms include the inability to perform routine tasks, loss of language skills, disorientation and personality changes. The diagnosis is largely based on an interview with the patient and family members and an examination of the patient, although brain imaging tests and blood tests may add helpful information.

The brain's cells communicate with each other through various chemicals called neurotransmitters. In Alzheimer's disease, levels of the neurotransmitter acetylcholine are decreased. Recently-released drugs which enhance the transmission of acetylcholine can cause at least limited improvement in memory during the early stages of Alzheimer's disease. A new drug, memantine, has been developed to slow the progression of advanced disease.

An extract of Ginkgo biloba may also slow memory loss and other symptoms. Some research suggests that certain activities that involve using the brain, such as reading and doing crossword puzzles, seem to reduce the risk. Because Alzheimer's disease severely affects both the patient and the family, proper planning, as well as medical and social programs tailored to the individual and to family members are essential. A well-structured and safe living environment is the best way to preserve the welfare and dignity of the person with Alzheimer's disease. See also *Aging*.

National Agencies & Associations

648 Alzheimer Society of Canada
20 Eglinton Avenue W
Toronto, Ontario, M4R-1K8
416-488-8772
800-618-8816
Fax: 416-322-6656
e-mail: info@alzheimer.ca
www.alzheimer.ca
Identified, develops and facilitates national priorities that enable its members to effectively alleviate the personal and social consequences of Alzheimer's disease and related disorders, promotes research and leads the search for a cure.
Richard Nakoneczny, President

649 Alzheimer's Disease Education and Referral Center
PO Box 8250
Silver Spring, MD 20907-8250
301-495-3311
800-438-4380
Fax: 301-495-3334
e-mail: adear@alzheimers.org
www.nia.nih.gov/alzheimers

A service of the National Institute on Aging the center distributes information on Alzheimer's disease on current research activities and on services available to patients and family members. Offers a free list of publications available upon request.

650 Alzheimer's Disease and Related Disorders Association
International Conference on Alzheimer's Disease
225 N Michigan Avenue
Chicago, IL 60601-7633
312-335-8700
800-272-3900
Fax: 866-699-1246
TTY: 312-335-5886
e-mail: icad@alz.org
www.alz.org
Dedicated to research for the prevention cure and treatment of Alzheimer's disease and related disorders and to providing support and assistance to the afflicted patients and their families.
Harry Johns, President and CEO
Angela Geiger, Chief Strategy Officer

651 Benjamin B Greenfield National Alzheimer's Center
225 N Michigan Avenue
Chicago, IL 60601-7633
312-335-700
800-272-3900
Fax: 866-699-1238
TTY: 312-335-5886
TDD: 312-335-8700
e-mail: icad@alz.org
www.alz.org
Located at the national Alzheimer's Association in Chicago this library offers a sizable collection of videos on a variety of subjects that may interest the Alzheimer's patient family members and caregivers.
Edward Berube, Chair
Harry Johns, President and CEO

652 Interior Alzheimer Society
#217, 1889 Springfield Road
Kelowna, BC, V1Y-5V5
250-762-3312
Fax: 250-762-3312
e-mail: ias@silk.net
www.alzheimer-society.ca
A registered, independent, charitable non-profit society that was founded in 1981. Mission is to support, educate, and advocate for all those affected by Alzheimer disease in the Central Okanagan area of British Columbia: the patients, caregivers, patients' families and the community.

653 John Douglas French Alzheimer's Foundation
11620 Wilshire Boulevard
Los Angeles, CA 90025-1781
310-445-4650
800-477-2243
Fax: 310-479-0516
e-mail: jdfaf@earthlink.net
www.jdfaf.org
Provides seed money for promising research including the cause cure and prevention of Alzheimer's disease. Also gives funding to scientists who might not otherwise be funded.
Michael M Minchin Jr, President
David Werthe, Director of Operations

State Agencies & Associations

Alabama

654 Alzheimer's Association: North Alabama Chapter
117A Longwood Drive SE
Huntsville, AL 35801-4872
256-880-1575
800-272-3900
Fax: 256-880-8596
e-mail: karen.motz@alz.org
www.alz.org/altn
Al Wiggins, Chair
Carolyn Rice, Vice Chair

655 Alzheimer's Association: Southeast Alabama Chapter
PO Box 609
Dothan, AL 36302
334-677-6799
800-272-3900
Fax: 334-671-3715
www.alz.org

Kay Jones, Executive Director

656 Alzheimer's Association: Southwest Alabama Chapter
PO Box 9272
Mobile, AL 36691

334-660-5661
800-272-3900
Fax: 334-660-5667
www.alz.org

Bunnie Sutton, Executive Director

Alaska

657 Alzheimer's Disease Resource Agency of Alaska
1750 Abbott Road
Anchorage, AK 99507

907-561-3313
800-478-1080
Fax: 907-561-3315
e-mail: dnobre@alzalaska.org
www.alzalaska.org

Jackie Brunton, President
Debbie Newsham, Vice President

Arizona

658 Alzheimer's Association: Desert Southwest Chapter
1028 E McDowell Road
Phoenix, AZ 85006-2622

602-528-0545
800-272-3900
Fax: 602-528-0546
e-mail: deborah.schaus@alz.org
www.alzdsw.org

Serving the state of Arizona and Southern Nevada offices in Phoenix, Tucson, Sun City, Prescott and Las Vegas.
Deborah Schaus, Executive Director
Dawn Boeck, Development Assistant

659 Alzheimer's Association: Northern Arizona
225 Grove Avenue
Prescott, AZ 86301-2911

928-771-9257
800-272-3900
Fax: 520-771-9297
e-mail: donald.connell@alz.org
www.alz.org

Don Connell, Regional Director

660 Alzheimer's Association: Northern Nevada
225 Grove Avenue
Prescott, AZ 86301

928-771-9257
Fax: 520-771-9297
e-mail: meg.fenzi@alz.org
www.alz.org/dsw

Meg Fenzi, Regional Director
Gail Schimberg, Office Manager

661 Alzheimer's Association: Southern Arizona
5132 East Pima Street
Tucson, AZ 85712

520-322-6601
800-272-3900
Fax: 520-322-6739
e-mail: tormay.newman@alz.org
www.alzdsw.org

Tormay Newman, Director

662 Alzheimer's Association: Southern Arizona Region
3003 S Country Club Road
Tucson, AZ 85713

520-322-6601
800-272-3900
Fax: 520-322-6739
e-mail: heribberto.contreras@alz.org
www.alz.org/dsw

Heriberto Contreras, Regional Director
Debra Anderson, Programs Manager

Arkansas

663 Alzheimer's Arkansas Programs and Services
10411 W Markham
Little Rock, AR 72205

501-224-0021
800-689-6090
Fax: 501-227-6303
e-mail: phyllis.watkins@alzark.org
www.alzark.org

Phyllis Watkins, Executive Director
Priscilla Pittman, Program Coordinator

664 Alzheimer's Association: Western Arkansas Chapter
320 N Greenwood Avenue
Fort Smith, AR 72901-3454

479-783-2022
800-272-3900
Fax: 479-782-3185
e-mail: ark@alzokar.org
www.alzokar.org

Rebecca Freeman, Executive Director

California

665 Alzheimer's Association San Diego/Imperial Chapter
6632 Convoy Court
San Diego, CA 92111

858-492-4400
800-272-3900
Fax: 858-492-4406
e-mail: lisa.bruner@sanalz.org
http://www.alz.org/sandiego/

The leading voluntary health organization in Alzheimer care, support and research. The mission is to eliminate Alzheimer's disease through the advancement of research; to provide and enhance care and support for all affected; to advocate for policy change; and to reduce the risk of dementia through the promotion of brain health.
Lisa Bruner, Executive Director
Anna King, Director of Programs

666 Alzheimer's Association: California Central Chapter: Ventura County Office
80 North Wood Road
Camarillo, CA 93010

80-4-4 60
800-272-3900
Fax: 805-485-4767
e-mail: nfeatherston@centralcoastalz.org
www.alz.org/cacentralcoast

The local chapter of the National Alzheimer's Association. The chapter stands by people with Alzheimer's disease, their families and professional caregivers through the following programs and services: a telephone help line, support groups, respite grants.
Norma Featherston, Area Director
Carol Swinney, Office Manager

667 Alzheimer's Association: Greater Sacramento
530 Bercut Dr.
Sacramento, CA 95811

916-930-9080
800-272-3900
Fax: 916-930-9085
e-mail: webmaster@alznorcal.org
www.alznorcal.org

Mary Gillon MPA, Regional Director

668 Alzheimer's Association: Greater North Valley Chapter
2105 Forest Avenue
Chico, CA 95928-3148

530-895-9661
800-272-3900
Fax: 530-872-7470
e-mail: info@alznorcal.org
www.alz.org/norcal

Herb Williams, President
Eduardo Salaz, Vice President

669 Alzheimer's Association: Los Angeles Chapter
133 N Sunol Drive
Los Angeles, CA 90063-5017

323-881-0574
800-272-3900
Fax: 323-938-1036
www.alz.org/californiasouthland

Earl Greinetz, President
Gary L Ferrell, Secretary/Treasurer

670 Alzheimer's Association: Monterey County Chapter
182 El Dorado Street
Monterey, CA 93940-5337

831-647-9890
800-272-3900
Fax: 831-655-9241
e-mail: info@alznorcal.org
www.alz.org/norcal

Herb Williams, President
Eduardo Salaz, Vice President

671 Alzheimer's Association: North Bay Chapter
4340 Redwood Highway
San Rafael, CA 94903

415-472-4340
800-272-3900
Fax: 415-472-4350
e-mail: info@alznorcal.org
www.alz.org/norcal

Provides a continuum of services for Alzheimer's families, education and referral in Marin, Sonoma and Napa counties. To provide

leadership and to eliminate Alzheimer's disease through the advancement of research while enhancing care and support services.
Herb Williams, President
Eduardo Salaz, Vice President

672   Alzheimer's Association: Orange County Chapter
17771 Cowan   949-955-9000
Irvine, CA 92614   800-272-3900
                                          Fax: 949-757-3700
                                    e-mail: helpoc@alz.org
                                          www.alz.org/oc
Dedicated to providing services, education and advocacy for individuals, families and the community affected by Alzheimer's disease and related memory disorders. Services include: 24/7 help line, support groups, family orientation program and care managers.
Norma Castellano, Program Specialist
Bobbie Babbage, Family Services Coordinator

673   Alzheimer's Association: Riverside/San Bernardino Counties Chapter
5900 Wilshire Boulevard   323-938-3379
Los Angeles, CA 90036   800-272-3900
                                          Fax: 323-938-1036
                              e-mail: la.webmaster@alz.org
                              www.alz.org/californiasouthland
Help line, support groups, information and education for caregivers and community.
400 Members
Earl Greinetz, President
Gary L Ferrell, Secretary/Treasurer

674   Alzheimer's Association: San Francisco Bay Area Chapter
1060 La Avenida   650-962-8111
Mountain View, CA 94043   800-272-3900
                                          Fax: 650-962-9644
                                  e-mail: info@alznorcal.org
                                        www.alz.org/norcal
Herb Williams, President
Eduardo Salaz, Vice President

675   Alzheimer's Association: Santa Barbara Central Coast Chapter
1528 Chapala Street   805-892-4259
Santa Barbara, CA 93101-8820   800-272-3900
                                          Fax: 805-892-4250
                          e-mail: rspiegel@centralcoastalz.org
                              www.alz.org/cacentralcoast
The Alzheimer's Association California Central Coast Chapter serves families caring for people with Alzheimer's disease and related dementia throughout San Luis Obispo, Santa Barbara and Ventura Counties, offering a variety of educational and supportive programs.
Rhonda Spiegel, Executive Director
Carrie Wanek, Director of Finance and Operations

676   Alzheimer's Association: Santa Cruz County Chapter
1777-A Capitola Road   831-464-9982
Santa Cruz, CA 95062   800-272-3900
                                          Fax: 831-464-8930
                                  e-mail: info@alznorcal.org
                                        www.alz.org/norcal
Herb Williams, President
Eduardo Salaz, Vice President

Colorado

677   Alzheimer's Association: Greater Grand Junction Area Chapter
2232 N 7th Street   970-256-1274
Grand Junction, CO 81501   800-272-3900
                                          Fax: 970-256-0569
                                          www.alz.org/co
Linda Mitchell, President/CEO
Laurie Frasier, Regional Director

678   Alzheimer's Association: Rocky Mountain Chapter
455 Sherman Street   303-813-1669
Denver, CO 80203   800-272-3900
                                          Fax: 303-813-1670
                                          www.alz.org/co
Linda Mitchell, President/CEO
Inge Holmes, Vice President of Administration

679   American Homes for the Aging: Western
5010 Aspen Drive   303-795-5465
Littleton, CO 80123   Fax: 303-794-0487
Part of the national association representing retirement communities, nursing homes and community services for the elderly.

Connecticut

680   Alzheimer's Association: Connecticut Chapter
96 Oak Street   860-956-9560
Hartford, CT 06106   800-356-5502
                                          Fax: 860-956-9590
                                          www.alzct.org
Works with all individuals and family members affected by Alzheimer's disease and related disorders; ensures humane systems of care and support and promotes research efforts to treat and cure Alzheimer's disease.
Christopher Rupp, Chairman
Daniel P Finke, Treasurer

681   Alzheimer's Association: South Central Connecticut Chapter
2911 Dixwell Avenue   203-230-1777
Hamden, CT 06518   800-356-5502
                                          Fax: 203-230-1712
                                          www.alz.org
Patricia Clark, Executive Director

Delaware

682   Alzheimer's Association: Delaware Chapter
240 N James Street   302-633-4420
Newport, DE 19804   800-272-3900
                                          Fax: 302-633-4494
                            e-mail: Wendy.Campbell@alz.org
                                    www.alz.org/desjsepa
Wendy L Campbell, President
Theresa Haenn, Vice President Development

Florida

683   Alzheimer's Association: Broward County Chapter
201 E Sample Road   800-861-7826
Deerfield Beach, FL 33407   800-272-3900
                                          Fax: 954-786-1538
                            e-mail: barbara.grasch@alz.org
                                    www.alz.org/seflorida
Barbara Grasch, Director of Program Services
Ellen Brown, CEO

684   Alzheimer's Association: East Central Florida Chapter
1250 South Harbor City Boulevard   407-729-8536
Melbourne, FL 32901   Fax: 407-729-8044
                                          www.alz.org

685   Alzheimer's Association: Florida Gulf Coast Chapter
9365 US Highway 19 N   727-578-2558
Pinellas Park, FL 33782   800-772-8672
                                          Fax: 727-578-2286
                                e-mail: milnel@alzflgulf.org
                                  www.alz.org/FLGulfCoast
Provides information and services to families and professionals dealing with memory related disorders.
Gloria JT Smith, President/CEO
Paul Anderson, Vice President Finance

686   Alzheimer's Association: Greater Miami Chapter
5200ÿNEÿ2nd Avenue   305-891-6228
Miami, FL 33137   800-861-7826
                                            Fax: 305-751-5551
                                    e-mail: reni.rizzo@alz.org
                                          www.alz.org/seflorida

Reni Rizzo, Community Education Coordinator
Ellen Brown, CEO

687   Alzheimer's Association: Greater Orlando Area Chapter
988 Woodcock Road   407-228-4299
Orlando, FL 32803   800-272-3900
                                            Fax: 407-228-4201
                                    e-mail: info@alzflorida.org
                                             www.alz.org/cnfl

Stu Gaines, Chair
Tish Sheesley, CEO

688   Alzheimer's Association: Greater Palm Beach Area Chapter
600 N Congress Avenue   561-478-3120
Delray Beach, FL 33445   800-861-7826
                                            Fax: 561-278-4910
                                                    www.alz.org

689   Alzheimer's Association: Northeast Florida
4237 Salisbury Rd   904-281-9077
Jacksonville, FL 32216   800-272-3900
                                            Fax: 866-281-9078
                                            www.alzorlando.org

690   Alzheimer's Association: Northern Central Florida Chapter
4510 NW 6th Place   352-372-6266
Gainesville, FL 32607   800-272-3900
                                            Fax: 352-372-2038
                                    e-mail: info@alzflorida.org
                                             www.alz.org/cnfl

Stu Gaines, Chair
Tish Sheesley, CEO

691   Alzheimer's Association: Northwest Florida Chapter
119 Hollywood Boulevard   850-302-0581
Ft. Walton Beach, FL 32548   800-302-0581
                                            Fax: 850-302-0583
                                                    www.alz.org

692   Alzheimer's Association: Southwest Florida Chapter
4075 Tamiami   941-235-7470
Port Charlotte, FL 33952   800-772-8672
                                            Fax: 941-235-7473
                                                    www.alz.org

693   Alzheimer's Association: Tampa Bay Chapter
14010 Roosevelt Blvd.   727-578-2558
Clearwater, FL 33762   800-772-8672
                                            Fax: 941-380-5701
                                    e-mail: milnel@alzflgulf.org
                                        www.alz.org/FLGulfCoast

Gloria JT Smith, President/CEO
Paul Anderson, Vice President Finance

694   Alzheimer's Association: Volusia/Flagler Branch
111 N Frederick Avenue   386-238-0066
Daytona Beach, FL 32114-5126   Fax: 386-238-8293
                                                    www.alz.org

695   Alzheimer's Association: West Central Florida Chapter
PO Box 2070   813-848-8888
New Port Richey, FL 34656-2070   800-841-6669
                                            Fax: 813-849-6124
                                                    www.alz.org

Georgia

696   Alzheimer's Association: Atlanta Chapter
1925 Century Boulevard   404-728-1181
Atlanta, GA 30345-4021   800-272-3900
                                            Fax: 404-636-9768
                                    e-mail: kim.franklin@alz.org
                                           www.alz.org/georgia

Bennett Watts, Chair
Bruce Flechter, Treasurer

697   Alzheimer's Association: Augusta Chapter
1899 Central Avenue   706-731-9060
Augusta, GA 30904-5755   800-272-3900
                                            Fax: 706-731-9099
                                    e-mail: kim.franklin@alz.org
                                           www.alz.org/georgia

Bennett Watts, Chair
Bruce Flechter, Treasurer

698   Alzheimer's Association: Central Georgia Chapter
277 Martin Luther King Jr Boulevard   478-746-7050
Macon, GA 31201-3498   800-272-3900
                                            Fax: 478-746-6679
                                    e-mail: kim.franklin@alz.org
                                           www.alz.org/georgia

Bennett Watts, Chair
Bruce Flechter, Treasurer

699   Alzheimer's Association: Greater Columbus Chapter
5900 River Road   706-327-6838
Columbus, GA 31904-0185   800-272-3900
                                            Fax: 706-494-0533
                                    e-mail: kim.franklin@alz.org
                                           www.alz.org/georgia

Bennett Watts, Chair
Bruce Flechter, Treasurer

700   Alzheimer's Association: Greater Georgia Chapter
1925 Century Boulevard   404-728-1181
Atlanta, GA 30345-4021   800-272-3900
                                            Fax: 404-636-9768
                                    e-mail: kim.franklin@alz.org
                                           www.alz.org/georgia

Bennett Watts, Chair
Bruce Flechter, Treasurer

701   Alzheimer's Association: Southeast Georgia Chapter
201 Television Circle   912-920-2231
Savannah, GA 31406   800-272-3900
                                            Fax: 912-921-7960
                                                    www.alzga.org

702   Alzheimer's Association: Southwest Georgia Chapter
1512-1 Gillionville Road   229-888-7676
Albany, GA 31707   Fax: 229-888-2620
                                                    www.alzga.org

Maggie Keenan, Office Volunteer
Jenny House, Director Programs and Development

Hawaii

703   Alzheimer's Association: Honolulu Chapter
1050 Ala Moana Boulevard   808-591-2771
Honolulu, HI 96814   800-272-3900
                                            Fax: 808-591-9071
                                    e-mail: alohainfo@alz.orgÿ
                                           www.alz.org/hawaii

Elizabeth Stevenson, Executive Director/CEO
Chris Shirai, Chairman

704   Alzheimer's Association: West Hawaii Chapter
PO Box 390247   808-322-4141
Kailua Kona, HI 96739-0247   Fax: 808-322-0008
                                                    www.alz.org

Idaho

705   Alzheimer's Association: Greater Idaho Chapter
1111 S Orchard   208-384-1788
Boise, ID 83705-2878   800-272-3900
                                            Fax: 208-385-7191
                            e-mail: suzette.albers-tunnell@alz.org
                                             www.alz.org/idaho

Suzette Albers-Tunne, Executive Director

706 Alzheimer's Association: Northern Idaho Chapter
2003ÿKootenai HealthÿWay
Coeur D Alene, ID 83814

208-666-2996
800-272-3900
Fax: 509-473-3389
e-mail: pjchristo@alz.org
www.alz.org/inlandnorthwest

PJ Christo, Outreach Coordinator
Joel Loiacono, Executive Director

Illinois

707 Alzheimer's Association: Central Illinois Chapter
606 W Glen Avenue
Peoria, IL 61614-4831

309-681-1100
800-272-3900
Fax: 309-681-1101
e-mail: nikki.vulgaris@alz.org
www.alz.org/illinoiscentral

Nikki Vulgaris, Executive Director
Brett Tilly, President

708 Alzheimer's Association: East Central Illinois Chapter
303 N. Hershey
Bloomington, IL 61704-7337

217-351-1726
888-686-1726
Fax: 217-351-2161
www.alz.org

Provides information, support, and referral services to families and individuals facing Alzheimer's disease. Includes newsletter, support groups, and education.

709 Alzheimer's Association: Four Rivers Chapter
401 N Wall Street
Kankakee, IL 60901

815-936-0464
800-332-4495
Fax: 815-936-9363
www.alz.org

710 Alzheimer's Association: Greater Illinois Chapter
4709 Golf Road
Skokie, IL 60076-1260

847-933-2413
800-272-3900
Fax: 847-933-2417
e-mail: info@alz.org
www.alzchi.org

711 Alzheimer's Association: Greater Illinois Chapter: Carbondale Office
402 E Plaza Drive
Carterville, IL 62918-1429

618-985-1095
800-272-3900
Fax: 618-457-7830
e-mail: GI.Chapter@alz.org
www.alz.org/illinois

Jill Schoenborn, Coordinator Outreach & Development

712 Alzheimer's Association: Land of Lincoln Chapter
2921 Greenbriar Drive
Springfield, IL 62704-4833

217-726-5184
800-272-3900
Fax: 217-726-5185
e-mail: GI.Chapter@alz.org
www.alz.org/illinois

Jane Field, Office Manager
James Dearing, Senior Program Manager

713 American Homes for the Aging: Midwest Regional Office
911 N Elm Street
Hinsdale, IL 60521-3641

630-323-6755
Fax: 630-325-0749

Regional office of the AHA, a national professional association of nonprofit nursing homes, retirement communities and homes for the aging.

Indiana

714 Alzheimer's Association: Central Indiana
50 East 91st Street
Indianapolis, IN 46240-1816

317-575-9620
800-272-3900
Fax: 317-582-0669
e-mail: Heather.Hershberger@alz.org
http://www.alz.org/indiana/

Heather Allen Hershberger, Executive Director
Wanda Lew, Director Finance and Operations

715 Alzheimer's Association: Central Indiana Chapter-Columbus Office
50 E 91st Street
Indianapolis, IN 46240-0547

317-575-9620
800-272-3900
Fax: 812-376-0541
e-mail: Heather.Hershberger@alz.org
www.alz.org/indiana

Help line, support groups, caregiver education, family care planning, safe return.
newsletter
Heather Alle Hershberger, Executive Director
Sarah Ferguson, Director of Development

716 Alzheimer's Association: Central Virginia
50 E 91st Street
Indianapolis, IN 46240

317-575-9620
Fax: 317-582-0669
e-mail: Heather.Hershberger@alz.org
www.alz.org/indiana

Heather Alle Hershberger, Executive Director
Wanda Lew, Director Finance and Operations

717 Alzheimer's Association: Northern Indiana Chapter
922 E Colfax Avenue
S Bend, IN 46617-3112

57- 2-2 41
888-303-0180
Fax: 57- 2-2 42
e-mail: AlzServicesNI@sbcglobal.net
www.alz-nic.org

Iowa

718 Alzheimer's Association: Big Sioux Chapter
201 Pierce Street
Sioux City, IA 51101-3716

712-279-5802
800-272-3900
Fax: 712-277-8076
e-mail: kim.mccormick@alz.org
www.alz.org/siouxland

Kim McCormick, Executive Director
Darla Vander Plaats, Vice President of Finance/Operations

719 Alzheimer's Association: East Central Iowa Chapter
1570 42nd Street NE
Cedar Rapids, IA 52402

319-294-9699
800-272-3900
Fax: 319-294-0068
e-mail: kelly.hauer@alz.org
www.alz.org/eci

Kelly Hauer, Executive Director
Tracey Robertson, Program Education & Outreach Coordinator

720 Alzheimer's Association: Greater Iowa Chapter
1730 28th Street
W Des Moines, IA 50266

515-440-2722
800-272-3900
Fax: 515-440-6385
e-mail: Carol.Sipfle@alz.org
www.alz.org/greateriowa

Carol Sipfle, Executive Director
Holly Bradford, Finance Director

721 Alzheimer's Association: Heart of Iowa Chapter
118 Hayward Avenue
Ames, IA 50014-7259

515-292-4109
800-407-5840
Fax: 515-292-0125
www.alz.org

722 Greater Iowa Chapter Alzheimer's Association Quadcity Office
736 Federal Street
Davenport, IA 52803-5750

563-324-1022
800-272-3900
Fax: 563-324-6267
e-mail: Jerry.Schroeder@alz.org
www.alz.org/greateriowa

Jerry Schroeder, Program Specialist
Julie Seier, Community Relations Coordinator

Kansas

723 Alzheimer's Association: Heart of America Chapter
3846 W 75th Street
Prairie Village, KS 66208-4126
913-831-3888
800-272-3900
Fax: 913-831-1916
e-mail: jan.horn@alz.org
www.alz.org/kansascity

Debra R Brook, Executive Director
Michelle Niedens, Education Director

724 Alzheimer's Association: Sunflower Chapter
347 S Laura
Wichita, KS 67211-4109
316-267-7333
800-272-3900
Fax: 316-267-6369
e-mail: marsha.hills@alz.org
www.alz.org/centralandwesternkansas

Marsha Hills, Executive Director
Kathy Sikes, Program Director

725 Alzheimer's Association: Topeka Regional Office, Heart of America Chapter
4125 SW Gage Center Drive
Topeka, KS 66604-1427
785-271-1844
800-272-3900
Fax: 785-271-1804
e-mail: cindy.miller@alz.org
www.alz.org/kansascity

Part of the national Alzheimer's Association, serving 16 counties in northeast Kansas representing approximately 10 500 Alzheimer's families. Basic services include family and professional support groups, information and referral, and caregiver's relief programs.
Debra R Brook, Executive Director
Cindy Miller, Outreach Coordinator

Kentucky

726 Alzheimer's Association: Lexington/ Bluegrass Chapter
465 E High Street
Lexington, KY 40507
859-266-5283
800-272-3900
Fax: 859-268-4764
e-mail: infoky-in@alz.org
www.alz.org/kyin

Debbie Lacy Goodman, VP Awareness & Community Relations
Tonya Cox, VP Programs & Education

727 Alzheimer's Association: Louisville Chapter
6100 Dutchmans Lane
Louisville, KY 40205
502-451-4266
Fax: 502-456-2701
e-mail: infoky-in@alz.org
www.alz.org/kyin

Teri Shirk, Chapter President & CEO
Ellen Kershaw, VP Public Policy

Louisiana

728 Alzheimer's Association: Northeast/Central Louisiana Chapter
2407 Ferrand Street
Monroe, LA 71201
318-322-2828
800-272-3900
Fax: 318-998-7360
www.alz.org

729 Alzheimer's Association: Greater New Orleans Chapter
DePaul Hospital
1040 Calhoun Street
New Orleans, LA 70118-5999
504-895-6223
800-272-3900
Fax: 504-895-0493

730 Alzheimer's Services of the Capital Area
3772 N Boulevard
Baton Rouge, LA 70806
225-334-7494
800-548-1211
Fax: 225-387-3664
e-mail: info@alzbr.org
www.alzbr.org

The mission of Alzheimer's Services of the Capital Area is to provide education and support services to memory impaired individuals as well as caregivers and professionals; and to enhance community awareness of Alzheimer's disease and related disorders.
Barbara Auten, Executive Director

Maine

731 Alzheimer's Association: Maine Chapter
383 U.S. Route 1
Scarborough, ME 04074-2419
207-772-0115
800-272-3900
Fax: 207-289-3705
e-mail: laurie.trenholm@alz.org
www.alz.org/maine

Joy Heptner, Executive Director
Liz Weaver, Program Director

732 Maine Alzheimer's Care Center
154 Dresden Avenue
Gardiner, ME 04345
207-626-1770

Maryland

733 Alzheimer's Association: Central Maryland Chapter
1850 York Road
Timonium, MD 21093-5122
410-561-9099
800-272-3900
Fax: 410-561-3433
e-mail: info.maryland@alz.org
www.alz.org/maryland

Cass Naugle, Executive Director
Teri Bennett, Helpline Coordinator

734 Alzheimer's Association: Eastern Shore Chapter
909 Progress Circle
Salisbury, MD 21804
410-543-1163
800-272-3900
Fax: 410-546-0184
e-mail: info.maryland@alz.org
www.alz.org/maryland

Cass Naugle, Executive Director
Elizabeth Marshall, Services Coordinator

735 Alzheimer's Association: Greater Washington DC Chapter
2524 Pensylvania Avenue Southeast
Washington, DC 20020
202-483-4258
Fax: 202-483-4164
www.alzheimersdc-md.org

Help line-telephone referral support groups, caregiver education, respite services. We have three offices serving DC and surrounding Maryland counties.

736 Alzheimer's Association: Western Maryland Chapter
108 Byte Drive
Frederick, MD 21702
301-696-0315
800-272-3900
Fax: 301-696-9061
e-mail: info.maryland@alz.org
www.alz.org/maryland

To eliminate Alzheimer's disease through the advancement of research and to enhance care and support for individuals their families and caregivers.
Cathy Hanson, Program Coordinator
Deborah Bauer, Education Coordinator

Massachusetts

737 Alzheimer's Association
473 S Street W
Raynham, MA 02767
508-880-0055
800-272-3900
Fax: 508-880-0056
www.alz.org/manh

Pam McCormack, Regional Manager

738 Alzheimer's Association: Massachusetts Chapter
311 Arsenal Street
Watertown, MA 02472
617-868-6718
800-272-3900
Fax: 617-868-6720
www.alz.org/manh

Nonprofit, national, voluntary health organization dedicated to Alzheimer research and care. Provides 24 hour help line, support groups, a wanderers prevention program early stage patient programs, family educators, professional training, and advocacy.
James Wessle MBA, President & CEO
Betsy Fitzgerald-Cam, Vice President Communications

739 Alzheimer's Association: Western Regional Office: Massachusetts Chapter
264 Cottage Street
Springfield, MA 01104

413-787-1113
800-272-3900
Fax: 413-787-1109
www.alz.org/manh

Nonprofit organization serving family and professional caregivers in seven counties in southwest Michigan. Provides information on Alzheimer's and other diseases, educational programs, resource libraries. Train-the-trainer agency referral, autopsy liaison, and other services.
Marcia McKen Med, Manager
Annie Clattenburg, Coordinator Administrative Services

Michigan

740 Alzheimer's Association: East Central Michigan Chapter
G-3287 Beecher Road
Flint, MI 48503

810-720-2791
800-337-3827
Fax: 810-720-3040
www.alzgmc.org

741 Alzheimer's Association: Greater Michigan Chapter
20300 Civic Center Drive
Southfield, MI 48076

248-351-0280
1 8-0 2-2 39
Fax: 248-351-0417
www.alzgmc.org

A national network of chapters, is the largest national voluntary health organization committed to finding a cure for Alzheimer's and helping those affected by the disease. Provides a wide range of services and programs for Alzheimer's and other dementia patients for their families and for the general public.

742 Alzheimer's Association: Greater Michigan Chapter: Upper Peninsula Region
710 Chippewa Square
Marquette, MI 49855-4521

906-228-3910
800-272-3900
Fax: 906-228-2455
TTY: 877-204-6924
www.alz.org/gmc

Pamela Parkkila, Director

743 Alzheimer's Association: Michigan Great Lakes Chapter: West Shore Region
1740 Village Drive
Muskegon, MI 49442-5546

231-780-1922
800-272-3900
Fax: 231-780-1494
e-mail: Barb.Betts@alz.org
www.alz.org/mglc

Providing caregiver support groups a help line informational materials community education and a quarterly newsletter.
Barb Betts, Program Coordinator
Valerie Hanson, Regional Coordinator

744 Alzheimer's Association: Mid-Michigan Chapter
4604 N Saginaw Road
Midland, MI 48640

989-839-9910
800-272-3900
Fax: 989-839-5910
TTY: 877-204-6924
www.alz.org/gmc

Dawn Spicer, Director

745 Alzheimer's Association: Northeast Michigan Chapter
ÿÿ526ÿW Chisholm St
Alpena, MI 49707

989-356-4087
800-272-3900
Fax: 989-354-7879
www.alzgmc.org

746 Alzheimer's Association: Northwest Michigan Chapter
921 W. 11th. Street
Traverse City, MI 49864

231-929-3804
800-272-3900
Fax: 231-922-1584
www.alz.nwmi.org

Minnesota

747 Alzheimer's Association: Minnesota/Dakotas
4550 W 77th Street
Minneapolis, MN 55435

952-830-0512
800-272-3900
Fax: 952-830-0513
e-mail: mary.birchard@alz.org
www.alz.org/mnnd

Mary Birchard, Executive Director
Michelle Barclay, Vice President Program Services

Mississippi

748 Alzheimer's Association: Mississippi Chapter
1900 Dunbarton Drive
Jackson, MS 39216

601-987-0020
800-272-3900
Fax: 601-987-9020
e-mail: info@msalz.org
www.alz.org/ms

Barb Dobrosky, Program Director
Patty Dunn, Director of Administration

749 Alzheimer's Foundation of the South: Mississippi Division
PO Box 2394
Gulfport, MS 39503

228-867-6251
800-950-6251
Fax: 228-864-8843
e-mail: alzms@cs.com
www.alzfoundation.com

Rosemary Hudgins, Executive Director

Missouri

750 Alzheimer's Association: Mid-Missouri Chapter
2400 Bluff Creek Drive
Columbia, MO 65201

573-443-8665
800-272-3900
Fax: 573-499-9701
e-mail: midmoinfo@alz.org
www.alz.org/mid-missouri

Linda Newkirk, Executive Director
Joetta Coen, Director of Programs

751 Alzheimer's Association: Northwest Missouri-Chapter
10th and Faraon
St. Joseph, MO 64502-1241

816-364-4467
800-272-3900
Fax: 816-364-2553
e-mail: brenda.gregg@alz.org
www.alz-heartofamerica.org

752 Alzheimer's Association: Southwest Missouri Chapter
1500 S Glenstone
Springfield, MO 65804

417-886-2199
800-272-3900
Fax: 417-886-0337
e-mail: rebecca.argilagos@alz.org
www.alz-swmo.org

Rebecca Argilagos, President/CEO
Annette West, Development Director

753 Alzheimer's Association: St. Louis Chapter
9370 Olive Boulevard
Saint Louis, MO 63132-3214

314-432-3422
800-272-3900
Fax: 314-432-3824
e-mail: Helpline@alzstl.orgÿÿÿÿ
www.alz.org/stl

Joan D'Ambrose, President
Jan Kraemer, Chair

Montana

754 Alzheimer's Association: Greater Billings Area Chapter
3010 11th Avenue N
Billings, MT 59101

406-252-3053
800-272-3900
Fax: 406-252-2933
e-mail: montana@alz.org
www.alz.org/montana

Kelly Donovan, President
Cindy Stevick, Vice President

Nebraska

755 **Alzheimer's Association: Lincoln/Greater Nebraska Chapter**
1500 S. 70th St.   402-420-2540
Lincoln, NE 68506   800-272-3900
Fax: 402-420-2541
e-mail: karen.noel@alz.org
alz.org/greatplains

Karen Noel, President/CEO
Gail McNair, Development Director

756 **Alzheimer's Association: Omaha/Eastern Nebraska Chapter**
1941 S 42nd Street   402-502-4301
Omaha, NE 68105-2167   800-272-3900
Fax: 402-502-7001
e-mail: bonnie.lingard@alz.org
www.alz.org/midlands

Duane Gross, President and CEO
Clayton Freeman, Program Director

Nevada

757 **Alzheimer's Association: Northern Nevada Chapter**
1301 Cordone Avenue   775-786-8061
Reno, NV 89502-6362   800-272-3900
Fax: 775-786-1920
e-mail: info@alznorcal.org
www.alz.org/norcal

Herb Williams, President
Eduardo Salaz, Vice President

758 **Alzheimer's Association: Southern Nevada Chapter**
5190 S Valley View Boulevard   702-248-2770
Las Vegas, NV 89118-6062   800-272-3900
Fax: 702-248-2771
e-mail: deborah.schaus@alz.org
www.alz.org/dsw

Luis Carrillo, Regional Director
Christine Terry, Program Manager

New Hampshire

759 **Alzheimer's Association of Vermont and New Hampshire**
10 Ferry Street   603-226-5868
Concord, NH 03301-5004   800-536-8864
Fax: 603-225-8126
www.alzvtnh.org

Robbie Nicol, Chair
Robert Dowd, First Vice Chair

New Jersey

760 **Alzheimer's Association: Greater New Jersey Chapter**
400 Morris Avenue   973-586-4300
Denville, NJ 07834   1 8-0 2-2 39
Fax: 973-586-4342
www.alznj.org

Provides programs and services to individuals with Alzheimer's disease, their families and caregivers, including education and training, support groups, a toll free telephone help line and respite assistance.

761 **Alzheimer's Association: South Jersey Chapter**
3 Eves Drive   856-797-1212
Marlton, NJ 08053   800-272-3900
Fax: 609-784-8486
e-mail: Wendy.Campbell@alz.org
www.alz.org/desjsepa

Wendy L Campbell, President & CEO
Theresa Haenn, Vice President Development

New Mexico

762 **Alzheimer's Association: New Mexico Chapter**
9500 Montgomery Boulevard NE   505-266-4473
Albuquerque, NM 87111   800-272-3900
Fax: 505-266-0108
e-mail: agnes.vallejos@alz.org
www.alz.org/newmexico

Agnes Vallejos, Executive Director
Mark Narvaez, Program Director

New York

763 **Alzheimer's Association: Sullivan/Delaware Chapter**
PO Box 911   941-794-3774
Monticello, NY 12701

764 **Alzheimer's Association: Central New York Chapter**
441 W Kirkpatrick Street   315-472-4201
Syracuse, NY 13204-1361   800-272-3900
Fax: 315-472-4206
e-mail: alzcny@alzcny.org
www.alz.org/centralnewyork

Larry Malfitano, President
Christina Hasemann, Vice President

765 **Alzheimer's Association: Hudson Valley/ Rockland/Westchester NY Chapter**
2 Jefferson Plaza   845-471-2655
Poughkeepsie, NY 12601-4027   800-872-0994
Fax: 845-471-8960
e-mail: info@alzhudsonvalley.org
www.alz.org/hudsonvalley

Elaine Sproat, President & CEO
Meg Boyce, Director of Programs & Services

766 **Alzheimer's Association: Long Island Chapter**
3281 Veterans Memorial Highway   631-580-5100
Ronkonkoma, NY 11779-3521   800-272-3900
Fax: 631-580-3100
e-mail: Info@alzheimersli.org
www.alz.org/hudsonvalley

Voluntary health agency that provides care and consultation, information and referral, education, national safe return program and support groups to individuals with Alzheimer's, their families and/or caregivers.
Mary Ann Malack-Ragona, Executive Director/CEO
Linda Cody, Director of Development

767 **Alzheimer's Association: New York City Chapter**
360 Lexington Avenue   646-744-2900
New York, NY 10017   800-272-3900
Fax: 212-490-6037
e-mail: helpline@alznyc.org
www.alznyc.org

Lou-Ellen Barkan, President/CEO
Jed A Levine, Executive Vice President

768 **Alzheimer's Association: Northeastern New York Chapter**
Washington Avenue Extension   518-867-4999
Albany, NY 12205-2083   800-272-3900
Fax: 518-867-4997
e-mail: infoeny@alz.org
www.alz.org/northeasternny

Regional affiliate of national association. Works to educate and support families, while raising funds in support of research.
Paul A Wajda, Chair
Warren E Garling, Vice Chair

769 **Alzheimer's Association: Putnam County Chapter**
Robin Hill Corporate Park
15 Mount Ebo Road S   845-278-0343
Brewster, NY 10509-2164   1 8-0 2-2 39
e-mail: info@alzhudsonvalley.org
www.alz.org/hudsonvalley

Stuart Greif, Program Development Specialist

770 Alzheimer's Association: Rochester Chapter
435 E Henrietta Road
Rochester, NY 14620
585-760-5400
800-272-3900
Fax: 585-760-5401
www.alz.org/rochesterny

Teresa A Galbier, President/CEO
Karen Lesperance, Chair

771 Alzheimer's Association: Southern Tier Chapter
401 Hayes Avenue
Endicott, NY 13760-5421
607-785-7852
800-272-3900
Fax: 607-785-4004
e-mail: alzcny@alzcny.org
www.alz.org/centralnewyork

L Jane Hudreck, Regional Director

772 Alzheimer's Association: Western New York Chapter
2805 Wehrle Drive
Williamsville, NY 14421
716-626-0600
800-272-3900
Fax: 717-626-2255
e-mail: Donna.McKenzie@alz.orgÿ
www.alz.org/wny

David Cascio, President
Linda Sabo, Executive Director

773 Alzheimer's Foundation of Staten Island
789 Post Avenue
Staten Island, NY 10310-6427
718-667-7110
877-574-7068
Fax: 718-667-8431
e-mail: info@sialzheimers.org
www.sialzheimers.org

Not-for-profit health and human services organization, serving people with Alzheimer's disease and related dementias.
Leilani Joven Pelletie, Executive Director
David Cascio, President

North Carolina

774 Alzheimer's Association: Eastern North Carolina Chapter
1305 Navaho Dr.
Raleigh, NC 27609
919-832-3732
800-228-8738
Fax: 919-832-7989
e-mail: awatkins@alznc.org
www.alznc.org

Dedicated to providing program services education for patients, families and professional caregivers, advocacy and research.
Alice Watkins, Executive Director
Rita Bhan, Developmental Director

775 Alzheimer's Association: Western Carolina Chapter
3800 Shamrock Drive
Charlotte, NC 28215
704-532-7390
800-272-3900
Fax: 704-532-5421
e-mail: infonc@alz.org
alz.org/northcarolina

A nonprofit voluntary organization dedicated to improving the quality of life for those with Alzheimer's and their families through a broad range of programs, including patient and family services, education, advocacy and support of research through national programs.
Beth Croom MA, Director of Programs/Education
Teresa Hoover, Program Associate/Helpline Coordinator

776 Alzheimer's Association: Western North Carolina Chapter
31 College Place
Asheville, NC 28801-1066
828-254-7363
800-272-3900
Fax: 828-255-0948
e-mail: infonc@alz.org
www.alz.org/northcarolina

Larry Reeves, Area Program Manager
Heidi Kimsey, Program Associate

North Dakota

777 Alzheimer's Association: Fargo/Moorhead Regional Center
4357 13th Avenue SW
Fargo, ND 58103
701-277-9757
800-272-3900
Fax: 701-277-9785
e-mail: gretchen.dobervich@alz.org
www.alz.org/mnnd

Gretchen Dobervich, Regional Center Director
Paulette Orth, Administrative Assistant

Ohio

778 Alzheimer's Association: Canton Chapter
408 Ninth St. SW
Canton, OH 44707
800-272-3900
Fax: 330-996-7757
e-mail: geoachl@alz.org
www.alz.org/akroncantonyoungt

Pam Schuellerman, Executive Director
Andy Junn, Development Director

779 Alzheimer's Association: Central Ohio Chapter
3380 Tremont Road
Columbus, OH 43221-2112
614-457-6003
800-272-3900
Fax: 614-457-6634
e-mail: helplinecentralohio@alz.org
www.alz.org/centralohio

Kenneth Strong, Executive Director
Joanie Johnson, President

780 Alzheimer's Association: Clark/Champaign, Miami Valley Chapter
3797 Summit Glen Drive
Dayton, OH 45449-2620
937-291-3332
800-272-3900
Fax: 937-323-9259
e-mail: eric.vanvlymen@alz.org.
www.alz.org/dayton

Judy Turner, Executive Director
Teresa Thomas, Development Director

781 Alzheimer's Association: Cleveland Area Chapter
23215 Commerce Park Drive
Beachwood, OH 44122-1013
216-721-8457
800-272-3900
Fax: 216-831-8585
e-mail: helpline@alzclv.org
www.alz.org/cleveland

Nancy B Udelson, Executive Director
Robert Bazzarelli, President

782 Alzheimer's Association: Greater Cincinnati Chapter
644 Linn Street
Cincinnati, OH 45203-1742
513-721-4284
800-272-3900
Fax: 513-345-8446
e-mail: clarissa.rentz@alz.org
http://www.alz.org/cincinnati

Committed to support education, advocacy and research on behalf of those affected by Alzheimer's disease.
Clarissa Rentz, Executive Director
Bob Luckerman, Operations Director

783 Alzheimer's Association: Greater East Ohio Chapter: Greater Youngstown Office
3695B Boardman-Canfield Rd
Canfield, OH 44406-0321
330-533-3300
800-272-3900
Fax: 330-533-3307
e-mail: geoachl@alz.org
www.alz.org

Pam Schuellerman, Executive Director
Andy Junn, Development Director

784 Alzheimer's Association: Miami Valley Chapter
3797 Summit Glen Drive
Dayton, OH 45449-3661
937-291-3332
800-272-3900
Fax: 937-291-0463
e-mail: judy.turner@alz.org
www.alz.org/dayton

Judy Turner, Executive Director
Teresa Thomas, Director of Development

785 Alzheimer's Association: Northwest Ohio Chapter
780 Park Avenue W   419-522-5050
Mansfield, OH 44906-7906   800-272-3900
Fax: 419-522-5318
e-mail: Alzheimers@nwoalz.org
www.alz.org/nwohio
Voluntary health organization committed to finding a cure for Alzheimer's and helping those affected by the disease.
Michael Malone, President
Jeffrey Cole, Vice President

786 Alzheimer's Association: West Central Ohio Chapter
200 East High Street   419-227-9700
Lima, OH 45801-3468   800-272-3900
Fax: 419-222-6212
e-mail: Alzheimers@nwoalz.org
www.alz.org/nwohio
A voluntary health agency providing information Alzheimer's disease and related dementias, serving 7 counties: Allen, Auglaize, Hancock, Hardin, Mercer, Putnam and Van Wert. Offers support group meetings in each county and provides a toll-free help line.
Salli Bollin, Executive Director
Renee Palacios, Development Coordinator

Oklahoma

787 Alzheimer's Association: Oklahoma Chapter
6465 S Yale   918-481-7741
Tulsa, OK 74136-7804   800-272-3900
Fax: 918-481-7745
TTY: 800-493-1411
e-mail: admin@alzokar.org
www.alz.org/alzokar
Dedicated to serving Alzheimer's patients, their families, and caregivers through education, outreach, programs, support services and public advocacy.
Judi A Ver Hoef, President/CEO
Mark Fried, Executive Vice President

Oregon

788 Alzheimer's Association: Columbia-Willamet Chapter
1650 Northwest Naito Parkway   503-416-0201
Portland, OR 97209-1610   800-272-3900
Fax: 503-413-6909
e-mail: infoalzoregon@alz.org
www.alzheimers-oregon.org
Judy McKellar, Executive Director
Karen Garst, President

789 Alzheimer's Association: Cascade/Coast Chapter
1238 Lincoln Street   541-345-8392
Eugene, OR 97401   800-272-3900
Fax: 541-345-5797
e-mail: infoalzoregon@alz.org
www.alz.org/oregon
Judy Clarke, Vice President
Karen Garst, President

790 Alzheimer's Association: Mary's Peak Chapter
1925 NW Circle Boulevard   541-752-1012
Corvallis, OR 97330-1312   Fax: 541-757-1395
www.alz.org

791 Alzheimer's Association: Mid-Willamette Chapter
PO Box 12768   503-371-7728
Salem, OR 97309-0768   Fax: 503-571-9842
e-mail: midwillamatte@alz.org
www.alz.org

Pennsylvania

792 Alzheimer's Association: Delaware Valley Chapter
399 Market Street   215-561-2919
Philadelphia, PA 19106   800-272-3900
Fax: 215-561-4663
e-mail: Wendy.Campbell@alz.org
www.alz.org/desjsepa
Wendy L Campbell, President
Theresa Haenn, Vice President Development

793 Alzheimer's Association: Greater Pennsylvania Chapter: SW Regional Office
Landmarks Building, 100 Station   412-261-5040
Pittsburgh, PA 15219   800-272-3900
Fax: 412-471-2722
www.alzpa.org
Education training, information, support groups, free newsletter, telephone support, services to caregivers and diagnosed individuals, as well as professionals.
Diane Balcom, President/CEO
Erica Hood, Director Of Programs

794 Alzheimer's Association: Greater Mid-Ohio
1100 Liberty Avenue   412-261-5040
Pittsburgh, PA 15222   800-272-3900
Fax: 412-471-2722
e-mail: bob.leroy@alz.org
www.alz.org/pa
Education training information support groups free newsletter telephone support services to caregivers and diagnosed individuals as well as professionals.
Bob LeRoy, President/CEO
Erica Hood, Vice President of Programs and Services

795 Alzheimer's Association: Laurel Mountains Chapter
1011 Old Salem Road
Greensburg, PA 15601-1095   800-652-3370
Fax: 724-837-4567
www.alz.org

796 Alzheimer's Association: Northeast Pennsylvania Chapter
63 North Franklin Street   717-822-4278
Wilkes Barre, PA 18701   800-272-3900
Fax: 717-822-9915
www.alzpa.org

797 Alzheimer's Association: Northwest Pennsylvania Chapter
1128 State Street   814-456-9200
Erie, PA 16501   800-272-3900
Fax: 814-454-0414
e-mail: bob.leroy@alz.org
www.alz.org/pa
Bob LeRoy, President/CEO
Erica Hood, Vice President of Programs and Services

798 Alzheimer's Association: South Central Pennsylvania Chapter
3544 North Progress Avenue   717-651-5020
Harrisburg, PA 17110   800-272-3900
Fax: 717-651-5066
e-mail: bob.leroy@alz.org
http://www.alz.org/pa/in_my_community_co
Bob LeRoy, President/CEO
Erica Hood, Vice President of Programs and Services

Rhode Island

799 Alzheimer's Association: Rhode Island Chapter
245 Waterman Avenue   401-421-0008
Providence, RI 02906   800-272-3900
Fax: 401-941-8988
e-mail: Donna.McGowan@alz.org
www.alz.org/ri
Elizabeth Morancy, Executive Director
Marge Angilly, Program Director

South Carolina

800 Alzheimer's Association: Low Country Chapter
2090 Executive Hall Road   843-571-2641
Charleston, SC 29407   800-860-1444
Fax: 843-571-6020
www.alz.org/sc
Ashton Houghton, VP of Development & Communications
Cawana Wilson, Program Director

801   Alzheimer's Association: Mid-State South Carolina Chapter
3223ÿSunset Blvd   803-791-3430
W Columbia, SC 29169-7044   800-636-3346
                                        Fax: 803-791-8388
                                        www.alz.org/sc

Adelle Stanley, Program Director
Lynee Moore, Director of Development

802   Alzheimer's Association: Upstate South Carolina Chapter
4124 Clemson Boulevard   864-224-3045
Anderson, SC 29621-5528   800-273-2555
                                        Fax: 864-225-1387
                                        e-mail: cindy.alewine@alz.org
                                        www.alz.org/sc

Cindy Alewine, President/CEO
Velma Haggan, VP of Finance & Operations

Tennessee

803   Alzheimer's Association: Eastern Tennessee Chapter
2200 Sutherland Avenue   865-544-6288
Knoxville, TN 37919   800-272-3900
                                        Fax: 865-544-6249
                                        e-mail: janice.wade@alz.org
                                        www.alz.org/tn

Janice Wade-Whitehea, Executive Director
Carolyn Jensen, Development Director

804   Alzheimer's Association: Highland Rim Chapter
201 W Lincoln Street   931-455-3345
Tullahoma, TN 37388-1004   800-272-3900
                                        Fax: 931-455-5396
                                        e-mail: tiffany.maicke@alz.org
                                        www.alz.org/altn

George Jensen, Chair
Bruce Duncan, Vice Chair

805   Alzheimer's Association: Memphis Area Office
326 Ellsworth   901-565-0011
Memphis, TN 38111   800-272-3900
                                        Fax: 901-565-9550
                                        e-mail: tammy.deniro@alz.org
                                        www.alz.org/altn

George Jensen, Chair
Bruce Duncan, Vice Chair

806   Alzheimer's Association: Middle Tennessee Chapter
4205 Hillsboro Pike   615-292-4938
Nashville, TN 37215-2859   800-272-3900
                                        Fax: 615-386-9768
                                        e-mail: tiffany.cloud-mann@alz.org
                                        www.alz.org/altn

George Jensen, Chair
Bruce Duncan, Vice Chair

807   Alzheimer's Association: Northeast Tennessee Chapter
207 North Boone Street   423-928-4080
Johnson City, TN 37604   800-272-3900
                                        Fax: 423-928-1152
                                        e-mail: tracey.kendall@alz.org
                                        www.alz.org/altn

Provide support, education, advocacy and research to those affected by Alzheimer's disease and their families.
George Jensen, Chair
Bruce Duncan, Vice Chair

808   Alzheimer's Association: Southeast Tennessee Chapter
7625 Hamilton Park Drive   423-265-3600
Chattanooga, TN 37421   800-272-3900
                                        Fax: 423-265-3611
                                        e-mail: amy.french@alz.org
                                        www.alz.org/altn

George Jensen, Chair
Bruce Duncan, Vice Chair

Texas

809   Alzheimer's Alliance of Smith County
211 Winchester   903-509-8323
Tyler, TX 75701-8732   800-789-0508
                                        Fax: 903-509-8373
                                        e-mail: jana@alzalliance.org
                                        www.alzalliance.org

Programs and services that help families and individuals affected by Alzheimers disease and related dementias.
Jana Humphrey, Executive Director
Sherlon Spurling, Client Services Coordinator

810   Alzheimer's Alliance: Texarkana Area
104 Cypress   903-223-8021
Texarkana, TX 75503-7812   877-312-8536
                                        Fax: 903-792-1792
                                        e-mail: lindanickersonalz@cableone.net
                                        www.alztexark.org

Linda Nickerson, Executive Director
Fran Long, Program Director

811   Alzheimer's Association: Capital of Texas Chapter
3429 Executive Center Drive   512-241-0420
Austin, TX 78731   800-367-2132
                                        Fax: 512-241-0430
                                        e-mail: TxChapterInfo@alz.org
                                        www.alz.org/texascapital

The Alzheimer Association Greater Austin Chapter is dedicated to providing leadership to enhance care and support services for individuals and their families while promoting the advancement of research eliminate Alzheimer's disease.
Daniel Hamilton, Chair
Christian Wells, Program Team Leader

812   Alzheimer's Association: El Paso Chapter
4687 N Mesa   915-544-1799
El Paso, TX 79912-1147   800-272-3900
                                        Fax: 915-544-8746
                                        e-mail: Luciana.murillo@alz.org
                                        www.alz-austin.org

Mitch Moss, Chair
Eddie Garcia, Chair Elect

813   Alzheimer's Association: Greater Beaumont Area Chapter
700 N Street   409-833-1613
Beaumont, TX 77701   800-272-3900
                                        Fax: 713-314-1315
                                        e-mail: richard.elbein@alz.org
                                        www.alz.org/texas

Richard Elbein, Chief Executive Officer
Deborah Coppola, Program Officer

814   Alzheimer's Association: Greater Dallas Chapter
4144 N Central Expressway   214-540-2400
Dallas, TX 75204-4228   800-272-3900
                                        Fax: 214-827-2064
                                        e-mail: Helpline@alzdallas.org
                                        www.alz.org/greaterdallas

Provides support and assistance to persons affected by Alzheimer's disease and related dementias and their families and caregivers. Serving Collin, Cooke, Dallas, Deaton, Ellis, Fanning, Grayson, Hunt, Kaufmau, Navarro and Rockwall counties.
John R Gilchrist Jr, Executive Director
Jack Broyles, Chairman

815   Alzheimer's Association: Greater East Texas Chapter
PO Box 630636   936-569-1325
Nacogdoches, TX 75963   800-272-3900
                                        Fax: 936-569-0514
                                        www.alz.org/texas

Phil King, Chief Financial Officer
Ana Guerrero, Development Officer

816   Alzheimer's Association: Greater Wichita Falls Chapter
901 Indiana   940-767-8800
Wichita Falls, TX 76301-3206   800-272-3900
                                                 Fax: 940-322-6259
                                e-mail: theresa.hocker@alz.org
                                www.alz.org/northcentraltexas

Theresa Hocker, Executive Director
Lyn Downing, Director of Development

817   Alzheimer's Association: Houston and Southeast Texas Chapter
2242 W Holcombe Boulevard   713-314-1313
Houston, TX 77030   800-272-3900
                                                 Fax: 713-314-1315
                                e-mail: alexis.eaton@alz.org
                       http://www.alz.org/texas/in_my_community

Richard Elbein, CEO
Alexis Eaton, Development Coordinator

818   Alzheimer's Association: Northeast Texas Chapter
211 Winchester   903-509-8323
Tyler, TX 75701-8732   800-789-0508
                                                 Fax: 903-509-8373
                                e-mail: jana@alzalliance.org
                                www.alzalliance.org

Jana Humphrey, Executive Director
Sherlon Spurling, Client Services Coordinator

819   Alzheimer's Association: Rio Grande Valley Region
222 E Van Buren   956-440-0636
Harlingen, TX 78550   800-272-3900
                                                 Fax: 956-440-9290
                                                 www.alztexas.org

A nonprofit organization designed to educate and support individuals with Alzheimer's, their families and caregivers.

820   Alzheimer's Association: STAR Chapter, Midland Region
4400 N Big Spring   432-570-9191
Midland, TX 79705   800-272-3900
                                                 Fax: 432-683-2345
                                e-mail: debbie.erdwurm@alz.org
                                www.alz.org/txstar

Mitch Moss, Chair
Eddie Garc¡a, Chair Elect

821   Alzheimer's Association: South Central Texas
7400 Louis Pasteur Drive   210-822-6449
San Antonio, TX 78229   800-272-3900
                                                 Fax: 210-824-8069
                                e-mail: anna.bridgman@alz.org
                                www.alz.org/txstar

Mitch Moss, Chair
Eddie Garc¡a, Chair Elect

822   Alzheimer's Association: Tarrant County Chapter
101 Summit Avenue   817-336-4949
Fort Worth, TX 76102   800-272-3900
                                                 Fax: 817-336-4966
                                e-mail: theresa.hocker@alz.org
                                www.alz.org/northcentraltexas

Offers support to those afflicted with Alzheimer's disease and their families through education, support groups, case management, telephone help line and referral to services (i.e. long term care, adult daycare, medical assistance, legal assistance etc.).
Theresa Hocker, Executive Director
Susanna Luk-Jones, Director of Program Services

Utah

823   Alzheimer's Association: Utah Chapter
855 E 4800 S   801-265-1944
Salt Lake City, UT 84107   800-272-3900
                                                 Fax: 801-269-1226
                                e-mail: utah.chapter@alz.org
                                www.alz.org/utah

Nick Sussman, Program Director
Paul Fairholm, President

Vermont

824   Alzheimer's Association: Vermont Chapter
300 Cornerstone Drive   802-316-3839
Williston, VT 05495-1139   800-272-3900
                                                 Fax: 802-229-5231
                                e-mail: ashley.witzenberger@alz.org
                                www.alz.org/vermont

Randy Brock, President and Chair
Ashley Witzenberg, Director of Development

Virginia

825   Alzheimer's Association: Central Virginia Chapter
1160 Pepsi Place   434-973-6122
Charlottesville, VA 22901   800-272-3900
                                                 Fax: 434-973-4224
                                e-mail: alzcwva@alz.org
                                www.alz.org/cwva

Sue Friedman, President and CEO
Brian Phelps, Chair

826   Alzheimer's Association: Greater Richmond Chapter
4600 Cox Road   804-967-2580
Glen Allen, VA 23060   800-272-3900
                                                 Fax: 804-967-2588
                                e-mail: sherry.peterson@alz.org
                                www.alz.org/grva

Alzheimer's Association provides support and services to those with Alzheimer's and their families services include: help line, support groups, educational programs for family and professional caregivers, monthly newsletter, lending library, and a speakers
Sherry Peterson, CEO
Marry Ann Johnson, Program Director

827   Alzheimer's Association: National Capital Area Chapter
3701 Pender Drive   703-359-4440
Fairfax, VA 22030   800-272-3900
                                                 Fax: 703-359-4441
                                e-mail: Danielle.Otsuka@alz.org
                                www.alz.org/grva

Provides support and services to those diagnosed with Alzheimer's disease and related disorders and their families. Services include information on the disease, care options, caregiving techniques and research, support groups, education and training, and advocacy.
Matthew B Aaron, Chair
Danielle Otsuka, Director of Development

828   Alzheimer's Association: Piedmont-Valley Area Chapter
1160 Pepsi Place   434-973-6122
Charlottesville, VA 22901   800-272-3900
                                                 Fax: 434-973-4224
                                e-mail: alzcwva@alz.org
                                www.alz.org/cwva

Sue Friedman, President and CEO
Brian Phelps, Chair

829   Alzheimer's Association: Roanoke Salem Chapter
3959 Electric Rd   540-345-7600
Roanoke, VA 24018   800-272-3900
                                                 Fax: 540-345-7900
                                e-mail: annette.clark@alz.org
                                www.alz.org/cwva

Sue Friedman, President and CEO
Brian Phelps, Chair

830   Alzheimer's Association: Southeastern Virginia Chapter
6350 Center Drive   757-459-2405
Norfolk, VA 23502   800-272-3900
                                                 Fax: 757-461-7902
                                e-mail: InfoSEVA@alz.org
                                www.alz.org/seva

Provides support to people with Alzheimer's disease or related dementia and their families; educates professionals and the public about Alzheimer's disease and related dementia; supports research into causes, improved diagnosis, therapies and cures.
Gino V Colombara, Executive Director
Patricia Far Lacey, Director of Education & Family Services

831   Alzheimer's Association: Southside Virginia Chapter
120 S Hill Avenue   434-447-3963
S Hill, VA 23970-0310   800-272-3900
                                            Fax: 434-447-9024
                              e-mail: gino.colombara@alz.org
                                                www.alz.org/seva
Gino V Colombara, Executive Director
June Rainey, Education & Family Services Coordinator

Washington

832   Alzheimer's Association: Inland Northwest Chapter
910 W. 5th Ave   509-473-3390
Spokane, WA 99204   800-272-3900
                                            Fax: 509-473-3389
                               e-mail: joel.loiacono@alz.org
                                         www.alz.org/inlandnorthwest
Joel Loiacono, Executive Director
Sandra Druffel, Development Director

833   Alzheimer's Association: Western & Central Washington Chapter
100 W. Harrison St   206-363-5500
Seattle, WA 98119   800-848-7097
                                            Fax: 206-363-5700
                               e-mail: InquiryWa@alz.org
                                            www.alz.org/alzwa
Nancy Dapper, Executive Director
Ellia Ryan, Development Director

West Virginia

834   Alzheimer's Association: Greater Mid-Ohio Valley Chapter
1218 Market Street   304-865-6775
Parkersburg, WV 26101   800-491-2717
                               e-mail: jane.marks@alz.org
                                                www.alz.org/wv
Jane Marks, Executive Director
Jane Siers, Development Director

835   Alzheimer's Association: N Central West Virginia Chapter
1299 Pineview Drive   304-599-1159
Morgantown, WV 26505-4543   800-491-2717
                                            Fax: 304-291-2577
                               e-mail: jane.marks@alz.org
                                                www.alz.org/wv
Jane Marks, Executive Director
Jane Siers, Development Director

836   Alzheimer's Association: South West Virginia Chapter
1111 Lee Street E   304-343-2717
Charleston, WV 25301   800-491-2717
                                            Fax: 304-343-2723
                               e-mail: jane.marks@alz.org
                                                www.alz.org/wv
Jane Marks, Executive Director
Jane Siers, Development Director

Wisconsin

837   Alzheimer's Association: Greater Wisconsin Chapter
1523 Rose Street   608-784-5011
La Crosse, WI 54603   80- 27- 390
                                            Fax: 608-784-4428
                               e-mail: GreaterWI@alz.org
                                                   www.alz.org
To eliminate Alzheimer's disease through the advancement of research; to provide and enhance care and support for all affected; and to reduce the risk of dementia through the promotion of brain health.
Brad Beckman, President

838   Alzheimer's Association: Indianhead Chapter
1227B Menomonie Street   715-835-7050
Eau Claire, WI 54703-5996   800-272-3900
                                            Fax: 715-835-0597
                               e-mail: Mary.Bouche@alz.org
                                                www.alz.org/gwwi
Mary B Bouche, Executive Director
Michael Furgiuele, Finance/Technical Director

839   Alzheimer's Association: Lake Superior Chapter
400 Chapple Avenue   715-682-3974
Ashland, WI 54806-1652   800-272-3900
                                            Fax: 715-682-6561
                               e-mail: GreaterWI@alz.org
                                                www.alz.org/gwwi
Kim Kinner, Executive Director
Diane Butz, Development and Marketing Director

840   Alzheimer's Association: Midstate Wisconsin Chapter
1000 N Oak Avenue   715-389-3200
Marshfield, WI 54449   Fax: 715-387-5727
                                                   www.alz.org

841   Alzheimer's Association: North Central Wisconsin Chapter
203 Schiek Plaza   715-362-7779
Rhinelander, WI 54501   800-272-3900
                                            Fax: 715-362-1879
                               e-mail: GreaterWI@alz.org
                                                   www.alz.org
Kim Kinner, Executive Director
Diane Butz, Development and Marketing Director

842   Alzheimer's Association: Northeast Wisconsin Chapter
2900 Curry Lane   920-469-2110
Green Bay, WI 54311   800-272-3900
                                            Fax: 920-498-2203
                               e-mail: GreaterWI@alz.org
                                                   www.alz.org
Kim Kinner, Executive Director
Diane Butz, Development and Marketing Director

843   Alzheimer's Association: South Central Wisconsin Chapter
10 E. Doty Street   608-239-7791
Madison, WI 53703   800-272-3900
                                            Fax: 608-232-3407
                               e-mail: tracy.earll@alz.org
                                                www.alz.org/scwisc
Provides support and assistance to the families of those impacted by Alzheimer's and related dementias, including educational programs, support groups, information and referral and advocacy.
150 Members
Paul Rusk, Executive Director
Danielle Luethje, Education Coordinator

844   Alzheimer's Association: Southeast Wisconsin Chapter
620 South 76th Street   414-479-8800
Milwaukee, WI 53214   800-922-2413
                                            Fax: 414-479-8819
                                            TTY: 414-479-8466
                               e-mail: info@alzheimers.sswi.org
                                                www.alz.org/sewi
To eliminate Alzheimer's disease through advancement of research and to enhance care and support for individuals, their families and caregivers. Individual consultation over the phone or in person. Extensive library of educational materials for loan or purchase.
Tom Hlavacek, Executive Director
Krista Scheel, Program Director

Wyoming

845   Alzheimer's Association: Wyoming Chapter
1500 S. 70th St   402-420-2540
Lincoln, NE 68506   800-272-3900
                               e-mail: bobbie.turner@alz.org
                                                www.alz.org/greatplains
The Alzheimer's Association of the Great Plains is dedicated to supporting those with Alzheimer's disease and their families and friends through specialized programs and services, educating families, communities, and health professionals about Alzheimer's disease.
Karen Noel, President/CEO
Teresa Stitcher- Fritz, Program Director

846   Alzheimer's Wyoming
900 Werner Court   307-265-7960
Casper, WY 82602   Fax: 307-265-7960
                               e-mail: alzawy@tribcsp.com
                                            www.alzheimerswyoming.org

Alzheimer's Affiliation of Wyoming is an independent organization that makes presentations about Alzheimer's Disease; assists Alzheimer support groups; provides funds for respite care; maintains a lending library; refers patients and their families to services.
Mary Hein, Executive Director

Foundations

847 Long Island Alzheimers Foundation
5 Channel Drive   516-767-6856
Port Washington, NY 11050   Fax: 516-767-6864
e-mail: info@liaf.org
www.liaf.org
To help lighten the burden and improve the quality of life for those suffering with Alzheimer's disease and related dementias, their caregivers and their families.
Fred Jenny, Executive Director

Research Centers

848 Aging and Alzheimer's Disease Center Oregon Health Sciences University
Oregon Health Sciences University
3181 SW Sam Jackson Park Road - CR1   503-494-6976
Portland, OR 97239-3098   Fax: 503-494-6695
e-mail: kaye@ohsu.edu
www.ohsu.edu/research/alzheimers
Researches causes and consequences of Alzheimer's disease and ways of clinical services. Publishes a newsletter twice a year.
Jeffrey Kaye, Director
Joan Benedict, Administrative Coordinator

849 Alzheimer's Disease Center Emory University/VA Medical Center
Wesley Woods Health Center 3rd Flo   404-728-6950
Atlanta, GA 30329   Fax: 404-286-55
e-mail: emoryadrc@emory.edu
www.med.emory.edu/ADRC
Researchers work to translate advances into improved care and diagnosis for Alzheimer's patients.
Allan Levey, Director
Stuart Zola, Co-Director

850 Alzheimer's Disease Center Kentucky University
Sanders-Brown Center on Aging
101 Sanders-Brown Building   859-257-1412
Lexington, KY 40536-0230   Fax: 859-323-2866
e-mail: rdavi3@email.uky.edu
/www.mc.uky.edu/coa
Researchers work to translate advances into improved care and diagnosis for Alzheimer's patients.
Lee T Todd Jr., President
Vince J Kellen, Chief Information Officer

851 Alzheimer's Disease Center Mayo Clinic Mayo Medical School
Mayo Medical School
200 First Street SW   507-284-2511
Rochester, MN 55905   Fax: 507-538-0161
TDD: 507-2849786
e-mail: mayoADC@mayo.edu
www.mayoresearch.mayo.edu
Researchers work to translate advances into improved care and diagnosis for Alzheimer's patients.
John H Noseworhty MD, President
William C Rupp MD, Vice President, CEO

852 Alzheimer's Disease Center Pennsylvania University School of Medicine
Ralston House
3615 Chestnut Street   215-662-7810
Philadelphia, PA 19104   e-mail: jason.karlawish@uphs.upenn.edu
www.uphs.upenn.edu/ADC
Researchers work to translate advances into improved care and diagnosis for Alzheimer's patients.
John Q Trojanowski, Director

853 Alzheimer's Disease Center: Boston University
Boston University School of Medicine

72 E Concord Street   617-638-5426
Boston, MA 02118   888-458-2823
Fax: 617-414-1197
e-mail: pfau@bu.edu
www.bu.edu/alzresearch
Researchers work to translate advances into improved care and diagnosis for Alzheimer's patients.
Neil W Kowall, Director
Richard Fine, Associate Director

854 Alzheimer's Disease Center: Johns Hopkins University School of Medicine
Johns Hopkins University Department of Pathology
720 Rutland Avenue   410-502-5164
Baltimore, MD 21205   Fax: 410-955-9777
e-mail: edelman1@jhmi.edu
www.alzresearch.org
Researchers work to translate advances into improved care and diagnosis for Alzheimer's patients.
Marilyn Albert, Director
Philip Wong, Associate Director

855 Alzheimer's Disease Center: University of California, Davis
4860 Y Street   916-734-5496
Sacramento, CA 95817   e-mail: wjjagust@lbl.gov
alzheimer.ucdavis.edu/
Researchers work to translate advances into improved care and diagnosis for Alzheimer's patients.
Charles DeCarli MD, Clinical Core Director

856 Alzheimer's Disease Center: University of Alabama at Birmingham
1720 7th Avenue S   205-934-3847
Birmingham, AL 35294-0017   Fax: 205-975-7365
e-mail: adbrain@uab.edu
www.main.uab.edu/adc
Researchers work to translate advances into improved care and diagnosis for Alzheimer's patients.
Daniel C Marson, Director
J Michael Wyss, Associate Director

857 Alzheimer's Disease Center: Washington University
1660 S Columbian Way   206-277-3281
Seattle, WA 98108-1597   800-317-5382
Fax: 206-768-5456
e-mail: wamble@u.washington.edu
www.depts.washington.edu/adrcweb
Researchers work to translate advances into improved care and diagnosis for Alzheimer's patients.
Murray A Raskind, Director
Elaine Peskind, Associate Director

858 Alzheimer's Disease Research Center Washington University School of Medicine
Washington University School of Medicine
4488 Forest Park Avenue   314-286-2683
St Louis, MO 63108   Fax: 314-286-2763
e-mail: morrisj@abraxas.wustl.edu
www.adrc.wustl.edu
Researchers work to translate advances into improved care diagnosis and treatment for Alzheimer's patients.
John Morris, Director
Virginia D Buckles, Executive Director

859 Alzheimer's Disease Research Center Duke University
Bryan ADRC
2200 W Main Street Suite A200   919-668-0820
Durham, NC 27705   866-444-2372
e-mail: kwe@duke.edu
adrc.mc.duke.edu
Researchers work to translate advances into improved care and diagnosis for Alzheimer's patients.
Kathleen A Welsh-Bohmer, Director
James Robert Burke, Associate Director

860 Cognitive Neurology and Alzheimer's Disease Center
CNADC

320 E Superior Street
Chicago, IL 60611
312-908-9339
Fax: 312-908-8789
e-mail: CNADC-Admin@northwestern.edu
www.brain.northwestern.edu
Researchers work to translate advances into improved care and diagnosis for Alzheimer's patients.
M -Marsel Mesulam, Director
Eileen H Bigio, Director of the Neuropathology Core

861   Cornell University: Winifred Masterson Burke Medical Research-Dementia
1300 York Avenue
New York, NY 10065
212-746-5454
Fax: 212-821-0576
e-mail: publicaffairs@med.cornell.edu
www.med.cornell.edu
Clinical and basic studies in metabolic aspects of the nervous system especially Alzheimer's disease.
David J Skorton MD, President
Thomas H Blair lll, Senior Director Administrator

862   Duke University Center for the Study of Aging and Human Development
duke Duke University
Box 3003
Durham, NC 27710
919-660-7500
Fax: 919-668-0453
e-mail: webmaster@geri.duke.edu
www.geri.duke.edu
Basic and clinical research into geriatrics and gerontology focusing on a number of chronic diseases in the elderly including osteoporosis cancer heart disease infectious diseases Alzheimer's disease and other disorders leading to dysmobility.
Harvey Jay Cohen MD, Director
Linda K George, Associate Director

863   Duke University Clinical Research Institute
Headquarters
2400 Pratt Street
Durham, NC 27705
919-668-8700
www.dcri.duke.edu
Multidisciplinary clinical research into the cause and prevention of human diseases such as Alzheimer's.
Robert A Harrington, Director
Elizabeth Be Reed, Chief Operating Officer

864   Indiana University Center for Aging Research
The Center for Aging Research
410 W 10th Street
Indianapolis, IN 46202-2872
317-423-5600
Fax: 317-423-5695
e-mail: nnienaber@regenstrief.org
iucar.iu.edu
Researchers work to translate advances into improved care and diagnosis for Alzheimer's patients.
Christopher Callahan, Director
Douglas K Miller, Associate Director

865   Indiana University: Human Genetics Center of Medical & Molecular Genetics
School of Medicine
340 West 10th Street
Indianapolis, IN 46202-3082
317-274-8157
e-mail: kcornett@iupui.edu
www.medicine.iu.edu
Comprised of a core group of scientists with primary appointments in the Department and a group of molecular biologists from other departments who hold joint appointments in Medical and Molecular Genetics.
D Craig Brater MD, Dean
Robert Aull, Associate Director

866   Institute for Basic Research in Developmental Disabilities
44 Holland Avenue
Albany, NY 12229-0001
866- 94- 973
TTY: 866- 933-488
www.omr.state.ny.us
James F Moran, Acting Commissioner

867   Long Island Alzheimers Foundation
5 Channel Drive
Port Washington, NY 11050
516-767-6856
Fax: 516-767-6864
e-mail: info@liaf.org
www.liaf.org

Researchers work to translate advances into improved care and diagnosis for Alzheimer's patients.
Fred Jenny, Executive Director
Anna Maria Warmuz, Executive Assistant

868   Massachusetts Alzheimers Disease Research Center
Massachusetts ADRC
Massachusetts General Hospital
Boston, MA 02114
617-726-3987
Fax: 617-726-7718
www.madrc.org
Multi-institutional consortium of Harvard affiliated facilities encompasses five Core units: an Administrative Core a Clinical Core a Database Management and Statistics Core a Neuropathology Core and an Education and Information Transfer Core. The ADRC also supports four specific research projects funded for 3-5 years and annually designates three or four pilot research projects that are funded for 1 year.
John H Growdon, Clinic Director
Bradley T Hyman, Center Director

869   Medical College of Georgia Alzheimers Research Center
1120 15th Street
Augusta, GA 30912
706-721-0211
Fax: 706-721-7063
e-mail: jbuccafu@mcg.edu
www.mcg.edu/centers/alz
Clinical and basic research of Alzheimer's disease.
Jerry Buccaf MD, Director
J Warren Beach, Member

870   Michigan Alzheimer's Disease Research Center
University of Michigan
1500 E Medical Center Drive
Ann Arbor, MI 48109-0316
734-936-4000
e-mail: sgilman@umich.edu
www.med.umich.edu/alzheimers
Researchers work to translate advances into improved care and diagnosis for Alzheimer's patients.
Sid Gilman MD, Director
Bruno Giordani Ph.D., Core Director

871   Mount Sinai School of Medicine: Alzheimers Disease Research Center
Alzheimer's Disease Research Center
One Gustave L Levy Place
New York, NY 10029-6574
212-241-6500
Fax: 212-369-2344
e-mail: mary.sano@mssm.edu
www.mssm.edu
Focuses on Alzheimer's disease research.
Mary Sano, Director
Samuel Gandy, Associate Director

872   Neurosciences Institute of the Neurosciences Research Program
The Neurosciences Institute
10640 John Jay Hopkins Drive
San Diego, CA 92121
858-626-2000
Fax: 858-626-2099
e-mail: info@nsi.edu
www.nsi.edu
Nonprofit organization focusing on Alzheimer's and related disorders.
Gerald M Edelman, President

873   Ohio State University Neuroscience Program
1835 Neil Avenue
Columbus, OH 43210
614-292-8185
Fax: 614-921-44
www.psy.ohio-state.edu
Specializes in brain disorders such as Alzheimer's disease.
Richard Petty, Chair
Scott Burch, Behavioral Neurosciences Area Assistant

874   Taub Institute For Research On Alzheimer's Disease and the Aging Brain
630 W 168th Street
New York, NY 10032
212-305-1818
Fax: 212-342-2849
e-mail: taubinstitute@columbia.edu.
www.cumc.columbia.edu/dept/taub
Studies Alzheimer's patients.
Richard Mayuex, Co-Director
Michael Shelanski, Co-Director

875 Taub Institute for Research on Alzheimers Disease and the Aging Brain
630 West 168th Street   212-305-1818
New York, NY 10032   Fax: 212-342-2849
e-mail: taubinstitute@columbia.edu
www.alzheimercenter.org
Researchers work to translate advances into improved care and diagnosis for Alzheimer's patients.
Michael L Shelanski, Co-Director
Richard Mayeux MD, Co-Director

876 The Alzheimer's Disease & Memory Disorders Center
ADMDC
One Baylor Plaza   713-798-5971
Houston, TX 77030   Fax: 713-798-7434
e-mail: neurons@bcm.edu
www.bcm.edu/neurology/admdc
Researchers work to translate advances into improved care and diagnosis for Alzheimer's Disease and other memory disorders.
Eli M Mizrahi, Chair, Department of Neurology
Keith Davis, Department Administrator

877 The Sam and Rose Stein Institute for Research on the Aging
University of California San Diego
9500 Gilman Drive   858-534-6299
La Jolla, CA 92093-0664   Fax: 858-534-5475
e-mail: steininstitute@ucsd.edu
www.sira.ucsd.edu
Research on aging and Alzheimer's disease.
Debra Kaine, Director
Maureen Halp MS, Executive Director

878 University Alzheimer Center University of Alabama at Birmingham
University of Alabama at Birmingham
1530 3rd Avenue S   205-934-4011
Birmingham, AL 35294-1150   800-333-6543
Fax: 205-975-7365
TTY: 205-934-4642
e-mail: adbrain@uab.edu
main.uab.edu
Researchers work to translate advances into improved care and diagnosis for Alzheimer's patients.
Dr. Carol Garrison, President
Kristen N Burdick, Director of Executive Affairs

879 University Alzheimer Center UHC: Case Western Reserve University
12200 Fairhill Road   216-844-6400
Cleveland, OH 44120   Fax: 216-844-6446
e-mail: Kathy.Shaw@Case.Edu
www.ohioalzcenter.org
Researchers work to translate advances into improved care and diagnosis for Alzheimer's patients.
Alan Lerner, Co-Director
Kathleen A Smyth, Administrator

880 University of Chicago Dept of Neurology University of Chicago Hospital
University of Chicago Hospital
5841 S Maryland Avenue   773-702-6390
Chicago, IL 60637-1470   Fax: 773-702-9076
e-mail: cgomez@neurology.bsd.uchicago.edu
neurology.uchicago.edu
Covers Translational Neuroscience Research and research programs in neuroimmunology neuromuscular disease and neurovirology provided the initial foundation and brought national recognition.
Kenneth Goodell, Senior Executive Administrator
Judith Maratea, Administrative Assistant

881 University of Illinois Health Services Research
University of Illinois College of Medicine
1601 Parkview Avenue   815-395-0600
Rockford, IL 61107   Fax: 815-395-5887
e-mail: prrockford@uic.edu
www.uirockford.com
A unit of the University of Illinois College of Medicine at Rockford serves faculty students health care providers human services agencies and other community organizations throughout Illi-

nois with demographic health social and economic data. The skills data and resources available to faculty and students at the college are also available to individuals and organizations needing assistance.
Joann Glacken, Research Support Services

882 University of Maryland: Division of Infectious Diseases
UM Baltimore Department of Medicine
725 W Lombard Street   410-706-4613
Baltimore, MD 21201   Fax: 410-706-4619
e-mail: rredfield@ihv.umaryland.edu
www.medschool.umaryland.edu
Focuses research on elderly studies including drug use treatments and infectious diseases of the aged.
Robert R Redfield, Head

883 University of Miami: Center on Aging Center on Aging
Center on Aging
1695 NW 9th Avenue   305-355-9080
Miami, FL 33136   Fax: 305-355-9076
e-mail: ajaret@med.miami.edu
centeronaging.med.miami.edu
Focuses on aged disorders such as Alzheimer's research.
Sara J Czaja, Co-Director
Carl Eisdorfer, Director

884 Yeshiva University: Resnick Gerontology Center
Albert Einstein College of Medicine
Jack and Pearl Resnick Campus   718-920-6722
Bronx, NY 10467   866-633-8255
Fax: 718-655-9672
e-mail: ljacobs@aecom.yu.edu
www.aecom.yu.edu
Alzheimer's disease and other dementia studies.
Allen M Spiegel MD, Dean
Amy R Ehrlich, Geriatrics Fellowship Program Director

Support Groups & Hotlines

885 Alzheimer's Association Autopsy Assistance Network
Alzheimer s Association
Western/Central Washington Chapter   206-363-5500
Seattle, WA 98125   800-848-7097
Fax: 206-363-5700
e-mail: rowena.rye@alz.org
http://alzwa.org/resources6.htm
The primary purposes of the Autopsy Assistance Network are: to provide families with information regarding autopsy; to assist in obtaining a confirmed diagnosis; provide tissue for Alzheimer's disease research; and establish diagnosis for purpose of clinical and epidemiological studies.
Nancy Dapper, Executive Director
Rowena Rye, Community Resources

886 Alzheimer's Support Group
Columbus Health Rehabilitation Center
2100 Midway Street   812-372-8447
Columbus, IN 47201   Fax: 812-375-5117
www.columbushrc.com/
The skilled Nursing Center includes a separate unit dedicated to the care of residents with Alzheimer's disease and other forms of dementia. The Alzheimer's program is designed to celebrate the spirit of their residents, striving to offer a comfortable and compassionate environment that emphasizes positive life experiences and active involvement in a daily routine.
Mike Spencer, Executive Director

887 National Health Information Center
PO Box 1133   310-565-4167
Washington, DC 20013   800-336-4797
Fax: 301-984-4256
e-mail: info@nhic.org
www.health.gov/nhic
Offers a nationwide information referral service, produces directories and resource guides.

Books

888 36-Hour Day
Hachette Book Group USA
3 Center Plaza
Boston, MA 02108
800-759-0190
Fax: 800-331-1664
e-mail: webmaster@hbgusa.com
www.hachettebookgroup.com
A family guide to caring for persons with Alzheimer's disease, related dementing illnesses, and memory loss later in life.
1999
ISBN: 0-446618-76-2

889 Alzheimer Early Stages
Daniel Kuhn MSW, author
Hunter House Publishers
1515 1/2 Park Street
Alameda, CA 94501
510-865-5282
800-266-5592
e-mail: ordering@hunterhouse.com
www.hunterhouse.com
First steps in caring and treatments. This book is for family members and friends of those recently diagnosed with Alzheimer's Disase.
288 pages Paperback
ISBN: 0-897933-97-4

890 Alzheimer's Disease
Springer Publishing Company
536 Broadway
New York, NY 10012-3955
212-431-4370
877-687-7476
Fax: 212-941-7842
e-mail: marketing@springerpub.com
www.springerpub.com
This volume presents the latest research and findings on Alzheimer's disease.
1996 224 pages Softcover
ISBN: 0-826196-22-5
Annette Imperati, Marketing Director

891 Alzheimer's Disease Orientation Kit
Alzheimer's Association
225 North Michigan Avenue
Chicago, IL 60611-1696
800-272-3900
Fax: 866-699-1246
TDD: 312-335-8700
e-mail: media@alz.org
www.alz.org
A collection of materials developed to familiarize the audience with Alzheimer's disease and its effects on the patient and family. Includes the Orientation to Alzheimer's Disease videotape, Learning Guide and Caregiver Packet.

892 Alzheimer's Disease: A Guide to Federal Programs
Alzheimer's Disease Education & Referral Center
PO Box 8250
Silver Spring, MD 20907-8250
800-438-4380
Fax: 301-495-3334
www.alzheimers.org
Directory of Alzheimer's disease programs sponsored by federal agencies. Lists agency by agency, it provides locations and telephone numbers for multisite activities and demonstration programs and lists information resources.

893 Alzheimer's Disease: Activity-Focused Care
Butterworth-Heinemann
225 Wildwood Avenue
Woburn, MA 01801
800-366-2665
Fax: 800-446-6520
www.bh.com
Information for professional and family caregivers on activity-focused care for Alzheimer's patients.
436 pages
ISBN: 0-750699-08-6

894 Alzheimer's Disease: Advances in Neurology
Raven Press

1185 Avenue of the Americas
New York, NY 10036-2601
212-930-9500
800-777-2295
304 pages
ISBN: 0-781700-81-7

895 Alzheimer's Disease: Questions and Answers
Merit Publishing International
5840 Corporate Way
West Palm Beach, FL 33407
561-697-1116
Fax: 561-477-4961
e-mail: meritpi@aol.com
www.meritpublishing.com
Answers questions about Alzheimer's, explains what it is, how it is diagnosed, causes, and how if affects functions of the brain.
1999
ISBN: 1-873413-52-1
Gene Evans, President
Martin Garrido, VP

896 Alzheimer's Disease: Thesaurus
Alzheimer's Disease Education & Referral Center
PO Box 8250
Silver Spring, MD 20907-8250
800-438-4380
Fax: 301-495-3334
www.alzheimers.org
To help librarians and others to save time and money when searing online for books, journal articles, videos and other materials related to Alzheimer's disease.
140 pages

897 Alzheimer's Disease: Treatment and Family Stress: Directions for Research
Superintendent of Documents
PO Box 371954
Pittsburgh, PA 15250-7954
202-512-2250
Presents a collection of papers giving current information on research investigations that increase the understanding of the nature and consequences of family caregiving.
486 pages

898 Alzheimer's, Stroke and 29 Other Neurological Disorders Sourcebook
Omnigraphics
615 Griswold Street
Detroit, MI 48226-3993
313-961-1340
800-234-1340
Fax: 800-875-1340
e-mail: customerservice@omnigraphics.com
www.omnigraphics.com
Provides vital information for the nontechnical reader focusing on Alzheimer's disease, stroke and various neurological disorders. Answers thousands of questions related to afflications of the central nervous system with each chapter reviwing a particular disorder and offers in-depth discussions.

ISBN: 0-780806-66-2
Georgiann Lauginiger, Customer Service Manager

899 Care That Works: A Relationship Approach to Persons with Dementia
John's Hopkins University Press
2715 N Charles Street
Baltimore, MD 21218-4319
410-516-6900
800-537-5487
Fax: 410-516-6998
www.press.jhu.edu
Focuses on building and improving the relationship between the caregiver and the person with Alzheimer's.
272 pages
ISBN: 0-801860-26-1

900 Care of Alzheimer's Patients: A Manual for Nursing Home Staff
Lisa P Gwyther, author
Alzheimer's Association
225 North Michigan Avenue
Chicago, IL 60611-1696
800-272-3900
Fax: 866-699-1246
TDD: 312-335-8700
e-mail: media@alz.org
www.alz.org
A care guide for nursing home staff. A useful resource for any caregiver or professional.
122 pages

901 Caregiver Helpbook
Legacy Health System
1015 NW 22nd Avenue   503-413-6778
Portland, OR 97210   Fax: 503-413-6911
                          e-mail: kshannon@lhs.org
                          www.legacyhealth.org
A helpful guide with useful self care tools for family caregivers of frail or ill older adults.
300 pages Paperback
ISBN: 0-937915-54-6
Kathy Shannon, Manager/Caregiver

902 Caring for Alzheimer's Patients: A Guide for Family & Healthcare Providers
Plenum Publishing Corporation
233 Spring Street   212-620-8460
New York, NY 10013-1522   800-221-9369
                          Fax: 212-463-0742
                          e-mail: books@plenum.com
Consists of five organizations that furnish information and resources concerning Alzheimer's Disease support groups and hospitals.
308 pages
ISBN: 0-306431-99-8

903 Complete Guide to Alzheimer's Proofing Your Home
Purdue University Press
509 Harrison Street   765-494-2038
West Lafayette, IN 47907-2025   800-247-6553
                          Fax: 765-496-2442
                          e-mail: pupress@purdue.edu
                          www.thepress.purdue.edu
Guide on how to modify homes of Alzheimer's patients to facilitate caregiving.
496 pages Paperback
ISBN: 1-557532-02-8

904 Confronting Alzheimer's Disease
American Assoc. of Homes and Services for Aging
2519 Connecticut Avenue NW   202-783-2242
Washington, DC 20008-2008   Fax: 202-783-2255
                          www.aahsa.org
A resource for administrators, professional caregivers and families dealing with Alzheimer's disease and related disorders.
225 pages

905 Court-Related Needs of the Elderly and Persons with Disabilities
Commission on the Mentally Disabled
1800 M Street NW   202-331-2240
Washington, DC 20036
Report of the National Conference, examines the barriers of the judicial system impeding access for the elderly and persons with disabilities.

906 Developing Support Groups for Individuals with Early-Stage Alzheimer's Disease
Robyn Yale, author
Health Professions Press
PO Box 10624   410-337-9585
Baltimore, MD 21285-0624   888-337-8808
                          Fax: 410-337-8539
                          www.healthpropress.com
This one-of-a-kind, step-by-step guidebook has been used as a national and international model to meet the needs of people just diagnosed with Alzheimer's disease. Clinical and administrative issues include selecting group participants, training facilitators and managing unique group topics, interactions and dynamics.
256 pages Paperback
ISBN: 1-878812-62-2

907 Directory of Alzheimer's Disease Treatment Facilities & Home Health Care
Oryx Press
4041 N Central Avenue   602-265-2651
Phoenix, AZ 85012-3397   800-279-4663
                          www.oryxpress.com
A compilation of 1,500 specialized facilities with day care, residential care, diagnosis and treatment facilities.

908 Ginny: A Love Remembered
Iowa State Press
2121 State Street   515-292-0155
Ames, IA 50014   800-862-6657
                          Fax: 515-292-3348
                          e-mail: orders@iowastatepress.com
                          iowastatepress.com
This book tells the story of midwest cartoonist Bob Artley's life with his beloved wife and their 10 year battle together against Alzheimer's disease, which finally claimed her.
278 pages Hardcover
ISBN: 0-813821-04-5
Brad Nobiling, Credit Manager

909 Hospice Alternative
Harper Collins Publishers/Basic Books
10 E 53rd Street   212-207-7057
New York, NY 10022-5299   800-242-7737
                          Fax: 212-207-7203
An account of the hospice experience. An innovative and humane way of caring for the terminally ill.
256 pages
ISBN: 0-465030-61-0

910 Hospice Care for Patients with Advanced Progressive Dementia
Springer Publishing Company
536 Broadway   212-431-4370
New York, NY 10012   877-687-7476
                          Fax: 212-941-7842
                          e-mail: marketing@springerpub.com
                          www.springerpub.com
Discusses adpating hospice care for terminally ill patients with dementia. Topics include infections, eating difficulties, and providing palliative care.
320 pages Hardcover
ISBN: 0-826111-62-9
Annette Imperati, Marketing Director

911 I'm Just Not Myself Anymore: A Family Guide to Alzheimer's Disease
Northwestern University Press
625 Colfax Street   847-491-5313
Evanston, IL 60208-4210   Fax: 847-491-8150
                          e-mail: nupress@nwu.edu
                          www.northwestern.edu
1993 283 pages Paperback
ISBN: 1-880416-72-7

912 Interventions for Alzheimer's Disease: A Caregiver's Complete Reference
Ruth M Tappen, author
Health Professions Press
PO Box 10624   410-337-9585
Baltimore, MD 21285-0624   888-337-8808
                          Fax: 410-337-8539
                          www.healthpropress.com
For professionals who plan, administer or provide services to Alzheimer's patients.
256 pages Paperback
ISBN: 1-878812-39-4

913 Key Elements of Dementia Care
Alzheimer's Association
225 North Michigan Avenue
Chicago, IL 60611-1696   800-272-3900
                          Fax: 866-699-1246
                          TDD: 312-355-8700
                          e-mail: media@alz.org
                          www.alz.org
Defines, describes, and illustrates dementia-capable care throughout the range of residential care settings.
1997 90 pages

914 Nursing Home and You: Partners in Caring for a Relative with Alzheimer's Disease
American Assn. of Homes & Services for the Aging
901 E Street NW   202-783-2242
Washington, DC 20004-2037   800-508-9442
                          Fax: 202-783-2255

Offers suggestions for families of nursing home residents on how to work with staff to foster smooth transitions.
32 pages

915 Occupational Therapy Practice Guidelines for Adults with Alzheimer's Disease
American Occupational Therapy Association
4720 Montgomery Lane 301-652-2682
Bethesda, MD 20824-1220 Fax: 301-652-7711
TDD: 800-377-8555
www.aota.org

21 pages
ISBN: 1-569001-46-4

916 Positive Interactions Program of Activities for People with Alzheimer's
Sylvia Nissenboim, author

Health Professions Press
PO Box 10624 410-337-9585
Baltimore, MD 21285-0624 888-337-8808
Fax: 410-337-8539
www.healthpropress.com
All interactions focus on preventing individual dignity and providing opportunities to experience meaningful involvement and satisfaction. Works in a variety of settings and promotes the OBRA quality of care guidelines.
176 pages 1997
ISBN: 1-878812-40-8
Christine Vroman, Editor

917 Rethinking Alzheimer's Care
Sam Fazio, Dorothy Seman, author

Health Professions Press
PO Box 10624 410-337-9585
Baltimore, MD 21285-0624 888-337-8808
Fax: 410-337-8539
www.healthpropress.com
Appropriate for all settings providing long-term care, adult day services, or assisted living, this fresh and humanistic approach to Alzheimer's care will encourage caregivers to rethink the disease experience and explore its possibilities, instead of its limitations.
200 pages Paperback
ISBN: 1-878812-62-9
Jane Stansell, Editor

918 Speaking Our Minds: Personal Reflections from Individuals with Alzheimer's
WH Freeman and Company
41 Madison Avenue 212-576-9400
New York, NY 10010 888-330-8477
Fax: 212-689-2383
www.whfreeman.com/generalreaders
Personal reflections of people with Alzheimer's disease.
161 pages Hardcover
ISBN: 0-716732-24-6

919 The Comfort of Home for Alheimer's Disease A Guide for Caregivers
M. Meyer, M. Mittelman, P. Derr, C. Epstein, author

CareTrust Publications LLC
PO Box 10283
Portland, OR 97296-0283 800-565-1533
Fax: 415-673-2005
e-mail: sales@comfortofhome.com
www.comfortofhome.com
Walks readers through all Alzheimer's stages and cover the basics from undarting the difference between AD and normal aging, to coping with the behavioral symptoms that come with the diminishing reasoning skills. Additionaly, Comfort talks about how to provide safe physical care around other medical conditions the Alzheimer's sufferer may have, due to normal aging. Not the least of all, Comfort provides self-care tips for the caregivers to remain emotionally and mentally healthy.
2008 288 pages
ISBN: 0-978790-30-8

920 Therapeutic Interventions in Alzheimer's
Aspen Publishers

7201 McKinney Circle 301-698-7100
Frederick, MD 21705-0990 800-638-8437
Fax: 301-695-7931
e-mail: customerservice@aspenpub.com
www.aspenpub.com
A program of functional skills for activities of daily living.
197 pages

921 Time for Alzheimer's: A True Story
Emerald Ink Publishing
7141 Office City Drive
Houston, TX 77087-3722 800-324-5663
www.emeraldink.com
Based on the author's personal experience in caring for her mother.
139 pages
ISBN: 1-885373-13-3

922 Understanding Alzheimer's Disease
University Press of Mississippi
3825 Ridgewood Road 601-432-6205
Jackson, MS 39211-6492 Fax: 601-432-6217
e-mail: press@ihl.state.ms.us
www.upress.state.ms.us
Aimed at people with Alzheimer's, family members, caregivers, health care and human service professionals. Describes Alzheimer's from early to advanced stages. Discusses the care of AD patients, ideas to help families care for the AD patient at home, reviews treatments for the psychiatric, behavioral and cognitive effects of AD and describes research efforts to better understand AD and develop effective therapies. Price $28 Hardcover, $12 Paperback.
1996 150 pages
ISBN: 0-878059-11-3
Kathy Burgess, Advertising/Marketing Services Manager

923 When We Become the Parent to Our Parents
MEA Productions
55 Binks Hill Road 603-536-2641
Plymouth, NH 03264 Fax: 603-536-4851
e-mail: me.allen@juno.com
www.maryemmallen.blogspot.com
Experiences of a woman who cared for her mother and aunt, both Alzheimer's patients.
62 pages
ISBN: 0-965167-51-8
Mary Emma Allen, Author

Children's Books

924 Grandpa Doesn't Know It's Me
Donna Guthrie, author

Alzheimer's Association
225 North Michigan Avenue
Chicago, IL 60611-1696 800-272-3900
Fax: 866-699-1246
TDD: 312-335-8700
e-mail: media@alz.org
www.alz.org
Geared to the concerns of a young child who has a relative with Alzheimer's disease.
26 pages

925 Grandpa's Music: A Story About Alzheimer's
Alison Acheson, author

Albert Whitman & Company
6340 Oakton Street 847-581-0033
Morton Grove, IL 60053-2723 800-255-7675
Fax: 847-581-0039
e-mail: mail@whitmanco.com
www.albertwhitman.com
Children's book using text and illustrations to show the effects of Alzheimer's disease.

ISBN: 0-807530-52-8
Pat McPartland, Sales
Joe Campbell, Customer Service

926 Just for Children: Helping You Understand Alzheimer's Disease
Alzheimer's Association
225 North Michigan Avenue
Chicago, IL 60611-1676   800-272-3900
                                      Fax: 866-699-1246
                                      TDD: 312-335-8700
                                  e-mail: media@alz.org
                                          www.alz.org
Information about Alzheimer's disease written especially for children.
1997 2 pages Pack of 100

927 Let's Talk About When Someone You Love Has Alzheimer's Disease
Rosen Publishing Group's PowerKids Press
29 E 21st Street   212-777-3017
New York, NY 10010   800-237-9932
                                      Fax: 888-436-4643
                          e-mail: customerservice@rosenpub.com
                                  www.rosenpublishing.com
This book sensitively helps children cope with this unsettling disease.

ISBN: 0-823923-06-1
Elizabeth Weitzman, Author

928 Through Tara's Eyes: Helping Children Cope with Alzheimer's Disease
American Health Assistance Foundation
15825 Shady Grove Road   301-948-3244
Rockville, MD 20850   800-437-2423
                                      Fax: 301-258-9454
                                          www.ahaf.org
Told from the perspective of Tara who has a grandmother with Alzheimer's disease but does not know anything is wrong with her grandmother.
36 pages

929 What's Wrong with Grandma? A Family Experience with Alzheimer's
Margaret Shawver, author
Prometheus Books
59 John Glenn Drive   716-691-0133
Amherst, NY 14228-2197   800-421-0351
                                      Fax: 716-691-0137
                      e-mail: marketing@prometheusbooks.com
                                  www.prometheusbooks.com
The story of a family's struggle with Alzheimer's disease as told by the youngest child.
62 pages Paperback
ISBN: 1-159011-74-2
Lisa Risio, Marketing Production Manager

930 Window of Time
Associated Publishers Group
1501 Country Hospital Road   615-254-2450
Nashville, TN 37218   800-327-5113
                                      Fax: 615-254-2405
                                  e-mail: vlill@apgbooks.com
                                          www.apgbooks.com
Illustrated book about the relationship between a grandfather with Alzheimer's and his grandson.
28 pages
ISBN: 0-963633-51-1

Magazines

931 Alzheimer Disease and Associated Disorders: An International Journal
Raven Press
1185 Avenue of the Americas   212-930-9500
New York, NY 10036-2601   800-777-2295
A leading international forum for reports of new research findings and new approaches to diagnosis and treatments. Contributions are offered from all scientific and medical fields.
Quarterly
ISBN: 0-89303H- -
Peter J Whitehouse

932 Mature Health
Haymarket Group, Ltd.
45 W 34th Street   212-239-0855
New York, NY 10001-3073
Magazine featuring articles on health aspects of aging, as well as articles on recreation and leisure.

933 Research & Practice
Alzheimer's Association
225 North Michigan Avenue
Chicago, IL 60611-1696   800-272-3900
                                      Fax: 866-699-1246
                                      TDD: 312-335-8700
                                  e-mail: media@alz.org
                                          www.alz.org
Provides practical information for healthcare professionals on the current status of prominent areas of Alzheimer research.
Quarterly
ISBN: 2-909342-84-0

Newsletters

934 Advances: Progress in Alzheimer Research and Care
Alzheimer's Association
225 North Michigan Avenue
Chicago, IL 60611-1696   800-272-3900
                                      Fax: 866-699-1246
                                      TDD: 312-335-8700
                                  e-mail: media@alz.org
                                          www.alz.org
Provides information related to research and caregiving.
Quarterly

935 Aging and Alzheimer's Disease Center Newsletter
Oregon Health Sciences University
3181 SW Sam Jackson Park Road   503-494-6976
Portland, OR 97201-3098   Fax: 503-494-7499
                                  e-mail: kaye@ohsu.edu
                          www.ohsu.edu/som-alzheimers
Researches causes and consequences of Alzheimer's disease and ways of clinical services.
2x Year
Jeffrey Kaye, Director

936 Alzheimer Disease and Associated Disorders
Charles Decarli, author
Lippincott Williams & Wilkins
16522 Hunters Green Parkway   301-223-2300
Hagerstown, MD 21740   800-638-3030
                                      Fax: 301-223-2398
                                  e-mail: orders@lww.com
                                          www.lww.com
A leading international forum for reports of new research findings and new approaches to diagnosis and treatment.
Quarterly Journal

937 Alzheimer's Association: Tarrant County Chapter
101 Summit Avenue   817-336-4949
Fort Worth, TX 76102   800-471-4422
                                      Fax: 817-336-4966
                          www.alz.org/northcentraltexas
Newsletter for those afflicted with Alzheimer's disease. Includes education, support groups, case management, telephone helpline and referral to services (i.e. long term care, adult daycare, medical assistance, legal assistance, etc.).
8 pages
Theresa Hocker, Executive Director
Susanna Luk-Jones, Director Services

938 LIAFLine Newsletter
Long Island Alzheimers Foundation
5 Channel Drive   516-767-6856
Port Washington, NY   Fax: 516-767-6864
                                  e-mail: info@liaf.org
                                          www.liaf.org
It is intended for caregivers, service providers and anyone interested in Alzheimer's Disease or the Foundation.
Fred Jenny, Executive Director

Pamphlets

939   10 Warning Signs of Alzheimer's Disease
Alzheimer's Association
225 N Michigan Avenue
Chicago, IL 60601-7633
312-335-8700
800-272-3900
Fax: 866-699-1246
TDD: 866-403-3073
e-mail: info@alz.org
www.alz.org

Contains a list of symptoms and answers to the most frequently asked questions.
Pack of 100
Harry Johns, President/CEO

940   Alzheimer's Disease
National Institutes of Health
5600 Fishers Lane
Rockville, MD 20857-0001
301-468-2600
www.nih.gov

Contains information on the diagnosis and treatment of Alzheimer's and on research that offers hope for the future. Included is a list of sources of help for both the patient and the family.

941   Alzheimer's Disease: The Basics
Alzheimer's Association
225 N Michigan Avenue
Chicago, IL 60601-7633
312-335-8700
800-272-3900
Fax: 866-699-1246
TDD: 312-335-5886
e-mail: info@alz.org
www.alz.org

Symptoms, diagnosis, treatments and more
32 pages
Harry Johns, President/CEO

942   Behaviors
Alzheimer's Association
225 N Michigan Avenue
Chicago, IL 60601-7633
312-335-8700
800-272-3900
Fax: 866-669-1246
TDD: 312-335-5886
e-mail: info@alz.org
www.alz.org

The most common behaviors and how to manage them.
12 pages
Harry Johns, President/CEO

943   Caregiver Stress
Alzheimer's Association
225 N Michigan Avenue
Chicago, IL 60601-7633
312-335-8700
800-272-3900
Fax: 866-699-1246
TDD: 312-335-5886
e-mail: info@alz.org
www.alz.org

Symptoms of caregiver stress and ways you can become a healthy caregiver.
6 pages
Harry Johns, President/CEO

944   Caring for Alzheimer's Patients
Human Sciences Press
233 Spring Street
New York, NY 10013-1522
212-620-8000
800-221-9369
This handbook is designed for families, friends, and health-care professionals coping with the myriad of problems encountered by those afflicted with Alzheimer's disease.
308 pages Cloth

945   Dementia Care Practice Recommendations Phases 1 and 2
Alzheimer's Association
225 N Michigan Avenue
Chicago, IL 60601-7633
312-335-8700
800-272-3900
Fax: 866-699-1246
TDD: 312-335-5886
e-mail: info@alz.org
www.alz.org

Covers fundamentals of dementia care and six key care practice areas: food and fluid consumption, pain management, social engagement, resident wandering, falls and physical restraint-free care.
32 pages
Harry Johns, President/CEO

946   Early-Onset Alzheimer's: I'M Too Young to Have Alzheimer's Disease
Alzheimer's Association
225 N Michigan Avenue
Chicago, IL 60601-7633
312-335-8700
800-272-3900
Fax: 866-699-1246
TDD: 312-335-5886
e-mail: info@alz.org
www.alz.org

Addresses unique challenges for diagnosed individuals who are younger than 65
12 pages
Harry Johns, President/CEO

947   Early-Stage Alzheimer's: If You Have Alzheimer's Disease What You Should Know
Alzheimer's Association
225 N Michigan Avenue
Chicago, IL 60601-7633
312-335-8700
800-272-3900
Fax: 866-669-1246
TDD: 312-335-5886
e-mail: info@alz.org
www.alz.org

Coping strategies and tips for living with Alzheimer's
16 pages
Harry Johns, President/CEO

948   Home Safety for People with Alzheimer's Disease
Alzheimer's Disease Education & Referral Center
PO Box 8250
Silver Spring, MD 20907
800-438-4380
Fax: 301-495-3334
e-mail: adear@nia.nih.gov
www.nia.nih.gov

For those who provide in-home care for people with Alzheimer's disease or related disorders. The goal is to improve home safety by identifying potential problems in the home and offering possible solutions to help prevent accidents.
32 pages

949   If You Have Alzheimer's Disease: What You Should Know, What You Should Do
Alzheimer's Association
225 North Michigan Avenue
Chicago, IL 60611-1696
800-272-3900
Fax: 866-699-1246
TDD: 312-335-8700
e-mail: media@alz.org
www.alz.org

Guide for the person with Alzheimer's disease. Includes suggestions of things to do that will help the person cope.
1994 Pack of 100

950   Just for Teens: Helping You Understand Alzheimer's Disease
Alzheimer's Association
225 North Michigan Avenue
Chicago, IL 60611-1696
800-272-3900
Fax: 866-699-1246
TDD: 312-335-8700
e-mail: media@alz.org
www.alz.org

Information about Alzheimer's disease aimed at teenagers.
Pack of 100

951   Late Stage Care
Alzheimer's Association
225 North Michigan Avenue
Chicago, IL 60611-1696
800-272-3900
Fax: 866-699-1246
TDD: 312-335-8700
e-mail: media@alz.org
www.alz.org

Suggestions for coping with caregiving problems that commonly occur late in the progression of Alzheimer's disease.
Pack of 100

952 Legal Plans
Alzheimer's Association
225 N Michigan Avenue   312-335-8700
Chicago, IL 60601-7633   800-272-3900
                                    Fax: 866-699-1246
                                    TDD: 312-335-5886
                                    e-mail: info@alz.org
                                    www.alz.org

Covers legal documents and how to find a lawyer.
16 pages
Harry Johns, President/CEO

953 MedicAlert & Alzheimer's Association Safe Return
Alzheimer's Association
225 N Michigan Avenue   312-335-8700
Chicago, IL 60601-7633   800-272-3900
                                    Fax: 866-699-1246
                                    TDD: 312-335-5886
                                    e-mail: info@alz.org
                                    www.alz.org

Enroll in the nationwide emergency response program that provides help when a person with dementia wanders or has a medical emergency.
1 pages
Harry Johns, President/CEO

954 Money Matters
Alzheimer's Association
225 N Michigan Avenue   312-335-8700
Chicago, IL 60601-7633   800-272-3900
                                    Fax: 866-699-1246
                                    TDD: 312-335-5886
                                    e-mail: info@alz.org
                                    www.alz.org

Identifies care costs and how to pay for them.
28 pages
Harry Johns, President/CEO

955 National Public Policy Program to Conquer Alzheimer's Disease
Alzheimer's Association
225 North Michigan Avenue
Chicago, IL 60611-1676   800-272-3900
                                    Fax: 866-699-1246
                                    TDD: 312-335-8700
                                    e-mail: media@alz.org
                                    www.alz.org

Summary of the Association's public policy goals, objectives and policies.
1997-Present 12 pages

956 Nutrition Screening Initiative
Nutrition Screening Initiative
2626 Pennsylvania Avenue NW   202-625-1662
Washington, DC 20037-1618   e-mail: nsi@gmmb.com
                                    www.cafp.org

Offers information on nutrition pertaining to older Americans and illnesses such as Alzheimer's disease.

957 Partnering with Your Doctor: A Guide for Persons with Memory Problems
Alzheimer's Association
225 N Michigan Avenue   312-335-8700
Chicago, IL 60601-7633   800-272-3900
                                    Fax: 866-699-1246
                                    TDD: 312-335-5886
                                    e-mail: info@alz.org
                                    www.alz.org

Tips on working with your doctor to get the best care.
20 pages
Harry Johns, President/CEO

958 Phase 3: Dementia Care Practice Recommendations
Alzheimer's Association

225 N Michigan Avenue   312-335-8700
Chicago, IL 60601-7633   800-272-3900
                                    Fax: 866-699-1246
                                    TDD: 312-335-5886
                                    e-mail: info@alz.org
                                    www.alz.org

Covers minimizing physical, emotional and spiritual distress; maximizing well-being; snsuring communication with the resident, family and care team.
28 pages
Harry Johns, President/CEO

959 Practice Recommendations for Home Care Professionals
Alzheimer's Association
225 N Michigan Avenue   312-335-8700
Chicago, IL 60601-7633   800-272-3900
                                    Fax: 866-699-1246
                                    TDD: 312-335-5886
                                    e-mail: info@alz.org
                                    www.alz.org

Covers concrete, evidence-based practice suggestions for addressing issues unique to people with dementia living in the community.
68 pages
Harry Johns, President/CEO

960 Report of the Panel on Alzheimer's Disease
National Clearinghouse for Alcohol and Drug Abuse
PO Box 2345
Rockville, MD 20857   800-729-6686
                                    www.health.org

52 pages

961 Respite Care Guide
Alzheimer's Association
225 N Michigan Avenue   312-335-8700
Chicago, IL 60601-7633   800-272-3900
                                    Fax: 866-699-1246
                                    TDD: 312-335-5886
                                    e-mail: info@alz.org
                                    www.alz.org

Find help when you need a break from caregiving.
19 pages
Harry Johns, President/CEO

962 Steps to Diagnosis
Alzheimer's Association
225 North Michigan Avenue
Chicago, IL 60611-1696   800-272-3900
                                    Fax: 866-699-1246
                                    TDD: 312-335-8700
                                    e-mail: media@alz.org
                                    www.alz.org

Educates individuals and their families on the importance of seeking a diagnosis, and the various test completed to obtain an accurate diagnosis.

963 Steps to Enhancing Communication
Alzheimer's Association
225 North Michigan Avenue
Chicago, IL 60611-1696   800-272-3900
                                    Fax: 866-699-1246
                                    TDD: 312-335-8700
                                    e-mail: media@alz.org
                                    www.alz.org

Offers caregivers techniques for improving their approach to listening to and communication with the individual with Alzheimer's disease.
1996 Pack of 100

964 Tax Credits and Deductions
Alzheimer's Association
225 N Michigan Avenue   312-335-8700
Chicago, IL 60601-7633   800-272-3900
                                    Fax: 866-669-1246
                                    TDD: 321-335-5886
                                    e-mail: info@alz.org
                                    www.alz.org

Outlines caregiving tax deductions and credits.
3 pages
Harry Johns, President/CEO

965 Terms & Tips: An Alzheimer Care Handbook
Marjorie Brandenburg, author

Alzheimer's Association
225 North Michigan Avenue
Chicago, IL 60611-1696
800-272-3900
Fax: 866-699-1246
TDD: 312-335-8700
e-mail: media@alz.org
www.alz.org

Offers an explanation for over 250 terms and offers practical caregiver ideas and tips. Primarily for people with dementia and their caregivers, family members, and all providers of hands-on assistance.
1995 84 pages

966 Treatments for Alzheimer's Disease
Alzheimer's Association
225 N Michigan Avenue
Chicago, IL 60601-7633
312-335-8700
800-272-3900
Fax: 866-699-1246
TDD: 312-335-5886
e-mail: info@alz.org
www.alz.org

Information about FDA-approved drugs.
3 pages
Harry Johns, President/CEO

967 Useful Information on Alzheimer's Disease
National Clearinghouse for Alcohol and Drug Abuse
PO Box 2345
Rockville, MD 20857-0001
800-729-6686
e-mail: www.webmaster@health.org
www.health.org

24 pages

968 You Are One of Us: Clergy/Church Connections to Alzheimer Families
Alzheimer's Disease Education & Referral Center
PO Box 8250
Silver Spring, MD 20907-8250
301-495-3311
800-438-4380
Fax: 301-495-3334
www.alzheimers.org

Describes how clergy and church members can help families by including patients and their relatives in church activities, visiting patients and developing church programs that support family caregivers.

Audio & Video

969 Alzheimer's Association Caregiver Resources
Alzheimer's Association
Western/Central Washington Chapter
Seattle, WA 98125
206-363-5500
800-848-7097
Fax: 206-363-5700
e-mail: rowena.rye@alz.org
http://alzwa.org/resources6.htm

A variety of numerous resources, materials and publications providing information for assisting those with Alzheimer's Disease including a documentation guide, informational fact sheets on topics such as bathing, dressing, eating and dealing with grief, in addition resources on long term care options and a newsletter.
Nancy Dapper, Executive Director
Rowena Rye, Community Resources

970 Alzheimer's Association Dementia Care Conference
Alzheimer's Association
225 North Michigan Avenue
Chicago, IL 60601-7633
312-335-5790
800-272-3900
Fax: 866-699-1246
TDD: 312-335-8700
e-mail: careconference@alz.org
www.alz.org/careconference/

Selected sessions from the conference discussing topics such as assisted living preconference, sexuality, intimacy and lifestyle changes, and activity intensive changing approaches to Alzheimer care.
Marisol Sukhu, Hotel/Events Information
Sheryl Trotz, Continuing Education & Presentations

971 Alzheimer's Association Safe Return Police Training Video
Alzheimer's Association Massachusetts Chapter
311 Arsenal Street
Watertown, MA 02472
617-868-6718
800-548-2111
Fax: 617-868-6720
e-mail: communications@alzmass.org
www.alzmass.org/

An educational package designed to help police officers recognize and respond appropriately to Alzheimer patients who may need assistance. Kit includes 1 videotape and 3 print pieces.
James Wessler, President/Chief Executive Officer
Betsy Fitzgerald, Director of Communications

972 Alzheimer's Association: Waves of Stone Video and Documentary
Alzheimer's Association Rhode Island Chapter
245 Waterman Street
Providence, RI 02906
401-421-3900
800-272-3900
Fax: 401-421-0115
e-mail: info@alz.org
http://www.alz-ri.org/Videoshtm.htm

PBS documentary on Alzheimer's disease that discusses both scientific research and caregiver issues.
1994 57 minutes
Elizabeth Morancy, Executive Director
Rita St Pierre, Program Director

973 Another Home for Mom
Lori Hope, author

Fanlight Productions
4196 Washington Street
Boston, MA 02131-1731
617-469-4999
800-937-4113
Fax: 617-469-3379
e-mail: fanlight@fanlight.com
www.fanlight.com

A gentle documentary following one couple as they confront the decision of whether to place the husbands mother, who has Alzheimer's disease, in a nursing home.
1989 27 Minutes
ISBN: 1-572950-77-3

974 Caring...Sharing: The Alzheimer's Caregiver
Fanflight Productions
47 Halifax Street
Boston, MA 02130
617-469-4949
800-937-4113
Fax: 617-469-3379
e-mail: fanlight@fanflight.com
www.fanlight.com

Examines what it means to be a caregiver. This program will be invaluable for any person or group involved in the care of the elderly.
38 minutes
ISBN: 1-572951-22-2

975 For Those Who Take Care: An Alzheimer's Disease Training Program for Nurses
Alzheimer's Disease Education & Referral Center
PO Box 8250
Silver Spring, MD 20907-8250
301-495-3311
800-438-4380
Fax: 301-495-3334
www.alzheimers.org

Guide for training nursing assistants and nurses' aides in long term care facilities, adult day care and private homes. Manual, text and student handouts. Produced by the University of Kentucky.

Web Sites

976 Alzheimer Research Forum
www.alzforum.org
The web's most dynamic scientific community dedicated to understanding alzheimer's disease and related disorders.

977 Alzheimer Support
www.alzheimersupport.com
Serves Alzheimer's sufferers and their loved ones by reporting the latest news in research and treatment, making hard-to-find, recommended nutritional supplements available at manufacturer-direct low prices, and, most importantly, donating profits from each purchase to fund Alzheimer's medical research.

978   Alzheimer's Association

www.alz.org

The leading, global voluntary health organization in Alzheimer care and support, and the largest private, nonprofit funder of Alzheimer research.

979   Alzheimer's Disease International

www.alz.co.uk/adi

The international federation of 73 Alzheimer associations around the world, in relations with the World Health Organization.

980   Healing Well

www.healingwell.com

A social network and support community for patients, caregivers, and families coping with the daily struggles of diseases, disorders and chronic illness.

981   Health Finder

www.healthfinder.gov

A government website where individuals can find information and tools to help you and those you care about stay healthy.

982   Healthlink USA

www.healthlinkusa.com

Health information concerning treatment, cures, prevention, diagnosis, risk factors, research, support groups, email lists, personal stories and much more. Updated regularly.

983   Helios Health

www.helioshealth.com

Online resource for your health information. Detailed information about specific health topics, access to expert advice from our Medical Advisory Board, and up-to-date health news.

984   MEDLINEplus Health Information

www.nlm.nih.gov/medlineplus

MedlinePlus has extensive information from the National Institutes of Health and other trusted sources on over 700 diseases and conditions.

985   MedicineNet

www.medicinenet.com

An online resource for consumers providing easy-to-read, authoritative medical and health information.

986   Medscape

www.medscape.com

Medscape offers specialists, primary care physicians, and other health professionals the Web's most robust and integrated medical information and educational tools.

987   Neurology Channel

www.neurologychannel.com

Find clearly explained, medically accurate information regarding conditions, including an overview, symptoms, causes, diagnostic procedures and treatment options. On this site it is possible to ask questions and get information from a neurologist and connect to people who have similar health interests.

988   WebMD

www.webmd.com

Information on Alzheimer's disease, including articles and resources.

Description

989 ## Amyotrophic Lateral Sclerosis

Amyotrophic Lateral Sclerosis, ALS, also called Lou Gehrig's disease, is a neurological disorder that affects the motor nerves in the brain and spinal cord. The cause of ALS is unknown. It is marked by progressive muscle weakness.

Initial symptoms may be subtle, but early signs of ALS can include twitching and cramping of muscles (particularly in the hands and feet), as well as difficulty in swallowing. As the disorder progresses, use of legs and arms, breathing, speaking, and swallowing become increasingly difficult.

Although the physical symptoms of ALS are most debilitating, the disease does not seem to impair intellectual functioning, although recent research indicates a significant number of people with ALS who have cognitive defects. Voluntary eye movement (blinking) and the senses also remain unaffected.

Currently, there is no cure for ALS. A regime of physical therapy and psychological support can help patients and their families.

National Agencies & Associations

990 **ALS Association National Office**
1275 K Street NW
Washington, DC 20005

818-880-9007
800-782-4747
Fax: 818-880-9006
e-mail: alsinfo@alsa-national.org
www.alsa.org

National nonprofit voluntary health organization dedicated solely to the fight against amyotrophic lateral sclerosis. Its mission: to find a cure for and improve living with ALS. The four fronts of battle are: encouraging identifying funding and monitor
Jane H Gilbert, President/CEO
Lucie Bruijn PhD, Chief Scientist

State Agencies & Associations

Arizona

991 **Arizona Chapter of the ALS Association**
4643 E Thomas Road
Phoenix, AZ 85018

602-297-3800
866-350-2572
Fax: 602-297-3804
e-mail: ken@alsaz.org
webaz.alsa.org

This chapter provides newsletters and other information to help patients and their families find sources of supplies, referrals or counseling as needed. Provides monthly support meetings, public awareness information and fundraising.
Ken Brissa, President

California

992 **ALS Association: Bay Area Chapter**
565 Commercial Street
San Francisco, CA 94111

415-904-2572
800-209-0433
Fax: 415-904-2573
e-mail: fightALS@alsabayarea.org
webaz.alsa.org

ALS Association chapters are multifaceted grass roots organizations that carry out ALSA's mission and strategic goals at the community level. The chapter, with supporting services from the national office, actively pursues the association's goals.
Fred Fisher, Executive Director
Madelon M Thomson, Director Patient/Family Services

993 **ALS Association: Greater Los Angeles Chapter**
28720 Roadside Drive
Agoura Hills, CA 91301

818-865-8067
866-750-2572
Fax: 818-865-8066
e-mail: webmaster@alsala.org
www.alsala.org

ALS Association chapters are multifaceted grass-roots organizations that carry out ALSA's mission and strategic goals at the community level. The chapter — with supporting services from the National Office — actively pursues the Association's goals.
Cameron Ward, Chairman
Barbara Frova, Vice Chair

994 **ALS Association: Greater Sacramento Chapter**
2717 Cottage Way
Sacramento, CA 95825

916-979-9265
Fax: 916-979-9271
e-mail: lou@alssac.org
www.alssac.org

ALS Association chapters are multifaceted grass roots organizations that carry out ALSA's mission and strategic goals at the community level. The chapter, with supporting services from the national office, actively pursues the association's goals.
Scott Ehlen, President
Richard Kline, Vice President

995 **ALS Association: Greater San Diego CIO**
7920 Silverton
San Diego, CA 92126-6350

858-271-5547
Fax: 858-271-5687
e-mail: info@alsasd.com
www.alsasd.com

ALS Association chapters are multifaceted grass-roots organizations that carry out ALSA's mission and strategic goals at the community level. The chapter — with supporting services from the National Office — actively pursues the Association's goals.
Jane Mitchell, Chairman
John Fieberg, Vice Chairman

996 **Orange County Chapter of the ALS Association**
1232 Village Way
Santa Ana, CA 92705-2334

714-285-1088
Fax: 714-285-0305
e-mail: information@alsaoc.org
weboc.alsa.org

Provides information to ALS patients families and caregivers; offers support groups, information and referrals, a loan closet and public awareness information.
Mark Hershey, President
Chad Kessler, Vice President

Colorado

997 **ALS Association: Rocky Mountain Chapter**
7403 Church Ranch Blvd.
Westminster, CO 80021

303-832-2322
866-ALS-3211
Fax: 303-832-3365
e-mail: info@alsaco.org
www.alscolorado.org

The ALS Association chapters are multifaceted grass-roots organizations that carry out ALSA's mission and strategic goals at the community level. The chapter — with supporting services from the National Office — actively pursues the Association's goals.
Pam Rush-Negri, Executive Director
Leslie Ryan, Patient Services Director

Connecticut

998 **Connecticut Chapter of the ALS Association**
4 Oxford Road
Milford, CT 06460

203-874-5050
877-257-2281
Fax: 203-874-7070
e-mail: Lauren@alsact.org
www.alsact.org

The central source in Connecticut for services and education of ALS patients, families and caregivers. Provides ALS patients with

information concerning medical care and facilities, support groups, daily living aids and other services.
Lauren D'Alessandro, Executive Director
Chris Capobianco, President

District of Columbia

999   ALS Association: National Capital Area Chapter
7507 Standish Place   301-978-9855
Rockville, MD 20855   Fax: 301-978-9854
                                 e-mail: info@ALSinfo.org
                                          www.alsinfo.org
Offers patient referrals, informational newsletters and brochures, patient support groups and meetings and fund raising for research into finding cures and treatments for ALS.
Ronnie Gunnerson, Executive Director
Wilson Krahnke, President

Florida

1000   ALS Association: Florida Chapter
3242 Parkside Center Circle   813-637-9000
Tampa, FL 33619   888-257-1717
                                     Fax: 813-637-9010
                          e-mail: cbright@als-florida.org
                                          webfl.alsa.org
ALS Association chapters are multifaceted grass-roots organizations that carry out ALSA's mission and strategic goals at the community level. The chapter — with supporting services from the National Office — actively pursues the Association's goals.
Nancy Baily, President

1001   ALS Association: Florida Chapter East Coast Regional Office
5005 W Laurel Street   813-637-9000
Tampa, FL 33607   888-257-1717
                                     Fax: 813-637-9010
                          e-mail: office@als-florida.org
                                          webfl.alsa.org
ALS Association chapters are multifaceted grass-roots organizations that carry out ALSA's mission and strategic goals at the community level. The chapter — with supporting services from the National Office — actively pursues the Association's goals.
Nancy Baily, President

Georgia

1002   ALS Association of Georgia
1955 Cliff Valley Way   404-636-9909
Atlanta, GA 30329   888-636-9940
                                     Fax: 404-636-9949
                               e-mail: info@alsaga.org
                                          www.alsaga.org
Offers meetings, local support groups, patient support equipment loan and research for persons suffering from ALS.
Kent Murphy, Chair
Candace Wood, Executive Director

Illinois

1003   Lois Insolia ALS Center at Northwestern Memorial Hospital
5550 West Touhyu   847-679-3311
Skokie, IL 60077   888-ALS-1107
                                     Fax: 847-679-9109
                            e-mail: info@lesturnerals.org
                                       www.lesturnerals.org
Utilizes a multidisciplinary approach in treating ALS. Trained specialists provide diagnostic, rehabilitative and supportive services that focus on assessment, care planning and education. Patients and loved ones are encouraged to attend the support groups offered. Provides in-home visits by ALS nurse consultants and social worker, support groups, a lending bank of equipment, and grant programs for financial aid.
Teepu Siddique MD, Director

Indiana

1004   ALS Association: Indiana Chapter
6525 E 82nd Street   317-915-9888
Indianapolis, IN 46250   888-508-3232
                                     Fax: 317-573-9889
                          e-mail: jlewellen@alsaindiana.org
                                          webin.alsa.org
ALS Association chapters are multifaceted grass-roots organizations that carry out ALSA's mission and strategic goals at the community level. The chapter — with supporting services from the National Office — actively pursues the Association's goals.
Melissa Pershing, Executive Director
Abbie Vollmar, Director of Patient Services

Kansas

1005   ALS Association: Keith Worthington Chapter
8340 Mission Road   913-648-2062
Prairie Village, KS 66206   800-878-2062
                                     Fax: 913-642-2431
                         e-mail: bcooper@alsa-midwest.org
                                       www.alsa-midwest.org
ALS Association chapters are multifaceted grass-roots organizations that carry out ALSA's mission and strategic goals at the community level. The chapter — with supporting services from the National Office — actively pursues the Association's goals.
Beckie Cooper, Executive Director

1006   ALS Association: Keith Worthington Chapter Central/Western Kansas Branch
526 South Market   316-612-0188
Wichita, KS 67202   800-878-2062
                                     Fax: 316-612-8768
                          e-mail: kwille@alsa-midwest.org
                                       www.alsa-midwest.org
ALS Association chapters are multifaceted grass-roots organizations that carry out ALSA's mission and strategic goals at the community level. The chapter — with supporting services from the National Office — actively pursues the Association's goals.
Kathleen Willie, Awareness and Development

Kentucky

1007   ALS Association: Kentucky CIO
2807 Amsterdam Road   85- 3-1 13
Villa Hills, KY 41017   800-406-7702
                                     Fax: 85- 3-1 19
                              e-mail: mbacon@alsaky.org
                                          webky.alsa.org
ALS Association chapters are multifaceted grass-roots organizations that carry out ALSA's mission and strategic goals at the community level. The chapter — with supporting services from the National Office — actively pursues the Association's goals.
Mary Bacon, Executive Director
Jennifer Lepa, Administrative Coordinator

Massachusetts

1008   ALS Association: Massachusetts Chapter, Wakefield Office
7 Lincoln Street   781-245-2133
Wakefield, MA 01880-3021   800-258-3323
                                     Fax: 781-245-5414
                                 e-mail: info@als-ma.org
                                          www.als-ma.org
Offers informational brochures and newsletters to promote public awareness, support groups and meetings for patients and their families, and referral information for members in the Massachusetts area.
Rick J Arrowood

Michigan

1009   ALS Association: Michigan Chapter
24359 Northwestern Highway   648-354-6100
Southfield, MI 48075   800-882-5764
                                     Fax: 248-354-6440
                               e-mail: sueb@alsofmi.org
                                       www.alsofmichigan.org

ALS Association chapters are multi-faceted grass-roots organizations that carry out ALSA's mission. and strategic goals at the community level. The chapter — with supporting services from the National Office — actively pursues the Association's goals.

Sue Burstein-Kahn, Executive Director
Lisa Alteri, President

1010 ALS Association: West Michigan Chapter
678 Front Street 616-459-1900
Grand Rapids, MI 49504 800-387-7121
Fax: 616-459-4522
e-mail: stacey@alsa-michigan.org
webmi.alsa.org

ALS Association chapters are multi-faceted grass-roots organizations that carry out ALSA's mission. and strategic goals at the community level. The chapter — with supporting services from the National Office — actively pursues the Association's goals.

Stacey Orsted, Executive Director
Katee Stahl, Administrative Assistant

Minnesota

1011 ALS Association: Minnesota Chapter
333 N Washington Avenue 612-672-0484
Minneapolis, MN 55401 888-672-0484
Fax: 612-672-9110
e-mail: info@alsmn.org
webmi.alsa.org

ALS Association chapters are multifaceted grass-roots organizations that carry out ALSA's mission and strategic goals at the community level. The chapter — with supporting services from the National Office — actively pursues the Association's goals.

Sue Spaulding, Executive Director
Sandy Judge, Development Director

Missouri

1012 ALS Association: Keith Worthington Chapter Central Missouri Branch Office
2025 E. Chestnut Expressway 417-886-5003
Springfield, MO 65802 888-386-1200
Fax: 417-886-5003
e-mail: springfield@alsa-midwest.org
www.alsa-midwest.org

ALS Association chapters are multifaceted grass-roots organizations that carry out ALSA's mission and strategic goals at the community level. The chapter — with supporting services from the National Office — actively pursues the Association's goals.

Paul Blackwell, Services Staff
Valerie Gustin, Awareness and Development

1013 ALS Association: St. Louis Regional Chapter
2258 Weldon Parkway 314-432-7257
Saint Louis, MO 63146 888-873-8539
Fax: 314-432-2991
e-mail: mhill@alsastl.org
webstl.alsa.org

A chapter serving the Eastern Missouri and Southern Illinois regions dedicated solely to finding the cause and cure of ALS through research, patient support, information and referrals and public awareness.

Maureen Barber-Hill, President
Richard Palank, Board Chair

Nebraska

1014 ALS Association: Keith Worthington Chapter Nebraska Branch Office
10730 Pacific at Shaker Place 402-991-8788
Omaha, NE 68114 866-762-6361
Fax: 402-991-3690
e-mail: nebraska@alsa-midwest.org
www.alsa-midwest.org

ALS Association chapters are multifaceted grass-roots organizations that carry out ALSA's mission and strategic goals at the community level. The chapter — with supporting services from the National Office — actively pursues the Association's goals.

Shannon Todd, Services Staff
Sherrie Hanneman, Awareness and Development

New Mexico

1015 ALS Association: New Mexico CIO
PO Box 16495 505-323-6348
Albuquerque, NM 87191-6495 e-mail: als@alsanm.org
www.alsa-nm.org

ALS Association chapters are multifaceted grass-roots organizations that carry out ALSA's mission and strategic goals at the community level. The chapter — with supporting services from the National Office — actively pursues the Association's goals.

Chuck Borgman, President
Terie Baker, Executive Director

New York

1016 ALS Association: Greater New York Chapter
42 Broadway 212-619-1400
New York, NY 10004 800-672-8857
Fax: 212-619-7409
e-mail: als@als-ny.org
www.als-ny.org

ALS Association chapters are multifaceted grass-roots organizations that carry out ALSA's mission and strategic goals at the community level. The chapter — with supporting services from the National Office — actively pursues the Association's goals.

Richard Rose, Chairman
Wendy Schriber, Vice Chairman

1017 ALS Association: Upstate New York CIO
890 7th N Street 315-413-0121
Liverpool, NY 13088 866-499-7257
Fax: 315-413-0508
e-mail: info@alsaupstateny.org
webuny.alsa.org

ALS Association chapters are multifaceted grass-roots organizations that carry out ALSA's mission and strategic goals at the community level. The chapter — with supporting services from the National Office — actively pursues the Association's goals.

Katharine Loomis, Executive Director
Shiann Atuegbu, Patient Services Coordinator

Ohio

1018 ALS Association: Northeast Ohio Chapter
2500 E 22nd Street 216-592-2572
Cleveland, OH 44115 888-592-2572
Fax: 216-592-2575
e-mail: alsa@alsaohio.org
webnoh.alsa.org

Offers telephone consultation services, support groups, caregivers support groups, equipment loan bank and a 24 hour telephone answering service for persons with ALS.

Lisa Bruening, Program Services Coordinator
Fred M DeGrandis, President

1019 ALS Association: Western Ohio Chapter
1170 Old Henderson Road 614-273-2572
Columbus, OH 43220 866-273-2572
Fax: 614-273-2573
e-mail: alsohio@alsohio.org
webcsoh.alsa.org

Offers telephone consultation services, support groups, caregivers support groups, equipment loan bank and a 24 hour telephone answering service for persons with ALS.

Marlin Seymour, Executive Director
Pinky Dressm LSW, Patient Services Coordinator

Oregon

1020 ALS Association: Oregon & SW Washington CIO
700 NE Multnomah 503-238-5559
Portland, OR 97232 800-681-9851
Fax: 503-296-5590
e-mail: info@alsa-or.org
webor.alsa.org

The ALS Association chapters are multifaceted grass-roots organizations that carry out ALSA's mission and strategic goals at the

community level. The chapter — with supporting services from the National Office — actively pursues the Association's goals.
Lance Christian, Executive Director

Pennsylvania

1021 ALS Association: Greater Philadelphia Chapter
321 Norristown Road   215-643-5434
Ambler, PA 19002   877-434-7441
                                                  Fax: 215-643-9307
                          e-mail: alsassoc@alsphiladelphia.org
                                        www.alsphiladelphia.org
To lead the fight to treat and cure ALS through global research and nationwide advocacy while also empowering people with Lou Gehrig's Disease and their families to live fuller lives by providing them with compassionate care and support.
Joan Borowsky, Development Coordinator

1022 ALS Association: Western Pennsylvania Chapter
416 Lincoln Avenue   412-821-3254
Pittsburgh, PA 15209   800-967-9296
                                                  Fax: 412-821-3549
                               e-mail: mbernarding@alswp.org
                                              webwpawv.alsa.org
The mission of this chapter is to provide services and education to ALS patients, families and caregivers through medical information, support groups, assisting health care providers and providing communication devices.
Michael Bernarding, Executive Director
Marie Folino, Patient Services Director

South Carolina

1023 ALS Association: Jim (Catfish) Hunter Chapter
120-101 Penmarc Drive   919-755-9001
Raleigh, NC 27603   877-568-4347
                                                  Fax: 919-755-0910
                              e-mail: jerry@catfishchapter.org
                                            www.catfishchapter.org
ALS association chapters are multifaceted grass roots organizations that carry out ALSA's mission and strategic goals at the community level. The chapter, with supporting services from the national office, actively pursues the association's goals.
Jerry Dawson RN BSN, President & CEO
Megan Gardner, Executive Director

Tennessee

1024 ALS Association: Middle Tennessee Chapter
522 E Iris Drive   61- 3-1 55
Nashville, TN 37204   877-216-5551
                                                  Fax: 615-331-5796
                             e-mail: cheri.sanders@alstn.org
                                                  webtn.alsa.org
ALS Association chapters are multifaceted grass-roots organizations that carry out ALSA's mission and strategic goals at the community level. The chapter — with supporting services from the National Office — actively pursues the Association's goals.
Cheri Sanders, Executive Director
Patty Lane, Patient Services Coordinator

Texas

1025 ALS Association: Greater Houston CIO
PO Box 271561   713-942-2572
Houston, TX 77277-1561   866-788-2572
                                                  Fax: 218-497-2572
                      e-mail: linda.richardson@alsa-houston.org
                                            www.alsa-houston.org
ALS Association chapters are multi-faceted grass roots organizations that carry out ALSA's mission and strategic goals at the community level. he chapter — with supporting services from the National Office — actively pursues the Association's goals.
Linda Richardson, President
Georgia Mclain, Patient Services

1026 ALS Association: North Texas Chapter
1231 Greenway Drive   972-714-0088
Irving, TX 75038   877-714-0088
                                                  Fax: 972-714-0066
                           e-mail: a.reid@alsanorthtexas.org
                                                  webntx.alsa.org
ALS Association chapters are multi-faceted grass roots organizations that carry out ALSA's mission and strategic goals at the community level. he chapter — with supporting services from the National Office — actively pursues the Association's goals.
Aleksei Reid, Executive Director
Leigh Craig, Development Director

1027 ALS Association: South Texas Chapter
8600 Wurzbach   210-733-5204
San Antonio, TX 78240   877-257-4673
                                                  Fax: 210-733-5206
                           e-mail: Information@alsasotx.org
                                                  www.alsasotx.org
ALS Association chapters are multi-faceted grass roots organizations that carry out ALSA's mission and strategic goals at the community level. he chapter — with supporting services from the National Office — actively pursues the Association's goals.
Bonnie Walsh, Executive Director
Julia Dyer, Development Associate

Vermont

1028 ALS Association: Northern New England Chapter
The Champlain Mill
10 Ferry Street   603-226-8855
Concord, NH 03301   866-257-6663
                                                  Fax: 603-226-8890
                     e-mail: executive.director@alsanne.org
                                                  www.alsanne.org
ALS Association chapters are multifaceted grass-roots organizations that carry out ALSA's mission and strategic goals at the community level. The chapter — with supporting services from the National Office — actively pursues the Association's goals.
Kathleen L Phillips, Executive Director
Christine Richards, Patient Services Director

Washington

1029 ALS Association: Evergreen Chapter
19115 68th Avenue   425-656-1650
Kent, WA 98032   866-786-7257
                                                  Fax: 425-656-1649
                        e-mail: BeckyMooreED@alsa-ec.org
                                                  webwa.alsa.org
The ALS Association chapters are multifaceted grass-roots organizations that carry out ALSA's mission and strategic goals at the community level. The chapter — with supporting services from the National Office — actively pursues the Association's goals.
Rebecca Moore, Executive Director
Sonja Zimmer, Patient Services Director

1030 ALS Association: Oregon & SW Washington CIO
700 NE Multnomah   503-238-5559
Portland, OR 97232   800-681-9851
                                                  Fax: 503-296-5590
                               e-mail: info@alsa-or.org
                                                  webor.alsa.org
The ALS Association chapters are multifaceted grass-roots organizations that carry out ALSA's mission and strategic goals at the community level. The chapter — with supporting services from the National Office — actively pursues the Association's goals.
Cindy Burdell, Director
Lance Christian, Executive Director

Wisconsin

1031 ALS Association: Southeast Wisconsin Chapter
2505 N 124th Street   262-784-5257
Brookfield, WI 53005   Fax: 262-784-5260
                                 e-mail: info@alsawi.org
                                                  webwi.alsa.org
Begun in 1987 as a support group this chapter is managed by a Board of Directors from all walks of life and disciplines. All mem-

bers share a dedication to carry out the mission of Hope Through Research and Support Through Caring. The goal is to help ALS
Melanie Roach-Bekos, Executive Director
Linda Lehmann, Office Manager

Research Centers

1032 ALS Center at UCSF
350 Parnassus Avenue
San Francisco, CA 94117
415-353-2108
Fax: 415-353-2524
e-mail: alscenter@ucsf.edu
www.ucsf.edu/brain/als
Research serves as a cornerstone for our patient programs allowing us to translate the most recent advancement in therapies drug development and clinical management into care for our patients.
Catherine Lomen-Hoer, Director
Carolyn Rodriguez, Clinical Coordinator

1033 ALS Clinic at Penn Neurological Institute ALS Association Greater Philadelphia Cha
ALS Association Greater Philadelphia Chapter
321 Norristown Road
Ambler, PA 19002
215-643-5434
Fax: 215-643-9307
e-mail: brenda@alsphiladelphia.org
www.pennhealth.com/als
A multidisciplinary center for the evaluation and treatment of amyotrophic lateral sclerosis (ALS) and related disorders.
Brenda Edelm LCSW BCD, Director of Patient Services
Lauren Elman, Associate Medical Director

1034 ALS Clinical Department of Neurology College of Medicine of the University of
College of Medicine of the University of Vermont
89 Beaumont Avenue
Burlington, VT 05405-3456
802-656-2154
Fax: 802-656-8577
e-mail: Rup.Tandan@uvm.edu
www.med.uvm.edu
Clinical care facility for ALS patients.
Daniel Mark Fogel, President
Robert Cioffi, Chair

1035 Center for ALS and Related Diorders The Cleveland Clinic DepartmentOf Neurol
The Cleveland Clinic DepartmentOf Neurology
9500 Euclid Avenue
Cleveland, OH 44195-5227
216-444-5538
800-223-2273
Fax: 216-445-4653
TTY: 216-444-0261
e-mail: andrewd@ccf.org
my.clevelandclinic.org
Clinical care and research facility for ALS patients.
Erik P Pioro, Director
Kathleen M Kelly, ALS Clinical Coordinator

1036 Les Turner Research Laboratory Northwestern University Medical School
Northwestern University Medical School
5550 W Touhy Avenue
Skokie, IL 60077
847-679-3311
888-ALS-1107
Fax: 847-679-9109
e-mail: info@lesturnerals.org
www.lesturnerals.org
Scientists and researchers dedicate their time to discover what causes ALS and find a cure for the disease. The international team of scientists at the Laboratory are internationally recognized for their accomplishments in the field of ALS research.
Harvey Gaffen, President
Wendy Abrams, Executive Director

1037 Mayo Clinic: Department of Neurology
200 First Street SW
Rochester, MN 55905
507-284-2511
Fax: 507-284-0161
TDD: 507-284-9786
www.mayo.edu
Ongoing research and treatment for ALS.
John H Noseworthy MD, President
William C Rupp, MD, Vice President, CEO

1038 Motor Neuron Disease Clinic University of Connecticut Health Center
University of Connecticut Health Center
263 Farmington Avenue
Farmington, CT 06030
860-679-2000
Fax: 860-679-1454
TTY: 860-679-2242
www.uchc.edu
Cato T Laurencin, MD, Vice President

1039 Motor Neuron Disease Program University of Michigan Health System
University of Michigan Health System
1500 E Medical Center Drive
Ann Arbor, MI 48109-316
734-936-6641
Fax: 734-153-53
www.med.umich.edu
Regional clinic that is dedicated to the diagnosis of Amyotrophic Lateral Sclerosis and improving the well-being of patients who have this disease.
Ora Hirsh Pescovitz MD, Vice President
Douglas L Strong, CEO

1040 Neuromuscular and ALS Center The Clinical Academic Building
The Clinical Academic Building
125 Patterson Street
New Brunswick, NJ 08901
732-235-7331
Fax: 732-235-7344
e-mail: nmalsweb@umdnj.edu
www2.umdnj.edu/nmalsweb
A multidisciplinary program for the diagnosis evaluation and long-term management of a host of neuromuscular diseases found in adults.
Jerry Belsh MD, Director
Annmarie Coyne-West, Patient Care Coordinator

1041 New England Medical Center: ALS Laboratory
800 Washington Street
Boston, MA 02111-1533
617-636-5000
Fax: 617-636-8568
www.tuftsmedicalcenter.org
Specializes in Amyotrophic Lateral Sclerosis research.
Ellen Zane, President, CEO
Margret Vosburgh, Chief Operating Officer

1042 Solomon Park Research Institute
12815 NE 124th Street
Kirkland, WA 98034
425-650-2020
800-470-1817
Fax: 425-650-2028
e-mail: pclapshaw@soloman.org
www.solomon.org
Amyotrophic lateral sclerosis research.
Patric Clapshaw, Director
Sheila Dunagan, Office Manager

1043 Stem Cell Research Program University of Wisconsin-Madison
University of Wisconsin-Madison
1500 Highland Avenue
Madison, WI 53705-2280
608-890-0173
Fax: 608- 26- 526
e-mail: gilbert@waisman.wisc.edu
www.waisman.wisc.edu/scrp
The mission of this program is to understand the molecular mechanisms responsible for the proliferation and differentiation of stem cells and assess their safety and efficacy following transplantation into various disease models.
Jacalyn McHugh, Research Program Manager
Anita Bhattacharyya, Principal Ivestigator

1044 Virginia Mason Medical Center Neuroscience Institute
Virginia Mason Medical Center
1100 9th Avenue
Seattle, WA 98101
206-341-1900
888-862-2737
www.virginiamason.org
Clinical care and research.
Gary Kaplan, Chairman, CEO

Support Groups & Hotlines

1045 ALS Association Free Standing Support Groups
ALS Association National Office

27001 Agoura Road
Calabasas Hills, CA 91301-5104

818-880-9007
800-782-4747
Fax: 818-880-9006
e-mail: alsinfo@alsa-national.org
www.alsa.org

We know of support groups in Alabama, California, Florida, Illinois, New York, Oklahoma, Oregon, Puerto Rico, Utah and Virginia.

1046 American Society of Human Genetics
9650 Rockville Pike
Bethesda, MD 20814-3998

301-634-7000
Fax: 301-634-7079
e-mail: estrass@genetics.faseb.org
www.faseb.org

This society will locate a genetic counselor in various areas across the United States for persons with ALS.

1047 Amyotrophic Lateral Sclerosis Toll Free Hotline
ALS Association
27001 Agoura Road
Calabasas Hills, CA 91301-5104

818-880-9007
800-782-4747
Fax: 818-880-9006
e-mail: alsinfo@alsanational.org
www.alsa.org

Informs individuals with ALS and their families of services available through the ALS Association.
Gary Leo, President
Sondi Scheck, VP Operations/Administration

1048 Les Turner Amyotrophic Lateral Sclerosis Foundation
5550 West Touhy
Skokie, IL 60077

847-679-3311
888-257-1107
Fax: 847-679-9109
e-mail: info@lesturnerals.org
www.lesturnerals.org

Support groups offer patients and family members a chance to not feel alone and frustrated in coping with ALS and offers them the support of professionals as well as others who are experiencing similar problems.
Claire Owen, Director Patient Services

1049 National Health Information Center
PO Box 1133
Washington, DC 20013

310-565-4167
800-336-4797
Fax: 301-984-4256
e-mail: info@nhic.org
www.health.gov/nhic

Offers a nationwide information referral service, produces directories and resource guides.

Books

1050 Amyotrophic Lateral Sclerosis: Guide for Patients and Families
Hiroshi Mitsumoto MD, author

Demos Medical Publishing
11 W 42nd Street
New York, NY 10036

212-683-0072
800-532-8663
e-mail: info@demosmedpub.com
www.demosmedpub.com

Covers every aspect of the management of ALS, from clinical features of the disease, to diagnosis, to an overview of symptom management. Major sections deal with medical and rehabilitative management, living with ALS, managing advanced disease, end-of-life issues and resources that can provide support and assistance in this time of need.
450 pages
ISBN: 1-932603-72-7

1051 Complete Bedside Companion: No-Nonsense Advice to Caring for the Seriously Ill
Rodger McFarlane, Philip Bashe, author

Simon & Shuster
1230 Avenue of the Americas
New York, NY 10020

212-698-7000
www.simonandschuster.com

Offers warmth, encouragement, and the medical, legal, financial, and emotional advice you need when caring for an ailing loved one.
1999 544 pages
ISBN: 0-684843-19-6

1052 Easy-to-Swallow, Easy-to-Chew Cookbook
Donna L Weihofen, JoAnne Robbins, Paula A Sullivan, author

Wiley Publishers
111 River Street
Hoboken, NJ 07030-5774

201-748-6000
Fax: 201-748-6088
e-mail: info@wiley.com
www.wiley.com

Presents a collection of more than 150 nutritious recipes that make eating enjoyable and satisfying for anyone who has difficulty chewing or swallowing. Also shares helpful tips and techniques to make eating easier for the elderly and those with such as Parkinson's, AIDS, or head and neck cancers.
256 pages
ISBN: 0-471200-74-1

1053 Journeys with ALS
DLRC Press
PO Box 61661
Virginia Beach, VA 23466

757-473-1130
800-776-0560
e-mail: mary@davidlawrence.com

Compiled by an ALS patient, this book contains 33 first person journeys with ALS. Some are hopeful, some are sad, a few are angry. All are powerful, real-life examples of people doing their best to cope, often with humor and high spirits.
1998
ISBN: 1-880731-58-4

1054 Learning to Fall: the Blessings of an Imperfect Life
Philip Simmons, author

Random House
1745 Broadway
New York, NY 10019

www.randomhouse.com

Philip Simmons was just thirty-five years old in 1993 when he learned that he had ALS, or Lou Gehrig's disease, and was told he had less than five years to live. As a young husband and father, and at the start of a promising literary career, he suddenly had to learn the art of dying. Nine years later, he has succeeded, against the odds, in learning the art of living.
176 pages

1055 Life on Wheels: for the Active Wheelchair User
Gary Karp, author

O'Reilly Media
1005 Gravenstein Highway N
Sebastopol, CA 95472

707-827-7000
800-998-9938
Fax: 707-829-0104
e-mail: orders@oreilly.com
www.oreilly.com

For people who want to take charge of their life experience. Describes medical issues (paralysis, circulation, rehab, cure research); day-to-day living (exercise, skin, bowel and bladder, sexuality, home access, maintaining a wheelchair); and social issues (self-image, adjustement, friends, family, cultural attitudes, activism)
565 pages
ISBN: 1-565922-53-2

1056 Non Chew Cookbook
Wilson Publishing Company
5708 Nicollet Avenue S
Minneapolis, MN 55419

800-843-2409
e-mail: nonchew@excite.com
www.nonchewcookbook.com

Soft food recipes good for the whole family.

1057 Realities in Coping with Progressive Neuromuscular Diseases
Charles Press Publishers
PO Box 15715
Philadelphia, PA 19103

215-561-2786
Fax: 215-561-0191
e-mail: mailbox@charlespresspub.com
www.charlespresspub.com

Focuses on this fundamental question by bringing together the work of 51 eminent authorities on neurology, nursing, psychology, social work, psychiarty, respiratory therapy, pastoral care and other related disciplines.
248 pages Hardcover only
ISBN: 0-914783-20-3

Newsletters

1058 ALS Today
Les Turner ALS Foundation
5550 West Touhy   847-679-3311
Skokie, IL 60077   888-257-1107
                                         Fax: 847-679-9109
                        e-mail: info@lesturnerals.org
                                         www.lesturnerals.org
Offers information on clinical trials, medical updates, recipes, resources and support groups available from the foundation.
3 per year

1059 LINK
ALS Association
27001 Agoura Road   818-880-9007
Calabasas Hills, CA 91301-5104   800-782-4747
                                         Fax: 818-880-9006
                        e-mail: alsinfo@alsa-national.org
                                         www.alsa.org
Offers information on a national level to all patients and chapter members of the ALS Association. Medical updates, loan equipment, resources, hotlines, support groups and news of charity and fundraising events are included as well.

1060 Massachusetts Chapter of the ALS Association Newsletter
Massachusetts Chapter of the ALS Association
7 Lincoln Street   781-245-2133
Wakefield, MA 01880-3021   800-258-3323
Offers information on activities, events, charity and fundraising activities, resources and more for members.
BiMonthly
Ginny DelVecchio, President

1061 Peach Lines
ALS Association of Georgia
3795 Manor House Drive   770-642-7962
Marietta, GA 30062-5147
Chapter newsletter offering information on support groups, meetings, hotlines, resources and reviews the newest technology and daily living aids for persons with ALS in the Georgia area.
BiMonthly

1062 Reaching Out
Orange County Chapter of the ALS Association
16787 Beach Boulevard   949-587-9700
Huntington Beach, CA 92647-4848
Offers information on support groups, meetings, charity events, fundraising activities and more for ALS members in the Orange County area.
BiMonthly

1063 South Texas Chapter of the ALS Association Newsletter
2389 W Military Highway   210-493-1311
San Antonio, TX 78231
Offers chapter information on events, charities, memorials, tributes and resources for persons with ALS and their families.
BiMonthly

1064 ALS News & Views
Western Pennsylvania Chapter-ALS Association
1323 Forbes Avenue   412-261-5940
Pittsburgh, PA 15219-4725
Offers information on resources, medical articles, events, charities, fundraising activities and more for patients with ALS, families and caregivers in the western Pennsylvania region.
8 pages BiMonthly
Rita Patchan, Editor

Pamphlets

1065 Basic Home Care for ALS Patients
ALS Association
1275 K Street NW   818-880-9007
Washington, DC 20005   800-782-4747
                                         Fax: 818-880-9006
                        e-mail: alsinfo@alsa-national.org
                                         www.alsa.org
Provides basic information about home care for people affected by ALS. This booklet is intended as an introductory guide and should be used along with professional medical care from one's physician, nurse and social worker.
Jane H Gilbert, President/CEO

1066 Maintaining Good Nutrition with ALS
ALS Association
1275 K Street NW
Washington, DC 20005   www.alsa.org
Helps people with ALS overcome the obstacles to eating well. Discusses the importance of nutrition to people with ALS and makes suggestions for dealing with various eating problems.
Jane H Gilbert, President/CEO

Audio & Video

1067 Driving Force: A Story of Life
Production House
811 St. John's   847-433-3172
Highland Park, IL 60035   Fax: 847-433-9383
Inspiring video featuring Dr. Frank de Leon Jones, a pychiatrist and ALS patient. Despite his disease and the need for continuous medical ventilation, Dr. de Leon Jones continues his challenging medical practice and physical education responsibilities. This is a film of courage, persistence and love of life. It offers poignant messages for ALS patients, family and caregivers as well as healthcare providers. Available in VHS or DVD.
Howie Samuelson, Executive Director

1068 Living with ALS: Adapting to Breathing Changes/Use of Non Invasive Ventilation
ALS Association
1275 K Street NW
Washington, DC 20005   www.alsa.org
Describes how ALS impacts this vital body function and what can be done to help the person with ALS.
Jane H Gilbert, President/CEO

1069 Living with ALS: Adjusting to Swallowing Difficulties & Good Nutrition
ALS Association
1275 K Street NW
Washington, DC 20005   www.alsa.org
In this video we look at the impact of ALS on swallowing and one's ability to maintain good nutrition. Health care professionals provide guidelines and tips for diet changes and for decision-making regarding a feeding tube; patients and their families share their own experiences and demonstrate their ingenuity in adapting to the changes that weakened swallowing muscles and structures can cause.
2003
Jane H Gilbert, President/CEO

1070 Living with ALS: Communication Solutions & Symptom Management
ALS Association
1275 K Street NW
Washington, DC 20005   www.alsa.org
Jane H Gilbert, President/CEO

1071 Living with ALS: Mobility, Activities of Daily Living, Home Adaptions
ALS Association
1275 K Street NW
Washington, DC 10005   www.alsa.org
This first video, Functioning When Your Mobility is Affected, covers a range of mobility issues that occur with ALS. Our goal is to help you maximize your mobility, independence, safety and

comfort. Health care professionals, persons with ALS and their families not only provide information in this video, but also demonstrate equipment and techniques that can help you maximize your function.
Jane H Gilbert, President/CEO

1072 Ventilation: Decision Making Process
Les Turner ALS Foundation
5550 West Touhy   847-679-3311
Skokie, IL 60077   888-257-1107
Fax: 847-679-9109
e-mail: info@lesturnerals.org
www.lesturnerals.org
Designed for ALS patients, their family members and health professionals. Includes interviews with three ventilator dependent ALS patients, family members and the medical staff from Lois Insolia ALS Center at Northwestern University Medical School. Available for loan to ALS patients.
20 Minutes

Web Sites

1073 Healing Well
www.healingwell.com
A social network and support community for patients, caregivers, and families coping with the daily struggles of diseases, disorders and chronic illness.

1074 Health Finder
www.healthfinder.gov
A government web site where individuals can find information and tools to help you and those you care about stay healthy.

1075 Healthlink USA
www.healthlinkusa.com
Health information concerning treatment, cures, prevention, diagnosis, risk factors, research, support groups, email lists, personal stories and much more. Updated regularly.

1076 Helios Health
www.helioshealth.com
Online resource for your health information. Detailed information about specific health topics, access to expert advice from our Medical Advisory Board, and up-to-date health news.

1077 MedWebPlus
www.medwebplus.com
An independently run site related to everything medical and a few things that aren't.

1078 MedicineNet
www.medicinenet.com
An online resource for consumers providing easy-to-read, authoritative medical and health information.

1079 Medscape
www.medscape.com
Medscape offers specialists, primary care physicians, and other health professionals the Web's most robust and integrated medical information and educational tools.

1080 Neurology Channel
www.neurologychannel.com
Find clearly explained, medically accurate information regarding conditions, including an overview, symptoms, causes, diagnostic procedures and treatment options. On this site it is possible to ask questions and get information from a neurologist and connect to people who have similar health interests.

1081 WebMD
www.webmd.com
Information on Amyotrophic Lateral Sclerosis, including articles and resources.

Description

1082 Arthritis

Arthritis is a nonspecific term meaning inflammation of one or more joints. There are over 100 kinds of arthritis, many of them associated with illnesses of other body systems, such as the skin, gut, or liver. Most cases of arthritis are chronic and involve multiple joints. The three most common are rheumatoid arthritis (RA), osteoarthritis (OA), sometimes called degenerative joint disease, and gouty arthritis, or gout. Juvenile Rheumatoid Arthritis (JRA) affects children.

Rheumatoid arthritis may strike either sex at any age, but typically affects women in the early adult years. It is marked by considerable inflammation, commonly of the hands and feet. RA may also involve the knee, elbow, shoulder, ankle and neck, as well as other body systems in addition to the joints. Osteoarthritis tends to occur later in life, related to repeated wear and tear most commonly on weight-bearing joints, such as the hip and knee. Osteoarthritis often occurs earlier in people who have injured their joints in sports. Gout, which typically affects men in midlife, reflects a disorder in the body's metabolism of uric acid. Its most common feature is excruciating pain in the big toe.

Joints affected by arthritis are typically painful, stiff, and swollen. Nonspecific treatment may be used for arthritis of any sort. This includes the nonsteroidal anti-inflammatory drugs (NSAIDs) and aspirin. Steroids can be injected into the knee in OA and be indicated in an oral form for RA. Severe casesof rheumatoid arthritis are generally treated with more specific drugs that attempt to alter the body's immune system. Gouty arthritis responds to drugs that alter the production and metabolism of uric acid. For any kind of arthritis, local application of heat and cold, as well as physical therapy, are often helpful. In certain cases, joint surgery is recommended.

National Agencies & Associations

1083 American Juvenile Arthritis Organization Arthritis Foundation
Arthritis Foundation
PO Box 7669
Atlanta, GA 30357-0669
404-872-7100
800-283-7800
Fax: 404-872-9559
e-mail: help@arthritis.org
www.arthritis.org
A council established by the Arthritis Foundation which serves the special needs of young people with arthritis and their families. Provides information, inspiration and advocacy by identifying the needs of children with arthritis and speaks out on their behalf.
David E Shuey, Chair
John H Klippel MD, President & CEO

1084 Arthritis & Autoimmunity Research Centre (AARC) Foundation
190 Elizabeth Street
Toronto, Ontario, M5G-2C4
416-340-3388
Fax: 416-340-4896
e-mail: aarc.foundation@aarcf-uhn.ca
uhn.info@uhn.on.ca
Increase awareness of this large family of diseases, which affects over four million Canadians.
Gerri Grant, Executive Director
Pippa Shaddick, Development Manager

1085 Arthritis Foundation
PO Box 7669
Atlanta, GA 30335-669
404-872-7100
800-283-7800
Fax: 404-872-0457
e-mail: help@arthritis.org
www.arthritis.org
A nonprofit organization that depends on volunteers to provide services to help people with arthritis. Supports research to find ways to cure and prevent arthritis and provides services to improve the quality of life for those affected by arthritis. Provides help through information, referrals, speakers bureaus, forums, self-help courses, and various support groups and programs nationwide.
David E Shuey, Chairman, CEO

1086 Arthritis Society
393 University Avenue
Toronto Ontario, M5G 1-1E6
416-979-7228
800-321-1433
Fax: 416-979-8366
e-mail: info@on.arthritis.ca
www.arthritis.ca
Promoting evaluating and funding research in the areas of causes prevention treatment and cures of arthritis.
Steven McNair, CEO/President
Sinead Canavan, Communications/Marketing Manager

1087 Myositis Association
1737 King Street
Alexandria, VA 22314
70- 29- 485
800-821-7356
Fax: 70- 53- 675
e-mail: tma@myositis.org
www.myositis.org
Involves swelling of the muscles. It is an inflammatory myopathies that is a disease of the muscle where there is swelling and loss of muscle.
Bob Goldberg, Executive Director
Theresa R Curry, Communications Manager

1088 National Arthritis and Musculoskeletal & Skin Diseases Information Clearinghouse
National Institutes of Health
31 Center Drive - MSC 2350
Bethesda, MD 20892-2350
301-496-8190
Fax: 301-480-2814
e-mail: niamsinfo@mail.nih.gov
www.niams.nih.gov
Our mission is to support research into the causes treatment and prevention of arthritis and musculoskeletal and skin diseases, the training of basic and clinical scientists to carry out this research and the dissemination of information on research programs.
Stephen I Katz MD PhD, Director
Robert H Carter, Deputy Director

1089 National Institute of Arthritis and Musculoskeletal and Skin Disease (NIAMS)
1 AMS Circle
Bethesda, MD 20892
301-495-4484
877-226-4267
Fax: 301-718-6366
TTY: 301-565-2966
e-mail: niamsinfo@mail.nih.gov
www.niams.nih.gov
The NIAMS Information Clearinghouse provides information about various forms of arthritis and rheumatic disease and bone, muscle, and skin diseases. It distributes patient and professional education materials and refers people to other sources of information.
Stephen I Katz MD, PhD, Director

State Agencies & Associations

Alabama

1090 Alabama Chapter of the Arthritis Foundation
2700 Hwy 280 E
Birmingham, AL 35223-3775
205-979-5700
800-879-7896
Fax: 205-979-4172
e-mail: info.al@arthritis.org
www.arthritis.org
Founded in 1948 this chapter affects thousands of lives through programs services information and referrals public and profes-

sional education and more for residents of Alabama. Research is a great priority of the chapter which supports the advancement
Kristin Whitehurst, Regional VP
Lisa Hemphill, Regional Development Director

Arizona

1091 **Arthritis Foundation: Central Arizona Chapter**
1313 E. Osborn Road   602-264-7679
Phoenix, AZ 85014   800-477-7679
Fax: 602-264-0563
e-mail: info.caz@arthritis.org
www.arthritis.org
A nonprofit health agency serving the needs of Arizona residents with arthritis. This chapter provides arthritis self-help courses, aquatic programs, foundation clubs, a juvenile arthritis parent group, exercise programs and informational brochures.
Warren Rizzo, Chair
Robert Leslie, Vice Chair

1092 **Arthritis Foundation: Greater Southwest Chapter**
1313 E Osborn Road   602-264-7679
Phoenix, AZ 85014   800-477-7679
Fax: 602-264-0563
e-mail: info.caz@arthritis.org
www.arthritis.org
A nonprofit health agency serving the needs of Arizona, New Mexico, El Paso residents with arthritis. This chapter provides self management workshops, aquatic programs, a juvenile arthritis parent and peer group, exercise programs and informational brochures.
Warren Rizzo, Chair
Robert Leslie, Vice Chair

Arkansas

1093 **Arthritis Foundation: Arkansas Chapter**
6213 Father Tribou Street   501-664-7242
Little Rock, AR 72205-3002   800-482-8858
Fax: 501-664-6588
e-mail: info.ar@arthritis.org
www.arthritis.org

Carla Davis, Secretary
Diane Denham, VP Finance/Administration

California

1094 **Arthritis Foundation: Northern California Chapter**
657 Mission Street   415-356-1230
San Francisco, CA 94105-4120   800-464-6240
Fax: 415-356-1240
e-mail: info.nca@arthritis.org
www.arthritis.org
Offers research into the causes of arthritis and more effective treatments; serves people in California with arthritis through information and referral services, exercise programs, self-help courses, education and other activities.
PJ Handelhand, President
Deborah Jackson, Senior VP

1095 **Arthritis Foundation: San Diego Area Chapter**
9089 Clairemont Mesa Boulevard   858-492-1090
San Diego, CA 92123-1288   800-422-8885
Fax: 858-492-9248
e-mail: info.sd@arthritis.org
www.arthritis.org
Offers various programs and services including professional seminars, a speakers bureau, public forums, exercise classes, patient and family support groups, arthritis self-help courses and medical research to the residents of the San Diego area living with arthritis.
Veronica Braun, President
Sandra Hayhurst, Director Health Promotion

1096 **Arthritis Foundation: Southern California Chapter**
800 W 6th Street   323-954-5750
Los Angeles, CA 90017-3775   800-954-2873
Fax: 323-954-5790
e-mail: info.sac@arthritis.org
www.arthritis.org
Cynthia Callihan, Administrative Assistant
Christeen Amloian, Assistant Controller

Colorado

1097 **Arthritis Foundation: Rocky Mountain Chapter**
2280 S Albion Street   303-756-8622
Denver, CO 80222-4906   800-475-6447
Fax: 303-759-4349
e-mail: info.rm@arthritis.org
www.arthritis.org
Serves Colorado, Montana, and Wyoming and is dedicated to finding solutions to over 100 forms of arthritis which affect 43 millions of people nationwide.
Kristie Archer, Programs Coordinator
Laura Rosseisen, President

Connecticut

1098 **Arthritis Foundation: Southern New England Chapter**
35 Cold Spring Road   860-563-1177
Rocky Hill, CT 06067   800-541-8350
Fax: 860-563-6018
e-mail: info.sne@arthritis.org
www.arthritis.org
A resource center for persons in Southern New England, Connecticut, Maine and Vermont with arthritis. Offers self-help courses, exercise programs, aquatic programs, Dial-A-Doctor help line, and physician referrals.
Stephen Evangelista, CEO
Gail Campbell, CFO

District of Columbia

1099 **Arthritis Foundation: Metropolitan Washington Chapter**
2011 Pennsylvania Avenue NW   202-537-6800
Washington, DC 20006   Fax: 202-537-6859
e-mail: info.mwa@arthritis.org
www.arthritis.org
The mission of the Arthritis Foundation is to improve lives through leadership in the prevention control and cure of arthritis and related conditions.
Calaneet Balas, President/CEO
Jacquelyn Hair, Director of Operations

Florida

1100 **Arthritis Foundation: Florida Chapter, Gulf Coast Branch**
3816 W Linebaugh Avenue   813-968-7000
Tampa, FL 33618   800-850-9455
Fax: 941-795-0348
e-mail: info.fl.b4@arthritis.org
www.arthritis.org
Dedicated to improving the quality of life for those in the seven county area of Pinellas, Pasco, Citrus, Levy, Hillsborough, Hernando and Polk, who have one or more of over 100 conditions that comprise the disease known as arthritis. Provides patient education and referral services.
Alexa Simpkins, Events Coordinator
Alvi McConahay, Regional Executive Director

Georgia

1101 **Arthritis Foundation: Georgia Chapter**
2790 Peachtree Road   404-237-8771
Atlanta, GA 30305   800-933-7023
Fax: 404-237-8153
e-mail: info.ga@arthritis.org
www.arthritis.org
A statewide health organization dedicated to reducing the devastating effects of arthritis by offering programs for people with ar-

thritis and their families, information and educational services for people with arthritis, medical professionals and the general public.
Andrea Collins, Vice President Mission Delivery
Christina Lennon, VP Resource Development

Illinois

1102 Arthritis Foundation: Greater Chicago Chapter
35 E Wacker Drive   312-372-2080
Chicago, IL 60601   800-795-0096
                                            Fax: 312-372-2081
                                       e-mail: info.gc@arthritis.org
                                                www.arthritis.org
Offers self-help courses, wellness workshops, educational seminars, aquatic programs, brochures and publications for persons with arthritis in the state of Illinois.
Roxanne Bartol, Information Systems Coordinator
Tom Fite, President

1103 Arthritis Foundation: Greater Illinois Chapter
2621 N Knoxville Avenue   309-682-6600
Peoria, IL 61604-3623   Fax: 309-682-6732
                                    e-mail: greaterillinois@arthritis.org
                                                www.arthritis.org
Craig Rogers, Area Director

Indiana

1104 Arthritis Foundation: Indiana Chapter
615 N Alabama   317-879-0321
Indianapolis, IN 46204   800-783-2342
                                            Fax: 317-876-5608
                                       e-mail: info.in@arthritis.org
                                                www.arthritis.org
Offers programs and services for the arthritis community of Indiana.
Jenny Conder, Area Vice President
BJ Farrell, Director of Development

Iowa

1105 Arthritis Foundation: Iowa Chapter
2600 72nd Street   515-278-0636
Des Moines, IA 50322-4724   866-378-0636
                                            Fax: 515-278-2603
                                       e-mail: info.ia@arthritis.org
                                                www.arthritis.org
Julie Dalrymple, Program Coordinator
Doyle Monsma CFRE, President/CEO

Kansas

1106 Arthritis Foundation: Kansas Chapter
1999 N Amidon Avenue   316-263-0116
Wichita, KS 67203-2122   800-362-1108
                                            Fax: 316-263-3260
                                                www.arthritis.org
Serves 103 counties and is governed by the Volunteer Board of Directors elected from throughout the state. Services offered include water exercise classes, arthritis support groups, children's summer camp, loan closet of hospital equipment and self-help programs.
Dennis Bender, Area VP
Valerie Fairchild, Program Director

Kentucky

1107 Arthritis Foundation: Kentucky Chapter
2908 Brownsboro Road   502-585-1866
Louisville, KY 40206   800-633-5335
                                            Fax: 502-585-1657
                                       e-mail: myoung@arthritis.org
                                                www.arthritis.org
Serves residents of 117 counties in Kentucky and the counties of Floyd and Clark in Indiana. This chapter is a resource center for funding research education programs for health professionals,

community education and support services for people with arthritis.
Barbara Perez, President/CEO
Annette Beach, Annual Giving Coordinator

Maryland

1108 Arthritis Foundation: Maryland Chapter
9505 Reisterstown Road   410-654-6570
Owings Mills, MD 21117   800-365-3811
                                            Fax: 410-654-9270
                                       e-mail: info.md@arthritis.org
                                                www.arthritis.org
This chapter supports research both locally and nationally to help find causes better treatments and ways to prevent the many forms of arthritis. Offers various educational booklets and brochures, a referral service for physician referrals, and other support services.
Barbara Newhouse, CEO
Gail Norman, COO

Massachusetts

1109 Arthritis Foundation: Massachusetts Chapter
29 Crafts Street   617-244-1800
Newton, MA 02458-1287   800-766-9449
                                            Fax: 617-558-7686
                                       e-mail: info.ma@arthritis.org
                                                www.arthritis.org
Offers essential information research programs and services for the close to one million Massachusetts residents with arthritis.
Suha Bekdash, Administrative Assistant
Carmen Quinonez, Finance Manager

Michigan

1110 Arthritis Foundation: Michigan Chapter Chapter and Metro Detroit
1050 Wilshire Drive   248-649-2891
Troy, MI 48084-1564   800-968-3030
                                            Fax: 248-649-2895
                                       e-mail: info.mi@arthritis.org
                                                www.arthritis.org
Supports research to prevent, control, and cure arthritis and related diseases. The Foundation also helps improve the lives of people with arthritis and their families by offering self-help classes, exercise programs, support groups, information and referrals.
Mary Sue Langen, Development Manager
Michelle Glazier, President/CEO

Minnesota

1111 Arthritis Foundation: North Central Chapter
1876 Minnehaha Avenue West   651-644-4108
Saint Paul, MN 55104   800-333-1380
                                            Fax: 651-644-4219
                                       e-mail: info.mn@arthritis.org
                                                www.arthritis.org
A nonprofit organization providing programs and services to anyone affected by arthritis in the Minnesota area. Offers aquatic programs support groups juvenile arthritis support groups, research, grants program and information and referrals.
Chris Davis, Community Development Coordinator
Deb Cassidy, Assistant to the President

Mississippi

1112 Arthritis Foundation: Mississippi Chapter
731 Avignon Drive   601-853-7556
Ridgeland, MS 39157   Fax: 601-853-7516
                                       e-mail: cbaker@arthritis.org
                                                www.arthritis.org
Many Mississippians volunteer their services to help the chapter with fund raising and program support. Programs include land and water based exercise classes, and support groups, direct assistance to needy individuals to purchase arthritis medications and services.
Cynthia Baker, Development Specialist
Pamela Snow, ProgramsÿDirector

Missouri

1113 Arthritis Foundation: Eastern Missouri Chapter
9433 Olive Boulevard
Saint Louis, MO 63132
314-991-9333
800-406-2491
Fax: 314-991-4020
e-mail: info.emo@arthritis.org
www.arthritis.org

Jan Bignall, Director of Development
Karen Shoulders, Director of Programs

1114 Arthritis Foundation: Western Missouri, Greater Kansas City
1900 W 75th Street
Prairie Village, KS 66208
913-262-2233
888-719-5670
Fax: 91- 26- 228
e-mail: info.wmo@arthritis.org
www.arthritis.org

The only organization in the area representing the National Office in support of its international research program and in providing services throughout the bi-state area. Offers a wide range of services and programs to deal with the needs of persons with arthritis.
Sherri Hayes, Director of Operations
Alyson Watkins, Special Events Coordinator

Nebraska

1115 Arthritis Foundation: Nebraska Chapter
600 N 93rd Street
Omaha, NE 68114
402-330-6130
800-642-5292
Fax: 402-330-6167
e-mail: mpuccioni@arthritis.org
www.arthritis.org

For close to 40 years the Arthritis Foundation has been the source for help and hope to the 263 000 Nebraskans and residents of Pottawattamie County Iowa with arthritis. Provides a wide variety of services designed to help people better cope with arthritis.
Cindy Doerr, Program Director/Editor
Marzia Pucci Shields, Executive Director

New Jersey

1116 Arthritis Foundation: New Jersey Chapter
555 Route 1 South
Iselin, NJ 08830
732-283-4300
888-467-3112
Fax: 732-283-4633
e-mail: info.nj@arthritis.org
www.arthritis.org

Offers various programs for the residents of New Jersey including support groups, self-help courses, water exercise and arthritis fitness classes and informational public forums.
Linda Gruskiewicz, President & CEO
Tanya Barbarics, Director

New Mexico

1117 Arthritis Foundation: New Mexico Chapter
1313 E Osborn Road
Phoenix, AZ 85014
602-264-7679
800-477-7679
Fax: 602-264-0563
e-mail: info.caz@arthritis.org
www.arthritis.org

Offers public education information, referrals, educational materials, chapter lending library, professional education resources and support groups for the residents of New Mexico.
Vikki Scarafiotti, President
Angela McTee, Director - New Mexico

New York

1118 Arthritis Foundation: Central New York Chapter
3300 Monroe Avenue
Rochester, NY 14618
585-264-1480
Fax: 585-264-1517
e-mail: info@uny@arthritis.org
www.arthritis.org

Melinda Merante, Executive Director
Nicole Mau, Director

1119 Arthritis Foundation: Long Island Chapter
501 Walt Whitman Road
Melville, NY 11747-2189
631-427-8272
Fax: 631-427-3546
e-mail: into.li@arthritis.org
www.arthritis.org

The mission of the Arthritis Foundation is to fund research to find the cause and cures for arthritis and to improve the quality of life for those affected. There is a wide range of programs available for patients.
Patrick T McAsey, President
Roshane Gillespie, Program Secretary

1120 Arthritis Foundation: New York Chapter
122 E 42nd Street
New York, NY 10168-1898
212-984-8700
Fax: 212-878-5960
e-mail: nfo.ny@arthritis.org
www.arthritis.org

Offers land exercise programs warm water resources and programs, self-help groups and courses, events and activities video clinics, peer support and a lending library to arthritis sufferers in the New York area.
Suzanne Bliss, President CEO

1121 Arthritis Foundation: Rockland/Orange Unit
Helen Hayes Hospital
Route 9W
W Haverstraw, NY 10993
845-947-3000
Fax: 845-429-9602
e-mail: ameyerowitz@arthritis.org
www.arthritis.org

Aviva Meyerowitz, Community Outreach Coordinator
Beatrice Jasanya, Community Outreach Coordinator

North Carolina

1122 Arthritis Foundation: Carolinas Chapter
4530 Park Road
Charlotte, NC 28209
704-529-5166
800-365-3811
Fax: 704-529-0626
e-mail: info.car@arthritis.org
www.arthritis.org

Barbara Newhouse, President CEO
Candy Fuller, Community Development Coordinator

Ohio

1123 Arthritis Foundation: Central Ohio Chapter
3740 Ridge Mill Drive
Hilliard, OH 43026
614-876-8200
Fax: 614-876-8363
e-mail: info.coh@arthritis.org
www.arthritis.org

Offers information and referral services, self-help courses, aquatics program equipment loans, clinics, home assessment and continuing education to help more than 350,000 people in Central Ohio, including over 5,000 children affected with the 100 types of arthritis
Stephanie Houck, Director of Special Events
David Painter, Director of Outreach

1124 Arthritis Foundation: Northeastern Ohio Chapter
4630 Richmond Road
Cleveland, OH 44128-5525
216-831-7000
800-245-2275
Fax: 216-831-1764
e-mail: info.neoh@arthritis.org
www.arthritis.org

Barb Cvelbar, Director of Health Promotion
Cheryl Carter, Director of Development

1125 Arthritis Foundation: Northwestern Ohio Chapter
35 E Wacker Drive
Chicago, IL 60601
31- 37- 208
800-735-0096
Fax: 31- 37- 208
e-mail: info.gc@arthritis.org
www.arthritis.org

Tom Fite, CEO

1126 Arthritis Foundation: Ohio River Valley Chapter
7124 Miami Avenue 513-271-4545
Cincinnati, OH 45243 800-383-6843
Fax: 513-271-4703
e-mail: info.orv@arthritis.org
www.arthritis.org

Barbara Perez, President/CEO
Edith Nixon, Chair

1127 Arthritis Foundation; Great Lakes Region, Northeastern Ohio
4630 Richmond Road 216-831-7000
Cleveland, OH 44128-5525 800-245-2275
Fax: 216-831-1764
e-mail: info.neoh@arthritis.org
www.arthritis.org

Mary L Kudasick, Regional VP

Oklahoma

1128 Arthritis Foundation: Oklahoma Chapter
710 W. Wilshire Blvd 405-936-3366
Oklahoma City, OK 73116 800-627-5486
Fax: 405-936-0617
e-mail: info.ok@arthritis.org
www.arthritis.org

Sherri O'Neil, Executive Director
Sherri Harris, Director Special Events

Pennsylvania

1129 Arthritis Foundation: Central Pennsylvania Chapter
3544 North Progress Avenue 717-763-0900
Harrisburg, PA 17110 800-776-0746
Fax: 717-763-0903
e-mail: info.cpa@arthritis.org
www.arthritis.org

Serves 28 counties in the central Pennsylvania area. More than 441,233 persons in the chapter area are affected with one of the forms of arthritis seriously enough to require medical care. The chapter offers research services, professional education and training, parent and community services and public health education.
Douglas Knepp, Interim Executive Director

Rhode Island

1130 Arthritis Foundation: Southern New England Chapter
35 Cold Spring Road 860-563-1177
Rocky Hill, CT 06067 800-541-8350
Fax: 860-563-6018
e-mail: info.sne@arthritis.org
www.arthritis.org

Offers programs and services for persons in the Rhode Island area who are living with arthritis.
Stephen Evangelista, CEO
Gail Campbell, CFO

Tennessee

1131 Arthritis Foundation: Southeast Region
421 Great Circle Road 615-254-6795
Nashville, TN 37228 800-454-4662
Fax: 615-254-8316
e-mail: info.tn@arthritis.org
www.arthritis.org

This chapter serves the residents of Tennessee by offering arthritis support through Life Improvement Series Classes, exercise programs, educational programs, free information, public forums and seminars.
David Popen Esq, CEO

Texas

1132 Arthritis Foundation: North Texas Chapter
4300 Macarthur 214-826-4361
Dallas, TX 75209-6524 800-442-6653
Fax: 214-824-5842
e-mail: info.ntx@arthritis.org
www.arthritis.org

With over 1.5 million people in the North Texas Chapter area with arthritis, the chapter's mission is to improve lives through leadership in the prevention, control and cure of arthritis and related diseases.
Carla Brandt, CFO/COO
Jane Hynes, Director Administration/Info Systems

Utah

1133 Arthritis Foundation: Utah/Idaho Chapter
448 E 400 S 801-536-0990
Salt Lake City, UT 84111 800-444-4993
Fax: 801-536-0991
e-mail: info.utid@arthritis.org
www.arthritis.org

A nonprofit organization serving individuals with arthritis and their families in Utah and Idaho by providing invaluable services, programs and activities.
Lisa B Fall, President
Leslie Nelson, Program Director

Vermont

1134 Arthritis Foundation: Northern New England Chapter
6 Chenell Drive 603-224-9322
Concord, NH 03301 800-639-2113
Fax: 603-224-3778
e-mail: info.sne@arthritis.org
www.arthritis.org

Stephen Evangelista, CEO
Margaret Duffy, Regional Program Director

Virginia

1135 Arthritis Foundation: Virginia Chapter
3805 Cutshaw Avenue 804-359-1700
Richmond, VA 23230 800-456-4687
Fax: 804-359-4900
e-mail: info.va@arthritis.org
www.arthritis.org

Founded in 1954 this chapter is a nonprofit voluntary health organization dedicated to finding the cause prevention and cure for the entire group of diseases called arthritis. Offered classes books and information to better manage arthritis.
Angela Courtney, Vice President Community Development
C Annie Magnant, President

Washington

1136 Arthritis Foundation: Washington/Alaska Chapter
3876 Bridge Way N 206-547-2707
Seattle, WA 98103 800-746-1821
Fax: 206-547-2707
e-mail: tzuehl@arthritis.org
www.arthritis.org

Offers arthritis help lines and information lines for residents of Washington state. Provides self-help courses arthritis aquatic programs and resources for persons living with various forms of arthritis.
Barbara Osen, North Puget Sound Branch Director
Kim Mellen, Campaign Coordinator

Wisconsin

1137 Arthritis Foundation: Wisconsin Chapter Foundation
1650 S 108th Street 414-321-3933
W Allis, WI 53214-4021 800-242-9945
Fax: 414-321-0365
e-mail: info@wi.arthritis.org
www.arthritis.org

Statewide programs offered. Including aquatics exercise programs, support groups, self-help courses, professional education, public education seminars, advocacy counsel, juvenile arthritis support programs and children's camp information and referral help.

Libraries & Resource Centers

1138   New York Chapter of the Arthritis Foundation
122 East 42nd Street
New York, NY 10168-1898   212-984-8700
                                         Fax: 212-878-5960
                                   e-mail: info.ny@arthritis.org
                                            www.arthritis.org
Offers people with arthritis, their families and all those with an interest in the rheumatic diseases, information on how to live every
day to its fullest, even when affected by a chronic disease.

Research Centers

1139   Affiliated Children's Arthritis Centers of New England
New England Medical Center
750 Washington Street   617-636-7285
Boston, MA 02111-1533   Fax: 617-350-8388
Research organization comprised of a network of 15 territory pedi-
atric centers throughout New England and based at the Floating
Hospital of New England Medical Center.
Jane G Schaller MD, Coordinator

**1140   Arthritis and Musculoskeletal Center: UAB Shelby
Interdisciplinary Biomedical Rese**
Shelby Interdisciplinary Biomedical Research Bldg
1825 University Boulevard   205-934-0245
Birmingham, AL 35294-2182   Fax: 205-934-1564
                                       e-mail: rpk@uab.edu
                                        www.main.uab.edu/amc
Arthritis and related rheumatic disorders are studied.
Robert Kimbe MD, Director
Jennifer A Croker, Executive Administrator

1141   Boston University Arthritis Center
580 Harrison Avenue   617-638-4590
Boston, MA 02118   Fax: 617-638-5226
                                     e-mail: mikyork@bu.edu
                                            www.bumc.bu.edu
The research efforts of the Rheumatology Section relate to basic
biologic mechanisms in the pathogenesis of scleroderma vasculitis
amyloidosis osteoarthritis and systemic lupus erythematosus.
There are concordant research efforts in clinical investigation of
these disorders including testing of novel therapies.
Karen H Antman, Dean
Paul Monach, Associate Fellowship Program Director

**1142   Boston University Medical Campus General Clinical Research
Center**
72 E Concord Street   617-638-4542
Boston, MA 02118   Fax: 617-638-8890
                                      e-mail: jkopp@bu.edu
                          dcc2.bumc.bu.edu/gcrcweb/GCRCcampus.htm
Integral unit of the University Hospital specializing in arthritis and
connective tissue studies.
Courtney Alpert, Administrative Coordinator
Janice Kopp, Executive Director

1143   Brigham and Women's Orthopedica and Arthritis Center
Brigham and Women's Hospital
75 Francis Street   617-732-5500
Boston, MA 02115   800-BWH-9999
                                         TTY: 617-732-6458
                                   www.brighamandwomens.org
Research studies into arthritis and rheumatic diseases.
Matthew Lian MD, Director

**1144   Central Missouri Regional Arthritis Center Stephen's College
Campus**
Stephen's College Campus
1507 E Broadway   573-882-8097
Columbia, MO 65215   Fax: 573-884-5509
                                                    TDD: 0
                                  e-mail: phelpsam@missouri.edu
                                          marrtc.missouri.edu
Research into arthritis and rheumatic diseases.
Amber Phelps, Health Program Specialist

1145   Department of Pediatrics, Division of Rheumatology
Duke University School of Medicine

T909 Children's Health Center   919-684-6575
Durham, NC 27710-1   Fax: 919-684-6616
                                   rheum.pediatrics.duke.edu
Clinical and laboratory pediatric rheumatoid studies.
Laura Schanberg MD, Cochairman
Egla Rabinovich MD, Co-Chairman

1146   Hahnemann University Hospital, Orthopedic Wellness Center
Hahnemann University Hospital
Broad and Vine   215-762-7000
Philadelphia, PA 19107-1511   Fax: 215-762-8109
                                     www.hahnemannhospital.com
Research activity at Hahnemann University into the areas of arthri-
tis.
Dr. Arnold Berman, Director

1147   Medical University of South Carolina
96 Jonathan Lucas Street   843-792-1991
Charleston, SC 29403   800-424-MUSC
                                         Fax: 843-792-7121
                                            www.muschealth.com
Offers basic and clinical research on various types of arthritis.
Richard M Silver, Division Director/Professor
Gary S Gilkeson, Vice Chairman Research

**1148   Medical University of South Carolina: Division of Rheumatology
& Immunology**
96 Jonathan Lucas Street   843-792-1991
Charleston, SC 29403   Fax: 843-792-7121
                                               www.musc.edu
Offers basic and clinical research on various types of arthritis.
Richard M Silver, Division Director/Professor
Gary S Gilkeson, Vice Chairman Research

1149   Multipurpose Arthritis and Musculoskeletal Disease Center
School of Medicine Rheumatology Division
1110 W Michigan Street   317-274-7177
Indianapolis, IN 46202   Fax: 317-274-7792
                                            medicine.iupui.edu
The mission of this center is to pursue major biomedical research
interests relevant to the rheumatic diseases. Current areas of emphasis include articular cartilage biology pathogenesis and treatment of various forms of amyloidosis the pathogenesis of
dermatomyositis and immunologic and biochemical markers of
cartilage breakdown and repair.
Steven Hugenburg MD, Division Director

1150   Oklahoma Medical Research Foundation
825 NE 13th Street   405-271-6673
Oklahoma City, OK 73104-5005   800-522-0211
                                         Fax: 405-271-OMRF
                                     e-mail: contact@omrf.org
                                          www.omrf.ouhsc.edu
Focuses on arthritis and muscoloskeletal disease research.
Dr Paul Kincade, Head of OMRF's Immunobiology
Philip M Silverman PhD, Member

1151   Rehabilitation Institute of Chicago
345 E Superior Street   312-238-1000
Chicago, IL 60611   800-354-7342
                                         TTY: 312-238-1059
                                               www.ric.org
Expertise in treating a range of conditions from the most complex
conditions including cerebral palsy spinal cord injury stroke and
traumatic brain injury to the more common such as arthritis
chronic pain and sports injuries.
Edward B Case, Executive Vice President and Chief Finan
Joanne C Smith, President and Chief Executive Officer

1152   Rosalind Russell Medical Research Center for Arthritis at UCSF
350 Parnassus Avenue   415-476-1141
San Francisco, CA 94117   Fax: 415-476-3526
                                  e-mail: rrac@medicine.ucsf.edu
                                  www.rosalindrussellcenter.ucsf.edu
Arthritis research and its probable causes.
Ephraim P Engelman MD, Director
David Wofsy, Associate Director

1153   University of Michigan: Orthopaedic Research Laboratories
University of Michigan Mott Hospital

109 Zina Pitcher Place
Ann Arbor, MI 48109-2200
734-936-7417
Fax: 734-647-0003
www.orl.med.umich.edu
Develops and studies the causes and treatments for arthritis including new devices and assistive aids.
Dr SA Goldstein, Director

1154 Warren Grant Magnuson Clinical Center
National Institute of Health
9000 Rockville Pike
Bethesda, MD 20892
301-496-2563
800-411-1222
Fax: 301-480-9793
TTY: 866-411-1010
e-mail: prpl@mail.cc.nih.gov
www.clinicalcenter.nih.gov
Established in 1953 as the research hospital of the National Institutes of Health. Designed so that patient care facilities are close to research laboratories so new findings of basic and clinical scientists can be quickly applied to the treatment of patients. Upon referral by physicians, patients are admitted to NIH clinical studies.
John Gallin, Director
David Henderson, Deputy Director for Clinical Care

Support Groups & Hotlines

1155 Arthritis Foundation Information Hotline
PO Box 7669
Atlanta, GA 30357-0669
800-283-7800
e-mail: contactus@arthritis.org
www.arthritis.org
Offers information and referrals, counseling, physicians information and more to persons living with arthritis.
John H Klippel, President/CEO

1156 Kids on the Block Arthritis Programs
Arthritis Foundation
PO Box 19000
Atlanta, GA 31126-1000
404-872-7100
800-283-7800
Fax: 404-872-0457
State and local programs that use puppetry to help children understand what it is like for children and adults who have arthritis.

1157 National Health Information Center
PO Box 1133
Washington, DC 20013
310-565-4167
800-336-4797
Fax: 301-984-4256
e-mail: info@nhic.org
www.health.gov/nhic
Offers a nationwide information referral service, produces directories and resource guides.

Books

1158 250 Tips for Making Life with Arthritis Easier
Arthritis Foundation Distribution Center
PO Box 6996
Alpharetta, GA 30023-6996
800-207-8633
Fax: 770-442-9742
www.arthritis.com
What do aerosol cooking spray and snow-shoveling have in common? Learn the answer to this question, and other clever and handy tips to make your life with or without arthritis easier. Plus learn about helpful serviced you didn't know were available through you bank, post office, phone company, grocery store, and other businesses you frequent.
88 pages

1159 Arthritis 101: Questions You Have, Answers You Need
Arthritis Foundation Distribution Center
PO Box 6996
Alpharetta, GA 30009-6996
800-207-8633
Fax: 770-442-9742
www.arthritis.com
Expert reviewers answer questions about basic arthritis facts, treatments, research, surgery and more. Also, specific information about six common conditions: rheumatoid arthritis, osteoarthritis, osteoporosis, fibromyalgia, lupus and gout.
144 pages

1160 Arthritis Helpbook: A Tested Self-Management Program for Coping
Kate Lorig and James Fries, author
Da Capo Press
Order Department
Jackson, TN 38301
800-343-4499
Fax: 800-351-5073
www.perseusbooksgroup.com/dacapo
This book teaches people proven techniques to reduce pain and increase dexterity, build a calcium-rich diet and maintain a healthy weight, design an exercise program that matches their needs, find tips and gadgets that solve common problems, overcome fatigue, depression, and other troubling feelings associated with these health issues, and learn about all available arthritis medications and surgeries.
2006 288 pages 6th Edition
ISBN: 0-201409-63-1

1161 Arthritis Self-Help Products
Aids for Arthritis
35 Wakefield Drive
Medford, NJ 08055-3204
609-654-6918
www.aidsforarthritis.com
Offers lists of arthritis self-help devices.

1162 Arthritis Self-Management
RA Rapaport Publishing
150 W 22nd Street
New York, NY 10011-2421
212-989-0200
800-234-0923
Fax: 212-989-4786
e-mail: editor@arthritis-self-mgmt.com
Publishes practical, how to information, focusing on the day-to-day and long term aspects of arthritis in a positive and upbeat style. Gives subscribers up-to-date news, facts and advice to help them maintain their wellness and make informed decisions regarding their health.
48+ pages Bi-Monthly
Christine Martin Grove, Editor
Ingrid Strauch, Executive

1163 Arthritis: What Exercises Work
Dava Sobel, Arthur C Klein, author
MacMillan
175 5th Avenue
New York, NY 10010
212-674-5151
800-221-7945
Fax: 212-420-9314
us.macmillan.com
The right exercises for your kind of arthritis, pain-level, age, occupation, and hobbies. The most effective exercises for arthritis available anywhere, supported by medical doctors and backed by the latest research.
200 pages
ISBN: 0-312130-25-1

1164 Arthritis: Your Complete Exercise Guide
Human Kinetics Press
PO Box 5076
Champaign, IL 61825-5076
217-351-5076
800-747-4457
Fax: 217-351-2674
www.humankinetics.com
1993 152 pages Paperback
ISBN: 0-873223-92-6
Steve Ruhlig, Marketing Director

1165 Bone Up on Arthritis
Arthritis Foundation
PO Box 6996
Alpharetta, GA 30009-6996
800-207-8633
Fax: 770-442-9742
www.arthritis.com
A self-help education packet designed for home-study use, this program can improve your pain and function levels by teaching proven self-help techniques.
w/Audio Tapes

1166 Clinical Care in the Rheumatic Disease
Arthritis Foundation Distribution Center

PO Box 6996
Alpharetta, GA 30023-6996 800-207-8633
Fax: 770-442-9742
www.arthritis.com
This book was written for all health professionals caring for people with rheumatic diseases and for students in these disciplines.
224 pages

1167 Educational Rights for Children with Arthritis: A Parents Manual
AJAO
1314 Spring Street NW
Atlanta, GA 30309-2810 404-872-7100
www.arthritis.org/
A self-instructional manual helping parents to identify and obtain school services needed by their child with arthritis. Covers laws and special services, explores strategies for working with school personnel and stresses good communication and advocacy techniques.

1168 Exercise Beats Arthritis
Bull Publishing Company
PO Box 1377
Boulder, CO 80306 800-676-2855
Fax: 303-545-6354
www.bullpub.com
Easy-to-follow program will help arthritis sufferers of all ages manage the problems of living with this condition. In depth look at minimizing the pain and limitations of arthritis, keep their joints mobile, increase muscle strength, strengthen bones and ligaments, perform daily tasks more easily.
1998 144 pages
ISBN: 0-923521-45-3

1169 Help Yourself Cookbook
Arthritis Foundation
PO Box 6996
Alpharetta, GA 30023-6996 800-207-8633
Fax: 770-442-9742
www.arthritis.com

158 pages

1170 Living With Rheumatoid Arthritis
John's Hopkins University Press
2715 N Charles Street
Baltimore, MD 21218-4319 410-516-6900
800-537-5487
Fax: 410-516-6998
www.press.jhu.edu
This book offers practical and usable answers to the questions of everyday life. The authors provide clear explanations of the causes, diagnosis and treatment of the disease and why medication, joint protection, physical activity and good nutrition are essential components of care.
1993 312 pages Paperback
ISBN: 0-801871-47-6

1171 Personal Guide to Living Well with Fibromyalgia
Arthritis Foundation Distribution Center
PO Box 6996
Alpharetta, GA 30023-6996 800-207-8633
Fax: 770-442-9742
www.arthritis.com
With this guide you'll learn the latest information about fibromyalgia, what researchers have uncovered about its causes, and an overview of the best treatment options available. Helpful worksheets and tables allow you to manage your condition and document your progress.
224 pages

1172 Primer on the Rheumatic Diseases
John H Klippel, author
Springer Publishing
233 Spring Street
New York, NY 10013 212-460-1500
Fax: 212-460-1575
e-mail: service-ny@springer.com
www.springer.com
Designed to provide up-to-date information about the major clinical syndromes. One of the most prestigious and comprehensive texts on arthritis and related diseases, including osteoarthritis,

rheumatoid arthritis, osteoporosis, lupus, and more than one hundred others.
724 pages
ISBN: 0-387356-64-8

1173 Toward Healthy Living: A Wellness Journal
Arthritis Foundation Distribution Center
PO Box 6996
Alpharetta, GA 30023-6996 800-207-8633
Fax: 770-442-9742
www.arthritis.com
This spiral-bound journal has ample pages where you can record your thoughts, plus scales to monitor your mood and pain. Throughout the book you will also find wisdom from a variety of famous and ordinary people - those who live with chronic ilness, and those whose life lessons can help you gain a more positive outlook on daily living.
144 pages

1174 Understanding Juvenile Rheumatoid Arthritis
American Juvenile Arthritis Organization
PO Box 19000
Atlanta, GA 31126-1000 800-283-7800
A manual for health professionals to use in teaching children with JRA and their families about disease management and self-care.
372 pages

1175 We Can: A Guide for Parents of Children with Arthritis
AJAO
1330 W Peachtree Street NW
Atlanta, GA 30309-2904 404-872-7100
www.arthritis.org/
Offers parents tips for daily living and practical points for helping their child toward independent adulthood.

Children's Books

1176 Arthritis
Franklin Watts Grolier
90 Old Sherman Turnpike
Danbury, CT 06816-0001 203-797-3500
800-621-1115
Fax: 203-797-3197
www.grolier.com
This book offers a clear explanation of the various forms and effects of the disease of arthritis and what treatments are available.
96 pages Grades 7-12
ISBN: 0-531108-01-5

1177 JRA and Me
American Juvenile Arthritis Organization
PO Box 19000
Atlanta, GA 31126-1000 800-283-7800
A workbook for school-aged children who have juvenile arthritis. This book offers a variety of educational games, puzzles and worksheets to teach children about their illness and how to take care of themselves.
57 pages

1178 Living with Arthritis
Franklin Watts Grolier
90 Old Sherman Turnpike
Danbury, CT 06816-0001 203-797-3500
800-621-1115
Fax: 203-797-3197
www.grolier.com
Shows how people with arthritis can overcome their pain and lead productive, full lives.
32 pages Grades 5-7

1179 Yard Sale Coloring Book
American Juvenile Arthritis Organization
PO Box 19000
Atlanta, GA 31126-1000 800-283-7800
A coloring/activity book based on a Kids on the Block script, written for third and fourth grade students. It can be used with Kids on the Block performances, as a stand-alone piece or with a free lesson plan packet.

Magazines

1180 Arthritis Today
Arthritis Foundation
1330 W Peachtree Street NW   404-872-7100
Atlanta, GA 30309-2922
Fax: 404-872-9559
The authoritative and respected source of information for persons with arthritis, their families and health professionals who manage their care. As the official magazine of the Arthritis Foundation, it is backed by the Foundation's experience of 44 years and leadership in the fight against arthritis. This magazine gives its readers the advice, information and inspiration they need to live better with arthritis.
Monthly

Newsletters

1181 AJAO Newsletter
American Juvenile Arthritis Organization
1330 W Peachtree Street NW
Atlanta, GA 31126-2904   404-872-7100
www.arthritis.org/answers
Offers information and updates about the organization's activities and events. Legislative information, medical updates, camp information and more for children living with arthritis.
Quarterly
Janet Austin MEd, Editor

1182 Arthritis Accent
Arthritis Foundation Southern N.E. Chapter
35 Cold Spring Road   860-563-1177
Rocky Hill, CT 06067-3166   800-541-8350
Fax: 860-563-6018
Information on chapter events and activities.
Quarterly

1183 Arthritis Foundation of Illinois
Greater Chicago Chapter
29 East Madison   312-372-2080
Chicago, IL 60602   800-735-0096
Fax: 312-372-2081
e-mail: info.gc@arthritis.org
www.arthritis.org
Marilynn J Cason, Chairman

1184 Arthritis Foundation: Newsletter of Nebraska Chapter
10846 Old Mill Road   402-330-6130
Omaha, NE 68154   800-642-5292
Fax: 402-330-6167
e-mail: mpuccioni@arthritis.org
www.arthritis.org
Contains information on research, medication, different types of arthritis and features on oustanding volunteers.
3x Year
Cindy Doerr, Program Director/Editor

1185 Arthritis Foundation: Southern Arizona Chapter
6464 E Grant Road   520-290-9090
Tucson, AZ 85715   800-444-5426
Offers updated information and news on chapter activities and events for persons with arthritis.
Monthly
Richard M Brown EdD, CFRE, President

1186 Arthritis News
Arthritis Foundation - WI Chapter
1650 S 108th Street   414-321-3933
West Allis, WI 53214   800-242-9945
Fax: 414-321-0365
e-mail: info.wi@arthritis.org
www.arthritis.org
Offers information on activities, events, medical research, information and referrals to persons living in the Wisconsin area that are afflicted with arthritis.
Quarterly
Judy Haugsland, CEO

1187 Arthritis Observer
Rocky Mountain Chapter of the Arthritis Foundation
2280 S Albion Street   303-756-8622
Denver, CO 80222-4906   800-475-6647
Fax: 303-759-4349
e-mail: info.m@arthritis.org
www.arthritis.org
Offers chapter information and educational programs to the community as well as updates on fund-raising events, resources, publications and medical updates for the arthritis community.
Quarterly

1188 Arthritis Reporter
New York Chapter of the Arthritis Foundation
122 E 42nd Street   212-984-8700
New York, NY 10168-0002   Fax: 212-878-5960
e-mail: info.ny@arthritis.org
www.arthritis.org
Chapter newsletter offering information on upcoming events, activities and groups for the arthritis community.
Quarterly

1189 Arthritis Update of Rhode Island
Arthritis Foundation Rhode Island Office
Airport Office Park   401-739-3773
Warwick, RI 02886   Fax: 401-739-8990
e-mail: info.sne@arthritis.org
www.arthritis.org
Offers information, activities, events and updates on the chapter.
Quarterly

1190 Arthritis Volunteer
Tennessee Chapter of the Arthritis Foundation
1719 W End Avenue   615-320-7626
Nashville, TN 37203-5123   Fax: 615-329-3982
Keeps members up-to-date on arthritis developments and on programs, services and special events in Tennessee.
Quarterly

1191 Factor Fax
Arthritis Foundation: Northeast California Chapter
3040 Explorer Drive   916-368-5599
Sacramento, CA 95827   800-571-3456
Fax: 916-368-5596
e-mail: info.neca@arthritis.org
www.arthritis.org
Offers information on all of the chapter's activites, events and resources for the arthritis community of central California.
Patrick Dunlap, VP Events/Programs/Services
Edward Kelley, Motion Coordinator

1192 Focus
Arthritis Foundation: Central Ohio Chapter
3740 Ridge Mill Drive   614-876-8200
Hilliard, OH 43026-9231   Fax: 614-876-8363
www.arthritis.org
Offers updated information on arthritis as well as news of the services and activities of the chapter.
Quarterly
Irene Baird, President

1193 Health Points
TyH Publications
17007 E Colony Drive
Fountain Hills, AZ 85268   800-801-1406
e-mail: editor@e-tyh.com
National newsletter with articles on complementary therapy, latest nutrition news, disability issues and much more. Focus is on fibromyalgia, chronic fatigue, arthritis and chronic pain.
Quarterly

1194 News Across Our Horizons
Northern & Southern New England Chapter
35 Cold Spring Road   860-563-1177
Rocky Hill, CT 06060   800-541-8350
Fax: 860-563-6018
e-mail: info.sne@arthritis.org
www.arthritis.org

Chapter newsletter offering information on programs, activities and events of the foundation, medical and research articles and resources for persons with arthritis.

1195   Newsletter of the Central Pennsylvania Chapter
Central Pennsylvania Chapter/Arthritis Foundation
17 S 19th Street   717-763-0900
Camp Hill, PA 17011-5459   800-776-0746
                                                                   Fax: 717-763-0903
                                              e-mail: info.cpa@arthritis.org
                                                                 www.arthritis.org
Offers information on activities and events of the Chapter.
Quarterly

1196   Spectrum
Michigan Chapter of the Arthritis Foundation
1050 Wilshire Drive   248-649-2891
Troy, MI 48084-1564   800-968-3030
                                                                  Fax: 248-649-2895
                                               e-mail: info.mi@arthritis.org
                                                                 www.arthritis.org
Promotes various activities and programs and provides current information about arthritis.

1197   Volunteer Voice
Kentucky Chapter of the Arthritis Foundation
410 W Chestnut Street   502-893-9771
Louisville, KY 40202-2368   800-633-5335
Newsletter offering information and updates on chapter activities, events, camps, juvenile programs and government/legislative information.

Pamphlets

1198   Americans with Disabilities Act Resource Manual
Arthritis Foundation
PO Box 7669   404-872-7100
Atlanta, GA 30357-0669   800-283-7800
                                                                  Fax: 404-872-0457

1199   Ankylosing Spondylitis
Arthritis Foundation
PO Box 7669   404-872-7100
Atlanta, GA 30357-0669   800-283-7800
                                                                  Fax: 404-872-0457

1200   Arthritis Answers: Basic Information About Arthritis
Arthritis Foundation
PO Box 7669   404-872-7100
Atlanta, GA 30357-0669   800-283-7800
                                                                  Fax: 404-872-0457

1201   Arthritis Foundation Services
Arthritis Foundation
PO Box 7669   404-872-7100
Atlanta, GA 30357-0669   800-283-7800
                                                                  Fax: 404-872-0457

1202   Arthritis Information: Advocacy and Government Affairs
Arthritis Foundation
PO Box 7669   404-872-7100
Atlanta, GA 30357-0669   800-283-7800
                                                                  Fax: 404-872-0457

1203   Arthritis Information: Children
Arthritis Foundation
PO Box 7669   404-872-7100
Atlanta, GA 30357-0669   800-283-7800
                                                                  Fax: 404-872-0457
List of materials for children with arthritis, their families and the health professionals who care for them.

1204   Arthritis and Diet Information Package
NAMSIC/National Institutes of Health
1 AMS Circle   301-495-4484
Bethesda, MD 20892-0001   877-226-4267
                                                                  Fax: 301-718-6366
                                                                  TTY: 301-565-2966
                                       e-mail: niamsinfo@mail.nih.gov
                                                                www.nih.gov/niams/

Offers information on nutrition and diet pertaining to the arthritis community.
16 pages

1205   Arthritis and Employment: You Can Get the Job You Want
Arthritis Foundation
PO Box 7669   404-872-7100
Atlanta, GA 30357-0669   800-283-7800
                                                                  Fax: 404-872-0457

1206   Arthritis and Inflammatory Bowel Disease
Arthritis Foundation
PO Box 7669   404-872-7100
Atlanta, GA 30357-0669   800-283-7800
                                                                  Fax: 404-872-0457

1207   Arthritis and Pregnancy
Arthritis Foundation
PO Box 7669   404-872-7100
Atlanta, GA 30357-0669   800-283-7800
                                                                  Fax: 404-872-0457
How arthritis affects pregnancy, managing pregnancy and a new baby.

1208   Arthritis and Vocational Rehabilitation
Arthritis Foundation
2970 Peachtree Road NW   404-237-8771
Atlanta, GA 30305   800-933-7023
                                                                  Fax: 404-237-8153
                                                e-mail: info.ga@arthritis.org
                                                                 www.arthritis.org

1209   Arthritis in Children Information Package
NAMSIC/National Institutes of Health
1 AMS Circle   301-495-4484
Bethesda, MD 20892-0001   877-226-4267
                                                                  Fax: 301-718-6366
                                                                  TTY: 301-565-2966
                                       e-mail: niamsinfo@mail.nih.gov
                                                                www.nih.gov/niams/

1210   Arthritis in Children and La Artritis Infantojuvenil
American Juvenile Arthritis Organization
PO Box 19000
Atlanta, GA 31126-1000   800-283-7800
A medical information booklet about juvenile rheumatoid arthritis. This booklet is written for parents or other adults and includes details about different forms of JRA, medications, therapies and coping issues.

1211   Arthritis on the Job: You Can Work With It
Arthritis Foundation
PO Box 7669   404-872-7100
Atlanta, GA 30357-0669   800-283-7800
                                                                  Fax: 404-872-0457

1212   Arthritis: Do You Know?
Arthritis Foundation
PO Box 7669   404-872-7100
Atlanta, GA 30357-0669   800-283-7800
                                                                  Fax: 404-872-0457
A brief overview of arthritis and the services of the Arthritis Foundation.

1213   Aspirin and Other Nonsteroidal Anti-Inflamatory Drugs
Arthritis Foundation
PO Box 7669   404-872-7100
Atlanta, GA 30357-0669   800-283-7800
                                                                  Fax: 404-872-0457

1214   Back Pain
Arthritis Foundation
PO Box 7669   404-872-7100
Atlanta, GA 30357-0669   800-283-7800
                                                                  Fax: 404-872-0457

1215   Behcet's Disease
Arthritis Foundation
PO Box 7669   404-872-7100
Atlanta, GA 30357-0669   800-283-7800
                                                                  Fax: 404-872-0457

**1216 Bursitis, Tendionitis and Other Soft Tissue Rheumatic
Syndromes**
Arthritis Foundation
PO Box 7669   404-872-7100
Atlanta, GA 30357-0669   800-283-7800
                                     Fax: 404-872-0457

1217 CPPD Crystal Deposition Disease
Arthritis Foundation
PO Box 7669   404-872-7100
Atlanta, GA 30357-0669   800-283-7800
                                     Fax: 404-872-0457

1218 Corticosteriod Medications
Arthritis Foundation
PO Box 7669   404-872-7100
Atlanta, GA 30357-0669   800-283-7800
                                     Fax: 404-872-0457

1219 Diet and Arthritis
Arthritis Foundation
PO Box 7669   404-872-7100
Atlanta, GA 30357-0669   800-283-7800
                                     Fax: 404-872-0457

1220 Ehlers-Danlos Syndrome
Arthritis Foundation
PO Box 7669   404-872-7100
Atlanta, GA 30357-0669   800-283-7800
                                     Fax: 404-872-0457

1221 Exercise and Your Arthritis
Arthritis Foundation
PO Box 7669   404-872-7100
Atlanta, GA 30357-0669   800-283-7800
                                     Fax: 404-872-0457
Types of exercise for people with arthritis and how to do them.

1222 Family
Arthritis Foundation
PO Box 7669   404-872-7100
Atlanta, GA 30357-0669   800-283-7800
                                     Fax: 404-872-0457
Effects of arthritis on family life and ways to cope.

1223 Family: Making the Difference
Arthritis Foundation
PO Box 7669   404-872-7100
Atlanta, GA 30357-0669   800-283-7800
                                     Fax: 404-872-0457

1224 Gold Treatment
Arthritis Foundation
PO Box 7669   404-872-7100
Atlanta, GA 30357-0669   800-283-7800
                                     Fax: 404-872-0457

1225 Gout
Arthritis Foundation
PO Box 7669   404-872-7100
Atlanta, GA 30357-0669   800-283-7800
                                     Fax: 404-872-0457

1226 Guide to Effective Volunteer Lobbying
Arthritis Foundation
PO Box 7669   404-872-7100
Atlanta, GA 30357-0669   800-283-7800
                                     Fax: 404-872-0457

1227 Health, Life and Disability Insurance for People with Arthritis
Arthritis Foundation
PO Box 7669   404-872-7100
Atlanta, GA 30357-0669   800-283-7800
                                     Fax: 404-872-0457
Information about these three types of insurance.

1228 Hydroxychloroquine
Arthritis Foundation
PO Box 7669   404-872-7100
Atlanta, GA 30357-0669   800-283-7800
                                     Fax: 404-872-0457

1229 Individuals with Arthritis
Mainstream
1030 5th Street NW   202-898-1400
Washington, DC 20001-2504
Mainstreaming individuals with arthritis into the workplace.
12 pages

1230 Juvenile Dermatomyositis
Arthritis Foundation
PO Box 7669   404-872-7100
Atlanta, GA 30357-0669   800-283-7800
                                     Fax: 404-872-0457
                                     www.arthritis.org

1231 Living and Loving: Information About Sexuality and Intimacy
Arthritis Foundation
PO Box 7669   404-872-7100
Atlanta, GA 30357-0669   800-283-7800
                                     Fax: 404-872-0457

1232 Managing Your Activities
Arthritis Foundation
PO Box 7669   404-872-7100
Atlanta, GA 30357-0669   800-283-7800
                                     Fax: 404-872-0457

1233 Managing Your Fatigue
Arthritis Foundation
PO Box 7669   404-872-7100
Atlanta, GA 30357-0669   800-283-7800
                                     Fax: 404-872-0457

1234 Managing Your Health Care
Arthritis Foundation
PO Box 7669   404-872-7100
Atlanta, GA 30357-0669   800-283-7800
                                     Fax: 404-872-0457

1235 Managing Your Pain
Arthritis Foundation
PO Box 7669   404-872-7100
Atlanta, GA 30357-0669   800-283-7800
                                     Fax: 404-872-0457

1236 Managing Your Stress
Arthritis Foundation
PO Box 7669   404-872-7100
Atlanta, GA 30357-0669   800-283-7800
                                     Fax: 404-872-0457

1237 Methotrexate
Arthritis Foundation
PO Box 7669   404-872-7100
Atlanta, GA 30357-0669   800-283-7800
                                     Fax: 404-872-0457

1238 Myositis
Arthritis Foundation
PO Box 7669   404-872-7100
Atlanta, GA 30357-0669   800-283-7800
                                     Fax: 404-872-0457

1239 Osteoarthritis
Arthritis Foundation
PO Box 7669   404-872-7100
Atlanta, GA 30357-0669   800-283-7800
                                     Fax: 404-872-0457
Offers introductions, examples, explanations and research pertaining to this type of arthritis.

1240 Osteonecrosis
Arthritis Foundation
PO Box 7669   404-872-7100
Atlanta, GA 30357-0669   800-283-7800
                                     Fax: 404-872-0457

1241 Overcoming Rheumatoid Arthritis
Michigan Chapter of the Arthritis Foundation

1050 Wilshire Drive
Troy, MI 48084-1564

248-649-2891
800-968-3030
Fax: 248-649-2895
e-mail: info.mi@arthritis.org
www.arthritis.org

Provides extensive information about the disease and treatment, with an emphasis on what you can do for yourself.

1242 Penicillamine
Arthritis Foundation
PO Box 7669
Atlanta, GA 30357-0669

404-872-7100
800-283-7800
Fax: 404-872-0457

1243 Polyarteritis Nodosa and Wegener's Granulomatosis
Arthritis Foundation
PO Box 7669
Atlanta, GA 30357-0669

404-872-7100
800-283-7800
Fax: 404-872-0457

1244 Polymyalgia Rheumatica and Giant Cell Arthritis
Arthritis Foundation
PO Box 7669
Atlanta, GA 30357-0669

404-872-7100
800-283-7800
Fax: 404-872-0457

1245 Pseudoxanthoma Elasticum Fact Sheet
Arthritis Foundation
PO Box 7669
Atlanta, GA 30357-0669

404-872-7100
800-283-7800
Fax: 404-872-0457

1246 Psoriatic Arthritis Information Package
NAMSIC/National Institutes of Health
1 AMS Circle
Bethesda, MD 20892-0001

301-495-4484
877-226-4267
Fax: 301-718-6366
TTY: 301-565-2966
e-mail: niamsinfo@mail.nih.gov
www.nih.gov/niams/

1247 Q&A's About Arthritis and Rheumatic Disease
NIH/National Institutes of Health
1 AMS Circle
Bethesda, MD 20892-0001

301-495-4484
877-226-4267
Fax: 301-718-6366
TTY: 301-565-2969
e-mail: niamsinfo@mail.nih.gov
www.nih.gov/niams

This pamphlet offers information, technical articles and research on arthritis and related disorders. Also included are referral organizations to help patients uncover more information.

1248 Reflex Sympathetic Dystrophy Syndrome Fact Sheet
Arthritis Foundation
PO Box 7669
Atlanta, GA 30357-0669

404-872-7100
800-283-7800
Fax: 404-872-0457

1249 Reiter's Syndrome
Arthritis Foundation
PO Box 7669
Atlanta, GA 30357-0669

404-872-7100
800-283-7800
Fax: 404-872-0457

1250 Rheumatoid Arthritis Information Package
NAMSIC/National Institutes of Health
1 AMS Circle
Bethesda, MD 20892-0001

301-495-4484
877-226-4267
Fax: 301-718-6366
TTY: 301-565-2966
e-mail: niamsinfo@mail.nih.gov
www.nih.gov/niams

Offers an introduction and definition of rheumatoid arthritis, treatments, causes, objectives, daily living, resources and medical information.

1251 Surgery: Information to Consider
Arthritis Foundation
PO Box 7669
Atlanta, GA 30357-0669

404-872-7100
800-283-7800
Fax: 404-872-0457

1252 Thinking About Tomorrow: A Career Guide for Teens with Arthritis
Arthritis Foundation
PO Box 7669
Atlanta, GA 30357-0669

404-872-7100
800-283-7800
Fax: 404-872-0457

1253 When Your Student Has Arthritis: A Guide for Teachers
Arthritis Foundation
PO Box 7669
Atlanta, GA 30357-0669

404-872-7100
800-283-7800
Fax: 404-872-0457

A medical information booklet written for teachers or other adults who have arthritis. The booklet describes different forms of juvenile arthritis, how arthritis might affect the child at school, and how to help the child work around these problems.

Audio & Video

1254 FIT Video
Arthritis Foundation
550 Pharr Road
Altlanta, GA 30023-6996

404-237-8771
800-933-7023
Fax: 404-237-8153
e-mail: info.ga@arthritis.org
www.arthritis.org

1255 In Control
Arthritis Foundation
1330 W Peachtree Street NW
Atlanta, GA 30309-2922

404-872-7100
800-283-7800
Fax: 404-872-0457

An excellent at-home program which includes video, audio cassettes and the Arthritis Helpbook. Provides tools to help meet the challenges of arthritis.

1256 PACE I
Arthritis Foundation
PO Box 6996
Alpharetta, GA 30023-6996

800-207-8633

1257 PACE II
Arthritis Foundation
PO Box 6996
Alpharetta, GA 30023-6996

800-207-8633
Fax: 770-442-9742
www.arthritis.com

1258 Pathways to Better Living
Arthritis Foundation
PO Box 6996
Alpharetta, GA 30023-6996

800-207-8633
Fax: 770-442-9742
www.arthritis.com

1259 Pool Exercise Program
Arthritis Foundation Distribution Center
PO Box 6996
Alpharetta, GA 30023-6996

800-207-8633
Fax: 770-442-9742
www.arthritis.com

This video features water exercises that will help you increase and maintain joint flexibility, strengthen and tone muscles, and increase endurance. All exercises are performed in water at chest level. No swimming skills are necessary.

Web Sites

1260 American Juvenile Arthritis Organization

www.arthritis.com

Serves the special needs of young people with arthritis and their families. Provides information, inspiration and advocacy.

1261 Arthritis Foundation

www.arthritis.org

Provide services to help through information, referrals, speakers bureaus, forums, self-help courses, and various support groups and programs nationwide.

1262 Healing Well

www.healingwell.com

An online health resource guide to medical news, chat, information and articles, newsgroups and message boards, books, disease-related web sites, medical directories, and more for patients, friends, and family coping with disabling diseases, disorders, or chronic illnesses.

1263 Health Finder

www.healthfinder.gov

Searchable, carefully developed web site offering information on over 1000 topics. Developed by the US Department of Health and Human Services, the site can be used in both English and Spanish.

1264 Healthlink USA

www.healthlinkusa.com

Health information concerning treatment, cures, prevention, diagnosis, risk factors, research, support groups, email lists, personal stories and much more. Updated regularly.

1265 Helios Health

www.helioshealth.com

Online resource for your health information. Detailed information about specific health topics, access to expert advice from our Medical Advisory Board, and up-to-date health news.

1266 MedicineNet

www.medicinenet.com

An online resource for consumers providing easy-to-read, authoritative medical and health information.

1267 Medscape

www.medscape.com

Medscape offers specialists, primary care physicians, and other health professionals the Web's most robust and integrated medical information and educational tools.

1268 National Arthritis & Musculoskeletal & Skin Diseases Information Clearinghouse

www.nih.gov/niams

Provides clinical and public information and research to increase understanding of the many rheumatic diseases and related disorders. Also provides lists and order forms for their resources and materials.

1269 WebMD

www.webmd.com

Information on arthritis, including articles and resources.

Description

1270 Asthma

Asthma is a respiratory disorder that causes shortness of breath, wheezing, coughing and chest tightness. About 12 million people in the U.S. have asthma, and its incidence is increasing. It is the leading cause of hospitalization for children; however, some children with asthma will outgrow the disorder by the time they are teenagers or adults. Asthma ranges from mild illness to life-threatening episodes.

Numerous environmental factors trigger an asthma attack including allergies, infections, exercise, cold weather and stress. Treatment consists of avoiding or minimizing factors that cause an asthma attack, for example pet dander and pollen.

In addition, several medications are used to relieve asthma symptoms by opening lung airways, known as bronchodilation. Many of these drugs can be inhaled so that they work directly on the lungs. Inhaled steroids may be used for long-term control. Research and new therapies are being directed at trying to find medications that will prevent asthma from occurring. See also *Lung Disease.*

National Agencies & Associations

1271 Allergy & Asthma Network Mothers of Asthmatics
2751 Prosperity Avenue   703-641-9595
Fairfax, VA 22031   800-878-4403
                                           Fax: 30- 40- 298
                                     e-mail: info@aanma.org
                                       www.breatherville.org
A national nonprofit network of families with a desire to overcome allergies and asthma by producing the most accurate timely practical and livable alternatives to suffering.
Nancy Sander, Founder/President
Hiwote Aberra, Database/Member Services Coordinator

1272 American Academy of Allergy, Asthma & Immunology
555 East Wells Street   414-272-6071
Milwaukee, WI 53202-3823   800-822-2762
                                           Fax: 414-272-6070
                                      e-mail: info@aaaai.org
                                             www.aaaai.org
Strives to serve the public through information on asthma and allergies, as well as referrals to allergists. Also offers pollen and mold statistics from the Committee on Pollen & Molds.
Thomas B Casale, Executive Vice President
Kay A Walen, Executive Director

1273 American Lung Association
1301 Pennsylvania Avenue NW   202-785-3355
Washington, DC 20004   800-LUN-GUSA
                                           Fax: 202-452-1805
                                     e-mail: info@lungusa.org
                                             www.lungusa.org
The mission of the American Lung Association is to prevent lung disease and promote lung health. Founded in 1904 to fight tuberculosis, the American Lung Association today fights disease in all its forms, with special emphasis on asthma, tobacco control and environmental health.
Charles Dean O'Conner, President, CEO
Don Awerkamp, Director

1274 Association of Birth Defect Children Birth Defect Research for Children
800 Celebration Avenue   407-566-8304
Celebration, FL 34747   Fax: 407-566-8341
                                 e-mail: staff@birthdefects.org
                                          www.birthdefects.org
Non-profit organization that provides parents and expectant parents with information about birth defects and support services for their children. Sponsors the National Birth Defect Registry, a research project that studies associations between birth defects and genetics.
Betty Mekdeci, Contact

1275 Asthma Society of Canada
4950 Yonge Street   416-787-4050
Toronto, Ontario, M2N-6K1   866-787-4050
                                           Fax: 416-787-5807
                                       e-mail: info@asthma.ca
                                               www.asthma.ca
A national registered healthcare charity, operating within a civil society business structure.
Christine Hampson, Ph.D., President, CEO
Dr. Oxana Latycheva, Ph.D., CAE, Vice President, Programming

1276 Asthma and Allergy Information Association
8201 Coprorate Drive   202-466-7643
Lanover, MD 20785   800-727-8462
                                           Fax: 202-466-8940
                                        e-mail: info@aafa.org
                                               www.aafa.org
A not-for-profit organization, is the leading patient organization for people with asthma and allergies, and the oldest asthma and allergy patient group in the world. AAFA provides practical information, community based services and support through a national network of chapters and support groups. AAFA develops health education, organizes state and national advocacy efforts and funds research to find better treatments and cures.
Christopher Cole, Chair

1277 National Advisory Allergic and Infectious Disease Council
6610 Rockledge Drive   301-496-5717
Bethesda, MD 20892-6612   866-284-4107
                                           Fax: 301-402-3573
                                           TTY: 800-877-8339
                                           TDD: 800-877-8339
                             e-mail: ocpostoffice@niaid.nih.gov
                             www.niaid.nih.gov/Pages/default.aspx
The National Institute of Allergy and Infectious Diseases (NIAID) conducts and supports basic and applied research to better understand treat and ultimately prevent infectious immunologic and allergic diseases.
Anthony S Fauci MD, Director
H Clifford Lane MD, Acting Deputy Director

State Agencies & Associations

Alaska

1278 Asthma and Allergy Foundation of America: Alaska Chapter
PO Box 201927
Anchorage, AK 99520-1927   e-mail: aafaalaska@gci.net
                                             www.aafaalaska.com
Formed in April, 2001, the AAFA Alaska chapter is moving quickly to provide educational programs and information about asthma and allergies through classes, workshops and educational materials. Focused not only on reaching children and adults with asthma information, but also health care professionals, caregivers, childcare providers and school personnel.
Suzi Jackson, Executive Director

California

1279 Asthma and Allergy Foundation of America: Southern California Chapter
5900 Wilshire Boulevard   323-937-7859
Los Angeles, CA 90036   800-624-0044
                                           Fax: 323-937-7815
                                     e-mail: aafasocal@aol.com
                                             www.aafasocal.com

Dedicated to controlling and curing asthma and allergic diseases through education, a network of support groups, the support of research and specialized training, increasing public awareness and providing medication and treatment to the under served. Program highlights include the Breathmobile, asthma camps and air power games for children.
Francene Lifson, Executive Director

Massachusetts

1280 Asthma and Allergy Foundation of America: New England Chapter
220 Boylston Street
Chestnut Hill, MA 02467

617-965-7771
877-227-8462
Fax: 617-965-8886
TTY: 877-227-8462
e-mail: info@asthmaandallergies.org
www.asthmaandallergies.org

Serves Massachusetts, Rhode Island, Connecticut, Maine, New Hampshire and Vermont. Program highlights include speakers and exhibits, telephone information and referrals, tobacco control program, scholarship essay contest for high school juniors, advocacy for safer environments and training programs for school, daycare and health professionals.
Patricia Goldman, Executive Director
Sharon Schumack, Health Education Coordinator

Michigan

1281 Asthma and Allergy Foundation of America: Michigan Chapter
17520 West 12 Mile Road
Southfield, MI 40876-8768

248-557-8050
888-444-0333
Fax: 248-557-8768
e-mail: aafamich@sbcglobal.net
www.aafa.org

Serves the state of Michigan through public forums, work place educational programs, patient advocacy, Asthma Camp and telephone referrals and information.
Karen Katz, Executive Director
Dr. Rola Bokhari-Panza, President

Missouri

1282 Asthma and Allergy Foundation of America: Greater Kansas City Chapter
9140 Ward Parkway
Kansas City, MO 64114

816-333-6608
888-542-8252
Fax: 816-333-6684
e-mail: info@aafakc.org
www.aafakc.org

Provides college scholarships, Family Asthma Education Day, adult discussion groups, Superkids Asthma Day Camp for grades 1-5, professional education, ACT, health fair participation, breathing machine, peak flow meter and spacer distribution programs. They also have a quarterly newsletter, an asthma action line, emergency medication assistance, assistance to local school districts, free educational materials, seminars for work site clinicians and daycare workers and the smoke-free dining group.
Noel Albert, Executive Director

1283 Asthma and Allergy Foundation of America: St. Louis Chapter
1500 South Big Bend
St. Louis, MO 63117

314-645-2422
Fax: 314-692-2022
e-mail: aafa@aafastl.org
www.aafastl.org/

The Asthma and Allergy Foundation of America (AAFA), St. Louis Chapter, was founded in 1981 by a group of volunteer board-certified allergists, including Dr. Phillip Korenblat of Washington University and Dr. Raymond Slavin of St. Louis University. AAFA St. Louis provides services to the community in helping children effectively manage their asthma through the provision of medical resources, equipment and education.
Robert Novelly, Executive Director
Amy Leipholtz, Development Director

New Jersey

1284 Asthma and Allergy Foundation of America: Southeast Pennsylvania Chapter
32 Caspertown Street
Gibbstown, NJ 08027

856-224-9547
Fax: 856-224-5893
e-mail: aafasepa@prodigy.net
www.aafa.org

In the process of establishing a vital, new program that will aid children with chronic asthma. Many parents, some who are without medical insurance coverage, are unaware of the availability of a medical support system that can help their children. The Children at Risk program will enable parents to have their children evaluated and also receive a free one month supply of medication. Parents will also receive information regarding available options for follow up care and prescription coverage.
Debi Maines, Executive Director

Oregon

1285 Asthma and Allergy Foundation of America
14530 SW 144th Avenue
Tigard, OR 97224

503-579-8375
Fax: 208-474-6839
e-mail: hensches@teleport.com

Serving the state of Oregon.
Sandra L Henschel, Executive Director

1286 Asthma and Allergy Foundation of America: Oregon Chapter
14530 Southwest 144th Avenue
Tigard, OR 97224-1445

503-579-8375
Fax: 208-474-6839
e-mail: hensches@teleport.com

Serving the state of Oregon.
Sandra L Henschel, Executive Director

Texas

1287 Asthma and Allergy Foundation of America
9101 Quarter Horse Lane
Fort Worth, TX 76123

817-297-3132
888-933-AAFA
Fax: 817-563-5696
e-mail: info@aafatexas.org
www.aafatexas.org

Offers many educational programs and services that touch patients, caregivers, physicians and allied health professionals, including: child care provider education programs, school nurse and respiratory therapist education programs, and work site allergy education.
Joan Hart, Executive Director
Jim Rosenthal, President

1288 Asthma and Allergy Foundation of America: North Texas Chapter
155 Southwood
Burleson, TX 76028

817-483-8131
888-933-AAFA
Fax: 817-563-5696
e-mail: aafantx@hotmail.com
www.aafa.org

Offers many educational programs and services that touch patients. caregivers, physicians and allied health professionals, including: child care provider education programs, school nurse and respiratory therapist education programs, work site allergy education programs, spacer and peak flow meter distribution to those in need, a toll free hotline, prescription assistance information, free educational materials in English and Spanish, an electronic newsletter, professional education, etc.
Joan Hart, Executive Director

Washington

1289 Ysthma and Allergy Foundation of America: Washington Chapter
1233 20th Street
Washington, DC 20036

206-368-2866
800-727-8462
Fax: 206-368-2941
e-mail: Info@aafa.org
www.aafa.org

Program highlights include trainings for health care professionals on asthma and allergy management, working collaboratively with other local and regional agencies to improve the quality of life for those affected by asthma and allergies, organizing health seminars and education programs.

Mary Brasle, Director of Programs and Services
Amy Patterson, Director Administration/Governance

Foundations

1290 Asthma and Allergy Foundation of America
1233 20th Street NW   202-466-7643
Washington, DC 20036   800-727-8462
Fax: 202-668-40
e-mail: info@aafa.org
www.aafa.org
AAFA provides practical information, community based services and support through a national network of chapters and support groups. AAFA develops health education, organizes state and national advocacy efforts and funds research to find better treatments and cures

William McLin, Executive Director

Research Centers

1291 Brigham and Women's Hospital: Rheumatology Immunology, and Allergy Division
75 Francis Street   61- 73- 550
Boston, MA 02115   Fax: 617-525-1001
TTY: 617-732-6458
www.brighamandwomens.org
Internationally renowned for excellence in clinical care clinical investigation and basic research. A faculty of 36 board certified rheumatologists and allergists provide eldtive urgent and emergency consultations as necessary.

Michael B Brenner MD, Division Chief
Jonathan S Coblyn, Clinical Director Rheumatology

1292 Childrens Hospital Immunology Division Children's Hospital
Children's Hospital
300 Longwood Avenue
Boston, MA 02115   61- 35- 600
www.childrenshospital.org
Organizational research unit of the Children's Hospital that focuses on the causes prevention and treatments of asthma infections and allergies.

Dr. James Mandell, CEO
Sandra Fenwick, President & COO

1293 Clinical Immunology, Allergy, and Rheumatology
Tulane Medical School
1700 Perdido Street   504-988-5187
New Orleans, LA 70112-1210   Fax: 504-988-3686
e-mail: medsch@tulane.edu
www.som.tulane.edu/medciar

Mauel Lopez MD, Director

1294 Duke Asthma, Allergy and Airway Center
4309 Medical Park Drive
Durham, NC 27704   919-620-7300
www.aaac.duhs.duke.edu/

Raffeal Rau, President
Dr Monica Kraft, Director

1295 Johns Hopkins University: Asthma and Allergy Center
5501 Hopkins Bayview Circle   410-550-2101
Baltimore, MD 21224-6801   Fax: 410-550-3256
e-mail: jhuallergy@jhmi.edu
www.hopkinsmedicine.org/allergy
Studies of allergic diseases and individuals with allergic disease pulmonary diseases and diseases involving inflammation and immunological processes.

Bruce S Bochner, Director
Peter S Creticos, Clinical Director

1296 National Jewish Division of Immunology National Jewish Medical and Research Cen
National Jewish Medical and Research Center

1400 Jackson Street   303-398-1337
Denver, CO 80206-2762   80- 42- 889
Fax: 303-270-2125
e-mail: harbeckr@njc.org
www.njc.org
The only medical center in the country whose research and patient care resources are dedicated to respiratory and immunologic diseases.

John Cambier, Chairman
Ronald J Harbeck, Medical Director

1297 Northwestern University: Division of Allergy and Immunology
The Feinberg School of Medicine
251 East Huron Street   312-926-6895
Chicago, IL 60611   Fax: 312-926-6905
e-mail: rpschleimer@northwestern.edu
www.medicine.northwestern.edu
A referral center of local regional and national stature.ÿ Areas of clinical excellence include asthma allergic bronchopulmonary aspergillosis idiopathic anaphylaxis drug allergy occupational immunologic lung disease and allergen immunotherapy.

Douglas E Vaughan MD, Chair
James Foody MD, Vice Chair Clinical Affairs

1298 University of Virginia: General Clinical Research Center
University of Virginia Health System
2515 Lee Street   434-924-2394
Charlottesville, VA 22908-0787   Fax: 434-924-9960
e-mail: gcrc@virginia.edu
www.healthsystem.virginia.edu/
Focuses on asthmatic disorders.

Arthur Garso Jr MD MPH, Principal Investigator
Eugene J Barrett, Program Director

1299 University of Wisconsin: Asthma, Allergy and Pulmonary Research Center
600 Highland Avenue   608-263-6400
Madison, WI 53792-2454   Fax: 608-263-6401
www.medicine.wisc.edu

Richard Hong, Head

Support Groups & Hotlines

1300 Allergy & Asthma Networks Hotline
Allergy and Asthma Network/Mothers of Asthmatics
2751 Prosperity Avenue   703-641-9595
Fairfax, VA 22031   800-878-4403
Fax: 703-573-7794
www.breatherville.org

Mary McGowan, Executive Director

1301 Asthma and Allergy Foundation of America
1233 20th Street NW   202-466-7643
Washington, DC 20036   Fax: 202-466-8940
e-mail: info@aafa.org
www.aafa.org
The foundation was formed to alleviate suffering and loss from asthma and allergy disorders. The foundation offers a nationwide network of chapters and support groups and provides education and emotional support for persons with allergies and asthma. Also funds research for improved treatments and ultimately a cure.

1302 National Health Information Center
PO Box 1133   310-565-4167
Washington, DC 20013   800-336-4797
Fax: 301-984-4256
e-mail: info@nhic.org
www.health.gov/nhic
Offers a nationwide information referral service, produces directories and resource guides.

1303 Physician Referral and Information Line
American Academy of Allergy Asthma and Immunology
611 East Wells Street   414-272-6071
Milwaukee, WI 53202-3889   800-822-2762
Fax: 414-272-6070
www.aaaai.org
Referral line offering information on allergy and asthma, referral to an allergy/immunology specialist.

1304 Support for Asthmatic Youth
Asthma and Allergy Foundation of America
1080 Glen Cove Avenue   516-625-5735
Glen Head, NY 11545-1565   Fax: 516-625-2976
A network of educational/support groups for adolescents between
the ages of 9 and 17. All meetings are free and feature guest speak-
ers, informational programs, games and other fun activities.
Renee Theodorakis MA, Director Adolescent Services

Books

1305 Asthma Care Training for Kids
Asthma and Allergy Foundation of America
1233 20th Street NW   202-466-7643
Washington, DC 20036   Fax: 202-466-8940
                                       e-mail: info@aafa.org
                                            www.aafa.org
Designed to help children ages 7-12 and their parents take charge
of their asthma. In a series of three action filled sessions, children
and their parents meet separately with their peers to learn about
asthma management.

1306 Asthma Organizer
Allergy and Asthma Network/Mothers of Asthmatics
2751 Prosperity Avenue   703-641-9595
Fairfax, VA 22031-4397   800-878-4403
                                     Fax: 703-573-7794
                               www.mothersofasthmatics.org
Includes daily symptom diary and forms to track medications, office visits and updates to your personal management plan. Information on peak flow monitoring, managing asthma at school,
understanding asthma activators, and allergy-proofing also included. Available in Spanish.
Loose Leaf
Mary McGowan, Executive Director

1307 Asthma Resources Directory
Allergy and Asthma Network/Mothers of Asthmatics
2751 Prosperity Avenue   703-641-9595
Fairfax, VA 22031-4397   800-878-4403
                                     Fax: 703-573-7794
                               www.mothersofasthmatics.org
Comprehensive listings of thousands of products, services, and re-
sources for allergy and asthma questions.
Mary McGowan, Executive Director

1308 Asthma Self-Help Book
Asthma and Allergy Foundation of America
1233 20th Street NW   202-466-7643
Washington, DC 20036   Fax: 202-466-8940
                                       e-mail: info@aafa.org
                                            www.aafa.org
A thorough, practical look at asthma that includes information
from the National Heart, Lung and Blood Institute's 1991 Asthma
Guidelines.

**1309 Asthma in the School: Improving Control with Peak Flow
Monitoring**
Asthma and Allergy Foundation of America
1233 20th Street NW   202-466-7643
Washington, DC 20036   Fax: 202-466-8940
                                       e-mail: info@aafa.org
                                            www.aafa.org
Comprehensive and practical guide to help the school nurse moni-
tor and assist students with asthma.

1310 Asthma in the Workplace
John H Dekker & Sons
2941 Clydon Street SW   616-538-5160
Grand Rapids, MI 49509   Fax: 616-538-0720
1993 664 pages
ISBN: 0-824787-99-4

1311 Asthma: The Complete Guide
Asthma and Allergy Foundation of America
1233 20th Street NW   202-466-7643
Washington, DC 20036-2330   800-727-8462
                                     Fax: 202-466-8940
                                            www.aafa.org

An excellent self-management guide for asthma and allergy patients and their families.
357 pages Paperback

1312 Breathing Disorders: Your Complete Exercise Guide
Human Kinetics
PO Box 5076   217-351-5076
Champaign, IL 61825-5076   800-747-4457
                                     Fax: 217-351-2674
                                       www.humankinetics.com
1993 144 pages Paperback
ISBN: 0-873224-26-4
Steve Ruhlig, Marketing Director

1313 Bronchial Asthma: Principles of Diagnosis and Treatment
Humana Press
999 Riverview Drive   973-256-1699
Totowa, NJ 07512   Fax: 973-256-8341
                               e-mail: humana@humanapr.com
                                       www.humanapress.com
2001 496 pages
ISBN: 0-896038-61-0

1314 Children with Asthma: A Manual for Parents
Allergy Control Products
PO Box 793   203-438-9580
Ridgefield, CT 06877-0793   800-422-3878
                                     Fax: 203-431-8963
                                   www.allergycontrol.com
Known as the asthma bible, this second edition is sprinkled with
anecdotes by patients and their parents.
296 pages Paperback

1315 Conquering Asthma
Michael Newhouse, MD, author
B.C Decker, Inc.
50 King Street E, Floor 2 PO Box620   905-522-7017
Ontario, Canada L8N 3K7,   800-568-7281
                                     Fax: 905-522-7839
                               e-mail: info@bcdecker.com
                                         www.bcdecker.com
This text shows asthmatics how to live a healthier and happier life
hardly aware that they have asthma.
1998 107 pages Paperback
ISBN: 1-896998-01-1

1316 Coping with Asthma
Rosen Publishing Group
29 E 21st Street   212-777-3017
New York, NY 10010   800-237-9932
                                     Fax: 888-436-4643
                            e-mail: customerservice@rosenpub.com
                                     www.rosenpublishing.com
This book prepares students by explaining to them the dangers of
asthma, a condition which, when properly treated, is completely
manageable.

ISBN: 0-823929-69-8
Carolyn Simpson, Author

1317 Understanding Asthma
Phil Lieberman, MD, author
University Press of Mississippi
3825 Ridgewood Road   601-432-6205
Jackson, MS 39211-6492   Fax: 601-432-6217
                            e-mail: kburgess@ihl.state.ms.us
                                     www.upress.state.ms.us
A guide to how the disease behaves and how the latest therapies
work.
1999 120 pages Paperback
ISBN: 1-578061-42-3
Kathy Burgess, Advertising/Marketing Services Manager

Children's Books

1318 All About Asthma
Asthma and Allergy Foundation of America

1233 20th Street NW
Washington, DC 20036-2330

202-466-7643
800-727-8462
Fax: 202-466-8940
www.aafa.org

Written by a 10-year-old with asthma, this cleverly illustrated book explains causes and symptoms, and ways to control asthma to lead a normal life.
39 pages Paperback

1319   Asthma
Franklin Watts Grolier
90 Old Sherman Turnpike
Danbury, CT 06816-0001

203-797-3500
800-621-1115
Fax: 203-797-3197
www.grolier.com

This book offers vital information on causes and treatments, plus advice on how to prevent flare-ups.
96 pages Grades 7-12
ISBN: 0-531106-97-7

1320   Asthma Challenge
Asthma and Allergy Foundation of America
1233 20th Street NW
Washington, DC 20036

202-466-7643
Fax: 202-466-8940
e-mail: info@aafa.org
www.aafa.org

An exciting new team game for large or small groups. Custom designed, full color, stand up board and two sets of pretested question cards. Teens and adults win AAFA Bucks as they test their knowledge in categories like Sneezes and Wheezes and Asthma Nuts and Bolts.

1321   Best of Superstuff Activity Booklet
American Lung Association
1740 Broadway
New York, NY 10019-4315

212-315-8700

For young children with asthma featuring a series of activities designed to help youngsters cope with asthma.
32 pages Ages 6-8

1322   Bronkie the Bronchiasaurus
Asthma and Allergy Foundation of America
1233 20th Street NW
Washington, DC 20036-2330

202-466-7643
800-727-8462
Fax: 202-466-8940
www.aafa.org

A Super Nintendo role-playing adventure in which players manage the asthma of two dinosaurs. They must avoid triggers, maintain their peak-flow and take daily medications. Only then can they use their strongest defense - the powerful breath blast. Designed for ages 7 to 15.

1323   Childhood Asthma: Learning to Manage
Asthma and Allergy Foundation of America
1233 20th Street NW
Washington, DC 20036-2330

202-466-7643
800-727-8462
Fax: 202-466-8940
www.aafa.org

Self-paced, entertaining activity books for home use featuring practical guidelines for managing childhood asthma with a focus on using peak flow meters.

1324   Clubhouse Kids Learn About Asthma
Asthma and Allergy Foundation of America
1233 20th Street NW
Washington, DC 20036-2330

202-466-7643
800-727-8462
Fax: 202-466-8940
www.aafa.org

Interactive CD-ROM helps children ages 4-12 learn about asthma at their own pace. Sound, animation and game-like features draw players into the life of Janie, who has just been diagnosed with asthma.

1325   I'm a Meter Reader
Allergy and Asthma Network/Mothers of Asthmatics
2751 Prosperity Avenue
Fairfax, VA 22031-4397

703-641-9595
800-878-4403
Fax: 703-573-7794
www.mothersofasthmatics.org

Provides expert advice on how a peak flow meter can help detect when an asthma attack can occur in an easy to understand format

with colorful illustrations. Available in Spanish. Companion video, I'm a Meter Reader, available as part of a set for $12.00.
Ages 4-9
Mary McGowan, Executive Director
Nancy Sander, Editor-in-Chief

1326   Let's Talk About Having Asthma
Rosen Publishing Group's PowerKids Press
29 E 21st Street
New York, NY 10010

212-777-3017
800-237-9932
Fax: 888-436-4643
e-mail: customerservice@rosenpub.com
www.rosenpublishing.com

This book talks about the cause and treatments for asthma as well as the precautions sufferers should take. Recommended for grades K-4.

ISBN: 0-823950-32-8

1327   Lion Who Had Asthma
Asthma and Allergy Foundation of America
1233 20th Street NW
Washington, DC 20036-2330

202-466-7643
800-727-8462
Fax: 202-466-8940
www.aafa.org

A beautifully illustrated book that encourages preschoolers to use their imaginations and take their asthma medications.
24 pages Hardcover

1328   Luke Has Asthma Too!
Allergy Control Products
PO Box 793
Ridgefield, CT 06877-0793

800-422-3878
Fax: 203-431-8963

This gentle book will make for good reading with children, whether they have asthma or not.

1329   Scorpions
Harper & Row
10 E 53rd Street
New York, NY 10022-5299

212-207-7000
www.harpercollins.com

This novel, while not wholly dedicated to examining the ramifications of asthma on a child's life, does incorporate the theme into a compelling narrative.
Grades 6-9

1330   So You Have Asthma Too!
Allergy and Asthma Network/Mothers of Asthmatics
2751 Prosperity Avenue
Fairfax, VA 22031-4397

703-641-9595
800-878-4403
Fax: 703-573-7794
www.mothersofasthmatics.org

A children's illustrated book, offering a clear description and understanding of childhood asthma. Available in Spanish. Also see companion video, SO YOU HAVE ASTHMA TOO!, available as part of a set for $12.00.
Mary McGowan, Executive Director
Nancy Sander, Editor-in-Chief

1331   Winning Over Asthma
Asthma and Allergy Foundation of America
1233 20th Street NW
Washington, DC 20036-2330

202-466-7643
800-727-8462
Fax: 202-466-8940
www.aafa.org

Simple coloring book explains asthma through a story about five-year-old Graham.
30 pages Paperback

Magazines

1332   Controlling Asthma
American Lung Association
1740 Broadway
New York, NY 10019-4315

212-315-8700

For parents of children with asthma, this newsmagazine tells how parents can help their child deal with the many problems presented by asthma.
16 pages

1333 Starting Strong-Staying Strong: A Resource Guide for Educational Support Groups
Asthma and Allergy Foundation of America
1233 20th Street NW   202-466-7643
Washington, DC 20036   800-727-8462
                                  Fax: 202-466-8940
                                e-mail: info@aafa.org
                                        www.aafa.org
A resource guide to help educational support groups get organized, publicize and remain successful. Great for people who want to start an asthma or allergy support group and for existing group leaders who want to strengthen their programs. Filled with stories of success and struggle from other group leaders, medical advisors and group members across the country. A companion CD-ROM provides additional tips.
Guide + CD-ROM
William McLin, Executive Director
Mike Tringale, Director Marketing/Communications

Newsletters

1334 Advance
Asthma and Allergy Foundation of America
1233 20th Street NW   202-466-7643
Washington, DC 20036-2330   800-727-8462
                                  Fax: 202-466-8940
                                        www.aafa.org
A bi-monthly , 8 page newsletter for patients and their families filled with timely and useful information about managing asthma and allergies.
BiMonthly

1335 Allergy & Asthma ADVOCATE Newsletter
American Academy of Allergy, Asthma and Immunology
611 E Wells Street   414-272-6071
Milwaukee, WI 53202   800-822-2762
                                  Fax: 414-272-6070
                                        www.aaaai.org
Offers tips and medical information on allergies and asthma via articles written by allied health and physician AAAAI members.
6 pages Quarterly

1336 BReATHE
Asthma and Allergy Foundation of America
8201 Corporate Drive
Landover, MD 20785   800-727-8462
                                e-mail: info@aafa.org
                                        www.aafa.org
E-newsletter filled with information on how to control asthma and allergies, with stories from patients who are living life without limits.
Bi-Monthly
William McLin, President/CEO
Angel Waldron, Sr Manager Marketing/Communications

1337 FreshAAIR
Asthma and Allergy Foundation of America
8201 Corporate Drive   202-466-7643
Landover, MD 20785   800-727-8462
                                  Fax: 202-466-8940
                                e-mail: info@aafa.org
                                        www.aafa.org
Filled with information about asthma, seasonal allergies, food allergies, back-to-school tips for parents, educational materials and more.
Bi-Monthly
William McLin, President/CEO
Angel Waldron, Sr Manager Marketing/Communications

1338 Leaders Link
Asthma and Allergy Foundation of America

8201 Corporate Drive
Landover, MD 20785   800-727-8462
                                e-mail: info@aafa.org
                                        www.aafa.org
Provides useful and timely insights on how to plan and lead asthma and allergy support group meetings, how to keep your support group active and strong, and useful ideas from other support groups.
Bi-Monthly
William McLin, President/CEO
Angel Waldron, Sr Manager Marketing/Communications

1339 MA Report
Allergy and Asthma Network/Mothers of Asthmatics
2751 Prosperity Avenue   703-641-9595
Fairfax, VA 22031-4397   800-878-4403
                                  Fax: 703-573-7794
                            www.mothersofasthmatics.org
Offers information on medical breakthroughs, patient care, public awareness, activities and events focusing on the allergy and asthma patient. This newsletter keeps a patient fully informed with medical articles written by experts in the field.
Monthly
Mary McGowan, Executive Director
Nancy Sander, Editor-in-Chief

Pamphlets

1340 About Asthma
American Lung Association
1740 Broadway   212-315-8700
New York, NY 10019-4315
A popular style pamphlet explaining symptoms, treatment and more for persons with asthma.
16 pages

1341 Adverse Reactions to Foods
American Academy of Allergy, Asthma and Immunology
611 E Wells Street   414-272-6071
Milwaukee, WI 53202-3889   800-822-2762
                                  Fax: 414-272-6070
                                        www.aaaai.org
A patient's guide to problem foods, food additives, diagnosis, and treatment.

1342 Allergies and You
American Lung Association
1740 Broadway   212-315-8700
New York, NY 10019-4315
Answers basic questions about allergy, particularly as it relates to asthma.

1343 Allergies to Animals
American Academy of Allergy, Asthma and Immunology
611 E Wells Street   414-272-6071
Milwaukee, WI 53202-3889   800-822-2762
                                  Fax: 414-272-6070
                                        www.aaaai.org

1344 Allergy & Asthma
American Academy of Allergy, Asthma and Immunology
611 E Wells Street   414-272-6071
Milwaukee, WI 53202-3889   800-822-2762
                                  Fax: 414-272-6070
                                        www.aaaai.org
An informational brochure discussing major topics of allerges and asthma.

1345 Allergy and Asthma: An Informational Brochure
American Academy of Allergy, Asthma and Immunology
611 E Wells Street   414-272-6071
Milwaukee, WI 53202-3889   800-822-2762
                                  Fax: 414-272-6070
                                        www.aaaai.org
Offers information on asthma, its symptoms, causes, diagnosis and treatments.

1346 Anaphylaxis
American Academy of Allergy, Asthma and Immunology

611 E Wells Street
Milwaukee, WI 53202-3889

414-272-6071
800-822-2762
Fax: 414-272-6070
www.aaaai.org

1347 Asthma Alert
American Lung Association
1740 Broadway
New York, NY 10019-4315

212-315-8700

Quick reference folders with information on asthma, the symptoms and what to do in an emergency.

1348 Asthma Handbook
American Lung Association
1740 Broadway
New York, NY 10019-4315

212-315-8700

Explains asthma, gives self-care methods for handling it and helps patients work more effectively with their doctor.
28 pages

1349 Asthma Lifelines
American Lung Association
1740 Broadway
New York, NY 10019-4315

212-315-8700

Promotional brochure providing descriptions of ALA asthma education materials.
12 pages

1350 Asthma and Allergies in Seniors
American Academy of Allergy, Asthma and Immunology
611 E Wells Street
Milwaukee, WI 53202

414-272-6071
800-822-2762
Fax: 414-272-6070
www.aaaai.org

1351 Asthma and Pregnancy
American Academy of Allergy, Asthma and Immunology
611 E Wells Street
Milwaukee, WI 53202-3889

414-272-6071
800-822-2762
Fax: 414-272-6070
www.aaaai.org

1352 Asthma and the School Child
American Academy of Allergy, Asthma and Immunology
611 E Wells Street
Milwaukee, WI 53202-3889

414-272-6071
800-822-2762
Fax: 414-272-6070
www.aaaai.org

1353 Atopic Dermatitis
American Academy of Allergy, Asthma and Immunology
611 E Wells Street
Milwaukee, WI 53202-3889

414-272-6071
800-822-2762
Fax: 414-272-6070
www.aaaai.org

This brochure offers information on symptoms, diagnosi, treatment, and prognosis.

1354 Being Close
National Jewish Center for Immunology
1400 Jackson Street
Denver, CO 80206-2762

303-388-4461

A booklet offering information to patients suffering from a respiratory disorder such as emphysema, asthma or tuberculosis, that discusses sexual problems and feelings.

1355 Childhood Asthma
American Academy of Allergy, Asthma and Immunology
611 E Wells Street
Milwaukee, WI 53202-3889

414-272-6071
800-822-2762
Fax: 414-272-6070
www.aaaai.org

1356 Childhood Asthma: A Guide for Parents
Asthma and Allergy Foundation of America
1233 20th Street NW
Washington, DC 20036-2330

202-466-7643
800-727-8462
Fax: 202-466-8940
www.aafa.org

This colorful booklet helps parents learn all about asthma in children.
32 pages

1357 Childhood Asthma: A Matter of Control
American Lung Association
1740 Broadway
New York, NY 10019-4315

212-315-8700

A guide for parents of children with asthma, this booklet covers topics such as identifying asthma signs and symptoms as well as controlling the condition.
28 pages

1358 Consumer Guide to Health Care Plans
American Academy of Allergy, Asthma and Immunology
611 E Wells Street
Milwaukee, WI 53202-3889

414-272-6071
800-822-2762
Fax: 414-272-6070
www.aaaai.org

Gives answers to some commonly asked questions on health care.

1359 Efficacy of Asthma Education, Selected Abstracts
American Lung Association
1740 Broadway
New York, NY 10019-4315

212-315-8700

Abstracts documenting the efficacy of asthma education programs for physicians and other health professionals.

1360 Exercise-Induced Asthma & Bronchospasm
American Academy of Allergy, Asthma and Immunology
611 E Wells Street
Milwaukee, WI 53202-3889

414-272-6071
800-822-2762
Fax: 414-272-6070
www.aaaai.org

This brochure covers testing, treatment, and other advice on how to deal with exercise-induced asthma.

1361 Facts About Asthma
American Lung Association
1740 Broadway
New York, NY 10019-4315

212-315-8700

Primary public information leaflet on asthma.
12 pages

1362 Facts About Peak Flow Meters
American Lung Association
1740 Broadway
New York, NY 10019-4315

212-315-8700

Discusses the use of a peak flow meter for adults and children with asthma.
8 pages

1363 Healthy Breathing
National Jewish Center for Immunology
1400 Jackson Street
Denver, CO 80206-2762

303-388-4461

Offers patients with lung or respiratory disorders information on exercise and healthy breathing.

1364 Helping Others Breathe Easier
Allergy and Asthma Network/Mothers of Asthmatics
2751 Prosperity Avenue
Fairfax, VA 22031-4397

703-641-9595
800-878-4403
Fax: 703-573-7794
www.mothersofasthmatics.org

Offers information on educational resources, support groups and the Network for persons afflicted with asthma or allergic disorders.
Mary McGowan, Executive Director
Nancy Sander, Editor-in-Chief

1365 Home Control of Allergies and Asthma
American Lung Association
1740 Broadway
New York, NY 10019-4315

212-315-8700

Discusses substances in the home that may trigger asthma and allergy problems and offers suggestions for controlling them.
12 pages

1366 Immunitherapy
American Academy of Allergy, Asthma and Immunology

611 E Wells Street
Milwaukee, WI 53202-3889

414-272-6071
800-822-2762
Fax: 414-272-6070
www.aaaai.org

This brochure offers information on administration, benefits, and potential side effects of immune therapy.

1367 Inhaled Medications for Asthma
American Academy of Allergy, Asthma and Immunology
611 E Wells Street
Milwaukee, WI 53202-3889

414-272-6071
800-822-2762
Fax: 414-272-6070
www.aaaai.org

This brochure gives helpful information on classes of inhaled medication, types of inhalation devices, spacers and holding chambers, how proper training is necessary.

1368 Latex Allergy
American Academy of Allergy, Asthma and Immunology
611 E Wells Street
Milwaukee, WI 53202-3889

414-272-6071
800-822-2762
Fax: 414-272-6070
www.aaaai.org

1369 Making the Most of Your Next Doctor Visit
American Academy of Allergy, Asthma and Immunology
611 E Wells Street
Milwaukee, WI 53202-3889

414-272-6071
800-822-2762
Fax: 414-272-6070
www.aaaai.org

A personal asthma management monitor. Includes personal tracking charts to help you along.
10 pages

1370 Many Faces of Asthma
American Lung Association
1740 Broadway
New York, NY 10019-4315

212-315-8700

Provides an overview of asthma as a major public health problem, describes what happens during asthma attacks and explains how asthma is treated and managed.
12 pages

1371 Nocturnal Asthma
National Jewish Center for Immunology
1400 Jackson Street
Denver, CO 80206-2762

303-388-4461

Offers information to patients about how to understand and manage asthma at night.

1372 Occupational Asthma
American Academy of Allergy, Asthma and Immunology
611 E Wells Street
Milwaukee, WI 53202-3889

414-272-6071
800-822-2762
Fax: 414-272-6070
www.aaaai.org

This brochure also contains a list of most common agents theat cause occupational asthma and who is at risk.

1373 Occupational Asthma: Lung Hazards on the Job
American Lung Association
1740 Broadway
New York, NY 10019-4315

212-315-8700

Discusses occupational asthma, a form of asthma in which airways overreact to various irritants in the workplace.

1374 Outpatient Treatment of Asthma
American Academy of Allergy, Asthma and Immunology
611 E Wells Street
Milwaukee, WI 53202-3889

414-272-6071
800-822-2762
Fax: 414-272-6070
www.aaaai.org

1375 Peak Flow Meter: A Thermometer for Asthma
American Academy of Allergy, Asthma and Immunology
611 E Wells Street
Milwaukee, WI 53202-3889

414-272-6071
800-822-2762
Fax: 414-272-6070
www.aaaai.org

1376 Pollen and Spores Around the World
American Academy of Allergy, Asthma and Immunology
611 E Wells Street
Milwaukee, WI 53202-3889

414-272-6071
800-822-2762
Fax: 414-272-6070
www.aaaai.org

Multi-paged brochure offering graphes and tables of pollen levels and different times of the year in different parts of the country.
10 pages

1377 Removing House Dust and Other Allergic Irritants From Your Home
American Academy of Allergy, Asthma and Immunology
611 E Wells Street
Milwaukee, WI 53202-3889

414-272-6071
800-822-2762
Fax: 414-272-6070
www.aaaai.org

This brochure covers some good ideas on how to reduce dust in the home.

1378 Role of the Allergist & Clinical Immunologist in Patient Care
American Academy of Allergy, Asthma and Immunology
611 E Wells Street
Milwaukee, WI 53202-3889

414-272-6071
800-822-2762
Fax: 414-272-6070
www.aaaai.org

An informational brochure containing definitions and addresses for further information.

1379 School Information Packet
Allergy and Asthma Network/Mothers of Asthmatics
2751 Prosperity Avenue
Fairfax, VA 22031-4397

703-641-9595
800-878-4403
Fax: 703-573-7794
www.mothersofasthmatics.org

Practical, medical, and legal information for school administrators and parents of students with asthma.
Mary McGowan, Executive Director
Nancy Sander, Editor-in-Chief

1380 Standards for the Diagnosis and Care of Patients with Asthma
American Lung Association
1740 Broadway
New York, NY 10019-4315

212-315-8700

Standards developed by the American Thoracic Society, the medical section of the ALA. For physicians.
24 pages

1381 Student Asthma Action Card
Asthma and Allergy Foundation of America
1233 20th Street NW
Washington, DC 20036-2330

202-466-7643
800-727-8462
Fax: 202-466-8940
www.aafa.org

Indispensable tool for familiarizing school personnel with asthma triggers, daily medications and emergency directions for each of their students with asthma.

1382 Superstuff
American Lung Association
1740 Broadway
New York, NY 10019-4315

212-315-8700

Kit specifically designed to help the elementary schoolchild with asthma to learn how to manage the condition. The kit contains teaching tools, puzzles, riddles, stories and games.

1383 Teens Talk to Teens About Asthma
Asthma and Allergy Foundation of America
1233 20th Street NW
Washington, DC 20036-2330

202-466-7643
800-727-8462
Fax: 202-466-8940
www.aafa.org

Quotes and thoughts from teens capture the essence of what it feels like to have asthma.

1384 There are Solutions for the Student with Asthma
American Lung Association
1740 Broadway
New York, NY 10017

212-315-8700

Leaflet telling how parents and school personnel can work together to make life easier for children with asthma.
4 pages

1385   Tips to Remember
American Academy of Allergy, Asthma and Immunology
611 E Wells Street   414-272-6071
Milwaukee, WI 53202-3889
A set of 23 tip sheets offering information on various topics including allergy and asthma treatments, pregnancy and asthma, animal allergies, sinusitis and more.

1386   Tips to Remember Brochures
American Academy of Allergy, Asthma and Immunology
611 E Wells Street   414-272-6071
Milwaukee, WI 53202-3889   800-822-2762
                                                   Fax: 414-272-6070
                                                       www.aaaai.org

Thirty three colorful brochures offered on numerous topics in allergy, asthma, and immunology.

1387   Triggers of Asthma
American Academy of Allergy, Asthma and Immunology
611 E Wells Street   414-272-6071
Milwaukee, WI 53202-3889   800-822-2762
                                                   Fax: 414-272-6070
                                                       www.aaaai.org

This brochure gives helpful information on what will cause an asthma attack.

1388   Understanding Asthma
National Jewish Center for Immunology
1400 Jackson Street   303-388-4461
Denver, CO 80206
Offers a brief introduction to asthma and then goes into the physiology of asthma, the triggers of asthma, and diagnosis and monitoring of asthma.
27 pages

1389   Understanding Immunology
National Jewish Center for Immunology
1400 Jackson Street   303-388-4461
Denver, CO 80206-2762
Offers information to patients and the public on the body's defenses. Explains how immunity develops, the basics of immunologic medicine and coping with respiratory disorders.

1390   Understanding Your Child with Asthma
National Jewish Center for Immunology
1400 Jackson Street   303-388-4461
Denver, CO 80206-2762   800-222-5264
Offers information on patient care, research, education and adult programs offered by the Association.

1391   Understanding the Pollen and Mold Season
American Academy of Allergy, Asthma and Immunology
611 E Wells Street   414-272-6071
Milwaukee, WI 53202-3889   800-822-2762
                                                   Fax: 414-272-6070
                                                       www.aaaai.org

1392   Unproven Methods in Diagnosing and Treating Allergies
Asthma and Allergy Foundation of America
1233 20th Street NW   202-466-7643
Washington, DC 20036-2330   800-727-8462
                                                   Fax: 202-466-8940
                                                        www.aafa.org

1393   Use of Steroids for Asthma and Allergies
American Academy of Allergy, Asthma and Immunology
611 E Wells Street   414-272-6071
Milwaukee, WI 53202-3889   800-822-2762
                                                   Fax: 414-272-6070
                                                       www.aaaai.org

1394   What Every Patient Should Know About Asthma & Allergy Medications
American Academy of Allergy, Asthma and Immunology

611 E Wells Street   414-272-6071
Milwaukee, WI 53202-3889   800-822-2762
                                                   Fax: 414-272-6070
                                                       www.aaaai.org

1395   What is an Allergic Reaction?
American Academy of Allergy, Asthma and Immunology
611 E Wells Street   414-272-6071
Milwaukee, WI 53202-3889   800-822-2762
                                                   Fax: 414-272-6070
                                                       www.aaaai.org

This brochure gives helpful information on what will cause an allergic reaction.

1396   Your Child and Asthma
National Jewish Center for Immunology
1400 Jackson Street   303-388-4461
Denver, CO 80206-2762
A booklet offering information to parents and family about their child with asthma. Offers information on diagnosis, treatments, triggers and family concerns.

Audio & Video

1397   Asthma Handbook Slides
American Lung Association
1740 Broadway   212-315-8700
New York, NY 10019-4315
Slides and script based on The Asthma Handbook for asthma patients and others.
Film

1398   Asthma Management
American Academy of Allergy, Asthma and Immunology
611 E Wells Street   414-272-6071
Milwaukee, WI 53202-3889   800-822-2762
                                                   Fax: 414-272-6070
                                                       www.aaaai.org

Although there is currently no cure for asthma, attacks can be controlled by appropriate asthma management. This video describes what happens during an asthma attack, how your allergists diagnoses asthma, and ways your allergist can help you to manage your condition.
10-13 minutes

1399   Asthma and the Athlete
American Academy of Allergy, Asthma and Immunology
611 E Wells Street   414-272-6071
Milwaukee, WI 53202   800-822-2762
                                                   Fax: 414-272-6070
                                                       www.aaaai.org

In the past, people with asthma were sometimes discouraged from exercising. Today we know that everyone, including asthmatics, can benefit from physical actilvity. This video details which exercises are best for those with asthma, and how an allergist can help asthmatic athletes to properly manage and treat their disease.
10-13 minutes

1400   Environmental Control Measures
American Academy of Allergy, Asthma and Immunology
611 E Wells Street   414-272-6071
Milwaukee, WI 53202-3889   800-822-2762
                                                   Fax: 414-272-6070
                                                       www.aaaai.org

By conrtolling your environment, you can reduce your exposure to substances called allergens that trigger your allergic symptoms. This program depicts common outdoor and indoor allergens, methods an allergist uses to diagnose which substances you're allergic to, and how to reduce your exposure to allergic triggers.
10-13 minutes

1401   I'm a Meter Reader
Allergy and Asthma Network/Mothers of Asthmatics
2751 Prosperity Avenue   703-641-9595
Fairfax, VA 22031-4397   800-878-4403
                                                   Fax: 703-573-7794
                                              www.mothersofasthmatics.org
Provides expert advice on how a peak flow meter can help detect when an asthma attack can occur in an easy to understand format.

Companion book, I'm a Meter Reader, available as part of a set for $12.00.
Video
Mary McGowan, Executive Director
Nancy Sander, Editor-in-Chief

1402 Immunotherapy
American Academy of Allergy, Asthma and Immunology
611 E Wells Street   414-272-6071
Milwaukee, WI 53202-3889   800-822-2762
                                        Fax: 414-272-6070
                                             www.aaaai.org
Immunotherapy, of allergy shots, is a long-term allergy and asthma treatment program that helps control allergic symptoms and reduces the need for medications. Learn more about immunotherapy through this video, which includes information on allergy testing and how your allergist determines if immunotherapy is right for you.
10-13 minutes

1403 Managing Asthma in School: An Action Plan
Asthma and Allergy Foundation of America
1233 20th Street NW   202-466-7643
Washington, DC 20036-2330   800-727-8462
                                        Fax: 202-466-8940
                                             www.aafa.org
Gives the basics of asthma and a plan for school nurses, parents and physicians to work together.
14 minutes

1404 Managing Childhood Asthma
American Lung Association
Box 596-COL   212-245-8000
New York, NY 10001   800-586-4872
                                        Fax: 312-440-9374
                                 e-mail: webmaster@ala.org
                                             www.ala.org
What parents need to know to manage asthma. 22 minutes.
Video

1405 Pharmacologic Therapy of Pediatric Asthma
American Lung Association
1740 Broadway   212-315-8700
New York, NY 10019-4315
A Learning Resource Program developed by a joint committee of the American Thoracic Society and the ALA.
Film

1406 Regular Kid
American Lung Association
1740 Broadway   212-315-8700
New York, NY 10019-4315
This film shows how families and children cope with asthma problems. Proven asthma management strategies are presented through the experiences of four children with asthma, ranging in age from toddler to teenager.
Film

1407 So You Have Asthma Too!
Allergy and Asthma Network/Mothers of Asthmatics
2751 Prosperity Avenue   703-641-9595
Fairfax, VA 22031-4397   800-878-4403
                                        Fax: 703-573-7794
                              www.mothersofasthmatics.org
Offers a clear description and understanding of childhood asthma. Also see companion book, So You Have Asthma Too!, available as part of a set for $12.00.
Video
Mary McGowan, Executive Director
Nancy Sander, Editor-in-Chief

1408 Stinging Insect Allergy
American Academy of Allergy, Asthma and Immunology
611 E Wells Street   414-272-6071
Milwaukee, WI 53202-3889   800-822-2762
                                        Fax: 414-272-6070
                                             www.aaaai.org
Although many people are afraid of stinging insects such as bees, the stings of these insects actually cause some people to have serious allergic reactions. This video tells how to recognize and avoid stinging insects, what to do if you are stung and how to identify symptoms of an allergic reaction and get medical help.
10-13 minutes

1409 Understanding Allergic Reactions
American Academy of Allergy, Asthma and Immunology
611 E Wells Street   414-272-6071
Milwaukee, WI 53202-3889   800-822-2762
                                        Fax: 414-272-6070
                                             www.aaaai.org
During an allergic reaction, your body responds to a substance generally considered harmless to most people. This video portrays what happens in you body's immune system during an allergic reaction, how to avoid allergic substances, and methods your allergist uses to treat your allergies.
10-13 minutes

1410 What School Personnel Should Know About Asthma
American Lung Association
1740 Broadway   212-315-8700
New York, NY 10019-4315
Professionally produced videotape discussing the triggers, symptoms and management of childhood asthma.
Videotape

1411 You're in Charge: Teens with Asthma
Asthma and Allergy Foundation of America
1233 20th Street NW   202-466-7643
Washington, DC 20036-2330   800-727-8462
                                        Fax: 202-466-8940
                                             www.aafa.org
Designed for young adults dealing with the daily challenges of asthma management. Teens share their experiences and use of peak flow meters and prescribed medications.
10 minutes

Web Sites

1412 American Academy of Allergy, Asthma and Immunology
                                             www.aaaai.org
The largest professional medical organization devoted to the allergy/immunology specialty. Represents asthma specialists, clinical immunologists, allied health professionals and others with a special interest in the research and treatment of allergic disease.

1413 American College of Allergy, Asthma and Immunology
                                             www.acaai.org
A professional association of more than 5,000 allergists/immunologists and allied health professionals whose mission is to promote excellence in the practice of the subspecialty of allergy and immunology.

1414 American Lung Association
                                             www.lungusa.org
To saave lives by improving lung health and preventing lung disease.

1415 Asthma and Allergy Foundation of America
                                             www.aafa.org
Dedicated to improving the quality of life for people with asthma and allergic diseases through education, advocacy and research.

1416 Gazoontite
                                             www.gazoontite.com
Provides links to websites involving asthma and also asthma-related products, such as books and guides.

1417 Healingwell
                                             www.healingwell.com
A social network and support community for patients, caregivers, and families coping with the daily struggles of diseases, disorders and chronic illness.

1418 Health Finder
                                             www.healthfinder.gov
A government web site where individuals can find information and tools to help you and those you care about stay healthy.

1419 Healthlink USA
                                             www.healthlinkusa.com

Health information concerning treatment, cures, prevention, diagnosis, risk factors, research, support groups, email lists, personal stories and much more. Updated regularly.

1420 Helios Health

www.helioshealth.com

Online resource for your health information. Detailed information about specific health topics, access to expert advice from our Medical Advisory Board, and up-to-date health news.

1421 MedicineNet

www.medicinenet.com

An online resource for consumers providing easy-to-read, authoritative medical and health information.

1422 Medscape

www.medscape.com

Medscape offers specialists, primary care physicians, and other health professionals the Web's most robust and integrated medical information and educational tools.

1423 WebMD

www.webmd.com

Provides links to over 100 articles involving asthma information.

Description

1424 Ataxia

Ataxia refers to a group of diseases that cause failure of muscular coordination, resulting in a staggered gait, the inability to stand or sit straight and the inability to make smooth, voluntary movements. All ataxias involve deterioration of the cerebellum and/or the brain and spinal structures that communicate with it. Conditions that are associated with ataxia may be hereditary or sporadic.

The most common hereditary ataxia is Friedreich's ataxia, which typically begins between 5 and 15 years of age. At first there is gait unsteadiness and slurred speech which progresses to weakness of the extremities. Some patients develop spinal deformity or cardiac problems. Other, less common hereditary ataxias generally begin during adult life. Sporadic cases also begin in adulthood and may be due to toxins, such as alcohol, or may be of unknown cause. Sporadic cases are often a symptom of some other disease, such as multiple sclerosis, stroke, or vitamin deficiencies. Although essentially all patients will become wheelchair-dependent at some point, the outlook for long-term survival is good.

Treatment for any of the ataxias is aimed at the underlying cause, but often supportive, with physical therapy, assistive devices, psychological support, career counseling and treatment of complications. Genetic counseling is appropriate for those with the hereditary forms and their families.

National Agencies & Associations

1425 National Ataxia Foundation
2600 Fernbrook Lane
Minneapolis, MN 55447
763-553-0020
Fax: 763-553-0167
e-mail: naf@ataxia.org
www.ataxia.org
The National Ataxia Foundation is dedicated to improving the lives of persons affected by ataxia through support education and research.
Michael Parent, Executive Director
Susan Hagen, Patient Services Director

Support Groups & Hotlines

1426 National Health Information Center
PO Box 1133
Washington, DC 20013
310-565-4167
800-336-4797
Fax: 301-984-4256
e-mail: info@nhic.org
www.health.gov/nhic
Offers a nationwide information referral service, produces directories and resource guides.

Alabama

1427 Alabama Ambassador: National Ataxia Foundation
123 Leigh Ann Road
Hazel Green, AL 35750
256-828-4858
e-mail: diannebw@aol.com
www.ataxia.org
Ambassadors are often in areas not served by a support group or chapter.
Dianne Blaine-Williamson, NAF Ambassador

1428 Alabama Support Group: National Ataxia Foundation
16 Oaks Circle
Birmingham, AL 35244
205-531-2514
e-mail: donnellyB6132@aol.com
www.ataxia.org
Becky Donnelly, Group Contact

Arizona

1429 Phoenix Area Support Group: National Ataxi Foundation
2322 W Sagebrush Drive
Chandler, AZ 85224-2155
480-726-3579
e-mail: rtg22@cox.net
www.ataxia.org
Rita Garcia, Director

1430 Tucson Support Group: National Ataxia Foundation
7665 E Placita Luna Preciosa
Tucson, AZ 85710
520-885-8326
e-mail: bbeck15@cox.net
Bart Beck, Director

California

1431 California Ambassador: National Ataxia Foundation
315 W Alamos
Clovis, CA 93612
559-281-9188
e-mail: mike betchel@yahoo.com
www.ataxia.org
Mike Betchel, NAF Ambassador

1432 Los Angeles Support Group: National Ataxia Foundation
339 W Palmer
Glendale, CA 91204
818-246-5758
e-mail: harryluther@sbcglobal.net
www.ataxia.org
Sid Luther, President

1433 Northern California Support Group: National Ataxia Foundation
26840 Eldridge Avenue
Hayward, CA 94544
510-783-3190
e-mail: rsisbig@aol.com
www.ataxia.com
Deborah Ominctin, Leader

1434 Orange County Support Group: National Ataxia Foundation
829 W Gary Ave
Montebello, CA 90640
323-788-7751
e-mail: dnavar@ucla.edu
www.ataxia.org
Daniel Navar, Group Leader

1435 San Diego Support Group: National Ataxia Foundation
2087 Granite Hills Drive
El Cajon, CA 92019
619-447-3753
e-mail: sdasg@cox.net
www.ataxia.org
Earl McLaughlin, Group Leader

Colorado

1436 Denver Support Group: National Ataxia Foundation
5902 W Maplewood Drive
Littleton, CO 80123
303-973-8035
e-mail: tom_sathre@acm.org
www.ataxia.org
Tom Sathre, Group Leader

Florida

1437 Florida Ambassador: National Ataxia Foundation
302 Beach Drive
Destin, FL 30541
850-654-2817
e-mail: csugars@cox.net
www.ataxia.org
Ambassadors are often in areas not served by a support group or chapter.
Christina Sugars, NAF Ambassador

1438 Northwest Florida Support Group: National Ataxia Foundation
54 Troon Terrace
Ponte Vedra, FL 32082-3321
904-273-4644
e-mail: jmcgranepvb@bellsouth.net
www.ataxia.org
June McGrane, Group Leader

1439 West Central FL Support Group: National Ataxia Foundation
9753 Elm Way
Tampa, FL 33635
813-453-1084
e-mail: flataxia@yahoo.com
www.ataxia.org
Crystal Frohna, Group Leader

Georgia

1440 Georgia Support Group: National Ataxia Foundation
320 Peters Street
Savannah, GA 30313
404-822-7451
e-mail: rookssgj@yahoo.com
www.ataxia.org

Greg Rooks, Group Leader

Illinois

1441 Chicago Area Support Group: National Ataxia Foundation
410 W Mahogany Ct
Palatine, IL 60067
847-496-7544
e-mail: caasg2@aol.com
www.ataxia.org

Craig Lisack, Group Leader

1442 Chicago Metro Support Group: National Ataxia Foundation
5633 N Kenmore
Chicago, IL 60660
773-334-1667
e-mail: cmarsh34@ameritech.net
www.ataxia.org

Chris Marsh, Group Leader

Indiana

1443 Southern Indiana Support Group: National Ataxia Foundation
1102 Ridgewood Drive
Huntingburg, IN 47542
812-630-4783
e-mail: monicasfaith@insightbb.com
www.ataxia.org

Monica Smith, Group Leader

Louisiana

1444 Louisiana Support Group: National Ataxia Foundation
2250 Gause Blvd
Slidell, LA 70431
985-643-0783
e-mail: ataxia1@earthlink.net
www.ataxia.org

Carla Hagler, Group Leader

Maine

1445 Maine Support Group: National Ataxia Foundation
PO Box 113
Bowdoinham, ME 04008
e-mail: rollins@gwi.net
www.ataxia.org

Kelly Rollins, Group Leader

Maryland

1446 Chesapeake Area Support Group: National Ataxia Foundation
3200 Baker Circle
Adamstown, MD 21710-9666
301-644-1836
e-mail: carljlauter@erols.com
www.ataxia.org

Carl J Lauter, Group Leader

Massachusetts

1447 New England Area Support Group: National Ataxia Foundation
45 Juliette Street
Andover, MA 01810
978-475-8072
www.ataxia.org

Donna Gorzela, Group Leader

Michigan

1448 Detroit Support Group: National Ataxia Foundation
20217 Wyoming
Detroit, MI 48221
313-736-2827
e-mail: tinyt48221@yahoo.cpom
www.ataxia.org

Tanya Tunstul, Group Leader

Minnesota

1449 Minnesota Ambassador: National Ataxia Foundation
5179 Meadow Drive SE
Rochester, MN 55904
504-282-7127
e-mail: logoetz@gmail.com
www.ataxia.org

Lori Goetzman, NAF Ambassador

1450 Twin Cities Area Support Group: National Ataxia Foundation
2549 32nd Avenue S
Minneapolis, MN 55406
612-724-3487
e-mail: lschultz@bitstream.net
www.ataxia.org

Lenore Healy Schultz, Group Leader

Mississippi

1451 Mississippi Area Support Group: National Ataxia Foundation
PO Box 17005
Hattisburg, MS 39404
e-mail: daglio1@bellsouth.net
www.ataxia.org

Camille Daglio, Group Leader

Missouri

1452 Kansas City Support Group: National Ataxia Foundation
17700 E 17th Terrace Court S
Independence, MO 64057
816-257-2428
www.ataxia.org

Lois Goodman, Group Leader

1453 Mid Missouri Support Group: National Ataxia Foundation
1609 Cocoa Court
Columbia, MO 65202
573-474-7232
e-mail: rogercooley@localnet.com
www.ataxia.org

Roger Cooley, Contact

New York

1454 Central NY Area Support Group: National Ataxia Foundation
2849 Bingley Road
Cazenovia, NY 13035
e-mail: johnsons@summitsolutions.net
www.ataxia.org

Linda Johnson, President

1455 New York Ambassador National Ataxia Foundation
36 W Redoubt Rd
Fishkill, NY 12524
763-553-0020
e-mail: vrabsolutely@aol.com
www.ataxia.org

Valerie Ruggiero, NAF Ambassador

1456 Tri-State Area Support Group: National Ataxia Foundation
Northgate 6C
Bronxville, NY 10708
212-844-8711
e-mail: markmeghan@aol.com
www.ataxia.org

Mark Mitchell, Group Leader

Ohio

1457 Central Ohio Support Group: National Ataxia Foundation
7852 Country Court
Mentor, OH 44060
440-255-8284
e-mail: wurbanski@oh.rr.com
www.ataxia.org

Cecilia Urbanski, Group Leader

1458 North East Ohio Support Group National Ataxia Foundation
Box 148
Mesopotamia, OH 44439
440-693-4454
e-mail: kakah@windstream.net
www.ataxia.org

Joe Miller, President

1459 Ohio Ambassador: National Ataxia Foundation
1283 Westfield SW
North Canton, OH 44720
330-499-4060
e-mail: jkardos@juno.com
www.ataxia.org

James Kardos, NAF Ambassador

Oklahoma

1460 Oklahoma Ambassador: National Ataxia Foundation
5700 SE Hazel Road
Bartlesville, OK 74006
918-331-9530
e-mail: droopydog36@hotmail.com
www.ataxia.org

Darrell Owens, NAF Ambassador

1461 **Willamette Valley Support Group: National Ataxia Foundation**
Albany General Hospital   541-812-4162
Albany, OR 97321   Fax: 541-812-4614
e-mail: malindam@samhealth.org
www.ataxia.org

Malinda Moore, President

1462 **South East Pennsylvania Support Group: National Ataxia Foundation**
610-272-1502
e-mail: lizout@aol.com
www.ataxia.org

Liz Nussear, Group Leader

1463 **Carolinas Support Group: National Ataxia National Ataxia Foundation**
1305 Cely Road   864-220-3395
Easley, SC 29642   e-mail: cecerussell@hotmail.com
www.ataxia.org

Cece Russell, Group Leader

1464 **Houston Support Group: National Ataxia Foundation**
9405 Highway 6 S   281-693-1826
Houston, TX 77083   e-mail: angelahcloud@aol.com
www.ataxia.org

Angela Cloud, Group Leader

1465 **North Texas Support Group: National Ataxia Foundation**
7 Wentworth Court
Trophy Club, TX 76262   e-mail: chevel1e@sbcglobal.net
www.ataxia.org

David Henry Jr, Group Leader

1466 **Texas Ambassador: National Ataxia Foundation**
356 Las Brisas Blvd   830-557-6050
Seguin, TX 78155-0193   e-mail: acemom@peoplepc.com
www.ataxia.org

Barbara Pluta, NAF Ambassador

1467 **Utah Support Group: National Ataxia Foundation**
Moran Eye Clinic   801-585-2213
Salt Lake City, UT 84132   e-mail: julia.kleinschmidt@hsc.utah.edu
www.ataxia.org

Dr Julia Kleinschmidt, Group Leader

1468 **Seattle Support Group: National Ataxia Foundation**
14104 107th Avenue   425-823-6239
Kirkland, WA 98034   e-mail: ataxiaseattle@comcast.net
www.ataxia.org

Milly Lewendon, Group Leader

1469 **Washington Ambassador National Ataxia Foundation**
PO Box 19045
Spokane, WA 99219   509-482-8501
www.ataxia.org

Linda Jacoy, Ambassador

Books

1470 **Directory of National Genetic Voluntary Organizations**
Genetic Alliance
4301 Connecticut Avenue NW   202-966-5557
Washington, DC 20008-2369   800-336-4363
Fax: 202-966-8553
e-mail: info@genticalliance.org
www.genticalliance.org

Lists hundreds of organizations and associations dealing with genetic conditions.

1471 **Hereditary Ataxia: Guidebook for Managing Speech & Swallowing**
National Ataxia Foundation
2600 Fernbrook Lane N   763-553-0020
Minneapolis, MN 55447-4752   Fax: 763-553-0167
e-mail: naf@mr.net
www.ataxia.org

1472 **Living with Ataxia**
National Ataxia Foundation
2600 Fernbrook Lane N   763-553-0020
Minneapolis, MN 55447-4752   Fax: 763-553-0167
e-mail: naf@mr.net
www.ataxia.org

Compassionate resource for people who have or may be at risk of having ataxia, and for their families. This book explains the nature and causes of ataxia, the basic genetics that underlie many kinds of ataxia, discusses medical management of ataxia, provides practical advice for everyday living, points the way to many useful resources and assures that living a good life is an entirely reasonable aspiration, even with ataxia.
112 pages

1473 **Ten Years to Live**
National Ataxia Foundation
2600 Fernbrook Lane N   763-553-0020
Minneapolis, MN 55447-4752   Fax: 763-553-0167
e-mail: naf@mr.net
www.ataxia.org

Struggles of the Schut family with hereditary ataxia.

ISBN: 0-962716-63-1

Newsletters

1474 **Alert**
Alliance of Genetic Support Groups
4301 Connecticut Avenue NW   301-652-5553
Washington, DC 20008-2304   800-336-4363
e-mail: alliance@capaccess.org
www.medhelp.org/www/agsg2.htm

Functions as a vehicle of communication between the Alliance and its constituency. Provides timely and useful information on genetics research.
Monthly

1475 **GENES Information Services**
Genetic Network of the Empire State
Empire State Plaza   518-474-7148
Albany, NY 12201   Fax: 518-474-8590

1476 **Generations**
National Ataxia Foundation
2600 Fernbrook Lane N   763-553-0020
Minneapolis, MN 55447-4752   Fax: 763-553-0167
e-mail: naf@mr.net
www.ataxia.org

Provides the latest in ataxia research, information on coping, reference material, updates on chapters and support groups and personal stories on living with ataxia. With a readership of more than 25,000, this publication is distributed throughout the US and the world. This publication is for ataxia families, the medical community, ataxia researchers and interested individuals. This publication is free to NAF members.
Quarterly

1477 **Genexus**
Great Plains Genetic Service Network
The University of Iowa   319-356-2674
Iowa City, IA 52242   Fax: 319-356-3347

1478 **Great Lakes Genetic News**
Great Lakes Regional Genetics Group
1500 Highland Avenue   608-266-2907
Madison, WI 53705-2274   Fax: 608-263-3496

1479 MARGIN
Mid-Atlantic Regional Human Genetics Network
260 S Broad Street   215-456-7910
Philadelphia, PA 19102-5021   Fax: 215-456-7911

1480 MSRGSN Newsletter
Mountain States Regional Genetics Service Network
4300 Cherry Creek Drive S   303-692-2423
Denver, CO 80246   Fax: 303-782-5576
                    e-mail: joyce.hooker@state.co.us
                                    www.mostgene.org

8-12 pages
Joyce Hooker, Coordinator

1481 NERG News
New England Regional Genetics Group
PO Box 670   207-839-5324
Mount Desert, ME 04660-0670   Fax: 207-839-8637

1482 SERGG
Southeast Regional Genetics Group
PO Box 1642   404-778-8551
Decatur, GA 30031-1642   Fax: 404-778-8562
                          e-mail: mlane@sergginc.org
                                        sergginc.org

Pamphlets

1483 Alliance Brochure
Genetic Alliance
4301 Connecticut Avenue NW   202-966-5557
Washington, DC 20008-2304   Fax: 202-966-8553
                    e-mail: info@geneticalliance.org
                                  www.geneticalliance.org
Explains the services and programs offered by the alliance.

1484 Ataxia Fact Sheet
National Ataxia Foundation
2600 Fernbrook Lane N   763-553-0020
Minneapolis, MN 55447-4752   Fax: 763-553-0167
                                    e-mail: naf@mr.net
                                        www.ataxia.org
Describes ataxia as a symptom and its association with other medical problems as well as the hereditary types.

1485 Familial Spastic Paraplegia
National Ataxia Foundation
2600 Fernbrook Lane N   763-553-0020
Minneapolis, MN 55447-4752   Fax: 763-553-0167
                                    e-mail: naf@mr.net
                                        www.ataxia.org
Defines this disorder and notes symptoms, causes and treatments.

1486 Frenkel's Exercises
National Ataxia Foundation
2600 Fernbrook Lane N   763-553-0020
Minneapolis, MN 55447-4752   Fax: 763-553-0167
                                    e-mail: naf@mr.net
                                        www.ataxia.org
Describes an exercise program designed for those with ataxia.

1487 Friedrich's Ataxia
National Ataxia Foundation
2600 Fernbrook Lane N   763-553-0020
Minneapolis, MN 55447-4752   Fax: 763-553-0167
                                    e-mail: naf@mr.net
                                        www.ataxia.org
Describes symptoms, diagnosis, genetics and hints on coping.

1488 Gene Testing for Ataxia
National Ataxia Foundation
2600 Fernbrook Lane N   763-553-0020
Minneapolis, MN 55447-4752   Fax: 763-553-0167
                                    e-mail: naf@mr.net
                                        www.ataxia.org
Describes the latest information about who should consider it and where to have it done.

1489 Health Insurance
National Ataxia Foundation
2600 Fernbrook Lane N   763-553-0020
Minneapolis, MN 55447-4752   Fax: 763-553-0167
                                    e-mail: naf@mr.net
                                        www.ataxia.org
Offers health insurance advice for persons with ataxia.

1490 Hereditary Ataxia: Brochure
National Ataxia Foundation
2600 Fernbrook Lane N   763-553-0020
Minneapolis, MN 55447-4752   Fax: 763-553-0167
                                    e-mail: naf@mr.net
                                        www.ataxia.org
Describes recessive and dominant ataxias, information on how hereditary ataxia is transmitted and explanations of the NAF's role in education, service and prevention.

1491 Hereditary Ataxia: Fact Sheets
National Ataxia Foundation
2600 Fernbrook Lane N   763-553-0020
Minneapolis, MN 55447-4752   Fax: 763-553-0167
                                    e-mail: naf@mr.net
                                        www.ataxia.org
Various ataxia fact sheets relating to specific forms of hereditary ataxia. Individual ataxia fact sheets include Friederich's ataxia and specific forms of spinocerebellar ataxias (SCAs).

1492 Incorporating Consumers into Regional Genetics Networks
Genetic Alliance
4301 Connecticut Avenue NW   202-966-5557
Washington, DC 20008-2304   Fax: 202-966-8553
                    e-mail: info@geneticalliance.org
                                  www.geneticalliance.org

1493 Informed Consent: Participation In Genetic Research Studies
Genetic Alliance
4301 Connecticut Avenue NW   202-966-5557
Washington, DC 20008-2304   Fax: 202-966-8553
                    e-mail: info@genticalliance.org
                                  www.geneticalliance.org
This booklet explains the nature of genetic research with its benefits and risks.

1494 Pen-Pal Directory
National Ataxia Foundation
2600 Fernbrook Lane N   763-553-0020
Minneapolis, MN 55447-4752   Fax: 763-553-0167
                                    e-mail: naf@mr.net
                                        www.ataxia.org
National, state and international directory of others who are affected by ataxia. Available to NAF Pen-Pal members only. Application available.

1495 Students with Friedreich's Ataxia
National Ataxia Foundation
2600 Fernbrook Lane N   763-553-0020
Minneapolis, MN 55447-4752   Fax: 763-553-0167
                                    e-mail: naf@mr.net
                                        www.ataxia.org
Worksheet for teachers, parents and others who need to understand the physical constraints of ataxia.

Audio & Video

1496 Together...There Is Hope
National Ataxia Foundation
2600 Fernbrook Lane N   763-553-0020
Minneapolis, MN 55447-4752   Fax: 763-553-0167
                                    e-mail: naf@mr.net
                                        www.ataxia.org
Video discussing ataxias genetic patterns of inheritance and the National Ataxia Foundation and its research efforts.

Web Sites

1497 Healing Well
                                  www.healingwell.com
An online health resource guide to medical news, chat, information and articles, newsgroups and message boards, books, disease-re-

111

lated web sites, medical directories, and more for patients, friends, and family coping with disabling diseases, disorders, or chronic illnesses.

1498 Health Finder

www.healthfinder.gov

Searchable, carefully developed web site offering information on over 1000 topics. Developed by the US Department of Health and Human Services, the site can be used in both English and Spanish.

1499 Healthlink USA

www.healthlinkusa.com

Health information concerning treatment, cures, prevention, diagnosis, risk factors, research, support groups, email lists, personal stories and much more. Updated regularly.

1500 Helios Health

www.helioshealth.com

Online resource for your health information. Detailed information about specific health topics, access to expert advice from our Medical Advisory Board, and up-to-date health news.

1501 MedicineNet

www.medicinenet.com

An online resource for consumers providing easy-to-read, authoritative medical and health information.

1502 Medscape

www.medscape.com

Medscape offers specialists, primary care physicians, and other health professionals the Web's most robust and integrated medical information and educational tools.

1503 National Ataxia Foundation

www.ataxia.org

Information on ataxia, ataxia research, listing of chapters and support groups and related links. Researchers may download NAF's ataxia reserch application guidelines and forms. Exerpts of articles in NAF's quarterly news publication, Generations. Online registration for NAF's annual membership meetings. Caladar of events on NAF activities. This site is for ataxia familes, the medical community, ataxia reserachers and interested individuals.

1504 WebMD

www.webmd.com

Information on Ataxia, including articles and resources.

Description

1505 Attention Deficit Hyperactivity Disorder

Attention Deficit-Hyperactivity Disorder, ADHD, and Attention Deficit Disorder, ADD, are neurologically based disorders. ADHD primarily affects children, with 2 to 4 percent of the school-age population in the United States having some symptoms. In about 25 percent of attention deficit cases, hyperactivity is not present, and it is thus labeled ADD. ADHD's three major symptoms are distractibility, impulsivity and hyperactivity. The dominant symptom of ADD is day dreaming or tuning out. ADHD is seen 10 times more frequently in boys than girls. Studies show that 90 percent have academic problems or are underachievers, although these difficulties may not begin until the middle school years.

While studies suggest that about 50 percent of children with these disorders will improve at puberty, both ADHD and ADD can exist throughout a lifetime and, in fact, may first be diagnosed in teen or adult years.

Often, an affected individual experiences difficulties that can impact learning, peer relations, family life, and self-esteem. These difficulties may manifest themselves through angry outbursts, self-imposed social isolation, blaming others, a quickness to fight, and a high sensitivity to criticism.

Treatment of ADHD and ADD include: education programs with resource or tutorial help; psychological programs to improve self-esteem and help families and individuals deal with associated stress; and medical therapy. Treatment must be individualized to address both intrinsic characteristics of the child and relevant environmental factors, and be coordinated with a variety of interventions within the school, home and community.

Many professionals agree that medication, when appropriate, combined with counseling, best controls symptoms. Stimulant medications, including the new longer active agents, are the drugs of choice. To identify children with this disorder and to develop the most appropriate treatment plan, parents will need to consult with a psychiatrist, pediatric neurologist, or pediatrician.

National Agencies & Associations

1506 Children & Adults with Attention Deficit Disorders
8181 Professional Place   301-306-7070
Landover, MD 20785   800-233-4050
Fax: 301-306-7090
www.chadd.org

CHADD's primary objectives are: to provide a support network for parents and caregivers; to provide a forum for continuing education; to be a community resource and disseminate accurate evidence-based information about AD/HD to parents, educators and adults.
E Clarke Ross, CEO
Ruth Hughes, Chief Program Officer Community Service

1507 Council for Exceptional Children
2900 Crystal Drive   703-620-3660
Arlington, VA 22202-3557   88- 23- 773
Fax: 703-264-9494
TTY: 866-915-5000
e-mail: service@cec.sped.org
www.cec.sped.org

Advocates appropriate policies standards and development for individuals with special needs. Provides professional development for special educators.
Bruce Ramirez, Executive Director
Joan Melner, Assistant Executive Director

1508 Feingold Association of the US
37 Shell Road   631-369-9340
Rocky Point, NY 11778   800-321-3287
Fax: 631-369-2988
e-mail: help@feingold.org
www.feingold.org

Helps families of children with learning and behavior problems including attention deficit disorder. Also helps chemically-sensitive and salicylate-sensitive adults. Program is based upon a diet which primarily eliminates certain synthetic food additives.

1509 Learning Disabilities Association of America
4156 Library Road   412-341-1515
Pittsburgh, PA 15234-1349   888-300-6710
Fax: 412-344-0224
e-mail: info@LDAAmerica.org
www.ldaamerica.org

An information and referral center for parents and professionals dealing with learning disabilities.
Barbara Lefler, Director of Affiliate Services
Patricia Lillie, President

1510 National Center for Learning Disabilities
381 Park Avenue S   212-545-7510
New York, NY 10016-8806   888-575-7373
Fax: 212-545-9665
www.ncld.org

One of the foremost nonprofit organizations committed to improving the lives of the estimated one in ten children with learning disabilities raising public awareness and understanding.
James H Wendorf, Executive Director
Sheldon H Horowitz EdD, Director/Professional Services

1511 National Dissemination Center for Children with Disabilities
1825 Connecticut Avenue NW   202-884-8200
Washington, DC 20009   800-695-0285
Fax: 202-884-8441
e-mail: nichcy@aed.org
www.nichcy.org

Publishes free, fact filled newsletters. Arranges workshops. Advises parents on the laws entitling children with disabilities to special education and other services.
Dr Suzanne Ripley, Contact

Libraries & Resource Centers

1512 HEATH Resource Center
George Washington University
2134 G Street NW   202-973-0904
Washington, DC 20052-0001   800-544-3284
Fax: 202-994-3365
e-mail: askheath@gwu.edu
http://www.heath.gwu.edu/

The HEATH Resource Center of The George Washington University, Graduate School of Education and Human Development, is the national clearinghouse on postsecondary education for individuals with disabilities.
Dr Lynda West, Principal Investigator
Dr Joel Gomez, Co-Principal Investigator

Support Groups & Hotlines

1513 Attention Deficit Information Network
475 Hillside Ave   617-455-9895
Needham, MA 02194

Offers support and information to families of children with attention deficit disorder, adults with ADD and professionals through an international network of 60 parent and adult chapters.

1514 National Federation of Families for Children's Mental Health
9605 Medical Center Drive 240-403-1901
Rockville, MD 20850 Fax: 240-403-1909
e-mail: ffcmh@ffcmh.org
www.ffcmh.org
Provides advocacy at the national level for the rights of children and youth with emotional, behavioral and mental health challenges and their families; provides leadership and technical assistance to a nation-wide network of family run organizations; and collaborates with family run and other child serving organizations to transform mental health care in America.
Sandra Spencer, Executive Director
Andrea Barnes, Policy & Research Assistant

1515 National Health Information Center
PO Box 1133 310-565-4167
Washington, DC 20013-1133 800-336-4797
Fax: 301-984-4256
e-mail: info@nhic.org
www.health.gov/nhic
A health information referral service sponsored by the Office of Disease Prevention and Health Promotion. Puts health professionals and consumers who have health questions in touch with those organizations that are best able to provide answers.

Books

1516 ADHD Parenting Handbook: Practical Advice for Parents from Parents
Colleen Alexander-Roberts, author

Taylor Trade Publishing
4501 Forbes Boulevard 301-459-3366
Lanham, MD 20706 Fax: 301-429-5743
e-mail: custserv@nbnbooks.com
www.rlpgtrade.com
A compilation of practical advice and tips for handling day-to-day activities that routinely become problematic for ADHD children, such as getting dressed for school, going to bed, performing chores, completing homework, and playing with other children.
Paperback
ISBN: 0-878338-62-4

1517 ADHD in Schools: Assessment and Intervention Strategies
George J DuPaul, Gary Stoner, author

Guilford Publications
72 Spring Street
New York, NY 10012 800-365-7006
Fax: 212-966-6708
e-mail: info@guilford.com
www.guilford.com
Provides essential guidance for school-based professionals meeting the challenges of ADHD at any grade level. Comprehensive and practical, includes several reproducible assessment tools and handouts.
330 pages Paperback
ISBN: 1-593850-89-0

1518 ADHD: Handbook for Diagnosis & Treatment
Western Psychological Services
12031 Wilshire Boulevard 310-478-2061
Los Angeles, CA 90025-1201 800-648-8857
Fax: 310-478-7838
www.wpspublish.com
This second edition helps clinicians diagnose and treat Attention Deficit Hyperactivity Disorder. Written by an internationally recognized authority in the field, it covers the history of ADHD, its primary symptoms, associated conditions, developmental course and outcome, and family context. A workbook companion manual is also available.
700 pages

1519 Attention Deficit Disorder: A Different Perception
Underwood-Miller

708 Westover Drive
Lancaster, PA 17601-1242 717-285-2255
www.vance.hw.nl/dbase/publisher
1993 180 pages Paperback
ISBN: 0-887331-56-4

1520 Attention Deficit Disorder: Learning Disabilities
Random House
25 Van Zant Street 410-848-1900
East Norwalk, CT 06855-1726 800-726-0600
Fax: 800-214-1438
www.randomhouse.com
Realities, myths, and controversial treatments. Section I tries to dispel the myths and discusses proven treatments for ADHD and LD. Section II explains how the scientific community evaluates new treatment methods, and Section III summarizes alternative treatments and discusses scientific evidence pertaining to its usefulness.
256 pages
ISBN: 0-385469-31-4

1521 Attention Deficit Hyperactivity Disorder: What Every Parent Wants to Know
Paul H Brookes Publishing Company
PO Box 10624 301-337-9580
Baltimore, MD 21285-0624 800-638-3775
Fax: 410-337-8539
e-mail: custserv@brookspublishing.com
www.brookespublishing.com
1993 320 pages Paperback
ISBN: 1-557661-41-3
Dante Washington, Customer Service Representative

1522 Coping with ADD/ADHD
Rosen Publishing Group
29 E 21st Street 212-777-3017
New York, NY 10010-6209 800-237-9932
Fax: 888-436-4643
e-mail: customerservice@rosenpub.com
www.rosenpublishing.com
At least 3.5 million American youngsters suffer from ADD. This book defines the syndrome and provides specific information about treatment and counseling.
150 pages Hardcover
ISBN: 0-823931-96-X

1523 Helping Your ADD Child With or Without Hyperactivity
John F Taylor PhD, author

Random House Inc.
Department of Library Marketing 800-733-3000
New York, NY 10017 800-726-0600
Fax: 212-940-7381
e-mail: crownpublicity@randomhouse.com
www.randomhouse.com
Inside this book you will find step-by-step tools for helping your ADD or ADHD child. From extensive screening for spotting the initial signs to the pros and cons of nutritional, psychological, and drug treatments.
2001
ISBN: 0-761527-56-7

1524 Hyperactive Children Grown Up
Gabrielle Weiss, Lily Trokenberg Hechtman, author

Guilford Publications
72 Spring Street
New York, NY 10012 800-365-7006
Fax: 212-966-6708
e-mail: info@guilford.com
www.guilford.com
Reports findings on the etiology, treatment, and outcome of attention deficits and hyperactivity at all stages of development.
473 pages Paperback
ISBN: 0-898625-96-7

1525 LD Child and the ADHD Child
Suzanne H Stevens, author

John F Blair Publishing

1406 Plaza Drive
Winston-Salem, NC 27103

336-768-1374
800-222-9796
Fax: 336-768-9194
e-mail: blairpub@aol.com
www.blairpub.com

Helps parents raise their LD and/or ADHD children so that they, too, can grow up to be okay-so that they will be happy, well-adjusted, and successful adults despite the learning and behavior patterns that make them different.
Paperback
ISBN: 0-895871-42-8

1526   Managing Attention Deficit Hyperactivity Disorder in Children:
Sam Goldstein, Michael Goldstein, author

Wiley Publishing
111 River Street
Hoboken, NJ 07030-5774

201-748-6000
Fax: 201-748-6088
e-mail: info@wiley.com
www.wiley.com

A proven approach to the diagnosis and management of one of the most challenging childhood disorders. In this book the authors describe a proven multidisciplinary approach to the diagnosis and treatment of childhood ADHD, developed at the prestigous Neurology, Learning and Behavior Center in Salt Lake City.
1998 896 pages
ISBN: 0-471121-58-9

1527   Maybe You Know My Kid: A Parent's Guide to Identifying ADHD

Birch Lane Press
120 Enterprise Avenue S
Secaucus, NJ 07094-1902   800-447-2665

The author writes about her family experiences with their son, David, who has attention deficit disorder. Contains a comprehensive review of important issues plus descriptions of some helpful management techniques.
222 pages

1528   Medications for Attention Disorders and Related Medical Problems

Specialty Press
300 NW 70th Avenue
Plantation, FL

954-792-8100
800-233-9273
Fax: 954-792-8545
e-mail: sales@addwarehouse.com
www.addwarehouse.com

A comprehensive handbook covering the history, characteristics, and causes of ADHD. The equal importance of appropriate academic programming, counseling, and medication are stressed throughout.
415 pages Hardcover

1529   Parents Helping Parents: A Directory of Support Groups for ADD

CibaGelgy, Pharmaceuticals Division
External Communications   908-277-5000
Summit, NJ 07901   Fax: 973-781-2601

1530   Parents' Hyperactivity Handbook: Helping the Fidgety Child

Plenum Press
233 Spring Street
New York, NY 10013-1578

212-620-8000
Fax: 212-463-0742
e-mail: info@plenum.com

1993 306 pages
ISBN: 0-306444-65-8

1531   Rethinking Attention Deficit Disorders
Miriam Cherkes-Julkowski, author

Brookline Books
PO Box 1209
Brookline, MA 02445

617-734-6772
800-666-2665
Fax: 617-734-3952
www.brooklinebooks.com

Gives the classroom teacher useful information that provides ideas and strategies for working with children suffering from ADD.
1997 Paperback
ISBN: 1-571290-37-0

1532   The New ADD in Adults Workbook
Lynn Weiss, PhD, author

Taylor Trade Publishing
4501 Forbes Boulevard
Lanham, MD 20706

301-459-3366
Fax: 301-429-5743
e-mail: custserv@nbnbooks.com
www.rlpgtrade.com

Not only touches on and dispels the most recent clinical findings, but also emphasizes the bigger perspective, focusing on the empowerment and diversity issues facing all of us on the A.D.D. continuum today. Persuades readers to work through their challenges with practical, prescriptive exercises and insights.
Paperback
ISBN: 0-878338-50-0

1533   You Mean I'm Not Lazy, Stupid or Crazy?

Tyrell & Jerem Press
PO Box 20089
Cincinnati, OH 45220-0089   800-622-6611

A new self-help book is the first written by ADD adults for ADD adults. This comprehensive guide provides accurate information, practical how-tos and moral support.

1534   Attention Deficit/Hyperactivity Disorder

Guilford Publications
72 Spring Street
New York, NY 10012-4068

212-431-9800
800-365-7006
Fax: 212-966-6708

A second edition that is the handbook on the diagnosis and treatment of ADHD in the 1990s. A companion workbook is also available with forms that may be photocopied.
747 pages Hardcover
ISBN: 0-898624-43-6

Children's Books

1535   Self-Control Games & Workbook

Western Psychological Services
12031 Wilshire Boulevard
Los Angeles, CA 90025-1201

310-478-2061
800-648-8857
Fax: 310-478-7838

This game is designed to teach self-control in academic and social situations. Addresses a total of 24 impulsive, inattentive and hyperactive behaviors. The companion workbook reinforces the use of positive self-statements, and problem-solving techniques, instead of expressing anger.
Game

1536   Shelley, the Hyperactive Turtle
Deborah Moss, author

Woodbine House
6510 Bells Mill Road
Bethesda, MD 20817

800-843-7323
Fax: 301-897-5838
e-mail: info@woodbinehouse.com
www.woodbinehouse.com

Reassures young children who are going through the diagnostic process or who are having problems behaving at school or making friends because of AD/HD.
20 pages
ISBN: 1-890627-75-1

Magazines

1537   Attention

Children & Adults with Attention Deficit Disorder
8181 Professional Place
Landover, MD 20785-7221

301-306-7070
800-233-4050
Fax: 301-306-7090
TTY: 301-429-0641

Quarterly

Newsletters

1538 ADHD Report
Guilford Publications
72 Spring Street
New York, NY 10012

800-365-7006
Fax: 212-966-6708
e-mail: info@guilford.com
www.guilford.com

Examines the nature, diagnosis, and outcomes associated with the disorder, and provides a single reliable guide to the latest developments in the fields of clinical management and education. Includes research findings, as well as ongoing coverage of ADHD in the news.
16 pages BiMonthly

1539 Chadder
Children & Adults with Attention Deficit Disorder
8181 Professional Place
Landover, MD 20785-7221

301-306-7070
800-233-4050
Fax: 301-306-7090
TTY: 301-429-0641

Quarterly

1540 Challenge
Challenge
PO Box 488
West Newbury, MA 01985-0688

978-462-0495
800-233-2322

National newsletter on ADD/ADHD that carries interviews with nationally-known scientists, as well as physicians, psychologists, social workers, educators, and other practitioners in the field of ADHD.
12 pages BiMonthly
Jean C Harrison, Executive Director

1541 Pure Facts
Feingold Association of the US
PO Box 6550
Alexandria, VA 22306-0550

703-768-3287

Monthly newsletter with articles on nutrition and behavior and lists of approved brand-name foods.

Pamphlets

1542 ADHD
Learning Disabilities Association of America
4156 Library Road
Pittsburgh, PA 15234-1349

412-341-1515
888-300-6710
Fax: 412-344-0224
e-mail: info@ldaamerica.org
www.ldaamerica.org

A booklet for parents offering information on Attention Deficit Hyperactivity Disorders and learning disabilities.
Sheila Buckley, Executive Director

1543 Attention Deficit Disorders and Hyperactivity
Council for Exceptional Children
1110 N Glebe Road
Arlington, VA 22201

703-620-3660
888-232-7733
Fax: 703-264-9494
e-mail: service@cec.sped.org
www.cec.sped.org

Published by the Council for Exceptional Children.

1544 COGREHAB
Life Science Associates
1 Fennimore Road
Bayport, NY 11705-2115

631-472-2111
Fax: 631-472-8146
e-mail: lifesciassoc@pipeline.com
lifesciassoc.home.pipeline.com

Divided into six groups for diagnosis and treatment of attention, memory and perceptual disorders to be used by and under the guidance of a professional.
$95 - $1,950

1545 Fact Sheet: Attention Deficit Hyperactivity Disorder
Learning Disabilities Association of America
4156 Library Road
Pittsburgh, PA 15234-1349

412-341-1515
888-300-6710
Fax: 412-344-0224
e-mail: info@ldaamerica.org
www.ldaamerica.org

A pamphlet offering factual information on ADHD.
Sheila Buckley, Executive Director

1546 Helping Adolescents with ADHD and Learning Disabilities
Learning Disabilities Association of America
4156 Library Road
Pittsburgh, PA 15234-1349

412-341-1515
888-300-6710
Fax: 412-344-0224
e-mail: info@ldaamerica.org
www.ldaamerica.org

Sheila Buckley, Executive Director

Audio & Video

1547 ADD Stepping Out of the Dark
ADD Videos
PO Box 622
New Paltz, NY 12561-0622

845-255-3612
Fax: 845-883-6452

A powerful, effective video, ideal for health professionals, educators and parents providing a visual montage designed to promote an understanding and awareness of attention deficit disorder. Based on actual accounts of those who have ADD, including a neurologist, an office worker, and parents of children with ADD. The video allows the viewer to feel the frustration and lack of attention that ADD brings to many.
Video
Lenae Madonna, Producer

1548 ADHD in Adults
Guilford Publications
72 Spring Street
New York, NY 10012-4068

212-431-9800
800-365-7006
Fax: 212-966-6708

This program integrates information on ADHD with the actual experiences of four adults who suffer from the disorder. Representing a range of professions, from a lawyer to a mother working at home, each candidly discusses the impact of ADHD on his or her daily life. These interviews are augmented by comments from family members and other clinicians who treat adults with ADHD.
Video

1549 ADHD in the Classroom: Strategies for Teachers
Rusell A Barkley, author

Guilford Publications
72 Spring Street
New York, NY 10012

800-365-7006
Fax: 212-966-6708
e-mail: info@guilford.com
www.guilford.com

Designed to help teachers create a learning environment that is responsive to the needs of all students, including those with ADHD.

1550 ADHD: What Do We Know?
Guilford Publications
72 Spring Street
New York, NY 10012-4068

212-431-9800
800-365-7006
Fax: 212-966-6708

An introduction for teachers and special education practitioners, school psychologists and parents of ADHD children. Topics outlined in this video include the causes and prevalence of ADHD, ways children with ADHD behave, other conditions that may accompany ADHD and long-term prospects for children with ADHD.
Video

1551 Around the Clock
Guilford Publications
72 Spring Street
New York, NY 10012-4068

212-431-9800
800-365-7006
Fax: 212-966-6708

This videotape provides both professionals and parents a helpful look at how the difficulties facing parents of ADHD children can be handled.

1552 Attention Deficit Disorder
Pro-Ed, Inc.
8700 Shoal Creek Boulevard   512-451-3246
Austin, TX 78757-6897   800-897-3202
                               Fax: 800-397-7633
                          e-mail: info@proedinc.com
                          www.proedinc.com/
A video and book providing helpful suggestions for both home and
classroom management of students with attention deficit disorder.
216 pages Paperback
ISBN: 0-890797-42-0
Krista Anderson, Technical Advisor
Matt Synatschk, Books & Materials Permissions Editor

1553 Educating Inattentive Children
Western Psychological Services
12031 Wilshire Boulevard
Los Angeles, CA 90025-1201   800-648-8857
                               Fax: 310-478-7838
An excellent resource for teachers who encounter inattention and
hyperactivity in the classroom. It helps teachers distinguish deliberate misbehavior from the incompetent, nonpurposeful behavior
of the inattentive child.
Video

1554 It's Just Attention Disorder
Western Psychological Services
12031 Wilshire Boulevard   310-478-2061
Los Angeles, CA 90025-1201   800-648-8857
                               Fax: 310-478-7838
This ground-breaking videotape takes the critical first steps in
treating attention-deficit disorder: it enlists the inattentive or hy-
peractive child as an active participant in his or her treatment.
Video

1555 Why Won't My Child Pay Attention?
Western Psychological Services
12031 Wilshire Boulevard   310-478-2061
Los Angeles, CA 90025-1201   800-648-8857
                               Fax: 310-478-7838
Practical and reassuring videotape, noted child psychologist tells
parents about two of the most common and complex problems of
childhood: inattention and hyperactivity.
Video

Web Sites

1556 Attention Deficit Information Network
                          www.addinfonetwork.com
Offers support and information to families of children and adults
with ADD and to professionals.

1557 Healing Well
                          www.healingwell.com
A social network and support community for patients, caregivers,
and families coping with the daily struggles of diseases, disorders
and chronic illness.

1558 Health Finder
                          www.healthfinder.gov
A government web site, where individuals can find information
and tools to help you and those you care about stay healthy.

1559 Healthlink USA
                          www.healthlinkusa.com
Health information concerning treatment, cures, prevention, diagnosis, risk factors, research, support groups, email lists, personal
stories and much more. Updated regularly.

1560 Helios Health
                          www.helioshealth.com
Online resource for your health information. Detailed information
about specific health topics, access to expert advice from our Medical Advisory Board, and up-to-date health news.

1561 MedicineNet
                          www.medicinenet.com
An online resource for consumers providing easy-to-read, authoritative medical and health information.

1562 Medscape
                          www.medscape.com
Medscape offers specialists, primary care physicians, and other
health professionals the Web's most robust and integrated medical
information and educational tools.

1563 WebMD
                          www.webmd.com
Information on Attention Deficit Disorder, including articles and
resources.

Description

1564 Autistic Spectrum Disorders

Autistic Spectrum Disorders, ASD, includes (from most to least severe) autism, high-functioning autism (HFA), Asperger's syndrome, and PDD-NOS (pervasive development disorder — not otherwise specified). ASD typically appear during the first three years of life. Autism involves severe impairment of social and communication development. HFA symptoms are less severe, but include delayed language development. Asperger's is similar to HFA, but with no speech delay. PPD-NOS describes autistic categories that do not fit into any of the above. ASD affects behavior, communication, social interaction and other neurological functions.

ASD has numerous symptoms, all of which reduce the child's ability to communicate and interact. Many autistic children have abnormal social relationships, impaired understanding, and uneven intellectual development with mental retardation in most cases. They may exhibit repetitive movement (i.e., rocking, spinning, and hand twisting), avoid making eye contact, and have impaired verbal skills. Occasionally, children with ASD will have decreased sensitivity to pain, and have abnormal responses to light, touch and sound. The disorder can include self-injury and bizarre behavior.

ASD is two to four times more common in boys than in girls. It is found in people of all ethnic backgrounds, and throughout the world. In 2009, nine in 1000 children were diagnosed with ASD, up from one in 500 just six years ago.

In some cases, ASD may be linked to damage to the brain or nervous system. Studies of twins with autism point to a possible genetic link. ASD has been associated with the following risk factors: pre- and perinatal birth complications; prenatal infections with certain viruses; abnormalities of the brain detected with a CT scan or MRI (although no specific defects in the brain structure have been consistently identified). More recently, usual childhood vaccines, environmental toxins, and pollutants are being questioned to explain the sharp rise in ASD cases in recent decades, but researchers have been unable to confirm these findings.

Although there are no known cures for ASD, experts advocate early and intense behavioral, developmental and speech therapy. Medications may alleviate some of the accompanying behavior problems, but provide minimal help for the disorder itself and are generally not used. There is strong emphasis on early diagnosis, early intervention, and individualized educational programs to provide the opportunity for maximum development for the child with Autistic Spectrum Disorder.

National Agencies & Associations

1565 ARRISE
9238 Parklane Avenue
Franklin Park, IL 60131-2836   847-451-2740

Provides information about autism.

1566 Autism Research Institute
4182 Adams Avenue   619-281-7165
San Diego, CA 92116-2536   866-366-3361
Fax: 619-563-6840
www.autism.com

A clearinghouse for research on autism and related disorders of learning and behavior. Conducts and compiles research findings to provide people with the latest research available.
Stephen M Edelson PhD, Director

1567 Autism Services Center
929 Fourth Avenue   304-525-8014
Huntington, WV 25701-0507   Fax: 304-525-8026
www.autismservicescenter.org

Provides educational information to the public and professional communities on autism provides case management activities and referrals for persons afflicted with autism and their families.
Ruth Christ Sullivan, Founder and Executive Director

1568 Autism Society of America
4740 East-West Hwy   301-657-0881
Bethesda, MD 20814   800-328-8476
Fax: 301-657-0869
e-mail: info@autism-society.org
www.autism-society.org

A national charitable organization with the mission of providing as much information as possible about autism and the various options, approaches, methods and systems available to parents of children with autism, family members and professionals.
Lee Grossman, President/CEO
Barbara Newhouse, Chief Operating Officer

1569 Autism Treatment Center of America
2080 S Undermountain Road   413-229-2100
Sheffield, MA 01257   877-766-7473
Fax: 413-229-3202
e-mail: correspondence@option.org
www.autismtreatmentcenter.org

Since 1983 the Autism Treatment Center of America has provided innovative training programs for parents and professionals caring for children challenged by Autism Autism Spectrum Disorders Pervasive Developmental Disorder (PDD) and other developmental disorders.
Barry Neil Kaufman, Co-Founder/Co-Creator Son-Rise Program
Bryn Hogan, Director Son-Rise Program

1570 Autism Treatment Center of America: Son-Rise Program
2080 South Undermountain Road   413-229-2100
Sheffield, MA 01257   877-766-7473
Fax: 413-229-3202
e-mail: correspondence@option.org
www.son-rise.org

Since 1983, the Autism Treatment Center of America has provided innovative training programs for parents and professionals caring for children challenged by Autism, Autism Spectrum Disorders, Pervasive Developmental Disorder (PDD) and other developmental difficulties. The Son-Rise Program teaches a specific yet comprehensive system of treatment and education designed to help families and caregivers enable their children to dramatically improve in all areas of learning.
Sean Fitzgerald, Assistant Director Son-Rise Program
Barry Neil Kaufman, Co-Founder

1571 Community Services for Autistic Adults & Children
8615 E Village Avenue   240-912-2220
Montgomery Village, MD 20886   Fax: 301-926-9384
e-mail: csaac@csaac.org
www.csaac.org

The Community Services for Autistic Adults & Children is a non-profit organization dedicated to helping those with autism. Since 1979 CSAAC has served over 150 individuals and helped people with autism find housing, employment and other community services.
Ian Paregol, Executive Director
Don Rodrick, Chief Financial Officer

1572 **National Institute of Neurological Disorders and Stroke**
NIH Neurological Institute 301-496-5751
Bethesda, MD 20824 800-352-9424
Fax: 301-402-2186
TTY: 301-468-5981
www.ninds.nih.gov

The mission of NINDS is to reduce the burden of neurological disease - a burden borne by every age group, by every segment of society, by people all over the world.
Story C Landis, PhD, Director
Walter J Koroshetz, Deputy Director

State Agencies & Associations

Alabama

1573 **Autism Society of Alabama**
Birmingham, AL 35243 205-951-1364
877-4AU-TISM
Fax: 205-967-8244
e-mail: info@autism-alabama.org
www.autism-alabama.org

Ryan Thomas, President
Jennifer Muller, Executive Director

1574 **Autism Society of North Alabama**
PO Box 2902 256-776-0505
Huntsville, AL 35801-2902 e-mail: sherron@northalabamaautism.org
www.northalabamaautism.org

Teresa White, President
Carol Wright, Vice President

Arizona

1575 **Autism Society of Pima County**
PO Box 44156 520-770-1541
Tucson, AZ 85733-4156 Fax: 520-319-5979
e-mail: az-pimacounty@autismsocietyofamerica.org
www.tucsonautism.org

Peter Earhart, President
Stephanie Hillÿ, Vice President

California

1576 **Autism Society of California**
PO Box 15247 562-943-3335
Long Beach, CA 90815-0600 800-700-0037
e-mail: brubin698@earthlink.net
www.autismsocietyca.org

Dean Wilson, President
Gregory Fletcher, First Vice President

Colorado

1577 **Autism Society of Colorado**
550ÿSÿWadsworth Boulevard 720-214-0794
Lakewood, CO 80226-4169 Fax: 720-274-2744
e-mail: co-colorado@autismsocietyofamerica.org
www.autismcolorado.org

Betty Lehman, Executive Director
Lorri Park, ProgramsÿDirector

Connecticut

1578 **Autism Society of Connecticut**
PO Box 1404
Guilford, CT 06437 888-453-4975
www.autismsocietyofct.org

Delaware

1579 **Autism Society of Delaware**
924 Old Harmony Road 302-224-6020
Newark, DE 19713 Fax: 302-224-6017
e-mail: delautism@delautism.org
www.delautism.org

Theda Ellis, Executive Director
Kim Siegel, Development Director

District of Columbia

1580 **Autism Society of District Columbia**
5167 7th Street NE 202-561-5300
Washington, DC 20011-2624 Fax: 202-561-8634
e-mail: dc-washington@autismsocietyofamerica.org
www.autism-society.org/chapter130

Sondra Cunningham, President
Rhoda McLees Smith

Florida

1581 **Autism Society of Greater Orlando**
4743 Hearthside Drive 407-855-0235
Orlando, FL 32837-5445 e-mail: contact@asgo.orgÿ
www.asgo.org

Donna Lorman, President
Marzena Batignani, Vice President

Georgia

1582 **Autism Society of Greater Georgia**
PO Box 3707 770-904-4474
Suwanee, GA 30024 Fax: 770-904-4476
www.asaga.com

Steve Doran, President
Cindy Pike, Executive Director

Hawaii

1583 **Autism Society of Hawaii**
PO Box 2995 808-282-3676
Honolulu, HI 96802-2995 e-mail: naomig122@hotmail.com
www.autismhawaii.org

Evelyn Akamine, President
Naomi Grossman

Idaho

1584 **Autism Society of Treasure Valley**
PO Box 44831 208-336-5676
Boise, ID 83711-9404 Fax: 202-884-5582
e-mail: Autism.asatvc@yahoo.com
www.asatvc.org

Illinois

1585 **Autism Society of Illinois**
2200 S Main Street 630-691-1270
Lombard, IL 60148-5366 888-691-1270
Fax: 630-932-5620
e-mail: info@autismillinois.org
www.autismillinois.org

Karen McDonough, Executive Director
Kym Bills, President

Indiana

1586 **Autism Society of Indiana**
4740 Kingsway Drive 317-695-0252
Indianapolis, IN 46205-0252 Fax: 317-815-0859
e-mail: info@inautism.org
www.inautism.org

Susan Pieples, President

Iowa

1587 **Autism Society of Iowa**
4549 Waterford Drive 515-327-9075
W Des Moines, IA 50265-2059 888-722-4799
Fax: 319-557-1169
e-mail: autism50ia@aol.com
www.autismia.org

Kansas

1588 **Autism Society of Kansas Autism Society of America**
Autism Society of America

PO Box 860984
Shawnee, KS 66286-2325
913-706-0042
Fax: 316-943-3292
e-mail: ks-johnsoncounty@autismsocietyofamerica.
www.autismsocietyoftheheartland.org

Bill Robinso, President
DeeDee Velasquez-Per, Board Member

Kentucky

1589 Autism Chapter of Bluegrass Chapter
243 Shady Lane
Lexington, KY 40503-2034
859-299-9000
www.asbg.org

Sara Spragens, President

1590 Autism Society of Western Kentucky
230 Second Street Suite 206
Henderson, KY 42419-1647
270-826-0510
e-mail: nboyett1956@yahoo.com
www.autism.org

Nancy Boyett, President

Louisiana

1591 Autism Society of Louisiana
5430 S Woodchase Court
Baton Rouge, LA 70808
800-955-3760
e-mail: pjmanco@cox.net
www.lastateautism.org

Pat Giamanco, President

Maine

1592 Autism Society of Maine
72B Main Street
Winthrop, ME 04364-1406
800-273-5200
Fax: 207-377-9434
e-mail: nancy@asmonline.org
www.asmonline.org

Kim Humphrey, President
Lynda Mazzola, Vice President

Maryland

1593 Autism Society of Baltimore-Chesapeake
PO Box 10822
Parkville, MD 21234-0822
410-655-7933
e-mail: questions@bcc-asa.org
www.bcc-asa.org

Massachusetts

1594 Autism Society of Massachusetts
47 Walnut Street
Wellesley Hills, MA 02481-2108
781-237-0272
Fax: 781-237-5020
e-mail: asamasschapter@hotmail.com
www.geocities.com/asamasschapter

Michigan

1595 Autism Society of Michigan
1213 Center Street
Lansing, MI 48906-5338
517-882-2800
800-223-6722
Fax: 517-862-2816
e-mail: mi-michigan@autismsocietyofamerica.org
www.autism-mi.org

Kathy Johnson, President
Penny Bearden, Vice President

Minnesota

1596 Autism Society of Minnesota
2380 Wycliff Street
St Paul, MN 55114-1257
651-647-1083
Fax: 651-642-1230
e-mail: info@ausm.org
www.ausm.org

Pam Erickson, Executive Director
Laurie Dixon, Associate Director

Mississippi

1597 Autism Society of Gateway Chapter
7777 Bonhomme Avenue
St Louis, MO 63105
314-863-0077
Fax: 314-863-7494
e-mail: PegiSues@aol.com
www.autism-society.org

Pegi Price, President

Nebraska

1598 Autism Society of Nebraska
1672 Van Dorn Street
Lincoln, NE 68502
402-472-4346
877-375-0120
e-mail: autismsociety@autismnebraska.org
www.autismnebraska.org

Shawn Neff, President
Georgann Albin, Executive Director

Nevada

1599 Autism Society of Northern Nevada
3490 Southampton Drive
Reno, NV 89509-8911
775-786-9315
Fax: 775-786-0984
www.autism-society.org/chapter547

Paul Deane, Vice President
Dinah Deane, President

New Hampshire

1600 Autism Society of New Hampshire
PO Box 68
Concord, NH 03302-0068
603-679-2424
Fax: 301-657-0869
e-mail: info@nhautism.com
www.nhautism.com

Stacey Shannon, President

New Jersey

1601 Autism Society of Southwest New Jersey
10 Shadow Oak Court
Mount Laurel, NJ 08054-2113
856-722-8518
e-mail: CMedo@aol.com
www.autism-society.org

New Mexico

1602 Autism Society of New Mexico
PO Box 30955
Albuquerque, NM 87190-0955
505-332-0306
e-mail: nmautism@nmautismsociety.org
www.nmautismsociety.org

New York

1603 Autism Society of Albany
PO Box 3487
Schenectady, NY 12303
518-355-2191
Fax: 518-355-2191
e-mail: info@albanyautism.org
www.albanyautism.org

Cindy Barkowski, Contact

North Carolina

1604 Autism Society of North Carolina
505 Oberlin Road
Raleigh, NC 27605-1345
919-743-0204
800-442-2762
Fax: 919-743-0208
e-mail: info@autismsociety-nc.org
www.autismsociety-nc.org

Scott Badesch, Chief Executive Officer
David Laxton, Director Communications

North Dakota

1605 Autism Society of North Dakota
628 6th Avenue
Alice, ND 58031
701-281-8254
e-mail: Jocelyn@AutismND.org
www.AutismND.org

Jocelyn Sloan, President

Ohio

1606 Autism Society of Greater Cincinnati
PO Box 43027
Cincinnati, OH 45243-0027
513-561-2300
Fax: 513-561-4748
e-mail: asgc@cinci.rr.com
www.autismcincy.org

Christi Carnahan, Secretary
Ken Jones, President

1607 Autism Society of Ohio Tri-County Chapter
1749 S Raccoon Road
330-720-2066
Austintown, OH 44515e-mail: TriCountyAutism_ASO@Yahoo.com
www.triautism.com

Terry Chapin, President
Jack Campbell, Vice President

Oklahoma

1608 Autism Society of Central Oklahoma
PO Box 720103
405-370-3220
Norman, OK 73070   e-mail: ASOCO-owner@yahoogroups.com
www.asofok.org

Jeremy Rand, Contact

Oregon

1609 Autism Society of Oregon
PO Box 396
Marylhurst, OR 97036-0396
503-636-1676
888-288-4761
Fax: 503-636-1696
e-mail: info@oregonautism.com
www.oregonautism.com

Jenny Schoonbee, President
Genevieve Athens, Executive Director

Pennsylvania

1610 Autism Society of Greater Harrisburg
PO Box 101
Enola, PA 17025-0856
717-732-8400
800-277-2425
e-mail: georgia.rackley@verizon.net
www.autismharrisburg.com

Georgia Rackley, President
Sherry Christian, Vice President

Rhode Island

1611 Autism Society of Rhode Island
PO Box 16603
Rumford, RI 02916
401-595-3241
e-mail: LRego@asa-ri.org
www.asa-ri.org

Lisa Rego, President

South Carolina

1612 Autism Society of South Carolina
806 Twelfth Street
W Columbia, SC 29169
803-750-6988
800-438-4790
Fax: 703-750-8121
e-mail: scas@scautism.org
www.scautism.org

Craig Stoxen, President & CEO
Tim Conroy, Chief Operating Officer & Vice President

South Dakota

1613 Autism Society of Black Hills
521 7th Street
Rapid City, SD 57701-4347
605-737-0377
e-mail: sheritony@rap.midco.net
www.autismsd.com

Sandy Burns, President
Sheri Perkins

Tennessee

1614 Autism Society of East Tennessee
PO Box 30015
Knoxville, TN 37930
865-824-2897
Fax: 865-824-2896
e-mail: asaetc@gmail.com
www.asaetc.org

John Thomas, President
Ron Bowling, Vice President

Texas

1615 Autism Society of Dallas
10503 Metric Drive
214-208-0792
Dallas, TX 75243   e-mail: autismsociety_dallas@yahoo.com
www.autism-society.org

Carolyn Garver, Contact
Pamela Lane, President

Vermont

1616 Autism Society of Vermont Autism Society of America
Autism Society of America
PO Box 978
White River Junction, VT 05001-0978
800-559-7398
e-mail: vt-vermont@autismsocietyofamerica.org
www.autism-info.org

Virginia

1617 Autism Society of Northern Virginia
PO Box 1334
Vienna, VA 22183-1334
703-495-8444
Fax: 703-571-8138
e-mail: info@asanv.org
www.asanv.org

Kymberly S DeLoatche, Executive Director
Christopher Waddell, President

Washington

1618 Autism Society of Washington
1101 Eastside Street SE
Olympia, WA 98501
888-ASW-4YOU
Fax: 253-503-1157
e-mail: info@autismsocietyofwa.org
www.autismsocietyofwa.org

Patty Gee, President & Executive Director

West Virginia

1619 Autism Socity of West Virginia
PO Box 1024
304-272-9834
Wayne, WV 25570e-mail: wv-westvirginia@autismsocietyofamerica.o
www.aswv.org

Kim Farley, President
Ginny Gattlieb, 1st VP

Wisconsin

1620 Autism Society of Wisconsin
1477 Kenwood Drive
Menasha, WI 54952
920-558-4602
888-428-8476
Fax: 920-553-0034
e-mail: asw@asw4autism.org
www.asw4autism.org

Nancy Alar, President
Dale Prahl, Vice President

Libraries & Resource Centers

1621 Autism Services Center
Keith Albee Building
929 4th Avenue
Huntington, WV 25701
304-525-8014
www.autismservicescenter.org

Serves people with autism, other developmental disabilities and those who care for and about them.

Dr Ruth Christ Sullivan, Director

1622 Emory Autism Resource Center
Emory University School of Medicine
Justin Tyler Traux Building   404-727-8350
Atlanta, GA 30322-0001   Fax: 404-727-3969
e-mail: michael.j.morrier@emory.edu
www.psychiatry.emory.edu/PROGRAMS/autism
The Emory Autism Resource Center is a component of the Department of Psychiatry and Behavioral Sciences of Emory University's School of Medicine. It is the only Georgia resource that provides a comprehensive continuum of services specially designed to meet the needs of children and adults with autism and their families.
Gail G McGee, PhD, Director
Michael J Morrier, MA, Asst Director Research Manager

1623 Indiana Resource Center for Autism (IRCA)
Indiana Institute on Disability & Community
Indiana University-Bloomington   812-855-6508
Bloomington, IN 47408-2696   800-825-4733
Fax: 812-855-9630
TTY: 812-855-9396
e-mail: prattc@indiana.edu
www.iidc.indiana.edu/irca
The Indiana Resource Center for Autism staff conduct outreach training and consultations, engage in research, and develop and disseminate information focused on building the capacity of local communities, organizations, agencies, and families to support children and adults across the autism spectrum in typical work, school, home, and community settings.
Dr Cathy Pratt PhD, Director

Research Centers

1624 Center for Neurodevelopmental Studies
5430 W Glenn Drive   623-915-0345
Glendale, AZ 85301   800-352-3792
Fax: 623-937-5425
e-mail: admin@ccnsaz.org
www.thechildrenscenteraz.org
Effective treatment methods for autism and developmental disabilities are subjects researched and studied at the Center.
Lorna Jean King, Founder

1625 Division TEACCH University of North Carolina at Chapel H
University of North Carolina at Chapel Hill
100 Renee Lynne Court   919-966-5156
Carrboro, NC 27510-6305   Fax: 919-966-4003
e-mail: teacch@unc.edu
www.teacch.com
This organization is the division for the treatment and education of Autistic and related communication handicapped children.
Catherine Jones, Office Manager/Parent Intake Coordinator
Elaine Coonrod, Clinical Director

1626 Institute for Basic Research in Developmental Disabilities
1050 Forest Hill Road   718-494-0600
Staten Island, NY 10314-6356   Fax: 718-494-0833
www.health.gov/NHIC/
Conducts research into neurodegenerative diseases, Alzheimer's disease, developmental disabilities, fragile X syndrome, Down's syndrome, autism, epilepsy and basic science issues underlying all developmental disabilities.

1627 Institute on Communication and Inclusion at Syracuse University
University of Syracuse
370 Huntington Hall   315-443-9379
Syracuse, NY 13244-2340   Fax: 315-443-2274
e-mail: icistaff@syr.edu
http://ici.syr.edu
College offering facilitated learning research into communication with persons who have autism or severe disabilities. Offers books videos and public awareness information on the research projects.
Dr Christine Ashby

1628 National Alliance for Autism Research
1 East 33rd Street   212-252-8584
New York, NY 10016   Fax: 212-252-8676
e-mail: contactus@autismspeaks.org
www.autismspeaks.org

The National Alliance for Autism Research has merged with Autism Speaks to further reach for the goal of finding the causes the best prevention and treatments and a cure for autism.
Peter H Bell, Executive Vice President
Mark Roithmayr, President

1629 State University of New York Health Sciences Center
SUNY Downstate Medical Center
450 Clarkson Avenue   718-270-1000
Brooklyn, NY 11203-2098   Fax: 718-270-1271
e-mail: health@downstate.edu
www.downstate.edu/
Child psychiatry research programs.
John C Larosa, President

1630 The West Virginia Autism Training Center Marshall University
Marshall University
1 John Marshall Drive   304-696-2332
Huntington, WV 25755   800-344-5115
e-mail: wvatc@marshall.edu
www.marshall.edu/coe/atc
The Autism Training Center was established through the efforts of parents of children with autism throughout West Virginia to provide education training and treatment programs for West Virginians who have Autism Pervasive Developmental Disorder (NOS) or Asperger's Disorder and have been formally registered with the Center.

Support Groups & Hotlines

1631 Autism Society of America
4340 East-West Highway   301-657-0881
Bethesda, MD 20814   800-328-8476
www.autism-society.org
Exists to improve the lives of all affected by autism by increasing public awareness about the day-to-day issues faced by people in the spectrum, advocating for apporopriate services for individuals across the lifespan, and providing the latest information regarding treatment, education, research and advocacy.
Lee Grossman, President/CEO

1632 Genetic Alliance
4301 Connecticut Avenue NW   202-966-5557
Washington, DC 20008-2369   800-336-4363
Fax: 202-668-8533
e-mail: info@geneticalliance.org
www.geneticalliance.org
A nonprofit health advocacy organization committed to transforming through genetics and promoting an environment of openness centered on the health of individuals, families and communities.
Sharon Terry, President/CEO

1633 National Autism Hotline Autism Services Center
Keith Albee Building
929 4th Avenue   304-525-8014
Huntington, WV 25710   Fax: 304-525-8026
www.autismservicescenter.org
Serving people with autism, other developmental disabilities anf those who care for and about them.

1634 National Health Information Center
PO Box 1133   310-565-4167
Washington, DC 20013-1133   800-336-4797
Fax: 301-984-4256
e-mail: info@nhic.org
www.health.gov/nhic
A health information referral service sponsored by the Office of Disease Prevention and Health Promotion. Puts health professionals and consumers who have health questions in touch with those organizations that are best able to provide answers.

Books

1635 A Miracle to Believe In
Option Indigo Press

2080 S Undermountain Road　413-229-2100
Sheffield, MA 01257　800-714-2779
　Fax: 413-229-8931
　optionindigo.com

A group of people from all walks of life come together and are transformed as they reach out, under the direction of the Kaufmans, to help a little boy the medical world had given up as hopeless.
379 pages
ISBN: 0-440201-08-2
Bears Kaufman, Founder
Samahria Kaufman, Founder

1636　A Parent's Guide to Asperger's Syndrome & High-Functioning Autism
Guilford Press
72 Spring Street
New York, NY 10012　800-365-7006
　Fax: 212-966-6708
　e-mail: info@guilford.com
　www.guilford.com

For parents of children on the higher end of the autistic spectrum. All educators, the authors provide the basic on diagnosis, causes, and treatment.
2002 278 pages
ISBN: 1-572307-67-6

1637　Activities for Developing Pre-Skill Concepts In Children with Autism
Toni Flowers, author
Autism Society of North Carolina Bookstore
505 Oberlin Road　919-743-0204
Raleigh, NC 27605-1345　800-442-2762
　Fax: 919-743-0208
　e-mail: info@autismsociety-nc.org
　www.autismsociety-nc.org
Chapters include auditory development, concept development, social development and visual-motor integration.

1638　Asperger Syndrome or High-Functioning Autism?
Eric Schopler, Gary B Mesibov, Linda J Kunce, author
Springer Publishing
233 Spring Street
New York, NY 10013　212-460-1550
　800-777-4643
　Fax: 212-460-1575
　e-mail: service-ny@springer.com
　www.springer.com

The precise relationship between high-functioning autism and Asperger Syndrome is still a subject of debate. Leaders in the field provide a general overview of the disorder and present diverse opinions on diagnosis and assessment-neuropsychological issues-treatment, and related conditions.
428 pages Hardcover
ISBN: 0-306457-45-3

1639　Asperger's Syndrome: A Guide for Parents and Professionals
taylor & Francis
325 Chestnut Street
Philadelphia, PA 19106　215-625-8900
　www.tonyattwood.com
Offers insight into the identification and treatment of children on the higher functioning end of ASD.
201 pages
ISBN: 1-853025-77-1

1640　Autism Society of North Carolina Bookstore
505 Oberlin Road　919-743-0204
Raleigh, NC 27605-1345　800-442-2762
　Fax: 919-743-0208
　e-mail: info@autismaociety-nc.org
　www.autismsociety-nc.org
Offers one of the largest selections of books about autism.

1641　Autism Through the Lifespan: The Eden Model
Woodbine House
6510 Bells Mill Road　301-897-3570
Bethesda, MD 20817-1636　800-843-7323
　Fax: 301-897-5838

Presents Eden's comprehensive model for helping children and adults with autism, offering services that extend over their entire lifespan. An overview of what is known about autism today, discussions about Eden's approach to behavior modification, placement and treatment, curriculum from early childhood to adulthood, staffing issues, integration, decision making, and parental roles. Also contains dozens of examples and case histories that illustrate the program's successes.
1998 383 pages Paperback
ISBN: 0-933149-28-x

1642　Autism Treatment Guide
Elizabeth King Gerlach, author
Autism Society of North Carolina Bookstore
505 Oberlin Road　919-743-0204
Raleigh, NC 27605-1345　800-442-2762
　Fax: 919-743-0208
　e-mail: info@autismsociety-nc.org
　www.autismsociety-nc.org
This 3rd edition offers many of the most current findings in treatments fo autism spectrum disorder. First published in 1993 and updated regularly, this concise handbook provides hundres of resource listings and suggested readings pertaining to ASD. This is a must-have reference book for parents and professionals
2003 157 pages Softcover

1643　Autism and Asperger Syndrome Preparing for Adulthood
Autism Society of North Carolina Bookstore
505 Oberlin Road　919-743-0204
Raleigh, NC 27605-1345　800-442-2762
　Fax: 919-743-0208
　e-mail: info@autismsociety-nc.org
　www.autismsociety-nc.org
Chapters include topics such as what becomes of adults with ASD, interventions for ASD, problems af communication, social functioning in adulthood, sterotyped, ritualistic, and obsessional behaviors, secondary education, post-secondary education, finding and coping with employment, pyschiatric disturbances in adulthood, leagal issues, sexual relationships and marriage, and enhancing independence.
2004 388 pages Softcover

1644　Autism in Adolescents and Adults
Eric Schopler, Gary B Mesibov, author
Springer Publishing
233 Spring Street
New York, NY 10013　121-460-1500
　800-777-4643
　Fax: 212-460-1575
　e-mail: service-ny@springer.com
　www.springer.com

456 pages Hardcover
ISBN: 0-306410-57-4

1645　Autism...Nature, Diagnosis and Treatment
Guilford Press
72 Spring Street
New York, NY 10012　800-365-7006
　Fax: 212-966-6708
　e-mail: info@guilford.com
　www.guilford.com

Covers perspectives, issues, neurobiological issues and new directions in diagnosis and treatment.
417 pages
ISBN: 0-898627-24-9

1646　Autism: Explaining the Enigma
Uta Frith, author
Wiley Publishing
111 River Street　201-748-6000
Hoboken, NJ 07030-5774　Fax: 201-748-6088
　e-mail: info@wiley.com
　www.wiley.com

Includes a new chapter outlining recent developments in neuropsycgological research, and overviews one of the most important theoretical and practical consequences of Frith's original insights into this puzzling condition.
264 pages
ISBN: 0-631229-01-8

1647 Autism: Identification, Education and Treatment
Dianne Zager, author

Lawrence Earlbaum Associates
10 Industrial Avenue   201-258-2200
Mahwah, NJ 07430   800-926-6579
                                    Fax: 201-236-0072
                                    www.erlbaum.com
Chapters include medical treatments, early intervention and communication development in autism.
2005 608 pages
ISBN: 0-805845-79-8

1648 Autism: The Facts
Simon Baron-Cohen, Patrick Bolton, author

Oxford University Press
2001 Evans Road
Cary, NC 27513   800-445-9714
                                    Fax: 919-677-1303
                              e-mail: custserv.us@oup.com
                                    www.oup-usa.org
Explains in a clear, straightforward manner what is known about the condition. Written first and foremost as a guide for parents, but required reading for interested professionals, it covers the recognition and diagnosis of autism, its biological and physiological causes, and the various treatments and educational techniques available.
128 pages
ISBN: 0-192623-27-3

1649 Autistic Adults at Bittersweet Farms

Haworth Press
10 Alice Street   607-722-5857
Binghamton, NY 13904-1580   800-429-6784
                                    Fax: 607-722-0012
                                    www.haworthpress.com
A touching view of an inspirational residential care program for autistic adolescents and adults.
205 pages Paperback
ISBN: 1-560240-57-0

1650 Beyond Gentle Teaching
J.J McGee and F.J Menolascino, author

Springer
233 Spring Street   212-460-1500
New York, NY 10013   800-777-4643
                                    Fax: 212-460-1575
                              e-mail: service-ny@springer.com
                                    www.springer.com
252 pages Hardcover
ISBN: 0-306438-56-1

1651 Biology of the Autistic Syndromes
Christopher Gillberg and Mary Coleman, author

Blackwell Publishing, Inc.
Commerce Place   781-388-8200
Malden, MA 02148   800-862-6657
                                    Fax: 781-388-8210
                              www.blackwellpublishing.com
Autism is not a disease but a syndrome of different diseases. In this completely reworked and updated 3rd edition, the authors adress the difficulties this presents for clinical diagnosis with diagnostic aids and clear guidlines for medical evaluation. This is an essential text text for clinicians and will also be of interest to parents of autistic children.
2000 340 pages
ISBN: 1-898683-22-0

1652 Children with Autism

Woodbine House
6510 Bells Mill Road
Bethesda, MD 20817   800-843-7323
                              e-mail: info@woodbinehouse.com
                                    www.woodbinehouse.com
A must-have reference if for the both the new parent coping with a child's recent diagnosis and one who's an experienced advocate. Available online only.
368 pages Paperback

1653 Communication Unbound: How Facilitated Communication Is Challenging Views

Teachers College Press
1234 Amsterdam Avenue   212-678-3929
New York, NY 10027   Fax: 212-678-4149
                              e-mail: tcpress@tc.columbia.edu
                                    www.teacherscollegepress.com
Addresses the ways in which we receive persons with autism in our society, our community and our lives.
1993 221 pages

1654 Diagnosis Autism: Now What? 10 Steps to Improve Treatment Outcomes
Lawrence P Kaplan, PhD, author

Autism Society of North Carolina Bookstore
505 Oberlin Road   919-743-0204
Raleigh, NC 27605-1345   800-442-2762
                                    Fax: 919-743-0208
                              e-mail: info@autismsociety-nc.org
                                    www.autismsociety-nc.org
This practical guide was written to help parents of children with autism spectrum disorder form successful pediatric partnerships with physicians and other healthcare practitioners involved in their child's diagnosis and treatment. Containing chrts and worksheets, sample questions, research resources, and numerous planning strategies, this guide will aid parents and caregivers as they strive to build collaborative relationships with their child's case management team.
2005

1655 Effective Teaching Methods for Autistic Children
Rosalind C Oppenheim, author

Charles C Thomas Publisher
2600 S 1st Street   217-789-8980
Springfield, IL 62704-4730   800-258-8980
                                    Fax: 217-789-9130
                              e-mail: books@ccthomas.com
                                    www.ccthomas.com
The Rimland School for Autistic Children in Evanston, Illinois, with a Foreward by Bernard Rimland. This enlightening monograph is seven chapters detailing the specific problems encountered in teaching autistic children. Anecdotal reports of seven such children bring to light the need for special training and provide an insight into their handling. Related research is reviewed and discussed.
1974 116 pages Paperback
ISBN: 0-398028-58-3

1656 Encounters with Autistic States

Jason Aronson
PO Box 15100
York, PA 17405-7100   800-782-0015
                                    Fax: 201-840-7242
                                    www.aronson.com
Hardcover
ISBN: 0-765700-62-

1657 Handbook of Autism and Pervasive Developmental Disorders

Autism Society of North Carolina Bookstore
505 Oberlin Road   919-743-0204
Raleigh, NC 27605-1345   800-442-2762
                                    Fax: 919-743-0208
                              e-mail: info@autismsociety-nc.org
                                    www.autismsociety.org
A list of contributors address such topics as characteristics of autistic syndromes and interventions.
2005 1317 pages 2 volumes

1658 Helping Children with Autism Learn: Treatment Approaches for Parents
Bryna Siegel, author

Oxford University Press

2001 Evans Road
Cary, NC 27513

800-445-9714
Fax: 919-677-1303
e-mail: custserv.us@oup.com
www.oup.com

512 pages
ISBN: 0-195325-06-0

1659   Hidden Child: The Linwood Method for Reaching the Autistic Child

Woodbine House
6510 Bells Mill Road
Bethesda, MD 20817-1636

301-897-3570
800-843-7323
Fax: 301-897-5838
e-mail: info@woodbinehouse.com
www.woodbinehouse.com

Chronicle of the Linwood Children's Center's successful treatment program for autistic children.
286 pages Paperback
ISBN: 0-933149-06-9

1660   I'm Not Autistic on the Typewriter

TASH
11201 Greenwood Avenue N
Seattle, WA 98133-8612

206-361-8870

An introduction to the facilitated communication training method.

1661   Keys to Parenting the Child with Autism

Marlene Targ Brill, M.Ed, author

Barrons Educational Series, Inc.
250 Wireless Boulevard
Hauppauge, NY 11788

800-645-3476
Fax: 631-434-3723
e-mail: fbrown@barronseduc.com
www.barronseduc.com

This book explains what autism is and how it is diagnosed.
2001 224 pages
ISBN: 0-764112-92-9

1662   Let Community Employment Be the Goal for Individuals with Autism

Autism Society of North Carolina Bookstore
505 Oberlin Road
Raleigh, NC 27605-1345

919-743-0204
800-442-2762
Fax: 919-743-0208
e-mail: info@autismsociaty-nc.org
www.autismsociety-nc.org

A guide designed for people who are responsible for preparing individuals with autism to enter the work force.
1993 66 pages Booklet

1663   Let Me Hear Your Voice A Family's Triumph Over Autism

Catherine Maurice, author

Autism Society of North Carolina Bookstore
505 Oberlin Road
Raleigh, NC 27605-1345

919-743-0204
800-442-2762
Fax: 919-743-0208
e-mail: info@autismsociety-nc.org
www.autismsociety-nc.org

The Maurice family's second and third children were diagnosed with autism. This book recounts their experience with a home program using behavior therapy.
1993 371 pages Softcover
ISBN: 0-679408-63-0

1664   Management of Autistic Behavior

Pro-Ed, Inc.
8700 Shoal Creek Boulevard
Austin, TX 78757-6897

512-451-3246
800-897-3202
Fax: 800-397-7633
e-mail: info@proedinc.com
www.proedinc.com

Comprehensive and practical book that tells what works best with specific problems.
450 pages Paperback
ISBN: 0-890791-96-1
Lindy Jordaan, Marketing Coordinator

1665   Navigating the Social World: A Curriculum for Individuals with Asperger's Syndrome

Jeanette McAfee, author

Future Horizons
721 W Abram Street
Arlington, TX 76013

800-489-0727
Fax: 817-277-2270
www.fhautism.com

Addresses the most urgent problems facing those with Asperger's Syndrome, high-functioning autism, and related disorders.
387 pages
ISBN: 1-885477-82-1

1666   Neurobiology of Autism

Johns Hopkins University Press
2715 N Charles Street
Baltimore, MD 21218-4319

410-516-6936
Fax: 410-516-6998
www.jhupbooks.com

This book discusses recent advances in scientific research that point to a neurobiological basis for autism and examines the clinical implications of this research.
272 pages
ISBN: 0-801856-80-9

1667   News from the Border: A Mother's Memoir of Her Autistic Son

Houghton Mifflin Company/Order Processing
222 Berkeley Street
Boston, MA 02116

617-351-5000
800-225-3362
www.hmco.com

A searingly honest account of the author's family experiences with autism. Raising an autistic child is the central, ongoing drama of her married life and this riveting account of acceptance and coping.
1993 384 pages Cloth

1668   Pervasive Developmental Disorders: Finding a Diagnosis and Getting Help

O'Reilly & Associates
1005 Gravenstein Highway N
Sebastopol, CA 95472-3858

707-829-0515
800-998-9938
Fax: 707-829-0104
www.oreilly.com

Published for parents and patients with PDD-NOS and atypical PDD.
Paperback
ISBN: 1-565925-30-0

1669   Please Don't Say Hello

Human Sciences Press
233 Spring Street
New York, NY 10013-1522

212-620-8000

Paul and his family moved into a new neighborhood. Paul's brother was autistic. The children thought that Eddie was retarded until they learned that there were skills that he could do better than they could.
1976 47 pages Paperback
ISBN: 0-898851-99-8

1670   Psychoeducational Profile (PEP-3): TEACCH Individualized Psychoeducational Assessm

Autism Society of North Carolina Bookstore
505 Oberlin Road
Raleigh, NC 27605-1345

919-743-0204
800-442-2762
Fax: 919-743-0208
e-mail: info@autismsociety-nc.org
www.autismsociety-nc.org

This is the revised edition of Psychoeducational Profile, a widely recognized assessment tool used to identify the learning strengths and weaknesses of children with autism spectrum disorder (ASD). Developed by Division TEACCH clinicians, this instrument has been updated in several ways, including improved psychometric properties, revised function domains, new items and sub-tests, within-group comparison data, and the addition of key documentation.
2005

1671   Raising a Child with Autism: A Guide to Applied Behavior Analysis for Parents

Taylor & Francis
325 Chestnut Street
Philadelphia, PA 19106

215-625-8900
Fax: 215-625-2940

Applied behavior analysis activities that parents can use with ASD children. Inlcuded is helpful guidance for toilet training, daily living, and increasing communication and sibling interaction.
173 pages
ISBN: 1-853029-10-6

1672 Reaching the Autistic Child: A Parent Training Program
Martin Kozloff, author

Brookline Books/Lumen Editions
PO Box 1209   617-734-6772
Brookline, MA 02445   800-666-2665
                                          Fax: 617-734-3952
                                          www.brooklinebooks.com
Detailed case studies of social and behavioral change in autistic children and their families show parents how to implement the principles for improved socialization and behavior.
1998 Softcover
ISBN: 1-571290-56-7

1673 Record Book for Individuals with Autism Spectrum Disorders
Marci Wheeler and Cathy Pratt, PhD, author

Autism Society of North Carolina Bookstore
505 Oberlin Road   919-743-0204
Raleigh, NC 27605-1345   800-442-2762
                                          Fax: 919-743-0208
                              e-mail: info@autismsociety-nc.org
                                          www.autismsociety-nc.org
This valuable resource provides a method for organizing and documenting information that will help parents track their child's development. This record book is divided into several categories, including: developmental and family history, sleeping and eating patterns, medical history, education history, behavior problems, skill development, and vital information. The book contains reproducible pages that will help parents keep important information up to date.
2000 44 pages Spiral Bound

1674 Riddle of Autism: A Psychological Analysis
Jason Aronson
PO Box 15100
York, PA 17405-7100   800-782-0015
                                          Fax: 201-840-7242
                                          www.aronson.com
Dr. Victor examines the myths that cloud an understanding of this disorder and describes the meanings of its specific behavioral symptoms.
356 pages Softcover
ISBN: 1-568215-73-8

1675 Siblings of Children with Autism: A Guide for Families
Woodbine House
6510 Bells Mill Road   301-897-3570
Bethesda, MD 20817   800-843-7323
                                          Fax: 301-897-5838
                                          www.woodbinehouse.com
Resource for families with autistic children and nonautistic siblings examines the perceptions, needs, compromises, and inevitable stresses that brothers and sisters face.
160 pages
ISBN: 1-890627-29-1

1676 TEACCH Transition Assessment Profile
Autism Society of North Carolina Bookstore
505 Oberlin Road   919-743-0204
Raleigh, NC 27605-1345   800-442-2762
                                          Fax: 919-743-0208
                              e-mail: info@autismsociety-nc.org
                                          www.autismsociety-nc.org
This new assessment profile is a major revision of the AAPEP. This comprehensive test was developed for older children and adolescents with autism spectrum disorder, particularly those who have transition needs. This assessment tool is structured to satisfy those provisions in the 2004 Individuals with Disabilities Education Act, which requires that adolescents be evaluated and also provided with a transition plan.
2007 Kit

1677 Targeting Autism: What We Know, Don't Know and Can Do to Help Young Children
University of California Press
1445 Lower Ferry Road   205-978-5000
Ewing, NJ 08618   800-777-4726
                                          Fax: 800-999-1958
                                          www.ucpress.com
Provides strong overviews of current work being done with autism and addresses the diferent life cycles of children with the condition through preschool, elementary school, and adolescence.
240 pages
ISBN: 0-520234-80-4

1678 Tasks Galore for the Real World
Laurie Eckenrode, Pat Fennell, and Kathy Hearsey, author

Autism Society of North Carolina Bookstore
505 Oberlin Road   919-743-0204
Raleigh, NC 27605-1345   800-442-2762
                                          Fax: 919-743-0208
                              e-mail: info@autismsociety-nc.org
                                          www.autismsociety-nc.org
These visually structured tasks are strategies that translate complex, everyday life skills into simpler, meaningful learning situations. The myriad of ideas in this guide will be valuable to anyone developing functional, daily living goals for a child or client.
2004

1679 Teach Me Language: A Language Manual for Children with Autism
Sabrina Freeman, PhD and Lorelei Dake, BA, author

Autism Society of North Carolina Bookstore
505 Oberlin Road   919-743-0204
Raleigh, NC 27605-1345   800-442-2762
                                          Fax: 919-743-0208
                              e-mail: info@autismsociety-nc.org
                                          www.autismsociety-nc.org
This book contains behaviorally based exercises and drills that adress common language weaknesses in children and incorporate professional speech pathology methods. These exercises were designed for children who are attentive, able to follow simple directions, have learned the basics of low-level language, and are visual learners. The activities and exercises are appropriate for children and young adults ages 5-18.
1997 410 pages Spiral Bound

1680 Teaching Children with Autism: Strategies to Enhance Communication and Socializing
Kathleen Ann Quill, author

Thomson Delmar Learning
Attn: Order Fullfillment
Florence, KY 41022   800-347-7707
                                          Fax: 800-487-8488
                                          www.delmarlearning.com
This book describes teaching strategies and instructional adaptations which promote communication and socialization in children with autism. It offers specific strategies that capitalize on the individual strengths and learning styles of the autistic child.
1996
ISBN: 0-827362-69-2

1681 Teaching Community Skills and Behaviors to Students with Autism or Related Problems
Indiana Resource Center for Autism
2853 East 10th Street   812-855-6508
Bloomington, IN 47408-2696   Fax: 812-855-9630
                                          TTY: 812-855-9396
                              e-mail: iidc@indiana.edu
                              www.iidc.indiana.edu/irca/fmain1.html
Emphasizing the needs of the person with autism and the philosophy of community integration, this book cover the process of successful community-based teaching.
1988 117 pages

1682 The Autism Sourcebook
Karen Siff Exkorn, author

Autism Society of North Carolina Bookstore

505 Oberlin Road
Raleigh, NC 27605-1345
919-743-0204
800-442-2762
Fax: 919-743-0208
e-mail: www.autismsociety-nc.org
www.autismsociety-nc.org

This comprehensive handbook is for parents of newly diagnosed children who are looking for information about ASD, its diagnosis, treatment options, and practical strategies in one in-depth text.
2005

1683   The Everything Parent's Guide to Children with Autism
Adelle Jameson Tilton, author

Autism Society of North Carolina Bookstore
505 Oberlin Road
Raleigh, NC 27605-1345
919-743-0204
800-442-2762
Fax: 919-743-0208
e-mail: info@autismsociety-nc.org
www.autismsociety-nc.org

This book offers a wealth of information and reassuring advice for parents of newly diagnosed children. It is filled with hundreds of helpful tips, unique insights, and real-life situations, this is an essential guide for parents and family members.
2004 285 pages Softcover

1684   Understanding the Nature of Autism A Guide to the Autism Spectrum Disorders
Janice E Janzen, author

Autism Society of North Carolina Bookstore
505 Oberlin Road
Raleigh, NC 27605-1345
919-743-0204
800-442-2762
Fax: 919-743-0208
e-mail: info@autismsociety-nc.org
www.autismsociety-nc.org

Straightforward and comprehensive information that can be used by parents and professionals to develop curricula and programs for children with autism spectrum disorder. This important resource is a standard text used by educators, parents, and caregivers.
2003 508 pages Softcover

1685   When Snow Turns to Rain
Woodbine House
6510 Bells Mill Road
Bethesda, MD 20817-1636
301-897-3570
800-843-7323
Fax: 301-897-5838
e-mail: info@woodbinehouse.com
www.woodbinehouse.com

A gripping personal account of one family's experiences with autism. Chronicles a family's journey from parental bliss to devastation, as they learn that their son has autism. This book delves into diagnosis, treatments and attitudes toward persons with autism.
1993 250 pages Paperback
ISBN: 0-933149-63-8

1686   Autism Spectrum Disorders: The Complete Guide
Chantal Sicile-Kira, author

Autism Society of North Carolina Bookstore
505 Oberlin Road
Raleigh, NC 27605-1345
919-743-0204
800-442-2762
Fax: 919-743-0208
e-mail: info@autismsociety-nc.org
www.autismsociety-nc.org

This reference guide was written to help parents, professionals, and other members of the community learn more about autism spectrum disorder, and it presents a thorough overview of the disorder, from diagnosis through adulthood.
2004 360 pages Softcover

Children's Books

1687   Joey and Sam
Illana Katz and Edward Ritvo, MD, author

Autism Society of North Carolina Bookstore
505 Oberlin Road
Raleigh, NC 27605-1345
919-743-0204
800-442-2762
Fax: 919-743-0208
e-mail: ASNC@aol.com

A unique and invaluable tool for teaching children about others who are different. This awrd-winning and heartwarming sibling storybook examines the similarities and differences in behavior and educational experiences of two brothers, one of whom has autism.
1993 Softcover
ISBN: 1-882388-00-3

1688   Kristy and the Secret of Susan
Scholastic
800-724-6527
www.scholastic.com

This book discusses Kristy and her new baby-sitting charge, Susan. Susan can't speak but sings beautifully. Susan is autistic. Part of the Babysitters Club series.

1689   Russell is Extra Special
Charles A Amenta III. MD, author

Autism Society of North Carolina Bookstore
505 Oberlin Road
Raleigh, NC 27605-1345
919-743-0204
800-442-2762
Fax: 919-743-0208
e-mail: info@autismsociety-nc.org
www.autismsociety-nc.org

A sensitive portrayal of an autistic boy written by his father.
Hardcover

1690   Wild Boy of Aveyron
Harlan Lane, author

Harvard University Press
79 Garden Street
Cambridge, MA 02138
800-405-1619
Fax: 800-406-9145
e-mail: contact_HUP@harvard.edu
www.hup.harvard.edu

A dramatic account of a wild boy of nature and a young French doctor who shaped the modern education of retarded, deaf, and preschool children.
368 pages
ISBN: 0-674953-00-2

Newsletters

1691   Autism Research Review International
Autism Research Institute
4182 Adams Avenue
San Diego, CA 92116-2536
619-281-7165
Fax: 619-563-6840
www.autismresearchchinstitute.com

A quarterly newsletter published by the Autism Research Institute.
8 pages Quarterly
Dr. Bernard Rimland, Director

Pamphlets

1692   Avoiding Unfortunate Situations
Autism Society of North Carolina Bookstore
505 Oberlin Road
Raleigh, NC 27605-1345
919-743-0204
800-442-2762
Fax: 919-743-0208
e-mail: info@autismsociety-nc.org
www.autismsociety-nc.org

A collection of tips and information from and about people with autism and other developmental disabilities and their encounters with law enforcement agencies.

1693   Developing a Functional and Longitudinal Individual Plan
Nancy Dalrymple, author

Autism Society of North Carolina Bookstore
505 Oberlin Road
Raleigh, NC 27605-1345
919-743-0204
800-442-2762
Fax: 919-743-0208
e-mail: info@autismspectrum-nc.org
www.autismspectrum-nc.org

It is the author's view that a functional, longitudinal approach should be taken when educating persons with autism spectrum dis-

order, and that the development of an individualized plan should incorporate school, home, and community. This guide discusses the importance of defining strengths, striving for independent functioning, and determining which activities should recieve priority in the areas of self-care, social and leisure activities, and employment.
1989 11 pages Booklet

1694   Enabling Communication in Children with Autism
Autism Society of North Carolina Bookstore
505 Oberlin Road   919-743-0204
Raleigh, NC 27605-1345   800-442-2762
                                    Fax: 919-743-0208
                        e-mail: info@autismsociety-nc.org
                              www.autismsociety-nc.org
Based on a 2 year research project, the goal of this book is to help teachers develop more communication-enabling enviroments for children with atuism spectrum disorder who use little or no speech. The authors illustrate many communication-enabling strategies, including the minimal speech approach, proximal communication, prompting, and multipointing.
2001 207 pages Softcover

1695   Job Seeker Involvment in Securing Employment
Nancy Kalina, author
Indiana Resource Center for Autism
2853 East 10th Street   812-855-6508
Bloomington, IN 47408-2696   Fax: 812-855-9630
                                    TTY: 812-855-9396
                            e-mail: iidc@indiana.edu
                      www.iidc.indiana.edu/irca/fmain1.html
A walk through the job development process, from identifying job options and writing a resume to negotiating workplace supports with a potential employer. Each step provides opportunities for the peronal with autism, or another disability, to become actively involved in their job search process.
1997 22 pages

1696   Learning to be Independent and Responsible
Nancy Dalrymple, author
Indiana Resource Center for Autism
2853 East 10th Street   812-855-6508
Bloomington, IN 47408-2696   Fax: 812-855-9630
                                    TTY: 812-855-9396
                            e-mail: iidc@indiana.edu
                      www.iidc.indiana.edu/irca/fmain1.html
People with autism build trust in people and environments through successful interactions. Individualized, supportive programs, utilizing positive instructional and environmental supports that lead to increased opportunities, chouse, and motivation are described in this booklet.
1989 11 pages

1697   Parents as Trainers of Legislators, Other Parents and Researchers
Autism Services Center
101 Richmond Street   304-525-8014
Huntington, WV 25702-1513   Fax: 304-525-8026
Reprint offering information on parents of autistic children that learn early in their child's life how little professionals know about autism.

1698   Sex, Sexuality, and the Autism Specrtum
Wendy Lawson, author
Autism Society of North Carolina Bookstore
505 Oberlin Road   919-743-0204
Raleigh, NC 27605-1345   800-442-2762
                                    Fax: 919-743-0208
                        e-mail: info@autismsociety-nc.org
                              www.autismsociety-nc.org
The author, a psychologist, who has Aspergers Syndrome, presents her unique perspective on sexuality and interpersonal relationships. Filled with honest insights and positive advice, this is a valuable guide for persons with ASD and the people who live and work with them.
2005 175 pages Softcover

1699   Son-Rise Method
Option Institute

2080 S Undermountain Road   413-229-2100
Sheffield, MA 01257-9643   Fax: 413-229-8931
                             e-mail: sonrise@option.org
                                    www.son-rise.org
Describes a program Barry and Samahria Kaufman developed to help heal their once-autistic son.

1700   What Is Autism
Autism Society of America
7910 Woodmont Avenue   301-657-0881
Bethesda, MD 20814-3065   800-328-8476
                                    Fax: 301-657-0869
                         e-mail: info@autism-society.org
                                www.autism-society.org
Offers a definition and introduction to autism, produces a wide range of autism information written for various audiences. Offers a quarterly magazine, national conference, nationwide chapter network and many other resources.

Audio & Video

1701   A Sense of Belonging: Including Students with Autism in their School Community
Indiana Resource Center for Autism
2853 East 10th Street   812-855-6508
Bloomington, IN 47408-2696   Fax: 812-855-9630
                                    TTY: 812-855-9396
                            e-mail: iidc@indiana.edu
                      www.iidc.indiana.edu/irca/fmain1.html
Highlights the efforts of two elementary and one middle school in Indiana in teaching students with autism in general education settings. Comments from parents, school administrators, classmates, and educators illustrate the role they each played in supporting students with autism in becoming active learners in their school community. Includes practical strategies for teaching the student with autism.
1997 20 minutes

1702   Autism: A Strange, Silent World
Filmakers Library
124 E 40th Street   212-808-4980
New York, NY 10016   Fax: 212-808-4983
                              e-mail: info@filmakers.com
                                    www.filmakers.com
A comprehensive view of autism by focusing on three children of different ages, with very different behaviors. Also introduces us to a remarkable group of parents, teachers and therapists who strive to maximize
VHS/DVD
Sue Oscar, Co-President
Linda Gottesman, Co-President

1703   Autism: A World Apart
Karen Cunninghame, author
Fanlight Productions
4196 Washington Street   617-469-4999
Boston, MA 02131-1731   800-937-4113
                                    Fax: 617-469-3379
                          e-mail: fanlight@fanlight.com
                                     www.fanlight.com
In this documentary, three families show us what the textbooks and studies cannot, what it's like to live with autism day after day, raise and love children who may be withdrawn and violent and unable to make personal connections with their families.
DVD
ISBN: 1-572959-50-9

1704   Developing IEPs Under the New Idea Regulations
LRP Publications
747 Dresher Road
Horsham, PA 19044-2247
                                         800-341-7874
                                    Fax: 215-784-9639
                             e-mail: custserve@lrp.com
                                         www.lrp.com
A practical, step-by-step approach makes it easy to understand the legal and educational issues surrounding IEPs.
26 minutes

1705 Discipline Under the New Idea: Practical Methods and Procedures
LRP Publications
747 Dresher Road
Horsham, PA 19044-2247   800-341-7874
                                          Fax: 215-784-9639
                                          e-mail: custserve@lrp.com
                                          www.lrp.com
Provides practical explanation of the discipline methods and procedures school officials are permitted to use for students with disabilities.
26 minutes

1706 Embracing Play: Teaching Your Child with Autism
Woodbine House
6510 Bells Mill Road   301-897-3570
Bethesda, MD 20817   800-843-7323
                                          Fax: 301-897-5838
                                          www.woodbinehouse.com
Guide for parents who incorporate applied behavior analysis with their child.
1993 47 minutes

1707 Functional Behavioral Assessments: How to Do Them Right!
LRP Publications
747 Dresher Road
Horsham, PA 19044-2247   800-341-7874
                                          Fax: 215-784-9639
                                          e-mail: custserve@lrp.com
                                          www.lrp.com
Assist you in understanding why a behavior problem has occured, so you can maximize the effectiveness of a planned intervention.
18 minutes

1708 Getting Started with Facilitated Communication
Syracuse University, Facilitated Communication Ins
370 Huntington Hall   315-443-9379
Syracuse, NY 13244-2340   Fax: 315-443-9218
                                          e-mail: fcstaff@syr.edu
                                          soeweb.syr.edu/thefci/
Describes in detail how to help individuals with autism and/or severe communication difficulties to get started with facilitated communication.
Videotape

1709 Going to School with Facilitated Communication
Syracuse University, School of Education
805 S Krouse   315-443-2693
Syracuse, NY 13244-0001
A video in which students with autism and/or severe disabilities illustrate the use of facilitated communication focusing on basic principles fostering facilitated communication.
Videotape

1710 I Want My Little Boy Back
Autism Treatment Center of America
2080 S Undermountain Road   413-229-2100
Sheffield, MA 01257   800-714-2779
                                          Fax: 413-229-8931
                                          e-mail: www.son-rise.org
                                          information@son-rise.org
This BBC documentary follows an English family with a child with autism before, during, and after their time at the Son-Rise Program. It uniquely captures the heart of the Son-Rise Program and is extremely useful in understanding the program's techniques.
Lauren Astor, Public Relations Manager

1711 I'm Not Autistic on the Typewriter
Syracuse University, School of Education
805 S Krouse   315-443-2693
Syracuse, NY 13244-0001
A video introducing facilitated communication, a method by which persons with autism express themselves.
Videotape

1712 Invisible Wall: Autism
PRIMEDIA/Films Media Group

Films for Humanities & Sciences
Princeton, NJ 08543   800-257-5126
                                          Fax: 609-671-0266
                                          e-mail: custserv@filmsmediagroup.com
                                          www.films.com/
It features interviews with Ivar Lovaas, the creator of applied behavior analysis therapy.
2001 52 minutes
Dean B Nelson, Chairman/President/CEO PRIMEMEDIA
Kevin Neary, Chief Financial Officer/PRIMEDIA

1713 Public Schools and Students with Autism: Components of a Defensible Program
LRP Publications
747 Dresher Road
Horsham, PA 19044-2247   800-341-7874
                                          Fax: 215-784-9639
                                          e-mail: custserve@lrp.com
                                          www.lrp.com
This video assists you in understanding transition planning, documentation of student progress and proven strategies you can implement in your program.
13 minutes

1714 Standards and Inclusion: Can We Have Both?
LRP Publications
747 Dresher Road
Horsham, PA 19044-2247   800-341-7874
                                          Fax: 215-784-9639
                                          e-mail: custserve@lrp.com
                                          www.lrp.com
Addresses the critical issues educators face when supporting students with disabilities in inclusive settings. Through dynamic, powerful presentations by two inclusion experts.
40 minutes

1715 Understanding Autism
Suzanne Newman, author
Fanlight Productions
4196 Washington Street   617-469-4999
Boston, MA 02131-1731   800-937-4113
                                          Fax: 617-469-3379
                                          e-mail: fanlight@fanlight.com
                                          www.fanlight.com
Parents of children with autism discuss the nature and symptoms of this lifelong disability and outlines a treatment program based on behavior modification principles.
1993 19 Minutes
ISBN: 1-572951-00-1

Web Sites

1716 Autism Research Institute
                                          www.autism.com/ari/
A clearinghouse for research on autism and related disorders of learning and behavior. Conducts and compiles research findings to provide people with the latest research available.

1717 Autism Resources
                                          www.autism-resources.com
Provides information and links regarding the developmental disabilities autism and Asperger's Syndrome.

1718 Autism Society of America
                                          www.autism-society.org
Exists to improve the lives of all affected by autism by increasing public awareness about the day-to-day issues faced by people on the spectrum, advocating for appropriate services for individuals across the lifespan, and providing the latest information regarding treatment, education, research and advocacy.

1719 Autism Treatment Center of America
                                          www.autismtreatment.com
the worldwide teaching center for The Son-Rise Program, a powerful and effective treatment for children and adults challenged by Autism, Autism Spectrum Disorders, Pervasive Developmental Disorder (PDD), Asperger's Syndrome, and other developmental difficulties.

1720 Community Services for Autistic Adults & Children

www.csaac.org

A private, non-profit agency which provides direct services to children and adults with autism across the lifespan. CSAAC's mission is to enable individuals with autism to reach their highest potential and contribute as confident individuals to their community.

1721 Healing Well

www.healingwell.com

A social network and support community for patients, caregivers, and families coping with the daily struggles of diseases, disorders and chronic illness.

1722 Health Finder

www.healthfinder.gov

A government web site there individuals can find information and tools to help you and those you care about stay healthy.

1723 Healthlink USA

www.healthlinkusa.com

Health information concerning treatment, cures, prevention, diagnosis, risk factors, research, support groups, email lists, personal stories and much more. Updated regularly.

1724 Helios Health

www.helioshealth.com

Online resource for your health information. Detailed information about specific health topics, access to expert advice from our Medical Advisory Board, and up-to-date health news.

1725 MedicineNet

www.medicinenet.com

An online resource for consumers providing easy-to-read, authoritative medical and health information.

1726 Medscape

www.medscape.com

Medscape offers specialists, primary care physicians, and other health professionals the Web's most robust and integrated medical information and educational tools.

1727 National Alliance for Autism Research

www.naar.org

The first organization in the United States dedicated to funding and accelerating biomedical research focusing on autism spectrum disorders.

1728 National Institute of Mental Health

www.nimh.nih.gov

Mission is to transform the understanding and treatment of mental illnesses through basic and clinical research, paving the way for prevention, recovery, and cure.

1729 Son Rise Program

www.autismtreatmentcenter.org

Describes an effective, loving and respectful method for treating children with autism. It teaches parents and healing professionals how to set up a home based program using the child's motivation to reach their special child.

1730 WebMD

www.webmd.com

Information on Autism, including articles and resources.

Description

1731 Birth Defects

Birth defects, or congenital abnormalities, occur in 3 to 4 percent of newborns and can include structural defects of the heart, major blood vessels, kidneys, urinary tract, gastrointestinal tract, skeleton and nervous system. The incidence of specific abnormalities varies with the type of defect. These defects may be single or several defects may occur together, often known as a syndrome.

Although in many instances the cause of the defect is unknown, genetic factors may cause many single malformations and syndromes. Some syndromes, such as Down syndrome, result from chromosomal abnormalities. Factors during the pregnancy can sometimes result in defects, such as taking certain drugs (Coumadin, Dilantin), maternal illness (diabetes), and various infections (German measles, Rubella).

Prior to birth, ultrasound evaluation of the fetus and testing of the amniotic fluid surrounding it can identify some defects. If a defect is identified and is serious, parents can decide how or if they wish the pregnancy to proceed. Other abnormalities may not be identified until birth. Treatment and outcome vary greatly, depending on the type and severity of the defect. Parents and other family members need honest information and emotional support when caring for a child born with congenital defects. If genetic factors are suspected, the parents should receive genetic counseling. See also *Spina Bifida and Congenital Heart Disease.*

National Agencies & Associations

1732 Birth Defect Research for Children
800 Celebration Avenue 407-566-8304
Celebration, FL 34747 Fax: 407-566-8341
e-mail: staff@birthdefects.org.
www.birthdefects.org
A nonprofit organization that provides information about birth defects of all kinds to parents and professionals. Offers a library of medical books and files of information on less common categories of birth defects and is involved in research to discover causes and prevention.
Betty Mekdeci, Executive Director
John Bragg, Administrative Assistant

1733 CAPP National Parent Resource Center
95 Berkeley Street 617-482-2915
Boston, MA 02116 800-331-0688
Fax: 617-695-2939
e-mail: cec@cec.sped.org
www.cec.sped.org
A parent-run resource system designed to further the needs and goals of family-centered community-based coordinated care for children with special health needs and their families. Offers written materials, training packages, workshops and presentations.
Marilyn Friend, President
Mark Innocenti, Associate Director

1734 Cleft Palate Foundation
1504 E Franklin Street 919-933-9044
Chapel Hill, NC 27514-2820 800-24C-LEFT
Fax: 919-933-9604
e-mail: info@cleftline.org
www.cleftline.org
Major services are provided through CLEFTLINE, a 24 hour toll free hotline for anyone affected by a facial birth defect. We provide free educational materials referrals to local treatment and support groups and hope.
Nancy C Smythe, Executive Director
Samantha Jennings MSW, Family Services Director

1735 Cornelia de Lange Syndrome Foundation
302 W Main Street 860-676-8166
Avon, CT 06001 800-223-8355
Fax: 860-676-8337
e-mail: info@cdlsusa.org
www.cdlsusa.org
Provides information about birth defects caused by Cornelia de Lange Syndrome.
Liana Garcia-Fresher, Executive Director
Barbara Koontz, Information Coordinator

1736 Easter Seals
233 South Wacker Drive 312-726-6200
Chicago, IL 60606 800-221-6827
Fax: 312-726-1494
TTY: 312-726-4258
e-mail: info@easter-seals.org
www.easter-seals.org
Provides services to children and adults with disabilities as well as support to their families.
Reenie Kavalor, VP Medical/Rehabilitation Services
Stephen F Rossman, Chair

1737 Federation for Children with Special Needs
1135 Tremont Street 617-236-7210
Boston, MA 02120 800-331-0688
Fax: 617-572-2094
e-mail: fcsninfo@fcsn.org
fcsn.org
A center for parents and parent organizations to work together on behalf of children with special needs.
Deborah Allen, Director
Peter Brenna CPA, Board of Director

1738 March of Dimes Birth Defects Foundation
1275 Mamaroneck Avenue
White Plains, NY 10605 914-997-4488
www.marchofdimes.com
Our mission is to improve the health of babies by preventing birth defects premature birth and infant mortality. The March of Dimes carries out this mission through programs of research community services education and advocacy to save babies' lives.

1739 National Early Childhood Technical Assistance Center
Campus Box 8040 UNC-CH 919-962-2001
Chapel Hill, NC 27599-8040 Fax: 919-966-7463
TDD: 919-843-3269
e-mail: nectac@unc.edu
www.nectac.org
Assists states and other designated governing jurisdictions as they develop multidisciplinary, coordinated and comprehensive services for children with special needs.
Lynn Kahn, Director
Beverly Payne-Betts, Administrative Assistant

1740 National Foundation for Facial Reconstruction
333 East 30th Street 212-263-6656
New York, NY 10016 Fax: 212-263-7534
e-mail: info@nffr.org
www.nffr.org
The National Foundation for Facial Reconstruction addresses the plight of children with a facial disfigurement by supporting state of the art treatment, innovative research, psychosocial support and medical training that inspires a new generation of pediatric doctors.
Whitney Burnett, Executive Director
Michele B Golombuski, MS, Associate Executive Director

1741 Parent Professional Advocacy League
45 Bromfield Street 617-542-7860
Boston, MA 02108 866-815-8122
Fax: 617-542-7832
e-mail: info@ppal.net
www.ppal.net

An organization of families of children with mental emotional or behavioral needs and concerned professionals. PALS support groups are run in many areas across the country.
Lisa Lambert, Executive Director

Research Centers

1742 Boston University Center for Human Genetics
715 Albany Street   617-638-4640
Boston, MA 02118-2394   Fax: 617-638-7092
                                   e-mail: amilunski@bu.edu
                                          www.bumc.bu.edu
Offers research into genetic disorders and growth disorders.
Dr Karen H Antman, Dean
Jeff Milunsky, Co-Director

1743 California Teratogen Information Service UC San Diego School of Medicine Dept of
UC San Diego School of Medicine Dept of Pediatrics
9500 Gilman Drive   619-294-6291
La Jolla, CA 92093-828   800-532-3749
                                       Fax: 619-220-0228
                               e-mail: ctispregnancy@ucsd.edu
                                        www.ctispregnancy.org
Statewide service operated by the California Teratogen Information Service (CTIS) and Clinical Research Program. Our goal is to promote healthy pregnancies through education and research.
Kenneth Lyon Jones MD, Medical Director
Christina D Chambers, Program Director

1744 Department of Reproductive Genetics: Magee Women's Hospital
200 Lothrop Street   412-647-8748
Pittsburgh, PA 15213-2582   800-533-8762
                                       Fax: 412-641-1032
                             e-mail: dbrucha@mail.magee.edu
                                            www.upmc.com
Obstetrical and gynecological teaching unit of the University of Pittsburgh School of Medicine. A full-service women's hospital and now has expanded to include a range of services for women and men.
W Allen Hogge, Clinical Investigator
Jie Hu, Assistant Investigator

1745 Division Of Developmental and Behavioral Pediatrics
Children's Hospital Medical Center of Cincinnati
3333 Burnet Avenue   513-636-4200
Cincinnati, OH 45229-3039   800-344-2462
                                       TTY: 513-636-4900
                                   www.cincinnatichildrens.org
The Division of Developmental and Behavioral Pediatrics provides services for infants children and adolescents from birth to age 21 who are experiencing developmental or behavioral problems.
David J Schonfeld, Director
Matthew W Zurad, Business Director

1746 Georgetown University Child Development Center
Box 571485   202-687-5000
Washington, DC 20057-1485   Fax: 202-687-8899
                              e-mail: gucdc@georgetown.edu
                                   www.gucchd.georgetown.edu
The mission of the GUCCHD is to bring together policy, research and clinical practice for the betterment of individuals and families, especially children youth and those with special needs including: development disabilities and special health care needs, mental health needs, young children and those in the child welfare system.
John De Gioia, President
Neal Horen, Co-Director Training and Technical Assis

1747 Louisiana State University Genetics Section of Pediatrics
200 Clay Avenue   504-896-9524
New Orleans, LA 70118   Fax: 504-894-3997
                                 e-mail: ylacas@lsuhsc.edu
                                     www.medschool.lsuhsc.edu
Yves Lacassie, Section Head
Mary Camille Fournet, Research Associate

1748 New England Regional Genetics Group
PO Box 920288   781-444-0126
Needham, MA 02492   Fax: 781-444-0127
                              e-mail: mfgnergg@verizon.net
                                            www.nergg.org
Human genetic services and educational planning pertaining to birth defects.
Mary-Frances Garber, Executive Director
Cindy Ingham, Co-Director

1749 Teratology OTIS
1295 N Martin   520-626-3547
Tucson, AZ 85721-202   866-626-6847
                             e-mail: contactus@otispregnancy.org
                                        www.otispregnancy.org
Teratology Information Services are comprehensive and multidisciplinary resources for medical consultation on prenatal exposures. TIS interpret information regarding known and potential reproductive risks into risk assessments that are communicated to individuals of reproductive age and health care providers.
Dee Quinn, Executive Director
Lori Wolfe, President

1750 Thomas Jefferson University: Daniel Baugh Institute
329 Jefferson Alumni Hall
1020 Locust Street   215-503-7823
Philadelphia, PA 19107   Fax: 215-503-2636
                          e-mail: James.Schwaber@mail.dbi.tju.edu
                                            www.dbi.tju.edu
Cares for both out and in-patients with complex problems involving a wide variety of infectious diseases. The Division has an active clinical research program bringing state-of-the-art treatments to patients.
James Schwaber, Director
Boris N Kholodenko, Director Computational Cell Biology

1751 University of Illinois at Chicago Craniofacial Center
College of Medicine
180 DENT M/C 588   312-996-7546
Chicago, IL 60612   Fax: 312-413-1157
                                   e-mail: dreisber@uic.edu
                                             www.uic.edu
David J Reisberg, Director

1752 University of Iowa Birth Defects and Genetic Disorders Unit
Iowa Registry for Congenital/Inherited Disorders
100 Oakdale Campus   319-335-3500
Iowa City, IA 52242-5000   866-274-4237
                                       Fax: 319-335-4030
                                   e-mail: ircid@uiowa.edu
                                            www.uiowa.edu
Established through the joint efforts of the University of Iowa the Iowa Department of Public Health and the Iowa Department of Human Services to monitor birth defects in the state.
Paul A Romitti, Director
Kim Keppler-Noreuil, Clinical Director for Birth Defects

1753 University of Miami: Mailman Center for Child Development
1601 NW 12th Avenue   305-243-6801
Miami, FL 33136-6820   Fax: 305-243-5978
                                       TTY: 305-243-5937
                                       TDD: 305-243-5937
                               peds2.med.miami.edu/mailman
Focuses on birth defects and children's illnesses.
Dr Robert Stempfel Jr, Director

1754 Wayne State University: CS Mott Center for Human Growth and Development
275 E Hancock Street   313-577-1485
Detroit, MI 48201   Fax: 313-577-8554
                                       home.med.wayne.edu
Human growth and development disorders.
Dr Robert Sokol, Director
Valerie M Parisi, Dean

1755 Wichita Medical Research & Education Foundation
3306 E Central Avenue   316-686-7172
Wichita, KS 67208-3104   Fax: 316-687-0033
                          e-mail: info@wichitamedicalresearch.org
                                   www.wichitamedicalresearch.org

The Wichita Medical Research Foundation promotes research for the development of new medical skills and knowledge which serve patients from Wichita and throughout Kansas.
Peggy L Johnson, Executive Director/COO
William Hendry PhD, President

Support Groups & Hotlines

1756 CUNY: Teratogen Information Service
People
1219 N Forest Road
Williamsville, NY 14221-3292
716-634-8132
888-773-0753
Fax: 716-634-3889
www.people-inc.org

Luther Robinson MD

1757 Connecticut Pregnancy Exposure Information Service
UConn Health Partners
Division of Human Genetics   860-523-6419
West Hartford, CT 06119   800-325-5391
humangenetics.uchc.edu
Provides up-to-date information on all types of exposures during pregnancy or breastfeeding for Connecticut residents or women who have Connecticut physicians.
Philip E Austin, President
James F Abromaitis, Commissioner

1758 Illinois Teratogen Information Service (IT IS)
680 N Lake Shore Drive   312-981-4354
Chicago, IL 60611   800-252-4847
e-mail: itis@fetal-exposure.org
www.fetal-exposure.org
A free statewide service that is financially supported by the Illinois Department of Public Health. Provides information regarding all types of exposures during pregnancy, and is available to women who are pregnant or planning a pregnancy, fathers, physicians, and other health care providers in the State of Illinois
Kristen L Dieter MS/CGC, Genetic Counselor/Coordinator ITIS
Eugene Pergament MD/Ph.D, Medical Geneticist

1759 Indiana Teratogen Information Service
Indiana University Medical Center
975 W Walnut Street
Indianapolis, IN 46202   317-274-2241
genetics.medicine.iu.edu
A telephone inquiry service that provides central, up-to-date, information from computersized sources, professional articles and expert consultants
David D Weaver MD, Director

1760 Missouri Teratogen Information Service
University of Missouri Health Care
1 Hospital Drive   573-882-7299
Columbia, MO 65212-1   Fax: 573-882-1593
e-mail: umhs-muhealth@missouri.edu
www.muhealth.org/
The Missouri Teratogen Information Services (MOTIS) helps promote healthy pregnancies by providing, counseling, education and information.
James Ross, Chief Executive Officer
James C Poehling, Chief Operating Officer

1761 National Health Information Center
PO Box 1133   310-565-4167
Washington, DC 20013-1133   800-336-4797
Fax: 301-984-4256
e-mail: info@nhic.org
www.health.gov/nhic
A health information referral service sponsored by the Office of Disease Prevention and Health Promotion. Puts health professionals and consumers who have health questions in touch with those organizations that are best able to provide answers.

1762 Nebraska Information Service
University of Nebraska Medical Center
985440 Nebraska Medical Center
Omaha, NE 68198-5440   402-559-5071
Fax: 402-559-7248

Teratogen Information Project
Beth Conover APRN, MS, Genetic Counselor
Kathleen Caldwell, Project Assistant

1763 New Jersey Pregnancy Risk Information Service
254 Easton Avenue   732-745-6659
New Brunswick, NJ 8901-1766
DebraLynn Day Salvatore, Medical Director

1764 PALS Support Groups
Parent/Professional Advocacy League
45 Bromfield Street   617-542-7860
Boston, MA 02108   866-815-8122
Fax: 617-542-7832
e-mail: info@ppal.net
ppal.net
Promotes a strong voice for families of children and adolescents with mental health needs. Advocates for supports, treatment and policies that enale families to live in their communities in an environment of stability and respect.
Lisa Lambert, Executive Director
Christopher Anselmo, Project Coordinator

1765 Pregnancy Healthline: Pennsylvania Hospital
8th & Spruce Streets   215-829-3601
Philadelphia, PA 19107
Betsy Schick-Boschetto MSN

1766 Pregnancy Risk Line
Utah Department of Health
PO Box 141010   801-328-2229
Salt Lake City, UT 84114-1010   800-822-2229
www.health.utah.gov/prl
Provides vaulable information to women who are pregnant, considering becoming pregnant, or breastfeeding, and to their healthcare providers.

1767 Pregnancy Safety Hotline
Western Pennsylvania Hospital
4800 Friendship Avenue
Pittsburgh, PA 15224-1722   412-687-7233
www.wphs.org

Michael Kerr MS

1768 Teratogen Information Services
University of Florida Health Science Center
PO Box 100296
Gainesville, FL 32610-0296   352-392-3050
www.health.ufl.edu

Donna H Poynor MA

1769 Teratogen and Birth Defects Information Project
University of South Dakota
414 E Clark Street   605-677-5011
Vermillion, SD 57069-2307   877-269-6837
Fax: 605-677-6534
e-mail: urelations@usd.edu
www.usd.edu
James Abbott, University President
Rod Parry, Dean of the Medical School

1770 University of Iowa Teratogen Information Service
University of Iowa Teratogen
200 Hakins Drive   319-353-7877
Iowa City, IA 52242   800-777-8442
www.uihealthcare.com
Donna Katen Bahensky, Chief Executive Officer
Anne Madenrice, Chief Operations Officer

1771 University of Nebraska Medical Center Tera Togen Project
Genetic Medicine-Munroe-Meyer Institute
985430 Nebraska Medical Center   402-559-6800
Omaha, NE 68198-5430   800-656-3937
Fax: 402-559-6688
e-mail: gbschaef@unmc.edu
www.unmc.edu/dept/mmi/
The section of Genetic Medicine provides comprehensive services for a variety of patients and their families. Direct services include diagnosis, interpretation of risks, supportive counseling, and suggestions/referrals for further management. The department partic-

ipates in clinics, inpatient consultation, and the Teratogen Information Project.
G Bradley Schaefer MD/FAAP/FACMG, Director Genetics Department

1772 Vermont Pregnancy Risk Information Service
Vermont Regional Genetics Center
1 Mill Street
Burlington, VT 05401-1530   800-932-4609
Alan E Guttmacher MD

Books

1773 Bendectin Report
930 Woodcock Road   407-245-7035
Orlando, FL 32812   800-313-2232
                                    www.birthdefects.org
Report on research connecting the anti-nausea medication, Bendectin, with birth defects. Includes latest judicial opinion confirming $24 million judgment in a Bendectin case.
90 pages

1774 Dursban Report
930 Woodcock Road   407-245-7035
Orlando, FL 32812   800-313-2232
                                    www.birthdefects.org
Report on research and latest EPA findings on Dursban and health problems, including MCS and birth defects.
90 pages

1775 Environmental Birth Defect Digest
930 Woodcock Road   407-245-7035
Orlando, FL 32812   800-313-2232
                                    www.birthdefects.org
Compendium of research briefs from the world medical literature, plus original articles covering birth defects associated with medications, radiation, chemicals, toxic sites, dioxin, pesticides, lead, mercury, Bendectin, aspartame and more.
42 pages

1776 Understanding Birth Defects
Franklin Watts Grolier
90 Old Sherman Turnpike   203-797-3500
Danbury, CT 06816-0001   800-621-1115
                                    Fax: 203-797-3197
                                    www.grolier.com
What birth defects are, their genetic and environmental origins and what can be done to help, plus the problems of low birth weight are discussed.
128 pages
ISBN: 0-531109-55-0

Children's Books

1777 Don't Feel Sorry for Paul
JB Lippincott
530 Walnut Street   215-521-8300
Philadelphia, PA 19105   Fax: 215-521-8902
                                    www.ilkins.com
Paul is seven and was born with deformities of both hands and feet. Paul must wear a prosthesis on both feet so that he can walk. He has a third prosthesis for his right hand. The third prosthesis has a pair of hooks Paul uses as fingers.
94 pages Hardcover
ISBN: 0-397315-88-0

1778 God, the Universe and Hot Fudge Sundaes
Houghton, Mifflin & Company
222 Berkeley Street
Boston, MA 02108-3107   617-351-5000
                                    www.hmco.com

Newsletters

1779 Birth Defect News
Birth Defect Research for Children

800 Celebration Ave   407-566-8304
Celebration, FL 34747   e-mail: staff@birthdefects.org
                                    www.birthdefects.org
8 pages Quarterly
Betty Mekdeci, Executive Director

1780 NewsLine
Federation for Children with Special Needs
95 Berkeley Street   617-482-2915
Boston, MA 02116-6230   800-331-0688
Offers information for parents and families on resources, medical updates, activities, fund-raising events and association news for their disabled children.
Quarterly

1781 PAL News
Parent Professional Advocacy League
95 Berkeley Street   617-482-2915
Boston, MA 02116-6264   800-331-0688
Offers information on medical and technological updates in the area of research on birth defects, support groups and family resources for persons with disabled children.
Quarterly

Pamphlets

1782 After School...Then What? The Transition to Adulthood
Federation for Children with Special Needs
95 Berkeley Street   617-482-2915
Boston, MA 02116-6230   800-331-0688
Preparing for the transition after high school for children with special needs.

1783 Agent Orange and Birth Defects
930 Woodcock Road   407-245-7035
Orlando, FL 32812   800-313-2232
                                    www.birthdefects.org
Research booklet, including the latest findings from the National Birth Defect Registry and government research connecting Agent Orange to birth defects.
42 pages

1784 Birth Defects & Genetics: The Genetics Revolution
March of Dimes Birth
233 Park Avenue South   212-353-8353
New York, NY 10003   Fax: 212-254-3518
                                    e-mail: NY639@marchofdimes.com
                                    www.marchofdimes.com
Offers information on genetic testing and what it means to the patient and family members.

1785 Childhood Illnesses in Pregnancy: Chicken Pox & Fifth Disease
March of Dimes
233 Park Avenue South   212-353-8353
New York, NY 10003   Fax: 212-254-3518
                                    e-mail: NY639@marchofdimes.com
                                    www.marchofdimes.com
Located on the March of Dimes website.

1786 Cleft Lip & Palate
March of Dimes
233 Park Avenue South   212-353-8353
New York, NY 10003   Fax: 212-254-3518
                                    e-mail: NY639@marchofdimes.com
                                    www.marchofdimes.com
Located on March of Dimes website.

1787 Club Foot and Other Foot Deformities
March of Dimes
233 Park Avenue South   212-353-8353
New York, NY 10003   Fax: 212-254-3518
                                    e-mail: NY639@marchofdimes.com
                                    www.marchofdimes.com

1788 Genetic Counseling
March of Dimes
233 Park Avenue South   212-353-8353
New York, NY 10003   Fax: 212-254-3518
                                    e-mail: NY639@marchofdimes.com
                                    www.marchofdimes.com

1789 Gulf War and Birth Defects
930 Woodcock Road
Orlando, FL 32812
407-225-7035
800-313-2232
www.birthdefects.org
Information booklet on recent data from the National Birth Defect Registry and other research related to Gulf War exposures and birth defects.
30 pages

1790 How to Find More About Your Child's Birth Defect or Disability
Association for Birth Defect Children
5400 Diplomat Circle
Orlando, FL 32810-5603
800-922-9234
www.birthdefects.org
An informational fact sheet that encourages parents who have a child with a birth defect or disability to become the expert on the child's disability with some suggestions on how to educate themselves.

1791 Low Birthweight
March of Dimes
233 Park Avenue South
New York, NY 10003
212-353-8353
Fax: 212-254-3518
e-mail: NY639@marchofdimes.com
www.marchofdimes.com
Fact Sheets: one or two page review written for the general public. Also available electronically on the website: www.marchofdimes.com

1792 PKU Quick Reference and Fact Sheet
March of Dimes
233 Park Avenue South
New York, NY 10003
212-353-8353
Fax: 212-254-3518
e-mail: NY639@marchofdimes.com
www.marchofdimes.com
Phenylketonuria (PKU) is an inherited disorder that affects the way the body is able to process food. If left untreated, it causes mental retardation. How PKU is passed on and how it is treated are outlined. The Information Fact Sheet is located on the March of Dimes website.

1793 Teaching Social Skills to Youngsters with Disabilities
Federation for Children with Special Needs
95 Berkeley Street
Boston, MA 02116-6230
617-482-2915
800-331-0688
Explains the importance of instruction and training to learn appropriate social behavior.

1794 Toxoplasmosis
March of Dimes
233 Park Avenue South
New York, NY 10003
212-353-8353
Fax: 212-254-3518
e-mail: NY639@marchofdimes.com
www.marchofdimes.com
Fact Sheets: one or two page review written for the general public. Also available electronically at the website: www.marchofdimes.com

Audio & Video

1795 Genetics and Inherited Traits
March of Dimes
233 Park Avenue South
New York, NY 10003
212-353-8353
Fax: 212-254-3518
e-mail: NY639@marchofdimes.com
www.marchofdimes.com

1796 Why My Child
5400 Diplomat Circle
Orlando, FL 32810-5603
407-629-1466
800-313-2232
www.birthdefects.org
A 9 1/2 minute video that explores the feelings every parent has when their child is born with a birth defect. Emmy-award-winning producer, Karen Dorsett, has created a compelling video that begins with the parents' question, Why my child? and follows through to concerns about links between birth defects and environmental exposures to drugs, pesticides, dioxin, radiation, hazardous wastes, etc.

Web Sites

1797 Association for Birth Defect Children
www.birthdefects.org
Provides parents and expectant parents with information about birth defects and support services for their children.

1798 Healing Well
www.healingwell.com
A social network and support community for patients, caregivers, and families coping with the daily struggles of diseases, disorders and chronic illness.

1799 Health Finder
www.healthfinder.gov
A government web site where individuals can find information and tools to help you and those you care about stay healthy.

1800 Healthlink USA
www.healthlinkusa.com
Health information concerning treatment, cures, prevention, diagnosis, risk factors, research, support groups, email lists, personal stories and much more. Updated regularly.

1801 Helios Health
www.helioshealth.com
Online resource for your health information. Detailed information about specific health topics, access to expert advice from our Medical Advisory Board, and up-to-date health news.

1802 March of Dimes Birth Defects Foundation
www.marchofdimes.com
Help moms have full-term pregnancies and research the problems that threaten the health of babies.

1803 MedicineNet
www.medicinenet.com
An online resource for consumers providing easy-to-read, authoritative medical and health information.

1804 Medscape
www.medscape.com
Medscape offers specialists, primary care physicians, and other health professionals the Web's most robust and integrated medical information and educational tools.

1805 WebMD
www.webmd.com
Information on birth defects, including articles and resources.

Description

1806 Brain Tumors

Brain tumors are either primary (originate in the brain) or metastatic (travel from other cancer sites). About 29,000 people in the United States are diagnosed with primary brain tumors each year; approximately 50 percent of those are benign (noncancerous). Cancerous brain tumors originating in the brain make up roughly 2 percent of all cancers. They may occur at any age but are most common in early adult and middle life. Metastatic brain tumors (those that spread from other cancers) occur in 20 to 40 percent of all cancers.

There are many different types of brain tumors, each with a distinctive appearance under the microscope and a characteristic pattern of onset, progression, location and response to treatment. Depending on the exact site and rate of growth of the tumor, symptoms may include change in personality, moodiness, impaired vision and hearing, headaches, nausea, vomiting, seizures, lethargy and a varying degree of weakness. Some cancers have a genetic basis. In most cases, the cause of an individual's brain tumor is not known.

The treatment of brain tumors, as in many other cancers, consists of a combination of surgical removal, chemotherapy and radiation therapy. Steroids reduce swelling, and antiseizure medication is commonly given. If the disease or its treatment has caused damage to the brain's functioning, the patient may also need physical therapy, speech therapy, or general supportive care. The prognosis depends on the patient's age and on the location, extent and precise type of the tumor. See also *Head Injuries.*

National Agencies & Associations

1807 American Brain Tumor Association
2720 River Road
Des Plaines, IL 60018-4117
847-827-9910
800-886-2282
Fax: 847-827-9918
e-mail: info@abta.org
www.abta.org
Services includes over 40 publications which address brain tumors their treatment and coping with the disease. Materials address brain tumors in all age groups. Provide free social service consultations and a mentorship program for new brain tumor support groups.
Elizabeth M Wilson, Executive Director
Geri Jo Duda RN, Patient Services

1808 Brain Tumor Society
124 Watertown Street
Watertown, MA 02472
617-924-9997
800-770-8287
Fax: 617-924-9998
e-mail: info@braintumor.org
www.tbts.org
Exists to find a cure for brain tumors and strives to improve the quality of life of brain tumor patients and their families. Disseminates educational information and provides access to psycho-social support and raises funds.
N Paul TonThat, Executive Director
Carrie Treadwell, Director of Research

1809 National Brain Tumor Foundation
22 Battery Street
San Francisco, CA 94111-5520
415-834-9970
800-934-2873
Fax: 415-834-9980
e-mail: info@braintumor.org
www.braintumor.org
Nonprofit health organization which raises funds for research and provides information and support to patients, their family members and friends and health professionals. Sponsors national and regional conferences, patient and caregiver programs.
Harriet Patt MPH, Director of Patient Services
N. Paul TonThat, Executive Director

1810 National Brain Tumor Society
22 Battery Street
San Francisco, CA 94111-5520
415-834-9970
800-934-2873
Fax: 415-834-9980
e-mail: info@braintumor.org
www.braintumor.org
Nonprofit health organization which raises funds for research and provides information and support to patients, their family members and friends and health professionals. Sponsors national and regional conferences, patient and caregiver programs.
Gerogre Gellert, Chief Medical Officer

1811 National Institute of Neurological Disorders and Stroke
NIH Neurological Institute
Bethesda, MD 20824
301-496-5751
800-352-9424
Fax: 301-402-2186
TTY: 301-468-5981
www.ninds.nih.gov
The mission of NINDS is to reduce the burden of neurological disease - a burden borne by every age group, by every segment of society, by people all over the world.
Story C Landis, PhD, Director
Walter J Koroshetz, Deputy Director

Foundations

1812 Brain Tumor Foundation for Children
6065 Roswell Road NE
Atlanta, GA 30328
404-252-4107
Fax: 404-252-4108
e-mail: bfc@bellsouth.net
www.braintumorkids.org
Provides information and emotional support for families of children with brain tumors. They also raise funds for brain tumor research and provide a telephone network system of parents who offer emotional support.
Rick Sauers, Chairman/Co-Founder
R Hal Meeks, Jr, President

1813 Children's Brain Tumor Foundation
274 Madison Avenue
New York, NY 10016
212-448-9494
866-228-HOPE
Fax: 212-448-1022
e-mail: info@cbtf.org
www.cbtf.org
Children's Brain Tumor Foundation (CBTF) is a national organization whose mission is to improve the treatment, quality of life and long-term outlook for children with brain and spinal cord tumors through research, support, education, and advocacy to families and survivors. CBTF provides research and quality of life grants, offers information and support via our toll free line, written educational material, meet the unique needs of childhood brain tumor survivors.
Robert Budlow, President
Joseph B Fay, Executive Director

1814 Pediatric Brain Tumor Foundation
302 Ridgefield Court
Asheville, NC 28806
828-665-6891
800-253-6530
Fax: 828-655-6894
e-mail: pbtfus@pbtfus.org
www.pbtfus.org
Dedicated to finding the cause and cure of childhood brain tumors through the support of medical research. Increases public awareness, aids in early detection and treatment, supports a national database on all primary brain tumors. Helps to provide hope and

emotional support for the thousands of children and families affected by this life threatening disease.
Michael Traynor, President
Glenn Wilcox, Vice President

Research Centers

1815 **Brain Research Center Children s Hospital National Medical Cen**
Children s Hospital National Medical Center
111 Michigan Avenue NW 202-476-3000
Washington, DC 20010 800-884-5433
Fax: 202-884-5226
e-mail: tbear@cnmc.org
www.dcchildrens.com

Edwin K Zechman Jr, President
Mark L Batshaw, Chief Medical Officer

1816 **Brain Research Foundation**
111 W Washington Street 312-759-5150
Chicago, IL 60602 Fax: 312-759-5151
e-mail: info@theBRF.org
www.thebrf.org
Supports cutting-edge neuroscience research that will lead to novel treatments and prevention of neurological disease and disorders in children and adults. Deliver this commitment through seed grants, which provide early stage fundinf for innovative research projects, as well as educational programs for researchers and the general public.
Nathan Hansom, President
Terre A Constantine PhD, Executive Director

1817 **Brain Tissue Resource Center McLean Hospital**
McLean Hospital
115 Mill Street 617-855-2000
Belmont, MA 02478 800-272-4622
Fax: 617-855-3199
e-mail: mcleaninfo@mclean.harvard.edu
www.brainbank.mclean.org
A centralized resource for the collection and distribution of human brain specimens for brain research.
Francine M Benes, Director
Edward D Bird, Director Emeritus

1818 **Central Brain Tumor Registry of the US**
244 E Ogden avenue 630-655-4786
Hinsdale, IL 60521 Fax: 630-655-1756
e-mail: cbtrus@aol.com
www.cbtrus.org
Nonprofit resource for gathering and distributing current statistics on all primary brain tumors for the entire US. Includes data on benign borderline and malignant primary brain tumors.
Carol Kruchko, President /Administrator
Jeri Dolan, Executive Administrator

1819 **University of California, San Francisco Brain Tumor Research Center**
Department of Neurological Surgery
505 Parnassus Avenue 415-353-7500
San Francisco, CA 94143-0112 Fax: 415-353-2889
e-mail: garritye@neurosurg.ucsf.edu
www.neurosurgery.ucsf.edu
Continuously funded by grants from the National Institutes of Health Since 1072, the Brain Tumor Research Center at UCSF is internationally recognized as a major research and treatment center for adults and children with tumors of the brain and spinal cord. This center emphasizes translational research into the biology and behavior of brain tumors - research in which scientists and health care clinicians work in partnership to translate laboratory findings of new or improved forms of therapy.
Charles B Wilson, Director
Michael Gillis, Administrative Director

Support Groups & Hotlines

1820 **National Health Information Center**
PO Box 1133 310-565-4167
Washington, DC 20013-1133 800-336-4797
Fax: 301-984-4256
e-mail: info@nhic.org
www.health.gov/nhic
A health information referral service sponsored by the Office of Disease Prevention and Health Promotion. Puts health professionals and consumers who have health questions in touch with those organizations that are best able to provide answers.

1821 **Parent-to-Parent Network**
Children's Brain Tumor Foundation
274 Madison Avenue 212-448-9494
New York, NY 10016 866-228-HOPE
Fax: 212-448-1022
e-mail: info@cbtf.org
www.cbtf.org
Allows families to share their experiences with those having similar concerns. Parents become better advocates for their children, and survivors become stronger advocates for themselves.
Robert Budlow, President
Joseph B Fay, Executive Director

Alabama

1822 **Pediatric Brain Tumor Support Group**
Children's Hospital
1600 7th Avenue S 205-939-9090
Birmingham, AL 35233-1785
Groups for parents and siblings of brain tumor patients. Related to Children's Hospital of Alabama. Babysitting available.
Paula Teague

Arizona

1823 **Arizona Brain Tumor Support Group**
Barrow Neurological Ins of St. Joe's Hospital
350 W Thomas Road
Phoenix, AZ 85013 623-205-6446
www.braintumorfoundation.org

Lanette Veres, Director

1824 **Southern Arizona Brain Tumor Support Group**
Arizona Cancer Cetner
1515 N Campbell Avenue 520-694-4605
Tucson, AZ e-mail: mdrozdoff@umcaz.edu
www.braintumorfoundation.org

Marsha Drozdoff, Contact

California

1825 **Bereavement Group for Children**
The Center for Attitudinal Healing
33 Buchanan Drive
Sausalito, CA 94965 415-331-6161
www.braintumor.org

Jimmy Pete, Contact

1826 **Brain Tumor Society**
National Brain Tumor Society
22 Battery Street 415-834-9970
San Francisco, CA 94111-5520 800-770-8287
Fax: 415-834-9980
e-mail: info@braintumor.org
www.braintumor.org

N Paul TonThat, Executive Director

1827 **Brain Tumor Support Group: Duarte**
City of Hope National Medical Center
1500 E Duarte Road
Duarte, CA 91010 626-256-4673
www.braintumor.org

Heather Ducksworth, Contact

1828 **Brain Tumor Support Group: Fresno**
Cancer Center at St. Agnes

7130 N Millbrook Avenue
Fresno, CA 93720

559-450-5528
e-mail: karen.kennedy@samc.com
www.braintumor.org

Karen Kennedy, Contact

1829 Brain Tumor Support Group: Fullerton
St. Jude Medical Plaza
2151 N Harbor Blvd
Fullerton, CA 92835

714-446-7182
e-mail: kathy.pearson@stjoe.org
www.braintumor.org

Kathy Pearson RN, Contact

1830 Brain Tumor Support Group: Newport Beach
Hoag Hospital
Advanced Technology Pavilion
Newport Beach, CA 92663

949-764-6036
e-mail: lberberet@hoaghospital.org
www.braintumor.org

Lori Berberet RN, Contact

1831 Brain Tumor Support Group: Orange
UC Irvine-Chao Family Comprehensive Cancer Center
101 The City Drive
Orange, CA 92868

714-456-8609
e-mail: bakerd@uci.edu
www.braintumor.org

Donna Baker LCSW, Contact

1832 Brain Tumor Support Group: Redding
American Cancer Society
3290 Bechelli Lane
Redding, CA 96002

530-222-1058
www.braintumor.org

1833 Brain Tumor Support Group: Sacramento
UC Davis Ambulatory Care Center
4860 Y Street
Sacramento, CA 95817

916-734-5613
e-mail: kksmith@ucdavis.edu
www.braintumor.org

Karen Smith RN, Contact
Carolyn Guadagnolo LCSW, Contact

1834 Brain Tumor Support Group: San Diego
Kaiser's Pt Loma Medical Facility
3250 Fordham
San Diego, CA 92117

619-515-9908
www.braintumor.org

Connie Campbell, Contact

1835 Brain Tumor Support Group: San Francisco
UCSF
521 Parnassus Avenue
San Francisco, CA 94143

415-990-4461
e-mail: mlovely@braintumor.org
www.braintumor.org

Sharon Lamb RN, Contact
Mary Lovely RN, Contact

1836 Brain Tumor Support Group: Santa Barbara
Cancer Center of Santa Barbara
300 W Pueblo Street
Santa Barbara, CA 93105

805-563-5852
www.braintumor.org

Rosario Campuzano, Contact

1837 Brain Tumor Support Group: Stanford
Stanford Cancer Center
875 Blake Wilbur Drive
Stanford, CA 94305

415-990-4461
e-mail: mlovely@braintumor.org
www.braintumor.org

Joanie Taylor RN, Contact
Sharon Lamb RN, Contact

1838 Brain Tumor Support Group: Westlake Village
The Wellness Community
530 Hampshire Road
Westlake Village, CA 91361

805-379-4777
e-mail: info@wellnesscommunityhope.org
www.braintumor.org

Rebecca Dekker MFT, Contact

1839 Brain Tumor/Pituitary Patient Support Group
John Wayne Cancer Institute

2200 Santa Monica Blvd
Santa Monica, CA 90404

949-515-9595
e-mail: pituitarybuddy@hotmail.com
www.braintumor.org

Sharmyn McGraw, Contact

1840 Children Living with Illness
The Center for Attitudinal Healing
33 Buchanan Drive
Sausalito, CA 94965

415-331-6161
Fax: 415-331-4545
www.healingcenter.org

Don Goewey, Executive Director

1841 Glendale Adventist Medical Center Brain Tumor Support Group
Cancer Services
381-A Merrill Avenue
Glendale, CA 91026

818-409-3530
www.braintumor.org

Connie Munoz LCSW, Contact

1842 Heads Up!
Northridge Hospital Medical Center
18300 Roscoe Blvd
Northridge, CA 91325

818-885-8500
e-mail: robert.salazar@chw.edu
www.braintumor.org

Wanda Martin, Contact
Robert Salazar, Additional Contact

1843 Neuro-Oncology Information and Support Group
Sister Mary Pia Regional Cancer Center
1800 N California Street
Stockton, CA 95204-6019

209-467-6550
www.stjosephscares.org

For patients and family members living with primary and metastatic brain tumors as well as spinal cord tumors. Free child care and refreshments are provided.
Jim Linderman

1844 Neuroscience Institute Brain Tumor Hotline
Hospital of the Good Samaritan
637 Lucas Avenue
Los Angeles, CA 90017-1912

800-762-1692
e-mail: info@goodsam.org
www.goodsam.org

Diana Selover, LCSW

1845 Patient Services
22 Battery Street
San Francisco, CA 94111-5520

415-834-9970
800-934-2873
Fax: 415-834-9980
e-mail: info@braintumor.org
www.braintumor.org

Quickly access brain tumor information and resources.
12 pages
George Gellert, Chief Medical Officer

1846 Peninsula Support & Education Group for Parents of Children with Brain Tumors
Parents Helping Parents
3041 Olcott Street
Santa Clara, CA 95054-3222

408-727-5775
866-747-4040
Fax: 408-727-0182
e-mail: info@php.com
www.php.com

A comprehensive family resource center providing information, training, guidance and support to families of children with special needs and the professionals who serve them.
Mary Ellen Peterson, Chief Executive Officer

1847 Support Group for Caregivers of Brain Tumor Patients
UCLA Medical Center
200 UCLA Medical Plaza
Los Angeles, CA 90095

310-206-6731
e-mail: cabe@mednet.ucla.edu
Cheryl Abe LCSW, Clinical Social Worker
Pamela Hoff LCSW, Clinical Social Worker

1848 Vital Options International
4419 Coldwater Canyon Avenue
Studio City, CA 91604-1479

818-508-5657
Fax: 818-788-5260
e-mail: info@vitaloptions.org
www.vitaloptions.org

A not-for-profit cancer communications, support, and advocacy organization with a mission, to facilitate a global cancer dialogue.
Selma R Schimmel, CEO/Founder
Juliana Lee, Production Manager

1849   Wellness Community Cancer Support Groups
San Francisco/East Bay
3276 Mc Nutt Avenue   925-933-0107
Walnut Creek, CA 94597   e-mail: emaslan@yahoo.com
                                            www.braintumor.org

Erika Maslan MFCC, Contact

1850   Wellness Community: South Bay Cities
109 W Torrance Blvd
Redondo Beach, CA 90277   www.braintumor.org
Tom May, Contact

1851   Wellness Community: West Los Angeles
2716 Ocean Park Blvd
Santa Monica, CA 90405   www.braintumor.org

1852   Support Group for Parents of Children with Brain Tumors
Oakland Children's Hospital
747 52nd Street   510-428-3885
Oakland, CA   800-400-PEDS
                                            www.kidsfirst.org

Contact can be reached at extension 2161.
Trish Murphy

Colorado

1853   Brain Tumor Resource and Vital Encouragement
Childrens Hospital
1056 19th Avenue   303-861-8888
Denver, CO   e-mail: webmaster@tchden.org
                                            www.tchden.org
Pediatric focus. Education and support. Retreats for parents of brain tumor patients.
Joanne Pearson, Outpatient Oncology

1854   Colorado Brain Tumor Support Group
Swedish Medical Center   303-806-7420
Englewood, CO 80113   e-mail: lgibson@thecni.org
                                    www.braintumorfoundation.org

Lorre Gibson, Contact

Connecticut

1855   Connecticut Brain Tumor Support Group
20 York Street   203-785-7528
New Haven, CT 06510   Fax: 203-688-2395
                                    www.braintumorfoundation.org

Angela Thomas LCSW, Contact

Delaware

1856   Pediatric Brain Tumor Support Group
Ronald McDonald House
PO Box 269   302-661-4077
Wilmington, DE 19899-3629 e-mail: izienberg@kidshealth.org
                                            www.kidshealth.org
Meets first Monday of each month from 7:30 to 9:30 p.m.
Niel Izienberg, Chief Executive Officer

District of Columbia

1857   Washington DC Metropolitan Area Support Group
George Washington University
2150 Pennsylvania Aveneu NW   202-994-4035
Washington, DC 20037-3201
Margaret Fiore, RN

Florida

1858   Angels in the Sun Brain Tumor Support Group
Wellness Community
3900 Clark Road
Sarasota, FL 34233   941-921-5539
                                    www.braintumorfoundation.org

John Kleinbaum, Program Director

1859   Brain Tumor Support Group
Miami Children's Hospital Foundation
3000 SW 62nd Avenue   305-662-8386
Miami, FL 33155   e-mail: maria.penate@mch.com
Call for schedule.
Maria Penate RN, Facilitator
Raquel Pasaron, Facilitator

1860   Florida Brain Tumor Association
PO Box 770182   954-755-4307
Coral Springs, FL 33077-0182   e-mail: sshetsky@fbta.info
                                            www.fbta.info

Provides hope, support and education to brain tumor survivors, their families and friends; conquers brain tumors by funding research into their causes and cures; and enriches the quality of life of those touched by brain tumors
Sheryl Shetsky, President
Gary L Kornfeld, VP

1861   Florida Brain Tumor Support Group
Healthpark Medical Ctr, Meeting Rm
Ft Meyers, FL 33919   239-433-4396
                                    www.braintumorfoundation.org

Dona Ross, Contact

1862   Florida Brain Tumor Support Group: Deerfield Beach
North Broward Medical Center   954-755-4307
Deerfield Beach, FL 33441   e-mail: sshetsky@fbta.info
                                            www.fbta.info

Sheryl Shetsky, President
Gary L Kornfeld, VP

1863   Hollywood Area Brain Tumor Support Group
Memorial Regional Hospital   954-265-4725
Hollywood, FL 33021   e-mail: csurloff@mhs.net
                                            www.fbta.info

Dr Cheri Surloff, Contact

1864   Sarasota Area Brain Tumor Support Group
Institute of Advanced Medicine
5880 Rand Avenue
Sarasota, FL   e-mail: sposin@fbta.info
                                            www.fbta.info

Sheryl R Shetsky, President
Gary L Kornfeld, VP

1865   West Palm Beach Area Brain Tumor Support Group
Good Samaritan Medical Center
West Palm Beach, FL 33401   561-655-5511
                                            www.fbta.info

Sheryl R Shetsky, President
Gary L Kornfeld, VP

Georgia

1866   All Ages Support Group
Brain Tumor Foundation for Children
6065 Roswell Road NE   404-252-4107
Atlanta, GA 30328-4015   Fax: 404-252-4108
                            e-mail: info@braintumorkids.org
                                        www.braintumorkids.org/
Patient Support Group Activities includes bowling, fishing, craft parties, picnics, sporting events, holiday parties, etc. These activities, social events and more are provided for children of all ages and their families.
Mary Campbell, Executive Director
R Hal Meeks Jr, President

1867   Emory Brain Tumor Support Group
Emory Clinic
Department of Neurosurgery
Atlanta, GA 30322   404-778-3091
                        www.neurosurgery.emory.edu/btsg/index
Meets the first Thursday of each month with the purpose of providing an opportunity for information-sharing and suport for brain tumor patients, as well as their family, friends and caregivers.
Maxine Brown, Contact

1868   Hearts and Minds
Piedmont Hospital

1968 Peachtree Road NW
Atlanta, GA

404-373-5202
Fax: 404-605-5000
www.piedmonthospital.org

Neal Kuhlhorst

1869 SBTF Brain Tumor Support Group
PO Box 422471
Atlanta, GA 30342

404-843-3700
e-mail: info@sbtf.org
www.sbtf.org

To improve the quality of life for brain tumor patients and their families.
Costas Hadjipanayis, President

Illinois

1870 Brain Tumor Support Group
Northwestern Memorial Hospital
675 N St. Clair
Chicago, IL 60611

312-695-8143
e-mail: mmaher@nmff.org

Mary Ellen Maher, Contact

1871 Parents of Children with Brain Tumors PCBT
Children's Memorial Hospital
2300 Children's Plaza
Chicago, IL 60614

773-880-4316

Meets quarterly and publishes a monthly newsletter. Library available at meetings (at CMH). Educational speakers and family functions.
Gina Baldacci LCSW, Contact

Indiana

1872 Brain Tumor Support Group
Community Hospital East
1500 North Ritter Avenue
Indianapolis, IN 46219

317-355-1411
e-mail: m.w.kemf@att.net
www.ecommunity.com/east

Meets the third Wednsday of each month from 6:30 to 7:30 p.m.
Michael Kemf, Facilitator
Marsha Cline, Facilitator

1873 Primary Brain Cancer Support Group
Women's Cancer Center at Lutheran Hospital
7950 W Jefferson Boulevard
Fort Wayne, IN 46804

260-435-7959

Meets on the first Tuesday of every month at 6:00 p.m.
Linda Jordan RN, Contact

Iowa

1874 Iowa Brain Tumor Support Group
University of Iowa Hospitals
Iowa City, IA 52242

319-356-2557

Lori Roetlin, Contact
Sue May, Additional Contact

1875 Neurological Center of Iowa
Iowa Clinic
1215 Pleasant Street
Des Moines, IA 50309-1418

515-241-5760
Fax: 515-241-6090
www.iowaclinic.com/

Networks people in similar situations.
Ed Brown, Chief Executive Officer

1876 Quad Cities Brain Tumor Support Group
Genesis Medical Center
1401 W Central Park
Davenport, IA 52804

563-421-1907
e-mail: ided@genesishealth.com

Meetings are on the 4th Monday of each month from 6:30 to 8:00 p.m.
Deb Ide, Contact

Kansas

1877 Gray Matters Support: Kansas City
24050 W 57th Street
Shawnee, KS 66226

e-mail: graymatters2007@yahoo.com

Debbie Stephenson, Contact

1878 Headstrong Brain Tumor Support Group
Victory in the Valley
3755 E Douglas
Wichita, KS 67218

316-682-7400
e-mail: info@victoryinthevalley.com

Kentucky

1879 Meningioma/Benign Brain Tumor Support Group
Michael Quinlan Brain Tumor Foundation
4012 Dupont Circle
Louisville, KY 40207

502-896-1701

Kathy Quinlan-Thompson, Contact

1880 Wellness Community: Kentucky
1717 Dixie Highway
Fort Wright, KY 41011

859-331-5568

Louisiana

1881 Brain Tumor Support Group
3939 Houma Boulevard, Doctor's Row
Metairie, LA 70005

504-835-5715
e-mail: gmom224@cox.net

Meets on the third Sunday of each month at 1:30 p.m., call to confirm.
Gayle Johnson, Contact Person

Maine

1882 Brain Tumor Support Group of Maine
Maine Medical Center
22 Bramhall Street
Portland, ME 04102

207-871-4527

Meets on the second Tuesday of each month from 7:00 to 9:00 p.m.
Nancy Fortier LCSW, Contact

Maryland

1883 Brain Tumor Networking Group
10628 Falls Road
Lutherville, MD 21022

410-832-2719
e-mail: cancerhelp@hopewellcancersupport.org

Carol Sharp, Contact

1884 Brain Tumor Support Group: Maryland
NIH Clinical Research Center
9000 Rockville Pike
Bethesda, MD 20892

301-496-6380
e-mail: garrenn@mail.nih.gov

Nancy Garren, Contact

1885 Brainiacs
Perryville Library
Perryville, MD 21903

410-459-8157

Liz Carrino, Contact

1886 Johns Hopkins Brain Tumor Education Group
Weinberg Building
Baltimore, MD 21231

410-502-2789

Liz Carrino, Contact

1887 Washington DC Metropolitan Area Brain Tumor Support Group
George Washington Ambulatory Center
I & 22nd Street
Middletown, MD 21769

301-371-8660

Lionel Chaiken, Contact
Jeff Schanz, Contact

Massachusetts

1888 Brain Tumor Patient and Caregiver Support Group
Dana Farber Cancer Institute
Boston, MA 02115

617-632-3634

Nancy Tharler LICSW, Contact

1889 Brain Tumor Support Group: Lahey
Lahey Clinic Medical Center
41 Mall Road
Burlington, MA 01805

617-726-1061
www.lahey.org

Michele Lucas MSW LICSW, Contact

1890 Brain Tumor Support Group: Worcester
UMass Memorial Medical Center-University Campus
55 Lake Avenue N 508-334-7595
Worcester, MA 01655 Fax: 800-697-2593
e-mail: ellen.sharenow@umassmemorial.org
Ellen Sharenow PhD, Contact

1891 Neurological Support Group of St. Luke's Hospital
101 Page Street 508-997-1515
New Bedford, MA 02740-3464
Contact can be reached at extension 2764.
Diane Robinson RN

1892 Parent Education/Support Group
Dana Farber Cancer Institute
44 Binney Street 617-632-3301
Boston, MA 2115 800-525-5068
e-mail: dana.farbercontactus@dfci.harvard.edu
www.dfci.harvard.edu
For parents of children with brain tumors. Please call for schedule.
Beverly Lavalley Run, Facilitator
Edward Benz Jr, President

Michigan

1893 Brain Tumor Networking Club
Gilda's Club Metro Detroit
3517 Rochester Road 248-577-0800
Royal Oak, MI 48073 Fax: 248-577-0898
Kristen Bernat, Contact

1894 Brain Tumor Support Group for Patients & Families
University of Michigan Medical Center
1500 E Medical Center Drive 734-936-9071
Ann Arbor, MI 48109-0316
Christina Crandall, Contact
Kathy Wilson, Contact

1895 Brain Tumor Support Group: Ann Arbor
St Joseph Mercy Hospital, Cancer Care Center
5301 E Huron River Drive
Ann Arbor, MI 48106 734-712-3658
www.sjmh.com
Paula Nedela RN, Contact

1896 Brain Tumor Support Group: West Bloomfield
Henry Ford Hospital
6777 W Maple 313-916-1796
West Bloomfield, MI 48322
Sandy Remer RN, Contact

Missouri

1897 Brain Cancer Support Group
St John's Hospital
Main Hospital 417-820-3157
Springfield, MO 65804 e-mail: laura.flowers@mercy.net
Laura Flowers, Contact

1898 Brain Tumor Support Group: Kansas City
St Luke's Hospital of Kansas City
4321 Washington Suite 4000 816-932-6015
Kansas City, MO 64111
Michelle Martin, Contact

1899 Brain Tumor Support and Networking Group
Wellness Community of Greater St. Louis
1058 Old Des Peres Road 314-238-2000
Saint Louis, MO 63131 e-mail: info@wellnesscommunitystl.org
www.wellnesscommunitystl.org/

Montana

1900 Cancer Patient/Caregiver Support Group
Wellness Community
1820 W Lincoln Street 406-582-1600
Bozeman, MT 59715 e-mail: twcmontana@qwest.net
Becky Robideaux, Contact

New Hampshire

1901 Brain Injury/Brain Tumor Support Group
Frisbie Memorial Hospital
Carroll Mitchell LMSW, Contact
Rochester, NH 03867

New Jersey

1902 Brain Tumor Support Group: New Jersey
90 Bergen Street 973-972-1164
Newark, NJ 07103 e-mail: mcclamls@umdnj.edu
LaDawn McClamb, Contact

1903 Brain Tumor Support Group: Toms River
Community Medical Center
99 Highway 37 W 732-557-8270
Toms River, NJ 08755 e-mail: slaniado@sbhcs.com
Sherry Laniado LCSW, Contact

1904 Central New Jersey Brain Tumor Support Group
St. Luke's Roman Catholic Church
300 Clinton Avenue 732-321-7000
North Plainfield, NJ 07063
Patty Anthony RN, Contact
Virginia Shrodo, Contact

New Mexico

1905 People Living Through Cancer Support Groups
3411 Candelaria NE 505-242-3263
Albuquerque, NM 87107 888-441-4439
Fax: 505-242-6756
e-mail: info@pltc.org
www.pltc.org
A not for profit organization that connects and supports cancer survivors and caregivers by transforming shared individual experiences into enduring hope.
Beth Brown, Executive Director
Mary Ellen Kurucz, Program Director

New York

1906 Brain Tumor Support Group for Patients and Families
Albany Medical Center
Office of NY Oncology/Hematology 845-338-4820
Albany, NY 12208-3412 e-mail: eehauser@gmail.com
Emilie Hauser, Contact

1907 Brain Tumor Support Group: Long Island
230 Main St. Emma Clark Library 516-747-8749
Setauket, NY
Billie Wilczek

1908 Long Island Brain Tumor Support Group
Old Bethpage Public Library
999 Old Country Road 516-996-3705
Plainview, NY 11803
Bob Crescenzo, Contact

1909 Mount Sinai Medical Center Brain Tumor Support Group
Ruttenberg Care Center-Guggenheim Pavilion
1190 Fifth Ave 212-717-3527
New York, NY 10029
Kathleen Maloney-Lutz RN, Contact

1910 New York Brain Tumor Support Group
525 E 68th Street 212-746-3986
New York, NY 10021 e-mail: wem9011@nyp.org
Wendy Mitchell LMSW, Contact

North Carolina

1911 Brain Tumor Support Group: Raleigh Area
Raleigh Community Hospital
3400 Wake Forest Road
Raleigh, NC 27609-7373 919-846-0923
www.raleighcommunity.com

Lectures, educational materials, and newsletter. Home and hospital visitation.
Louise Clark, Director

1912 Duke Pediatric Brain Tumor Family Support Program
Preston Robert Tisch Brain Tumor Center
Duke University Medical Center 919-668-2327
Durham, NC 27710 Fax: 919-668-2485
e-mail: korpi001@mc.duke.edu
www.cancer.duke.edu/btc/
Assists the families of pediatric patients with identifying strengths and supports available for coping with the emotional and social impact of the brain tumor on the family, offering information about resources in the community in addition to both individual and group supportive counseling.
Darell D. Binger, MD, PhD, Director

1913 Preston Robert Tisch Brain Tumor Center at Duke
Cornucopia Cancer Support Center
5517 Durham Chapel Hill Blvd 919-668-6178
Durham, NC 27707 e-mail: stephanie.english@duke.edu
Stephanie English MSW LCSW, Contact

Ohio

1914 Brain Tumor Support Group: Cincinnati
Wellness Community
4918 Cooper Road 513-791-4060
Cincinnati, OH 45242 Fax: 513-791-8239

1915 Southwest Ohio Brain Tumor Support Group
Kettering Medical Center
3535 Southern Boulevard 937-298-3399
Kettering, OH 45429-1221 e-mail: jean.ruppert@kmcnetwork.org
Jean Ruppert MS CNRN RN, Contact

1916 Support Group for Parents of Children with Brain Tumors
Cincinnati Childrens Hospital Medical Center
Childrens Hospital Medical Center 513-636-4200
Cincinnati, OH 45229-3039 800-344-2462
www.cincinnatichildrens.org/default.htm
Thomas Boat, Director
Stephen Daniels, Associate Chair

Oregon

1917 Brain Tumor Education & Support Group
Legacy Good Samaritan Hospital Cancer Center
1130 NW 22nd Ave 503-413-7921
Portland, OR 97210
Wendy Talbot MSW LCSW, Contact
Selma Annala RT CLC, Contact

1918 Central Oregon Brain Tumor Support Group
900 SW 23rd Place 541-350-7243
Redmond, OR 97756 e-mail: rgklug@crestviewcable.com
Rubyanne Klug, Contact

Pennsylvania

1919 Brain Tumor Community Group
Lancaster General Health Campus
Wellness Conference Room 800-860-9949
Lancaster, PA 17601
Christine Burfete RN, Contact

1920 Brain Tumor Support Group: Johnstown
John P Murtha Neuroscience and Pain Institute
1450 Scalp Avenue 814-534-3797
Johnstown, PA 15904 e-mail: dlehew@conemaugh.org
Denise LeHew RN CNRN, Contact

1921 Brain Tumor Support Group: Philadelphia
University of PA Hospital-Neurological Institute
3400 Spruce Street 215-615-5240
Philadelphia, PA 19104
Alisha Amendt MSN CRNP, Contact
Arbena Merolli MSW, Contact

1922 Brain Tumor Support Group: Pittsburgh
Cancer Caring Center

4117 Liberty Avenue 412-622-1212
Pittsburgh, PA 15224 e-mail: indo@cancercaring.org

1923 Delware Valley Brain Tumor Support Group at Jefferson
Jefferson Health System
Bluemle Life Sciences Building 215-955-4429
Philadelphia, PA 19107
Ann Marie DiBona RN, Contact
Janis Haaf RN, Contact

1924 Pediatric Cancer Foundation of the Lehigh Valley
Camelot for Children
2354 W Emmaus Avenue 610-393-9215
Allentown, PA 18103
Nicole Ronco, Contact

Rhode Island

1925 Brain Tumor Support Group: Providence
Brown University Campus
BioMedical Center 401-789-0126
Providence, RI 02912
Judy Allenson, Contact
Betty Bentley, Contact

1926 Rhode Island Brain & Spine Tumor Foundation
Bethany Home
229 Medway Street 401-272-4177
Providence, RI 02906 e-mail: ribstf@gmail.com
Colin Shaw, Contact

South Carolina

1927 Brain Tumor Support Group: Charleston
Hollings Cancer Center
86 Jonathon Lucas Street 843-792-8257
Charleston, SC 29445 e-mail: lizzic@musc.edu
Christa Lizzi RN, Contact

1928 Brain Tumor Support Group: Florence
Florence Neurosurgery and Spine
1204 E Cheves Street 843-206-1910
Florence, SC 29506 e-mail: info@florenceneurosurgery.com

South Dakota

1929 Cancer Support Group
Sanford Cancer Cetner Oncology Clinic
1020 W 18th Street 605-328-8000
Sioux Falls, SD 57104
Sue Halbritter RN NP, Contact

Tennessee

1930 Cancer Support Group: Knoxville
Wellness Community of East Tennessee
702 Lindsay Place 865-546-4661
Knoxville, TN 37919 e-mail: info@wellnesscommunitytn.org

1931 Cancer Support Group: Nashville
Gilda's Club Nashville
1707 Division Street 615-329-1124
Nashville, TN 37203 e-mail: info@gildasclubnashville.org

1932 Memphis Regional Brain Tumor Survivors Group
Methodist University Hospital
1265 Union Ave 904-757-0806
Memphis, TN 38104 e-mail: cherrywel2@comcast.net
Cherry Welborn, Contact

Texas

1933 Brain Tumor Support Group: El Paso
Rio Grande Cancer Foundation
10460 Vista Del Sol Drive 915-562-7660
El Paso, TX 79925 e-mail: juttar@rgcf.org
Jutta Ramirez, Contact
Robert Lefferts, Contact

1934 Central Texas Brain Tumor Support Group
Brain and Spine Center at Brackenridge Hospital

3rd Floor Boardroom   512-636-1578
Austin, TX 78701
Thomas Lewman, Contact

1935 **Houston Area Brain Tumor Network**
MD Anderson Cancer Center Brain & Spine Center
1515 Holcombe Blvd   713-794-1777
Houston, TX 77030   e-mail: spanju@mdanderson.org
Mark Anderson, Contact
Suki Panju, Contact

1936 **South Texas Brain Tumor Foundation Support Group**
San Antonio Employees Federal Credit Union
6000 NW Loop 410   210-670-9323
San Antonio, TX 78201
Susie Soriano, Contact

Utah

1937 **Cancer Wellness House**
59 S 1100 E   801-236-2294
Salt Lake City, UT 84102
Karen Elliott

Virginia

1938 **Brain Tumor Support Group: Richmond**
St Mary's Hospital
Education Center   877-284-3905
Richmond, VA 23226   e-mail: curebt@hotmail.com
Carol Roberts RN MS, Contact

1939 **Valley Brain Tumor Support Group**
Rehab2Health
Shenandoah Memorial Hospital   540-984-4921
Woodstock, VA 22664   e-mail: vbtsg@shentel.net
Valorie Hockman, Contact

Washington

1940 **Brain Cancer Support Group: Port Orchard**
2186 Yukon Harbor Rd SE   360-536-5042
Port Orchard, WA 98366   e-mail: ideas56@msn.com
Victoria Tierney MA RC, Contact

1941 **Brain Cancer Support Group: Seattle**
Northwest Hospital
Professional Building   206-297-2500
Seattle, WA 98133

1942 **Virginia Mason Brain Tumor Support Group**
1201 Terry Avenue   206-223-7552
Seattle, WA 98111
Michelle Handler RN, Contact

1943 **Wenatchee Valley Brain Tumor Support Group**
Wellness Place
1610 Fifth Street   509-679-9574
Wenatchee, WA 98801   e-mail: hastings9@charter.net
Jeff Hastings, Contact
Mary Lowe, Contact

West Virginia

1944 **Brain Tumor Support Group: Southern West Virginia**
First Presbyterian Church
16 Broad Street   304-744-0393
Charleston, WV 25301-2487
Jeri McDonald

Wisconsin

1945 **Brain Tumor Support Group: John Sierzant Lutheran Hospital, Gunderson Clinic**
1836 S Avenue   608-791-9862
LaCrosse, WI
Esther Lindeman RN

1946 **LODAT: Brain Tumor Support Group**
Children's Hospital of Wisconsin

Room 888
Milwaukee, WI   414-962-8984
www.braintumor.org
Living One Day At a Time is a parent support group for families of chidren with cancer. Monthly newsletter, informational meetings, social activities for families, and bereavement support.
Frances Swigart

Books

1947 **Brain Tumor Resource Directory**
National Brain Tumor Foundation
22 Battery Street   415-834-9970
San Francisco, CA 94111-5520   800-934-2873
      Fax: 415-834-9980
e-mail: nbtf@braintumor.org
www.braintumor.org
Comprehensive reference for healthcare providers, the directory contains the names and phone numbers of various organizations that offer services and products of particular interest to brain tumor patients and their families.
Rob Tufel, Director Patient Services

1948 **Death Be Not Proud: A Memoir**
Harper Collins
10 E 53rd Street
New York, NY 10022   212-207-7000
      www.harpercollins.com
The father of a young man diagnosed with glioblastoma multiforme wrote this 50-year-old classic.

ISBN: 0-060929-89-8

1949 **Resource Guide for Parents of Children with Brain and Spinal Cord Tumors**
Children's Brain Tumor Foundation
274 Madison Avenue   212-448-9494
New York, NY 10016   866-228-HOPE
      Fax: 212-448-1022
e-mail: info@cbtf.org
www.cbtf.org
Contains practical information to sort out the complexities of medical procedures, interruptions in school and social life, and uncertainty about the future.
Robert Budlow, President
Joseph B Fay, Executive Director

1950 **Support Group Directory**
National Brain Tumor Foundation
22 Battery Street   415-834-9970
San Francisco, CA 94111-5520   800-934-2873
      Fax: 415-834-9980
e-mail: nbtf@braintumor.org
www.braintumor.org
Directory listing support groups in the US and Canada, pediatric support groups, online support groups and additional resources on the North American Brain Tumor Coalition. Available online only.
Rob Tufel, Director Patient Services

1951 **That's Unacceptable: Surviving a Brain Tumor: My Personal Story**
Rebecca L Libutti, author

Krystal Publishing
PO Box 221   908-889-6038
Martinsville, NJ 08836   800-833-9327
      Fax: 908-889-6038
e-mail: RLibutti@aol.com
www.krystalpublishing.com
Written by a ten-year survivor of glioblastoma multiforme, the book's title was the author's first response to the initial discouragement she received about pursuing aggressive treatment.
198 pages Paperback
RL Libutti

1952 **The Essential Guide to Brain Tumors**
National Brain Tumor Foundation

22 Battery Street
San Francisco, CA 94111-5520

415-834-9970
800-934-2873
Fax: 415-834-9980
e-mail: nbtf@braintumor.org
www.braintumor.org

Full of information concerning the brain, how it functions, what causes tumors, types of brain tumors, managing symptoms, and even surviving brain tumorrs.
80 pages
Rob Tufel, Director Patient Services

1953   Understanding and Coping with Your Child's Brain Tumor
National Brain Tumor Foundation
22 Battery Street
San Francisco, CA 94111-5520

415-834-9970
800-934-2873
Fax: 415-834-9980
e-mail: nbtf@braintumor.org
www.braintumor.org

Guide for families contains information for parents of children with brain tumors, including information about diagnosis, tumor types, treatment methods, social and emotional support and more. It also contains a glossary, along with listings of organizations and resources.
52 pages
Rob Tufel, Director Patient Services

Children's Books

1954   My Name is Buddy
Dave Bauer, author
National Brain Tumor Foundation
22 Battery Street
San Francisco, CA 94111-5520

415-834-9970
800-934-2873
Fax: 415-834-9980
e-mail: nbtf@braintumor.org
www.braintumor.org

Unique book for children with brain tumors. The reader follows Buddy, a Golden Retriever, on his journey through a brain tumor diagnosis and treatment. This true story uses photographs and narrative to describe Buddy's experiences before and after surgery and talks about his feelings and fears as a brain tumor patient.
Rob Tufel, Director Patient Services

Newsletters

1955   Butterfly Bulletin
Brain Tumor Foundation for Children
6065 Roswell Road NE
Atlanta, GA 30328-4015

404-252-4107
Fax: 404-252-4108
e-mail: info@braintumorkids.org
www.braintumorkids.org

Reporting on news and events of the Brain Tumor Foundation for Children.
Quarterly
Rick Sauers, Chairman/Co-Founder
R Hal Meeks, Jr, President

1956   Caring Hand
Pediatric Brain Tumor Foundation
302 Ridgefield Court
Asheville, NC 28806

828-665-6891
800-253-6530
Fax: 828-655-6894
e-mail: pbtfus@pbtfus.org
www.pbtfus.org

The Caring Hand is a regular newsletter, distributed free of charge to patient families, caregivers and medical/social work professionals.
Michael Traynor, President
Glenn Wilcox, Vice President

1957   Childhood Brain Tumor Foundation Newsletter
Childhood Brain Tumor Foundation
20312 Watkins Meadow Drive
Germantown, MD 20876-4259

310-515-2900
877-217-4166
e-mail: cbtf@childhoodbraintumor.org
www.childhoodbraintumor.org

Seeking second opinions, access to healthcare, and combating discrimination.

1958   Helping Hand
Pediatric Brain Tumor Foundation
302 Ridgefield Court
Asheville, NC 28806

828-665-6891
800-253-6530
Fax: 828-655-6894
e-mail: pbtfus@pbtfus.org
www.pbtfus.org

The Helping Hand is a regular newsletter, distributed free of charge to Ride for Kids®and supporters.
Michael Traynor, President
Glenn Wilcox, Vice President

1959   Message Line Newsletter
American Brain Tumor Association
2720 S River Road
Des Plaines, IL 60018-4117

847-827-9910
800-886-2282
Fax: 847-827-9918
e-mail: info@abta.org
www.abta.org

Describes research advances and announces updates to publications.
TriAnnual
Elizabeth Wilson, Executive Director
Geri Jo Duda, RN, Patient Services

1960   SEARCH
National Brain Tumor Foundation
22 Battery Street
San Francisco, CA 94111-5520

415-834-9970
800-934-2873
Fax: 415-834-9980
e-mail: nbtf@braintumor.org
www.braintumor.org

Newsletter that covers topics of current interest to brain tumor survivors and their families.
Quarterly
Rob Tufel, Director Patient Services

1961   TLC (Tips for Living And Coping)
American Brain Tumor Association
2720 S River Road
Des Plaines, IL 60018-4117

847-827-9910
800-886-2282
Fax: 847-827-9918
e-mail: info@abta.org
www.abta.org

E-bulletin of news, research and development finds, support and treatment information.

ISBN: 0-944093-37-X
Elizabeth Wilson, Executive Director
Geri Jo Duda, RN, Patient Services

Pamphlets

1962   Clinical Trial Fact Sheet
National Brain Tumor Foundation
22 Battery Street
San Francisco, CA 94111-5520

415-834-9970
800-934-2873
Fax: 415-834-9980
e-mail: nbtf@braintumor.org
www.braintumor.org

Lists of clinical trial by state, tumor type and/or treatment type.

1963   Coping with Your Loved One's Brain Tumor
National Brain Tumor Foundation
22 Battery Street
San Francisco, CA 94111-5520

415-834-9970
800-934-2873
Fax: 415-834-9980
e-mail: nbtf@braintumor.org
www.braintumor.org

Describes important coping stategies for caregivers and family members of a loved one with a brain tumor.
12 pages Booklet

1964   Dictionary for Brain Tumor Patients
American Brain Tumor Association

2720 S River Road
Des Plaines, IL 60018-4117

847-827-9910
800-886-2282
Fax: 847-827-9918
e-mail: info@abta.org
www.abta.org

Offers a dictionary of terms used in the diagnosis and everday living with brain tumors.
Paperback
ISBN: 0-944093-27-2
Elizabeth Wilson, Executive Director
Geri Jo Duda, RN, Patient Services

1965 Ependymoma
American Brain Tumor Association
2720 S River Road
Des Plaines, IL 60018-4117

847-827-9910
800-886-2282
Fax: 847-827-9918
e-mail: info@abta.org
www.abta.org

ISBN: 0-944093-40-X
Elizabeth Wilson, Executive Director
Geri Jo Duda, RN, Patient Services

1966 Glioblastoma Multiforme and Anaplastic Astrocytoma
American Brain Tumor Association
2720 S River Road
Des Plaines, IL 60018-4117

847-827-9910
800-886-2282
Fax: 847-827-9918
e-mail: info@abta.org
www.abta.org

ISBN: 0-944093-36-1
Elizabeth Wilson, Executive Director
Geri Jo Duda, RN, Patient Services

1967 Living with A Brain Tumor
American Brain Tumor Association
2720 S River Road
Des Plaines, IL 60018-4117

847-827-9910
800-886-2282
Fax: 847-827-9918
e-mail: info@abta.org
www.abta.org

A guide for brain tumor patients.
2004
ISBN: 0-944093-54-X
Elizabeth Wilson, Executive Director
Geri Jo Duda, RN, Patient Services

1968 Medulloblastoma
American Brain Tumor Association
2720 S River Road
Des Plaines, IL 60018-4117

847-827-9910
800-886-2282
Fax: 847-827-9918
e-mail: info@abta.org
www.abta.org

Paperback
ISBN: 0-944093-33-7
Elizabeth Wilson, Executive Director
Geri Jo Duda, RN, Patient Services

1969 Meningioma
American Brain Tumor Association
2720 S River Road
Des Plaines, IL 60018-4117

847-827-9910
800-886-2282
Fax: 847-827-9918
e-mail: info@abta.org
www.abta.org

ISBN: 0-944093-23-X
Elizabeth Wilson, Executive Director
Geri Jo Duda, RN, Patient Services

1970 Metastatic Brain Tumors
American Brain Tumor Association

2720 S River Road
Des Plaines, IL 60018-4117

847-827-9910
800-886-2282
Fax: 847-827-9918
e-mail: info@abta.org
www.abta.org

ISBN: 0-944093-26-4
Elizabeth Wilson, Executive Director
Geri Jo Duda, RN, Patient Services

1971 Oligodendroglioma and Mixed Glioma
American Brain Tumor Association
2720 S River Road
Des Plaines, IL 60018-4117

847-827-9910
800-886-2282
Fax: 847-827-9918
e-mail: info@abta.org
www.abta.org

Pamphlet
ISBN: 0-944093-43-4
Elizabeth Wilson, Executive Director
Geri Jo Duda, RN, Patient Services

1972 Organizing a Support Group
American Brain Tumor Association
2720 S River Road
Des Plaines, IL 60018-4117

847-827-9910
800-886-2282
Fax: 847-827-9918
e-mail: info@abta.org
www.abta.org

Elizabeth Wilson, Executive Director
Geri Jo Duda, RN, Patient Services

1973 Pituitary Tumors
American Brain Tumor Association
2720 S River Road
Des Plaines, IL 60018-4117

847-827-9910
800-886-2282
Fax: 847-827-9918
e-mail: info@abta.org
www.abta.org

Pamphlet
ISBN: 0-944093-44-2
Elizabeth Wilson, Executive Director
Geri Jo Duda, RN, Patient Services

1974 Primer of Brain Tumors
American Brain Tumor Association
2720 S River Road
Des Plaines, IL 60018-4117

847-827-9910
800-886-2282
Fax: 847-827-9918
e-mail: info@abta.org
www.abta.org

A patient's reference manual offering information on brain tumors.

ISBN: 0-944093-35-3
Elizabeth Wilson, Executive Director
Geri Jo Duda, RN, Patient Services

1975 Radiation Therapy of Brain Tumors: A Basic Guide
American Brain Tumor Association
2720 S River Road
Des Plaines, IL 60018-4117

847-827-9910
800-886-2282
Fax: 847-827-9918
e-mail: info@abta.org
www.abta.org

ISBN: 0-944093-28-0
Elizabeth Wilson, Executive Director
Geri Jo Duda, RN, Patient Services

1976 Returning to Work: Strategies for Brain Tumor Patients
National Brain Tumor Foundation
22 Battery Street
San Francisco, CA 94111-5520

415-834-9970
800-934-2873
Fax: 415-834-9980
e-mail: nbtf@braintumor.org
www.braintumor.org

Reviews brain tumor survivors rights with respect to returning to work and suggests several strategies to make it an easier transition to go back into the workplace.
16 pages Brochure
Rob Tufel, Director Patient Services

1977 Stereotactic Radiosurgery
American Brain Tumor Association
2720 S River Road   847-827-9910
Des Plaines, IL 60018-4117   800-886-2282
                                    Fax: 847-827-9918
                                    e-mail: info@abta.org
                                    www.abta.org

ISBN: 0-944093-42-6
Elizabeth Wilson, Executive Director
Geri Jo Duda, RN, Patient Services

1978 Understanding Brain Tumors: Glioblastoma Multiforme
National Brain Tumor Foundation
22 Battery Street   415-834-9970
San Francisco, CA 94111-5520   800-934-2873
                                    Fax: 415-834-9980
                                    e-mail: nbtf@braintumor.org
                                    www.braintumor.org
Helps patients and caregivers understand more about the diagnosis and treatment of glioblastoma multiforme.
16 pages
Rob Tufel, Director Patient Services

1979 Using A Medical Library
American Brain Tumor Association
2720 S River Road   847-827-9910
Des Plaines, IL 60018-4117   800-886-2282
                                    Fax: 847-827-9918
                                    e-mail: info@abta.org
                                    www.abta.org

Elizabeth Wilson, Executive Director
Geri Jo Duda, RN, Patient Services

1980 What You Need to Know About Brain Tumors
National Cancer Institute
Building 31   301-435-3848
Bethesda, MD 20892-0001   800-422-6237
                                    www.nci.nih.gov
Offers factual information about brain tumors, possible causes, primary and secondary tumors, symptoms, diagnosis, treatment, side effects, followup care, support and medical terms.

1981 When Your Child Returns to School
American Brain Tumor Association
2720 S River Road   847-827-9910
Des Plaines, IL 60018-4117   800-886-2282
                                    Fax: 847-827-9918
                                    e-mail: info@abta.org
                                    www.abta.org
Guides parents and teachers through a successful return to school when a child has had a brain tumor.
Paperback
ISBN: 0-944093-21-3
Elizabeth Wilson, Executive Director
Geri Jo Duda, RN, Patient Services

Audio & Video

1982 Conference Audiotapes
National Brain Tumor Foundation
22 Battery Street   415-834-9970
San Francisco, CA 94111-5520   800-934-2873
                                    Fax: 415-834-9980
                                    e-mail: nbtf@braintumor.org
                                    www.braintumor.org
Audiotapes of keynote addresses and conference workshops from NBTF's biennial National Brain Tumor Conferences where leading researchers, physicians and health professionals address a range of issues affecting brain tumor survivors, such as new approaches to radiation and surgery, research and coping skills for families.
Rob Tufel, Director Patient Services

1983 Strategies for Healing
National Brain Tumor Foundation
414 13th Street   510-839-9777
Oakland, CA 94612   800-934-2873
                                    Fax: 510-839-9779
                                    e-mail: nbtf@braintumor.org
                                    www.braintumor.org
CD-Rom contains vital information about treatment options and self-care for newly diagnosed patients and their families.
Rob Tufel, Director Patient Services

Web Sites

1984 American Brain Tumor Association
                                    www.abta.org
Provide free social service consultations; a mentorship program for new brain tumor support group leaders; a nationwide database of established support groups; the Connections pen-pal program; networking with organizations that provide services to patients and families; a resource listing of physicians offering investgative treatments.

1985 Brain Tumor Society
124 Watertown Street   617-924-9997
Watertown, MA 02472   800-770-8287
                                    Fax: 617-924-9998
                                    e-mail: info@tbts.org
                                    www.tbts.org
Disseminates educational information and provides access to psycho-social support and raises funds to advance carefully selected scientific research projects, improve clinical care and find a cure.

1986 Healing Well
                                    www.healingwell.com
An online health resource guide to medical news, chat, information and articles, newsgroups and message boards, books, disease-related web sites, medical directories, and more for patients, friends, and family coping with disabling diseases, disorders, or chronic illnesses.

1987 Health Finder
                                    www.healthfinder.gov
Searchable, carefully developed web site offering information on over 1000 topics. Developed by the US Department of Health and Human Services, the site can be used in both English and Spanish.

1988 Healthlink USA
                                    www.healthlinkusa.com
Health information concerning treatment, cures, prevention, diagnosis, risk factors, research, support groups, email lists, personal stories and much more. Updated regularly.

1989 Helios Health
                                    www.helioshealth.com
Online resource for your health information. Detailed information about specific health topics, access to expert advice from our Medical Advisory Board, and up-to-date health news.

1990 MedicineNet
                                    www.medicinenet.com
An online resource for consumers providing easy-to-read, authoritative medical and health information.

1991 Medscape
                                    www.medscape.com
Medscape offers specialists, primary care physicians, and other health professionals the Web's most robust and integrated medical information and educational tools.

1992 National Brain Tumor Foundation
                                    www.braintumor.org
Nonprofit health organization which raises funds for research and provides information and support to patients, their family members and friends and health professionals. Sponsors national and regional conferences, patient and caregiver programs, support groups, special patient programs including a teleconference series, a newsletter, a medical advice nurse and a wide variety of patient information about treatments, tumor types and coping. Also has a web site listing patient resources.

1993   Pediatric Brain Tumor Foundation of the US

www.ride4kids.org

Goal is to create an awareness about this growing disease among children and adults so that fundraising programs may continue to expand in increased laboratory research.

1994   WebMD

www.webmd.com

Information on Brain Tumors, including articles and resources.

Description

Cancer

Cancer is a general term for more than 100 diseases characterized by abnormal or uncontrolled growth of cells. The resulting mass, or disease, can invade and destroy surrounding normal tissue. Cancer cells from the tumor can also spread (metastasize) through the blood or lymph (plasmatic fluid) to start new cancers in other parts of the body. In 2010, about 1,529,560 new cancer cases were diagnosed, and about 569,490 Americans died from their disease. Cancer is the second leading cause of death in the U.S., exceeded only by heart disease. Although these figures seem bleak, most cancers are potentially curable if detected at an early stage.

Cancer, also called a malignancy (from Latin, meaning bad), can be either a solid tumor (carcinoma), such as lung cancer, or a disorder of blood cell formation, such as leukemia.

Cancer is caused by an interplay of internal and external factors, individually or in combination. Abnormal genes can cause multiple changes that affect cell growth. Environmental factors, such as cigarette smoke, (also called a carcinogen – causing cancer) and exposure to radiation, play a role. Many cancers can be prevented by health awareness. For example, 90 percent of the over one million skin cancers that will be diagnosed this year could be drastically reduced by protection from solar rays. Lung cancer, one of the most prevalent and hazardous cancers could be drastically reduced by eliminating tobacco use. The American Cancer Society estimates that 30 percent of all cancer deaths are related to cigarette smoking.

Cancer treatment may be curative – removes the tumor in the hope that it will not reoccur, or palliative – prolongs life and minimize discomfort when a cure is not possible. A treatment program typically includes a combination of surgery, radiation therapy, and chemotherapy. Immunotherapy is the newest form of treatment and uses agents known as biologic-response modifiers (BRM), to alter the immune system in its response to malignant growth. Brief descriptions of the more common cancers follow.

Brain Cancer

Brain cancer occurs at varying rates but overall it comprises approximately 5.6 cases per 100,000 populations each year. They are most common in early or middle adult life and incidence in the elderly population is increasing. Overall incidence is about equal in males and females.

The seriousness of brain tumors is determined by their size, location, and rate of growth. While brain cancer does not normally spread to others areas, many other cancers have the propensity of spreading throughout the nervous system and producing metastatic tumors in the brain. In adults, these tumors are most commonly from cancer of the lung, breast, or skin (melanoma). Symptoms include headaches, seizures, behavior problems, changes in eating or sleeping habits, lethargy and clumsiness. See also Brain Tumors.

Breast Cancer

Breast cancer is the most common malignant tumor in women in the western hemisphere. Approximately 207,090 new cases of breast cancer in women were diagnosed in 2010. As many as one in nine women will develop breast cancer during her lifetime. Incidence of breast cancer increases under the following conditions: age; (two-thirds of cases develop after age 55); a close relative (mother, sister) with breast cancer; a previous history of breast cancer; a previous history of breast cancer; exposure to radiation. Other risk factors include not having children, early onset of menstruation, and estrogen replacement therapy.

Early detection can be lifesaving. Many breast cancers are self-diagnosed. More than 80 percent of breast cancers occur as a painless mass. Monthly breast self-examination for women of all ages is crucial. The American Cancer Society recommends that women aged 20-39 have a clinical breast examination performed every three years. Depending on the presence of known risk factors, patients should undergo mammography either yearly or every other year between 40 and 50 years, and yearly after age 50.

Warning signs that can aid women in detecting breast cancer include lumps, swelling, skin irritation, tenderness of the nipple, and dimpling of the skin. Treatments vary, depending on when the cancer is discovered and whether it has spread. Research has shown that the traditional radical mastectomy (removal of the entire breast) canoften be replaced by lumpectomy (removal of just the tumor), coupled with radiation therapy. Chemotherapy or hormonal manipulation is also prescribed in some cases. The five year survival rate for localized (not spread) breast cancer has improved in recent years from 78 percent to 97 percent.

Colon and Rectal Cancer

In western countries, colon and rectal (colorectal) cancer account for more new cases of cancer per year than any other anatomic site except the lung. The incidence begins to rise at age 40 and peaks at age 60 to 75. Incidence of colorectal cancer increases in people who eat low-fiber diets that are high in animal protein, fat, and refined carbohydrates.

Symptoms vary, depending on the location and size of the tumor. Vague signs include weight loss, reduced appetite, and general malaise. More specific signs include rectal bleeding, blood in the stool, or a change in bowel habits.

A digital rectal examination and testing the stool for the presence of blood are important screening tests. Flexible sigmoidoscopy in which the doctor inserts a thin, flexible tube into the rectum shows tumors in 60 percent of cases. A colonoscopy is performed when a tumor is believed to be higher up the colon. These procedures are used to visualize abnormalities and take tissue samples (biopsy).

Treatment consists of surgical removal of the tumor, followed by radiotherapy and/or chemotherapy.

Leukemia

Leukemia is a disorder characterized by uncontrolled growth of abnormal and immature white or red blood cells, and is divided into acute and chronic forms. Although leukemia is often thought of as a childhood disease, it strikes 10 times as many adults as children. New treatment, especially for acute leukemia in children has resulted in dramatic improvements in the 5- year survival rates. Today, the likelihood of disease remission is greater than 95 percent, with 30 percent chance of the disease reappearing.

Warning signs of leukemia are related to the disruption of the different cells in the blood: weakness and fatigue are caused by anemia (decreased red blood cells); easy bruising and hemorrhages (e.g. nosebleeds) from reduced clotting cells (platelets); and repeated infections from abnormal white cells. Generalized symptoms include weight loss and malaise.

Treatment for leukemia includes chemotherapy with a wide variety of anticancer drugs. Transfusions restore red cells and platelets, and frequent infections are treated with antibiotics. Bone marrow transplants, in which new blood cells are provided, are one of the most recent and successful advances in the treatment of this disease.

Liver Cancer

Liver cancer comprises only about 0.6 percent of all cancers diagnosed in the United States. Risk include hepatitis B infection, hepatitis C infection, and exposure to any agent that causes liver damage, including alcohol. The remaining patients have no underlying liver disorder.

Symptoms include abdominal pain, weight loss, and a mass on the upper right side of the abdomen. The outlook for patients with liver cancer is usually grim. Surgery provides the best hope, but is suitable in only a few cases. Most experts remain wary of the benefit of liver transplantation. See also Liver Disease.

Lung Cancer

Lung cancer is one of the most prevalent cancers with an estimated 170,000 new cases each year. The frequency is increasing rapidly. Originally a disease that primarily affected men older than 60, lung cancer has become the second most common cause of cancer in women.

Cigarette smoking and exposure to industrial substances, such as asbestos, are strongly linked to lung cancer. Recent research has shown that exposure to secondhand smoke increases the risk for this disease.

Warning signs of lung cancer are persistent coughing, shortness of breath, sputum streaked with blood, chest pain, and reoccurring pneumonia or bronchitis. Early detection is difficult, as symptoms do not appear until the disease is in advanced stages. Treatment includes surgical removal of the lung if the cancer has not spread (metastasized) and/or chemotherapy and radiation therapy. Survival rates depend on tumor size, location, and whether or not the disease has spread. Because lung cancer is so difficult to treat, public health efforts are focused on prevention. See also Lung Disease.

Oral Cancer

Oral cancer represents approximately 2 percent of all newly diagnosed cancers, and 1.5 percent of cancer deaths. Incidence is more than twice as high in men as in women, and is most frequently found in men over age 40. Risk factors include cigarette, pipe, and cigar smoking, as well as the use of chewing tobacco and excessive intake of alcohol.

Oral cancer symptoms include a sore that bleeds easily, or a lump, thickening, or persistent red or white patch in the mouth. Difficulties in chewing and swallowing are symptoms of progressive disease.

Oral cancer can affect any part of the mouth, and primary care physicians and dentists often detect the disease during routine check-ups. Treatment consists of surgical removal (frequently disfiguring), radiation therapy, or a combination of both.

Ovarian Cancer

Ovarian cancer develops in 1 in 70 women and accounts for 4 percent of cancers in women. Despite its low incidence, it is the cause of more deaths in women than any other female reproductive cancer. Incidence rates are highest in the industrialized nations.

Risk factors include prior history of breast cancer and not having had children. Women who become pregnant at an early age, who have early menopause, and who use oral contraceptives are at less risk.

Ovarian cancer symptoms usually do not appear until the disease is well developed. The most common sign is an enlarging abdomen from of accumulated fluid; digestive disturbance such as discomfort, gas and distention, may also occur.

Often an abdominal mass is discovered during a routine pelvic examination in women who are symptom free. Therefore, women age 18 or older, or earlier if they are sexually active should have annual check-ups. (The Pap smear detects cervical cancer, not ovarian cancer.) Once diagnosed, 78 percent of ovarian cancer patients survive longer than one year and more than 52 percent survive longer than five years. If the disease is diagnosed before it has spread to the other parts of the body, the five-year survival rate is 95 percent.

Treatment includes surgical removal, followed by varying combinations of chemotherapy. As in all cancers, early detection is the key to effective therapy.

Pancreatic Cancer

Pancreatic cancer is one of the most dangerous cancers because it is difficult to detect and responds poorly to anticancer therapy. The incidence of this tumor has been increasing during the 21st century with 43,140 cases diagnosed in 2010. Men are affected more commonly than women, and the average age of diagnosis is from 55 to 65 years.

There is an increased incidence in those who smoke, consume a fatty diet and, to a lesser extent, who are diabetics. Chronic inflammation of the pancreas, especially among alcoholics, is also a predisposing cause.

Pancreatic cancer runs a particularly silent course, with no symptoms until it has significant advanced. The overall 5- year survival rate for patients with pancreatic cancer is less than 5 percent. Surgery is the mainstay of therapy, but only is appropriate for 15 percent of patients; radiation and/or chemotherapy are often part of treatment.

Prostate Cancer

Approximately 1 in 6 men will develop prostate cancer by 85. Incidencerates are higher among blacks and increases with age.

Early prostate cancer is symptom free. Pain and difficulty urinating, are late signs of prostate cancer. More than 50 percent of patients have a nodule that can be felt by a digital examination.

The American Cancer Society recommends that beginning at age 50, the digital rectal examination and PSA (prostatespecific antigen) blood test should be performed annually to men with a life expectancy of at least 10 years, due to the slow growth of prostate cancer. African- American males, who are at a greater risk of developing prostate cancer, should start screening at age 45, as should men with a close relative (father, brother) was diagnosed with prostate cancer at a young age.

Surgery, radiation and hormones are all used to treat prostate cancer, depending on age and health of the patient and how far the disease has progressed.

Skin Cancer

There are over one million cases of skin cancer that are diagnosed each year. The vast majority of these cases, called basal cell or squamous cell cancers, appear on areas that are most exposed to the sun and are highly curable. Melanoma is the most serious skin cancer and accounts for 4 percent of cases. Diagnosis of melanomas has more than doubled since the mid-70s and is estimated now to develop in 1 of 50 Americans. Similar to the more benign skin cancers, melanoma develops as the result of excessive exposure to the sun and has a higher incidence among those who work outdoors. Persons with fair complexions are at particular risk.

The warning signs of skin cancer include a persistent skin lesion, especially those that change in the size, color or shape. Other signs include scaliness, oozing, bleeding, pain or spread of pigmentation.

Prevention plays a key role in the development of melanoma, especially avoiding the sun's ultraviolet rays between 10 a.m. and 3 p.m. Sunscreens and protective clothing should be worn by those who spend the majority of their time outside, those who easily sunburn, and all children. In addition, early detection is critical because, despite advances in treatment, including the use of biologic response modifiers, melanoma is difficult to cure.

Stomach Cancer

Stomach (or gastric) cancer is most common among those living in northern areas of the U.S., and poor African-American populations. Its incidence increases with age; more than 75 percent of patients are over 50 years of age.

Diet and infection are believed to play a role in the development of stomach cancer. It is also more common in persons with vitamin B12 deficiency (pernicious anemia). Other causes are under investigation.

Symptoms of stomach cancer are usually vague, and include indigestion, abdominal discomfort, bloating, heartburn, and weight loss.

Removal of the tumor when possible offers the only hope of cure. The prognosis is good if the tumor is limited, but most patients are not diagnosed until their disease has spread.

Testicular Cancer

Cancer of the testes accounts for approximately 1 percent of all male cancers. However, unlike most cancers, testicular cancer usually occurs in the 15 to 40 age group; with the average age at diagnosis is 32 years.

The cause of testicular cancer is uncertain, but the incidence is increased in men with cogenital crytorochidism (a failure of one or both testes to descend). Some researchers believe that getting an infection with a virus, such as mumps, may play a role.

Fortunately, testicular cancer is one of the most curable of all cancers, In order to discover it early, men must perform self examination at regular intervals to feel for local abnormal growths such as lumps or nodules. Pain in the scrotal sac can also occur, although more than 90 percent of patients have a painless, solid testicular swelling.

Treatment of testicular cancer may include surgical removal, radiation, and chemotherapy.

Urinary Tract Cancer

Urinary tract cancers comprise about 9 percent of new cancer cases each year in men and 4 percent in women. The two most common urinary tract cancers are of the bladder and kidney.

Overall, the incidence rate is three times greater among men than women, and usually occurs in patients who are 40-70 years of age. Smoking is the greatest risk factor, with smokers having twice the incidence of nonsmokers. African-Americans, those living in urban areas, and workers exposed to dye, rubber, or leather are also at higher risk.

Common symptoms of bladder cancer include microscopic or observable blood in the urine and painful, increased, and urgent urination. Pain the lower back may also be present. Bladder cancer may be treated by surgical removal of the tumor combined with chemotherapy.

Risk factors for kidney (renal) cancer are cigarette smoking (most important) and obesity in women. Symptoms are similar to those in bladder cancer and may also include weight loss, nausea, and vomiting.

Total removal of the cancerous kidney is the treatment of choice and is used in nearly 90 percent of cases; radiation therapy and chemotherapy are relatively ineffective. Biologic response modifiers are promising but must responses are limited in duration.

Uterine and Cervical Cancer

The overall incidence of cervical cancer has decreased over the past 40 years, due mainly to regular checkups and the use of the Pap smear test for early detection. Risk factors include intercourse at an early age, cigarette smoking, multiple sex partners, and history of a sexually transmitted disease. Infection with the virus that causes genital warts (HPV), is responsible for half of all cases of cervical cancer.

Warning signs include bleeding outside the normal menstrual cycle or after menopause. Cervical cancer in most patients is treated with surgery, radiation, or a combination of both. Due to a recently developed vaccine that is 100 percent effective against HPV, the rates of cervical cancer have sharply decreased.

The American Cancer Society recommends that all women who are, or have been, sexually annual Pap test and pelvic examination. After three or more consecutive satisfactory examinations with normal findings, the Pap test may be performed less frequently, after being discussed with your health care provider.

Uterine cancer has been increasing since the 1970s. Risk factors include obesity, diabetes, high blood pressure, late onset of menopause, and estrogen-only hormone replacement therapy. Symptoms for most women include some form of abnormal bleeding from the uterus. Treatment for uterine and cervical cancers include surgery, radiation therapy, hormone therapy and, occasionally, chemotherapy.

National Agencies & Associations

1995   **American Bone Marrow Donor Registry**
PO Box 8841
Mandeville, LA 70470-8841

985-626-1749
800-745-2452
Fax: 985-626-7414
e-mail: jakabmdr@bellsouth.net
www.abmdr.org

A registry of bone marrow donors. Provides information on donor searches and recruitment.

1996   **American Cancer Society**
1599 Clifton Road NE
Atlanta, GA 30329-4250

404-320-3333
800-ACS-2345
TTY: 800-228-4327
www.cancer.org

A nationwide community based voluntary health organization dedicated to eliminating cancer as a major health problem by preventing saving lives and diminishing suffering through research education advocacy and services. Provides free printed materials.
Stephen F Sener, President
J. Lenard Lichtenfeld, MD, MACP, Deputy Chief Medical Officer

1997   **American Prostate Society**
PO Box 870
Hanover, MD 21076-3117

410-859-3735
877-859-3735
Fax: 410-850-0818
e-mail: ameripros@mindspring.com
www.americanprostatesociety.com

The only organization dedicated exclusively to using existing medical capabilities to reduce death due to prostate cancer and to reduce unnecessary or ineffective prostate therapies for prostate growth.

1998   **American Society of Colon and Rectal Surgeons**
85 W Algonquin Road
Arlington Heights, IL 60005-4460

847-290-9184
Fax: 847-290-9203
e-mail: ascrs@facsrs.org
www.fascrs.org

ASCRS Represents more than 1000 board certified colon and rectal surgeons and other surgeons dedicated to advancing and promoting the science and practice of the treatment of patients with cancer and other diseases affecting the colon and related areas.
David Beck MD, President
Steven Wexner MD, President Elect

1999   **Americas Association for the Care of the Children**
P.O. Box 2154
Boulder, CO 80306-2154

303-527-2742
www.aaccchildren.net

Carries out a variety of programs to promote the health of children. Publishes educational materials on child health of interest to parents, educators and health professionals.
Laurene Philips, President
Douglas Johnson, Vice President

2000   **Association for Research of Childhood Cancer**
PO Box 251
Buffalo, NY 14225-0251

716-681-4433
e-mail: president@arocc.org
www.arocc.org

A nonprofit organization staffed by volunteers and formed in 1971 by parents who had lost children to pediatric cancer. Charter members raise funds by various projects in order to provide seed money to various pediatric research centers.
Anne O'Donnell, President

2001   **Association for the Cure of Cancer of the Prostate**
1250 4th Street
Santa Monica, CA 90401

310-570-4700
800-757-2873
Fax: 310-570-4701
e-mail: info@pcf.org
www.capcure.org

Goal is to find better treatments and a cure for recurrent prostate cancer. Pursues the mission by reaching out to individuals corpora-

tions and others to harness society's resources - both financial and human - to fight this deadly disease.
Mike Milken, Founder/Chairman
Jonathan W Simmons, President, CEO

2002 Bone Marrow Foundation
30 E End Avenue   212-838-3029
New York, NY 10128   800-365-1336
                                   Fax: 21-22- 008
                  e-mail: theBMF@BoneMarrow.org
                                cmgm.stanford.edu
Goal is to improve the quality of life for bone marrow and stem cell transplant patients and their families by providing financial aid education and emotional support.
Christina Merrill, Founder and Executive Director
Lee Kozer, Director

2003 Breast Cancer Action
55 New Montgomery Street   415-243-9301
San Francisco, CA 94105   877-2ST-OPBC
                                   Fax: 415-243-3996
                         e-mail: info@bcaction.org
                                  www.bcaction.org
Breast Cancer Action carries the voices of people affected by breast cancer to inspire and compel the changes necessary to end the breast cancer epidemic.
Joyce Bichier, Deputy Director

2004 Breast Cancer Society of Canada
118 Victoria Street N   519-336-0746
Sarnia, Ontario, N7T-6Y5   800-567-8767
                                   Fax: 519-336-5725
                             e-mail: bcsc@bcsc.ca
                                       www.bcsc.ca
Is a registered charitable organization established in 1991 in Point Edwards Ontario. Our mandate is to fund vital Canadian research into improving the detection, prevention and treatment of breast cancer as well as to ultimately find a cure and create awareness through education.
Marsha Davidson, Executive Director
Dawn Hamilton, Fundraising & Administrative Coordinator

2005 Burger King Cancer Caring Center
4117 Liberty Avenue   412-622-1212
Pittsburgh, PA 15224   Fax: 412-622-1216
                      e-mail: info@cancercaring.org
                                 www.cancercaring.org
Provides a wide variety of support services to cancer patients their families and friends including support groups, education classes, personal counseling and telephone help line.
Rebecca Whitlinger, Executive Director
Stephanie Samolovitch, MSW, LSW, Director Support Services

2006 Canadian Breast Cancer Network (CBCN)
300-331 Cooper Street   613-230-3044
Ottawa, Ontario, K2P-0G5   800-685-8820
                                   Fax: 613-230-4424
                            e-mail: cbcn@cbcn.ca
                                       www.cbcn.ca
Is a survivor-directed, national network of organizations and individuals. CBCN is a national link between all groups and individuals concerned about breast cancer, and represents the concerns of all Canadians affected by breast cancer and those at risk.
Jackie Manthorne, CEO
Chantale Lavoie, Program Coordinator

2007 Canadian Cancer Society
10 Alcorn Avenue   416-961-7223
Toronto, ON, M4V-3B1   Fax: 416-488-2872
                              e-mail: info@cancer.ca
                                       www.cancer.ca
A national community-based organization of volunteers whose mission is the eradication of cancer and the enhancement of the quality of life of people living with cancer.
Peter Goodhand, President/CEO

2008 CancerCare
Public Information Associates

275 7th Avenue   212-302-2400
New York, NY 10001   800-813-4673
                                   Fax: 212-712-8495
                          e-mail: info@cancercare.org
                                   www.cancercare.org
National nonprofit organization that provides free, professional support services for anyone affected by a cancer diagnosis.
Helen H Miller LCSW, Executive Director

2009 Candlelighters Childhood Cancer Foundation
10400 Connecticut Avenue   301-962-3520
Kensington, MD 20895   800-366-2223
                                   Fax: 301-962-3521
                             e-mail: staff@acco.org
                                 www.candlelighters.org
Founded by parents of children with cancer. Candlelighters helps families of pediatric and adolescent cancer patients cope with the educational and emotional needs of the disease. The organization is the largest distributor of free childhood cancer books and other materials.
Ruth Hoffman MPH, Executive Director
Amber Masso, Program Director

2010 Colon Cancer Canada
5915 Leslie Street   416-785-0449
Toronto, On, M2H-1J8   888-571-8547
                                   Fax: 416-785-0450
                   e-mail: info@coloncancercanada.ca
                              www.coloncancercanada.ca
Raise public awareness for this deadly disease and to raise money for vital research.
Bunnie Schwartz, Co-Founder & President
Leah Archambault, Executive Officer Coordinator

2011 Colorectal Cancer Association of Canada
5 Place Ville Marie   514-875-7745
Montreal, QC, H3B-2G2   Fax: 514-875-7746
                          e-mail: admin@ccac-accc.ca
                                   www.ccac-accc.ca
Non-profit organization dedicated to improving the quality of life of patients and increasing awareness of the disease.
Barry D Stein, President
Heidi Watts, Program Director

2012 ENCORE YWCA-National Board
YWCA-National Board
726 Broadway   212-614-2827
New York, NY 10003-9502   800-953-7587
The YWCA's discussion and exercise program for women who have had breast cancer surgery. Designed to restore physical strength and emotional well-being.

2013 Foundation for Dignity
37 S 20th Street   215-567-2828
Philadelphia, PA 19103
Offers counseling and seminars concerning the employment rights of cancer patients and for human services workers. The society offers an extensive list of publications dealing with all aspects of cancer prevention and care.
Barbara Hoffman, Staff Attorney

2014 International Association of Laryngectomees
American Cancer Society
Box 691060   757-888-0324
Stockton, CA 95269-1060   866-425-3678
                                   Fax: 209-472-0516
                      e-mail: ialhq@larynxlink.com
                                       www.theial.com
Consists of local clubs worldwide that provides services and information to patients who have undergone laryngectomies and their families. Members are given information on first aid, postoperative care, rehabilitation, esophageal speech and other speech alternatives. Directories of speech instructors and self-care supplies for the surgical site are distributed.
Jack Henslee, Executive Director

2015 International Society for Dermatologic Surgery
Rosenparkklinik GmbH   212-213-5439
Germany,   e-mail: info@isdsworld.org
                                   www.isdsworld.com

Goals of this organization are to promote high standards of patient care, provide continuing education and research in dermatologic surgery and encourage public interest in this field.
C. William Hanke MD, Executive Director

2016   Leukemia and Lymphoma Society
1311 Mamaroneck Avenue   914-949-5213
White Plains, NY 10605   800-955-4572
                                     Fax: 914-949-6691
                                          www.lls.org
The Leukemia and Lymphoma Society is the world's largest voluntary health organization dedicated to funding blood cancer research education and patient services.
John Walter, President & CEO

2017   Make Today Count
1235 E Cherokee   417-885-3324
Springfield, MO 65804-2263   800-432-2273
                                     Fax: 417-888-7426
                                smsu.edu/nursing/community
An organization that helps patients and their families cope with cancer and other serious diseases and improve their quality of life.
Connie Zimmerman, Director

2018   National Alliance of Breast Cancer Organizations
9 E 37th Street
New York, NY 10016   888-806-2226
                                     Fax: 212-689-1213
                               e-mail: nabcoinfo@aol.com
                                          www.nabco.org
A network of breast cancer organizations that provides information assistance and referral to anyone with questions about breast cancer and acts as a voice for the interests and concerns of breast cancer survivors and women at risk.

2019   National Cancer Institute
6116 Executive Boulevard
Bethesda, MD 20892-8322   800-422-6237
                          e-mail: cancergovstaff@mail.nih.gov
                                          www.cancer.gov
One of the largest organizations dealing solely with cancer in its many forms. Offers educational information public awareness research grants and more for patients their families and health care professionals. Information specialists answer cancer-related questions by phone, LiveHelp instant messaging, and e-mail.
Deborah Pearson RN MPH, Chief Public Inquiries Office

2020   National Cancer Institute of Canada
10 Alcorn Avenue   416-961-7223
Toronto, Ontario, M4V-3B1   Fax: 416-961-4189
                               e-mail: research@cancer.ca
                                        www.ncic.cancer.ca
Was formed through a joint initiative of the Department of National Health and Welfare and the Canadian Cancer Society.
Dr Elizabeth Eisenhauer, President

2021   National Coalition for Cancer Survivorship
1010 Wayne Avenue   301-650-9127
Silver Spring, MD 20910   888-650-9127
                                     Fax: 301-565-9670
                           e-mail: info@canceradvocacy.org
                                      www.canceradvocacy.org
Survivor led advocacy organization working exclusively on behalf of people with all types of cancer and their families. Dedicated to assuring quality and care for all Americans.
Thomas P Sellers, President/CEO

2022   National Foundation for Cancer Research
4600 EW Highway   301-654-1250
Bethesda, MD 20814   800-321-2873
                                     Fax: 301-654-5824
                                e-mail: info@nfcr.org
                                          www.nfcr.org
Contracts with major universities for basic science cancer research in the fields of biophysics, theoretical physics and biochemistry.
William Potter, President
David M Sotsky, Director

2023   National Hospice & Palliative Care Organization (NHPCO)
1731 King Street   703-837-1500
Alexandria, VA 22314   800-658-8898
                                     Fax: 703-837-1233
                              e-mail: nhpcoinfo@nhpco.org
                                          www.nhpco.org
The nation's only advocate for terminally ill patients and their families. Founded in 1978, the NHPCO is the only organization devoted to hospice in the United States. Support is included from state hospice organizations, patients, families, communities, provider program members and professional/volunteer members. Represents hospice care interests to Congress, regulatory agencies, courts, voluntary organizations and the public.
Donald Schumacher, PsyD, President/CEO

2024   National Hospice & Palliative Care Org.
1731 King Street   703-837-1500
Alexandria, VA 22314   800-658-8898
                                     Fax: 703-837-1233
                             e-mail: nhpco_info@nhpco.org
                                          www.nhpco.org
The nation's only advocate for terminally ill patients and their families. Founded in 1978, the NHPCO is the only organization devoted to hospice in the United States. Support is included from state hospice organizations, patients, families and communities.
Donald Schum PsyD, President/CEO
Galen Miller PhD, Executive Vice President

2025   National Institute on Aging Information Center
31 Center Drive MSC 2292   301-496-1752
Bethesda, MD 20892   800-222-2225
                                     Fax: 301-496-1072
                                     TTY: 800-222-4225
                                        www.nih.gov/nia
Concerned with the health problems of older Americans. The Center offers free printed materials including fact sheets about going to the hospital and about prostate problems.
Richard J Hodes MD, Director

2026   National Kidney and Urologic Diseases Information Clearinghouse
31 Center Drive,MSC 2560   301-496-3583
Bethesda, MD 20892-2560   800-891-5390
                                     Fax: 301-907-8906
                          e-mail: nkudic@info.niddk.nih.gov
                                          www.niddk.nih.gov
A service of the Federal Government's National Institute for Diabetes and Digestive and Kidney Diseases. Offers free information about benign prostate enlargement and other non-cancerous urinary tract problems.
Griffin P Rodgers, Director

2027   National Marrow Donor Program
3001 Broadway Street NE   612-627-5800
Minneapolis, MN 55413-1763   800-627-7692
                                          www.marrow.org
Created to improve the effectiveness of the search for bone marrow donors so that a greater number of bone marrow transplants can be carried out.
Jeffrey W Chell MD, CEO
Patricia A Coppo MS, COO

2028   National Ovarian Cancer Coalition
2501 Oak Lawn Avenue   214-273-4200
Dallas, TX 75219   888-OVA-RIAN
                                     Fax: 561-393-7275
                              e-mail: NOCC@ovarian.org
                                          www.ovarian.org
Our mission is to raise awareness about ovarian cancer and to promote education about this disease. By dispelling myths and misunderstandings the coalition is committed to improve the overall survival rate and quality of life for women with ovarian cancer.
Elizabeth Isham Cory, President

2029   New Brunswick Innovation Foundation
440 King Street, Suite 602   506-452-2884
Fredericton, NB, E3B-5H8   877-554-6668
                                     Fax: 506-452-2886
                                e-mail: info@nbif.ca
                                          www.nbif.ca

An independent corporation, has the mission to contribute to building the province's innovation capacity.
Alfred W Lacey, President/CEO

2030 Rethink Breast Cancer
215 Spadina Avenue   416-920-0980
Toronto, Ontario, M5T-2C7   Fax: 416-920-5798
e-mail: hello@rethinkbreastcancer.com
www.rethinkbreastcancer.com
Is a charity helping young people who are concerned about and affected by breast cancer through innovative breast cancer education, research and support programs.
MJ DeCoteau MA, Executive Director

2031 Skin Cancer Foundation
149 Madison Avenue   212-725-5176
New York, NY 10016-8728   800-754-6490
Fax: 212-725-5751
e-mail: info@skincancer.org
www.skincancer.org
Conducts public and medical education programs to help reduce skin cancer. Major goals are to increase public awareness of the importance of taking protective measures against the damaging rays of the sun and to teach people how to recognize the early signs.
Perry Robins MD, President

2032 Support for People with Oral and Head and Neck Cancer
PO Box 53   516-759-5333
Locust Valley, NY 11560-0053   800-377-0928
Fax: 516-671-8794
e-mail: info@spohnc.org
www.spohnc.org
Nonprofit organization founded in 1991 to address the broad emotional physical and humanistic needs of oral and head and neck cancer patients.
Nancy E Leupold, President/Founder

2033 Y-ME National Breast Cancer Organization
135 S LaSalle Street   312-986-8338
Chicago, IL 60603   800-221-2141
Fax: 312-294-8597
e-mail: askyme@y-me.org
www.y-me.org
Provides support information and education to anyone touched by breast cancer. Support and information are available 24 hours through the National Breast Cancer Hotline which is staffed by breast cancer survivors who are trained peer counselors.
Cindy Geoghegan, CEO

State Agencies & Associations

Alabama

2034 American Cancer Society: Alabama
1100 Ireland Way   205-879-2242
Birmingham, AL 35205   Fax: 205-930-8895
e-mail: scarlet.thompson@cancer.org
www.cancer.org/docroot/com/com_0.asp
The American Cancer Society is the nationwide community-based voluntary health organization dedicated to eliminating cancer as a major health problem by preventing cancer, saving lives and diminishing suffering from cancer, through research and education.
Scarlet Thom (205-930-8889), Media/Public Relations Alabama

2035 Leukemia and Lymphoma Society: Alabama Chapter
Leukemia Society of America
100 Chase Park S   205-989-0098
Birmingham, AL 35244   888-560-9700
Fax: 205-989-0099
www.leukemia-lymphoma.org
Dedicated to finding cures for leukemia and related cancers and to improving the quality of life for patients and their families.
Valerie Hunton, Executive Director

Alaska

2036 American Cancer Society: Alaska
3851 Piper Street   907-277-8696
Anchorage, AK 99508   Fax: 907-263-2073
e-mail: leslie.jones@cancer.org
www.cancer.org
The American Cancer Society is the nationwide community-based voluntary health organization dedicated to eliminating cancer as a major health problem by preventing cancer saving lives and diminishing suffering from cancer through research and education.
Leslie Jones (251-414-1303), Media/Public Relations Alaska

Arizona

2037 American Cancer Society: Arizona
4212 N 16th Street   602-224-0524
Phoenix, AZ 85016   800-227-2345
Fax: 602-778-7699
e-mail: meg.kondrich@cancer.org
www.cancer.org
The American Cancer Society is the nationwide community-based voluntary health organization dedicated to eliminating cancer as a major health problem by preventing cancer saving lives, and diminishing suffering from cancer through research and education.
Meg Kondrich (602-381-3092), Media/Public Relations Arizona

2038 International Holistic Center
PO Box 15103   928-771-2826
Phoenix, AZ 85060-5103   e-mail: ihcinc@cox.net
www.holisticresources.org
Provides information and referrals concerning holistic health care in Arizona and beyond.
Stan Kalson, Director

2039 Leukemia and Lymphoma Society: Mountain States Chapter
Leukemia Society of America
3877 N 7th Street   602-567-7600
Phoenix, AZ 85014   800-568-1372
Fax: 602-567-7601
www.leukemia-lymphoma.org
Dedicated to finding cures for leukemia and related cancers and to improving the quality of life for patients and their families. Serves New Mexico and the Greater El Paso, TX area.
Tim Metzer, Executive Director

Arkansas

2040 American Cancer Society: Arkansas
901 N University   501-664-3480
Little Rock, AR 72207   Fax: 501-603-5223
e-mail: jodie.spears@cancer.org
www.cancer.org
The American Cancer Society is the nationwide community-based voluntary health organization dedicated to eliminating cancer as a major health problem by preventing cancer, saving lives, and diminishing suffering from cancer, through research and education.
Jodie Spears (501-603-5210), Media/Public Relations Arkansas

2041 Health Resource
933 Faulkner Street   501-329-5272
Conway, AR 72034   800-949-0090
Fax: 501-329-9489
e-mail: research@thehealthresource.com
www.thehealthresource.com
A medical information service which provides clients with an individualized, in depth research report on his or her specific health problem. Reports include latest treatment options, mainstream, experimental and alternative and top specialists.
Janice Guthrie, Director/Researcher
Shirley Effinger, Researcher

California

2042 American Cancer Society Santa Clara County / Silicon Valley / Central Coast Region
747 Camden Avenue   408-871-1062
Campbell, CA 95008   Fax: 408-871-2993
e-mail: angie.carrillo@cancer.org
www.cancer.org

The American Cancer Society is the nationwide community-based voluntary health organization dedicated to eliminating cancer as a major health problem by preventing cancer, saving lives and diminishing suffering from cancer, through research and education.
Angie Carril (408-688-0106), Media/Public Relations Silicon Valley

2043 American Cancer Society: Central Los Angeles
3333 Wilshire Boulevard   213-386-6102
Los Angeles, CA 90010   Fax: 213-480-0806
          e-mail: katherine.spangle@cancer.org
                              www.cancer.org
The American Cancer Society is the nationwide community-based voluntary health organization dedicated to eliminating cancer as a major health problem by preventing cancer, saving lives, and diminishing suffering from cancer, through research and education.
Katie Spangl (213-736-5075), Media/Public Relations Los Angeles Area

2044 American Cancer Society: East Bay/Metro Region
1700 Webster Street   510-832-7012
Oakland, CA 94612   Fax: 510-763-8826
          e-mail: patty.guinto@cancer.org
                              www.cancer.org
The American Cancer Society is the nationwide community-based voluntary health organization dedicated to eliminating cancer as a major health problem by preventing cancer, saving lives, and diminishing suffering from cancer, through research and education.
Patty Guinto (510-452-5229), Media/Public Relations East Bay Area

2045 American Cancer Society: Fresno/Madera Counties
2222 W Shaw Avenue   559-451-0722
Fresno, CA 93711   Fax: 559-451-0744
          e-mail: erica.jones@cancer.org
                              www.cancer.org
The American Cancer Society is the nationwide community-based voluntary health organization dedicated to eliminating cancer as a major health problem by preventing cancer, saving lives, and diminishing suffering from cancer, through research and education.
Erica Jones (559-451-0163), Media/Public Relations Fresno CA

2046 American Cancer Society: Inland Empire
1240 Palmyrita Avenue   951-683-6415
Riverside, CA 92507   Fax: 951-682-6804
          e-mail: beckie.mooreflati@cancer.org
                              www.cancer.org
The American Cancer Society is the nationwide community-based voluntary health organization dedicated to eliminating cancer as a major health problem by preventing cancer, saving lives, and diminishing suffering from cancer, through research and education.
Beckie Moore Flati 714-779-8104, Media/Public Relations Riverside Region

2047 American Cancer Society: Orange County
1940 E Deere Avenue   949-261-9446
Santa Ana, CA 92705-5718   Fax: 949-261-9419
          e-mail: jennifer.horspool@cancer.org
                              www.cancer.org
The American Cancer Society is the nationwide community-based voluntary health organization dedicated to eliminating cancer as a major health problem by preventing cancer, saving lives, and diminishing suffering from cancer, through research and education.
Jennifer Hor (949-567-0637), Media/Public Relations Orange County

2048 American Cancer Society: Sacramento County
1765 Challenge Way   916-446-7933
Sacramento, CA 95815   Fax: 916-64 -977
          e-mail: maria.robinson@cancer.org
                              www.cancer.org
The American Cancer Society is the nationwide community-based voluntary health organization dedicated to eliminating cancer as a major health problem by preventing cancer, saving lives, and diminishing suffering from cancer, through research and education.
Maria Robins (916-446-7933), Media/Public Relations Sacramento County

2049 American Cancer Society: San Diego County
2655 Camino Del Rio N   619-299-4200
San Diego, CA 92108   800-227-2345
                                 Fax: 619-296-0928
          e-mail: robin.brown@cancer.org
                              www.cancer.org
The American Cancer Society is the nationwide community-based voluntary health organization dedicated to eliminating cancer as a major health problem by preventing cancer, saving lives, and diminishing suffering from cancer, through research and education.
Robin Brown (619-682-7439), Media/Public Relations San Diego CA

2050 American Cancer Society: San Francisco County
201 Mission Street   415-394-7100
San Francisco, CA 94105   Fax: 415-495-1877
          e-mail: patty.guinto@cancer.org
                              www.cancer.org
The American Cancer Society is the nationwide community-based voluntary health organization dedicated to eliminating cancer as a major health problem by preventing cancer, saving lives and diminishing suffering from cancer, through research and education.
Patty Guinto (510-452-5229), Media/Public Relations San Francisco

2051 American Cancer Society: Santa Maria Valley
426 E Barcellus   805-922-2354
Santa Maria, CA 93454   Fax: 805-925-1424
          e-mail: jeb.baird@cancer.org
                              www.cancer.org
The American Cancer Society is the nationwide community-based voluntary health organization dedicated to eliminating cancer as a major health problem by preventing cancer, saving lives and diminishing suffering from cancer, through research and education.
Jeb Baird (805-560-6819), Media/Public Relations Santa Maria

2052 American Cancer Society: Sonoma County
1451 Guerneville Road   707-545-6720
Santa Rosa, CA 95403   Fax: 707-545-3179
          e-mail: angie.carrillo@cancer.org
                              www.cancer.org
The American Cancer Society is the nationwide community-based voluntary health organization dedicated to eliminating cancer as a major health problem by preventing cancer, saving lives and diminishing suffering from cancer, through research and education.
Angie Carril (408-688-0106), Media/Public Relations Central Coast

2053 Cancer Control Society and Cancer Book House
2043 N Berendo Street   213-663-7801
Los Angeles, CA 90027   Fax: 323-663-7757
                      www.cancercontrolsociety.com
An informational organization offering books, films, videos, clinic tours and lists of patients with cancer.
Lorraine Rosenthal, Co-Founder
Frank Cousineau, President

2054 City of Hope National Medical Center Beckman Research Institute
Beckman Research Institute
1500 E Duarte Road   626-256-4673
Duarte, CA 91010   800-826-4673
          e-mail: tpogue@coh.org
                              www.cityofhope.org
City of Hope is an innovative biomedical research, treatment and educational institution dedicated to the prevention and cure of cancer and other life-threatening illness.
Stephen J Foreman, Chair

2055 Leukemia & Lymphoma Society: Orange, Riverside, And San Bernadino Counties
2020 E 1st Street   714-881-0610
Santa Ana, CA 92705   888-535-9300
                                 Fax: 714-881-0616
                      www.leukemia-lymphoma.org
Dedicated to finding cures for leukemia and related cancers and to improving the quality of life for patients and their families.

2056 Leukemia and Lymphoma Society: San Diego/Hawaii Chapter
Leukemia Society of America

155

8575 Gibbs Drive
San Diego, CA 92123
858-277-1800
888-535-9300
Fax: 858-277-1748
www.leukemia.org
Dedicated to finding cures for leukemia and related cancers and to improving the quality of life for patients and their families.
Keith Turner, Executive Director

2057 Leukemia and Lymphoma Society: Greater Sacramento Area Chapter
Leukemia Society of America
4604 Roseville Road
North Highlands, CA 95660
916-348-1793
Fax: 916-348-7864
www.leukemia.org
Dedicated to finding cures for leukemia and related cancers and to improving the quality of life for patients and their families.
Tracy Latino, Executive Director

2058 Leukemia and Lymphoma Society: Greater Los Angeles Chapter
Leukemia Society of America
6033 W Century Boulevard
Los Angeles, CA 90045
310-342-5800
Fax: 310-342-5801
www.leukemia-lymphoma.org
Dedicated to finding cures for leukemia and related cancers and to improving the quality of life for patients and their families.
Donna Lynch, Executive Director

2059 Leukemia and Lymphoma Society: Northern California Chapter
Leukemia Society of America
1390 Market Street
San Francisco, CA 94102
415-625-1100
Fax: 415-625-1155
www.leukemia.org
Dedicated to finding cures for leukemia and related cancers and to improving the quality of life for patients and their families.

2060 Leukemia and Lymphoma Society: Orange, Riverside, And San Bernadino Counties
2020 E 1st Street
Santa Ana, CA 92705
714-881-0610
888-535-9300
Fax: 714-881-0616
www.leukemia-lymphoma.org
Dedicated to finding cures for leukemia and related cancers and to improving the quality of life for patients and their families.

2061 Leukemia and Lymphoma Society: Tri-County Chapter
Leukemia Society of America
2020 E 1st Street
Santa Ana, CA 92705
714-881-0610
888-535-9300
Fax: 714-881-0616
www.leukemia-lymphoma.org
Dedicated to finding cures for leukemia and related cancers and to improving the quality of life for patients and their families.
Sam Thomas, Executive Director

2062 National Health Federation
PO Box 688
Monrovia, CA 91017
626-357-2181
Fax: 626-303-0642
e-mail: contact-us@thenhf.com
www.thenhf.com
A nonprofit consumer-oriented organization devoted to health matters. Dedicated to preserving freedom of choice in health care issues, prevention of diseases and the promotion of wellness.
Scott Tips, President
Sylvia Provenza, Vice-President

2063 Regional Cancer Foundation
1200 Gough Street
San Francisco, CA 94109
415-775-9956
Fax: 415-346-8652
e-mail: mail@regionalcancerfoundation.org
www.regionalcancerfoundation.org
This foundation offers, at no charge, a second opinion consultation to individuals diagnosed with cancer. The patient and a family member or friend meet with an interdisciplinary panel of local cancer specialists with expertise in radiation therapy, chemotherapy, and cancer treatment plans.
William Gillis, CEO
Arhur J Inerfield, Chairman

Colorado

2064 American Cancer Society: Colorado
2255 S Oneida Street
Denver, CO 80224
303-758-2030
Fax: 303-759-1615
e-mail: lynda.solomon@cancer.org
www.cancer.org
The American Cancer Society is the nationwide community-based voluntary health organization dedicated to eliminating cancer as a major health problem by preventing cancer, saving lives and diminishing suffering from cancer, through research and education.
Lynda Solomo 720-524-5470, Media/Public Relations Colorado
Joel Quevill 719-636-5101, Media/Public Relations Colorado

Connecticut

2065 American Cancer Society: Connecticut
Meriden Executive Park
Meriden, CT 06450
203-379-4700
Fax: 203-379-5060
e-mail: simone.upsey@cancer.org
www.cancer.org
The American Cancer Society is the nationwide community-based voluntary health organization dedicated to eliminating cancer as a major health problem by preventing cancer, saving lives and diminishing suffering from cancer, through research and education.
Simone Upsey (203-379-4717), Media/Public Relations NH/MS/NL Counties
Christian Me (203-563-1510), Media/Public Relations LF/FF Counties

2066 Leukemia and Lymphoma Society: Connecticut Chapter
Leukemia Society of America
300 Research Parkway
Meriden, CT 06450
203-379-0445
888-282-9465
Fax: 203-379-0451
www.leukemia.org
Founded in 1949 to help serve and educate the communities and residents who have been touched by leukemia, lymphoma, multiple myeloma and Hodgkin's disease.

2067 Leukemia and Lymphoma Society: Central Connecticut Chapter
Leukemia Society of America
300 Research Parkway
Meriden, CT 06450
203-379-0445
888-282-9465
Fax: 203-379-0451
www.leukemia.org
Founded in 1971 to help serve the residents of the counties of New Haven, New London and parts of Middlesex and Litchfield who have been touched by leukemia, lymphoma, multiple myeloma and Hodgkin's disease.

2068 Leukemia and Lymphoma Society: Fairfield County Chapter
Leukemia Society of America
25 Third Street
Stamford, CT 06905
203-967-8326
Fax: 203-325-8559
www.leukemia.org
Dedicated to finding cures for leukemia and related cancers and to improving the quality of life for patients and their families.

Delaware

2069 American Cancer Society: Delaware
92 Reads Way
New Castle, DE 19720
302-324-4427
Fax: 302-324-4233
e-mail: dawn.ward@cancer.org
www.cancer.org
The American Cancer Society is the nationwide community-based voluntary health organization dedicated to eliminating cancer as a major health problem by preventing cancer, saving lives, and diminishing suffering from cancer, through research and education.
Dawn Ward (410-933-5134), Media/Public Relations Delaware

2070 Leukemia & Lymphoma Society Leukemia Society of America
100 W 10th Street
Wilmington, DE 19801
302-661-7300
800-220-1617
Fax: 302-661-0363
www.leukemia-lymphoma.org
Our mission is to cure leukemia, lymphoma, Hodgkin's disease and myeloma and to improve the quality of life of patients and their families.

2071 Leukemia and Lymphoma Society: Delaware Chapter
Leukemia Society of America
100 W 10th Street   302-661-7300
Wilmington, DE 19801   800-220-1617
                                         Fax: 302-661-0363
                                www.leukemia-lymphoma.org
Our mission is to cure leukemia, lymphoma, Hodgkin's disease
and myeloma and to improve the quality of life of patients and their
families.

District of Columbia

2072 American Cancer Society: District of Columbia
1875 Connecticut Avenue NW   202-483-2600
Washington, DC 20009   Fax: 202-483-1174
                         e-mail: angela.collins@cancer.org
                                              www.cancer.org
The American Cancer Society is the nationwide community-based
voluntary health organization dedicated to eliminating cancer as a
major health problem by preventing cancer, saving lives, and diminishing suffering from cancer, through research and education.
*Angela Colli (202-483-2600), Media/Public Relations Washington
DC*

2073 American Institute for Cancer Research
1759 R Street NW   202-328-7744
Washington, DC 20009   800-843-8114
                                         Fax: 202-328-7226
                              e-mail: aicrweb@aicr.org
                                                www.aicr.org
Not-for-profit research and educational organization. Provides
grants for research into the causes, development, prevention and
treatment of cancer through diet and nutrition. Offers publications,
research results, conferences and various public services.

2074 Center for Science in the Public Interest
1875 Connecticut Avenue NW   202-332-9110
Washington, DC 20009   Fax: 202-265-4954
                              e-mail: cspi@cspinet.org
                                            www.cspinet.org
The nation's leading consumer group concerned with food and nutrition issues. Focuses on diseases that result from consuming too
many calories, too much fat, sodium and sugar such as cancer and
heart disease.
William Corr, Board of Directors
Tom Gegax, Board of Directors

Florida

2075 American Cancer Society: Florida
2006 W Kennedy Boulevard   813-254-3630
Tampa, FL 33606   Fax: 813-349-4431
                          e-mail: cynthia.dunlap@cancer.org
                                              www.cancer.org
The American Cancer Society is the nationwide community-based
voluntary health organization dedicated to eliminating cancer as a
major health problem by preventing cancer, saving lives, and diminishing suffering from cancer, through research and education.
C. Dunlap (941-365-2858), Media/Public Relations Tampa Region
Kristen Redd (727-546-9822), Media/Public Relations Tampa Region

2076 Leukemia & Lymphoma Society: Suncoast Chapter
3507 E Frontage Road   813-963-6461
Tampa, FL 33607   800-436-6889
                                         Fax: 813-963-1306
                                              www.leukemia.org
Serves patients with leukemia, lymphoma, multiple myeloma and
Hodgkin's disease in Charlotte, Citrus, Collier, DeSoto, Hardee,
Hernando, Hillsborough, Lee, Manatee, Pasco, Pinellas and
Sarasota counties.

2077 Leukemia and Lymphoma Society: Southern Florida Chapter
Leukemia Society of America
3325 Hollywood Boulevard   954-961-3234
Hallandale, FL 33021   Fax: 954-961-7376
                                              www.leukemia.org
Dedicated to finding cures for leukemia and related cancers and to
improving the quality of life for patients and their families.

2078 Leukemia and Lymphoma Society: Central Florida Chapter
Leukemia Society of America
3319 Maguire Boulevard   407-898-0733
Orlando, FL 32803-3720   Fax: 407-896-8645
                                              www.leukemia.org
Dedicated to finding cures for leukemia and related cancers and to
improving the quality of life for patients and their families.

2079 Leukemia and Lymphoma Society: Northern Florida Chapter
Leukemia Society of America
9143 Phillips Highway   904-538-0721
Jacksonville, FL 32256   800-868-0072
                                         Fax: 904-538-9245
                                              www.leukemia.org
Dedicated to finding cures for leukemia and related cancers and to
improving the quality of life for patients and their families.

2080 Leukemia and Lymphoma Society: Palm Beach Area Chapter
Leukemia Society of America
4360 Northlake Boulevard   561-775-9954
Palm Beach Gardens, FL 33410   888-478-8550
                                         Fax: 561-775-0930
                                              www.leukemia.org
Dedicated to finding cures for leukemia and related cancers and to
improving the quality of life for patients and their families.

2081 Leukemia and Lymphoma Society: Suncoast Chapter
Leukemia Society of America
3507 E Frontage Road   813-963-6461
Tampa, FL 33607   800-436-6889
                                         Fax: 813-963-1306
                                              www.leukemia.org
Serves patients with leukemia, lymphoma, multiple myeloma and
Hodgkin's disease in Charlotte, Citrus, Collier, DeSoto, Hardee,
Hernando, Hillsborough, Lee, Manatee, Pasco, Pinellas and
Sarasota counties.

Georgia

2082 American Cancer Society: Georgia
50 Williams Street   404-315-1123
Atlanta, GA 30303   Fax: 404-315-9348
                          e-mail: elissa.mccrary@cancer.org
                                              www.cancer.org
The American Cancer Society is the nationwide community-based
voluntary health organization dedicated to eliminating cancer as a
major health problem by preventing cancer, saving lives, and diminishing suffering from cancer, through research and education.
E. McCrary (404-949-6418), Media/Public Relations Georgia

2083 Kidscope
2045 Peachtree Road
Atlanta, GA 30309   404-892-1437
                                              www.kidscope.org
A nonprofit organization formed to help families and children
better understand the effects from cancer in a parent. The name can
also be read as Kids Cope - one of the goals being to improve the
chances that a child will successfully cope with the diagnosis.
H Elizabeth King PhD, Board Member
Carol Webb PhD, Board Member

2084 Leukemia and Lymphoma Society: Georgia Chapter
Leukemia Society of America
3715 Northside Parkway   404-720-7900
Atlanta, GA 30327   800-399-7312
                                         Fax: 404-720-7878
                                e-mail: dick.brown@lls.org
                                www.leukemia-lymphoma.org
Dedicated to finding cures for leukemia and related cancers and to
improving the quality of life for patients and their families.
Dick Brown, Executive Director
Maureen Quin Davidson, Director TNT

Hawaii

2085 **American Cancer Society: Hawaii**
2370 Nuuanu Avenue
Honolulu, HI 96817

808-595-7544
800-ACS-2345
Fax: 808-595-7545
TTY: 866-228-4327
e-mail: milton.hirata@cancer.org
www.cancer.org

The American Cancer Society is the nationwide community-based voluntary health organization dedicated to eliminating cancer as a major health problem by preventing cancer, saving lives, and diminishing suffering from cancer, through research and education.
Milton Hirata, Media Relations Contact - Hawaii

Idaho

2086 **American Cancer Society: Idaho**
2676 Vista Avenue
Boise, ID 83705

208-345-2184
800-ACS-2345
Fax: 208-343-9922
TTY: 866-228-4327
e-mail: jim.ryan@cancer.org
www.cancer.org

The American Cancer Society is the nationwide community-based voluntary health organization dedicated to eliminating cancer as a major health problem by preventing cancer, saving lives, and diminishing suffering from cancer, through research and education.
Jim Ryan, Media Relations Contact - Idaho

Illinois

2087 **American Cancer Society: Illinois**
225 N Michigan Avenue
Chicago, IL 60601

312-372-0471
800-ACS-2345
Fax: 312-372-0910
TTY: 866-228-4327
e-mail: melissa.leeb@cancer.org
www.cancer.org

The American Cancer Society is the nationwide community-based voluntary health organization dedicated to eliminating cancer as a major health problem by preventing cancer, saving lives, and diminishing suffering from cancer, through research and education.
Melissa Leeb, Media Relations Contact - Illinois

2088 **Leukemia and Lymphoma Society: Illinois Chapter**
Leukemia Society of America
651 W Washington Boulevard
Chicago, IL 60661

312-651-7350
800-742-6595
Fax: 312-463-0980
e-mail: pam.swenk@lls.org
www.leukemia.org

Dedicated to finding cures for leukemia and related cancers and to improving the quality of life for patients and their families.
Pam Swenk, Executive Director
Jennifer Hufnagel, Director Donor Development

Indiana

2089 **American Cancer Society: Indiana**
5635 W 96th Street
Indianapolis, IN 46278

317-344-7800
800-ACS-2345
Fax: 317-344-7810
TTY: 866-228-4327
e-mail: leslie.smith@cancer.org
www.cancer.org

The American Cancer Society is the nationwide community-based voluntary health organization dedicated to eliminating cancer as a major health problem by preventing cancer, saving lives, and diminishing suffering from cancer, through research and education.
Leslie Smith Babione, Media Relations Contact - Indianapolis
Katie Burton (317-280-6643), Media/Public Relations Indiana

2090 **Leukemia and Lymphoma Society: Indiana Chapter**
Leukemia Society of America
941 E 86th Street
Indianapolis, IN 46240

317-726-2270
800-846-7764
Fax: 317-726-2280
e-mail: amy.kwas@lls.org
www.leukemia.org

Dedicated to finding cures for leukemia and related cancers and to improving the quality of life for patients and their families.
Amy Kwas, Executive Director
Sarah Moore, Deputy Executive Director

Iowa

2091 **American Cancer Society: Iowa**
8364 Hickman Road
Des Moines, IA 50325

515-253-0147
800-ACS-2345
Fax: 515-253-0806
TTY: 866-228-4327
e-mail: chaarles.reed@cancer.org
www.cancer.org

The American Cancer Society is the nationwide community-based voluntary health organization dedicated to eliminating cancer as a major health problem by preventing cancer, saving lives, and diminishing suffering from cancer, through research and education.
Chuck Reed, Media Relations Contact - Iowa

2092 **People Against Cancer**
604 E Street
Otho, IA 50569-0010

515-972-4444
800-662-2326
Fax: 515-972-4415
e-mail: info@PeopleAgainstCancer.net
www.peopleagainstcancer.com

A nonprofit grassroots organization whose mission is to find the best cancer therapy for people with cancer worldwide.
Frank Wiewel, Executive Director

Kansas

2093 **American Cancer Society: Kansas City**
6700 Antioch
Merriam, KS 66024

913-432-3277
800-ACS-2345
Fax: 913-432-1732
TTY: 866-228-4327
e-mail: christine.winter@cancer.org
www.cancer.org

The American Cancer Society is the nationwide community-based voluntary health organization dedicated to eliminating cancer as a major health problem by preventing cancer, saving lives, and diminishing suffering from cancer, through research and education.
Christine Winter, Media Relations Contact

2094 **Leukemia and Lymphoma Society: Mid-America Chapter**
Leukemia Society of America
6811 W 63rd Street
Shawnee Mission, KS 66202

913-262-1515
800-256-1075
Fax: 913-262-2167
e-mail: janna.lacock@lls.org
www.leukemia.org

Dedicated to finding cures for leukemia and related cancers and to improving the quality of life for patients and their families.
Janna LaCock, Executive Director
Jill Ring, Development Director

2095 **Leukemia and Lymphona Society: Kansas Chapter**
Leukemia Society of America
300 N Main
Wichita, KS 67202

316-266-4050
800-779-2417
Fax: 316-266-4960
e-mail: kelly.gerstenkorn@lls.org
www.lls.org/ks

Cure leukemia, lymphoma, Hodgkin's disease and myeloma and improve the quality of life for patients and their families.
Kelly Gerstenkorn, Executive Director

Kentucky

2096 **American Cancer Society: Kentucky**
701 W Muhammad Ali Boulevard
Louisville, KY 40203

502-584-6782
800-ACS-2345
Fax: 502-584-6767
TTY: 866-228-4327
e-mail: doug.dressman@cancer.org
www.cancer.org

The American Cancer Society is the nationwide community-based voluntary health organization dedicated to eliminating cancer as a

major health problem by preventing cancer, saving lives, and diminishing suffering from cancer, through research and education.
Doug Dressman, Executive Director-Louisville

2097 Leukemia and Lymphoma Society: Kentucky Chapter
Leukemia Society of America
600 E Main Street   502-584-8490
Louisville, KY 40202-2661   800-955-2566
                                            Fax: 502-589-5316
                              e-mail: karyl.ferman@lls.org
                                            www.leukemia.org
Founded in 1975 to serve Kentucky and Southern Indiana residents touched by leukemia and its related cancers. Goal is to find a cure for leukemia and its related cancers and to improve the quality of life for patients and their families.
Karyl D Ferman, Executive Director
Katie Anderson, Director Team in Training

Louisiana

2098 American Cancer Society: Louisiana
2605 River Road   504-469-0021
New Orleans, LA 70121   800-ACS-2345
                                            Fax: 504-219-2290
                                            TTY: 866-228-4327
                              e-mail: jewel.m.bush@cancer.org
                                            www.cancer.org
The American Cancer Society is the nationwide community-based voluntary health organization dedicated to eliminating cancer as a major health problem by preventing cancer, saving lives, and diminishing suffering from cancer, through research and education.
Jewel M Bush, Media Relations Contact

Maine

2099 American Cancer Society: Maine
1 Bowdoin Mill Island   207-373-3700
Topsham, ME 04086   800-ACS-2345
                                            Fax: 207-725-6680
                                            TTY: 866-228-4327
                              e-mail: susan.clifford@cancer.org
                                            www.cancer.org
The American Cancer Society is the nationwide community-based voluntary health organization dedicated to eliminating cancer as a major health problem by preventing cancer, saving lives, and diminishing suffering from cancer, through research and education.
Susan Clifford, Media Relations Contact - Maine

Maryland

2100 American Cancer Society: Maryland
8219 Town Center Drive   410-931-6850
Baltimore, MD 21236   800-ACS-2345
                                            Fax: 410-931-6875
                                            TTY: 866-228-4327
                              e-mail: dawn.ward@cancer.org
                                            www.cancer.org
The American Cancer Society is the nationwide community-based voluntary health organization dedicated to eliminating cancer as a major health problem by preventing cancer, saving lives, and diminishing suffering from cancer, through research and education.
Dawn Ward, Media Relations Contact - Baltimore Area

2101 Leukemia and Lymphoma Society: Maryland Chapter
Leukemia Society of America
11350 McCormick Road   410-527-0220
Hunt Valley, MD 21031-2001   800-242-4572
                                            Fax: 410-527-0510
                              e-mail: sharon.yateman@lls.org
                                            www.leukemia.org
Dedicated to finding cures for leukemia and related cancers and to improving the quality of life for patients and their families.
Sharon E Yateman MSW LCSW, Executive Director
Allyson Yospe, Deputy Executive Director

2102 Rose Kushner Breast Cancer Advisory Center
PO Box 757   301-897-3445
Malaga Cove, CA 90274   Fax: 301-897-3444
                              e-mail: lkkushner@yahoo.com
                                            www.rkbcac.org

Provides a mail service offering referrals to health professionals as well as information about detection, diagnosis, treatment and physical and psychological rehabilitation for patients with breast cancer.

Massachusetts

2103 American Cancer Society: Boston
18 Tremont Street   617-556-7400
Boston, MA 02108   800-ACS-2345
                                            Fax: 617-263-6825
                                            TTY: 866-228-4327
                              e-mail: kate.langstone@cancer.org
                                            www.cancer.org
The American Cancer Society is the nationwide community-based voluntary health organization dedicated to eliminating cancer as a major health problem by preventing cancer, saving lives, and diminishing suffering from cancer, through research and education.
Kate Langstone, Media Relations Contact - Boston Area

2104 American Cancer Society: Central New England Region-Weston MA
9 Riverside Road   781-894-6633
Weston, MA 02493   800-ACS-2345
                                            Fax: 781-314-2699
                                            TTY: 866-228-4327
                              e-mail: jessica.saporetti@cancer.org
                                            www.cancer.org
The American Cancer Society is the nationwide community-based voluntary health organization dedicated to eliminating cancer as a major health problem by preventing cancer, saving lives, and diminishing suffering from cancer, through research and education.
Jessica Saporetti, Media Relations Contact

Michigan

2105 Leukemia and Lymphoma Society: Michigan Chapter
1421 E 12 Mile Road   248-581-3900
Madison Heights, MI 48071   800-456-5413
                                            Fax: 248-581-3901
                              e-mail: peggy.shriver@lls.org
                                            www.leukemia.org

Peggy Shriver, Executive Director
Robin R Rhea, Director Operations

Minnesota

2106 American Cancer Society: Duluth
130 W Superior Street   218-727-7439
Duluth, MN 55802   800-ACS-2345
                                            Fax: 218-727-8069
                                            TTY: 866-228-4327
                              e-mail: janis.rannow@cancer.org
                                            www.cancer.org
The American Cancer Society is the nationwide community-based voluntary health organization dedicated to eliminating cancer as a major health problem by preventing cancer, saving lives, and diminishing suffering from cancer, through research and education.
Janis Rannow, Media Relations Contact

2107 American Cancer Society: Mendota Heights Mendota Heights
Mendota Heights
2520 Pilot Knob Road   651-255-8100
Mendota Heights, MN 55120   800-ACS-2345
                                            Fax: 651-255-8133
                                            TTY: 866-228-4327
                              e-mail: lou.harvin@cancer.org
                                            www.cancer.org
The American Cancer Society is the nationwide community-based voluntary health organization dedicated to eliminating cancer as a major health problem by preventing cancer, saving lives, and diminishing suffering from cancer, through research and education.
Lou Harvin, Media Relations Contact
Janis Rannow, Media Relations Contact

2108 American Cancer Society: Rochester
2900 43 Street NW
Rochester, MN 55901
507-287-2044
800-ACS-2345
Fax: 507-287-2178
TTY: 866-228-4327
e-mail: janis.rannow@cancer.org
www.cancer.org

The American Cancer Society is the nationwide community-based voluntary health organization dedicated to eliminating cancer as a major health problem by preventing cancer, saving lives, and diminishing suffering from cancer, through research and education.
Janis Rannow, Media Relations Contact

2109 American Cancer Society: Saint Cloud
3721 23rd Street S
Saint Cloud, MN 56301
320-255-0220
800-239-7028
Fax: 320-255-5517
TTY: 866-228-4327
e-mail: janis.rannow@cancer.org
www.cancer.org

The American Cancer Society is the nationwide community-based voluntary health organization dedicated to eliminating cancer as a major health problem by preventing cancer, saving lives, and diminishing suffering from cancer, through research and education.
Janis Rannow, Media Relations Contact

2110 Leukemia and Lymphoma Society: Minnesota Chapter
5217 Wayzata Boulevard
Golden Valley, MN 55426
763-852-3000
888-220-4440
Fax: 763-852-3001
e-mail: Murray.Schmidt@lls.org
www.leukemia.org

Murray Schmidt, Executive Director
Vickie Shaw, Deputy Executive Director

Mississippi

2111 American Cancer Society: Jackson
1380 Livingston Lane
Jackson, MS 39213
601-362-8874
800-ACS-2345
Fax: 601-362-8876
TTY: 866-228-4327
e-mail: kelly.lindsay@cancer.org
www.cancer.org

The American Cancer Society is the nationwide community-based voluntary health organization dedicated to eliminating cancer as a major health problem by preventing cancer, saving lives, and diminishing suffering from cancer, through research and education.
Kelly Lindsay, Media Relations Contact

2112 Leukemia and Lymphoma Society: Mississippi Chapter
408 Fontaine Place
Ridgeland, MS 39157
601-956-7447
877-538-5364
Fax: 601-956-6957
e-mail: Travis.Lee@lls.org
www.leukemia.org

Travis Lee, Campaign Director Team in Training
Natalie Michael, Campaign Director Team in Training

Missouri

2113 American Cancer Society: Saint Louis
4207 Lindell Boulevard
Saint Louis, MO 63108
314-286-8100
800-ACS-2345
Fax: 314-286-8160
TTY: 866-228-4327
e-mail: christine.winter@cancer.org
www.cancer.org

The American Cancer Society is the nationwide community-based voluntary health organization dedicated to eliminating cancer as a major health problem by preventing cancer, saving lives, and diminishing suffering from cancer, through research and education.
Christine Winter, Media Relations Contact

Montana

2114 American Cancer Society: Montana
3550 Mullan Road
Missoula, MT 59808
406-542-2191
800-ACS-2345
Fax: 406-327-0146
TTY: 866-228-4327
e-mail: jim.ryan@cancer.org
www.cancer.org

The American Cancer Society is the nationwide community-based voluntary health organization dedicated to eliminating cancer as a major health problem by preventing cancer, saving lives, and diminishing suffering from cancer, through research and education.
Jim Ryan, Media Relations Contact

Nebraska

2115 American Cancer Society: Nebraska
9850 Nicholas Street
Omaha, NE 68114
402-393-5800
800-ACS-2345
Fax: 402-393-7790
TTY: 866-228-4327
e-mail: mike.lefler@cancer.org
www.cancer.org

The American Cancer Society is the nationwide community-based voluntary health organization dedicated to eliminating cancer as a major health problem by preventing cancer, saving lives, and diminishing suffering from cancer, through research and education.
Mike Lefler, Media Relations Contact

2116 Leukemia and Lymphoma Society: Nebraska Chapter
10832 Old Mill Road
Omaha, NE 68154
402-344-2242
888-847-4974
Fax: 402-344-2422
e-mail: pattie.gorham@lls.org
www.leukemia.org

Pattie Gorham, Executive Director
Tonya Schroeder, Patient Services Manager - Portland Area

Nevada

2117 American Cancer Society: Nevada
6165 S Rainbow Boulevard
Las Vegas, NV 89118
702-798-6877
800-ACS-2345
Fax: 702-798-0530
TTY: 866-228-4327
e-mail: paulette.anderson@cancer.org
www.cancer.org

The American Cancer Society is the nationwide community-based voluntary health organization dedicated to eliminating cancer as a major health problem by preventing cancer, saving lives, and diminishing suffering from cancer, through research and education.
Paulette Anderson, Media Relations Contact

New Hampshire

2118 American Cancer Society: New Hampshire Gail Singer Memorial Building
Gail Singer Memorial Building
2 Commerce Drive
Bedford, NH 03110
603-472-8899
800-ACS-2345
Fax: 603-472-7093
TTY: 866-228-4327
e-mail: peter.davies@cancer.org
www.cancer.org

The American Cancer Society is the nationwide community-based voluntary health organization dedicated to eliminating cancer as a major health problem by preventing cancer, saving lives, and diminishing suffering from cancer, through research and education.
Peter Davies, Media Relations Contact

2119 New Hampshire Cancer Pain Initiative
125 Airport Road
Concord, NH 03301
603-225-0900
e-mail: info@nhpain.org
www.nhpain.org

Made up of concerned people who have joined together to promote the alleviation of cancer pain through education, research and advisory activities.

New Jersey

2120 American Cancer Society: New Jersey
2600 US Highway 1   732-297-8000
N Brunswick, NJ 08902   800-ACS-2345
                                 Fax: 732-297-9043
                                 TTY: 866-228-4327
                          e-mail: marjorie.kaplan@cancer.org
                                 www.cancer.org
The American Cancer Society is the nationwide community-based
voluntary health organization dedicated to eliminating cancer as a
major health problem by preventing cancer, saving lives, and diminishing suffering from cancer, through research and education.
Marjorie Kaplan, Media Relations Contact

**2121 Leukemia and Lymphoma Society: Northern New Jersey
Chapter**
Leukemia Society of America
116 South Euclid Avenue   908-654-9445
Westfield, NJ 07090   Fax: 908-654-9496
                                 www.leukemia.org
Dedicated to finding cures for leukemia and related cancers and to
improving the quality of life for patients and their families.

2122 Leukemia and Lymphoma Society: Southern New Jersey Chapter
Leukemia Society of America
216 Haddon Avenue   856-869-0200
Westmont, NJ 08108-2811   888-920-8557
                                 Fax: 856-869-7383
                                 www.leukemia.org
Dedicated to finding cures for leukemia and related cancers and to
improving the quality of life for patients and their families.

New Mexico

2123 American Cancer Society: New Mexico
10501 Montgomery Boulevard NE   505-260-2105
Albuquerque, NM 87111   800-ACS-2345
                                 Fax: 505-266-9513
                                 TTY: 866-228-4327
                          e-mail: john.weisgerber@cancer.org
                                 www.cancer.org
The American Cancer Society is the nationwide community-based
voluntary health organization dedicated to eliminating cancer as a
major health problem by preventing cancer, saving lives, and diminishing suffering from cancer, through research and education.
John Weisgerber, Media Relations Contact

2124 Leukemia and Lymphoma Society: Mountain States Chapter
Leukemia Society of America
3411 Candelaria NE   505-872-0141
Albuquerque, NM 87107   888-286-7846
                                 Fax: 505-872-2480
                                 www.leukemia.org
Dedicated to finding cures for leukemia and related cancers and to
improving the quality of life for patients and their families. Serves
New Mexico and the Greater El Paso, TX area.
Deborah Hoffman, Executive Director
Mikki Aronoff, Patient Services Manager - Portland Area

New York

**2125 American Cancer Society: Central New York Region/East
Syracuse**
6725 Lyons Street   315-437-7025
E Syracuse, NY 13057   800-ACS-2345
                                 Fax: 315-437-8233
                                 TTY: 866-228-4327
                          e-mail: kim.mcmahon@cancer.org
                                 www.cancer.org
The American Cancer Society is the nationwide community-based
voluntary health organization dedicated to eliminating cancer as a
major health problem by preventing cancer, saving lives, and diminishing suffering from cancer, through research and education.
Kim McMahon, Media Relations Contact

2126 American Cancer Society: Long Island
75 Davids Drive   631-436-7070
Hauppauge, NY 11788   800-ACS-2345
                                 Fax: 631-436-5380
                                 TTY: 866-228-4327
                          e-mail: jennifer.cucurullo@cancer.org
                                 www.cancer.org
The American Cancer Society is the nationwide community-based
voluntary health organization dedicated to eliminating cancer as a
major health problem by preventing cancer, saving lives, and diminishing suffering from cancer, through research and education.
Jennifer Cucurullo, Media Relations Contact

2127 American Cancer Society: New York City
132 W 32nd Street   212-586-8700
New York, NY 10001-3983   800-ACS-2345
                                 Fax: 212-237-3855
                                 TTY: 866-228-4327
                          e-mail: jennifer.cucurullo@cancer.org
                                 www.cancer.org
The American Cancer Society is the nationwide community-based
voluntary health organization dedicated to eliminating cancer as a
major health problem by preventing cancer, saving lives, and diminishing suffering from cancer, through research and education.
Jennifer Cucurullo, Media Relations Contact

2128 American Cancer Society: Queens Region / Rego Park
97-99 Queens Boulevard   718-263-2224
Rego Park, NY 11374   800-ACS-2345
                                 Fax: 718-261-0758
                                 TTY: 866-228-4327
                          e-mail: jennifer.cucurullo@cancer.org
                                 www.cancer.org
The American Cancer Society is the nationwide community-based
voluntary health organization dedicated to eliminating cancer as a
major health problem by preventing cancer, saving lives, and diminishing suffering from cancer, through research and education.
Jennifer Cucurullo, Media Relations Contact

2129 American Cancer Society: Westchester Region/White Plains
2 Lyon Place   914-949-4800
White Plains, NY 10601   800-ACS-2345
                                 Fax: 914-397-8851
                                 TTY: 866-228-4327
                          e-mail: jennifer.cucurullo@cancer.org
                                 www.cancer.org
The American Cancer Society is the nationwide community-based
voluntary health organization dedicated to eliminating cancer as a
major health problem by preventing cancer, saving lives, and diminishing suffering from cancer, through research and education.
Jennifer Cucurullo, Media Relations Contact

2130 Foundation for Advancement in Cancer Therapy
Old Chelsea Station
New York, NY 10113   212-741-2790
                                 www.fact-ltd.org
Distributes information on cancer prevention and nontoxic thera-
pies for cancer.
Ruth Sackman, President/Co-founder

2131 Leukemia & Lymphoma Society Chapter: New York City
475 Park Avenue S   212-376-7100
New York, NY 10016   800-955-4572
                                 Fax: 212-448-9214
                          e-mail: ossom@lls.org
                                 www.leukemia-lymphoma.org
Dedicated to finding cures for leukemia and related cancers and to
improving the quality of life for patients and their families. Educational materials, support services and financial aid available. Volunteer opportunities.
Michael Osso, Executive Director
Sara Lipsky, Deputy Executive Director

**2132 Leukemia & Lymphoma Society: Westchester/ Hudson Valley
Chapter**
1311 Mamaroneck Avenue   914-949-0084
White Plains, NY 10605   Fax: 914-949-0391
                                 www.lls.org/wch

Mission is to cure leukemia, lymphoma, Hodgkin's disease and myeloma, and to improve the quality of life of patients and their families.
Dennis P Chillemi, Executive Director
Diandra Kodl, Deputy Executive Director

2133 Leukemia and Lymphoma Society Chapter: New York City
475 Park Avenue S
New York, NY 10016
212-376-7100
800-955-4572
Fax: 212-448-9214
e-mail: ossom@lls.org
www.leukemia-lymphoma.org
Dedicated to finding cures for leukemia and related cancers and to improving the quality of life for patients and their families. Educational materials, support services and financial aid available. Volunteer opportunities.
Michael Osso, Executive Director
Sara Lipsky, Deputy Executive Director

2134 Leukemia and Lymphoma Society: Central New York Chapter
Leukemia Society of America
401 N Salina Street
Syracuse, NY 13203
315-471-1050
800-690-8944
Fax: 315-471-6434
e-mail: chip.lockwood@lls.org
www.leukemia.org
Dedicated to finding cures for leukemia and related cancers and to improving the quality of life for patients and their families.
Chip Lockwood, Executive Director
Kristen Duggleby, Campaign Director Donor Relations

2135 Leukemia and Lymphoma Society: Long Island Chapter
Leukemia Society of America
555 Broadhollow Road
Melville, NY 11747
631-752-8500
Fax: 631-752-9066
e-mail: tammy.philie@lls.org
www.leukemia.org
Established to serve Long Islanders with leukemia, lymphoma, Hodgkin's disease and myeloma, their families and friends.
Tammy Philie, Executive Director
Nicole Kowaleski, Deputy Executive Director

2136 Leukemia and Lymphoma Society: Upstate New York Chapter
Leukemia Society of America
5 Computer Drive W
Albany, NY 12205
518-438-3583
866-255-3583
Fax: 518-438-6431
e-mail: Maureen.Thornton@lls.org
www.leukemia.org
Dedicated to finding cures for leukemia and related cancers and to improving the quality of life for patients and their families.
Maureen O'Brien-Thor, Executive Director
Raechel Hunt, Patient Services Manager - Portland Area

2137 Leukemia and Lymphoma Society: Western New York & Finger Lakes Chapter
Leukemia Society of America
4053 Maple Road
Amherst, NY 14226
716-834-2578
800-784-2368
Fax: 716-837-0335
e-mail: nancy.hails@lls.org
www.leukemia.org
Dedicated to finding cures for leukemia and related cancers and to improving the quality of life for patients and their families.
Nancy Hails, Executive Director
Luann Burgio, Deputy Executive Director

North Carolina

2138 American Cancer Society: North Carolina
8300 Health Park
Raleigh, NC 27615
919-334-5218
800-ACS-2345
Fax: 919-841-1422
TTY: 866-228-4327
e-mail: jbright@cancer.org
www.cancer.org
The American Cancer Society is the nationwide community-based voluntary health organization dedicated to eliminating cancer as a major health problem by preventing cancer, saving lives, and diminishing suffering from cancer, through research and education.
Jeff Bright, Media Relations Contact

2139 Leukemia and Lymphoma Society: Eastern North Carolina Chapter
Flagship Building
401 Harrison Oaks Boulevard
Cary, NC 27513
919-677-3993
800-936-9337
Fax: 919-677-3992
e-mail: tiffany.armstrong@lls.org
www.leukemia.org
Tiffany Armstrong, Executive Director
Loreal Massiah, Patient Services Manager - Portland Area

2140 Leukemia and Lymphoma Society: North Carolina Chapter
Leukemia Society of America
5950 Fairview Road
Charlotte, NC 28210
704-998-5012
800-888-9934
Fax: 704-998-5010
Dedicated to finding cures for leukemia and related cancers and to improving the quality of life for patients and their families.

2141 Leukemia and Lymphoma Society: North Texas
5950 Fairview Road
Charlotte, NC 28210
704-998-5012
Fax: 704-998-5010
e-mail: jane.weaver@lls.org
www.leukemia.org
Dedicated to finding cures for leukemia and related cancers and to improving the quality of life for patients and their families.
Jane Weaver, Executive Director
Keri Norris, Office Manager

North Dakota

2142 American Cancer Society: North Dakota
4646 Amber Valley Parkway
Fargo, ND 58104
701-232-1385
800-ACS-2345
Fax: 701-232-1109
TTY: 866-228-4327
e-mail: jim.ryan@cancer.org
www.cancer.org
The American Cancer Society is the nationwide community-based voluntary health organization dedicated to eliminating cancer as a major health problem by preventing cancer, saving lives, and diminishing suffering from cancer, through research and education.
Jim Ryan, Media Relations Contact

Ohio

2143 American Cancer Society: Ohio
870 Michigan Avenue
Columbus, OH 43215
888-227-6446
Fax: 877-227-2838
TTY: 866-228-4327
e-mail: robert.paschen@cancer.org
www.cancer.org
The American Cancer Society is the nationwide community-based voluntary health organization dedicated to eliminating cancer as a major health problem by preventing cancer, saving lives, and diminishing suffering from cancer, through research and education.
Robert Paschen, Media Relations Contact

2144 Leukemia and Lymphoma Society: Central Ohio Chapter
Leukemia Society of America
2225 City Gate Drive
Columbus, OH 43219
614-476-7194
800-686-CURE
Fax: 614-476-7189
e-mail: phil.tanner@lls.org
www.leukemia.org
Dedicated to finding cures for leukemia and related cancers and to improving the quality of life for patients and their families.
Phil Tanner, Executive Director
Dan Swisher, Office Manager

2145 Leukemia and Lymphoma Society: Northern Ohio Chapter
Leukemia Society of America

23297 Commerce Park
Cleveland, OH 44122
216-910-1200
800-589-5721
Fax: 216-910-1201
e-mail: frank.canning@lls.org
www.leukemia.org
Dedicated to finding cures for leukemia and related cancers and to improving the quality of life for patients and their families.
Frank Canning, Field Director
Nancy Toghill, Office Manager

2146 Leukemia and Lymphoma Society: Southern Ohio Chapter
Leukemia Society of America
2300 Wall Street
Cincinnati, OH 45212
513-361-2100
Fax: 513-361-2109
e-mail: michelle.steed@lls.org
www.leukemia.org
Dedicated to finding cures for leukemia and related cancers and to improving the quality of life for patients and their families. This chapter serves a 22-county geographic area.
Michelle Steed, Executive Director

Oklahoma

2147 American Cancer Society: Oklahoma
6525 N Meridian
Oklahoma City, OK 73116
405-843-9888
800-ACS-2345
Fax: 405-848-0795
TTY: 866-228-4327
e-mail: christina.lindholm@cancer.org
www.cancer.org
The American Cancer Society is the nationwide community-based voluntary health organization dedicated to eliminating cancer as a major health problem by preventing cancer, saving lives, and diminishing suffering from cancer, through research and education.
Christina Li (816-218-7171), Media/Public Relations

2148 Leukemia and Lymphoma Society: Oklahoma Chapter
Leukemia Society of America
500 N Broadway
Oklahoma City, OK 73102
405-943-8888
888-828-4572
Fax: 405-943-8355
e-mail: sherry.martin@lls.org
www.leukemia.org
Dedicated to finding cures for leukemia and related cancers and to improving the quality of life for patients and their families.
Sherry Marti MSW LCSW, Patient Services Manager - Portland Area
Jill Hull, Campaign Director Team in Training

Oregon

2149 American Cancer Society: Oregon
0330 SW Curry Street
Portland, OR 97239
503-295-6422
800-ACS-2345
Fax: 503-228-1062
TTY: 866-228-4327
e-mail: gretchen.rosenberger@cancer.org
www.cancer.org
The American Cancer Society is the nationwide community-based voluntary health organization dedicated to eliminating cancer as a major health problem by preventing cancer, saving lives, and diminishing suffering from cancer, through research and education.
Gretchen Rosenberger, Media Relations Contact

2150 Leukemia and Lymphoma Society: Oregon Chapter
Leukemia Society of America
9320 SWBarbur Boulevard
Portland, OR 97219
503-245-9866
800-466-6572
Fax: 503-245-9865
e-mail: Sarah.Varner@lls.org
www.leukemia.org
Dedicated to finding cures for leukemia and related cancers and to improving the quality of life for patients and their families.
Sarah Varner, Executive Director
Sue Sumpter, Patient Services Manager - Portland Area

Pennsylvania

2151 American Cancer Society: Harrisburg Capital Area Unit
Capital Area Unit

3211 N Front Street
Harrisburg, PA 17110
215-985-5336
888-227-5445
Fax: 717-231-5784
TTY: 866-228-4327
e-mail: john.held@cancer.org
www.cancer.org
The American Cancer Society is the nationwide community-based voluntary health organization dedicated to eliminating cancer as a major health problem by preventing cancer, saving lives, and diminishing suffering from cancer, through research and education.
Colleen Fitz (215-985-5357), Media Relations Contact
John Held, Media Relations Contact

2152 American Cancer Society: Philadelphia
1626 Locust Street
Philadelphia, PA 19103
215-985-5336
888-227-5445
Fax: 215-985-5406
TTY: 866-228-4327
e-mail: john.held@cancer.org
www.cancer.org
The American Cancer Society is the nationwide community-based voluntary health organization dedicated to eliminating cancer as a major health problem by preventing cancer, saving lives, and diminishing suffering from cancer, through research and education.
John Held, Media Relations Contact
Colleen Fitz 215-985-5357, Media/Public Relations

2153 American Cancer Society: Pittsburgh
320 Bilmar Drive
Pittsburgh, PA 15205
215-985-5336
888-227-5445
Fax: 412-919-1101
TTY: 866-228-4327
e-mail: dcatena@cancer.org
www.cancer.org
The American Cancer Society is the nationwide community-based voluntary health organization dedicated to eliminating cancer as a major health problem by preventing cancer, saving lives, and diminishing suffering from cancer, through research and education.
Dan Catena, Media Relations Contact

2154 Leukemia and Lymphoma Society: Central Pennsylvania Chapter
800 Corporate Circle
Harrisburg, PA 17110
717-652-6520
800-822-2873
Fax: 717-652-8614
e-mail: beth.mihmet@lls.org
www.leukemia.org
Elizabeth Mihmet, Executive Director
Danielle Bubnis, Patient Services Manager

2155 Leukemia and Lymphoma Society: Eastern Pennsylvania Chapter
555 N Lane
Conshohocken, PA 19428
610-238-0360
800-482-CURE
Fax: 484-530-0833
e-mail: ursula.raczak@lls.org
www.leukemia.org
Lydia Hernandez-Vele, Executive Director
Ursula Raczak, Deputy Executive Director

2156 Leukemia and Lymphoma Society: Western Pennsylvania/West Virginia Chapter
Leukemia Society of America
333 E Carson Street
Pittsburgh, PA 15219-1439
412-395-2873
800-726-2873
Fax: 412-395-2888
e-mail: massaric@lls.org
www.leukemia.org
Tina Massari, Executive Director
Jeanne Caliguiri, Development Director

Rhode Island

2157 American Cancer Society: Rhode Island
931 Jefferson Boulevard
Warwick, RI 02886
401-722-8480
800-ACS-2345
Fax: 401-421-0535
TTY: 866-228-4327
e-mail: jim.beardsworth@cancer.org
www.cancer.org

The American Cancer Society is the nationwide community-based voluntary health organization dedicated to eliminating cancer as a major health problem by preventing cancer, saving lives, and diminishing suffering from cancer, through research and education.
Jim Beardsworth, Media Relations Contact

2158 Leukemia and Lymphoma Society: Rhode Island Chapter
1150 Pontiac Avenue   401-943-8888
Cranston, RI 02920   Fax: 401-943-1377
e-mail: koconisb@lls.org
www.leukemia.org

Bill Koconis, Executive Director
Gloria Hincapie, Patient Services Manager

South Carolina

2159 American Cancer Society: South Carolina
128 Stonemark Lane   803-750-1693
Columbia, SC 29210   800-ACS-2345
Fax: 803-750-4000
TTY: 866-228-4327
e-mail: mjwardle@cancer.org
www.cancer.org
The American Cancer Society is the nationwide community-based voluntary health organization dedicated to eliminating cancer as a major health problem by preventing cancer, saving lives, and diminishing suffering from cancer, through research and education.
Mary Jane Wardle, Media Relations Contact

2160 Leukemia and Lymphoma Society: South Carolina Chapter
1247 Lake Murray Boulevard   803-749-4299
Irmo, SC 29063   Fax: 803-749-4088
www.leukemia.org

2161 Leukemia and Lymphoma Society: South/West
107 Westpark Boulevard   803-731-4060
Columbia, SC 29210   Fax: 803-731-4066
e-mail: paul.jeter@lls.org
www.leukemia.org

Paul Jeter, Executive Director
Cassandra Wineglass, Patient Services Manager

South Dakota

2162 American Cancer Society: South Dakota
4904 S Technopolis Drive   605-361-8277
Sioux Falls, SD 57106   800-ACS-2345
Fax: 605-361-8537
TTY: 866-228-4327
e-mail: charlotte.hofer@cancer.org
www.cancer.org
The American Cancer Society is the nationwide community-based voluntary health organization dedicated to eliminating cancer as a major health problem by preventing cancer, saving lives, and diminishing suffering from cancer, through research and education.
Charlotte Ho (605-376-3758), Media Relations Contact

Tennessee

2163 American Cancer Society: Tennessee
2000 Charlotte Avenue   615-327-0991
Nashville, TN 37203   800-ACS-2345
Fax: 615-341-7335
TTY: 866-228-4327
e-mail: brian.gillespie@cancer.org
www.cancer.org
The American Cancer Society is the nationwide community-based voluntary health organization dedicated to eliminating cancer as a major health problem by preventing cancer, saving lives, and diminishing suffering from cancer, through research and education.
Brian Gillespie, Media Relations Contact

2164 Leukemia & Lymphoma Society: Tennessee Chapter
404 BNA Drive   615-331-2980
Nashville, TN 37217   800-332-2980
Fax: 615-331-2941
e-mail: winslowm@tn.leukemia-lymphoma.org
www.leukemia-lymphoma.org
Founded in 1982 to better serve the needs of Tennesseans. Offers contribution funded community services, family support groups,

free educational materials and financial assistance for those affected by leukemia, Hodgkin's disease, myeloma and lymphomas.
Colleen Grady, Executive Director
Mary Winslow, Patient Services Manager

Texas

2165 American Cancer Society: Texas
2433 Ridgepoint Drive   512-919-1800
Austin, TX 78754   800-ACS-2345
Fax: 512-919-1846
TTY: 866-228-4327
e-mail: justine.hall@cancer.org
www.cancer.org
The American Cancer Society is the nationwide community-based voluntary health organization dedicated to eliminating cancer as a major health problem by preventing cancer, saving lives, and diminishing suffering from cancer, through research and education.
Justin Hall, Media Relations Contact

2166 Leukemia and Lymphoma Society: North Texas Chapter
Leukemia Society of America
8111 LBJ Freeway   972-239-0959
Dallas, TX 75251   800-800-6702
Fax: 972-239-0892
e-mail: Tina.Garcia@lls.org
www.leukemia.org
Dedicated to finding cures for leukemia and related cancers and to improving the quality of life for patients and their families.
Tina Garcia, Executive Director
Sarah Bayley, Donor Development Director

2167 Leukemia and Lymphoma Society: South/West Texas Chapter
Leukemia Society of America
431 Isom Road   210-377-1775
San Antonio, TX 78216-4170   800-683-2458
Fax: 210-344-3717
www.leukemia.org
Dedicated to finding cures for leukemia and related cancers and to improving the quality of life for patients and their families.
Jon Walter, President/CEO
Jimmy Nangle, CFO

2168 Leukemia and Lymphoma Society: Texas Gulf Coast Chapter
Leukemia Society of America
5005 Mitchelldale   713-680-8088
Houston, TX 77092   Fax: 713-683-9504
e-mail: BillieSue.Parris@lls.org
www.leukemia.org
Dedicated to finding cures for leukemia and related cancers and to improving the quality of life for patients and their families.
Billie Sue Parris, Executive Director
Jane Thompson, Office Manager

Utah

2169 American Cancer Society: Utah
941 E 3300 S   801-483-1500
Salt Lake City, UT 84106   800-ACS-2345
Fax: 801-483-1558
TTY: 866-228-4327
e-mail: patricia.monsoor@cancer.org
www.cancer.org
The American Cancer Society is the nationwide community-based voluntary health organization dedicated to eliminating cancer as a major health problem by preventing cancer, saving lives, and diminishing suffering from cancer, through research and education.
Patricia Monsoor, Media Relations Contact

Vermont

2170 American Cancer Society: Vermont
121 Connor Way   802-872-6300
Williston, VT 05495   800-ACS-2345
Fax: 802-872-6399
TTY: 866-228-4327
e-mail: chris.falk@cancer.org
www.cancer.org
The American Cancer Society is the nationwide community-based voluntary health organization dedicated to eliminating cancer as a

major health problem by preventing cancer, saving lives, and diminishing suffering from cancer, through research and education.
Chris Falk, Media Relations Contact

Virginia

2171 American Cancer Society: Virginia
4240 Park Place Court   804-527-3700
Glen Allen, VA 23060   800-ACS-2345
                                       Fax: 804-527-3797
                                       TTY: 866-228-4327
e-mail: domenick.casuccio@cancer.org
                                       www.cancer.org
The American Cancer Society is the nationwide community-based voluntary health organization dedicated to eliminating cancer as a major health problem by preventing cancer, saving lives, and diminishing suffering from cancer, through research and education.
Domenick Casuccio, Media Relations Contact

2172 Arlin J Brown Information Center
PO Box 251
Fort Belvoir, VA 22060-0251   540-752-9511
An information clearinghouse on types of cancer health methods and nontoxic cancer therapies.

2173 Leukemia and Lymophoma Society: National Capital Area Chapter
Leukemia Society of America
5845 Richmond Highway   703-399-2900
Alexandria, VA 22303   Fax: 703-399-2901
e-mail: donna.mckelvey@lls.org
                                       www.leukemia.org
Serves the greater Washington DC metropolitan area including Northern Virginia Prince George's and Montgomery counties.
Donna Mckelvey, Executive Director
Beth Rather Gorman, Deputy Executive Director

Washington

2174 American Cancer Society: Washington
728 134th Street SW   425-741-8949
Everett, WA 98204   Fax: 425-741-9638
e-mail: liz.lamb-ferro@cancer.org
                                       www.cancer.org
The American Cancer Society is the nationwide community-based voluntary health organization dedicated to eliminating cancer as a major health problem by preventing cancer, saving lives, and diminishing suffering from cancer, through research and education.
Liz Lamb-Ferro, Media Relations Contact

2175 CanHelp
PO Box 1678
Livingston, NJ 07039   800-364-2341
                                       Fax: 888-800-0201
e-mail: joan@canhelp.com
                                       www.canhelp.com
Offers reports for cancer patients on orthodox and alternative therapies and coaching/counseling to help with treatment decision-making and coping.
Patrick M McGrady, Founder
Joan Runfola LCSW, Director

2176 Washington Leukemia and Lymphoma Society: Alaska Chapter
Leukemia Society of America
530 Dexter Avenue N   206-628-0777
Seattle, WA 98109   888-345-4572
                                       Fax: 206-292-9791
e-mail: wachapter@lls.org
                                       www.leukemia-lymphoma.org
Dedicated to finding cures for leukemia and related cancers and to improving the quality of life for patients and their families.
Anne Gillingham, Executive Director
Kimberly Conn, Deputy Executive Director

West Virginia

2177 American Cancer Society: West Virginia
301 RHL Boulevard   304-746-9950
Charleston, WV 25309   800-ACS-2345
                                       Fax: 304-746-9962
                                       TTY: 866-228-4327
e-mail: amy.wentz@cancer.org
                                       www.cancer.org
The American Cancer Society is the nationwide community-based voluntary health organization dedicated to eliminating cancer as a major health problem by preventing cancer, saving lives, and diminishing suffering from cancer, through research and education.
Amy Wentz Berner, Media Relations Contact

Wisconsin

2178 American Cancer Society: Wisconsin
N19 W24350 Riverwood Drive   262-523-5500
Waukesha, WI 53188   800-ACS-2345
                                       Fax: 262-523-5533
                                       TTY: 866-228-4327
e-mail: peter.balistrieri@cancer.org
                                       www.cancer.org
The American Cancer Society is the nationwide community-based voluntary health organization dedicated to eliminating cancer as a major health problem by preventing cancer, saving lives, and diminishing suffering from cancer, through research and education.
Peter Balistrieri, Media Relations Contact

2179 Leukemia and Lymphoma Society: Wisconsin Chapter
Leukemia Society of America
200 S Executive Drive   262-790-4701
Brookfield, WI 53005   800-261-7399
                                       Fax: 262-790-4706
e-mail: bede.barthpotter@lls.org
                                       www.leukemia.org
Founded in 1963 to serve Wisconsites touched by leukemia, lymphoma, Hodgkin's disease and myeloma.
Bede Barth Potter, Executive Director
Karen Ropel, Deputy Executive Director

Wyoming

2180 American Cancer Society: Wyoming
333 S Beech Street   307-577-4892
Casper, WY 82601   800-ACS-2345
                                       Fax: 307-234-0926
                                       TTY: 866-228-4327
e-mail: joel.quevillon@cancer.org
                                       www.cancer.org
The American Cancer Society is the nationwide community-based voluntary health organization dedicated to eliminating cancer as a major health problem by preventing cancer, saving lives, and diminishing suffering from cancer, through research and education.
Joel Quevillon, Media Relations Contact

Foundations

2181 Chemotherapy Foundation
183 Madison Avenue   212-213-9292
New York, NY 10016   Fax: 212-133-31
                                       www.chemotheraphyfoundation.org
The Chemotherapy Foundation is dedicated to developing more effective methods of treatment for the control and cure of cancer. They provide educational materials and provide funds for innovative chemotherapy research, and sponsor professional and public educational symposia.
Shirley Cox, Executive Director

2182 Dermatology Foundation
1560 Sherman Avenue   847-328-2256
Evanston, IL 60201-4808   Fax: 847-328-0509
e-mail: dfgen@dermatologyfoundation.org
                                       www.dermfnd.org

The Foundation focuses on funding research that will advance patient care, and help develop and retain tomorrow's teachers and clinical leaders in the specialty.

Sandra Rahn Benz, Executive Director

2183 National Children's Cancer Society
One South Memorial Drive   314-241-1600
Saint Louis, MO 63102   800-882-6227
                                  Fax: 314-241-1996
                         e-mail: pbeck@children-cancer.org
                                  www.children-cancer.org

Our mission is to improve the quality of life for children with cancer and their families worldwide. We serve as a financial, emotional, educational, and medical resource for those in need, at every stage of their illness and recovery. The NCCS provides direct financial assistance to families for expenses not covered by insurance during their treatment; including transportation, lodging, gas money, medical assistance, health insurance premiums, and phone cards.

Mark Slocomb, Chairman
Mark Stolze, President/CEO

Libraries & Resource Centers

2184 Cancer Federation
PO Box 1298   951-849-4325
Banning, CA 92220   Fax: 951-849-0156
                            e-mail: info@cancerfed.org
                                  www.cancerfed.com

The Federation is a not-for-profit organization that provides information, counseling, educational materials and meetings for the cancer patients, their families and friends. Also, they fund research and scholarships.

John Steinbacher, Executive Director

2185 Cancer Information Service
National Cancer Institute
6116 Executive Boulevard   301-435-3848
Bethesda, MD 20892-8322   800-422-6237
                                  TTY: 800-332-8615
                                  http://cis.nci.nih.gov/

The National Cancer Institute's Cancer Information Service is a national resource for information and education about cancer. The CIS provides the latest and most accurate cancer information to patients and their families, the public, and health professionals by talking with people one-on-one through its Telephone Service, working with organizations through its Partnership Program, participating in research efforts to find the best ways to help people.

2186 Patient Advocates for Advanced Cancer Treatments (PAACT)
PO Box 141695   616-453-1477
Grand Rapids, MI 49514-1695   Fax: 616-453-1846
                            e-mail: paact@paactusa.org
                                  www.paactusa.org

Provides support and advocacy for prostate cancer patients, their families, and the general public at risk. Information relative to the advancements in the detection, diagnosis, evaluation, and treatment of prostate cancer. Information, referrals, phone help, conferences, newsletter.

Richard H. Profit, Jr., President

Research Centers

2187 Purdue Cancer Center Purdue University
Purdue University
201 S University Street   765-494-9129
W Lafayette, IN 47907-2064   Fax: 765-494-9193
                         e-mail: cancerresearch@purdue.edu
                                  www.cancer.purdue.edu

Provide a forum for 75 of Purdue's best and brightest scientists to collaborate across campus and nationwide to prevent cancer to ease its detection and to cure it.

Timothy Ratliff, Director
Andrea Gregory-Kreps, Operations Manager

Alabama

2188 Birmingham VA Medical Center: Research and Development
700 S 19th Street   205-933-8101
Birmingham, AL 35233   866-487-4243
                                  Fax: 205-933-4484
                                  www.birmingham.va.gov

An acute tertiary care facility with particularly strong programs in both medicine and surgery andÿserves as the primary referral center for the state. We provide health care services to eligible veterans in the VA Southeast Network .

John R Gingrich, Chief of Staff
Rica Lewis-Payton, Medical Center Director

2189 Breast Cancer Resource Foundation of Alabama
PO Box 531225   205-871-4653
Birmingham, AL 35253   Fax: 205-975-2432
                    e-mail: Jennifer.Galbreath@ccc.uab.edu
                                  www.bcrfa.org

Dedicated to finding a cure for breast cancer.

Dianne Mooney, President
Jennifer Galbreath, Program Director

2190 University of Alabama At Birmingham Comprehensive Cancer Center
UAB Comprehensive Cancer Center
1802 6th Avenue S   205-934-5077
Birmingham, AL 35294-3300   800-UAB-0933
                              e-mail: info@ccc.uab.edu
                                  www3.ccc.uab.edu

The Center provides advanced cancer care research and education based on stringent peer-reviewed data.

Edward E Partridge, Director and Associate Director for Comm
Kirby I Bland, Deputy Director

Arizona

2191 Southwest Association for Education in Biomedical Research
PO Box 210101   520-621-3931
Tucson, AZ 85721-0101   Fax: 520-621-3355
                        e-mail: swaebr@ahsc.arizona.edu
                                  www.swaebr.org

The mission of the Southwest Association for Education in Biomedical Research is to develop and implement a strong proactive campaign to educate school children as well as the general public in the vital role biomedical research plays in their everyday lives.

Charles Atkinson, President

2192 University of Arizona Cancer Center
3838 N Campbell Avenue   520-694-2873
Tucson, AZ 85719-1454   800-327-2873
                                  www.azcc.arizona.edu

Comprehensive cancer center for diagnosis treatment and prevention.

David S Alberts, Director

California

2193 Burnham Institute Cancer Center The Burnham Institute for Medical Resear
The Burnham Institute for Medical Research
10901 N Torrey Pines Road   858-646-3100
La Jolla, CA 92037   Fax: 858-646-3199
                         e-mail: info@sanfordburnham.org
                                  www.burnham.org

Known for world-class capabilities in stem cell research and drug discovery technologies. Dedicated to revealing the fundamental molecular causes of disease and devising the innovative therapies of tomorrow.

Kristiina Vu MD PhD, Director
John Reed, President and Chief Executive Officer

2194 City of Hope Comprehensive Cancer Research Center
1500 E Duarte Road   626-256-4673
Duarte, CA 91010   800-256-4673
                                  Fax: 626-930-5394
                              e-mail: tkronitis@coh.org
                                  www.cityofhope.org

Excellence in biomedical research patient-centered medical care and community outreach.
Theodore G Krontiris MD, Director
Richard Jove, Deputy Director

2195   Geraldine Brush Cancer Research Institute California Pacific Medical Center
California Pacific Medical Center
2330 Clay Street #201   415-600-6000
San Francisco, CA 94115   e-mail: cpmcadmin@sutterhealth.org
                                            www.cpmc.org

Martin Brotman, President

2196   Ida and Joseph Friend Cancer Resource Center
Box 0981, UCSF   415-885-3693
San Francisco, CA 94143-981   800-444-2559
                                         Fax: 415-885-3701
            e-mail: cancerresource@ucsfmedctr.org
                        communications@cc.ucsf.edu
The Cancer Resource Center supports wellness and the healing process by providing patients and their loved ones with information emotional support and community resources. The CRC maintains a multimedia library provides access to specialized health databases and offers research assistance. We host diverse support groups and classes and direct people to other community resources. All CRC programs are free.
Frank Mccorm PhD, Director

2197   Jonsson Comprehensive Cancer Center University of California At Los Angeles
University of California At Los Angeles
8-684 Factor Building   310-825-5268
Los Angeles, CA 90095-1781   888-662-8252
                                         Fax: 310-206-5553
            e-mail: jcccinfo@mednet.ucla.edu
                    www.cancer.mednet.ucla.edu
UCLA's Jonsson Comprehensive Cancer Center (JCCC) has established an international reputation for developing new cancer therapies providing the best in experimental treatments and expertly guiding and training the next generation of medical researchers.
Judith Gasson, Director
James Economou, Executive Director

2198   Melanoma Research Foundation
1411 K Street NW   202-347-9675
Washington, DC 20005   800-673-1290
                                         Fax: 202-347-9678
            e-mail: info@melanoma.org
                    www.melanoma.org
Founded in October 1996 by melanoma patients and their families to support research which will lead to cure for melanoma. Strictly a volunteer organization - not one person will receive compensation for his or her efforts.
Peggy L Cheirrett, Director

2199   Northern California Cancer Center
2201 Walnut Avenue   510-608-5000
Fremont, CA 94538-2334   800-511-2300
                                         Fax: 510-608-5095
                                            www.nccc.org
The North California Cancer Center is dedicated to understanding the causes prevention and detection of cancer and to improving the quality of life for individuals living with cancer.
Saul Rosenberg MD, Director Emeritus
Sally Glaser PhD, CEO

2200   Pediatric Cancer Research Laboratory Children's Hospital of Orange County
Children's Hospital of Orange County
455 S Main Street   714-997-3000
Orange, CA 92868-3874   Fax: 714-532-8380
                                            www.choc.org
CHOC is the first hospital devoted exclusively to caring for children in Orange County.
Dr Mitchell Cairo, Director

2201   Rebecca and John Moores UCSD Cancer Center
3855 Health Sciences Drive   585-534-7600
La Jolla, CA 92093-0658   Fax: 858-534-7628
                                e-mail: dedavis@ucsd.edu
                                        www.cancer.ucsd.edu
One of the just 39 centers in the US to hold a National Cancer Institute designation as a Comprehensive Cancer Center. As such it ranks among the top centers in the nation conducting basic and clinical cancer research providing advanced patient care and serving the community through outreach and education programs.
John Alksne, Professor Surgery
Michael Andre, Adjunct Professor Radiology

2202   Salk Institute Cancer Center Salk Institute for Biological Studies
Salk Institute for Biological Studies
PO Box 85800   858-453-4100
San Diego, CA 92186-5800   Fax: 858-453-8534
                        e-mail: communications@salk.edu
                                            www.salk.edu
The Cancer Center was established in 1970. It is one of only eight basic research cancer centers in the country designated by the National Cancer Institute. The center includes 22 faculty members 150 postdoctoral researchers 45 graduate students and 80 research assistants. It comprises about half of the research at the Salk Institute.
Walter Eckhart, Professor and Laboratory Head
William R Brody, President

2203   Salk Institute for Biological Studies
PO Box 85800   858-453-4100
San Diego, CA 92186-5800   Fax: 858-453-8534
                        e-mail: communications@salk.edu
                                            www.salk.edu
Cellular and molecular biology research focusing mainly on cancer.
William R Brody, President
Marsha A Chandler, Executive Vice President

2204   Santa Barbara Breast Cancer Institute
5333 Hollister Avenue   805-964-8883
Santa Barbara, CA 93111-2341
Otto Sartorius, Director

2205   Stanford University: Beckman Center for Molecular and Genetic Medicine
School of Medicine, Department of Biochemistry
291 Campus Drive Rm LK3C02
Stanford, CA 94305-5101   650-725-3900
                                        cmgm.stanford.edu

Dr Paul Berg, Emeritus Professor Biochemistry
Philip A Pizzo MD, Dean

2206   USC/Norris Comprehensive Cancer Center
1441 Eastlake Avenue
Los Angeles, CA 90033-1048   323-865-3000
                                        uscnorriscancer.usc.edu
Major regional and national resource for cancer research treatment prevention and education.
Peter A Jones, Director
Robert W Haile, Associate Director for Cause & Preventio

2207   University of California Berkeley Cancer Research Laboratory
447 Life Science Addition   510-642-4711
Berkeley, CA 94720-2751   Fax: 510-642-5741
                                e-mail: crl@berkeley.edu
                                    biology.berkeley.edu/crl
Basic research with a special emphasis on mammary cancer and tumor immunotherapy.
Astar Winoto, Director
Judith Yee, Manager

2208   University of California: Los Angeles Bone Marrow Transplantation Program
200 UCLA Medical Plaza
Los Angeles, CA 90024   310-206-6889
                                www.healthcare.ucla.edu/transplant
Treatment of leukemia and anemia.
David W Golde MD, Director
Gabriel Danovitch, M.D., Medical Director, Proffesor of Medicine

Colorado

2209 AMC Cancer Research Center
1600 Pierce Street
Denver, CO 80214
303-233-6501
800-321-1557
Fax: 303-239-3400
e-mail: contactus@amc.org
www.amc.org
Offers research activities publications meetings educational activities public services testing services community-based cancer control programs and knowledge of cancer mortality rates.
Alice Norton, Executive Director
Gail Eckhardt, Clinical Science

2210 Colorado Cancer Research Program
2253 S Oneida Street
Denver, CO 80224
303-777-2663
888-785-6789
Fax: 303-777-2642
e-mail: ccrp@co-cancerresearch.org
www.co-cancerresearch.org
A nonprofit community-based cancer program established to provide community hospitals and physicians access to a wide range of cancer research trials in order to provide their patients with greater options for the treatment control and prevention.
Jane Hajovsky, Executive Director
Eduardo Pajon, Principal Investigator

2211 University of Colorado Cancer Center
13001 E 17th Place
Aurora, CO 80045
303-724-3155
800-473-2288
Fax: 303-724-3162
e-mail: CancerCenter.Webmaster@uchsc.edu
www.uccc.info
UCCC consortium is the hub for cancer research in Colorado. With eight programs 17 shared core resources and nearly 400 members from three universities and six institutions UCCC is responsible for the majority of cancer research in the Rocky Mountain region.
Dan Theodorescu MD PhD, Director
Laurie Gasper MD, Associate Director for Clinical Research

Connecticut

2212 Yale University Comprehensive Cancer Center
333 Cedar Street
New Haven, CT 06520-8028
203-785-4095
866-925-3226
Fax: 203-785-4116
www.yalecancercenter.org
A National Cancer Institute designated comprehensive cancer center for over 30 years Yale Cancer Center is one of only 40 Centers in the nation and the only comprehensive center in Southern New England.
Thomas Lynch, Director
Kevin Vest, PT, MBA, FACHE, Deputy Director

District of Columbia

2213 Georgetown University: Vincent T Lombardi Cancer Research Center
3800 Reservoir Road NW
Washington, DC 20057
202-444-4000
lombardi.georgetown.edu
Established in 1970 the Lombardi Comprehensive Cancer Center is named for the legendary Green Bay Packers and Washington Redskins coach Vince Lombardi who was treated for cancer at Georgetown University Hospital.
Louis M Weiner, Director
Peter G Shields, Deputy Director

2214 Howard University Cancer Center
2041 Georgia Avenue NW
Washington, DC 20060-0001
202-806-7697
Fax: 202-462-8928
e-mail: ladams-campbell@howard.edu
cancer.howard.edu
Reduce the burden of cancer through research education and service with emphasis on the unique ethnic and cultural aspects of minority and underserved populations.
Lucile Adams-Campbel, Director
Wayne A I Frederick, Interim Director

Florida

2215 Rambaugh-Goodwin Institute for Cancer Research
1850 NW 69th Avenue
Plantation, FL 33313
954-587-9020
Fax: 954-587-6378
e-mail: info@rgicr.org
www.rgicr.org
RGI is committed to rapidly developing anti-cancer therapies in conjunction with industrial and academic partners using efficient models of cancer growth and metastasis with the aim of moving novel compounds to market in the shortest time possible.
Claire Thuning-Robin, Director

2216 UM/Sylvester Comprehensive Cancer Center
1475 NW 12th Avenue
Miami, FL 33136
305-243-1000
800-545-2292
www.sylvester.org
UMHC offers an outpatient clinic a 40-bed inpatient unit a comprehensive treatment unit the Mohs surgery center/dermatology clinic the Rosenfield GI Center a cardiology lab and clinic a radiology/imaging suite an interventional radiology clinic the Spine Institute clinics on-site laboratory and pharmacy the Courtelis Center for Psychosocial Oncology the Jill Selevan Chapel a cafeteria as well as administrative offices.
W Jarrard Goodwin, Director
Glen Barbar PhD, Executive Director

Georgia

2217 Emory University: Georgia Center for Cancer Statistics
Rollins School of Public Health
201 Dowman Drive
Atlanta, GA 30322
404-727-6123
Fax: 404-727-7261
e-mail: gccs@sph.emory.edu
www.sph.emory.edu/gccs
Serves as a cancer registry for five counties of metropolitan Atlanta and ten rural counties of central Georgia.
James W Wagner, President

2218 Emory University: Winship Cancer Institute
1365-C Clifton Road NE
Atlanta, GA 30322
404-778-1900
888-946-7447
www.cancer.emory.edu
A clinical cancer center coordinating basic and clinical cancer research.
Walter Currans, Executive Director
Fadlo Khuri MD, Deputy Directory for Basic Research

Hawaii

2219 Pacific Health Research Institute
700 Bishop Street
Honolulu, HI 96813
808-524-4411
Fax: 808-524-5559
e-mail: info@phrei.org
www.phrihawaii.org
Located in Honolulu Hawaii Pacific Health Research Institute (PHRI) is the largest independent biomedical research institute in the state. Since its founding on 1960 as an independent not for profit 501(c)(3) research institute PHRI today has become a leader in biomedical research in the Pacific. Indeed its researchers are performing complex investigations aimed at conquering some of the most debilitating and lethal diseases that afflict humankind.
Vicki L Shambaugh, MA, MPH, Director
Helen Petrovitch, Executive Director

2220 University of Hawaii: Cancer Research Center
1236 Lauhala Street
Honolulu, HI 96813
808-586-2985
Fax: 808-586-2982
e-mail: cvogel@crch.hawaii.edu
www.crch.org
The mission of the Cancer Research Center of Hawaii is to reduce the burden of cancer through research education and service with an emphasis on the unique ethnic culture and environmental characteristics of Hawaii and the Pacific.
Carl-Wilhelm Vogel, Professor (Researcher)
Michele Carbone, Interim Cancer Center Director

Illinois

2221 Kellogg Cancer Care Center Evanston Hospital
Evanston Hospital
2650 Ridge Avenue   847-570-2000
Evanston, IL 60201   888-364-6400
      www.enh.org
Integral unit of the Evanston Hospital this center researches treatment and diagnosis of cancer including phase 1 and phase 2 studies.
Mark R Neaman, President, CEO
Jeffery H Hillebrand, COO

2222 Leukemia Research Foundation
3520 Lake Avenue   847-424-0600
Wilmette, IL 60091-1064   888-558-5385
      Fax: 847-424-0606
      e-mail: info@lrfmail.org
      www.leukemia-research.org
To conquer leukemia lymphoma and myelodysplastic syndromes by funding research into their causes and cures and to enrich the quality of life of those touched by these diseases.
Kevin Radelet, Executive Director
Cindy Kane, Senior Director of Development

2223 Oncology Hematology Associates of Central Illinois
8940 N Wood Sage Road   309-243-3000
Peoria, IL 61615-7828   866-662-6564
      www.illinoiscancercare.com
Research into cancer treatments.
Robert Cooper, Director
Paul A S Fishkin, Hematology Internal Medicine Medical O

2224 Robert H Lurie Comprehensive Cancer Center of Northwestern University
Galter Pavilion 675 N Street Clair   312-695-0990
Chicago, IL 60611   866-587-4322
      Fax: 312-695-1352
      e-mail: cancer@northwestern.edu
      www.lurie.northwestern.edu
Lurie Cancer Center is a founding member of the National Comprehensive Cancer Network an exclusive alliance of 21 of the nation's leading cancer centers.
Steven T Rosen, Director
Leonidas Platanias, Deputy Director

2225 University of Chicago Cancer Research Center
5841 S Maryland Avenue   773-702-6180
Chicago, IL 60637   877-824-0600
      e-mail: cancerresources@uccrc.org
      uccrc.uchicago.edu
The University of Chicago Cancer Research Center (UCCRC) employs a wealth of intellectual technological and financial resources to pursue a comprehensive collaborative research program involving more than 200 renowned scientists and clinicians.
Mary Ellen Connellan, Executive Director
Justin Ullman, President

2226 University of Chicago: Clinical Nutrition Research Unit
5841 S Maryland Avenue   773-702-6180
Chicago, IL 60637-1463   877-824-0600
      e-mail: feedback@bsd.uchicago.edu
      www.uchicago.edu
Provide superior healthcare in a compassionate manner ever mindful of each patient's dignity and individuality.
Michael M Le Beau PhD, Director
James L Madara, CEO

Indiana

2227 Mary Margaret Walther Program Walther Cancer Institute
Walther Cancer Institute
9292 N Meridian Street   317-708-6101
Indianapolis, IN 46260   Fax: 317-708-6102
      e-mail: info@walther.org
      www.walther.org
Focuses research on all types of cancer studies.
Leonard J Betley, Chairman
James E Ruckle, President/CEO

Iowa

2228 Iowa Oncology Research Association
300 E Locust   515-244-7586
Des Moines, IA 50309   888-244-6061
      Fax: 515-244-3037
      e-mail: sherrijr@iora.org
      www.iora.org
Clinical cancer studies and research.
Sherri Rickabaugh, Administrator
Becky Berrett, Research Assistants

2229 University of Iowa: Holden Comprehensive Cancer Center
UI Hospitals and Clinics
University of Iowa   319-353-8620
Iowa City, IA 52242-1002   800-777-8442
      Fax: 319-353-8988
      e-mail: cancer-center@uiowa.edu
      www.uihealthcare.com/depts/cancercenter
The Holden Cancer Center promotes interactive high-quality cancer research high-quality health care related to the prevention detection and treatment of cancer and educates cancer professionals and the citizens of Iowa about cancer.
Jean E Robillard, Vice President for Medical Affairs
Kenneth P Kates, CEO

Kansas

2230 Kansas State University: Terry C Johnson Center for Basic Cancer Research
Center for Basic Cancer Research
1 Chalmers Hall   785-532-6705
Manhattan, KS 66506   Fax: 785-532-6707
      e-mail: marcia@k-state.edu
      www.k-state.edu/cancer.center
The mission of the Terry C. Johnson Center for Basic Cancer Research is to further the understanding of cancers by funding basic cancer research and supporting higher education training and public outreach.
Rob Denell, Director
S Keith Chapes, Associate Director

Kentucky

2231 Henry Vogt Cancer Research Institute James Graham Brown Cancer Center
James Graham Brown Cancer Center
2301 S 3rd Street   502-852-5555
Louisville, KY 40208   800-334-8635
      e-mail: info@ulh.org
      www.louisville.edu/hsc/centers
The overall goal of the scientists in the Henry Vogt Cancer Research Institute is to study mechanisms relevant to tumor cell biology at the basic and translational level in order to provide insights that will contribute to the ultimate prevention and cure of malignant diseases.
Donald M Miller, Director
John W Eaton, Deputy Director

2232 Kentucky Cancer Program
2365 Harrodsburg Road   859-219-0772
Lexington, KY 40504-3381   Fax: 859-219-0548
      e-mail: dka@kcp.uky.edu
      www.kcp.uky.edu
The KCP provides a variety of cancer programs and services to health professionals the public patients and survivors.
Debra Armstong, Director
Diane Frasure, Administrative Associate

2233 University of Kentucky: Children Cancer Study Group
Markey Cancer Center
800 Rose Street   859-257-4500
Lexington, KY 40536-93   800-333-8874
      Fax: 859-323-2074
      www.ukhealthcare.uky.edu/markey/
Kentucky Children's Hospital is the only children's hospital in the region. Patients range in age from infants through adolescents and have a variety of illness and injuries.
Michael Karpf, Executive Vice President for Health Affa
Frank Butler, VP for Medical Center Operations

2234 University of Kentucky: Lucille Parker Markey Cancer Center
800 Rose Street
Lexington, KY 40536
859-247-4500
800-333-8874
Fax: 859-323-2074
www.ukhealthcare.uky.edu/markey/
The Markey Cancer Center mission is to eliminate the morbidity and mortality of cancer through a comprehensive program of research education clinical care and community outreach.
Alfred M Cohen MD FACS, Director
Michael Karpf, Executive Vice President for Health Affa

Louisiana

2235 Baton Rouge Regional Tumor Registry Mary Bird Perkins Cancer Center
Mary Bird Perkins Cancer Center
4950 Essen Lane
Baton Rouge, LA 70809
225-767-0847
Fax: 225-215-1215
www.marybird.org
The Louisiana Tumor Registry is composed of a central office and regional registries that collect and process cancer incidence data from the state's eight established geographic regions. These eight geographic areas are based on Louisiana's historic health districts.
Todd D Stevens, President, CEO
J Gerald Jolly, Chairman

2236 Tulane University Pulmonary Diseases Critical Care and Enviromental Medicine
School of Medicine
1430 Tulane Avenue
New Orleans, LA 70112
504-988-5187
800-588-5300
e-mail: medsch@tulane.edu
www.som.tulane.edu/pulmdis/facilities
Provides state-of-the-art care to patients and teaching to trainees through several areas of academic excellence that include: Interstitial Lung Diseases; Asthma; Cystic Fibrosis; Sleep Disorders; Interventional Pulmonology; Lung Cancer; Smoking Cessation; Critical Care; and Environmental Medicine.
Mary Brown, Vice President Health Science Systems
Roy Weiner, Associate Dean for Clinical Research

Maryland

2237 Frederick Cancer Research Center
PO Box B
Frederick, MD 21702-1201
301-846-1000
Fax: 301-846-1108
web.ncifcrf.gov
Direct research into the causes treatment and prevention of cancer AIDS and related diseases.
Craig W Reynolds, Associate Director
Jo Anne Barb, Secretary

2238 Johns Hopkins University: Sydney Kimmel Comprehensive Cancer Center
The Harry and Jeanette Weinberg Buidling
401 N Broadway
Baltimore, MD 21231-0005
410-955-5222
www.hopkinskimmelcancercenter.org
Johns Hopkins Kimmel Cancer Center has active programs in clinical research laboratory research education community outreach and prevention and control.
Ronald J Danielles, President
Edward Miller MD, Dean of Medical Faculty, CEO

2239 National Foundation for Cancer Research National Foundation for Cancer Research
National Foundation for Cancer Research
4600 E W Highway
Bethesda, MD 20814-3206
301-654-1250
800-321-2873
Fax: 301-654-5824
e-mail: info@nfcr.org
www.nfcr.org
NFCR promotes and facilitates collaboration among scientists to accelerate the pace of discovery from bench to bedside. NFCR is committed to Research for a Cure - cures for all types of cancers.
Sujuan Ba MD, COO
Franklin C Salisbury Jr, President

2240 Warren Grant Magnuson Clinical Center
National Institute of Health

9000 Rockville Pike
Bethesda, MD 20892
301-496-4000
800-411-1222
Fax: 301-480-9793
TTY: 866-411-1010
e-mail: prpl@mail.cc.nih.gov
clinicalcenter.nih.gov/index.html
Established in 1953 as the research hospital of the National Institutes of Health. Designed so that patient care facilities are close to research laboratories so new findings of basic and clinical scientists can be quickly applied to the treatment of patients. Upon referral by physicians, patients are admitted to NIH clinical studies.
John Gallin, Director
David Henderson, Deputy Director for Clinical Care

Massachusetts

2241 Boston University Cancer Research Center
820 Harrison Avenue
Boston, MA 02118
617-638-8265
Fax: 617-638-6518
e-mail: sfenness@bu.edu
www.bumc.bu.edu/clinicaltrials
The Office of Clinical Research (OCR) was established on July 1 1998 to serve as the central focus for clinical research support conduct and training at Boston University Medical Center.
Douglas V Faller, Director
Salli Fennessey, Manager

2242 Dana-Farber Institute: Department of Biostatistics and Computational Biology
450 Brookline Avenue
Boston, MA 02115-5450
617-632-3000
Fax: 617-632-2444
e-mail: biostatistics@jimmy.harvard.edu
www.dana-farber.org
Integral unit of the Institute organized into laboratories of biostatistics computing and epidemiology.
Marvin Zelen, Researcher
Edward J Benz, President, CEO

2243 Massachusetts Institute of Technology Center for Cancer Research
MIT Center for Cancer
Koch Institute at MIT 76-158
Cambridge, MA 02142
617-253-6403
Fax: 617-324-2238
e-mail: cancer@mit.edu
web.mit.edu/ccr
The mission of MIT Cancer Center is to apply tools of basic science and technology to determine how cancer is caused progresses and responds to treatment. Through this effort they have developed an increasingly complete understanding of the nature of cancer cells which has led directly to improved treatments for the disease.
Dr Tyler Jacks, Director
Dr Jaqueline Lees, Associate Director

2244 Massachusetts Institute of Technology: Center for Cancer Research
Koch Institute at MIT 76-158
Cambridge, MA 02142
617-253-6403
Fax: 617-324-2238
e-mail: cancer@mit.edu
web.mit.edu/ccr
The Koch Institute includes over 40 laboratories and more than 500 researchers located at headquarters and across the MIT campus. Koch Institute will continue the CCR's tradition of scientific excellence while also seeking to directly promote innovative ways to diagnose monitor and treat cancer through advanced technology.
Tyler Jacks, Director
Dr Jaqueline Lees, Associate Director

Michigan

2245 Gershenson Radiation Oncology Center Barbara Ann Karmanos Cancer Institute
Barbara Ann Karmanos Cancer Institute
4100 John Road
Detroit, MI 48201
313-745-9191
800-527-6266
Fax: 313-745-2314
e-mail: info@karmanos.org
www.karmanos.org
Radiation therapy and cancer treatment and research.
Gerold Bepler, President

2246 Meyer L Prentis Comprehensive Cancer Center of Metropolitan Detroit
Barbara Ann Karmanos Cancer Institute
4100 John Road
Detroit, MI 48201

313-745-9191
800-527-6266
Fax: 313-745-2314
e-mail: info@karmanos.org
www.karmanos.org

Gerald Bepler, President

2247 Meyer L Prentis Comprehensive Cancer Cente Barbara Ann Karmanos Cancer Institute
4100 John Road
Detroit, MI 48201

313-745-9191
800-527-6266
Fax: 313-745-2314
e-mail: info@karmanos.org
www.karmanos.org

Gerald Bepler, President

2248 University of Michigan: Cancer Center Cancer Research Committee
Cancer Research Committee
1500 E Medical Center Drive
Ann Arbor, MI 48109-094

734-764-0039
800-865-1125
Fax: 734-936-9582
www.cancer.med.umich.edu

The U-M Comprehensive Cancer Center provides its patients diagnostic treatment and support services in a collaborative environment focused on excellence in patient care.
Eric R Fearon, Associate Director for Science
Max S Wicha, Director

2249 Wayne State University Center for Molecular Medicine and Genetics
Wayne State University School of Medicine
3127 Scott Hall
Detroit, MI 48201

313-577-5323
Fax: 313-577-5218
e-mail: sshaw@wayne.edu
www.genetics.wayne.edu

Research focusing on human conditions such as cancer and neuromuscular disorders.
Lawrence I Grossman, Professor/Director
Jeffrey A Loeb, Associate Director

Minnesota

2250 Mayo Comprehensive Cancer Center
200 First Street SW
Rochester, MN 55905-0001

507-284-2511
Fax: 507-284-0161
TTY: 507-284-9786
www.mayo.edu

Scientists and physician investigators conduct wide-ranging research to improve patient care while training the next generation of medical scholars.
Denis Cortese, President/Chief Executive Officer
Robert A Rizza, Director

2251 University of Minnesota Masonic Cancer Center
Division of Oncology
420 Delaware Street SE
Minneapolis, MN 55455

612-624-8484
800-226-2376
Fax: 612-626-3069
e-mail: ccinfo@umn.edu
www.cancer.umn.edu

The Masonic Cancer Center fosters this mission by creating a collaborative research environment focused on the causes prevention detection and treatment of cancer; applying that knowledge to improve quality of life for patients and survivors; and sharing its discoveries with other scientists students professionals and the community.
Brian Steeves, Deputy Director
Ann D Cieslak, Executive Director

Missouri

2252 Cancer Research Center
3501 Berrywood Drive
Columbia, MO 65201

573-875-2255
Fax: 873-443-1202
www.cancerresearchcenter.org

Not only does the Cancer Research Center offer research they also offer community outreach programs to educate church groups civic clubs and other organizations about their research and cancer prevention.
Abe Eisenstark, Research Director
Jack Bozarth, Director

Nebraska

2253 Lincoln Cancer Center
4600 Valley Road
Lincoln, NE 68510-4844

402-483-2827
Fax: 402-483-4184
Barb Morton, Director

2254 University of Nebraska at Omaha Eppley Institute for Research in Cancer
University of Nebraska
985950 Nebraska Medical Center
Omaha, NE 68198-5950

402-559-4090
e-mail: hmmaurer@unmc.edu
www.unmc.edu/eppley

To improve the health of Nebraska through premier educational programs innovative research the highest quality patient care and outreach to underserved populations.
Harold M Maurer, Chancellor
Thomas H Rosenquist, Vice Chancellor

New Hampshire

2255 Cancer and Leukemia Group B
230 W Monroe
Chicago, IL 60606

773-702-9171
Fax: 312-345-0117
e-mail: marciak@uchicago.edu
www.calgb.org

Integral unit of the Institute specializing in leukemia research and prevention.
Marcia Kelly, Administrative Coordinator
Michael Kelly, Director Protocol Operations

2256 Norris Cotton Cancer Center Dartmouth-Hitchcock Medical Center
Dartmouth-Hitchcock Medical Center
One Medical Center Drive
Lebanon, NH 03756

603-653-9000
800-639-6918
Fax: 603-653-9003
e-mail: cancercenter@dartmouth.edu
www.cancer.dartmouth.edu

The Cancer Center provides a positive environment for treatment cure and recovery for patients with all forms of cancer.
Mark Israel MD, Director
Burton L Eisenberg, Deputy Director

New Jersey

2257 Melanoma Research Foundation
1411 K Street NW
Washington, DC 20005

202-347-9675
800-673-1290
Fax: 202-347-9678
e-mail: info@melanoma.org
www.melanoma.org

Founded in October 1996 by melanoma patients and their families to support research which will lead to cure for melanoma. Strictly a volunteer organization - not one person will receive compensation for his or her efforts.
Peggy Cheirrett, Director

New Mexico

2258 University of New Mexico Cancer Research and Treatment Center
University of New Mexico
1201 Camino de Salud NE
Albuquerque, NM 87131-0001

505-272-4946
800-432-6806
Fax: 505-925-0100
www.cancer.unm.edu

One of the nation's 60 premier National Cancer Institute (NCI)-Designated Cancer Centers and we have been named one of America's Best Cancer Hospitals by U.S. News & World Report. UNM Cancer Center provides cancer diagnosis and treatment to

over 40% of the adults and virtually all of the children diagnosed with cancer each year in New Mexico.
Cheryl Willman, Director/CEO
John A Trotter, Deputy EVP for Health Sciences

2259 University of New Mexico: Cancer Research and Treatment Center
1201 Camino de Salud NE
Albuquerque, NM 87131-5001
505-272-4946
800-432-6806
Fax: 505-925-0100
www.cancer.unm.edu
One of the nation's 60 premier National Cancer Institute (NCI)-Designated Cancer Centers and we have been named one of America's Best Cancer Hospitals by U.S. News & World Report. UNM Cancer Center provides cancer diagnosis and treatment to over 40% of the adults and virtually all of the children diagnosed with cancer each year in New Mexico.
Cheryl Willman, Director/CEO
John A Trotter, Deputy EVP for Health Sciences

2260 University of New Mexico: Center for Non-Invasive Diagnosis
Mind Imaging Center/University of New Mexico
1101 Yale Boulevard NE
Albuquerque, NM 87131-0001
505-277-0111
Fax: 505-272-4056
hsc.unm.edu
Cardiology and cancer research.
David Lepre, Executive Director

2261 University of New Mexico: Center for Non-I Mind Imaging Center/University of New Me
1101 Yale Boulevard NE
Albuquerque, NM 87131
505-272-5774
Fax: 505-272-4056
hsc.unm.edu
Cardiology and cancer research.
David Lepre, Executive Director

New York

2262 Ackerman Institute for the Family
149 E 78th Street
New York, NY 10075
212-879-4900
Fax: 212-744-0206
e-mail: ackerman@ackerman.org
www.ackerman.org
Independent nonprofit research organization specializing in family therapy teaching and clinical services.
Lois Braverman, President/CEO
Evan Imber-B PhD, Director

2263 Albany Medical College Joint Center for Cancer and Blood Disorders
43 New Scotland Avenue
Albany, NY 12208
518-262-3125
877-AMC-8008
Fax: 518-262-3165
TTY: 518-262-1180
www.amc.edu
Offers research in the fields of cancer and blood disorders focusing on radiotherapy pathology and surgery.
Herbert Abbott, General Pediatric
Kevin Costello, Internal Medicine

2264 Albert Einstein Cancer Center Albert Einstein College of Medicine
Albert Einstein College of Medicine
1300 Morris Park Avenue
Bronx, NY 10461
718-430-2302
Fax: 718-430-2000
e-mail: aecc@aecom.yu.edu
www.aecom.yu.edu/cancer
The goal of AECC is to foster basic clinical population-based and translational research that addresses all aspects of the cancer problem.
Allen M Spiegel MD, Dean
Miriam W Turkel, Director of Administration

2265 Association for Research of Childhood Cancer
PO Box 251
Buffalo, NY 14225-0251
716-681-4433
e-mail: president@arocc.org
www.arocc.org

The Association was chartered by New York State in that year as a not-for-profit corporation whose primary purpose was to fund the major pediatric research centers in Western New York.
Larry Lorenz, Vice President
Anne O'Donnel, President

2266 Bassett Research Institute
One Atwell Road
Cooperstown, NY 13326
607-547-3456
800-227-7388
e-mail: research.institute@bassett.org
www.bassett.org
Research institute committed to seeking new information and new strategies for preventing detecting and treating disease.
Wiliiam F Streck MD, President/CEO

2267 Cancer Institute of Brooklyn
927 49th Street
Brooklyn, NY 11219-2923
718-972-5816
Fax: 718-972-8693
Jo-Ann Hertz, Executive Director

2268 Cancer Research Institute: New York
One Exchange Plaza 55 Broadway
New York, NY 10006
212-688-7515
800-992-2623
Fax: 212-832-9376
e-mail: info@cancerresearch.org
www.cancerresearch.org
The Cancer Research Institute is the world's only non-profit organization dedicated exclusively to the support and coordination ofÿlaboratory and clinical efforts that will lead to the immunological treatment control and prevention of cancer.
Jill O'Donnel-Tormey, Executive Director
Leslie Anson, Assistant to the Executive Director

2269 Columbia University Comprehensive Cancer Center
630 W 168th Street
New York, NY 10032
212-305-4186
Fax: 212-305-6889
/www.cumc.columbia.edu/
Lee Goldman, President

2270 Medical Foundation of Buffalo Hauptman-Woodward Medical Research Insti
Hauptman-Woodward Medical Research Institute
700 Ellicott Street
Buffalo, NY 14203-1102
716-898-8600
Fax: 716-898-8660
www.hwi.buffalo.edu
Nonprofit organization devoted to cancer research.
Herbert A Hauptman PhD, President/Nobel Laureate
Eaton E Lattman, Executive Director & CEO

2271 Memorial Sloan-Kettering Cancer Center
1275 York Avenue
New York, NY 10065
212-639-2000
888-675-7722
e-mail: publicaffairs@mskcc.org
www.mskcc.org
Sloan-Kettering Institute has endeavored to lead the way in basic science research oftentimes translating those advances into clinical treatments.
Harold Varmus, President, CEO
Paul A Marks, President Emeritus

2272 New York University Cancer Institute New York University Medical Center
New York University Medical Center
530 First Avenue
New York, NY 10016
212-263-7300
888-769-8633
Fax: 212-263-0715
www.nyucancerinstitute.org
The mission of the NYU Cancer Institute is to decrease and eliminate cancer as a significant health problem throughout New York the national and the world by developing and maintaining excellent programs in patient care research education and prevention.
William Carroll, Director
Lauren E Hackett, Executive Director of Administration

2273 Roswell Park Cancer Institute National Cancer Institute
Elm & Carlton Streets
Buffalo, NY 14263
716-845-2300
877-275-7724
e-mail: askrpci@roswellpark.org
www.roswellpark.org
Roswell Park Cancer Institute has made fundamental contributions to reducing the cancer burden and has successfully main-

tained an exemplary leadership role in setting the national standards for cancer care research and education.
Donald L Trump MD, Director
Ann Gioia, Director

2274 State University of New York Health Science Center At Brooklyn
450 Clarkson Avenue
Brooklyn, NY 11203   718-270-1000
                                          www.downstate.edu
Downstate includes Colleges of Medicine Nursing and Health Related Professions and a School of Graduate Studies as well as its own teaching hospital an M.P.H. Program and extensive research facilities.
John C LaRosa, President
John B Clark, Interim Chancellor

2275 University of Rochester: James P Wilmot Cancer Center
601 Elmwood Avenue   585-275-5823
Rochester, NY 14642   866-494-5668
                                          Fax: 585-276-0158
                          www.stronghealth.com/services/cancer
To use education science and technology to improve health transforming the patient experience with fresh ideas and approaches steeped in disciplined science and delivered by health care professionals who innovate take intelligent risks and care about the lives they touch.
Richard I Fisher MD, Director

North Carolina

2276 Cancer Center of Wake Forest University at Bowman Gray School of Medicine
Wake Forest University School Of Medicine
Medical Center Boulevard   336-716-2011
Winston-Salem, NC 27157   800-446-2255
                                          Fax: 336-716-9593
                          e-mail: medadmit@wfubmc.edu
                                   www1.wfubmc.edu/cancer
Provide a superb education as well as personal support. Beyond the academic experiences offered at our medical school we encourage the development of our students as caring physicians dedicated to providing the very best care professionally and personally to all patients.
William B Applegate M D M P, Dean
John D McConnell, CEO

2277 Duke Comprehensive Cancer Center
2424 Erwin Road   919-684-3377
Durham, NC 27705   888-ASK-DUKE
                                          Fax: 919-684-5653
                                          www.cancer.duke.edu
One of only 39 centers in the country designated by the National Cancer Institute (NCI) as a 'comprehensive cancer center ' Duke combines cutting-edge research with compassionate care. Our team of nationally recognized physicians and staff treat nearly 6 000 new patients per year giving them the extensive experience that yields better results. In fact U.S. News & World Report rates Duke #7 in the nation for cancer care and best in the Southeast.
H Kim Lyerly, Director
Anthony Means, Deputy Director

2278 University of North Carolina UNC Lineberger Comprehensive Cancer Center
School of Medicine
101 Manning Drive   919-966-0000
Chapel Hill, NC 25414   866-869-1856
                                          Fax: 919-962-2621
                          e-mail: lccc@med.unc.edu
                                   cancer.med.unc.edu
The Center provides multidisciplinary programs for most cancers giving patients the benefit of many medical specialists in one place often in one visit.
H Shelton Earp, Director
Michael O'Malley, Associate Director

Ohio

2279 Case Western Reserve University: Ireland Cancer Center
University Hospitals of Cleveland
11100 Euclid Avenue   216-844-1529
Cleveland, OH 44106   888-844-8447
                          www.uhhospitals.org/irelandcancer
Thomas F Senty, CEO

2280 Case Western Reserve University: Ireland C University Hospitals of Cleveland
11100 Euclid Avenue   21- 84- 152
Cleveland, OH 44106   888-844-8447
                          www.uhhospitals.org/irelandcancer
Information and support to patients, families and the public.
Thomas F Senty, CEO

2281 Children's Hospital Research Foundation
700 Childrens Drive   614-722-2000
Columbus, OH 43205-2696   800-792-8401
                                          Fax: 61- 35- 079
                e-mail: CommunityLink@NationwideChildrens.org
                                   www.nationwidechildrens.org
Offers research activities into Reye's Syndrome genetics and children's cancer chemotherapy.
Richard McClead, Medical Director
Richard J Brilli, Chief Medical Officer

2282 Medical College of Toledo: Cancer Research Division
Department of Pathology
3000 Arlington Avenue   419-383-3470
Toledo, OH 43614-2595   800-321-8383
                                          Fax: 419-383-6130
                          e-mail: utmc.webmaster@utoledo.edu
                                          utmc.utoledo.edu
Researches into all aspects of cancer.
Jill Zyrek-Betts, Assistant Professor

2283 Ohio State University Comprehensive Cancer Center
Arthur G James Cancer Hospital
300 W 10th Avenue   614-293-7521
Columbus, OH 43210-1240   e-mail: michael.caligiuri@osumc.edu
                                   www.osuccc.osu.edu
A national and international leader in research,ÿwhich translates to high-quality patient care and educational programs for residents of Ohio and beyond.
Michael A Caligiuri M D, Director
John C Byrd, Associate Director

2284 Ohio State University General Clinical Research Center
The Ohio State University Davis Me   614-293-8750
Columbus, OH 43210   Fax: 614-293-3796
                          e-mail: william.malarkey@osumc.edu
                                   www.crc.osu.edu
Provides facilities and financial support for inpatient and outpatient cancer research.
William Malaykey, Program Director
David Phillips, Administrative Director

2285 The Cancer Prevention Institute
601 W Riverview Avenue   937-227-9400
Dayton, OH 45406   877-274-4543
                                          Fax: 937-293-7652
                          e-mail: info@pch-dayton.org
                                   www.cancerpreventioninstitute.org
Nonprofit organization focusing research activities primarily on cancer prevention anti-cancer drugs early diagnosis of cancer and bone marrow toxicity. previously known as the Hipple Cancer Research Center.

Oklahoma

2286 Natalie Warren Bryant Cancer Center St. Francis Hospital
St. Francis Hospital
6600 S Yale Avenue   918-488-6688
Tulsa, OK 74136   e-mail: webadministrator@saintfrancis.com
                                   www.saintfrancis.com/locations/nwbcc
Jake Henry Jr, President/Chief Executive Officer
Barry Steichen, Executive Vice President/Chief Administr

2287 Oklahoma Medical Research Foundation Immunobiolgy & Cancer Research
Oklahoma Medical Research Foundation

825 North East 13th Street
Oklahoma City, OK 73104-5005

405-271-7430
800-522-0211
Fax: 405-271-7016
e-mail: OMRF-President@omrf.org
www.omrf.ouhsc.edu

Dr. Stephen Prescott, President

2288 Oklahoma Medical Research Foundation: Oklahoma Medical Research Foundation
825 N E 13th Street
Oklahoma City, OK 73104

40- 27- 743
800-522-0211
Fax: 405-271-7016
e-mail: OMRF-President@omrf.org
www.omrf.ouhsc.edu

Conducting basic research to benefit society and integrity in research is essential to expanding our knowledge of the basic biological processes fundamental to life.
Paul W Kincade Ph D, Program Chair
Stephen M Prescott, President

2289 Samuel Roberts Noble Foundation Biomedical Division
Samuel Roberts Noble Foundation
2510 Sam Noble Parkway
Ardmore, OK 73401

580-223-5810
Fax: 580-224-6217
www.noble.org

One of the largest international offshore drilling contractors in the world.
Michael A Cawley, CEO/President
Bill Goddard, Trustee

Pennsylvania

2290 Abramson Cancer Center of the University of Pennsylvania
3535 Market Street
Philadelphia, PA 19104-3309

800-789-PENN
Fax: 215-349-5445
e-mail: craig@mail.med.upenn.edu
www.penncancer.com

National leader in cancer research patient care and education.
Douglas L Fraker MD, Deputy Director
Caryn Lerman, Interim Director

2291 Allegheny Singer Research Institute West Penn Allegheny Health System
West Penn Allegheny Health System
4800 Friendship Avenue
Pittsburgh, PA 15224

412-362-8677
877-284-2000
Fax: 412-359-8610
e-mail: tchakurd@wpahs.org
www.wpahs.org

Christopher Olivia MD, President, CEO

2292 Fox Chase Cancer Center
333 Cottman Avenue
Philadelphia, PA 19111-2497

215-728-6900
888-369-2427
www.fccc.edu

Linda Fliescher MPH PhD, Assistant Vice President for Communicati
Theresa Berger MBE, Project Manager

2293 Temple University FELS Institute for Cancer Research
School of Medicine
3500 N Broad Street
Philadelphia, PA 19140

215-707-7000
Fax: 215-707-7000
www.temple.edu/medicine

Policies and programs are oriented toward research and training in cancer-related basic biological and biochemical sciences with progressive extension into the areas of molecular developmental and chemical biology to advance knowledge of the etiology and pathogenesis of cancer. A major goal of the Institute is to utilize the advances made in basic science programs to develop novel targeted therapies for the treatment of cancer.
John M Daly MD, Dean
Diane Omdal, Director, Research Administration

2294 University of Pittsburgh Cancer Institute
5150 Centre Avenue
Pittsburgh, PA 15232

412-647-2811
e-mail: PCI-INFO@upmc.edu
www.upci.upmc.edu

Since 1985 the UPCI has been committed to improving the understanding of how cancer develops; to characterizing new lifesaving approaches for cancer prevention detection diagnosis and treatment; and to educating future generations of scientists and clinicians.
Nancy E Davidson MD, Committee Chair
Adam Brufsky MD PhD, Associate Director

Rhode Island

2295 Brown University Division of Biology and Medicine
BioMed Research Admin, Brown Medical School
The Warren Alpert Medical School of
Providence, RI 02912-0001

401-863-3330
Fax: 401-863-2660
bms.brown.edu

Interdisciplinary studies in biological and medical sciences including studies in health care problems and fields of research such as cancer and diabetes.
John Perry, Senior Associate Dean
Edward J Wing, Medicine / Biological Sciences

2296 Roger Williams Clinical Cancer Research Center
Roger Williams General Hospital
825 Chalkstone Avenue
Providence, RI 02908

401-456-2000
www.rwmc.com

Kenneth Belcher, President

2297 Roger Williams Clinical Cancer Research Ce Roger Williams General Hospital
825 Chalkstone Avenue
Providence, RI 02908

401-456-2000
www.rwmc.com

Provides the most advanced specialty care.
Kenneth H Belcher, President

South Carolina

2298 Children's Center for Cancer and Blood Disorders
University of South Carolina School of Medicine
7 Richland Medical Park
Columbia, SC 29203

803-434-7000
www.palmettohealth.org

Joint clinical and basic research of juvenile cancer and blood disorders.
Charles D Beaman Jr, CEO

2299 Children's Center for Cancer and Blood Dis University of South Carolina School of M
7 Richland Medical Park
Columbia, SC 29203

803-434-7000
800-775-2287
www.palmettohealth.org

Joint clinical and basic research of juvenile cancer and blood disorders.
Charles D Beaman Jr, CEO

Tennessee

2300 St. Jude Children's Research Hospital
262 Danny Thomas Place
Memphis, TN 38105

901-495-3300
Fax: 901-495-4011
e-mail: donors@stjude.com
www.stjude.org

One of the world's premier pediatric cancer research centers.
Harvey J Cohen, Chair
William Evan PharmD, Director/CEO

2301 University of Tennessee Memphis: Cancer Center
N327 Van Vleet Building 3 N Dunlap
Memphis, TN 38163-0001

901-448-5150
Fax: 901-528-5033

Alvin M Mauer MD, Director

Texas

2302 Baylor University Bone Marrow Transplantation Research Center
Baylor Research Institute
3500 Gaston Avenue
Dallas, TX 75246

214-820-2687
800-422-9567
www.baylorhealth.com

Offers bone marrow transplantation research in leukemia studies.
John B McWhorter, President
Irving D Prengler, VP Medical Staff Affairs

2303   Baylor University Bone Marrow Transplantat Baylor Research Institute
3500 Gaston Avenue   214-820-2687
Dallas, TX 75246   800-422-9567
                                           Fax: 800-922-9567
                                        www.baylorhealth.com
Offers bone marrow transplantation research in leukemia studies.
John B McWhorter, President
Irving D Prengler, VP Medical Staff Affairs

2304   Cancer Therapy and Research Center
7979 Wurzbach Road   210-450-1000
San Antonio, TX 78229   800-340-2872
                                                www.ctrc.net
The mission of the Cancer Therapy & Research Center is to conquer cancer through research prevention and treatment.
Ian M Thompson MD, Director

2305   San Antonio Cancer Institute
7703 Floyd Curl Drive   210-567-7000
San Antonio, TX 78229-3900   Fax: 210-567-2709
                                          www.uthscsa.edu/
Dr Tyler J Curiel, Director
William L Henrich MD MACP, President

2306   Southwest Foundation for Biomedical Research
PO Box 760549
San Antonio, TX 78245-0549   210-258-9400
                                                www.sfbr.org
Advancing the health of our global community through innovative biomedical research.
John R Hurd, Chairman
Lewis J Moorman III, Vice-Chairman

2307   University of Texas: MD Anderson Cancer Center
1515 Holcombe Boulevard   713-792-2121
Houston, TX 77030-4009   800-392-1611
                                           www.mdanderson.org
To eliminate cancer in Texas the nation and the world through outstanding programs that integrate patient care research and prevention and through education for undergraduate and graduate students trainees professionals employees and the public.
John Mendelsohn, President -Executive Committee
Raymond DuBois, Executive Vice President

2308   University of Texas: Medical Branch at Galveston Cancer Center
301 University Boulevard   409-772-1011
Galveston, TX 77555   Fax: 409-747-1938
                                          TTY: 409-772-4200
                                  e-mail: public.affairs@utmb.edu
                                                www.utmb.edu
The mission of The University of Texas Medical Branch at Galveston is to provide scholarly teaching innovative scientific investigation and state-of-the-art patient care in a learning environment to better the health of society.
B Mark Evers, Director
David L Calender, President

Utah

2309   Brigham Young University Cancer Research Center
E181 Benson Science Building   801-422-3913
Provo, UT 84602   e-mail: cancer_research@byu.edu
                                          cancerresearch.byu.edu
Provide a rigorous research training program for students.
Daniel L Simmons, Director
Merrill J Christensen, Board Member

2310   Huntsman Cancer Institute University of Utah School of Medicine
University of Utah School of Medicine
2000 Circle of Hope   801-585-0303
Salt Lake City, UT 84112   877-585-0303
                                           Fax: 801-585-5886
                                  e-mail: public.affairs@hci.utah.edu
                                          www.huntsmancancer.org

Understand cancer from its beginnings to use that knowledge in the creation and improvement of cancer treatments to relieve the suffering of cancer patients and to provide education about cancer risk prevention and care.
Mary C Beckerle, Executive Director
Wallace Akerley, Senior Director of Clinical Research

Vermont

2311   University of Vermont Cancer Center University of Vermont
University of Vermont
E-213 Given Buildinge   802-656-4414
Burlington, VT 05405   877-540-4673
                                           Fax: 802-656-8788
                                  e-mail: info@vermontcancer.org
                                          www.vermontcancer.org
Richard Branda, Interim Director
Marianne Baggs, Assistant to the Director

Virginia

2312   Cancer Research Foundation of America
1600 Duke Street   703-836-4412
Alexandria, VA 22314-3421   800-227-2732
                                           Fax: 703-836-4413
                                  e-mail: mmcleod@crfa.org
                                          www.preventcancer.org
Prevention and early detection of cancer through research education and community outreach to all populations including children and the underserved.
Carolyn R Aldige, President and Founder
Marcia Myers Carlucci, Chairman

2313   Virginia Commonwealth University: Massey Cancer Center
401 College Street   804-828-0450
Richmond, VA 23298-5017   877-4MA-SSEY
                                           Fax: 804-828-8453
                                  e-mail: massey@vcu.edu
                                          www.massey.vcu.edu
The mission of the University of Central Arkansas is to maintain the highest academic quality and to ensure that its programs remain current and responsive to the diverse needs of those it serves.
Gordon D Ginder MD, Director
Steven Grant MD, Associate Director

Washington

2314   Fred Hutchinson Cancer Research Center
1100 Fairview Avenue N   206-288-7222
Seattle, WA 98109-1024   800-804-8824
                                           Fax: 206-288-1025
                                  e-mail: hutchdoc@fhcrc.org
                                                www.fhcrc.org
At Fred Hutchinson Cancer Research Center our interdisciplinary teams of world-renowned scientists and humanitarians work together to prevent diagnose and treat cancer HIV/AIDS and other diseases.
Lee Hartwell, Director/President
Mark Groudine, Executive Vice President and Deputy Dire

West Virginia

2315   West Virginia University: Mary Babb Randolph Cancer Center
Mary Babb Randolph Cancer Center Clinic
One Medical Center Drive   304-293-4500
Morgantown, WV 26506   877-427-2894
                                           Fax: 304-598-4553
                                          www.hsc.wvu.edu/mbrcc
Premier cancer facility with a national reputation of excellence in cancer treatment prevention and research.
Augusto Ochoa, Director

Wisconsin

2316   Eastern Cooperative Oncology Group
1818 Market Street   215-789-3645
Philadelphia, PA 19103   800-4 C-NCER
                                           Fax: 267-256-5291
                                          ecog.dfci.harvard.edu

Studies into cancer including biological response modifiers and cancer studies.

2317 University of Wisconsin Paul P Carbone Comprehensive Cancer Center
600 Highland Avenue   608-263-6400
Madison, WI 53792-6164   800-622-8942
                                     Fax: 608-263-8613
                          e-mail: gxw@medicine.wisc.edu
                                     www.cancer.wisc.edu
The University of Wisconsin Paul P. Carbone Comprehensive Cancer Center is the only comprehensive cancer center in Wisconsin as designated by the National Cancer Institute. An integral part of the UW School of Medicine and public Health this cancer center unites more than 250 physicians and scientists who work together in translating discoveries from research laboratories into new treatments that benefit cancer patients.
George Wildi MD, Director
Kelly Sitkin, Development Director

Support Groups & Hotlines

2318 American Cancer Society: San Jose Prostate Cancer Support Group
3369 Union Avenue
San Jose, CA 95124-2033   408-559-8553
                                          www.cancer.org

2319 American Foundation for Urologic Disease: Us Too Line
1128 N Charles Street   301-727-2908
Baltimore, MD 21201-5506   800-828-7866
                                    e-mail: admin@afud.org
                                          www.afud.org
Provides information and referrals for family members, victims and other individuals concerned with prostate cancer.

2320 American Institute for Cancer Research
1759 R Street NW   202-328-7744
Washington, DC 20009   800-843-8114
                                     Fax: 202-328-7226
                               e-mail: aicrweb@aicr.org
                                          www.aicr.org

2321 Cancer Information Service
National Cancer Institute
Fhch 1100 Fairview Avenue North J24   206-667-4675
Seattle, WA 98109-1024   800-422-6237
                                     Fax: 206-667-7792
                                     TTY: 800-332-8615
                                          www.cancer.gov
Provides the latest and most accurate cancer information to patients, their families, the public, and health professionals. Also provides personalized responses to specific questions about cancer and assistance to smokers who want to quit.
Nancy Zbaren, Program Director

2322 Cancer Support Community
401 Laurel Street   415-929-7400
San Francisco, CA 94118-1909
Offers understanding, support and guidance to people with cancer and those who care about them.
Victoria Wells, Executive Director

2323 Cancervive
11636 Chayote Street   310-203-9232
Los Angeles, CA 90049   800-486-2873
                                     Fax: 310-471-4618
                             e-mail: cancervivr@aol.com
                                          www.cancervive.org
Dedicated to providing support, public education and advocacy to those who have experienced this disease. The mission of Cancervive is to assist survivors to reclaim their lives after cancer.
Susan Nessim Keeney, Founder/President

2324 Center for Cancer Survival
104 W Anapamu Street   805-962-6221
Santa Barbara, CA 93101-3126

Nonprofit, nonmedical outreach education program teaching specific emotional, mental and spiritual skills for survival on their journey of recovery from cancer.
Richard Sheldon, Founder

2325 Collaborative Medicine Center
10 Willow Street   415-383-3197
Mill Valley, CA 94941-2895
Not specifically a cancer treatment center but works with cancer patients by using a variety of supportive modalities. The emphasis at the center is on helping people learn to support and activate their own healing processes.
Martin L Rossman MD

2326 Commonwealth Cancer Help Program
451 Mesa Road   415-868-0970
Bolinas, CA 94924   Fax: 415-868-2230
                       e-mail: commonweal@commonweal.org
                  www.commonweal.org/programs/cancer-help/
An educational program designed to help participants reduce the stress of cancer, explore health habits, be with others experiencing the same difficulties and consider information on established and complementary therapeutic options.
Michael Lerner, President
Susan Braun, Executive Director

2327 Corporate Angel Network
Westchester County Airport
One Loop Road   914-328-1313
White Plains, NY 10604-1215   866-328-1313
                                     Fax: 914-328-3938
                        e-mail: info@corpangelnetwork.org
                                     www.corpangelnetwork.org
To ease the emotional stress, physical discomfort and financial burden of travel for cancer patients by arranging free flights to treatment cetners, using the empty seats on corporate aircraft flying on routine business.
Peter H. Fleiss, Executive Director

2328 Exceptional Cancer Patients/ECaP
532 Jackson Park Drive   814-337-8192
Meadville, CT 16335   Fax: 814-337-0699
          e-mail: info@ecap-online.org, info@mind-body.org
                               www.ecap-online.org/home.htm
The mission of EcaP/Exceptional Cancer Patients is to provide exceptional resources, comprehensive professional training programs and extraordinary interdisciplinary retreats that help people facing the challenges of cancer and other chronic illnesses discover their inner healing resources.
Bernie Siegal MD, Founder
Barry Bittman MD, Chief Executive Officer

2329 Gilda's Club: Grand Rapids
1806 Bridge Street NW   616-453-8300
Grand Rapids, MI 49504   Fax: 616-453-8355
                             e-mail: info@gildasclubgr.org
                                          www.gildasclubgr.org
A free cancer support community of children, adults, families and friends.
Leann Arkema, President/CEO

2330 Gilda's Club: New York City
502 Eigth Avenue   718-788-1600
Brooklyn, NY 11215   Fax: 718-788-0322
                            e-mail: info@gildasclubnyc.org
                                          www.gildasclubnyc.org
Creates welcoming communities of free support for everyone living with cancer - men, women, teens and children - along with their families and friends. The innovative program is an essential complement to medical care, providing networking and support groups, workshops, lectures and social activities, all free of charge.
Robert Easton, Chairman of the Board
Lily Safani, CEO

2331 Gilda's Club: Quad Cities
1234 E River Drive   319-326-7504
Davenport, IA 52803   877-926-7504
                                    Fax: 563-323-1658
                            e-mail: qc@gildasclubqc.org
                                    www.gildasclubqc.org
A cancer support community providing people living with cancer, and all who touch their lives, access to other people going through the same experience.
Claudia Robinson, CEO

2332 Gilda's Club: South Florida
119 Rose Drive   954-763-6776
Fort Lauderdale, FL 33316   Fax: 954-763-6761
                    e-mail: info@gildasclubsouthflorida.org
                                www.gildasclubsouthflorida.org
A free cancer support community for women, men, children, and teens with all types of cancer and their families and friends. Offer networking groups, lectures, workshops, specialized children's and teen programs, and social events in a nonresidential, non-medical, home-like setting.
Shelley Goren, CEO

2333 I Can Cope
American Cancer Society
1599 Clifton Road NE   404-320-3333
Atlanta, GA 30329-4250   800-227-2345
                                          www.cancer.org
An educational program for people facing cancer, either personally, or as a friend or family caregiver. Helps dispel cancer myths by presenting straightforward facts and answers to your cancer-related questions

2334 International Association of Cancer Victors and Friends
7740 W Manchester Avenue   310-822-5032
Playa del Rey, CA 90293-8449   Fax: 310-822-4193
                            e-mail: IACUF@Inetworld.net
Offers reports and information on alternative therapies and recent cancer studies.
Ann Cinquina

2335 JamesCare For Life Support Groups & Services
James Cancer Hospital & Solove Research Institute
300 W 10th Avenue   614-293-5066
Columbus, OH 43210   800-293-5066
                                    Fax: 614-293-2565
                            e-mail: jamesline@osumc.edu
                                          cancer.osu.edu
JamesCare for Life Cancer Support Groups and Services provides a wide range of resources and services to assist patients and families on their journey. This group offers support for patients and families to share experiences, express concerns, and learn more about the impact of cancer and available treatments.
Michael A Caligiuri MD, CEO

2336 Look Good... Feel Better
American Cancer Society
1599 Clifton Road NE   404-320-3333
Atlanta, GA 30329-4250   800-227-2345
A community-based, free, national service. Teaches female cancer patients beauty tips to look better and feel good about how they look during chemotherapy and radiation treatments

2337 Lung Cancer Alliance Support Group
88 16th Street NW   202-463-2080
Washington, DC 20006   800-298-2436
                        e-mail: info@lungcanceralliance.org
                                www.lungcanceralliance.org
Dedicated solely to support and advocacy for all those living with or at risk for lung cancer.
Laurie Ambrose, President/CEO

2338 National Foundation for Cancer Research Hotline
4600 E W Highway   301-654-1250
Bethesda, MD 20814   800-321-2873
                                    Fax: 301-654-5824
                                    e-mail: info@nfcr.org
                                          www.nfcr.org
To support cancer research and public education relating to prevention, earlier diagnosis, better treatments and ultimately, a cure

for cancer. Promotes and facilitates collaboration among scientists to accelerate the pace of discovery from bench to bedside.
Silas Deane, VP Marketing/Communications

2339 National Health Information Center
PO Box 1133   310-565-4167
Washington, DC 20013-1133   800-336-4797
                                    Fax: 301-984-4256
                                    e-mail: info@nhic.org
                                        www.health.gov/nhic
A health information referral service sponsored by the Office of Disease Prevention and Health Promotion. Puts health professionals and consumers who have health questions in touch with those organizations that are best able to provide answers.

2340 National Hospice Helpline
1700 Diagonal Road   703-837-1500
Alexandria, VA 22314   800-658-8898
                                    Fax: 703-525-5762
                            e-mail: nhcpo_info@nhpco.org
                                          www.nhpco.org
Offers more information on hospice in general and offers referrals to a hospice program in your area.
Scott Vickers, Director

2341 PDQ
National Cancer Institute
6116 Executive Boulevard   301-402-5874
Bethesda, MD 20892-8322   800-422-6237
                                          www.cancer.gov
An NCI database that contains the latest information about cancer treatment, screening, prevention, genetics, supportive care, and complementary and alternative medicine, plus clinical trials.
Mark Greene MD, Editor-in-Chief

2342 Reach to Recovery
American Cancer Society
1599 Clifton Road NE   404-320-3333
Atlanta, GA 30329-4250   800-227-2345
                                          www.cancer.org
Provides support for people recentlry diagnosed with breast cancer; people facing a possible diagnosis of breast cancer; those interested in or who have undergone a lumpectomy or mastectomy; those considering breast reconstruction; those who have lymphedema; those who are undergoing or who have completed treatment such as chemotherapy and radiation therapy; people facing breast cancer recurrence or metastasis

2343 United Ostomy Associations of America Advocacy Hotline
PO Box 512
Northfield, MN 55057-0512   800-826-0826
                                    e-mail: info@uoaa.org
                                          www.ostomy.org
A national network for bowel and urinary diversion support groups in the United States. The goal is to provide a nonprofit association that will serve to unify and strengthen its member support groups, which are organized for the benefit of people who have, or will have intestinal or urinary diversions and their caregivers.
Dave Rudzin, President

2344 Wainwright House Cancer Support Programs
260 Stuyvesant Avenue   914-967-6080
Rye, NY 10580-3115
Weeklong residential retreats offered four times a year to cancer patients. Retreats are devoted to cancer patient education, health promotion and stress management.
Richard Grossman, Program Director

2345 Women's Suffrage for Prostate Cancer Awareness
743 Caribou Court
Sunnyvale, CA 94087-4229   800-776-2262
                                e-mail: info@pcawomen.org
                                          www.pcawomen.org
Women have banded together here to help people cope with the effects of prostate cancer on their lives and educate others about it. Members understand problems of patients and families and are here to support and educate.

Books

2346 3rd Opinion: International Directory to Complementary Therapy Centers
Avery Publishing Group
120 Old Broadway   516-741-2155
New Hyde Park, NY 11040-5000
Discusses over 300 alternative treatment cancer centers, educational centers, support groups and other research services.

2347 A Breast Cancer Journey: Your Personal Guidebook
American Cancer Society
1599 Clifton Road NE   404-320-3333
Atlanta, GA 30329-4250   800-227-2345
Helps women steer through the maze of information, empowering them to take control of their disease, treatment choices, health care team and life. Guidebook format encourages the reader to organize her information in a logical, easily accessible manner, record personal feelings and concerns and understand the details of practical matters such as paperwork and insurance, legal and sexual issues, side effects of treatment, and helping the entire family with support.
440 pages paperback
ISBN: 0-944235-20-4

2348 American Cancer Society Cancer Book
Doubleday & Company
666 5th Avenue
New York, NY 10103-0001   212-765-6500
www.randomhouse.com
Publishes 135 cancer organizations, centers, support services and various programs.

2349 American Cancer Society's Guide to Complementary/Alternative Cancer Methods
American Cancer Society
1599 Clifton Road NE   404-320-3333
Atlanta, GA 30329-4250   800-227-2345
Helps the public, the consumer and patients and their families understand what works, what's dangerous, and how best to evaluate the hundreds of claims that can be found on the internet and in the popular press. Each entry is researched and based on scientific evidence. Possible problems or complications are identified and clearly highlighted for easy reference. Covers a broad range, including herbs, vitamins, minerals, diet, manual healing and biological methods. Clear, understandable language.
464 pages hardcover
ISBN: 0-944235-20-4

2350 American Cancer Society's Guide to Pain Control
American Cancer Society
1599 Clifton Road NE   404-320-3333
Atlanta, GA 30329-4250   800-227-2345
Provides a wealth of information, including talking to your health care team about pain, understanding what pain is and where it comes from, current drug and non-drug treatments and dealing with the financial burden of pain treatment. Includes information on how to record, chart and rate pain, guidelines for pain management, a comprehensive list of medications and other methods of pain relief and an informative resource guide.
400 pages paperback
ISBN: 0-944235-20-4

2351 American Cancer Society's Healthy Eating Cookbook: A Celebration of Food...
American Cancer Society
1599 Clifton Road NE   404-320-3333
Atlanta, GA 30329-4250   800-227-2345
More than 200 pages of irresistable recipes that turn healthy eating into a celebration of good food. Features photos and recipes from a host of the American Cancer Society's celebrity friends and fans. Includes hundreds of recipes, celebrity photos and essays, a handy Smart Substitution reference section and numerous tips for healthy cooking, including smart shopping, using leftovers and eating out.
216 pages hardcover
ISBN: 0-944235-20-4

2352 Bowel Cancer
Oxford University Press
2001 Evans Road   212-726-6000
Cary, NC 27513-2010   800-451-7556
                                        Fax: 919-677-1303
                                        www.oup-usa.org
Offers information and public awareness on the disease of bowel cancer.
152 pages

2353 Breast Cancer
Branden Publishing Company
17 Station Street   617-734-2045
Brookline Village, MA 02147   Fax: 617-734-2046
                                        www.branden.com
Paperback
ISBN: 0-828319-49-9

2354 Cancer Dictionary
Facts on File
11 Penn Plaza   212-967-8800
New York, NY 10001   800-322-8755
                                        Fax: 800-678-3633
352 pages Paperback

2355 Cancer Facts and Figures
American Cancer Society
1599 Clifton Road NE   404-320-3333
Atlanta, GA 30329-4250   800-227-2345
Publishes over 57 treatment centers.

2356 Cancer Rates and Risks
National Cancer Institute
Building 31
Bethesda, MD 20892-0001   800-422-6237
This book is a compact guide to statistics, risk factors, and risks for major cancer sites.
136 pages

2357 Cancer Sourcebook
Karen Bellenir, author
Omnigraphics
Penobscot Building   313-961-1340
Detroit, MI 48226-4105   800-234-1340
                                        Fax: 800-875-1340
                                        www.omnigraphics.com/
Offers basic information on cancer types, symptoms, diagnostic methods, and treatments. Includes statistics on cancer occurrences worldwide and the risks associated with known carcinogens and activities.
2003 1119 pages
ISBN: 0-780806-33-6

2358 Cancer Therapy: Ind. Consumer's Guide to Non-Toxic Treatment & Prevention
Ralph W. Moss, author
Equinox Press
Cancer Decisions   814-238-3367
Lemont, PA 16851   800-980-1234
                                        Fax: 814-238-5865
                                        www.cancerdecisions.com
A must for cancer patients and their families who want: Practical information on the most promising non-toxic treatments; Scientific evidence in readable language; Well-documented resource lists and medical references.
523 pages
ISBN: 1-881025-06-3

2359 Cancer in the Family: Helping Children Cope with a Parent's Illness
American Cancer Society
1599 Clifton Road NE   404-320-3333
Atlanta, GA 30329-4250   800-227-2345
A diagnosis of cancer changes a family forever. Ordinary responsibilities become more demanding, and parents sometimes need assistance in balancing all of their children's needs. This book outlines steps to take to help children understand what happens when a parent has been diagnosed with cancer. Offers suggestions for talking to children, helping them cope, answering difficult

questions, managing role changes and disruptions in routines, recognizing signs that your child needs help.
272 pages paperback
ISBN: 0-944235-20-4

2360   Caregiving: A Step-By-Step Resource for Caring for the Person w/Cancer at Home
American Cancer Society
1599 Clifton Road NE   404-320-3333
Atlanta, GA 30329-4250   800-227-2345
This practical guide offers manageable solutions to the myriad conditions and situations the caregiver may face, from physical to emotional conditions and dealing with health care providers and insurance carriers, to taking care of his or her own needs as well as those of the patient. East to use, this handy reference offers thorough, concise check-lists, questions to ask, signs and symptoms to note, and where to turn for more help.
336 pages paperback
ISBN: 0-944235-20-4

2361   Celebrate! Healthy Entertaining for Any Occasion
American Cancer Society
1599 Clifton Road NE   404-320-3333
Atlanta, GA 30329-4250   800-227-2345
You can celebrate in style without taking a break from healthy eating or delicious food. This book combines 20 festive, fun theme menus with easy recipes that don't sacrifice taste. Each menu offers a combination of approximately 8 manageable recipes, including appetizers, main dishes, side dishes, desserts and even beverages. Activities and decorating ideas in each section help make entertaining a breeze.
272 pages paperback
ISBN: 0-944235-20-4

2362   Choices: Realistic Alternatives in Cancer Treatment
Harper Collins
Avenue of the Americas
New York, NY 10019   800-331-3761
                                                                   Fax: 800-822-4090
Covers a wide gamut of information that includes treatment centers, associations, research groups, and other facilities that are equipped to assist cancer patients and their families.

2363   Colorectal Cancer: A Compassionate Resource for Patients and Their Families
American Cancer Society
1599 Clifton Road NE   404-320-3333
Atlanta, GA 30329-4250   800-227-2345
Addresses the full range of issues that colorectal cancer patients and their families may face- from what to do when confronted with a diagnosis to the latest medical data, treatment and procedures. Describes the process of the digestive system and the organs involved when the body is affected by colorectal cancer. Dietary factors for preventing colorectal cancer are explained and information about surgery, chemotherapy and radiation treatment follows. Includes easy recipes and a diet plan.
290 pages paperback
ISBN: 0-944235-20-4

2364   Consumer's Guide to Cancer Drugs
American Cancer Society
1599 Clifton Road NE   404-320-3333
Atlanta, GA 30329-4250   800-227-2345
Created for patients, cancer survivors and caregivers. Provides detailed information for the more than 200 medicines used to treat cancer or the symptoms of cancer. Drugs are listed alphabetically by generic name and described in depth. Detailed descriptions include common side effects, precautions and other important facts. All generic and trade names are listed in the index for easy cross-reference. Easy-to-understand language.
448 pages paperback
ISBN: 0-944235-20-4

2365   Coping: A Young Woman's Guide to Breast Cancer Prevention
Rosen Publishing Group
29 E 21st Street   212-777-3017
New York, NY 10010   800-237-9932
                                                                   Fax: 888-436-4643
                                         e-mail: customerservice@rosenpub.com
                                                             www.rosenpublishing.com

Breast cancer research has revealed the genetic predisposition of some cancers. This guide explains the nature of cancer, the risk of cancer and the ways to reduce that risk, especially for young women with a family history of breast cancer.

ISBN: 0-825929-67-1

2366   Everyone's Guide to Cancer Therapy
Andrews McMeel Publishing, LLC
c/o Simon & Schuster, Inc.
Riverside, NJ 08075   800-943-9839
                                                              Fax: 800-943-9831
                                   e-mail: MPrzybylski@amuniversal.com
                                                           www.andrewsmcmeel.com
How cancer is diagnosed, treated, and managed day to day.
2002 960 pages Paperback
ISBN: 0-740718-56-8

2367   Health Consequences of Smoking: Cancer & Chronic Lung Disease in the Workplace
DIANE Publishing Company
330 Pusey Avenue, Unit #3 Rear   610-461-6200
Darby, PA 19023   800-782-3833
                                                              Fax: 610-461-6130
                                   e-mail: dianepublishing@gmail.com
                                                           www.dianepublishing.net
Examines the relationship between cigarette smoking and occupational exposures. Establishes that in order to protect the workers fully, forces of labor, management, insurers and government must become as engaged in attempts to reduce the prevalence of cigarette smoking as they are in occupational exposure. Tables and figure. Extensive bibliography, index.
542 pages Paperback
ISBN: 0-788123-11-4
Herman Baron, Publisher

2368   Healthy and Hearty Diabetic Cooking
Diabetes Self-Management Books
PO Box 11477
Des Moines, IA 50381-0001   800-664-9269
James Hazlett, Editor
Melissa Glim, Associate Editor

2369   Home Care Guide for Cancer
John's Hopkins University Press
2715 N Charles Street   410-516-6900
Baltimore, MD 21218-4319   800-537-5487
                                                              Fax: 410-516-6998
                                                              www.press.jhu.edu
This easy to use workbook was designed for home caregivers, patients, support groups and education programs; it features easy to read type and index for quick reference and advice on twenty common cancer caregiving problems.
1996 260 pages Paperback
ISBN: 0-943126-30-4

2370   I Choose to Fight: Tom Harper's Courageous Victory Over Cancer
Prentice Hall
15 Columbus Circle
New York, NY 10023-7707   212-373-8000
                                                              www.prenhall.com
A semi, auto-biographical account of Tom Harper's ordeal with testicular cancer, an afflication in young men.

2371   Informed Decisions: The Complete Book of Cancer Diagnosis, Treatment and Recovery
American Cancer Society
1599 Clifton Road NE   404-320-3333
Atlanta, GA 30329-4250   800-227-2345
Offers the latest information on every aspect of cancer, from detection to recovery. Covers everything from cancer causes and risk, screening and diagnostic tests, and treatment strategies to coping tips and questions to ask your doctor. Includes tips on how to effectively deal with the system and get the most advanced care in the country. Helps cancer patients and families make the right kinds of decisions- decisions that suit your particular needs and desires, and help you feel in control.
690 pages hardcover
ISBN: 0-944235-20-4

2372 Kid's 1st Cookbook: Delicious-Nutritious Treats to Make Yourself
American Cancer Society
1599 Clifton Road NE
Atlanta, GA 30329-4250
404-320-3333
800-227-2345
Do creepy spiders, sloppy dogs and tornado swirls sound edible to you? They will to kids. Inside this beautifully illustrated hardcover edition are activities, colorful recipes and cooking tips that will turn meal preparation into exciting family fun. Kids of all ages can take charge, don a chef's hat and create delicious and nutricious snacks and dishes for every meal.
96 pages hardcover
ISBN: 0-944235-20-4

2373 Love Knot
Jones & Bartlett Publishers
40 Tall Pine Drive
Sudbury, MA 01776
978-443-5000
800-832-0034
Fax: 978-443-8000
e-mail: aberry@jbpub.com
www.jbpub.com
232 pages Paperback
ISBN: 0-763714-12-7
Joy Stark, Associate Marketing Manager

2374 My Prostate and Me: Dealing with Prostate Cancer
Addison Books
2719 Houston Avenue
Houston, TX 77009-7607
800-829-9653

2375 National Cancer Institute Fact Book
National Cancer Institute
Building 31
Bethesda, MD 20892-0001
800-422-6237
This book presents general information about the National Cancer Institute including budget data, grants and contracts and historical information.

2376 No Less a Woman
Firestone Touchstone Paperbacks/Simon & Schuster
200 Old Tappan Road
Old Tappan, NJ 07675-7005
800-999-5479
Offers intimate interviews that explore the major issues of coping and surviving breast cancer, from diagnosis and treatment to physical and psychological recovery. In their own words, ten women describe how they successfully adjusted to the changes in their bodies and their feelings about themselves.
288 pages
ISBN: 0-671868-99-3

2377 Organizing and Maintaining Support Groups for Parents
Candlelighters' Childhood Cancer Foundation
7910 Woodmont Avenue
Bethesda, MD 20814-3015
301-657-8401
800-366-2223
Benefits of self-help support groups, activities, referral systems and parent/professional relations.

2378 Prostate Cancer: A Survivor's Guide
Don Kaltenbach and Tim Richards, author
Dattoli Cancer Foundation
2803 Fruitville Road
Sarasota, FL 24237
941-365-5599
800-915-1001
Fax: 941-366-3786
e-mail: info@dattolifoundation.org
www.dattolifoundation.org
Written with the aid of leading prostate cancer specialists, this book clearly explains tests, the latest statistics and how to interpret them.
updated 2003 256 pages
ISBN: 0-964008-89-0

2379 Prostate Cancer: What Every Man and His Family Needs to Know
American Cancer Society
1599 Clifton Road NE
Atlanta, GA 30329-4250
404-320-3333
800-227-2345
Written by a team of internationally known and respected medical experts, this newly revised edition explains everything a man needs to know about prostate cancer, the most common form of cancer (excluding skin cancer) among American men.
322 pages paperback
ISBN: 0-944235-20-4

2380 Prostate Health Workbook
Newton Malerman, author
Hunter House Publishing
PO Box 2194
Alameda, CA 94501
510-865-5282
800-266-5592
Fax: 510-865-4295
e-mail: ordering@hunterhouse.com
www.hunterhouse.com
A practical guide for the prostate cancer patients.
2002 160 pages Paperback
Cristina Sverdrup, Customer Service Manager

2381 Singing from the Soul
Bone Marrow Foundation
981 1st Avenue
New York, NY 10022-5102
212-838-3029
800-365-1336
e-mail: thebmf@aol.com
www.bonemarrow.org
Jose Carreras' autobiography describes in eloquent detail his bone marrow transplant experience.

2382 Teratologies: A Cultural Study of Cancer
Routledge
270 Madison Avenue
New York, NY 10016
212-216-7800
Fax: 212-563-2269
www.routledge.com
A distinctively feminist look at how cancer is perceived, experienced and theorized in contemporary society. Beginning with powerful personal accounts of her own illness, as well as self-help manuals and patients' personal stories, Jackie Stacey explores changing beliefs about the causes and treatments of cancer in both biomedecine and its increasingly popular alternative counterparts.
304 pages

2383 The Mountain You've Climbed: A Parent's Guide to Childhood Cancer Survivorship
1015 Locust Street
Saint Louis, MO 63101
314-241-1600
Fax: 314-241-1996
e-mail: krudd@children-cancer.org
www.nationalchildrenscancersociety.org
This guide is designed to answer parent's questions regarding childhood cancer, address issues related to diagnosis and offer suggestions on how to integrate the cancer experience into all areas of the family's life. It addresses issues beginning from the time of diagnosis through the completion of treatment and beyond.
Mark Slocomb, Chairman
Mark Stolze, President/CEO

2384 Understanding Breast Cancer Genetics
Barbara T Zimmerman, PhD, author
University Press of Mississippi
3825 Ridgewood Road
Jackson, MS 39211-6492
601-432-6205
Fax: 601-432-6217
e-mail: kburgess@ihl.state.ms.us
www.upress.state.ms.us
Clinical explanations for the genetic causes of the disease women most greatly fear.
2004 128 pages Paperback
ISBN: 1-578065-79-8
Kathy Burgess, Advertising/Marketing Services Manager

2385 Understanding Cancer Therapies
Helen S L Chan, MD, author
University Press of Mississippi
3825 Ridgewood Road
Jackson, MS 39211-6492
601-432-6205
Fax: 601-432-6217
e-mail: kburgess@ihl.state.ms.us
www.upress.state.ms.us
A practical and hopeful guide to the many treatments available.
2006 144 pages Paperback
ISBN: 1-578066-89-1
Kathy Burgess, Advertising/Marketing Services Manager

2386 Understanding Colon Cancer
A Richard Adrouny, MD; FACP, author

University Press of Mississippi
3825 Ridgewood Road   601-432-6205
Jackson, MS 39211-6492   Fax: 601-432-6217
                              e-mail: kburgess@ihl.state.ms.us
                                      www.upress.state.ms.us
For the general reader a concise manual of facts, warnings, prevention, treatments, and forecasts.
2002 168 pages Paperback
ISBN: 1-578062-03-9
Kathy Burgess, Advertising/Marketing Services Manager

2387 When a Parent Has Cancer: A Guide to Caring for Your Children

Harper Collins
10 E 53rd Street
New York, NY 10022   212-207-7000
                                    www.harpercollins.com

ISBN: 0-060187-09-3

2388 Women and Cancer: A Compassionate Reource for Patients and Their Families

American Cancer Society
1599 Clifton Road NE   404-320-3333
Atlanta, GA 30329-4250   800-227-2345
Concise, thorough and up-to-date, this book provides women who have been diagnosed with cancer information about the four most common cancers of the reproductive system- breast, cervical, endometrial and ovarian cancer. Each chapter describes how each organ is structured and how it functions, and the risks and benefits of new drug therapies, radiation and chemotherapy, and surgical procedures. Includes patient stories and addresses the full range of issues faced by patients and their families.
290 pages paperback
ISBN: 0-944235-20-4

2389 Young People with Cancer: A Handbook for Parents
Barry Leonard, author

DIANE Publishing Company
330 Pusey Avenue, Unit #3 Rear   610-461-6200
Darby, PA 19023   800-782-3833
                                  Fax: 610-461-6130
                        e-mail: dianepublishing@gmail.com
                                  www.dianepublishing.net
Gives you information on all stages of your child's cancer. It tells you what to expect and suggests ways to prepare for different situations.
109 pages Paperback
ISBN: 0-756736-59-5
Herman Baron, Publisher

Children's Books

2390 Cancer

Franklin Watts Grolier
90 Old Sherman Turnpike   203-797-3500
Danbury, CT 06816-0001   800-621-1115
                                  Fax: 203-797-3197
                                      www.grolier.com
Discusses causes such as chemicals, viruses, radiation and oncogenes, as well as diagnosis, types of cancers, immune defenses and common treatments.
96 pages Grades 7-12
ISBN: 0-531108-03-1

2391 Cancer: Overview Series

Lucent Books
Thomson Gale
Farmington Hills, MI 48333-9187   800-877-4253
                                  Fax: 800-414-5043
                  e-mail: gale.customerservice@thomson.com
                                    www.gale.com/lucent

Questions are answered for young adults on the issues of cancer prevention and treatment.
1999 112 pages
ISBN: 1-560063-63-7

2392 Help Yourself: Tips for Teenagers with Cancer

National Cancer Institute
Building 31
Bethesda, MD 20892-0001   800-422-6237
This magazine-style booklet is designed to provide information and support adolescents with cancer.
37 pages

2393 Hospital Days: Treatment Ways

National Cancer Institute
Building 31
Bethesda, MD 20892-0001   800-422-6237
Coloring book helping to orient children with cancer to hospital and treatment procedures.
26 pages

2394 Kathy's Hats: A Story of Hope
Trudy Krisher, author

Albert Whitman & Company
6340 Oakton Street   847-581-0033
Morton Grove, IL 60053-2723   800-255-7675
                                  Fax: 847-581-0039
                          e-mail: mail@awhitmanco.com
                                    www.albertwhitman.com
When Kathy turns nine she learns she has cancer. When she loses her hair due to the chemotherapy, she feels ugly and awkward. This is a matter-of-fact book about a tough time and subject, and its calm and respectable treatment well serves a story that is indeed one of hope.
32 pages Hardcover
ISBN: 0-807541-16-6
Pat McPartland, Sales
Joe Campbell, Customer Service

2395 Kemo Shark

Kidscope
3400 Peachtree Road NE
Atlanta, GA 30326-1107   404-233-0001
                                      www.kidscope.org
Color comic book designed to help children with the psychological and physiological changes in a family where a parent has cancer and chemotherapy.

2396 Living with Cancer

Franklin Watts Grolier
90 Old Sherman Turnpike   203-797-3500
Danbury, CT 06816-0001   800-621-1115
                                  Fax: 203-797-3197
                                      www.grolier.com
Shows how persons with cancer can overcome their illness and lead productive lives.
32 pages Grades 5-7
ISBN: 0-531108-59-7

2397 My Book for Kids with Cancer

Waterfront Books
98 Brookes Avenue
Burlington, VT 05401-3326   800-639-6063
                                www.waterfrontbooks.com/
Frustrated because he couldn't find any books about kids who survived cancer, Jason decided to write his own.
32 pages

2398 Our Mom Has Cancer

American Cancer Society
1599 Clifton Road NE   404-320-3333
Atlanta, GA 30329-4250   800-227-2345
When Abigail and Adrienne's mom told them she had cancer, they were afraid. But when the girls couldn't find any books that explained what might happen to their mother and what they might expect, they wrote one themselves. The girls, ages 9 and 11, tell readers that when their mother was tired during treatment, friends and family pitched in to help cook and to push her in her wheel-

chair. When chemotherapy made their mom's hair fall out, they threw a hat party for her.

32 pages hardcover
ISBN: 0-944235-20-4

2399 Sammie's New Mask: A Coloring Book for Friends of Children with Cancer
1015 Locust Street
Saint Louis, MO 63101
314-241-1600
Fax: 314-241-1996
e-mail: krudd@children-cancer.org
www.nationalchildrenscancersociety.org
Sammie's New Mask is about a young girl named Sammie and her friend, Jack, who has cancer. This story addresses Sammie's concerns and common misconceptions about cancer. This coloring book is designed for children in kindergarten through third grade.

K-3rd Grade
Mark Slocomb, Chairman
Mark Stolze, President/CEO

2400 Sammy's Mommy Has Cancer: For Children Who Have a Loved One with Cancer
Sherry Kohlenberg, author
Magination Press (American Psychological Assoc.)
750 First Street NE
Washington, DC 20002-4242
202-336-5510
800-374-2721
Fax: 202-336-5502
TDD: 202-336-6123
e-mail: magination@apa.org
www.apamaginationpress.apa.org
Sherry Kohlenberg wrote this book after she was diagnosed with breast cancer for her son. It is a warm, sensitive, straightforward story that will help young children understand and accept the changes in their lives when a parent is diagnosed with a life threatening illness. Parents will welcome this valuable aid in explaining the illness to their children. Both the story and the introduction offer useful suggestions for involving children in the jiys and sorrows of good and bad days.

1993 32 pages Softcover
ISBN: 0-945354-55-X

2401 Silver Kiss
Delacorte
1540 Broadway
New York, NY 10036-4039
212-354-6500
This moving tale describes the feelings of Zoe as her mother dies of cancer and her family attempts to shield her from seeing the slow decline in her mother.

Grades 8-12

2402 Silver Linings: Living with Cancer
Vantage Press
516 W 34th Street
New York, NY 10001-1395
212-736-1767
Fax: 212-736-2273
Highly personal journey of one woman's battle with breast cancer for over thirty-five years. From operations, radiation treatments, and hormone therapy and her faith and hope while induring them.

ISBN: 0-533113-52-0

2403 The Mountain You've Climbed: A Young Adult Guide to Childhood Cancer Survivorship
1015 Locust Street
Saint Louis, MO 63101
314-241-1600
Fax: 314-241-1996
e-mail: krudd@children-cancer.org
www.nationalchildrenscancersociety.org
This guide is designed to answer questions and address issues related to cancer survivorship for people ages 15 to 24. As survivorship rates continue to increase, the knowledge regarding late-effects also continues to increase. This survivorship guide will answer questions as well as address healthy living styles for your future.

Ages 15-24
Mark Slocomb, Chairman
Mark Stolze, President/CEO

2404 They Never Want to Tell You: Children Talk About Cancer
Harvard University Press

79 Garden Street
Cambridge, MA 02138
617-495-2480
800-448-2242
Fax: 800-962-4983
www.hup.harvard.edu
A comprehensive book that focuses on eight children who share their various experiences with cancer.

Grades 7-12
ISBN: 0-674883-70-5

2405 Waiting for Johnny Miracle
Harper & Row
10 E 53rd Street
New York, NY 10022-5299
212-207-7000
This powerful book focuses on Becky, a 17-year-old girl who must face the fear of cancer after being diagnosed with a malignant tumor. This book brings up the painful issues that come with the pain, treatment and death of cancer.

Grades 8-12

2406 Why God Gave Me Pain
Loyola University Press
3441 N Ashland Avenue
Chicago, IL 60657-1355
773-281-1818
Using a girl's diary entries, this book expounds on the side effects of cancer as well as the psychological ramifications of the debilitating disease.

Magazines

2407 American Journal of Clinical Oncology: Cancer Clinical Trials
Raven Press
1185 Avenue of the Americas
New York, NY 10036-2601
212-930-9500
800-777-2295
Offers outstanding coverage of ongoing research in cancer treatment. This journal is the primary source for timely updates covering all aspects of cancer management.

BiMonthly
ISBN: 0-277373-2 -
Luther W Brady, Editor

2408 Cancer Detection and Prevention Journal
Elsevier
Journals Customer Service Dept.
Orlando, FL 32887-4800
877-839-7126
Fax: 407-363-1354
e-mail: usjcs@elsevier.com
www.elsevier.com
A peer-refereed journal devoted to cancer prevention by predictive and preventitive oncology. It is uniquely focused on advances in genetics, molecular medicine and biotechnologies that have an impact on clinical oncology modalities.

2002-present

2409 Cancer Nursing: An International Journal for Cancer Care
Lippincott Williams & Wilkins
PO Box 1600
Hagerstown, MD 21741-1600
800-638-3030
Fax: 301-223-2400
e-mail: orders@lww.com
www.lww.com
Addresses the whole spectrum of problems arising in the care and support of cancer patients- prevention and early detection, geriatric and pediatric cancer nursing, medical and surgical oncology, ambulatory care, nutritional support, psychosocial aspects of cancer, patient responces to all treatment modalities, and specific nursing interventions.

BiMonthly
ISBN: 0-162220-X -

2410 Diseases of the Colon and Rectum
American Society of Colon and Rectal Surgeons
85 W Algonquin Road
Arlington Heights, IL 60005
847-290-9184
Fax: 847-290-9203
e-mail: ascrs@fascrs.org
www.fascrs.org
Diseases of the Colon and Rectum (DCR) is the official journal of the American Society of Colon and Rectal Surgeons and is mailed

to all members on a mothly basis as a member benefit. Non-member subscribers have access to the online version of DCR.
journal

2411   Pancreas
Raven Press
1185 Avenue of the Americas   212-930-9500
New York, NY 10036-2601   800-777-2295
Provides a central forum for communication of original works involving both basic and clinical research on the exocrine and endocrine pancreas and their consequences in the disease state.
8x Year
ISBN: 0-885317-7 -
Vay Liang W Go, Editor

2412   Practice Parameters
American Society of Colon and Rectal Surgeons
85 W Algonquin Road   847-290-9184
Arlington Heights, IL 60005   Fax: 847-290-9203
                                     e-mail: ascrs@fascrs.org
                                     www.fascrs.org
Parameters that have been published in the scientific journal Diseases of the Colon and Rectum, along with other scientific journals. They can be found on the website under Professionals.

2413   Roswellness Magazine
Roswell Park Cancer Institute
Elm & Carlton Streets   716-845-2300
Buffalo, NY 14263   877-275-7724
                                     e-mail: askrpci@roswellpark.org
                                     www.roswellpark.org
A consumer magazine promoting good health habits, cancer prevention and early detection, and the services of Roswell Park Cancer Institute.
2x/year
Donald L Trump MD, FACP, President/CEO
Candace Johnson PhD, Deputy Director

2414   Skin Cancer Foundation Journal
Skin Cancer Foundation
245 5th Avenue   212-725-5176
New York, NY 10016-8728   800-754-6490
                                     Fax: 212-725-5751
                                     e-mail: info@skincancer.org
                                     www.skincancer.org
A collection of articles by physicians, scientists and lay writers on the subject.

Newsletters

2415   Candlelighters' Quarterly
Childhood Cancer Foundation
7910 Woodmont Avenue   301-657-8401
Bethesda, MD 20814   800-366-2223
Artlices on living with and treating pediatric/adolescent cancer, written by and for parents and professionals in the field. Includes reviews, resources, pen pal column, and more.

2416   Candlelighters' Youth Newsletter
Childhood Cancer Foundation
7910 Woodmont Avenue   301-657-8401
Bethesda, MD 20814-3015   800-366-2223
Offers information to teenagers and young adults on cancer issues, medical information, camps and programs.
Quarterly

2417   Exceptional Cancer Patients/ECaP Newsletter
Exceptional Cancer Patients/ECaP
532 Jackson Park Drive   814-337-8192
Meadville, CT 16335   Fax: 814-337-0699
                                     e-mail: info@ecap-online.org, info@mind-body.org
                                     www.ecap-online.org/home.htm
E-newsletter with inspirational articles
2x/year
Bernie Siegal MD, Founder
Barry Bittman MD, Chief Executive Officer

2418   Melanoma Newsletter
Skin Cancer Foundation

245 5th Avenue   212-725-5176
New York, NY 10016-8728   800-754-6490
                                     Fax: 212-725-5751
                                     e-mail: info@skincancer.org
                                     www.skincancer.org
For medical investigators and practitioners.

2419   Nutrition Action Healthletter
Center for Science in the Public Interest
1875 Connecticut Avenue NW   202-332-9110
Washington, DC 20009-5736   Fax: 202-265-4954
                                     e-mail: cspi@cspinet.org
                                     www.cspinet.org
The nation's leading consumer group concerned with food and nutrition issues. Focuses on diseases that result from consuming too many calories, too much fat, sodium and sugar such as cancer and heart disease.
16 pages 10 per year
Stephen Schmidt, Editor

2420   Oncology Times: The News Center for the Cancer Care Team
Lippincott Williams & Wilkins
PO Box 1600
Hagerstown, MD 21741-1600   800-638-3030
                                     Fax: 301-223-2400
                                     e-mail: orders@lww.com
                                     www.lww.com
Reports on breaking clinical news in oncology, radiology, surgery, chemotherapy, and biological and gene therapy, as well as the professional, political, reimbursement, and practice management issues that affect those treating cancer patients.
2x Monthly

2421   Options: New Directions in the War on Cancer
People Against Cancer
614 E Street   515-972-4444
Otho, IA 50569-0010   Fax: 515-972-4415
                                     e-mail: info@peopleagainstcancer.com
                                     www.peopleagainstcancer.com
Published by People Against Cancer.
8 pages
Frank Wiewel, Executive Director

2422   Phoenix: Newsletter
Candlelighters' Childhood Cancer Foundation
7910 Woodmont Avenue   301-657-8401
Bethesda, MD 20814-3015   800-366-2223
For adult survivors of childhood cancer.

2423   Sun and Skin News
Skin Cancer Foundation
245 5th Avenue   212-725-5176
New York, NY 10016-8728   800-754-6490
                                     Fax: 212-725-5751
                                     e-mail: info@skincancer.org
                                     www.skincancer.org
Deals with skin cancer and related subjects in nontechnical terms.

2424   Support for People with Oral and Head and Neck Cancer
PO Box 53   516-759-5333
Locust Valley, NY 11560-0053   800-377-0928
                                     Fax: 516-671-8794
                                     e-mail: info@spohnc.org
                                     www.spohnc.org
This a patient run support program. Other services include patient networking oportunities, a national newsletter, a resource library and insurance information and assistance.
Nancy E Leupold, President/Founder

2425   The Phoenix
United Ostomy Associations of America, Inc.
The Phoenix Magazine   949-600-7296
Mission Viejo, CA 92690   800-826-0826
                                     e-mail: publisher@uoaa.org
                                     www.uoaa.org
The Phoenix magazine is the official publication of the United Ostomy Associations of America, Inc. and is published four times a year- December, March, June, and September.
Quarterly

2426 Voice of Hope
National Children's Cancer Society
1015 Locust Street   314-241-1600
Saint Louis, MO 63101   Fax: 314-241-1996
e-mail: krudd@children-cancer.org
www.nationalchildrenscancersociety.org
It educates donors on how their support is furthering the N.C.C.S. mission, and acknowledges supporters. Distributed to donors of the N.C.C.S.
3x/year
Mark Slocomb, Chairman
Mark Stolze, President/CEO

Pamphlets

2427 Advanced Cancer: Living Each Day
National Cancer Institute
Building 31
Bethesda, MD 20892-0001   800-422-6237
Booklet delving into all aspects of everyday living with cancer. Offers information on coping, how children react, facing the unknown, living wills, additional resources and making treatment decisions.
30 pages

2428 After Breast Cancer: A Guide to Followup Care
National Cancer Institute
Building 31
Bethesda, MD 20892-0001   800-422-6237
Explains the importance of checking for possible signs of recurring cancer by receiving regular mammograms, getting breast exams from a doctor, and continuing monthly breast self-exams.
15 pages

2429 Basic Family Library
Candlelighters' Childhood Cancer Foundation
7910 Woodmont Avenue   301-657-8401
Bethesda, MD 20814-3015   800-366-2223
A bibliography of materials on childhood cancers, medical support, death and bereavement and materials for children.

2430 Brachytherapy and IMRT
Michael Dattoli, Jennifer Cash, and Don Kaltenbach, author
Dattoli Cancer Foundation
2803 Fruitville Road   941-365-5599
Sarasota, FL 34237   800-915-1001
Fax: 941-366-3786
e-mail: info@dattolifoundation.org
www.dattolifoundation.org
A primer on seed implants and Intensity Modulated Radiation Therapy (IMRT). This booklet provides a comprehensive overview of prostate cancer treatment protocols that utilize brachytherapy and IMRT either with or without hormonal therapy.
50 pages Booklet

2431 Breast Biopsy: What You Should Know
National Cancer Institute
Building 31   301-496-4000
Bethesda, MD 20892-0001
Offers information on what happens before, during and after a breast biopsy.

2432 Breast Cancer: Understanding Treatment Options
National Cancer Institute
Building 31
Bethesda, MD 20892-0001   800-422-6237
Summarizes the biopsy procedure and examines the pros and cons of various types of breast surgery. It discusses lumpectomy and radiation therapy as primary treatment.
19 pages

2433 Breast Exams: What You Should Know
National Cancer Institute
Building 31
Bethesda, MD 20892-0001   800-422-6237

Provides answers to questions about breast cancer and breast screening methods.
10 pages

2434 Camps for Children with Cancer and their Siblings
Candlelighters' Childhood Cancer Foundation
7910 Woodmont Avenue   301-657-8401
Bethesda, MD 20814-3015   800-366-2223
A listing by state of day and overnight camp programs, children served and programs.

2435 Cancer Tests You Should Know About: A Guide for People 65 and Over
National Cancer Institute
Building 31
Bethesda, MD 20892-0001   800-422-6237
Describes the cancer tests important for people age 65 and older. Informs men and women of the exams they should be requesting when they schedule checkups with their doctors.
14 pages

2436 Cancer of the Bladder: Research Report
National Cancer Institute
Building 31
Bethesda, MD 20892-0001   800-422-6237
Offers information on the types of bladder cancer, mortality rates, diagnosis, symptoms, therapies, rehabilitation, clinical trials, and selected references.

2437 Cancer of the Colon and Rectum: Research Report
National Cancer Institute
Building 31
Bethesda, MD 20892-0001   800-422-6237
Informative pamphlet offering factual statistics on causes and prevention, detection, diagnosis, staging, treatment, followup, clinical trials and selected references.

2438 Cancer of the Ovary: Research Report
National Cancer Institute
Building 31
Bethesda, MD 20892-0001   800-422-6237

2439 Cancer of the Pancreas: Research Report
National Cancer Institute
Building 31
Bethesda, MD 20892-0001   800-422-6237
Offers information on the various types of pancreatic cancer, treatments, surgical procedures, chemotherapy, biological therapy, hormone therapy, clinical trials and selected references.

2440 Cancer of the Uterus: Endometrial Cancer
National Cancer Institute
Building 31
Bethesda, MD 20892-0001   800-422-6237
Offers information on the description and function of the uterus, incidence and mortality, possible causes and prevention, detection, diagnosis, staging, treatment, clinical trials and selected references.

2441 Cancer of the Uterus: Research Report
National Cancer Institute
Building 31
Bethesda, MD 20892-0001   800-422-6237

2442 Candlelighters Guide to Bone Marrow Transplants in Children
Candlelighters' Childhood Cancer Foundation
7910 Woodmont Avenue   301-657-8401
Bethesda, MD 20814-3015   800-366-2223
For parents who are contemplating a BMT or harvest for their child or whose child is undergoing the procedure.

2443 Chemotherapy and You: A Guide to Self-Help During Treatment
National Cancer Institute
Building 31
Bethesda, MD 20892-0001   800-422-6237
Explains chemotherapy and addresses problems and concerns of patients undergoing this treatment.

2444 Chew or Snuff is Real Bad Stuff
National Cancer Institute

Building 31 301-435-3848
Bethesda, MD 20892-2580 800-422-6237
www.nci.nih.gov
Designed for young adults, this brochure describes the health and social effects of using smokeless tobacco products.

2445 Clearing the Air: A Guide to Quitting Smoking
National Cancer Institute
Building 31
Bethesda, MD 20892-0001 800-422-6237
Offers hints on quitting smoking and cancer prevention.
24 pages

2446 Cutaneous Melanoma of the Head and Neck
American Academy of Otolaryngology
1 Prince Street 703-836-4444
Alexandria, VA 22314-3357 Fax: 703-683-5100
www.entnet.org

Self-instruction package.
Paperback
ISBN: 1-567720-22-6

2447 Diet, Nutrition and Cancer Prevention: The Good News
National Cancer Institute
Building 31
Bethesda, MD 20892-0001 800-422-6237
Provides an overview of dietary guidelines that may assist individuals in reducing their risks for some cancers.
16 pages

2448 Diet, Nutrition and Cancer Prevention: A Guide to Food Choices
National Cancer Institute
Building 31
Bethesda, MD 20892-0001 800-422-6237
Describes what is known about diet, nutrition and cancer prevention. Provides information about foods that contain components like fiber, fat and vitamins that may affect a person's risk of getting certain cancers.

2449 Dilemmas of Providing Help in a Crisis: The Role of Friends & Parents
Candlelighters' Childhood Cancer Foundation
7910 Woodmont Avenue 301-657-8401
Bethesda, MD 20814-3015 800-366-2223

2450 Do the Right Thing: Get a Mammogram
National Cancer Institute
Building 31
Bethesda, MD 20892-0001 800-422-6237
Targets black women age 40 and older. Describes the importance of regular mammograms in the early detection of breast cancer.

2451 Eating Hints: Recipes and Tips for Better Nutrition During Cancer Treatment
National Cancer Institute
Building 31
Bethesda, MD 20892-0001 800-422-6237
Provides recipes that help patients meet their needs for good nutrition during treatment.

2452 Facing Forward: A Guide for Cancer Survivors
National Cancer Institute
Building 31
Bethesda, MD 20892-0001 800-422-6237
Presents a concise overview of important survivor issues, including ongoing health needs, psychosocial concerns, insurance and employment.
43 pages

2453 Facts About Lung Cancer
American Lung Association
1740 Broadway 212-315-8700
New York, NY 10019-4315

2454 Facts About Radon
American Lung Association
1740 Broadway 212-315-8700
New York, NY 10019-4315

2455 Help, Hope, Believe
National Children's Cancer Society

1015 Locust Street 314-241-1600
Saint Louis, MO 63101 Fax: 314-241-1996
e-mail: krudd@children-cancer.org
www.nationalchildrenscancersociety.org
N.C.C.S. Informational Brochure
3x/year
Mark Slocomb, Chairman
Mark Stolze, President/CEO

2456 Helping Children Cope While a Sibling Undergoes Bone Marrow Transplant
Bone Marrow Foundation
981 1st Avenue 212-838-3029
New York, NY 10022-5102 e-mail: thebmf@aol.com
www.bonemarrow.org
Discusses the wide array of emotions felt by the entire family as a child receives a bone marrow transplant.

2457 If You've Thought About Breast Cancer
Rose Kushner Breast Cancer Advisory Center
PO Box 224
Kensington, MD 20895-0224 Fax: 301-897-3444

2458 Immune System: How it Works
National Cancer Institute
Building 31
Bethesda, MD 20892-0001 800-422-6237
Written for the high school level, this booklet explains the human immune system for the general public. It describes the sophistication of the body's immune responses, the impact of immune disorders and the relation of the immune system to cancer therapies.
28 pages

2459 Informed Consent: Does the Current Process Reflect Current Treatments
Candlelighters' Childhood Cancer Foundation
7910 Woodmont Avenue 301-657-8401
Bethesda, MD 20814-3015 800-366-2223

2460 Insurance Articles
Candlelighters' Childhood Cancer Foundation
7910 Woodmont Avenue 301-657-8401
Bethesda, MD 20814-3015 800-366-2223
Includes: Tips on securing health insurance for childhood cancer survivors and patients, Stay a step ahead of you insuruer, and others.

2461 Interpreting Your PSA and Related Prostate Cancer Blood Tests
Michael Dattoli, Jennifer Cash, and Don Kaltenbach, author
Dattoli Cancer Foundation
2803 Fruitville Road 941-365-5599
Sarasota, FL 34237 800-915-1001
Fax: 941-366-3786
e-mail: info@dattolifoundation.org
www.dattolifoundation.org
Provides a comprehensive overview of the PSA (prostate specific antigen) blood test and other related lab tests including the PSA velocity, free and bound PSA, and the PAP (prostatic Acid Phosphatase) blood test.
2006 50 pages Booklet

2462 Leading Self-Help Groups: Report on Workshop for Leaders of Groups
Candlelighters' Childhood Cancer Foundation
7910 Woodmont Avenue 301-657-8401
Bethesda, MD 20814-3015 800-366-2223

2463 Letter to a Friend Whose Child is Newly Diagnosed with Cancer
Candlelighters' Childhood Cancer Foundation
7910 Woodmont Avenue 301-657-8401
Bethesda, MD 20814-3015 800-366-2223

2464 Managing Your Child's Eating Problems During Cancer Treatment
National Cancer Institute
Building 31
Bethesda, MD 20892-0001 800-422-6237

Contains information about the importance of nutrition, side effects of cancer and its treatment.
32 pages

2465 **Mastectomy: A Treatment for Breast Cancer**
National Cancer Institute
Building 31
Bethesda, MD 20892-0001   800-422-6237
Presents information about the different types of breast surgery, explains what to expect at the hospital and during the recovery period.
25 pages

2466 **Melanoma: Research Report**
National Cancer Institute
Building 31
Bethesda, MD 20892-0001   800-422-6237
Offers information on types of skin cancer, detection, diagnosis, staging, treatment, clinical trials, selected references and additional information for patients with skin cancer.

2467 **Nutrition for Patients Receiving Chemotherapy/Radiation Treatment**
National Cancer Institute
Building 31
Bethesda, MD 20892-0001   800-422-6237
Describes the importance of maintaining nutritional intake while receiving chemotherapy and radiation.

2468 **Once a Year for a Lifetime**
National Cancer Institute
Building 31
Bethesda, MD 20892-0001   800-422-6237
Targets all women age 40 and older describing the importance of regular mammograms in the early detection of breast cancer.

2469 **Oral Cancers: Research Report**
National Cancer Institute
Building 31
Bethesda, MD 20892-0001   800-422-6237
Describes types of oral cancer, causes and risk factors, symptoms, prevention, detection, diagnosis, treatment, staging, methods of treatments, followup care, clinical trials and selected references for more information.

2470 **Pap Test: It Can Save Your Life**
National Cancer Institute
Building 31
Bethesda, MD 20892-0001   800-422-6237
Easy-to-read pamphlet tells women of the importance of getting a Pap test, how often to get it done and where to go to get it.

2471 **Preparing your Child for a Bone Marrow Transplant**
Bone Marrow Foundation
981 1st Avenue   212-838-3029
New York, NY 10022-5102   e-mail: thebmf@aol.com
                                                    www.bonemarrow.org
Discusses the wide array of emotions felt by the entire family as a child receives a bone marrow transplant.

2472 **Questions and Answers About Breast Lumps**
National Cancer Institute
Building 31
Bethesda, MD 20892-0001   800-422-6237
Describes some of the most common noncancerous breast lumps and what can be done about them.
22 pages

2473 **Questions and Answers About Choosing a Mammography Facility**
National Cancer Institute
Building 31
Bethesda, MD 20892-0001   800-422-6237
Lists questions to ask in selecting a quality mammography facility.

2474 **Questions and Answers About DES Exposure During Pregnancy and Before Birth**
National Cancer Institute
Building 31
Bethesda, MD 20892-0001   800-422-6237

2475 **Questions and Answers About Metastatic Cancer**
National Cancer Institute
Building 31
Bethesda, MD 20892-0001   800-422-6237
Presents information on detection, treatment methods and common areas of reoccurrence.

2476 **Questions and Answers About Pain Control**
National Cancer Institute
Building 31
Bethesda, MD 20892-0001   800-422-6237
Discusses pain control using both medical and nonmedical methods.

2477 **Radiation Therapy and You: A Guide To Self-Help During Treatment**
National Cancer Institute
Building 31
Bethesda, MD 20892-0001   800-422-6237
Explains radiation therapy and addresses concerns of patients receiving radiation treatment.

2478 **Recurrence: What Do I Do Now?**
Dattoli Cancer Foundation
2803 Fruitville Road   941-365-5599
Sarasota, FL 34237   800-915-1001
                                              Fax: 941-366-3786
                          e-mail: info@dattolifoundation.org
                                      www.dattolifoundation.org
This booklet offers comprehensive information on the issues surrounding ruccurence: detection, risk categories, treatment options including radiation, brachytherapy, and hormone therapy.
58 pages Booklet

2479 **Research Report: Adult Kidney Cancer and Wilms' Tumor**
National Cancer Institute
Building 31
Bethesda, MD 20892-0001   800-422-6237

2480 **Skin Cancers, Basal Cell and Squamous Cell Carcinomas: Research Report**
National Cancer Institute
Building 31
Bethesda, MD 20892-0001   800-422-6237
Offers information on types of skin cancer, incidence and mortality, risk factors, prevention, symptoms, detection, diagnosis, staging, treatment, followup care and clinical trials.

2481 **Students with Cancer: A Resource for the Educator**
National Cancer Institute
Building 31
Bethesda, MD 20892-0001   800-422-6237
Designed for teachers who have students with cancer in their classrooms or schools.
22 pages

2482 **Sunlight, Ultraviolet Radiation and the Skin**
National Cancer Institute
Building 31
Bethesda, MD 20892-0001   800-422-6237

2483 **Support Systems for Parents of Children with Cancer**
Candlelighters' Childhood Cancer Foundation
7910 Woodmont Avenue   301-657-8401
Bethesda, MD 20814-3015   800-366-2223

2484 **Taking Time: Support for People with Cancer & People Who Care for Them**
National Cancer Institute
Building 31
Bethesda, MD 20892-0001   800-422-6237
Discusses the emotional sides of cancer. how to deal with the disease and learn to talk with friends, family members and others about cancer.

2485 **Talking with Your Child About Cancer**
National Cancer Institute
Building 31
Bethesda, MD 20892-0001   800-422-6237

Designed for the parent whose child has been diagnosed with cancer.
16 pages

2486 Testicular Cancer: Research Report
National Cancer Institute
Building 31
Bethesda, MD 20892-0001   800-422-6237

2487 Testicular Self-Examination
National Cancer Institute
Building 31
Bethesda, MD 20892-0001   800-422-6237
Contains information about risks and symptoms of testicular cancer and provides instructions on how to perform testicular self-examination.

2488 What You Need to Know About Bladder Cancer
National Cancer Institute
Building 31   301-496-4000
Bethesda, MD 20892-0001
Offers information on the history, symptoms, diagnosis, treatment, followup care, support groups, medical terms and resources for more information.

2489 What You Need to Know About Cancer
National Cancer Institute
Building 31
Bethesda, MD 20892-0001   800-422-6237
Offers information on signs and symptoms, diagnosis, treatment, early detection and advances in medical technology.

2490 What You Need to Know About Cancer of The Colon and Rectum
National Cancer Institute
Building 31
Bethesda, MD 20892-0001   800-422-6237
Offers information on symptoms, diagnosis, treatments, and support for cancer patients.

2491 What You Need to Know About Cervical Cancer
National Cancer Institute
Building 31
Bethesda, MD 20892-0001   800-422-6237
Areas covered include early detection, symptoms, treatments, diagnosis, followup care, support, medical terms and resources.

2492 What You Need to Know About Esophagal Cancer
National Cancer Institute
Building 31
Bethesda, MD 20892-0001   800-422-6237
Offers information on symptoms, causes, preventions, diagnosis, support, medical terms and available resources.

2493 What You Need to Know About Kidney Cancer
National Cancer Institute
Building 31
Bethesda, MD 20892-0001   800-422-6237
Offers factual information on diagnosis, symptoms, prevention, treatment and referral sources.

2494 What You Need to Know About Larynx Cancer
National Cancer Institute
Building 31
Bethesda, MD 20892-0001   800-422-6237
Offers information on what cancer is, symptoms, diagnosis, treatment options, side effects of medication, rehabilitation, learning to speak again, living with cancer, causes and preventions, medical terms and resources.

2495 What You Need to Know About Lung Cancer
National Cancer Institute
Building 31
Bethesda, MD 20892-0001   800-422-6237
Offers information on types of lung cancer, symptoms, diagnosis, treatments, support, medical terms and resources.

2496 What You Need to Know About Oral Cancers
National Cancer Institute
Building 31
Bethesda, MD 20892-0001   800-422-6237

Offers information on symptoms, diagnosis, treatments, rehabilitation, followup care, support, medical terms and resources for cancer patients.

2497 What You Need to Know About Ovarian Cancer
National Cancer Institute
Building 31
Bethesda, MD 20892-0001   800-422-6237
Early detection, symptoms, diagnosis, treatments, medical terms and resources for further information.

2498 What You Need to Know About Pancreatic Cancer
National Cancer Institute
Building 31
Bethesda, MD 20892-0001   800-422-6237
Offers information on symptoms, diagnosis, treatment, support, medical terms and resources.

2499 What You Need to Know About Prostate Cancer
National Cancer Institute
Building 31
Bethesda, MD 20892-0001   800-422-6237
Offers information on symptoms, diagnosis, treatment options, side effects of medications, followup care, living with cancer and support resources for patients.

2500 What You Need to Know About Skin Cancer
National Cancer Institute
Building 31
Bethesda, MD 20892-0001   800-422-6237
Offers information on types of skin cancer, symptoms, causes, prevention, treatment planning, treating skin cancer, research and medical terms.

2501 What You Need to Know About Testicular Cancer
National Cancer Institute
Building 31
Bethesda, MD 20892-0001   800-422-6237
Offers information on the symptoms, diagnosing of testicular cancer, side effects of treatments, followup care, support for patients, cancer research, medical terms and resources.

2502 What You Need to Know About Uterine Cancer
National Cancer Institute
Building 31
Bethesda, MD 20892-0001   800-422-6237
Offers information on symptoms, diagnosing cancer of the uterus, treatments, followup care, support for patients, medical terms and resources.

2503 What You Need to Know About...
National Cancer Institute
Building 31
Bethesda, MD 20892-0001   800-422-6237
This is a series of booklets, broken down in this directory. Each provides information about a specific type of cancer. These booklets discuss emotional issues, treatment, diagnosis, symptoms and questions to ask the doctor about cancer.

2504 What are Clinical Trials All About?
National Cancer Institute
Building 31
Bethesda, MD 20892-0001   800-422-6237
Explains clinical trials (studies of new cancer treatments) to help patients decide if they want to take part in a trial.

2505 When Cancer Recurs: Meeting the Challenge Again
National Cancer Institute
Building 31
Bethesda, MD 20892-0001   800-422-6237
Offers information on why cancer can recur, where cancers can recur, diagnosing recurrent cancer, treatment methods and resources that offer more help.

2506 When Someone in Your Family Has Cancer
National Cancer Institute
Building 31
Bethesda, MD 20892-0001   800-422-6237
Written for young people whose parent or sibling has cancer.
28 pages

2507 Who is This Person Who Helped Save My Life
Bone Marrow Foundation
981 1st Avenue
New York, NY 10022-5102
212-838-3029
e-mail: thebmf@aol.com
www.bonemarrow.org
Discusses the wide range of emotions for a patient in the process of searching for and identifying a donor.

2508 Why Do You Smoke?
National Cancer Institute
Building 31
Bethesda, MD 20892-0001
800-422-6237
Contains a self-test to determine why people smoke and suggest alternatives that can help them stop and prevent cancer.

2509 Wish Fulfillment Organizations
Candlelighters' Childhood Cancer Foundation
7910 Woodmont Avenue
Bethesda, MD 20814-3015
301-657-8401
800-366-2223
A list of groups granting wishes of children with life-threatening, chronic or terminal illnesses, with criteria and contacts.

2510 Young People with Cancer: A Handbook for Parents
National Cancer Institute
Building 31
Bethesda, MD 20892-0001
800-422-6237
Discusses the most common types of childhood cancer, treatments, and side effects and issues that may arise when a child is diagnosed with cancer.
86 pages

Audio & Video

2511 Beyond the Loss of the Breast
Sherry Thomas-Zon, author

Fanlight Productions
4196 Washington Street
Boston, MA 02131-1731
617-469-4999
800-937-4113
Fax: 617-469-3379
e-mail: fanlight@fanlight.com
www.fanlight.com
This video addresses breast cancer throught the personal narratives and poetry of two women living with recurrent breast cancer and the film maker, whose mother died from metastatic disease.
1994 25 Minutes
ISBN: 1-572951-68-0

2512 Living with Ovarian Cancer
National Ovarian Cancer Coalition
500 NE Spanish River Blvd
Boca Raton, FL 33431
561-393-0005
888-682-7426
Fax: 561-393-7275
e-mail: nocc@ovarian.org
www.ovarian.org
Videotape for women who have been recently diagnosed with ovarian cancer. Created to orient and inform patients and their families; describes the experiences of individuals intimately connected with the disease.
Suzy Lockwood-Rayermann RN, Chair
Julene Fabrizio, President

2513 Not Just a Cancer Patient
Fanlight Productions
4196 Washington Street
Boston, MA 02131-1731
617-469-4999
800-937-4113
Fax: 617-469-3379
e-mail: fanlight@fanlight.com
www.fanlight.com
Focuses on several articulate teenagers who are undergoing cancer treatment to help caregivers understand the needs and feelings of this population.
1991 23 Minutes
ISBN: 1-572950-86-2

2514 Skin Cancer: Preventable and Curable
Skin Cancer Foundation

245 5th Avenue
New York, NY 10016-8728
212-725-5176
800-754-6490
Fax: 212-725-5751
e-mail: info@skincancer.org
www.skincancer.org

Web Sites

2515 American Academy of Dermatology
www.aad.org
An organization of doctors who specialize in diagnosing and treating skin problems.

2516 American Cancer Society
www.cancer.org
Provides free printed materials, offers a range of services to patients and their families.

2517 American Lung Association
www.lungusa.org
A voluntary organization interested in the prevention and control of lung disease.

2518 American Prostate Society
www.ameripros.org
Organization dedicated exclusively to using existing medical capabilities to reduce death due to prostate cancer and to reduce unnecessary or ineffective prostate surgery.

2519 American Society of Colon and Rectal Surgeons
www.fascrs.org
Represents more than 1000 board certified colon and rectal surgeons and other surgeons dedicated to advancing and promoting the science and practice of the treatment of patients with diseases and disorders affecting the colon, rectum and anus.

2520 Association for the Cure of Cancer of the Prostate
www.capcure.org

2521 Bone Marrow Foundation
www.bonemarrow.org

2522 Healing Well
www.healingwell.com
An online health resource guide to medical news, chat, information and articles, newsgroups and message boards, books, disease-related web sites, medical directories, and more for patients, friends, and family coping with disabling diseases, disorders, or chronic illnesses.

2523 Health Finder
www.healthfinder.gov
Searchable, carefully developed web site offering information on over 1000 topics. Developed by the US Department of Health and Human Services, the site can be used in both English and Spanish.

2524 Healthlink USA
www.healthlinkusa.com
Health information concerning treatment, cures, prevention, diagnosis, risk factors, research, support groups, email lists, personal stories and much more. Updated regularly.

2525 Helios Health
www.helioshealth.com
Online resource for your health information. Detailed information about specific health topics, access to expert advice from our Medical Advisory Board, and up-to-date health news.

2526 International Association of Eating Disorders Professionals
www.iaedp.com
Supplies printed information and sponsors meetings and other activities. Publishes a directory of speech instructors and maintains a list of sources for supplies for laryngectomee.

2527 Leukemia and Lymphoma Society
www.leukemia.org
A national voluntary health agency dedicated to curing leukemia, lymphoma, Hodgkin's disease and myeloma and to improving the quality of life of patients and their families.

2528   MedicineNet

www.medicinenet.com

An online resource for consumers providing easy-to-read, authoritative medical and health information.

2529   Medscape

www.medscape.com

Medscape offers specialists, primary care physicians, and other health professionals the Web's most robust and integrated medical information and educational tools.

2530   National Alliance of Breast Cancer Organizations

www.nabco.org

A network of breast cancer organizations that provides information, assistance and referral to anyone with questions about breast cancer and acts as a voice for the interests and concerns of breast cancer survivors and women at risk.

2531   National Ovarian Cancer Coalition

www.ovarian.org

Our mission is to raise awareness about ovarian cancer and to promote education about the disease.

2532   Support for People with Oral and Head and Neck Cancer

www.spohnc.org

Nonprofit organization founded in 1991 to address the broad emotional, physical and humanistic needs of oral and head and neck cancer patients.

2533   United Ostomy Association

www.uoa.org

A national network for bowel and urinary diversion support groups in the United States. Its goal is to provide a nonprofit association that will serve to unify and strengthen its member support groups, which are organized for the benefit of people who have, or will have intestinal or urinary diversions and their caregivers.

2534   WebMD

www.webmd.com

Information on Cancer, including articles and resources.

2535   Webhelp

www.webhelp.com

Provides links to information, including research, treatment, prevention, support, and more.

Description

2536 Carpal Tunnel Syndrome

Carpal Tunnel Syndrome, CTS, is a painful, often debilitating condition caused by compression of the median nerve as it passes through the wrist (carpal tunnel) to the hand. CTS most commonly occurs in women aged 30 to 50 years. The incidence is highest among keyboard users, secretaries, musicians, assembly-line workers, and others who engage in repetitive handwork.

An initial indication of CTS is a feeling that the hand is asleep. Typically, the patient wakes at night with numbness and tingling of the affected hand. The most serious functional problem occurs when it becomes difficult or impossible to move the thumb into a grasping position with the other fingers. In advanced cases, pain associated with CTS may radiate up the arm to the shoulder. While job-related movement is the most common cause of CTS, people with underlying conditions, such as diabetes, gout, rheumatoid arthritis, obesity and pregnancy, are more prone to experience symptoms. Although less common, the onset of CTS can stem from trauma, such as a blow to the hand or wrist.

Diagnosis involves the Phalen Test, in which the hands are placed together, back to back and the wrist is flexed. This maneuver generally produces tingling of the hand in a patient with CTS. Diagnosis is confirmed by testing how quickly an impulse is transmitted along the median nerve.

The condition can most often be successfully treated based on an understanding of workplace movement issues — ergonomics. keyboard users, and those engaged in similar activities, should adjust their seats and backrests to assure that their arms are positioned comfortably during work sessions. For mild cases of CTS, a lightweight brace, especially worn at night, can decrease symptoms by holding the wrist stable. Marked improvement may arise from wearing a brace for a week or two. However, in many cases, it is recommended that the sufferer cease working until symptoms have improved. Exercises and deep-tissue massage can strengthen the wrist and hand.

Over-the-counter anti-inflammatory medications, such as ibuprofen and aspirin, can also reduce symptoms of mild Carpal Tunnel Syndrome. In more acute conditions, cortisone injections may be administered. When symptoms are severe and persistent, surgery may be required to reduce pressure on the nerves. The most common surgery is an open incision technique called open carpal tunnel release, which usually improves the condition dramatically. A newer and less invasive procedure is endoscopic carpal tunnel release, which uses a smaller incision and visualizes the operative field using a fiber optic camera.

National Agencies & Associations

2537 American Academy of Orthopaedic Surgeons
6300 N River Road
Rosemont, IL 60018-4262
847-823-7186
800-346-2267
Fax: 847-823-8125
e-mail: custserv@aaos.org
www.aaos.org
The American Academy of Orthopaedic Surgeons provides education and practice management services for orthopaedic surgeons and allied health professionals. The Academy also serves as an advocate for improved patient care and to inform the public.
Daniel J Berry MD, President
John R Tongue MD, Vice President

2538 American Chronic Pain Association
PO Box 850
Rocklin, CA 95677
800-533-3231
Fax: 916-632-3208
e-mail: ACPA@pacbell.net
www.theacpa.org
ACPA mission is: (1) to facilitate peer support and education for individuals with chronic pain and their families so that these individuals may live more fully in spite of their pain; (2) to raise awareness among the health care community and policy makers.
Penny Cowan, Executive Director

2539 American Society for Surgery of the Hand
6300 N River Road
Rosemont, IL 60018
847-384-8300
Fax: 847-384-1435
e-mail: info@assh.org
www.assh.org
The mission of the ASSH is to advance the science and practice of hand and upper extremity surgery through education research and advocacy on behalf of patients and practitioners.
Mark C Anderson CAE, Executive VP, CEO
Robert Szabo MD MPH, President

2540 Arthritis Trust of America
7376 Walker Road
Fairview, TN 37602-8141
615-799-1002
e-mail: admin@arthritistrust.org
www.arthritistrust.org
The Arthritis Trust of America provides information about auto-immune or collagen tissue diseases such as Rheumatoid Arthritis and related diseases. They provide publications and physician referrals and when funds are available they fund research.
Perry A Chapdelaine BA MA, Executive Director
Cheryl Jacobsen, President

2541 National Institute of Arthritis and Musculoskeletal and Skin Disease (NIAMS)
1 AMS Circle
Bethesda, MD 20892-3675
301-495-4484
888-226-4267
Fax: 301-718-6366
TTY: 301-565-2966
e-mail: niamsinfo@mail.nih.gov
www.niams.nih.gov
The NIAMS Information Clearinghouse provides information about various forms of arthritis and rheumatic disease and bone, muscle, and skin diseases. It distributes patient and professional education materials and refers people to other sources of information.
Stephen I Katz MD, PhD, Director

Research Centers

2542 Center for Neurology & Stroke Baptist Hospital Office
Baptist Hospital Office
333 West Thomas Road
Pheonix, AZ 85015
602-335-0300
Fax: 602-249-3118
e-mail: info@cnsaz.com
www.cnsaz.com
Providing comprehensive testing and consulting for neurological disorders.

2543 **Michigan Hand Center**
1111 Leffingwell Avenue NE
Grand Rapids, MI 49525
616-459-7101
800-582-7244
Fax: 616-957-0444
e-mail: info@michiganhandcenter.com
www.michiganhand.com

Janid Pike, Director

2544 **National Institute of Arthritis & Musculoskeletal Skin Diseases**
National Institutes of Health
I AMS Circle
Bethesda, MD 20892-3675
301-495-4484
Fax: 301-718-6366
TTY: 301-565-2966
e-mail: niamsinfo@mail.nih.gov
www.niams.nih.gov

Support Groups & Hotlines

2545 **National Health Information Center**
PO Box 1133
Washington, DC 20013-1133
310-565-4167
800-336-4797
Fax: 301-984-4256
e-mail: info@nhic.org
www.health.gov/nhic
A health information referral service sponsored by the Office of Disease Prevention and Health Promotion. Puts health professionals and consumers who have health questions in touch with those organizations that are best able to provide answers.

Books

2546 **Occupational Therapy Practice Guidelines for Adults with Carpal Tunnel Syndrome**
American Occupational Therapy Association
4720 Montgomery Lane
Bethesda, MD 20824-1220
301-652-2682
Fax: 301-652-7711
TDD: 800-377-8555
www.aota.org

13 pages Paperback
ISBN: 1-569001-47-2

2547 **Pain Free Typing Techniques: Simple Solutions to Prevent Strain Injury**
Howard Richman, author
Sound Feelings Publishing
18375 Ventura Boulevard
Tarzana, CA 91356
818-757-0600
e-mail: information@soundfeelings.com
www.soundfeelings.com
This 12 page booklet provides drug-free treatments and suggestions for repetitive motion disorder and cumulative trauma disorders. Unconventional concepts for increasing human performance are revealed, which help prevent computer-related illnesses including hand pain, wrist pain, and other keyboard ergonomics. Most repetitive motion disorders and overuse injuries can be improved by correcting certain angles and positions.
1999 12 pages Booklet
ISBN: 1-882060-80-6

Pamphlets

2548 **Carpal Tunnel Syndrome**
Arthritis Foundation
PO Box 7669
Atlanta, GA 30357-0669
404-872-7100
800-283-7800
Fax: 404-872-0457
Offers an introduction to Carpal Tunnel, causes, symptoms, diagnosis and resources.

Web Sites

2549 **Avoiding Carpal Tunnel Syndrome**
www.indiana.edu/~ucsstaff/cts.html
A guide for computer keyboard users, by Mark Sheehan, reprinted from the University Computing Times.

2550 **CTD Resource Network**
www.ctdrn.org
This is an organization providing educational material and charitable assistance related to the prevention and treatment of cumulative trauma disorders, also known as repetitive strain injuries.

2551 **Carpal Tunnel Syndrome Home Page**
www.ctsplace.com
Information about carpal tunnel syndrome (CTS) and how to prevent it.

2552 **Computer-Related Repetitive Strain Injury**
www.unl.edu/ee/eeshop/rsi.html#PREVENT
Contains advice on proper posture and equipment from Paul Marxhausen, an engineering electronics technician.

2553 **Health Finder**
www.healthfinder.gov
Searchable, carefully developed web site offering information on over 1000 topics. Developed by the US Department of Health and Human Services, the site can be used in both English and Spanish.

2554 **MedicineNet**
www.medicinenet.com
An online resource for consumers providing easy-to-read, authoritative medical and health information.

2555 **Neurology Channel**
www.neurologychannel.com
Find clearly explained, medically accurate information regarding conditions, including an overview, symptoms, causes, diagnostic procedures and treatment options. On this site it is possible to ask questions and get information from a neurologist and connect to people who have similar health interests.

2556 **RSI Resources**
www.geocities.com/HotSprings/1702
Information on carpal tunnel and other repetitive strain injuries.

Description

2557 Celiac Disease

Celiac disease, also called celiac sprue, is a chronic disease in which the small bowel cannot absorb most nutrients. This inability, called malabsorption, is caused by inflammation of the bowel triggered by a sensitivity to gluten, a cereal protein found in wheat and rye, and less so in barley and oats.

The disease may appear when a child is first given wheat products, generally in the second year of life. Some cases, however, do not appear until a person is in their twenties, or later, with women showing symptoms 10 to 15 years earlier than men. Affected children will fail to grow normally. Adults may lose weight despite a voracious appetite. There is no typical presentation of celiac disease. However, painful abdominal distention and passage of large, loose stools are common; iron deficiency anemia and vitamin deficiencies may appear.

Family incidence is a valuable clue. Celiac disease is more common in people with Type I diabetes and certain forms of thyroid and skin disease. Blood tests are helpful in making the diagnosis, but the most definitive test is examination of a small sample of the inflamed bowel.

Withdrawal of dietary gluten is the treatment for celiac disease; eating even small amounts of gluten-containing foods can prevent remission and cause relapse. Vitamins and minerals may also have to be supplemented. See also *Gastrointestinal Disorders* and *Crohn's Disease*.

National Agencies & Associations

2558 American Celiac Society
PO Box 23455
New Orleans, LA 70183

504-737-3293
Fax: 973-669-8808
e-mail: americanceliacsociety@yahoo.com
www.americanceliacsociety.org

Nonprofit tax exempt organization that supports efforts in education research and mutual support. Helps to set up support groups sponsors conferences seek funding for education and research identify ingredients in foods and educate the public.
Annette Bentley, President
Jim Bentley Vice President

2559 Canadian Celiac Association
5025 Orbitor Drive Building 1
Mississauga, ON, L4W-4Y5

905-507-6208
800-363-7296
Fax: 905-507-4673
www.celiac.ca

A national organization dedicated to providing services and support to persons with celiac disease and dermatitis herpetiformis through programs of awareness, advocacy, education and research.
Janet Dalziel, President
Cathy Morris, VP

2560 Celiac Sprue Association: USA
PO Box 31700
Omaha, NE 68131-700

402-558-0600
877-CSA-4CSA
Fax: 402-643-4108
e-mail: celiacs@csaceliacs.org
www.csaceliacs.org

Member based nonprofit support organization dedicated to helping individuals with celiac disease and dermatitis herpetiformis

worldwide through education information and research. Includes over 150 support contacts nationwide and Cel-Kids Network.
Mary Schluckebier, Executive Director
Diane Craig, President

2561 Gluten Intolerance Group: GIG
31214 124th Avenue SE
Auburn, WA 98092-3667

253-833-6655
Fax: 253-833-6675
e-mail: info@gluten.net
www.gluten.net

Provides instructional and general information materials as well as counseling and access to gluten-free products and ingredients to persons with celiac sprue and their families, operates telephone information and referral service and conducts educational seminars.
Cynthia Kupp RDCD, Executive Director

Support Groups & Hotlines

2562 American Celiac Society Hotline
Dietary Support Coalition
PO BOX 23455
New Orleans, LA 70183-455

504-737-3293
e-mail: americanceliacsociety@yahoo.com

Provides practical assistance to members and individuals with celiac disease and information about the disease to the public.
Annette Bentley, President
James Bentley, Vice President

2563 Celiac Disease Foundation
13251 Ventura Boulevard
Studio City, CA 91604-1838

818-990-2354
Fax: 818-990-2379
e-mail: cdf@celiac.org
www.celiac.org/

Provides services and support to persons with celiac disease and dermatitis herpetiformis, through programs of awareness, education, advocacy and research; telephone information and referral services; medical advisory board annual educational conference and quarterly newsletters.
Rita T Hopkins, Executive Director

2564 National Health Information Center
PO Box 1133
Washington, DC 20013

310-565-4167
800-336-4797
Fax: 301-984-4256
e-mail: info@nhic.org
www.health.gov/nhic

Offers a nationwide information referral service, produces directories and resource guides.

Books

2565 CSA/USA Cookbook Series
Celiac Sprue Association/USA
PO Box 31700
Omaha, NE 68131

402-558-0600
877-272-4272
Fax: 402-643-4108
e-mail: celiacs@csaceliacs.org
www.csaceliacs.org

Three cookbooks compiled from CSA members' contributions. Each contains a section of cooking hints, information on adapting recipes and a variety of special topics related to cooking gluten-free.
34 pages Annual
Mary Schluckebier, Executive Director

2566 Cooperative Gluten-Free Commercial Products Listing
Celiac Sprue Association/USA
PO Box 31700
Omaha, NE 68131

402-558-0600
877-272-4272
Fax: 402-643-4108
e-mail: celiacs@csaceliacs.org
www.csaceliacs.org

Listing of gluten-free products compiled from written documentation recieved by the Celiac Sprue Association from manufacturers and distributors. Also includes vendor information for companies

specializing in gluten-free products and phone numbers of companies.
2006 Annual
Mary Schluckebier, Executive Director

2567 Diets to Help Gluten and Wheat Allergy
HarperCollins Canada Limited/Order Department
1995 Markham Road
Scarborough, M1B 5M8,   800-387-0117
                             Fax: 800-668-5788
This book offers sound and practical advice on gluten allergy wheat sensitivity and Celiac disease.
96 pages
ISBN: 0-722529-10-4

2568 Gluten Intolerance
American Dietetic Association
1120 Connecticut Avenue NW   202-775-8277
Washington, DC 20036   800-877-1600
                           www.eatright.org
Resource and recipe book.

2569 The Gluten-Free Gourmet
Bette Hagman, author
Gluten Intolerance Group: GIG
31214 124th Avenue SE   253-833-6655
Auburn, WA 98092-3667   Fax: 253-833-6675
                     e-mail: info@gluten.net
                           www.gluten.net
225 recipes.
272 pages
ISBN: 0-805064-84-2
Cynthia Kupper RDCD, Executive Director

Newsletters

2570 GIG Quarterly Magazine
Gluten Intolerance Group: GIG
31214 124th Avenue SE   253-833-6655
Auburn, WA 98092-3667   Fax: 253-833-6675
                     e-mail: info@gluten.net
                           www.gluten.net
Member magazine. Offers updated medical and technological information for patients with celiac disease, their families and healthcare professionals.
Quarterly
Cynthia Kupper RDCD, Executive Director

2571 Lifeline
Celiac Sprue Association/USA
PO Box 31700   402-558-0600
Omaha, NE 68131   877-272-4272
                    Fax: 402-643-4108
          e-mail: celiacs@csaceliacs.org
                    www.csaceliacs.org
Quarterly newsletter for members; contains up-to-date research information, personal stories from celiacs, cooking tips, recipes and contact information for support chapters and resource units.
Mary Schluckebier, Executive Director

2572 Whooo's Report
American Celiac Society
PO Box 23455   504-737-3293
New Orleans, LA 70183   e-mail: amerceliacsoc@netscape.net
Provides practical assistance to members and individuals with celiac disease and information about the disease to the public.

Pamphlets

2573 Celiac Disease
Gluten Intolerance Group: GIG
31214 124th Avenue SE   253-833-6655
Auburn, WA 98092-3667   Fax: 253-833-6675
                     e-mail: info@gluten.net
                           www.gluten.net
Offers facts and statistics on celiac disease.
Cynthia Kupper RDCD, Executive Director

2574 Celiac Disease: A Hidden Epidemic
Peter Greene, MD, author
Harper Collins Publishers
10 East 53rd Street
New York, NY 10022   212-207-7000
                     www.harpercollins.com
An inside-out examination and explanation of Celiac Disease.
2006 352 pages
ISBN: 0-060766-93-X
Cynthia Kupper RDCD, Executive Director

2575 Dermatitis Herpetiformis
Gluten Intolerance Group: GIG
31214 124th Avenue SE   253-833-6655
Auburn, WA 98092-3667   Fax: 253-833-6675
                     e-mail: info@gluten.net
                           www.gluten.net
Offers facts and statistics on dermatitis herpetformis.
Cynthia Kupper RDCD, Executive Director

2576 Grains and Flours
Celiac Sprue Association/USA
PO Box 31700   402-558-0600
Omaha, NE 68131   877-272-4272
                    Fax: 402-643-4108
          e-mail: celiacs@csaceliacs.org
                    www.csaceliacs.org
A variety of different gluten-free flour mixtures, to experiment with and discover your favorite!
Mary Schluckebier, Executive Director

2577 Guide to Gluten-Free Diets
American Allergy Association
PO Box 7273   650-322-1663
Menlo Park, CA 94026-7273
Offers information on safe substitutes for baking and cooking. Differentiates celiac disease from wheat allergy. Sources of gluten in diet with warnings on when to check with the manufacturer.

2578 Patient Packet
Celiac Sprue Association/USA
PO Box 31700   402-558-0600
Omaha, NE 68131   877-272-4272
                    Fax: 402-643-4108
          e-mail: celiacs@csaceliacs.org
                    www.csaceliacs.org
A basic information packet for the newly-diagnosed celiac. Provided free of charge to individuals, physicians, dietitians, and family members.
Mary Schluckebier, Executive Director

2579 Quick Start Diet Guide
Gluten Intolerance Group: GIG
31214 124th Avenue SE   253-833-6655
Auburn, WA 98092-3667   Fax: 253-833-6675
                     e-mail: info@gluten.net
                           www.gluten.net
Packet available to download on website.
Cynthia Kupper RDCD, Executive Director

Audio & Video

2580 CD-A NIH Consensus Conference
Celiac Sprue Association/USA
PO Box 31700   402-558-0600
Omaha, NE 68131   877-272-4272
                    Fax: 402-643-4108
          e-mail: celiacs@csaceliacs.org
                    www.csaceliacs.org
Celiac Disease - A NIH Consensus Conference - Reaching Out to Improve the Health of Millions.
Mary Schluckebier, Executive Director

Web Sites

2581 Celiac Disease & Gluten-Free Diet Online Resource Center
                           www.celiac.com

Internet based support organization that provides important resources and information for people on gluten-free diets due to celiac disease, gluten intolerance or wheat allergy.

2582 Celiac Disease Foundation

www.celiac.org/

Provides services and support to persons with celiac disease and dermatitus herpetiformis, through programs of awareness, education, advocacy and research; telephone information and referral services; medical advisory board; and special educational seminars and quarterly meetings.

2583 Celiac Sprue Association: USA

www.csaceliacs.org

Member based, nonprofit support organization dedicated to helping individuals with celiac disease and dermatitis herpetiformis worldwide through education, information and research. Includes over 90 support chapters, 50 resource units, and Cel-Kids Network. Sponsors an annual conference, publishes educational materials, conducts a summer youth camp and provides phone and on-line counseling.

2584 Gluten Intolerance Group: GIG

www.gluten.net

Provides instructional and general information materials, as well as counseling and access to gluten-free products and ingredients to persons with celiac sprue and their families, operates telephone information and referral service, conducts educational seminars for health professionals, conducts and supports research, offers leadership and assistance to contacts and provides for a gluten-free kids camp.

2585 Healing Well

www.healingwell.com

An online health resource guide to medical news, chat, information and articles, newsgroups and message boards, books, disease-related web sites, medical directories, and more for patients, friends, and family coping with disabling diseases, disorders, or chronic illnesses.

2586 Health Finder

www.healthfinder.gov

Searchable, carefully developed web site offering information on over 1000 topics. Developed by the US Department of Health and Human Services, the site can be used in both English and Spanish.

2587 Healthlink USA

www.healthlinkusa.com

Health information concerning treatment, cures, prevention, diagnosis, risk factors, research, support groups, email lists, personal stories and much more. Updated regularly.

2588 Helios Health

www.helioshealth.com

Online resource for your health information. Detailed information about specific health topics, access to expert advice from our Medical Advisory Board, and up-to-date health news.

2589 MedicineNet

www.medicinenet.com

An online resource for consumers providing easy-to-read, authoritative medical and health information.

2590 Medscape

www.medscape.com

Medscape offers specialists, primary care physicians, and other health professionals the Web's most robust and integrated medical information and educational tools.

2591 WebMD

www.webmd.com

Provides links to over 20 articles involving Celiac disease.

Description

2592 Cerebral Palsy

Cerebral palsy, CP, applies to disorders of voluntary movement resulting from damage to areas in the brain. CP can be caused by birth trauma, insufficient oxygen supplied to the infant at or before birth, premature birth or a severe systemic disease, such as meningitis, during early infancy. However, the exact cause is often difficult to establish.

Children with cerebral palsy may not be identified until they reach 1-2 years of age and may show only lagging motor development. Therefore, children known to be at risk should be followed closely. Increased spastic movements are the most common symptoms, but children may also show weakness, poor sense of balance, involuntary movements and abnormal walking. In more severe cases, difficulty in speaking and mental retardation may also be present.

Since there is no known cure for cerebral palsy, the goal of treatment is to develop maximal independence. Therapy may include physical and occupational rehabilitation, the use of leg braces, speech training and special orthopedic surgery. Parents need assistance and guidance in understanding their child's status and potential.

National Agencies & Associations

2593 American Academy for Cerebral Palsy and Developmental Medicine
555 E Wells   414-918-3014
Milwaukee, WI 53202   Fax: 414-276-2146
e-mail: info@aacpdm.org
www.aacpdm.org
A multidisciplinary scientific society devoted to the study of cerebral palsy and other childhood onset disabilities, promoting professional education for the treatment and management of these conditions and to improving the quality of life for people with the condition.
1550 members
Scott Hoffinger, President

2594 Canadian Cerebral Palsy Sports Association
Box 41009   613-748-1430
Ottawa, Ontario, K1G-5K9   866-247-9934
Fax: 613-748-1355
e-mail: info@ccpsa.ca
www.ccpsa.ca
Is an athlete focused national organization administering and governing sport opportunities targeted to athletes with CP and related disabilities.
Sandy Hermiston, President

2595 Easter Seals
233 S Wacker Drive   312-726-6200
Chicago, IL 60606   800-221-6827
Fax: 312-726-1494
TTY: 312-726-4258
e-mail: info@easter-seals.org
www.easter-seals.org
Provides services to children and adults with disabilities as well as support to their families.
Stephen F Rossman, Chairman

2596 Independent Living Research Utilization Project
2323 S Shepherd   713-520-0232
Houston, TX 77019   Fax: 713-520-5785
TTY: 713-520-0232
e-mail: ilru@ilru.org
www.ilru.org
A national center for information training research and technical assistance in independent living. Goal is to expand the body of knowledge in independent living and to improve utilization of results of research programs and demonstration projects.
Lex Frieden, Director
Linda CoVan, Grant Coordinator

2597 National Rehabilitation Information Center
8201 Corporate Drive   301-459-5900
Landover, MD 20785   800-346-2742
Fax: 301-459-4263
TTY: 301-459-5984
e-mail: narincinfo@heitechservices.com
www.naric.com/
One of the three components of the office of Special Education and Rehabilitative Services. Operates in concert with the Rehabilitation Services Administration and the Office of Special Education Programs.
Mark Odum, Director

2598 United Cerebral Palsy Associations
1660 L Street NW   202-776-0406
Washington, DC 20036   800-872-5827
Fax: 202-776-0414
TTY: 202-973-7197
e-mail: info@ucp.org
www.ucp.org
A network of approximately 119 state and local voluntary agencies which provide services conduct public and professional education programs and support research in cerebral palsy.
Stephen Bennett, President, CEO
Michael E Hill, Senior Vice President

State Agencies & Associations

Alabama

2599 United Cerebral Palsy of Alabama
301 EA Darden Drive   256-237-8203
Anniston, AL 36202   Fax: 256-235-2388
e-mail: executivedirector@ecaucp.org
www.ecaucp.org
United Cerebral Palsy provides information, advocacy, referral services for persons with disabilities and/or their families. UCP also operates an equipment loan program, conducts parent workshops, disseminates written literature on topics of interest.
Linda Johns, Executive Director
Shannon Priddy, Development Director

2600 United Cerebral Palsy of East Central Alabama
301 EA Darden Drive   256-237-8203
Anniston, AL 36202   Fax: 256-235-2388
e-mail: executivedirector@ecaucp.org
www.ucpa.org
United Cerebral Palsy provides information, advocacy, referral services for persons with disabilities and/or their families. UCP also operates an equipment loan program, conducts parent workshops, disseminates written literature on topics of interest to people with disabilities.

2601 United Cerebral Palsy of Greater Birmingha m
120 Oslo Circle   205-944-3900
Birmingham, AL 35211   800-654-4483
Fax: 205-944-3990
e-mail: gedwards@ucpbham.com
www.ucpbham.com
United Cerebral Palsy provides information, advocacy, referral services for persons with disabilities and/or their families. UCP also operates an equipment loan program, conducts parent workshops, disseminates written literature on topics of interest to people with disabilities.
Gary Edwards, Executive Director
Jennifer H Ellison, Chief Development Officer

2602 United Cerebral Palsy of Huntsville & Tennessee Valley
2075 Max Luther Drive   256-852-5600
Huntsville, AL 35810   Fax: 256-852-6722
e-mail: tracyc@ucphuntsville.org
www.ucp.org
United Cerebral Palsy provides information, advocacy, referral services for persons with disabilities and/or their families. UCP also operates an equipment loan program, conducts parent workshops, disseminates written literature on topics of interest.
Cheryl Smith, Executive Director
Tim Reeves, President

2603 United Cerebral Palsy of Mobile
3058 Dauphin Square Connector   251-479-4900
Mobile, AL 36607   Fax: 251-479-4998
e-mail: info@ucpmobile.org
www.ucp.org
United Cerebral Palsy provides information, advocacy, referral services for persons with disabilities and/or their families. UCP also operates an equipment loan program, conducts parent workshops, disseminates written literature on topics of interest.
Glenn Harger, President/CEO
Susan Watson, VP/COO

2604 United Cerebral Palsy of Northwest Alabama
4212 Jackson Highway   256-381-4310
Sheffield, AL 35660   Fax: 256-381-4378
e-mail: alison@ucpshoals.org
www.ucpshoals.org
United Cerebral Palsy provides information, advocacy, referral services for persons with disabilities and/or their families. UCP also operates an equipment loan program, conducts parent workshops, disseminates written literature on topics of interest.
Alison Isbell, Director
Linda Williamson, Development Director/WEE-CARE Director

2605 United Cerebral Palsy of West Alabama
1100 UCP Parkway   205-345-3031
Northport, AL 35476   Fax: 205-345-3035
e-mail: lisasucp@comcast.net
www.ucpa.org
United Cerebral Palsy provides information, advocacy, referral services for persons with disabilities and/or their families. UCP also operates an equipment loan program, conducts parent workshops, disseminates written literature on topics of interest.
Lisa D Skelton, Executive Director
Brenda Ewart, Development Director

Alaska

2606 United Cerebral Palsy of Alaska/PARENTS
4743 E Northern Lights Boulevard   907-337-7678
Anchorage, AK 99508   800-478-7678
Fax: 907-337-7671
TTY: 907-337-7629
e-mail: parents@parentsinc.org
www.ucpa.org
Provides information, advocacy, referral services for persons with disabilities and/or their families. UCP also operates an equipment loan program, conducts parent workshops, disseminates written literature on topics of interest to people with disabilities.

Arizona

2607 United Cerebral Palsy of Central Arizona
1802 Parkside Lane   602-943-5472
Phoenix, AZ 85027   Fax: 602-943-4936
e-mail: info@ucpofaz.org
www.ucpa.org
United Cerebral Palsy provides information, advocacy, referral services for persons with disabilities and/or their families. UCP also operates an equipment loan program, conducts parent workshops, disseminates written literature on topics of interest.
Dan Rossi, Executive Director
Perry Bramlett, Chief Human Resources Officer

2608 United Cerebral Palsy of Southern Arizona
635 N Craycroft Road   520-795-3108
Tucson, AZ 85711   Fax: 520-795-3196
e-mail: staff@ucpsa.org
www.ucpsa.org
United Cerebral Palsy provides information, advocacy, referral services for persons with disabilities and/or their families. UCP also operates an equipment loan program, conducts parent workshops, disseminates written literature on topics of interest.
Cindy Mars, Executive Director
Gary Bahman, Finance Director

Arkansas

2609 United Cerebral Palsy of Central Arkansas
9720 N Rodney Parham Road   501-224-6067
Little Rock, AR 72227   Fax: 501-227-5591
e-mail: general@ucpcark.org
www.ucpark.org
United Cerebral Palsy provides information, advocacy, referral services for persons with disabilities and/or their families. UCP also operates an equipment loan program, conducts parent workshops, disseminates written literature on topics of interest.

2610 United Cerebral Palsy of South Arkansas
9720 N Rodney Parham Road   501-224-6067
Little Rock, AR 72227   800-228-6174
Fax: 501-227-5591
e-mail: general@ucpcark.org
www.ucpark.org
United Cerebral Palsy provides information, advocacy, referral services for persons with disabilities and/or their families. UCP also operates an equipment loan program, conducts parent workshops, disseminates written literature on topics of interest.

California

2611 United Cerebral Palsy of Central California
4224 North Cedar Avenue   559-221-8272
Fresno, CA 93726-3700   Fax: 559-221-9347
e-mail: lauriea@ccucp.org
www.ucpa.org
United Cerebral Palsy provides information, advocacy, referral services for persons with disabilities and/or their families. UCP also operates an equipment loan program, conducts parent workshops, disseminates written literature on topics of interest to people with disabilities.

2612 United Cerebral Palsy of Greater Sacrament o
191 Lathrop Way   916-565-7700
Sacramento, CA 95815   Fax: 916-565-7773
e-mail: ucp@ucpsacto.org
www.ucpsacto.org
UCP provides programs and services for people with all types of developmental disabilities. These services include: day programs for adults, an in-home respite service, transportation, independent living services, information and referral services.
Doug Bergman, President/CEO
Tanya Hartle, COO

2613 United Cerebral Palsy of Los Angeles & Ventura Counties
6430 Independence Avenue   818-782-2211
Woodland Hills, CA 91367   Fax: 818-909-9106
e-mail: mail@ucpla.com
www.ucpla.org
United Cerebral Palsy provides information, advocacy, referral services for persons with disabilities and/or their families. UCP also operates an equipment loan program, conducts parent workshops, disseminates written literature on topics of interest to people with disabilities.
Ronald S Cohen, Chief Executive Officer
Clark Jensen, Chief Operating Officer

2614 United Cerebral Palsy of Orange County
980 Roosevelt   949-333-6400
Irvine, CA 92602   Fax: 949-333-6400
e-mail: info@ucp-oc.org
www.ucp-oc.org
United Cerebral Palsy provides information, advocacy, referral services for persons with disabilities and/or their families. UCP

also operates an equipment loan program, conducts parent workshops, disseminates written literature on topics of interest.
Paul Pulver, Executive Directorÿ
Lauren Mille Beeler, Director of Therapy Services

2615   United Cerebral Palsy of San Diego County
8525 Gibbs Drive   858-571-7803
San Diego, CA 92123   Fax: 858-571-0919
                                                    e-mail: ucp@ucpsd.org
                                                                www.ucpa.org
United Cerebral Palsy provides information, advocacy, referral services for persons with disabilities and/or their families. UCP also operates an equipment loan program, conducts parent workshops, disseminates written literature on topics of interest.
David Carucci, Executive Director
Mary Krieger, Associate Executive Director

2616   United Cerebral Palsy of San Joaquin, Calaveras & Amador Counties
333 W Benjamin Holt Drive   209-956-0290
Stockton, CA 95207   Fax: 209-956-0294
                                                    e-mail: slarson@ucpsj.org
                                                                www.ucp.org
United Cerebral Palsy provides information, advocacy, referral services for persons with disabilities and/or their families. UCP also operates an equipment loan program, conducts parent workshops, disseminates written literature on topics of interest to people with disabilities.
Leslie Heier, Interim Executive Director
Theresa Galano-Burke, Executive Assistant

2617   United Cerebral Palsy of San Luis Obispo
3620 Sacramento Drive   805-543-2039
San Luis Obispo, CA 93401   877-UCP-CAR1
                                                    Fax: 805-543-2045
                                                    e-mail: shaftmt@aol.com
                                                                www.ucp-slo.org
United Cerebral Palsy provides information, advocacy, referral services for persons with disabilities and/or their families. UCP also operates an equipment loan program, conducts parent workshops, disseminates written literature on topics of interest to people with disabilities.
Mark Shaffer, UCP Executive Director
Karl Winkler, UCPÿAdministrative Assistant

2618   United Cerebral Palsy of Santa Barbara County
6430 Independence Avenue   818-782-2211
Woodland Hills, CA 91367   888-733-4227
                                                    Fax: 818-909-9106
                                                    e-mail: mail@ucpla.org
                                                                www.ucpla.org
United Cerebral Palsy provides information, advocacy, referral services for persons with disabilities and/or their families. UCP also operates an equipment loan program, conducts parent workshops, disseminates written literature on topics of interest.
Ellen Kessler, Chairperson
Nick Roxborough, President

2619   United Cerebral Palsy of Santa Clara & San Mateo Counties
512 E Maude Avenue   650-917-6900
Sunnyvale, CA 94085-4431   Fax: 650-948-8503
                                                    e-mail: info@ucpscsm.org
                                                                www.ucpscsm.org/
United Cerebral Palsy provides information, advocacy, referral services for persons with disabilities and/or their families. UCP also operates an equipment loan program, conducts parent workshops, disseminates written literature on topics of interest.
Stephen Bennett, President/CEO National Office (DC)
Armetta Parker, Marketing/Communications Director (DC)

2620   United Cerebral Palsy of Stanislaus County
1213 13th Street   209-577-2122
Modesto, CA 95353   Fax: 209-577-2392
                                                    e-mail: rlonczak@ucpstan.org
                                                                www.ucpstan.org
United Cerebral Palsy provides information, advocacy, referral services for persons with disabilities and/or their families. UCP also operates an equipment loan program, conducts parent work-

shops, disseminates written literature on topics of interest to people with disabilities.
Robert S Lonczak, Executive Director
Jeanette Jones, ProgramÿCoordinator

2621   United Cerebral Palsy of the Golden Gate
1970 Broadway   510-832-7430
Oakland, CA 94612   Fax: 510-839-1329
                                                    e-mail: info@ucpgg.org
                                                                www.ucp.org
United Cerebral Palsy provides information, advocacy, referral services for persons with disabilities and/or their families. UCP also operates an equipment loan program, conducts parent workshops, disseminates written literature on topics of interest.
Karen Glatze, Administrator
Dori Maxon, SNAP Program Director

2622   United Cerebral Palsy of the Inland Empire
35-325 Date Palm Drive   760-321-8184
Cathedral City, CA 92234   877-512-2224
                                                    Fax: 760-321-8284
                                                    e-mail: info@ucpie.org
                                                                www.ucpie.org
United Cerebral Palsy provides information, advocacy, referral services for persons with disabilities and/or their families. UCP conducts parent workshops, disseminates written literature on topics of interest to people with disabilities.
Roger M Alexander, Chair
Micki James, Vice Chair

2623   United Cerebral Palsy of the North Bay
3835 Cypress Drive   707-766-9990
Petaluma, CA 94954   800-872-5827
                                                    Fax: 202-776-0414
                                                    e-mail: info@ucpnb.org
                                                                www.ucp.org
United Cerebral Palsy's mission is to advance the independence, productivity and full citizenship of people with disabilities through an affiliate network.
Margaret Farman, Executive Director
Ron Hamilton, Chief of Operations

Colorado

2624   United Cerebral Palsy of Colorado
801 Yosemite Street   303-691-9339
Denver, CO 80230-5708   866-701-2277
                                                    Fax: 303-691-0846
                                                                www.cpco.org
United Cerebral Palsy provides information, advocacy, referral services for persons with disabilities and/or their families. UCP also operates an equipment loan program, conducts parent workshops, disseminates written literature on topics of interest.
Jim Reuter, Chairman of the Board
Judith I Ham, President/CEO

Connecticut

2625   United Cerebral Palsy of Eastern Connecticut
42 Norwich Road   860-447-3800
Quaker Hill, CT 06375   Fax: 860-443-8272
                                                    e-mail: email@ucpect.org
                                                                www.ucp.org
United Cerebral Palsy provides information, advocacy, referral services for persons with disabilities and/or their families. UCP also operates an equipment loan program, conducts parent workshops, disseminates written literature on topics of interest to people with disabilities.
Margaret Morrison, Executive Director
Patricia Mansfield, Executive Director

2626   United Cerebral Palsy of Greater Hartford
80 Whitney Street   860-236-6201
Hartford, CT 06105   Fax: 860-218-2454
                                                    e-mail: jmcmahon@sunrisegroup.org
                                                                www.ucp.org
United Cerebral Palsy provides information, advocacy, referral services for persons with disabilities and/or their families. UCP also operates an equipment loan program, conducts parent work-

shops, disseminates written literature on topics of interest to people with disabilities.

2627   United Cerebral Palsy of Southern Connecticut
94-96 South Turnpike Road
Wallingford, CT 06492   203-269-3511
                                      Fax: 203-269-7411
e-mail: ucpasouthernct@yahoo.com
www.ucpa.org
United Cerebral Palsy provides information, advocacy, referral services for persons with disabilities and/or their families. UCP also operates an equipment loan program, conducts parent workshops, disseminates written literature on topics of interest to people with disabilities.

Delaware

2628   United Cerebral Palsy of Delaware
700 A River Road   302-764-2400
Wilmington, DE 19809-2746   Fax: 302-764-8713
e-mail: wmccool@ucpde.org
www.ucp.org/ucp_local.cfm/52
United Cerebral Palsy provides information, advocacy, referral services for persons with disabilities and/or their families. UCP also operates an equipment loan program, conducts parent workshops, disseminates written literature on topics of interest.
Michelle Welch, President
D Bruce McClenathan, Vice President

District of Columbia

2629   United Cerebral Palsy of Washington DC & Northern Virginia
1818 New York Avenue NE   202-526-0146
Washington, DC 20002   Fax: 202-526-0519
e-mail: webmaster@ucpdcnova.org
www.ucpa.org
United Cerebral Palsy provides information, advocacy, referral services for persons with disabilities and/or their families. UCP also operates an equipment loan program, conducts parent workshops, disseminates written literature on topics of interest to people with disabilities.

Florida

2630   United Cerebral Palsy of Central Florida
3305 S Orange Avenue   407-852-3300
Orlando, FL 32806   Fax: 407-852-3301
e-mail: mbetts@ucpcfl.org
www.ucpcfl.org
United Cerebral Palsy provides information, advocacy, referral services for persons with disabilities and/or their families. UCP also operates an equipment loan program, conducts parent workshops, disseminates written literature on topics of interest.
Ilene E Wilkins, President & Chief Executive Officer
Jill Wisth, Chief Financial Officer

2631   United Cerebral Palsy of East Central Florida
1100 Jimmy Ann Drive   386-274-6474
Daytona Beach, FL 32117   Fax: 386-274-6532
e-mail: info@ucpecf.org
www.ucp.org
Barry Pollack, President/CEO
Kelly Johanessen, VP of Operations

2632   United Cerebral Palsy of Florida
1830 Buford Court   850-922-5630
Tallahassee, FL 32308   Fax: 850-922-1258
e-mail: gloriawe@earthlink.net
www.ucp.org
United Cerebral Palsy provides information, advocacy, referral services for persons with disabilities and/or their families. UCP also operates an equipment loan program, conducts parent workshops, disseminates written literature on topics of interest.

2633   United Cerebral Palsy of North Florida: Tender Loving Care
1241 NE Avenue   850-769-7960
Panama City, FL 32401   Fax: 850-769-1060
e-mail: kimberly.mcmanus@comcast.net
www.ucp.org
United Cerebral Palsy provides information, advocacy, referral services for persons with disabilities and/or their families. UCP

also operates an equipment loan program, conducts parent workshops, disseminates written literature on topics of interest to people with disabilities.

2634   United Cerebral Palsy of Northeast Florida
3311 Beach Boulevard   904-396-1462
Jacksonville, FL 32207   Fax: 904-396-1199
e-mail: cpnefagency@hotmail.com

2635   United Cerebral Palsy of Northwest Florida
2912 North East Street   850-432-1596
Pensacola, FL 32501-1324   Fax: 850-432-1930
e-mail: information@ucpnwfl.org
www.ucp.org
The number one service provider in Northwest Florida for individuals with cerebral palsy and other developmental disabilities, UCP provides information ,advocacy and referral services for persons with disabilities and/or their families. Additionally, UCP offers individuals assistance with daily living skills training, computer training, basic education, speech, physical and occupational therapy, residential, supported living and finding long-term employment.

2636   United Cerebral Palsy of Sarasota-Manatee
1090 S Tamiami Trail   941-957-3599
Sarasota, FL 34236   Fax: 947-957-3499
e-mail: ucpwendy@aol.com
www.ucpsarasota.org
United Cerebral Palsy provides information, advocacy, referral services for persons with disabilities and/or their families. UCP also operates an equipment loan program, conducts parent workshops, disseminates written literature on topics of interest.
Barnett A Greenberg, Chairperson
Mark Famiglio, President

2637   United Cerebral Palsy of South Florida
2700 W 81st Street   305-325-1080
Hialeah, FL 33016   Fax: 305-325-1313
e-mail: info@ucpsouthflorida.org
www.ucp.org
United Cerebral Palsy provides information, advocacy, referral services for persons with disabilities and/or their families. UCP also operates an equipment loan program, conducts parent workshops, disseminates written literature on topics of interest.
Joseph Aniello, President & CEO
Linda Gluck, Vice President & CFO

2638   United Cerebral Palsy of Tallahassee
1830 Buford Court   850-878-2141
Tallahassee, FL 32308   Fax: 850-922-1258
e-mail: gloriawe@earthlink.net
www.ucp.org
United Cerebral Palsy provides information, advocacy, referral services for persons with disabilities and/or their families. UCP also operates an equipment loan program, conducts parent workshops, disseminates written literature on topics of interest.

2639   United Cerebral Palsy of Tampa Bay
2215 E Henry Avenue   813-239-1179
Tampa, FL 33610   800-749-5155
                                      Fax: 813-237-3091
e-mail: kryals@advanceability.org
www.achievetampabay.org
United Cerebral Palsy provides information, advocacy, referral services for persons with disabilities and/or their families. UCP also operates an equipment loan program, conducts parent workshops, disseminates written literature on topics of interest to people with disabilities.
David W Brooks, Executive Director
William Chisholm, Program Director

Georgia

2640   United Cerebral Palsy of Georgia
3300 NE Expressway   770-676-2000
Atlanta, GA 30341   Fax: 770-455-8040
e-mail: info@ucpga.org
www.ucp.org
United Cerebral Palsy provides information, advocacy, referral services for persons with disabilities and/or their families. UCP

also operates an equipment loan program, conducts parent workshops, disseminates written literature on topics of interest to people with disabilities.

Diane Wilush, Executive Director
Kevin Walton, Associate Executive Director

Hawaii

2641 **United Cerebral Palsy of Hawaii**
414 Kuwili Street
Honolulu, HI 96817-5050

808-532-6744
800-606-5654
Fax: 808-532-6747
e-mail: ucpa@diverseabilities.org
www.ucpahi.org

United Cerebral Palsy provides information, advocacy, referral services for persons with disabilities and/or their families. UCP also operates an equipment loan program, conducts parent workshops, disseminates written literature on topics of interest.

Jerry Pupillo, President
Stephen Hink, 1st Vice President

Idaho

2642 **United Cerebral Palsy of Idaho**
5420 W Franklin Road
Boise, ID 83705

208-377-8070
888-289-3281
Fax: 208-322-7133
e-mail: info@ucpidaho.org
www.ucp.org

United Cerebral Palsy provides information, advocacy and referral services for persons with disabilities and/or their families.

Kim Kane, Executive Director
Kathy Griffin, Program Director

Illinois

2643 **United Cerebral Palsy Land of Lincoln**
101 N 16th Street
Springfield, IL 67203

217-525-6522
Fax: 217-525-9017
e-mail: info@ucpll.org
www.ucp.org

United Cerebral Palsy provides information, advocacy, referral services for persons with disabilities and/or their families. UCP also operates an equipment loan program, conducts parent workshops, disseminates written literature on topics of interest.

Brenda L Yarnell, President/CEO
Kathy Leuelling, Chief Operating Officer

2644 **United Cerebral Palsy of East Central Illinois**
1023 N Water
Decatur, IL 62523

217-428-5033
Fax: 217-428-5094
ww.ucpa.org

United Cerebral Palsy provides information, advocacy, referral services for persons with disabilities and/or their families. UCP also operates an equipment loan program, conducts parent workshops, disseminates written literature on topics of interest.

2645 **United Cerebral Palsy of Greater Chicago**
547 W Jackson
Chicago, IL 60661

312-765-0419
Fax: 312-765-0503
TTY: 312-368-0179
e-mail: pdulle@ucpnet.org
www.ucpnet.org

United Cerebral Palsy provides information, advocacy, referral services for persons with disabilities and/or their families. UCP also operates an equipment loan program, conducts parent workshops, disseminates written literature on topics of interest to people with disabilities.

Paul J Dulle, President/CEO
Peggy Childs, Executive Vice President

2646 **United Cerebral Palsy of Illinois**
310 E Adams
Springfield, IL 62701

877-550-8274
877-550-8274
Fax: 217-528-9739
TTY: 877-550-8274
e-mail: cpil@sbcglobal.net
www.ucpillinois.org

United Cerebral Palsy provides information, advocacy, referral services for persons with disabilities and/or their families. UCP

also operates an equipment loan program, conducts parent workshops, disseminates written literature on topics of interest to people with disabilities.

Don Moss, Executive Director
Alice Foss, Associate Director

2647 **United Cerebral Palsy of Southern Illinois**
9 Cusumano Professional Plaza Drive
Mount Vernon, IL 62864

618-244-2505
Fax: 618-244-3568
e-mail: ucpsi@onemain.com
www.ucpa.org

United Cerebral Palsy provides information, advocacy, referral services for persons with disabilities and/or their families. UCP also operates an equipment loan program, conducts parent workshops, disseminates written literature on topics of interest to people with disabilities.

2648 **United Cerebral Palsy of Will County**
311 S Reed Street
Joliet, IL 60436

815-744-3500
Fax: 815-744-3504
e-mail: ucpwill@ucpwill.org
www.ucp.org

United Cerebral Palsy provides information, advocacy, referral services for persons with disabilities and/or their families. UCP also operates an equipment loan program, conducts parent workshops, disseminates written literature on topics of interest to people with disabilities.

Samuel Mancuso, President & Chief Executive Officer
Stephanie Bergner, Family Support/Respite Administrator

2649 **United Cerebral Palsy of the Blackhawk Region**
7399 Forest Hills Road
Rockford, IL 61111

815-636-7132
Fax: 815-282-8835
e-mail: ucpbr@aol.com
www.ucpa.org

United Cerebral Palsy provides information, advocacy, referral services for persons with disabilities and/or their families. UCP also operates an equipment loan program, conducts parent workshops, disseminates written literature on topics of interest to people with disabilities.

2650 **United Cerebral Palsy: Eastern Seals**
230 W Monroe Street
Chicago, IL 60606

312-726-6200
800-221-6827
Fax: 312-726-1494
stsweb.indstate.edu

United Cerebral Palsy provides information, advocacy, referral services for persons with disabilities and/or their families. UCP also operates an equipment loan program, conducts parent workshops, disseminates written literature on topics of interest.

Indiana

2651 **United Cerebral Palsy Association of Indiana**
1915 West 18th Street
Indianapolis, IN 46202-1016

317-632-3561
Fax: 317-632-3338
e-mail: donnar@ucpaindy.org
www.ucpa.org

United Cerebral Palsy provides information, advocacy, referral services for persons with Cerebral Palsy and/or their families. UCP also provides funding for equipment and operates an equipment loan program, disseminates written literature on topics of interest to people with disabilities.

Donna L Roberts, Executive Director

2652 **United Cerebral Palsy Associations**
6100 N Keystone Avenue
Indianapolis, IN 46220

317-632-3561
Fax: 317-632-3338
e-mail: donnar@ucpaindy.org
www.ucpaindy.org

United Cerebral Palsy provides information, advocacy, referral services for persons with Cerebral Palsy and/or their families. UCP also provides funding for equipment and operates an equipment loan program, disseminates written literature on topics of interest.

Donna L Roberts, Executive Director
Beth Allison, Case Manager

2653 United Cerebral Palsy of the Wabash Valley
621 Poplar Street
Terre Haute, IN 47807
812-232-6305
Fax: 812-234-3683
e-mail: ucp.wv@verizon.net
stsweb.indstate.edu
United Cerebral Palsy provides information, advocacy, referral services for persons with disabilities and/or their families. UCP also operates an equipment loan program, conducts parent workshops, disseminates written literature on topics of interest to people with disabilities.
Jacquie Denehie, Executive Director

Kansas

2654 United Cerebral Palsy of Kansas
5111 E 21st Street
Wichita, KS 67208
316-688-1888
Fax: 316-688-5687
e-mail: davej@cprf.org
www.ucp.org
United Cerebral Palsy provides information, advocacy, referral services for persons with disabilities and/or their families. UCP also operates an equipment loan program, conducts parent workshops, disseminates written literature on topics of interest.
Dave Jones, Executive Director
Amelia Ornelas, Office Manager

Louisiana

2655 United Cerebral Palsy of Baton Rouge McMains Children's Developmental Center
1805 College Drive
Baton Rouge, LA 70808
225-923-3420
Fax: 225-922-9316
e-mail: jketcham@mcmainscdc.org
www.mcmainscdc.org
United Cerebral Palsy provides information, advocacy, referral services for persons with disabilities and/or their families. UCP also operates an equipment loan program, conducts parent workshops, disseminates written literature on topics of interest.
Janet Ketcham, Director
Norman Landry, President

2656 United Cerebral Palsy of Greater New Orleans
1000 Leonidas St & Leake Avenue
New Orleans, LA 70118
504-865-0003
Fax: 504-865-0300
e-mail: info@ucpgno.com
www.ucpa.org
United Cerebral Palsy provides information, advocacy, referral services for persons with disabilities and/or their families. UCP also operates an equipment loan program, conducts parent workshops, disseminates written literature on topics of interest to people with disabilities.

Maine

2657 United Cerebral Palsy of Northeastern Maine
700 Mount Hope Avenue
Bangor, ME 04401
207-941-2952
877-603-0030
Fax: 207-941-2955
e-mail: office@ucpofmaine.org
www.ucp.org
United Cerebral Palsy provides information, advocacy, referral services for persons with disabilities and/or their families. UCP also operates an equipment loan program, conducts parent workshops, disseminates written literature on topics of interest to people with disabilities.
Bobbi-Jo Yeager, Executive Director
Tricia Kail, Director of Services

Maryland

2658 United Cerebral Palsy of Central Maryland
1700 Reistertown Road
Baltimore, MD 21208-2935
410-484-4540
Fax: 410-484-1807
TTY: 800-451-2452
e-mail: info@ucp-cm.org
www.ucp.org
United Cerebral Palsy provides information, advocacy, referral services for persons with disabilities and/or their families. UCP

also operates an equipment loan program, conducts parent workshops, disseminates written literature on topics of interest.
Diane Coughlin, President and CEO
Judy Cox, Assistant to the President

2659 United Cerebral Palsy of Prince Georges & Montgomery Counties
4409 Forbes Boulevard
Lanham, MD 20706
301-459-0566
Fax: 301-459-7691
TTY: 301-459-7691
TDD: 301-262-4982
e-mail: ucppgmc@aol.com
www.ucppgmc.com
Provides information, advocacy, referral services for persons with disabilities and/or their families. UCP also operates an equipment loan program, conducts parent workshops, disseminates written literature on topics of interest to people with disabilities.
Charles McNelly, Executive Director
Diane Dekoladenu, Program Director

2660 United Cerebral Palsy of Southern Maryland
221 Chinquapin Round Road
Annapolis, MD 21401
410-280-2003
Fax: 410-269-5757
e-mail: ucpinfo@ucpsm.org
www.ucpsm.org
United Cerebral Palsy provides information, advocacy, referral services for persons with disabilities and/or their families. UCP also operates an equipment loan program, conducts parent workshops, disseminates written literature on topics of interest to people with disabilities.

Massachusetts

2661 United Cerebral Palsy of Berkshire County
208 W Street
Pittsfield, MA 01201
413-442-1562
Fax: 413-499-4077
e-mail: info@ucpberkshire.org
www.ucp.org
United Cerebral Palsy provides information, advocacy, referral services for persons with disabilities and/or their families. UCP also operates an equipment loan program, conducts parent workshops, disseminates written literature on topics of interest to people with disabilities.
Christine Singer, Executive Director
Joni Thomas, Director of Development

2662 United Cerebral Palsy of MetroBoston
71 Arsenal Street
Watertown, MA 02472
617-926-5480
Fax: 617-926-3059
e-mail: ucpboston@ucpboston.org
www.ucp.org
United Cerebral Palsy provides information, advocacy, referral services for persons with disabilities and/or their families. UCP also operates an equipment loan program, conducts parent workshops, disseminates written literature on topics of interest.
Todd Kates, Executive Director
Roberta Jaro, Associate Executive Director

Michigan

2663 United Cerebral Palsy of Metropolitan Detroit
23077 Greenfield
Southfield, MI 48075
248-557-5070
Fax: 248-557-0224
e-mail: main@ucpdetroit.org
www.ucp.org
United Cerebral Palsy provides information, advocacy, referral services for persons with disabilities and/or their families. UCP also operates an equipment loan program, conducts parent workshops, disseminates written literature on topics of interest.
Leslynn Angel, President & CEO
Latoya Jones, Chief Financial Officer

2664 United Cerebral Palsy of Michigan
4970 Northwind Drive
E Lansing, MI 48823
517-203-1200
800-828-2714
Fax: 517-203-1203
e-mail: ucp@ucpmichigan.org
www.ucp.org
United Cerebral Palsy provides information, advocacy, referral services for persons with disabilities and/or their families. UCP

also operates an equipment loan program, conducts parent workshops, disseminates written literature on topics of interest.
Linda Potter, Executive Director
Linda Carey, Office Manager

Minnesota

2665   United Cerebral Palsy of Central Minnesota
510 25th Avenue North   320-253-0765
St. Cloud, MN 56303-3255   Fax: 320-253-6753
e-mail: info@ucpcentralmn.org
www.ucpcentralmn.org
Provides information, advocacy, referral services for persons with disabilities and/or their families. UCP conducts parent workshops, disseminates free newsletter. Computers go round recycles quality used computers to persons with disabilities. UCP awards scholarship for post secondary education.

2666   United Cerebral Palsy of Central Ohio
510 25th Avenue N   320-253-0765
St Cloud, MN 56303   Fax: 320-253-6753
TTY: 320-253-0765
e-mail: info@ucpcentralmn.org
www.ucpcentralmn.org
Provides information, advocacy, referral services for persons with disabilities and/or their families. UCP conducts parent workshops, disseminates information in a free newsletter.
Judy K Moening, Executive Director
Alison Pauly, Program & Development Coordinator

2667   United Cerebral Palsy of Minnesota
1821 University Avenue W   651-646-7588
St Paul, MN 55104-2892   877-528-5678
Fax: 651-646-3045
e-mail: ucpmnStacey@hotmail.com
www.ucp.org
United Cerebral Palsy provides information, advocacy, referral services for persons with disabilities and/or their families. UCP also operates an equipment loan program, conducts parent workshops, disseminates written literature on topics of interest.
Stacey Vogele, Executive Director
Ramsey Lee, Events Coordinator

Missouri

2668   United Cerebral Palsy of Greater Kansas City
1044 Main Street   816-531-4454
Kansas City, MO 64105   Fax: 816-531-3383
e-mail: bscott@ucpkc.org
www.ucp.org
Provides information, advocacy, referral services for persons with disabilities and/or their families. UCP also operates residential programs and care management for seniors.
Bruce A Scott, President & CEO
Sam T Switzer, Senior Vice President & CFO

2669   United Cerebral Palsy of Greater St. Louis
8645 Old Bonhomme Road   314-994-1600
St. Louis, MO 63132-3999   Fax: 314-994-0179
e-mail: forkoshr@ucpstl.org
www.ucpa.org
United Cerebral Palsy provides information, advocacy, referral services for persons with disabilities and/or their families. UCP also operates an equipment loan program, conducts parent workshops, disseminates written literature on topics of interest to people with disabilities.

2670   United Cerebral Palsy of Northwest Missouri
3303 Frederick Avenue   816-364-3836
St. Joseph, MO 64506   Fax: 816-390-8546
e-mail: ucpnwmo@ccp.com
www.ucpa.org
United Cerebral Palsy provides information, advocacy, referral services for persons with disabilities and/or their families. UCP also operates an equipment loan program, conducts parent workshops, disseminates written literature on topics of interest to people with disabilities.

2671   United Cerebral Palsy of Northwestern
3303 Frederick Avenue   816-364-3836
St Joseph, MO 64506   Fax: 816-390-8546
e-mail: ucp@ucpnwmo.org
www.ucp.org
United Cerebral Palsy provides information, advocacy, referral services for persons with disabilities and/or their families. UCP also operates an equipment loan program, conducts parent workshops, disseminates written literature on topics of interest to people with disabilities.
Teresa Gagliano, Executive Director
Carmen Bartlett, Program Director

Nebraska

2672   United Cerebral Palsy of Nebraska
920 S 107th Avenue   402-502-3572
Omaha, NE 68114   800-729-2556
Fax: 402-502-6791
e-mail: jennyh@ucpnebraska.org
www.ucp.org
United Cerebral Palsy provides information, advocacy, referral services for persons with disabilities and/or their families. UCP also operates an equipment loan program, conducts parent workshops, disseminates written literature on topics of interest.
Carol Hahn, Executive Director
Anne Brodin, Financial & Services Director

Nevada

2673   United Cerebral Palsy of Northern Nevada
4068 S McCarran Boulevard   775-331-3323
Reno, NV 89502-7532   Fax: 775-331-7913
e-mail: upcnn@ucpnn.org
www.ucpa.org
United Cerebral Palsy provides information, advocacy, referral services for persons with disabilities and/or their families. UCP also provides employment and supported living services and disseminates written literature on topics of interest.

New Jersey

2674   United Cerebral Palsy of Hudson County
721 Broadway   201-436-2200
Bayonne, NJ 07002   Fax: 201-436-6642
e-mail: kkearney@ucpofhudsoncounty.org
www.ucp.org
United Cerebral Palsy provides information, advocacy, referral services for persons with disabilities and/or their families. UCP also operates an equipment loan program, conducts parent workshops, disseminates written literature on topics of interest to people with disabilities.
Nick Starita, Executive Director
Keith J Kearney, Associate Executive Director

2675   United Cerebral Palsy of Morris-Somerset
245 Main Street   908-879-2243
Chester, NJ 07930   Fax: 908-879-8363
e-mail: info@ucpnj.org
www.ucpa.org
United Cerebral Palsy provides information, advocacy, referral services for persons with disabilities and/or their families. UCP also operates an equipment loan program, conducts parent workshops, disseminates written literature on topics of interest.

2676   United Cerebral Palsy of New Jersey
1005 Whitehead Road Extension   609-392-4004
Ewing, NJ 08638   888-322-1918
Fax: 609-882-4054
TTY: 609-882-0620
e-mail: info@cpofnj.org
www.cpofnj.org
United Cerebral Palsy provides information, advocacy, referral services for persons with disabilities and/or their families. UCP also operates an equipment loan program, conducts parent workshops, disseminates written literature on topics of interest.

2677 Center for the Disabled
314 S Manning Boulevard
Albany, NY 12208
518-437-5700
e-mail: bulgaro@cftd.org
www.cfdsny.org
United Cerebral Palsy provides information, advocacy, referral services for persons with disabilities and/or their families. UCP also operates an equipment loan program, conducts parent workshops, disseminates written literature on topics of interest to people with disabilities.
Alan Krafchin, CEO/President
Patrick J Rielly, Chief Operating Officer

2678 Cerebral Palsy Associations of New York State
90 State Street
Albany, NY 12207
518-436-0178
Fax: 518-436-8619
e-mail: AffiliateServices@cpofnys.org
www.cpofnys.org
Provides information, advocacy, referral services for persons with disabilities and/or their families. CP also operates an equipment loan program, conducts parent workshops and disseminates written literature on topics of interest to people with disabilities.
Michael Alvaro, Executive Vice President
Susan Constantino, President & CEO

2679 Niagara Cerebral Palsy
9812 Lockport Road
Niagara Falls, NY 14304
716-297-0798
Fax: 716-297-0998
e-mail: info@niagaracp.org
www.ucpaofniagara.com
Provides educational, residential, vocational and recreational programs.

2680 Prospect Child And Family Center
133 Aviation Road
Queensbury, NY 12804
518-798-0170
Fax: 518-798-0533
e-mail: pcfccent@prospectcenter.com
www.prospectcenter.com
United Cerebral Palsy provides information, advocacy, referral services for persons with disabilities and/or their families. UCP also operates an equipment loan program, conducts parent workshops, disseminates written literature on topics of interest to people with disabilities.

2681 United Cerebral Palsy of Chemung County
1118 Charles Street
Elmira, NY 14901
607-734-7107
Fax: 607-734-7334
www.chemungcp.com
United Cerebral Palsy provides information, advocacy, referral services for persons with disabilities and/or their families. UCP also operates an equipment loan program, conducts parent workshops, disseminates written literature on topics of interest to people with disabilities.
Mark Peters, Executive Director
Leisa Alger, Associate Executive Director

2682 United Cerebral Palsy of Fulton & Montgomery Counties
67 Division Street
Amsterdam, NY 12010
518-842-3511
Fax: 518-843-6042
www.ucpa.org
United Cerebral Palsy provides information, advocacy, referral services for persons with disabilities and/or their families. UCP also operates an equipment loan program, conducts parent workshops, disseminates written literature on topics of interest to people with disabilities.

2683 United Cerebral Palsy of Greater Suffolk
250 Marcus Boulevard
Hauppauge, NY 11788
631-232-0011
Fax: 631-232-4422
e-mail: info@ucp-suffolk.org
www.ucp-suffolk.org
United Cerebral Palsy provides information, advocacy, referral services for persons with disabilities and/or their families. UCP also operates an equipment loan program, conducts parent workshops, disseminates written literature on topics of interest.
Stephen H Friedman, President & CEO
James Monnier, Board of Directors

2684 United Cerebral Palsy of Nassau County
380 Washington Avenue
Roosevelt, NY 11575
516-378-2000
Fax: 516-868-4089
e-mail: info@ucpn.org
www.ucpn.org
United Cerebral Palsy provides information, advocacy, referral services for persons with disabilities and/or their families. UCP also operates an equipment loan program, conducts parent workshops, disseminates written literature on topics of interest to people with disabilities.
Robert Masterson, President
Thomas Connolly, Executive Vice President

2685 United Cerebral Palsy of New York City
80 Maiden Lane
New York, NY 10038-4811
212-683-6700
800-GIV-EUCP
Fax: 212-685-8394
e-mail: info@ucpnyc.org
www.ucpnyc.org
United Cerebral Palsy provides information, advocacy, referral services for persons with disabilities and/or their families. UCP also operates an equipment loan program, conducts parent workshops, disseminates written literature on topics of interest.

2686 United Cerebral Palsy of Orange County
980 Roosevelt
Irvine, CA 92620
949-333-6400
Fax: 949-333-6440
e-mail: info@ucp-oc.org
www.ucp-oc.org
United Cerebral Palsy provides information, advocacy, referral services for persons with disabilities and/or their families. UCP also operates an equipment loan program, conducts parent workshops, disseminates written literature on topics of interest.
Paul Pulver, Executive Directory
Lauren Mille Beeler, Director of Therapy Services

2687 United Cerebral Palsy of Putnam & Southern Dutchess Counties
40 John Barrett Road
Patterson, NY 12563
845-878-9078
Fax: 845-878-3203
e-mail: hvcs@aol.com
www.ucpa.org
United Cerebral Palsy provides information, advocacy, referral services for persons with disabilities and/or their families. UCP also operates an equipment loan program, conducts parent workshops, disseminates written literature on topics of interest to people with disabilities.

2688 United Cerebral Palsy of Queens: Queens Centers for Progress
81-15 164th Street
Jamaica, NY 11432
718-380-3000
Fax: 718-380-0483
TTY: 718-969-0270
e-mail: info@queenscp.org
www.queenscp.org
Provides information advocacy and referral services for persons with disabilities and/or their families. Offers an equipment loan program parent workshops and written literature on topics of interest to people with disabilities. Comprehensive services i
Charles Houston, Executive Director

2689 United Cerebral Palsy of Westchester County
1186 King Street
Rye Brook, NY 10573
914-937-3800
Fax: 914-937-0967
www.cpwestchester.org
United Cerebral Palsy provides information advocacy referral services for persons with disabilities and/or their families. UCP also operates an equipment loan program conducts parent workshops disseminates written literature on topics of interest to p
Richard Osterer, President
Richard Eising, Executive Vice President

2690 United Cerebral Palsy of Western New York
7 Community Drive
Buffalo, NY 14225
716-894-0130
Fax: 716-894-8257
e-mail: ucpawny1@aol.com
www.ucpa.org
United Cerebral Palsy provides information advocacy referral services for persons with disabilities and/or their families. UCP also operates an equipment loan program conducts parent workshops disseminates written literature on topics of interest to p

2691 United Cerebral Palsy of the North Country
4 Commerce Lane   315-379-9667
Canton, NY 13617   Fax: 315-379-9388
                                        e-mail: ucpa@imcnet.net
                                                   www.ucpa.org
United Cerebral Palsy provides information advocacy referral services for persons with disabilities and/or their families. UCP also operates an equipment loan program conducts parent workshops disseminates written literature on topics of interest to p

North Carolina

2692 Easter Seals UCP North Carolina & Virginia
2315 Myron Drive   919-783-8898
Raleigh, NC 27607   800-662-7119
                                              Fax: 919-782-5486
                               e-mail: QM@nc.eastersealsucp.com
                                               nc.easterseals.com
A lifelong partner to families managing disabilities and mental health challenges. Serves more than 20,000 individuals and their families annually through an array of services. Enhances the quality of life for individuals and maximizes their potential for engaging in their communities.
Connie L Cochran, President/CEO

Ohio

2693 United Cerebral Palsy of Central Ohio
440 Industrial Mile Road   614-279-0109
Columbus, OH 43228-2411   Fax: 914-279-2527
                            e-mail: tfitch@ucpofcentralohio.org
                                         www.ucpofcentralohio.org
United Cerebral Palsy provides information advocacy referral services for persons with disabilities and/or their families. UCP also operates an equipment loan program conducts parent workshops disseminates written literature on topics of interest to p
Charles Dyas, President/Executive Committee Chair
Diane Dierna, Vice-President

2694 United Cerebral Palsy of Cincinnati
3601 Victory Parkway   513-221-4606
Cincinnati, OH 45229   Fax: 513-872-5262
                              e-mail: sschiller@ucp-cincinnati.org
                                             www.ucp-cincinnati.org
United Cerebral Palsy provides information advocacy referral services for persons with disabilities and/or their families. UCP also operates an equipment loan program conducts parent workshops disseminates written literature on topics of interest to p
Susan Schiller, Executive Director, Development Director

2695 United Cerebral Palsy of Greater Cleveland
10011 Euclid Avenue   216-791-8363
Cleveland, OH 44106   Fax: 216-721-3372
                                e-mail: sdean@ucpcleveland.org
                                                   www.ucpa.org
United Cerebral Palsy provides information, advocacy, referral services for persons with disabilities and/or their families. UCP also operates an equipment loan program, conducts parent workshops, disseminates written literature on topics of interest to people with disabilities.

2696 United Cerebral Palsy of Greater Dane
10011 Euclid Avenue   216-791-8363
Cleveland, OH 44106   Fax: 216-721-3372
                                e-mail: sdean@ucpcleveland.org
                                             www.ucpcleveland.org
United Cerebral Palsy provides information advocacy referral services for persons with disabilities and/or their families. UCP also operates an equipment loan program conducts parent workshops disseminates written literature on topics of interest to p
Robert J Darden, President
Douglas A Neary, Vice President

Oklahoma

2697 United Cerebral Palsy of Oklahoma
10400 Greenbriar Place   405-759-3562
Oklahoma City, OK 73159   Fax: 405-917-7082
                                        e-mail: info@ucpok.org
                                                   www.ucpok.org

United Cerebral Palsy provides information advocacy referral services for persons with disabilities and/or their families. UCP also operates an equipment loan program conducts parent workshops disseminates written literature on topics of interest to p

Oregon

2698 United Cerebral Palsy of Oregon & SW Washington
11731 NE Glenn Widing Drive   503-777-4166
Portland, OR 97220   800-473-4581
                                              Fax: 503-771-8048
                                    e-mail: ucpa@ucpaorwa.org
                                                     www.ucp.org
United Cerebral Palsy provides information advocacy referral services for persons with disabilities and/or their families. UCP also operates an equipment loan program conducts parent workshops disseminates written literature on topics of interest to p
Bud Thoune, Executive Director
Doug Taylor, Development and Marketing Director

Pennsylvania

2699 United Cerebral Palsy Central PA
44 S 38th Street   717-975-0611
Camp Hill, PA 17011   Fax: 717-975-0839
                            e-mail: kidscenter@ucpcentralpa.org
                                                     www.ucp.org
United Cerebral Palsy provides information advocacy referral services for persons with disabilities and/or their families. UCP also operates an equipment loan program conducts parent workshops disseminates written literature on topics of interest to p
Jeffrey W Cooper, President/CEO
Jennifer Brubakerÿÿ, Director of Administrative Services

2700 United Cerebral Palsy of Beaver, Butler & Lawrence Counties
101 Hindman Lane   724-482-4765
Butler, PA 16001   Fax: 724-283-5945
                                                   www.ucpa.org
United Cerebral Palsy provides information, advocacy, referral services for persons with disabilities and/or their families. UCP also operates an equipment loan program, conducts parent workshops, disseminates written literature on topics of interest to people with disabilities.

2701 United Cerebral Palsy of Northwestern Pennsylvania
3745 W 12th Street   814-836-9113
Erie, PA 16505   Fax: 814-833-3919
                                    e-mail: leaton@mecaup.com
                                                   www.ucpa.org
United Cerebral Palsy provides information advocacy referral services for persons with disabilities and/or their families. UCP also operates a wheelchair ramp building program conducts parent workshops offers adaptive recreation activities disseminate
Laura Eaton, Executive Director

2702 United Cerebral Palsy of Pennsylvania
908 N Second Street   717-441-6044
Harrisburg, PA 17102   866-761-6129
                                              Fax: 717-236-2046
                         e-mail: kimberlycossar@wannarassoc.com
                                                     www.ucp.org
United Cerebral Palsy provides information advocacy referral services for persons with disabilities and/or their families. UCP also operates an equipment loan program conducts parent workshops disseminates written literature on topics of interest to p
Joan Martin, Executive Director
Vini Portzline, Policy Information Exchange

2703 United Cerebral Palsy of Philadelphia Vicinity
102 E Mermaid Lane   215-242-4200
Philadelphia, PA 19118   Fax: 215-247-4229
                                              TTY: 215-248-7620
                                    e-mail: ucpkravitz@aol.com
                                                 www.ucpphila.org
United Cerebral Palsy provides information advocacy referral services for persons with disabilities and/or their families. UCP also operates an equipment loan program conducts parent workshops disseminates written literature on topics of interest to p
Gary J Weyhmuller, President
David J Barnhart, Vice President

2704 United Cerebral Palsy of Pittsburgh
4638 Centre Avenue   412-683-7100
Pittsburgh, PA 15213   Fax: 412-683-4160
                                      e-mail: info@ucppittsburgh.org
                                      www.ucp.org
United Cerebral Palsy provides information advocacy referral services for persons with disabilities and/or their families. UCP also operates an equipment loan program conducts parent workshops disseminates written literature on topics of interest to p
Al Condeluci, CEO
Joyce Redmerski, Chief Financial Officer

2705 United Cerebral Palsy of South Central Pennsylvania
788 Cherry Tree Court   717-632-5552
Hanover, PA 17331   800-333-3873
                                      Fax: 717-632-2315
                                      e-mail: phoughton@ucpsouthcentral.org
                                      www.ucp.org
Provides early intervention, in home personal care and community integration services for children and adults with disabilities in York, Adams and Franklin counties.
Paulette Houghton, Executive Director
William Long, Director of Operations

2706 United Cerebral Palsy of Southern Alleghenies Region
119 Jari Drive   814-262-9600
Johnstown, PA 15904   877-371-1110
                                      Fax: 814-262-9650
                                      e-mail: info@ucpsar.org
                                      www.alucp.org
United Cerebral Palsy provides information, advocacy, referral services for persons with disabilities and/or their families. UCP also operates an equipment loan program, conducts parent workshops, disseminates written literature on topics of interest.
Marie Polinsky, CEO
Mark Malzi, CFO

2707 United Cerebral Palsy of Southwestern Pennsylvania
190 N Main Street   724-229-0851
Washington, PA 15301   Fax: 724-229-9252
                                      e-mail: info@ucpswpa.org
                                      www.ucp.org
United Cerebral Palsy provides information, advocacy, referral services for persons with disabilities and/or their families. UCP also operates an equipment loan program, conducts parent workshops, disseminates written literature on topics of interest.

2708 United Cerebral Palsy of Western Pennsylvania
2904 Seminary Drive   724-832-8272
Greensburg, PA 15601   Fax: 724-837-8278
                                      e-mail: ucp@ucpofwesternpa.org
                                      www.ucpa.org
United Cerebral Palsy provides information, advocacy, referral services for persons with disabilities and/or their families. UCP also operates an equipment loan program, conducts parent workshops, disseminates written literature on topics of interest.

Rhode Island

2709 United Cerebral Palsy of Rhode Island
200 Main Street   401-728-1800
Pawtucket, RI 02862   Fax: 401-728-0182
                                      e-mail: ucprisupport@ucpri.org
                                      www.ucpa.org
United Cerebral Palsy provides information, advocacy, referral services for persons with disabilities and/or their families. UCP also operates an equipment loan program, conducts parent workshops, disseminates written literature on topics of interest to people with disabilities.

Tennessee

2710 United Cerebral Palsy of Middle Tennessee
1200 9th Avenue N   615-242-4091
Nashville, TN 37208   Fax: 615-242-3582
                                      e-mail: request@ucpnashville.org
                                      www.ucpa.org
United Cerebral Palsy provides information, advocacy, referral services for persons with disabilities and/or their families. UCP also operates an equipment loan program, conducts parent workshops, disseminates written literature on topics of interest to people with disabilities.

2711 United Cerebral Palsy of the Mid-South
4189 Leroy   901-761-4277
Memphis, TN 38108   Fax: 901-761-7876
                                      e-mail: ucp@ucpmemphis.org
                                      www.ucpa.org
United Cerebral Palsy provides information, advocacy, referral services for persons with disabilities and/or their families. UCP also operates an equipment loan program, conducts parent workshops, disseminates written literature on topics of interest to people with disabilities

Texas

2712 United Cerebral Palsy of Greater Houston
4500 Bissonet   713-838-9050
Bellaire, TX 77401   Fax: 713-838-9098
                                      e-mail: ucp@ucphouston.org
                                      www.ucpa.org
United Cerebral Palsy provides information, advocacy, referral services for persons with disabilities and/or their families. UCP also operates an equipment loan program, conducts parent workshops, disseminates written literature on topics of interest to people with disabilities.

2713 United Cerebral Palsy of Metropolitan Dallas
8802 Harry Hines Boulevard   214-247-4505
Dallas, TX 75235   800-999-1898
                                      Fax: 214-351-2610
                                      e-mail: billknudsen@ucpdallas
                                      www.ucpdallas.org
United Cerebral Palsy provides information, advocacy, referral services for persons with disabilities and/or their families. UCP also operates an equipment loan program, conducts parent workshops, disseminates written literature on topics of interest to people with disabilities.
Bill Knudsen, President / Chief Executive Officer
Becky Adams, Chief Operations Officer

2714 United Cerebral Palsy of Tarrant County
1555 Merrimac Circle   817-332-7171
Fort Worth, TX 76107   Fax: 817-332-7601
                                      e-mail: info@ucptc.org
                                      www.ucpa.org
United Cerebral Palsy provides information, advocacy, referral services for persons with disabilities and/or their families. UCP also operates an equipment loan program, conducts parent workshops, disseminates written literature on topics of interest to people with disabilities.

2715 United Cerebral Palsy of Texas
1016 La Posada Drive   512-472-8696
Austin, TX 78752   800-798-1492
                                      Fax: 512-472-8026
                                      e-mail: info@ucptexas.org
                                      www.ucpa.org
United Cerebral Palsy provides information, advocacy, referral services for persons with disabilities and/or their families. UCP also operates an equipment loan program, conducts parent workshops, disseminates written literature on topics of interest.

Utah

2716 United Cerebral Palsy of Utah
PO Box 65219   801-266-1805
S Salt Lake, UT 84165   Fax: 801-266-2404
                                      e-mail: shellyp@ucputah.org
                                      www.ucpa.org
United Cerebral Palsy provides information, advocacy, referral services for persons with disabilities and/or their families. UCP also operates an equipment loan program, conducts parent workshops, disseminates written literature on topics of interest.

Virginia

2717 **Cerebral Palsy of Virginia**
5825 Arrowhead Drive 757-497-7474
Virginia Beach, VA 23462 Fax: 757-497-0868
e-mail: kap@cerebralpalsyofvirginia.org
www.cerebralpalsyofvirginia.org
Cerebral Palsy provides information, advocacy, referral services for persons with disabilities and/or their families. Cerebral Palsy also operates an equipment loan program, summer computer camp, art works job training program and much more.
Kathy Prendergast, Executive Director
Michelle Majority, Associate Executive Director

2718 **United Cerebral Palsy of Washington DC**
1818 New York Avenue 202-526-0146
Washington, DC 20002 Fax: 202-526-0519
e-mail: dcarter@ucpdc.org
www.ucpdc.org
United Cerebral Palsy provides information, advocacy, referral services for persons with disabilities and/or their families. UCP also operates an equipment loan program, conducts parent workshops, disseminates written literature on topics of interest.
Mark A Simione ÿ, ÿBoard President
Roderick Johnson, ÿBoard Secretary

Washington

2719 **United Cerebral Palsy of Pierce County**
6315 S 19th Street 253-565-1463
Tacoma, WA 98466-6217 Fax: 253-565-1463
e-mail: info@ucp-sps.org
www.ucpa.org
United Cerebral Palsy provides information, advocacy, referral services for persons with disabilities and/or their families. UCP also operates an equipment loan program, conducts parent workshops, disseminates written literature on topics of interest to people with disabilities.

Wisconsin

2720 **United Cerebral Palsy of Greater Dane County**
2801 Coho Street 608-273-4434
Madison, WI 53713 Fax: 608-273-3426
e-mail: ucpgdc@ucpdane.org
www.ucpa.org
Provides information, advocacy, referral services for persons with disabilities and/or their families. UCP also conducts parent workshops and disseminates written literature on topics of interest to people with disabilities.
Susan Knox, Administrative Assistant

2721 **United Cerebral Palsy of North Central Wisconsin**
108 Scott Street 715-842-8700
Wausau, WI 54401 800-472-4408
www.ucpa.org
United Cerebral Palsy provides information, advocacy, referral services for persons with disabilities and/or their families. UCP also operates an equipment loan program, conducts parent workshops, disseminates written literature on topics of interest to people with disabilities.

2722 **United Cerebral Palsy of Southeastern Wisconsin**
7519 W Oklahoma Avenue 414-329-4500
Milwaukee, WI 53219 888-482-7739
Fax: 414-329-4510
TTY: 414-329-4511
e-mail: info@ucpsew.org
www.ucpa.org
United Cerebral Palsy provides information, advocacy, referral services for persons with disabilities and/or their families. UCP also operates an equipment loan program, conducts parent workshops, disseminates written literature on topics of interest to people with disabilities.

2723 **United Cerebral Palsy of West Central Wisconsin**
206 Water Street 715-832-1782
Eau Claire, WI 54703 Fax: 715-832-8203
e-mail: ucp1ruth@sbcglobal net
www.ucpa.org

United Cerebral Palsy provides information, advocacy, referral services for persons with disabilities and/or their families. UCP also operates an equipment loan program, conducts parent workshops, disseminates written literature on topics of interest to people with disabilities.

2724 **United Cerebral Palsy of Wisconsin**
206 Water Street 715-832-1782
Eau Claire, WI 54703 800-261-1895
Fax: 715-832-8203
e-mail: ucp1ruth@sbcglobal net
www.ucpa.org
United Cerebral Palsy provides information, advocacy, referral services for persons with disabilities and/or their families. UCP also operates an equipment loan program, conducts parent workshops, disseminates written literature on topics of interest.

Research Centers

2725 **Orthopaedic Biomechanics Laboratory Shriners Hospital for Crippled Children**
Shriners Hospital for Crippled Children
2181 Westlawn Building 319-335-7529
Iowa City, IA 52242-1100 Fax: 319-335-7530
Offers research and studies into cerebral palsy.
Stephen R Skinner, Clinical Director

Support Groups & Hotlines

2726 **Family Support Network**
215 Centennial Mall S 402-477-2992
Lincoln, NE 68508-1813 800-245-6081

2727 **National Health Information Center**
PO Box 1133 310-565-4167
Washington, DC 20013-1133 800-336-4797
Fax: 301-984-4256
e-mail: info@nhic.org
www.health.gov/nhic
A health information referral service sponsored by the Office of Disease Prevention and Health Promotion. Puts health professionals and consumers who have health questions in touch with those organizations that are best able to provide answers.

Books

2728 **An Introduction to Your Child Who Has Cerebral Palsy**
Medic Publishing Company
PO Box 89 425-881-2883
Redmond, WA 98073-0089
Information and answers to questions for parents of children with cerebral palsy.

2729 **Children with Cerebral Palsy**
Woodbine House
6510 Bells Mill Road 301-897-3570
Bethesda, MD 20817-1636 800-843-7323
Fax: 301-897-5838
e-mail: info@woodbinehouse.com
www.woodbinehouse.com
Explains what Cerebral Palsy is, and discusses its diagnosis and treatment. Also offers information and advice concerning daily care, early intervention, therapy, educational options and family life.
432 pages Paperback
ISBN: 0-933149-15-8

2730 **Discovery Book**
United Cerebral Palsy Association
1660 L Street NW 202-776-0406
Washington, DC 20036-5602 800-872-5827
Fax: 202-776-0414
ucpnatl@ucpa.org

2731 **Individuals with Cerebral Palsy**
Mainstream

1030 5th Street NW
Washington, DC 20001-2504
202-898-1400
e-mail: info@mainstreaminc.org
www.mainstreaminc.org
Mainstreaming individuals with cerebral palsy into the workplace.
12 pages

2732 **Occupational Therapy Practice Guidelines for Adults with Cerebral Palsy**
American Occupational Therapy Association
4720 Montgomery Lane
301-652-2682
Bethesda, MD 20824-1220
Fax: 301-652-7711
TDD: 800-377-8555
www.aota.org
15 pages
ISBN: 1-569001-59-6

Children's Books

2733 **Can't You Be Still?**
Gemma B Publishing
776 Corydon Avenue
204-452-7566
Winnipeg, MB, R3M 0Y1,
Fax: 204-475-9903
e-mail: gempub@mts.net
www.gemmab.mb.ca
On Ann's first day at school, the other students are both fascinated and horrified by her cerebral palsy. She wins them over by helping them jump into the water and swim. Available in Braille.
24 pages Paperback
ISBN: 0-969647-70-0
Sarah Yates, President

2734 **Cerebral Palsy**
Franklin Watts Grolier
90 Old Sherman Tpke
203-797-3500
Danbury, CT 06816-0001
800-621-1115
Fax: 203-797-3197
www.grolier.com
A look at the causes, detection, prevention, effects and treatment of Cerebral Palsy.
112 pages Grades 7-12
ISBN: 0-531125-29-7

2735 **Here's What I Mean To Say**
Gemma B Publishing
776 Corydon Avenue
204-452-7566
Winnipeg, MB, R3M 0Y1,
Fax: 204-475-9903
e-mail: gempub@mts.net
www.gemmab.mb.ca
In this books Ann's battle to read is assisted by an angel, who helps her read the directions in Jay's computer game. Is the angel read or is this the magic of reading? Available in Braille.
32 pages Paperback
ISBN: 0-969647-72-7
Sarah Yates, President

2736 **Mine for Keeps**
Little, Brown & Company
34 Beacon Street
617-227-0730
Boston, MA 02108-1415
800-343-9204
Sarah Jean Copeland was born with cerebral palsy. At four years of age she was placed in a school for handicapped children but made such good progress that she could return home. Coming home for Sarah meant a new school, and new adjustments to her parents, two sisters, and her brother. At first Sarah was scared and didn't think she could do all the things she needed to do, but she soon learned her fears were not well-founded.
186 pages Hardcover

2737 **My Brother Matthew**
Woodbine House
6510 Bells Mill Road
Bethesda, MD 20817-1636
800-843-7323
A book written from the point of view of the brother of Matthew, a boy with multiple disabilities, David describes the incidents characterizing how life in his family changes.
28 pages Grades K-5
Sarah Strickler

2738 **Nobody Knows!**
Gemma B Publishing
776 Corydon Avenue
204-452-7566
Winnipeg, MB, R3M 0Y1,
Fax: 204-475-9903
e-mail: gempub@mts.net
www.gemmab.mb.ca
Is an adventure during which a frustrated Ann goes out to find someone who understand what she wants. She meets a turtle and an alligator, who like her don't use words to communicate. Available in Braille.
24 pages Paperback
ISBN: 0-969647-71-9
Sarah Yates, President

Newsletters

2739 **Family Support Bulletin**
United Cerebral Palsy Associations
1660 L Street NW
202-842-1266
Washington, DC 20036-1202
800-872-5827

Pamphlets

2740 **Cerebral Palsy: Facts & Figures**
United Cerebral Palsy Associations
1660 L Street NW
Washington, DC 20036
800-872-5827
Fax: 202-776-0414
www.ucp.org
Offers information on what cerebral palsy is, the effects, causes, types, and prevention.

Audio & Video

2741 **A Day At A Time**
Filmakers Library
124 E 40th Street
212-808-4980
New York, NY 10016-1798
Fax: 212-808-4983
e-mail: info@filmakers.com
www.filmakers.com
The story of twin girls with Cerebral Palsy, whose family is determined that they have every opportunity to participate in and lead normal lives. Winner of a number of awards. DVD or VHS $195, Classroom Rental $75
VHS or DVD
Sue Oscar, Co-President

Web Sites

2742 **American Academy for Cerebral Palsy and Developmental Medicine**
AACPDM.org
A multidisciplinary scientific society devoted to the study of cerebral palsy and other childhood onset disabilities, to promoting professional education for the treatment and management of these conditions, and to improving the quality of life for people with these disabilities.

2743 **Healing Well**
www.healingwell.com
An online health resource guide to medical news, chat, information and articles, newsgroups and message boards, books, disease-related web sites, medical directories, and more for patients, friends, and family coping with disabling diseases, disorders, or chronic illnesses.

2744 **Health Finder**
www.healthfinder.gov
Searchable, carefully developed web site offering information on over 1000 topics. Developed by the US Department of Health and Human Services, the site can be used in both English and Spanish.

2745 **Healthlink USA**
www.healthlinkusa.com

Health information concerning treatment, cures, prevention, diagnosis, risk factors, research, support groups, email lists, personal stories and much more. Updated regularly.

2746 Helios Health

www.helioshealth.com

Online resource for your health information. Detailed information about specific health topics, access to expert advice from our Medical Advisory Board, and up-to-date health news.

2747 MedicineNet

www.medicinenet.com

An online resource for consumers providing easy-to-read, authoritative medical and health information.

2748 Medscape

www.medscape.com

Medscape offers specialists, primary care physicians, and other health professionals the Web's most robust and integrated medical information and educational tools.

2749 National Institute of Neurological Disorders and Stroke

www.ninds.nih.gov

The mission of NINDS is to reduce the burden of neurological disease - a burden borne by every age group, by every segment of society, by people all over the world.

2750 National Rehabilitation Information Center

www.naric.com/

One of the three components of the office of Special Education and Rehabilitative Services.

2751 Neurology Channel

www.neurologychannel.com

Find clearly explained, medically accurate information regarding conditions, including an overview, symptoms, causes, diagnostic procedures and treatment options. On this site it is possible to ask questions and get information from a neurologist and connect to people who have similar health interests.

2752 United Cerebral Palsy Associations

www.ucpa.org

A network of approximately 119 state and local voluntary agencies which provide services, conduct public and professional education programs and support research in cerebral palsy.

2753 WebMD

www.webmd.com

Provides links to over 20 articles involving cerebral palsy.

Description

2754 Chronic Fatigue Syndrome

Chronic Fatigue Syndrome, CFS, is an illness characterized by longstanding fatigue that impairs daily functioning. It may be accompanied by sore throat, swollen glands, muscle and joint pain, headaches, sleeplessness, and impaired memory or concentration. Profound or life-altering fatigue—the disease's hallmark—usually comes on suddenly and persists for at least six months, and often for years.

The cause of CFS is controversial. One theory is that a chronic viral infection is involved. Allergic reactions have also been proposed, and various immunologic abnormalities have been reported. Another theory involves proposed disturbances in the hormonal (endocrine) system. Psychological factors may be the cause, although CFS is distinct from typical depression or anxiety. Because the cause is unknown, there is no single test or group of tests that can diagnose CFS. Therefore, the goal in evaluating an individual with presumed CFS is to exclude other treatable illnesses.

Given the difficulty in proving a diagnosis or understanding the cause of CFS, it is not surprising that many treatments have been offered for it. Antidepressants appear to be the most successful treatment studied so far; as many as 80 percent of patients report benefit. Other therapies, including nutritional supplements, hormones, antiviral drugs and steroids have been mostly disappointing.

Patients with CFS need emotional support from physicians and family, due to the debilitating nature of the disease. Individual and group therapy may help some individuals. See also *Fibromyalgia*.

National Agencies & Associations

2755 American Academy of Sleep Medicine
2510 North Frontage Road   630-737-9700
Darien, IL 60561   Fax: 630-737-9790
                                         www.aasmnet.org
A unique multi-disciplinary organization for both individual members and center members. The individual member branch includes clinicians involved in the diagnosis and treatment of patients with disorders of sleep and alertness.
Jerome Barrett, Executive Director

2756 International Association for Chronic Fatigue
27 N Wacker Drive   847-258-7248
Chicago, IL 60606   Fax: 847-579-0975
                                         e-mail: Admin@iacfs.net
                                         www.IACFS.net
A nonprofit organization of research scientists, physicians, licensed medical healthcare professionals and other individuals and institutions interested in promoting the stimulation, coordination and exchange of ideas for CFS research and patient care.
Newsletter
Fred Friedbe PhD, President

2757 National CFS Association
PO Box 18426   816-737-1343
Kansas City, MO 64133   e-mail: information@ncfsa.org
                                         www.ncfsfa.org

Provides information on different brochures journals books magazines and pamphlets on the Chronic Fatigue Syndrome.
Orvalene Prewitt, President

2758 National Chronic Fatigue Syndrome and Fibromyalgia Association
PO Box 18426   816-737-1343
Kansas City, MO 64133-8426   e-mail: information@ncfsfa.org
                                         www.ncfsfa.org
Compiles and provides peer reviewed, scientifically accurate educational materials to inform the public, health professionals, patients and their families about the nature and impact of chronic fatigue syndrome, fibromyalgia and related disorders. Offers a support group.
Orvalene Prewitt, President

2759 National Chronic Fatigue Syndrome and Fibr
PO Box 18426   816-737-1343
Kansas City, MO 64133   Fax: 816-524-6782
                                         e-mail: information@ncfsfa.org
                                         www.ncfsfa.org
Compiles and provides peer reviewed scientifically accurate educational materials to inform the public health professionals, patients and their families about the nature and impact of chronic fatigue syndrome, fibromyalgia and related disorders.
Orvalene Prewitt, President

2760 National Institute of Allergy and Infectious Diseases
Office of Communications
6610 Rockledge Drive   301-496-5717
Bethesda, MD 20892-6612   866-284-4107
                                         Fax: 301-402-3573
                                         TDD: 800-877-8339
                                         e-mail: af10r@nih.gov
                                         www.niaid.nih.gov
Offers information and educational materials on Chronic Fatigue Syndrome and other disorders.
Anthony S Fauci, MD, Director

2761 Option Institute
2080 South Undermountain Road   413-229-2100
Sheffield, MA 01257   800-714-2779
                                         Fax: 413-229-8931
                                         e-mail: participantsupport@option.org
                                         www.option.org
Self-defeating beliefs, along with attitudes and judgments, can lead to a host of physical and psychological challenges, including Chronic Fatigue Syndrome. The Option Institute offers programs designed to help you gain new perspectives on the attitudes and judgments that may be affecting your life, especially those regarding and surrounding Chronic Fatigue Syndrome.
Barry Kaufman, Co-Founder
Samahria Ltye Kaufman, Co-Founder

Foundations

2762 National CFIDS Foundation
103 Aletha Road   781-449-3535
Needham, MA 02492   Fax: 781-449-8606
                                         e-mail: info@ncf-net.org
                                         www.ncf-net.org
The goals of the Foundation are to help fund medical research to find a cause, expedite treatments and eventually a cure for this devastating disease. The NCF also strives to provide information, education, and support to those people who have CFIDS (also known as chronic fatigue syndrome (CFS), myalgic encephalomyelitis (ME) and many other names)— as well as related illnesses such as Gulf War Illness (GWI) and Multiple Chemical Sensitivities (MCS). Provides guides, articles, and newsletters.
Gail Kansky, President
Prof. Alan Cocchetto, Medical Advisor

Support Groups & Hotlines

2763 CDC AIDS/STD Hotline

404-639-3534
800-342-2437
TTY: 800-243-7889
www.cdc.gov

Hotline

2764 Centers for Disease Control and Prevention
1600 Clifton Road
Atlanta, GA 30333
800-232-4636
TTY: 888-232-6348
e-mail: cdcinfo@cdc.gov
www.cdc.gov

Collaborating to create the expertise, information, and tools that people and their communities need to protect their health - through health promotion, prevention of disease, injury and disability, and preparedness for new health threats.
Thomas R Frieden MD MPH, Director

2765 Chronic Fatigue Syndrome & Fibromyalgia Support
7250 Clearvista Dr
Indianapolis, IN 46256
317-252-9223
Offers emotional support, education and information about CFS and FMS through statewide monthly meetings and a quarterly newsletter. Provides 24-hour hotline and physician/attorney referrals. Financial assistance for members. Support group meets twice a month at Community Hospital North Professional Building and at other locations throughout Indiana.

2766 National Chronic Fatigue Syndrome and Fibromyalgia Association
PO Box 18426
Kansas City, MO 64133
816-737-1343
Fax: 816-524-6782
e-mail: information@ncfsfa.org
www.ncfsfa.org

To educate and inform the public about the nature and impact of Chronic Fatigue Syndrome and Fibromyalgia and related disorders.
Orvalene Prewitt, President

2767 National Health Information Center
PO Box 1133
Washington, DC 20013-1133
310-565-4167
800-336-4797
Fax: 301-984-4256
e-mail: info@nhic.org
www.health.gov/nhic

A health information referral service sponsored by the Office of Disease Prevention and Health Promotion. Puts health professionals and consumers who have health questions in touch with those organizations that are best able to provide answers.

Books

2768 CFIDS in Children Packet
CFIDS Association of America
PO Box 220398
Charlotte, NC 28222-0398
800-442-3437
This packet contains articles about CFIDS and children.
60 pages

2769 CFS Cookbook
CFIDS Association of America
PO Box 220398
Charlotte, NC 28222-0398
800-442-3437
Gourmet recipes designed to combat the monotony associated with CFIDS, allergy and immune-compromised diets.
218 pages

2770 Chronic Fatigue Syndrome Cookbook: Delicious & Wellness-Enhancing Recipes
DIANE Publishing Company
330 Pusey Avenue, Unit #3 Rear
Darby, PA 19023
610-461-6200
800-782-3833
Fax: 610-461-6130
e-mail: dianepublishing@gmail.com
www.dianepublishing.net

These recipes help combat the boredom of the CFS diet usually recommended and still satisfy all of your nutritional requirements as a CFS sufferer. In addition, the book includes a comprehensive look at the do's and don't's of a CFS diet, quick recipes for those days when you are too tired to cook and an insightful medical introduction.
218 pages Hardcover
ISBN: 0-756753-28-7
Herman Baron, Publisher

2771 Chronic Fatigue Syndrome and the Yeast Connection
CFIDS Association of America
PO Box 220398
Charlotte, NC 28222-0398
800-442-3437
Dr. Crook explains the possible role of multiple entities, including yeast overgrowth, allergies and chemical sensitivities, in CFS and how each contributes to immune dysregulation.
386 pages

2772 Chronic Fatigue Syndrome: Information for Physicians
Barry Leonard, author
DIANE Publishing Company
330 Pusey Avenue, Unit #3 Rear
Darby, PA 19023
610-461-6200
800-782-3833
Fax: 610-461-6130
e-mail: dianepublishing@gmail.com
www.dianepublishing.net

Includes a historical perspective on chronic fatigue syndrome; epidemiology; clinical picture; evaluation of patients; patient management; etiologic theories; public health service resources; fact sheet; resources for patients, overview of the CFS research program; NIAID and NIAID/Johns Hopkins hospital study, which seeks volunteers, management strategies for CFS; the relationship between nuerally mediatec hypotension and CFS and fibromyalgia and CFS; solving diagnostic and therapeutic dilemmas.
60 pages Paperback
ISBN: 0-788143-78-6
Herman Baron, Publisher

2773 Chronic Fatigue Syndrome: The Limbic Hypothesis
CFIDS Association of America
PO Box 220398
Charlotte, NC 28222-0398
800-442-3437
A detailed thesis proposing CFS as a limbic system encephalopathy in the context of a dysregulated neuroimmune system.
259 pages

2774 Chronic Fatigue: Your Complete Exercise Guide
Human Kinetics Press
PO Box 5076
Champaign, IL 61825-5076
217-351-5076
800-747-4457
Fax: 217-351-2674
www.humankinetics.com

1993 144 pages Paperback
ISBN: 0-873223-93-4
Steve Ruhlig, Marketing Director

2775 Coping With CFS
CFIDS Association of America
PO Box 220398
Charlotte, NC 28222-0398
704-365-2343
800-442-3437
Fax: 704-365-9755
e-mail: info@cfids.org
www.cfids.org

Offers practical, established coping strategies for living better with CFIDS. Based on Dr. Friedberg's experiences as a person with CFIDS and a counselor to PWCs.
176 pages
Jon Sterling, Chairman
Kim Kenny, President/CEO

2776 Disability and Chronic Fatigue Syndrome
The Haworth Press
10 Alice Street
Binghamton, NY 13904-1580
607-722-5857
800-429-6784
Fax: 800-895-0582
e-mail: getinfo@haworthpressinc.com
www.haworthpressinc.com

Discusses the difficult subject of how to diagnose disability in chronic fatigue syndrome patients, how to determine the severity of a patient's disability, and how new disability guidelines would make more chronic fatigue patients eligible to apply for disability benefits.
121 pages Paperback
ISBN: 0-789005-01-8
Bill Cohen, Publisher
Sandy Jones, VP Marketing

2777 Doctor's Guide to Chronic Fatigue Syndrome
CFIDS Association of America
PO Box 220398
Charlotte, NC 28222-0398   800-442-3437
Written by one of the world's leading experts on CFIDS.
275 pages

2778 Fifty Things You Should Know About the Chronic Fatigue Syndrome Epidemic
St. Martin's Press
175 5th Avenue   212-674-5151
New York, NY 10010-7848   800-221-7945
    Fax: 212-420-9314
1993
ISBN: 0-312950-43-8

2779 Hope and Help for Chronic Fatigue Syndrome
CFIDS Association of America
PO Box 220398
Charlotte, NC 28222-0398   704-365-2343
    800-442-3437
    Fax: 704-365-9755
    e-mail: info@cfids.org
    www.cfids.org
Insight into the experience of having CFIDS, the physical and emotional impact, difficulty in obtaining a diagnosis, available methods of treatment and key strategies for regaining control over your life.
216 pages
Jon Sterling, Chairman
Kim Kenny, President/CEO

2780 International Classification of Sleep Disorders
American Academy of Sleep Medicine
One Westbrook Corporate Center   708-492-0930
Westchester, IL 60154   Fax: 708-492-0943
    www.aasmnet.org
A comprehensive manual for physicians and other healthcare professionals containing information on 84 sleep disorders. The extensive text describes the diagnostic features of each disorder and includes specific diagnostic and severity criteria for each disorder.
396 pages Paperback

2781 Living with CFS: A Personal Story of the Struggle for Recovery
CFIDS Association of America
PO Box 220398
Charlotte, NC 28222-0398   800-442-3437
Describes the pain associated with the author's loss of livelihood, impaired physical and mental functioning and the strain on his marriage and friendships, while maintaining hope for recovery.
224 pages
ISBN: 1-560250-75-5

2782 Living with ME
CFIDS Association of America
PO Box 220398
Charlotte, NC 28222-0398   800-442-3437
    Fax: 704-365-9755
The author describes M.E. (mylagic encephalomyelitis - the British term for chronic fatigue syndrome), and discusses practical methods for coping and comments on various treatments.

2783 Music Appreciation
CFIDS Association of America
PO Box 220398
Charlotte, NC 28222-0398   800-442-3437
A full-length collection of poems by Skloot who has been disabled by CFIDS since 1988.
105 pages

2784 Night-Side: CFS and the Illness Experience
CFIDS Association of America

PO Box 220398   704-365-2343
Charlotte, NC 28222-0398   800-442-3437
    Fax: 704-365-9755
    e-mail: info@cfids.org
    www.cfids.org
An honest and ultimately hopeful exploration of what it means to have your life shattered by disease.
190 pages
Jon Sterling, Chairman
Kim Kenny, President/CEO

2785 Recovering From the Chronic Fatigue Syndrome: A Guide to Self-Empowerment
Berkley Books
200 Madison Avenue
New York, NY 10016-3903   212-951-8800
    www.penguinputman.com
This book teaches persons with CFIDS to take control of their illness and to help themselves find the road to recovery.
1993 224 pages Paperback
ISBN: 0-399518-07-0

2786 Running on Empty
CFIDS Association of America
PO Box 220398   704-365-2343
Charlotte, NC 28222-0398   800-442-3437
    Fax: 704-365-9755
    e-mail: info@cfids.org
    www.cfids.org
Landmark guide to CFIDS has just been revised and re-released. A must read for the newly disgnosed.
315 pages
Jon Sterling, Chairman
Kim Kenny, President/CEO

2787 Self-Caring Fatigue
Rodale Press
33 E Minor Street   610-967-5171
Emmaus, PA 18098-0099   800-441-7761
    Fax: 610-967-8963
    e-mail: info@rodale.com
    www.rodale.com
A step-by-step plan to uncover and eliminate the causes of chronic fatigue.
1993 320 pages
ISBN: 0-875961-61-4

2788 Solving the Puzzle of CFS
2730 Wilshire Boulevard   310-453-4424
Santa Monica, CA 90403-4724   Fax: 310-966-9196

Magazines

2789 CFIDS Chronicle
CFIDS Association of America
PO Box 220398   704-362-2343
Charlotte, NC 28222-0398   800-442-3437
    Fax: 704-365-9755
The largest and most comprehensive periodical specifically pertaining to chronic fatigue syndrome information in the world.

2790 Feel Good Catalog
2895 W Oxford Avenue   303-790-1045
Englewood, CO 80110-4370   800-997-6789
Variety of items to ease pain.

2791 Journal SLEEP
American Academy of Sleep Medicine
One Westbrook Corporate Center   708-492-0930
Westchester, IL 60154   Fax: 708-492-0943
    www.journalslep.org
Publishes articles ranging from clinical investigations of sleep/wake disorders and medical problems during sleep, to investigations of the basic physiological and biochemical events and anatomical structures involved in normal and abnormal sleep. Includes psychological and psycho-physiological research, as

well as research in relevant areas of circadian and biological rhythms.
10x Year
ISBN: 0-161810-5 -

2792   Journal of the Chronic Fatigue Syndrome
Haworth Medical Press
10 Alice Street   607-722-5857
Binghamton, NY 13904-1503   800-429-6784
Fax: 607-722-0012
www.haworth.org
Peer reviewed medical journal containing CFIDS scientific abstract information. Appropriate for patients as well as medical professionals.
Quarterly
Nancy Klimas MD, Founding Co-Editor

Newsletters

2793   Health Points
TyH Publications
17007 E Colony Drive
Fountain Hills, AZ 85268   800-801-1406
e-mail: editor@e-tyh.com
National newsletter with articles on complementary therapy, latest nutrition news, disability issues and much more. Focus is on fibromyalgia, chronic fatigue, arthritis and chronic pain.
Quarterly

2794   Heart of America News
National Chronic Fatigue Syndrome & Fibromyalgia
PO Box 18426   660-313-2000
Kansas City, MO 64133-8426
Offers scientifically accurate information, medical updates, informational references, articles on coping and living with Chronic Fatigue Syndrome and more, based on peer-reviewed materials.
Quarterly

2795   National Forum
103 Aletha Road   781-449-3535
Needham, MA 02492   Fax: 781-449-8606
e-mail: info@ncf-net.org
www.ncf-net.org
The Forum's focus: CFIDS/ME, FMS, GWI, MCS and related illnesses.
Gail Kansky, President

2796   Syndrome Sentinel
Massachusetts CFIDS Association
808 Main Street
Waltham, MA 02451-8533   781-893-4415
www2.shore.net
This quarterly newsletter contains articles written by health-care professionals working with these conditions. Contributors include traditional and alternative experts, as well as personal stories from people with these chronic syndromes and their significant others.

2797   The National Forum
The National CFIDS Foundation
103 Aletha Road   781-449-3535
Needham, MA 02492   Fax: 781-449-8606
e-mail: info@ncf-net.org
www.ncf-net.org
Offers the latest information on CFIDS treatments being tried throughout the United States.

Pamphlets

2798   Americans with Disabilities Act: CFS and Employment
National Chronic Fatigue Syndrome & Fibromyalgia
PO Box 18426   660-313-2000
Kansas City, MO 64133-8426

2799   CFIDS Membership Packet
CFIDS Association of America
PO Box 220398
Charlotte, NC 28222-0398   800-442-3437
Fax: 704-365-9755

Offers pamphlets, brochures, information on local support groups for members.

2800   CFIDS in Children
CFIDS Association of America
PO Box 220398
Charlotte, NC 28222-0398   800-442-3437
Describes the special difficulties faced by children with CFIDS.

2801   CFS in the Workplace
National Chronic Fatigue Syndrome & Fibromyalgia
PO Box 18426   660-313-2000
Kansas City, MO 64133

2802   Chronic Fatigue Syndrome & School Success
National Chronic Fatigue Syndrome & Fibromyalgia
PO Box 18426   660-313-2000
Kansas City, MO 64133-8426

2803   Chronic Fatigue Syndrome in Children
National Chronic Fatigue Syndrome & Fibromyalgia
PO Box 18426   660-313-2000
Kansas City, MO 64133

2804   Chronic Fatigue Syndrome in Men
National Chronic Fatigue Syndrome & Fibromyalgia
PO Box 18426   660-313-2000
Kansas City, MO 64133-8426

2805   Chronic Fatigue Syndrome: A Pamphlet for Physicians
National Institute of Allergy & Infectious Disease
Building 31, Room 7A50
Bethesda, MD 20892-2520   301-496-5717
www.niaid.nih.gov
Offers information on epidemiology, clinical procedures, evaluations, patient management, neuropsychologic features and etiologic theories.

2806   Chronic Fatigue Syndrome: The Thief of Vitality
National Chronic Fatigue Syndrome & Fibromyalgia
PO Box 18426   660-313-2000
Kansas City, MO 64133-8426

2807   Coping Skills
National Chronic Fatigue Syndrome & Fibromyalgia
PO Box 18426   660-313-2000
Kansas City, MO 64133-8426

2808   Disability Packet
CFIDS Association of America
PO Box 220398
Charlotte, NC 28222-0398   800-442-3437
Includes nine Chronicle articles about disability benefits and how persons with CFIDS can secure Social Security Disability Insurance benefits.
42 pages

2809   Facts About Chronic Fatigue Syndrome
Centers for Disease Control & Prevention
Division of Viral Diseases   404-639-3311
Atlanta, GA 30333

2810   Fibromyalgia
National Chronic Fatigue Syndrome & Fibromyalgia
PO Box 18426   660-313-2000
Kansas City, MO 64133-8426

2811   March is Chronic Fatigue Syndrome Awareness Month Tips
National Chronic Fatigue Syndrome & Fibromyalgia
PO Box 18426   660-313-2000
Kansas City, MO 64133

2812   Neuropsychological Rehabilitation Suggestions/Techniques
National Chronic Fatigue Syndrome & Fibromyalgia
PO Box 18426   660-313-2000
Kansas City, MO 64133-8426

2813   School's Guide for Students with CFS
National Chronic Fatigue Syndrome & Fibromyalgia
PO Box 18426   660-313-2000
Kansas City, MO 64133-8426

2814 Social Security Disability Benefits Information
National Chronic Fatigue Syndrome & Fibromyalgia
PO Box 18426   660-313-2000
Kansas City, MO 64133-8426

2815 Understanding CFIDS
CFIDS Association of America
PO Box 220398
Charlotte, NC 28222-0398   800-442-3437
Provides an extensive overview of CFIDS and answers the most
commonly asked questions about the disease.

2816 Understanding the Emotions Surrounding CFS
National Chronic Fatigue Syndrome & Fibromyalgia
PO Box 18426   660-313-2000
Kansas City, MO 64133-8426

Audio & Video

**2817 Behavioral and Circadian Sleep Problems of Infancy and
Childhood**
American Academy of Sleep Medicine
One Westbrook Corporate Center   708-492-0930
Westchester, IL 60154   Fax: 708-492-0943
                                            www.aasmnet.org
Addresses the problems of sleep disorders in children and outlines
the types of disturbances, both of a medical and behavioral nature,
that are commonly identified.
66 slides

2818 CFS and Self-Esteem
CFIDS Association of America
PO Box 220398
Charlotte, NC 28222-0398   800-442-3437
Addresses the sources of low self-esteem in persons with CFIDS
and offers reassurance and practical techniques for increasing
self-confidence.
Audiotape

2819 CFS: Addressing the Realities of a Chronic Illness
National Chronic Fatigue Syndrome & Fibromyalgia
PO Box 18426   660-313-2000
Kansas City, MO 64133-8426
This video offers reliable information featuring patients and a
medical professional.

2820 CFS: Unraveling the Mystery
CFIDS Association of America
PO Box 220398
Charlotte, NC 28222-0398   800-442-3437
An excellent videotape for convincing skeptics that CFIDS is a real
disease.
Videotape

2821 Chronic Fatigue Syndrome: For Those Who Care
CFIDS Association of America
PO Box 220398
Charlotte, NC 28222-0398   800-442-3437
An audiotape designed for friends and family of persons with
CFIDS.
Audiotape

**2822 Chronic Fatigue Syndrome: Information, Relaxation/Healing
Exercise**
CFIDS Association of America
PO Box 220398
Charlotte, NC 28222-0398   800-442-3437
Includes a comprehensive overview of CFS and relaxation/healing
and imagery/stress reduction exercises for persons with CFIDS.
Audiotape

2823 Fibromyalgia
National Chronic Fatigue Syndrome & Fibromyalgia
PO Box 18426   660-313-2000
Kansas City, MO 64133
Videotape

**2824 HHS Satelite Video on Chronic Fatigue Syndrome and
Fibromyalgia Association**
National Chronic Fatigue Syndrome and Fibromyalgia

PO Box 18426   660-313-2000
Kansas City, MO 64133-8426

2825 Living Hell: The Real World of Chronic Fatigue Syndrome
CFIDS Association of America
PO Box 220398
Charlotte, NC 28222-0398   800-442-3437
An emotional exposure of the tragedy of CFIDS.
Videotape

2826 Neurocognitive Aspects of CFS
CFIDS Association of America
PO Box 220398
Charlotte, NC 28222-0398   800-442-3437
A description of CFIDS-associated neurocognitive deficits and
strategies for coping with them and the embarrassment and frustra-
tion they cause.
Audiotape

Web Sites

2827 American Association for Chronic Fatigue Syndrome
                                            www.aacfs.org
A non profit organization of research scientists, physicians, licensed medical healthcare professionals, and other indviduals and
institutions interested in promoting the stimulation, coordination,
and exchange of ideas for CFS research and patient care.

2828 CFIDS Association of America
                                            www.cfids.org
The nation's leading charitable organization devoted to conquering chronic fatigue syndrome by supporting research, education
and public policy programs.

2829 Centers for Disease Control and Prevention
                                            www.cdc.gov
Offers information and educational materials on CFS.

2830 Healing Well
                                            www.healingwell.com
An online health resource guide to medical news, chat, information
and articles, newsgroups and message boards, books, disease-related web sites, medical directories, and more for patients, friends,
and family coping with disabling diseases, disorders, or chronic
illnesses.

2831 Health Finder
                                            www.healthfinder.gov
Searchable, carefully developed web site offering information on
over 1000 topics. Developed by the US Department of Health and
Human Services, the site can be used in both English and Spanish.

2832 Healthlink USA
                                            www.healthlinkusa.com
Health information concerning treatment, cures, prevention, diagnosis, risk factors, research, support groups, email lists, personal
stories and much more. Updated regularly.

2833 Helios Health
                                            www.helioshealth.com
Online resource for your health information. Detailed information
about specific health topics, access to expert advice from our Medical Advisory Board, and up-to-date health news.

2834 Journal of Chronic Fatigue Syndrome
                                            www.cfs-news.org/jcfs.htm
Offers multidisciplinary original research, practical clinical management, case reports, and literature reviews to keep the entire
health care delivery team well informed.

2835 MedicineNet
                                            www.medicinenet.com
An online resource for consumers providing easy-to-read, authoritative medical and health information.

2836 Medscape
                                            www.medscape.com
Medscape offers specialists, primary care physicians, and other
health professionals the Web's most robust and integrated medical
information and educational tools.

2837 Option Institute

www.option.org/cfs.shtml

Self-defeating beliefs, along with attitudes and judgments, can lead to a host of physical and psychological challenges, including Chronic Fatigue Syndrome. The Option Institute offers programs designed to help you gain new perspectives on the attitudes and judgments that may be affecting your life, especially those regarding and surrounding Chronic Fatigue Syndrome.

2838 Sleepnet

www.sleepnet.com

Links all the sleep information located on the internet. Provides a place for everyone to read and post questions, or responses.

2839 WebMD

www.webmd.com

Information on Chronic Fatigue Syndrome, including articles and resources.

Description

2840 Chronic Pain

Chronic pain is defined as pain persisting for more than one month after resolution of an acute injury or pain that persists or recurs for more than three months. The pain may begin for unknown reasons, or may begin with some injury or illness but persist long after the triggering event is gone. Human pain has physiological causes but also has psychological components differing for each person. Many Americans suffer from chronic pain. The annual cost, including treatment and lost work days, now hovers around $100 billion in the US.

Doctors and patients have tried almost every conceivable type of therapy for chronic pain. Drug treatments include narcotics (codeine and morphine), non-narcotic painkillers such as acetaminophen, and nonsteroidal anti-inflammatory drugs such as ibuprofen. Use of antidepressants, either alone or in conjunction with pain medications, can be beneficial. Doctors may inject drugs to block the nerves that carry the pain signal, or may even cut the nerve. Physical measures include heat or cold application, application of electrical stimuli (TENS), stretching, and general conditioning exercises. Psychological treatment includes psychotherapy, meditation, hypnosis and biofeedback-relaxation. Because of the complexity of chronic pain and its treatment, some doctors have begun to specialize in management of pain, and have organized multidisciplinary pain clinics which offer expertise from anesthesiology, rheumatology, neurosurgery, psychology and physical therapy.

A realistic goal of therapy is to improve one's daily functioning; for instance, being able to return to work or pleasurable activities. Those able to achieve this status will often state that the pain is still there but that it does not bother them like it once did. Whatever the stage of one's condition, peer support is important, and is available from local in-person support groups or from Internet chat rooms and bulletin boards.

National Agencies & Associations

2841 American Chronic Pain Association
PO Box 850
Rocklin, CA 95677
800-533-3231
Fax: 916-632-3208
e-mail: ACPA@pacbell.net
www.theacpa.org
ACPA mission is: (1) to facilitate peer support and education for individuals with chronic pain and their families so that these individuals may live more fully in spite of their pain; and (2) to raise awareness among the health care community and policy makers.
Penny Cowan, Executive Director

2842 American Pain Society
4700 W Lake Avenue
Glenview, IL 60025
847-375-4715
866-574-2654
Fax: 847-375-6479
e-mail: info@ampainsoc.org
www.ampainsoc.org
A multidisciplinary organization of basic and clinical scientists practicing clinicians policy analysts and others. Mission is to ad-

vance pain-related research education treatment and professional practice.
Catherine H Underwood, Executive Director
Seddon R Savage MD, MS, President

2843 International Association for the Study of Pain
111 Queen Anne Avenue N
Seattle, WA 98109-4955
206-283-0311
Fax: 206-283-9403
e-mail: iaspdesk@iasp-pain.org
www.iasp-pain.org
The International Association for the Study of Pain is the leading professional forum for science practice and education in the field of pain.
Eija Anneli Kalso MD,, President
Judith A Paice PhD, RN, President Elect

2844 International Pelvic Pain Society Women's Medical Plaza
Women's Medical Plaza
1100 E Woodfield Road
Schaumburg, IL 60173
847-517-8712
800-624-9676
Fax: 847-517-7229
e-mail: info@pelvicpain.org
www.pelvicpain.org
Short range goal is to recruit organize and educate health care professionals actively involved with the treatment of patients who have chronic pelvic pain.
Fred Marion Howard, Chairman of the Board
Richard P Marvel MD, President

2845 Reflex Sympathetic Dystrophy Syndrome Association (RSDSA)
PO Box 502
Milford, CT 06460
203-877-3790
877-662-7737
Fax: 203-882-8362
e-mail: info@rsds.org
www.rsds.org
Nonprofit professional and consumer organization founded to support research into the cause, treatment and cure of reflex sympathetic dystrophy syndrome. RSDSA also organizes support groups, promote awareness among health professionals and develop educational programs.
Paul R Charlesworth, President
James E Tyrrell Jr, Chairman of the Board

Support Groups & Hotlines

2846 National Health Information Center
PO Box 1133
Washington, DC 20013-1133
310-565-4167
800-336-4797
Fax: 301-984-4256
e-mail: info@nhic.org
www.health.gov/nhic
A health information referral service sponsored by the Office of Disease Prevention and Health Promotion. Puts health professionals and consumers who have health questions in touch with those organizations that are best able to provide answers.

Books

2847 ACPA Facilitator Guide & Materials
American Chronic Pain Association
PO Box 850
Rocklin, CA 95677
916-632-0922
800-533-3231
Fax: 916-632-3208
e-mail: acpa@pacbell.net
www.theacpa.org
This guide will help you and others in your community organize an ACPA chapter. The manual contains how-to information on organizing an ACPA chapter, sharing responsibility for the group with others, finding a meeting place, conducting the first meeting, and generating public interest in your area. You must be an ACPA member to purchase this manual.
Penny Cowan, Executive Director

2848 ACPA Family Manual
Penny Cowan, author

American Chronic Pain Association

PO Box 850
Rocklin, CA 95677

916-632-0922
800-533-3231
Fax: 916-632-3208
e-mail: acpa@pacbell.net
www.theacpa.org

A manual designed with the needs of those who live with a person who has chronic pain.
149 pages
ISBN: 0-967387-82-5
Penny Cowan, Executive Director

2849   ACPA Journal Reflections of You
American Chronic Pain Association
PO Box 850
Rocklin, CA 95677

916-632-0922
800-533-3231
Fax: 916-632-3208
e-mail: acpa@pacbell.net
www.theacpa.org

A daily meditation and personal journal book which provides positive and motivating thoughts to stimulate your thinking and challenge you to personal growth. Your daily entries in the journal will help track your progress and show when you have reached your personal goal.
Penny Cowan, Executive Director

2850   ACSM's Exercise Management for Persons with Chronic Disease & Disabilities
Human Kinetics Press
PO Box 5076
Champaign, IL 61825-5076

217-351-5076
800-747-4457
Fax: 217-351-2674
www.humankinetics.com

1993 384 pages Hardcover
ISBN: 0-736038-72-8
Steve Ruhlig, Marketing Director

2851   Essential Guide to Chronic Illness: The Active Patient's Handbook
James W Long, author
DIANE Publishing Company
330 Pusey Avenue, Unit #3 Rear
Darby, PA 19023

610-461-6200
800-782-3833
Fax: 610-461-6130
e-mail: dianepublishing@gmail.com
www.dianepublishing.net

A comprehensive guide to dealing with nearly 50 chronic illness and conditions from acne to Zollinger-Ellison syndrome, including diabetes, menopause, migraines, rheumatoid arthritis and psoriasis.
625 pages Paperback
ISBN: 0-788169-03-3
Herman Baron, Publisher

2852   From Patient to Person: First Steps
American Chronic Pain Association
PO Box 850
Rocklin, CA 95677

916-632-0922
800-533-3231
Fax: 916-632-3208
e-mail: acpa@pacbell.net
www.theacpa.org

A workbook designed to help anyone who has a chronic pain problem to gain a better understanding of how one can begin to cope with all the problems that their pain creates.

ISBN: 0-967387-80-9
Penny Cowan, Executive Director

2853   Occupational Therapy Practice Guidelines for Adults with Low Back Pain
American Occupational Therapy Association
4720 Montgomery Lane
Bethesda, MD 20824-1220

301-652-2682
Fax: 301-652-7711
TDD: 800-377-8555
www.aota.org

15 pages
ISBN: 1-569001-49-9

2854   Occupational Therapy Practice Guidelines for Adults with Hip Fracture/Replacement
American Occupational Therapy Association

4720 Montgomery Lane
Bethesda, MD 20824-1220

301-652-2682
Fax: 301-652-7711
TDD: 800-377-8555
www.aota.org

10 pages
ISBN: 1-569001-48-0

2855   Staying Well: Advanced Pain Management for ACPA Members
American Chronic Pain Association
PO Box 850
Rocklin, CA 95677

916-632-0922
800-533-3231
Fax: 916-632-3208
e-mail: acpa@pacbell.net
www.theacpa.org

This workbook is designed for those who have a working knowledge of the basics of pain management. This workbook provides additional skills necessary to continue to move forward in the journey to wellness.

ISBN: 0-969387-81-7
Penny Cowan, Executive Director

2856   Understanding Chronic Pain
Angela Koestler, PhD; Ann Myers, MD, author
University Press of Mississippi
3825 Ridgewood Road
Jackson, MS 39211-6492

601-432-6205
Fax: 601-432-6217
e-mail: kburgess@ihl.state.ms.us
www.upress.state.ms.us

A handbook for people coping with chronic pain and suffering and for those who seek to understand and support them.
2002 184 pages Paperback
ISBN: 1-578064-40-6
Kathy Burgess, Advertising/Marketing Services Manager

2857   Your Pain is Real: Free Yourself from Chronic Pain, Breakthrough Med. Trtmnt.
DIANE Publishing Company
330 Pusey Avenue, Unit #3 Rear
Darby, PA 19023

610-461-6200
800-782-3833
Fax: 610-461-6130
e-mail: dianepublishing@gmail.com
www.dianepublishing.net

A complete, authoritative and hopeful book on the subject of chronic pain relief. Offers revolutionary ways to relieve all types and degrees of painful conditions. Also offers breakthrough medical treatments, clear guidelines for seeking expert care and the latest scientific findings on pain management.
252 pages Hardcover
ISBN: 0-756753-70-8
Herman Baron, Publisher

Newsletters

2858   American Chronic Pain Association
PO Box 850
Rocklin, CA 95677-0850

916-632-0922
800-533-3231
Fax: 916-632-3208
e-mail: ACPA@pacbell.net
www.theacpa.org

A nonprofit organization with over 400 chapters in the US, Canada, Australia, New Zealand and Russia. The purpose of this organization is to provide a support system for those suffering chronic pain through group activities.
Quart w/ mbrshp
Penny Cowan, Executive Founder & Director

2859   Health Points
TyH Publications
17007 E Colony Drive
Fountain Hills, AZ 85268

800-801-1406
e-mail: editor@e-tyh.com

National newsletter with articles on complementary therapy, latest nutrition news, disability issues and much more. Focus is on fibromyalgia, chronic fatigue, arthritis and chronic pain.
Quarterly

Pamphlets

2860 Suicide is Not an Option
National Chronic Fatigue Syndrome
PO Box 18426   660-313-2000
Kansas City, MO 64133-8426

Audio & Video

2861 ACPA Relaxation Tapes
American Chronic Pain Association
PO Box 850   916-632-0922
Rocklin, CA 95677   800-533-3231
                        Fax: 916-632-3208
                        e-mail: acpa@pacbell.net
                        www.theacpa.org
Audio tapes offering information on pain relief, breath relaxation and autogenic relaxation. These tapes are designed to help persons regain control of their bodies through exercises in relaxation techniques. $10.00-$25.00.
Audio Tapes
Penny Cowan, Executive Director

2862 ACPA Video: 10 Steps from Patient to Person
American Chronic Pain Association
PO Box 850   916-632-0922
Rocklin, CA 95677   800-533-3231
                        Fax: 916-632-3208
                        e-mail: acpa@pacbell.net
                        www.theacpa.org
The video, featuring Penny Cowan, founder of the ACPA, discussed the value of a multidisiplinary pain management program and what is necessary to maintain wellness long term.
Penny Cowan, Executive Director

2863 Affirmation Tape
American Chronic Pain Association
PO Box 850   916-632-0922
Rocklin, CA 95677   800-533-3231
                        Fax: 916-632-3208
                        e-mail: ACPA@pacbell.net
                        www.theacpa.org
Designed to help you focus on positive things about yourself and builds self-esteem.
Penny Cowan, Executive Director

2864 Relaxation Tape
American Chronic Pain Association
PO Box 850   916-632-0922
Rocklin, CA 95677   800-533-3231
                        Fax: 916-632-3208
                        e-mail: ACPA@pacbell.net
                        www.theacpa.org
Tape one includes pain relief and breath relaxation. Tape two includes general relaxation and autogenic relaxation.
Penny Cowan, Executive Director

Web Sites

2865 American Chronic Pain Association
                        www.theacpa.org
Facilitating peer support and education for individuals with chronic pain and their families so that these individuals may live more fully in spite of their pain.

2866 American Pain Society
                        ampainsoc.org
Multidisciplinary organization of basic and clinical scientists, practicing clinicians, policy analysts, and others.

2867 Discovery Health
                        health.discovery.com
A source of information on various health topics, including chronic pain and its symptoms and treatments.

2868 Healing Well
                        www.healingwell.com
An online health resource guide to medical news, chat, information and articles, newsgroups and message boards, books, disease-related web sites, medical directories, and more for patients, friends, and family coping with disabling diseases, disorders, or chronic illnesses.

2869 Health Finder
                        www.healthfinder.gov
Searchable, carefully developed web site offering information on over 1000 topics. Developed by the US Department of Health and Human Services, the site can be used in both English and Spanish.

2870 Healthlink USA
                        www.healthlinkusa.com
Health information concerning treatment, cures, prevention, diagnosis, risk factors, research, support groups, email lists, personal stories and much more. Updated regularly.

2871 Helios Health
                        www.helioshealth.com
Online resource for your health information. Detailed information about specific health topics, access to expert advice from our Medical Advisory Board, and up-to-date health news.

2872 International Pelvic Pain Society
                        www.pelvicpain.org/
Short range goal is to recruit, organizae, and educate health care professionals actively invlved with the treatment of patients who have chronic opelvic pain.

2873 MedicineNet
                        www.medicinenet.com
An online resource for consumers providing easy-to-read, authoritative medical and health information.

2874 Medscape
                        www.medscape.com
Medscape offers specialists, primary care physicians, and other health professionals the Web's most robust and integrated medical information and educational tools.

2875 WebMD
                        www.webmd.com
Information on chronic pain, including articles and resources.

Description

2876 Congenital Heart Disease

Congenital Heart Disease (CHD) represents the most common group of congenital (present from birth) anomalies. CHD can be thought of as a group of disorders that result from the abnormal formation of the heart in utero. The heart develops between the 2nd and 6th week of gestation, and may be affected by genetic mutation, maternal systemic medications or toxins (e.g. alcohol abuse). The incidence of CHD in the population is about 8 cases in 1,000 live births, or just under 1%. About half of these cardiac defects are considered to be minor and can be followed clinically while the other half fall into the categories of major CHD. This latter group often requires surgery early in life to either completely repair the heart defect or in some cases, to redirect blood through the cardiovascular system to palliate the structural abnormality.

CHD can be divided into three major categories: left to right shunting lesions, left heart obstructive lesions and those that lead to marked cyanosis (decreased oxygen delivery to the organs and tissues), the so called cyanotic heart diseases.

The left to right shunting lesions are the most common of the three groups and include the ventricular septal defect (VSD), the atrial septal defect (ASD), the atrioventricular septal defect (also referred to as the AV canal), and the patent ductus arteriosus. In all of these left to right shunting lesions, there is a progressive increase in the amount of blood sent from the left side of the heartacross the given defect (hole) into the right side that delivers blood to the lungs. There is as a result, too much blood entering the pulmonary circuit and this can lead to problems with breathing and feeding for infants in the first few months of life.

The more common left heart obstructive diseases include aortic stenosis, coarctation of the aorta and the hypoplastic left heart syndrome. Each of these can lead to a marked reduction in the amount of blood flow that is able to leave the left side of the heart and can be delivered to the organs and tissues. This leads to marked abnormalities in the way the organs and tissues function and can cause serious and emergent problems for infants in the first week or two of life.

Cyanotic heart disease are those cardiac malformations that lead to a bluish discoloration of the baby as there is insufficient oxygenated blood that is delivered to the body with or without inadequate blood delivered to the lungs to pick up oxygen. The more common disorders in this group are tetralogy of Fallot, Transposition of the great arteries, tricuspid atresia and truncus arteriosus.

With the remarkable advances in neonatal cardiac surgery and interventional cardiac catheterization, almost all of the cardiac malformations can be aggressively addressed with excellent results, even in the youngest and smallest of patients. Overall, survival from all cardiac surgeries in children with CHD is greater than 95%, and even for the most complex of CHD it is approaching 90%. These children often require long-term follow-up from a pediatric cardiologist, but the vast majority lead healthy active lives. See also *Birth Defects*.

National Agencies & Associations

2877 Adult Congenital Heart Association
6757 Greene Street
Philadelphia, PA 19119-3508
215-849-1260
888-921-ACHA
Fax: 215-849-1261
e-mail: Info@achaheart.org
www.achaheart.org
The Adult Congenital Heart Association (ACHA) is a nonprofit organization which seeks to improve the quality of life and extend the lives of adults with congenital heart defects through education, outreach, advocacy and promotion of research.
Amy Verstappen, President
Paula Miller, Membership Service Manager

2878 Congenital Heart Information Network
101 N Washington Avenue
Margate City, NJ 08402-1195
609-822-1572
Fax: 609-822-1574
e-mail: mb@tchin.org
www.tchin.org
C.H.I.N. is a national organization that provides reliable information support services, financial assistance and resources to families of children with congenital heart defects and acquired heart disease and adults with congenital heart defects.
Mona Barmash, President

2879 Kids with Heart National Association for Children's Heart Disorders
1578 Careful Drive
Green Bay, WI 54307-2504
920-498-0058
800-538-5390
e-mail: michelle@kidswithheart.org
www.kidswithheart.org
Kids with Heart is a nonprofit organization founded in 1985 dedicated to providing support for families affected by congenital heart defects through surgical care packages.
Michelle Rin BA, President
Dean Rintamaki, Vice President

2880 Schneeweiss Adult Congenital Heart Disease Center
New York Presbyterian Hospital
161 Fort Washington Avenue
New York, NY 10032
212-305-6936
Fax: 212-305-0490
congenitalheart.hs.columbia.edu
We provide such diagnostic services such as echocardiography cardiac MRI and cardiac catheterization. Highly specialized care is provided by a team of physicians specifically interested in the problems of adults with congenital heart disease.
Marlon S Rosenbaum MD, Director

Web Sites

2881 Heartpoint
www.heartpoint.com
Heartpoint provides information about specific heart defects.

2882 MedicineNet
www.medicinenet.com
An online resource for consumers providing easy-to-read, authoritative medical and health information.

2883 Medline Plus
www.nlm.nih.gov/medlineplus
This website includes information about congenital heart disease and includes links regarding support and treatment.

2884 Yale: Congenital Heart Disease
info.med.yale.edu/intmed/cardio/chd
This web site provides in-depth information regarding various types of heart conditions.

Description

2885 Cooley's Anemia (Thalassemia)

Cooley's anemia, or beta-Thalassemia major, is an inherited disorder characterized by abnormal production of hemoglobin in the red blood cells. There are two forms of beta-Thalassemia: beta-Thalassemia minor, in which the person has no symptoms, and beta-Thalassemia major, or Cooley's anemia, which is a severe, debilitating disease. Although a baby who has Cooley's anemia appears normal at birth, growth rates are impaired, and puberty may be significantly delayed or absent. Without therapy, there is a general decline. The skin becomes pale or jaundiced, facial bones become more prominent and pronounced, and the spleen becomes enlarged.

While there is no cure for Cooley's anemia, there are treatments such as blood transfusions, which can reduce some symptoms of the disease. However, children with Cooley's anemia should receive as few transfusions as possible because of the danger of iron overload from the "heme" portion of hemoglobin. Chelation, or binding, of the excess iron associated with multiple, repetitive transfusions is important, and is accomplished with deferoxamine. Removal of the spleen may reduce transfusion requirements.

Because there is no cure for beta-Thalassemia major, genetic screening of at-risk populations is very important, notably for persons of Mediterranean, African and Southeast Asian ancestry. Prenatal diagnosis can also be performed.

National Agencies & Associations

2886 American Hellenic Educational Progressive Association
1909 Q Street NW   202-232-6300
Washington, DC 20009   Fax: 202-232-2140
e-mail: ahepa@ahepa.org
www.ahepa.org
The mission of the AHEPA Family is to promote Hellenism Education Philanthropy Civic Responsibility and Family and Individual Excellence.
Basil N Mossaidis, Executive Director

2887 Fanconi Anemia Research Foundation
1801 Willamette Street   541-687-4658
Eugene, OR 97401   888-326-2664
Fax: 541-687-0548
e-mail: info@fanconi.org
www.fanconi.org
Funds research and provides education and support services worldwide to families affected with Fanconi anemia a rare genetic aplastic anemia that leads to bone marrow failure acute myelogenous leukemia and squamous cell carcinomas.

State Agencies & Associations

California

2888 Cooley's Anemia Foundation (CAF): California
2629 Foothill Boulevard
La Crescenta, CA 91214   800-601-2821
Fax: 212-279-5999
e-mail: info@cooleysanemia.org
www.cooleysanemia.org
The Cooley's Anemia Foundation (CAF) is dedicated to serving people afflicted with various forms of thalassemia, most notably the major form of this genetic blood disease, Cooley's anemia/thalassemia major. CAF's mission is advancing the treatment and curing the disease.
Christine Giannamore, Coordinator
Gina Cioffi Esq, National Office Executive Director

Illinois

2889 Cooley's Anemia Foundation (CAF): Illinois Oakbrook Towers
Oakbrook Towers
40 N Tower Road   847-602-2616
Altbrook, IL 62503   800-522-7222
Fax: 212-279-5999
e-mail: info@cooleysanemia.org
www.cooleysanemia.org
The Cooley's Anemia Foundation (CAF) is dedicated to serving people afflicted with various forms of thalassemia most notably the major form of this genetic blood disease Cooley's anemia/thalassemia major. CAF's mission is advancing the treatment and curing the disease.
Bruce Rod, President Illinois Office
Gina Cioffi, National Office Executive Director

Maryland

2890 Cooley's Anemia Foundation (CAF): Capital Area
15321 Peach Orchard Avenue   301-989-8947
Silver Spring, MD 20905   800-522-7222
Fax: 212-279-5999
e-mail: info@cooleysanemia.org
www.cooleysanemia.org
The Cooley's Anemia Foundation (CAF) is dedicated to serving people afflicted with various forms of thalassemia most notably the major form of this genetic blood disease Cooley's anemia/thalassemia major. CAF's mission is advancing the treatment and curing the disease.
Carl C Vitaliti, President Capital Area Office
Gina Cioffi Esq, National Office Executive Director

Massachusetts

2891 Cooley's Anemia Foundation (CAF): Massachusetts Chapter
44 Joseph Road   617-332-5952
Newton, MA 02460-1122   800-522-7222
Fax: 212-279-5999
e-mail: info@cooleysanemia.org
www.cooleysanemia.org
The Cooley's Anemia Foundation (CAF) is dedicated to serving people afflicted with various forms of thalassemia most notably the major form of this genetic blood disease Cooley's anemia/thalassemia major. CAF's mission is advancing the treatment and curing the disease.
Rudi Viscomi, President Massachusetts Office
Gina Cioffi, National Office Executive Director

New Jersey

2892 Cooley's Anemia Foundation (CAF): New Jersey Chapter
29 Alyson Place   732-688-2279
Bloomfield, NJ 07003   800-522-7222
Fax: 212-279-5999
e-mail: info@cooleysanemia.org
www.cooleysanemia.org
The Cooley's Anemia Foundation (CAF) is dedicated to serving people afflicted with various forms of thalassemia most notably the major form of this genetic blood disease Cooley's anemia/thalassemia major. CAF's mission is advancing the treatment and curing the disease.
Christine Somma, President New Jersey Office
Gina Cioffi, National Office Executive Director

New York

2893 Cooley's Anemia Foundation (CAF): Rochester
585-482-5587
800-522-7222
Fax: 212-279-5999
e-mail: info@cooleysanemia.org
www.cooleysanemia.org

The Cooley's Anemia Foundation (CAF) is dedicated to serving people afflicted with various forms of thalassemia most notably the major form of this genetic blood disease Cooley's anemia/thalassemia major. CAF's mission is advancing the treatment and curing the disease.
Shirley Cammilleri, President Rochester Office
Gina Cioffi Esq, National Office Executive Director

2894 Cooley's Anemia Foundation (CAF): Buffalo
135 Wellington Road   716-834-8903
Buffalo, NY 14216   800-522-7222
                                                    Fax: 212-279-5999
                                e-mail: info@cooleysanemia.org
                                          www.cooleysanemia.org
The Cooley's Anemia Foundation (CAF) is dedicated to serving people afflicted with various forms of thalassemia most notably the major form of this genetic blood disease Cooley's anemia/thalassemia major. CAF's mission is advancing the treatment and curing the disease.
Dennis Locurto, President Buffalo Office
Gina Cioffi Esq, National Office Executive Director

2895 Cooley's Anemia Foundation (CAF): Long Island
111 Cherry Valley Avenue   516-358-9100
Garden City, NY 11530   800-522-7222
                                                    Fax: 516-358-9101
                                e-mail: info@cooleysanemia.org
                                          www.cooleysanemia.org
The Cooley's Anemia Foundation (CAF) is dedicated to serving people afflicted with various forms of thalassemia most notably the major form of this genetic blood disease Cooley's anemia/thalassemia major. CAF's mission is advancing the treatment and curing the disease.
Thomas Rotolo, President Long Island Office
Janice Cenzoprano, Vice President Long Island Office

2896 Cooley's Anemia Foundation (CAF): Queens
157-26 9th Avenue   718-746-7677
Beachurst, NY 11357   800-522-7222
                                                    Fax: 718-746-7678
                                e-mail: info@cooleysanemia.org
                                          www.cooleysanemia.org
The Cooley's Anemia Foundation (CAF) is dedicated to serving people afflicted with various forms of thalassemia most notably the major form of this genetic blood disease Cooley's anemia/thalassemia major. CAF's mission is advancing the treatment and curing the disease.
Paul Tucci, President Queen Office
Abbey Chakalis, Events Manager

2897 Cooley's Anemia Foundation (CAF): Staten Island
16B Dreyer Avenue   718-761-5380
Staten Island, NY 10314   800-522-7222
                                                    Fax: 718-761-5381
                                e-mail: info@cooleysanemia.org
                                          www.cooleysanemia.org
The Cooley's Anemia Foundation (CAF) is dedicated to serving people afflicted with various forms of thalassemia most notably the major form of this genetic blood disease Cooley's anemia/thalassemia major. CAF's mission is advancing the treatment and curing the disease.
Gina Cioffi Esq, National Office Executive Director
Craig Butler, National Office Communications Director

2898 Cooley's Anemia Foundation (CAF): Suffolk Chapter Office
740 Smithtown Bypass   631-863-0532
Smithtown, NY 11787   800-522-7222
                                                    Fax: 631-863-0535
                                e-mail: info@cooleysanemia.org
                                          www.cooleysanemia.org
The Cooley's Anemia Foundation (CAF) is dedicated to serving people afflicted with various forms of thalassemia most notably the major form of this genetic blood disease Cooley's anemia/thalassemia major. CAF's mission is advancing the treatment and curing the disease.
Gina Cioffi Esq, National Office Executive Director
Craig Butler, National Office Communications Director

2899 Cooley's Anemia Foundation (CAF): Westchester/Rockland Chapter
3 Samuel Purdy Lane   914-232-1808
Katonah, NY 10536   800-522-7222
                                                    Fax: 212-279-5999
                                e-mail: info@cooleysanemia.org
                                          www.cooleysanemia.org
The Cooley's Anemia Foundation (CAF) is dedicated to serving people afflicted with various forms of thalassemia most notably the major form of this genetic blood disease Cooley's anemia/thalassemia major. CAF's mission is advancing the treatment and curing the disease.
Peter Chieco, President Westchester/Rockland Office
Janet Manning, Executive Director

Texas

2900 Cooley's Anemia Foundation (CAF): Texas
4504 Astor Road   214-324-6147
Mesquite, TX 75150-2320   800-522-7222
                                                    Fax: 214-324-0612
                                e-mail: info@cooleysanemia.org
                                          www.cooleysanemia.org
The Cooley's Anemia Foundation (CAF) is dedicated to serving people afflicted with various forms of thalassemia most notably the major form of this genetic blood disease Cooley's anemia/thalassemia major.
Mateen Shah, President
Gina Cioffi Esq, National Office Executive Director

Foundations

2901 Cooleys Anemia Foundation
330 Seventh Avenue
New York, NY 10001   800-522-7222
                                                    Fax: 212-279-5999
                                e-mail: info@cooleysanemia.org
                                          www.cooleysanemia.org
Our mission is advancing the treatment and cure for this fatal blood disease, enhancing the quality of life of patients and educating the medical profession, trait carriers and the public about Cooley's anemia/thalassemia major.
Gina Cioffi, Esq, National Executive Director
Craig Butler, Communications Director

Support Groups & Hotlines

2902 National Health Information Center
PO Box 1133   310-565-4167
Washington, DC 20013   800-336-4797
                                                    Fax: 301-984-4256
                                          e-mail: info@nhic.org
                                             www.health.gov/nhic
A health information referral service sponsored by the Office of Disease Prevention and Health Promotion. Puts health professionals and consumers who have health questions in touch with those organizations that are best able to provide answers.

Books

2903 Genes, Blood & Courage
129-09 26th Avenue   212-598-0911
Flushing, NY 11354   800-522-7222
                                          www.cooleysanemia.org

2904 What is Cooley's Anemia
129-09 26th Avenue   718-321-2873
Flushing, NY 11354   800-522-7222
                                                    Fax: 718-321-3340
                                e-mail: info@cooleysanemia.org
                                          www.cooleysanemia.org
Patient and family handbook.
Jayne Restivo, National Executive Director

2905 What is Thalassemia?
Cooley's Anemia Foundation

129-09 26th Avenue
Flushing, NY 11354

718-321-2873
800-522-7222
Fax: 718-321-3340
e-mail: info@cooleysanemia.org
www.cooleysanemia.org

A guide to help thalassemics and their parents understand thalassemia, the reasons for treatment and the hope for the future.
Jayne Restivo, National Executive Director

Children's Books

2906   Coloring Book on Thalassemia
129-09 26th Avenue
Flushing, NY 11354

718-321-2873
800-522-7222
Fax: 718-321-3340
e-mail: info@cooleysanemia.org
www.cooleysanemia.org

Available in English, Italian, Greek and Chinese.
Jayne Restivo, National Executive Director

Magazines

2907   AHEPAN Magazine
American Hellenic Educational Progressive Assn
1909 Q Street NW
Washington, DC 20009

202-232-6300
Fax: 202-232-2140
e-mail: ahepa@ahepa.org
www.ahepa.org

This magazine includes all of the AHEPA organizations.
Quarterly
Basil N Mossaidis, Executive Director

Newsletters

2908   Lifeline
Cooley's Anemia Foundation
129-09 26th Avenue
Flushing, NY 11354

718-321-2873
800-522-7222
Fax: 718-321-3340
e-mail: info@cooleysanemia.org
www.cooleysanemia.org

A newsletter published by Cooley's Anemia Foundation.
Jayne Restivo, National Executive Director

Pamphlets

2909   Desferal Q&A
129-09 26th Avenue
Flushing, NY 11354

718-321-2873
800-522-7222
Fax: 718-321-3340
e-mail: info@cooleysanemia.org
www.cooleysanemia.org

Guideline for home infusion.
Jayne Restivo, National Executive Director

2910   What is Thalassemia Trait?
Cooley's Anemia Foundation
129-09 26th Avenue
Flushing, NY 11354

718-321-2873
800-522-7222
Fax: 718-321-3340
e-mail: info@cooleysanemia.org
www.cooleysanemia.org

This booklet offers information on the thalassemia trait.
1995
Jayne Restivo, National Executive Director

Audio & Video

2911   TAG Annual Patient/Family Conference Video
Cooley's Anemia Foundation

Thalassemia Action Group
New York, NY 10001

800-522-7222
Fax: 212-279-5999
e-mail: TAG@cooleysanemia.org
www.cooleysanemia.org/

Video from the Thalassemia Action Group/TAG Annual Patient/Family Conference held in March of each year.
Gina Cioffi Esq, National Executive Director
Craig Butler, Communications Director

2912   To Live
Cooley's Anemia Foundation
330 Seventh Avenue
New York, NY 10001

800-522-7222
Fax: 212-279-5999
e-mail: info@cooleysanemia.org
www.cooleysanemia.org/

An informative and educational video from Cooley's Anemia Foundation.
Gina Cioffi Esq, National Executive Director
Craig Butler, Communications Director

2913   You're Not Alone
Cooley's Anemia Foundation
330 Seventh Avenue
New York, NY 10004

800-522-7222
Fax: 212-279-5999
e-mail: info@cooleysanemia.org
www.cooleysanemia.org

An informative and educational video from Cooley's Anemia Foundation.
Gina Cioffi Esq, National Executive Director
Craig Butler, Communications Director

Web Sites

2914   Healing Well
www.healingwell.com
An online health resource guide to medical news, chat, information and articles, newsgroups and message boards, books, disease-related web sites, medical directories, and more for patients, friends, and family coping with disabling diseases, disorders, or chronic illnesses.

2915   Health Finder
www.healthfinder.gov
Searchable, carefully developed web site offering information on over 1000 topics. Developed by the US Department of Health and Human Services, the site can be used in both English and Spanish.

2916   Healthlink USA
www.healthlinkusa.com
Health information concerning treatment, cures, prevention, diagnosis, risk factors, research, support groups, email lists, personal stories and much more. Updated regularly.

2917   Helios Health
www.helioshealth.com
Online resource for your health information. Detailed information about specific health topics, access to expert advice from our Medical Advisory Board, and up-to-date health news.

2918   MedicineNet
www.medicinenet.com
An online resource for consumers providing easy-to-read, authoritative medical and health information.

2919   Medscape
www.medscape.com
Medscape offers specialists, primary care physicians, and other health professionals the Web's most robust and integrated medical information and educational tools.

2920   WebMD
www.webmd.com
Information on Cooley's Anemia (Thalassemia), including articles and resources.

Description

2921 Crohn's Disease

Crohn's disease is a chronic inflammation in the lining of the digestive tract, generally in the small bowel or part of the colon. The cause is unknown, although the disease is more common in some families and racial groups. Although not a proven cause, periods of emotional stress have been linked with flare-ups of the disease. Onset is typically before age 30, with the peak incidence between 14 and 24 years.

Common symptoms include diarrhea, weight loss, fever, abdominal pain and loss of appetite. If the disease is extensive it may cause deficiencies of essential vitamins and other nutrients. Sometimes inflammation occurs outside the gut, attacking the eyes, joints or skin. Local complications include bowel perforation with formation of abscesses or fistulas which drain out to the skin. Established chronic Crohn's disease is characterized by lifelong exacerbations. These patients carry an increased risk of cancer of the small bowel and colon/rectum.

Therapy depends on the location of the disease and on its severity. Although no specific therapy is known, drug treatment can range from simple anti-diarrheal medications to anti-inflammatory drugs and immunosuppressives. Surgery may be necessary to treat complications. In all cases, careful attention should be paid to the patient's nutritional status and psychological well-being. See also *Gastrointestinal Disorders* and *Celiac Disease.*

National Agencies & Associations

2922 CCFA Camps Across America Crohn's & Colitis Foundation of America
Crohn's & Colitis Foundation of America
386 Park Avenue S   212-685-3440
New York, NY 10016   800-932-2423
Fax: 212-779-4098
e-mail: info@ccfa.org
www.ccfa.org
A chance for children with Crhon's disease or ulcerative colitis to have a camping experience. Because CCFA camps are offered by chapters across the country every camp has its own flavor and style. Activities, as well as the length of stay may vary from child to child.
Richard Geswell, President

2923 Crohn's & Colitis Foundation of America
386 Park Avenue S   212-685-3440
New York, NY 10016   800-932-2423
Fax: 212-779-4098
e-mail: info@ccfa.org
www.ccfa.org
CCFA's mission is to cure and prevent Crohn's disease and ulcerative colitis through research and to improve the quality of life of children and adults affected by this disease through education and support. The foundation offers patient and professional support.
Richard Geswell, President

2924 Ileitis and Colitis Educational Foundation
Central DuPage Hospital
25 N Winfield Road   630-933-1600
Winfield, IL 60190   Fax: 630-933-1300
TTY: 630-933-4833
e-mail: cdh_information@cdh.org
www.cdh.org

Offers support groups fund-raising activities educational materials and public awareness campaigns pertaining to these disorders.
Luke McGuinness, President, CEO
Richard A Mark, Vice Chair

2925 International Foundation for Functional Gastrointestinal Disorders (IFFGD)
PO Box 170864   414-964-1799
Milwaukee, WI 53217-8076   888-964-2001
Fax: 414-964-7176
e-mail: iffgd@iffgd.org
www.iffgd.org
Nonprofit education, support and research organization devoted to increasing awareness and understanding of functional gastrointestinal disorders, including irritable bowel syndrome (IBS), constipation, diarrhea, pain, and incontinence. Mission is to inform, assist and support people affected by these disorders.
Nancy J Norton, President

2926 National Institute of Diabetes, Digestive & Kidney Diseases
National Institutes of Health
1 Information Way   301-496-4000
Bethesda, MD 20892-3560   800-860-8747
Fax: 703-738-4929
TTY: 866-569-1162
e-mail: ndic@info.niddk.nih.gov
www.diabetes.niddk.nih.gov
Conducts and supports research on many of the most serious diseases affecting public health. The Institute supports much of the clinical research on the diseases of internal medicine and related subspecialty fields as well as many basic science disciplines.
Dr. Griffin Rodgers, Acting Director

2927 Pediatric Crohn's and Colitis Association
PO Box 188   617-489-5854
Newton, MA 02468   e-mail: questions@pcca.hypermart.net
www.pcca.hypermart.net
Focuses on all aspects of pediatric and adolescent Crohn's disease and ulcerative colitis, including medical, nutritional, psychological and social factors. Activities include information sharing, educational forums, newsletters and hospital outreach programs.

2928 Reach Out for Youth with Ileitis and Colitis
PO Box 857   631-293-3102
Bellmore, NY 11710   e-mail: info@reachoutforyouth.org
www.reachoutforyouth.org
Provides educational seminars and individual and group support to patients and their families. Fundraising efforts support the center's programs, clinical and laboratory research, and purchase of state-of-the-art equipment.
Susan Spellman, Founder and Executive Director

2929 United Ostomy Association
PO Box 512
Northfield, MN 55057   800-826-0826
Fax: 507-645-5168
e-mail: info@uoa.org
www.uoa.org
A national network for bowel and urinary diversion support groups in the United States. Its goal is to provide a nonprofit association that will serve to unify and strengthen its member support groups, which are organized for the benefit of people who have, or will have intestinal or urinary diversions and their caregivers.
David Rudzin, President

2930 World Ostomy and Continence Nurses Society
15000 Commerce Parkway
Mt Laurel, NJ 08054   888-224-9626
Fax: 856-439-0525
e-mail: info@wocn.org
www.wocn.org
Membership comprises nurses that specialize in enterostomal therapy.
Phyllis Bonham PhD, President
Kathleen Lawrence, President-Elect

State Agencies & Associations

Alabama

2931 CCFA Alabama Chapter
244 Goodwin Crest Drive
Birmingham, AL 35209
205-941-9900
800-249-1993
Fax: 205-941-1411
e-mail: ptalty@ccfa.org OR info@ccfa.org
www.ccfa.org/chapters/alabama
Crohn's and Colitis Foundation of America is a non-profit, volunteer-driven organization dedicated to finding the cure for Crohn's disease and ulcerative colitis.
Pat Talty, Executive Director

Arizona

2932 CCFA Southwest Chapter: Arizona
8098 Via de Negocio
Scottsdale, AZ 85258
480-246-3676
877-259-2104
Fax: 480-246-3679
e-mail: southwest@ccfa.org
www.ccfa.org/chapters/southwest
Crohn's and Colitis Foundation of America is a non-profit volunteer-driven organization dedicated to finding the cure for Crohn's disease and ulcerative colitis.
Kathie Gadberry, Executive Director
Bernadette Sewer, Development Coordinator

California

2933 CCFA California: Greater Bay Area Chapter
386 Park Avenue S
New York, NY 10016-2722
650-578-6590
800-932-2423
Fax: 650-578-6599
e-mail: ccfagba@pacbell.net
www.ccfa.org
To cure and prevent Crohn's disease and ulcerative colitis through research, and to improve the quality of life of children and adults affected by these digestive diseases through education and support.
Carol Gerstein, Executive Director
Bernadette Sewer, Development Coordinator

2934 CCFA California: Greater Los Angeles Chapter
1640 S Sepulveda Boulevard
Los Angeles, CA 90025
310-478-4500
866-831-9157
Fax: 310-478-4546
e-mail: losangeles@ccfa.org
www.ccfa.org/chapters/losangeles
Crohn's and Colitis Foundation of America is a non-profit volunteer-driven organization dedicated to finding the cure for Crohn's disease and ulcerative colitis.
Iyad Zabaneh, Development Coordinator
Kerri Yoder, Education Manager

Colorado

2935 CCFA Rocky Mountain Chapter: Colorado
1777 S Bellaire Street
Denver, CO 80222
303-639-9163
866-768-2232
Fax: 303-693-9166
e-mail: rockymountain@ccfa.org
www.ccfa.org/chapters/rockymountain
Crohn's and Colitis Foundation of America is a non-profit volunteer-driven organization dedicated to finding the cure for Crohn's disease and ulcerative colitis.
Nancy Freimuth, Walk Manager
Mackenzie Lyle, Interim Executive Director

Connecticut

2936 CCFA Central Connecticut Chapter
P O Box 275
Branford, CT 06405
203-208-3130
e-mail: mgrande@ccfa.org
www.ccfa.org/chapters/centralct

Crohn's and Colitis Foundation of America is a non-profit volunteer-driven organization dedicated to finding the cure for Crohn's disease and ulcerative colitis.
Sally Connolly, Board President

2937 CCFA Northern Connecticut Affiliate Chapter
PO Box 370614
W Hartford, CT 06137-0614
212-679-1570
800-932-2423
Fax: 212-679-3567
e-mail: info@ccfa.org
www.ccfa.org/chapters/northernct
Crohn's and Colitis Foundation of America is a non-profit volunteer-driven organization dedicated to finding the cure for Crohn's disease and ulcerative colitis.
Marilyn Hagg Blohm, Executive Director National Headquarters
Jeff Neale, Public Relations National Headquarters

Florida

2938 CCFA Florida Chapter
21301 Powerline Road
Boca Raton, FL 33433-2391
561-218-2929
877-664-2929
Fax: 516-218-2240
e-mail: kkeohane@ccfa.org
www.ccfa.org/chapters/florida
Crohn's and Colitis Foundation of America is a non-profit volunteer-driven organization dedicated to finding the cure for Crohn's disease and ulcerative colitis.
Deborah Barnard, Development Manager
Lacy Woods, Administrator

Georgia

2939 CCFA Georgia Chapter
2250 N Druid Hills Road
Atlanta, GA 30329
404-982-0616
800-472-6795
Fax: 404-982-0656
e-mail: georgia@ccfa.org
www.ccfa.org/chapters/georgia
Crohn's and Colitis Foundation of America is a non-profit volunteer-driven organization dedicated to finding the cure for Crohn's disease and ulcerative colitis.
Marcia Greenburg, Executive Director
Karen Rittenbaum, Development Director

Illinois

2940 CCFA Illinois: Carol Fisher Chapter
2250 E Devon Avenue
Des Plaines, IL 60018
847-827-0404
800-886-6664
Fax: 847-827-6563
e-mail: Illinois@ccfa.org
www.ccfa.org/chapters/illinois
Crohn's and Colitis Foundation of America is a non-profit volunteer-driven organization dedicated to finding the cure for Crohn's disease and ulcerative colitis.
Marianne Floriano, Executive Director
Kristina Sickles, Development Coordinator

Indiana

2941 CCFA Indiana Chapter
931 E 86th Street
Indianapolis, IN 46240
317-259-8071
800-332-6029
Fax: 317-259-8091
e-mail: indiana@ccfa.org
www.ccfa.org/chapters/indiana
Crohn's and Colitis Foundation of America is a non-profit volunteer-driven organization dedicated to finding the cure for Crohn's disease and ulcerative colitis.
Scott Baumruck, Development Director
Dawn Drinkut, Development Assistant

2942   CCFA Iowa Chapter
PO Box 1184   515-664-8961
Johnston, IA 50131-0016   Fax: 319-277-6293
e-mail: iowa@ccfa.org
www.ccfa.org/chapters/iowa
Crohn's and Colitis Foundation of America is a non-profit volunteer-driven organization dedicated to finding the cure for Crohn's disease and ulcerative colitis.
Tony Kline, Chapter President
Abbie Hansen, Vice President Communications

2943   CCFA Mid-America Chapter: Kansas
1034 S Brentwood   314-863-4747
St Louis, MO 63117   800-783-8006
Fax: 314-863-4749
e-mail: sskodak@ccfa.org
www.ccfa.org/chapters/midamerica
Crohn's and Colitis Foundation of America is a non-profit volunteer-driven organization dedicated to finding the cure for Crohn's disease and ulcerative colitis.
Steve Skodak, Executive Director
Andi Harrington, Development Manager

2944   CCFA Kentucky Chapter c/o CCFA Indiana Chapter
c/o CCFA Indiana Chapter
95 White Bridge Road   615-356-0444
Nashville, TN 37205   866-814-CCFA
Fax: 615-356-0445
e-mail: tennessee@ccfa.org
www.ccfa.org/chapters/kentucky
Crohn's and Colitis Foundation of America is a non-profit volunteer-driven organization dedicated to finding the cure for Crohn's disease and ulcerative colitis.
Steve Picton, President
Erskine Courtenay, Vice President

2945   CCFA Louisiana Chapter
7611 Maple Street   504-861-3433
New Orleans, LA 70118   866-382-2232
Fax: 504-861-3466
e-mail: lams@ccfa.org
www.ccfa.org/chapters/louisiana
Crohn's and Colitis Foundation of America is a non-profit volunteer-driven organization dedicated to finding the cure for Crohn's disease and ulcerative colitis.
David Lee Thomas, Development Director
Gail C Smith, Development Assistant

2946   CCFA Maryland Chapter
10400 Little Patuxent Parkway   443-276-0861
Columbia, MD 21044   800-618-5583
Fax: 443-276-0865
e-mail: maryland@ccfa.org
www.ccfa.org/chapters/md-southde
Crohn's and Colitis Foundation of America is a non-profit volunteer-driven organization dedicated to finding the cure for Crohn's disease and ulcerative colitis.
Robert J Milanchus, Regional Executive Director
Mary Glagola, President

2947   CCFA New England Chapter: Massachusetts
280 Hillside Avenue   781-449-0324
Needham, MA 02494   800-314-3459
Fax: 781-449-0325
e-mail: ne@ccfa.org
www.ccfa.org/chapters/ne

Crohn's and Colitis Foundation of America is a non-profit volunteer-driven organization dedicated to finding the cure for Crohn's disease and ulcerative colitis.
Jess Adani, Development Manager
Kristin Patmos, Education Manager

2948   CCFA Michigan Chapter: Farmington Hills
31313 N Western Highway   248-737-0900
Farmington Hills, MI 78334   Fax: 248-737-0904
e-mail: michigan@ccfa.org
www.ccfa.org/chapters/michigan
Crohn's and Colitis Foundation of America is a non-profit volunteer-driven organization dedicated to finding the cure for Crohn's disease and ulcerative colitis.
Bernard L Riker, Executive Director
Gilda Hauser, Development Manager

2949   CCFA Minnesota Chapter
1885 University Avenue W   651-917-2424
Saint Paul, MN 55104   888-422-3266
Fax: 651-917-2425
e-mail: Minnesota@ccfa.org
www.ccfa.org/chapters/minnesota
Crohn's and Colitis Foundation of America is a non-profit volunteer-driven organization dedicated to finding the cure for Crohn's disease and ulcerative colitis.
Maggie Brown, Take Steps Manager
Ruby Lanoux, Development Manager

2950   CCFA Mississippi Chapter c/o Louisiana Chapter
c/o Louisiana Chapter
7611 Maple Street   504-861-3433
New Orleans, LA 70118   866-382-2232
Fax: 504-861-3466
e-mail: lams@ccfa.org
www.ccfa.org/chapters/louisiana
Crohn's and Colitis Foundation of America is a non-profit volunteer-driven organization dedicated to finding the cure for Crohn's disease and ulcerative colitis.
David Lee Thomas, Development Director Louisiana Office
Gail C Smith, Development Assistant Louisiana Office

2951   CCFA Mid-America Chapter: Missouri
1034 S Brentwood   314-863-4747
Saint Louis, MO 63117   800-783-8006
Fax: 314-863-4749
e-mail: info@ccfa.org
www.ccfa.org/chapters/midamerica
Crohn's and Colitis Foundation of America is a non-profit volunteer-driven organization dedicated to finding the cure for Crohn's disease and ulcerative colitis.
Steve Skodak, Executive Director
Andi Harrington, Development Manager

2952   CCFA New Jersey Chapter
45 Wilson Avenue   732-786-9960
Manalapan, NJ 07726   Fax: 732-786-9964
e-mail: newjersey@ccfa.org
www.ccfa.org/chapters/newjersey
Crohn's and Colitis Foundation of America is a non-profit volunteer-driven organization dedicated to finding the cure for Crohn's disease and ulcerative colitis.
Rosemarie Golombos, Executive Director
Barbara Fedorchak, Chapter Development Manager

New York

2953 CCFA Greater New York Chapter: National Headquarters
386 Park Avenue S
New York, NY 10016-8804
800-932-2423
800-932-2423
Fax: 212-679-3567
e-mail: info@ccfa.org
www.ccfa.org
Crohn's and Colitis Foundation of America is a non-profit volunteer-driven organization dedicated to finding the cure for Crohn's disease and ulcerative colitis.
Marilyn Hagg Blohm, Executive Director
Jeff Neale, Public Relations/Media Director

2954 CCFA Long Island Chapter
585 Stewart Avenue
Garden City, NY 11530
516-222-5530
Fax: 516-222-5535
e-mail: longisland@ccfa.org
www.ccfa.org/chapters/longisland
Crohn's and Colitis Foundation of America is a non-profit volunteer-driven organization dedicated to finding the cure for Crohn's disease and ulcerative colitis.
Marilyn Hagg Blohm, Executive Director National Office
Jeff Neale, Public Relations/Media National Office

2955 CCFA Rochester/Southern Tier Chapter
2117 Buffalo Road
Rochester, NY 14624
585-617-4771
800-932-2423
e-mail: rochester@ccfa.org
www.ccfa.org/chapters/rochester
Crohn's and Colitis Foundation of America is a non-profit volunteer-driven organization dedicated to finding the cure for Crohn's disease and ulcerative colitis.
Marilyn Hagg Blohm, Executive Director National Headquarters
Jeff Neale, Public Relations

2956 CCFA Upstate/Northeastern New York Chapter
4 Normanskill Boulevard
Delmar, NY 12054
518-439-0252
e-mail: upstateny@ccfa.org
www.ccfa.org/chapters/upstateny
Crohn's and Colitis Foundation of America is a non-profit volunteer-driven organization dedicated to finding the cure for Crohn's disease and ulcerative colitis.
Linda Winston, Chapter President
Peter Purcel MD, Medical Advisory Chair

2957 CCFA Western New York Chapter
2714 Sheridan Drive
Tonawanda, NY 14150-0224
716-833-2870
800-932-2423
e-mail: jpetri@ccfa.org
www.ccfa.org/chapters/westernny
Crohn's and Colitis Foundation of America is a non-profit volunteer-driven organization dedicated to finding the cure for Crohn's disease and ulcerative colitis.
Marilyn Hagg Blohm, Executive Director National Headquarters
Jeff Neale, Public Relations

North Carolina

2958 CCFA Carolinas Chapter
2901 N Davidson Street
Charlotte, NC 28205
704-332-1611
877-332-1611
Fax: 704-332-1612
e-mail: carolinas@ccfa.org
www.ccfa.org/chapters/carolinas
Crohn's and Colitis Foundation of America is a non-profit volunteer-driven organization dedicated to finding the cure for Crohn's disease and ulcerative colitis.
Angela Parks, Development Director
Julie Perkins, Special Events/Development Manager

Ohio

2959 CCFA Central Ohio Chapter
5008 Pine Creek Drive
Westerville, OH 43081
614-865-1933
800-625-5977
Fax: 614-865-1934
e-mail: centralohio@ccfa.org
www.ccfa.org/chapters/centralohio

Crohn's and Colitis Foundation of America is a non-profit volunteer-driven organization dedicated to finding the cure for Crohn's disease and ulcerative colitis.
Janelle Gasaway, Take Steps Manager
Kelly Bush, Development Coordinator

2960 CCFA Northeast Ohio Chapter
23775 Commerce Park Road
Beachwood, OH 44122
216-831-2692
866-345-2232
Fax: 216-831-2792
e-mail: neohio@ccfa.org
www.ccfa.org/chapters/neohio
Crohn's and Colitis Foundation of America is a non-profit volunteer-driven organization dedicated to finding the cure for Crohn's disease and ulcerative colitis.
Kristin Knipp, Development Coordinator
Patty Kaplan, Development Manager NE Ohio Chapter

2961 CCFA Southwest Ohio Chapter
8 Triangle Park Drive
Cincinnati, OH 45246
513-772-3550
877-283-7513
Fax: 513-772-7599
e-mail: SWOhio@ccfa.org
www.ccfa.org/chapters/swohio
Crohn's and Colitis Foundation of America is a non-profit volunteer-driven organization dedicated to finding the cure for Crohn's disease and ulcerative colitis.
Rachel Spradlin, Take Steps Manager
Jenny Southers, Development Manager SE Ohio Chapter

Oklahoma

2962 CCFA Oklahoma Chapter
4504 E 67th Street
Tulsa, OK 74136
918-523-8540
800-658-1533
Fax: 918-523-8560
e-mail: jsummers@ccfa.org
www.ccfa.org/chapters/oklahoma
Crohn's and Colitis Foundation of America is a non-profit volunteer-driven organization dedicated to finding the cure for Crohn's disease and ulcerative colitis.
Judy Summers, Regional Executive Director
Christopher Woods, President

Pennsylvania

2963 CCFA Philadelphia/Delaware Valley Chapter
367 E Street Road
Trevose, PA 19053
215-396-9100
888-340-4744
Fax: 215-396-1170
e-mail: Philadelphia@ccfa.org
www.ccfa.org/chapters/philadelphia
Crohn's and Colitis Foundation of America is a non-profit volunteer-driven organization dedicated to finding the cure for Crohn's disease and ulcerative colitis.
Barbara Berman, Executive Director
Suzanne Rhodeside, Development Director

2964 CCFA Western Pennsylvania/West Virginia Chapter
300 Penn Center Boulevard
Pittsburgh, PA 15235
412-823-8272
877-823-8272
Fax: 412-823-8276
e-mail: wpawv@ccfa.org
www.ccfa.org/chapters/wpawv
Crohn's and Colitis Foundation of America is a non-profit volunteer-driven organization dedicated to finding the cure for Crohn's disease and ulcerative colitis.
10-12 pages
Jamie Rhoades, Development Manager
Susan Kukic, Executive Director

South Carolina

2965 CCFA South Carolina Chapter
2901 N Davidson Street
Charlotte, NC 28205
704-332-1611
877-632-1611
Fax: 704-332-1612
e-mail: carolinas@ccfa.org
www.ccfa.org/chapters/carolinas

Crohn's and Colitis Foundation of America is a non-profit volunteer-driven organization dedicated to finding the cure for Crohn's disease and ulcerative colitis.
Angela Parks, Development Manager
Tewanna Sanders, Education & Support Manager

Tennessee

2966   CCFA Tennessee Chapter
95 White Bridge Road   615-356-0444
Nashville, TN 37205   866-814-2232
                                         Fax: 615-356-0445
                                 e-mail: tennessee@ccfa.org
                             www.ccfa.org/chapters/tennessee
Crohn's and Colitis Foundation of America is a non-profit volunteer-driven organization dedicated to finding the cure for Crohn's disease and ulcerative colitis.
Michelle J Chianese, Education & Support Manager
Nicole Boisvert, Walk Manager

Texas

2967   CCFA Houston Gulf Coast/South Texas Chapter
5120 Woodway   713-572-2232
Houston, TX 77056   800-785-2232
                                         Fax: 713-572-2433
                                 e-mail: infohouston@ccfa.org
                              www.ccfa.org/chapters/houston
Crohn's and Colitis Foundation of America is a non-profit volunteer-driven organization dedicated to finding the cure for Crohn's disease and ulcerative colitis.
Brandy Bendele, Walk Manager
Erin Fagan, Development Manager

2968   CCFA North Texas Chapter
12801 N Central Expressway   972-386-0607
Dallas, TX 75243   Fax: 972-386-0509
                                   e-mail: ntexas@ccfa.org
                               www.ccfa.org/chapters/ntexas
Crohn's and Colitis Foundation of America is a non-profit volunteer-driven organization dedicated to finding the cure for Crohn's disease and ulcerative colitis.
Rachel Wallace, Development Manager
Sharon Seagraves, Executive Director

Virginia

2969   CCFA Greater Washington DC/Virginia Chapter
4085 Chain Bridge Road   703-865-6130
Fairfax, VA 22314   877-807-5271
                                         Fax: 703-865-8873
                              e-mail: washingtondc@ccfa.org
                          www.ccfa.org/chapters/washingtondc
Crohn's and Colitis Foundation of America is a non-profit volunteer-driven organization dedicated to finding the cure for Crohn's disease and ulcerative colitis.
Eileen Pugh, Executive Director
Stephanie Campbell, Development Coordinator

Washington

2970   CCFA Washington State Chapter
9 Lake Bellevue Drive   425-451-8455
Bellevue, WA 98005   877-703-6900
                                         Fax: 425-451-1708
                                 e-mail: northwest@ccfa.org
                             www.ccfa.org/chapters/northwest
Crohn's and Colitis Foundation of America is a non-profit volunteer-driven organization dedicated to finding the cure for Crohn's disease and ulcerative colitis.
Linda Huse, Executive Director
Jennifer Simmons, Development Manager

Wisconsin

2971   CCFA Wisconsin Chapter
1126 S 70th Street   414-475-5520
W Allis, WI 53214   877-586-5588
                                         Fax: 414-475-5502
                                  e-mail: wisconsin@ccfa.org
                             www.ccfa.org/chapters/wisconsin
Crohn's and Colitis Foundation of America is a non-profit volunteer-driven organization dedicated to finding the cure for Crohn's disease and ulcerative colitis.
Jan Lenz, Executive Director
Nadine Davis, Development Coordinator

Libraries & Resource Centers

2972   National Digestive Diseases Information Clearinghouse
2 Information Way
Bethesda, MD 20892-3570   800-891-5389
                                         Fax: 703-738-4929
                                        TTY: 866-569-1162
                             e-mail: nddic@info.niddk.nih.gov
                               http://digestive.niddk.nih.gov/
Established to increase knowledge and understanding about digestive diseases among people with these conditions and their families, health care professionals, and the general public. To carry out this mission, NDDIC works closely with a coordinating panel of representatives from Federal agencies, voluntary organizations on the national level, and professional groups to identify and respond to informational needs about digestive diseases.
Kathy Kranzfelder, Director

Research Centers

2973   Hahnemann University, Krancer Center for Inflammatory Bowel Disease Research
Broad & Vine Streets   215- 76- 700
Philadelphia, PA 19102   Fax: 215-762-8109
                                     www.hahnemannhospital.com
Research into the causes and treatments of ulcerative colitis and Crohn's disease.
Dr. Harris Clearfield, Director

Support Groups & Hotlines

2974   Crohn's & Colitis Foundation of America Hotline
Crohn's & Colitis Foundation of America
386 Park Avenue S
New York, NY 10016   800-932-2423
                                       e-mail: info@ccfa.org
                                             www.ccfa.org
Our mission is to cure and prevent Crohn's disease and ulcerative colitis through research and to improve the quality of life of children and adults affected by these digestive disease through education and support. Known collectively as inflammatory bowel disease (IBD), these painful chronic illnesses affect up to one million Americans, including approximately 100,000 children under the age of 18.

2975   National Health Information Center
PO Box 1133   310-565-4167
Washington, DC 20013   800-336-4797
                                         Fax: 301-984-4256
                                       e-mail: info@nhic.org
                                          www.health.gov/nhic
A health information referral service sponsored by the Office of Disease Prevention and Health Promotion. NHIC puts health professionals and consumers who have health questions in touch with those organizations that are best able to provide answers.

Books

2976   Crohn's Disease and Ulcerative Colitis Fact Book
Crohn's & Colitis Foundation of America

386 Park Avenue S
New York, NY 10016-8804

212-685-3440
800-932-2423
Fax: 212-779-4098
e-mail: info@ccfa.org
www.ccfa.org

Written in layman's language, this first complete guide is helpful in understanding and coping with inflammatory bowel diseases.

2977 Managing Your Child's Crohn's Disease or Ulcerative Colitis
Crohn's & Colitis Foundation of America
386 Park Avenue S
New York, NY 10016-8804

212-685-3440
800-932-2423
Fax: 212-779-4098
e-mail: info@ccfa.org
www.ccfa.org

Full-length book on Crohn's disease and ulcerative colitis, specifically targeted for parents of children and teenagers; includes topics on cause and diagnosis, treatment, surgery, hospitalization, diet and nutrition, school and social issues and resources for the patient.
$16.95 Members

2978 Ostomy Book: Living Comfortably with Colostomies, Ileostomies and Urostomies
Barbara Dorr Mullen and Kerry Anne McGinn, author
Bull Publishing Company
PO Box 1377thur Boulevard
Boulder, CO 80306

800-676-2855
Fax: 303-545-6354
www.bullpub.com

This book provides complete information on everything from details of surgery to the management of the appliances. Just as importantly, it is a beautifully told story of the entire expereince from diagnosis through rehabilitation to looking forward to a full and happy life.

ISBN: 0-923521-12-7

2979 People...Not Patients: Source Book for Living with Bowel Disease
Chron's & Colitis Foundation of America
386 Park Avenue S
New York, NY 10016-8804

212-685-3440
800-932-2423
Fax: 212-779-4098
e-mail: info@ccfa.org
www.ccfa.org

Contains the essential information you need to help you cope with Chron's disease and ulcerative colitis after you leave the doctor's office.

2980 Special Kind of Cookbook
Canadian Foundation for Ileitis and Colitis
Box 961, Sta T, Calgary
Alberta, Canada, T2H 2H4,

403-263-2425

Presents guidelines for good nutrition to help maintain one's body during a period of inflammatory bowel disease and to maintain health during periods of remission.

2981 Treating IBD
Crohn's & Colitis Foundation of America
386 Park Avenue S
New York, NY 10016-8804

212-685-3440
800-932-2423
Fax: 212-779-4098
e-mail: info@ccfa.org
www.ccfa.org

Patient's guide to the medical and surgical management of Inflammatory Bowel Disease, this book gives information on treating crohn's disease and ulcerative colitis, including drug therapies, advances in nutritional care, and recently developed surgical alternatives.

2982 Understanding Crohn Disease and Ulcerative Colitis
Jon Zonderman, Ronald S Vender, MD, author
University Press of Mississippi
3825 Ridgewood Road
Jackson, MS 39211-6492

601-432-6205
Fax: 601-432-6217
e-mail: kburgess@ihl.state.ms.us
www.upress.state.ms.us

For patients and caregivers an overview of the nature and treatments of inflammatory bowel disease.
2000 128 pages Paperback
ISBN: 1-578062-03-9
Kathy Burgess, Advertising/Marketing Services Manager

Magazines

2983 Colon and Rectal Surgery
International Academy of Proctology
PO Box 1716
Martinsville, IN 46151

765-342-3686
Fax: 765-342-4173

Information for professionals involved with colon and rectal surgery.
George Donnally MD

2984 Digestive Health Matters
Intl. Foundation for Gastrointestinal Disorders
PO Box 170864
Milwaukee, WI 53217-0864

414-964-1799
888-964-2001
Fax: 414-964-7176
e-mail: iffgd@iffgd.org

Quarterly journal focuses on upper and lower gastrointestinal disorders in adults and children. Educational pamphlets and factsheets are available. Patient and professional membership.

2985 Foundation Focus
Crohn's & Colitis Foundation of America
386 Park Avenue S
New York, NY 10016-8804

212-685-3440
800-932-2423
Fax: 212-779-4098
e-mail: info@ccfa.org
www.ccfa.org

Magazine for CCFA supporters.

2986 Phoenix Magazine
United Ostomy Association of America
PO Box 512
Northfield, MN 55057

800-826-0826
Fax: 507-645-5168
e-mail: info@uoaa.org
www.uoa.org

America's leading ostomy patient magazine providing colostomy, ileostomy, urostomy and continent diversion information, management techniques, new products and much more.
Quarterly
David Rudzin, President

Newsletters

2987 Crohn's Disease, Ulcerative Colitis, and School
Pediatric Crohn's & Colitis Association
PO Box 188
Newton, MA 02468

617-489-5854
e-mail: questions@pcca.hypermart.net
pcca.hypermart.net

Information on Crohn's Disease and Ulcerative Colitis, including medical, nutritional, psychological and social factors.

2988 IBD File
Crohn's & Colitis Foundation of America
386 Park Avenue S
New York, NY 10016-8804

212-685-3440
800-932-2423
Fax: 212-779-4098
e-mail: info@ccfa.org
www.ccfa.org

Offers updated information and the latest medical news about Crohn's Disease and Colitis.

2989 Inflammatory Bowel Disease
Gastro-Intestinal Research Foundation
70 E Lake Street
Chicago, IL 60601

312-332-1350
Fax: 312-332-4757
e-mail: girf@girf.org
www.girf.org

Newsletter and patient pamphlet.

2990 Inner Circle
Reach Out for Youth with Ileitis and Colitis
84 Northgate Circle   516-293-3102
Melville, NY 11747   Fax: 516-293-3103
Provides information to patients with ileitis and colitis and their families.

2991 Inside Story
Reach Out for Youth with Ileitis and Colitis
84 Northgate Circle   516-293-3102
Melville, NY 11747   Fax: 516-293-3103
Provides information to patients with ileitis and colitis and their families.

Pamphlets

2992 ABC's of Pediatric Inflammatory Bowel Disease
Pediatric Crohn's & Colitis Association
PO Box 188   617-489-5854
Newton, MA 02468   e-mail: questions@pcca.hypermart.net
                                       pcca.hypermart.net
Information on Pediatric Inflammatory Disease, including medical, nutritional, psychological and social factors.

2993 CCFA: A Case for Support
Crohn's & Colitis Foundation of America
386 Park Avenue S   212-685-3440
New York, NY 10016-8804   800-932-2423
                                  Fax: 212-779-4098
                              e-mail: info@ccfa.org
                                       www.ccfa.org
Reviews the work of the Crohn's and Colitis Foundation of America, sponsors a nationally recognized research program, which seeks to improve treatment and ultimately find the cure for inflammatory bowel disease.

2994 Coping with Crohn's and Colitis is Tough
Crohn's & Colitis Foundation of America
386 Park Avenue S   212-685-3440
New York, NY 10016-8804   800-932-2423
                                  Fax: 212-779-4098
                              e-mail: info@ccfa.org
                                       www.ccfa.org
Offers information on the Crohn's and Colitis Association. Also offers factual information and statistics on the diseases.

2995 Crohn's Disease
NDDIC
2 Information Way   301-654-3810
Bethesda, MD 20892-0001   800-891-5389
                                  Fax: 301-907-8906
                      e-mail: nddic@info.niddlc.nin.gov
                                       www.niddk.nih.gov

October 1992

2996 Guide for Children and Teenagers to Crohn's Disease/Ulcerative Colitis
Crohn's & Colitis Foundation of America
386 Park Avenue S   212-685-3440
New York, NY 10016-8804   800-932-2423
                                  Fax: 212-779-4098
                              e-mail: info@ccfa.org
                                       www.ccfa.org
Offers important information on these illnesses to children and teens.

2997 Ileostomy Guide
United Ostomy Associations of America, Inc.
PO Box 66
Fairview, TN 37062-0066   800-826-0826
                              e-mail: info@uoaa.org
                                       www.uoaa.org
Written for persons who have recently had an ileostomy, this guidebook covers a spectrum of topics including basic facts about ileostomies, information for patients, helpful ideas and practical tips.
28 pages

2998 Questions & Answers About Diet and Nutrition
Crohn's & Colitis Foundation of America
386 Park Avenue S   212-685-3440
New York, NY 10016-8804   800-932-2423
                                  Fax: 212-779-4098
                              e-mail: info@ccfa.org
                                       www.ccfa.org
Raises important facts about how diet and nutrition affect persons with Crohn's Disease.

2999 Questions and Answers About Complications
Crohn's & Colitis Foundation of America
386 Park Avenue S   212-685-3440
New York, NY 10016-8804   800-932-2423
                                  Fax: 212-779-4098
                              e-mail: info@ccfa.org
                                       www.ccfa.org
Medical facts and complications from surgery.

3000 Questions and Answers About Crohn's Disease & Ulcerative Colitis
Crohn's & Colitis Foundation of America
386 Park Avenue S   212-685-3440
New York, NY 10016-8804   800-932-2423
                                  Fax: 212-779-4098
                              e-mail: info@ccfa.org
                                       www.ccfa.org
Offers information on the illness and answers the most frequently asked questions about Crohn's Disease. Also includes a glossary of IBD terms.

3001 Questions and Answers About Emotional Factors in Ileitis and Colitis
Crohn's & Colitis Foundation of America
386 Park Avenue S   212-685-3440
New York, NY 10016-8804   800-932-2423
                                  Fax: 212-779-4098
                              e-mail: info@ccfa.org
                                       www.ccfa.org
Answers some of the most commonly asked questions about ileitis and colitis and the role of emotional factors in their cause and course.

3002 Questions and Answers About Pregnancy in Ileitis and Colitis
Crohn's & Colitis Foundation of America
386 Park Avenue S   212-685-3440
New York, NY 10016-8804   800-932-2423
                                  Fax: 212-779-4098
                              e-mail: info@ccfa.org
                                       www.ccfa.org
Answers questions about inflammatory bowel disease concerning conception, pregnancy, delivery and nursing.

3003 Questions and Answers About Surgery
Crohn's & Colitis Foundation of America
386 Park Avenue S   212-685-3440
New York, NY 10016-8804   800-343-3637
                                  Fax: 212-779-4098
                              e-mail: info@ccfa.org
                                       www.ccfa.org
Answers questions and offers basic facts about surgery for persons suffering from Crohn's Disease and Ulcerative Colitis.

3004 Teacher's Guide to Crohn's Disease and Ulcerative Colitis
Crohn's & Colitis Foundation of America
386 Park Avenue S   212-685-3440
New York, NY 10016-8804   800-932-2423
                                  Fax: 212-779-4098
                              e-mail: info@ccfa.org
                                       www.ccfa.org
The purpose of this brochure is to increase the support and encouragement given to young people with Crohn's disease and ulcerative colitis by teachers who understand their illness.

3005 Crohn's Disease, Ulcerative Colitis and Your Child
Crohn's & Colitis Foundation of America
386 Park Avenue S   212-685-3440
New York, NY 10016-8804   800-932-2423
                                  Fax: 212-779-4098
                              e-mail: info@ccfa.org
                                       www.ccfa.org

Answers questions about IBD in children, providing information on early signs, growth and developments, treatments and special problems in school.

Web Sites

3006 Crohn's & Colitis Foundation of America

www.ccfa.org

CCFA provides educational and patient support services to both the lay and medical communities and plans to provide grants dedicated to pediatric research.

3007 Healing Well

www.healingwell.com

An online health resource guide to medical news, chat, information and articles, newsgroups and message boards, books, disease-related web sites, medical directories, and more for patients, friends, and family coping with disabling diseases, disorders, or chronic illnesses.

3008 Health Finder

www.healthfinder.gov

Searchable, carefully developed web site offering information on over 1000 topics. Developed by the US Department of Health and Human Services, the site can be used in both English and Spanish.

3009 Healthlink USA

www.healthlinkusa.com

Health information concerning treatment, cures, prevention, diagnosis, risk factors, research, support groups, email lists, personal stories and much more. Updated regularly.

3010 MedicineNet

www.medicinenet.com

An online resource for consumers providing easy-to-read, authoritative medical and health information.

3011 Medscape

www.medscape.com

Medscape offers specialists, primary care physicians, and other health professionals the Web's most robust and integrated medical information and educational tools.

3012 National Digestive Diseases Information Clearinghouse

www.niddk.nih.gov

Offers various educational information, resources and reprints focusing on Colitis, Ulcerative Colitis and Crohn's disease.

3013 Pediatric Crohn's and Colitis Association

pcca.hypermart.net/

Focuses on all aspects of pediatric and adolescent Crohn's disease and ulcerative colitis, including medical, nutritional, psychological and social factors. Activities include information sharing, educational forums, newsletters and hospital outreach programs, as well as support of research.

3014 United Ostomy Association

www.uoa.org

A national network for bowel and urinary diversion support groups in the United States. Its goal is to provide a nonprofit association that will serve to unify and strengthen its member support groups, which are organized for the benefit of people who have, or will have intestinal or urinary diversions and their caregivers.

3015 WebMD

www.webmd.com

Information on Crohn's disease, including articles and resources.

Description

3016 Cystic Fibrosis

Cystic fibrosis, CF, is an inherited disease of the exocrine (mucus-producing) glands, primarily affecting the gastrointestinal and respiratory tracts. The mucus that is secreted by persons with the disease is especially thick, thus blocking, rather than lubricating, passageways in the lungs and digestive tract. CF is the most common life-shortening genetic disease in the white population, occurring in 1 in 3,000 live births in the United States, but it occurs in people of all ethnic and racial backgrounds.

In the newborn with CF, thick fecal material may cause partial obstruction of the intestine, which then may contort and rupture. Later in life, blockage of secretions from the pancreas results in frequent, foul-smelling, fatty stools, distention of the abdomen and slowed growth. Damage to the lung occurs as thick mucus secretions plug airways. Fifty percent of all patients develop breathing problems marked by a chronic cough, wheezing and repeated lung infections.

The course of CF is usually determined by the degree to which the lungs are affected, and varies greatly from patient to patient. The prognosis is poor, but advances in therapy have helped many survive well into adulthood. Treatment usually includes aggressive use of antibiotics and other drugs to prevent lung complications, physical therapy, adequate nutrition and psychosocial support.

The first CF gene therapy research began in 1993, and scientists have identified mutations in a CF regulator genethat cause cells to produce abnormally thick mucus. Gene therapy to replace the defective gene with a functional copy is currently under study. Genetic screening is now available.

National Agencies & Associations

3017 Cystic Fibrosis Worldwide
50 Elm Street
Southbridge, MA 01550
508-764-2730
Fax: 508-765-8883
e-mail: information@cfww.org
www.cfww.org

IACFA is a non profit organization headquartered in Zurich Switzerland. The purpose and direction of the organization is to assist in improving the quality of life by identifying common problems and attempting to define possible solutions.
Christine Noke, Executive Director
Mitch Messer, President

Foundations

3018 Cystic Fibrosis Foundation
6931 Arlington Road
Bethesda, MD 20814
301-951-4422
800-344-4823
Fax: 301-951-6378
e-mail: info@cff.org
www.cff.org

The mission of the Cystic Fibrosis Foundation is to assure the development of the means to cure and control cystic fibrosis and to improve the quality of life for those with the disease.
Robert J Beall, PhD, President/CEO

Libraries & Resource Centers

3019 Children's Hospital of Orange County
455 S Main Street
Orange, CA 92868-3874
714-997-3000
e-mail: mail@choc.org
www.choc.org

Our mission is to nuture, advance and protect the health and well-being of children.
Kimberly C Cripe, President/CEO

Research Centers

Alabama

3020 Cystic Fibrosis Foundation
6931 Arlington Road
Bethesda, MD 20814
301-951-4422
800-344-4823
Fax: 301-951-6378
e-mail: info@cff.org
www.cff.org

The mission of the Cystic Fibrosis Foundation a nonprofit donor-supported organization is to assure the development of the means to cure and control cystic fibrosis and to improve the quality of life for those with the disease.
Robert J Beall, President and CEO

Arizona

3021 Cystic Fibrosis Center: Phoenix Childrens Hospital
A, author
1919 E Thomas Road
Phoenix, AZ 85016
602-546-1000
888-908-5437
Fax: 602-460-23
www.phoenixchildrens.com
Robert Meyer, President and Chief Executive Officer
Bruce Morgenstern, Medical Staff President

Arkansas

3022 Arkansas Cystic Fibrosis Center Arkansas Children's Hospital
Arkansas Children's Hospital
1 Children's Way
Little Rock, AR 72202
501-364-1100
Fax: 501-364-3930
TTY: 501-364-1184
e-mail: pedspulmonary@uams.edu
www.arpediatrics.org

Provide high-quality specialized care to patients from comprehensive diagnosis to ongoing treatment.
John L Carroll MD, Division Chief
Dennis E Schellhase, Director

California

3023 Children's Hospital of Los Angeles
4650 Sunset Boulevard
Los Angeles, CA 90027
323-660-2450
e-mail: webmaster@chla.usc.edu
www.childrenshospitalla.com

Provides the highest quality healthcare for children who are the sickest and most seriously injured in our region and beyond.
Richard D Cordova, President/CEO
Rodney B Hanners, Senior Vice President & Chief Operating

3024 Childrens Hospital at Oakland
747 52nd Street
Oakland, CA 94609
510-428-3000
www.childrenshospitaloakland.org

The mission of Children's Hospital Oakland is to ensure the delivery of the highest quality pediatric care for all children through regional primary and subspecialty networks; a strong education and teaching program a diverse workforce state of the art research programs and facilities; and nationally recognized child advocacy efforts.
Bertram Lubin MD, President and Chief Executive Officer
Kathleen Hogue Gonzalez, Vice President, Research Administration

3025 Cystic Fibrosis Center: Cedars-Sinai Medical Center
Cedars-Sinai Medical Center

8700 Beverly Boulevard
Los Angeles, CA 90048

310-423-3277
800-233-2771
Fax: 310-423-4131
www.cedars-sinai.edu

3026 Cystic Fibrosis Center: Cedars-Sinai Medic Cedars-Sinai Medical Center
8700 Beverly Boulevard
Los Angeles, CA 90048

310-423-3277
800-233-2771
Fax: 310-423-4131
www.cedars-sinai.edu

3027 Cystic Fibrosis Center: University of California at San Francisco
400 Parnassus Avenue
San Francisco, CA 94122-0106

415-353-2961
Fax: 415-476-9278
e-mail: ucsf.org?
pulmonary.ucsf.edu

Provides comprehensive evaluation as well as inpatient and outpatient care for patients with cystic fibrosis.
Mary Ellen Kleinhenz MD, Adult CF Director
Dennis Niels MD, Pediatric CF Director

3028 Cystic Fibrosis Research
2672 Bayshore Parkway
Mountain View, CA 94043

650-404-9975
Fax: 650-404-9981
e-mail: cfri@cfri.org
www.cfri.org

Cystic Fibrosis Research exists to fund research to provide educational and personal support and spread awareness of Cystic Fibrosis a life threatening genetic disease.
Carroll Jenkins, Executive Director
David Soohoo, Director of Programs

3029 Memorial Miller Children's Hospital Cystic Fibrosis Center
2801 Atlantic Avenue
Long Beach, CA 90806

562-933-2000
Fax: 562-933-8501
e-mail: enussbaum@memorialcare.org
www.memorialcare.org/miller

provides a multidisciplinary approach to asthma cystic fibrosis sleep disorders and the entire spectrum of chronic and acute lung and airway disorders in children.
Eliezer Nuss MD, Medical Director
Barry Arbuckle PhD, President

3030 Stanford CF Center Packard Children's Hospital At Stanford
Packard Children's Hospital At Stanford
725 Welch Road
Palo Alto, CA 94304-1601

650-497-8000
e-mail: jkirby@leland.stanford.edu
cfcenter.stanford.edu

Colorado

3031 Denver Childrens Hospital
1830 Franklin Street
Denver, CO 80218

72-77-136
800-624-6553
Fax: 303-832-9245
TTY: 720-777-9390
www.thechildrenshospital.org

Frank Accurs MD, Director
Jim Schmerling, President, CEO

Connecticut

3032 University of Connecticut Health Center
263 Farmington Avenue
Farmington, CT 06030-0001

860-679-2000
TTY: 860-679-2242
TDD: 860-679-2242
e-mail: president@uconn.edu
www.uchc.edu

Philip E Austin, President
Cato T Laurencin MD, Vice President for Health Affairs

3033 Yale University Cystic Fibrosis Research Center
Yale Pediatrics
333 Cedar Street
New Haven, CT 06510

203-432-4771
e-mail: sheila.rivera@yale.edu
www.yalepediatrics.org

One of only two in the state of Connecticut the CF Center in the Children's Hospital at the Yale-New Haven Hospital offers a multidisciplinary team approach to provide the most comprehensive state of the art care of CF patients.
Marie Egan MD, Director
Richard C Levin, President

District of Columbia

3034 Metropolitan DC Cystic Fibrosis Center Children s Hospital National Medical Cen
Children s Hospital National Medical Center
111 Michigan Avenue NW
Washington, DC 20010-2970

202-476-2327
888-884-2327
e-mail: tbear@cnmc.org
www.dcchildrens.com

An active clinical and basic science research program that exists within the center.

Florida

3035 Cystic Fibrosis Center: All Children's Hospital
Department of Pulmonology
501 6th Street S
Saint Petersburg, FL 33701

727-898-7451
800-456-4543
Fax: 727-767-4218
www.allkids.org

Anthony D Kriseman MD, Pulmonology
Joseph (Jay) Fleece lll, Chair

3036 Miami Childrens Hospital Division of Pulmonology
3100 SW 62nd Avenue
Miami, FL 33155-3309

305-666-6511
800-432-6837
Fax: 305-663-8417
e-mail: info@mch.com
www.mch.com

Division evaluates and treats many respiratory disorders including asthma chronic lung disease cystic fibrosis pneumonia and tuberculosis. The Division is strongly committed to a multidisciplinary medical approach to these complex disorders.
Moises Simps MD, Director
M Narendra Kini, President, CEO

3037 Nemours Childrens Clinic
807 Childrens Way
Jacksonville, FL 32207

904-390-3600
Fax: 904-390-3699
www.nemours.org

Nemours Children's Clinic is one integrated multispecialty group practice with locations in four states seeing patients from across the US and the world.
David J Bailey, President, CEO

Georgia

3038 Department of Pediatrics Medical College of Georgia
1120 15th Street
Augusta, GA 30912

706-721-3466
Fax: 706-721-7311
e-mail: pwalling@ georgiahealth.edu
www.mcg.edu/pediatrics

Dr William Kanto Jr, Chairperson Pediatrics

3039 Emory University: Cystic Fibrosis Center
201 Dowman Drive
Atlanta, GA 30322-1028

404-727-6123
Fax: 404-727-4828
e-mail: lwolfen@emory.edu
www.emory.edu

Lindy Wolfen MD, Director
Jim Wagner, President

Illinois

3040 Comer Children's Hospital at the University of Chicago
5841 S Maryland Avenue
Chicago, IL 60637

773-702-1000
888-824-0200
www.uchospitals.edu

3041 Comer Children's Hospital at the Universit
5841 S Maryland Avenue
Chicago, IL 60637

773-702-1000
888-824-0200
www.uchicagokidshospital.org

To provide superior healthcare in a compassionate manner ever mindful of each patient's dignity and individuality.

3042   Cystic Fibrosis Center: Childrens Memorial Hospital
2300 Childrens Plaza   773-880-4000
Chicago, IL 60614-3363   800-543-7362
                                 e-mail: cf@childrensmemorial.org
                                         www.childrensmemorial.org
The Cystic Fibrosis Center at Children's Memorial Hospital has
been a CFF-accredited CF care center since 1963. It is committed
to providing exemplary care to each patient and family focused on
individualized preventative care active management of lung health
and nutrition and patient family education.
Susanna McCo MD, Director
Patrick M Magoon, President, CEO

**3043   Cystic Fibrosis Center: Park Ridge Lutheran General Children's
Hospital**
Lutheran General Children's Hospital
1775 Dempster Street   847-723-154
Park Ridge, IL 60068   Fax: 847-696-3041
                                     www.advocatehealth.com/lgch
James H Skogsbergh, President, CEO

3044   Loyola University Medical Center: Department of Pediatrics
2160 S 1st Avenue   708-327-9120
Maywood, IL 60153   888-584-7888
                                                     www.luhs.org
Vicki PhD, R Keough, Dean and Professor

3045   Loyola University Medical Center: Departme
2160 S 1st Avenue
Maywood, IL 60153   708-327-9120
                                                www.stritch.luc.edu
Provides a comprehensive array of general tertiary and
subspecialty care for children.
Vicki PhD, R Keough, Dean and Professor

3046   Saint Francis Medical Center Peoria Pulmonary Association
214 NE Glen Oak Avenue
Peoria, IL 61637   309-655-2000
                                             www.osfsaintfrancis.org
Dr. Denise Mammolito, President

3047   Saint Francis Medical Center Peoria Pulmon
530 NE Glen Oak Avenue
Peoria, IL 61637   309-672-2000
                                             www.osfsaintfrancis.org
Dr. Denise Mammolito, President

Indiana

3048   The Riley Cystic Fibrosis Center
702 Barnhill Drive   317-944-2060
Indianapolis, IN 46202   800-248-1199
                                     www.rileychildrenshospital.com
The Riley Cystic Fibrosis Center is the only Cystic Fibrosis Foundation accredited Cystic Fibrosis Center in the state. The Center
provides state-of-the-art CF care at Riley and across the state.
Daniel Fink, President, CEO

Iowa

3049   Blank Childrens Hospital Pediatric Pulmonology Clinic
Children's Health Center 1
1212 Pleasant Street
Des Moines, IA 50309   515-241-6548
                                            www.blankchildrens.org
David Starke, President, CEO
Ken Cheyne, Medical Director

**3050   Pediatric Allergy & Pulmonary Division University of Iowa
Healthcare**
University of Iowa Healthcare
200 Hawkins Drive   319-356-2296
Iowa City, IA 52242   e-mail: allerpulm@uiowa.edu
                              www.uihealthcare.com/depts/med/pediatric
The Division of Allergy and Pulmonology offers evaluation and
management of allergic disorders in children with too many infec-
tions and acute and chronic breathing disorders of childhood and
adolescence.
Jody Kurtt RN, Director

Kansas

3051   Kansas University Medical Center: Cystic Fibrosis Center
3901 Rainbow Boulevard   913-588-5000
Kansas City, KS 66160   800-332-4199
                                             Fax: 913-588-7963
                                       e-mail: gperry@kumc.edu
                                                  www2.kumc.edu
Barbara F Atkinson MD, Executive Vice Chancellor

**3052   St. Joseph Medical Center Cystic Fibrosis Care and Teaching
Center**
929 N. St. Francis   316-268-5000
Wichita, KS 67214   Fax: 316-583-90
                                     e-mail: contact@viachristi.org
                                              www.viachristi.org
Kay Glasner, Director
Maria Loving, Public Relations Specialist

Kentucky

3053   Kentucky University: Cystic Fibrosis Center
800 Rose Street   859-257-1000
Lexington, KY 40536-0298   800-333-8874
                                             Fax: 859-257-7706
                                     www.ukhealthcare.uky.edu
The cystic fibrosis team works with more than 175 patients and is
dedicated to working with the most advanced therapies to improve
the life of every patient.
Jamshed F Kanga MD, Director
Dr. Michael Karpf, Executive Vice President

3054   Kosair Childrens Cystic Fibrosis Center
Suite 201   502-629-6000
Louisville, KY 40202-2021 e-mail: contactcenter@nortonhealthcare.org
                                       www.nortonhealthcare.com
The Cystic Fibrosis Center is one of 120 centers in the United
States accredited by the National Cystic Fibrosis Foundation. Spe-
cialists provide diagnosis and multidisciplinary care for cystic fi-
brosis patients of all ages. Professional education and training is
also provided.
Nemie Eid, Medical Director
Stephen A Williams, President, CEO

Louisiana

3055   Ernest N Morial Asthma, Allergy & Respiratory Disease Center
Louisiana State University School of Medicine
1901 Perdido Street   504-568-4634
New Orleans, LA 70112-3932   888-695-8647
                                             Fax: 504-568-4295
                                     e-mail: dthoma2@lsumc.edu
                                                  www.lsuhsc.edu
Warren R Summer MD, Director

Maine

3056   Central Maine Cystic Fibrosis Center
300 Main Street   207-795-0111
Lewiston, ME 04240-7027   Fax: 207-795-2303
                                                   www.cmhc.org
Ralph V Harder, Director
Peter Chkale, Chief Executive Officer

3057   Maine Medical Center: Cystic Fibrosis Clinical Center
22 Bramhall Street   207-662-0111
Portland, ME 04102-3175   Fax: 207-775-6024
                                                    www.mmc.org
Richard W Peterson, President, CEO

3058   Maine Medical Center: Cystic Fibrosis Clin
22 Bramhall Street   207-662-0111
Portland, ME 04102-3175   877-339-3107
                                             Fax: 207-775-6024
                                             TTY: 207-662-4900
                                                    www.mmc.org
Richard W Peterson, President, CEO

Maryland

3059 Cystic Fibrosis Center: National Institute of Health NIDDK
Building 31 Room 9A06
Bethesda, MD 20892-2560   301-496-3583
www2.niddk.nih.gov
Dr Griffin Rodgers, Acting Director

Massachusetts

3060 Baystate Medical Center Wesson Memorial Unit
Wesson Memorial Unit
759 Chestnut Street   413-794-0000
Springfield, MA 01199   e-mail: Marian.Panto@bhs.org
www.baystatehealth.com
BMC serves as a regional resource for specialty medical care and
research while providing comprehensive primary medical services
to the community.
Mark R Tolosky, President & Chief Executive Officer
Paula S Dennison, Senior Vice President Human Resources

3061 Childrens Hospital Medical Center Cystic Fibrosis Center
300 Longwood Avenue   617-355-6000
Boston, MA 02115   Fax: 617-730-0373
TTY: 617-730-0152
www.childrenshospital.org
The Cystic Fibrosis Center at Children's Hospital Boston is one of
the oldest and largest cystic fibrosis centers in the United States
and was founded by Dr. Harry Schwachman one of the earliest physician investigators to help characterize the disorder.
Terry Spence MD, Director
Sandra Fenwick, President, CEO

3062 Cystic Firbrosis Center: Tufts New England Medical Center
Pediatric Pulmonology and Allergy Department
800 Washington Street
Boston, MA 02111   617-636-5000
www.nemc.org
We strive to heal to comfort to teach to learn and to seek the knowl-
edge to promote health and prevent disease.
Ellen Zane, President and Chief Executive Officer
Margaret Vosburgh, Chief Operating Officer

3063 Massachusetts General Hospital
55 Fruit Street   617-726-2000
Boston, MA 02114-2622   Fax: 617-726-6989
TTY: 617-724-8800
TDD: 617-724-8800
www.massgeneral.org
Peter L Slavin MD, President
David Torchi MD, Chairman and Chief Executive Officer

3064 University of Massachusetts Memorial Medical Center
55 Lake Avenue N
Worcester, MA 01655   508-334-1000
www.umassmemorial.org
UMass Memorial Medical Center is the region's trusted academic
medical center committed to improving the health of the people of
Central New England through excellence in clinical care service
teaching and research.
Walter Ettinger, President
George Brenckle, Senior Vice President and Chief Informat

Michigan

3065 East Lansing Cystic Fibrosis Center Michigan State University
Michigan State University
1200 E Michigan Avenue   517-364-5440
Lansing, MI 48912   Fax: 517-364-5413
phd.msu.edu
Eliane F Eakin MD, Director
H Dele Davies MD, Department Chair

3066 Kalamazoo Center for Medical Studies Michigan State University
Michigan State University
1000 Oakland Drive   269-337-4400
Kalamazoo, MI 49008-1202   800-275-5267
Fax: 269-337-4234
e-mail: programs@kcms.msu.edu
www.kcms.msu.edu

3067 University of Michigan: Cystic Fibrosis Center
A Alfred Taubman Health Care Center
1500 E Medical Center Drive   734-936-4000
Ann Arbor, MI 48109-0318   Fax: 734-936-7635
TTY: 800-649-3777
TDD: 800-649-3777
www.med.umich.edu
Samya Z Nasr MD, Director
Douglas L Strong, CEO

Minnesota

3068 University of Minnesota: Cystic Fibrosis Center
University of Minnesota Hospital
420 Delaware Street SE   612-624-0962
Minneapolis, MN 55455   800-688-5252
Fax: 612-624-0696
e-mail: cfcenter@umn.edu
www.med.umn.edu/peds/cfcenter/home.html
The mission was to develop approaches to understanding and treat-
ing the complications of CF.
Warren E Regelmann MD, Co-Director
Jordan M Dunitz MD, Co-Director

Mississippi

3069 University of Mississippi Medical Center
2500 N State Street   601-984-5046
Jackson, MS 39216-4500   Fax: 601-984-1973
www.umc.edu
Suzanne Mill MD, Director
Daniel W Jones MD, Chancellor

Missouri

3070 Children's Mercy Hospital Children's Mercy Hospitals & Clinics
Children's Mercy Hospitals & Clinics
2401 Gilham Road   816-234-3000
Kansas City, MO 64108   866-512-2168
Fax: 816-842-6107
TTY: 816-234-3816
e-mail: webmaster@cmh.edu
www.childrensmercy.org
Children's Mercy Hospital provides the highest level of medical
care technology services equipment and facilities in promoting the
health and well-being of children in the region from birth through
adolescence.
Randall L O'Donnell PhD, President/CEO
V Fred Burry MD, Executive Medical Director/Executive Vic

3071 University of Missouri Columbia Cystic Fibrosis Center
University of Missouri/Dept of Child Health
One Hospital Drive N712   573-882-6882
Columbia, MO 65212-1   Fax: 573-821-54
e-mail: clarksonb@health.missouri.edu
www.ch.missouri.edu/cysticfibrosis.htm
Peter Konig, Director
Melissa Lawson MD, Division Director

3072 Washington University: Cystic Fibrosis Center
St. Louis Children's Hospital
One Children's Place   314-454-2694
Saint Louis, MO 63110   888-678-4357
Fax: 314-454-2515
peds.wustl.edu
Dedicated to the treatment of patients with cystic fibrosis (CF) for
more than 4 decades. The Cystic Fibrosis Clinical Center and affil-
iated programs has developed into a premier clinical and research
program.
Thomas Ferko MD, Director

Nebraska

3073 University of Nebraska Medical Center Cystic Fibrosis Center
The Nebraska Medical Center 402-552-2000
Omaha, NE 68198-5190 800-922-0000
Fax: 402-559-7062
e-mail: necfcntr@unmc.edu
www.unmc.edu

Harold M Maurer MD, Chancellor
Hari Bandla MD, Associate Professor

Nevada

3074 Children's Lung Specialists
3838 Meadow Lane 702-598-4411
Las Vegas, NV 89107 Fax: 702-598-1988
e-mail: cls@childrens-lung-specialists.com
www.childrens-lung-specialists.com
The certified Cystic Fibrosis Center of Southern Nevada.
Ruben Diaz MD, Director/President/Owner
Craig Nakamu MD, Assistant Director

New Hampshire

3075 New Hampshire Cystic Fibrosis Care Teaching and Research Center
DarthmouthHitchcock Medical Center
One Medical Center Drive 603-650-5000
Lebanon, NH 03756-1 Fax: 603-500-07
TTY: 603-650-8034
www.dhmc.org

William Boyl Jr MD, Director
Dennis Stoke MD, Director

New Jersey

3076 Monmouth Medical Center: Cystic Fibrosis & Pediatric Pulmonary Center
Monmouth Medical Center
368 Lakehurst Road 732-222-5200
Toms River, NJ 08755 888-724-7123
Fax: 908-222-4472
e-mail: info@sbhcs.com
www.sbhcs.com

Peri Kamalakar, Director of Pediatric Hematology/Oncolog

3077 Monmouth Medical Center: Cystic Fibrosis & Monmouth Medical Center
368 Lakehurst Road 732-222-5200
Toms River, NJ 08755 888-724-7123
Fax: 908-222-4472
e-mail: info@sbhcs.com
www.sbhcs.com

Peri Kamalakar, Director of Pediatric Hematology/Oncolog

3078 New Jersey Medical School
185 S Orange Avenue 973-972-4595
Newark, NJ 07101-1709 Fax: 973-972-5965
e-mail: webnjms@umdnj.edu
njms.umdnj.edu
The mission of New Jersey Medical School is to educate students physicians and scientists to meet society's current and future healthcare needs through patient-centered education; pioneering research; innovative clinical rehabilitative and preventive care; and collaborative community outreach.
Maria Soto-G MD, Vice Dean
Robert L Johnson MD, Interim Dean

New York

3079 Albany Medical College Pediatric Pulmonary & Cystic Fibrosis Center
Department of Pediatrics
43 New Scotland Avenue 518-262-3125
Albany, NY 12208 877-262-8008
Fax: 518-262-6884
www.amc.edu

Scott Scroed MD, Division Chief

3080 Armond V Mascia Cystic Fibrosis Center NY Medical College
Division of Pediatrics Pulmonology
New York Medical College 914-594-4000
Valhalla, NY 10595 Fax: 914-594-4336
e-mail: pedpulm@nymc.edu
www.nycmc.edu
Provides comprehensive inpatient and outpatient consultation and management for children suffering from a broad variety of respiratory problems. They are the only accredited Cystic Fibrosis center in the Hudson Valley. The center is dedicated to teaching research and patient care.
Allen Dozer MD, Chief
Karl P Alder MD, President, CEO

3081 CF & Pediatric Pulmonary Care Center The Pediatric Pulmonary Care Center at M
The Pediatric Pulmonary Care Center at Mount Sinai
One Gustave L Levy Place 212-241-6500
New York, NY 10029-6574 800-637-4624
Fax: 212-876-3255
www.mssm.edu
Center staff perform outpatient and inpatient consultations with an integrated multidisciplinary team of professionals who are dedicated specifically to the practice of Pediatric Pulmonary Medicine.
Dennis S Charney MD, Dean, Executive Vice President

3082 Childrens Lung and Cystic Fibrosis Center
Women and Children's Hospital of Buffalo
140 Hodge Avenue 716-878-7000
Buffalo, NY 14222-2099 Fax: 716-888-3945
e-mail: AMTaylor@kaleidahealth.org
www.wchob.org
Services for infants children and teenagers with cystic fibrosis and other chronic respiratory conditions.
Annise Taylor, Manager
Cheryl Klass, President

3083 Cystic Fibrosis Center St. Vincent's Hospital & Medical Center
St. Vincent's Hospital & Medical Center of NY
36 7th Avenue 212-604-8895
New York, NY 10011-6600 Fax: 212-604-3899
www.svcmc.org

Maria Berdel MD, Co-Director
Patricia Wal MD, Co-Director

3084 Pulomonolgy Morgan Stanley Children's Hospital
Morgan Stanley Children's Hospital
3959 Broadway 212-305-5437
New York, NY 10032-3702 877-NYP-WELL
www.childrensnyp.org

Meyer Kattan MD, Director

3085 State University of NY Hospital: Upstate Medical Center
750 E Adams Street 315-464-5540
Syracuse, NY 13210-1834 877-464-5540
TDD: 315-464-5769
www.upstate.edu/uh

Dr Stephen R Goodman, Vice President

3086 State University of NY Hospital: Upstate M
750 E Adams Street 315-464-5540
Syracuse, NY 13210 877-464-5540
TTY: 315-464-5769
www.upstate.edu/uh

Dr Stephen R Goodman, Vice President

North Carolina

3087 Duke University Medical Center: Division of Pulmonary and Critical Care Medicine
350 Hanes House 919-684-3364
Durham, NC 27710 888-275-3853
Fax: 919-684-2292
www.pulmonary.duke.edu
Provides primary and consultative care for patients with various lung diseases on an inpatient and outpatient basis.
Judith Voynow MD, Chief

3088 UNC Cystic Fibrosis Center Department of Pediatrics
Department of Pediatrics

7011 Thurston-Bowles Building   919-966-1077
Chapel Hill, NC 27599-7248   Fax: 919-966-7524
www.med.unc.edu/cystfib/CFcent.htm
A large multidisciplinary group focused on the pathogenesis and other lung diseases.
Richard C Boucher MD, Director
Margaret Lei MD, Director

North Dakota

3089 **St. Alexius Medical Heart and Lung Clinic**
900 E Broadway Avenue   701-530-7000
Bismarck, ND 58501   877-530-5550
Fax: 701-530-8984
TTY: 701-530-5555
TDD: 701-530-5555
www.st.alexius.org
Specializes in services such as cardiac consultation cardiac surgery cardiac catheterization electrophysiology angioplasty intracoronary stents rotoblade asthma emphysema cystic fibrosis chronic lung disease. lung cancer allergy and anesthesia.
Richard Shider, Director

Ohio

3090 **Case Western Reserve University: Cystic Fibrosis Center**
10900 Euclid Avenue   216-368-2000
Cleveland, OH 44106-2624   Fax: 216-844-5916
e-mail: Mds11@case.edu
www.case.edu
Barbara Snyder, President

3091 **Case Western Reserve University: Cystic Fi**
10900 Euclid Avenue   216-368-2000
Cleveland, OH 44106   Fax: 216-844-5916
e-mail: Mds11@case.edu
www.case.edu
Babara Snyder, President

3092 **Columbus Children's Hospital: Cystic Fibrosis Center**
700 Childrens Drive   614-722-2000
Columbus, OH 43205-0296   Fax: 614-722-4755
www.nationwidechildrens.org
Dr Steve Allen, CEO
Elizabeth D Allen MD, Physician

3093 **Lewis H Walker MD: Cystic Fibrosis Center Children's Hospital Medical Center of Ak**
Children's Hospital Medical Center of Akron
One Perkins Square   330-543-1000
Akron, OH 44308-1062   800-262-0333
TTY: 330-543-8080
www.akronchildrens.org/respiratory
One of six CF centers in the state of Ohio providing comprehensive care for patients who suffer from this disease. The center which is part of the Robert T. Stone Respiratory Center actively participates in clinical trials to research new drug therapies to manage cystic fibrosis.
Nathan Krayn MD, Director Cystic Fibrosis Center
William H Considine, President, CEO

3094 **Pediatric Pulmonary Center The Children's Medical Center of Dayton**
The Children's Medical Center of Dayton
1 Children's Plaza   937-641-3000
Dayton, OH 45404-1815   800-228-4055
Fax: 937-641-4500
www.childrensdayton.org
Robert Fink MD, Medical Director
David Kinsaul, President, CEO

3095 **University of Cincinnati College of Medicine Division of Pediatrics**
Children s Hospital Medical Center
3333 Burnet Avenue   513-636-4200
Cincinnati, OH 45229-3039   800-344-2462
Fax: 513-636-0345
TTY: 513-636-4900
e-mail: thomas.boat@cchmc.org
www.cincinnatichildrens.org

The University of Cincinnati Department of Pediatrics consists entirely of staff members from Cincinnati Children's Hospital Medical Center one of the nation's leading pediatric research and teaching institutions.
Thomas F Boat MD, Professor of Pediatrics
Michael Fisher, President, CEO

Oklahoma

3096 **University of Oklahoma: Cystic Fibrosis Center**
Department of Pediatrics
940 NE 13th Street   405-271-4401
Oklahoma City, OK 73104   Fax: 405-271-8710
e-mail: brenda-freese@ouhsc.edu
www.oumedicine.com
James A Royall MD, Professor/Chief Pediatric Pulmonology
Terrence L Stull MD, Chairman

Oregon

3097 **Oregon Health & Science University**
3181 SW Sam Jackson Park Road   503-494-8311
Portland, OR 97239-3098   e-mail: contactus@ohsuhealth.com
www.ohsuhealth.com
Oregon Health & Science University is a leading health and research university that strives for excellence in patient care education research and community service.
Joseph Rober Jr MD MBA, President
Steven D Stadum JD, Executive Vice President

Pennsylvania

3098 **Cystic Fibrosis Center: Polyclinic Medical Center**
Polyclinic Medical Center
PO Box 8700   717-231-8900
Harrisburg, PA 17105-8700   800-334-1007
Fax: 717-782-4679
www.pinnaclehealth.org
Muttiah Gane MD, Director

3099 **Pediatric Pulmonary and Cystic Fibrosis Center**
St. Christopher's Hospital for Children
3601 A Street   215-427-5000
Philadelphia, PA 19134   888-STC-RIS
Fax: 215-427-5555
www.stchristophershospital.com
A team of pediatric pulmonary medicine experts treats children with a wide range of acute and chronic lung diseases such as cystic fibrosis bronchopulmonary dysplasia apnea respiratory infections bronchiolitis congenital malformations including chest wall deformities and pneumonia.
Laurie Varlo MD, Director

3100 **University of Pennsylvania: Penn Lung Center**
Hospital of The University of Pennsylvania
3 Ravdin Suite F   215-662-4000
Philadelphia, PA 19104   800-789-7366
www.pennhealth.com
Penn Lung Center of the University of Pennsylvania Health System is a multidisciplinary resource for consultation second opinion diagnosis and ongoing treatment of patients with lung disease.
Leslie A Litzky MD, Associate Professor of Pathology and Lab
Maryl Kreide MD MSCE, Assistant Professor of Medicine

3101 **University of Pittsburgh Cystic Fibrosis Center: Children's Hospital**
Department of Cell Biology And Physiology
S362 BST   412-648-9362
Pittsburgh, PA 15261   Fax: 412-648-8330
e-mail: cdpweb@pitt.edu
www.cbp.pitt.edu/centers/cfrc.html
The primary goal of the Center is to focus the attention of new and established investigators on multidisciplinary approaches designed to improve the understanding and treatment of cystic fibrosis (CF).
Raymond A Frizzell PhD, Director
Carol A Bertrand PhD, Research Assistant Professor

Rhode Island

3102 Rhode Island Hospital: Cystic Fibrosis Center
Department of Pediatrics
593 Eddy Street   401-444-4000
Providence, RI 02903   Fax: 401-444-2168
                                      e-mail: mschechter@lifespan.org
                                                    www.lifespan.org

Michael S Schechter MD, Director
George A Vecchione, President, CEO

South Carolina

3103 Medical University of South Carolina: Cystic Fibrosis Center
Department of Pediatrics
171 Ashley Avenue   803-792-1414
Charleston, SC 29403   800-424-6872
                                                Fax: 843-876-1435
                                                www.musc.edu/cfcenter

Isabel Virella-Lowell, MD, Director
W Stuart Smith, Vice President, Executive Director

3104 Medical University of South Carolina: Cyst Department of Pediatrics
171 Ashley Avenue   803-792-1414
Charleston, SC 29403   800-424-6872
                                                Fax: 843-876-1435
                                                www.musc.edu/cfcenter
The objectives of the Cystic Fibrosis Center at MUSC are to offer unsurpassed care to patients with cystic fibrosis to teach medical students house staff medical care providers and general public about cystic fibrosis and to learn about cystic fibrosis through clinical and laboratory research.

Isabel Virella-Lowell, MD, Director
W Stuart Smith, Vice President, Executive Director

Tennessee

3105 Memphis Cystic Fibrosis Center LeBonheur Children's Medical Center
LeBonheur Children's Medical Center
50 N Dunlap Street   901-287-5437
Memphis, TN 38103   e-mail: info@lebonheur.org
                                                www.lebonheur.org

Meri Armour, President, CEO

3106 Vanderbilt Children's Hospital
2200 Childrens Way   615-936-1000
Nashville, TN 37232   866-936-7811
                                                www.vanderbiltchildrens.com
Children's Hospital provides top-level care while including the family as an essential element of a child's treatment plan.

Luke Gregory, Chief Executive Officer
Jonathan Gitlin MD, Vice Chancellor

Texas

3107 Cook Children's Medical Center: Cystic Fibrosis Clinic
4214 Andrews Highway
Midland, TX 79701   432-570-5693
                                                www.cookchildrens.org

James C Cunningham MD, Director
Paula Webb RN MSN CNAA B, Vice President of Nursing Services

3108 Cystic Fibrosis Care and Teaching Center Children's Medical Center
Children's Medical Center
1935 Medical District Dr   214-456-7000
Dallas, TX 75235   Fax: 214-456-2563
                                                www.childrens.com
The Dallas Cystic Fibrosis Care and Teaching Center manages the outpatient and inpatient care of approximately 400 infants children adolescents and adults.

Claude Prest MD, Director
Brenda Urbanczyk, Practice Administrator

3109 Cystic Fibrosis-Lung Disease Center: Santa Rosa Children's Hospital
CHRISTUS Center for Children and Families

333 N Santa Rosa   210-704-2011
San Antonio, TX 78207   Fax: 210-704-2651
                                                www.santarosahealth.org
Serving more than 150 000 children each year CSRCH is a 200-plus bed facility and is the only academic Children's hospital in San Antonio partnering with The University of Texas Health Science Center at San Antonio while collaborating with private pediatricians to provide comprehensive pediatric services at one location since 1959.

Donna Beth Willey-Courand MD, Director
Patrick Carrier, President, CEO

3110 Texas Childrens Cystic Fibrosis Care Center
Texas Children's Clinical Care Center
6701 Fannin Street   832-824-1000
Houston, TX 77030   800-364-5437
                                                Fax: 832-825-3072
            e-mail: pulmonarymedicine@texaschildrenshospital
                                                www.texaschildrenshospital.org
Provides comprehensive clinical services to help patients families and referring physicians deal with the many problems cystic fibrosis causes.

Dan K Seilheimer MD, Director
Peter W Hiatt MD, Chief of Service

3111 Tri-Services Military Cystic Fibrosis Center
Brooke Army Medical Center/Pediatrics Department
3851 Roger Brooke Drive   210-916-3400
Fort Sam Houston, TX 78234-6320   Fax: 210-916-3076
                                e-mail: ted.cieslak@cen.amedd.army.mil
                                                www.bamc.amedd.army.mil

COL Ted Cieslak, Chief of Pediatrics
Joseph Caravalho, Commanding Officer

Utah

3112 University of Utah Intermountain Cystic Fibrosis Center
University Hospital & Clinics
50 N. Medical Drive   801-581-2121
Salt Lake City, UT 84132   800-824-2073
                                                Fax: 801-585-5350
                                  e-mail: judy.carle@hsc.utah.edu
                                                www.med.utah.edu

Barbara A Chatfield MD, Director Pediatric Program
Loris Betz, Senior VP, Executive Dean

Vermont

3113 Medical Center Hospital of Vermont Cystic Fibrosis Center
Cystic Fibrosis Center
111 Colchester Avenue   802-847-0000
Burlington, VT 05401-7152   800-358-1144
                                                Fax: 802-555-2323
                                                www.fahc.org

Tom Lahiri MD, Director
Melinda L Estes MD, President, CEO

Virginia

3114 Eastern Virginia Medical School Children's Hospital of The King's Daught
Children's Hospital of The King's Daughters
601 Children's Lane   757-668-7000
Norfolk, VA 23507   e-mail: healthinfo@chkd.org
                                                www.chkd.org
Provider of quality children's health services

Leslie Acakpo-Satchi, Neurosurgery
Maria Aguiar, Pathology

3115 University of Virginia School of Medicine Cystic Fibrosis Center
Department of Pediatrics
PO Box 800793   434-924-2250
Charlottesville, VA 22908   800-251-3627
                                                Fax: 434-243-6618
                                                www.healthsystem.virginia.edu
Comprehensive care for children and adults with cystic fibrosis.

Steven T DeKosky MD, Vice President, Dean
Sharon L Hostler, Senior Associate Dean

Washington

3116 University of Washington: Cystic Fibrosis Center
University of Washington Medical Center/Adult Prog
1959 NE Pacific Street   206-598-6116
Seattle, WA 98195   Fax: 206-598-4610
www.washington.edu
UW Medicine works to improve the health of the public by advancing medical knowledge
Ronald Gibson, Center Director
Ronald Gibson, Professor and Center Director

West Virginia

3117 West Virginia University Cystic Fibrosis Center
Pediatrics Department
PO Box 9214   304-293-1201
Morgantown, WV 26506-9214   Fax: 304-293-1216
e-mail: kmoffett@hsc.wvu.edu
www.hsc.wvu.edu
The Hospital providing the full range of services including allergy/immunology cardiology child development critical care cystic fibrosis endocrinology adolescent medicine gastroenterology genetics and metabolic disease hematology/oncology neonatology nephrology neurology and apnea evaluation. Services provided by faculty with joint appointments include ophthalmology urology orthopedics psychiatry surgery and cardiothoracic surgery.
Kathryn S Moffett MD, Director
Giovanni Piedimonte, Chair

Wisconsin

3118 Medical College of Wisconsin: Cystic Fibrosis Clinic
Children's Hospital of Wisconsin
PO Box 1997   414-266-2000
Milwaukee, WI 53201-1997   877-266-8989
www.chw.org
Children's Hospital and Health System is an independent health care system dedicated solely to the health and well-being of children.
Robert Kliegman MD, Executive VP
Peter J Bartz, Cardiology Pediatric

3119 University of Wisconsin-Madison: Cystic Fibrosis/Pulmonary Center
Clinical Science Center
600 Highland Avenue   608-263-6400
Madison, WI 53792   800-323-8942
www.uwhealth.org
UW Health represents the academic medical care providers of the University of Wisconsin-Madison and its affiliated organizations.
Michael J Rock, Faculty
Prasad S Dalvie, Radiology

Support Groups & Hotlines

3120 National Health Information Center
PO Box 1133   310-565-4167
Washington, DC 20013-1133   800-336-4797
Fax: 301-984-4256
e-mail: info@nhic.org
www.health.gov/nhic
A health information referral service sponsored by the Office of Disease Prevention and Health Promotion. Puts health professionals and consumers who have health questions in touch with those organizations that are best able to provide answers.

Books

3121 Cystic Fibrosis: A Guide for Patient and Family
Raven Press
1185 Avenue of the Americas   212-930-9500
New York, NY 10036-2601   800-777-2295
253 pages Softcover
ISBN: 0-397516-53-3

3122 Understanding Cystic Fibrosis
Karen Hopkin, PhD, author
University Press of Mississippi
3825 Ridgewood Road   601-432-6205
Jackson, MS 39211-6492   Fax: 601-432-6217
e-mail: kburgess@ihl.state.ms.us
www.upress.state.ms.us
A useful guide for families and patients.
1998 128 pages Paperback
ISBN: 0-878059-67-9
Kathy Burgess, Advertising/Marketing Services Manager

Children's Books

3123 Give Me One Wish
Norton Publishers
500 5th Avenue   212-354-5500
New York, NY 10110-0002   800-233-4830
www.scholastic.com/
This book reads like a novel because it re-enacts the author's daughter's bout with cystic fibrosis.
Grades 10-12

3124 Robyn's Book: A True Diary
Scholastic
730 Broadway   212-505-3000
New York, NY 10003-9511   800-325-6149
This book chronicles the life of the author and her battle with cystic fibrosis.
Grades 7-12

3125 Toothpick
Holiday
40 E 49th Street   212-688-0085
New York, NY 10017-1105
This book uses relationships between two different teenagers to parallel the life of a person with cystic fibrosis.
Grades 6-9

Newsletters

3126 Better Breathing Bulletin
American Lung Association of Connecticut
45 Ash Street   860-289-5401
East Hartford, CT 06108-3294   800-586-4872
Fax: 860-289-5405
www.alact.org
This newsletter is aimed at persons with chronic lung problems.
John E Zinn, President/CEO

3127 Commitment
Cystic Fibrosis Foundation
6931 Arlington Road   301-951-4422
Bethesda, MD 20814-5231   800-344-4823
Fax: 301-951-6378
e-mail: info@cff.org
www.cff.org
Offers general information on cystic fibrosis, fund-raising features, public policy and news from across the nation on cystic fibrosis.

Pamphlets

3128 Consumer Fact Sheet
Cystic Fibrosis Foundation
6931 Arlington Road   301-951-4422
Bethesda, MD 20814-5231   800-344-4823
Fax: 301-951-6378
e-mail: info@cff.org
www.cff.org
Offers a brief introduction to cystic fibrosis, symptoms, causes, treatments and offers illustrations pertaining to drainage positions.

3129 Cystic Fibrosis: A Guide for Parents
American Lung Association

1740 Broadway
New York, NY 10019-4315 — 212-315-8700
Comprehensive booklet covering topics such as treatment, social aspects, inheritance, genetics and outlook for the future.
24 pages

3130 **For Adults with Cystic Fibrosis: Facts on Reproduction**
National Maternal and Child Health Clearinghouse
2070 Chain Bridge Road — 703-442-9051
Vienna, VA 22182-2588 — 888-275-4772
Fax: 703-821-2098
e-mail: ask@hrsa.gov
www.ask.hrsa.gov

The purpose of this booklet is to review the reproductive issues that are unique to individuals with cystic fibrosis.

3131 **Foundation Facts**
Cystic Fibrosis Foundation
6931 Arlington Road — 301-951-4422
Bethesda, MD 20814-5231 — 800-344-4823
Fax: 301-951-6378
e-mail: info@cff.org
www.cff.org

Offers information on the fund-raising and grants offered and supported by the foundation.

3132 **Here's Everything You'll Need to Save Money with the CFF Health Services**
CFF Home Health & Pharmacy Services
6931 Arlington Road
Bethesda, MD 20814-5223 — 800-342-6967
Fax: 800-233-3504

Offers information on the Cystic Fibrosis Foundation's home health services.

3133 **Home Line**
Cystic Fibrosis Foundation
6931 Arlington Road — 301-951-4422
Bethesda, MD 20814-5231 — 800-344-4823
Fax: 301-951-6378
e-mail: info@cff.org
www.cff.org

Offers information on services and programs offered by the foundation.

Audio & Video

3134 **Alex: The Life of a Child**
Cystic Fibrosis Foundation
6931 Arlington Road — 301-951-4422
Bethesda, MD 20814 — 800-344-4823
Fax: 301-951-6378
e-mail: info@cff.org
www.cff.org

The story of Alexandra Deford, a young girl who lost her battle with CF at the age of 8, has touched the hearts of millions and has helped to put a face to this disease. Alex's courage and strength is a true inspiration, and in the decades since her death, much progress has been made in the fight against CF. VHS only.
1986 1 Hr 35 Minutes
Robert J Beall, PhD, President/CEO

3135 **Embers of the Fire**
Mary Kondrat, author
Fanlight Productions
4196 Washington Street — 617-469-4999
Boston, MA 02131-1731 — 800-937-4113
Fax: 617-469-3379
e-mail: fanlight@fanlight.com
www.fanlight.com

Offers a straight forward explanation of the disease with a primary focus on the stories of several courageous young people with cystic fibrosis during a week at summer camp. Addresses their fears of rejection, isolation and death while demonstrating the ways they have learned to lead fulfilling lives.
1992 28 Minutes
ISBN: 1-572950-98-6

3136 **Expanding the Horizon of Hope: 50 Years of Progress**
Cystic Fibrosis Foundation
6931 Arlington Road — 301-951-4422
Bethesda, MD 20814 — 800-344-4823
Fax: 301-951-6378
e-mail: info@cff.org
www.cff.org

This film highlights the progress that has been made in CF research and care over the past 50 years, as well as the challenges that still lie ahead. It pays tribute to all who are involved in the CF effort—from researchers and clinicians, to patients and their families, to volunteers, donors and staff. DVD only.
2005 60 Minutes
Robert J Beall, PhD, President/CEO

3137 **Faces of Cystic Fibrosis**
Cystic Fibrosis Foundation
6931 Arlington Road — 301-951-4422
Bethesda, MD 20814 — 800-344-4823
Fax: 301-951-6378
e-mail: info@cff.org
www.cff.org

Through the words of people with CF and their family members, hear the story of how the fight against CF has evolved into a story of hope and optimism that was never possible before...and how none of this would be possible without the dedication and efforts of volunteers. Available in VHS/DVD.
2001 11 Minutes
Robert J Beall, PhD, President/CEO

3138 **Information About the Sweat Test**
Cystic Fibrosis Foundation
6931 Arlington Road — 301-951-4422
Bethesda, MD 20814 — 800-344-4823
Fax: 301-951-6378
e-mail: info@cff.org
www.cff.org

See and hear some basic information about the sweat test, the standard diagnostic test for CF. It is intended to help families better understand the sweat testing procedure and what to expect when the test is conducted. VHS only.
3.47 Minutes
Robert J Beall, PhD, President/CEO

Web Sites

3139 **Healing Well**
www.healingwell.com
An online health resource guide to medical news, chat, information and articles, newsgroups and message boards, books, disease-related web sites, medical directories, and more for patients, friends, and family coping with disabling diseases, disorders, or chronic illnesses.

3140 **Health Finder**
www.healthfinder.gov
Searchable, carefully developed web site offering information on over 1000 topics. Developed by the US Department of Health and Human Services, the site can be used in both English and Spanish.

3141 **Healthlink USA**
www.healthlinkusa.com
Health information concerning treatment, cures, prevention, diagnosis, risk factors, research, support groups, email lists, personal stories and much more. Updated regularly.

3142 **Helios Health**
www.helioshealth.com
Online resource for your health information. Detailed information about specific health topics, access to expert advice from our Medical Advisory Board, and up-to-date health news.

3143 **MedicineNet**
www.medicinenet.com
An online resource for consumers providing easy-to-read, authoritative medical and health information.

3144 **Medscape**
www.medscape.com

Medscape offers specialists, primary care physicians, and other health professionals the Web's most robust and integrated medical information and educational tools.

3145 WebMD

www.webmd.com

Provides links to over 45 articles involving cystic fibrosis.

Description

3146 # Diabetes Mellitus

Diabetes mellitus is a condition in which the body lacks enough insulin to control its own blood glucose (sugar) level. Ordinarily, the pancreas releases enough of this hormone to let the body's cells absorb and metabolize glucose. In Type I diabetes (formerly called juvenile-onset diabetes and affecting 10 percent of diabetic patients), the pancreas simply stops producing insulin. In Type II, commonly affecting overweight individuals older than 40, the pancreas might release normal, reduced, or even elevated levels of insulin, but the body's cells are resistant to the insulin's action. In either case, blood glucose levels rise (hyperglycemia) until the kidney starts to dump sugar into the urine. The patient may experience excessive thirst and urination, hunger, weakness and weight loss. In extreme cases, when there is either insufficient insulin or the body undergoes stress, or strenuous exercise, some components of the blood become seriously altered and the patient may lapse into a coma. Long-term complications include an increased risk of coronary heart disease and other vascular diseases, such as stroke, vision loss and kidney failure.

Type I appears to be caused by a genetic predisposition that may express itself after an acute insult, often a viral infection. Genetic factors are important in Type II diabetes which runs strongly in families. It is much more common in obese people, as well as among African-Americans, Hispanics and Native Americans.

Prevention of acute and long-term complications requires careful management including maintaining the proper diet and exercise, blood glucose monitoring and medications. Thorough education of the patient and relevant family members is absolutely critical.

Some individuals with Type II diabetes can control their disease through diet, exercise and weight loss alone. Some will have to take oral medication that helps the pancreas make more insulin or makes the body more sensitive to insulin. Some Type II diabetics, and all Type I diabetics, need to take insulin. Research has shown that tight control of diabetes through frequent blood testing and proper adjustment of the dosage of insulin is most beneficial. Insulin is generally given in multiple injections throughout the day, with preparations varying by length of effectiveness. Closest control of glucose levels is achieved by giving insulin through a continuously-connected insulin pump. Pancreas transplantation is considered only for patients who also need some other organ, generally a kidney.

National Agencies & Associations

3147 **American Association of Diabetes Educators**
200 W Madison Street
Chicago, IL 60606   800-338-3633
                                 e-mail: aade@aadenet.org
                                      www.aadenet.org

An independent multidisciplinary organization of health professionals involved in teaching persons with diabetes. The mission is to enhance the competence of health professionals who teach persons with diabetes and advance the specialty practice of diabetes.
Donna Tomky, President
Tami Ross, VP

3148 **American Diabetes Association**
1701 N Beauregard Street   804-225-8038
Alexandria, VA 22311   888-342-2383
                                  Fax: 804-225-8211
                           e-mail: askada@diabetes.org
                                      www.diabetes.org

The nation's leading voluntary organization concerned with diabetes and its complications. The mission of the organization is to prevent and cure diabetes and to improve the lives of persons with diabetes. Offers a network of offices nationwide.
Julie Heverly, Area Director
Larry Hausner, CEO

3149 **Diabetes Exercise and Sports Association**
310 West Liberty   502-581-0207
Louisville, KY 40202   800-898-4322
                                  Fax: 502-581-0206
                     e-mail: desa@diabetes-exercise.org
                              www.diabetes-exercise.org

Exists to enhance the quality of life for people with diabetes through exercise and physical fitness.
Paula Harper, Founder
Guy Hornsby PhD, Chair

3150 **Juvenile Diabetes Foundation: International**
26 Broadway
New York, NY 10004   800-533-2873
                                  Fax: 212-785-9595
                                e-mail: info@jdrf.org
                                         www.jdf.org

Focuses energies on fund-raising, referrals, educational materials and information pertaining to juvenile diabetes.
Jeffery Brewer, President

3151 **National Certification Board for Diabetes Educators**
330 E Algonquin Road   847-228-9795
Arlington Heights, IL 60005   877-239-3233
                                  Fax: 847-228-8469
                                e-mail: info@ncbde.org
                                        www.ncbde.org

The Board for Diabetes Educators is dedicated to promoting excellence in the field of diabetes education through the development maintenance and protection of the certified Diabetes Educator credential and the certification process.
Samuel Abbate, Chair
Lance Hoxie, Chief Executive Officer

3152 **National Diabetes Action Network for the Blind**
National Federation of the Blind
200 East Wells Street   410-659-9314
Baltimore, MD 21230   Fax: 410-685-5653
                                  e-mail: nfb@nfb.org
                                         www.nfb.org

Leading support and information organization of persons losing vision due to diabetes. Provides personal contact and resource information with other blind diabetics about non-visual techniques of independently managing diabetes and monitoring glucose levels.
Marc Maurer, President
Fredric Schroeder, First Vice President

3153 **National Institute of Diabetes, Digestive & Kidney Diseases**
National Institutes of Health
1 Information Way   301-496-4000
Bethesda, MD 20892-2560   800-860-8747
                                  Fax: 703-738-4929
                                   TTY: 866-569-1162
                          e-mail: NIHInfo@OD.NIH.GOV
                             www.diabetes.niddk.nih.gov

Conducts and supports research on many of the most serious diseases affecting public health. The Institute supports much of the

clinical research on the diseases of internal medicine and related subspecialty fields as well as many basic science disciplines.
Dr. Griffin Rodgers, Acting Director

State Agencies & Associations

Alabama

3154 American Diabetes Association: Alabama
3918 Montclair Road
Birmingham, AL 35213
205-870-5172
888-DIA-BETE
Fax: 205-879-2903
e-mail: acasey@diabetes.org
www.diabetes.org
Aimee Casey, Executive Director
Stephanie Willis, Director

3155 Juvenile Diabetes Research Foundation: Birmingham
14 Office Park Circle
Birmingham, AL 35223
205-871-0333
Fax: 205-871-0355
e-mail: alabama@jdf.org
www.jdrf.org/alabama
Karin Scott, Executive Director
Sarah Hendren, Special Events Manager

Alaska

3156 American Diabetes Association: Alaska
801 W Fireweed Lane
Anchorage, AK 99503
907-272-1424
888-DIA-BETE
Fax: 907-272-1428
e-mail: mcassano@diabetes.org
www.diabetes.org
Michelle Cassano, Executive Director
Phoebe O'Connell, Manager

Arizona

3157 American Diabetes Association: Arizona
8125 N 23rd Avenue
Phoenix, AZ 85021
602-861-4731
Fax: 602-995-1344
www.diabetes.org

3158 American Diabetes Association: Arizona, Border Area
333 W Ft Lowell Rd
Tucson, AZ 85705
520-795-3711
888-DIA-BETE
Fax: 520-795-1179
e-mail: fgomez@diabetes.org
www.diabetes.org
Fred Gomez, Executive Director
Heidi Goldsmith, Manager

3159 American Diabetes Association: Atlanta Met
8125 N 23rd Avenue
Phoenix, AZ 85021
602-861-4731
Fax: 602-995-1344
e-mail: kbisko@diabetes.org
www.diabetes.org
Karen Bisko, Executive Director
Suzanne Miller, Director

3160 American Diabetes Association: Northern Arizona
5333 N 7th Street
Phoenix, AZ 85014
602-861-4731
Fax: 602-995-1344
e-mail: llandon@diabetes.org
www.diabetes.org
Laura Landon, Executive Director
Suzanne Miller, Programs Director

3161 Juvenile Diabetes Research Foundation: Phoenix Chapter
4343 E Camelback Road
Phoenix, AZ 85018
602-224-1800
Fax: 602-224-1801
e-mail: desertsouthwest@jdrf.org
www.jdrf.org/arizona
Marci Zimmerman, Executive Director
Valerie Jones, Associate Executive Director

Arkansas

3162 American Diabetes Association: Arkansas
320 Executive Court
Little Rock, AR 72205
501-221-7444
888-DIA-BETE
Fax: 501-221-3138
e-mail: rselig@diabetes.org
www.diabetes.org
Rick Selig, Director
Charlotte Williams, Associate Manager

3163 Juvenile Diabetes Research Foundation: Northwest Arkansas Branch
440 N College Avenue
Fayetteville, AR 72701
479-443-9190
Fax: 479-443-2692
e-mail: nwarkansas@jdrf.org
www.jdrf.org/nwark
Deb Euculano, Special Events Manager

California

3164 American Diabetes Association: California
2720 Gateway Oaks Drive
Sacramento, CA 95833
916-924-3232
888-DIA-BETE
Fax: 916-924-0529
e-mail: AskADA@diabetes.org
www.diabetes.org/
The American Diabetes Association is a nonprofit health organization providing diabetes research, information and advocacy. Founded in 1940, the American Diabetes Association conducts programs in all 50 states and the District of Columbia.
Michael D Farley CFRE, Chief Community Relations Officer
Richard Kahn PhD, Chief Scientific/Medical Officer

3165 Diabetes Society of Santa Clara Valley
4040 Moorpark Avenue
San Jose, CA 95117
408-241-1922
888-DIA-BETE
Fax: 408-241-1972
e-mail: Info@thediabetessociety.org
www.diabetes.org
The Diabetes Society is dedicated to providing education and information to those who have diabetes educating the general public about the seriousness of this disease, and supporting research aimed at preventing complications and finding a cure.
Douglas Metz DPM/MPH, Executive Director
Thomas Smith, Program/Camp Director

3166 Juvenile Diabetes Research Foundation: Bakersfield Chapter
712 19th Street
Bakersfield, CA 93301
661-636-1305
Fax: 661-636-1307
e-mail: Bakersfield@jdrf.org
www.jdrf-bakersfield.org
The Juvenile Diabetes Research Foundation International (JDRF) is a charitable funder and advocate of type 1 (juvenile) diabetes research worldwide. The mission of JDRF is to find a cure for diabetes and its complications through the support of research.
Allison Perkins Thomas, Bakersfield Branch Manager
Arnold Donald, President/CEO Corporate Office (NY)

3167 Juvenile Diabetes Research Foundation: Gre ater Bay Area Chapter
49 Stevenson Street
San Francisco, CA 94105
415-977-0360
Fax: 415-977-0355
e-mail: greaterbay@jdf.org
www.jdrf.org/greaterbay
The Juvenile Diabetes Research Foundation International (JDRF) is a charitable funder and advocate of type 1 (juvenile) diabetes research worldwide. The mission of JDRF is to find a cure for diabetes and its complications through the support of research.
Vicki Weiland, Executive Director
Mavie Mendelson, Special Events Director

3168 Juvenile Diabetes Research Foundation: Inl and Empire Chapter
1001 East Cooley Drive
Colton, CA 92324
909-424-0100
Fax: 909-424-0044
e-mail: inlandempire@jdrf.org
www.jdrf.org/index.cfm?page_id=100614
The Juvenile Diabetes Research Foundation International (JDRF) is a charitable funder and advocate of type 1 (juvenile) diabetes re-

search worldwide. The mission of JDRF is to find a cure for diabetes and its complications through the support of research.
Jamie Brunelle, Board of Directors
Evelyn Edinin, Board of Directors

3169 Juvenile Diabetes Research Foundation: Los Angeles Chapter
800 West Sixth Street   213-233-9901
Los Angeles, CA 90017   Fax: 213-622-6276
e-mail: losangeles@jdrf.org
www.jdrf.org/losangeles
The Juvenile Diabetes Research Foundation International (JDRF) is a charitable funder and advocate of type 1 (juvenile) diabetes research worldwide. The mission of JDRF is to find a cure for diabetes and its complications through the support of research.
Mark Rieck, Executive Director
Dennis Ellman Esq, Board of Directors President

3170 Juvenile Diabetes Research Foundation: Nor thern California Inland Chapter
1329 Howe Avenue   916-920-0790
Sacramento, CA 95825   Fax: 916-920-0367
e-mail: northernca@jdrf.org
www.jdrf.org/norcal
The Juvenile Diabetes Research Foundation International (JDRF) is a charitable funder and advocate of type 1 (juvenile) diabetes research worldwide. The mission of JDRF is to find a cure for diabetes and its complications through the support of research.
Victoria Webster, Executive Director
Molly Atkinson, Special Events Coordinator

3171 Juvenile Diabetes Research Foundation: Ora nge County Chapter
17872 Mitchell North   949-553-0363
Irvine, CA 92614   Fax: 949-553-8813
e-mail: orangecounty@jdrf.org
www.jdf.org/chapters/CA/Orange-County
The Juvenile Diabetes Research Foundation International (JDRF) is a charitable funder and advocate of type 1 (juvenile) diabetes research worldwide. The mission of JDRF is to find a cure for diabetes and its complications through the support of research.
Louise Cummings, Executive Director
Jennifer Walker, Special Events Manager

3172 Juvenile Diabetes Research Foundation: San Diego Chapter
5677 Oberlin Drive   858-597-0240
San Diego, CA 92121   Fax: 858-597-2072
e-mail: sandiego@jdrf.org
www.jdrf-sandiego-news.org
The Juvenile Diabetes Research Foundation International (JDRF) is a charitable funder and advocate of type 1 (juvenile) diabetes research worldwide. The mission of JDRF is to find a cure for diabetes and its complications through the support of research.
Linda Riley, Executive Director
Katherine Griswold, Special Events Manager

Colorado

3173 American Diabetes Association: Denver
2480 W 26th Avenue   720-855-1102
Denver, CO 80211   Fax: 720-855-1302
e-mail: AskADA@diabetes.org
www.diabetes.org/
The American Diabetes Association is a nonprofit health organization providing diabetes research, information and advocacy. Founded in 1940 the American Diabetes Association conducts programs in all 50 states and the District of Columbia.
Michael D Farley CFRE, Chief Community Relations Officer
Richard Kahn PhD, Chief Scientific/Medical Officer

3174 Juvenile Diabetes Research Foundation: Colorado Springs Chapter
3710 Sinton Road   719-633-8110
Colorado Springs, CO 80907   Fax: 719-633-8155
e-mail: lpage@jdrf.org
www.jdrfcoloradosprings.org
The Juvenile Diabetes Research Foundation International (JDRF) is a charitable funder and advocate of type 1 (juvenile) diabetes re-

search worldwide. The mission of JDRF is to find a cure for diabetes and its complications through the support of research.
Lynn Page, Branch Manager
Andi Chernushin, President

3175 Juvenile Diabetes Research Foundation: Roc ky Mountain Chapter
5613 DTC Parkway   303-779-0525
Greenwood Village, CO 80111   Fax: 303-720-1630
e-mail: RockyMountain@jdrf.org
www.jdrf.org/rockymountain
The Juvenile Diabetes Research Foundation International (JDRF) is a charitable funder and advocate of type 1 (juvenile) diabetes research worldwide. The mission of JDRF is to find a cure for diabetes and its complications through the support of research.
James Buckles, Executive Director
Nancy L Walters, Special Events Director

Connecticut

3176 American Diabetes Association: Connecticut
306 Industrial Park Road   203-639-0385
Middletown, CT 06457   888-DIA-BETE
Fax: 860-632-5098
e-mail: AskADA@diabetes.org
www.diabetes.org
The American Diabetes Association is a nonprofit health organization providing diabetes research, information and advocacy. Founded in 1940 the American Diabetes Association conducts programs in all 50 states and the District of Columbia.
Michael D Farley CRFE (Corpora, Chief Community Relations Officer
Richard Kahn PhD, Chief Scientific/Medical Officer

3177 Juvenile Diabetes Research Foundation: Greater New Haven Chapter
2969 Whitney Avenue   203-248-1880
Hamden, CT 06518   Fax: 203-248-1820
e-mail: newhaven@jdf.org
www.jdrf.org/greaternewhaven
The Juvenile Diabetes Research Foundation International (JDRF) is a charitable funder and advocate of type 1 (juvenile) diabetes research worldwide. The mission of JDRF is to find a cure for diabetes and its complications through the support of research.
Mary K Kessler, Executive Director
Will Martinez, Board of Directors President

3178 Juvenile Diabetes Research Foundation: Fai rfield County Chapter
200 Connecticut Avenue   203-854-0658
Norwalk, CT 06854   Fax: 203-854-0798
e-mail: fairfield@jdrf.org
www.jdrf.org/fairfieldcounty
The Juvenile Diabetes Research Foundation International (JDRF) is a charitable funder and advocate of type 1 (juvenile) diabetes research worldwide. The mission of JDRF is to find a cure for diabetes and its complications through the support of research.
Barbara Rose, Executive Director
Michelle Tighe, Special Events Coordinator

3179 Juvenile Diabetes Research Foundation: Nor th Central CT and Western MA
18 North Main Street   860-561-1153
West Hartford, CT 06107   Fax: 860-561-3440
e-mail: northcentralct@jdrf.org
www.jdrf.org/index.cfm?page_id=100619
The Juvenile Diabetes Research Foundation International (JDRF) is a charitable funder and advocate of type 1 (juvenile) diabetes research worldwide. The mission of JDRF is to find a cure for diabetes and its complications through the support of research.
Mary Ann Slomski, Executive Director
Ellen Kellie, Special Events Coordinator

Delaware

3180 American Diabetes Association: Delaware
100 W 10th Street   302-656-0030
Wilmington, DE 19801   888-342-2383
                                            Fax: 302-656-7331
                                    e-mail: AskADA@diabetes.org
                                               www.diabetes.org
The American Diabetes Association is a nonprofit health organization providing diabetes research, information and advocacy. Founded in 1940 the American Diabetes Association conducts programs in all 50 states and the District of Columbia.
Michael D Farley CFRE (Corpora, Chief Community Relations Officer
Richard Kahn PhD, Chief Scientific/Medical Officer

3181 Juvenile Diabetes Research Foundation: Del aware
100 West 10th Street   302-888-1117
Wilmington, DE 19801   Fax: 302-888-1878
                                      e-mail: delaware@jdrf.org
                                             www.jdrf.org/delaware
The Juvenile Diabetes Research Foundation International (JDRF) is a charitable funder and advocate of type 1 (juvenile) diabetes research worldwide. The mission of JDRF is to find a cure for diabetes and its complications through the support of research.
Ellen Rubesin, Executive Director
Stephanie Bucksner, Special Events Coordinator

District of Columbia

3182 American Diabetes Association: District of Columbia
1025 Connecticut Avenue NW   202-331-8303
Washington, DC 20036   888-342-2383
                                            Fax: 202-331-1402
                                    e-mail: AskADA@diabetes.org
                                               www.diabetes.org
The American Diabetes Association is a nonprofit health organization providing diabetes research, information and advocacy. Founded in 1940 the American Diabetes Association conducts programs in all 50 states and the District of Columbia.
Michael D Farley CFRE (Corpora, Chief Community Relations Officer
Richard Kahn PhD, Chief Scientific/Medical Officer

3183 Juvenile Diabetes Research Foundation: Cap itol Chapter
1400 K Street NW   202-371-0044
Washington, DC 20005   Fax: 202-371-0046
                                      e-mail: capitol@jdrf.org
                                             www.jdrfcapitol.org
The Juvenile Diabetes Research Foundation International (JDRF) is a charitable funder and advocate of type 1 (juvenile) diabetes research worldwide. The mission of JDRF is to find a cure for diabetes and its complications through the support of research.
Pam Gatz, Executive Director
Carrie Hamilton, Special Events Director

Florida

3184 American Diabetes Association: Northeast F lorida/Southeast Georgia
8384 Baymeadows Road   904-730-7200
Jacksonville, FL 32256   888-342-2383
                                            Fax: 940-730-7933
                                    e-mail: AskADA@diabetes.org
                                               www.diabetes.org
The American Diabetes Association is a nonprofit health organization providing diabetes research, information and advocacy. Founded in 1940 the American Diabetes Association conducts programs in all 50 states and the District of Columbia.
Sheri Criswell, Executive Director
Richard Kahn PhD, Chief Scientific/Medical Officer

3185 American Diabetes Association: Seattle
1101 N Lake Destiny Road   407-660-1926
Maitland, FL 32751   Fax: 407-660-1080
                                    e-mail: AskADA@diabetes.org
                                               www.diabetes.org
The American Diabetes Association is a nonprofit health organization providing diabetes research, information and advocacy.

Founded in 1940 the American Diabetes Association conducts programs in all 50 states and the District of Columbia.
Pauline Lowe, Executive Director
Richard Kahn PhD, Chief Scientific/Medical Officer

3186 American Diabetes Association: South Coast Regional/Central Florida
1101 North Lake Destiny Road   407-660-1926
Maitland, FL 32751   888-342-2383
                                            Fax: 407-660-1080
                                    e-mail: AskADA@diabetes.org
                                               www.diabetes.org
The American Diabetes Association is a nonprofit health organization providing diabetes research, information and advocacy. Founded in 1940, the American Diabetes Association conducts programs in all 50 states and the District of Columbia, reaching hundreds of communities.
Michael D Farley CFRE (Corporate), Chief Community Relations Officer
Richard Kahn Ph.D (Corporate), Chief Scientific/Medical Officer

3187 Juvenile Diabetes Research Foundation: Cen tral Florida Chapter
279 Douglas Avenue   407-774-2166
Altamonte Springs, FL 32714   Fax: 407-774-2168
                                    e-mail: centralflorida@jdrf.org
                                          www.jdrf.org/centralflorida
The Juvenile Diabetes Research Foundation International (JDRF) is a charitable funder and advocate of type 1 (juvenile) diabetes research worldwide. The mission of JDRF is to find a cure for diabetes and its complications through the support of research.
Kendra Presley, Special Events Manager
Gwen Bell, Office Manager

3188 Juvenile Diabetes Research Foundation: Flo rida Sun Coast Chapter
3333 Clark Road   941-929-0621
Sarasota, FL 34231   Fax: 941-929-0602
                                    e-mail: floridasuncoast@jdrf.org
                                             www.jdrf.org/index.cfm
The Juvenile Diabetes Research Foundation International (JDRF) is a charitable funder and advocate of type 1 (juvenile) diabetes research worldwide. The mission of JDRF is to find a cure for diabetes and its complications through the support of research.
Sara Rankin, Executive Director
Jeannie Kawcak, Special Events Coordinator

3189 Juvenile Diabetes Research Foundation: Gre ater Palm Beach County Chapter
1450 Centrepark Boulevard   561-686-7701
West Palm Beach, FL 33401   Fax: 561-686-7702
                                    e-mail: greaterpalmbeach@jdrf.org
                                          www.jdrf.org/greaterpalmbeach
The Juvenile Diabetes Research Foundation International (JDRF) is a charitable funder and advocate of type 1 (juvenile) diabetes research worldwide. The mission of JDRF is to find a cure for diabetes and its complications through the support of research.
Lora Hazelwood, Executive Director
Esther Swann, Special Events Coordinator

3190 Juvenile Diabetes Research Foundation: Nor th Florida Chapter
8400 Baymeadows Way   904-739-2101
Jacksonville, FL 32256   Fax: 904-739-2693
                                    e-mail: northflorida@jdrf.org
                                          www.jdrf.org/northflorida
The Juvenile Diabetes Research Foundation International (JDRF) is a charitable funder and advocate of type 1 (juvenile) diabetes research worldwide. The mission of JDRF is to find a cure for diabetes and its complications through the support of research.
Brooks Biagini, Executive Director
Wendy Smit, Special Events Assistant

3191 Juvenile Diabetes Research Foundation: Sou th Florida Chapter
3411 NW 9th Avenue   954-565-4775
Fort Lauderdale, FL 33309   Fax: 954-565-4767
                                    e-mail: southflorida@jdrf.org
                                    www.jdrf.org/chapters/FL/South-Florida
The Juvenile Diabetes Research Foundation International (JDRF) is a charitable funder and advocate of type 1 (juvenile) diabetes re-

search worldwide. The mission of JDRF is to find a cure for diabetes and its complications through the support of research.
Ingrid Velarde, Special Events Coordinator
Katelyn Tolzien, Special Events Coordinator

3192   Juvenile Diabetes Research Foundation: Tam pa Bay Chapter
5959 Central Avenue   727-344-2873
Saint Petersburg, FL 33710   Fax: 727-384-9009
                                       e-mail: tampabay@jdrf.org
                                       www.jdf.org
The Juvenile Diabetes Research Foundation International (JDRF) is a charitable funder and advocate of type 1 (juvenile) diabetes research worldwide. The mission of JDRF is to find a cure for diabetes and its complications through the support of research.
Arnold Donald, President/CEO Corporate Office
Robin Harding, EVP Development & COO

Georgia

3193   American Diabetes Association: Atlanta Met ro
17 Executive Park   404-320-7100
Atlanta, GA 30329   888-342-2383
                                       Fax: 404-320-0025
                                       e-mail: AskADA@diabetes.org
                                       www.diabetes.org
The American Diabetes Association is a nonprofit health organization providing diabetes research, information and advocacy. Founded in 1940 the American Diabetes Association conducts programs in all 50 states and the District of Columbia, reaching hundreds of communities
Michael Gault, Senior Executive Director
Richard Kahn PhD, Chief Scientific/Medical Officer

3194   American Diabetes Association: Savannah
5105 Paulsen Street   912-353-8110
Savannah, GA 31405   888-343-2383
                                       Fax: 912-353-9114
                                       e-mail: AskADA@diabetes.org
                                       www.diabetes.org
The American Diabetes Association is a nonprofit health organization providing diabetes research, information and advocacy. Founded in 1940 the American Diabetes Association conducts programs in all 50 states and the District of Columbia.
Maria Center, Director
Richard Kahn PhD, Chief Scientific/Medical Officer

3195   Juvenile Diabetes Research Foundation: Geo rgia Chapter
400 Perimeter Center Terrace   404-420-5990
Atlanta, GA 30346   Fax: 404-420-5995
                                       e-mail: georgia@jdrf.org
                                       www.jdrfgeorgia.org/
The Juvenile Diabetes Research Foundation International (JDRF) is a charitable funder and advocate of type 1 (juvenile) diabetes research worldwide. The mission of JDRF is to find a cure for diabetes and its complications through the support of research.
Rob Shaw, Executive Director
Scott Whiteside, EVP/General Manager

Hawaii

3196   American Diabetes Association: Hawaii
1500 S Beretania Street   808-947-5979
Honolulu, HI 96826   888-342-2383
                                       Fax: 808-947-5978
                                       e-mail: AskADA@diabetes.org
                                       www.diabetes.org
The American Diabetes Association is a nonprofit health organization providing diabetes research, information and advocacy. Founded in 1940 the American Diabetes Association conducts programs in all 50 states and the District of Columbia.
Majken Mechling, Executive Director
Richard Kahn PhD, Chief Scientific/Medical Officer

3197   Juvenile Diabetes Research Foundation: Haw aii Chapter
1019 Waimanu Street   808-988-1000
Honolulu, HI 96814   Fax: 808-597-8758
                                       e-mail: hawaii@jdrf.org
                                       www.jdf.org
The Juvenile Diabetes Research Foundation International (JDRF) is a charitable funder and advocate of type 1 (juvenile) diabetes re-

search worldwide. The mission of JDRF is to find a cure for diabetes and its complications through the support of research.
Arnold Donald, President/CEO Corporate
Robin Harding, EVP/Develpment & COO Corporate

Illinois

3198   American Diabetes Association: Greater Ill inois
2580 Federal Drive   217-875-9011
Decatur, IL 62526   888-342-2383
                                       Fax: 217-875-6849
                                       e-mail: AskADA@diabetes.org
                                       www.diabetes.org
The American Diabetes Association is a nonprofit health organization providing diabetes research, information and advocacy. Founded in 1940 the American Diabetes Association conducts programs in all 50 states and the District of Columbia, reaching hundreds of communities.
Donna Scott, Executive Director
Richard Kahn PhD, Chief Scientific/Medical Officer

3199   American Diabetes Association: Northern Il linois
30 North Michigan Avenue   312-346-1805
Chicago, IL 60602   888-343-2383
                                       Fax: 312-346-5342
                                       e-mail: AskADA@diabetes.org
                                       www.diabetes.org
The American Diabetes Association is a nonprofit health organization providing diabetes research, information and advocacy. Founded in 1940, the American Diabetes Association conducts programs in all 50 states and the District of Columbia, reaching hundreds of communities.
Michael D Farley CFRE (Corporate), Chief Community Relations Officer
Richard Kahn Ph.D (Corporate), Chief Scientific/Medical Officer

3200   Juvenile Diabetes Research Foundation: Gre ater Chicago Chapter
500 North Dearborn Street   312-670-0313
Chicago, IL 60610   Fax: 312-670-0250
                                       e-mail: illinois@jdrf.org
                                       www.jdrfillinois.org
The Juvenile Diabetes Research Foundation International (JDRF) is a charitable funder and advocate of type 1 (juvenile) diabetes research worldwide. The mission of JDRF is to find a cure for diabetes and its complications through the support of research.
Amy Franze, Executive Director
Janine Tobola, Director Office Operations

Indiana

3201   American Diabetes Association: Northern In diana/Northern Ohio
6415 Castleway W Drive   317-352-9226
Indianapolis, IN 46250   888-342-2383
                                       Fax: 317-594-0748
                                       e-mail: AskADA@diabetes.org
                                       www.diabetes.org
The American Diabetes Association is a nonprofit health organization providing diabetes research, information and advocacy. Founded in 1940 the American Diabetes Association conducts programs in all 50 states and the District of Columbia.
Jennifer Pferrer, Executive Director
Richard Kahn PhD, Chief Scientific/Medical Officer

3202   Diabetes Youth Foundation of Indiana
7311 Tousley Drive   317-750-9310
Indianapolis, IN 46256-9212   Fax: 317-243-4418
                                       e-mail: dyfjulie@yahoo.com
                                       www.dyfofindiana.org
This nonprofit group whose mission is to improve the lives of children with diabetes and their families.
Julie Shutt, Executive Director
Rick Crosslin, Camp Director

3203   Juvenile Diabetes Research Foundation: Ind iana State Chapter
8465 Keystone Crossing   317-202-0352
Indianapolis, IN 46240   Fax: 317-202-0357
                                       e-mail: indianastate@jdrf.org
                                       www.jdrf.org/indiana

The Juvenile Diabetes Research Foundation International (JDRF) is a charitable funder and advocate of type 1 (juvenile) diabetes research worldwide. The mission of JDRF is to find a cure for diabetes and its complications through the support of research.
Henry Rodriguez MD, Chapter President

3204 Juvenile Diabetes Research Foundation: Nor thern Indiana Chapter
2004 Ironwood Circle 574-273-1810
South Bend, IN 46635 Fax: 574-273-1870
e-mail: northernindiana@jdrf.org
www.jdrf.org
The Juvenile Diabetes Research Foundation International (JDRF) is a charitable funder and advocate of type 1 (juvenile) diabetes research worldwide. The mission of JDRF is to find a cure for diabetes and its complications through the support of research.
Arnold Donald, President/CEO Corporate
Robin Harding, EVP/Development & COO Corporate

Iowa

3205 American Diabetes Association: Cedar Rapid s District
St Luke's Resource Center 319-247-5124
Cedar Rapids, IA 52406 888-342-2383
Fax: 319-247-5125
e-mail: AskADA@diabetes.org
www.diabetes.org
The American Diabetes Association is a nonprofit health organization providing diabetes research, information and advocacy. Founded in 1940 the American Diabetes Association conducts programs in all 50 states and the District of Columbia.
Jennifer Petsche, Manager
Richard Kahn PhD, Chief Scientific/Medical Officer

3206 Juvenile Diabetes Research Foundation: Eas tern Iowa Chapter
701 10th Street SE 319-393-3850
Cedar Rapids, IA 52403 Fax: 319-393-3852
e-mail: easterniowa@jdrf.org
www.jdrf.org/easterniowa
The Juvenile Diabetes Research Foundation International (JDRF) is a charitable funder and advocate of type 1 (juvenile) diabetes research worldwide. The mission of JDRF is to find a cure for diabetes and its complications through the support of research.
Ann Elise Walsh, Special Events Manager
Mary Henry, Special Events Coordinator

3207 Juvenile Diabetes Research Foundation: Gre ater Iowa Chapter
5444 NW 96th Street 515-986-1512
Johnston, IA 50131 Fax: 515-986-1513
e-mail: greateriowa@jdif.org
www.jdrf.org/greateriowa
The Juvenile Diabetes Research Foundation International (JDRF) is a charitable funder and advocate of type 1 (juvenile) diabetes research worldwide. The mission of JDRF is to find a cure for diabetes and its complications through the support of research.
Jean Howieson, Special Events Director
Judy Greaves, Office Administrator

Kansas

3208 American Diabetes Association: Kansas
837 S Hillside 316-684-6091
Wichita, KS 67211 888-342-2383
Fax: 316-684-5675
e-mail: AskADA@diabetes.org
www.diabetes.org
The American Diabetes Association is a nonprofit health organization providing diabetes research, information and advocacy. Founded in 1940 the American Diabetes Association conducts programs in all 50 states and the District of Columbia.
Sarah Beth Webb, Director
Richard Kahn PhD, Chief Scientific/Medical Officer

Kentucky

3209 American Diabetes Association: Kentucky
161 St Matthews Avenue 502-452-6072
Louisville, KY 40207 888-342-2383
Fax: 502-893-2698
e-mail: AskADA@diabetes.org
www.diabetes.org
The American Diabetes Association is a nonprofit health organization providing diabetes research, information and advocacy. Founded in 1940 the American Diabetes Association conducts programs in all 50 states and the District of Columbia.
Samantha Carroll, Associate Director
Richard Kahn PhD, Chief Scientific/Medical Officer

3210 Juvenile Diabetes Research Foundation: Kentuckiana Chapter
133 Evergreen Road 502-485-9397
Louisville, KY 40243 866-485-9397
Fax: 502-485-9591
e-mail: kentuckiana@jdrf.org
www.jdf.org/chapters/ky/kentuckiana
The Juvenile Diabetes Research Foundation International (JDRF) is a charitable funder and advocate of type 1 (juvenile) diabetes research worldwide. The mission of JDRF is to find a cure for diabetes and its complications through the support of research.
Twynette S Davidson, Executive Director
Joe Salvagne, Chapter President

Louisiana

3211 American Diabetes Association: Louisana
2644 S Sherwood Forest Boulevard 225-216-3980
Baton Rouge, LA 70816 888-342-2383
Fax: 225-295-7005
e-mail: AskADA@diabetes.org
www.diabetes.org
Paige Grogan, Associate Manager
Lori Koonce, Associate Manager

3212 Juvenile Diabetes Research Foundation: Bat on Rouge Chapter
9457 Brookline Avenue 225-932-9511
Baton Rouge, LA 70809 Fax: 225-932-9514
e-mail: batonrouge@jdrf.org
www.jdrf.org/batonrouge
Kristy Andries, President/Development Chair
Danielle Graham, Special Events Assistant

3213 Juvenile Diabetes Research Foundation: Lou isiana Chapter
2201 Veterans Memorial Bouelvard 504-828-2873
Metairie, LA 70002 Fax: 504-828-4922
e-mail: louisiana@jdrf.org
www.jdrf.org/louisiana
Sam Robinson, President Board of Directors
Becky Spinnato, Vice President Fundraising

3214 Juvenile Diabetes Research Foundation: Shr eveport Chapter
2001 East 70th Street 318-798-1195
Shreveport, LA 71105 Fax: 318-798-1194
e-mail: jburns@jdrf.org
www.jdrf.org/shreveport
Jeff Knutson, President Board of Directors
Craig Floyd, Vice President Fundraising

Maine

3215 American Diabetes Association: Maine
80 Elm Street 207-774-7717
Portland, ME 04101 888-342-2383
Fax: 207-774-7714
e-mail: AskADA@diabetes.org
www.diabetes.org
Emily Silevinac, Associate Manager
Ryan Williams, Associate Manager

3216 Juvenile Diabetes Research Foundation: New England/Maine Chapter
33 Silver Street   207-761-0133
Portland, ME 04101   Fax: 207-761-1687
e-mail: maine@jdrf.org OR eburgo@jdrf.org
www.jdrf.org/maine
Heidi Daniels, New England Chapter Executive Director
Emily Hampton Burgo, Branch Manager

Maryland

3217 American Diabetes Association: Maryland
800 Wyman Park Drive   410-265-0075
Baltimore, MD 21211   888-342-2383
Fax: 410-235-4048
e-mail: AskADA@diabetes.org
www.diabetes.org
Kathy Rogers, Executive Director
Dotty Raynor, Director

3218 Juvenile Diabetes Research Foundation: Maryland Chapter
200 East Joppa Road   410-823-0073
Towson, MD 21286   Fax: 410-823-0416
e-mail: maryland@jdrf.com
www.jdrf.org/maryland/
Rebecca Maude, Executive Director
Dotty Raynor, Outreach Manager

Massachusetts

3219 American Diabetes Association: Boston
330 Congress Street   617-482-4580
Boston, MA 02210   888-342-2383
Fax: 617-482-1824
e-mail: AskADA@diabetes.org
www.diabetes.org
Christopher Boynton, Executive Director
Lori Glowacki, Director of Special Events

3220 Juvenile Diabetes Research Foundation: New England/Bay State Chapter
20 Walnut Street   781-431-0700
Wellesley, MA 02481   Fax: 781-431-8836
e-mail: baystate@jdrf.org
www.jdrf.org/baystate
Heidi Daniels, New England Chapter Executive Director
Virginia Irving, Associate Executive Director

Michigan

3221 American Diabetes Association: Michigan
3940 Broadmoor Avenue SE   616-458-9341
Grand Rapids, MI 49512   888-342-2383
Fax: 616-575-9930
e-mail: AskADA@diabetes.org
www.diabetes.org
Darla Hill, Coordinator
Sharice Purman, Director

3222 Juvenile Diabetes Research Foundation: Metropolitan Detroit/SE Michigan
24359 Northwestern Highway   248-355-1133
Southfield, MI 48075-2020   Fax: 248-355-1188
e-mail: metrodetroit@jdrf.org
www.jdrfdetroit.org
Rita L Combest, Development Director
Susan Kossik, Development Manager

3223 Juvenile Diabetes Research Foundation: West Michigan Chapter
5075 Cascade Road SE   616-957-1838
Grand Rapids, MI 49546   Fax: 616-957-1169
e-mail: westmichigan@jrdf.org
www.jdrf.org/westmichigan
Annette Guilfoyle, Executive Director
Maxine Gray, Special Events Coordinator

Minnesota

3224 American Diabetes Association: Minnesota
Parkdale Center   763-593-5333
Saint Louis Park, MN 55416   888-342-2383
Fax: 952-582-9000
e-mail: AskADA@diabetes.org
www.diabetes.org
Jenni Hargraves, Executive Director
Becky Barnett, Associate Manager

3225 Juvenile Diabetes Research Foundation: Minnesota Chapter
2626 East 82nd Street   952-851-0770
Bloomington, MN 55425   800-663-1860
Fax: 952-851-0766
e-mail: minnesota@jdrf.org
www.jdrf.org/minnesota
Jackie Casey, Executive Director
Angie McCarthy, Special Events Manager

Mississippi

3226 American Diabetes Association: Mississippi
16 Northtown Drive   601-932-1118
Jackson, MS 39211   888-342-2383
Fax: 601-932-1988
e-mail: AskADA@diabetes.org
www.diabetes.org

The nation's leading voluntary health organization providing diabetes research, information and advocacy. Our mission is to prevent and cure diabetes and to improve the lives of all people affected by diabetes.
Mary D Fortune, Executive Vice President
Stephanie J Coghlan MBA, Senior Regional Director

Missouri

3227 American Diabetes Association: Missouri
1944-A Sunshine   417-890-8400
Springfield, MO 65804   888-342-2383
Fax: 417-890-8484
e-mail: AskADA@diabetes.org
www.diabetes.org
Renee Paulsell, Executive Director
Jennifer Cotner-Jone, Associate Director

3228 Juvenile Diabetes Research Foundation: St. Louis Chapter
225 S Meramec Avenue   314-726-6778
Clayton, MO 63105   Fax: 314-726-6778
e-mail: metrostlouis@jdrf.org
www.jdrfstl.org
M Marie Davis, Executive Director
William Schmitt, Corporate Development

Montana

3229 American Diabetes Association: Montana
3203 3rd Avenue N   406-256-0616
Billings, MT 59101   888-342-2383
Fax: 406-896-0289
e-mail: AskADA@diabetes.org
www.diabetes.org
Trina Adams, Associate Manager

Nebraska

3230 American Diabetes Association: Nebraska
14216 Dayton Circle   402-571-1101
Omaha, NE 68137   888-342-2383
Fax: 402-572-8141
e-mail: AskADA@diabetes.org
www.diabetes.org
Shawn Murphy, Executive Director
Kortney Krill, Associate Manager

3231 Juvenile Diabetes Research Foundation: Lin coln Chapter
1540 S 70th Street
Lincoln, NE 68506 402-484-8300
Fax: 402-484-8302
e-mail: lincoln@jdrf.org
www.jdrf.org/lincoln

Deb Gokie, Executive Director
Maggie Pavelka, Special Events Assistant

3232 Juvenile Diabetes Research Foundation: Oma ha Council Bluffs Chapter
9202 W Dodge Road
Omaha, NE 68114 402-397-2873
Fax: 402-572-3343
e-mail: omaha@jdrf.org
www.jdrf.org/omaha

Shawn Reynolds, Executive Director
Melissa Shapiro, Special Events Coordinator

Nevada

3233 American Diabetes Association: Nevada
2785 E Desert Inn Road
Las Vegas, NV 89121 702-369-9995
888-342-2383
Fax: 702-369-3717
e-mail: AskADA@diabetes.org
www.diabetes.org

Mary Stokes, Manager
Carly Rohrer, Associate Manager

3234 Juvenile Diabetes Research Foundation: Nevada Chapter
5542 S Fort Apache Road
Las Vegas, NV 89148 702-732-4795
Fax: 702-732-1635
e-mail: nevada@jdf.org
www.jdrf.org/nevada

Stuart Mason, Nevada Chapter Co-Founder
Flora Mason, Nevada Chapter Co-Founder

3235 Juvenile Diabetes Research Foundation: Nor thern Nevada Branch
5335 Kietzke Lane
Reno, NV 89511 775-786-1881
Fax: 775-827-0131
e-mail: northernnevada@jdrf.org
www.jdrf.org/northernnevada

Molly Dillon, Branch Manager
Arnie Pitts MD, Board of Directors President

New Hampshire

3236 American Diabetes Association: New Hampshire
249 Canal Street
Manchester, NH 03101 603-627-9579
888-342-2383
Fax: 603-669-1477
www.diabetes.org

3237 Juvenile Diabetes Research Foundation: New England/New Hampshire Chapter
2 Wellman Avenue
Nashua, NH 03064 603-595-2595
Fax: 603-595-2073
e-mail: newhampshire@jdrf.org
www.jdrf.org/newhampshire

Brooke Edwards, Special Events Coordinator
Heidi Daniels, New England Chapter Executive Director

New Jersey

3238 American Diabetes Association: New Jersey
CentrePoint II Suite 103
Bridgewater, NJ 08807 732-469-7979
888-342-2383
Fax: 732-469-4887
e-mail: AskADA@diabetes.org
www.diabetes.org

James Roberts, Executive Director
Pamela Hooper, Director

3239 Juvenile Diabetes Research Foundation: South Jersey Chapter
1415 Route 70 E
Cherry Hill, NJ 08034 856-429-1101
Fax: 856-429-1105
e-mail: southjersey@jdrf.org
www.jdrf.org/southjersey

Stephen Blocher, Executive Director
Robin Berger, Special Events Coordinator

3240 Juvenile Diabetes Research Foundation: Cen tral Jersey Chapter
740 Broad Street
Shrewsbury, NJ 07702 732-219-6654
Fax: 732-219-8722
e-mail: centraljersey@jdrf.org
www.jdrf.org/chapters/NJ/Central-Jersey

Lori McLane, Executive Director
Beckie Burlew, Special Events Coordinator

3241 Juvenile Diabetes Research Foundation: Mid -Jersey Chapter
28 Kennedy Boulevard
East Brunswick, NJ 08816 732-296-7171
Fax: 732-296-1433
e-mail: midjersey@jdrf.org
www.jdrf.org/NJ/Mid-Jersey

Elizabeth Giardina Preston, Chapter Executive Director
Sandra Hilsenrath, Special Events Coordinator

3242 Juvenile Diabetes Research Foundation: Roc kland County/Northern New Jersey
560 Sylvan Avenue
Englewood Cliffs, NJ 07632 201-568-4838
Fax: 201-568-5360
e-mail: rockland@jdrf.org
www.jdrf.org/northernnj

Douglas Rouse, Executive Director
Allison Hartstone, Special Events Coordinator

New Mexico

3243 American Diabetes Association: New Mexico
2625 Pennsylvania NE
Albuquerque, NM 87110 505-266-5716
888-342-2383
Fax: 505-268-4533
e-mail: AskADA@diabetes.org
www.diabetes.org

Betsey Robinson, Associate Director
Lisa Johnson, Manager

3244 Juvenile Diabetes Research Foundation: Albuquerque
2501 San Pedro NE
Albuquerque, NM 87110 505-255-4005
Fax: 505-260-1430
e-mail: newmexico@jdrf.org
www.jdrf.org/newmexico

Joann Perrine, Branch Manager
Elizabeth Romero, Fundraising Assistant

New York

3245 American Diabetes Association: New York
Pine W Plaza Building 2
Albany, NY 12205 518-218-1755
888-342-2383
Fax: 518-218-0114
e-mail: AskADA@diabetes.org
www.diabetes.org

Amy R Young, District Director
Karen Dooley, Associate Manager

3246 Juvenile Diabetes Research Foundation Executive Office/Corporate Headquarters
Executive Office/Corporate Headquarters
120 Wall Street
New York, NY 10005-4001 212-725-4925
800-533-2873
Fax: 212-785-9595
e-mail: info@jdrf.org
www.jdrf.org/

Allan J Lewis, President/Chief Executive Officer
Amy C Franze, EVP Development

3247 Juvenile Diabetes Research Foundation: Long Island/South Shore Chapter
532 Broadhollow Road
Melville, NY 11747 631-414-1126
Fax: 631-414-1133
e-mail: longisland@jdrf.org
www.jdrf.org/longisland

Barbara Rogus, Executive Director
Christina Colandro, Special Events Manager

3248 Juvenile Diabetes Research Foundation: Buf falo/Western New York Chapter
331 Alberta Drive
Buffalo, NY 14226
716-833-2873
Fax: 716-833-0199
e-mail: westernny@jdrf.org
www.jdrf.org/westernny

Karen Swierski, Executive Director
Jennifer Hickok, Special Events Manager

3249 Juvenile Diabetes Research Foundation: Hud son Valley Chapter
Hollowbrook Office Park
Wappinger Falls, NY 12590
845-297-8600
Fax: 845-297-7887
e-mail: hudsonvalley@jdrf.org
www.letscurediabetes.com

Charlie Lawrence, Branch Manager
Linda Delia, Events Assistant

3250 Juvenile Diabetes Research Foundation: New York Chapter
432 Park Avenue S
New York, NY 10016
212-689-2860
Fax: 212-689-4038
e-mail: newyorkchapter@jdrf.org
www.jdrf.org/nyc

Mania Boyder, New York City Chapter Executive Director

3251 Juvenile Diabetes Research Foundation: Nor theastern New York
6 Greenwood Drive
East Greenbush, NY 12061
518-477-2873
Fax: 518-477-7004
e-mail: northeastny@jdrf.org
www.jdrf.org/NortheasternNY

Bev Kennedy, Executive Director
Darlene Robbiano, Special Events Manager

3252 Juvenile Diabetes Research Foundation: Roc hester Branch/Western New York Chapter
1200-A Scottsville Road
Rochester, NY 14624
585-546-1390
Fax: 585-546-1404
e-mail: rochester@jdrf.org
www.jdrf.org/rochester

Mary Anne Fox, Executive Director
Anne Blythe, Special Events Coordinator

3253 Juvenile Diabetes Research Foundation: Wes tchester County Chapter
30 Glenn Street
White Plains, NY 10603
914-686-7700
Fax: 914-686-7701
e-mail: westchester@jdrf.org
www.jdrf.org/westchester

Katherine Cintron, Executive Director
Dejan Popovich, Special Events Coordinator

North Carolina

3254 American Diabetes Association: Eastern North Carolina
1701 N Beauregard Street
Alexandria, VA 22311
919-743-5400
888-342-2383
Fax: 919-783-7838
e-mail: AskADA@diabetes.org
www.diabetes.org

The American Diabetes Association is the nation's leading non-profit health organization providing diabetes research, information and advocacy.
Larry Hausner, CEO
Richard Kahn PhD, Chief Scientific & Medical Officer

3255 American Diabetes Association: North Carolina
222 South Church Street
Charlotte, NC 28202
704-373-9111
888-342-2383
Fax: 704-373-9113
www.diabetes.org

Dianne Roth, Executive Director

3256 Juvenile Diabetes Research Foundation: Triangle/Eastern North Carolina Chapter
2210 Millbrook Road
Raleigh, NC 27604
919-431-8330
Fax: 919-431-8373
e-mail: triangle@jdrf.org
www.jdrftriangle.org

Jim Burson, Chapter President
Courtney Davies, Executive Director

3257 Juvenile Diabetes Research Foundation: Cha rlotte Chapter
9140 ArrowPoint Boulevard
Charlotte, NC 28273
704-561-0828
Fax: 704-561-9920
e-mail: charlotte@jdrf.org
www.jdrf.org/charlotte

Brenning Johnston, Volunteer Coordinator

3258 Juvenile Diabetes Research Foundation: Pie dmont Triad Chapter
1401-B Old Mill Circle
Winston-Salem, NC 27103
336-768-1027
Fax: 336-768-1029
e-mail: piedmont@jdrf.org
www.jdrf.org/triad

Brad Calloway, President Board of Directors
Tom Brinkley, VP Fundraising & Development

North Dakota

3259 American Diabetes Association: Nashville
1323 23rd Street S
Fargo, ND 58103
701-234-0123
Fax: 701-235-3080
e-mail: AskADA@diabetes.org
www.diabetes.org

Stephanie Chimeziri, Associate Director

3260 American Diabetes Association: North Dakota
1323 23rd Street South
Fargo, ND 58103
701-234-0123
888-342-2383
Fax: 701-235-3080
www.diabetes.org

Ohio

3261 American Diabetes Association: Ohio
4500 Rockside Road
Independence, OH 44131
216-328-9989
888-342-2383
Fax: 216-328-0007
e-mail: AskADA@diabetes.org
www.diabetes.org

Jill Pupa, Executive Director
Patti Clair, Associate Director

3262 Juvenile Diabetes Research Foundation/JDRF
1293-H Lyons Road
Dayton, OH 45458
937-439-2873
Fax: 937-439-4086
e-mail: dayton@jdrf.org
www.jdrf.org/dayton

Karen Myers, Executive Director
Vicky Williams, Office Manager

3263 Juvenile Diabetes Research Foundation: Mid-Ohio Chapter
950 Michigan Avenue
Columbus, OH 43215
614-464-2873
Fax: 614-464-2877
e-mail: midohio@jdrf.org
www.jdrf.org/midohio

Staci Perkins, Executive Director
Roberta Smedes, Office Manager

3264 Juvenile Diabetes Research Foundation: Akr on/Canton Chapter
5000 Rockside Road
Canton, OH 44131
888-718-3061
Fax: 216-328-8340
e-mail: jcallahan@jdrf.org
www.jdrf.org/chapters/OH/Northeast-Ohio

Laura E Maciag, Executive Director
Danielle Thompson, Special Events Manager

3265 Juvenile Diabetes Research Foundation: Gre ater Cincinnati Chapter
8041 Hosbrook Road
Cincinnati, OH 45236-3830
513-793-3223
Fax: 513-936-5333
e-mail: cincinnati@jdrf.org
www.jdrf.org/cincinnati

Bill Rice, Executive Director
Bethe Ferguson, Special Events Coordinator

3266 Juvenile Diabetes Research Foundation: Tol edo/Northwest Ohio Chapter
3450 W Central Avenue
Toledo, OH 43606
419-873-1377
800-533-2873
Fax: 419-720-6339
e-mail: northwestohio@jdrf.org
www.jdrf.org/northwestohio
Megan Meyer, Executive Director
Marna Cousino, Special Events Coordinator

Oklahoma

3267 American Diabetes Association: Oklahoma
3000 United Founders Boulevard
Oklahoma City, OK 73112
405-840-3881
888-342-2383
Fax: 405-840-3899
e-mail: AskADA@diabetes.org
www.diabetes.org
Diane Sarantakos, Executive Director
Andrea Barnett, Associate Manager

3268 Juvenile Diabetes Research Foundation: Cen tral Oklahoma Chapter
2601 NW Expressway
Oklahoma City, OK 73112
405-810-0070
888-533-9255
Fax: 405-810-0078
e-mail: oklahoma@jdrf.org
www.jdrf.org/centralok
Renee MacDonald, Executive Director
Shannon Scott, Special Events Coordinator

3269 Juvenile Diabetes Research Foundation: Tul sa Green County Chapter
4606 E 67th Street
Tulsa, OK 74136
918-481-5807
Fax: 918-481-5823
e-mail: tulsa@jdrf.org
www.jdrf.org/tulsa-green
Brandi Sullivan, Executive Director
Angela Peterson, Special Events Coordinator

Oregon

3270 American Diabetes Association: Oregon
2350 Oakmont Way
Eugene, OR 97401
541-343-0735
888-342-2383
Fax: 541-342-1491
e-mail: AskADA@diabetes.org
www.diabetes.org
Cynthia Benton, Associate Director

3271 Juvenile Diabetes Research Foundation: Ore gon/SW Washington Chapter
7460 SW Hunziker Street
Portland, OR 97223
503-643-1995
866-598-9074
Fax: 503-598-9087
e-mail: oregon-washington@jdrf.org
www.jdrf.org/oregon
Ashleigh Farleigh, Special Events Manager
Debbie Secor, Special Events Assistant

Pennsylvania

3272 American Diabetes Association: Pennsylvania
3544 Progress Avenue
Harrisburg, PA 17110
717-657-4310
888-342-2383
Fax: 717-657-4320
www.diabetes.org

3273 American Diabetes Association: Western Pennsylvania
300 Penn Center Boulevard
Pittsburgh, PA 15235
412-824-1181
888-342-2383
Fax: 412-824-2191
e-mail: AskADA@diabetes.org
www.diabetes.org
Terri Seidman, Area Manager
Steven Shivak, Executive Director

3274 Juvenile Diabetes Research Foundation: Central Pennsylvania Chapter
119 Aster Drive
Harrisburg, PA 17112
717-901-6489
Fax: 717-901-6573
e-mail: centralpa@jdrf.org
www.jdrf.org/centralpa
Susan Harral, Executive Director
Kate Severs, Special Events Assistant

3275 Juvenile Diabetes Research Foundation: Ber ks County Chapter
619 Wellington Avenue
West Lawn, PA 19609
610-775-4169
Tammy A. Edwards, Contact

3276 Juvenile Diabetes Research Foundation: Nor thwestern Pennsylvania Chapter
1700 Peach St
Erie, PA 16501
814-452-0635
Fax: 814-452-0645
e-mail: northwestpa@jdrf.org
www.jdrf.org/northwestpa
Douglas K White, Executive Director
Amy Bement, Special Events Assistant

3277 Juvenile Diabetes Research Foundation: Phi ladelphia Chapter
225 City Line Avenue
Bala Cynwyd, PA 19004
610-664-9255
Fax: 610-664-9585
e-mail: philadelphia@jdrf.org
www.jdrf.org/philadelphia
Ellen Rubesin, Executive Director
Kathy Farren, Special Events Director

3278 Juvenile Diabetes Research Foundation: Wes tern Pennsylvania
960 Penn Avenue
Pittsburgh, PA 15222
412-471-1414
888-528-8788
Fax: 412-471-1417
e-mail: westernpa@jdrf.org
www.jdrf.org/westernpa
David R Donahue, Executive Director
Kimberly A McElroy, Office Manager

Rhode Island

3279 American Diabetes Association: Central Virginia Office
222 Richmond Street
Providence, RI 02903
401-351-0498
Fax: 401-351-1674
e-mail: AskADA@diabetes.org
www.diabetes.org/richmond
The nation's leading voluntary health organization concerned with diabetes and its complications. The mission of the Association is to prevent and cure diabetes and improve the lives of all people with diabetes.
Nancy Castrina, Director
Elisabeth King, Associate Manager

3280 American Diabetes Association: Rhode Island
222 Richmond Street
Providence, RI 02903
401-351-0498
888-342-2383
Fax: 401-351-1674
www.jdf.org

3281 American Diabetes Association: Richmond
222 Richmond Street
Providence, RI 02903
401-351-0498
Fax: 401-351-1674
e-mail: AskADA@diabetes.org
www.diabetes.org
Liana Ahrens, Associate Manager
Matthew Netto, Associate Manager

South Carolina

3282 American Diabetes Association: South Carolina
2711 Middleburg Drive
Columbia, SC 29204
803-799-4246
888-342-2383
Fax: 803-799-5792
www.diabetes.org

3283 American Diabetes Association: South Coast
2711 Middleburg Drive
Columbia, SC 29204
803-799-4246
Fax: 803-799-5792
e-mail: AskADA@diabetes.org
www.diabetes.org

3284 **Juvenile Diabetes Research Foundation: Palmetto Chapter**
3608 Landmark Drive 803-782-1477
Columbia, SC 29204 Fax: 803-782-8975
e-mail: palmetto@jdrf.org
http://palmettojdrf.org

Jack Douglas, President Executive Committee
David Campbell, Vice President Executive Committee

3285 **Juvenile Diabetes Research Foundation: Low Country Chapter**
520 Folly Road 843-345-0369
Charleston, SC 29412 Fax: 843-406-7957
e-mail: dmenefee@jdrf.org
www.jdrf.org/lowcountry

Pam Nestor McAdams, Events/Walk Director South Coastal Chptr

South Dakota

3286 **Juvenile Diabetes Research Foundation: Sio ux Falls Chapter**
PO Box 88540 605-338-2295
Sioux Falls, SD 57109-8540

Tennessee

3287 **American Diabetes Association: Nashville**
4205 Hillsboro Road 615-298-3066
Nashville, TN 37215 888-342-2383
Fax: 615-292-5357
e-mail: AskADA@diabetes.org
www.diabetes.org

Glenda Berry, Executive Director
Harlyn Hardin, Director of Programs

3288 **American Diabetes Association: Tennessee**
5583 Murray Road 901-682-8232
Memphis, TN 38119 888-342-2383
Fax: 901-682-8170
e-mail: AskADA@diabetes.org
www.diabetes.org

John Carroll, Director
Daniele Cain, Coordinator

3289 **Juvenile Diabetes Research Foundation: East Tennessee Chapter**
355 Trane Lane 865-544-0768
Knoxville, TN 37919 Fax: 865-544-4312
e-mail: EastTennessee@jdrf.org
www.jdf.org/chapters/tn/ecsh-tennessee

3290 **Juvenile Diabetes Research Foundation: Mid dle Tennessee Chapter**
105 Westpark Drive 615-383-6781
Nashville, TN 37027 Fax: 615-383-4284
e-mail: MidTennessee@jrdf.org
www.jdf.org/chapters/tn/middle-tennessee

Texas

3291 **American Diabetes Association: Texas**
4150 International Plaza 817-332-7110
Fort Worth, TX 76109 888-342-2383
Fax: 817-732-6244
www.diabetes.org

3292 **Juvenile Diabetes Research Foundation: South Central Texas Chapter**
8700 Crownhill Boulevrad 210-822-5336
San Antonio, TX 78209 Fax: 210-822-1443
e-mail: scentraltexas@jrdf.org
www.jdf.org

3293 **Juvenile Diabetes Research Foundation: Dal las Chapter**
9400 North Central Expressway 214-373-9808
Dallas, TX 75231-5063 Fax: 214-373-6337
e-mail: dallas@jrdf.org
www.jdf.org/chapters/tx/

3294 **Juvenile Diabetes Research Foundation: Gre ater Fort Worth/ Arlington Chapter**
3840 Hulen Street 817-332-2601
Fort Worth, TX 76107-2127 Fax: 817-332-5641
e-mail: grfortworth@jrDRF.org
www.jdf.org

3295 **Juvenile Diabetes Research Foundation: Hou ston/Gulf Coast Chapter**
2425 Fountain View 713-334-4400
Houston, TX 77057 Fax: 713-334-4040
e-mail: houston@jdrf.org
www.jdf.org

3296 **Juvenile Diabetes Research Foundation: Wes t Texas Chapter**
Clay Desta Towers, 10 Desta Drive 432-570-5643
Midland, TX 79705 Fax: 432-682-0765
e-mail: westtexas@jdrf.org
www.jdf.org

Utah

3297 **American Diabetes Association: Utah**
1245 E Brickyard Road 801-363-3024
Salt Lake City, UT 84106 888-342-2383
Fax: 801-363-3031
www.diabetes.org

Vermont

3298 **American Diabetes Association: Vermont**
1 Kennedy Drive 802-654-7716
S Burlington, VT 05403 888-342-2383
Fax: 802-658-9145
www.diabetes.org

Virginia

3299 **American Diabetes Association: Richmond**
4335 Cox Road 804-225-8038
Glen Allen, VA 23060 888-342-2383
Fax: 804-270-4742
www.diabetes.org

3300 **American Diabetes Association: Virginia**
870 Greenbrier Circle 757-424-6662
Chesapeake, VA 23320 888-342-2383
Fax: 757-420-0490
www.diabetes.org

3301 **Juvenile Diabetes Research Foundation: Gre ater Blue Ridge Chapter**
3959 Electric Road 540-772-1975
Roanoke, VA 24018 888-849-0510
Fax: 540-772-6672
e-mail: greaterblueridge@jdrf.org
www.jdf.org

Washington

3302 **American Diabetes Association: Seattle**
Metropolitan Park E 206-282-4616
Seattle, WA 98101 888-342-2383
Fax: 206-903-8107
www.diabetes.org

Linda Henderson, Executive Director
Sarah Popelka, Director

3303 **American Diabetes Association: Washington**
1200 Sixth Avenue 509-624-7478
Spokane, WA 99204 888-342-2383
Fax: 509-624-7212
www.diabetes.org

3304 **Juvenile Diabetes Research Foundation: Seattle Guild**
1215 Fourth Avenue 206-343-0873
Seattle, WA 98161-1101 Fax: 206-343-7015
e-mail: terickson@jdrf.org
http://www.jdrf.org/index.cfm

3305 **Juvenile Diabetes Research Foundation: Sea ttle Chapter**
1333 N Northlake Way 206-545-1510
Seattle, WA 98103-8900 Fax: 206-545-1511
www.jdf.org

3306 Juvenile Diabetes Research Foundation: Spo kane County Area Chapter
9 South Washington
Spokane, WA 99201
509-459-6307
Fax: 509-459-6392
e-mail: inlandnw@jdrf.org
http://www.jdrf.org/index.cfm

Kay C Dightman, Contact

West Virginia

3307 American Diabetes Association: West Virginia
PO Box 238
Hurricane, WV 25526
304-768-2596
888-342-2383
Fax: 304-562-1887
e-mail: rahearn@diabetes.org
diabetes.org

Roberta Ahearn, Executive Director

3308 American Diabetes Association: Wisconsin
PO Box 238
Hurricane, WV 25526
304-768-2596
Fax: 304-562-1887
e-mail: rahearn@diabetes.org
www.diabetes.org

Roberta Ahearn, Executive Director

3309 Juvenile Diabetes Research Foundation: Hun tington Chapter
PO Box 2903
Huntington, WV 25728
304-525-4533

Wisconsin

3310 American Diabetes Association: Wisconsin
1701 North Beauregard Street Alexan
Monona, WI 53713
608-222-7785
888-342-2383
Fax: 608-222-7795
e-mail: bfolco@diabetes.org
www.diabetes.org

Barb Folco, Manager
Jay Kemp, Coordinator

3311 Juvenile Diabetes Research Foundation: Southeastern Chapter
3333 North Mayfair Road
Wauwatosa, WI 53222
414-453-4673
Fax: 414-453-4919
e-mail: southeastwi@jdrf.org
http://www.jdrf.org/sewi

3312 Juvenile Diabetes Research Foundation: Gre ater Madison Chapter
434 S. Yellowstone Drive
Madison, WI 53719
60- 83- 287
Fax: 60- 83- 921
e-mail: westernwi@jdrf.org
http://www.jdrf.org/index.cfm

3313 Juvenile Diabetes Research Foundation: Nor theast Wisconsin Chapter
1800 Appleton Road
Menasha, WI 54952-0101
920-997-0038
Fax: 920-997-0039
e-mail: northeastwi@jdrf.org
www.jdrf.org

Julie Kersten, Executive Director
Dana Paschen, Special Events Coordinator

Libraries & Resource Centers

3314 Diabetes Control Program
California Department of Health Services
PO Box 997413
Sacramento, CA 95899-7413
916-552-9888
Fax: 916-552-9988
http://www.caldiabetes.org/
Our mission is to prevent diabetes and its complications in California's diverse communities.
Susan Lopez-Payan, Interim Chief

3315 Division of Diabetes Translation
National Center for Chronic Disease Prevention
4770 Buford Highway NE
Atlantia, GA 30341-3717
770-488-5000
Fax: 770-488-5966
e-mail: cdcinfo@cdc.gov
www.cdc.gov/diabetes

The Division of Diabetes Translation's (DDT) goal is to reduce the burden of diabetes in the United States. The division works to achieve this goal by combining support for public health-oriented diabetes prevention and control programs (DPCPs) and translating diabetes research findings into widespread clinical and public health practice.

3316 Health Science Library
Marshall University
1600 Medical Center Drive
Huntington, WV 25701
304-691-1700
www.musom.marshall.edu/library
The Health Sciences Library's primary mission is serving the informational needs of the students, faculty, and staff at Marshall University and the Cabell-Huntington Hospital. The Library also plays an important role in providing information services to hospitals and healthcare professionals in the Huntington and the Tri-State area.
Edward Dzierzak, Director

3317 Joslin Center at University of Maryland Medicine
22 S Greene Street
Baltimore, MD 21201
800-492-5538
TDD: 800735225800
e-mail: joslin@umms001.ab.umd.edu
www.umm.edu/joslindiabetes
The Joslin Center at University of Maryland Medicine meets the highest standards of care for people with diabetes. Its programs reflect a philosophy which have been the hallmark of Joslin's care — a comprehensive team approach to diabetes treatment with programs designed to help children and adults with diabetes take charge of their own health and well-being.
Thomas W Donner, MD, Director

3318 Naomi Berrie Diabetes Center at Columbia University Medical Center
Russ Berrie Medical Science Pavillion
1150 St. Nicholas Avenue
New York, NY 10032
212-851-5494
Fax: 212-851-5459
e-mail: diabetes@columbia.edu
nbdiabetes.org
The special focus of the Naomi Berrie Diabetes Center is on families — a concept that differentiates it from almost every other diabetes treatment facility in America. People with diabetes are strongly encouraged to involve their entire families in the treatment process.
Robin Goland, MD, Co-Director
Rudolph Liebel, MD, Co-Director

3319 National Diabetes Information Clearinghous e
One Information Way
Bethesda, MD 20892-3560
800-860-8747
Fax: 703-738-4929
e-mail: ndic@info.niddk.nih.gov
diabetes.niddk.nih.gov
To serve as a diabetes informational, educational, and referral resource for health professionals and the public. NDIC is a service of the NIDDK.

3320 Schulze Diabetes Institute
University of Minnesota
420 Delaware Street SE
Minneapolis, MN 55455
612-626-3016
e-mail: diitinfo@umn.edu
www.med.umn.edu
Formerly the Diabetes Institute for Immunology and Transplantation
David Sutherland MD, PhD, Director
Bernard Hering MD, Director

3321 Tallahassee Memorial Diabetes Center
Tallahassee Memorial Health Care
1981-2 Capital Circle NE
Tallahassee, FL 32308
850-431-5404
800-662-4278
Fax: 850-431-6325
www.tmh.org/diabetes
TMH provides comprehensive, patient-centered services to both children and adults. The Diabetes Center uses a team approach that involves the patient, physicians, nurse educators, registered dieti-

tians with access to a diabetes counselor and registered pharmacists and social worker.
Richard M Bergenstal, MD, Medical Director

Research Centers

3322 Barbara Davis Center for Childhood Diabetes
13001 E 17th Place   303-724-2323
Aurora, CO 80045-6511   Fax: 303-724-6839
e-mail: george.eisenbarth@uchsc.edu
www.uchsc.edu/misc/diabetes
Research and educational organization.
Marian Rewers, Clinical Director
George S Eisenbarth, Executive Director

3323 Baylor College of Medicine: Children's General Clinical Research Center
One Baylor Plaza   713-798-4780
Houston, TX 77030   Fax: 713-790-1345
e-mail: pedi-webmaster@bcm.edu
www.bcm.edu/pediatrics
Offers research into juvenile aspects of immunology and infectious diseases including diabetes research activities.
Lisa Bomgaars, Medical Director
Mark A Ward, Director

3324 Benaroya Research Institute Virginia Mason Medical Center
Virginia Mason Medical Center
1201 9th Avenue   206-583-6525
Seattle, WA 98101-2795   Fax: 206-223-7543
e-mail: info@benaroyaresearch.org
www.benaroyaresearch.org
Immunology and diabetes research.
Robert B Lemon, Chair
Gerald Nepom, Director

3325 Diabetes Education and Research Center The Franklin House
The Franklin House
PO Box 897   215-829-3426
Philadelphia, PA 19105   Fax: 215-829-5807
e-mail: webmaster@dibeteseducationandresearchcen
www.diabeteseducationandresearchcenter.o
Is a non-profit organization serving the needs of people living in Philadelphia PA and surrounding communities. The goal of the Foundation is to improve the health of people with diabetes.

3326 Diabetes Research and Training Center: University of Alabama at Birmingham
Department of Medicine
1530 3rd Avenue S   205-934-4011
Birmingham, AL 35294-1150   Fax: 205-934-4389
TTY: 205-934-4642
www.main.uab.edu
The DRTC works to develop and evaluate new models of diabetes care and to facilitate translational diabetes research.
Dr Carol Garrison, President
Dr. William Ferniany PhD, CEO

3327 Division on Endocrinology Northwestern University Feinberg School
Northwestern University Feinberg School of Medicin
251 East Huron Street   312-926-6895
Chicago, IL 60611   Fax: 312-503-7757
e-mail: help@medicine.northwestern.edu
www.medicine.northwestern.edu
Nonprofit organization focusing research activities on endocrinology metabolism nutrition and specializing in diabetes.
James Foody MD, Vice Chair
J Larry Jameson, Professor Division of Endocrinology

3328 Endocrinology Research Laboratory Cabrini Medical Center
Cabrini Medical Center
227 E 19th Street   212-222-7464
New York, NY 10003-7457   e-mail: info@cabrininty.org
www.cabrininy.org
Focuses on the effects of insulin and insulin-like growth factors on human body functions.
Dr Leonid Poretsky, Director

3329 Indiana University: Area Health Education Center
714 N Senate Avenue   317-278-8893
Indianapolis, IN 46202   Fax: 317-278-0392
e-mail: ahec@iupui.edu
www.ahec.iupui.edu
A collaborative statewide system for community-based primary health care professions education that fosters the continuing improvement of health care services for all citizens in Indiana.
Richard D Kiovsky, Director
Jonathan C Barclay, Associate Director

3330 Indiana University: Center for Diabetes Research
340 West 10th Street   317-274-8157
Indianapolis, IN 46202-3082   Fax: 317-274-1437
e-mail: rconsidi@iupui.edu
www.medicine.iu.edu
Our goal is to promote the training of scientists whose research will develop new understandings of the basis of the disease and its complications and to cultivate basic science research that can speed the discovery of more effective therapies.
Robert Considine, Associate Professor of Medicine
D Craig Brater MD, Dean

3331 Indiana University: Pharmacology Research Laboratory
Division of Clinical Pharmacology
1001 W 10th Street   317-630-8795
Indianapolis, IN 46202   Fax: 317-630-8185
e-mail: tamllewi@iupui.edu
www.medicine.iupui.edu/clinpharm
We will train highly skilled compassionate and altruistic professionals both generalists and specialists to be future leaders in medical practice academia and industry.
David A Flockhart, Division Director
John T Callaghan, Associate Professor of Medicine

3332 International Diabetes Center at Nicollet
3800 Park Nicollet Boulevard   952-993-3393
Saint Louis Park, MN 55416-2533   888-825-6315
Fax: 952-993-1302
e-mail: idcdiabetes@parknicollet.com
www.parknicollet.com/diabetes
Research center which improves the quality of life of individuals with diabetes and those at risk of developing diabetes by undertaking clinical care education research and outreach activities that stimulate and support health.
Richard Berg MD, Executive Director

3333 Joslin Diabetes Center
One Joslin Place   617-732-2400
Boston, MA 02215-5306   800-567-5461
Fax: 617-322-40
e-mail: diabetes@joslin.harvard.edu
www.joslin.org
An internationally recognized leader in diabetes and endocrine disease treatment research and patient and professional education affiliated with Harvard Medical School. In addition to its headquarters in Boston's Longwood Medical area Joslin has affiliated treatment centers across the nation. Established in 1898.
John L Brooks, Chairman of the Board
Martin J Abrahamson MD, Senior VP, Medical Director

3334 Metabolic Research Institute
1515 N Flagler Drive   561-802-3060
West Palm Beach, FL 33401   Fax: 561-802-3260
e-mail: moreinformation@metabolic-institute.com
www.metabolic-institute.com
The Metabolic Research Institute specializes in clinical studies involving endocrinology disorders complications of endocrinology disorders metabolic problems and selected renal disease.
William A Kaye, Co-Director
Barry Horowitz, Co-Director

3335 Sansum Diabetes Research Institute
2219 Bath Street   805-682-7638
Santa Barbara, CA 93105-4321   Fax: 805-682-3332
e-mail: info@sansum.org
www.sansum.org

A research institute devoted to the prevention treatment and cure of diabetes.
Lois Jovanovich, CEO & Chief Scientific Officer of Sansum
Wendy Bevier, Associate Investigator

3336 University of Chicago: Comprehensive Diabetes Center
5841 S Maryland Avenue 773-702-2371
Chicago, IL 60637 800-989-6740
e-mail: diabetes@uchospitals.edu
www.kovlerdiabetescenter.org
The University of Chicago Kovler Diabetes Center offers a unique fully comprehensive approach to diagnosing and treating diabetes. Focuses on children adolescents and adults with diabetes as well as individuals at the highest risk for serious complications.
Louis H Philipson, Medical Director
Christopher Rhodes, Kovler Diabetes Center Pediatric Program

3337 University of Colorado: General Clinical Research Center, Pediatric
13001 E 17th Place 720-777-2957
Aurora, CO 80045 Fax: 72- 77- 727
e-mail: CTRCAdmin@tchden.org
www.uchsc.edu/pedsgcrc
Focuses on developmental studies and diabetes research.
Ronald J Sokol, Program Director
Philip S Zeitler, Associate Program Director

3338 University of Iowa: Diabetes Research Center
Department of Internal Medicine
200 Hawkins Drive
Iowa City, IA 52242 319-353-7842
www.int-med.uiowa.edu
The Diabetes Research Center combines the talents of experienced clinical investigators molecular biologists and vascular physiologists in an integrated multidisciplinary approach toward the study and treatment of abnormalities of vascular reactivity which characterize diabetes mellitus.
Ken Kates, Associate Vice President and Chief Execu
John Swenning, Associate Director

3339 University of Kansas Cray Diabtetes Center
3901 Rainbow Boulevard 913-588-5000
Kansas City, KS 66160-7376 Fax: 913-588-4023
TTY: 913-588-7963
e-mail: geaks@kumc.edu
www.kumc.edu
The KU Medical Center is a complex institution whose basic functions include research education patient care and community service involving multiple constituencies at state and national levels.
Timothy Kestermont, Division of Clinical Research Administra
Barbara F Atkinson MD, Executive Vice Chancellor

3340 University of Massachusetts: Diabetes and Endocrinology Research Center
55 Lake Avenue N 508-856-8989
Worcester, MA 01655 e-mail: evelyn.vignola@umassmed.edu
www.umassmed.edu
UMMS has exploded onto the national scene as a major center for research, and in the past four decades, UMMS researchers have made pivotal advances in HIV, cancer, diabetes, infectious disease and in understanding the molecular basis of disease.
Micheal F Collins MD, Senior VP
Michael P Czech PhD, Professor and Chair

3341 University of Miami: Diabetes Research Institute
200 S Park Road 954-964-4040
Hollywood, FL 33021 800-321-3437
Fax: 954-964-7036
e-mail: info@drif.org
www.diabetesresearch.org
The Diabetes Research Institute (DRI) is an innovator in many fields of diabetes research but one of its primary strengths lies in islet cell transplantation, a cellular therapy that restores insulin production to normalize blood sugar control.
Thomas D Stern, Chairman
Camillo Ricordi, DRI Scientific Director

3342 University of New Mexico General Clinical Research Center
University of New Mexico Hospital

The University of New Mexico 505-277-0111
Albuquerque, NM 87131-2240 Fax: 505-272-0266
e-mail: mburge@salud.unm.edu
hsc.unm.edu/som/gcrc
Diabetes research.
Steve McKernan, CEO
Richard Larson MD, Vice President for Research

3343 University of Pennsylvania Diabetes and Endocrinology Research Center
700 Clinical Research Building (CRB 215-898-4365
Philadelphia, PA 19104 Fax: 215-898-5408
e-mail: gburgese@mail.med.upenn.edu
www.med.upenn.edu/idom/derc
The Penn Diabetes and Endocrinology Research Center (DERC) participates in the nationwide inter-disciplinary program established over two decades ago by the NIDDK to foster research and training in the areas of diabetes and related endocrine and metabolic disorders.
Mitchell A Lazar, Director
Morris J Birnbaum MD, Co Director

3344 University of Pittsburgh: Department of Molecular Genetics and Biochemistry
200 Lothrop Street 412-648-9570
Pittsburgh, PA 15261 Fax: 412-624-8997
e-mail: info@mmg.pitt.edu
www.mgb.pitt.edu
MMG students and fellows routinely publish their research in outstanding journals, present their science at international conferences and go on to achieve positions at prestigious laboratories and institutions.
J Richard Chaillet, Associate Professor
Bruce A McClane, Professor

3345 University of Tennessee: General Clinical Research Center
1265 Union Avenue 901-516-2212
Memphis, TN 38104 Fax: 901-516-7013
e-mail: bsalpert@utmem.edu
www.utmem.edu/crc
Congress directed the National Institutes of Health to establish clinical research centers throughout the United States to launch an all-out attack on human diseases.
Bruce S Alpert MD, Program Director
Teresa Carr, Research Nurses

3346 University of Texas General Clinical Research Center
7400 Merton Minter Boulevard 409-772-1950
San Antonio, TX 78229 Fax: 409-772-8097
e-mail: public.affairs@utmb.edu
www.utmb.edu/gcrc
Focuses on diabetes and infectious disease research.
Michael Lich MD, Program Director
Garland D Anderson, Principal Investigator

3347 University of Washington Diabetes: Endocrinology Research Center
DVA Puget Sound Health Care System
1660 S Columbian Way
Seattle, WA 98108 206-616-4860
Fax: 206-764-2693
e-mail: derc@u.washington.edu
www.depts.washington.edu/diabetes
The primary purpose of the DERC is to facilitate and enhance the diabetes-related research of approximately 100 Affiliate Investigators at the University of Washington
Jerry P Palmer MD, Director
David E Cummings MD, Deputy Director and Associate Director f

3348 Vanderbilt University Diabetes Center
1211 Medical Center Drive 615-322-5000
Nashville, TN 37232 Fax: 615-936-1667
e-mail: dc.brown@vanderbilt.edu
www.mc.vanderbilt.edu/diabetes/vdc
The Vanderbilt Diabetes Center provides complete care for children and adults with diabetes under one roof
Joe C Davis, Chair in Biomedical Sciences
Alvin C Powers, Director Vanderbilt Diabetes Center

3349 Veterans Affairs Medical Center: Research Service
500 Foothill Drive   801-582-1565
Salt Lake City, UT 84148   Fax: 801-584-1289
                                                                        www.va.gov
Diabetes and cancer research.
James Floyd, Director
Byron Bair, Director

3350 Warren Grant Magnuson Clinical Center
National Institute of Health
9000 Rockville Pike   301-496-4000
Bethesda, MD 20892   800-411-1222
                                                              Fax: 301-480-9793
                                                              TTY: 866-411-1010
                                                  e-mail: prpl@mail.cc.nih.gov
                                                            clinicalcenter.nih.gov
Established in 1953 as the research hospital of the National Institutes of Health. Designed so that patient care facilities are close to research laboratories so new findings of basic and clinical scientists can be quickly applied to the treatment of patients. Upon referral by physicians, patients are admitted to NIH clinical studies.
John Gallin, Director
David Henderson, Deputy Director for Clinical Care

3351 Washington University: Diabetes Research and Training Center
School of Medicine
660 S Euclid Avenue   314-362-0558
Saint Louis, MO 63110   Fax: 314-747-2692
                                                  e-mail: apermutt@wustl.edu
                                                              drtc.im.wustl.edu
DRTC investigators were involved in conducting 60 investigator-initiated diabetes-related clinical research protocols on the WU GCRC
Jean Schaffer MD, Professor of Medicine
Kristin E Mondy MD, Medicine/Infectious Diseases

Support Groups & Hotlines

3352 American Diabetes Association National Center
1701 N Beauregard Street
Alexandria, VA 22311   800-342-2383
                                                              Fax: 703-549-6995
                                                  e-mail: askada@diabetes.org
                                                              www.diabetes.org
To prevent and cure diabetes and to improve the lives of all people affected by diabetes.
John W Griffin Jr, Chair of the Board
Larry Hausner MBA, CEO

3353 Diabetes Society
1165 Lincoln Avenue   408-287-3785
San Jose, CA 95125   Fax: 408-287-2701
                                      e-mail: ckassouf@diabetessociety.org
                                                            www.diabetessociety.org
The Diabetes Society was organized in 1963 as the result of efforts by a group of mothers of children with diabetes. Today, the Diabetes Society offers its services to the estimated 140,000 people with diabetes in the Santa Clara Valley.
Greg Price, Board President
Carol Kassouf, CEO

3354 Juvenile Diabetes International Hotline
Juvenile Diabetes Research Foundation Int'l
26 Broadway
New York, NY 10004   800-533-2873
                                                              Fax: 212-785-9595
                                                  e-mail: info@jdrf.org
                                                              www.jdf.org
The leading charitable funder and advocate of type 1 (juvenile) diabetes research worldwide.
Robert Wood Johnson IV, Chairman
Jeffrey Brewer, President/CEO

3355 National Health Information Center
PO Box 1133   310-565-4167
Washington, DC 20013   800-336-4797
                                                              Fax: 301-984-4256
                                                  e-mail: info@nhic.org
                                                              www.health.gov/nhic

A health information referral service sponsored by the Office of Disease Prevention and Health Promotion. Puts health professionals and consumers who have health questions in touch with those organizations that are best able to provide answers.

Books

3356 101 Tips for Improving Your Blood Sugar
American Diabetes Association
1660 Duke Street
Alexandria, VA 22314-3447   800-232-3472
                                                              Fax: 703-549-6995
                                                              www.diabetes.org
Tips for 101 common situations and questions to reduce the risk of complications from blood sugar at the wrong level.
122 pages

3357 Balance Your Act: A Book for Adults with Diabetes
Pritchett & Hull
3440 Oakcliff Road
Atlanta, GA 30340-3079   800-774-1124
1993 96 pages Paperback
ISBN: 0-939838-14-1

3358 Buyer's Guide
American Diabetes Association
1660 Duke Street
Alexandria, VA 22314-3447   800-232-3472
                                                              Fax: 703-549-6995
                                                              www.diabetes.org
A catalog listing all manufacturers of insulin, syringes, pumps, test strips, monitors and more.

3359 Caring for the Diabetic Soul
American Diabetes Association
1660 Duke Street
Alexandria, VA 22314-3447   800-232-3472
                                                              Fax: 703-549-6995
                                                              www.diabetes.org
Restoring emotional balance for yourself and your family.
213 pages

3360 Clinical Practice Recommendations
American Diabetes Association
1660 Duke Street
Alexandria, VA 22314-3447   800-232-3472
                                                              Fax: 703-549-6995
                                                              www.diabetes.org
Features all current position and consensus statements of the American Diabetes Association.

3361 Complete Weight Loss Workbook
American Diabetes Association
1660 Duke Street
Alexandria, VA 22314-3447   800-232-3472
                                                              Fax: 703-549-6995
                                                              www.diabetes.org
A unique, brisk, practical workbook that offers a series of fresh, memorable tests, checklists, worksheets, mini-cases, calculation exercises, mental reminders, and other practical aids to losing weight and staying fit for good.
252 pages

3362 Computer Planned Menus for Health Professionals
American Diabetes Association
1660 Duke Street
Alexandria, VA 22314-3447   800-232-3472
                                                              Fax: 703-549-6995
                                                              www.diabetes.org
Input a patient's dietary prescription, food preferences, and budget, and the program produces individualized menus. Professional version includes license to distribute these customized menus.

3363 Control Diabetes the Easy Way
Random House Trade Books

400 Hahn Road
Westminster, MD 21157-4663

800-733-3000
Fax: 800-659-2436

ISBN: 0-679778-03-9

3364   Convenience Food Facts
American Diabetes Association
1660 Duke Street
Alexandria, VA 22314-3447

800-232-3472
Fax: 703-549-6995
www.diabetes.org

Helps to serve appetizing convenience foods low in sodium, cholesterol, and fat.
459 pages Softcover

3365   Cooking a la Heart
American Diabetes Association
1660 Duke Street
Alexandria, VA 22314-3447

800-232-3472
Fax: 703-549-6995
www.diabetes.org

Recipes that include a complete nutrient profile with diabetic exchanges.

3366   Diabetes & Pregnancy: What to Expect
American Diabetes Association
1660 Duke Street
Alexandria, VA 22314-3447

800-232-3472
Fax: 703-549-6995
www.diabetes.org

Information concerning an unborn baby's development, tests to expect, labor and delivery, birth control, and more.

3367   Diabetes A to Z
American Diabetes Association
1660 Duke Street
Alexandria, VA 22314-3447

800-232-3472
Fax: 703-549-6995
www.diabetes.org

Dictionary-style guidebook discussing basic terms and issues concerning diabetes. Third edition.
202 pages

3368   Diabetes Care Made Easy
Chronimed Publishing
PO Box 59032
Minneapolis, MN 55459-0032

612-513-6475
800-848-2793
Fax: 612-443-2806

Written and designed for both adults and for children with limited reading skills, this easy-to-read book explains how to exercise and eat for better health, prevent foot problems, test blood sugar, cope with emotions, take insulin, and more. Also available in Spanish.
180 pages Paperback
ISBN: 1-885115-31-8

3369   Diabetes Education Goals
American Diabetes Association
1660 Duke Street
Alexandria, VA 22314-3447

800-232-3472
Fax: 703-549-6995
www.diabetes.org

Features advice on how to assess, plan, and evaluate patient education and counseling programs. Covers both short-term and in-depth goals. Focuses on the education process and assessing the unique needs of each patient.
64 pages Softcover

3370   Diabetes Low-Fat & No-Fat Meals in Minutes
John Wiley and Sons, Inc.
Customer Service-Consumer Accounts
Indianapolis, IN 46256

877-762-2974
Fax: 800-597-3299
e-mail: consumers@wiley.com
www.wiley.com

Includes more than 250 recipes, 60 days of diabetic menus, and 16 pages of full-color photographs. Each recipe features a complete nutrition analysis, including diabetic exchanges.
1998 352 pages
ISBN: 1-565610-84-9

3371   Diabetes Medical Nutrition Therapy
American Diabetes Association
1660 Duke Street
Alexandria, VA 22314-3447

800-232-3472
Fax: 703-549-6995
www.diabetes.org

A professional guide to management and nutrition education resources. Provides in-depth coverage of nutrition assessment, goal setting, intervention, and outcome evaluation. Information is provided on specific resources and case studies are cited for practical examples.
Softcover

3372   Diabetes Mellitus: A Practical Handbook
Bull Publishing Company
PO Box 1377
Boulder, CO 80306

800-676-2855
Fax: 303-545-6354
www.bullpub.com

This helpful and user friendly practical guide adresses the everyday concerns of all diabetics.
2002 Paperback
ISBN: 0-923521-72-0

3373   Diabetes Self-Management
RA Rapaport Publishing
150 W 22nd Street
New York, NY 10011-2421

212-989-0200
800-234-0923
Fax: 212-989-4786
e-mail: editor@diabetes-self-mgmt-com

Publishes practical, how to information, focusing on the day-to-day and long term aspects of diabetes in a positive and upbeat style. Gives subscribers up-to-date news, facts and advice to help them maintain their wellness and make informed decisions regarding their health.
Ingird Strauch, Executive
Richard A. Rapaport, Publisher

3374   Diabetes Sourcebook
Dawn D Matthews, author
Omnigraphics
615 Griswold
Detroit, MI 48226-4105

313-961-1340
800-234-1340
Fax: 800-875-1340
www.omnigraphics.com

This Sourcebook contains information for people seeking to understand the risk factors, complications, and management of the different types of diabetes. It includes information about testing, diagnosis, medications, and other topics related to living with diabetes.
2003 622 pages
ISBN: 0-780806-29-8

3375   Diabetes Teaching Guide for People Who Use Insulin
Joslin Diabetes Center
1 Joslin Place
Boston, MA 02215-5306

617-732-2400
Fax: 617-732-2562
e-mail: diabetes@joslin.harvard.edu
www.joslin.org

Discusses the causes of diabetes, the role of diet and exercise, meal planning and complications. Also provide information on drawing blood, mixing and injecting insulin.

3376   Diabetes Youth Curriculum: A Toolbox for Educators
Chronimed Publishing
PO Box 59032
Minneapolis, MN 55459-0032

612-513-6475
800-848-2793
Fax: 612-443-2806

Program consisting of two volumes: the Curriculum and the Resource and Activities Guide (listed separately). Divided into sections dealing with general development concepts and specific guidelines for ages 6 to 8, 9 to 11, and 12 to 16.
136 pages Paperback
ISBN: 0-937721-49-2

3377   Diabetes: A Guide to Living Well
American Diabetes Association

7 Washington Square
Albany, NY 12205

518-218-1755
888-342-2383
Fax: 518-218-0114
e-mail: ADAorders@pbd.com
www.diabetes.org

Offers a guide to helping the person with diabetes design a program of individualized self-care and gain the willingness to follow it. Also tells how to deal with diet, exercise, stress, emotions, negative beliefs, and self-image.
242 pages Paperback
ISBN: 1-580402-09-7

3378   Diabetes: Your Complete Exercise Guide
Human Kinetics Publishers
PO Box 5076
Champaign, IL 61825-5076

217-351-1549
800-747-4457
Fax: 217-351-5076

Part of the Cooper Clinic and Research Institute Fitness Series providing exercise rehabilitation for persons with diabetes.
144 pages Paperback
ISBN: 0-873224-27-2

3379   Diabetes: Your Questions Answered
Paul Drury and Wendy Gatling, author

Elsevier
Book Customer Service Department
St. Louis, MO 63146

800-545-2522
Fax: 800-535-9935
e-mail: usbkinfo@elsevier.com
www.elsevier.com

This new volume in the popular Your Questions Answered series uses a question-and-answer format to provide easy access to hands-on guidance on the management of diabetes. Its succinct, practical coverage explores the latest evidence-based practice guilines and their interpretation. Case vignettes illustrate the clinical relevance of the material.
2004 380 pages Softcover
ISBN: 0-443073-89-9

3380   Diabetic Gourmet
Diabetes Self-Management Books
PO Box 10676
Des Moines, IA 50336-0676

800-664-9269

3381   Diabetic's Guide to Health and Fitness
Human Kinetics Publishers
PO Box 5076
Champaign, IL 61825-5076

217-351-1549
800-747-4457
Fax: 217-351-5076

272 pages Paperback
ISBN: 0-880113-47-2

3382   Direct and Indirect Costs of Diabetes in the US
American Diabetes Association
1660 Duke Street
Alexandria, VA 22314-3447

800-232-3472
Fax: 703-549-6995
www.diabetes.org

Examines the specific costs of diabetes, as well as all the costs of health care for people with diabetes and compares those costs with the total cost of health care for the US population without diabetes.
32 pages Softcover

3383   Dr. Bernstein's Diabetes Solution
Richard K Bernstein, MD, author

Little, Brown and Company
Publicity Department
New York, NY 10020

800-759-0190
e-mail: publicity@littlebrown.com
www.hachettebookgroupusa.com

A complete guide to achieving normal blood sugars with strong emphasis on diet and up-to-date information on products, insulins, and oral agents.
512 pages Hardcover
ISBN: 0-316099-06-6

3384   Easy & Elegant Entrees
American Diabetes Association

1660 Duke Street
Alexandria, VA 22314-3447

800-232-3472
Fax: 703-549-6995
www.diabetes.org

Recipes that are low in fat and calories.

3385   Exchanges for All Occasions
American Diabetes Association
1660 Duke Street
Alexandria, VA 22314-3447

800-232-3472
Fax: 703-549-6995
www.diabetes.org

Meal planning suggestions for traveling, entertaining, camping, dining out, and more.

3386   Family Cookbook: Volumes I-IV
American Diabetes Association
1660 Duke Street
Alexandria, VA 22314-3447

800-232-3472
Fax: 703-549-6995
www.diabetes.org

Unforgettable recipes for the whole family. Great for diabetics.

3387   Fitness Book: For People with Diabetes
American Diabetes Association
1660 Duke Street
Alexandria, VA 22314-3447

800-232-3472
Fax: 703-549-6995
www.diabetes.org

Advice on learning to exercise to lose weight, exercise safely, increase your competitive edge, get your mind and body ready to exercise, and more.
149 pages

3388   Great Starts & Fine Finishes
American Diabetes Association
1660 Duke Street
Alexandria, VA 22314-3447

800-232-3472
Fax: 703-549-6995
www.diabetes.org

Healthy select cookbook offering great meals in minutes.

3389   Healthy Eater's Guide to Family & Chain Restaurants
American Diabetes Association
1660 Duke Street
Alexandria, VA 22314-3447

800-232-3472
Fax: 703-549-6995
www.diabetes.org

Advice on safe choices from fast-food menus, complete with nutrition values and exchanges.

3390   Healthy Homestyle Cookbook
American Diabetes Association
1660 Duke Street
Alexandria, VA 22314-3447

800-232-3472
Fax: 703-549-6995
www.diabetes.org

Lay-flat binding for hands-free reference.
181 pages

3391   How to Cook for People with Diabetes
American Diabetes Association
1660 Duke Street
Alexandria, VA 22314-3447

800-232-3472
Fax: 703-549-6995
www.diabetes.org

One hundred and fifty recipes featuring unusual techniques.
205 pages

3392   If Your Child Has Diabetes: An Answer Book for Parents
Putnam Publishing Group
200 Madison Avenue
New York, NY 10016-3903

212-951-8400

Provides information and recommendations for parents of children with diabetes on subjects such as school, recreation, medical and life insurance and employment as well as general information about diabetes.

3393   Intensified Insulin Management for You
Chronimed Publishing

PO Box 59032
Minneapolis, MN 55459-0032

612-513-6475
800-848-2793
Fax: 612-443-2806

Manual helping those with diabetes to understand and use an intensified insulin regimen under the guidance of their health care provider. A personalized program for advanced diabetes self-care that focuses on emotional and intellectual goals as well as on how diet and exercise fit into an intensified regimen.
85 pages Paperback
ISBN: 0-937721-84-0

3394   Intensive Diabetes Management
American Diabetes Association
1660 Duke Street
Alexandria, VA 22314-3447

800-232-3472
Fax: 703-549-6995
www.diabetes.org

Delivers practical advice on how to help your patients achieve better glucose control through intensified management.
128 pages Softcover

3395   Learning to Live Well with Diabetes
Chronimed Publishing
PO Box 59032
Minneapolis, MN 55459-0032

612-513-6475
800-848-2793
Fax: 612-443-2806

Updated and revised edition reflects the latest medical advances, technologies, and research. In straight-forward language, it explains how to take charge of your diabetes and live an active, healthy life.
525 pages Paperback
ISBN: 0-937721-79-4

3396   Life with Diabetes: A Series of Teaching Outlines
American Diabetes Association
1660 Duke Street
Alexandria, VA 22314-3447

800-232-3472
Fax: 703-549-6995
www.diabetes.org

Presents a comprehensive curriculum for diabetes education. Each outline includes a statement of purpose, prerequisites for attending the session, materials needed for teaching the session, recommended teaching method, a content outline, instructor notes, an evaluation and documentation plan, and suggested readings related to each topic.

3397   Managing Type II Diabetes
Chronimed Publishing
PO Box 59032
Minneapolis, MN 55459-0032

612-513-6475
800-848-2793
Fax: 612-443-2806

Revised and updated guide for people with Type II diabetes. Offers the latest medical advances and practical advice. Includes tips on dealing with emotions, finding motivation to manage diabetes, preventing and treating complications, monitoring blood glucose, and more.
192 pages Paperback
ISBN: 1-885115-26-1

3398   Managing Your Gestational Diabetes
Chronimed Publishing
PO Box 59032
Minneapolis, MN 55459-0032

612-513-6475
800-848-2793
Fax: 612-443-2806

Gives answers to questions on weight gain, injecting insulin, and preventing complications.
128 pages Paperback
ISBN: 1-565610-52-0

3399   Manual of Pediatric Nutrition
Kristy Hendricks RD, MS, ScD (Editor), author
B.C Decker, Inc.
50 King Street E, Floor 2 PO Box620
Ontario, Canada L8N 3K7,

905-522-7017
800-568-7281
Fax: 905-522-7839
e-mail: info@bcdecker.com
www.bcdecker.com

A comprehensive guide that provides an overview of nutritional care for both healthy and ill pediatric patients.
2005 500 pages
ISBN: 1-550093-08-8

3400   Maximizing the Role of Nutrition in Diabetes Management
American Diabetes Association
1660 Duke Street
Alexandria, VA 22314-3447

800-232-3472
Fax: 703-549-6995
www.diabetes.org

Integrates medical, nutritional, and behavioral sciences and recognizes the importance of each in total diabetes care.
64 pages Softcover

3401   Medical Management of Pregnancy Complicated by Diabetes
American Diabetes Association
1660 Duke Street
Alexandria, VA 22314-3447

800-232-3472
Fax: 703-549-6995
www.diabetes.org

Information on every aspect of pregnancy and diabetes, providing precise protocols for treatment. Techniques for managing blood glucose levels from the time of conception through every stage of pregnancy.
136 pages Softcover

3402   Medical Management of Type I Diabetes
American Diabetes Association
1660 Duke Street
Alexandria, VA 22314-3447

800-232-3472
Fax: 703-549-6995
www.diabetes.org

Instruction on all issues impacting patients with Type 1 diabetes, including: blood glucose regulation, nutrition, exercise, blood pressure, blood lipid levels, and other key elements.
176 pages Softcover

3403   Medical Management of Type II Diabetes
American Diabetes Association
1660 Duke Street
Alexandria, VA 22314-3447

800-232-3472
Fax: 703-549-6995
www.diabetes.org

Complete overview of Type II diabetes, including diagnosis and classification, pathogenesis, and prevention/treatment of complications.
112 pages Softcover

3404   Month of Meals Set of 5
American Diabetes Association
1660 Duke Street
Alexandria, VA 22314-3447

800-232-3472
Fax: 703-549-6995
www.diabetes.org

Each planner offers twenty-eight day's worth of tasty selections including a holiday planner, ethnic meals, fast foods, meat and potatoes, and vegetarian dishes. Available individually.
5 planners

3405   Outsmarting Diabetes
Richard S Beaser, author
John Wiley and Sons, Inc.
Customer Service-Consumer Accounts
Indianapolis, IN 46256

877-762-2974
Fax: 800-597-3299
e-mail: consumers@wiley.com
www.wiley.com

Shows how intensive control can dramatically reduce the effects of insulin-dependent diabetes and the risk of long-term complications.
256 pages Paperback
ISBN: 0-471346-94-4

3406   Pumping Insulin
John Walsh PA, CDE and Ruth Roberts, MA, author
Torrey Pines Publishing

The Diabetes Mall
San Diego, CA 92103

619-497-0900
800-988-4772
Fax: 619-497-0900
www.diabetesnet.com

Features information for achieving excellent blood sugar control, correcting pump problems quickly, and lowering risks for complications.
322 pages Paperback

3407 Quick and Easy Meals and Menus
Diabetes Self-Management Books
PO Box 11066
Des Moines, IA 50380-0001

800-664-9269

3408 Quick and Healthy Recipes & Ideas
American Diabetes Association
1660 Duke Street
Alexandria, VA 22314-3447

800-232-3472
Fax: 703-549-6995
www.diabetes.org

More than 190 recipes with complete nutrition information for each.

3409 Quick and Hearty Main Dishes
American Diabetes Association
1660 Duke Street
Alexandria, VA 22314-3447

800-232-3472
Fax: 703-549-6995
www.diabetes.org

Offers recipes for main courses.

3410 Raising a Child with Diabetes: A Guide for Parents
American Diabetes Association
1660 Duke Street
Alexandria, VA 22314-3447

800-232-3472
Fax: 703-549-6995
www.diabetes.org

You'll learn how to help your child adjust to insulin to allow for favorite foods, have a busy schedule and still feel healthy and strong, negotiate the twists and turns of being different, and much more.

3411 Real Life Parenting of Kids with Diabetes
Virginia Nasmyth Loy, author

McGraw-Hill Companies
Returns Department
Dubuque, IA 52002

877-833-5524
Fax: 609-308-4484
e-mail: pbg.ecommerce_custserv@mcgraw-hill.com
www.mcgraw-hill.com

Virginia Loy had engineered successful management of her two sons' diabetes for 12 years at the time of publication. She is offering her organized, experienced, and practical advice to parents, for helping children to cope with and manage their diabetes from elementary school through college.
2001 188 pages Paperback
ISBN: 1-580400-83-3

3412 Resource and Activities Guide
Chronimed Publishing
PO Box 59032
Minneapolis, MN 55459-0032

612-513-6475
800-848-2793
Fax: 612-443-2806

For use with the Diabetes Youth Curriculum. Contains 300 educational activities that correspond with the text in the Curriculum and can easily be removed for photocopying.
260 pages Loose Leaf
ISBN: 0-937721-50-6

3413 Right from the Start
American Diabetes Association
1660 Duke Street
Alexandria, VA 22314-3447

800-232-3472
Fax: 703-549-6995
www.diabetes.org

Addresses issues such as: learning to take charge, coping, changing one's eating habits, getting fit, self-testing, family issues, preventive care, finances, as well as resources to turn to for further information and support. Available for both Type 1 and Type 2.
Pkg. of 25

3414 Savory Soups and Salads
American Diabetes Association
1660 Duke Street
Alexandria, VA 22314-3447

800-232-3472
Fax: 703-549-6995
www.diabetes.org

Offers exciting recipes for quick and healthy side dishes.

3415 Simple and Tasty Side Dishes
American Diabetes Association
1660 Duke Street
Alexandria, VA 22314-3447

800-232-3472
Fax: 703-549-6995
www.diabetes.org

Healthy recipes for the diabetic.

3416 Special Celebrations and Parties Cookbook
American Diabetes Association
1660 Duke Street
Alexandria, VA 22314-3447

800-232-3472
Fax: 703-549-6995
www.diabetes.org

Offers a list of more than 150 holiday recipes.

3417 Take-Charge Guide to Type I Diabetes
American Diabetes Association
1660 Duke Street
Alexandria, VA 22314-3447

800-232-3472
Fax: 703-549-6995
www.diabetes.org

Offers answers to the most important questions regarding Type 1 diabetes.

3418 Therapy for Diabetes Mellitus and Related Disorders
American Diabetes Association
1660 Duke Street
Alexandria, VA 22314-3447

800-232-3472
Fax: 703-549-6995
www.diabetes.org

Guides through the treatment of specific problems of persons with diabetes. Represents the views and experience of leading clinicians in a concise, practical approach to treatment.
384 pages

3419 Type 2 Diabetes: Your Healthy Living Guide
American Diabetes Association
1660 Duke Street
Alexandria, VA 22314-3447

800-232-3472
Fax: 703-549-6995
www.diabetes.org

A thorough guide to staying healthy with Type 2. Includes everything from choosing a health care team and eating and exercising properly to self-monitoring, insulin, dealing with complications, and keep mentally fit.
180 pages

3420 Using Insulin
Torrey Pines Press
The Diabetes Mall
San Diego, CA 92103

619-497-0900
800-988-4772
Fax: 619-497-0900
www.diabetesnet.com

How to take charge of your blood sugars in diabetes. Information on feeling better, improving your health, and achieving peace of mind.
316 pages Paperback

3421 Voice of the Diabetic
811 Chern Street
Columbia, MO 65201

573-875-8911
e-mail: epc@roudley.com
www.nfb.org

Personal stories and practical guidelines by blind diabetics and medical professionals, medical news, resource column and a recipe corner.

3422 Weight Management for Type II Diabetes
John Wiley and Sons, Inc.

Customer Service-Consumer Accounts
Indianapolis, IN 46256

877-762-2974
Fax: 800-597-3299
e-mail: consumers@wiley.com
www.wiley.com

An interactive, personalized guide that helps you manage your weight and your diabetes by making gradual lifestyle changes. Details how to set reasonable goals, keep pace with an exercise program, design your own meal plan, manage stress, and more.
1997 224 pages Paperback
ISBN: 0-471347-50-7

3423 **When Diabetes Complicates Your Life**
Chronimed Publishing
PO Box 59032
Minneapolis, MN 55459-0032

612-513-6475
800-848-2793
Fax: 612-443-2806

Directly addresses the subject of diabetic complications. This revised edition includes chapters on nerves and circulation, kidneys, and eyes. Enhancements to the new edition include a chapter on vitamins, herbs, and supplements, and reference to the latest research.
Feb 1998 208 pages Paperback
ISBN: 1-565611-27-6

Children's Books

3424 **Diabetes**
Franklin Watts Grolier
90 Old Sherman Turnpike
Danbury, CT 06816-0001

203-797-3500
800-621-1115
Fax: 203-797-3197
www.grolier.com

Looks at the differences between juvenile and adult-onset diabetes, discusses the history of the disease, causes, complications and treatments.
128 pages Grades 7-12
ISBN: 0-531108-82-1

3425 **Dinosaur Tamer**
American Diabetes Association
1660 Duke Street
Alexandria, VA 22314-3447

800-232-3472
Fax: 703-549-6995
www.diabetes.org

Twenty-five fictional stories that will entertain, enlighten, and ease your child's frustrations about having diabetes. Each tale evaporates the fear of insulin shots, blood tests, going to diabetes camp, and more.
Ages 8-12

3426 **Even Little Kids Get Diabetes**
Connie Pirner, author

Albert Whitman & Company
6340 Oakton Street
Morton Grove, IL 60053-2723

847-581-0033
800-255-7675
Fax: 847-581-0039
e-mail: mail@awhitmanco.com
www.albertwhitman.com

A preschooler tells how it was discovered when she was only two, that she has this common disease and describes her daily treatment and the precautions her family must observe.
24 pages Hardcover
ISBN: 0-807521-58-8
Pat McPartland, Sales
Joe Campbell, Customer Service

3427 **Everyone Likes to Eat**
John Wiley and Sons, Inc.
Customer Service-Consumer Accounts
Indianapolis, IN 46256

877-762-2974
Fax: 800-597-3299
e-mail: consumers@wiley.com
www.wiley.com

Revised and up-to-date second edition. How children can eat most of the foods they enjoy and still take care of their diabetes. In-

tended for elementary-school-age children, this guide is filled with activities, puzzles, and problem-solving exercises.
128 pages Paperback
ISBN: 0-471346-82-1

3428 **Grilled Cheese**
American Diabetes Association
1660 Duke Street
Alexandria, VA 22314-3447

800-232-3472
Fax: 703-549-6995
www.diabetes.org

Story designed to ease children's fears and frustrations of having diabetes.

3429 **Kiss the Candy Days Good-bye**
Delacorte Press
1540 Broadway
New York, NY 10036-4039

212-354-6500

This book focuses on Jimmy who is surprised to learn he has diabetes after seeming so healthy and fit. The story contains information on symptoms and the dangers of untreated diabetes.
Grades 6-8

3430 **Living with Diabetes**
Franklin Watts Grolier
90 Old Sherman Turnpike
Danbury, CT 06816-0001

203-797-3500
800-621-1115
Fax: 203-797-3197
www.grolier.com

Shows how persons with diabetes can control their illness and lead productive lives.
32 pages Grades 5-7
ISBN: 0-531108-44-9

3431 **Shira: A Legacy of Courage**
Doubleday
666 5th Avenue
New York, NY 10103-0001

212-354-6500

A biographical account of Shira Putter's fight with a rare form of diabetes. Using the victim's diary, this book is both powerful and poignant, as well as an educational resource for all people struggling with diabetes.
Grades 4-9

3432 **Sun, the Rain and the Insulin**
American Diabetes Association
1660 Duke Street
Alexandria, VA 22314-3447

800-232-3472
Fax: 703-549-6995
www.diabetes.org

Author chronicles a week at a summer diabetes camp, using her expertise and experience to capture the journey and the fight to cope that all people go through when diabetes hits the family.

Magazines

3433 **Countdown**
Juvenile Diabetes Foundation International
432 Park Avenue S
New York, NY 10016-8013

212-889-7575
Fax: 212-725-7259

Offers the latest news and information in diabetes research and treatment to everyone from an international arena of diabetes investigators to parents of small children with diabetes, from physicians to school teachers, from pharmacists to corporate executives.
Sandy Dylak, Editor

3434 **Diabetes**
American Diabetes Association
1660 Duke Street
Alexandria, VA 22314-3447

800-232-3472
Fax: 703-549-6995
www.diabetes.org

A peer-reviewed journal focusing on laboratory research.
Monthly

3435 **Diabetes Care**
American Diabetes Association

1660 Duke Street
Alexandria, VA 22314-3447   800-232-3472
Fax: 703-549-6995
www.diabetes.org
A peer-reviewed journal emphasizing reviews, commentaries and original research on topics of interest to clinicians.
Monthly

3436 Diabetes Forecast
American Diabetes Association
1660 Duke Street
Alexandria, VA 22314-3447   800-232-3472
Fax: 703-549-6995
www.diabetes.org
The monthly lifestyle magazine for people with diabetes, featuring complete, in-depth coverage of all aspects of living with diabetes.
Monthly

3437 Diabetes Spectrum: From Research to Practice
American Diabetes Association
1701 N Beauregard Street
Alexandria, VA 22311   800-232-3472
Fax: 703-549-6995
www.diabetes.org
A journal translating research into practice and focusing on diabetes education and counseling.
Quarterly

3438 Joslin Magazine
Joslin Diabetes Center
1 Joslin Place   617-732-2400
Boston, MA 02215-5306   Fax: 617-732-2562
e-mail: diabetes@joslin.harvard.edu
www.joslin.org

3439 Voice of the Diabetic
Ed Bryant, author
National Federation of the Blind
1800 Johnson Street   410-659-9314
Baltimore, MD 21230-4998   Fax: 410-685-5653
e-mail: subscribe@diabetes.nfb.org
www.nfb.org
The leading publication in the diabetes field. Each issue addresses the problems and concerns of diabetes, with a special emphasis for those who have lost vision due to diabetes. Available in print and on cassette.
28 pages Quarterly
Eileen Ley, Director of Publishing
Elizabeth Lunt, Editor

Newsletters

3440 Clinical Diabetes
American Diabetes Association
1660 Duke Street
Alexandria, VA 22314-3447   800-232-3472
Fax: 703-549-6995
www.diabetes.org
A bimonthly newsletter providing practical treatment information for primary care physicians.
BiMonthly

3441 Diabetes Advisor
American Diabetes Association
1701 N Beauregard Street   703-549-1500
Alexandria, VA 22311   800-232-3472
Fax: 703-836-7439
e-mail: askada@diabetes.org
www.diabetes.org
Offers informative articles and research in the area of diabetes for professionals and patients. Offers facts and research on diagnosis, symptoms, technology and the newest devices for persons with diabetes, as well as referral and hotline numbers.
Bi-Monthly
John G Graham IV, CEO

3442 Diabetes Dateline
National Diabetes Information Clearinghouse

1 Information Way   301-654-3327
Bethesda, MD 20205   800-860-8747
Fax: 301-907-8906
e-mail: ndic@info.niddck.nih.gov
www.niddk.nih.gov
BiAnnually

3443 Diabetes Educator
American Association of Diabetes Educators
444 N Michigan Avenue   312-644-2233
Chicago, IL 60611-3959   Fax: 312-644-4411
Offers information to health professionals working with persons with diabetes.
James J Balija, Executive Director

3444 Kid's Corner
American Diabetes Association
1660 Duke Street
Alexandria, VA 22314-3447   800-232-3472
Fax: 703-549-6995
www.diabetes.org
A mini-magazine for kids that offers word searches, puzzles and jokes - plus an encouraging story in each issue about kids with diabetes.
8 pages Quarterly

Pamphlets

3445 Dental Tips for Diabetics
National Diabetes Information Clearinghouse
1 Information Way   301-654-3327
Bethesda, MD 20892-0001   800-860-8747
Fax: 301-907-8906
e-mail: ndic@info.niddk.nih.gov
www.niddk.nih.gov
Discusses the relationship between diabetes and periodontal disease. Describes the symptoms of periodontal problems and preventive measures.

3446 Diabetes Dateline
National Diabetes Information Clearinghouse
1 Information Way   301-654-3327
Bethesda, MD 20892-0001   Fax: 301-907-8906
e-mail: ndic@aerie.com
This bulletin features news about current issues in diabetes research and control, special events, patient and professional meeting, and new publications available from NDIC and other organizations.
Quarterly

3447 Diabetes and Brief Illness
Chronimed Publishing
PO Box 59032   612-513-6475
Minneapolis, MN 55459-0032   800-848-2793
Fax: 612-443-2806
This booklet gives self-care instructions and eating suggestions to prevent development of ketoacidosis during brief illness that disrupts normal eating.
12 pages 10-pack

3448 Diabetes and Exercise
Chronimed Publishing
PO Box 59032   612-513-6475
Minneapolis, MN 55459-0032   800-848-2793
Fax: 612-443-2806
Exercise and weight loss tips and precautions for those with both insulin and non-insulin-dependent diabetes.
36 pages Pack of 10

3449 Diabetes in Pregnancy
March of Dimes
233 Park Avenue South   212-353-8353
New York, NY 10003   Fax: 212-254-3518
e-mail: NY639@marchofdimes.com
www.marchofdimes.com
Fact Sheets: one or two page review written for the general public. Also available electronically on the website: www.marchofdimes.com.

3450 Diabetic Foot Care
American Diabetes Association
1660 Duke Street
Alexandria, VA 22314-3447
800-232-3472
Fax: 703-549-6995
www.diabetes.org
Booklet discussing early detection and prompt treatment of diabetic foot problems.
12 pages

3451 Gestational Diabetes: What To Expect
American Diabetes Association
7 Washington Square
Albany, NY 12205
518-218-1755
888-342-2383
Fax: 518-218-0114
e-mail: ADAorders@pbd.com
www.diabetes.org
A complete comprehensive guide for women with gestational diabetes. Explains the stages in your baby's development, the types of prenatal testing you may recieve, and what to expect during labor, delivery, and beyond.
100 pages
ISBN: 1-580402-33-X

3452 Healthy Eating
Chronimed Publishing
PO Box 59032
Minneapolis, MN 55459-0032
612-513-6475
800-848-2793
Fax: 612-443-2806
Offers simple guidelines for choosing healthful foods, lowering fat intake, and timing meals and snacks. Available in Spanish.
Pack of 10

3453 Healthy Food Choices
American Diabetes Association
1660 Duke Street
Alexandria, VA 22314-3447
800-232-3472
Fax: 703-549-6995
www.diabetes.org
Pamphlet containing the basics of good nutrition.

3454 Hypoglycemia The Other Sugar Disease
Anita Flegg, author
Book Coach Press
3-390 MacKay Street
Ontario, Canada K1M 2C4,   e-mail: info@bookcoachpress.com
www.bookcoachpress.com
This book is filled with dozens of real-life practical tips and will give you the tools to feel better and take control of your life.

3455 Insulin-Dependent Diabetes
National Diabetes Information Clearinghouse
1 Information Way
Bethesda, MD 20892-0001
301-654-3327
Fax: 301-654-3327
e-mail: ndic@aerie.com
Explains diabetes and how it develops and describes the differences between the two major forms of diabetes, insulin-dependent and noninsulin-dependent.

3456 Low Blood Sugar
Chronimed Publishing
PO Box 59032
Minneapolis, MN 55459-0032
612-513-6475
800-848-2793
Fax: 612-443-2806
Pack of 10

3457 Noninsulin-Dependent Diabetes
National Diabetes Information Clearinghouse
1 Information Way
Bethesda, MD 20892-0001
301-654-3327
Fax: 301-907-8906
e-mail: ndic@aerie.com
Describes the symptoms and diagnosis of noninsulin-dependent diabetes; diabetes management, including diet, oral drugs, and insulin; glucose monitoring; and complications.
1992 35 pages

3458 Recognizing and Treating Low Blood Sugar (Hypoglycemia)
Chronimed Publishing
PO Box 59032
Minneapolis, MN 55459-0032
612-513-6475
800-848-2793
Fax: 612-443-2806
The causes, symptoms, and treatment of low blood sugar are clearly presented in this booklet, including guidelines for using glucagon.
12 pages Pack of 10

3459 Taking Care of Gestational Diabetes
International Diabetes Center at Park Nicollet
3800 Park Nicollet Boulevard
Minneapolis, MN 55416-2699
952-993-3874
888-637-2675
Fax: 952-993-0501
e-mail: idccustsvc@parknicollet.com
www.idcpublishing.com
Available in Spanish. Empowering women to make healthy choices for a healthy pregnancy, a healthy baby, and a healthy lifestyle. This book covers food planning, testing, targets, medications and more.
242 pages

3460 Understanding Gestational Diabetes
National Diabetes Information Clearinghouse
1 Information Way
Bethesda, MD 20892-0001
301-654-3327
Fax: 301-907-8906
e-mail: ndic@aerie.com
A guide for women who develop diabetes during pregnancy. It discusses symptoms and diagnosis of gestational diabetes, risk factors, tests during pregnancy and daily management including the use of insulin and blood gluclose monitoring.
44 pages

Audio & Video

3461 ADA Clinical Education Series on CD-Rom
American Diabetes Association
1660 Duke Street
Alexandria, VA 22314-3447
800-232-3472
Fax: 703-549-6995
www.diabetes.org
Features complete texts of Medical Management of Type 1 Diabetes, Medical Management of Type 2 Diabetes, Therapy for Diabetes Mellitus and Related Disorders, 2nd Ed., and Medical Management of Pregnancy Complicated by Diabetes, 2nd Ed.
CD-Rom

3462 Black Experience
American Diabetes Association
300 Research Parkway
Meriden, CT 06450-7137
203-639-0385
800-342-2383
Fax: 203-639-0292
www.diabetes.org/
Designed to increase awareness of diabetes in the black community.
L Butcher, District Director

3463 Diabetes & Exercise Video
American Diabetes Association
1660 Duke Street
Alexandria, VA 22314-3447
800-232-3472
Fax: 703-549-6995
www.diabetes.org
A video offering information on how to maintain good health and exercise in controlling diabetes.

3464 Label Reading and Shopping
American Diabetes Association/Conn. Affiliate
300 Research Parkway
Meriden, CT 06450-7137
203-639-0385
800-842-6323
Fax: 203-639-0292
www.diabetes.org/
Provides practical information on how to shop and what to look for on labels.
Videotape

3465 Living Well with Diabetes
American Diabetes Association/Conn. Affiliate

300 Research Parkway
Meriden, CT 06450-7137

203-639-0385
800-842-6323
Fax: 203-639-0292
www.diabetes.org/

Presents two patient role models who are successfully following a treatment plan for noninsulin dependent diabetes.
Videotape

3466 **On Top of My Game: Living with Diabetes**
American Diabetes Association/Conn. Affiliate
300 Research Parkway
Meriden, CT 06450-7137

203-639-0385
800-842-6323
Fax: 203-639-0292
www.diabetes.org/

Six patients and their families share their day-to-day frustrations and successes in managing diabetes.
Videotape

3467 **Physicians Guide to Type I Diabetes**
American Diabetes Association/Conn. Affiliate
300 Research Parkway
Meriden, CT 06450-7137

203-639-0385
800-842-6323
Fax: 203-639-0292
www.diabetes.org/

Principles of good care in the diagnosis and management of Type I.
Videotape

3468 **Survival Skills for Diabetic Children**
Ajn Company
555 W 57th Street
New York, NY 10019-2961

212-582-8820
800-226-6256
Fax: 212-586-5462

How to provide insulin-dependent children with education, supervision, and support.
1988 28 minutes

3469 **Understanding Diabetes: A User's Guide to Novolin**
American Diabetes Association/Conn. Affiliate
300 Research Parkway
Meriden, CT 06450

203-639-0385
800-842-6323
Fax: 203-639-0292
www.diabetes.org/

Basic information about diabetes and the role insulin plays in blood glucose control.
Videotape

Web Sites

3470 **American Association of Diabetes Educators**

www.aabenet.org

The mission is to enhance the competence of health professionals who teach persons with diabetes, advance the specialty practice of diabetes education, and to improve the quality of diabetes education and care for all those affected by diabetes.

3471 **American Diabetes Association**

www.diabetes.org

Offers a network of 52 affiliates with over 55,000 volunteers, including a professional membership of more than 10,000 physicians, social workers, nutritionists, educators and nurses.

3472 **Diabetes Dictionary**

www.niddk.nih.gov

Provides research funding and support for basic and clinical research in the areas of type 1 and type 2 diabetes and other metabolic disprders.

3473 **Diabetes Exercise and Sports Association**

www.diabetes-exercise.org

Exists to enhance the quality of life for people with diabetes through exercise and physical fitness.

3474 **Healing Well**

www.healingwell.com

An online health resource guide to medical news, chat, information and articles, newsgroups and message boards, books, disease-related web sites, medical directories, and more for patients, friends, and family coping with disabling diseases, disorders, or chronic illnesses.

3475 **Health Finder**

www.healthfinder.gov

Searchable, carefully developed web site offering information on over 1000 topics. Developed by the US Department of Health and Human Services, the site can be used in both English and Spanish.

3476 **Healthlink USA**

www.healthlinkusa.com

Health information concerning treatment, cures, prevention, diagnosis, risk factors, research, support groups, email lists, personal stories and much more. Updated regularly.

3477 **Helios Health**

www.helioshealth.com

Online resource for your health information. Detailed information about specific health topics, access to expert advice from our Medical Advisory Board, and up-to-date health news.

3478 **MedicineNet**

www.medicinenet.com

An online resource for consumers providing easy-to-read, authoritative medical and health information.

3479 **Medscape**

www.medscape.com

Medscape offers specialists, primary care physicians, and other health professionals the Web's most robust and integrated medical information and educational tools.

3480 **National Diabetes Information Clearinghous e**

www.niddk.nih.gov/health/diabetes/ndic

Offers various materials, resources, books, pamphlets and more for persons and families in the area of diabetes.

3481 **WebMD**

www.webmd.com

Information on diabetes, including articles and resources.

Description

3482 Down Syndrome

Down syndrome is a collection of inherited abnormalities caused by an extra chromosome. Instead of having the normal number of chromosomes (46), children with Down syndrome have an extra chromosome 21. (Because there are three copies of chromosome 21 instead of the normal two, Down syndrome is often called trisomy 21). This chromosomal abnormality results in altered growth and development. Approximately 4,000 children are born with Down syndrome every year in the United States. The overall incidence is about 1 in every 700 live births, but there is a marked variability depending on maternal age. In the early childbearing years, the incidence is about 1/2000 live births; for mothers over 40, it rises to at least 1/100 if not more frequent with advancing age.

Down syndrome is associated with a wide variety of clinical signs, although most individuals do not possess all of them. Common findings include decreased muscle tone, slanting eyes with folds of skin in the inside corners, white spots appearing in the irises of the eyes, and single creases across the palms of one or both hands. Physically, children with Down syndrome have broad feet with short toes, short ears and necks, small heads and small oral cavities. Mental development in the child with Down syndrome is impaired; the mean IQ is approximately 50. Hearing and speech abilities may also be hampered. However, many children with Down syndrome can reach surprisingly high levels of achievement. Congenital heart disease is found in nearly half of patients, and there is an increased susceptibility to acute leukemia. Today, most patients survive well into adulthood, although problems such as Alzheimer's Disease and psychiatric illness may increase with age.

It is essential that parents enroll their with Down syndrome in an infant development program. These programs advise parents on how to help a child with Down syndrome in language, cognitive, social and motor skills.

National Agencies & Associations

3483 ARC The ARC of the United States
The ARC of the United States
1660 L Street NW   301-565-3842
Washington, DC 20036   800-433-5255
                               Fax: 301-565-3843
                        e-mail: info@thearc.org
                                www.thearc.org
Works to include all children and adults with cognitive intellectual and developmental disabilities in every community.
Mohan Mehra, President
Nancy Webster, Vice President

3484 Aleh Foundation Aleh Institutions USA
Aleh Institutions USA
5317 13th Avenue   718-851-4596
Brooklyn, NY 11219   800-317-2534
                               Fax: 718-851-4597
                   e-mail: shlomo@alehfoundation.com
                            www.alehfoundation.org
Founded in 1983, the Aleh Rehabilitation Center has served as a residential facility to close to 200 children with multiple, physical and mental disabilities. These children and their families benefit from a wide range of services in a caring, supportive atmosphere.
Rabbi Shlomo Braun, Founder & Director

3485 Canadian Down Syndrome Society
5005 Dalhousie Drive NW   403-270-8500
Calgary Alberta, T3N-5R8   800-883-5608
                               Fax: 403-270-8291
                          e-mail: info@cdss.ca
                                   www.cdss.ca
Resource linking parents and professionals through advocacy education and providing information.
Krista J Flint, Executive Director

3486 National Association for Down Syndrome
PO Box 206   630-325-9112
Wilmette, IL 60091   e-mail: info@nads.org
                                   www.nads.org
A non-for-profit organization founded in Chicago in 1961 by parents of children with Down syndrome who felt a need to create a better environment and bring about understanding and acceptance of people with Down syndrome.
Jackie Rotondi, President
Diane Urhausen, Executive Director

3487 National Dissemination Center for Children with Disabilities
1825 Connecticut Avenue NW   202-884-8200
Washington, DC 20009   800-695-0285
                               Fax: 202-884-8441
                        e-mail: nichcy@aed.org
                                  www.nichcy.org
Publishes free, fact filled newsletters. Arranges workshops. Advises parents on the laws entitling children with disabilities to special education and other services.
Dr Suzanne Ripley, Contact

3488 National Down Syndrome Congress
1370 Center Drive   770-604-9500
Atlanta, GA 30338   800-232-6372
                               Fax: 770-604-9898
                     e-mail: info@ndsccenter.org
                              www.NDSCcenter.org
The mission of the NDSC is to provide information, advocacy, and support concerning all aspects of life for individuals with Down Syndrome.
Brooks Robertson, President
Sue Joe, Resources Specialist

3489 National Down Syndrome Society
666 Broadway   212-460-9330
New York, NY 10012   800-221-4602
                               Fax: 212-979-2873
                         e-mail: info@ndss.org
                                   www.ndss.org
NDSS supports researchers seeking the causes of and answers to many of the medical genetic behavioral and learning problems associated with Down syndrome. Also sponsors symposia and conferences for parents and professionals provides advocacy.
Jon Colman, President
Betsy Goodwin, Founder

3490 National Early Childhood Technical Assistance System
University of North Carolina, Chapel Hill
Campus Box 8040 UNC-CH   919-962-2001
Chapel Hill, NC 27599-0001   Fax: 919-966-7463
                         e-mail: nectac@unc.edu
                                  www.nectac.org
Assists states and other entities in developing comprehensive services for children with special needs through the age of eight and their families.
Lynne Kahn, Director & Principal Investigator
Joan Danaher, Associate Director Information Resources

State Agencies & Associations

California

3491 Down Syndrome Association of Los Angeles
16461 Sherman Way   818-786-0001
Van Nuys, CA 91406   Fax: 818-786-0004
                           e-mail: info@dsala.org
                                  www.dsala.org

Offers information on Down syndrome, counseling, resources, facts, laws and other forms of information.
Gail Williamson, Executive Director
Sandra Baker, Office Administrator/Spanish Coordinator

Colorado

3492 Mile High Down Syndrome Association
2121 S Oneida Street   303-797-1699
Denver, CO 80224   Fax: 303-756-6144
                          e-mail: info@mhdsa.org
                                 www.mhdsa.org

Mac Macsovits, Executive Director
Melissa Davis, Volunteer Coordinator

Connecticut

3493 Connecticut Down Syndrome Congress
263 Farmington Avenue   205-351-1157
Farmington, CT 06030-0485   888-486-8537
               e-mail: manager@ctdownsyndrome.org
                         www.ctdownsyndrome.org

Sheryl Knapp, Secretary
Walter Glomb, President

Florida

3494 Gold Coast Down Syndrome Organization
2255 Glades Road   561-912-1231
Boca Raton, FL 33431   Fax: 561-912-1232
                      e-mail: gcdso@bellsouth.net
                     www.goldcoastdownsyndrome.org

Gold Coast Down syndrome Organization is a private nonprofit corporation dedicated to making the future brighter for people with Down syndrome in Palm Beach County, Florida.

3495 Goodwill Industries-Suncoast
Goodwill Industries-Suncoast
10596 Gandy Boulevard   727-523-1512
St. Petersburg, FL 33702   888-279-1988
                                Fax: 727-577-2749
            e-mail: gw.marketing@goodwill-suncoast.rog
                       www.goodwill-suncoast.org

A nonprofit community based organization whose purpose is to improve the quality of life for people who are disabled, disadvantaged and/or aged. This mission is accomplished through a staff of over 1,200 employees providing independent living skills, affordable housing, career assessment and planning, job skills, training, placement, and job retention assistance with useful employment. Annually, Goodwill Industries-Suncoast serves over 30,000 people in Citrus, Hernando, Levy, Marion and more.
Martin W Gladysz, Chair
R Lee Waits, President/CEO

Georgia

3496 Down Syndrome Association of Atlanta
4355 J Cobb Parkway   404-320-3233
Atlanta, GA 30339   Fax: 770-946-9687
              e-mail: contactus@AtlantaDSAA.org
                            www.atlantadsaa.org

Hawaii

3497 Hawaii Down Syndrome Congress
419 Keoniana Street   808-949-1999
Honolulu, HI 96815   e-mail: Conkay@AOL.com
                               www.downscity.com

Constance K Smith, President

Indiana

3498 Indiana Down Syndrome Foundation
2625 N. Meridian Street #49   317-925-7617
Indianapolis, IN 46208   888-989-9255
                                Fax: 317-925-7619
                      e-mail: info@dsindiana.org
                                www.indianadsf.org

Lisa Tokarz-Guiterre, Executive Director
Jeff Huffman, President

Massachusetts

3499 Massachusetts Down Syndrome Congress
20 Burlington Mall Road   781-221-0024
Melrose, MA 02176   800-664-MDSC
                                Fax: 781-221-0011
                         e-mail: mdsc@mdsc.org
                                   www.mdsc.org

Maureen Gallagher, Executive Director
Sarah Cullen, Outreach Coordinator

Minnesota

3500 Down Syndrome Association of Minnesota
656 Transfer Road   651-603-0720
St Paul, MN 55114   800-511-3696
                                Fax: 651-603-0726
                       e-mail: dsamn@dsamn.org
                                  www.dsamn.org

A non-profit organization dedicated to ensuring that all individuals with Down syndrome and their families receive the support necessary to participate in, contribute to and achieve the fulfillment of life in their community.
Craig Parker, President
Kathleen Forney, Executive Director

New York

3501 Association for Children with Down Syndrome
4 Fern Place   516-933-4700
Plainview, NY 11803   Fax: 516-933-9524
                        e-mail: msmith@acds.org
                                   www.acds.org

Nonprofit educational program that combines national information and research dissemination with direct services at the local level. Services include early intervention, pre-school, recreation programs and residential homes.
Michael M Smith, Executive Director
Cecilia Barry, Principal

Ohio

3502 Down Syndrome Association of Greater Cinci nnati
644 Linn Street   513-761-5400
Cincinnati, OH 45203-1734   Fax: 513-761-5401
                        e-mail: dsagc@dsagc.com
                                   www.dsagc.com

The mission of the Down Syndrome Association of Greater Cincinnati is to provide information resources and support to individuals with Down syndrome, their families, and their communities.
Janet Gora, Executive Director
Nora Lindsay Quinn, Event Coordinator

Tennessee

3503 Down Syndrome Association of Middle Tennessee
111 N Wilson Boulevard   615-386-9002
Nashville, TN 37205-2411   Fax: 615-386-9754
                       e-mail: dsamt@bellsouth.net
                                   www.dsamt.org

A nonprofit organization of families whose mission is to enhance the quality of life for all individuals with Down Syndrome by providing information and support to families professionals and the community.
Sheila Moore, Executive Director
Erin Kice, Program Coordinator

Texas

3504 Down Syndrome Guild of Dallas
701 N Central Expressway   214-267-1374
Richardson, TX 75080-1174   Fax: 972-234-2510
                                       www.downsyndromedallas.org

Kelly Drablos, President
Tamara White, Secretary

3505 Texas Association on Mental Retardation
TAMR Headquarters   512-349-7470
Austin, TX 78755   Fax: 512-349-2117
                               e-mail: pat.holder@tamr-web.com
                                       www.tamr-web.com
An organization made up of professionals, parents, consumers and advocates. Our goal is to create an accessible system of services and resources which support personal choice and promotes lives of dignity and self-determination.
Pat Holder

Virginia

3506 Down Syndrome Association of Hampton Roads
The Endependence Center   757-466-3696
Norfolk, VA 23502   e-mail: DSAHR@verizon.net
                                       www.dsahr.org
The Down Syndrome Association of Hampton Roads is a not-for-profit organization serving the needs of individuals with Down Syndrome and their families. The association is supported by a board of directors, an advisory board and dedicated volunteers.
Andrea Anderson, President
Florence Thacker, Secretary

Wisconsin

3507 Down Syndrome Association of Wisconsin
3211 South Lake Drive   414-327-3729
Milwaukee, WI 53235   866-327-3729
                                   Fax: 414-327-1329
                                 e-mail: info@dsaw.org
                                       www.dsaw.org
An organization created by families for families of individuals and for individuals with Down Syndrome. Our primary mission is to provide each person with Down Syndrome the support needed to achieve personal goals and develop self-esteem.
Tom Oday, President
Nicole Cook, Treasurer

Libraries & Resource Centers

3508 Adult Down Syndrome Center of Lutheran General Hospital
1999 Dempster Street
Park Ridge, IL 60068   847-318-2303
                                       www.advocatehealthc.com
The Adult Down Syndrome Center is a comprehensive medical resource providing multidisciplinary medical and psychosocial care for adults with Down syndrome, with an emphasis on health promotion.
Brian Chicoine MD, Medical Director

3509 Ann Whitehill Down Syndrome Program
Riley Hospital for Children
702 Barnhill Drive
Indianapolis, IN 46202   800-248-1199
                                       rileychildrenshospital.com
Brings together specialists from many areas to address the medical and psychosocial needs of children with Down Syndrome. We also refer the family to local resources for therapy and developmental programs.

3510 Blick Clinic for Developmental Disabilities
640 W Market Street   330-762-5425
Akron, OH 44303-1465   Fax: 330-762-4019
                            e-mail: blickclinic@blickclinic.com
                                       www.blickclinic.com
Blick Clinic is a private, non-profit outpatient clinic which began by a group of parents of children with developmental disabilities and a few volunteer professionals. Together, they developed the

Clinic into a single, comprehensive source of diagnostic, evaluation, treatment, and support group services to persons with developmental disabilities.

3511 Dartmouth-Hitchcock Medical Center - Genetics and Development
One Medical Center Drive   603-653-6044
Lebanon, NH 03756-0001   Fax: 603-653-3585
                                       www.dhmc.org
Dartmouth-Hitchcock Clinic is committed to a regional, integrated, comprehensive healthcare system, which can evolve under physician leadership, lay administrative support and public trustee guidance. DHC and its partnering DHMC organizations are recognized as leaders in using scientific methods to improve health care delivery.
Carol B Andrew EdD, MS
Mary Beth Dinulos, MD

3512 Developmental Evaluation Clinic
Westchester Institute for Human Development
Cedarwood Hall   914-493-8150
Valhalla, NY 10595-1681   e-mail: wihd@wihd.org
                                       www.wihd.org
WIHD envisions a future where all people, including children and adults living with disabilities, fully participate in society, live healthy and productive lives, and have access to culturally appropriate services and supports, emerging technologies, competent professionals, caring families, caregivers, and communities.

3513 Developmental Medicine Center (DMC)
Children's Hospital Boston
300 Longwood Avenue
Boston, MA 02115   617-355-7025
                                       www.childrenshospital.org
Provides developmental evaluation and treatment services for children aged birth to adolescence with a wide range of developmental, behavioral and learning difficulties
Leonard A Rappaport MD, MS, Program Director

3514 Down Syndrome Center of Western Pennsylvania
3420 5th Avenue   412-692-7963
Pittsburgh, PA 15213-2524   Fax: 412-692-5723
                                       www.chp.edu
The Down Syndrome Center of Western Pennsylvania has a lending library of books, videos, audio cassettes and periodicals; provides current information about Down syndrome to families and professionals; maintains a file of articles on issues relating to Down Syndrome and publishes a quarterly newsletter in conjunction with the Down Syndrome Group of Western Pennsylvania.
Dr William Cohen, MD, Director

3515 Down Syndrome Clinic of Houston
6701 Fannin Street, 16th Floor   832-822-3478
Dallas, TX 75235-7701   Fax: 832-825-3399
               e-mail: downsyndrome@texaschildrenshospital.org
                                       www.texaschildreshospital.org
The mission of the Down Syndrome Clinic of Houston is to help individuals with Down syndrome reach his or her fullest potential. We accomplish our goal by offering a clinic where children receive complete evaluations by a multidisciplinary team. Families will obtain needed strategies for management of common concerns.
Nirupama Madduri, MD, Chief of Service
Jennifer Chung, Clinic Coordinator

3516 Dr. Gertrude A Barber National Institute
136 E Avenue   814-453-7661
Erie, PA 16507-1899   Fax: 814-455-1132
                           e-mail: BNIerie@barberinstitute.org
                                       www.barberinstitute.org
We believe that all persons have the capacity for growth and fulfillment, and to that end they must be afforded every opportunity to attain the greatest use of thier potential within themselves and their community.
John Barber, JD, President/CEO
Maureen Barber-Carey, EdD, Executive Vice President

3517 Jane and Richard Thomas Center for Down Syndrome
Cincinnati Center for Developmental Disorders
3333 Burnet Avenue
Cincinnati, OH 45229-3039   513-636-0520
                                  Fax: 513-636-0527
                                       www.cincinnatichildrens.org

The Jane and Richard Thomas Center for Down Syndrome conducts research and offers interdisciplinary evaluations and intervention for infants, children, adolescents and young adults with Down syndrome. By providing a range of comprehensive services within one center, families can now spend less time pursuing services through multiple agencies and professionals.
David J Schonfeld MD, Division Head

3518 Kennedy Krieger Institute
707 N Broadway   443-923-9200
Baltimore, MD 21205-1888   800-873-3377
                                     Fax: 410-550-9292
                            e-mail: info@kennedykrieger.org
                                     www.kennedykrieger.org
Kennedy Krieger Institute is an internationally recognized facility located in Baltimore, Maryland dedicated to improving the lives of children and adolescents with pediatric developmental disabilities through patient care, special education, research, and professional training. Our clinical programs offer an interdisciplinary approach in treatment tailored to the individual needs of each child.
Gary W Goldstein, President

3519 Marcus Institute for Development and Learning
1920 Briarcliff Road   404-727-9450
Atlanta, GA 30329   Fax: 404-727-9598
                          e-mail: Marcus_Info@MarcusInstitute.org
                                     www.marcus.org
Our mission is to provide information, services and programs to people with developmental disabilities and their families, as well as those who live and work with them. We offer integrated state-of-the-art clinical, behavioral, educational and family support services through a single organization to reduce the stress and aggravation for families who may have a child with mild to severe disabilities.
Charles M Shaffer, Jr, President/CEO
Dr Claire Coles, Director Fetal Alcohol Center

3520 MeritCare Children's Hospital Down Syndrome Outpatient Service
Coordinated Treatment Center
736 Broadway   701-234-6600
Fargo, ND 58122-4420   800-828-2901
                                     Fax: 701-234-6965
                                     www.meritcare.com
MeritCare Children's Hospital offers a multidisciplinary outpatient service to help accommodate the special medical developmental, behavioral, family and community needs of patients with Down Syndrome.

3521 Santa Rosa Medical Center
PO Box 7330   210-228-2386
San Antonio, TX 78207-0330
Dr. Robert Clayton

3522 UCSF Children's Hospital Health Library
505 Parnassus Avenue
San Francisco, CA 94143   415-476-1000
                                     www.ucsfhealth.org
This Health Library is an online resource to supplement information your doctors, nurses and pharmacists may provide. Our library includes a medical dictionary and an online calendar of our health events. We have news about our research advances and treatments, patient education materials and listings of other helpful Web sites.

3523 University of Maryland: Department of Pediatrics
22 South Greene Street   410-328-8667
Baltimore, MD 21201   Fax: 410-328-3981
                            http://www.umm.edu/pediatrics/
Recognized throughout Maryland and the mid-Atlantic region as a valuable resource for critically and chronically ill children, the University of Maryland Hospital for Children combines state-of-the-art medicine with family-centered care.

3524 University of Washington: Experimental Education Unit
Box 357925   206-543-4011
Seattle, WA 98195-7925   Fax: 206-543-8480
                                     www.eeuweb.org
The Experimental Education Unit (EEU) is a state-certified special education school that serves children from birth to age 7 with diverse abilities. Faculty at the EEU conduct research projects, and provide training opportunities to undergraduate and graduate students, educators, and other professionals.
Rick Neel, Director

Illinois

3525 LaRabida Children's Hospital: Developmental Disabilities & Delays
East 65th Street at Lake Michigan   773-363-6700
Chicago, IL 60649   e-mail: info@larabida.org
                                     www.larabida.org
La Rabida Children's Hospital is dedicated to excellence in caring for children with chronic illness, disabilities, or who have been abused, allowing them to achieve their fullest potential through expertise and innovation within the health care and academic communities.
Paula Kienberger Jaudes, MD, President/CEO

Iowa

3526 Center for Disabilities and Development
University of Iowa Hospitals and Clinics
100 Hawkins Drive   319-353-6900
Iowa City, IA 52242-1011   877-686-0031
                                     Fax: 319-356-8284
                                     TTY: 877-686-0032
                            e-mail: CDD-Webmaster@uiowa.edu
                              www.healthcare.uiowa.edu/cdd
Provides comprehensive health care and services to people with disabilities of all ages and their families through a combination of outpatient, impatient, and community based programs. UHS provides information, evaluation, treatment recommendations, and training related to aging and disabilities. UHS provides both preservice and inservice training programs for service providers and others who provide services to individuals with disabilities.

Maryland

3527 Mt. Washington Pediatric Clinic
1708 W Rogers Avenue   410-578-8600
Baltimore, MD 21209-4596   Fax: 410-466-1715
                                     www.mwph.org
The primary purpose of the Mt. Washington Pediatric Hospital and its affiliates is to sponsor and promote the provision of the highest quality pediatric health care services in a nurturing environment.
Sheldon J Stein, President/CEO
Robert H Imhoff, III, VP Development

Pennsylvania

3528 Children's Hospital of Philadelphia
34th St & Civic Center Boulevard
Philadelphia, PA 19104-4399   215-590-1000
                                     www.chop.edu
The oldest hospital dedicated exclusively to pediatrics, strives to be the world leader in the advancement of healthcare for children by integrating excellent patient care, innovative research and quality professional education into all of its programs.

Rhode Island

3529 Children's Neurodevelopment Center
Hasbro Children's Hospital
593 Eddy Street
Providence, RI 02903   401-444-5685
                            www.hasbrochildrenshosptial.org
The Children's Neurodevelopment Center (CNDC) at Hasbro Children's Hospital provides evaluation and treatment of children with neurological, genetic, developmental, metabolic and behavioral disorders.
David Mandelbaum MD, PhD, Director

Research Centers

3530 **Institute for Basic Research in Developmental Disabilities**
44 Holland Avenue   718-494-0600
Albany, NY 12229-0001   866-946-9733
                                           Fax: 718-494-0833
                                           TTY: 866-933-4889
                                         www.omr.state.ny.us
Conducts research into neurodegenerative diseases Alzheimer's disease developmental disabilities fragile X syndrome Down's Syndrome autism epilepsy and basic science issues underlying all developmental disabilities.
W Ted Brown, Director
Raju K Pullarkat PhD, Chair Developmental Biochemistry

3531 **Kennedy Krieger Institute - Down Syndrome**
10 Center Drive   301-496-4000
Bethesda, MD 20892   888-554-2080
                                           Fax: 443-923-9138
                                           TTY: 443-923-2645
                         e-mail: webmaster@kennedykrieger.org
                                         clinicalcenter.nih.gov
Dedicated to improving the lives of children and adolescents with pediatric developmental disabilities through patient care special education research and professional training.
John Gallin, Director
Char Koller, Research

3532 **National Institute of Child Health and Human Development**
PO Box 3006
Rockville, MD 20847   800-370-2943
                                           Fax: 301-984-1473
                                           TTY: 888-320-6942
           e-mail: NICHDInformationResourceCenter@mail.nih.
                                         www.nih.gov/nichd

Support Groups & Hotlines

3533 **Down Syndrome Association of Greater Cinci nnati**
644 Linn Street
Cincinnati, OH 45203-1734   513-761-5400
                                           Fax: 513-761-5401
                                   e-mail: janet@dsagc.com
                                              www.dsagc.com
Janet Gora, Executive Director
Collette Maddy, Office Coordinator

3534 **National Down Syndrome Congress**
1370 Center Drive   770-604-9500
Atlanta, GA 30338   800-232-6372
                                           Fax: 770-604-9898
                              e-mail: info@ndsccenter.org
                                         www.ndsccenter.org
Provides information, advocacy and support concerning all aspects of life for individuals with Down syndrome.
David Tolleson, Executive Director

3535 **National Down Syndrome Society Hotline**
666 Broadway   212-460-9330
New York, NY 10012   800-221-4602
                                           Fax: 212-979-2873
                                    e-mail: info@ndss.org
                                               www.ndss.org
NDSS supports researchers seeking the causes of and answers to many of the medical, genetic, behavioral and learning problems associated with Down syndrome; sponsors symposia and conferences for parents and professionals; performs advocacy; provides information and refferal through a toll-free number; and develops and disseminates educational materials.
Jon Colman, President
Patricia Baker, Program Manager

3536 **Parents of Children with Down Syndrome**
Arc of Montgomery County
11600 Nebel Street
Rockville, MD 20852-2538   301-984-5777
                                           Fax: 301-816-2429
                                           TTY: 301-881-1548
                            e-mail: asachs@arcmontmd.org
                                         www.arcmontmd.org/

Activities include formal and informal meetings, parent-to-parent support, contacting new parents of down syndrome children to offer support and information on community resources, providing information on doctors, hospitals and professionals.
Petere Holden, Executive Director
John Slavcoff, President of the Board

Books

3537 **ACDS Infant, Toddler & Pre-school Curriculum for Children**
Association for Children with Down Syndrome
4 Fern Place   516-933-4700
Plainview, NY 11803   Fax: 516-933-9524
                                  e-mail: msmith@acds.org
                                               www.acds.org
This curriculum is user friendly for parents, educators, related service professionals and other caregivers. It provides checklists and teaching strategies to facilitate aquisition of skills in cognition, self-help, socialization, speech and language, gross and fine motor skills plus much more.
Michael M. Smith, Executive Director

3538 **Babies with Down Syndrome**
Woodbine House
6510 Bells Mill Road
Bethesda, MD 20817-1636   800-843-7323
Praised as the finest book ever written for new parents, this book covers everything they need to know about rearing these beautiful and special children in a loving environment.
237 pages Paperback
ISBN: 0-933149-02-6

3539 **Bethy and the Mouse: God's Gifts in Special Packages**
Faith and Life Press
718 Main Street   316-283-5100
Newton, KS 67114-0344
A father's account of his special children, Bethy with Down Syndrome and The Mouse who has been born with microcephaley. A tender story of a father's love.
164 pages Paperback
ISBN: 0-873031-11-3

3540 **Breast Feeding the Baby with Down Syndrome**
LaLeche League International
957 Plum Grove Road   847-519-7730
Schaumburg, IL 60173-4048   Fax: 847-963-0460
                                    e-mail: llli@llli.org
                                               www.llli.org
16 pages Pamphlet

3541 **Cara: Growing with a Retarded Child**
Temple University Press
USB Room 305, Broad & Oxford
Philadelphia, PA 19122   215-204-8787
                                   www.temple.edu/tempress
The author offers information and experiences on raising her daughter, Cara, who has Down syndrome.

3542 **Communication Skills in Children with Down Syndrome**
Woodbine House
6510 Bells Mill Road
Bethesda, MD 20817   800-843-7323
Offers parents a chance to learn what to expect as communication skills progress from infancy through early teenage years. Discussions are included on speech and language therapy, hearing problems, school performance and intelligibility issues.
150 pages Paperback
ISBN: 0-933149-53-0

3543 **Current Approaches to Down's Syndrome**
Greenwood Publishing Group, Inc/Praeger Publishers
PO Box 6926
Portsmouth, NH 03802-6926   800-225-5800
                                           Fax: 877-231-6980
                            e-mail: service@greenwood.com
                                         www.greenwood.com

An exploration of current initiatives relating to Down syndrome in the medical, educational and social fields.
447 pages
ISBN: 0-275902-12-9
David Lane, Editor
Brian Stratford, Editor

3544 Differences in Common: Straight Talk on Mental Retardation/Down Syndrome
Woodbine House
6510 Bells Mill Road
Bethesda, MD 20817   800-843-7323
A collection of essays by the mother of an adult son who has Down syndrome. Focuses on mainstreaming, terminology, parent groups and advocacy.
M Trainer, Editor

3545 Down Syndrome: A Review of Current Knowledge
Jean-Adolphe Rondal, Juan Perera, and Lynn Nadek, author
John Wiley and Sons, Inc.
Customer Service-Consumer Accouts
Indianapolis, IN 46256   877-762-2974
                                          Fax: 800-597-3299
                                          e-mail: consumers@wiley.com
                                          www.wiley.com
1999 350 pages Hardcover
IT Lott, Editor
E McCoy, Editor

3546 Down Syndrome: An Update and Review for Primary Care Physicians
Dartmouth-Hitchcock Medical Center
1 Medical Center Drive   603-650-5000
Lebanon, NH 03756-0001
An excellent medical review of Down syndrome intended for physicians.
WC Cooley, Editor

3547 Down Syndrome: The Facts
Oxford University Press
2001 Evans Road   212-726-6000
Cary, NC 27513-2010   800-451-7556
                                          Fax: 919-677-1303
                                          www.oup-usa.org
A book for parents who have a child with Down syndrome written by a pediatrician who works with Down syndrome children.
M Selikowitz, Editor

3548 From 17 Months to 17 Years...A Look at Down Syndrome
Bonnie Lavender
RR-1, Box 102C   315-287-2973
Richville, NY 13681
Includes profiles of six families who have children with Down syndrome. Offers photographs and accompanying text that detail each family's experiences with Down syndrome.
B Lavender, Editor
GJ Lega, Editor

3549 Medical and Surgical Care for Children with Down Syndrome
Woodbine House
6510 Bells Mill Road
Bethesda, MD 20817-1636   800-843-7323
Provides detailed and easy-to-understand information for parents on a wide range of medical conditions and treatments including: heart disease, recurrent infections, thyroid problems, eye problems, skin conditions, ear, nose and throat problems, orthopedic conditions, leukemia, facial and dental concerns and neurological problems.
320 pages Paperback
ISBN: 0-933149-54-9

3550 Parent's Guide to Down Syndrome: Toward a Brighter Future
Siegfried M Pueschel, MD, PhD, JD, MPH, author
Brookes Publishing Company

Customer Service Department
Baltimore, MD 21285-0624   800-638-3775
                                          Fax: 410-337-8539
                                          e-mail: custserv@brookespublishing.com
                                          www.brookespublishing.com
A comprehensive reference book especially for new parents but useful and informative to seasoned parents as well. Range of topics include a history of Down syndrome, physical characterisitcs, developmental expectations, early intervention, feeding the young child and the school years.
2001 338 pages Paperback
ISBN: 1-557664-52-8

3551 Parents of Children with Down Syndrome
11600 Nebel Street   301-984-5792
Rockville, MD 20852-2538   Fax: 301-816-2429
Activities include formal and informal meetings, parent-to-parent support, contacting new parents of down syndrome children to offer support and information on community resources, providing information on doctors, hospitals and professionals.

3552 Paul
Miriam Perrone
440 Park Avenue   912-638-8551
Saint Simons Island, GA 31522-4357
How a determined mother carved a semi-independent life for her now-grown Down's syndrome child.

3553 Show Me No Mercy
Cokesbury
PO Box 801 a young adult man with Down syndrome relates the experience of how he will be reunited with his son after a family tragedy separates them.
R Perske, Editor

3554 Since Owen
Johns Hopkins University Press
2715 N Charles Street   410-516-6900
Baltimore, MD 21211-2105   Fax: 410-516-6968
                                          www.press.jhu.edu
A well written book displaying understanding from a veteran parent communicating with other parents of children with disabilities.
466 pages
Charles R Callanan, Editor

3555 Teaching the Infant with Down Syndrome: A Guide for Parents & Professionals
Pro-Ed, Inc.
8700 Shoal Creek Boulevard   512-451-3246
Austin, TX 78757-6897   800-897-3202
                                          Fax: 800-397-7633
                                          e-mail: info@proedinc.com
                                          www.proedinc.com
A manual providing teaching ideas and activities that can be used to assist an infant's development.
MJ Hanson, Editor

3556 To Give an Edge: A Guide for New Parents of Children with Down's Syndrome
Viking Press
7000 Washington Avenue S   612-941-8780
Eden Prairie, MN 55344-3580
A guide for new parents designed to provide information about the disorder and how other parents of children with Down syndrome have coped.
JE Rynders, Editor
JM Horrobin, Editor

3557 Understanding Down's Syndrome An Introduction for Parents
Brookline Books
PO Box 1209   617-734-6772
Brookline, MA 02445   800-666-2665
                                          Fax: 617-734-3952
                                          www.brooklinebooks.com
The author provides answers and explanations to the countless questions directed to him during his twenty years' involvement with Down syndrome individuals and their families.
Softcover
ISBN: 1-571290-09-5

Children's Books

3558 Our Brother Has Down's Syndrome: An Introduction for Children
Firefly Books
250 Sparks Avenue
Willowdale, M2H 2S4,   416-499-8412
                                   e-mail: service@fireflybooks.com
                                              www.fireflybooks.com
Two young sisters tell about their little brother with Down syndrome in this color picture book.
21 pages
S Cairo, Editor

3559 Secret Place of the Stairs
Harper & Row
10 E 53rd Street
New York, NY 10022-5299   212-207-7000
A story that weaves many themes, including the institutionalizing of the protagonist's sister, her parents' divorce and her own expectations.
Grades 7-10

3560 We Can Do It!
Macmillan
866 3rd Avenue
New York, NY 10022-6221   212-702-7865
                                              www.macmillan.com
A colorful book of photographs that show the daily activities of young children with different developmental delays, including Down syndrome.
L Dwight, Editor

Magazines

3561 Down Syndrome, Papers and Abstracts for Professionals
200 Rabbit Road
Gaithersburg, MD 20878   301-963-1857
Quarterly review of research literature pertaining to Down syndrome.
Monthly

3562 Exceptional Parent Magazine
209 Harvard Street   617-730-5800
Brookline, MA 02446-5071   Fax: 617-730-8742
A publication dealing with many issues affecting exceptional children and their families.
Monthly

Newsletters

3563 Down Syndrome News
National Down Syndrome Congress
7000 Peachtree Dunwoody Rd NE   770-604-9500
Atlanta, GA 30328-1655   800-232-6372
                              e-mail: NDSC.center@aol.com
                                        www.ndsccenter.org
Contains book reviews, articles and items of interest to those touched by Down syndrome.
10x Annually
Frank J Murphy, Executive Director

3564 Down Syndrome Today
Down Syndrome Today Publications
PO Box 212   516-654-3242
Holtsville, NY 11742-0212
Offers information, articles, resources and materials for the parent and professional working and nurturing patients and persons with Downs syndrome.
Debra Hoeft, Publisher

3565 National Down Syndrome Society Update
666 Broadway   212-460-9330
New York, NY 10012-2317   800-221-4602
                                                    Fax: 212-979-2873
                                                       www.ndss.org
Offers information on the activities of the society, new breakthroughs in medical technology, articles offering state of the art in-

formation to families and individuals with Down syndrome, and answers to questions about the illness.
12 pages Quarterly
Fran Goldstein, Editor

3566 On the Up with Down Syndrome
Carole Shafer, author
Down Syndrome Association of Wisconsin
9401 West Beloit Road   414-327-3729
Milwaukee, WI 53227   866-327-3729
                                                    Fax: 414-327-1329
                                      e-mail: thomtalent@aol.com
                                                       www.dsaw.org
Offers the exchange of ideas and experiences. Free to our members. Membership is $20.00/year.
Quarterly
Ron Irwin, Board President
Robbin Lyons, Newsletter Contact

Pamphlets

3567 Alzheimer's Disease and Down Syndrome
National Down Syndrome Society
666 Broadway   212-460-9330
New York, NY 10012-2317   800-221-4602
                                                       www.ndss.org
1995

3568 Down Syndrome
March of Dimes
233 Park Avenue South   212-353-8353
New York, NY 10003   Fax: 212-254-3518
                              e-mail: NY639@marchofdimes.com
                                             www.marchofdimes.com

3569 Heart and Down Syndrome
National Down Syndrome Society
666 Broadway   212-460-9330
New York, NY 10012-2317   800-221-4602
                                                       www.ndss.org
1995

3570 Life Planning and Down Syndrome
National Down Syndrome Society
666 Broadway   212-460-9330
New York, NY 10012-2317   800-221-4602
                                                       www.ndss.org

3571 Neurology of Down Syndrome
National Down Syndrome Society
666 Broadway   212-460-9330
New York, NY 10012-2317   800-221-4602
                                                       www.ndss.org
1995

3572 New Parents
Association for Children with Down Syndrome
4 Fern Place   516-933-4700
Plainview, NY 11803   Fax: 516-933-9524
                                      e-mail: msmith@acds.org
                                                       www.acds.org
Bibliography compiled for parents who have just given birth to a child with Down syndrome. Free upon reciept of a stamped, self-addressed envelope.
Michael Smith, Executive Director

3573 Sexuality in Down Syndrome
National Down Syndrome Society
666 Broadway   212-460-9330
New York, NY 10012-2317   800-221-4602
                                                       www.ndss.org
1995

3574 Speech and Language in Children and Adolescents with Down Syndrome
National Down Syndrome Society

666 Broadway
New York, NY 10012-2317

212-460-9330
800-221-4602
www.ndss.org

1995

Audio & Video

3575 Adaptation to the Initial Crisis
Lawren Productions
930 Pitner Avenue
Evanston, IL 60202-1556

847-328-6700
800-421-2363

A family learns to adapt to the birth of a child with a handicap.

3576 Bernardsville Beginnings
National Down Syndrome Society
666 Broadway
New York, NY 10012-2317

212-460-9330
800-221-4602
Fax: 212-979-2873
www.ndss.org

Follows Alison through her first full year in a first grade inclusion program. Step-by-step account of teaching staff preparation, classroom experiences, a portrayal of one girl's successful adjustment, and a whole class matured by the experience.
23 minutes

3577 Bittersweet Waltz
National Down Syndrome Society
666 Broadway
New York, NY 10012-2317

212-460-9330
800-221-4602
Fax: 212-979-2873
e-mail: info@ndss.org
www.ndss.org

Experience of Alec and his first year included in a regular fifth grade class. From a point of view of a parent, a child, and the school administration.
18 minutes

3578 Colin and Ricky
Lawren Productions
930 Pitner Avenue
Evanston, IL 60202-1556

847-328-6700
800-421-2363

A young boy comes to deal with his disappointment surrounding the birth of his baby brother with Down syndrome.

3579 Congratulations: An Introduction to Down Syndrome for Parents/Family/Friends
New Challenges
96 Ogden Avenue
White Plains, NY 10605

914-287-0723

Film for parents which addresses some of the most commonly asked questions about raising a child with Down syndrome.

3580 Daddy's Girl
Carle Media
110 W Main Street
Urbana, IL 61801-2715

217-384-4838

A film starring a twelve-year-old actress with Down syndrome, dealing with her divorced father's inability to accept the fact that his daughter has Down syndrome.
Carolyn Baxley

3581 Down Syndrome: See the Potential
Down Syndrome Association of Charlotte
PO Box 3136
Charlotte, NC 28210

800-232-6372

Video highlighting the capability of children with Down syndrome.

3582 Gifts of Love
National Down Syndrome Society
666 Broadway
New York, NY 10012-2317

212-460-9330
800-221-4602
Fax: 212-979-2873
www.ndss.org

Four families of children with Down syndrome talk about their feelings and experiences with their children, particularly during the first six years. All the children live at home and attend programs in their communities.
25 minutes

3583 Infant Motor Development: A Look at the Phases
Communication Skill Builders/Therapy Skill Builder
3830 E Bellevue
Tucson, AZ 85733

520-323-7500

A video depicting development in and activities for infants birth through 12 months.

3584 New Expectations
Lawren Productions
930 Pitner Avenue
Evanston, IL 60202-1556

800-421-2363

Focuses on the emotional and technical aspects of Down syndrome. Highlights four persons at various life stages from infancy to adulthood in the areas of education and employment.

3585 New Set of Fears, a New Set of Hopes
Meyer Children's Rehabilitation Institute
Resource Center, 444 S 44th Street
Omaha, NE 68131

402-559-7467
800-232-6372

Explores the way a family adjusts as they go through the life cycle with their child who has Down syndrome.

3586 Opportunities to Grow
National Down Syndrome Society
666 Broadway
New York, NY 10012-2317

212-460-9330
800-221-4602
Fax: 212-979-2873
e-mail: info@ndss.org
www.ndss.org

Sequel to Gifts of Love video shows how people with Down syndrome, ages 6 to 26, participate equally in all phases of community life. Vignettes of 15 young men and women illustrate how inclusion, education, computer facilitation, socialization programs, and employment training help them to fulfill their potential.
25 minutes

3587 Stepping Stones
AIT
PO Box A
Bloomington, IN 47402-0120

800-457-4509

Series of video programs on teaching basic skills to at-risk, special needs and normally developed children.

3588 Thanks Mom and Dad: Profiles of Patrick
University of Washington
CDMRC Mail Stop WJ-10
Seattle, WA 98195-0001

206-543-4011
800-232-6372

Documentary on the life of Patrick, a young man with Down syndrome from birth through his graduation from high school.

3589 You Don't Outgrow Down Syndrome
National Association for Down Syndrome
PO Box 4542
Oak Brook, IL 60522-4542

630-325-9112
800-232-6372
www.nads.org

Winner of the second annual International Rehabilitation Film Festival.

Web Sites

3590 Aleh Foundation

www.aleh.org

Aleh Rehabilitation Center has served as a residential facility to close to 200 children with multiple, physical and mental disabilities.

3591 Down Syndrome

www.downsyn.com

A resource for new paretns of children with Down syndrome. Provides a personnel perspective from parents who also have children with Down syndrome.

3592 Healing Well

www.healingwell.com

An online health resource guide to medical news, chat, information and articles, newsgroups and message boards, books, disease-related web sites, medical directories, and more for patients, friends, and family coping with disabling diseases, disorders, or chronic illnesses.

3593 Health Finder

www.healthfinder.gov

Searchable, carefully developed web site offering information on over 1000 topics. Developed by the US Department of Health and Human Services, the site can be used in both English and Spanish.

3594 Healthlink USA

www.healthlinkusa.com

Health information concerning treatment, cures, prevention, diagnosis, risk factors, research, support groups, email lists, personal stories and much more. Updated regularly.

3595 Helios Health

www.helioshealth.com

Online resource for your health information. Detailed information about specific health topics, access to expert advice from our Medical Advisory Board, and up-to-date health news.

3596 MedicineNet

www.medicinenet.com

An online resource for consumers providing easy-to-read, authoritative medical and health information.

3597 Medscape

www.medscape.com

Medscape offers specialists, primary care physicians, and other health professionals the Web's most robust and integrated medical information and educational tools.

3598 National Down Syndrome Society

www.ndss.org

NDSS works to obtain a better understanding of Down syndrome, the potential of people with Down syndrome, to support research about the condition, and to provide information and referral services for families and professionals.

3599 WebMD

www.webmd.com

Information on Down Syndrome, including articles and resources.

Description

3600 ## Eating Disorders (Anorexia Nervosa, Bulimia)

Anorexia nervosa and bulimia nervosa are eating disorders characterized by a disturbed sense of body image and an irrational fear of obesity. They are manifested by abnormal patterns relating to food and by self-induced, marked weight loss.

Anorexia is a psychiatric disorder in which dieting and a desire for thinness leads to excessive weight loss. About 95 percent of persons with this disorder are female, although males can be affected. The onset usually occurs during adolescence and some sufferers are in their 60s. Anorexia nervosa is characterized by self-starvation, food preoccupation and rituals, compulsive exercising, and often a resulting absence of menstrual cycles. The cause is unknown, although social factors appear to play an important role, including advertisements that equate thinness with desirability. Denial is a prominent feature, and sufferers usually resist treatment.

Bulimia is characterized by recurring episodes of binge eating followed by efforts to avoid weight gain, such as purging through self-induced vomiting or abuse of laxatives and/or diuretics (water pills). Unlike patients with anorexia, those with bulimia usually have normal weight. Binges are often triggered by psychological stress and carried out in secret. Warning signs of bulimia include eating uncontrollably, frequent use of the bathroom, erosion of dental enamel of the front teeth (from vomiting), and painless swollen salivary glands. Bulimia may coexist with anorexia.

Anorexia nervosa is associated with a 10 percent death rate, generally from a sudden disturbance of heart rhythm. Fortunately, most sufferers will eventually return to a normal or near-normal body weight, although many continue to struggle with body image and unhealthy eating patterns. Treatment for both illnesses is similar, beginning with the need to restore body weight. Initial treatment may require hospitalization for physical stabilization. Long-term psychological treatment and behavior modification is often necessary and focuses on behavioral and emotional growth for both the individual with the eating disorder and their family. See also *Obesity*.

National Agencies & Associations

3601 **Academy for Eating Disorders**
111 Deer Lake Road
Deerfield, IL 60015-1577
847-498-4274
Fax: 847-480-9282
e-mail: info@aedweb.org
www.aedweb.org
AED is an association of multidisciplinary professionals promoting effective treatment, developing prevention initiatives, advocating for the field, stimulating research and sponsoring an annual conference.
Debra K Katzman, President
Debbie Truebold, Executive Director

3602 **American Dietetic Association**
120 S Riverside Plaza
Chicago, IL 60606-6995
312-899-0040
800-877-1600
e-mail: media@eatright.org
www.eatright.org
ADA offers nutrition information consumer tips nutrition fact sheets consumer frequently asked questions and referrals to registered dieticians.
Patricia M Babjak, Chief Executive Officer
Judith C Rodriguez, President

3603 **Anna Westin Foundation**
PO Box 268
Chaska, MN 55318
952-361-3051
e-mail: kitty@annawestinfoundation.org
www.annawestinfoundation.org
The Anna Westin Foundation is dedicated to the prevention and treatment of eating disorders. They are committed to preventing the tragic loss of life to anorexia nervosa and bulimia and to raising public awareness of those dangerous illnesses.
Kitty Westin, President

3604 **Anorexia Nervosa & Bulimia Association**
767 Bayridge Drive
Kingston Ontario, K7P-1C0
www.phe.queensu.ca
Facilitate advocate and coordinate support for any individual directly or indirectly affected by eating disorders and to raise public awareness through improved communication and the provision of education within our community.

3605 **Dads and Daughters**
34 E Superior Street
Duluth, MN 55802
218-772-3942
888-824-DADS
Fax: 218-728-0314
e-mail: info@dadsanddaughters.org
www.thedadman.com
Provides tools to strengthen father-daughter relationships and transform pervasive cultural messages that value daughters more for how they look than who they are.
Gregg Rutter, Development Director

3606 **Eating Disorders Action Group**
6156 Quinpool Road
Halifax Nova Scotia, B3L 1-3Z9
902-443-9944
e-mail: reception@edag.ca
www.edag.ca
A community based charitable organization dedicated to promoting healthy body image and self esteem and to supporting individuals who experience disordered eating.

3607 **Eating Disorders Anonymous**
PO Box 55876
Phoenix, AZ 85078-5876
e-mail: info@eatingdisordersanonymous.org
www.4eda.org
EDA provides information about local support group meetings.

3608 **Eating Disorders Coalition for Research, Policy and Action**
720 7th Street NW
Washington, DC 20001-4303
202-543-9570
Fax: 202-543-9570
e-mail: manager@eatingdisorderscoalition.org
www.eatingdisorderscoalition.org
Advocates at the federal level on behalf of people with eating disorders their families and professionals working with these populations. Promotes federal support for improved access to care.
David Jaffe, Executive Director
Jeanine Cogan, Policy Director

3609 **Healthy Weight Network**
402 S 14th Street
Hettinger, ND 58639
701-567-2646
Fax: 701-567-2602
e-mail: hwj@healthyweight.net
www.healthyweight.net
Promotes information and resources pertaining to the Health at Any Size paradigm.
Frances M Berg MS, Founder/Editor

3610 **International Association of Eating Disorders Professionals**
PO Box 1295
Pekin, IL 61555-1295
309-346-3341
800-800-8126
Fax: 309-346-2874
e-mail: iaedpmembers@earthlink.net
www.iaedp.com

IAEDP Offers professional counseling and assistance to the medical community, courts, law enforcement officials and social welfare agencies.
Mary Bellofatto, President
Emmett R Bishop MD CEDS, Immediate Past President

3611   Jessie's Hope Society
11739 23rd Street   604-466-4877
Maple Ridge, BC, V2X-5X8   877-288-0877
                                          Fax: 604-466-4897
                                     e-mail: info@jessieshope.org
                                          www.jessieshope.org
Promote positive body image by fostering in youth within communities and across cultures throughout British Columbia.
Brian W Chittock, Executive Director

3612   National Association of Anorexia Nervosa and Associated Disorders
PO Box 640   63- 57- 133
Naperville, IL 60566   Fax: 847-433-4632
                                      e-mail: anadhelp@anad.org
                                              www.anad.org
Works to prevent eating disorders and provides numerous programs — all free — to help victims and families including hotlines, support groups, referrals, information packets and newsletters. Educational/prevention programs include presentations and early detection.
Vivian Hanse Meehan, Founder/President
Laura Discipio, Executive Director

3613   National Eating Disorder Information Centr e
ES 7-421, 200 Elizabeth Street   416-340-4156
Toronto, Ontario, M5G-2C4   866-633-4220
                                          Fax: 416-340-4736
                                        e-mail: nedic@uhn.on.ca
                                              www.nedic.ca
Promotes healthy lifestyles, including both healty eating and appropriate, enjoyable exercise.
Merryl Bear MEd, Director
Jessica Rust, Administrative Coordinator

3614   National Eating Disorders Association
603 Stewart Street   206-382-3587
Seattle, WA 98101   800-931-2237
                                          Fax: 206-829-8501
                             e-mail: info@NationalEatingDisorders.org
                                     www.nationaleatingdisorders.org
Our mission is to eliminate eating disorders and body dissatisfaction through prevention efforts education referral and support services advocacy training and research.
Lynn S Grefe MA, Chief Executive Officer
Molly Bauthues, Communications Manager

3615   National Eating Disorders Screening Program
One Washington Street   781-239-0071
Wellesley Hills, MA 02481   Fax: 781-431-7447
                             e-mail: smhinfo@mentalhealthscreening.org
                                     www.mentalhealthscreening.org
Offers eating disorders screening.
Douglas G Jacobs MD, President & CEO

3616   National Women's Health Information Center
8270 Willow Oaks Corporate Drive
Fairfax, VA 22031   800-994-9662
                                          Fax: 703-560-6598
                                          TTY: 888-220-5446
                                          TDD: 888-220-5446
                                    e-mail: Wanda.jones@hhs.gov
                                              www.4woman.gov
Government agency with free health information for women.
Wanda K Jones PhD, Deputy Assistant Secretary for Health
Frances E Ashe-Goins RN, Deputy Director

3617   Weight-control Information Network National Institutes of Health
National Institutes of Health

1 WIN Way   202-828-1025
Bethesda, MD 20892-3665   877-946-4627
                                          Fax: 202-828-1028
                                    e-mail: win@info.niddk.nih.gov
                                     www.win.niddk.nih.gov/index.htm
Information on obesity weight-control and nutrition.
BiAnnual

State Agencies & Associations

Connecticut

3618   Renfrew Center of Connecticut
1445 E. Putnam Avenue
Wilton, CT 06897   800-736-3739
                                          Fax: 203-563-9936
                                   e-mail: foundation@renfrew.org
                                          www.renfrewcenter.com

Florida

3619   Renfrew Center of Miami
151 Majorca Avenue
Coral Gables, FL 33134   800-REN-FREW
                                          Fax: 305-445-2729
                                   e-mail: info@renfrewcenter.com
                                          www.renfrewcenter.com

3620   Renfrew Center of South Florida
7700 Renfrew Lane
Coconut Creek, FL 33073   800-736-3739
                                          Fax: 954-698-9007
                                   e-mail: info@renfrewcenter.com
                                          www.renfrewcenter.com

Maryland

3621   St. Joseph's Medical Center
7601 Osler Drive
Towson, MD 21204   410-337-1000
                                          www.sjmcmd.org
John Tolmie, President/CEO

Massachusetts

3622   Massachusetts Eating Disorder Association
92 Pearl Street   617-558-1881
Newton, MA 02458   866-343-MEDA
                                          Fax: 617-558-1771
                                     e-mail: info@medainc.org
                                          www.medainc.org
A nonprofit organization dedicated to the treatment and prevention of eating disorders. MEDA provides help line resource and referral, assessments, client consultations, individual therapy, support groups and an intensive evening treatment program.
100+ Members
Rebecca Manley, Founder
Beth Mayer, CEO

New Jersey

3623   American Anorexia Bulimia Association: New Jersey Chapter
10 Station Place   732-549-6886
Metuchen, NJ 09940   800-522-2230
                                          Fax: 609-688-1544
                                     e-mail: njaaba@NJAABA.org
                                              www.njaaba.org

3624   Renfrew Center of Northern New Jersey
174 Union Street
Ridgewood, NJ 07450   800-736-3739
                                          Fax: 201-652-6253
                                   e-mail: info@renfrewcenter.org
                                          www.renfrewcenter.com

New York

3625 National Eating Disorders Association Long Island
603 Stewart Street 206-382-3587
Seattle, WA 98101 800-931-2237
Fax: 206-829-8501
e-mail: info@NationalEatingDisorders.org
www.nationaleatingdisorders.org
Nonprofit organization devoted to prevention, education and support on the issue of eating disorders. As the number of eating disorder sufferers has grown significantly in our local community, the council was developed to deal with the needs of those suffering with eating disorders.
Robbie Munn, President
Lynn Grefe, CEO

3626 Renfrew Center of New York
11 E 36th Street
New York, NY 10016 800-736-3739
Fax: 212-686-1865
e-mail: info@renfrewcenter.org
www.renfrewcenter.com

3627 Westchester Task Force on Eating Disorders/American Anorexia Bulimia
3 Mount Joy Avenue 914-472-3701
Scarsdale, NY 10583-2632

Pennsylvania

3628 American Anorexia Bulimia Association of Philadelphia
PO Box 1287 215-221-1864
Langhorne, PA 19047 Fax: 215-702-8944
www.aabaphila.org

3629 American Anorexia Bulimia Association:
PO Box 1287 215-221-1864
Langhorne, PA 19047 Fax: 215-702-8944
www.aabaphila.org

3630 Pennsylvania Educational Network for Eating Disorders
4801 McKnight Road
Pittsburgh, PA 15101 412-215-7967
www.pened.org
PENED is a nonprofit organization providing education, support, and referral information to the general and professional public.

3631 Renfrew Center of Bryn Mawr
735 Old Lancaster Road
Bryn Mawr, PA 19010 800-736-3739
Fax: 610-527-9361
e-mail: info@renfrewcenter.org
www.renfrewcenter.com

3632 Renfrew Center of Philadelphia
475 Spring Lane
Philadelphia, PA 19128 800-REN-FREW
Fax: 215-482-7390
e-mail: info@renfrew.org
www.renfrewcenter.com

Research Centers

3633 Academy for Eating Disorders
111 Deer Lake Road 847-498-4274
Deerfield, IL 60015-1577 Fax: 847-480-9282
e-mail: info@aedweb.org
www.aedweb.org
Disseminate knowledge regarding eating disorders to members of the Academy other professionals and the general public
Debra Katzman, President
Susie Orbach, Board of Advisor

3634 Center for the Study of Anorexia and Bulimia
1841 Broadway at 60th Street 212-333-3444
New York, NY 10023 Fax: 212-333-5444
www.icpnyc.org
The Institute is composed of a group of 150 professionally trained licensed psychotherapists who offer a full range of psychotherapeutic services including individual and group psy-

chotherapy and psychoanalysis in addition to more specialized treatment services
Jim M Pollack CSW, Executive Director/Director of Treatment
Ron Taffel PhD, Chair

3635 Division of Digestive & Liver Diseases of Cloumbia University
630 W 168th Street 212-305-5960
New York, NY 10032-3784 Fax: 212-305-8466
e-mail: hjw14@columbia.edu
www.cumc.columbia.edu
The Division's faculty members are devoted to research and the clinical care of patients with gastrointestinal liver and nutritional disorders. The Division is also responsible for the Gastroenterology Training Program at the medical center and for teaching medical students interns residents fellows and attending physicians aspects of gastrointestinal and liver diseases
Howard J Worman MD, Division Director
Karen Wisdom, Director

3636 Harris Center for Education and Advocacy in Eating Disorders
2 Longfellow Place 617-726-8470
Boston, MA 02114 Fax: 617-726-1595
e-mail: dherzog@partners.org
www.harriscentermgh.org
Conducts research provides a newsletter and information.
David B Herzog MD, Director
David B Herzog MD, Director

Support Groups & Hotlines

3637 AABA Support Group
Tucker Pavilion
Richmond, VA 23225 804-320-3911
Chippenham Medical Center, Tucker Pavillion, 7101 Jahnke Road. Every 1st and 3rd Tuesday of the month, 7:30 p.m.
Elliot Spanier, Contact

3638 About Kids GI Disorders
IFFGD
PO Box 170864 414-964-1799
Milwaukee, WI 53217-8076 888-964-2001
Fax: 414-964-7176
e-mail: iffgd@iffgd.org
www.aboutkidsgi.org
ABOUT KIDS is the pediatric branch of the International Foundation for Functional Gastrointestinal Disorders (IFFGD), a registered nonprofit education and research organization founded in 1991. Their mission is to inform, assist, and support those affected by gastrointestinal (GI) disorders, addressing issues of digestive health in children through support of education and research. IFFGD promotes awareness among the public, health care providers, researchers, and regulators.
Nancy J Norton, President/Founder

3639 Association of Gastrointestinal Motility D isorders
AGMD International Corporate Headquarters
12 Roberts Drive 781-275-1300
Bedford, MA 01730 Fax: 781-275-1304
e-mail: digestive.motility@gmail.com
www.agmd-gimotility.org
A non-profit international organization which serves as an integral educational resource concerning digestive motility diseases and disorders. Also functions as an important information base for members of the medical and scientific communities. Also provides a forum for patients suffering from digestive motility diseases and disorders as well as their families and members of the medical, scientific, and nutritional communities.
Mary Angela DeGrazia-DiTucci, President/Patient/Founder

3640 Coconut Creek Eating Disorders Support Group
Renfrew Center
7700 NW 48th Avenue 954-698-9222
Coconut Creek, FL 33073-3508 877-367-3383
Fax: 954-698-9007
www.renfrew.org

Samuel Menagad, Director

3641 Eating Disorder Resource Center
330 W 58th Street
New York, NY 10019
212-989-3987
e-mail: info@edrcnyc.org
www.edrcnyc.org

A specialized treatment program for women and men who were suffering from bulimia. Now EDRC treats eating disorders of all kinds, offering individual, group, family and couples treatment for those challenged by bulimia, binge eating disorder, anorexia and other kinds of body dysmorphia.

3642 Eating Disorders Association of New Jersey
10 Station Place
Metuchen, NJ 08840
800-522-2230
Fax: 732-906-9307
e-mail: info@edanj.org
www.edanj.org

A non-profit state organization whose mission is to provide supportive services and resources to indivudals affected by eating disorders, including family members and friends.

3643 First Presbyterian Church in the City of New York Support Groups
First Presbyterian Church in the City of New York
12 West 12th Street
New York, NY 10011
212-675-6150
e-mail: fpcnyc@fpcnyc.org
www.fpcnyc.org

The First Presbyterian Church in the City of New York provides numerous programs and supports groups for both adults and children including an educational program for autistic children.
Jon M Walton, Senior Pastor

3644 Holliswood Hospital Psychiatric Care, Serv ices and Self-Help/Support Groups
87-37 Palermo Street
Holliswood, NY 11423
718-776-8181
800-486-3005
Fax: 718-776-8572
e-mail: HolliswoodInfo@libertymgt.com
www.holliswoodhospital.com/

The Holliswood Hospital, a 110-bed private psychiatric hospital located in a quiet residential Queens community, is a leader in providing quality, acute inpatient mental health care for adult, adolescent, geriatric and dually diagnosed patients. Holliswood Hospital treats patients with a broad range of psychiatric disorders. Additionally, specialized services are available for patients with psychiatric diagnoses compounded by chemical dependency, or a history of physical or sexual abuse.
Susan Clayton, Support Group Coordinator
Angela Hurtado, Support Group Coordinator

3645 National Health Information Center
PO Box 1133
Washington, DC 20013
310-565-4167
800-336-4797
Fax: 301-984-4256
e-mail: info@nhic.org
www.health.gov/nhic

A health information referral service sponsored by the Office of Disease Prevention and Health Promotion. Puts health professionals and condumers who have health questions in touch with those organizations that are best able to provide answers.

3646 Pediatric/Adolescent Gastroesophageal Reflux Association
PO Box 7728
Silver Spring, MD 20901
301-601-9541
e-mail: gergroup@aol.com
www.reflux.org

Provides information and support to parents, patients and doctors about Gastroesophageal Reflux.
Beth Anderson, Director

3647 Richmond Support Group
Warwick Medical & Professional Ctr
Richmond, VA
804-320-7881

Books

3648 Anorexia Nervosa & Recovery: A Hunger for Meaning
The Haworth Press

10 Alice Street
Binghamton, NY 13904
607-722-5857
800-429-6784
e-mail: getinfo@haworth.com
www.haworth.com

1993 146 pages Paperback
ISBN: 0-918393-95-7

3649 Bearly Any Fat Cookbook
Obesity Foundation
5600 S Quebec Street
Englewood, CO 80111-2202
303-850-0328
e-mail: editor@obesity.org
www.obesity.org

Perfect cookbook to assist anyone in a weight reduction program.

3650 Body Betrayed
American Psychiatric Press
1400 K Street NW
Washington, DC 20005-2403
202-682-6268
Fax: 202-789-2648

A book concentrating on women, eating disorders and treatments.
440 pages Hardcover
ISBN: 0-880485-22-1

3651 Bulimia: A Guide to Recovery
Gurze Books
PO Box 2238
Carlsbad, CA 92018-9883
800-756-7533
Fax: 760-434-5476
e-mail: gzcatl@aol.com
www.bulimia.com

This intimate guidebook offers a complete understanding of bulimia and a plan for recovery. It includes a two-week program to stop bingeing, things-to-do instead of bingeing, a two-week guide for support groups, specific advice for loved ones and Eating Without Fear, Hall's story of self-cure which has inspired thousands of other bulimics.
280 pages Paperback
ISBN: 0-936077-31-X

3652 Conversations with Anorexics
Jason Aronson
PO Box 15100
York, PA 17405-7100
800-782-0015
Fax: 201-840-7242
www.aronson.com

A Compassionate and Hopeful Journey through the Therapeutic Process.
238 pages
ISBN: 1-568212-61-5

3653 Coping with Eating Disorders
Rosen Publishing Group
29 E 21st Street
New York, NY 10010
212-777-3017
800-237-9932
Fax: 888-436-4643
e-mail: customerservice@rosenpub.com
www.rosenpublishing.com

This book offers practical suggestions on coping with eating disorders.

ISBN: 0-823929-74-4
Barbara Moe, Author

3654 Cult of Thinness
Oxford University Press
2001 Evans Road
Cary, NC 27513-2010
212-726-6000
800-451-7556
Fax: 919-677-1303
www.oup-usa.org

1996 256 pages
ISBN: 0-195082-41-9

3655 Deadly Diet: Recovering from Anorexia & Bulimia
New Harbinger Publications
5674 Shattuck Avenue
Oakland, CA 94609-1662
800-748-6273
Fax: 510-652-5472
www.newharbinger.com

1993 265 pages Paperback
ISBN: 1-879237-42-3

3656 Eating Diorders Resource Catalogue
Gurze Books
PO Box 2238
Carlsbad, CA 92018-9883   800-756-7533
Fax: 760-434-5476
www.bulimia.com

This catalogue of resources contains over 140 books, videos and audiotapes, lists of national organizations and treatment facilities and basic facts about eating disorders. It is widely distributed by individuals who are suffering, their loved ones, the health care professionals who treat them and educators who are working towards prevention.
24 pages Annual

3657 Eating Disorder Sourcebook
Gurze Books
PO Box 2238
Carlsbad, CA 92018-2238   800-756-7533
Fax: 760-434-5476
e-mail: gzcatl@aol.com
www.bulimia.com

An ideal book for someone with a loved one who has an eating disorder but who knows little about this subject, this new release presents a clear overview of basic issues.
222 pages Paperback

3658 Eating Disorders Resource Catalogue
Gurze Books
PO Box 2238
Carlsbad, CA 92018-9883   800-756-7533
Fax: 760-434-5476
www.bulimia.com

This catalogue of resources contains over 140 books, videos and audiotapes, lists of national organizations and treatment facilities and basic facts about eating disorders. It is widely distributed by individuals who are suffering, their loved ones, the health care professionals who treat them and educators who are working towards prevention.
28 pages Annual

3659 Eating Disorders-Overview Series
Lucent Books
Thomson Gale
Farmington Hills, MI 48333-9187   800-877-4253
Fax: 800-414-5043
e-mail: gale.customerservice@thomson.com
www.gale.com/lucent

This book examines how eating disorders can be identified, who is affected by them, and how they can be treated.
2001
ISBN: 1-560066-59-8

3660 Eating Disorders: When Food Turns Against You
Franklin Watts Grolier
90 Old Sherman Tpke
Danbury, CT 06816-0001   203-797-3500
Fax: 203-797-3197
www.grolier.com

1993 96 pages
ISBN: 0-531111-75-0

3661 Emotional Eating: A Practical Guide to Taking Control
Free Press
866 3rd Avenue
New York, NY 10022   800-223-7445
Fax: 800-943-9831
www.simonsays.com

1003 200 pages
ISBN: 0-029002-15-0

3662 Encyclopedia of Obesity and Eating Disorders
Facts on File
11 Penn Plaza
New York, NY 10001   212-967-8800
800-322-8755
Fax: 800-678-3633

From abdominoplasty to Zung Rating Scale, this volume defines and explains these disorders, along with medical and other problems associated with them.
272 pages Hardcover

3663 Endorphins: Eating Disorders & Other Addictive Behavior
WW Norton & Company
500 5th Avenue   212-354-5500
New York, NY 10110-0054   800-233-4830
Fax: 800-458-6515
www.wwnorton.com

1993 320 pages
ISBN: 0-393701-56-5

3664 Etiology and Treatment of Bulimia Nervosa
Jason Aronson
PO Box 15100
York, PA 17405-7100   800-782-0015
Fax: 201-767-1576
www.aronson.com

352 pages Softcover
ISBN: 1-568213-39-5

3665 Evaluation and Management of Eating Disorders
Human Kinetics Publishers
PO Box 5076   217-351-1549
Champaign, IL 61825-5076   800-747-4457
Fax: 217-351-5076

368 pages Cloth
ISBN: 0-873229-11-8

3666 Fear of Being Fat
Jason Aronson
PO Box 15100
York, PA 17405-7100   800-782-0015
Fax: 201-840-7242
www.aronson.com

366 pages
ISBN: 0-876688-99-7

3667 Getting Better Bit(e) by Bit(e)
Gurze Books
PO Box 2238
Carlsbad, CA 92018-2238   800-756-7533
Fax: 760-434-5476
e-mail: gzcatl@aol.com
www.bulimia.com

This practical book on recovery from bulimia and binge eating is packed with lists, exercises, case studies, discussions, insights and specific things to do. This book also addresses the day-to-day problems faced by eating disorder sufferers and concentrates on key behavior changes necessary for progress.
143 pages Paperback

3668 Going Backwards
Scholastic
730 Broadway   212-505-3000
New York, NY 10003-9511   800-325-6149
A story that weaves the themes of acceptance, death, mortality and family loyalty to present a controversial plot.
Grades 7-10

3669 Golden Cage: The Enigma of Anorexia Nervosa
Gurze Books
PO Box 2283
Carlsbad, CA 92018-2283   800-756-7533
Fax: 760-434-5476
e-mail: gzcatl@aol.com
www.bulimia.com

3670 Group Psychotherapy for Eating Disorders
American Psychiatric Press
1400 K Street NW   202-682-6268
Washington, DC 20005-2403   Fax: 202-789-2648
The first book to fully explore the use of group therapy in the treatment of eating disorders.
353 pages Hardcover
ISBN: 0-880484-19-5

3671 Helping Athletes with Eating Disorders
Human Kinetics Publishers
PO Box 5076   217-351-1549
Champaign, IL 61825-5076   800-747-4457
Fax: 217-351-5076

Gives readers the information they need to identify and address major eating disorders such as: anorexia, bulimia nervosa, and eating disorders not otherwise specified.
208 pages Cloth
ISBN: 0-873223-83-7

3672   Hope and Recovery: A Mother-Daughter Story About Anorexia Nervosa & Bulimia
Franklin Watts Grolier
90 Old Sherman Tpke
Danbury, CT 06816-0001
　　　　　　　　　　　　　　　800-621-1115
　　　　　　　　　　　　　　Fax: 800-374-4329
Mother and daughter tell a story of a young woman's recovery from the horror of an eating disorder. This compelling account shows how anorexia and bulimia can affect an entire family.
192 pages
ISBN: 0-531111-40-7

3673   Hungry Self: Women, Eating and Identity
Gurze Books
PO Box 2283
Carlsbad, CA 92018-2283
　　　　　　　　　　　　　　　800-756-7533
　　　　　　　　　　　　　　Fax: 760-434-5476
　　　　　　　　　　　e-mail: gzcatl@aol.com
　　　　　　　　　　　　　www.bulimia.com

3674   Insights in the Dynamic Psychotherapy of Anorexia and Bulimia
Jason Aronson
400 Keystone Industrial Park
Dunmore, PA 18512-1523
　　　　　　　　　　　　　　　800-782-0015
　　　　　　　　　　　　　　Fax: 201-840-7242
　　　　　　　　　　　　　　www.aronson.com

320 pages Hardcover
ISBN: 0-876685-68-8

3675   It's Not Your Fault
Gurze Books
PO Box 2238
Carlsbad, CA 92018-2238
　　　　　　　　　　　　　　　800-756-5476
　　　　　　　　　　　　　　Fax: 760-434-5476
　　　　　　　　　　　e-mail: gzcatl@aol.com
　　　　　　　　　　　　　www.bulimia.com
In this comprehensive, medically sound guide to overcoming eating disorders, Dr. Marx defines the warnings signs of eating disorders, explores causes, at risk populations, the role of drug therapy and advises patients and families where and how they can find help.

3676   Making Peace with Food
Gurze Books
PO Box 2238
Carlsbad, CA 92018-2238
　　　　　　　　　　　　　　　800-756-7533
　　　　　　　　　　　　　　Fax: 760-434-5476
　　　　　　　　　　　e-mail: gzcatl@aol.com
　　　　　　　　　　　　　www.bulimia.com
This unique, full sized workbook is designed to help anyone who experienced compulsive eating, yo-yo dieting, food and body anxiety, or associated eating disorders. Filled with ideas, workbook pages, exercises and resources, Kano's book is an excellent aid to clarifying and overcoming your personal diet/weight struggle.
224 pages Paperback

3677   Meals Without Squeals Sense
Bull Publishing
PO Box 1377
Boulder, CO 80306
　　　　　　　　　　　　　　　800-676-2855
　　　　　　　　　　　　　　Fax: 303-545-6354
　　　　　　　　　　　　　　www.bullpub.com
Straight forward information on childrens growth accompanies age specific, child tested recipes. Explained is how common feeding problems can be solved and show ways to offer children positive experiences with food.
2006 288 pages
ISBN: 1-933503-00-4

3678   My Name is Caroline
Doubleday
666 Fifth Avenue
New York, NY 10103
　　　　　　　　　　　　　　212-354-6500

A poignant tale of one woman's battle with bulimia throughout her life as a successful student, athlete, scholar and musician.
Grades 10-12

3679   Obesity: Theory and Therapy
Raven Press
1185 Avenue of the Americas　　　　　212-930-9500
New York, NY 10036-2601　　　　　　800-777-2295
A classic reference for clinicians dealing with obesity, this volume provides the most up-to-date research, preclinical and clinical information.
500 pages
ISBN: 0-881678-84-8

3680   Practice Guidelines for Eating Disorders
American Psychiatric Press
1400 K Street NW　　　　　　　　　202-682-6268
Washington, DC 20005-2403　　　Fax: 202-789-2648
Designed for health care professionals, this guideline includes information on all aspects of anorexia nervosa and bulimia nervosa, including self-induced vomiting, use of laxatives and vigorous exercise to prevent weight gain.
38 pages Paperback
ISBN: 0-890423-00-8

3681   Psychodynamic Technique in the Treatment of the Eating Disorders
Jason Aronson
PO Box 15100
York, PA 17405-7100
　　　　　　　　　　　　　　　800-782-0015
　　　　　　　　　　　　　　Fax: 201-840-7242
　　　　　　　　　　　　　　www.aronson.com

440 pages Hardcover
ISBN: 0-876686-22-6

3682   Self-Starvation
Jason Aronson
PO Box 15100
York, PA 17405-7100
　　　　　　　　　　　　　　　800-782-0015
　　　　　　　　　　　　　　Fax: 201-840-7242
　　　　　　　　　　　　　　www.aronson.com

312 pages Softcover
ISBN: 1-568218-22-2

3683   Starving to Death in a Sea of Objects
Jason Aronson
PO Box 15100
York, PA 17405-7100
　　　　　　　　　　　　　　　800-782-0015
　　　　　　　　　　　　　　Fax: 201-840-7242
　　　　　　　　　　　　　　www.aronson.com
How emancipation becomes security for anorexics.
464 pages Softcover
ISBN: 0-876684-35-5

3684   Surviving an Eating Disorder: Perspectives & Strategies
Gurze Books
PO Box 2238
Carlsbad, CA 92018-2238
　　　　　　　　　　　　　　　800-756-7533
　　　　　　　　　　　　　　Fax: 760-434-5476
　　　　　　　　　　　e-mail: gzcatl@aol.com
　　　　　　　　　　　　　www.bulimia.com
Parents, spouses and friends of individuals with food problems will find practical guidelines in this book for helping themselves and their loved ones.
222 pages Paperback

3685   Treating Bulimia: A Psychoeducational Approach
American Anorexia/Bulimia Association
165 W 46th Street　　　　　　　　　212-575-6200
New York, NY 10036-2501　　e-mail: amanbu@aol.com
　　　　　　　　　　　www.members.aol.com/amanbu

3686   When Food is Love
Gurze Books
PO Box 2238
Carlsbad, CA 92018-2238
　　　　　　　　　　　　　　　800-756-7533
　　　　　　　　　　　　　　Fax: 760-434-5467
　　　　　　　　　　　e-mail: gzcatl@aol.com
　　　　　　　　　　　　　www.gurze.com
Drawing on her own personal experience, Roth explores similarities between eating and loving such as fantasizing, wanting the for-

bidden, creating drama, control issues, and the experience of relationship.
205 pages Paperback

3687 Withering Child
University of Georgia Press
330 Research Drive
Athens, GA 30602

404-542-2830
800-266-5842
Fax: 709-369-6131
e-mail: books@ugapress.uga.edu
www.uga.edu/ugapress

1993 288 pages
ISBN: 0-820315-60-5

Children's Books

3688 Billy's Story
Metro Intergroup of Overeaters Anonymous
117 W 26th Street
New York, NY 10001

212-206-8621

3689 I Was a Fifteen-Year-Old Blimp
Harper & Row
10 E 53rd Street
New York, NY 10022-5299

212-207-7000

This story focuses on Gabby, a teenage girl who overhears others discuss her weight and takes radical steps to become popular.
Grades 6-9

Magazines

3690 BASH Magazine
Bulimia Anorexia Self-Help/Behavior Adaptation
PO Box 39903
Saint Louis, MO 63139-8903

800-762-3334

A journal of eating and mood disorders.
Monthly

Newsletters

3691 AABA Newsletter
American Anorexic and Bulemic Association
165 W 46th Street
New York, NY 10036-2501

212-575-6200

This newsletter is published three times a year and is mailed to the members of the AABA. The AABA is a tax-exempt, nonprofit organization with a membership of professionals, sufferers of eating disorders, and their family and friends.

3692 Eating Disorders Review
Gurze Books
PO Box 2238
Carlsbad, CA 92018-9883

800-756-7533
Fax: 760-434-5476
e-mail: gzcatl@aol.com
www.bulimia.com

Presents current clinical information for the professional treating eating disorders. Features summeries of relevant research from journals and unpublished studies, abstracts, nutritional notes, questions and answers, book reviews and reproducible client handouts.
8 pages BiMonthly
Joel Yager MD, Editor-in-Chief
Liegh Cohn, Publisher

3693 National Association of Anorexia Nervosa and Associated Disorders Newsletter
PO Box 7
Highland Park, IL 60035

847-831-3438
Fax: 847-433-4632
e-mail: anad20@aol.com
www.anad.org

2 pages Quarterly
Vivian Hansen Meehan, President
Dawn Ries, Administrator

3694 WIN Notes
Weight-control Information Network

1 WIN Way
Bethesda, MD 20892-3665

202-828-1025
877-946-4627
Fax: 202-828-1028
e-mail: win@mathewsgroup.com
www.niddk.nih.gov/health/nutrit/win.htm

Addresses the health information needs of individuals with weight-control problems. Available on the WIN web site.
BiAnnual

3695 Working Together
Anorexia Nervosa and Associated Disorders
PO Box 7
Highland Park, IL 60035-0007

847-831-3438
Fax: 847-433-4632

Designed for individuals, families, group leaders and professionals concerned with eating disorders. Provides updates on treatments, resources, conferences, programs, articles by therapists, recovered victims, group members and leaders.
Quarterly
Dawn Ries, Administrator

Pamphlets

3696 Applying New Attitudes & Directions
Anorexia Nervosa and Associated Disorders
PO Box 7
Highland Park, IL 60035-0007

847-831-3438
Fax: 847-433-4632
e-mail: anad20@aol.com

Self-help booklet offering an eight-step program to recovery with suggestions, information and recovery stories.
Dawn Ries, Administrator

Audio & Video

3697 Bulimia: A Guide to Recovery
Gurze Books
PO Box 2238
Carlsbad, CA 92018-2238

800-756-7533
Fax: 760-434-5476
e-mail: gzcatl@aol.com
www.bulimia.com

This newly rediscovered tape is an inspirational talk by Lindsey Hall on the relationship between bulimia, self-esteem and love. This was one of Lindsey's last public appearances, where she addressed a 1991 eating disorers conference in Colorado Springs.
Audio tape

Web Sites

3698 Anorexia Nervosa & Related Eating Disorders

www.anred.com

Comprehensive site on eating disorders and related issues.

3699 GERD Information Resource Center

www.gerd.com

A resource center with educational resources on Gastroesophageal Reflux Disease (GERD).

3700 Gastroenterology Therapy Online

www.gastrotherapy.com

An informational website with resources for many kinds of diseases.

3701 Healing Well

www.healingwell.com

An online health resource guide to medical news, chat, information and articles, newsgroups and message boards, books, disease-related web sites, medical directories, and more for patients, friends, and family coping with disabling diseases, disorders, or chronic illnesses.

3702 Health Finder

www.healthfinder.gov

Searchable, carefully developed web site offering information on over 1000 topics. Developed by the US Department of Health and Human Services, the site can be used in both English and Spanish.

3703 Healthlink USA

www.healthlinkusa.com

Health information concerning treatment, cures, prevention, diagnosis, risk factors, research, support groups, email lists, personal stories and much more. Updated regularly.

3704 Helios Health

www.helioshealth.com

Online resource for your health information. Detailed information about specific health topics, access to expert advice from our Medical Advisory Board, and up-to-date health news.

3705 MedicineNet

www.medicinenet.com

An online resource for consumers providing easy-to-read, authoritative medical and health information.

3706 Medscape

www.medscape.com

Medscape offers specialists, primary care physicians, and other health professionals the Web's most robust and integrated medical information and educational tools.

3707 National Association for Anorexia Nervosa and Associated Disorders

www.anad.org

ANAD provides educational/prevention programs include presentations and early detection packets for schools and community groups, sponsoring local and national training conferences for health professionals, and working with electronic and print media. Undertakes and encourages research, fights insurance discrimination.

3708 National Eating Disorders Association

www.NationalEatingDisorders.org

National nonprofit organization dedicated to increasing the awareness and prevention of eating disorders.

3709 WebMD

www.webmd.com

Information on Eating Disorders, including articles and resources.

3710 Weight-control Information Network

www.niddk.nih.gov/health/nutrit/win.htm

WIN addresses the health information needs of individuals through the production and dissemination of educational materials. In addition, WIN is developing communication strategies for a pilot program to encourage at-risk individuals to achieve and maintain a healthy weight by making changes in their lifestyle.

Description

3711 Endometriosis

Endometriosis is a hormonal condition in which the tissue that normally lines the inside of the uterus (endometrium) is also found outside the uterus, generally on the outer surface of pelvic organs. These cells respond to the woman's hormonal cycles, and swell and bleed at the time of menses. This causes pain, generally worse with each period, pelvic masses and alterations of the menstrual cycle. The pain may be aggravated by intercourse or defecation. Although the reported incidence varies, endometriosis is commonly found in 10 to 15 percent of women between the ages of 25 and 44 years. It is estimated that 25 to 50 percent of infertile women have this disorder.

Treatment depends on the severity of the symptoms and the age and reproductive wishes of the patient. The pain associated with mild cases may be treated with non-steroidal anti-inflammatory drugs. More severe cases may respond to suppression of ovarian function. Laparoscopic surgery may destroy some of the collection of tissue, and is often used in hopes of improving fertility. Hysterectomy (removal of the uterus) is used for intractable cases, especially in women who do not desire future pregnancy.

National Agencies & Associations

3712 American Association of Gynecologic Laproscopists
6757 Katella Avenue
Cypress, CA 90630-4505
714-503-6200
800-554-2245
Fax: 714-503-6201
e-mail: lmichels@aagl.org
www.aagl.com

Our global commitment to women's healthcare is embodied in our continuing medical education of physicians and professionals to further promote the well documented high standards of minimally invasive gynecologic surgery.
Linda Michels, Executive Director
Franklin D Loffer MD, EVP/Medical Director

3713 American Society for Reproductive Medicine
1209 Montgomery Highway
Birmingham, AL 35216-2809
205-978-5000
Fax: 205-978-5005
e-mail: asrm@asrm.com
www.asrm.com

A private, nonprofit medical organization devoted to advancing the knowledge, understanding and expertise in all phases of reproductive medicine and biology. Offers patient education brochures, recommended readings and support. Publishes professional journal and consumer publications.
Robert W Rebar, MD, Executive Director
Andrew LaBarbera, PhD, Scientific Director

3714 Endometriosis Association
630 Ibis Drive
Delray Beach, FL 33444
561-274-7442
800-239-7280
Fax: 561-274-0931
e-mail: exec-comm@endocenter.org
www.endocenter.org

Nonprofit international organization dedicated to helping women and girls suffering from endometriosis. Services include chapter and support groups, crisis/counseling assistance, education of the public and medical community materials including books and videos.
Ann Koerner, Operations Manager

3715 Endometriosis Association International
8585 N 76th Place
Milwaukee, WI 53223
414-355-2200
800-992-3636
Fax: 414-355-6065
www.endometriosisassn.org

Offers a 24 hour crisis call hotline, support groups, education in the form of literature including fact sheets, brochures, newsletters, articles educational videos, books and research.
Mary Lou Ballweg, President/Executive Director
Carolyn Keith, Co-Founder

3716 Hysterectomy Educational Resources & Services (HERS) Foundation
422 Bryn Mawr Avenue
Bala Cynwyd, PA 19004
610-667-7757
888-750-4377
Fax: 610-677-8096
e-mail: hersfdn@earthlink.net
www.hersfoundation.com

A nonprofit foundation which provides information about the alternatives to hysterectomy, the risks of the alternatives, and the consequences of the surgery. HERS provides telephone counseling by appointment for a fee of $5.00 per quarter hour. The fee can be waived if necessary. HERS also provides copies of a medical journals, a quarterly newsletter, and a free lending library of books, videos and audio tapes.

3717 International Pelvic Pain Society Women's Medical Plaza
Women's Medical Plaza
1100 E Woodfield Road
Schaumburg, IL 60173
847-517-8712
800-624-9676
Fax: 847-517-7229
e-mail: info@pelvicpain.org
www.pelvicpain.org

Short range goal is to recruit organize and educate health care professionals actively involved with the treatment of patients who have chronic pelvic pain.
Fred Marion Howard, Chairman of the Board
Howard Taylo Sharp MD, President

3718 National Women's Health Network
1413 K Street
Washington, DC 20005
202-682-2640
Fax: 202-682-2648
e-mail: nwhn@nwhn.org
www.womenshealthnetwork.org

Nonprofit organization that does not accept financial support from pharmaceutical or tobacco companies or medical device manufacturers. Advocates for national policies that protect and promote all women's health and provides evidence-based independent information.
Bindiya Patel, Chairperson
Malika Redmond, Action Vice Chair

Foundations

3719 Fertility Research Foundation
877 Park Avenue
New York, NY 10021
212-744-5500
Fax: 212-744-6536
e-mail: info@frfbaby.com
www.frfbaby.com

Offers information on treatment and the latest research on male and female infertility.
Masood Khatamee MD, Executive Director

Libraries & Resource Centers

3720 National Womens Health Resource Center
157 Broad Street
Red Bank, NJ 07701
877-986-9472
Fax: 732-249-4671
e-mail: info@healthywomen.org
www.healthywomen.org

The not-for-profit National Women's Health Resource Center (NWHRC) is the leading independent health information source for women. NWHRC develops and distributes up-to-date and ob-

jective women's health information based on the latest advances in medical research and practice.
Elizabeth Battaglino Cahill, Executive Vice President
Amber McCracken, Director Communications

Research Centers

3721 Dartmouth Medical School: Microbiology Department
Department of Microbiology & Immunology
1 Rope Ferry Road   603-650-1200
Hanover, NH 03755-1404   877-DMS-1797
Fax: 603-650-1202
e-mail: microbiology@dartmouth.edu
www.dms.dartmouth.edu
Dartmouth Medical School is a beacon of discovery and learning stimulating inquiry and harnessing ingenuity for new solutions and better health
Ann Hill, Administrative Assistant
Gregory J MacDonald MD, Assistant Professor of Medicine

3722 Endometriosis Association Research Program : Vanderbuilt University
1211 22nd Avenue S   615-322-5000
Nashville, TN 37232   Fax: 615-343-8881
www.mc.vanderbilt.edu

Heather Arnold, Senior Secretary

3723 Endometriosis Reseach Center and Women's Hospital
The Endometriosis Research Center
630 Ibis Drive   561-274-7442
Delray Beach, FL 33444   800-239-7280
Fax: 561-274-0931
www.endocenter.org
A nonprofit organization dedicated to establishing a center to conduct research and provide women education and treatment.

3724 Endometriosis Reseach Center and Women's H The Endometriosis Research Center
630 Ibis Drive   561-274-7442
Delray Beach, FL 33444   800-239-7280
Fax: 561-274-0931
e-mail: exec-comm@endocenter.org
www.endocenter.org
A nonprofit organization dedicated to establishing a center to conduct research and provide women education and treatment.

3725 Endometriosis Research Center 0
630 Ibis Drive   561-274-7442
Delray Beach, FL 33444   800-239-7280
Fax: 561-274-0931
e-mail: endofl@aol.com
www.endocenter.org
Endometriosis is a reproductive and immunological illness affecting millions of women and girls around the world Mistakenly stigmatized as merely painful periods, Endometriosis is a far more than a killer cramp the far- reaching effects of this Endometriosis can negatively impact all of society.

3726 Endometriosis Research Center 0
630 Ibis Drive   561-274-7442
Delray Beach, FL 33444   800-239-7280
Fax: 561-274-0931
e-mail: exec-comm@endocenter.org
www.endocenter.org
Endometriosis is a reproductive and immunological illness affecting millions of women and girls around the world Mistakenly stigmatized as merely painful periods Endometriosis is a far more than a killer cramp the far- reaching effects of this Endometriosis can negatively impact all of society.

3727 University of Tennessee: Division of Reproductive Endocrinology
956 Court Avenue
Memphis, TN 38163   901-528-5859
www.utmem.edu/obgyn/reproductive.htm
Studies into endometriosis.
Dr. Jon Buster, Chief

Support Groups & Hotlines

3728 National Health Information Center
PO Box 1133   310-565-4167
Washington, DC 20013   800-336-4797
Fax: 301-984-4256
e-mail: info@nhic.org
www.health.gov/nhic
A helath information referral service sponsored by the Office of Disease Prevention and Health Promotion. Puts health professionals and consumers who have health questions in touch with those organizations that are best able to provide answers.

3729 RESOLVE Helpline
1760 Old Meadow Road   703-556-7172
McLean, VA 22102   Fax: 703-506-3266
www.resolve.org
A nationwide network mandated to promote reproductive health and to ensure equal access to all family building options for men and women experienceing infertility or other reproductive disorders.
Barbara Collura, Executive Director

Books

3730 Alternatives for Women with Endometriosis Guide by Women for Women
Third Side Press
225 W Farragut   773-271-3029
Chicago, IL 60625-1863   Fax: 773-271-0459
e-mail: thirdside@aol.com
174 pages
ISBN: 1-879427-12-5

3731 Coping with Endometriosis
Avery Putnam Penguin
375 Hudson Street   212-366-2000
New York, NY 10014   800-847-5515
Fax: 800-775-4829
e-mail: online@penguinputnam.com
www.penguinputnam.com
Educates readers about the disease, focusing on the particular psychological and emotional concerns that those suffering from endometriosis may have.
322 pages
ISBN: 1-583330-74-7

3732 Endometriosis Sourcebook
Endometriosis Association
8585 N 76th Place   414-355-2200
Milwaukee, WI 53223   800-992-3636
Fax: 414-355-6065
e-mail: endo@endometriosisassn.org
www.EndometriosisAssn.org
Comprehensive, authorative and up-to-date resource that includes information about treatment options, strategies for coping with the disease and its effects on you and those around you.
473 pages Paperback
ISBN: 0-809232-63-4
Mary Lou Ballweg, Founder/Executive Director

3733 Endometriosis and Infertility and Traditio nal Chinese Medicine
Blue Poppy Press
5441 Western Avenue   303-447-8372
Boulder, CO 80301   800-487-9296
Fax: 303-245-8362
e-mail: honora@bluepoppy.com
www.bluepoppy.com/press
An easy to understand guide to Chinese medicine as it relates to endometriosis and infertility.
105 pages Paperback
ISBN: 0-936185-14-7
Honora Wolfe, Marketing Director

3734 Endometriosis: A Key to Healing through Nutrition
Endometriosis Association

8585 N 76th Place
Milwaukee, WI 53223

414-355-2200
800-992-3636
Fax: 414-355-6065
e-mail: endo@endometriosisassn.org
www.endometriosisassn.org

An excellent resource tool to help patients begin making changes in their diets.
Mary Lou Ballweg, Founder/Executive Director

3735 Endometriosis: A Natural Approach
Ulysses Press
PO Box 3440
Berkeley, CA 94703

510-601-8301
800-377-2542
Fax: 510-601-8307
e-mail: ulysses@ulyssespress.com
www.ulyssespress.com

This is a solid resource, written in a clear, basic tone, for anyone who needs information about the widespread disease known as endometriosis. Chapters cover all aspects of endometriosis, from what it is and what causes it, to diagnosis, natural therapies, and conventional treatments.
120 pages
ISBN: 1-569750-88-2

3736 Endometriosis: Advanced Management and Surgical Techniques
Springer Verlag
175 5th Avenue
New York, NY 10010

212-460-1500
800-777-4643
Fax: 212-473-6272
e-mail: service@springer-ny.com
www.springer-ny.com

This book provides a practical, clinical, and thorough examination of both the medical and surgical treatment of this disease.

3737 Endometriosis: Complete Reference for Taking Charge of Your Health
Contemporary Books/McGraw-Hill Companies
130 E Randolf Street
Chicago, IL 60601

312-233-7596
Fax: 312-233-7570

An authoritative guide on endometriosis, including its prevention and relationship with other diseases. Special sections are dedicated to endo and menopause, endo and teenagers, endo and nutrition, endo and cancer as well as endo and environmental toxins.

Newsletters

3738 Endometriosis Association Newsletter
Endometriosis Association
8585 N 76th Place
Milwaukee, WI 53223

414-355-2200
800-992-3636
Fax: 414-355-6065
e-mail: endo@endometriosisassn.org
www.EndometriosisAssn.org

Contains research updates and latest health news that affects women and girls with endometriosis. Regular features such as crisis call helpers, news and announcements, and request for contact provide networking and support assistance.
10 pages Bi-Monthly
Mary Lou Ballweg, Executive Director

Pamphlets

3739 Infertility: Causes and Treatment
American College/Obstetricians and Gynecologists
409 12th Street SW
Washington, DC 20024

304-725-8410
800-762-2264
Fax: 304-728-2171
www.acog.com

To obtain a free copy of this publication, please send a self-addressed stamped #10 envelope and request by title.

Audio & Video

3740 Monroe Institute Surgical Support Tapes
Endometriosis Association

8585 N 76th Place
Milwaukee, WI 53223-2633

414-355-2200
800-992-3636
Fax: 414-355-6065
e-mail: endo@endometriosisassn.org
www.EndometriosisAssn.org

Anxiety is normal for women before surgery, so women with endometriosis will be happy to hear this wonderful series of audiotapes specifically developed for relaxation.
Audiotape
Mary Lou Ballweg, Founder/Executive Director

Web Sites

3741 American Society for Reproductive Medicine
www.asrm.com
Devoted to advancing the knowledge, understanding and expertise in all phases of reproductive medicine and biology. Offers patient education brochures, recommended readings and support.

3742 Endometriosis Association
www.EndometriosisAssn.org
Nonprofit organization dedicated to helping women and girls suffering from endometriosis. Services include chapter and support groups, crisis/counseling assistance, education of the public and the medical community. Materials, including books, video/audiotapes, CDs, newsletters and articles mostly based on data from the Association's research registries and its extensive research program, including a flagship scientific team at Vanderbuilt University School of Medicine.

3743 Endometriosis Research Center
www.endocenter.org
Maintain and offer a vast database of unbased and fact-based materials on every aspect of Endometriosis to practitioners, researchers, patients and all those interested in the disease.

3744 Endometriosis Support Group
www.geocities.com/HotSprings/5422
Online support group and question forum for endometriosis.

3745 Healing Well
www.healingwell.com
An online health resource guide to medical news, chat, information and articles, newsgroups and message boards, books, disease-related web sites, medical directories, and more for patients, friends, and family coping with disabling diseases, disorders, or chronic illnesses.

3746 Health Finder
www.healthfinder.gov
Searchable, carefully developed web site offering information on over 1000 topics. Developed by the US Department of Health and Human Services, the site can be used in both English and Spanish.

3747 Healthlink USA
www.healthlinkusa.com
Health information concerning treatment, cures, prevention, diagnosis, risk factors, research, support groups, email lists, personal stories and much more. Updated regularly.

3748 Helios Health
www.helioshealth.com
Online resource for your health information. Detailed information about specific health topics, access to expert advice from our Medical Advisory Board, and up-to-date health news.

3749 International Pelvic Pain Society
www.pelvicpain.org/
Short range goal is to recruit, organize, and educate health care professionals actively involved with the treatment of patients who have chronic pelvic pain.

3750 MedicineNet
www.medicinenet.com
An online resource for consumers providing easy-to-read, authoritative medical and health information.

3751 Medscape
www.medscape.com

Medscape offers specialists, primary care physicians, and other health professionals the Web's most robust and integrated medical information and educational tools.

3752 Universe of Women's Health

www.obgyn.net

A comprehensive website dedicated to women's health.

3753 WebMD

www.webmd.com

Information on Endometriosis, including articles and resources.

Description

3754 Fabry Disease

Fabry disease is an inherited fat storage disorder caused by deficiency of an enzyme involved in the biodegradation of lipids (fats). As abnormal storage of the fatty compound increases with time, blood vessels become narrowed, leading to decreased blood flow. The problem occurs in all blood vessels in the body, but affects in particular the skin, kidneys, heart, brain and nerves.

In children, Fabry begins with pain and burning sensations in hands and feet that is worse with exercise and hot weather. Other symptoms include a dark red rash around the waist, decreased ability to perspire and cloudiness of the cornea, which usually does not affect vision.

As those with Fabry's grow older, they may have impaired circulation, leading to early heart attacks and strokes. As kidneys become more involved, many patients require kidney transplants or dialysis. Gastrointestinal symptoms include frequent bowel movements shortly after eating. Patients with Fabry disease usually survive into adulthood but have a reduced life expectancy.

Currently, there is no cure for Fabry disease and treatment typically deals with controlling its symptoms. Pain in hands and feet respond to several medications. Gastrointestinal hyperactivity may be controlled by taking a nutritional supplement. Enzyme replacement therapy was given a dramatic boost in 2003 when the FDA approved a new synthetic enzyme. It is given intravenously and reduces lipid (fat) accumulation in many types of cells.

National Agencies & Associations

3755 Association for Neuro-Metabolic Disorders
3901 Rainbow Boulevard 913-588-5000
Kansas City, KS 66160 800-334-7980
TTY: 913-588-7963
e-mail: VOLK4OLKS@aol.com
www.kumc.edu
Serves as an advocate organization for families of patients with neuro-methabolic disorders such as phenylketonuria, maple syrup urine disease, galactosemia and biotinidase. Provides educational information for parents and children and provides networking.
Barbara F Atkinson MD, Executive Vice Chancellor

3756 Genetic and Rare Diseases Information Center
PO Box 8126 301-251-4925
Gaithersburg, MD 20898-8126 888-205-2311
Fax: 301-251-4911
TTY: 888-205-3223
e-mail: GARDinfo@nih.gov
www.rarediseases.info.nih.gov/GARD
Provides free and immediate access to accurate, reliable information about genetic and rare diseases. Also provides assistance to patients and families, health professionals and other interested parties.

3757 International Center for Fabry Disease Mt. Sinai School of Medicine
Mt. Sinai School of Medicine

One Gustave L Levy Place 212-241-6500
New York, NY 10029 866-322-7963
e-mail: fabry.disease@mssm.edu
www.mssm.edu
Clinical research center attended by a staff of physicians and nurses specially trained to understand and meet the needs of individuals with Fabry disease. Services offered to both men and women of all ages include diagnosis, evaluation and treatment consultation.
Robert J Desnick PhD MD, Professor and Chair
Dennis Charney MD, Executive VP

3758 National Institute of Neurological Disorders and Stroke (NINDS)
NIH Neurological Institute 301-496-5751
Bethesda, MD 20824 800-352-9424
Fax: 301-496-0296
TTY: 301-468-5981
www.ninds.nih.gov
The mission of NINDS is to reduce the burden of neurological disease - a burden borne by every age group, by every segment of society, by people all over the world.
Story C Landis PhD, Director
Walter J Koroshetz, Deputy Director

3759 National Organization for Rare Disorders (NORD)
55 Kenosia Avenue 203-744-0100
Danbury, CT 06813-1968 800-999-6673
Fax: 203-798-2291
TDD: 203-797-9590
e-mail: orphan@rarediseases.org
www.rarediseases.org
The National Organization for Rare Disorders(NORD), a 501(c)3 organization, is a unique federation of voluntary health organizations dedicated to helping people with rare orphan diseases and assisting the organizations that serve them. NORD is committed to the identification, treatment, and cure of rare disorders through programs of education, advocacy, research, and service.
Frank Sasinowski, Chair
Carolyn Asbury, PhD, Vice Chair

3760 National Tay-Sachs and Allied Disease Association
2001 Beacon Street 800-906-8723
Brighton, MA 02135 800-906-8723
Fax: 617-277-0134
e-mail: info@ntsad.org
www.ntsad.org
A mutual support group coordinated by staff and volunteers who are parents of affected children of affected adults. One of several programs supported and sponsored by the association.
Bradley L Campbell, President
Stewart Altman, Vice President

Research Centers

3761 Lysosomal Disease Center at the University of Pittsburgh
E1650 Biomedical Science Tower
Pittsburgh, PA 15261 800-334-7980
pitt.edu
Offers diagnosis management treatment and genetic counseling for people with or at risk for lysosomal storage disease and their families.
John A Barrenger MD PhD, Director
Erin O'Rourk MS CGC, Manager

3762 National Gaucher Disease Foundation
2227 Idlewood Road 770-934-2910
Tucker, GA 30084 800-504-3189
Fax: 770-934-2911
e-mail: rhonda@gaucherdisease.org
www.gaucherdisease.org
Provides information and assistance for those affected by Gaucher disease.
Rhonda P Buyers, CEO/Executive Director
Barbara Lichtenstein, Programs Director National Gaucher Care

Support Groups & Hotlines

3763 Fabry Support & Information Group
108 NE 2nd Street Suite C
Concordia, MO 64020

660-463-1355
Fax: 660-463-1356
e-mail: info@fabry.org
www.fabry.org

To raise awareness of Fabry disease and its symptoms. The website provides mutual self-help by linking patients and family members/caregivers. In this way they can support and encourage one another.
J Johnson, Founder

Web Sites

3764 A World of Genetic Societies

www.faseb.org/genetics

Listing of genetic professional societies, many with searchable databases.

3765 Alliance of Genetic Support Groups

www.geneticalliance.org

Coalition of individuals, professionals and genetic support organizations.

3766 Fabry Support & Information Group

www.fabry.org

Discussion page, information about disease, newsletters, patient biographies, links.

3767 Gene Clinics

www.geneclinics.org

Searchable, expert-authored, peer reviewed disease database.

3768 International Center for Fabry Disease

www.mssm.edu/crc/Fabry/fabry.html

Associated with Mt. Sinai, with information about Fabry including a program to family tree.

3769 International Storage Disease Collaborative

www.pediatrics.med.umn/edu/isdcsg/

This study group focuses on stem cell and bone marrow transplantation. Has discussion page/general information.

3770 MedicineNet

www.medicinenet.com

An online resource for consumers providing easy-to-read, authoritative medical and health information.

3771 Morbus Fabry

home.t-online.de

Fabry information and links to other sites.

3772 NIH's National Institute of Neurological Disorders & Strokes

www.ninds.nih.gov

Description of disease, therapies.

3773 National Organization for Rare Disorders (NORD)

www.rarediseases.org

The NORD is a unique federation of voluntary health organizations dedicated to helping people with rare orphan diseases and assisting the organization that serve them.

3774 National Society of Genetic Counselors

nsgc.org

Society website with searchable membership database.

3775 OMIM: Fabry Disease

www.ncbi.nlm.nih.gov

Description of disease and links to research papers written.

3776 Pediatric Database: Fabry Disease

www.icondata.com

Description of disease.

3777 Support-Group.Com: Fabry Disease

www.support-group.com

Fabry Disease discussion forum.

Description

3778 Fibromyalgia Syndrome

Fibromyalgia syndrome, FMS, also called fibrositis or fibromyositis, is a condition of widespread muscular pain and fatigue. It strikes mostly women between the ages of 20 and 50, and may affect as many as one in 20 adult females. The pain ranges from mild discomfort to complete disability and may vary from day to day. Physical over-exertion, changes in weather, drafty environments, stress, depression, and hormonal changes can all contribute to flare-ups in FMS symptoms.

In addition to widespread pain, FMS also causes a decreased sense of energy, disturbances of sleep, and varying degrees of anxiety and depression. Other medical conditions sometimes associated with fibromyalgia include tension headaches, migraine, irritable bowel syndrome, premenstrual tension syndrome, chronic fatigue syndrome, cold intolerance, and restless leg syndrome.

A physician's diagnosis of FMS is usually based on the following criteria: widespread musculoskeletal pain; tenderness at 11 or more of 18 specific tender points, which are exquisitely more tender than adjacent sites; and scans of the brain. Fibromyalgia may remit spontaneously with decreased stress but can recur at frequent intervals or become chronic.

There is currently no commonly accepted cure for this condition. Aspirin and other drugs used to treat musculoskeletal pain partially improve symptoms. Antidepressant drugs, taken in low doses, have been shown to provide restorative sleep. Patients may also benefit from regular aerobic exercises, local applications of heat, gentle massage and reduced stress in their lives. See also *Chronic Fatigue Syndrome.*

National Agencies & Associations

3779 American Fibromyalgia Syndrome Association
6380 East Tanque Verde   520-733-1570
Tucson, AZ 85715   Fax: 520-290-5550
e-mail: kthorson@afsafund.org
www.afsafund.org
Nonprofit organization whose primary mission is to seed research in FMS and CFS. We acknowledge that patient and physician education, public awareness and advocacy are all important ingredients in aiding the lives of people with FMS and CFS.
Kristen Thorson, President
Steve Thorson, VP

3780 FM-CFS Canada
99 Fifth Avenue
Ottawa, Ontario, K1S-5P5   www.fm-cfs.ca
Dedicated to advancing Fibromyalgia (FM) and Chronic Fatigue Syndrome (CFS) education, research and treatment.
Graham Mayes, President/Director
Ed Napke MD PhD, VP/Director

3781 National Chronic Fatigue Syndrome and Fibromyalgia Association
PO Box 18426   816-737-1343
Kansas City, MO 64133   Fax: 816-524-6782
e-mail: information@ncfsfa.org
www.ncfsfa.org

Offering a support group, medical and patient information plus research.
Orvalene Prewitt, President

3782 National Chronic Fatigue Syndrome and Fibr
PO Box 18426   816-737-1343
Kansas City, MO 64133   Fax: 816-524-6782
e-mail: information@ncfsfa.org
www.ncfsfa.org
Offering a support group medical and patient information plus research.
Orvalene Prewitt, President

3783 National Fibromyalgia Association
2121 S Towne Centre Place   714-921-0150
Anaheim, CA 92806   Fax: 714-921-6920
e-mail: kfox@fmaware.org
www.fmaware.org
Develops and extends programs dedicated to improving the quality of life for people with Fibromyalgia by increasing the awareness of the public media government and medical communities. Supports an ongoing media presence and assist local support groups.
Lynne Matallana, Founder/President
Rae Marie Gleason, Executive Director

3784 National Fibromyalgia Partnership (NFP)
PO Box 160
Linden, VA 22642   866-725-4404
Fax: 866-666-2727
e-mail: mail@fmpartnership.org
www.fmpartnership.org
The NFP is a 501(c)(3) non-profit, membership organization which publishes medically accurate information on Fibromyalgia to patients, health care professionals and the public. Information and resources not listed in this volume are available in print and/or on the NFP Web site. It also provides support and start-up information to support groups. Additional Web site: www.frontiersnews.org
Tamara K Liller, President & Director of Publications
Jacqueline M Yencha, Vice-President, Asst Dir of Publications

3785 National Hemophilia Foundation/Hemophilia and AIDS/HIV Network (HANDI)
116 W 32nd Street   212-328-3700
New York, NY 10001   Fax: 212-328-3777
www.hemophilia.org
Dedicated to the treatment and the cure of hemophilia AIDS and other blood related disorders. This foundation wished to improve the quality of life of all those affected through promotion and support of research education and other services.
Val Bias, CEO
Neil Frick, Vice President

3786 National ME/FM Action Network
National ME/FM Action Network   613-829-6667
Nepean, Ontario, K2H- 8V7   Fax: 613-829-8518
www.mefmaction.net
A non-profit organization dedicated to advancing the recognition and understanding of Myalgic Encephalomyelitis/Chronic Fatigue Syndrome (ME/CFS) and Fibromyalgia Syndrome (FMS) through education, advocacy, support, and research.
Lydia Neilson, Contact

3787 Option Institute
2080 S Undermountain Road   413-229-2100
Sheffield, MA 01257   800-714-2779
Fax: 413-229-8931
e-mail: participantsupport@option.org
www.option.org
Self-defeating beliefs along with attitudes and judgments can lead to a host of physical and psychological challenges, including Fibromyalgia. The Option Institute offers programs designed to help you gain new perspectives on the attitudes and judgments that can hamper progress.
Barry Kaufman, Co-Founder
Samahria Lyt Kaufman, Co-Founder

Libraries & Resource Centers

3788 Fibromyalgia Resources Group
103 Sherwood Hill Road
Brewster, NY 10509
845-278-5944
Fax: 845-278-2641
e-mail: kindness@fibrobetsy.com
Personalized patient service searches and distributes information on patient recommended, fibromyalgia literate doctors world wide. Information packet is included with each doctor list emailed. Doctor recommendations are welcome.
Betsy Jacobson, President

Support Groups & Hotlines

3789 National Chronic Fatigue Syndrome and Fibr omyalgia Association Support Group
PO Box 18426
Kansas City, MO 64133
816-737-1343
Fax: 816-524-6782
e-mail: information@ncfsfa.org
www.ncfsfa.org
To educate and inform the public about the nature and impact of Chronic Fatigue Syndrome and Fibromyalgia and related disorders.
Orvalene Prewitt, President

3790 National Health Information Center
PO Box 1133
Washington, DC 20013
310-565-4167
800-336-4797
Fax: 301-984-4256
e-mail: info@nhic.org
www.health.gov/nhic
A health information referral service sponsored by the Office of Disease Prevention and Health Promotion. Puts health professionals and consumers who have health questions in touch with those organizations that are best able to provide answers.

3791 Rocky Mountain CFIDS/FMS Association
7020 E Girard Avenue
Denver, CO 80224
303-423-7367
e-mail: link@rmcfa.org
www.rmcfa.org
An educational resource for patients, medical professionals and those affected by these diseases.
Tim Smith, President

Arizona

3792 Fibromyalgia Network
PO Box 31750
Tucson, AZ 85751-1750
520-290-5508
800-853-2929
Fax: 520-290-5550
e-mail: inquiry@fmnetnews.com
www.fmnetnews.com
Provides individuals with ad-free, patient-focused information that can be use today.

Books

3793 All About Fibromyalgia
Oxford University Press
198 Madison Avenue
New York, NY 10016-4314
212-726-6033
800-451-7556
Fax: 212-726-6447
www.oup-usa.org

ISBN: 0-195147-53-7

3794 Delicate Balance: Living Successfully with Chronic Illness
Perseus Books Group
5500 Central Avenue
Boulder, CO 80301
800-386-5656
Fax: 303-449-3356
e-mail: info@perseuspublishing.com
www.perseuspublishing.com
Up to date and practical advice and inspiration for the millions of Americans who struggle daily against chronic illness. From locating a suitable healthcare provider and making sense of the powerful emotions that accompany chronic illness, to seeking accomodations from the Americans with Disabilities Act, this book is helpful and hopeful.
312 pages
ISBN: 0-738203-23-8

3795 Fibromyalgia
NAMSIC/National Institutes of Health
1 AMS Circle
Bethesda, MD 20892-0001
301-495-4484
877-226-4267
Fax: 301-718-6366
TTY: 301-565-2966
e-mail: niamsinfo@mail.nih.gov
www.nih.gov/niams

3796 Fibromyalgia & Other Central Pain Syndromes
Daniel Wallace, Daniel Clauw, author
Lippincott Williams & Wilkins
16522 Hunters Green Parkway
Hagerstown, MD 21740-2116
800-638-3030
Fax: 301-223-2400
www.lww.com
Devoted to fibromyalgia and other centrally mediated chronic pain syndromes. Leading experts examine the latest research findings on these syndromes and present evidence-based reviews of current controversies.
2005
ISBN: 0-781752-61-2

3797 Fibromyalgia Guidelines: The Concensus Diagnosis & Treatment Protocols
FM-CFS Canada
99 Fifth Avenue
Ottawa ON CANADA K1S 5P5,
www.fm-cfs.ca/fm
This entire special issue of the Journal of Musculoskeletal Pain [JMP] is devoted to presentation of what will likely to be called the Canadian Consensus Document on Fibromyalgia Syndrome (FMS). The document encompasses a very broad scope, involving a clinical case definition, diagnosis, and management of FMS.
130 pages Volume 11, #4

3798 Fibromyalgia Relief Book: 213 Ideas for Improving Your Quality of Life
Walker & Company
435 Hudson Street
New York, NY 10014
212-727-8300
Fax: 212-727-0984
e-mail: orders@walkerbooks.com
www.walkerbooks.com

208 pages Paperback
ISBN: 0-802775-53-5
Josh Wood, Sales Director

3799 Fibromyalgia Supporter
Anadem Publishing Company
3620 N High Street
Columbus, OH 43214
800-633-0055
Fax: 614-262-6630
e-mail: anadem@anadem.com
www.anadem.com

3800 Fibromyalgia Survivor
Anadem Publishing Company
3620 N High Street
Columbus, OH 43214
800-633-0055
Fax: 614-262-6630
e-mail: anadem@anadem.com
www.anadem.com

ISBN: 0-964689-12-X

3801 Fibromyalgia Syndrome and Chronic Fatigue Syndrome in Young People
Fibromyalgia Network
PO Box 31750
Tucson, AZ 85751-1750
800-853-2929
Fax: 520-290-5550
www.fmnetnews.com
Guide for parents.

3802 Fibromyalgia and Chronic Myofascial Pain Syndrome: a Survivor Manual
New Harbinger Publishers
5674 Shattuck Avenue
Oakland, CA 94609
800-748-6273
Fax: 510-652-5472
www.newharbinger.com
Written from the perspective of myofacial pain syndrome.
432 pages

3803 Fibromyalgia, Managing the Pain
Anadem Publishing Company
3620 N High Street
Columbus, OH 43214-3611
800-633-0055
Fax: 614-262-6630
e-mail: anadem@anadem.com
www.anadem.com
Comprehensive guide to the syndrome, including chapters on diagnosis, medication, physical medicine treatments, occupational adjustments, advice on flare ups and some medical and legal aspects of FMS.

3804 Inside Fibromyalgia
Anadem Publishing Company
3620 N High Street
Columbus, OH 43214
614-262-2539
800-633-0055
Fax: 614-262-6630
e-mail: anadem@anadem.com
www.anadem.com
Written by a physician who has fibromyalgia. From the newest medications to alternative therapies and everything in between, Dr. Pellegrino helps you develop a plan for healing today and tomorrow.
Paperback
ISBN: 1-890018-36-8

3805 Laugh at Your Muscles
Anadem Publishing Company
3620 N High Street
Columbus, OH 43214-3611
800-633-0055
Fax: 614-262-6630
e-mail: anadem@anadem.com
www.anadem.com

3806 Occupational Therapy Practice Guidelines for Adults with Rheumatoid Arthritis
American Occupational Therapy Association
4720 Montgomery Lane
Bethesda, MD 20824-1220
301-652-2682
Fax: 301-652-7711
TDD: 800-377-8555
www.aota.org

20 pages
ISBN: 1-569001-12-X

3807 Taking Charge of Fibromyalgia
FMS Educational Systems
500 Bushway Road
Wayzata, MN 55391
419-841-3435
Fax: 419-841-3435
e-mail: info@fmsedsys.com
www.fmsedsys.com
Written by three professionals who have fibromyalgia and who often update the book.

3808 Taking Control of TMJ: Your Total Wellness Program
Robert O Uppgaard, DDS, author

New Harbinger Publications
5674 Shattuck Avenue
Oakland, CA 94609
800-748-6273
Fax: 510-652-5472
www.newharbinger.com
Six-step wellness program helps readers understand what TMJ is and provides exercises to improve jaw functioning, relieve pain and deal with trigger points, eliminate harmful habits, deal with contributing stress, and evaluate and improve your diet and exercise habits. Additional chapters cover the connection between TMJ, whiplash, and fibromyalgia.
2004 200 pages Paperback
ISBN: 1-572241-26-8

3809 Understanding Post-Traumatic Fibromyalgia
Anadem Publishing Company
3620 N High Street
Columbus, OH 43214-3611
800-633-0055
Fax: 614-262-6630
e-mail: anadem@anadem.com
www.anadem.com
Anyone with post-traumatic fibromyalgia will benefit from reading this book focusing exclusively on this condition.

Magazines

3810 FM Monograph
National Fibromyalgia Partnership
PO Box 160
Linden, VA 22642
866-725-4404
Fax: 866-666-2727
e-mail: mail@fmpartnership.org
www.fmpartnership.org
Publishes a print quarterly (available online and in booklet form in English, Spanish, and French) which provides information on fibromyalgia symptoms, diagnosis, treatment, and research. Comprehensive resource packets and reprints are also available on a variety of subjects. Technical support is provided to fibromyalgia support organizations worldwide.
Quarterly
Tamara Liller, President

3811 Fibromyalgia AWARE
National Fibromyalgia Association
2238 N Glassell Street
Orange, CA 92865
714-921-0150
Fax: 714-921-6920
e-mail: nfa@FMaware.org
www.FMaware.org
Official publication of the National Fibromyalgia Association. Available to members and contributors.

3812 Fibromyalgia Frontiers
National Fibromyalgia Partnership (NFP)
PO Box 160
Linden, VA 22642
866-725-4404
Fax: 866-666-2727
e-mail: mail@fmpartnership.org
www.fmpartnership.org
Publishes a print quarterly (available online and in booklet form in English, Spanish, and French) which provides information on fibromyalgia symptoms, diagnosis, treatment, and research. Comprehensive resource packets and reprints are also available on a variety of subjects. Technical support is provided to fibromyalgia support organizations worldwide. Included with membership into NFP.
Quarterly
Tamara Liller, President

3813 Journal of Musculoskeletal Pain
Haworth Medical Press
10 Alice Street
Binghamton, NY 13904-1503
607-722-5857
800-429-6784
Fax: 607-722-0012
e-mail: getinfo@haworthpress.com
www.haworthpress.com
Peer reviewed medical journal containing FMS scientific abstract information. Appropriate for medical professionals as well as amateur.
Quarterly

Newsletters

3814 Fibromyalgia Clinic Kentfield Rehabilitation Newsletter
Fibromyalgia Clinic
25 Sir Francis Drake Boulevard
Kentfield, CA 94904
415-485-3530

3815 Florida Fibromyalgia News
FMS Association of Florida
PO Box 14848
Gainesville, FL 32604-4848
352-371-2750
Quarterly newsletter.

3816 Health Points
TyH Publications
17007 E Colony Drive
Fountain Hills, AZ 85268
800-801-1406
e-mail: editor@e-tyh.com
National newsletter with articles on complementary therapy, latest nutrition news, disability issues and much more. Focus is on fibromyalgia, chronic fatigue, arthritis and chronic pain.
Quarterly

3817 Healthwatch
CFIDS and Fibromyalgia Health Resource
2040 Alameda Padre Serra
Santa Barbara, CA 93103
800-366-6056
Fax: 805-965-0042
e-mail: cutomerservice@prohealthinc.com
www.immunesupport.com
Healthwatch serves fibromyalgia and chronic fatigue syndrome sufferers by focusing on reporting the latest news in research and treatment, making hard-to-find nutritional supplements available at low prices, and raising needed funds for medical research.

3818 Journal of Musculoskeletal Medicine
Cliggott Publishing Company
55 Holly Hill Lane
Greenwich, CT 06830-6074
203-661-0600
This journal provides a unique and efficient monthly update on the management of musculoskeletal disorders. Offers articles regarding orthopedics, rheumatology, sports medicine, etc.

3819 Tender Points
The Arthritis Society
393 University Avenue
Ontario, Canada M5G 1E6,
416-979-7228
800-321-1433
Fax: 416-979-8366
e-mail: info@on.erthritis.ca
Newsletter of The Arthritis Society.
Quarterly

3820 To Your Health and Healthpoints
To Your Health
17007 E Colony Drive
Fountain Hills, AZ 85268
800-801-1406
Fax: 480-837-1875
www.e-tyh.com
Resource catalogue and newspaper for FMS, CFIDS, arthritis, and chronic pain. Features vitamins and health products developed specifically for FMS and CFIDS making hard-to-find, recommended nutritional supplements available to fibromyalgia and chronic fatigue syndrome sufferers at a manufacturer-direct low price.

Audio & Video

3821 Audio Cassette Program on Fibromyalgia
Arthritis Foundation/Research Cassettes
111 E Wacker Drive
Chicago, IL 60601-3713
312-616-3470
Covers treatment and research taped during a patient education forum.

3822 Fibromyalgia Interval Training
Arthritis Foundation Distribution Center
PO Box 6996
Alpharetta, GA 30023-6996
800-207-8633
Fax: 770-442-9742
www.arthritis.com
Designed for people with fibromyalgia, the video features warm water exercises in shallow and deep water, including warmup, stretching, upper and lower body exercises, aerobics, strengthing, cool-down and relaxation. Designed to help you manage the pain, stiffness and fatigue of fibromyalgia.

3823 Fibromyalgia Stretch Video & Strength and Toning Video
Oregon Fibromyalgia Foundation
1221 SW Yamhill
Portland, OR 97205
503-228-3217
www.myalgia.com

These videos offer comprehensive stretching and strength and toning regimens developed by exercise physiologist Sharon Clark PhD, FNP, specifically for people with FMS. Fibromyalgia patients are shown demonstrating these unique stretching and strength and toning programs. Prices are per video and do not include shipping and handling.

3824 Fibromyalgia: Face to Face
Ontario Fibromyalgia Association
250 Cloor Street E
Toronto, Ontario, M4W
416-979-7228
A 14 minute insight into living with FMS from people, including children, who are coping with this syndrome.

3825 Improving Muscle Tone and Strength
Oregon Fibromyalgia Foundation
1221 SW Yamhill
Portland, OR 97205
503-228-3217
A video developed by exercise physiologist Sharon Clark, PhD, RN, specifically for people with fibromyalgia.

Web Sites

3826 American Fibromyalgia Research Association
www.afsafund.org
Charitable organization whose primary mission is to seed research in FMS and CFS. We acknowledge that patient and physician education, public awareness and advocacy are all important ingredients in aiding the lives of people with FMS and CFS.

3827 FM/CFS Canada
www.fm-cfs.ca
Dedicated to advancing Fibromyalgia (FM) and Chronic Fatigue Syndrome (CFS) education, research and treatment.

3828 Healing Well
www.healingwell.com
An online health resource guide to medical news, chat, information and articles, newsgroups and message boards, books, disease-related web sites, medical directories, and more for patients, friends, and family coping with disabling diseases, disorders, or chronic illnesses.

3829 Health Finder
www.healthfinder.gov
Searchable, carefully developed web site offering information on over 1000 topics. Developed by the US Department of Health and Human Services, the site can be used in both English and Spanish.

3830 Healthlink USA
www.healthlinkusa.com
Health information concerning treatment, cures, prevention, diagnosis, risk factors, research, support groups, email lists, personal stories and much more. Updated regularly.

3831 Helios Health
www.helioshealth.com
Online resource for your health information. Detailed information about specific health topics, access to expert advice from our Medical Advisory Board, and up-to-date health news.

3832 MedicineNet
www.medicinenet.com
An online resource for consumers providing easy-to-read, authoritative medical and health information.

3833 Medscape
www.medscape.com
Medscape offers specialists, primary care physicians, and other health professionals the Web's most robust and integrated medical information and educational tools.

3834 My Fibromyalgia & Chronic Fatigue Syndrome
www.fms-help.com
A woman's personal story about her battle with fibromyalgia.

3835 National Fibromyalgia Association
www.fmaware.org
Information for fibromyalgia patients and the general public.

3836 **National Fibromyalgia Partnership (NFP)**
PO Box 160
Linden, VA 22642
866-725-4404
Fax: 866-666-2727
e-mail: mail@fmpartnership.org
www.fmpartnership.org

The NFP is a 501(c)(3) non-profit, membership organization which publishes medically accurate information on fibromyalgia to patients, health care professionals and the public. Information and resources not listed in this volume are available in print and/or on the NFP website. It also provides support and start-up informaiton to support groups. Additional website: www.frontiersnews.org

Tamara K Liller, President & Director of Publications
Jacqueline M Yencha, Vice-President, Asst Dir of Publications

3837 **Neurology Channel**
www.neurologychannel.com

Find clearly explained, medically accurate information regarding conditions, including an overview, symptoms, causes, diagnostic procedures and treatment options. On this site it is possible to ask questions and get information from a neurologist and connect to people who have similar health interests.

3838 **Option Institute**
Option Institute
www.option.org/fibromyalgia.html

Self-defeating beliefs, along with attitudes and judgments, can lead to a host of physical and psychological challenges, including Fibromyalgia. The Option Institute offers programs designed to help you gain new perspectives on the attitudes and judgments that may be affecting your life, especially those regarding and surrounding Fibromyalgia.

3839 **WebMD**
www.webmd.com

Information on Fibromyalgia Syndrome, including articles and resources.

Description

3840 Gastrointestinal Disorders

The digestive tract is responsible for taking food into the body, processing it into simple chemicals that can be absorbed to nourish the body, and expelling the remainder.

Motility disorders of the gastrointestinal (GI) tract are conditions in which there is a failure of normal top-to-bottom movement of gastric contents. In reflux, the food content moves from the stomach back into the esophagus, irritating that organ and causing heartburn, the most common symptom. This is known as GERD, or gastro-esophageal reflux disease, and sometimes causes choking or coughing. Complications include inflammation and even ulceration of the esophagus. It is a problem in infants, but also occurs in adults especially with advancing age. Occasionally, an ulcer may develop in a segment of the GI tract, typically in the stomach or duodenum. An infectious agent, H. pylori, plays a central role in peptic ulcer disease. In achalasia, the normal movement of food down the GI tract by peristalsis is disrupted, and contents of the esophagus are unable to move into the stomach. As a result, the person chokes on food or liquid. Chest pain and coughing at night may also occur.

Other motility disorders reflect the bowel's inability to move its contents forward properly. Children may be born with Hirschprung's disease in which peristalsis is absent or abnormal in the large bowel, resulting in partial or complete obstruction. The most common motility disorder in adults is called irritable bowel syndrome; also known as functional bowel or spastic colitis, it causes variable degrees of abdominal pain and bloating, diarrhea and/or constipation.

Outpouchings in the walls of the lower GI tract, called diverticula, sometimes trap nutrient waste, and may become infected, bleed, and rupture. Finally, the digestive tract may fail in its primary task of absorbing nutrients, known as malabsorption syndromes. Rarely it will absorb too much of something. In hemochromatosis, for instance, the bowel takes in too much iron from the diet, and the excess is stored in and damages the liver, pancreas, heart, and gonads. More commonly, the body absorbs too little nutrient rather than too much. For instance, celiac disease, or sprue, is a disorder caused by intolerance to gluten, a cereal protein in wheat rye, barley, and oats. Lactose intolerance is an inability to digest a carbohydrate in dairy products. Treatment for malabsorption syndromes includes dietary modifications and, in more serious cases, supplementation with intravenous feedings known as parenteral nutrition.

National Agencies & Associations

3841 American College of Gastroenterology
PO Box 342260
Bethesda, MD 20827-2260
301-263-9000
www.acg.gi.org

ACG serves clinical and scientific information needs of member physicians and surgeons who specialize in digestive and related disorders. Emphasis is on scholarly practice, teaching and research.
Delbert H Chumley MD, President
Edgar Achkar MD, Director

3842 American Dietetic Association
120 S Riverside Plaza
Chicago, IL 60606-6995
312-899-0040
800-877-1600
e-mail: media@eatright.org
www.eatright.org

ADA serves the public through the promotion of optimal nutrition health and well-being.
Patricia M Babjak, Chief Executive Officer
Judith Rodriguez, President

3843 American Gastroenterological Association National Office
National Office
4930 Del Ray Avenue
Bethesda, MD 20814
301-654-2055
Fax: 301-654-5920
e-mail: member@gastro.org
www.gastro.org

AGA fosters the development and application of the science of gastroenterology by providing leadership and aid including patient care, research, teaching, continuing education, scientific communication and matters of national health policy.
Ian L Taylor MD, President
Loren Lane MD, Vice President

3844 American Hemochromatosis Society
4044 W Lake Mary Boulevard
Lake Mary, FL 32746-2012
407-829-4488
888-655-4766
Fax: 407-333-1284
e-mail: mail@americanhs.org
www.americanhs.org

Educates the public, the medical community and the media by distributing the most current information available on hereditary hemochromatosis (HH) including DNA screening for HH and pediatric HH; also facilitates patient empowerment through an online network.
Sandra Thomas, President/Founder

3845 American Motility Society
45685 Harmony Lane
Belleville, MI 48111
734-699-1130
Fax: 734-699-1136
e-mail: admin@motilitysociety.org
www.motilitysociety.org

Promotes research and sponsors professional education seminars about gastrointestinal motility topics including disorders of esophageal, gastric, small intestinal, and colonic function; and sponsors biennial meetings (even years), syposia and courses.
Michael Cami MD, President
Lori Ennis, Executive Director

3846 American Pancreatic Association
PO Box 14906
Minneapolis, MN 55414
612-626-9797
Fax: 612-625-7700
e-mail: apa@umn.edu
www.american-pancreatic-association.org

Provides forum for presentation of scientific research related to the pancreas.
Suresh Chari, President

3847 American Pseudo-Obstruction and Hirschsprung's Disease Society
1825 Connecticut Avenue NW
Washington, DC 20009
202-884-8200
Fax: 20- 88- 844
TTY: 800-695-0285
e-mail: nichcy@aed.org
www.nichcy.org

Promotes public awareness of gastrointestinal motility disorders in particular intestinal pseudo-obstruction and Hirschsprung's disease; provides education and support to individuals and families of children who have been diagnosed with these disorders.

3848 **American Society for Gastrointestinal Endoscopy**
1520 Kensington Road 630-573-0600
Oak Brook, IL 60523 800-353-2743
Fax: 630-573-0691
e-mail: info@asge.org
www.asge.org
ASGE provides information training and practice guidelines about
gastrointestinal endoscopic techniques.
M Brian Fennerty, President
Gregory G Ginsberg, President-Elect

3849 **American Society for Parenteral and Enteral Nutrition (ASPEN)**
8630 Fenton Street 301-587-6315
Silver Spring, MD 20910-3805 Fax: 301-587-2365
e-mail: aspen@nutr.org
www.nutritioncare.org
Offers information and continuing medical education to professionals involved in the care of parenterally and enterally fed patients. Membership includes complimentary subscriptions to two
peer reviewed journals.
Charles Ston Vanway, President
Tom Jaksic MD, Vice President

3850 **American Society of Adults with Pseudo-Obstruction**
International Corporate Headquarters
19 Carrol Road 781-935-9776
Woburn, MA 01801-6161 Fax: 781-933-4151
ASAP educates the general public and medical community about
chronic intestinal pseudo-obstruction (CIP) and other related digestive motility disorders; serves as an integral source of information for patients of all ages with CIP and related disorders.

3851 **Center for Digestive Disorders: Central**
25 N Winfield Road 630-933-1600
Winfield, IL 60190 877-933-4234
Fax: 630-933-1300
TTY: 630-933-4833
e-mail: cdh_information@cdh.org
www.cdh.org
Multifaceted program to meet the needs of people who suffer from
gastrointestinal problems; offers literature, videotapes and educational meetings and, if medical care is needed, appropriate referrals are made.
Luke McGuinness, President/CEO
Jim Spear, Executive Vice President/CFO

3852 **Cyclic Vomiting Syndrome Association**
10520 W Bluemound Road 414-342-7880
Milwaukee, WI 53226 Fax: 414-342-8980
e-mail: cvsa@cvsaonline.org
www.cvsaonline.org
CVSA provides opportunities for patients, families and professionals to offer and receive support and share knowledge about cyclic vomiting syndrome; actively promotes and facilitates medical
research about nausea and vomiting.
Kathleen Adams, President, Co Founder

3853 **Digestive Disease National Coalition**
507 Capitol Court NE 202-544-7497
Washington, DC 20002 Fax: 202-546-7105
e-mail: ddnc@hmcw.org
www.ddnc.org
Informs the public and the health care community about digestive
disorders; seeks Federal funding for research education and training; and represents members' interests regarding Federal and State
legislation that affects digestive diseases research.
Linda Aukett, Chairperson
James DeGerome MD, President

3854 **International Academy of Proctology**
2209 John R Wooden Drive 765-342-3686
Martinsville, IN 46151 Fax: 765-342-4173
Encourages study of diseases of the colon and accessory organs of
digestion and conducts seminars.
George Donna MD

3855 **International Foundation for Functional Gastrointestinal Disorders**
PO Box 170864 414-964-1799
Milwaukee, WI 53217-8076 888-964-2001
Fax: 414-964-7176
e-mail: iffgd@iffgd.org
www.iffgd.org
IFFGD is a nonprofit education support and research organization
devoted to increasing awareness and understanding of functional
gastrointestinal disorders, including irritable bowel syndrome
(IBS), constipation, diarrhea, pain, and incontinence.
Nancy J Norton, President

3856 **Iron Overload Diseases Association**
525 Mayflower Road 561-586-8246
W Palm Beach, FL 33405 866-768-8629
Fax: 561-842-9881
e-mail: iod@ironoverload.org
www.ironoverload.org
Conducts professional education symposiums and exhibits at medical meetings; serves and counsels hemochromatosis patients and
families; offers doctor referrals; promotes patient advocacy concerning insurance, Medicare, blood banks, and the FDA.
Roberta Crawford, Founder/President

3857 **National Digestive Diseases Information Clearinghouse**
Two Information Way
Bethesda, MD 20892-3570 800-891-5389
Fax: 703-738-4929
TTY: 866-569-1162
e-mail: nddic@info.niddk.nih.gov
www.digestive.niddk.nih.gov
Offers various educational information, public resources and re-
prints, public awareness materials and more on digestive disor-
ders.
Griffin P Rodgers MD MACP, Director

3858 **North American Society for Pediatric Gastroenterology and Nutrition**
PO Box 6 215-233-0808
Flourtown, PA 19031 Fax: 215-233-3918
e-mail: naspghan@naspghan.org
www.naspghan.org
Promotes research and provides a forum for professionals in the ar-
eas of pediatric GI liver disease, gastroenterology, and nutrition.
Associated with fellow organizations in Europe and Australia
(ESPGAN, AUSPGAN).
Margaret K Stallings, Executive Director
Philip M Sherman, MD, FRCPC, President

3859 **Pediatric Adolescent Gastroesophageal Reflux Association**
PO Box 7728 301-601-9541
Silver Spring, MD 20907 888-887-7729
e-mail: gergroup@aol.com
www.reflux.org
PAGER's mission is to: (l) gather and disseminate information on
pediatric gastroesophageal reflux (GER) and related disorders; (2)
provide educational and emotional support to patients with GER,
their families, and professionals; (3) promote awareness of GER
within both the medical community and the general public; and (4)
promote research into the causes, treatments and eventual cure for
pediatric GER.
Beth Anderson, Director

3860 **Pediatric Adolescent Gastroesophageal Asso ciation**
PO Box 7728 301-601-9541
Silver Spring, MD 20907 e-mail: gergroup@aol.com
www.reflux.org
PAGER's mission is to: (l) gather and disseminate information on
pediatric gastroesophageal reflux (GER) and related disorders; (2)
provide educational and emotional support to patients with GER,
their families and professionals; (3) promote awareness.
Beth Anderson, Director
Jennifer Rackley, Associate Director

3861 **Pediatric/Adolescent Gastroesophageal Reflux Association**
PO Box 7728 301-601-9541
Silver Spring, MD 20907-1153 888-887-7729
e-mail: gergroup@aol.com
www.reflux.org

PAGER gathers and disseminates information on pediatric gastroesophageal reflux and related disorders; provides support and education to patients their families and the public; promotes the general welfare of patients, their families and the public.
Beth Anderson, Director
Jennifer Rackley, Associate Director

3862 Society for Surgery of the Alimentary Tract
900 Cummings Center   978-927-8330
Beverly, MA 01915   Fax: 978-524-8890
                                        www.ssat.com
SSAT provides a forum for exchange of information among physicians specializing in alimentary tract surgery.
David W Rattner, President
David M Mahvi MD, President-Elect

3863 Society of American Gastrointestinal Endoscopic Surgeons
11300 W Olympic Boulevard   310-437-0544
Los Angeles, CA 90064   Fax: 310-437-0585
                                        www.sages.org
SAGES encourages study and practice of gastrointestinal endoscopy laparoscopy and minimal access surgery.
Jo Buyske, President
Steven D Schwaitzberg MD, President-Elect

3864 Society of Gastroenterology Nurses and Associates
401 N Michigan Avenue   312-321-5165
Chicago, IL 60611-4267   800-245-7462
                                   Fax: 312-673-6694
                          e-mail: sgna@smithbucklin.com
                                        www.sgna.org
SGNA provides members with continuing education opportunities practice and training guidelines and information about trends and development in the field of gastroenterology.
Peggy Gauthier, President
Leslie Stewart, President-Elect

3865 United Ostomy Association
PO Box 512
Northfield, MN 55057   800-826-0826
                                   Fax: 507-645-5168
                             e-mail: info@uoaa.org
                                        www.uoaa.org
A national network for bowel and urinary diversion support groups in the United States. Its goal is to provide a nonprofit association that will serve to unify and strengthen its member support groups, which are organized for the benefit of people who have, or will have intestinal or urinary diversions and their caregivers.
David Rudzin, President

Foundations

3866 American Porphyria Foundation
PO Box 22712   713-266-9617
Houston, TX 77227   Fax: 713-840-9552
                             e-mail: porphyrus@aol.com
                          www.porphyriafoundation.com
The APF is dedicated to improving the health and well-being of individuals and families affected by porphyria. Our mission is to enhance public awareness about porphyria, develop educational programs and distributing educational material for patients and physicians and support research to improve treatment and ultimately lead to a cure.
Desiree H Lyon, Executive Director

3867 Gastro-Intestinal Research Foundation
70 East Lake Street   312-332-1350
Chicago, IL 60601-5907   Fax: 312-332-4757
                              e-mail: girf@girf.org
                                        www.girf.org
Provides funds for equipment, laboratories and the support of investigators and young physicians in the University of Chicago Gastroenterology Section, a group of full-time dedicated doctors who seek solutions to all kinds of gastrointestinal illnesses, affecting the esophagus, the stomach, the small intestine, the large intestine, the liver, the gallbladder, and the pancreas.
Jennifer Wright, Executive Director

3868 Oley Foundation
Albany Medical Center   518-262-5079
Albany, NY 12208-3478   800-776-6539
                                   Fax: 518-262-5528
                                        www.oley.org
Promotes and advocates education and research in home parenteral and enteral nutrition; provides support and networking to patients through information clearinghouse and regional volunteer networks; sponsors meetings and conferences, including annual patient/clinician conference; maintains speakers bureau.
Joan Bishop, Executive Director

Research Centers

3869 Baylor College of Medicine: General Clinical Research Center for Adults
One Baylor Plaza   713-798-4951
Houston, TX 77030   e-mail: dbier@bcm.edu
                              www.bcm.edu/pediatrics
Endocrinology, genetics and gastroenterology research.
Dennis M Bier MD, Program Director
Paul Klotman, President

3870 Digestive Disorders Associates Ridgely Oaks Professional Center
Ridgely Oaks Professional Center
621 Ridgely Avenue   41- 22- 488
Annapolis, MD 21401   800-273-0505
                                   Fax: 410-224-6971
                                   TTY: 800-735-2258
                                        www.dda.net
Specialize in the diagnosis and treatment of diseases of the entire digestive system including esophagus stomach small and large intestine colon liver pancreas and gall bladder.
Michael S Epstein, Founder
Charles E King, Doctor

3871 Gastrointestinal Research Foundation
70 E Lake Street   312-332-1350
Chicago, IL 60601-5915   Fax: 312-332-4757
                              e-mail: info@girf.org
                                        www.girf.org
Founded to help combat gastrointestinal diseases. Raises funds to support research at the Center for study of the Digestive Diseases at the University of Chicago Medical Center and to support advanced training for scientists. Sponsors educational activities for the public.
Martin N Sandler, Co-Founder
Steven R Davidson, Co-Chairman

3872 University of California: Davis Gastroenterology & Nutrition Center
Pediatric GI Medical Center
4301 X Street   916-453-3750
Sacramento, CA 95817-2214
Research into gastrointestinal mobility and electro-physiology nutrition support and references for the public and patient evaluations.
Robert A Cannon MD, Director

3873 University of California: Los Angeles Center for Ulcer Research
LA Medical Center
Building 115 Room 117   310-312-9284
Los Angeles, CA 90073   Fax: 310-268-4963
                       e-mail: cureadmn@mednet.ucla.edu
                                 www.cure.med.ucla.edu
Offers basic and clinical research related to peptic ulcer disease including causes checks and balances and stress-ulcer relationships.
Enrique Rozengurt, Director
Emeran Mayer, Co-Director

3874 University of Michigan Michigan Gastrointestinal Peptide Research Ctr.
U-M Health System
1500 E Medical Center Drive   734-936-4000
Ann Arbor, MI 48109   Fax: 734-763-2535
                          e-mail: GutPeptide@umich.edu
                                 www.med.umich.edu/mgpc

Research into gastroenterology including chemistry of gut hormones is studied.
Chung Owyang MD, Director
Juanita Merc MD PhD, Associate Director

3875 University of Pennsylvania: Harrison Department of Surgical Research
3400 Spruce Street
Philadelphia, PA 19104

215-662-4000
800-789-PENN
Fax: 215-615-0471
e-mail: julie.koehler@uphs.upenn.edu
www.uphs.upenn.edu/surgery/res/harrisonr

Offers research and studies on surgical transplantations gastrointestinal physiology.
Julie Hagan Koehler MBA, Business Director
Georgina Suarez, Administrative Assistant

Support Groups & Hotlines

3876 National Health Information Center
PO Box 1133
Washington, DC 20013

310-565-4167
800-336-4797
Fax: 301-984-4256
e-mail: info@nhic.org
www.health.gov/nhic

A health information referral service sponsored by the Office of Disease Prevention and Health Promotion. Puts health professionals and consumers who have health questions in touch with those organizations that are best able to provide answers.

3877 Pull-thru Network
2312 Savoy Street
Hoover, AL 35226-1528

205-978-2930
e-mail: ptnmail@charter.net
www.pullthrough.org

Dedicated to the needs of those born wutith anorectal malformation or colon disease and any of the associated diagnoses.

Magazines

3878 ASAP Forum
ASAP International Corporate Headquarters
19 Carroll Road
Woburn, MA 01801

781-935-9776
Fax: 781-933-4151
e-mail: asapgi@sprynet.com

Educates the general public and medical community about chronic intestinal pseudo-obstruction (CIP) and other related digestive motility disorders; serves as an integral source of information for patients of all ages with CIP and related disorders, their families, and members of the medical community.

3879 American Journal of Gastroenterology
American College of Gastroenterology
4900B 31st St S
Arlington, VA 22206-1656

703-820-7400
Fax: 703-931-4520
www.acg.gi.org

Serves clinical and scientific information needs of member physicians and surgeons, who specialize in digestive and related disorders. Emphasis is on scholarly practice, teaching, and research.
Thomas F Fise, Executive Director

3880 American Journal of Gastrointestinal Surgery
Society for Surgery of the Alimentary Tract
13 Elm Street
Manchester, MA 01944

978-526-8330
Fax: 978-526-4018
e-mail: ssat@prri.com
www.ssat.com

Provides information for physicians specializing in gastrointestinal surgery.

3881 Clinical Perspectives in Gastroenterology
American Gastroenterological Association
7910 Woodmont Avenue
Bethesda, MD 20814

301-654-2055
Fax: 301-654-5920
e-mail: aga001@801.com
www.gastro.org

Focuses on research, medical and professional developments in the science of gastroenterology.
Robert Greenberg, Executive VP

3882 Digestive Health Matters
Intl. Foundation for Gastrointestinal Disorders
PO Box 170864
Milwaukee, WI 53217-0864

414-964-1799
888-964-2001
Fax: 414-964-7176
e-mail: iffgd@iffgd.org
www.iffgd.org

Quarterly journal focuses on upper and lower gastrointestinal disorders in adults and children. Educational pamphlets and factsheets are available. Patient and professional membership.

3883 Gastroenterology
American Gastroenterological Association
7910 Woodmont Avenue
Bethesda, MD 20814-3002

301-654-2055
Fax: 301-654-5920
e-mail: aga001@801.com
www.gastro.org

Focuses on research, medical and professional developments in the science of gastroenterology.
Robert Greenberg, Executive VP

3884 Gastroenterology Nursing
Society of Gastroenterology Nurses and Associates
401 N Michigan Avenue
Chicago, IL 60611

312-321-5165
800-245-7462
Fax: 312-321-5194
e-mail: sgna@sba.com
www.sgna.org

Provides members with information about trends and development in the field of gastroenterology nursing.

3885 Gastrointestinal Endoscopy
American Society for Gastrointestinal Endoscopy
1520 Kensington Road
Oak Brook, IL 60523

630-573-0600
Fax: 630-573-0691
www.asge.org

Provides information, training, and practice guidelines about gastrointestinal endoscopic techniques.

3886 Journal of Parenteral and Enteral Nutrition
ASPEN
8630 Fenton Street
Silver Spring, MD 20910-3805

301-587-6315
Fax: 301-587-2365
e-mail: aspen@nutr.org
www.nutritioncare.org

Offers information to professionals involved in the care of parenterally and enterally fed patients.
100 pages BiMonthly
Adrian Nickel, Director Communications/Marketing

3887 Journal of Pediatric Gastroenterology and Nutrition
N American Society for Pediatric Gastroenterology
6900 Grove Road
Thorofare, NJ 08086

609-848-1000
Fax: 609-848-5274
www.jpgn.org/

Provides information for professionals in the areas of pediatric GI liver disease, gastroenterology, and nutrition.

3888 Journal of the American Dietetic Association
American Dietetic Association
216 W Jackson Boulevard
Chicago, IL 60606-6995

312-899-0040
800-877-1600
Fax: 312-899-1979
www.eatright.org

Professional journal of the ADA.

3889 Nutrition in Clinical Practice
ASPEN
8630 Fenton Street
Silver Spring, MD 20910-3805

301-587-6315
Fax: 301-587-2365
e-mail: aspen@nutr.org
www.nutritioncare.org

Offers information to professionals involved in the care of parenterally and enterally fed patients.
100 pages BiMonthly
Adrian Nickel, Director Communications/Marketing

3890 Pancreas
American Pancreatic Association

10833 LeConte Avenue
Los Angeles, CA 90095-6904
310-825-4976
Fax: 310-206-2472
e-mail: hreber@surgery.medch.ucla.edu
Provides information on scientific research related to the pancreas.
Howard A Reber MD

3891 Phoenix Magazine
United Ostomy Association of America
PO Box 512
Northfield, MN 55057
800-826-0826
Fax: 507-645-5168
e-mail: info@uoaa.org
www.uoa.org
America's leading ostomy patient magazine providing colostomy, ileostomy, urostomy and continent diversion information, management techniques, new products and much more.
Quarterly
David Rudzin, President

Newsletters

3892 ADA Courier
American Dietetic Association
216 W Jackson Boulevard
Chicago, IL 60606-6995
312-899-0040
800-877-1600
Fax: 312-899-1979
www.eatright.org
Information for the public on the promotion of optimal nutrition, health, and well-being.

3893 APF Newsletter
PO Box 22712
Houston, TX 77227
713-266-9617
Fax: 713-840-9552
e-mail: porphyrus@aol.com
www.porphyriafoundation.com
Provides updates on treatment and research, as well as informative articles on patients and specialists who treat porphyria. It's mailed to all Sponsors of the APF.
Desiree H Lyon, Executive Director

3894 ASAP Capsule
ASAP International Corporate Headquarters
19 Carroll Road
Woburn, MA 01801
781-935-9776
Fax: 781-933-4151
e-mail: asapgi@sprynet.com
Professional membership newsletter for ASAP, an organization which educates the general public and medical community about chronic intestinal pseudo-obstruction (CIP) and other related digestive motility disorders; serves as an integral source of information for patients of all ages with CIP and related disorders, their families, and members of the medical community.

3895 ASAP Digest
ASAP International Corporate Headquarters
19 Carroll Road
Woburn, MA 01801
781-935-9776
Fax: 781-933-4151
e-mail: asapgi@sprynet.com
General membership newsletter for ASAP. Educates the general public and medical community about chronic intestinal pseudo-obstruction (CIP) and other related digestive motility disorders; serves as an integral source of information for patients of all ages with CIP and related disorders, their families, and members of the medical community.

3896 Clinical Updates
American Society for Gastrointestinal Endoscopy
1520 Kensington Road
Oak Brook, IL 60523
630-573-0600
Fax: 630-573-0691
www.asge.org
Provides information, training, and practice guidelines about gastrointestinal endoscopic techniques.
Quarterly

3897 Code V
Cyclic Vomiting Syndrome Association (CVSA)
13180 Caroline Court
Elm Grove, WI 53122-1732
614-837-2586
Fax: 614-837-6543
e-mail: drwaites@infinet.com
www.beaker.iupui.edu/cvsa

Newsletter for members of the CVSA.

3898 Hemochromatosis Awareness
Hemochromatosis Foundation
PO Box 8569
Albany, NY 12208
518-489-0972
Fax: 518-489-0227
www.hemochromatosis.org
Provides information to the public, families, professionals and government agencies about hereditary hemochromatosis (HH); conducts and raises funds for research; encourages early screening for HH; holds symposiums and meetings; and offers genetic counseling along with support for patients, families, and professionals.
Margit Krikker MD, Medical Director

3899 Ironic Blood
Iron Overload Diseases Association
433 Westward Drive
North Palm Beach, FL 33408-5123
561-840-8512
Fax: 561-842-9881
e-mail: iod@ironoverload.org
www.ironoverload.org
Information for hemochromatosis patients and families.

3900 Lifeline Letter
Oley Foundation
Albany Medical Center
Albany, NY 12208-3478
518-262-5079
800-776-6539
Fax: 518-262-5528
e-mail: bishopj@mail.amc.edu
www.oley.org
Information on home parenteral and enteral nutrition for patients and the public.
16 pages Bi-Monthly
Joan Bishop, Executive Director

3901 Ostomy Quarterly
United Ostomy Association
PO Box 66
Fairview, TN 37062
800-826-0826
e-mail: info@uoa.org
www.uoa.org
First person stories, ostomy management advice from an ET and MD, organization news and ostomy product information.
72 pages Quarterly

3902 Pull-thru Network News
Pull-thru Network
4 Woody Lane
Westport, CT 06880
203-221-7530
e-mail: Pullthrunw@aol.com
members.aol.com/pullthrunw/Pullthru.html
Provides information to patients and families of children who have had or will have pull-through surgery to correct an imperforate anus or associated malformation, Hirschsprung's disease, or other fecal incontinence problems.

3903 SGNA News
Society of Gastroenterology Nurses and Associates
401 N Michigan Avenue
Chicago, IL 60611
312-321-5165
800-245-7462
Fax: 312-321-5194
e-mail: sgna@sba.com
www.sgna.org
Provides members with information about trends and development in the field of gastroenterology.

3904 WIN Notes
Weight-control Information Network
1 WIN Way
Bethesda, MD 20892-3665
202-828-1025
877-946-4627
Fax: 202-828-1028
e-mail: win@mathewsgroup.com
www.niddk.nih.gov/health/nutrit/win.htm
Addresses the health information needs of individuals with weight-control problems. Available on the WIN web site.
BiAnnual

Pamphlets

3905 Acute Intermittent Porphyria
American Prophyria Foundation

PO Box 22712
Houston, TX 77227 713-266-9617
www.enterprise.net
An informational brochure published by the American Porphyria Foundation.

3906 Common Questions About Porphyria
American Prophyria Foundation
PO Box 22712
Houston, TX 77227 713-266-9617
www.enterprise.net
An informational brochure published by the American Porphyria Foundation.

3907 Diet and Nutrition in Porphyria
American Prophyria Foundation
PO Box 22712
Houston, TX 77227 713-266-9617
www.enterprise.net
An informational brochure published by the American Porphyria Foundation.

3908 Drugs and Porphyria
American Prophyria Foundation
PO Box 22712
Houston, TX 77227 713-266-9617
www.enterprise.net
An informational brochure published by the American Porphyria Foundation.

3909 Erythropoietic Protoporphyria
American Prophyria Foundation
PO Box 22712
Houston, TX 77227 713-266-9617
www.enterprise.net
An informational brochure published by the American Porphyria Foundation.

3910 Hematin
American Prophyria Foundation
PO Box 22712
Houston, TX 77227 713-266-9617
www.enterprise.net
An informational brochure published by the American Porphyria Foundation.

3911 Iron Overload Alert
Iron Overload Diseases Association
433 Westward Drive 561-840-8512
North Palm Beach, FL 33408-5123 Fax: 561-842-9881
e-mail: iod@ironoverload.org
www.ironoverload.org
Information for hemochromatosis patients and families.

3912 Issues in Women's Gastrointestinal Health
Gastro-Intestinal Research Foundation
70 E Lake Street 312-332-1350
Chicago, IL 60601 Fax: 312-332-4757
e-mail: girf@girf.org
www.girf.org
Patient education pamphlet.

3913 Porphyria Cutanea Tarda
American Prophyria Foundation
PO Box 22712
Houston, TX 77227 713-266-9617
www.enterprise.net
An informational brochure published by the American Porphyria Foundation.

Audio & Video

3914 A Day in the Life of a Child
Albany Medical Center 518-262-5079
Albany, NY 12208-3478 800-776-6539
Fax: 518-262-5528
www.oley.org
In this video you are welcomed into the household of the Miller family. The Millers have three children, one of whom is tube fed. Jessica has been dependent on tube-feedings since birth, and her family is prepared to show you just what that means. They share tips for keeping a sterile environment in a house with three children, and tips for helping Jessica fit in with her peers.
Joan Bishop, Executive Director

3915 Cleveland Clinic Teaching Conference
Hemochromatosis Foundation
PO Box 8569 518-489-0972
Albany, NY 12208 Fax: 518-489-0227
www.hemochromatosis.org
Provides information to the public, families, and professionals about hereditary hemochromatosis.

3916 Family Teaching Conference
Hemochromatosis Foundation
PO Box 8569 518-489-0972
Albany, NY 12208 Fax: 518-489-0227
www.hemochromatosis.org
Provides information to the public, families, and professionals about hereditary hemochromatosis.
2 3/4 hours

3917 Life with Mic-Key
Albany Medical Center 518-262-5079
Albany, NY 12208-3478 800-776-6539
Fax: 518-262-5528
www.oley.org
Serves as an informative and introductory guide for adapting to life with a Mic-key low profile feeding tube. Low profile means that the Mic-key tube lies very close to the patient's body and does not stick out. It's slim design allows more air to circulate around the stoma site and makes it easy to care for. The Mic-key tube uses a balloon to hold it in place and comes with several important accessories, including two types of extensions sets and an anti-reflux valve.
10 Minutes
Joan Bishop, Executive Director

3918 Mealtime Notions - The 'Get Permission' Approach to Mealtimes and Oral Motor
Marsha Dunn Klein, MED, OTR/L, author
Albany Medical Center 518-262-5079
Albany, NY 12208-3478 800-776-6539
Fax: 518-262-5528
www.oley.org
This video explores the development of trusting feeding relationships, understanding the child's pace, and strategies for increasing permissive behavior. Tools discussed in this video include an introduction to the sensory continuum, a description of the around the bowl technique, and tips for removing the stress from your child's mealtime.
10 Minutes
Joan Bishop, Executive Director

Web Sites

3919 American College of Gastroenterology (ACG)
www.acg.gi.org
Serves clinical and scientific information needs of member physicians and surgeons, who specialize in digestive and related disorders. Emphasis is on scholarly practice, teaching, and research.

3920 American Gastroenterological Association (AGA)
www.gastro.org
Fosters the development and application of the science of gastroenterology by providing leadership and aid, including patient care, research, teaching, continuing education, scientific communication, and matters of national health policy pertaining to gastroenterology.

3921 American Hemochromatosis Society
www.americanhs.org
Educates the public, the medical community, and the media by distributing the most current information available on hereditary hemochromatosis (HH), including DNA screening for HH and pediatric HH; also facilitates patient empowerment through an online network.

3922 American Porphyria Foundation
PO Box 22712
Houston, TX 77227   713-266-9617
       Fax: 713-840-9552
e-mail: porphyrus@aol.com
www.porphyriafoundation.com
Advances awareness, research, and treatment of the porphyrias; provides self-help services for members; and provides referrals to porphyria treatment specialists.
Karl E Anderson, MD, Chairman

3923 American Pseudo-Obstruction and Hirschsprung's Disease Society
Promotes public awareness of gastrointestinal motility disorders, in particular intestinal pseudo-obstruction and Hirschsprung's Disease; provides education and support to individuals and families of children who have been diagnosed with these disorders through parent-to-parent contact, publications, and educational symposia; and encourages and supports medical research in the area of gastrointestinal motility disorders.

3924 American Society for Gastrointestinal Endoscopy
www.asge.org
ASGE provides information, training, and practice guidelines about gastrointestinal endoscopic techniques.

3925 American Society of Abdominal Surgeons
www.gis.net/~absurg/
ASAS sponsors extensive continuing education program for physicians in the field of abdominal surgery and maintains library.

3926 Background on Functional Gastrointestinal Disorders
www.med.unc.edu
Statistical background information on gastrointestinal disorders.

3927 Children's Motility Disorder Foundation
www.motility.org
CMDF works to increase awareness of pediatric motility disorders in the general public and among the physicians most likely to encounter children suffering from these conditions, such as pediatricians and family practice doctors. Supports medical research regarding the causes, treatment, and potentially life-threatening disorders.

3928 Cyclic Vomiting Syndrome Association
www.cvsaonline.org/
CVSA provides opportunities for patients, families, and professionals to offer and receive support and share knowledge about cyclic vomiting syndrome; actively promotes and facilitates medical research about nausea and vomiting; increases worldwide public and professional awareness; and serves as a resource center for information.

3929 Gastrointestinal Research Foundation
www.girf.org
Founded to help combat gastrointestinal diseases. Raises funds to support research at the Center for the study of the Digestive Diseases at the University of Chicago Medical Center and to support advanced training for scientists. Sponsors educational activities for the public.

3930 Healing Well
www.healingwell.com
An online health resource guide to medical news, chat, information and articles, newsgroups and message boards, books, disease-related web sites, medical directories, and more for patients, friends, and family coping with disabling diseases, disorders, or chronic illnesses.

3931 Health Finder
www.healthfinder.gov
Searchable, carefully developed web site offering information on over 1000 topics. Developed by the US Department of Health and Human Services, the site can be used in both English and Spanish.

3932 Healthlink USA
www.healthlinkusa.com
Health information concerning treatment, cures, prevention, diagnosis, risk factors, research, support groups, email lists, personal stories and much more. Updated regularly.

3933 Helios Health
www.helioshealth.com
Online resource for your health information. Detailed information about specific health topics, access to expert advice from our Medical Advisory Board, and up-to-date health news.

3934 Hemochromatosis Foundation
www.hemochromatosis.org
Provides information to the public, families, and professionals about hereditary hemochromatosis (HH); conducts and raises funds for research; encourages early screening for HH; holds symposiums and meetings; and offers genetic counseling along with support for patients, families, and professionals.

3935 International Foundation for Functional Gastrointestinal Disorders
www.iffgd.org
IFFGD is a nonprofit education, support and research organization devoted to increasing awareness and understanding of functional gastrointestinal disorders, including irritable bowel syndrome (IBS), constipation, diarrhea, pain, and incontinence. Mission is to inform, assist and support people affected by these disorders.

3936 MedicineNet
www.medicinenet.com
An online resource for consumers providing easy-to-read, authoritative medical and health information.

3937 Medscape
www.medscape.com
Medscape offers specialists, primary care physicians, and other health professionals the Web's most robust and integrated medical information and educational tools.

3938 National Digestive Diseases Information Clearinghouse
www.niddk.nih.gov
Offers various educational information, public resources and reprints, public awareness materials and more on digestive disorders.

3939 North American Society for Pediatric Gastroenterology and Nutrition
www.naspgn.org
Promotes research and provides a forum for professionals in the areas of pediatric GI liver disease, gastroenterology, and nutrition. Associated with fellow organizations in Europe and Australia (ESPGAN, AUSPGAN).

3940 Nutrition in Clinical Practice
www.clinnutr.org
Offers information to professionals involved in the care of parenterally and enterally fed patients.

3941 Oley Foundation
www.wizvax.net/oleyfdn
Promotes and advocates education and research in home parenteral and enteral nutrition; provides support and networking to patients through information clearinghouse and regional volunteer networks; sponsors meetings and conferences, including annual patient/clinician conference; maintains speakers bureau.

3942 Pediatric Adolescent Gastroesophageal Assn
www.reflux.org
Discussions led by local experts, family medical histories and check swabs, supervised nap room and separate activity room for kids, trained babysitters available.

3943 Pediatric/Adolescent Gastroesophageal Reflux Association
www.reflux.org
PAGER gathers and disseminates information on pediatric gastroesophageal reflux and related disorders; provides support and education to patients, their families, and the public; promotes the general welfare of patients, their families, and the public; promotes the general welfare of patients with gastroesophageal reflux and their families; and promotes public awareness of the condition.

3944 Pull-thru Network
members.aol.com/pullthrunw/Pullthru.html
Provides emotional support and information to patients and families of children who have had or will have pull-through surgery to correct an imperforate anus or associated malformation,

Hirschsprung's disease, or other fecal incontinence problems; sponsors online discussion groups. A chapter of the United Ostomy Association.

3945 Society for Surgery of the Alimentary Tract

www.ssat.com

SSAT provides a forum for exchange of information among physicians specializing in alimentary tract surgery.

3946 Society of American Gastrointestinal Endoscopic Surgeons

www.sages.org

SAGES encourages study and practice of gastrointestinal endoscopy, laparoscopy, and minimal acces surgery.

3947 WebMD

www.webmd.com

Information on Gastrointestinal Disorders, including articles and resources.

Description

3948 Gaucher's Disease

Gaucher's disease is an inherited disorder of metabolism of fats. These metabolic products can not be broken down properly because of a deficiency of an enzyme called glucocerebroside. Symptoms can include fatigue, anemia, bleeding problems (such as nosebleeds and easy bruising), enlargement of the spleen and/or liver, bone pain, easily fractured bones and brown pigmentation of the skin. The degree of symptoms and complications vary by age of onset and the degree of involvement of the disorder's clinical forms. Diagnosis is based on finding Gaucher's typical cells in the bone marrow.

The treatment for Gaucher's disease is enzyme replacement, called Cerezyme, administered intravenously. Removal of the spleen and blood transfusions may be necessary. Current research is aimed at genetic therapy.

National Agencies & Associations

3949 National Foundation for Jewish Genetic Diseases
One Gustave L Levy Place   212-241-6500
New York, NY 10029-6574   Fax: 212-241-6947
www.mssm.edu/jewish_genetics
This foundation was created to raise funds for and to inform the public about genetic diseases which afflict descendants of eastern and central European Jews. It sponsors medical symposia from time to time.
R J Desnick PhD MD, Center Director
Dennis S Charney, Executive VP

3950 National Gaucher Foundation
2227 Idlewood Road
Tucker, GA 33008   800-504-3189
Fax: 770-934-2911
e-mail: ngf@gaucherdisease.org
www.gaucherdisease.org
National foundation providing information and assistance for those affected by Gaucher disease as well as education and outreach to increase public awareness.
Robin A Ely MD, President/Medical Director
Rhonda P Buyers, CEO/Executive Director

3951 National Organization for Rare Disorders (NORD)
55 Kenosia Avenue   203-744-0100
Danbury, CT 06813-1968   800-999-6673
Fax: 203-798-2291
TDD: 203-797-9590
e-mail: orphan@rarediseases.org
www.rarediseases.org
The NORD is a unique federation of voluntary health organizations dedicated to helping people with rare orphan diseases and assisting the organizations that serve them.
Frank Sasinowski, Chair
Carolyn Asbury, PhD, Vice Chair

Research Centers

3952 Children's Gaucher Research Fund
8110 Warren Court   916-797-3700
Granite Bay, CA 95746-2123   Fax: 916-797-3707
e-mail: research@childrensgaucher.org
www.childrensgaucher.org
A nonprofit organization that raises funds to coordinate support research to find a cure for Type 2 and Type 3 Gaucher Disease.
Roscoe Brady, Scientific Advisory Board
Gregory Grabowski, Scientific Advisory Board

3953 Comprehensive Gaucher Treatment Center at Tower Hematology Oncology
9090 Wilshire Boulevard   310-888-8680
Beverly Hills, CA 90211   888-248-4456
Fax: 310-285-7298
e-mail: info@gaucherwest.com
www.gaucherwest.com
The Comprehensive Gaucher Treatment Center at Tower Hematology Oncology under the direction of Dr. Barry Rosenbloom provides clinical evaluations for the diagnosis and treatment of patient's with Gaucher disease. We provide a multi-disciplinary program that includes Hematology Genetics Orthopedics and Radiology. To ensure continuity of care we provide assistance to other physicians regarding testing diagnosis evaluation and management of the Gaucher patient.
Barry Rosenbloom, Director
Cheryl Elzinga, Gaucher Coordinator

3954 LAC/USC Imaging Science Center
1975 Zonal Avenue   323-442-1900
Los Angeles, CA 90089-9034   Fax: 323-442-2722
e-mail: nestrada@usc.edu
www.usc.edu/schools/medicine
Provides a Gaucher Disease radiology consultant: Michael R Terk MD.and Muskuloskeletal Imaging.
Coreen Rodgers, COO
Sherri Sammon, Associate Director

Support Groups & Hotlines

3955 Brave Kids
151 Sawgrass Corners Drive   904-280-1895
Ponte Vedra Beach, FL 32082   800-568-1008
Fax: 904-280-1897
e-mail: info@bravekids.org
www.bravekids.org
An organization that offers support for parents and children suffering from serious health problems.
Kristen Fitzgerald, Founder

3956 National Health Information Center
PO Box 1133   310-565-4167
Washington, DC 20013   800-336-4797
Fax: 301-984-4256
e-mail: info@nhic.org
www.health.gov/nhic
Offers a nationwide information referral service, produces directories and resource guides.

Newsletters

3957 Gaucher Disease Newsletter
National Gaucher Foundation
11140 Rockville Pike   301-816-1515
Rockville, MD 20852-3151   800-925-8885
Offers information on the latest research, treatments and technology for persons affected by Gaucher Disease. Also includes legislative and medical information.
Quarterly

Pamphlets

3958 Gaucher Disease Fact Sheet
National Gaucher Foundation
11140 Rockville Pike   301-816-1515
Rockville, MD 20852-3151   800-925-8885
Offers information on what Gaucher Disease is, the symptoms, risks, treatments and the workings of the National Gaucher Foundation.

3959 Living with Gaucher Disease
National Gaucher Foundation
11140 Rockville Pike   301-816-1515
Rockville, MD 20852-3151   800-925-8885

A guide for parents, families and relatives that teach them how to deal with and cope with a diagnosis of Gaucher Disease.
24 pages

Audio & Video

3960 Pain & Hope
National Gaucher Foundation
11140 Rockville Pike   301-816-1515
Rockville, MD 20852-3151   800-925-8885
A patient and family perspective on Gaucher Disease.

Web Sites

3961 Gaucher Disease Homepage
www.gaucherdisease.org
Information on Gaucher disease, including symptoms, treatment, prevalence, resources, support, and news.

3962 Healing Well
www.healingwell.com
An online health resource guide to medical news, chat, information and articles, newsgroups and message boards, books, disease-related web sites, medical directories, and more for patients, friends, and family coping with disabling diseases, disorders, or chronic illnesses.

3963 Health Finder
www.healthfinder.gov
Searchable, carefully developed web site offering information on over 1000 topics. Developed by the US Department of Health and Human Services, the site can be used in both English and Spanish.

3964 Healthlink USA
www.healthlinkusa.com
Health information concerning treatment, cures, prevention, diagnosis, risk factors, research, support groups, email lists, personal stories and much more. Updated regularly.

3965 Helios Health
www.helioshealth.com
Online resource for your health information. Detailed information about specific health topics, access to expert advice from our Medical Advisory Board, and up-to-date health news.

3966 MedicineNet
www.medicinenet.com
An online resource for consumers providing easy-to-read, authoritative medical and health information.

3967 Medscape
www.medscape.com
Medscape offers specialists, primary care physicians, and other health professionals the Web's most robust and integrated medical information and educational tools.

3968 WebMD
www.webmd.com
Information on Gaucher's disease, including articles and resources.

Description

3969 Growth Disorders

There are many conditions that make a child grow more slowly than average. Any sort of severe chronic illness, especially one involving the digestive system, may cause this. Certain genetic conditions such as Turner syndrome, a sex chromosome abnormality or achondroplasia (skeletal maldevelopment) will predictably limit growth and eventual adult height. Endocrine, or hormonal, causes of short stature include underactivity of the thyroid gland (hypothyroidism) or pituitary gland, where growth hormone (GH) is normally formed. Finally, there are many cases where the child's height is significantly below that of peers, yet none of these conditions is present. This may reflect two parents who are themselves quite short, or may be completely unexplained.

If slow growth is related to low levels of GH, therapy with synthetic GH is extremely effective. Regular injections will be necessary for a prolonged period until an acceptable height is reached.

Regardless of the underlying cause, a child whose disorder is recognized at birth or who is not growing as quickly as the rest of his or her peers should receive a complete evaluation by a pediatric endocrinologist or other growth specialist.

National Agencies & Associations

3970 Dwarf Athletic Association of America
708 Gravenstein Highway N
Sebastopol, CA 95472

972-317-8299
888-598-3222
Fax: 972-966-0184
e-mail: daaa@flash.net
www.daaa.org

Develops, promotes and provides quality amateur level athletic opportunities for dwarf athletes in the US. Our mission is to encourage people with dwarfism to participate in sports regardless of their level of skill.
Amy B Andrews, Board President
Mike Cekanor, Board VP

3971 Genetic Alliance
4301 Connecticut Avenue NW
Washington, DC 20008

202-966-5557
Fax: 202-966-8553
e-mail: info@geneticalliance.org
www.geneticalliance.org

Improves health through the authentic engagement of communities and individuals. The goal is to build capacity within the genetics community. Transform health through genetics, and promote an environment of openness cetnered on the health of individuals, families and communities.
Sharon F Terry MA, President/CEO

3972 Little People of America
250 El Camino Real
Tustin, CA 92780

714-368-3689
888-LPA-2001
Fax: 714-368-3367
e-mail: info@lpaonline.org
www.lpaonline.org

Focuses research, support and information on persons who are short in stature.
Lois Gerage-Lamb, President
Bill Bradford, Senior VP

3973 Little People's Research Fund (LPRF)
616 Old Edmondson Avenue
Catonsville, MD 21228

410-747-1100
800-232-LPRF
Fax: 410-747-1374
e-mail: lprf@lprf.org
www.lprf.org

LPRF supports research into the disabling conditions of skeletal dysplasia (dwarfism), promotes patient care and education of the medical community as well as the general public. It assists families by sponsoring clinics in various states.
Steven E Kopits MD, Medical Advisor

3974 National Institute of Child Health and Human Development
PO Box 3006
Rockville, MD 20847

800-370-2943
Fax: 866-760-5947
TTY: 888-320-6942
e-mail: NICHDInformationResourceCenter@mail.nih.
www.nichd.nih.gov

Duane Alexander MD, Director

Foundations

3975 Human Growth Foundation
997 Glen Cove Avenue
Glen Head, NY 11545

516-671-4041
800-451-6434
Fax: 516-671-4055
e-mail: hgf1@hgfound.org
www.hgfound.org

Our mission is to help children, and adults with disorders of growth and growth hormone through research, education, support, and advocacy. The Foundation is dedicated to helping medical science to better understand the process of growth. It is composed of concerned parents and friends of children, and adults, with growth problems; and, interested health professionals.
Patricia D Costa, Executive Director

3976 MAGIC Foundation for Children's Growth
6645 West North Avenue
Oak Park, IL 60302

708-383-0808
800-362-4423
Fax: 708-383-0899
e-mail: dianne@magicfoundation.org
www.magicfoundation.org

Provides support services for the families of children afflicted with a wide variety of chronic and/or critical disorders, syndromes and that affect a child's growth.
Dianne Tamburrino, Executive Director
Susan Smith, RN, Director Medical Education

3977 March of Dimes Birth Defects Foundation
1275 Mamaroneck Avenue
White Plains, NY 10605

914-997-4488
www.marchofdimes.com

Our mission is to improve the health of babies by preventing birth defects, premature birth, and infant mortality.

Research Centers

3978 Case Western Reserve University: Bolton Brush Growth Study Center
2123 Abington Road
Cleveland, OH 44106-4905

216-368-4649
Fax: 216-368-3204
e-mail: mgh4@po.cwru.edu
dental.cwru.edu/bolton-brush

Investigations and research into the growth and development of the human body. Extensive collection of longitudinal human growth data.
Mark G Hans, Director
Aaron Weinbe DMD PhD, Associate Professor and Chairman

3979 International Skeletal Dysplasia Registry Medical Genetics Institute
Medical Genetics Institute
8700 Beverly Boulevard
Los Angeles, CA 90048

310-423-3277
800-233-2771
Fax: 310-423-0462
www.csmc.edu

Provides patient services for skeletal dysplasia patients particularly research in dwarfism.
David L Rimoin MD PhD, Director
Xiao-Ning Chen, Research Scientist

3980 New Jersey Institute of Technology Center for Biomedical Engineering
University Heights
Newark, NJ 07102-1982
973-596-8449
Fax: 973-596-6056
e-mail: william.c.hunter@njit.edu
www.njit.edu

Offers research into facial and bone disorders.
Robert A Altenkirch, President
Joel Bloom, Vice President

3981 WM Krogman Center for Research in Child Growth and Development
3101 Walnut Street
Philadelphia, PA 19104-6003
215-898-1470
e-mail: mannj@upenn.edu
www.upenn.edu

Focuses research and studies on growth disorders and birth defects.
Dr Solomon Katz, Director

Support Groups & Hotlines

3982 National Health Information Center
PO Box 1133
Washington, DC 20013
310-565-4167
800-336-4797
Fax: 301-984-4256
e-mail: info@nhic.org
www.health.gov/nhic

Offers a nationwide information referral service, produces directories and resource guides.

Books

3983 Growing Children: A Parent's Guide
Human Growth Foundation
997 Glen Cove Avenue
Glen Head, NY 11545
516-671-4041
800-451-6434
Fax: 516-671-4055
e-mail: hgf1@hgfound.org
www.hgfound.org

Offers parents information on the normal pattern of their child's growth, growth charts, recognition of growth problems, evaluation of growth problems and resources for more information.
Patricia D Costa, Executive Director

3984 Short and OK
Human Growth Foundation
997 Glen Cove Avenue
Glen Head, NY 11545
516-671-4041
800-451-6434
Fax: 516-671-4055
e-mail: hgf1@hgfound.org
www.hgfound.org

Guide for parents of short children offering information on behavior issues, medical issues and psychological warning signs.
54 pages
Patricia D Costa, Executive Director

Pamphlets

3985 Achondroplasia
Human Growth Foundation
997 Glen Cove Avenue
Glen Head, NY 11545
516-671-4041
800-451-6434
Fax: 516-671-4055
e-mail: hgf1@hgfound.org
www.hgfound.org

Signs, causes and prevention of achondroplasia.
Patricia D Costa, Executive Director

3986 Growth Hormone Testing
Human Growth Foundation
997 Glen Cove Avenue
Glen Head, NY 11545
516-671-4041
800-451-6434
Fax: 516-671-4055
e-mail: hgf1@hgfound.org
www.hgfound.org

What to expect during the testing period.
Patricia D Costa, Executive Director

3987 Intrauterine Growth Retardation
Human Growth Foundation
997 Glen Cove Avenue
Glen Head, NY 11545
516-671-4041
800-451-6434
Fax: 516-671-4055
e-mail: hgf1@hgfound.org
www.hgfound.org

Explains some of the reasons for an infant's failure to grow normally in intrauterine life.
Patricia D Costa, Executive Director

3988 Most Frequently Asked Questions with Growth Hormone Deficiency
Human Growth Foundation
997 Glen Cove Avenue
Glen Head, NY 11545
516-671-4041
800-451-6434
Fax: 516-671-4055
e-mail: hgf1@hgfound.org
www.hgfound.org

Provides a brief overview for parents about Growth Hormone Deficiency.
Patricia D Costa, Executive Director

3989 Septo-Optic Dysplasia
Human Growth Foundation
997 Glen Cove Avenue
Glen Head, NY 11545
516-671-4041
800-451-6434
Fax: 516-671-4055
e-mail: hgf1@hgfound.org
www.hgfound.org

Also known as DeMorsier Syndrome. Describes the disease and the different treatments that can lead to the significant improvement in the quality of life.
Patricia D Costa, Executive Director

Web Sites

3990 Alliance of Genetic Support Groups
A coalition of voluntary genetic support groups, consumers and professionals addressing the needs of individuals and families affected by genetic disorders from a national perspective.

3991 Atomz
www.pediatricservices.com
A search engine providing over 60 links to sites involving various growth disorders.

3992 Healing Well
www.healingwell.com
An online health resource guide to medical news, chat, information and articles, newsgroups and message boards, books, disease-related web sites, medical directories, and more for patients, friends, and family coping with disabling diseases, disorders, or chronic illnesses.

3993 Health Finder
www.healthfinder.gov
Searchable, carefully developed web site offering information on over 1000 topics. Developed by the US Department of Health and Human Services, the site can be used in both English and Spanish.

3994 Healthlink USA
www.healthlinkusa.com
Health information concerning treatment, cures, prevention, diagnosis, risk factors, research, support groups, email lists, personal stories and much more. Updated regularly.

3995 Helios Health
www.helioshealth.com
Online resource for your health information. Detailed information about specific health topics, access to expert advice from our Medical Advisory Board, and up-to-date health news.

3996   Human Growth Foundation

www.HGFound.org

Organization committed to expanding and accelerating research into growth hormone deficiency. Provides education and support to those affected by growth disorders and their families and fosters the exchange of information with the medical community.

3997   MedicineNet

www.medicinenet.com

An online resource for consumers providing easy-to-read, authoritative medical and health information.

3998   Medscape

www.medscape.com

Medscape offers specialists, primary care physicians, and other health professionals the Web's most robust and integrated medical information and educational tools.

3999   OHSU Homepage Search

www.ohsu.edu

A search which provides several links for information on growth disorders.

4000   WebMD

www.webmd.com

Information on growth disorders, including articles and resources.

Description

4001 Head Injuries

Head Injuries, or Traumatic Brain Injuries, cover a range of severity. Currently, there are 5.3 million Americans living with a disability because of a head or brain injury. Concussion, the most common injury, is the momentary loss of consciousness. It usually resolves without any major complications. Damage can result from penetration of the skull or from acceleration/deceleration of the brain that occurs in severe automobile accidents. Injuries can include brain bruising and bleeding into the brain, resulting in swelling that can be life threatening because the skull, as a rigid structure, cannot expand.

Postconcussion syndrome commonly follows a mild injury and can include temporary headaches, dizziness, mild mental slowing and sleepiness. A moderate head or brain injury results in loss of consciousness usually lasting from minutes to a few hours, followed by a few days or weeks of confusion. Loss of consciousness for greater than two minutes implies a worse outcome. Cognitive and psychological impairments lasting many months or even permanently are usual consequences of moderate injury. A severe injury almost always results in prolonged unconsciousness or coma lasting days to weeks or longer. People who sustain a severe head or brain injury often have brain contusions, hematomas (a collection of blood) and/or damage to the nerve fibers or axons. Many people who sustain a severe brain injury make significant improvements in the first year or two. After that improvement tends to slow down, but may continue for years. Some physical and/or cognitive impairments are permanent. See also *Brain Tumors*.

National Agencies & Associations

4002 American Brain Tumor Association
2720 River Road
Des Plaines, IL 60018-4117
847-827-9910
800-886-2282
Fax: 847-827-9918
e-mail: info@abta.org
www.abta.org

Services includes over 40 publications which address brain tumors their treatment and coping with the disease. Materials address brain tumors in all age groups. Provide free social service consultations and a mentorship program for new brain tumor support groups.
Elizabeth M Wilson, Executive Director
Geri Jo Duda RN, Patient Services

4003 Brain Injury Association
1608 Spring Hill Road
Vienna, VA 22182
703-761-0750
800-444-6443
Fax: 703-761-0755
e-mail: info@biausa.org
www.biausa.org

The BIA's mission is to create a better future through brain injury prevention research education and advocacy. Offers information on state and national offices treatment and rehabilitation conferences prevention financial development and more.
Susan H Connors, President/CEO
Mary S Reitter CAE, EVP/COO

4004 Dynamic Rehab
1800 W Big Beaver Road
Troy, MI 48084
281-485-4144
888-DYN-MIC
Fax: 281-485-4196
e-mail: dynmaicrehab@sbcglobal.net
www.dynamicrehab.net

Primary focus is the production and distribution of motivational videotapes and workshops.
Greta Ludwig PT, Owner/Physical Therapist
Teresa Turner, Owner/Physical Therapist

4005 FASST, Friends & Survivors Standing Together
21100 W. Capitol Drive
Pewaukeeille, WI 53072
Fax: 262-790-9670
Nonprofit organization supporting brain injured people and their caregivers. Information, support groups and more.

4006 Family Caregiver Alliance/National Center on Caregiving
180 Montgomery Street
San Francisco, CA 94104
415-434-3388
800-445-8106
Fax: 415-434-3508
e-mail: info@caregiver.org
www.caregiver.org

Caregiver information and assistance via phone or e-mail; fact sheets and publications describing and documenting caregiver needs and services.
Kathleen Kelly, Executive Director
Ping Hao, President

4007 International Brain Injury Association
5909 Ashby Manor Place
Alexandria, VA 22313
703-960-0027
Fax: 703-960-6603
e-mail: chaynes@hdipub.com
www.internationalbrain.org

Provides scientific and medical leadership worldwide in the field of brain injury.
Nathan Zasler, Chairman
Margaret Roberts, Executive Director/Administration

4008 Rainbow House
4149 W 26th Street
Chicago, IL 60623
773-521-1815
www.rainbow-house.org

Rainbow House is a Chicago-based nonprofit organization whose mission is to end domestic violence. Rainbow House has offered domestic violence prevention programs support and outreach services and resources to survivors across the City of Chicago.
Angel Beltran, Chair
Rosy Mares, Vice Chair

4009 TPN: The Perspective Network
PO Box 121012
W Melbourne, FL 32912-1012
770-844-6898
Fax: 770-844-6898
e-mail: TPN@tbi.org
www.tbi.org

The Perspective Network provides forums and resources for persons with families, caregivers, friends and the professionals who serve them. Their goals are to promote a sense of community and to increase public awareness of brain injury.

State Agencies & Associations

Alabama

4010 Alabama Head Injury Foundation
3100 Lorna Road
Hoover, AL 5216-
205-823-3818
800-433-8002
Fax: 205-823-4544
e-mail: ahifl@bellsouth.net
http://www.ahif.org

Services provided to Alabamians with traumatic brain injury or spinal cord injury include information, housing, respite care, recreation programs, resource coordination.
Keith Belt, President
Charles D Priest, Executive Director

Alaska

4011 Brain Injury Association of America's National Family Helpline
1608 Spring Hill Road 703-761-0750
Vienna, VA 22182 800-444-6443
Fax: 703-761-0755
e-mail: FamilyHelpline@biausa.org
www.biausa.org

Greg Oshanick, Chairman
Susan Conners, President and CEO

Arizona

4012 Brain Injury Association of Arizona
5025 E. Washington Street 602-508-8024
Phoenix, AZ 85034 888-500-9165
Fax: 602-508-8285
e-mail: info@biaaz.org
www.biaaz.org

Services provided by BIAAZ: camp for adults age 18+ with brain injuries; one-to-one phone and/or mail peer support program for individuals affected by brain injury and their families.

Mattie Cummins, Executive Director
Lisa Counters, Board President

Arkansas

4013 Brain Injury Association of Arkansas
PO Box 26236 501-374-3585
Little Rock, AR 72221-6236 800-444-6443
Fax: 501-918-6595
e-mail: info@brainassociation.org
www.brainassociation.org

Dana Austen, President
Kortney Coats, Vice President

Colorado

4014 Brain Injury Association of Colorado
4200 W Conejos Place 303-355-9969
Denver, CO 80204 800-955-2443
Fax: 303-355-9968
e-mail: informationreferral@biacolorado.org
www.biacolorado.org

William Levis, President
Gavin Attwood, Executive Director

Connecticut

4015 Brain Injury Association of Connecticut
200 Day Hill Road 86- 2-9 02
Windsor, CT 06095 800-278-8242
Fax: 86- 2-9 05
e-mail: general@biact.org
www.biact.org

500 Members
Paul A Slager, President
Julie Peters, Executive Director

Delaware

4016 Brain Injury Association of Delaware
840 Walker Road 302-346-2083
Dover, DE 19904 800-411-0505
Fax: 888-258-3694
e-mail: biadresourcecenter@cavtel.net
www.biausa.org/Delaware

Devon Dorman, President
Esther Curtis, Executive Director

Florida

4017 Brain Injury Association of Florida
1637 Metropolitan Boulevard 850-410-0103
Tallahassee, FL 32308 800-992-3442
Fax: 850-410-0105
e-mail: biaftalla@biaf.org
www.biaf.org

Valerie E Breen, President/CEO

4018 Choices for Work Program Goodwill Industries-Suncoast
Goodwill Industries-Suncoast
10596 Gandy Boulevard 727-523-1512
St Petersburg, FL 33702 888-279-1988
Fax: 727-563-9300
e-mail: gw.marketing@goodwill-suncoast.com
www.goodwill-suncoast.org

A nonprofit community based organization whose purpose is to improve the quality of life for people who are disabled, disadvantaged and/or aged. This mission is accomplished through a staff of over 1,200 employees providing independent living skills, affordable housing, career assessment and job skills training and opportunities.

R Lee Waits, President/Chief Executive Officer
Martin W Gladysz, Chair

4019 Goodwill Industries-Suncoast
Goodwill Industries-Suncoast
10596 Gandy Boulevard 727-523-1512
St. Petersburg, FL 33702 888-729-1988
Fax: 727-563-9300
e-mail: gw.marketing@goodwill-suncoast.org
www.goodwill-suncoast.org

A nonprofit community based organization whose purpose is to improve the quality of life for people who are disabled, disadvantaged and/or aged. This mission is accomplished through a staff of over 1,200 employees providing independent living skills, affordable housing, career assessment and planning, job skills, training, placement, and job retention assistance with useful employment. Annually, Goodwill Industries-Suncoast serves over 30,000 people in Citrus, Hernando, Levy, Marion and more.

R Lee Waits, President/CEO
Martin W Gladysz, Chair

4020 Pensacola Brain Injury TBI/ABI Support Group
TBI/ABI Support Group
2001 N E Street 850-457-2870
Pensacola, FL 32507 e-mail: hens8250@bellsouth.net
pensacolabrainnetwork.com/sys-tmpl/door

Survivors and caregivers oriented association. Publishes monthly magazine.

Peggy Henshall, Support Group Coordinator

Hawaii

4021 Brain Injury Association of Hawaii
420 Kuwili Street 808-791-6942
Honolulu, HI 96817-1474 Fax: 808-454-1975
e-mail: biahi@hawaiiantel.net
www.biausa.org/Hawaii

Ian Mattoch, President
Mary Wilson, Executive Director

Idaho

4022 Brain Injury Association of Idaho
PO Box 414 208-342-0999
Boise, ID 83701-0414 888-374-3447
Fax: 208-333-0026
e-mail: info@biaid.org
www.biaid.org

Michelle Featherston, President

Illinois

4023 Brain Injury Association of Illinois
PO Box 64420 312-726-5699
Chicago, IL 60664-0420 800-699-6443
Fax: 312-630-4011
e-mail: info@biail.org
www.biail.org

Philicia L Deckard, Executive Director
Irene Pedersen, Founder

Indiana

4024 Brain Injury Association of Indiana
9531 Valparaiso Court
Indianapolis, IN 46268

317-356-7722
866-854-4246
Fax: 31- 8-2 17
e-mail: info@biai.org
www.biausa.org/Indiana

Anna Garrett, Executive Director
Laura C Trexler, TBI Grant Program Director

Iowa

4025 Brain Injury Association of Iowa
7025 Hickman Road
Urbandale, IA 50322

319-466-7455
800-444-6443
Fax: 800-381-0812
e-mail: info@biaia.org
www.biaia.org

Geoffrey Lauer, Executive Director

Kansas

4026 Brain Injury Association of Kansas and Greater Kansas City
6405 Metcalf Avenue
Overland Park, KS 66202

913-754-8883
800-444-6443
Fax: 816-842-1531
e-mail: info@biaks.org
www.biaks.org

Rob Flores, President
Betsy Johnson, Executive Director

Kentucky

4027 Brain Injury Association of Kentucky
7410 New Lagrange Roadd
Louisville, KY 40222

502-493-0609
800-592-1117
Fax: 502-426-2993
www.biak.us

Chell Austin, Executive Director
Wes Wilkinson, Development Director

Maine

4028 Brain Injury Association of Maine
13 Washington Street
Waterville, ME 04901

207-861-9900
800-275-1233
Fax: 207-861-4617
e-mail: info@biame.org
www.biame.org

Mary Lombardo, President
Leslie DuVall, Director of Operations

Maryland

4029 Brain Injury Association of Maryland
2200 Kernan Drive
Baltimore, MD 21207

410-448-2924
800-221-6443
Fax: 410-448-3541
e-mail: info@biamd.org
www.biamd.org

Patricia Janus, President
Diane Tripplet, Executive Director

Massachusetts

4030 Brain Injury Association of Massachusetts
30 Lyman Street
Westborough, MA 01581

508-475-0032
800-242-0030
Fax: 508-475-0400
e-mail: biama@biama.org
www.biama.org

Shahriar Khaksari, President
Arlene Korab, Executive Director

Michigan

4031 Brain Injury Association of Michigan
7305 Grand River
Brighton, MI 48114-2334

810-229-5880
800-444-6443
Fax: 810-229-8947
e-mail: info@biami.org
www.biami.org

Our mission is to enhance the lives of those affected by brain injury through education, advocacy, research and local support groups and to reduce the incidence of brain injury through prevention.
Katie Knight, Program Coordinator
Michael F Dabbs, President

Minnesota

4032 Brain Injury Association of Minnesota
34 13th Avenue NE
Minneapolis, MN 55413

612-378-2742
800-669-6442
Fax: 612-378-2789
e-mail: info@braininjurymn.org
www.braininjurymn.org

20-24 pages
Andrew Kiragu, Board Chairman

Mississippi

4033 Brain Injury Association of Mississippi
2727 Old Canton
Jackson, MS 39296-5912

601-981-1021
800-444-6443
Fax: 601-981-1039
e-mail: info@msbia.org
www.msbia.org

Howard T Katz, Chairman
Lee Jenkins, Executive Director

Missouri

4034 Brain Injury Association of Missouri
10270 Page Avenue
Saint Louis, MO 63132-1322

314-426-4024
800-444-6443
Fax: 314-426-3290
e-mail: info@biamo.org
www.biamo.org

Information and referral services and support groups through the state of Missouri.
John Bennett, President of the Board
Terrie Price, VP

Montana

4035 Brain Injury Association of Montana
1280 S 3rd W
Missoula, MT 59801

406-541-6442
800-241-6442
Fax: 406-541-4360
e-mail: biam@biamt.org
www.biamt.org

Bobbi Perkins, President
Kristen Morgan, Program Director

New Hampshire

4036 Brain Injury Association of New Hampshire
109 N State Street
Concord, NH 03301

603-225-8400
800-773-8400
Fax: 603-228-6749
e-mail: mail@bianh.org
www.bianh.org

Brant Elkind, President
Steven Wade, Executive Director

New Jersey

4037 Brain Injury Association of New Jersey
825 Georges Road
N Brunswick, NJ 08902
732-745-0200
800-669-4323
Fax: 732-745-0211
e-mail: info@bianj.org
www.bianj.org

Barbara Parker, President

New Mexico

4038 Brain Injury Association of New Mexico
3234 Candelaria NE
Albuquerque, NM 87107
505-292-7414
88- 2-2 74
Fax: 505-271-8983
e-mail: info@braininjurynm.org
www.braininjurynm.org

John Tiwald, Board President
Mark Pedrotty, VP

4039 Brain Injury Association of New Mexico Hel
3234 Candelaria NE
Albuquerque, NM 87107
505-292-7414
88- 2-2 74
Fax: 505-271-8983
e-mail: info@braininjurynm.org
www.braininjurynm.org

John Tiwald, Board President
Mark Pedrotty, VP

New York

4040 Brain Injury Association of New York State
10 Colvin Avenue
Albany, NY 12206-1242
518-459-7911
800-228-8201
Fax: 518-482-5285
e-mail: info@bianys.org
www.bianys.org

Marie Cavallo, President
Judith Avner, Executive Director

4041 RRTC on Community Integration of Persons with TBI
2323 S Shepherd
Houston, TX 77019
713-630-0526
800-732-8124
Fax: 713-630-0529
e-mail: terri.hudler-hull@memorialhermann.org
www.tbicommunity.org

Karen A Hart PhD, Director Of Training
Sunil Kothari, Medical Director

North Carolina

4042 Brain Injury Association of North Carolina
2113 Cameron Street
Raleigh, NC 27605
919-833-9634
800-377-1464
Fax: 919-833-5415
e-mail: bianc@bianc.net
www.tbicommunity.org

Cindy Boyd, Board Chairman
Sandra Farmer, President

4043 Brain Injury Association of North Dakota H
2113 Cameron Street
Raleigh, NC 27605
919-833-9634
800-377-1464
Fax: 919-833-5415
e-mail: bianc@bianc.net
www.bianc.net/

Cindy Boyd, Board Chairman
Sandra Farmer, President

Ohio

4044 Brain Injury Association of Ohio
855 Grand View Avenue
Columbus, OH 43215-1123
614-481-7100
866-644-6242
Fax: 614-481-7103
e-mail: help@biaoh.org
www.biaoh.org

Jon Fishpaw, President
Suzanne Minnich, Executive Director

Oklahoma

4045 Brain Injury Association of Oklahoma
PO Box 88
Hillsdale, OK 73743-0088
580-233-4363
800-444-6443
Fax: 580-233-4546
e-mail: brainhelp@braininjuryoklahoma.orgÿ
www.braininjuryoklahoma.org

Tracy Grammer, President

Oregon

4046 Brain Injury Association of Oregon
PO Box 549
Molalla, OR 97038
503-740-3155
800-544-5243
Fax: 503-961-8730
e-mail: info@biaoregon.org
www.biaoregon.org

Tootie Smith, President
Sherry Stock, Executive Director

Pennsylvania

4047 Brain Injury Association of Pennsylvania
950 Walnut Bottom Road
Carlisle, PA 17015
717-657-3601
866-635-7097
Fax: 717-692-5567
e-mail: info@biapa.org
www.biapa.org

Drew Nagele, Chairman of Board Development Committee
Stewart L Cohen, Chairman

Rhode Island

4048 Brain Injury Association of Rhode Island
935 Park Avenue
Cranston, RI 02910-2743
401-461-6599
Fax: 401-461-6561
e-mail: braininjuryctr@biaofri.org
www.biaofri.org

Michael Baker, Co-President
Colleen McCarthy, Co-President

4049 Brain Injury Association of Rhode Island H
935 Park Avenue
Cranston, RI 02910
401-461-6599
Fax: 401-461-6561
e-mail: braininjuryctr@biaofri.org
www.biaofri.org

Michael Baker, Co-President
Colleen McCarthy, Co-President

South Carolina

4050 Brain Injury Association of South Carolina
800 Dutch Square Boulevard
Columbia, SC 29210
803-731-9823
877-TBI-FACT
Fax: 803-731-4804
e-mail: scbraininjury@bellsouth.net
www.biausa.org/sc

Elaine Phillips, President
Joyce Davis, Executive Director

Tennessee

4051 Brain Injury Association of Tennessee
955 Woodland St
Nashville, TN 37206
615-248-5878
877-757-2428
Fax: 615-383-1176
e-mail: biaoftn@yahoo.com
www.biaoftn.org

Guynn Edwards, President

4052 Brain Injury Association of Tennessee Help
955 Woodland St
Nashville, TN 37206
615-248-2541
877-757-2428
Fax: 615-383-1176
e-mail: biaoftn@yahoo.com
www.biaoftn.org

Guynn Edwards, President
Pam Bryan, Executive Director

Texas

4053 **Brain Injury Association of Texas**
316 W 12th Street
Austin, TX 78701

512-326-1212
800-392-0040
Fax: 512-478-3370
e-mail: info@biatx.org
www.biatx.org

Jane Boutte, President

Utah

4054 **Brain Injury Association of Utah**
1800 S W Temple
Salt Lake City, UT 84115

801-484-2240
800-281-8442
Fax: 801-484-5932
e-mail: biau@sisna.com
www.biau.org

Teresa Such-Niebar, President
Ron S Roskos, Executive Director

Vermont

4055 **Brain Injury Association of Vermont**
92 S Main Street
Waterbury, VT 05676

802-244-6850
877-856-1772
Fax: 802-244-4005
e-mail: support1@biavt.org
www.biavt.org

Marsha Bancroft, President
Trevor Squirrell, Executive Director

Virginia

4056 **Brain Injury Association of Virginia**
1506 Willow Lawn Drive
Richmond, VA 23230

804-355-5748
800-444-6443
Fax: 804-355-6381
e-mail: info@biav.net
www.biav.net

Anne McDonnell, Executive Director
Lynette Scott, Program Director

Washington

4057 **Brain Injury Association of Washington**
800 Jefferson Street
Seattle, WA 98104

206-388-0900
800-523-5438
Fax: 206-388-0901
e-mail: info@biawa.org
www.biawa.org

Richard Adler, President
Gene van den Bosch, Executive Director

4058 **Brain Injury Association of Washington Hel**
3516 S 47th Street
Tacoma, WA 98409

253-238-6085
Fax: 253-238-1042
e-mail: info@biawa.org

Richard Adler, President
Mary Spielma Chapman, Interim Executive Director

West Virginia

4059 **Brain Injury Association of West Virginia**
PO Box 574
Institute, WV 25112-0574

304-766-4892
800-356-6443
Fax: 304-766-4940
e-mail: mdavis@brainman.com
www.biausa.org/WVirginia

Michael W Davis, Board of Director
Linda Arthur, Board of Director

Wisconsin

4060 **Brain Injury Association of Wisconsin**
21100 W Capitol Drive
Pewaukee, WI 53072

262-790-9660
800-882-9282
Fax: 262-790-9670
e-mail: admin@execpc.com
www.biaw.org

Advocacy, education, prevention, information, resources, and support groups in regards to traumatic brain injury.
David Voss, President
Mark Warhus, Executive Director

Wyoming

4061 **Brain Injury Association of Wyoming**
111 W 2nd Street
Casper, WY 82601

307-473-1767
800-643-6457
Fax: 307-237-5222
e-mail: biaw@tribcsp.com
www.biausa.org/Wyoming

Larry Plemmons, President
Jack Nokes, Director

Foundations

4062 **Brain Trauma Foundation**
708 Third Avenue
New York, NY 10017-4201

212-772-0608
Fax: 212-772-2035
e-mail: info@braintrauma.org
www.braintrauma.org

Our goal at the Brain Trauma Foundation is to improve the outcome of TBI patients through Guideline development, clinical research, professional education, and quality improvement programs.
Quarterly
Jamshid Ghajar, MD, President
Pamela Drexel, Executive Director

Research Centers

4063 **Brady Institute Jamaica Hospital Medical Center**
Jamaica Hospital Medical Center
8900 Van Wyck Expressway
Jamaica, NY 11418-2897

718-206-6000
Fax: 718-206-6559
www.jamaicahospital.org

The James and Sarah Brady Institute for Traumatic Brain Injury.
David P Rosen, President & CEO
Neil Foster Phillips, Chairman

4064 **Dana Alliance for Brain Initiatives**
745 Fifth Avenue
New York, NY 10151

212-223-4040
Fax: 212-317-8721
e-mail: danainfo@dana.org
www.dana.org

A non-profit organization of more than 250 neuroscientists which was formed to help provide information about the personal and public benefits of brain research.
Jane Nevins, Vice President
Edward F Rover, President

4065 **Institute for Rehabilitation and Research**
21720 Kingsland Blvd.
Katy, TX 77450

28- 57- 555
800-447-3422
Fax: 713-874-1798
e-mail: tirr.referrals@memorialhermann.org
www.tirr.org

John Kajander, President

4066 **New York University Medical Center Head Trauma Program**
Reet
New York, NY 10010-4020

212-998-9819
Fax: 212-340-7158

Research pertaining to young adults suffering from head injuries.
Dr Yehuda Ben-Yishay, Coordinator

4067 **Ohio State University Laboratory of Psychobiology**
1885 Neil Avenue
Columbus, OH 43210-1222

614-292-8185
Fax: 614-292-4537
www.psy.ohio-state.edu/labs

Studies done on recovery of function after brain damage.
Laura Peterson, Lab Coordinator
James Walton, Research Associate

4068 Rehabilitation Institute of Michigan
261 Mack Avenue
Detroit, MI 48201
313-745-1203
Fax: 313-745-2376
www.rimrehab.org

Physical medicine and rehabilitation medicine.
William H Restum PhD, President
Horacio Varg Jr, Interim Executive Director

4069 Thomas Jefferson University Ischemia-Shock Research Center
1020 Locust Street
Philadelphia, PA 19107-6731
215-503-1272
Fax: 215-955-2073
Promotes research into head injuries and clinical studies.

4070 Thomas Jefferson University Ischemia-Shock
1020 Walnut Street
Philadelphia, PA 19107
215-955-6000
Fax: 215-923-7932
www.jefferson.edu/main
Promotes research into head injuries and clinical studies.

4071 Tulane University: US-Japan Biomedical Research Laboratories
1430 Tulane Avenue
New Orleans, LA 70112
504-988-5462
Fax: 504-394-7169
e-mail: medsch@tulane.edu
www.som.tulane.edu/labs/usjamed
Focuses research efforts on neuroendocrinology and neurosciences.
Benjamin Sachs, Senior Vice President, Dean
Patrice Dela MD, Vice Chair

4072 UCLA Neuropsychiatric Institute
760 Westwood Plaza
Los Angeles, CA 90095
310-825-2631
Fax: 310-825-9179
www.semel.ucla.edu
Devote to teach research and patient care in psychiatry neuroscience and related fields.
Peter C Whybrow MD, Professor and Executive Chair
Peter Whybrow, Director

4073 University of California: Irvine Brain Imaging Center
101 The City Drive S
Irvine, CA 92697-3960
949-824-5011
Fax: 949-824-7873
e-mail: BIC@msx.hsis.uci.edu
www.bic.uci.edu
Offers PET scan analysis of brain functions focusing on brain damage brain tumors and head injuries.
Steven G Potkin MD, Director

4074 University of California: San Francisco Laboratory for Neurotrauma
1001 Potrero Avenue
San Francisco, CA 94110-3518
415-206-8313
Research done into traumatic brain and head injuries.
Lawrence H Pitts MD

4075 University of Tennessee: Memphis State University of Neuropsychology Lab
Memphis State University
202 Psychology Building
Memphis, TN 38152
901-678-2145
Fax: 901-678-2579
e-mail: contactus@mail.psyc.memphis.edu
www.memphis.edu/psychology/
Evaluation and development of assessment and treatment procedures for neurologically impaired persons.
Guy Mittleman, Professor Director of CAPR
Frank Andrasik, Professor, Chair

4076 Virginia Commonwealth University: Rehab Research and Training Center
1314 W Main Street
Richmond, VA 23284-2011
804-828-1851
Fax: 804-828-2193
TTY: 804-828-2494
www.worksupport.com
Focuses research on traumatic brain and head injuries.
Paul Wehman, Director
Jeanne Dalton, Public Relations Assistant Specialist

Michigan

4077 Wayne State University: Gurdjian-Lissner Biomechanics Laboratory
Department of Neurological Surgery
4160 John R Street
Detroit, MI 48201
313-831-0777
Fax: 313-966-0368
e-mail: jont@med.wayne.edu
www.med.wayne.edu/neurosurgery
Head and neck injury research.
Murali Guthi MD FA CS, Professor (Clinician-Educator) and Chair
Kenneth Case MD, Associate Professor

Support Groups & Hotlines

4078 National Health Information Center
PO Box 1133
Washington, DC 20013
310-565-4167
800-336-4797
Fax: 301-984-4256
e-mail: info@nhic.org
www.health.gov/nhic
Offers a nationwide information referral service, produces directories and resource guides.

Alabama

4079 Alabama Head Injury Foundation Helpline
3100 Lorna Road
Hoover, AL 35216-5451
205-823-3818
800-433-8002
Fax: 205-823-4544
e-mail: ahif1@bellsouth.net
www.ahif.org/
The Alabama Head Injury Foundation (AHIF) was founded by professionals and families in 1983 to increase public awareness of Traumatic Brain Injury (TBI) and to stimulate the development of supportive services. AHIF provides accessible resources, services and programs that meet the unique needs of individuals with traumatic brain injury (TBI) as well as spinal cord injury (SCI) in certain programs.
Charles D Priest, Executive Director
Sandra Koplon, Director Community Outreach

Arizona

4080 Brain Injury Association of Arizona
777 E Missouri
Phoenix, AZ 85014
602-508-8024
888-500-9165
Fax: 602-508-8285
e-mail: info@biaaz.org
www.biaaz.org
Information and resources for brain injury survivors and their families. Support group listings available.
Mattie Cummins, Executive Director
Mary Bradley, Board President

Arkansas

4081 Brain Injury Association of Arkansas Helpline
PO Box 26236
North Little Rock, AR 72221-6236
501-374-3585
800-235-2443
Fax: 501-918-6595
e-mail: info@brainassociation.org
www.brainassociation.org
Founded in 1980, the Brain Injury Association of America (BIAA) is a national organization serving and representing individuals, families and professionals who are touched by a life-altering, often devastating, traumatic brain injury (TBI). BIAA provides information, education and support through its network of chartered state affiliates, local chapters and support groups across the country to assist the 5.3 million Americans currently living with traumatic brain injury and their families.
Dianne Gutierrez, President Arkansas State Office
Dana Gonzales Ph.D, Vice President

California

4082 Brain Injury Association of California Hel pline
2658 Mt Vernon Avenue   661-872-4903
Bakersfield, CA 93306   Fax: 661-873-2508
                                         e-mail: calbiainfo@yahoo.com
                                         www.calbia.org/
Founded in 1980, the Brain Injury Association of America (BIAA) is a national organization serving and representing individuals, families and professionals who are touched by a life-altering, often devastating, traumatic brain injury (TBI). BIAA provides information, education and support through its network of chartered state affiliates, local chapters and support groups across the country to assist the 5.3 million Americans currently living with traumatic brain injury and their families.
Paula Daoutis, Executive Director
Richard Adams MD, Board of Directors

4083 Jodi House
1235 C Veronica Springs Road   805-563-2882
Santa Barbara, CA 93105   Fax: 805-563-3982
                                         e-mail: info@jodihouse.org
                                         www.jodihouse.org
Jodi House is a community-based, post-rehabilitation day program that provides opportunities for social interaction, life skill training, recreation, and support for adults living with acquired brain injury (i.e. from head trauma, tumor, and stroke) and their families.
Jim Kearns, President
Luciana Cramer, Executive Director

Colorado

4084 Brain Injury Association of Colorado Helpline
6825 E Tennessee Avenue   303-355-9969
Denver, CO 80224   800-955-2443
                                         Fax: 303-355-9968
                                         e-mail: biacolo@aol.com
                                         www.BIAColorado.org
Judy Dettmer, President
Helen O Kellogg, Exececutive Director

Connecticut

4085 Brain Injury Association of Connecticut Helpline
1800 Silas Deane Highway   860-721-8111
Rocky Hill, CT 6067-1304   800-278-8242
                                         Fax: 860-721-9008
                                         e-mail: general@biact.org
                                         www.biact.org
Supports persons with brain injuries and their families by promoting services to facilitate full inclusion within their local community and to increase awareness and understanding of brain injury and its prevention through community education.
500 Members
David Bush, Chairman
Julia Peterson, Executive Director

4086 TBI Support Group
Gaylord Hospital
PO Box 400   203-284-2800
Wallingford, CT 06492
Christine Wilson

Delaware

4087 Brain Injury Association of Delaware Helpl ine
32 West Loockerman Street   302-346-2083
Dover, DE 19904   800-411-0505
                                         Fax: 302-678-3183
                                         e-mail: biadresourcecenter@cavdel.net
                                         www.biausa.org/Delaware/bia.htm
Founded in 1980, the Brain Injury Association of America (BIAA) is a national organization serving and representing individuals, families and professionals who are touched by a life-altering, often devastating, traumatic brain injury (TBI). BIAA provides information, education and support through its network of chartered state affiliates, local chapters and support groups across the country to assist the 5.3 million Americans currently living with traumatic brain injury and their families.
John Goodier, President Delaware State Office
Howard H Hitch, Vice President

Florida

4088 Brain Injury Association of Florida
1637 Metropolitan Blvd   850-410-0103
Tallahassee, FL 32308   800-992-3442
                                         Fax: 850-410-0105
                                         e-mail: biaftalla@biaf.org
                                         www.biaf.org
Valerie E Breen, President/CEO

Hawaii

4089 Brain Injury Association of Hawaii
420 Kuwili Street   808-791-6942
Honolulu, HI 96817   e-mail: biahi@hawaiiantel.net
                                         www.biausa.org/Hawaii
Dedicated to serving those affected by brain injury throughgh advocacy, prevention, and support
Mary Wilson, Executive Director

Illinois

4090 American Brain Tumor Association Patient Line
2720 S River Road   847-827-9910
Des Plaines, IL 60018-4117   800-886-2282
                                         Fax: 847-827-9918
                                         e-mail: info@abta.org
                                         www.abta.org
Offers emergency support, information and referrals for patients and their families.
Naomi Berkowitz, Director

4091 Brain Injury Association of Illinois Helpline
Chicago, IL 60664-420   312-726-5699
                                         800-699-6443
                                         Fax: 312-630-4011
                                         e-mail: info@biail.org
                                         www.biail.org
Works with all people with brain inquiries and their families with professionals who serve them. Provides camp oppurtunities, support groups, educational seminars, information and referrals and a quarterly newsletter.
Irene Pedersen, Founder
Philicia Deckard, Executive Director

Indiana

4092 Brain Injury Association of Indiana Helpli ne
9531 Valparaiso Court   317-356-7722
Indianapolis, IN 46268   800-407-4246
                                         Fax: 317-808-7770
                                         e-mail: info@biai.org
                                         www.biausa.org/Indiana
Founded in 1980, the Brain Injury Association of America (BIAA) is a national organization serving and representing individuals, families and professionals who are touched by a life-altering, often devastating, traumatic brain injury (TBI). BIAA provides information, education and support through its network of chartered state affiliates, local chapters and support groups across the country to assist the 5.3 million Americans currently living with traumatic brain injury and their families.
Stacey Payne, Executive Director Indiana State Office
Laura C Trexler, TBI Grant Program Director

Iowa

4093 Brain Injury Association of Iowa Helpline
Brain Injury Association of America

2101 Kimball Avenue LL7
Waterloo, IA 50702

319-272-2312
800-475-4442
Fax: 319-272-2109
e-mail: diaia@cedarnet.org
www.biaia.org

Julie Dixon, President
Ed Boll, Program Manager

Kentucky

4094 Brain Injury Association of Kentucky Helpl ine
7410 New LaGrange Road
Louisville, KY 40222

502-493-0609
800-592-1117
Fax: 502-426-2993
e-mail: Melinda.Mast@biak.us
www.biak.us

Founded in 1980, the Brain Injury Association of America (BIAA) is a national organization serving and representing individuals, families and professionals who are touched by a life-altering, often devastating, traumatic brain injury (TBI). BIAA provides information, education and support through its network of chartered state affiliates, local chapters and support groups across the country to assist the 5.3 million Americans currently living with traumatic brain injury and their families.

Debbie Nelson, President Kentucky State Office
Melinda Mast, Executive Director

Louisiana

4095 Brain Injury Association of Louisiana Help line
c/o National Headquarters Office
8201 Greensboro Drive
McLean, VA 22102

703-761-0750
800-444-6443
Fax: 703-761-0755
e-mail: familyhelpline@biausa.org
www.biausa.org/

Founded in 1980, the Brain Injury Association of America (BIAA) is a national organization serving and representing individuals, families and professionals who are touched by a life-altering, often devastating, traumatic brain injury (TBI). BIAA provides information, education and support through its network of chartered state affiliates, local chapters and support groups across the country to assist the 5.3 million Americans currently living with traumatic brain injury and their families.

Susan H Connors, President/Chief Executive Officer (VA)
Mary S Reitter CAE, EVP/Chief Operations Officer (VA)

Maine

4096 Brain Injury Association of Maine Helpline
325 Main Street
Waterville, ME 04901

207-681-9900
800-275-1233
Fax: 207-861-4617
e-mail: info@biame.org
www.biame.org

Founded in 1980, the Brain Injury Association of America (BIAA) is a national organization serving and representing individuals, families and professionals who are touched by a life-altering, often devastating, traumatic brain injury (TBI). BIAA provides information, education and support through its network of chartered state affiliates, local chapters and support groups across the country to assist the 5.3 million Americans currently living with traumatic brain injury and their families.

Bev Bryant, President Maine State Office
John Bott, Executive Director

Maryland

4097 Brain Injury Association of Maryland Helpl ine
Kernan Hospital
2200 Kernan Drive
Baltimore, MD 21207

410-448-2924
800-221-6443
Fax: 410-448-3541
e-mail: info@biamd.org
www.biamd.org

Founded in 1980, the Brain Injury Association of America (BIAA) is a national organization serving and representing individuals, families and professionals who are touched by a life-altering, often devastating, traumatic brain injury (TBI). BIAA provides informa-

tion, education and support through its network of chartered state affiliates, local chapters and support groups across the country to assist the 5.3 million Americans currently living with traumatic brain injury and their families.

Patricia Janus, President Maryland State Office
Dianne Tripp, Executive Director

Massachusetts

4098 Brain Injury Association of Massachusetts Helpline
30 Lyman Street
Westborough, MA 01581

508-475-0032
800-242-0030
Fax: 508-475-0400
e-mail: biama@biama.org
www.biama.org

Founded in 1980, the Brain Injury Association of America (BIAA) is a national organization serving and representing individuals, families and professionals who are touched by a life-altering, often devastating, traumatic brain injury (TBI). BIAA provides information, education and support through its network of chartered state affiliates, local chapters and support groups across the country to assist the 5.3 million Americans currently living with traumatic brain injury and their families.

Gregory L Zagloba, President Massachusetts State Office
Arlene Korab, Executive Director

4099 VALT Support Group (Vital Active Life After Trauma)
53 Linden Street
Brookline, MA 02149

617-277-6327

Michigan

4100 Brain Injury Association of Michigan Helpline
8619 W Grand River
Brighton, MI 48116-2334

810-229-5880
800-444-6443
Fax: 810-229-8947
e-mail: info@biami.org
www.biami.org

James Tuinstra, Chair
Michael F Dabbs, President

Minnesota

4101 Brain Injury Association of Minnesota Helpline
34 13th Avenue North East
Minneapolis, MN 55413

612-378-2742
800-669-6442
Fax: 612-378-2789
e-mail: biam@protocom.com
www.braininjurymn.org

Tom Gode, Executive Director

Mississippi

4102 Brain Injury Association of Mississippi Helpline
PO Box 55912
Jackson, MS 39296-5912

601-981-1021
800-641-6642
Fax: 601-981-1039
e-mail: biaofms@aol.com
www.members.aol.com/biaofms

Howard Katz PhD, Chair

Missouri

4103 Brain Injury Association of Kansas and Greater Kansas City Helpline
1100 Pennsylvania Avenue
Kansas City, MO 64105

816-842-8607
800-783-1356
Fax: 816-842-1531
www.braininjuryresource.org

Mark Thompson, President
Leigh Liggett, Executive Director

4104 Brain Injury Association of Missouri Helpline
10270 Page Avenue
St Louis, MO 63132-1322

314-426-4024
800-377-6442
Fax: 314-426-3290
e-mail: brainInJry@aol.com
www.biausa.org/bia

Information and referral services and support groups throughout the state of Missouri.
Terrie Price, Board President
Scott Gee, Executive Director

Montana

4105 **Brain Injury Association of Montana Helpline**
52 Corbin Hall
Missoula, MT 59812
406-243-5973
800-241-6442
Fax: 406-243-2349
e-mail: biam@selway.umt.edu

Dr. MV Morton, President
Rose Davis, Office Manager

Nevada

4106 **Brain Injury Association of Nevada Helplin e**
c/o National Office Headquarters
8201 Greensboro Drive
McLean, VA 22102
703-761-0750
Fax: 702-591-0755
e-mail: FamilyHelpline@biausa.org
www.biausa.org/contactinfo.htm
Founded in 1980, the Brain Injury Association of America (BIAA) is a national organization serving and representing individuals, families and professionals who are touched by a life-altering, often devastating, traumatic brain injury (TBI). BIAA provides information, education and support through its network of chartered state affiliates, local chapters and support groups across the country to assist the 5.3 million Americans currently living with traumatic brain injury and their families.
Susan H Connors, President/Chief Executive Officer
Mary S Reitter CAE, EVP/Chief Operations Officer

New Hampshire

4107 **Brain Injury Association of New Hampshire**
Brain Injury Association of America
109 N State Street
Concord, NH 3301-4447
603-225-8400
800-773-8400
Fax: 603-228-6749
e-mail: mail@bianh.org
www.bianh.org

Newton Kersaw, President
Steven Wade, Executive Director

New Jersey

4108 **Brain Injury Association of New Jersey Helpline**
Brain Injury Association of America
1090 King George Post Road
Edison, NJ 8837
732-738-1002
800-669-4323
Fax: 732-738-1132
e-mail: info@bianj.org
www.bianj.org

Albert Pressler, President
Barbara Geigerparker, Executive Director

New Mexico

4109 **Brain Injury Association of New Mexico Hel pline**
121 Cardenas NE
Albuquerque, NM 87108
505-292-7414
888-292-7415
Fax: 505-271-8983
e-mail: braininjurynm@msn.com
www.braininjurynm.org
Founded in 1980, the Brain Injury Association of America (BIAA) is a national organization serving and representing individuals, families and professionals who are touched by a life-altering, often devastating, traumatic brain injury (TBI). BIAA provides information, education and support through its network of chartered state affiliates, local chapters and support groups across the country to assist the 5.3 million Americans currently living with traumatic brain injury and their families.
Mark Pedrotty Ph.D, Board President New Mexico State Office
Clara Holguin, Executive Director

New York

4110 **Brain Injury Association of New York State Helpline**
10 Colvin Avenue
Albany, NY 12206-1242
518-459-7911
800-228-8201
Fax: 518-482-5285
e-mail: info@bianys.org
www.bianys.org

Michael Kaplen, President
Judy Avner, Executive Director

4111 **Cafe Plus**
216 W Manlius Street
East Syracuse, NY 13057
315-446-3124
www.dreamscape.com/cafeplus
For people who have survived a head-injury or some type of head trauma.
David Listowski, Manager

4112 **Hy Feinstein Clubhouse**
Long Island Head Injury Association
65 Austin Boulevard
Commack, NY 11725
631-543-2245
Fax: 631-543-2261
www.lihia.org
The LIHIA provides a place for people with head injury to participate in meaningful work, to have the opportunity to meet and build friendships and ultimately seek employment within the community.

North Carolina

4113 **Brain Injury Association of North Carolina Helpline**
PO Box 748
Raleigh, NC 27602
919-833-9634
800-377-1464
Fax: 919-833-5415
e-mail: biaofnc@aol.com
www.bianc.net/

Bob Gauldin, President
Cecil Greene Jr, Executive Director

North Dakota

4114 **Brain Injury Association of North Dakota H elpline**
209 2nd Street SE
Valley City, ND 58072
701-845-1124
Fax: 701-845-1175
e-mail: FamilyHelpline@biausa.org
www.biausa.org/contactinfo.htm
Founded in 1980, the Brain Injury Association of America (BIAA) is a national organization serving and representing individuals, families and professionals who are touched by a life-altering, often devastating, traumatic brain injury (TBI). BIAA provides information, education and support through its network of chartered state affiliates, local chapters and support groups across the country to assist the 5.3 million Americans currently living with traumatic brain injury and their families.
Mary Simonson, President
Ken Moliter, Vice President

Ohio

4115 **Brain Injury Association of Ohio**
1335 Dublin Road
Columbus, OH 43215-1000
614-481-7100
866-644-6242
Fax: 614-481-7103
e-mail: help@biaoh.org
www.biaoh.org

Suzanne Minnich, Executive Director

Oklahoma

4116 **Brain Injury Association of Oklahoma Helpl ine**
PO Box 88
Hillsdale, OK 73743-0088
580-233-4363
800-765-6809
Fax: 580-233-4546
e-mail: information@braininjuryoklahoma.org
www.braininjuryoklahoma.org
Founded in 1980, the Brain Injury Association of America (BIAA) is a national organization serving and representing individuals, families and professionals who are touched by a life-altering, often devastating, traumatic brain injury (TBI). BIAA provides informa-

tion, education and support through its network of chartered state affiliates, local chapters and support groups across the country to assist the 5.3 million Americans currently living with traumatic brain injury and their families.

Tracy Grammer, President Oklahoma State Office
Mary S Reitter CAE, COO/National Headquarters (703-761-0750)

Oregon

4117 Brain Injury Association of Oregon Helpline
Brain Injury Association of America
2145 NW Overton Street   503-413-7707
Portland, OR 97210   800-544-5243
                           Fax: 503-413-6849
                    e-mail: biaor@biaoregon.org
                           www.biaoregon.org

Non-profit providing information and referral, support groups, prevention, education, training, and advocacy for those with brain injury, families, and professionals.
Sherry Stock, Executive Director

Rhode Island

4118 Brain Injury Association of Rhode Island H elpline
935 Park Avenue   401-461-6599
Cranston, RI 02910-2743   Fax: 401-461-6561
                    e-mail: braininjuryctr@biaofri.org
                                    biaofri.org

Founded in 1980, the Brain Injury Association of America (BIAA) is a national organization serving and representing individuals, families and professionals who are touched by a life-altering, often devastating, traumatic brain injury (TBI). BIAA provides information, education and support through its network of chartered state affiliates, local chapters and support groups across the country to assist the 5.3 million Americans currently living with traumatic brain injury and their families.

Paula O'Connor, President Rhode Island State Office
Sharon Brinkworth, Executive Director

Tennessee

4119 Brain Injury Association of Tennessee Help line
151 Athens Way   615-248-5878
Nashville, TN 37228   877-757-2428
                           Fax: 615-248-5879
                    e-mail: biaoftn@yahoo.com
                           www.biaoftn.org

Founded in 1980, the Brain Injury Association of America (BIAA) is a national organization serving and representing individuals, families and professionals who are touched by a life-altering, often devastating, traumatic brain injury (TBI). BIAA provides information, education and support through its network of chartered state affiliates, local chapters and support groups across the country to assist the 5.3 million Americans currently living with traumatic brain injury and their families.

Guynn Edwards, President Tennessee State Office
Stephanie Pruitt, Executive Director

Utah

4120 Brain Injury Association of Utah Helpline
Brain Injury Association of America
1800 SW Temple Suite 203   801-484-2240
Salt Lake City, UT 84115   800-281-8442
                           Fax: 801-484-5932
                    e-mail: biau@sisna.com
                www.starpage.com/braininjury/

Barbara Hayward, President
Ron Roskos, Executive Director

Vermont

4121 Brain Injury Association of Vermont Helpli ne
PO Box 226   802-985-8440
Shelburne, VT 05482   877-856-1772
                           Fax: 802-985-8440
                    e-mail: biavtinfo@adelphia.net
                                    www.biavt.org

Founded in 1980, the Brain Injury Association of America (BIAA) is a national organization serving and representing individuals, families and professionals who are touched by a life-altering, often devastating, traumatic brain injury (TBI). BIAA provides information, education and support through its network of chartered state affiliates, local chapters and support groups across the country to assist the 5.3 million Americans currently living with traumatic brain injury and their families.

Bob Luce, President Vermont State Office
Trevor Squirrell, Executive Director

Virginia

4122 Brain Injury Association of Virginia Helpline
3212 Cutshaw Avenue   804-355-5748
Richmond, VA 23230-5018   800-334-8443
                           Fax: 804-355-6381
                    e-mail: info@biav.net
                           www.biav.net

Nonprofit organization providing information and resources related to brain injury to individuals with brain injuries, their families and professionals who deal with brain injury.
Harry Weinstock, Executive Director

4123 Brain Injury Association of Virginia Helpl ine
3212 Cutshaw Avenue   804-355-5748
Richmond, VA 23230   800-334-8443
                           Fax: 804-355-6381
                    e-mail: info@biav.net
                           www.biav.net

Founded in 1980, the Brain Injury Association of America (BIAA) is a national organization serving and representing individuals, families and professionals who are touched by a life-altering, often devastating, traumatic brain injury (TBI). BIAA provides information, education and support through its network of chartered state affiliates, local chapters and support groups across the country to assist the 5.3 million Americans currently living with traumatic brain injury and their families.

Irv Cantor, President Virginia State Office
Anne McDonnell, Executive Director

Washington

4124 Brain Injury Association of Washington Hel pline
800 Jefferson Street   206-388-0900
Seattle, WA 98104   800-523-5438
                           Fax: 206-388-0901
                    e-mail: info@biawa.org
                           www.biawa.org

Founded in 1980, the Brain Injury Association of America (BIAA) is a national organization serving and representing individuals, families and professionals who are touched by a life-altering, often devastating, traumatic brain injury (TBI). BIAA provides information, education and support through its network of chartered state affiliates, local chapters and support groups across the country to assist the 5.3 million Americans currently living with traumatic brain injury and their families.

Richard Adler, President Washington State Office
Gene Van Den Bosch, Executive Director

4125 Head Injury Hotline
Brain Injury Resource Center
PO Box 84151   206-621-8558
Seattle, WA 98124-5451   Fax: 206-329-4355
                    e-mail: brain@headinjury.com
                           www.headinjury.com

Disseminates head injury information and provides referrals to facilitate adjustment to life following head injury. Organizes seminars for professionals, head injury survivors, and their families.
Constance Miller MA, Founder/President
B Parker Lindner MPA, Communications Specialist

West Virginia

4126 Brain Injury Association of West Virginia Helpline
Brain Injury Association of America

PO Box 574
Institute, WV 25112-574

304-766-4892
800-356-6443
Fax: 304-766-4940
e-mail: biawv@aol.com

Michael W Davis, President

Wisconsin

4127   Brain Injury Association of Wisconsin Help line
21100 W Capitol Drive
Pewaukee, WI 53072

262-790-9660
800-882-9282
Fax: 262-790-9670
e-mail: admin@execpc.com
www.biaw.org

Founded in 1980, the Brain Injury Association of America (BIAA) is a national organization serving and representing individuals, families and professionals who are touched by a life-altering, often devastating, traumatic brain injury (TBI). BIAA provides information, education and support through its network of chartered state affiliates, local chapters and support groups across the country to assist the 5.3 million Americans currently living with traumatic brain injury and their families.

Kalli Reinheimer, President Wisconsin State Office
Mark Warhus, Executive Director

Wyoming

4128   Brain Injury Association of Wyoming
111 West 2nd Street
Casper, WY 82601

307-473-1767
800-643-6457
Fax: 307-237-5222
www.biausa.org.wy

Dorothy Cronin, Director

Books

4129   An Educational Challenge: Meeting the Needs of Students with Brain Injury
Brain Injury Association
105 N Alfred Street
Alexandria, VA 22314

703-236-6000
800-444-6443
Fax: 703-236-6001

4130   Brain Injury Glossary
HDI Publishers
10600 NW Freeway, Suite 202
Houston, TX 77219

800-321-7037
Fax: 713-956-2288

Contains glossary and descriptions of health care providers.

4131   Brainlash
Demos Medical Publishing
386 Park Avenue S
New York, NY 10016

212-683-0072
Fax: 212-683-0118
e-mail: orderdept@demospub.com
www.demosmedpub.com

Maximize your recovery from mild brain injury.
376 pages
ISBN: 1-888799-37-4
Dr. Diana M Schneider

4132   Coming Home: A Discharge Manual for Families of Persons with a Brain Injury
HDI Publishers
10600 NW Freeway, Suite 202
Houston, TX 77219

800-321-7037
Fax: 713-956-2288

4133   Communication Disorders Following Traumatic Brain Injury
Pro-Ed, Inc.
8700 Shoal Creek Boulevard
Austin, TX 78757-6897

512-451-3246
800-897-3202
Fax: 800-397-7633
e-mail: info@proedinc.com
www.proedinc.com

For graduates and professionals, this text takes a holistic approach toward treating the client with traumatic brain injury.
439 pages Paperback
ISBN: 0-890792-95-X
Lindy Jordaan, Marketing Coordinator

4134   Dano Cerebral: Guia Para Familias y Cuidadores
Brain Injury Association/HDI Publishers/Catalogue
PO Box 131401
Houston, TX 77219

800-321-7037
Fax: 713-526-7787

This book, written in Spanish, is a thorough, well-researched guide for people with brain injury, their families and caregivers. Up-to-date information covers such topics as Intensive Care- admittance and discharge; Mechanics of brain injury; Coma; Consequences of brain injury; Mental and Emotional symptoms among many others.
158 pages 1994

4135   From the Ashes
Phoenix Project
PO Box 84151
Seattle, WA 98124-5451

206-329-1371

A self-help book that addresses the trauma that comes with a head injury and introduces methods of building a fulfilling and productive life.
108 pages

4136   Handbook of Head Truma: Acute Care to Recovery
Plenum Publishing Corporation
233 Spring Street
New York, NY 10013-1522

212-620-8000
800-221-9369
Fax: 212-463-0742
e-mail: books@plenum.com

466 pages
ISBN: 0-306439-47-6

4137   Head Injury and the Family: A Life and Living Perspective
St. Lucie Press
100 E Linton Boulevard
Delary Beach, FL 33483

407-274-9906
Fax: 407-274-9927

One of the best books written in this area. Easy to read, written with family, caregivers and patients in mind. Includes exercises and vignettes.

4138   Integrating Community Resources
HDI Publishers
10600 NW Freeway, Suite 202
Houston, TX 77219

800-321-7037
Fax: 713-956-2288

4139   Living with Brain Injury: A Guide for Families
Brain Injury Association/HDI Publishers/Catalogue
PO Box 131401
Houston, TX 77219

800-321-7037
Fax: 713-526-7787

This book will help readers- families, persons with brain injury and professionals alike- through this uncharted territory. topics include: How brain injury is caused and how it can be treated: Physical, cognitive and behavioral symptoms; Questions family members commonly ask.
145 pages 1998

4140   National Directory of Brain Injury Rehabilitatiom
Brain Injury Association
105 N Alfred Street
Alexandria, VA 22314

703-236-6000
800-444-6443
Fax: 703-236-6001

Desk reference for professionals listing brain injury rehabilitation programs and individual service providers nationwide.

4141   National Directory of Head Injury Rehabilitation Services
Brain Injury Association
105 N Alfred Street
Alexandria, VA 22314

703-236-6000
800-444-6443
Fax: 703-236-6001

4142   Planning for the Future
Brain Injury Association

105 N Alfred Street
Alexandria, VA 22314
703-236-6000
800-444-6443
Fax: 703-236-6001
This book provides a meaningful life for a child with a disability after your death.

4143 Recovery from Brain Damage in the Elderly
Aspen Publishers
PO Box 990
Frederick, MD 21705-0990
800-638-8437
Recovery and rehabilitation techniques in the area of brain damage in the elderly.

4144 Sexuality and the Person with Traumatic Brain Injury
Brain Injury Association
105 N Alfred Street
Alexandria, VA 22314
703-236-6000
800-444-6443
Fax: 703-236-6001

4145 Stress Management Following Head Injury: Strategies for Families and Caregivers
Brain Injury Association
105 N Alfred Street
Alexandria, VA 22314
703-236-6000
800-444-6443
Fax: 703-236-6001

4146 TBI Tool Kit
HDI Publishers
10600 NW Freeway, Suite 202
Houston, TX 77219
800-321-7037
Fax: 713-956-2288

4147 Traumatic Brain Injury Rehabilitation: Brain Injury Consortium Monograph Series
St. Lucie Press
100 E Linton Boulevard
Delray Beach, FL 33483
407-274-9906
Fax: 407-274-9927
Assistive technology, under the Americans with Disabilities Act, is that designed for and used by individuals with the intent of eliminating, ameliorating, or compensating for functional limitations. Coverage includes impaired functions that limit vocational outcome, behavior concerns in the workplace, maximizing a client's residual knowledge skills, use of computers and adapting work environments.

4148 Traumatic Head Injury: Cause, Consequence and Challenge
Brain Injury Association/HDI Publishers/Catalogue
PO Box 131401
Houston, TX 77219
800-321-7037
Fax: 713-526-7787
A resource book on traumatic brain injury which translates technical medical information on brain injury into simple, easy-to-understand language for persons with brain injury and their families. Covered topics: a general overview of brain injury; similarities and differences among people with brain injury; types and consequences of brain injury; recovery and rehabilitation; accepting and coping with change.
60 pages 1993

4149 Why Did it Happen on a School Day: My Family's Experience with Brain Injury
Brain Injury Association
105 N Alfred Street
Alexandria, VA 22314
703-236-6000
800-444-6443
Fax: 703-236-6001

4150 Working After Brain Injury
HDI Publishers
10600 NW Freeway, Suite 202
Houston, TX 77219
800-321-7037
Fax: 713-956-2288

Magazines

4151 Journal of Head Trauma Rehabilitation
Aspen Publishers
1600 Research Boulevard
Rockville, MD 20850-3129
301-251-8500
800-638-8437
www.aspenpub.com

Scholarly journal designed to provide information on clinical management and rehabilitation of the head-injured for the practicing professional.

4152 Mouth Magazine
PO Box 558
Topeka, KS 66601-0558
785-272-2578
Fax: 785-272-7348
www.mouthmag.org
Bi-monthly magazine with subscription.

Newsletters

4153 BIAW News
Brain Injury Association of Wisconsin
21100 W Capitol Drive
Pewaukee, WI 53072
262-790-9660
800-882-9282
Fax: 262-790-9670
e-mail: admin@execpc.com
www.biaw.org
David Voss, President
Mark Warhus, Executive Director

4154 Brain Injury Source
Brain Injury Association
105 N Alfred Street
Alexandria, VA 22314
703-236-6000
Fax: 703-236-6001
e-mail: BIAV@visi.net
www.biausa.org
Written for and by professionals in the field. Blends professionally written articles on information and research in brain injury with a user friendly format that incorporates graphics and charts to effectively deliver the messages. Full color.
50+ pages Quarterly

4155 TBI Challenge!
Brain Injury Association of America
105 N Alfred Street
Alexandria, VA 22314-3010
703-236-6000
Fax: 703-236-6001
www.biausa.org
Exclusively for and about persons with brain injury. Provides information to individuals with brain injury and their families. Professionals will benefit from the perspectives provided in Kid's Corner, Relatively Speaking, Ask the Lawyer, Information and Resources and Ask the Doctor.
bimonthly

Arizona

4156 Brainstorm
Brain Injury Association of Arizona
777 E Missouri
Phoenix, AZ 85014
602-323-9165
888-500-9165
Fax: 602-508-8285
e-mail: info@biaaz.org
www.biaaz.org
A newsletter serving persons with brain injury, their families and professionals.
8 pages Quarterly
Mary Bradley, Board President
Mattie Cummins, Executive Director

Florida

4157 Brain Waves
Brain Injury Association of Florida
1637 Metropolitan Boulevard
Tallahassee, FL 32308
850-410-0103
800-992-3442
Fax: 850-410-0105
e-mail: biaftalla@biaf.org
www.biaf.org
Each issue highlights a topic related to TBI and TBI resources.
Bi-Annually
Valerie E Breen, President/CEO

Pamphlets

4158 A Survey of Accredited and Other Rehabilitation Facilities
Brain Injury Association
105 N Alfred Street   703-236-6000
Alexandria, VA 22314   800-444-6443
                                        Fax: 703-236-6001
Education, training and cognitive rehabilitation in barin injury programs.

4159 About Head Injuries
Channing L Bete Company
200 State Road
South Deerfield, MA 01373   800-628-7733
Covers basic information including identifying the members of the treatment team and how to take care of yourself as a caregiver.

4160 Adolescents with Closed Head Injuries: A Report of Initial Cognitive Deficits
Brain Injury Association
105 N Alfred Street   703-236-6000
Alexandria, VA 22314   800-444-6443
                                        Fax: 703-236-6001

4161 Basic Questions About Head Injury & Disability
Brain Injury Association
105 N Alfred Street   703-236-6000
Alexandria, VA 22314   800-444-6443
                                        Fax: 703-236-6001

4162 Behavioral and Psychosocial Sequelae of Pediatric Head Injury
Brain Injury Association
105 N Alfred Street   703-236-6000
Alexandria, VA 22314   800-444-6443
                                        Fax: 703-236-6001

4163 Brain Damage is a Family Affair
Brain Injury Association
105 N Alfred Street   703-236-6000
Alexandria, VA 22314   800-444-6443
                                        Fax: 703-236-6001

4164 Brain Injuries: A Guide for Families & Caretakers
Brain Injury Association
105 N Alfred Street   703-236-6000
Alexandria, VA 22314   800-444-6443
                                        Fax: 703-236-6001

4165 Brain Injury: A Home Based Cognitive Rehabilitation Program
HDI Publishers
10600 NW Freeway, Suite 202
Houston, TX 77219   800-321-7037
                                        Fax: 713-956-2288

4166 Catastrophic Injury Cases: The Relationship of Traumatic Brain Injury
Brain Injury Association
105 N Alfred Street   703-236-6000
Alexandria, VA 22314   800-444-6443
                                        Fax: 703-236-6001

4167 Children with Disabilities: Understanding Sibling Issues
Brain Injury Association
105 N Alfred Street   703-236-6000
Alexandria, VA 22314   800-444-6443
                                        Fax: 703-236-6001

4168 Counseling Head Injured Patients: Guidelines for Community Health Workers
Brain Injury Association
105 N Alfred Street   703-236-6000
Alexandria, VA 22314   800-444-6443
                                        Fax: 703-236-6001

4169 Education Concerns for the Traumatically Head Injured Student
Brain Injury Association
105 N Alfred Street   703-236-6000
Alexandria, VA 22314   800-444-6443
                                        Fax: 703-236-6001

4170 From One Family Member to Another
Brain Injury Association
105 N Alfred Street   703-236-6000
Alexandria, VA 22314   800-444-6443
                                        Fax: 703-236-6001
A mother tells the story of her son's injury and recovery. Gives suggestions for structuring the home environment.

4171 Guide to Selecting and Monitoring Head Injury Rehabilitation Services
Brain Injury Association
105 N Alfred Street   703-236-6000
Alexandria, VA 22314   800-444-6443
                                        Fax: 703-236-6001

4172 Head Injury Survivor on Campus: Issues & Resources
Brain Injury Association
105 N Alfred Street   703-236-6000
Alexandria, VA 22314   800-444-6443
                                        Fax: 703-236-6001

4173 Head Injury: A Booklet for Families
Brain Injury Association
105 N Alfred Street   703-236-6000
Alexandria, VA 22314   800-444-6443
                                        Fax: 703-236-6001

4174 Head Injury: A Guide for Families
HDI Publishers
10600 NW Freeway, Suite 202
Houston, TX 77219   800-321-7037
                                        Fax: 713-956-2288
Structured by problem with examples and practical coping strategies.

4175 Hearing Loss Following Head Injury
Brain Injury Association
105 N Alfred Street   703-236-6000
Alexandria, VA 22314   800-444-6443
                                        Fax: 703-236-6001

4176 Hiring Persons with a Brain Injury: What to Expect
HDI Publishers
10600 NW Freeway, Suite 202
Houston, TX 77219   800-321-7037
                                        Fax: 713-956-2288

4177 Individual Psychotherapy with the Brain Injured Adult
Brain Injury Association
105 N Alfred Street   703-236-6000
Alexandria, VA 22314   800-444-6443
                                        Fax: 703-236-6001
Review of literature on substance abuse and head injury. Includes statistics, and treatment options, strategies and extensive bibliography.

4178 Information General Sobre: Lesion Cerebral
Brain Injury Association
105 N Alfred Street   703-236-6000
Alexandria, VA 22314   800-444-6443
                                        Fax: 703-236-6001

4179 Introductory Information for Families
Brain Injury Association
105 N Alfred Street   703-236-6000
Alexandria, VA 22314   800-444-6443
                                        Fax: 703-236-6001
A collection of readings on basic information about TBI and a guide for selecting rehabilitation facilities.

4180 Know Your Brain
Nat'l Institute of Neurological Disorders & Stroke
PO Box 5801
Bethesda, MD 20824   800-352-9424
                                        Fax: 301-402-2186
                                        www.ninds.nih.gov
Basic information about the brain, neuroscience research, and disorders of the brain.

4181 Legal and Financial Issues for Families
Brain Injury Association
105 N Alfred Street   703-236-6000
Alexandria, VA 22314   800-444-6443
                                        Fax: 703-236-6001

Packet designed for families that explores some of the legal and financial issues faced after TBI.

4182   Life After Brain Injury: Who am I
HDI Publishers
10600 NW Freeway, Suite 202
Houston, TX 77219   800-321-7037
                                     Fax: 713-956-2288
A well-structured book. Dicusses specific problems areas. Includes good examples and gives lists of practical coping strategies.

4183   Mild Brain Injury: Damage and Outcome
Brain Injury Association
105 N Alfred Street   703-236-6000
Alexandria, VA 22314   800-444-6443
                                     Fax: 703-236-6001

4184   Neuropsychology of Attention and Memory
Brain Injury Association
105 N Alfred Street   703-236-6000
Alexandria, VA 22314   800-444-6443
                                     Fax: 703-236-6001

4185   Persisting Problems After Mild Head Injury: A Review of the Syndrome
Brain Injury Association
105 N Alfred Street   703-236-6000
Alexandria, VA 22314   800-444-6443
                                     Fax: 703-236-6001

4186   Post-Traumatic Headaches: Subtypes & Behavioral Treatments
Brain Injury Association
105 N Alfred Street   703-236-6000
Alexandria, VA 22314   800-444-6443
                                     Fax: 703-236-6001

4187   Recovery and Cognitive Retraining After Craniocerebral Trauma
Brain Injury Association
105 N Alfred Street   703-236-6000
Alexandria, VA 22314   800-444-6443
                                     Fax: 703-236-6001

4188   Relationships Between Personality Disorders
Brain Injury Association
105 N Alfred Street   703-236-6000
Alexandria, VA 22314   800-444-6443
                                     Fax: 703-236-6001
Social Disturbances and physical disability following TBI.

4189   Resources List of Organizations
Brain Injury Association
105 N Alfred Street   703-236-6000
Alexandria, VA 22314   800-444-6443
                                     Fax: 703-236-6001

4190   Severe Brain Injury
Brain Injury Association
105 N Alfred Street   703-236-6000
Alexandria, VA 22314   800-444-6443
                                     Fax: 703-236-6001
This pamphlet is in hand out format and would be appropriate for use in clinic or hospital setting.

4191   Spouses of Persons Who Are Brain Injured: Overlooked Victims
Brain Injury Association
105 N Alfred Street   703-236-6000
Alexandria, VA 22314   800-444-6443
                                     Fax: 703-236-6001

4192   Stress Management Following Head Injury: Strategies for Families & Caregivers
Brain Injury Association
105 N Alfred Street   703-236-6000
Alexandria, VA 22314   800-444-6443
                                     Fax: 703-236-6001

4193   Subarachnoid Hemorrhage & Aneurysm
University Hospital & Clinics
One Hosptial Drive   314-882-4141
Columbia, MO 65212

This pamphlet includes easy to read, general information plus a glossary and schematic diagrams. This pamphlet would be most appropriate for use with recently head injured patients.

4194   Substance Abuse Task Force White Paper
Brain Injury Association
105 N Alfred Street   703-236-6000
Alexandria, VA 22314   800-444-6443
                                     Fax: 703-236-6001
Review of literature on substance abuse and head injury. Includes statistics, and treatment options, strategies and extensive bibliography.

4195   Susan's Dad: A Child's Story of Head Injury
Brain Injury Association
105 N Alfred Street   703-236-6000
Alexandria, VA 22314   800-444-6443
                                     Fax: 703-236-6001

4196   Teaching Persons with A Brain Injury: What to Expect
HDI Publishers
10600 NW Freeway, Suite 202
Houston, TX 77219   800-321-7037
                                     Fax: 713-956-2288

4197   Unseen Injury: Minor Head Injury
Brain Injury Association
105 N Alfred Street   703-236-6000
Alexandria, VA 22314   800-444-6443
                                     Fax: 703-236-6001

4198   What is Anoxic Brain Injury
Brain Injury Association
105 N Alfred Street   703-236-6000
Alexandria, VA 22314   800-444-6443
                                     Fax: 703-236-6001

4199   When Your Child Goes to School After an Injury
Brain Injury Association
105 N Alfred Street   703-236-6000
Alexandria, VA 22314   800-444-6443
                                     Fax: 703-236-6001

4200   When Your Child is Seriously Injured: The Emotional Impact on Families
Brain Injury Association
105 N Alfred Street   703-236-6000
Alexandria, VA 22314   800-444-6443
                                     Fax: 703-236-6001

4201   Working After A Head Injury
HDI Publishers
10600 NW Freeway, Suite 202
Houston, TX 77219   800-321-7037
                                     Fax: 713-956-2288

Audio & Video

4202   A Fate Better than Death
Brain Injury Association
105 N Alfred Street   703-236-6000
Alexandria, VA 22314   800-444-6443
                                     Fax: 703-236-6001
Video features 4 young adults with traumatic brain injury. Focuses on support groups.

4203   Neuropsychological Assessment: What it Does & Does Not Do
Brain Injury Association
105 N Alfred Street   703-236-6000
Alexandria, VA 22314   800-444-6443
                                     Fax: 703-236-6001
This pamphlet is in hand out format and would be appropriate for use in clinic or hospital setting.

4204   Peter Wegner Is Alive and Well and Living in Providence
Filmakers Library
124 E 40th Street   212-808-4980
New York, NY 10016-1798   Fax: 212-808-4983
                                     e-mail: info@filmakers.com
                                     www.filmakers.com

Peter Wegner was a professor at Brown University when he recveived an award in London and was hit by a bus there. The film follows the challenges and decisions faced by his family, in dealing with the serious brain injuries sustained. Comatose, brain surgery, how can a person decide the right path for their loved one? Winner of American Psychology Award. DVD or VHS $195, Classroom Rental $55

VHS or DVD
Sue Oscar, Co-President

4205   Unseen Injury: Minor Head Injury
Brain Injury Association
105 N Alfred Street   703-236-6000
Alexandria, VA 22314   800-444-6443
                                      Fax: 703-236-6001
Designed specifically for viewing by family members.

4206   Surviving Coma: The Journey Back
Brain Injury Association
105 N Alfred Street   703-236-6000
Alexandria, VA 22314   800-444-6443
                                      Fax: 703-236-6001

21 minutes

Web Sites

4207   Agency for Healthcare: Research Facility
                                      www.ahcpr.gov
Mission is to improve quality, safety, efficiency, and effectiveness of healthcare for all Americans.

4208   American Brain Tumor Association
                                      www.abta.org
Provides a mentorship program for new brain tumor support group leaders; a nationwide database of established support groups; the Connections pen-pal program; networking with organizations that provide services to patients and families; a resource listing of physicians offering investgative treatments.

4209   Brain Injury Association
                                      www.biausa.org
Seeking to improve the quality of life for people with brain injuries and their families through information and resource referral, legislative advocacy, prevention awareness, and professional education. BIA's mission is to create a better future through brain injury prevention, research, education and advocacy.

4210   Brain Research Institute: Medicine School University of California, Los Angeles
                                      medicine.ucsd.edu
BRI is an organized research unit.

4211   Headinjury.Com
                                      www.headinjury.com
Maintained by the Head Injury Hotline, a non-profit clearinghouse founded and operated by head injury activist. The primary goal are to empower through education, resources and support. The basic premise is that the medical system is deeply flawed and that the brain injury rehab industry is no exception. The site integrates resources from diverse organizations including support groups, rehabilitation and research sites.

4212   Healing Well
                                      www.healingwell.com
An online health resource guide to medical news, chat, information and articles, newsgroups and message boards, books, disease-related web sites, medical directories, and more for patients, friends, and family coping with disabling diseases, disorders, or chronic illnesses.

4213   Health Finder
                                      www.healthfinder.gov
Searchable, carefully developed web site offering information on over 1000 topics. Developed by the US Department of Health and Human Services, the site can be used in both English and Spanish.

4214   Healthlink USA
                                      www.healthlinkusa.com

Health information concerning treatment, cures, prevention, diagnosis, risk factors, research, support groups, email lists, personal stories and much more. Updated regularly.

4215   Helios Health
                                      www.helioshealth.com
Online resource for your health information. Detailed information about specific health topics, access to expert advice from our Medical Advisory Board, and up-to-date health news.

4216   MedicineNet
                                      www.medicinenet.com
An online resource for consumers providing easy-to-read, authoritative medical and health information.

4217   Medscape
                                      www.medscape.com
Medscape offers specialists, primary care physicians, and other health professionals the Web's most robust and integrated medical information and educational tools.

4218   Neurology Channel
                                      www.neurologychannel.com
Find clearly explained, medically accurate information regarding conditions, including an overview, symptoms, causes, diagnostic procedures and treatment options. On this site it is possible to ask questions and get information from a neurologist and connect to people who have similar health interests.

4219   Road Less Traveled
                                      www.lesstravel.org
Dedicated to survivors and families of victims of Traumatic Brain Injury.

4220   TBI Help
                                      www.tbihelp.com
Information concerning head injury.

4221   Traumatic Brain Injury
                                      community-2.webtv.net
This site is dedicated to survivors and all who wish to learn more about traumatic brain injury.

Description

4222 Hearing Impairment

Approximately 21 million Americans have some degree of hearing impairment or Deafness. This common problem affects people of all ages, and the loss can range from mild to severe.

Hearing loss is divided into four categories: conductive, sensorineural, mixed and central. Conductive hearing loss is caused by a defect in the external ear canal or middle ear, and can be helped by hearing aids, medical treatment or surgery. Sensorineural hearing loss results from damage to the inner ear and to the primary nerve that transmits sound waves to the brain. Mixed hearing loss is a combination of conductive and sensorineural defects. Central hearing loss results from impairment of brain function.

Hearing loss may be present at birth or begin later in life. Causes include infections (such as meningitis), injury, prolonged noise exposure, hereditary diseases and side effects of certain drugs. Amplification of sound with hearing aids helps almost all persons with mild-to-severe conductive or sensorineural hearing loss. Profoundly deaf persons who cannot be helped by hearing aids may benefit from a cochlear implant, a specialized device inserted into the inner ear. Children with hearing impairments may have slow or inaccurate speech development, or problems with concentration. Early diagnosis usually helps children improve their auditory ability, through the use of hearing aids, educational programs and speech therapy. Hearing loss in adults, if moderate or severe, is usually obvious to the patient family members. In young children, however, the problem is easily overlooked and the opportunity for early intervention can be lost.

National Agencies & Associations

4223 ABLEDATA
8630 Fenton Street
Silver Spring, MD 20910

301-608-8998
800-227-0216
Fax: 301-608-8958
TTY: 301-608-8912
e-mail: abledata@macrointernational.com
www.abledata.com

An information and referral service that uses computer listings and a large file system to answer requests related to assistive devices. Houses a large file system library and contacts with other sources which enables them to answer just about any question.
Katherine Belknap, Project Director
Steve Lowe, Associate Project Manager/Webmaster

4224 ADARA
PO Box 480
Myersville, MD 21773

501-224-6678
Fax: 501-868-8812
TTY: 501-868-8850
e-mail: adaraorg@comcast.net
www.adara.org

Professional networking for excellence in service delivery with individuals who are deaf or hard of hearing. A partnership of national organizations, local affiliates, professional sections and individual members working together to support social services.
Tim Beatty, President
Doug H Dittfurth, Vice President

4225 Academy of Dispensing Audiologists
1020 Monarch Street
Lexington, KY 40513

866-493-5544
Fax: 859-271-0607
www.audiologist.org

Encourages audiology training programs to include pertinent aspects of hearing aid dispensing in their curriculum.
Bruce Vircks, President
Eric Hagberg, President-Elect

4226 Academy of Rehabilitative Audiology
PO Box 952
DeSoto, TX 75123

e-mail: ara@audrehab.org
www.audrehab.org

Provides professional education research and interest in programs for hearing handicapped persons.
Joseph J Montano, President

4227 Alexander Graham Bell Association for the Deaf and Hard of Hearing
3417 Volta Place NW
Washington, DC 20007

202-337-5220
Fax: 202-337-8314
TTY: 202-337-5221
e-mail: info@agbell.org
www.agbell.org

The world's oldest and largest membership organization promoting the use of spoken language by children and adults who are hearing impaired. Members include parents of children with hearing loss, adults who are deaf or hard of hearing and educators.
Alexander T Graham, Executive Director/CEO
John R Wyant, President

4228 American Academy of Audiology
11730 Plaza America Drive
Reston, VA 20190

703-790-8466
800-222-2336
Fax: 703-790-8631
e-mail: nfo@audiology.org
www.audiology.org

A professional organization of individuals dedicated to providing high quality hearing care to the public. Provides professional development education and research and provides increased public awareness of hearing disorders and audiologic services.
Cheryl Kreid Carey CAE, Executive Director
Edward A M Sullivan, Deputy Executive Director

4229 American Academy of Otolaryngology: Head
1650 Diagonal Road
Alexandria, VA 22314-3357

703-836-4444
TTY: 703-519-1585
e-mail: executiveservices@entnet.org
www.entnet.org

The missions of the AAO-HNS and its foundation are to advance the art and science of otolaryngology-head and neck surgery through state-of-the-art education, research and learning; and to unite, serve and represent the interests of its members and their families.
J Regan Thomas MD, President

4230 American Association of the Deaf-Blind
8630 Fenton Street
Silver Spring, MD 20910-3803

301-495-4403
Fax: 301-495-4404
TTY: 301-495-4402
e-mail: AADB-Info@aadb.org
www.aadb.org

Promotes better opportunities and services for deaf-blind people. The mission of this organization is to assure that a comprehensive, coordinated system of services is accessible to all deaf-blind people, enabling them to achieve their maximum potential.
600 Members
Timothy Jackson, President
Jill Gaus, Vice President

4231 American Auditory Society
19 Mantua Road
Mt. Royal, NJ 08061

856-423-3118
Fax: 856-423-3420
e-mail: aas@talley.com
www.amauditorysoc.org

Publishes Ear & Hearing and The Bulletin of the American Auditory Society.
Karen Jo Doyle MD, President

4232 American Hearing Research Foundation
8 S Michigan Avenue   312-726-9670
Chicago, IL 60603-4539   Fax: 312-726-9695
                    e-mail: sparmet@american-hearing.org
                              www.american-hearing.org
Supports medical research and education into the causes preven-
tion and cures of deafness, hearing losses and balance disorders.
Also keeps physicians and the public informed of the latest devel-
opments in hearing research and education.
Sharon Parmet, Executive Director
Sharon Parmet, Associate Director

4233 American Society for Deaf Children
800 Florida Avenue NE, #2047   717-703-0073
Washington, DC 20002-3695   800-942-2732
                                   Fax: 410-795-0965
                                   TTY: 717-334-8808
                       e-mail: asdc@deafchildren.org
                              www.deafchildren.org
A nonprofit parent-helping-parent organization promoting a positive attitude toward signing and deaf culture. Also provides support encouragement and current information about deafness to
families with deaf and hard of hearing children.
Beth S Benedict PhD, President
Joseph Finnegan, VP

4234 American Speech-Language-Hearing Association
2200 Research Boulevard   301-296-5700
Rockville, MD 20850   80- 63- 825
                                   Fax: 301-296-8580
                                   TTY: 301-296-5650
                       e-mail: actioncenter@asha.org
                                   www.asha.org
A professional and scientific organization for speech-language pathologists and audiologists concerned with communication disorders. Provides informational materials and a toll-free HELPLINE
number for consumers to inquire about speech, language or hearing disorders.
Arlene A Pietranton PhD CAE, Executive Director
Paul R Rao, President

4235 American Tinnitus Association
522 SW Fifth Avenue   503-248-9985
Portland, OR 97204-0005   800-634-8978
                                   Fax: 503-248-0024
                          e-mail: tinnitus@ata.org
                                   www.ata.org
Provides information about tinnitus and referrals to local con-
tacts/support groups nationwide. Also provides a bibliography service, funds scientific research related to tinnitus and offers
workshops to professionals. Works to promote public education.
Michael Malusevic, Chief Executive Officer
Wes Breazeale, Chief Development Officer

4236 Association of Late-Deafened Adults
8038 MacIntosh Lane   815-332-1515
Rockford, IL 61107   866-402-2532
                                   Fax: 877-907-1738
                                   TTY: 815-332-1515
                           e-mail: info@alda.org
                                   www.alda.org
Serves as a resource and information center for late-deafened
adults and works to increase public awareness of the special needs
of late-deafened adults.
Cynthia Amerman, President
Brenda Estes, President-Elect

4237 Auditory-Verbal International
1390 Chain Bridge Road   703-739-1049
McLean, VA 22101   Fax: 703-739-0395
                                   TTY: 703-739-0874
                       e-mail: audiverb@aol.com
                              www.auditory-verbal.org
Dedicated to helping children who have hearing losses learn to listen and speak. Promotes the Auditory-Verbal Therapy approach
which is based on the belief that the overwhelming majority of
these children can hear and talk by using their residual hearing
ability.
Chellie Lisenby, Executive Director
Steven R Rech, President

4238 Better Hearing Institute
1444 I Street NW   202-449-1100
Washington, DC 20005   800-327-9355
                                   Fax: 202-216-9646
                                   TTY: 703-642-0580
                       e-mail: mail@betterhearing.org
                              www.betterhearing.org
A nonprofit educational organization that implements national
public information programs on hearing loss and available medical, surgical, hearing aid and rehabilitation assistance for millions
with uncorrected hearing problems.
Sergei Kochk PhD, Executive Director
Renee La Mura, Administrative Director

4239 CAPCOM
6707 Old Dominion Drive   202-363-0535
McLean, VA 22101   800-241-2232
                                   TTY: 703-749-1876
Conducts research on the special needs of the hearing impaired including senior citizens. Presents workshops on law and the deaf
and on promoting productive working relationships for the hearing
impaired employees of agencies and corporations.

4240 Canine Assistance for the Disabled CADI
CADI
3958 Union Road   314-892-2554
Saint Louis, MO 63125   e-mail: supportdogs@MSN.com
The mission of Support Dogs Inc. is to give people with disabilities
greater independence and improve lives through the help of a support or touch dog and promote canines as partners through abilities
education.

4241 Center on Employment: Rochester Institute of Technology
National Technical Institute for the Deaf
52 Lomb Memorial Drive   505-475-6219
Rochester, NY 14623-5604   Fax: 585-475-7570
                                   TTY: 505-475-6219
                           e-mail: ntidcoe@rit.edu
                              www.rit.edu/ntid/coops/jobs
Operated by the National Technical Institute for the Deaf at Roch-
ester Institute of Technology, the NTIC Center on employment was
established to promote successful employment of RIT's deaf students and graduates.
John Macko, Director
Lorie Fidurko, Office Assistant

4242 Cochlear Implant Association
5335 Wisconsin Avenue NW   202-895-2781
Washington, DC 20015-2052   Fax: 202-895-2782
                          e-mail: CIAIinfo@cici.org
                                   www.cici.org
Provides information and support to implant users and their fami-
lies, professionals and the general public.
John McCelland, President
Lorie Singer, VP

4243 Convention of American Instructors of the Deaf
PO Box 377   817-354-8414
Bedford, TX 76095-0377   TTY: 817-354-8414
                           e-mail: caid@swbell.net
                                   www.caid.org
An organization that promotes professional development commu-
nication and information among educators of deaf individuals and
other interested people.
Helen Lovato, Office Manager

4244 Council on Education of the Deaf College of Education
College of Education
800 Florida Avenue NE   330-672-0735
Washington, DC 20002-0001   Fax: 330-672-2498
                                   TTY: 330-672-2396
                           e-mail: ced@gallaudet.edu
                    www.deafed.net/PageText.asp?hdnPageId=58
Offers information and referral services to the hearing impaired.
Dr Karen Dilka, Executive Director
Dr Carmel Collum Yarger, President

4245 Deaf Artists of America
302 Goodman Street N
Rochester, NY 14607-1148   Fax: 315-244-3690
                                  TTY: 315-224-3460
Organized to bring support and recognition to deaf and hard of
hearing artists. The goals are to publish information about deaf artists, provide cultural and educational opportunities, exhibit and
market deaf artists' work and collect and disseminate information.
Tom Willard, Executive Director

4246 Deaf REACH
3521 12th Street NE
Washington, DC 20017   202-832-6681
                              Fax: 202-832-8454
                              TTY: 202-832-6681
                              www.deaf-reach.org
Offers group homes for mentally ill adults, day programs for the
developmentally disabled deaf, referrals case management and
housing placement. Serves adults with disabilities, specifically
deaf and/or low-income.
Annette Reichman, President
Johnathan Tomar, VP

4247 Deafness Research Foundation
641 Lexington Avenue   212-328-9480
New York, NY 10022   866-454-3924
                              Fax: 212-328-9484
                              TTY: 888-435-6104
                              e-mail: info@drf.org
                              www.drf.org
The nation's largest voluntary health organization entirely committed to public awareness and support for basic and clinical research into deafness and hearing disabilities. Sponsors a broad
program of innovative research and education.
Elizabeth Thorp, President, CEO
Clifford Tallman, Principal

4248 Deafness and Communicative Disorders Branch
Department of Education
400 Maryland Ave., SW   202-205-8730
Washington, DC 20202-2736   800-872-5327
                               Fax: 202-437-0833
                               TTY: 202-205-8352
                               e-mail: annette.reichman@ed.gov
                               www.ed.gov/offices/OSERS/RSA.html
Promotes improved and expanded rehabilitation services for deaf
and hard of hearing people and individuals with speech or language
impairments.
Annette Reichman, Branch Chief

4249 Dogs for the Deaf
10175 Wheeler Road   541-826-9220
Central Point, OR 97502   Fax: 541-826-6696
                              TTY: 541-826-9220
                              TDD: 541-826-9220
                              e-mail: info@dogsforthedeaf.org
                              www.dogsforthedeaf.org
Trains ear dogs to alert deaf persons to certain sounds. Dogs are
chosen from pet adoption shelters and assigned on the basis of a
prioritized waiting list. Four to five months of training teaches
them to alert their masters to a number of sounds.
Robin Dickson, President/CEO

4250 EAR Foundation
1817 Patterson Street   615-627-2724
Nashville, TN 37203   800-545-4327
                              Fax: 615-627-2728
                              TTY: 615-627-2724
                              TDD: 615-627-2724
                              e-mail: info@earfoundation.org
                              www.earfoundation.org
A national non-profit organization committed to the goal of better
hearing and balance through public and professional education
programs including The Meniere's Network and the Young Ears
program. The Meniere's Network is a national network of patient
outreach.
Amy Nielsen, Associate Director

**4251 Hands Organization: Advocacy Network for the Deaf and
Hearing Impaired**
Advocacy Network For The Deaf And Hearing Impaired

PO Box 17755   773-978-8552
Chicago, IL 60617-0755   TTY: 773-978-8552
Advocacy for the deaf and hearing impaired; information and referrals educational events sign language summer youth camps and
newsletters.

4252 Hear Now: Starkey Hearin Foundation
The Starkey Hearing Foundation
6700 Washington Avenue S
Eden Prairie, MN 55344   866-354-3254
                              Fax: 952-828-6900
                              e-mail: shf_contact@starkey.com
                              www.sotheworldmayhear.org
Committed to making technology accessible to deaf and hard of
hearing individuals throughout the United States. Also raises
funds to provide hearing aids, cochlear implants and related ser-
vices to children and adults who have hearing losses.
Peter Lecy, President
Brady Forseth, Executive Director

4253 Hearing Education and Awareness for Rocker s
1405 Lyon Street   415-409-3277
San Francisco, CA 94115   Fax: 415-552-4296
                              TTY: 415-476-7600
                              e-mail: hear@hearnet.com
                              www.hearnet.com
Educates the public about the real dangers of hearing loss resulting
from repeated exposure to excessive noise levels.
Kathy Peck, Executive Director

4254 Helen Keller National Center for Deaf/Blind Youth and Adults
141 Middle Neck Road   516-944-8900
Sands Point, NY 11050-1299   Fax: 516-944-7302
                              TTY: 516-944-8637
                              e-mail: hkncinfo@hknc.org
                              www.hknc.org
The national center and its 10 regional offices providing diagnostic
evaluations comprehensive vocational and personal adjustment
training and job preparation and placement for people who are
deaf/blind from every state and territory.

4255 House Ear Institute
2100 W 3rd Street   213-483-4431
Los Angeles, CA 90057   800-388-8612
                              Fax: 213-483-8789
                              TTY: 213-484-2642
                              TDD: 213-484-2642
                              e-mail: info@hei.org
                              www.hei.org
A national non-profit otologic research and educational institute
that provides information on hearing and balance disorders.
John W House MD, President
James D Boswell, CEO

4256 International Hearing Dog
5901 E 89th Avenue   303-287-3277
Henderson, CO 80640   Fax: 303-287-3425
                              TTY: 303-287-3277
                              e-mail: ihdi@aol.com
                              www.ihdi.org
Trains dogs to hear for deaf persons - telephones, doorbells, babies
etc.
Valerie Foss Brugger, President

4257 International Hearing Society
16880 Middlebelt Road   734-522-7200
Livonia, MI 48154   800-521-5247
                              Fax: 734-522-0200
                              e-mail: amarkey@ihsinfo.org
                              www.ihsinfo.org
A nonprofit professional association which represents Hearing Instrument Specialists in the United States, Canada and several other
countries. The society is recognized for promoting and maintaining the highest possible standards for its members.
Allen Lowell, President
Kathleen Mennillo, Executive Director

4258 John Tracy Clinic
806 W Adams Boulevard
Los Angeles, CA 90007-2505

213-748-5481
800-522-4582
Fax: 213-749-1651
TTY: 213-747-2924
www.johntracyclinic.org

An educational facility for preschool age children who have hearing losses and their families. In addition to on-site services worldwide correspondence courses in English and Spanish are offered to parents whose children are of preschool age and are hard of hearing.
Maria E Garay, President, CEO
Jill Muhs, VP Programs

4259 National Association of the Deaf
8630 Fenton Street
Silver Spring, MD 20910-4500

301-587-1788
Fax: 301-587-1791
e-mail: nad.info@nad.org
www.nad.org

The nation's largest constituency organization safeguarding the accessibility and civil rights of 28 million deaf and hard of hearing Americans in education, employment, health care and telecommunications. A private, nonprofit organization.
Howard A Rosenblum, CEO

4260 National Association of the Deaf Law and Advocacy Center
8630 Fenton Street
Silver Spring, MD 20910-4500

301-587-1788
Fax: 301-587-1791
TTY: 301-587-1789
e-mail: NADinfo@nad.org
www.nad.org

Represents deaf and hard of hearing individuals in cases of discrimination on the basis of deafness under federal laws such as the ADA, IDEA and the Rehabilitation Act. Provides legal information about how these laws affect deaf people in jobs, education and more.
Nancy J Bloch, CEO/Ex-Officio Board Member
Rosaline H Crawford, Director-Law and Advocacy Center

4261 National Captioning Institute
3725 Concorde Parkway
Chantilly, VA 20151

703-917-7600
Fax: 703-917-9853
TTY: 703-917-7600
e-mail: jagudelo@ncicap.org
www.ncicap.org

Advocates captioned television for people who want to see, as well as hear, the dialogue of a television program. It not only enables deaf and hard-of-hearing people to understand all of a program's content but it is also beneficial for new Americans learning English.
Gene Chao, President, CEO
Marc Okrand, Director, Administration

4262 National Center for Voice and Speech: Univ ersity of Iowa
The University Of Iowa
250 Hawkins Drive
Iowa City, IA 52242

319-335-6600
Fax: 319-335-6603
e-mail: julie-ostrem@uiowa.edu
www.ncvs.org

This is a consortium of institutions focusing on voice and speech disorders. The members of this consortium are the University of Iowa, the Denver Center for Performing Arts, the University of Wisconsin-Madison and the University of Utah.
Eric Hunter, Deputy Executive Director
Ingo Titze PhD, Executive Director

4263 National Dissemination Center for Children
1825 Connecticut Avenue NW
Washington, DC 20009

202-884-8200
800-695-0285
Fax: 202-884-8441
TTY: 202-884-8200
e-mail: nichcy@aed.org
www.nichcy.org

Publishes free fact filled newsletters. Arranges workshops. Advises parents on the laws entitling children with disabilities to special education and other services.
Dr Suzanne Ripley, Executive Director
Stephen D Luke, Director of Research

4264 National Family Association for Deaf-Blind
141 Middle Neck Road
Sands Point, NY 11050

800-225-0411
Fax: 516-883-9060
e-mail: NFADB@aol.com
www.nfadb.org

NFADB advocates for all persons who are deaf-blind of any chronological age and cognitive ability, supports national policy to benefit people who are deaf-blind, encourages the founding and strengthening of family organizations in each state and shares information.
Linda Syler, President

4265 National Fraternal Society of the Deaf
1118 S 6th Street
Springfield, IL 62703

217-289-7429
Fax: 217-789-7489
TTY: 217-789-7438
e-mail: thefrat@nfsd.com
www.nfsd.com

This organization is comprised of over 80 divisions across the country that work in the area of life insurance and advocacy for deaf people.
Al Van Nevel, Grand President

4266 National Information Clearinghouse on Children Who are Deaf-Blind
Teaching Research
345 N Monmouth Avenue
Monmouth, OR 97361

800-438-9376
Fax: 503-838-8150
TTY: 800-854-7013
e-mail: info@nationaldb.org
www.nationaldb.org

Collects organizes and disseminates information related to children and youth who are deaf-blind and connects consumers of deaf-blind information to sources of information about deaf-blindness assistive technology and deaf-blind people.
John Reiman PhD, Associate Research Professor
Kathy McNulty

4267 National Institute on Deafness and other Communication Disorders
National Institutes Of Heath
31 Center Drive
Bethesda, MD 20892-2320

301-496-7243
800-241-1044
Fax: 301-402-0018
TTY: 800-241-1055
e-mail: nidcdinfo@nidcd.nih.gov
www.nidcd.nih.gov

A national resources center for information about hearing, balance, smell, taste, voice, speech and language.
James Battey Jr MD PhD, Director
Marin Allen PhD, Chief Office of Health Communication

4268 National Organization for Hearing Research
225 Haverford Avenue
Narberth, PA 19072

610-664-3135
Fax: 610-668-1428
TTY: 610-664-3135
e-mail: info@nohrfoundation.org
www.nohrfoundation.org

This organization is a nonprofit private foundation seeking to fund exceptional researchers with $5 000 seed money grants.

4269 Rainbow Alliance of the Deaf
309 Millside Drive
Columbus, OH 43230

e-mail: president@rad.org
www.rad.org

A national organization serving the deaf gay and lesbian community. Represents approximately 24 chapters throughout the United States Canada and Europe.
Larry Pike, President
Steven Schumacher, Secretary

4270 Registry of Interpreters for the Deaf
333 Commerce Street
Alexandria, VA 22314

703-838-0030
Fax: 703-838-0454
TTY: 703-838-0459
e-mail: 72620.3143@compuserve.com
www.RID.org

A membership organization with almost 4 000 members including professional interpreters and translators persons with deafness or hearing impairments and professionals in related fields.
Clay Nettles, Executive Director
Cheryl Moose, President/Board of Directors

4271　Self-Help for Hard of Hearing People
7910 Woodmont Avenue　　　　　301-657-2248
Bethesda, MD 20814-3079　　　　Fax: 301-913-9413
　　　　　　　　　　　　　　TTY: 301-657-2248
　　　　　　　　　　　e-mail: info@hearingloss.org
　　　　　　　　　　　　　　www.hearingloss.org
Promotes awareness and information about hearing loss communication assistive devices and alternative communication skills through publications exhibits and presentations.
Pete Frackler, President
Deb Charlea Baker, Vice President

4272　Society of Hearing Impaired Physicians
1999 Mowry Avenue　　　　　　510-797-2939
Fremont, CA 94538-1622　　　　Fax: 510-797-0168
　　　　　　　　　　　e-mail: fphship@aol.com
This Society aids and assists physicians medical students and prospective medical students whose hearing impairment may necessitate different tools and/or approaches to medical practice and training.

4273　Telecommunications for the Deaf
8630 Fenton Street　　　　　　301-589-3786
Silver Spring, MD 20910　　　　Fax: 301-589-3797
　　　　　　　　　　　　　　TTY: 301-589-3006
　　　　　　　　　　　e-mail: info@tdi-online.org
　　　　　　　　　　　　　　www.tdi-online.org
A nonprofit consumer advocacy organization promoting full visual and other access to information and telecommunications for people who are deaf, hard of hearing, deaf-blind and speech impaired.
Claude Stout, Executive Director
Scott Recht, Business Manager

4274　Tripod
1727 W Burbank Boulevard　　　818-972-2080
Burbank, CA 91506　　　　　　Fax: 818-972-2090
　　　　　　　　　　　　　　TTY: 818-972-2080
　　　　　　　　　　　e-mail: info@tripod.org
　　　　　　　　　　　　　　www.tripod.org
TRIPOD is a nonprofit organization dedicated to providing support and services for deaf and hard of hearing children and their families. TRIPOD offers model local educational programs, Montessori, bilingual parent, infant, toddler and preschool programs.

4275　USA Deaf Sports Federation
PO Box 910338　　　　　　　605-367-5760
Lexington, KY 40591-0338　　　Fax: 605-782-8441
　　　　　　　　　　　　　　TTY: 605-367-5761
　　　　　　　　e-mail: HomeOffice@usdeafsports.org
　　　　　　　　　　　　　　www.usdeafsports.org
A governing body for all deaf sports and recreation in the United States.
Lawrence R Fleischer, President
Robert C Steele, VP of Financial Affairs

State Agencies & Associations

Alabama

4276　Alabama Association of the Deaf
1002 Tomahawk Drive
Talladega, AL 35160
　　　　　　　　　　　　　　Fax: 256-362-1495
　　　　　　　　　　　　　　TTY: 256-362-1415
　　　　　　　e-mail: kochie.matt@aidb.state.al.us
　　　　　　　　　　　　　　www.aldeaf.org

Mike Lozynsky, President
Ricky Clemons, VP

Arizona

4277　Arizona Association of the Deaf
5025 N Central Avenue
Phoenix, AZ 85012
　　　　　　　　　　　e-mail: tposedly@aol.com
　　　　　　　　　　　　　　www.azadinc.org
This organization shall be organized and operated exclusively to promote the welfare of deaf and hard of hearing residents of the state of Arizona in education, economic, security, social equality, and just rights and privileges as citizens.
James Oster, President
Tom Buell, Vice President

Arkansas

4278　Arkansas Association of the Deaf
26 Corporate Hill Drive
Little Rock, AR 72205
　　　　　　　　　　　e-mail: president@arkad.org
　　　　　　　　　　　　　　www.arkad.org
The mission of the Arkansas Association of the Deaf is to promote the educational, economic, and social welfare of Arkansans who are deaf or hard of hearing.
Holly Ketchum, President
Tommy Walker, Trustee

District of Columbia

4279　Shiloh Senior Center for the Hearing Impaired
913 P Street NW　　　　　　　202-232-1425
Washington, DC 20001　　　　TTY: 202-667-9779
Senior programs, sponsored by the DC Office on Aging in co-ordination with grantee: Shiloh Baptist Church serving the entire Metro Washington area's deaf and hard-of-hearing senior citizens.

Florida

4280　Florida Association of the Deaf
7852 Mansfield Hollow Rd.
Delray Beach, FL 33446
　　　　　　　　　　　e-mail: alange@fadcentral.org
　　　　　　　　　　　　　　www.fadcentral.org
The mission of the Florida Association of the Deaf is to promote, protect, and preserve the rights and quality of life of Deaf and hard of hearing individuals in the state of Florida.
June McMahon, President
Lissette Molina, Vice President

4281　Goodwill Industries-Suncoast
Goodwill Industries-Suncoast
10596 Gandy Boulevard　　　　727-523-1512
St. Petersburg, FL 33702　　　888-279-1988
　　　　　　　　　　　　　　Fax: 727-563-9300
　　　　　e-mail: gw.marketing@goodwill-suncoast.com
　　　　　　　　　　　　　www.goodwill-suncoast.org
A nonprofit community based organization whose purpose is to improve the quality of life for people who are disabled, disadvantaged and/or aged. This mission is accomplished through a staff of over 1,200 employees providing independent living skills, affordable housing, career assessment and planning, job skills, training, placement, and job retention assistance with useful employment. Annually, Goodwill Industries-Suncoast serves over 30,000 people in Citrus, Hernando, Levy, Marion and more.
R Lee Waits, President/Chief Executive Officer
Martin W Gladysz, Chair

Georgia

4282　Georgia Association of the Deaf
PO Box 1616
Stockbridge, GA 30281-1616　e-mail: turqcat9992000@yahoo.com
　　　　　　　　　　　　　　www.gadeaf.org

Ray Williams, President
Sandra Dukes, Vice President

Illinois

4283 Illinois Association of the Deaf
PO Box 1275   773-237-1877
Oak Park, IL 60304   Fax: 847-740-2319
                                           TTY: 847-740-2319
                                        e-mail: info@iadeaf.org
                                               www.iadeaf.org

The Illinois Association of the Deaf is a non-profit, political, educational, social economic, welfare of the deaf, and cultural organization made up of deaf, hard of hearing, and hearing members.
Sara Bianco, President
Marietta Coufal, Vice-President

Kansas

4284 Kansas Association of the Deaf
PO Box 10085   785-273-0612
Olathe, KS 66051   Fax: 785-273-9063
                                       e-mail: legalnetwk@aol.com
                                             www.deafkansas.org

The mission of the Kansas Association of the Deaf a state-wide, non-profit organization is to assure that an extensive, organized system of services is accessible to all deaf or hard of hearing people in Kansas.
Ann Cooper, President
Shane Dundas, Vice-President

Kentucky

4285 Kentucky Association of the Deaf
1707 Richmond Drive
Louisville, KY 40205-1407   Fax: 606-272-7747
                                           TTY: 606-223-3999
                                    e-mail: j.k.martin@insightbb.com
                                               www.kydeaf.org

The mission of the Kentucky Association of the Deaf is to advocate for the deaf and hard of hearing in Kentucky by promoting equality, accessibility, and quality of life through employment, services, education and welfare.
Rick Pittman, Board of Director
J Kevin Martin, President

Louisiana

4286 Louisiana Association of the Deaf
3112 Valley Creek Drive   225-923-1266
Baton Rouge, LA 70808   Fax: 225-923-1235
                                           TTY: 225 923-1266
                                      e-mail: kathylad@lad1908.org
                                              www.lad1908.org

Randall Pippins, President
Edward Wood, VP

Massachusetts

4287 Massachusetts State Association of the Deaf
PO Box 276   781-388-9114
Reading, MA 01867   Fax: 781-388-9015
                                           TTY: 781-388-9115
                                      e-mail: MSADeaf@aol.com
                                                www.msad.org

The Massachusetts State Association of the Deaf is a statewide nonprofit organization serving the estimated 350 000 deaf and hard of hearing Massachusetts citizens and their families.
Justine Barros, President
Michelle Donatello, Vice President

Michigan

4288 Michigan Deaf Association
49063 Churchill St
Mattawan, MI 49071   Fax: 586-775-0906
                                       e-mail: dimckitty@aol.com
                                               www.mideaf.org

MDA is a non-profit, tax exempt organization with a mission to help improve the lives of Deaf and Hard of Heating citizens of Michigan. MDA is affiliated with he National Association of the

Deaf whose mission is to promote, protect, and preserve the rights of the deaf and hearing impaired communities.
Scott Pott, President

New York

4289 League for the Hard of Hearing
50 Broadway   917-305-7700
New York, NY 10004   Fax: 917-305-7888
                                           TTY: 917-305-7999
                                         e-mail: inf@lhh.org
                                                 www.lhh.org

A private not-for-profit rehabilitation agency for infants, children and adults who are hard of hearing and deaf. The League's mission is to improve the quality of life for people with all degrees of hearing loss.
Laurie Hanin, Executive Director
Anita Stein-Meyers, Assistant Director Audiology

North Carolina

4290 North Carolina Association of the Deaf
1200 Revolution Mill Drive   919-773-2974
Greensboro, NC 27405   Fax: 919-834-0127
                                       e-mail: ncadeaf@gmail.com
                                               www.ncadeaf.org

Frank Griffin, President

North Dakota

4291 North Dakota Association of the Deaf
1115 11th Avenue North
Fargo, ND 58102   e-mail: rolewitz @ hotmail.com
                                               www.nddeaf.org

The North Dakota Association of the Deaf is actively involved in issues affecting Deaf citizens in North Dakota.
Michele Rolewitz, President
Jeremy Sebelius, Secretary

Oklahoma

4292 Oklahoma Association of the Deaf
2737 Sunnybrook Lane
Enid, OK 73703   www.ok-oad.org

The purpose of Oklahoma Association of the Deaf is to promote the interests of the deaf and to advance the social, educational, cultural and economic well-being of the deaf.
Glenna Cooper, President

Oregon

4293 Oregon Association of the Deaf
999 Locust Street NE
Salem, OR 97301   e-mail: contact@deaforegon.com
                                            www.deaforegon.com

The Oregon Association of the Deaf is a non-profit organization working toward a better life for the deaf. Their mission is to create an opportunity for the Deaf of Oregon to join together in planning, devising, conducting and participating in activities.
Daniel Sloan, Committee
Wendy Stanley, Committee

Rhode Island

4294 Rhode Island Association of the Deaf
PO Box 40853
Providence, RI 02940   e-mail: CwFuller@aol.com
                                     http://riadeaf.blogspot.com/

Jeannie Valdez, President

Texas

4295 Texas Association of the Deaf
PO Box 1982
Manchaca, TX 78652-3570   e-mail: steve@deaftexas.org
                                              www.deaftexas.org

Texas Association of the Deaf is an organization for persons who are deaf or hard of hearing. It is a membership organization to provide information and education including surveys and studies to

bring the viewpoint on various issues affecting the lives of the deaf and hearing impaired.
Steve C Baldwin, President
Chris Kearney, VP

Virginia

4296   Virginia Association of the Deaf
5251 College Drive
Dublin, VA 24084   757-587-9555
                                    Fax: 757-461-5376
                                    TTY: 757-461-7527
                        e-mail: rbavister@comcast.net
                                    www.vad.org

Rachel Bavister, President
LaDonna Larsen, VP

Wisconsin

4297   Wisconsin Association of the Deaf
519 Heatherstone Ridge
Sun Prairie, WI 53590-4230   608-825-9791
                                    TTY: 414-607-3297
                        e-mail: wad@wi-deaf.org
                                    www.wi-deaf.org
The mission of the Wisconsin Association of the Deaf is to ensure that a comprehensive and coordinated system of resources is accessible to Wisconsin people who are deaf or hard of hearing, enabling them to achieve their maximum potential.
Jerrod Keim, President
Jeffrey Cucinotta, Vice President

Wyoming

4298   Deaf Association of Wyoming
PO Box 20107
Cheyenne, WY 82003   307-635-1125
                    e-mail: president@dawyoming.org
                                    www.dawyoming.org
The Deaf Association of Wyoming is a state non-profit organizations; which is associated with the Association of the Deaf. Membership is open to all deaf persons, parents of deaf children, interpreters, professionals who work with deaf and all interested parties.
Heather Parsons, President
Bill Bitner, VP

Libraries & Resource Centers

4299   Alexander Graham Bell Association for the Deaf and Hard of Hearing
3417 Volta Place NW
Washington, DC 20007-2737   202-337-5220
                                    Fax: 202-337-8314
                                    TTY: 202-337-5221
                            e-mail: info@agbell.org
                                    www.agbell.org
Contains one of the world's largest historical collections of publications, documents and information on deafness. In addition to the main collection, which includes books, periodicals and indexed clipping files dating from the turn of the century, the library also houses a significant archival collection dealing with the history of deafness since the 16th century.
Todd Houston, PhD, Executive Director/CEO
Jessica Ripper, Senior Dir Marketing/Communications

4300   Captioned Films/Videos
National Association of the Deaf
8630 Fenton Street
Silver Spring, MD 20910-4500   301-587-1788
                                    Fax: 301-587-1791
                                    TTY: 301-587-1789
                                    www.nad.org
The mission of the National Association of the Deaf is to promote,protect,and preserve the rights and quality of life of eaf and hard of hearing individuals in the United States of America.
Bill Stark, Project Director
Donna Morris, Publications Manager

4301   Captioned Media Program
National Association of the Deaf

8630 Fenton Street   301-587-1788
Spartanburgng, SC 29307-4500   Fax: 301-587-1791
                                    TTY: 301-587-1789
                                    www.nad.org
Free loans of educational and entertainment captioned films and videos for deaf and hard of hearing people.
Bill Stark, Project Director
Donna Morris, Publications Manager

4302   Friends of Libraries for Deaf Action USA
2930 Craiglawn Road
Silver Spring, MD 20904-1816   202-727-2255
                                    Fax: 301-572-5168
                                    TTY: 301-572-5168
                            e-mail: folda86@aol.com
                                    http://www.folda.net/
Library services for people with disabilities.
Alice L Hagemeyer, President

4303   Wallace Memorial Library
Rochester Institute of Technology
90 Lomb Memorial Drive
Rochester, NY 14623   585-475-2562
                                    www.rit.edu
Information on physical disabilities and deafness.
Chandra McKenzie, Assistant Provost/Director

District of Columbia

4304   Library Services to the Deaf Community
District of Columbia Public Library
901 G Street NW   202-727-2145
Washington, DC 20001   TTY: 202-727-2255
                    e-mail: library_deaf_dc@yahoo.com
                                    www.dclibrary.org
Assures that the deaf community is aware of existing library and information services by the District of Columbia Public Library; promotes public awareness about the deaf community, deaf history and culture, American Sign Language, and assistive technology for people with hearing loss.
John W Hill Jr, President
Bonnie R Cohen, VP

Research Centers

4305   Boys Town National Research Hospital
555 N 30th Street
Omaha, NE 68131   402-498-6511
                                    800-320-1171
                                    Fax: 402-498-6331
                                    TTY: 800 320-1171
                                    www.boystownhospital.org
An internationally recognized center for state-of-the-art research diagnosis treatment of patients with ear diseases hearing and balance disorders cleft lip and palate and speech/language problems. Also includes programs such as Parent/Child Workshops Center for Childhood Deafness Register for Heredity Hearing Loss Center for Hearing research Center for Abused Handicapped and summer programs for gifted deaf teens and college students.
Patrick E Brookhouser MD, Executive VP
Walt Jestead PhD, Director of Research

4306   Center for Hearing Loss in Children Boystown National Research Hospital
Boystown National Research Hospital
555 N 30th Street   402-498-6511
Omaha, NE 68131-2136   800-282-6657
                                    Fax: 402-498-6331
                                    TTY: 800 320-1171
                            e-mail: chilic@boystown.org
                                    www.boystown.org
The Center for Hearing Loss in Children unites professionals from a variety of disciplines to focus on research training information dissemination and continuing education in the area of childhood deafness.
Patrick Brookhouser, Director
Walt Jestead PhD, Director of Research

4307   Central Institute for the Deaf
825 S Taylor Avenue   314-977-0132
Saint Louis, MO 63110-1502   877-444-4574
                                                  Fax: 314-977-0023
                                                  TTY: 314-977-0037
                                            e-mail: rfeder@cid.edu
                                                       www.cid.edu
Central Institute for the Deaf is a private nonprofit auditory-oral
school for children who have hearing impairments. We teach chil-
dren with hearing loss birth-12 to listen talk and succeed in the
mainstream.
Robin Feder MS CFRE, Executive Director
Christine Cl MAEd CED, Joanne Parrish Knight Family Center Coor

**4308   City University of New York Center for Research in Speech and
Hearing**
365 Fifth Avenue   212-817-7000
New York, NY 10016-4309   877-428-6942
                                                  Fax: 212-817-1537
                                       e-mail: strangepin@aol.com
                                                   www.gc.cuny.edu
Programmable research of digital and auditory hearing aids and
sensory aids for the speech and hearing impaired person.
Dr. William Kelly, President
Marilyn Marzolf, Chief of Staff

4309   Civitan International Research Center
1530 3rd Avenue S   205-934-8900
Birmingham, AL 35294-0001   800-822-2472
                                                  Fax: 205-975-6330
                                                  www.circ.uab.edu
Studies of deaf children.
Dr Harald Sontheimer, Director
Dr Alan Percy, Medical Director

4310   Cleveland Hearing and Speech Center
11635 Euclid Avenue   216-231-0787
Cleveland, OH 44106-4319   Fax: 216-231-2135
                                                  TTY: 216-231-5266
                                      e-mail: webmaster@chsc.org
                                                      www.chsc.org
Offers research and studies into speech language and hearing dis-
orders.
Bernard P Henri PhD, Executive Director
Hilary F Beatrez, Director Finance

4311   David T Siegel Institute for Communicative Disorders
Humana Hospital-Michael Reese
3033 S Cottage Grove Avenue   773-791-2900
Chicago, IL 60616-3346   Fax: 773-791-4014
Conducts behavioral research on language development and sign
language for the deaf.
Edward Applebaum, Chief Service

4312   Eaton-Peabody Laboratory of Auditory Physiology
Massachusetts Eye & Ear Institute
243 Charles Street   617-573-7900
Boston, MA 02114-3002   Fax: 617-720-4408
                                         research.meei.harvard.edu/EPL
Auditory system and auditory information processing including
ear-brain interactions in normal and pathologic hearing.
John Fernandez, President, CEO
Thane Benson, Consultant

4313   Gallaudet University Cued Speech Team
800 Florida Avenue NE   202-651-5000
Washington, DC 20002-3660   866-637-0102
                                                  Fax: 202-651-5508
                                                  TTY: 202-651-5005
                                  e-mail: publicrelations@gallaudet.edu
                                                   www.gallaudet.edu
Transmission of spoken languages are researched.
Dr T Allen Hurwitz, President
Deborah DeStefano, Special Assistant to the President

4314   Gallaudet University: Center for Auditory and Speech Sciences
800 Florida Avenue NE   202-651-5000
Washington, DC 20002-3660   866-637-0102
                                                  Fax: 202-651-5295
                                                  TTY: 202-651-5005
                                                   www.gallaudet.edu
Develops new hearing tests that use speech sounds to measure
hearing loss.
Dr T Allen Hurwitz, President
Deborah DeStefano, Special Assistant to the President

4315   Hear Center
301 E Del Mar Boulevard   626-796-2016
Pasadena, CA 91101   Fax: 626-796-2320
                                         e-mail: info@hearcenter.org
                                                   www.hearcenter.org
Auditory and verbal program designed to help hearing impaired
children infants and adults lead normal and productive lives. Seeks
to develop auditory techniques to aid people who have communication problems due to deafness.
Josephine Wilson, Executive Director

4316   Houston Ear Research Foundation
7737 SW Freeway   713-771-9966
Houston, TX 77074-1867   800-843-0807
                                                  Fax: 713-771-0546
                                                  TTY: 800-843-0807
                                    e-mail: info@houstoncochlear.org
                                               www.houstoncochlear.org
Aims to improve health care and education for deaf and hearing-impaired children.

4317   Loyola University of Children: Parmly Hearing Institute
1032 W Sheridan Road   773-274-3000
Chicago, IL 60666   Fax: 773-508-2719
                                           e-mail: rfay@luc.edu
                                                       www.luc.edu
Engage in the comparative study of sensory systems including
hearing vision speech perception vestibular function and the spe-
cial senses of the lateral-line organ and electroreception in fish.
Richard Fay PhD, Director
Dr William Yost, Professor of Psychology

**4318   Memphis State University Center for the Communicatively
Impaired**
Memphis State University
101 Wilder Tower   901-678-2111
Memphis, TN 38152-3520   800-669-2678
                                                  Fax: 901-251-82
                                                   www.memphis.edu/ausp
Offers research into hearing loss and deafness as well as speech im-
pairments.
Shirley Raines, President
Walt Manning, Associate Director

4319   Northern Illinois University Research and Training Center
1425 W Lincoln Highway   815-753-0446
DeKalb, IL 60115-2825   800-892-3050
                                                  Fax: 815-753-6520
                                                       www.niu.edu
Conducts research resource development and training/technical
assistance projects geared toward enhancing the employment independent living and quality of life outcomes for traditionally
underserved people who are deaf.
Sue E Ouellette PhD, Project Director

4320   Ohio State University Otological Research Laboratories
410 W 10th Avenue   614-293-8103
Columbus, OH 43210   800-293-5123
                                                  Fax: 614-293-5506
                                               www.medicalcenter.osu.edu
Clinical and basic research in otology.
Steven G Gabbe MD, CEO

**4321   Ohio University Therapy Associates: Hearing, Speech and
Language Clinic**
W218 Grover Center   740-593-1000
Athens, OH 45701   Fax: 740-593-0287
                                        e-mail: webteam@ohio.edu
                                              www.ohio.edu/hearingspeech

Focuses on hearing and speech impairments.
Brooke Hallowell, Director
Davida Parsons, Clinical Director

4322   Oregon Health Sciences University Oregon Hearing Research Center Tinnitus Clinic
3181 S W Sam Jackson Park Road   503-494-8311
Portland, OR 97239-3098   Fax: 503-945-5656
      TTY: 503-494-0910
      e-mail: ohrc@ohsu.edu
      www.ohsu.edu/ohrc/tinnitusclinic
The first medical clinic in the world established exclusively for the treatment of chronic tinnitus. During the last 25 years we have successfully treated more than 7 000 patients with severe tinnitus. The Clinic also treats patients with hyperacusis (hypersensitivity to sounds).
William H Martin PhD, Director
John V Brigande, Faculty Member

4323   Regional Resource Center on Deafness Western Oregon State College
Western Oregon State College
345 N Monmouth Avenue   503-838-8000
Monmouth, OR 97361   877-877-1593
      TTY: 503-838-8000
      e-mail: wolfgram@wou.edu
      www.wou.edu
Improve the employment and independent living status of deaf and hard-of-hearing people by increasing the number of rehabilitation professionals and their community partners nationwide who have the necessary knowledge and communication skills to serve this population.
Dr. John P Minahan, President
Cheryl Davis, Director

4324   Rehabilitation Engineering Center for Technological Aids for the Deaf
Lexington Center
800 Florida Avenue NE   202-651-5335
Washington, DC 20002   Fax: 202-651-5324
      e-mail: info@hearingresearch.org
      www.hearingresearch.org
A federally funded center that conducts research into hearing aid technology and alternate technologies.
Matthew H Bakke Ph D, Director
Arlene C Neuman Ph D, Director

4325   Research and Training Center for Persons Who are Deaf or Hard of Hearing
University of Arkansas
26 Corporate Hill Drive   501-686-9691
Little Rock, AR 72205-3822   Fax: 501-686-9698
      TTY: 501-686-9691
      e-mail: dwatson@uark.edu
      www.uark.edu/depts/rehabres
Rehabilitation of deaf and hearing impaired individuals.
Douglas Watson, Director
Glenn B Anderson, Professor Director of Training

4326   Rochester Institute of Technology: Natn'l Technical Institute for the Deaf
Lyndon Baines Johnson Building
52 Lomb Memorial Drive   585-475-6400
Rochester, NY 14623   Fax: 585-475-5978
      TTY: 585-475-6400
      e-mail: ntidmc@rit.edu
      www.ntid.rit.edu
Provides technical and professional education and training for deaf students.
Steve Nolan, Director
Gerard Buckley, President

4327   Scottish Rite Center for Childhood Language Disorders
2800 - 16th Street NW   202-232-8155
Washington, DC 20009-3602   Fax: 209-483-8169
      dcsr.org

Association offering speech-language evaluations and treatment hearing screening and consultation and referrals to children ages birth to 18 years with hearing or speech disorders.
Ronald A Seale, Sovereign Grand Commander/Supreme Counci
Leonard Proden, Sovereign Grand Inspector General

4328   Speech Simulation Research Foundation
PO Box 824   757-442-2755
Nassawadox, VA 23413-0824
Focuses on hearing and speech disorders.
Monte Penney, Director

4329   State University College at Fredonia Youngerman Clinic
280 Central Avenue   716-673-3111
Fredonia, NY 14063   Fax: 716-673-3332
      e-mail: Business.School@fredonia.edu
      www.fredonia.edu
Studies communication disorders including hearing and speech.
Dennis L Hefner, President
Denise Szalkowski, Assistant to the President

4330   State University College at Plattsburgh Auditory Research Laboratory
101 Broad Street
Plattsburgh, NY 12901-2170   518-564-2000
      www.plattsburgh.edu
Roger Hamernik, Professor of Biological Sciences
Delbert Hart, Lecturer of Computer Science

4331   Syracuse University Institute for Sensory Research
Syracuse University
621 Skytop Road   315-443-4164
Syracuse, NY 13244-1   Fax: 315-443-1184
      e-mail: rlsmith@syr.edu
      www.isr.syr.edu
Sensory processing and hearing disorders.
Robert Smith, Director

4332   Temple University Speech and Hearing Science Laboratories
1801 N Broad Street
Philadelphia, PA 19122   215-204-7000
      www.temple.edu
Speech and hearing studies.
Ann Weaver Hart, President
William T Bergan, Vice President

4333   Temple University: Section of Auditory Research
1801 N Broad Street   215-204-7000
Philadelphia, PA 19140   Fax: 215-707-6417
      www.temple.edu
Wasyl Szerem MD, Residency Program Director
William T Bergan, Vice President

4334   Trace Center University of Wisconsin: Madison
University of Wisconsin: Madison
1550 Engineering Drive   608-262-6966
Madison, WI 53706-2274   Fax: 608-262-8848
      TTY: 608-263-5408
      e-mail: info@trace.wisc.edu
      trace.wisc.edu
Research and development center working with communication control and computer access technologies for people with disabilities.
Peter Borden, Communication Director
Gregg Vanderheiden, Center Director

4335   University of Alabama Speech and Hearing Center
5721 USA Drive N   251-445-9378
Mobile, AL 36688-2   Fax: 251- 44- 937
      e-mail: sh-cntr@jaguar1.usouthal.edu
      www.southalabama.edu/speechandhearing
Providing undergraduate master's and doctoral programs that challenge the student to achieve the highest standards of academic learning scientific inquiry and clinical excellence.
Robert E Moore, Chair
Elizabeth M Adams, Assistant Professor of Audiology

4336 University of Chicago: Temporal Bone Laboratory for Ear Research
5841 S Maryland Avenue
Chicago, IL 60637-1463
773-702-1000
Fax: 773-702-6809
www.uchospitals.edu
Focuses on hearing impairments and deafness research.
Dr Raul Hinojasa, Director

4337 University of Maine: Conley Speech and Hearing Center
5724 Dunn Hall
Orono, ME 04469-5724
207-581-2006
Fax: 207-581-2060
e-mail: mboyd@maine.edu
www.umaine.edu/comscidis
Speech disorders of adults and children including hearing impairments and deafness.
Judy Stickles, Clinic Director
Amy Engler Booth, Audiologist

4338 University of Michigan Communicative Disorders Clinic
412 Maynard Street
Ann Arbor, MI 48109-2054
734-764-1817
Fax: 734-764-7084
e-mail: kkellogg@chartermi.net
www.umich.edu/comdis
Focuses on communicative disorders including hearing impairments and speech disorders.
Mary Sue Coleman, President
Joerg Lahann, Assistant Professor of Biomedical Engine

4339 University of Michigan: Kresge Hearing Research Institute
1150 W Medical Center Drive
Ann Arbor, MI 48109-0500
734-764-8110
Fax: 734-764-0014
TTY: 734-764-8110
e-mail: josef@umich.edu
www.khri.med.umich.edu
Focuses on hearing and auditory disorders.
Josef M Miller, Director
Sue Kelch, Research Administrator

4340 University of Nebraska: Lincoln Barkley Memorial Center
1400 R Street
Lincoln, NE 68588
402-472-7211
Fax: 402-472-7697
e-mail: jbernthal1@unl.edu
www.unl.edu
Focuses on hearing impairments and deaf research.
Harvey Perlman, Chancellor
Marjorie Kostelnik, Dean Education Human Science

4341 University of North Carolina at Chapel Hill Division of Speech & Hearing
CB 7190
Chapel Hill, NC 27599-1
919-966-1007
Fax: 919-966-0100
e-mail: jroush@med.unc.edu
www.med.unc.edu/ahs/sphs
The Division of Speech and Hearing Sciences prepares clinical practitioners in speech-language pathology and audiology to be scholars teachers and researchers in both the theoretical and applied aspects of human communication sciences and disorders.
William M Roper, Dean, CEO
Terry Magnuson, Vice Dean for Research

4342 University of Oklahoma Speech & Hearing Center
University of Oklahoma
1100 N Lindsey
Oklahoma City, OK 73104
405-271-4000
Fax: 405-713-60
www.ouhsc.edu

David L Boren, President

4343 University of Texas at Dallas Callier Center for Communication Disorders
1966 Inwood Road
Dallas, TX 75235-7205
214-905-3000
Fax: 214-905-3022
TDD: 214-905-3012
e-mail: roeser@callier.utdallas.edu
www.callier.utdallas.edu
Focuses on communication and behavioral disorders including hearing impairments and deafness research.
Tom Campbell, Executive Director
Phillip L Wilson, Head of Audiology

4344 University of Washington Department of Speech & Hearing Sciences
1417 NE 42nd Street
Seattle, WA 98105-6246
206-685-7400
Fax: 206-543-1093
e-mail: sphscadv@u.washington.edu
depts.washington.edu
Communication sciences and disorders.
Joan Hanson, Clinic Manager
Mary Wood, Assistant to the Chair

4345 University of Washington Speech and Hearing Clinic
1417 NE 42nd Street
Seattle, WA 98105-6246
206-685-7400
Fax: 206-543-1093
e-mail: shclinic@u.washington.edu
depts.washington.edu/sphsc/clinic.htm
Normal speech language and hearing processes development and disorders research.
Nancy B Alarcon, Clinic Director
Joan Hanson, Clinic Manager

4346 University of Wisconsin: Auditory Physiology Center
273 Medical Sciences Building
Madison, WI 53706
608-263-2400
www.wisc.edu
Activities include studies in hearing loss and deafness.
Dr John Brugge, Director

4347 Yeshiva University: Institute of Communication Disorders
Montefiore Medical Center
500 West 185th Street
New York, NY 10033
212-960-5400
Fax: 718-515-8235
e-mail: mfried@montefiore.org
www.yu.edu
Studies on communicative disorders including speech and hearing.
Richard M Joel, President
Josh Joseph, VP, Chief of Staff

Support Groups & Hotlines

4348 Aurora of Central New York
518 James Street
Syracuse, NY 13203-2282
315-422-7263
Fax: 315-229-46
TDD: 315-422-4792
e-mail: auroracny@auroraofcny.org
Professional counseling services helps to assist individuals and their families deal with the trauma of hearing or vision loss.
Debra Chaken, Executive Director

4349 Beginnings for Parents of Children Who are Deaf or Hard of Hearing
3714 Benson Drive
Raleigh, NC 27609
919-850-2746
800-541-4327
Fax: 919-850-2804
TTY: 919-850-2746
e-mail: raleigh@beginningssvcs.com
www.ncbegin.org/
Beginnings provides support to parents of deaf and hard-of-hearing children in an unbiased, family-centered atmosphere. In addition, Beginnings also offers impartial information on communication options, placement and educational programs, and workshops for professional personnel who work with deaf and hard-of-hearing children. Advocacy and support for young people from birth to age 21 is available.
Joni Y Alberg Ph.D, Executive Director
Christene A Tashjian, Research/Development Asst Exec Director

4350 Children of Deaf Adults
PO Box 30715
Santa Barbara, CA 93130-0715
805-682-0997
www.coda-international.org
Promotes family awareness and individual growth in hearing children of deaf parents.
Carmel Batson, President
Millie Brother, Founder

4351 Children's Rights Program
Alexander Graham Bell Association

3417 Volta Place NW
Washington, DC 20007

202-337-5220
866-337-5220
Fax: 202-337-8314
e-mail: info@agbell.org
www.agbell.org

Actively advocates for the legal rights of children with hearing impairments and for legislation to upgrade the delivery of services to children and adults who are hearing impaired.
Gerri A Hanna, Director Advocacy/Policy

4352   Dial-a-Hearing Screening Test
PO Box 1880
Media, PA 19063

610-544-7700
800-222-3277
Fax: 610-543-2802
e-mail: dahst@aol.com

Hearing help information center. Provides local phone number for Dial-a-Hearing Screening Test and hearing information.
George Biddle, Executive Director

4353   Hearing Aid Helpline
International Hearing Society (IHS)
16880 Middlebelt Road
Livonia, MI 48154

734-522-7200
800-521-5247
Fax: 734-522-0200
e-mail: chelms@ihsinfo.org
http://ihsinfo.org/IhsV2/Home/Index.cfm

Hearing Aid Helpline, a service of International Hearing Society (IHS), provides a referral service for locating qualified hearing healthcare professionals. IHS is a professional association representing Hearing Instrument Specialists worldwide engaged in the practice of testing human hearing, selecting, fitting and dispensing of hearing instruments. Founded in 1951, the Society conducts programs in competency accreditation, education, training promoting specialty-level certification.
Cindy Helms, Executive Director
Phyllis Wilson, Associate Director

4354   John Tracy Clinic on Deafness
806 W Adams Boulevard
Los Angeles, CA 90007-2599

800-522-4582
Fax: 213-749-1651
www.jpc.org

Hotline.
Barbara Hecht, President
Eska Wilson, Vice President

4355   National Health Information Center
PO Box 1133
Washington, DC 20013

310-565-4167
800-336-4797
Fax: 301-984-4256
e-mail: info@nhic.org
www.health.gov/nhic

Offers a nationwide information referral service, produces directories and resource guides.

4356   Project Eyes and Ears
1844 T Street SE
Washington, DC 20020-4635

202-889-7045
Fax: 202-889-6312

Disseminates information about resources to families and service providers, provides transition services for pre-kindergarten children who are deaf-blind and integrates children into normalized settings.
Janice Wellborn

Books

4357   A Child with Hearing Loss in Your Classroom? Don't Panic!
Alexander Graham Bell Association
3417 Volta Place NW
Washington, DC 20007-2737

202-337-5220
Fax: 202-337-8270
TTY: 202-337-5220

Designed for mainstream teachers, this booklet discusses educational needs for students with hearing impairments. It especially focuses on students' language skills and their abilities to follow directions, learn new concepts, and comprehend reading. Candid advice about getting support from professionals, implementing and mantaining an IEP, improving classroom acoustic environments and using the PATERR approach.
1993 25 pages

4358   A New Civil Right: Telecommunications Equality for Deaf and Hard of Hearing
Karen Peltz Strauss, author
Hearing Loss Association of America
7910 Woodmont Avenue
Bethesda, MD 20814-3079

301-657-2248
Fax: 301-913-9413
TTY: 301-657-2249
e-mail: info@hearingloss.org
www.hearingloss.org

This book provides a compelling picture of the challenges and the realization that FCC regulation is required for people with hearing loss to receive the functional equivalence of what everyone else takes for granted.
2006 Hardcover
Jerry Portis, Executive Director
Brenda Battat, Assistant Executive Director

4359   A Quiet World: Living with Hearing Loss
David G Myers, author
Hearing Loss Association of America
7910 Woodmont Avenue
Bethesda, MD 20814-3079

301-657-2248
Fax: 301-913-9413
TTY: 301-657-2249
e-mail: info@hearingloss.org
www.hearingloss.org

A social psychologist, teacher, and author. The Author's gradual hearing loss caused serious trouble in his career and in his relationships with loved ones as he approached 50. He tells the story of his journey from denial to acceptance to an exploration of the technologies that offer help.
2000 Hardcover
Jerry Portis, Executive Director
Brenda Battat, Assistant Executive Director

4360   ASL PAH! Deaf Students' Essays About their Language
Sign Media
4020 Blackburn Lane
Burtonsville, MD 20866-1167

301-421-0268
800-475-4756
Fax: 301-421-0270
TTY: 301-421-4460
e-mail: signmedia@aol.com
www.signmedia.com

Tape/text combination featuring student essays on the role of ASL in their lives. The tape offers additional insights from the student authors. The text is not a transcript of the tape.
1979 Paperback/Video
ISBN: 0-932130-14-3
Barabara Olmert, Director Marketing

4361   ASL in Schools: Policies and Curriculum
Gallaudet University
11030 S Langley Avenue
Chicago, IL 60628-3819

800-621-2736
Fax: 800-621-8476
TTY: 888-630-9347
www.gallaudet.edu

Conference participants questioned experts on bilingual education for deaf students and discussed policy issues faced by educators across the United States.
139 pages

4362   Academic Acceptance of ASL
Gallaudet University
11030 S Langley Avenue
Chicago, IL 60628-3819

800-621-2736
Fax: 800-621-8476
TTY: 888-630-9347
www.gallaudet.edu

This monograph presents a dozen articles that demonstrate clearly and convincingly that the study of ASL affords the same educational values and the same intellectual rewards as the study of any other foreign language.
196 pages

4363   Access for All: Integrating Deaf, Hard of Hearing and Hearing Preschoolers
Gallaudet University

11030 S Langley Avenue
Chicago, IL 60628-3819 800-621-2736
Fax: 800-621-8476
TTY: 888-630-9347
www.gallaudet.edu
Describes a model program for integrating the Deaf and hard of hearing children in early education.
150 pages Book & Video

4364 American Deaf Culture
Gallaudet University
11030 S Langley Avenue
Chicago, IL 60628-3819 800-621-2736
Fax: 800-621-8476
TTY: 888-630-9347
www.gallaudet.edu
This book presents a collection of classic articles which have been selected to provide a variety of perspectives on language and culture of deaf people in America.
132 pages

4365 American Deaf Culture: An Anthology
Sign Media
4020 Blackburn Lane 301-421-0268
Burtonsville, MD 20866-1167 800-475-4756
Fax: 301-421-0270
TTY: 301-421-4460
e-mail: signmedia@aol.com
www.signmedia.com
Features deaf and hearing authors offering their experience and perspectives on cultural values, ASL, social interaction in the Deaf community, education, folklore and more.
Paperback
ISBN: 0-932130-09-7
Barbara Olmert, Director Marketing
Sherman Wilcox, Editor

4366 American Sign Language: A Beginning Course
National Association of the Deaf
8630 Fenton Street 301-587-1788
Silver Spring, MD 20910-4500 Fax: 301-587-1791
TTY: 301-587-1789
www.nad.org
An interactive approach to teaching and learning American Sign Language, with 700 sign illustrations, each accompanied by an object drawing.
199 pages Paperback
ISBN: 0-913072-64-8
Donna Morris, Publications Manager

4367 An Invisible Condition: The Human Side of Hearing Loss
SHHH Publications
7910 Woodmont Avenue 301-657-2248
Bethesda, MD 20814-3572 Fax: 301-913-9413
Offers editorials from the SHHH Journal that have shaped the past decade of self help with their focus on the plight and hopes and the aspirations of hard of hearing people everywhere.

4368 Angels and Outcasts: An Anthology of Deaf Characters in Literature
Gallaudet University
11030 S Langley Avenue
Chicago, IL 60628-3819 800-621-2736
Fax: 800-621-8476
TTY: 888-630-9347
www.gallaudet.edu
Collection of writings by and about deaf people revealing attitudes and prejudices common to western cultures.
375 pages

4369 Approaching Equality
TJ Publishers
817 Silver Spring Avenue 301-585-4440
Silver Spring, MD 20910-4617 800-999-1168
Fax: 301-585-5930
TTY: 301-585-4441
e-mail: tjpubinc@aol.com

Written by the former chair of the Commission on the Education of the deaf, this book reviews the dramatic developments in the education of deaf children.
112 pages Softcover
ISBN: 0-932666-39-6
Angela K Thames, President
Jerald A Murphy, VP

4370 Assessment & Management of Mainstreamed Hearing-Impaired Children
Pro-Ed, Inc.
8700 Shoal Creek Boulevard 512-451-3246
Austin, TX 78757-6897 800-897-3202
Fax: 800-397-7633
e-mail: info@proedin.com
www.proedinc.com
The theoretical and practical considerations of developing appropriate programming for hearing-impaired children who are being educated in mainstream educational settings are presented in this book.
415 pages Hardcover
ISBN: 0-890794-58-8
Lindy Jordaan, Marketing Coordinator

4371 Assessment of Hearing Impaired People
Gallaudet University
11030 S Langley Avenue
Chicago, IL 60628-3819 800-621-2736
Fax: 800-621-8476
TTY: 888-630-9347
www.gallaudet.edu
This is a comprehensive review of 62 tests used by educational institutions, rehabilitation agencies, and mental health centers.
128 pages Softcover

4372 At Home Among Strangers
Gallaudet University
11030 S Langley Avenue
Chicago, IL 60628-3819 800-621-2736
Fax: 800-621-8476
TTY: 888-630-9347
www.gallaudet.edu
Details the history and culture of the deaf community.
336 pages

4373 Basic Course in Manual Communication
National Association of the Deaf
8630 Fenton Street 301-587-1788
Silver Spring, MD 20910-4500 Fax: 301-587-1791
TTY: 301-587-1789
www.nad.org
Over 700 signs are grouped according to shape, location, and movement. Also includes dialogues for practice.
158 pages Paperback
Donna Morris, Publications Manager

4374 Basic Sign Communication: Student Materials
National Association of the Deaf
8630 Fenton Street 301-587-1788
Silver Spring, MD 20910-4500 Fax: 301-587-1791
TTY: 301-587-1789
www.nad.org
Includes study and reference materials for all three levels of Basic Sign Communication.
232 pages Paperback
ISBN: 0-913072-56-7
Donna Morris, Publications Manager

4375 Basic Sign Communication: Vocabulary
National Association of the Deaf
8630 Fenton Street 301-587-1788
Silver Spring, MD 20910-4500 Fax: 301-587-1791
TTY: 301-587-1789
www.nad.org
Features sections on Sign Vocabulary, Numbers, and Classifiers. Contains 1000 illustrated signs, organized alphabetically by gloss for quick reference.
162 pages Paperback
ISBN: 0-913072-55-9
Donna Morris, Publications Manager

4376 Basic Vocabulary and Language Thesaurus for Hearing Impaired Children
Alexander Graham Bell Association
3417 Volta Place NW   202-337-5220
Washington, DC 20007-2737   Fax: 202-337-8270
                                   TTY: 202-337-5220
This simple thesaurus lists spontaneous vocabulary used by normally hearing children and lets patients and teachers check so that children with hearing losses have mastered these words.
1977 76 pages

4377 Basic Vocabulary: American Sign Language for Parents and Children
TJ Publishers
817 Silver Spring Avenue   301-585-4440
Silver Spring, MD 20910-4617   800-999-1168
                                   Fax: 301-585-5930
                                   TTY: 301-585-4441
                                   e-mail: tjpubinc@aol.com
Carefully selected words and signs include those families use every day. Alphabetically organized vocabulary incorporates developmental lists helpful to both deaf and hearing children and over 1,000 clear sign language illustrations.
240 pages Softcover
ISBN: 0-932666-00-0
Angela K Thames, President
Jerald A Murphy, VP

4378 Being in Touch
Gallaudet University
11030 S Langley Avenue
Chicago, IL 60628-3819   800-621-2736
                                   Fax: 800-621-8476
                                   TTY: 888-630-9347
                                   www.gallaudet.edu
Provides information on hearing and vision loss.
80 pages

4379 Best Practices in Educational Interpreting
Sign Enhancers
2625 SE Hawthorne Boulevard   503-304-4501
Portland, OR 97214-2941   Fax: 503-304-1063
                                   TTY: 503-304-4501
                                   e-mail: sign@signenhancers.com
                                   www.signenhancers.com
Specific recommendations of best practices for working in preschool through graduate school. Case studies focus on real-life situations with suggested solutions and questions for further thought.
269 pages
ISBN: 0-205263-11-9

4380 Between Friends
Beltone Electronics Corporation
4201 W Victoria Street
Chicago, IL 60646-6772   773-583-3600
                                   www.beltone.com
For hearing aid wearers: quizzes, jokes, health, recipes and financial items.
6 pages
Renee Rockoff, Editor

4381 Black and Deaf in America
TJ Publishers
817 Silver Spring Avenue   301-585-4440
Silver Spring, MD 20910-4617   800-999-1168
                                   Fax: 301-585-5930
                                   TTY: 301-585-4441
                                   e-mail: tjpubinc@aol.com
An in depth look at some of the problems of the black deaf community, including undereducation and underemployment. This book includes an important chapter on signs used in the black community and presents interviews with prominent Black deaf individuals who share their joys, fears and hope for the future.
91 pages Softcover
ISBN: 0-932666-18-3
Angela K Thames, President
Jerald A Murphy, VP

4382 Blueprint for Conversational Competence
Alexander Graham Bell Association

3417 Volta Place NW   202-337-5220
Washington, DC 20007-2737   Fax: 202-337-8270
                                   TTY: 202-337-5220
A book that develops conversational skills in children with hearing impairments.
175 pages

4383 Book of Name Signs
Gallaudet University
11030 S Langley Avenue
Chicago, IL 60628-3819   800-621-2736
                                   Fax: 800-621-8476
                                   TTY: 888-630-9347
                                   www.gallaudet.edu
This text discusses the rules for ASL name sign formulation and their appropriate uses and presents a list of over 400 name signs.
112 pages

4384 Broken Ears: Wounded Hearts
Gallaudet University
11030 S Langley Avenue
Chicago, IL 60628-3819   800-621-2736
                                   Fax: 800-621-8476
                                   TTY: 888-630-9347
                                   www.gallaudet.edu
An intimate journey into the lives of a deaf, multihandicapped child and her young hearing parents.
186 pages Hardcover

4385 CUED Speech Resource Book for Parents of Deaf Children
Alexander Graham Bell Association
3417 Volta Place NW   202-337-5220
Washington, DC 20007-2737   Fax: 202-337-8270
                                   TTY: 202-337-5220
A comprehensive book describing cued speech, getting started, your child's rights in and out of school and families expectations with special attention on siblings and peer relationships.
832 pages Hardcover

4386 Can't Your Child Hear?
Gallaudet University
11030 S Langley Avenue
Chicago, IL 60628-3819   800-621-2736
                                   Fax: 800-621-8476
                                   TTY: 888-630-9347
                                   www.gallaudet.edu
Is deafness a difference to be accepted or a defect to be corrected? This comprehensive reference will help parents, as well as educators and other professionals, recognize their options in understanding and handling a child who is deaf.
340 pages Softcover

4387 Chelsea: The Story of a Signal Dog
Gallaudet University
11030 S Langley Avenue
Chicago, IL 60628-3819   800-621-2736
                                   Fax: 800-621-8476
                                   TTY: 888-630-9347
                                   www.gallaudet.edu
A story of a young deaf couple and their dog who acts as their ears.
169 pages

4388 Choices in Deafness
Woodbine House
6510 Bells Mill Road
Bethesda, MD 20817-1636   800-843-7323
Serving as an invaluable guide to the world of deaf education, this expanded edition covers a wide variety of communication options for children with hearing impairments. By providing medical, audiological, and educational information. It also contains numerous case studies. This indispensible book is an outstanding resource for parents.
1996 212 pages
ISBN: 0-933149-09-3

4389 Chuck Baird
Gallaudet University

11030 S Langley Avenue
Chicago, IL 60628-3819   800-621-2736
                                Fax: 800-621-8476
                                TTY: 888-630-9347
                                www.gallaudet.edu

Contains 35 full-color plates of the artwork of the deaf artist.
55 pages

4390   Classroom Notetaker
Alexander Graham Bell Association
3417 Volta Place NW   202-337-5220
Washington, DC 20007-2737   Fax: 202-337-8270
                                 TTY: 202-337-5220

This detailed manual for instructors, administrators and staff note takers promotes classroom notetaking within long-term educational programs as vital for students who are deaf and hard of hearing from elementary school to college. This book will help readers to sell a notetaking program to schools and will give a good foundation for designing and implementing a notetaking program in a school or college.
1996 150 pages

4391   Closer Look: The English Program at the Model Secondary School for the Deaf
Gallaudet University
11030 S Langley Avenue
Chicago, IL 60628   800-621-2736
                                Fax: 800-621-8476
                                TTY: 888-630-9347
                                www.gallaudet.edu

Program highlighting student-centered activities using carefully selected novels and literature texts to enhance students' reading comprehension and writing abilities through interaction with real literature.
67 pages

4392   Cochlear Implant Auditory Training Guidebook
Alexander Graham Bell Association
3417 Volta Place NW   202-337-5220
Washington, DC 20007-2737   Fax: 202-337-8270
                                 TTY: 202-337-5220

This guidebook full of reproducible masters was designed for parents and professionals working with children ages four and up who have cochlear implants. It includes an easy to follow hierarchy for listening goals and a quick placement test to help you find where to start.
236 pages

4393   Cochlear Implantation for Infants and Children
Alexander Graham Bell Association
3417 Volta Place NW   202-337-5220
Washington, DC 20007-2737   Fax: 202-337-8270
                                 TTY: 202-337-5220

This comprehensive text presents the surgical, medical, audiological speech and language and habilitation aspects of cochlear implants in infants and children.
1997 263 pages

4394   Cognition, Education and Deafness
Gallaudet University
11030 S Langley Avenue
Chicago, IL 60628-3819   800-621-2736
                                Fax: 800-621-8476
                                TTY: 888-630-9347
                                www.gallaudet.edu

The work of 54 authors is gathered in this definitive collection of current research on deafness and cognition. The articles are grouped into seven sections: cognition, problem solving, thinking processes, language development, reading methodologies, measurement of potential and intervention programs.
260 pages Hardcover

4395   Communicate with Me: Conversation Skills for Deaf Students
Gallaudet University
11030 S Langley Avenue
Chicago, IL 60628-3819   800-621-2736
                                Fax: 800-621-8476
                                TTY: 888-630-9347
                                www.gallaudet.edu

Students learn how to begin and end conversations, choose appropriate topics and maintain subjects.
160 pages

4396   Communication Access for Persons with Hearing Loss
Mark Ross, author
Hearing Loss Association of America
7910 Woodmont Avenue   301-657-2248
Bethesda, MD 20814-3079   Fax: 301-913-9413
                                 TTY: 301-657-2249
                                 e-mail: info@hearingloss.org
                                 www.hearingloss.org

Communication access for persons with hearing loss covers both visual and hearing techniques devoted to persons with hearingloss, ranging from mild to profound.
Jerry Portis, Executive Director
Brenda Battat, Assistant Executive Director

4397   Communication Issues Among Deaf People
Gallaudet University
11030 S Langley Avenue
Chicago, IL 60628-3819   800-621-2736
                                Fax: 800-621-8476
                                TTY: 888-630-9347
                                www.gallaudet.edu

Monograph discussing important aspects of communication including total communication and the value of ASL.
138 pages

4398   Communication Issues Among Deaf People: Eyes, Hands and Voices
National Association of the Deaf
8630 Fenton Street   301-587-1788
Silver Spring, MD 20910-4500   Fax: 301-587-1791
                                 TTY: 301-587-1789
                                 www.nad.org

Includes over thirty relevant articles reflecting a wide range of perceptions and attitutes on communication among deaf people.
145 pages
Donna Morris, Publications Manager

4399   Communication Rules for Hard of Hearing People
Hearing Loss Association of America
7910 Woodmont Avenue   301-657-2248
Bethesda, MD 20814-3079   Fax: 301-913-9413
                                 TTY: 301-657-2249
                                 e-mail: info@hearingloss.org
                                 www.hearingloss.org

To open the world of communication to people with hearing loss through education, information, support and advocacy.
Jerry Portis, Executive Director
Brenda Battat, Assistant Executive Director

4400   Communication and Adult Hearing Loss
Alexander Graham Bell Association
3417 Volta Place NW   202-337-5220
Washington, DC 20007-2737   Fax: 202-337-8270
                                 TTY: 202-337-5220

This informative book was written for anyone who wants to communicate more effectively with a person with adult hearing loss.
1993 136 pages

4401   Comprehensive Signed English Dictionary
Harris Communications
6541 City W Parkway   612-906-1180
Eden Prairie, MN 55344-3248   Fax: 612-946-0924

Complete dictionary offers 3100 signs, including signs reflecting contemporary vocabulary.
457 pages

4402   Consumer Handbook on Dizziness and Vertigo
Dennis Poe, MD, author
Hearing Loss Association of Amercia
7910 Woodmont Avenue   301-657-2248
Bethesda, MD 20814-3079   Fax: 301-913-9413
                                 TTY: 301-657-2249
                                 e-mail: info@hearingloss.org
                                 www.hearingloss.org

Learn the differences between dizziness and vertigo.
Hardcover
ISBN: 0-966182-64-2

4403 Conversational Sign Language II: An Intermdiate Advanced Manual
Harris Communications
6541 City W Parkway
Eden Prairie, MN 55344-3248
612-906-1180
Fax: 612-946-0924
This book presents English words and their American Sign Language equivalents.
218 pages

4404 Dancing Without Music
Gallaudet University
11030 S Langley Avenue
Chicago, IL 60628-3819
800-621-2736
Fax: 800-621-8476
TTY: 888-630-9347
www.gallaudet.edu
Investigates being deaf and its social ramifications.
320 pages

4405 Deaf Children in Public Schools Placement, Context, and Consequences
Gallaudet University
11030 S Langley Avenue
Chicago, IL 60628-3819
800-621-2736
Fax: 800-621-8476
TTY: 888-630-9347
www.gallaudet.edu
Assesses the progress of three second-grade deaf students to demonstrate the importance of placement, context, and language in their development.
August 1997 250 pages
ISBN: 1-563680-62-9

4406 Deaf Culture, Our Way
Gallaudet University
11030 S Langley Avenue
Chicago, IL 60628-3819
800-621-2736
Fax: 800-621-8476
TTY: 888-630-9347
www.gallaudet.edu
A revised edition of Silence is Golden, Sometimes, this new edition contains sections on Classic Humor, Bathroom Tales, Classic Hazards and New Technology.
115 pages

4407 Deaf Empowerment, Emergence, Struggle and Rhetoric
Gallaudet University
11030 S Langley Avenue
Chicago, IL 60628-3819
800-621-2736
Fax: 800-621-8476
TTY: 888-630-9347
www.gallaudet.edu
Examines the rhetorical foundation that motivated Deaf people to work for social change during the past two centuries. Assesses the goal of a multicultural society and offers suggestions for community building through a new humanitarianism.
July 1997 192 pages Hardcover
ISBN: 1-563680-61-0

4408 Deaf Heritage: A Narrative History of Deaf America
National Association of the Deaf
8630 Fenton Street
Silver Spring, MD 20910-4500
301-587-1788
Fax: 301-587-1791
TTY: 301-587-1789
www.nad.org
In-depth history of Deaf America contains pictures, vignettes, and biographical profiles.
483 pages Paperback
Donna Morris, Publications Manager

4409 Deaf Heritage: Student Text and Workbook
National Association of the Deaf
8630 Fenton Street
Silver Spring, MD 20910-4500
301-587-1788
Fax: 301-587-1791
TTY: 301-587-1789
www.nad.org

Each chapter is followed by a vocabulary section and workbook activities including questions and follow-up activities for students.
115 pages Paperback
Donna Morris, Publications Manager

4410 Deaf History Unveiled: Interpretations from the New Scholarship
Gallaudet University
11030 S Langley Avenue
Chicago, IL 60628-3819
800-621-2736
Fax: 800-621-8476
TTY: 888-630-9347
www.gallaudet.edu
Essays written by internationally renowned deaf studies scholars.
316 pages

4411 Deaf Like Me
Gallaudet University
11030 S Langley Avenue
Chicago, IL 60628-3819
800-621-2736
Fax: 800-621-8476
TTY: 888-630-9347
www.gallaudet.edu
Written by the uncle and father of a deaf girl, this is an account of parents coming to terms with deafness.
292 pages

4412 Deaf President Now! The 1988 Revolution at Gallaudet University
Gallaudet University
11030 S Langley Avenue
Chicago, IL 60628-3819
800-621-2736
Fax: 800-621-8476
TTY: 888-630-9347
www.gallaudet.edu
This book chronicles the events leading up to the revolution in which deaf people won social change for themselves and all disabled people.
240 pages

4413 Deaf Sport: The Impact of Sports Within the Deaf Community
Gallaudet University
11030 S Langley Avenue
Chicago, IL 60628-3819
800-621-2736
Fax: 800-621-8476
TTY: 888-630-9347
www.gallaudet.edu
Describes the full ramifications of athletics for deaf people.
224 pages

4414 Deaf Students and the School-to-Work Transition
Gallaudet University
11030 S Langley Avenue
Chicago, IL 60628-3819
800-621-2736
Fax: 800-621-8476
TTY: 888-630-9347
www.gallaudet.edu
Studies severely and profoundly hearing impaired students as they leave high school and enter the work force.
278 pages

4415 Deaf Studies Curriculum Guide
Gallaudet University
11030 S Langley Avenue
Chicago, IL 60628-3819
800-621-2736
Fax: 800-621-8476
TTY: 888-630-9347
www.gallaudet.edu
Designed to help students explore the history, language and culture of deaf people.
250 pages

4416 Deaf Women: A Parade Through the Decades
Gallaudet University
11030 S Langley Avenue
Chicago, IL 60628-3819
800-621-2736
Fax: 800-621-8476
TTY: 888-630-9347
www.gallaudet.edu

A compilation of information, history, anecdotes and research that showcases many deaf women from all walks of American life.
192 pages

4417 Deaf and Hard of Hearing Individuals
Mainstream
1030 5th Street NW   202-898-1400
Washington, DC 20001-2504
Mainstreaming deaf individuals into the workplace.
12 pages

4418 Deaf in America: Voices from a Culture
Gallaudet University
11030 S Langley Avenue
Chicago, IL 60628-3819   800-621-2736
                                       Fax: 800-621-8476
                                       TTY: 888-630-9347
                                       www.gallaudet.edu
Written by authors who are themselves deaf.
134 pages

4419 Deafness and Child Development
Gallaudet University
11030 S Langley Avenue
Chicago, IL 60628-3819   800-621-2736
                                       Fax: 800-621-8476
                                       TTY: 888-630-9347
                                       www.gallaudet.edu
Provides rational, informed and balanced approaches to the effects of deafness in child development.
236 pages

4420 Deafness: 1993-2013
National Association of the Deaf
8630 Fenton Street   301-587-1788
Silver Spring, MD 20910   Fax: 301-587-1791
                                       TTY: 301-587-1789
                                       www.nad.org
Over 30 articles cover such topics as magnet schools, deaf identity, technology, multicultural education, communication, leadership, and sign language research.
Paperback
Donna Morris, Publications Manager

4421 Deafness: A Personal Account
Faber & Faber
19 Union Square W   781-721-1427
New York, NY 10003-3304   e-mail: contact@faber.co.uk
                                       www.faber.co.uk
Poet, critic and translator David Wright's enduring memoir (now with a substantial new introduction by the author) describes with humor and insight his early life, his development as a poet, and little-known history of deaf education.
202 pages

4422 Deafness: An Autobiography
Gallaudet University
11030 S Langley Avenue
Chicago, IL 60628-3819   800-621-2736
                                       Fax: 800-621-8476
                                       TTY: 888-630-9347
                                       www.gallaudet.edu/~gupress
This book is intended to explore the author's own experiences with deafness, and satisfy the curiosity about the condition of deaf people.
238 pages

4423 Deafness: Historical Perspectives
National Association of the Deaf
8630 Fenton Street   301-587-1788
Silver Spring, MD 20910   Fax: 301-587-1791
                                       TTY: 301-587-1789
                                       www.nad.org
Focuses on the history of deaf people. Topics cover a spectrum from a history of deaf theaters, to a genealogy of our first deaf families, to a conversation with a ghost.
Paperback
Donna Morris, Publications Manager

4424 Deafness: Life and Culture II
National Association of the Deaf
8630 Fenton Street   301-587-1788
Silver Spring, MD 20910   Fax: 301-587-1791
                                       TTY: 301-587-1789
                                       www.nad.org
Continues to explore the variety and diversity of the deaf experience.
133 pages Paperback
ISBN: 0-913072-79-6
Donna Morris, Publications Manager

4425 Directory of Auditory-Oral Programs
Alexander Graham Bell Association
3417 Volta Place NW   202-337-5220
Washington, DC 20007-2737   Fax: 202-337-8270
                                       TTY: 202-337-5220
This directory lists auditory/oral programs in public and private schools, auditory-oral programs in speech and hearing centers and therapists who offer private tutoring and auditory-oral therapy.
67 pages

4426 Discovering Sign Language
Gallaudet University
11030 S Langley Avenue
Chicago, IL 60628-3819   800-621-2736
                                       Fax: 800-621-8476
                                       TTY: 888-630-9347
                                       www.gallaudet.edu/~gupress
Here is a book of information about deaf people and sign communication.
104 pages Softcover

4427 Douglas Tilden, the Man and His Legacy
Gallaudet University
11030 S Langley Avenue
Chicago, IL 60628-3819   800-621-2736
                                       Fax: 800-621-8476
                                       TTY: 888-630-9347
                                       www.gallaudet.edu/~gupress
A beautiful tribute to the Deaf sculptor, Douglas Tilden.
216 pages

4428 Ear Book
Gallaudet University
11030 S Langley Avenue
Chicago, IL 60628-3819   800-621-2736
                                       Fax: 800-621-8476
                                       TTY: 888-630-9347
                                       www.gallaudet.edu/~gupress
A how-to book on obtaining and using an otoscope, recognizing and managing common ear disorders, when to call the doctor and when your child needs ear tubes.
136 pages Softcover

4429 Ear Gear: A Student Workbook on Hearing and Hearing Aids
Gallaudet University
11030 S Langley Avenue
Chicago, IL 60628-3819   800-621-2736
                                       Fax: 800-621-8476
                                       TTY: 888-630-9347
                                       www.gallaudet.edu/~gupress
Attractive workbook designed to teach elementary-age children about hearing loss and the use of hearing aids.
75 pages

4430 Educating Deaf Children Bilingually
Gallaudet University
11030 S Langley Avenue
Chicago, IL 60628-3819   800-621-2736
                                       Fax: 800-621-8476
                                       TTY: 888-630-9347
                                       www.gallaudet.edu/~gupress
Discusses perspectives and practices of educating deaf children with goals of age-level achievement.
120 pages

4431 Educating the Deaf: Psychology, Principles and Practices
Gallaudet University

11030 S Langley Avenue
Chicago, IL 60628-3819 800-621-2736
Fax: 800-621-8476
TTY: 888-630-9347
www.gallaudet.edu/~gupress
Offers extensive coverage of the background and history of the education of the deaf, as well as specific information on working with multihandicapped students.
383 pages

4432 Education and Deafness
Longman Publishing Group
95 Church Street 914-993-5000
White Plains, NY 10601-1515
This comprehensive introduction to educating students with hearing impairments provides extensive coverage of the interrelated issues that affect the teaching of these students. It concentrates on the severely to profoundly hearing impaired but includes an entire chapter devoted to students whose impairments are less severe (hard-of-hearing students).
320 pages Paperback
ISBN: 0-801300-26-6

4433 Educational and Development Aspects of Deafness
Gallaudet University
11030 S Langley Avenue
Chicago, IL 60628-3819 800-621-2736
Fax: 800-621-8476
TTY: 888-630-9347
www.gallaudet.edu/~gupress
Book detailing the ongoing revolution in the education of deaf children.
415 pages

4434 Empowerment and Black Deaf Persons
Gallaudet University
11030 S Langley Avenue
Chicago, IL 60628-3819 800-621-2736
Fax: 800-621-8476
TTY: 888-630-9347
www.gallaudet.edu/~gupress
Conference proceedings focusing on the guidance and training of African American deaf individuals.
175 pages

4435 Encyclopedia of Deafness and Hearing Disorders
Facts on File
11 Penn Plaza 212-967-8800
New York, NY 10001 800-322-8755
Fax: 800-678-3633
A comprehensive guide to all aspects of hearing impairments.

4436 Eye-Centered: A Study of Spirituality of Deaf People
NCOD
814 Thayer Avenue 301-587-7992
Silver Spring, MD 20910-4500
The findings of the five-year De Sales Project conducted by The National Catholic Office for the Deaf.

4437 FM Auditory Trainers: A Winning Choice for Students, Teachers and Parents
Alexander Graham Bell Association
3417 Volta Place NW 202-337-5220
Washington, DC 20007-2737 Fax: 202-337-8270
TTY: 202-337-5220
A practical guide to the selection and use of FM trainers in class or at home.
67 pages

4438 For Teachers of the Hearing Impaired
Gallaudet University
11030 S Langley Avenue
Chicago, IL 60628-3819 800-621-2736
Fax: 800-621-8476
TTY: 888-630-9347
www.gallaudet.edu/~gupress
Contains practical articles by and for teachers of hearing impaired children.

4439 Foundations of Spoken Language for Hearing Impaired Children
Alexander Graham Bell Association
3417 Volta Place NW 202-337-5220
Washington, DC 20007-2737 Fax: 202-337-8270
TTY: 202-337-5220
This guide traces the individual progress of a child's speech development.
1978 87 pages

4440 Free Hand: Education of the Deaf
TJ Publishers
817 Silver Spring Avenue 301-585-4440
Silver Spring, MD 20910-4617 800-999-1168
Fax: 301-585-5930
TTY: 301-585-4441
e-mail: tjpubinc@aol.com
Based on the proceedings of a 1990 symposium on the educational uses of ASL, A Free Hand presents papers by prominent educators, researchers and linguists in the changing role of American sign language in the classroom.
204 pages Softcover
ISBN: 0-932666-40-X
Angela K Thames, President
Jerald A Murphy, VP

4441 GA and SK Etiquette
Gallaudet University
11030 S Langley Avenue
Chicago, IL 60628-3819 800-621-2736
Fax: 800-621-8476
TTY: 888-630-9347
www.gallaudet.edu/~gupress
This booklet presents guidelines for proper usage of the TDD.
53 pages

4442 Gallaudet Encyclopedia of Deaf People and Deafness
Gallaudet University
11030 S Langley Avenue
Chicago, IL 60628-3819 800-621-2736
Fax: 800-621-8476
TTY: 888-630-9347
www.gallaudet.edu/~gupress
Three-volume set of research and information on deaf people and deafness.
1400 pages

4443 Growing Together: Information for Parents of Deaf & Hard of Hearing Children
Gallaudet University
11030 S Langley Avenue
Chicago, IL 60628-3819 800-621-2736
Fax: 800-621-8476
TTY: 888-630-9347
www.gallaudet.edu/~gupress
This publication answers questions often asked by parents of children with a hearing loss.
92 pages

4444 Handtalk Zoo
Macmillan Publishing Company
866 3rd Avenue 212-702-2000
New York, NY 10022-6221 800-257-5755
www.mcp.com
Wonderful photographs are used to show children at the zoo communicating with sign language.
28 pages Hardcover
ISBN: 0-027008-01-0

4445 Hearing Aid Handbook
Gallaudet University
11030 S Langley Avenue
Chicago, IL 60628-3819 800-621-2736
Fax: 800-621-8476
TTY: 888-630-9347
www.gallaudet.edu/~gupress
A complete guide for wearers and clinicians for the use and maintenance of hearing aids.
172 pages Paperback

4446 **Hearing Impaired Children and Youth and Developmental Disabilities**
Gallaudet University
11030 S Langley Avenue
Chicago, IL 60628-3819   800-621-2736
                                                        Fax: 800-621-8476
                                                        TTY: 888-630-9347
                                                        www.gallaudet.edu/~gupress
Offers insights from 24 experts to help clarify relationships between hearing impairments and developmental difficulties.
416 pages

4447 **Hearing Loss Help**
Impact Publications
9104 Manassas Drive   703-361-7300
Manassas Park, VA 20111-5211   Fax: 703-335-9469
                                        e-mail: info@impactpublications.com
                                                www.impactpublications.com
Self-help guide provides factual information on how we hear, and on the causes and symptoms of hearing loss. Gives practical information on ways to improve everyday communication and create better listening conditions, and covers assistive listening devices.

4448 **Hearing Loss and Hearing Aids: A Bridge to Healing**
Richard Carmen, author
Hearing Loss Association of America
7910 Woodmont Avenue   301-657-2248
Bethesda, MD 20814-3079   Fax: 301-913-9413
                                                        TTY: 301-657-2249
                                        e-mail: info@hearingloss.org
                                                www.hearingloss.org
The Consumer Handbook on hearing loss and hearing aids.
Softcover
ISBN: 0-966182-61-8
Jerry Portis, Executive Director
Brenda Battat, Assistant Executive Director

4449 **Hispanic Deaf**
Gallaudet University
11030 S Langley Avenue
Chicago, IL 60628-3819   800-621-2736
                                                        Fax: 800-621-8476
                                                        TTY: 888-630-9347
                                                        www.gallaudet.edu/~gupress
Hispanic students now make up the largest minority in education for deaf students. This timely collection includes articles by many of the professionals most closely involved with the education of this very special population.
213 pages Hardcover

4450 **History of Special Education: From Isolation to Integration**
Gallaudet University
11030 S Langley Avenue
Chicago, IL 60628-3819   800-621-2736
                                                        Fax: 800-621-8476
                                                        TTY: 888-630-9347
                                                        www.gallaudet.edu/~gupress
Comprehensive volume examining the facts and events that shaped this field in Western Europe, United States and Canada.
464 pages

4451 **Hollywood Speaks**
Gallaudet University
11030 S Langley Avenue
Chicago, IL 60628-3819   800-621-2736
                                                        Fax: 800-621-8476
                                                        TTY: 888-630-9347
                                                        www.gallaudet.edu/~gupress
How deafness has been treated in movies and how it provides yet another window onto social history in addition to a fresh angle from which to view Hollywood.
167 pages Hardcover

4452 **Hometown Heroes: Successful Deaf Youth in America**
Gallaudet University
11030 S Langley Avenue
Chicago, IL 60628-3819   800-621-2736
                                                        Fax: 800-621-8476
                                                        TTY: 888-630-9347
                                                        www.gallaudet.edu/~gupress

A lively book showcasing more than 40 deaf and hard-of-hearing teenagers in the United States.
108 pages

4453 **How Hearing Impacts Relationships**
Richard Carmen, author
Hearing Loss Association of America
7910 Woodmont Avenue   301-657-2248
Bethesda, MD 20814-3079   Fax: 301-913-9413
                                                        TTY: 301-657-2249
                                        e-mail: info@hearingloss.org
                                                www.hearingloss.org
At last families of loved ones with untreated hearing loss can know they are not alone and what options are available.
Softcover
ISBN: 0-966182-63-4
Jerry Portis, Executive Director
Brenda Battat, Assistant Executive Director

4454 **How the Student with Hearing Loss Can Succeed in College**
Alexander Graham Bell Association
3417 Volta Place NW   202-337-5220
Washington, DC 20007-2737   Fax: 202-337-8270
                                                        TTY: 202-337-5220
This revised book details how students who are deaf or hard of hearing and professionals must work together for students in college to be successful.
1996 304 pages

4455 **How to Survive a Hearing Loss**
Gallaudet University
11030 S Langley Avenue
Chicago, IL 60628-3819   800-621-2736
                                                        Fax: 800-621-8476
                                                        TTY: 888-630-9347
                                                        www.gallaudet.edu/~gupress
This book presents the results of the author's intensive research about hearing and the ear.
241 pages

4456 **Hug Just Isn't Enough**
Gallaudet University
11030 S Langley Avenue
Chicago, IL 60628-3819   800-621-2736
                                                        Fax: 800-621-8476
                                                        TTY: 888-630-9347
                                                        www.gallaudet.edu/~gupress
Photos of deaf children and excerpts from interviews with parents of deaf youngsters.

4457 **I Didn't Hear the Dragon Roar**
Gallaudet University
11030 S Langley Avenue
Chicago, IL 60628-3819   800-621-2736
                                                        Fax: 800-621-8476
                                                        TTY: 888-630-9347
                                                        www.gallaudet.edu/~gupress
The remarkable true story of a deaf woman's journey from Hong Kong to Katmandu.
251 pages

4458 **IDEA Advocacy for Children Who are Deaf or Hard of Hearing**
Alexander Graham Bell Association
3417 Volta Place NW   202-337-5220
Washington, DC 20007-2737   Fax: 202-337-8270
                                                        TTY: 202-337-5220
This book offers up to date information about the 1997 Individuals with Disabilities Education Act which affects children who are deaf or hard of hearing.
1997 96 pages

4459 **Implications and Complications for Deaf Students of Full Inclusion Movement**
Gallaudet University
11030 S Langley Avenue
Chicago, IL 60628-3819   800-621-2736
                                                        Fax: 800-621-8476
                                                        TTY: 888-630-9347
                                                        www.gallaudet.edu/~gupress

A collection of papers discussing the full inclusion movement.
80 pages

4460   In Silence: Growing Up Hearing in a Deaf World
Gallaudet University
11030 S Langley Avenue
Chicago, IL 60628-3819   800-621-2736
                                     Fax: 800-621-8476
                                     TTY: 888-630-9347
                                     www.gallaudet.edu/~gupress
Author's story of growing up as a hearing child of deaf parents.
335 pages

4461   In This Sign
Gallaudet University
11030 S Langley Avenue
Chicago, IL 60628-3819   800-621-2736
                                     Fax: 800-621-8476
                                     TTY: 888-630-9347
                                     www.gallaudet.edu/~gupress
A modern classic following a family of deaf parents and their hearing impaired child through several decades of growth and pain, tragedy and triumph.
275 pages

4462   Inclusion?
Gallaudet University
11030 S Langley Avenue
Chicago, IL 60628-3819   800-621-2736
                                     Fax: 800-621-8476
                                     TTY: 888-630-9347
                                     www.gallaudet.edu/~gupress
This book defines quality education for deaf and hard of hearing students.
213 pages

4463   International Directory of Periodicals Related to Deafness
Gallaudet University
11030 S Langley Avenue
Chicago, IL 60628-3819   800-621-2736
                                     Fax: 800-621-8476
                                     TTY: 888-630-9347
                                     www.gallaudet.edu/~gupress
Offers information on more than 500 magazines and journals related to deafness.
150 pages

4464   International Telephone Directory for TDD Users
Gallaudet University
11030 S Langley Avenue
Chicago, IL 60628-3819   800-621-2736
                                     Fax: 800-621-8476
                                     TTY: 888-630-9347
                                     www.gallaudet.edu/~gupress
Offers 12,000 TDD members and organizations serving deaf people.
190 pages

4465   Introduction to Communication
Gallaudet University
11030 S Langley Avenue
Chicago, IL 60628-3819   800-621-2736
                                     Fax: 800-621-8476
                                     TTY: 888-630-9347
                                     www.gallaudet.edu/~gupress
Curriculum materials exploring the areas of sound, hearing and interpersonal communication.
100 pages

4466   Invisible Condition: The Human Side of Hearing Loss
Howard E Stone, author

Hearing Loss Association of America
7910 Woodmont Avenue   301-657-2248
Bethesda, MD 20814-3079   Fax: 301-913-9413
                                     TTY: 301-657-2249
                                     e-mail: info@hearingloss.org
                                     www.hearingloss.org

A collection of 14 years of editorials by the author from the SHHH Journal. An inspiration book that transcends hearing loss.
1993
Jerry Portis, Executive Director
Brenda Battat, Assistant Executive Director

4467   Its Your Turn Now: Using Dialogue Journals with Deaf Students
Gallaudet University
11030 S Langley Avenue
Chicago, IL 60628-3819   800-621-2736
                                     Fax: 800-621-8476
                                     TTY: 888-630-9347
                                     www.gallaudet.edu/~gupress
Based on years of experience, this book reviews teachers' questions and answers.
130 pages

4468   Journey Into the Deaf World
DawnSignPress
6130 Nancy Ridge Drive   858-625-0600
San Diego, CA 92121-3223   800-549-5350
                                     Fax: 858-625-2336
                                     TTY: 858-625-0600
                                     e-mail: comments@dawnsign.com
                                     www.dawnsign.com
Provides explanation about the nature and meaning of the deaf world. Comprehensive work discusses latest findings and theories for deaf studies students and professionals working with deaf people.
528 pages Paperback
ISBN: 0-915035-63-4
Barry Howland, Marketing Director

4469   Journey Out of Silence
Dora Tinglestad Weber, author

Hearing Loss Association of America
7910 Woodmont Avenue   301-657-2248
Bethesda, MD 20814-3079   Fax: 301-913-9413
                                     TTY: 301-657-2249
                                     e-mail: info@hearingloss.org
                                     www.hearingloss.org
Dora Weber, who made a long and arduous journey out of silence, shares her experiences in an effort to encourage those who are hearing impaired and to increase the sensitivity of those who are not.
Softcover
ISBN: 1-890676-30-6
Jerry Portis, Executive Director
Brenda Battat, Assistant Executive Director

4470   Joy of Signing
Gospel Publishing House
1445 N Boonville Avenue   417-862-2781
Springfield, MO 65802-1894   Fax: 417-862-7566
                                     e-mail: jclore@ag.org
                                     www.GospelPublishing.com
Illustrated sign language text with descriptions of the origin of selected signs and examples of how each is used. Second edition.
352 pages
Judy Clore, Promotions Coordinator

4471   Kaleidoscope of Deaf America
Harris Communications
6541 City W Parkway   612-906-1180
Eden Prairie, MN 55344-3248   Fax: 612-946-0924
Puts you in touch with the trends, the events and the thinking that is shaping your future.
79 pages

4472   Kendall Demonstration Elementary School Curriculum Guides
Gallaudet University
11030 S Langley Avenue
Chicago, IL 60628-3819   800-621-2736
                                     Fax: 800-621-8476
                                     TTY: 888-630-9347
                                     www.gallaudet.edu/~gupress

These guides provide detailed information to help teachers organize curriculum, structure classes and develop individualized education programs.
18 months+

4473   Kid-Friendly Parenting with Deaf and Hard of Hearing Children
Gallaudet University
11030 S Langley Avenue
Chicago, IL 60628-3819   800-621-2736
                                      Fax: 800-621-8476
                                      TTY: 888-630-9347
                               www.gallaudet.edu/~gupress
A step-by-step guide offering parents hundreds of ideas and play activities for children ages 3 to 12.
336 pages

4474   Learning to Hear Again
Alexander Graham Bell Association
3417 Volta Place NW   202-337-5220
Washington, DC 20007-2737   Fax: 202-337-8270
                                   TTY: 202-337-5220
This audiologic rehabilitation curriculum guide is designed to help audiologists and speech language pathologist provide rehabilitation and education for adults with hearing losses. The authors are practicing audiologists and have used these methods successfully in individual and group sessions. This comprehensive manual comprises lesson plans, activities and materials ready to be duplicated and distributed to clients.
1996 224 pages

4475   Learning to See: American Sign Language as a Second Language
Gallaudet University
11030 S Langley Avenue
Chicago, IL 60628-3819   800-621-2736
                                      Fax: 800-621-8476
                                      TTY: 888-630-9347
                               www.gallaudet.edu/~gupress
Provides a comprehensive introduction to the history and structure of ASL to the deaf community.
134 pages

4476   Least Restrictive Environment: The Paradox of Inclusion
LRP Publications
PO Box 980
Horsham, PA 19044-0980   800-341-7874
                                      Fax: 215-784-9639
                               e-mail: custserv@lrp.com
                                      www.lrp.com
Analyzes relevant federal law and the inclusion reform movement, and discusses the premise that an effort to force one generic placement on all children will create more problems than thought imaginable.
Paperback

4477   Legal Rights for the Deaf and Hard of Hearing
Hearing Loss Association of America
7910 Woodmont Avenue   301-657-2248
Bethesda, MD 20814-3079   Fax: 301-913-9413
                                    TTY: 301-657-2249
                            e-mail: info@hearingloss.org
                                 www.hearingloss.org
A comprehensive analysis of recent laws passed to protect the rights of and guarantee equal access for people with hearing loss. The book explains in layman's terminology how legislation affects individuals with disabilities in everyday life.
2002 Softcover
Jerry Portis, Executive Director
Brenda Battat, Assistant Executive Director

4478   Legal Rights of Hearing-Impaired People
Gallaudet University
11030 S Langley Avenue
Chicago, IL 60628-3819   800-621-2736
                                      Fax: 800-621-8476
                                      TTY: 888-630-9347
                               www.gallaudet.edu/~gupress
Includes updated interpretations of legislation affecting hearing-impaired people, including chapters dealing with the ADA.
297 pages

4479   Lessons in Laughter: The Autobiography of a Deaf Actor
Gallaudet University
11030 S Langley Avenue
Chicago, IL 60628-3819   800-621-2736
                                      Fax: 800-621-8476
                                      TTY: 888-630-9347
                               www.gallaudet.edu/~gupress
Born deaf of deaf parents, Bernard Bragg dreamed of using sign language to act. This book recounts how he starred in his own television show.
237 pages

4480   Let's Learn About Deafness
Gallaudet University
11030 S Langley Avenue
Chicago, IL 60628-3819   800-621-2736
                                      Fax: 800-621-8476
                                      TTY: 888-630-9347
                               www.gallaudet.edu/~gupress
Hands-on school classroom activities for the deaf student.
82 pages

4481   Listen to Me: Auditory Exercises for Adults
Alexander Graham Bell Association
3417 Volta Place NW   202-337-5220
Washington, DC 20007-2737   Fax: 202-337-8270
                                   TTY: 202-337-5220
Helps hard of hearing teenagers and adults to listen, lip read, pick up clues from conversations and remember what they have heard.
65 pages

4482   Listen with the Heart: Relationships and Hearing Loss
Hearing Loss Association of America
7910 Woodmont Avenue   301-657-2248
Bethesda, MD 20814-3079   Fax: 301-913-9413
                                    TTY: 301-657-2249
                            e-mail: info@hearingloss.org
                                 www.hearingloss.org
Written for family and friends as well as professionals. It is an excellent text for college and graduate level courses in psychology, mental health counseling, speech and hearing, special education, and deaf education.
Jerry Portis, Executive Director
Brenda Battat, Assistant Executive Director

4483   Listening
National Catholic Office for the Deaf
7201 Buchnan Street   301-577-1684
Landover Hills, MD 20784-4500   e-mail: nco@erols.com
                                      www.ncod.org
Published as a pastoral service for the hearing impaired.

4484   Listening & Talking
Alexander Graham Bell Association
3417 Volta Place NW   202-337-5220
Washington, DC 20007-2737   Fax: 202-337-8270
                                   TTY: 202-337-5220
This guide promotes spoken language in young hearing-impaired children.
191 pages

4485   Listening to Learn: A Handbook for Parents with Hearing-Impaired Children
Alexander Graham Bell Association
3417 Volta Place NW   202-337-5220
Washington, DC 20007-2737   Fax: 202-337-8270
                                   TTY: 202-337-5220
Developed by teachers, this handbook provides parents with the essential steps necessary to develop effective spoken communication with their children.
98 pages

4486   Listening: Ways of Hearing in a Silent World
Hannah Merker, author
Hearing Loss Association of America

7910 Woodmont Avenue
Bethesda, MD 20814-3079
301-657-2248
Fax: 301-913-9413
TTY: 301-657-2249
e-mail: info@hearingloss.org
www.hearingloss.org

This book is about one woman's evocative account of her perceptions and rememberance of sound.
1999
Jerry Portis, Executive Director
Brenda Battat, Assistant Executive Director

4487 Literature Journal
Gallaudet University
11030 S Langley Avenue
Chicago, IL 60628-3819
800-621-2736
Fax: 800-621-8476
TTY: 888-630-9347
www.gallaudet.edu/~gupress

This book includes extensive examples of student and teacher entries taken from actual journals of deaf high school students.
44 pages

4488 Living with Hearing Loss
Marcia B Dugan, author
Hearing Loss Association of America
7910 Woodmont Avenue
Bethesda, MD 20814-3079
301-657-2248
Fax: 301-913-9413
TTY: 301-657-2249
e-mail: info@hearingloss.org
www.hearingloss.org

Living with Hearing Loss takes the reader from A to Z on the kinds and causes of hearing loss and its common early signs. Topics Include: Seeking Professional Evaluations, Hearing Aids, Assistive Technology, Speechreading, Communication Tips, Cochlear Implants, Dealing with Tinnitus, and resources.
2003
ISBN: 1-563681-34-0
Jerry Portis, Executive Director
Brenda Battat, Assistant Executive Director

4489 Looking Back: A Reader on the History of Deaf Communities & Sign Language
Gallaudet University
11030 S Langley Avenue
Chicago, IL 60628-3819
800-621-2736
Fax: 800-621-8476
TTY: 888-630-9347
www.gallaudet.edu/~gupress

Renowned researchers from around the world present provocative findings in six areas relating to the deaf culture.
558 pages

4490 Loss for Words
Gallaudet University
11030 S Langley Avenue
Chicago, IL 60628-3819
800-621-2736
Fax: 800-621-8476
TTY: 888-630-9347
www.gallaudet.edu/~gupress

The author's touching story of her life as an interpreter for her parents, head of her household by the age of eight and a teacher and helper to both of her deaf parents.
208 pages

4491 Mainstreaming Deaf and Hard of Hearing Students
Gallaudet University
800 Florida Avenue NE
Washington, DC 20002-3695
202-651-5000
800-621-2736
Fax: 800-621-8476
TTY: 888-630-9347
www.gallaudet.edu/~gupress

Gallaudet University is the world leader in liberal education and career development for deaf and hard-of-hearing undergraduate students.
40 pages

4492 Man Without Words
Gallaudet University

11030 S Langley Avenue
Chicago, IL 60628-3819
800-621-2736
Fax: 800-621-8476
TTY: 888-630-9347
www.gallaudet.edu/~gupress

Author relates her experiences teaching sign language to a 27 year old deaf Mexican man who had no education and no language.
203 pages

4493 Martimer
APSEA-RCHI
Box 308
Amherst, NS, B4H 3Z6,
902-667-3808
Fax: 902-667-0893

Periodical describing programs and services provided by the APSEA Resource Center for the Hearing Impaired.
Phyllis Cameron, Editor

4494 Mask of Benevolence: Disabling the Deaf Community
Gallaudet University
11030 S Langley Avenue
Chicago, IL 60628-3819
800-621-2736
Fax: 800-621-8476
TTY: 888-630-9347
www.gallaudet.edu/~gupress

Written by a doctor who does not view deafness as a handicap but rather a different state of hearing.
310 pages

4495 Meeting Halfway in ASL
MSM Productions
PO Box 23380
Rochester, NY 14692-3380
716-442-6370
Fax: 716-442-6371
TTY: 716-442-6370
e-mail: Books@deaflife.com
www.deaflife.com

Illustrated photographic sign-language book containing 1,300 photos.

ISBN: 0-963401-67-
Matthew Moore, Publisher

4496 Meeting the Challenge: Hearing-Impaired Professionals in the Workplace
Gallaudet University
11030 S Langley Avenue
Chicago, IL 60628-3819
800-621-2736
Fax: 800-621-8476
TTY: 888-630-9347
www.gallaudet.edu/~gupress

Provides information on communication methods, educational backgrounds and job search tactics used by more than 1500 participants and their current employment conditions.
236 pages

4497 Mental Health Services for Deaf People
Gallaudet University
11030 S Langley Avenue
Chicago, IL 60628-3819
800-621-2736
Fax: 800-621-8476
TTY: 888-630-9347
www.gallaudet.edu/~gupress

Contains information on over 350 mental health programs and services for deaf people across the United States.
210 pages

4498 Missing Words: The Family Handbook on Adult Hearing Loss
Gallaudet University
11030 S Langley Avenue
Chicago, IL 60628-3819
800-621-2736
Fax: 800-621-8476
TTY: 888-630-9347
www.gallaudet.edu/~gupress

Written by a mother who lost her hearing and her daughter, learning to cope.
304 pages

4499 Mother Father Deaf: Living Between Sound and Silence
Harvard University Press

79 Garden Street
Cambridge, MA 02138-1423

617-495-2480
800-448-2242
Fax: 800-962-4983
www.hup.harvard.edu

Based on interviews with 150 adult hearing children of deaf parents who chart the sometimes difficult middle ground between spoken and signed language.

4500 Moving Toward the Standards
Gallaudet University
11030 S Langley Avenue
Chicago, IL 60628-3819

800-621-2736
Fax: 800-621-8476
TTY: 888-630-9347
www.gallaudet.edu/~gupress

A national action plan for mathematics education reform for the deaf.
55 pages

4501 Music in Motion
Modern Signs Press
PO Box 1181
Los Alamitos, CA 90720-1181

562-596-8548
800-572-7332
Fax: 562-795-6614
TTY: 562-493-4168
e-mail: modsigns@aol.com
www.modsigns.com

Includes guitar notes and glossary of sign descriptions for 325-word vocabulary.
109 pages
ISBN: 0-916708-07-1

4502 NAD Deaf Awareness Kit
National Association of the Deaf
8630 Fenton Street
Silver Spring, MD 20910

301-587-1788
Fax: 301-587-1791
TTY: 301-587-1789
www.nad.org

Includes information that can be used both during Deaf Awareness Week and year-round to recognize the accomplishments and heritage of the deaf community.
Donna Morris, Publications Manager

4503 Never the Twain Shall Meet: The Communications Debate
Gallaudet University
11030 S Langley Avenue
Chicago, IL 60628-3819

800-621-2736
Fax: 800-621-8476
TTY: 888-630-9347
www.gallaudet.edu/~gupress

Should sign language be used in the education of Deaf children or should they be forced to deal with a hearing, speaking world on its own terms?.
129 pages

4504 Next Step
Gallaudet University
11030 S Langley Avenue
Chicago, IL 60628-3819

800-621-2736
Fax: 800-621-8476
TTY: 888-630-9347
www.gallaudet.edu/~gupress

A national conference focusing on issues related to substance abuse in the deaf and hard of hearing population.
209 pages

4505 No Sound
Harris Communications
6541 City W Parkway
Eden Prairie, MN 55344-3248

612-906-1180
Fax: 612-946-0924

A moving, highly informative autobiography of Julius Wiggins, founder and president of the newspaper Silent News. Second edition.
211 pages

4506 No Walls of Stone: An Anthology of Literature by Deaf Writers
Gallaudet University

11030 S Langley Avenue
Chicago, IL 60628-3819

800-621-2736
Fax: 800-621-8476
TTY: 888-630-9347
www.gallaudet.edu/~gupress

Short fiction, essays, verse and drama written by the deaf and hard of hearing writer.
240 pages
Jill Jepson, Editor

4507 None So Deaf
Gallaudet University
11030 S Langley Avenue
Chicago, IL 60628-3819

800-621-2736
Fax: 800-621-8476
TTY: 888-630-9347
www.gallaudet.edu/~gupress

A student history of education of deaf people and the development of sign language.
51 pages Paperback

4508 Odyssey of Hearing Loss: Tales of Triumph
Michael A Harvey, PhD, author

Hearing Loss Association of America
7910 Woodmont Avenue
Bethesda, MD 20814-3079

301-657-2248
Fax: 301-913-9413
TTY: 301-657-2249
e-mail: info@hearingloss.org
www.hearingloss.org

A glimpse into the lives of 10 people; each showing how sharing insights about hearing loss helps people on the road to healing and a life well examined.
Jerry Portis, Executive Director
Brenda Battat, Assistant Executive Director

4509 Okada Hearing Ear Guide
RR 1 Box 640F
Fontana, WI 53125-9714

414-275-5226

Trains dogs to aid hearing-impaired persons.

4510 On My Own
Gallaudet University
11030 S Langley Avenue
Chicago, IL 60628-3819

800-621-2736
Fax: 800-621-8476
TTY: 888-630-9347
www.gallaudet.edu/~gupress

Book examining doorbell devices, alarm clocks, telephone amplifiers and other assistive devices for the deaf.
50 pages Teacher's Guide

4511 Oral Interpreting Selections from Papers from Kirsten Gonzales
Alexander Graham Bell Association
3417 Volta Place NW
Washington, DC 20007-2737

202-337-5220
Fax: 202-337-8270
TTY: 202-337-5220

These six easy to read articles discuss speech reading and oral interpreting. The articles answer questions that are frequently asked by professionals and the general public.
30 pages

4512 Other Side of Silence
Gallaudet University
11030 S Langley Avenue
Chicago, IL 60628-3819

800-621-2736
Fax: 800-621-8476
TTY: 888-630-9347
www.gallaudet.edu/~gupress

Explores the deaf community through interviews from across the country.
256 pages

4513 Our Forgotten Children: 3rd Edition
Alexander Graham Bell Association
3417 Volta Place NW
Washington, DC 20007-2737

202-337-5220
Fax: 202-337-8270
TTY: 202-337-5220

This simple book describes characteristics of hard-of-hearing children in the school and discusses their educational requirements, psychological and social needs and amplification options.
68 pages

4514 Our Forgotten Children: Hard of Hearing Pupils in the Schools
Julia M Davis, PhD, author
Hearing Loss Association of America
7910 Woodmont Avenue   301-657-2248
Bethesda, MD 20814-3079   Fax: 301-913-9413
                                TTY: 301-657-2249
                          e-mail: info@hearingloss.org
                                www.hearingloss.org
Important resource about the educational environment.
2001
Jerry Portis, Executive Director
Brenda Battat, Assistant Executive Director

4515 Outsiders in a Hearing World
Gallaudet University
11030 S Langley Avenue
Chicago, IL 60628-3819   800-621-2736
                                Fax: 800-621-8476
                                TTY: 888-630-9347
                          www.gallaudet.edu/~gupress
The author gives a sociologist's view of what it is like to be deaf.
240 pages

4516 Parents and Teachers: Partners in Language Development
Alexander Graham Bell Association
3417 Volta Place NW
Washington, DC 20007-2737   202-337-5220
                                Fax: 202-337-8270
                                TTY: 202-337-5220
Outlines the essential role of the teacher and parent in the development of language in the school aged child with hearing impairment.
386 pages

4517 Perigee Visual Dictionary of Signing
Harris Communications
6541 City W Parkway   612-906-1180
Eden Prairie, MN 55344-3248   Fax: 612-946-0924
An A-to-Z guide to American Sign Language vocabulary.
450 pages

4518 Perspectives Folio: Mainstreaming
Gallaudet University
11030 S Langley Avenue
Chicago, IL 60628-3819   800-621-2736
                                Fax: 800-621-8476
                                TTY: 888-630-9347
                          www.gallaudet.edu/~gupress
Presents 14 articles from Perspectives magazine that offer practical, experience-based advice on mainstreaming for parents and students themselves.
39 pages

4519 Perspectives on Deafness
National Association of the Deaf
8630 Fenton Street   301-587-1788
Silver Spring, MD 20910   Fax: 301-587-1791
                                TTY: 301-587-1789
                                      www.nad.org
Focuses on the many perspectives which constitute diversity within the deaf community.
Paperback
Donna Morris, Publications Manager

4520 Place of Their Own: Creating the Deaf Community in America
Gallaudet University Press
11030 S Langley Avenue
Chicago, IL 60628-3819   800-621-2736
                                TTY: 888-630-9347
                                www.gallaudet.edu
Traces the history of deaf people and views deafness not from the perspective of a pathology, but of culture, not as a disease or disability to overcome or be cured, but as the distinguishing characteristic of a distinct community of individuals whose history and achievement are worthy of study.

4521 Politics of Deafness
Gallaudet University
11030 S Langley Avenue
Chicago, IL 60628   800-621-2736
                                Fax: 800-621-8476
                                TTY: 888-630-9347
                          www.gallaudet.edu/~gupress
Embarks upon a postmodern examination of the search for identity in deafness and its relationship to the prevalent Hearing culture that has marginalized Deaf people.
June 1997 304 pages Softcover
ISBN: 1-563680-58-0

4522 Possible Dream: Mainstream Experiences of Hearing-Impaired Students
Alexander Graham Bell Association
3417 Volta Place NW   202-337-5220
Washington, DC 20007-2737   Fax: 202-337-8270
                                TTY: 202-337-5220
This collection highlights the experiences of auditory-oral children who are Bell Association financial aid winners and their families.
66 pages
Mildred L Oberkotter, Editor

4523 Post Milan
Gallaudet University
11030 S Langley Avenue
Chicago, IL 60628-3819   800-621-2736
                                Fax: 800-621-8476
                                TDD: 800-621-8476
                          www.gallaudet.edu/~gupress
Timely issues covering trends in ASL and ASL/English literacy.
323 pages

4524 PreReading Strategies
Gallaudet University
11030 S Langley Avenue
Chicago, IL 60628-3819   800-621-2736
                                Fax: 800-621-8476
                                TTY: 888-630-9347
                          www.gallaudet.edu/~gupress
Here is a wealth of good advice for preparing students to understand what they read, building comprehension and enjoyment.
65 pages

4525 Psychoeducational Assessment of Hearing-Impaired Students
Pro-Ed, Inc.
8700 Shoal Creek Boulevard   512-451-3246
Austin, TX 78757-6897   Fax: 512-451-8542
                          e-mail: info@proedinc.com
                                www.proedinc.com
This book includes a comprehensive presentation of issues and procedures related to the assessment of hearing-impaired students.
251 pages Paperback
ISBN: 0-890794-55-3
Lindy Jordaan, Marketing Coordinator

4526 Reading and Deafness
Pro-Ed, Inc.
8700 Shoal Creek Boulevard   512-451-3246
Austin, TX 78757-6897   800-897-3202
                                Fax: 800-397-7633
                          e-mail: info@proedinc.com
                                www.proedinc.com
Three areas are looked at in this book: deaf children's prereading development of real-world knowledge; cognitive abilities and linguistic skills.
422 pages Hardcover
ISBN: 0-887441-07-6
Lindy Jordaan, Marketing Coordinator

4527 Rebuilt: My Journey Back to the Hearing World
Michael Chorost, author
Hearing Loss Association of America

7910 Woodmont Avenue   301-657-2248
Bethesda, MD 20814-3079   Fax: 301-913-9413
                                    TTY: 301-657-2249
                          e-mail: info@hearingloss.org
                                    www.hearingloss.org

Brimming with insight and written with charm and self-deprecating humor, Rebuilt unveils, in personal terms, the astounding possibilities of a new technological age.
240 pages Paperback
ISBN: 0-618717-60-9
Jerry Portis, Executive Director
Brenda Battat, Assistant Executive Director

4528   Say That Again, Please
Gallaudet University
11030 S Langley Avenue
Chicago, IL 60628-3819   800-621-2736
                                    Fax: 800-621-8476
                                    TTY: 888-630-9347
                          www.gallaudet.edu/~gupress

This book serves to enlighten those who are interested.
370 pages

4529   Schedules of Development for Hearing Impaired Infants and their Parents
Alexander Graham Bell Association
3417 Volta Place NW   202-337-5220
Washington, DC 20007-2737   Fax: 202-337-8270
                                    TTY: 202-337-5220

Written for parents and teachers, this assessment record of verbal learning will help to evaluate each child's language development.
1977 14 pages

4530   Science of Sound
Gallaudet University
11030 S Langley Avenue
Chicago, IL 60628-3819   800-621-2736
                                    Fax: 800-621-8476
                                    TTY: 888-630-9347
                          www.gallaudet.edu/~gupress

This exciting book is carefully designed to help hearing-impaired students understand, use and enjoy the principles of sound.
32 pages

4531   Seeds of Disquiet: One Deaf Woman's Experience
Gallaudet University
11030 S Langley Avenue
Chicago, IL 60628-3819   800-621-2736
                                    Fax: 800-621-8476
                                    TTY: 888-630-9347
                          www.gallaudet.edu/~gupress

This book relates to the story of how Cheryl Heppner reacted to two severe losses in her hearing.
192 pages

4532   Seeing Voices: A Journey Into the World of the Deaf
Gallaudet University
11030 S Langley Avenue
Chicago, IL 60628-3819   800-621-2736
                                    Fax: 800-621-8476
                                    TTY: 888-630-9347
                          www.gallaudet.edu/~gupress

Dr. Sacks takes us into the world of deaf people.
180 pages

4533   Sign Communication: A Family Affair
Gallaudet University
11030 S Langley Avenue
Chicago, IL 60628-3819   800-621-2736
                                    Fax: 800-621-8476
                                    TTY: 888-630-9347
                          www.gallaudet.edu/~gupress

Book designed to help hearing parents communicate effectively with their deaf children on issues of good health and personal growth.
132 pages

4534   Sign Language Feelings
Gallaudet University

11030 S Langley Avenue
Chicago, IL 60628-3819   800-621-2736
                                    Fax: 800-621-8476
                                    TTY: 888-630-9347
                          www.gallaudet.edu/~gupress

Worksheets teach signs for happy, sad and all of the feelings in between.

4535   Sign Language Interpreters and Interpreting
Gallaudet University
11030 S Langley Avenue
Chicago, IL 60628-3819   800-621-2736
                                    Fax: 800-621-8476
                                    TTY: 888-630-9347
                          www.gallaudet.edu/~gupress

This monograph presents articles about personal characteristics and abilities of interpreters, the effects of lag time on interpreter errors, and the interpretation of register.
161 pages

4536   Sign Language Made Simple
Gospel Publishing House
1445 N Boonville Avenue   417-862-2781
Springfield, MO 65802-1894   Fax: 417-862-7566
                               e-mail: jclore@ag.org
                          www.GospelPublishing.com

Illustrated sign language text with descriptions of the origin of selected signs and examples of how each is used. Second edition.
240 pages
Judy Clore, Promotions Coordinator

4537   Sign Language Talk
Franklin Watts Grolier
90 Old Sherman Tpke   203-797-3500
Danbury, CT 06816-0001   800-843-3749
                                    Fax: 203-797-3197
                                        www.grolier.com

Using 300 easy-to-follow illustrations, this book introduces the structure of sign language, shows how sentences are formed and how signed conversations differ from spoken ones.
96 pages
ISBN: 0-531105-97-0

4538   Sign Language and the Deaf Community: Essays in Honor of William Stokoe
National Association of the Deaf
8630 Fenton Street   301-587-1788
Silver Spring, MD 20910   Fax: 301-587-1791
                                    TTY: 301-587-1789
                                            www.nad.org

Collection of essays, written by professionals in the field of sign language research and usage, describing how information has dramatically altered society's understanding of deaf people and their culture.
267 pages Paperback
Donna Morris, Publications Manager

4539   Signed English Starter
Harris Communications
6541 City W Parkway   612-906-1108
Eden Prairie, MN 55344-3248   Fax: 612-946-0924

The first book to use when learning Signed English.
208 pages

4540   Signing Exact English
Modern Signs Press
PO Box 1181   562-596-8548
Los Alamitos, CA 90720-1181   800-572-7332
                                    Fax: 562-795-6614
                                    TTY: 562-493-4168
                          e-mail: modsigns@aol.com
                                    www.modsigns.com

A reference manual containing manual signs representing nearly 4,000 words, plus signs for letters, numbers, prefixes and suffixes.
1993 479 pages Softcover
ISBN: 0-196708-23-3

4541   Signing Illustrated
Gallaudet University

11030 S Langley Avenue
Chicago, IL 60628-3819
800-621-2736
Fax: 800-621-8476
TTY: 888-630-9347
www.gallaudet.edu/~gupress
A guide presenting illustrations of over 1,350 signs.
85 pages

4542 Signing Naturally: Teacher's Curriculum Guide-Level 1
DawnSignPress
6130 Nancy Ridge Drive
San Diego, CA 92121-3223
619-625-0600
800-549-5350
Fax: 619-625-2336
e-mail: DawnSign@aol.com
Guide and video.
336 pages 22 minutes
ISBN: 0-915035-07-3

4543 Signs Everywhere
Modern Signs Press
PO Box 1181
Los Alamitos, CA 90720-1181
562-596-8548
800-572-7332
Fax: 562-795-6614
TTY: 562-493-4168
e-mail: modsigns@aol.com
www.modsigns.com
Includes signs for cities, towns and states through United States, Canada and Mexico. Drawings and descriptions of the signs accompany maps showing locations of states and cities.
280 pages
ISBN: 0-916708-05-5

4544 Signs for Computing Terminology
National Association of the Deaf
8630 Fenton Street
Silver Spring, MD 20910-4500
301-587-1788
Fax: 301-587-1791
TTY: 301-587-1789
www.nad.org
Contains over 600 computer related sign illustrations used by deaf and hearing computer specialists.
182 pages Paperback
ISBN: 0-913072-63-X
Donna Morris, Publications Manager

4545 Silent Alarm: On the Edge with a Deaf EMT
Gallaudet University
11030 S Langley Avenue
Chicago, IL 60628-3819
800-621-2736
Fax: 800-621-8476
TTY: 888-630-9347
www.gallaudet.edu/~gupress
Silent Alarm tells the gripping story of survival and the good that the author did as a topnotch EMT.
160 pages

4546 Silent Garden: Raising Your Deaf Child
Gallaudet University
11030 S Langley Avenue
Chicago, IL 60628
800-621-2736
Fax: 800-621-8476
TTY: 888-630-9347
www.gallaudet.edu/~gupress
Provides parents with a firm foundation for making the difficult decisions necessary for their deaf child's future. Includes information on critical concerns, communication, technological alternative, and reassurance through case studies and interviews.
304 pages Softcover
ISBN: 1-563680-58-0

4547 Simultaneous Communication, ASL and Other Communication Modes
Gallaudet University
11030 S Langley Avenue
Chicago, IL 60628-3819
800-621-2736
Fax: 800-621-8476
TTY: 888-630-9347
www.gallaudet.edu/~gupress
This monograph presents four major articles that examine issues surrounding communications in an educational environment.
236 pages

4548 Sing Praise
Sunday School Board of the Southern Baptists
127 9th Avenue N
Nashville, TN 37234-0001
800-458-2772
For use by interpreters to the deaf.

4549 Sociolinguistics in Deaf Communities
Gallaudet University
11030 S Langley Avenue
Chicago, IL 60628-3819
800-621-2736
Fax: 800-621-8476
TTY: 888-630-9347
www.gallaudet.edu/~gupress
The first volume in a series offering assessments and up-to-date information on sign language linguistics.
280 pages

4550 Software to Go
Gallaudet University
11030 S Langley Avenue
Chicago, IL 60628-3819
800-621-2736
Fax: 800-621-8476
TTY: 888-630-9347
www.gallaudet.edu/~gupress
Lists and describes commercial software that may be borrowed by educators of hearing impaired students.
100 pages

4551 Sound and Sign, Childhood Deafness and Mental Health
Gallaudet University
11030 S Langley Avenue
Chicago, IL 60628-3819
800-621-2736
Fax: 800-621-8476
TTY: 888-630-9347
www.gallaudet.edu/~gupress
Presents research to support beliefs that deaf children should be educated using a combination manual and oral communication in residual hearing and speech.
265 pages

4552 Speak to Me
Gallaudet University
11030 S Langley Avenue
Chicago, IL 60628-3819
800-621-2736
Fax: 800-621-8476
TTY: 888-630-9347
www.gallaudet.edu/~gupress
A story of a single mother confronted with the deafness of her son.
160 pages

4553 Speech and the Hearing-Impaired Child
Alexander Graham Bell Association
3417 Volta Place NW
Washington, DC 20007-2737
202-337-5220
Fax: 202-337-8270
TTY: 202-337-5220
Provides a systematic approach to the teaching of speech and a challenge to all involved in the development of spoken language skills in hearing-impaired children.
402 pages

4554 Speechreading in Context
Gallaudet University
11030 S Langley Avenue
Chicago, IL 60628-3819
800-621-2736
Fax: 800-621-8476
TTY: 888-630-9347
www.gallaudet.edu/~gupress
This useful guide for teachers and therapists approaches speechreading instruction with the help of context cues.
32 pages

4555 Speechreading: A Way to Improve Understanding
Gallaudet University
11030 S Langley Avenue
Chicago, IL 60628-3819
800-621-2736
Fax: 800-621-8476
TTY: 888-630-9347
www.gallaudet.edu/~gupress

Designed for a wide audience, this book presents valuable information on the nature and process of speechreading and its benefits.
152 pages

4556 Speechreading: A Way to Improve Understand ing
Harriet Kaplan, author
Hearing Loss Association of America
7910 Woodmont Avenue   301-657-2248
Bethesda, MD 20814   Fax: 301-913-9413
                                   TTY: 3016572249
                             e-mail: info@hearingloss.org
                                   www.hearingloss.org
Discusses the nature and process of speechreading, its benefits, and its limitations. This useful book clarifies commonly-held misconceptions about speechreading. The beginning chapters address difficult communication situations and problems related to the speaker, the speechreader, and the environment It then offers strategies to manage them.
160 pages Paperback
Jerry Portis, Executive Director
Brenda Battat, Assistant Executive Director

4557 Study of American Deaf Folklore
Gallaudet University
11030 S Langley Avenue
Chicago, IL 60628-3819   800-621-2736
                                   Fax: 800-621-8476
                                   TTY: 888-630-9347
                             www.gallaudet.edu/~gupress
Presents a discussion of the different functions that folklore serves in the community.
156 pages

4558 Substance Abuse and Recovery: Empowerment of Deaf Persons
Gallaudet University
11030 S Langley Avenue
Chicago, IL 60628-3819   800-621-2736
                                   Fax: 800-621-8476
                                   TTY: 888-630-9347
                             www.gallaudet.edu/~gupress
Professionals in the field of substance abuse and deafness present their views on abuse.
217 pages

4559 Talk with Me
Alexander Graham Bell Association
3417 Volta Place NW   202-337-5220
Washington, DC 20007-2737   Fax: 202-337-8270
                                   TTY: 202-337-5220
Written by a clinical psychologist and mother, this book educates parents and professionals about crucial early decisions that affect the speech, language, auditory, social and emotional development of children with hearing impairments.
222 pages

4560 Teaching English to the Deaf as a Second Language
Depart. of English, Gallaudet University
800 Florida Avenue NE   202-651-5000
Washington, DC 20002   e-mail: janice-johnson@gallaudet.edu
                                   eli.gallaudet.edu/
Publishes articles of practical interest to classroom teachers of hearing impaired and second language students.

Kendall Green

4561 There's a Hearing Impaired Child in my Class
Gallaudet University
11030 S Langley Avenue
Chicago, IL 60628-3819   800-621-2736
                                   Fax: 800-621-8476
                                   TTY: 888-630-9347
                             www.gallaudet.edu/~gupress
This complete package provides basic facts about deafness, practical strategies for teaching hearing impaired children, and the question-and-answer information for all students.
44 pages

4562 Thirteen Keys to A Successful High School Experience
Alexander Graham Bell Association

3417 Volta Place NW   202-337-5220
Washington, DC 20007-2737   Fax: 202-337-8270
                                   TTY: 202-337-5220
In this booklet, three students who have profound hearing losses share their mainstream education experiences. This booklet is great for teachers of any age child and many of the suggestions to make mainstreaming easier are practical and easy to implement.
1996 28 pages

4563 Toward Effective Public School Programs for Deaf Students
Thomas N. Kluwin, Donald F. Moores, Gonter Gaustad, author
Teachers College Press
1234 Amsterdam Avenue   212-678-3929
New York, NY 10027   Fax: 212-678-4149
                             e-mail: tcpress@tc.columbia.edu
                                   www.teacherscollegepress.com
Examining various options for providing effective education-including the highly controversial practice of mainstreaming-the editors base their study on one of the largest and longest-running studies ever of public school programs for the deaf.
272 pages
ISBN: 0-807731-59-5
Martha Gonter Gaustad, Editors

4564 Understanding Deafness Socially
Gallaudet University
11030 S Langley Avenue
Chicago, IL 60628-3819   800-621-2736
                                   Fax: 800-621-8476
                                   TTY: 888-630-9347
                             www.gallaudet.edu/~gupress
Articles on the social dynamics of deafness.
196 pages

4565 Understanding Ear Infections
Alexander Graham Bell Association
3417 Volta Place NW   202-337-5220
Washington, DC 20007-2737   Fax: 202-337-8270
                                   TTY: 202-337-5220
Based on medical research, this clinical aid for medical and hearing professionals explains ear infections and their complications to patients and their families. Sturdily designed of cardboard and spiral-bound, each page has photos and diagrams that explain each topic and answer commonly asked questions about ear infections.
1993 27 pages

4566 Viewpoints on Deafness
National Association of the Deaf
8630 Fenton Street   301-587-1788
Silver Spring, MD 20910   Fax: 301-587-1791
                                   TTY: 301-587-1789
                                   www.nad.org
Monograph presents a collection of viewpoints on deafness.
157 pages Paperback
Donna Morris, Publications Manager

4567 Visible Speech
SRC Software Research Corporation
Box 4277, Station A   250-727-3744
Victoria, BC, V8X 3X8,
Computerized speech culture, analysis and computer-based speech training.
6 pages
AE Wright, Publisher

4568 Voyage to an Island
Gallaudet University
11030 S Langley Avenue
Chicago, IL 60628-3819   800-621-2736
                                   Fax: 800-621-8476
                                   TTY: 888-630-9347
                             www.gallaudet.edu/~gupress
This book recounts the story of how the author, a deaf woman from Finland, adjusts to moving to the exotic island of St. Lucia.
248 pages

4569 Week the World Heard Gallaudet
Gallaudet University

11030 S Langley Avenue
Chicago, IL 60628-3819
800-621-2736
Fax: 800-621-8476
TTY: 888-630-9347
www.gallaudet.edu/~gupress

This book gives the readers a day-by-day description of the Deaf President Now movement as it unfolded from March 6 to 13, 1988.
176 pages Paperback

4570 What is an Audiogram?
Gallaudet University
11030 S Langley Avenue
Chicago, IL 60628-3819
800-621-2736
Fax: 800-621-8476
TTY: 888-630-9347
www.gallaudet.edu/~gupress

Here's a cheery friend to solve the mysteries of the audiogram.
16 pages

4571 What's that Pig Outdoors? A Memoir of Deafness
Henry Kisor, author

Pengiuin Group
375 Hudson Street
New York, NY 10014-3657
800-526-0275
Fax: 212-366-2952
e-mail: ecommerce@us.penguin.com
www.us.penguin.com

Life of a journalist who is deaf and lives in a hearing world lipreading. Discusses some of the technical advances which help the deaf.
288 pages Hardcover
ISBN: 0-140148-99-2

4572 When Your Child is Deaf: A Guide for Parents
Alexander Graham Bell Association
3417 Volta Place NW
Washington, DC 20007-2737
202-337-5220
Fax: 202-337-8270
TTY: 202-337-5220

This book gives encouragement and advice to parents on their essential roles in teaching speech to their child.
182 pages

4573 When the Mind Hears
Gallaudet University
11030 S Langley Avenue
Chicago, IL 60628-3819
800-621-2736
Fax: 800-621-8476
TTY: 888-630-9347
www.gallaudet.edu/~gupress

Told largely from the vantage point of Laurent Clerc.
460 pages

4574 Who Speaks for the Deaf Community?
National Association of the Deaf
8630 Fenton Street
Silver Spring, MD 20910
301-587-1788
Fax: 301-587-1791
TTY: 301-587-1789
www.nad.org

Paperback
Donna Morris, Publications Manager

4575 Wired for Sound
Gallaudet University
11030 S Langley Avenue
Chicago, IL 60628-3819
800-621-2736
Fax: 800-621-8476
TTY: 888-630-9347
www.gallaudet.edu/~gupress

Secondary school edition of Ear Gear, this attractive workbook is designed to give older students an in-depth understanding of hearing and hearing aids.
156 pages

4576 Working with Deaf People: Accessibility and Accommodation in the Workplace
2600 S 1st Street
Springfield, IL 62704-4730
217-789-8980
Fax: 217-789-9130
e-mail: books@ccthomas.com
www.ccthomas.com

Reveals the kinds of patterns of work adjustment problems that can surface among deaf employees, including the points of view of both supervisors an deaf people.
250 pages Paperback
ISBN: 0-398061-26-2
Charles C Thomas, Publisher

4577 Working with Deaf Persons in Sunday School
Sunday School Board of the Southern Baptists
127 9th Avenue N
Nashville, TN 37234-0001
800-458-2772

Provides guidance for organizing and conducting Sunday School classes/departments for deaf children, youth and adults.

4578 Writer's Workshop
Gallaudet University
11030 S Langley Avenue
Chicago, IL 60628-3819
800-621-2736
Fax: 800-621-8476
TTY: 888-630-9347
www.gallaudet.edu/~gupress

Offers suggestions to teachers who are interested in turning the classroom into an environment where students learn to express themselves in writing.
95 pages

4579 You Just Don't Understand
Deborah Tannen, author

Hearing Loss Association of America
7910 Woodmont Avenue
Bethesda, MD 20814-3079
301-657-2248
Fax: 301-913-9413
TTY: 301-657-2249
e-mail: info@hearingloss.org
www.hearingloss.org

Studded with lively and entertaining examples of real conversations, this book gives you the tools to understand what went wrong — and to find a common language in which to strengthen relationships at work and at home. A classic in the field of interpersonal relations, this book will change forever the way you approach conversations.
Softcover
ISBN: 0-060959-62-2
Jerry Portis, Executive Director
Brenda Battat, Assistant Executive Director

4580 You and Your Deaf Child
Gallaudet University
11030 S Langley Avenue
Chicago, IL 60628-3819
800-621-2736
Fax: 800-621-8476
TTY: 888-630-9347
www.gallaudet.edu/~gupress

This guide for parents explores how families interact to deal with the special impact of a child who is hearing impaired.
1997 224 pages 2nd edition

Children's Books

4581 ABC's of Finger Spelling
Modern Signs Press
PO Box 1181
Los Alamitos, CA 90720-1181
562-596-8548
800-572-7332
Fax: 562-795-6614
TTY: 562-493-4168
e-mail: modsigns@aol.com
www.modsigns.com

Helps teach upper and lower case letters of the alphabet. Includes printed letters and easy-to-follow drawings of the hand shapes.
60 pages
ISBN: 0-916708-13-6

4582 Alphabet of Animal Signs
Garlic Press
605 Powers Street
Eugene, OR 97402-5337
541-345-0063
Fax: 541-345-0063
e-mail: garlicpress@mindspring.com
www.garlicpress.com

Presents animal illustrations and associated signs for each letter of the alphabet.
16 pages Paperback
ISBN: 0-931993-65-2
SH Collins, Contact

4583   Animal Signs: A First Book of Sign Language
Gallaudet University
11030 S Langley Avenue
Chicago, IL 60628-3819   800-621-2736
                                          Fax: 800-621-8476
                                          TTY: 888-630-9347
                                   www.gallaudet.edu/~gupress
Full-color photos of animals and their signs.
16 pages Ages 1-4

4584   Another Handful of Stories
Gallaudet University
11030 S Langley Avenue
Chicago, IL 60628-3819   800-621-2736
                                          Fax: 800-621-8476
                                          TTY: 888-630-9347
                                   www.gallaudet.edu/~gupress
Second book contains a series of 37 stories told by deaf individuals.
124 pages

4585   At Grandma's House
Modern Signs Press
PO Box 1181   562-596-8548
Los Alamitos, CA 90720-1181   800-572-7332
                                          Fax: 562-795-6614
                                          TTY: 562-493-4168
                                     e-mail: modsigns@aol.com
                                          www.modsigns.com
Pictures, signs and printed words tell the tale of April, a cuddly little rabbit who loves to play with her beloved Grandma.
28 pages

4586   Be Happy, Not Sad
Modern Signs Press
PO Box 1181   562-596-8548
Los Alamitos, CA 90720   800-572-7332
                                          Fax: 562-795-6614
                                          TTY: 562-493-4168
                                     e-mail: modsigns@aol.com
                                          www.modsigns.com
These books help children understand hard to explain emotions through signing. Includes Be Happy Not Sad coloring workbook.
2 Book Set

4587   Belonging
Gallaudet University
11030 S Langley Avenue
Chicago, IL 60628-3819   800-621-2736
                                          Fax: 800-621-8476
                                          TTY: 888-630-9347
                                   www.gallaudet.edu/~gupress
Gustie Blaine loses her hearing after an illness and must now learn to accept her loss and understand the changes it brings.
176 pages

4588   Chris Gets Ear Tubes
Gallaudet University
11030 S Langley Avenue
Chicago, IL 60628-3819   800-621-2736
                                          Fax: 800-621-8476
                                          TTY: 888-630-9347
                                   www.gallaudet.edu/~gupress
A helpful book for parents and children to share concerning ear tubes and hospitals.
44 pages

4589   Clerc: The Story of His Early Years
Gallaudet University
11030 S Langley Avenue
Chicago, IL 60628-3819   800-621-2736
                                          Fax: 800-621-8476
                                          TTY: 888-630-9347
                                   www.gallaudet.edu/~gupress

A novel by Laurent Clerc, a deaf teacher who helped Gallaudet establish schools to educate deaf Americans.
208 pages

4590   Come Sign with Us: Sign Language Activities for Children
Gallaudet University
11030 S Langley Avenue
Chicago, IL 60628-3819   800-621-2736
                                          Fax: 800-621-8476
                                          TTY: 888-630-9347
                                   www.gallaudet.edu/~gupress
Revised version, offering more follow-up activities, including many in context, to teach children sign language. Features more than 300 line drawings of both adults and children signing familiar words, phrases, and sentences using ASL. Shows how to form each sign exactly and also presents the origins of ASL, facts about deafness, and the deaf community.
160 pages Softcover
ISBN: 1-563680-51-3

4591   Day We Met Cindy
Gallaudet University
11030 S Langley Avenue
Chicago, IL 60628-3819   800-621-2736
                                          Fax: 800-621-8476
                                          TTY: 888-630-9347
                                   www.gallaudet.edu/~gupress
A picture storybook telling the story of Cindy, the hearing impaired aunt of one of the students of a first grade class.
32 pages

4592   Finger Alphabet
Gallaudet University
11030 S Langley Avenue
Chicago, IL 60628-3819   800-621-2736
                                          Fax: 800-621-8476
                                          TTY: 888-630-9347
                                   www.gallaudet.edu/~gupress
Includes activities for improving fingerspelling.
30 pages

4593   Flying Fingers Club
Gallaudet University
11030 S Langley Avenue
Chicago, IL 60628-3819   800-621-2736
                                          Fax: 800-621-8476
                                          TTY: 888-630-9347
                                   www.gallaudet.edu/~gupress
Three young friends, one deaf and two hearing find they can communicate secretly in sign language.
104 pages

4594   Gift of the Girl Who Couldn't Hear
Alexander Graham Bell Association
3417 Volta Place NW   202-337-5220
Washington, DC 20007-2737   Fax: 202-337-8270
                                          TTY: 202-337-5220
This fictional novel for middle school readers introduces Eliza, a gifted singer and Lucy, her best friend who has been deaf since birth.
79 pages

4595   Goldilocks and the Three Bears
Gallaudet University
11030 S Langley Avenue
Chicago, IL 60628-3819   800-621-2736
                                          Fax: 800-621-8476
                                          TTY: 888-630-9347
                                   www.gallaudet.edu/~gupress
Offers children ages 3-8 the classic story with new words and matching signs in Signed English.
48 pages Casebound
ISBN: 1-563680-57-2

4596   Grandfather Moose
Modern Signs Press

PO Box 1181
Los Alamitos, CA 90720-1181

562-596-8548
800-572-7332
Fax: 562-795-6614
TTY: 562-493-4168
e-mail: modsigns@aol.com
www.modsigns.com

Offers exciting and beautifully illustrated rhymes, games and chants in sign language.
32 pages

4597 Handful of Stories
Gallaudet University
11030 S Langley Avenue
Chicago, IL 60628-3819

800-621-2736
Fax: 800-621-8476
TTY: 888-630-9347
www.gallaudet.edu/~gupress

Sometimes incredible, moving and amusing, these stories are based on the personal experiences of deaf storytellers.
118 pages

4598 Handmade Alphabet
Gallaudet University
11030 S Langley Avenue
Chicago, IL 60628-3819

800-621-2736
Fax: 800-621-8476
TTY: 888-630-9347
www.gallaudet.edu/~gupress

This book presents 26 beautiful color drawings showing a hand forming a letter of the manual alphabet.
26 pages

4599 Hasta Luego, San Diego
Gallaudet University
11030 S Langley Avenue
Chicago, IL 60628-3819

800-621-2736
Fax: 800-621-8476
TTY: 888-630-9347
www.gallaudet.edu/~gupress

A Flying Fingers Club mystery.
104 pages

4600 Hearing Loss
Franklin Watts Grolier
90 Old Sherman Tpke
Danbury, CT 06816-0001

203-797-3500
800-621-1115
Fax: 203-797-3197
www.grolier.com

Offers a concise explanation of how and why hearing losses occur, how the ear works and how to protect your hearing.
144 pages Grades 7-12
ISBN: 0-531125-19-0

4601 I Have a Sister, My Sister is Deaf
TJ Publishers
817 Silver Spring Avenue
Silver Spring, MD 20910-4617

301-585-4440
800-999-1168
Fax: 301-585-5930
TTY: 301-585-4441
e-mail: tjpubinc@aol.com

An emphatic, affirmative look at the relationship between siblings, as a young deaf child is affectionately described by her older sister. This Coretta Scott King honor award winner helps young children develop an understanding that deaf children share the same interests as hearing children.
1977 32 pages Softcover
ISBN: 0-064430-59-6
Angela K Thames, President
Jerald A Murphy, VP

4602 I Was So Mad!
Modern Signs Press
PO Box 1181
Los Alamitos, CA 90720-1181

562-596-8548
800-572-7332
Fax: 562-795-6614
TTY: 562-493-4168
e-mail: modsigns@aol.com
www.modsigns.com

Includes manual alphabet and glossary of signs.
40 pages
ISBN: 0-916708-16-0

4603 In Our House
Modern Signs Press
PO Box 1181
Los Alamitos, CA 90720-1181

562-596-8548
800-572-7332
Fax: 562-795-6614
TTY: 562-493-4168
e-mail: modsigns@aol.com
www.modsigns.com

This colorful picturebook tells the story of Joy and Jason helping Mom and Dad around the house. Has a 140-word vocabulary listed in an alphabetical glossary.
32 pages
ISBN: 0-191670-81-1

4604 Invisible Inc #4
Alexander Graham Bell Association
3417 Volta Place NW
Washington, DC 20007-2737

202-337-5220
Fax: 202-337-8270
TTY: 202-337-5220

The intrepid trio accept an invitation to doom as they solve the mystery behind their school's haunted computer.
1996 42 pages

4605 King Midas With Selected Sentences in ASL
Gallaudet University
11030 S Langley Avenue
Chicago, IL 60628-3819

800-621-2736
Fax: 800-621-8476
TTY: 888-630-9347
www.gallaudet.edu/~gupress

Fairytale retold with full color illustrations and American Sign Language sentences.
72 pages Casebound
ISBN: 0-930323-75-0

4606 Learning to Sign in my Neighborhood
Gallaudet University
11030 S Langley Avenue
Chicago, IL 60628-3819

800-621-2736
Fax: 800-621-8476
TTY: 888-630-9347
www.gallaudet.edu/~gupress

Here are signs to learn and pictures to color, all in one friendly book.
32 pages

4607 Little Green Monsters
Modern Signs Press
PO Box 1181
Los Alamitos, CA 90720-1181

562-596-8548
800-572-7332
Fax: 562-795-6614
TTY: 310-493-4168

Forty-five word vocabulary in signs and printed words introduces concept of directionality. Includes manual alphabet and glossary of signs.
36 pages

4608 Little Red Riding Hood
Gallaudet University
11030 S Langley Avenue
Chicago, IL 60628-3819

800-621-2736
Fax: 800-621-8476
TTY: 888-630-9347
www.gallaudet.edu/~gupress

A beloved folktale that is told in American Sign Language format.
48 pages

4609 Living with Deafness
Franklin Watts Grolier
90 Old Sherman Tpke
Danbury, CT 06816-0001

203-797-3500
800-621-1115
Fax: 203-797-3197
www.grolier.com

Shows how deaf persons can overcome their disability and live happy, productive lives.
32 pages Grades 5-7
ISBN: 0-531108-42-2

4610   Mandy
Gallaudet University
11030 S Langley Avenue
Chicago, IL 60628-3819   800-621-2736
                                                    Fax: 800-621-8476
                                                    TTY: 888-630-9347
                                                    www.gallaudet.edu/~gupress
A beautiful story about a young deaf girl's relationship with her grandmother.
32 pages

4611   Matthew Pinkowski's Special Summer
Gallaudet University
11030 S Langley Avenue
Chicago, IL 60628-3819   800-621-2736
                                                    Fax: 800-621-8476
                                                    TTY: 888-630-9347
                                                    www.gallaudet.edu/~gupress
Matthew begins his special summer by moving to Minnesota, where he meets some special friends.
150 pages

4612   Messy Monsters, Jungle Joggers and Bubble Baths
Alexander Graham Bell Association
3417 Volta Place NW   202-337-5220
Washington, DC 20007-2737   Fax: 202-337-8270
                                                    TTY: 202-337-5220
This child's work book is filled with poems, stories and delightful drawings that make speaking lip reading and using residual hearing fun for the elementary school aged child.
97 pages

4613   Mother Goose in Sign
Garlic Press
605 Powers Street   541-345-0063
Eugene, OR 97402-5337   Fax: 541-345-0063
                                    e-mail: garlicpress@mindspring.com
                                                    www.garlicpress.com
Fully illustrated Mother Goose nursery rhymes in sign language.
16 pages Paperback
ISBN: 0-931993-66-0
SH Collins, Contact

4614   My ABC Signs of Animal Friends
DawnSignPress
6130 Nancy Ridge Drive   619-625-0600
San Diego, CA 92121-3223   800-549-5350
                                                    Fax: 619-625-2336
                                           e-mail: DawnSign@aol.com
Sign language primer for both hearing and deaf children from birth to age five.
32 pages
ISBN: 0-915035-31-6

4615   My First Book of Sign
Gallaudet University
11030 S Langley Avenue
Chicago, IL 60628-3819   800-621-2736
                                                    Fax: 800-621-8476
                                                    TTY: 888-630-9347
                                                    www.gallaudet.edu/~gupress
This book makes signing fun for children from three to eight.
76 pages

4616   My Signing Book of Numbers
Gallaudet University
11030 S Langley Avenue
Chicago, IL 60628-3819   800-621-2736
                                                    Fax: 800-621-8476
                                                    TTY: 888-630-9347
                                                    www.gallaudet.edu/~gupress
Picture book helps children learn their numbers in sign language.
56 pages

4617   Nick's Mission
Alexander Graham Bell Association
3417 Volta Place NW   202-337-5220
Washington, DC 20007-2737   Fax: 202-337-8270
                                                    TTY: 202-337-5220
Twelve-year-old Nick plans to spend his summer vacation at the lake, snorkeling and playing with Wags, his dog, not at speech therapy as his mother has planned. But the summer will embroil Nick and Wags in an exciting mystery that includes kidnapping, smuggling, stolen macaws and maybe even speech therapy.
1996 148 pages

4618   Now I Understand
Gallaudet University
11030 S Langley Avenue
Chicago, IL 60628-3819   800-621-2736
                                                    Fax: 800-621-8476
                                                    TTY: 888-630-9347
                                                    www.gallaudet.edu/~gupress
Explores what happens when a hard-of-hearing boy is mainstreamed.
56 pages

4619   Number and Letter Games
Gallaudet University
11030 S Langley Avenue
Chicago, IL 60628-3819   800-621-2736
                                                    Fax: 800-621-8476
                                                    TTY: 888-630-9347
                                                    www.gallaudet.edu/~gupress
A fascinating way to learning sign language with games, riddles and map skills for children and adults.
30 pages

4620   Nursery Rhymes from Mother Goose
Gallaudet University
11030 S Langley Avenue
Chicago, IL 60628-3819   800-621-2736
                                                    Fax: 800-621-8476
                                                    TTY: 888-630-9347
                                                    www.gallaudet.edu/~gupress
The complete nursery rhyme is presented in Signed English.
64 pages

4621   Popsicles are Cold
Modern Signs Press
PO Box 1181   562-596-8548
Los Alamitos, CA 90720-1181   800-572-7332
                                                    Fax: 562-795-6614
                                                    TTY: 562-493-4168
                                           e-mail: modsigns@aol.com
                                                    www.modsigns.com
Colorful pictures and rhyming words highlight this storybook with a 33-word vocabulary in signs and printed words.
32 pages

4622   Season of Change
Gallaudet University
11030 S Langley Avenue
Chicago, IL 60628-3819   800-621-2736
                                                    Fax: 800-621-8476
                                                    TTY: 888-630-9347
                                                    www.gallaudet.edu/~gupress
A cheerful teenager tired of having people treat her as a problem just because she does not hear very well.
108 pages

4623   Secret Signing: A Sign Language Activity Book
Gallaudet University
11030 S Langley Avenue
Chicago, IL 60628-3819   800-621-2736
                                                    Fax: 800-621-8476
                                                    TTY: 888-630-9347
                                                    www.gallaudet.edu/~gupress
Children will enjoy this activity book with signs.
64 pages Level K-1

4624   Secret in the Dorm Attic
Gallaudet University

11030 S Langley Avenue
Chicago, IL 60628-3819
800-621-2736
Fax: 800-621-8476
TTY: 888-630-9347
www.gallaudet.edu/~gupress

Susan, Donald and Matt are back, as the Flying Fingers Club solving yet another mystery.
104 pages

4625 Sesame Street Sign Language ABC
Gallaudet University
11030 S Langley Avenue
Chicago, IL 60628-3819
800-621-2736
Fax: 800-621-8476
TTY: 888-630-9347
www.gallaudet.edu/~gupress

Muppets learn words and letters signed by Linda Bove.
30 pages

4626 Sesame Street Sign Language Fun
Gallaudet University
11030 S Langley Avenue
Chicago, IL 60628-3819
800-621-2736
Fax: 800-621-8476
TTY: 888-630-9347
www.gallaudet.edu/~gupress

This book uses the Muppets to explain concepts such as opposites, words and feelings.
62 pages

4627 Sign Numbers
Modern Signs Press
PO Box 1181
Los Alamitos, CA 90720-1181
562-596-8548
800-572-7332
Fax: 562-795-6614
TTY: 562-493-4168
e-mail: modsigns@aol.com
www.modsigns.com

A manual teaching sign language and written numbers that includes printed numbers and easy-to-follow drawings of the number hand shapes.
60 pages

4628 Sign-Me-Fine
Gallaudet University
11030 S Langley Avenue
Chicago, IL 60628-3819
800-621-2736
Fax: 800-621-8476
TTY: 888-630-9347
www.gallaudet.edu/~gupress

Written for young adults, this book introduces American Sign Language and how it differs from English.
120 pages

4629 Signed Language Coloring Books
Gallaudet University
11030 S Langley Avenue
Chicago, IL 60628-3819
800-621-2736
Fax: 800-621-8476
TTY: 888-630-9347
www.gallaudet.edu/~gupress

Six coloring books made up of easy-to-color pictures that include the printed, signed and fingerspelled words for each image.
16 pages

4630 Signing for Kids
Gallaudet University
11030 S Langley Avenue
Chicago, IL 60628-3819
800-621-2736
Fax: 800-621-8476
TTY: 888-630-9347
www.gallaudet.edu/~gupress

Contains 17 chapters dealing with special areas of interest to children like pets, family, friends and people.
142 pages

4631 Signs for Me: Basic Vocabulary for Children, Parents and Teachers
DawnSignPress

6130 Nancy Ridge Drive
San Diego, CA 92121-3223
619-625-0600
800-549-5350
Fax: 619-625-2336
e-mail: DawnSign@aol.com

ASL/English vocabulary primer filled with all the basics for pre-schoolers. The focus is on learning ASL signs and English words for better language development. Illustrates the meaning of the sign, the sign itself, and the English word in bold print.
112 pages
ISBN: 0-915035-27-8

4632 Silent Dances
Gallaudet University
11030 S Langley Avenue
Chicago, IL 60628-3819
800-621-2736
Fax: 800-621-8476
TTY: 888-630-9347
www.gallaudet.edu/~gupress

Space adventure story featuring a deaf graduate of Gallaudet University.
275 pages

4633 Silent Garden: Raising Your Deaf Child
Alexander Graham Bell Association
3417 Volta Place NW
Washington, DC 20007-2737
202-337-5220
Fax: 202-337-8270
TTY: 202-337-5220

This book provides parents of deaf children with crucial information on the possibilities afforded their children. Ogden, deaf since birth and a professor of deaf studies offers parents the foundation for making the difficult decisions necessary to start their children on the road to realizing their full potential.
1996 313 pages

4634 Silent Observer
Gallaudet University
11030 S Langley Avenue
Chicago, IL 60628-3819
800-621-2736
Fax: 800-621-8476
TTY: 888-630-9347
www.gallaudet.edu/~gupress

Lovely illustrations tell the story of an affectionate memoir of childhood presented through the eyes of a deaf girl.
48 pages

4635 Simple Signs
Gallaudet University
11030 S Langley Avenue
Chicago, IL 60628-3819
800-621-2736
Fax: 800-621-8476
TTY: 888-630-9347
www.gallaudet.edu/~gupress

Charming, full-color pictures and hints introducing ASL to children.
32 pages

4636 Sleeping Beauty
Gallaudet University
11030 S Langley Avenue
Chicago, IL 60628-3819
800-621-2736
Fax: 800-621-8476
TTY: 888-630-9347
www.gallaudet.edu/~gupress

Classic story with full-color illustrations and line drawings of more than 30 sentences rendered in ASL, offering new dimensions of imagination while also strengthening young readers' language skills.
64 pages
ISBN: 0-930323-97-1

4637 Songs in Sign
Gallaudet University
11030 S Langley Avenue
Chicago, IL 60628-3819
800-621-2736
Fax: 800-621-8476
TTY: 888-630-9347
www.gallaudet.edu/~gupress

Fully illustrated sign English.
30 pages

4638 Very Special Sister
Gallaudet University
11030 S Langley Avenue
Chicago, IL 60628-3819   800-621-2736
                               Fax: 800-621-8476
                               TTY: 888-630-9347
                               www.gallaudet.edu/~gupress
Tells the story of Laura who is deaf and her delight at the fact that
she will soon have a brother.
36 pages

4639 Where Is Spot?
Gallaudet University
11030 S Langley Avenue
Chicago, IL 60628-3819   800-621-2736
                               Fax: 800-621-8476
                               TTY: 888-630-9347
                               www.gallaudet.edu/~gupress
A Signed English edition of a childhood favorite.
20 pages

4640 Word Signs: A First Book of Sign Language
Gallaudet University
11030 S Langley Avenue
Chicago, IL 60628-3819   800-621-2736
                               Fax: 800-621-8476
                               TTY: 888-630-9347
                               www.gallaudet.edu/~gupress
Full-color photos of basic words and their signs.
16 pages Ages 1-4

Magazines

4641 American Annals of the Deaf
Convention of American Instructors of the Deaf
800 Florida Avenue NE   202-651-5530
Washington, DC 20002-3660   Fax: 202-651-5860
                               TTY: 202-651-5530
                               e-mail: mary.carew@galludet.edu
                               gupress.gallaudet.edu/annals/
Scholarly journal at the forefront of research related to the educa-
tion of deaf people. Annual reference Issue identifies programs
and services for deaf people nationwide.
64 pages 5x Year
Donald Moores, Editor
Mary E Carew, Managing Editor

4642 American Journal of Audiology
American Speech-Language-Hearing Association
10801 Rockville Pike   301-897-5700
Rockville, MD 20852-3226   800-638-8255
                               e-mail: actioncenter@asha.org
                               www.asha.org
Russell L Malone PhD, Editor

4643 American Journal of Speech-Language Pathology
American Speech-Language-Hearing Association
10801 Rockville Pike   301-897-5700
Rockville, MD 20852-3226   800-638-8255
Russell L Malone PhD, Editor

4644 Audiology Today
1735 N Lynn Street   703-524-1923
Arlington, VA 22209-2019   Fax: 703-524-2303
Jerry Northern PhD, Editor

4645 Auricle
Auditory-Verbal International
2121 Eisenhower Avenue   703-739-1049
Alexandria, VA 22314-4688   Fax: 703-739-0395
                               TTY: 703-739-0874
                               e-mail: audiverb@aol.com
                               www.auditory-verbal.org
To provide the choice of listening and speaking as the way of life
for children and adults who are deaf on hard of hearing.
Magazine
Sara Lake, Executive Director/CEO/Publisher
Mary Benson, Executive Assistant

4646 Deaf Life
MSM Productions
PO Box 23380   716-442-6370
Rochester, NY 14692-3380   Fax: 716-442-6371
                               www.deaflife.com
This magazine focuses on profiles, news, controversial issues, cul-
tural topics and more relating to the Deaf community.
50 pages Monthly
Matthew Moore, Publisher

4647 Deaf Sports Review
American Athletic Association of the Deaf
3607 Washington Boulevard   801-393-8710
Ogden, UT 84403-1737   Fax: 801-393-2263
                               TTY: 801-393-7916
A magazine that describes deaf athletes and past and upcoming
events.
Quarterly
Shirley Platt, Editor

4648 Deaf USA
Eye Festival Communications
6917B Woodley Avenue   818-902-9800
Van Nuys, CA 91406-4844   Fax: 818-902-9840
Provides news coverage on all activities and issues of interest to
deaf and hard of hearing readers as well as professionals and asso-
ciates within this specialized market.
Monthly
David Rosenbaum, Editor

4649 Deaf-Blind American
American Association of the Deaf-Blind
814 Thayer Avenue
Silver Spring, MD 20910-4500   800-735-2258
                               Fax: 301-588-8705
                               TTY: 301-588-6545
                               e-mail: aadb@erols.com
A journal of the American Association of the Deaf-Blind with arti-
cles on new technology, legislation news affecting deaf-blind
Americans, success stories on deaf-blind, conference news, and
many other topics of interest to deaf-blind people.
4x Year
Jamie McNamara, Editor

4650 Hearing Health
1050 17th Street NW   209-289-5850
Washington, DC 20036   e-mail: info@hearinghealthmag.com
A publication for deaf and hard-of-hearing people, as well as hear-
ing health care professionals, libraries, agencies, schools and orga-
nizations.
BiMonthly
Paula Bartone-Bonillas, Editor

4651 JADARA
ADARA
PO Box 251554   501-868-8850
Little Rock, AR 72225-1554   Fax: 501-868-8812
A journal for professionals networking for excellence in service
delivery with individuals who are deaf or hard of hearing. The jour-
nal is a vehicle for dissemination and exchange of information
which has a large bearing on the quality of service delivery to the
deaf and hearing impaired populations.
Quarterly
Gerry Walter, Editor

4652 Journal of AAA
American Academy of Audiology
1735 N Lynn Street   703-524-1923
Arlington, VA 22209-2019   800-222-2336
                               Fax: 703-524-2303
James Jerger, Editor

4653 Journal of Speech-Language-Hearing Research
American Speech-Language-Hearing Association
10801 Rockville Pike   301-897-5700
Rockville, MD 20852-3226   800-638-8255
Russell L Malone PhD, Editor

4654 Language, Speech and Hearing Services in the Schools
American Speech-Language-Hearing Association

10801 Rockville Pike 301-897-5700
Rockville, MD 20852 800-638-8255
Professional journal for clinicians, audiologists and speech-language pathologists.

Russell L Malone PhD, Editor

4655 NADmag
National Association of the Deaf
8630 Fenton Street 301-587-1788
Silver Spring, MD 20910 Fax: 301-587-1791
TTY: 301-587-1789
www.nad.org/nadmagadrates
Each NADmag focuses on a specific theme, such as technology and telecommunications, human services, deaf culture, education, and interpreting.
32 pages Bi-Monthly
Donna Morris, Publications Manager

4656 Perspectives in Education and Deafness
Gallaudet University
11030 S Langley Avenue
Chicago, IL 60628-3819 800-621-2736
Fax: 800-621-8476
TTY: 888-630-9347
www.gallaudet.edu/~gupress
A practical, reader-friendly magazine, offering help and advice in and beyond the classroom, tuned to the needs of today's students, teachers, and families.
5x Annually
Mary Abrams Perica, Editor

4657 SHHH Journal
Self Help For Hard of Hearing People
7910 Woodmont Avenue 301-657-2248
Bethesda, MD 20814-3079 Fax: 301-913-9413
TTY: 301-657-2249
An educational journal about hearing loss for hard-of-hearing people.
BiMonthly
Barbara G Harris, Editor

4658 Silent News
1425 Jefferson Road 716-272-4900
Rochester, NY 14623-3139 Fax: 716-272-4904
TTY: 716-272-4900
Covers news and events of interest to deaf and hard-of-hearing people all over the world.
Monthly
Tom Willard, Editor

4659 Silent News Job Bulletin
1425 Jefferson Road 716-272-4900
Rochester, NY 14623-3139 Fax: 716-272-4904
TTY: 716-272-4900
Lists current job openings and career opportunities working with deaf and hard-of-hearing people.
BiAnnually

4660 Tinnitus Today
American Tinnitus Association
PO Box 5
Portland, OR 97207-0005 503-248-9985
800-634-8978
Fax: 503-248-0024
www.ata.org
A quarterly magazine published by the American Tinnitus Association.
28 pages Quarterly
ISBN: 1-530656-9 -
David P. Fagerlie, Chief Executive Officer
Terri Baltus, Chief Development Officer

4661 USA Deaf Sports Federation
3607 Washington Boulevard 801-393-8710
Ogden, UT 84403-1737 Fax: 801-393-2263
TTY: 801-393-7916
e-mail: homeoffice@usadsf.org
www.usadsf.org

A glossy magazine called Deaf Sports Review featuring articles on all deaf sports and recreation.
Dr. Bobbie Beth Scoggins, President
Valerie Kinney, Adminstrative Assistant

4662 Volta Review
Alexander Graham Bell Association
3417 Volta Place NW 202-337-5220
Washington, DC 20007-2737 Fax: 202-337-8270
TTY: 202-337-5220
A professionally reviewed journal highlighting research and studies in the field of deafness.
5x Year
Michelle Vanderhoff, Managing Editor

4663 Volta Voices
Alexander Graham Bell Association
3417 Volta Place NW 202-337-5220
Washington, DC 20007-2737 Fax: 202-337-8270
TTY: 202-337-5220
A magazine highlighting inspirational stories from parents of children who are deaf, legislative news, technology update and stories pertaining to speech, speech reading, and the use of residual hearing.
BiMonthly
Michelle Vanderhoff, Managing Editor

4664 World Around You
Gallaudet University
11030 S Langley Avenue
Chicago, IL 60628-3819 800-621-2736
Fax: 800-621-8476
TTY: 888-630-9347
www.gallaudet.edu/~gupress
A current events magazine directed at keeping junior high and high school deaf and hard-of-hearing students informed about deaf people and the deaf community.
5x Year
Cathryn Carroll, Editor

Newsletters

4665 AAAD Bulletin
American Athletic Association of the Deaf
3607 Washington Boulevard 801-393-8710
Ogden, UT 84403-1737 Fax: 801-393-2263
TTY: 801-393-7916
A newsletter describing deaf athletes and upcoming events.
Quarterly
Shirley Platt, Editor

4666 ADARA Updated
ADARA
PO Box 251554 501-868-8850
Little Rock, AR 72225-1554 Fax: 501-868-8812
Updates readers on events, resources, legislation, information of national interest, conferences, workshops and employment opportunities. Information from and about local chapters, special interest sections, and national organizations is included in this publication.
Quarterly
Nanncy Long PhD, Editor

4667 ALDA News
Association of Late-Deafened Adults
1131 Lake Street 877-907-1738
Oak Park, IL 60301 Fax: 877-907-1738
TTY: 708-358-0135
www.alda.org
Marilyn Howe, Publisher

4668 Adult Bible Lessons for the Deaf
Sunday School Board of the Southern Baptists
127 9th Avenue N
Nashville, TN 37234-0001 800-458-2772
Bible study quarterly that relates to the needs of deaf and hearing impaired persons.
Quarterly

4669 Audiology Express
American Academy of Audiology
1735 N Lynn Street   703-524-1923
Arlington, VA 22209-2019   800-222-2336
                                 Fax: 703-524-2303

4670 Better Hearing News
Better Hearing Institute
5021B Backlick Road   703-642-0580
Annandale, VA 22003-6043   800-327-9355
                                 Fax: 703-750-9302

Quarterly
Jerry J Rizzo, Executive Director

4671 Canine Listener
Dogs for the Deaf
10175 Wheeler Road   541-826-9220
Central Point, OR 97502   800-990-3647
                                 Fax: 541-826-6696
                                 TTY: 541-826-9220
                                 TDD: 541-826-9220
                     e-mail: info@dogsforthedeaf.org
                           www.dogsforthedeaf.org
Offers information on various dogs for the deaf that are available, hotlines, support groups and articles on the newest technology for the hard of hearing person.
Quarterly
Robin Dickson, President/CEO

4672 Caption Center News
Caption Center
125 Western Avenue   617-429-9225
Boston, MA 02134-1008   Fax: 617-562-0590
Reports developments in closed captioning for persons with hearing impairments.

4673 Deaf Artists of America
302 Goodman Street N   716-244-3460
Rochester, NY 14607-1148   Fax: 716-244-3690
                                 TTY: 716-244-3460

Tom Willard, Editor

4674 Deaf Episcopalian
Episcopal Conference of the Deaf
PO Box 27459   215-247-1059
Philadelphia, PA 19118-0459   e-mail: Bmose@aol.com
                                 www.ecdeaf.com/

Rev. Virginia Nagel, Editor

4675 Deaf Work
Baptist Sunday School Board
127 9th Avenue N   615-251-2000
Nashville, TN 37234-0002
Offers information for religious workers and church educators who teach the handicapped.

4676 Deafpride Advocate
Deafpride
1350 Potomac Avenue SE   202-675-6700
Washington, DC 20003-4412

4677 Endeavor
American Society for Deaf Children
PO Box 3355   717-334-7922
Gettysburg, PA 17325-1373   800-942-2732
                                 Fax: 717-334-8808
                                 TTY: 717-334-7922
                           e-mail: asdc1@aol.com
                           www.deafchildren.org

Newsletter for parents of deaf children.
36 pages Quarterly
Linda Zumbrun, Operations Manager

4678 Frat
National Fraternal Society of the Deaf
1300 W NW Highway   847-392-9282
Mt Prospect, IL 60056-2217   Fax: 847-392-9298
                                 TTY: 708-392-1409

Offers fraternal insurance information and news about members.
BiMonthly
Wayne D Shook, Editor

4679 GA-SK Newsletter
Telecommunications for the Deaf
8630 Fenton Street   301-589-3786
Silver Spring, MD 20910-3822 Fax: 301-589-3797
                                 TTY: 301-589-3006
A newsletter focusing on issues for the deaf and hearing impaired person.
Quarterly
Barry Solomon, Editor
Alfred Sonnenstrahl, Manager

4680 Gallaudet Today
Gallaudet University
575 5th Avenue   212-599-0027
Washington, DC 20002   Fax: 212-599-0039
                                 www.drf.org
A university publication with both general and special issues on deafness-related topics.
Quarterly
Vickie Walter, Editor

4681 Hear
Deafness Research Foundation
15 W 39th Street   212-768-1181
New York, NY 10018-3806
Offers information on the Foundation's activities and events, technical updates on assistive devices, legislative and medical information on the latest breakthroughs and laws for the hearing impaired, book reviews and resources.
Monte H Jacoby, Executive Director

4682 NTID Focus
National Technical Institute for the Deaf
52 Lomb Memorial Drive   716-475-6906
Rochester, NY 14623-5604   Fax: 716-475-5623
                           e-mail: ntidmc@rit.edu
                           www.rit.edu/ntid
A college publication featuring news and stories about NTID programs and community members.
TriAnnual
Kathryn Shwartz, Editor

4683 Newsletter of American Hearing Research
American Hearing Research Foundation
8 S Michigan Avenue   312-726-9670
Chicago, IL 60603-4539   Fax: 312-726-9695
               e-mail: blederer@american-hearing.org
                    www.american-hearing.org
Concerned with hearing research and education.
6-8 pages 3 per year
William L Lederer, Executive Director
Sharon Parmet, Development/Communications Associate

4684 Newsline
Sertoma Foundation
1912 E Meyer Boulevard   816-333-8300
Kansas City, MO 64132-1141   Fax: 816-333-4320
                           e-mail: info@sertoma.org
                                 www.sertoma.org
Reports on activities of the Sertoma Foundation in the field of speech and hearing impairments.

4685 Otoscope
EAR Foundation
1817 Patterson Street   615-329-7807
Nashville, TN 37203   800-545-4327
                                 Fax: 615-329-7935
                                 TTY: 615-329-7849
                           e-mail: ear@earfoundation.org
                           www.earfoundation.org

8-14 pages Quarterly
Amy Nielsen, Director Educational Progams

4686 Research at Gallaudet
Gallaudet University

11030 S Langley Avenue
Chicago, IL 60628-3819

800-621-2736
Fax: 800-621-8476
TTY: 888-630-9347
www.gallaudet.edu/~gupress

Newsletter reporting research and activities of the Institute.

4687 Speech and Deafness Newsletter
Hearing, Speech
1620 18th Avenue   206-323-5770
Seattle, WA 98122-2798
Agency newsletter for membership and community.
8 pages
Patty Tumberg, Editor

4688 Tech Talk
Caption Center
125 Western Avenue   617-492-9225
Boston, MA 02134-1008   Fax: 617-562-0590

4689 USA Deaf Sports Federation
3607 Washington Boulevard   801-393-8710
Ogden, UT 84403-1737   Fax: 801-393-2263
                                         TTY: 801-393-7916
                             e-mail: homeoffice@usadsf.org
                                             www.usadsf.org
A matte newsletter called USADSF Bulletin featuring articles on
all deaf sports and recreation.
Dr. Bobbie Beth Scoggins, President
Valerie Kinney, Adminstrative Assistant

4690 World Federation of the Deaf News
Ilkantie 4, PO Box 65   358-058-0583
SF-00401 Helsinki Finland,   Fax: 358-058-0377
The official magazine of the World Federation of the Deaf, features
information on the work of the EFD, the latest news and interviews
with people active in the Deaf communities throughout the world.
Quarterly
Antti Makipaa, Editor

Pamphlets

**4691 25 Ways to Promote Spoken Language in Your Child with a
Hearing Loss**
Alexander Graham Bell Association
3417 Volta Place NW   202-337-5220
Washington, DC 20007-2737   Fax: 202-337-8270
                                         TTY: 202-337-5220
This pamphlet teaches twenty-five golden rules about preparing
your child to listen and to speak.
1995 62 pages

4692 Aging and Hearing Loss: Some Commonly Asked Questions
National Information Center on Deafness
800 Florida Avenue NE   202-651-5051
Washington, DC 20002-3660   Fax: 202-651-5054
                                         TTY: 202-651-5052
Discusses the hearing evaulation, tests used to determine type and
extent of hearing loss and what an audiogram tells us.

**4693 Alerting and Communication Devices for Deaf and Hard of
Hearing People**
National Information Center on Deafness
800 Florida Avenue NE   202-651-5051
Washington, DC 20002   Fax: 202-651-5054
                                         TTY: 202-651-5052
Describes general communication in everyday life.

4694 Alexander Graham Bell's Life
Alexander Graham Bell Association
3417 Volta Place NW   202-337-5220
Washington, DC 20007-2737   Fax: 202-337-8270
                                         TTY: 202-337-5220
This pamphlet highlights Alexander Gram Bell's professional and
personal involvement with deafness as a teacher of the deaf; a
friend of many notable persons, including Helen Keller; a scientist

interested in acoustics; the inventor of the telephone; and the
founder of the Bell Association.
1996

4695 All About the New Generation of Hearing Aids
National Information Center on Deafness
800 Florida Avenue NE   202-651-5051
Washington, DC 20002-3660   Fax: 202-651-5054
                                         TTY: 202-651-5052
Explains the terms digital hearing aid, and digitally controlled
hearing aid.

4696 Assistive Devices Demonstration Centers
National Information Center on Deafness
800 Florida Avenue NE   202-651-5051
Washington, DC 20002-3660   Fax: 202-651-5054
                                         TTY: 202-651-5052
A resource list identifying demonstration centers across the United
States.

4697 Books for Parents of Deaf and Hard of Hearing Children
National Information Center on Deafness
800 Florida Avenue NE   202-651-5051
Washington, DC 20002   Fax: 202-651-5054
                                         TTY: 202-651-5052
Identifies books written for parents and everday experiences of
deaf and hard of hearing children.

4698 Care of the Ears and Hearing for Health
American Hearing Research Foundation
8 S Michigan Avenue   312-726-9670
Chicago, IL 60603-4539   Fax: 312-726-9695
                     e-mail: blederer@american-hearing.org
                                     www.american-hearing.org
Offers information on ear infections relating to chronic progres-
sive deafness.
William L Lederer, Executive Director
Sharon Parmet, Development/Communications Associate

4699 Consumer's Guide to Hearing Aids
Hearing Loss Association of America
7910 Woodmont Avenue   301-657-2248
Bethesda, MD 20814-3079   Fax: 301-913-9413
                                         TTY: 301-657-2249
                             e-mail: info@hearingloss.org
                                         www.hearingloss.org
Color booklet illustrating the different styles of hearing aids and
comparing different models and features. Illustrates the technol-
ogy pyramid and hearing aid pricing.
2006 24 pages
Jerry Portis, Executive Director
Brenda Battat, Assistant Executive Director

4700 Deaf Culture Videotapes
National Information Center on Deafness
800 Florida Avenue NE   202-651-5051
Washington, DC 20002-3660   Fax: 202-651-5054
                                         TTY: 202-651-5052
This list identifies deaf culture and deaf history videotapes available from the Historic Film Collection of the National Association
of the Deaf.

4701 Deaf Culture: Suggested Readings
National Information Center on Deafness
800 Florida Avenue NE   202-651-5051
Washington, DC 20002-3660   Fax: 202-651-5054
                                         TTY: 202-651-5052
A selected reading list providing annotations for 62 books high-
lighting the community, and history of deaf people.

4702 Deafness: A Fact Sheet
National Information Center on Deafness
800 Florida Avenue NE   202-651-5051
Washington, DC 20002-3660   Fax: 202-651-5054
                                         TTY: 202-651-5052

4703 Developing Cognition in Young Children Who are Deaf
Hope
55 E 100 N   435-752-9533
Logan, UT 84321-4648   Fax: 435-752-9533

Presents interesting, updated information on the importance of early cognition development in young children who are deaf. Contains many ideas for ways to promote early thinking skills, especially those that promote and enhance early communication and language development.

4704 Ear and Hearing
National Information Center on Deafness
800 Florida Avenue NE   202-651-5051
Washington, DC 20002-3660   Fax: 202-651-5054
                                                      TTY: 202-651-5052
An illustrated publication of the ear and what can go wrong with it.

4705 Educating Deaf Children: An Introduction
National Information Center on Deafness
800 Florida Avenue NE   202-651-5051
Washington, DC 20002-3660   Fax: 202-651-5054
                                                      TTY: 202-651-5052
Describes the different settings in which deaf children are currently educated.

4706 Facts About Hearing Aids
Alexander Graham Bell Association
3417 Volta Place NW   202-337-5220
Washington, DC 20007-2737   Fax: 202-337-8270
                                                      TTY: 202-337-5220
This brochure describes defferent types of hearing aids, factors to consider when choosing a hearing aid, the best way to go about purchasing a hearing aid. It also addresses cost and provides information on hearing conservation.

4707 Facts and Fancies About Hearing Aids
American Hearing Research Foundation
8 S Michigan Avenue   312-726-9670
Chicago, IL 60603-4539   Fax: 312-726-9695
                              e-mail: blederer@american-hearing.org
                                        www.american-hearing.org
Offers information on types of hearing aids and hearing aid evaluations.
William L Lederer, Executive Director
Sharon Parmet, Development/Communications Associate

4708 Genetics and Deafness
National Information Center on Deafness
800 Florida Avenue NE   202-651-5051
Washington, DC 20002-3660   Fax: 202-651-5054
                                                      TTY: 202-651-5052
Written for deaf people and their families who wish to learn more about the relationship between heredity and deafness.

4709 Hearing Loss: Information for Professionals in the Aging Network
National Information Center on Deafness
800 Florida Avenue NE   202-651-5051
Washington, DC 20002-3660   Fax: 202-651-5054
                                                      TTY: 202-651-5052
Introduces professionals in the aging network to the realities of hearing loss.

4710 How Does Your Child Hear and Talk?
American Speech-Language-Hearing Association
10801 Rockville Pike   301-897-8682
Rockville, MD 20852-3226   800-638-8255
                              e-mail: actioncenter@asha.org
                                        www.asha.org
Offers a chart to parents on children's growth pertaining to their hearing and speech.

4711 Late-Deafened Adults: A Selected Annotated Bibliography
National Information Center on Deafness
800 Florida Avenue NE   202-651-5051
Washington, DC 20002-3660   Fax: 202-651-5054
                                                      TTY: 202-651-5052
A selected reading list of books and articles for late-deafened people and their families.

4712 Leading National Publications of and for Deaf People
National Information Center on Deafness
800 Florida Avenue NE   202-651-5051
Washington, DC 20002   Fax: 202-651-5054
                                                      TTY: 202-651-5052

Identifies publications with national circulations to deaf audiences.

4713 Making New Friends
National Information Center on Deafness
800 Florida Avenue NE   202-651-5051
Washington, DC 20002-3660   Fax: 202-651-5054
                                                      TTY: 202-651-5052
Identifies resources that offer opportunities for deaf people.

4714 Meniere's Disease: Hearing Loss & Inner Ear Blood Flow
Self Help for Hard of H
7910 Woodmont Avenue   301-657-2248
Bethesda, MD 20814-3079   Fax: 301-913-9413
                                                      TTY: 301-657-2249
                              e-mail: national@shhh.org
                                        www.shhh.org
Includes a personal narrative.

4715 National Information Center on Deafness Brochure
National Information Center on Deafness
800 Florida Avenue NE   202-651-5051
Washington, DC 20002   Fax: 202-651-5054
                                                      TTY: 202-651-5052
A description of services offered by NICD.

4716 Noise Can Be Harmful to Your Health
Deafness Research Foundation
15 W 39th Street   212-768-1181
New York, NY 10018-3806
Offers information, including a chart of noise levels, low to harmful, and the effects these noise levels have on your hearing.

4717 Otitis Media
Deafness Research Foundation
15 W 39th Street   212-768-1181
New York, NY 10018-3806
Offers information on Otitis Media, prevention, causes, treatments and symptoms.

4718 Perspectives Folio: Parent-Child
Gallaudet University
11030 S Langley Avenue
Chicago, IL 60628-3819   800-621-2736
                                                 Fax: 800-621-8476
                                                 TTY: 888-630-9347
                              www.gallaudet.edu/~gupress
Seven articles emphasizing family communication while providing important information for parents about deafness and the deaf culture.
29 pages

4719 Publications from the National Information Center on Deafness
National Information Center on Deafness
800 Florida Avenue NE   202-651-5051
Washington, DC 20002-3660   Fax: 202-651-5054
                                                      TTY: 202-651-5052
Order form and explanations of NICD publications.

4720 Questions and Answers About Employment of Deaf People
National Information Center on Deafness
800 Florida Avenue NE   202-651-5051
Washington, DC 20002-3660   Fax: 202-651-5054
                                                      TTY: 202-651-5052

4721 Questions and Answers on Hearing Loss
Self Help for Hard of H
7910 Woodmont Avenue   301-657-2248
Bethesda, MD 20814-3079   Fax: 301-913-9413
                                                      TTY: 301-657-2249
                              e-mail: national@shhh.org
                                        www.shhh.org

4722 So You Have Had an Ear Operation...What Next?
American Hearing Research Foundation
8 S Washington Avenue   312-726-9670
Chicago, IL 60603-4539   Fax: 312-726-9695
                              e-mail: blederer@american-hearing.org
                                        www.american-hearing.org

Offers information on ear infections and surgery.
William L Lederer, Executive Director
Sharon Parmet, Development/Communications Associate

4723 Statewide Services for Deaf and Hard of Hearing People
National Information Center on Deafness
800 Florida Avenue NE   202-651-5051
Washington, DC 20002   Fax: 202-651-5054
                                  TTY: 202-651-5052
A resource list of states that have established commissions and
other offices to serve deaf people.

4724 Travel Resources for Deaf and Hard of Hearing People
National Information Center on Deafness
800 Florida Avenue NE   202-651-5051
Washington, DC 20002   Fax: 202-651-5054
                                  TTY: 202-651-5052
A publication list of travel industry resources for deaf and hard of
hearing people.

4725 What are TTY's? TDDs? TTs?
National Information Center on Deafness
800 Florida Avenue NE   202-651-5051
Washington, DC 20002-3660   Fax: 202-651-5054
                                  TTY: 202-651-5052
Discusses text telephones used by deaf people.

4726 World of Sound
International Hearing Society
16880 Middlebelt Road   313-478-2610
Livonia, MI 48154-3367   Fax: 313-478-4520
The purpose of this booklet is to provide basic information for
those with questions about hearing loss, hearing aids and Hearing
Instrument Specialists.

**4727 You Don't Have to Hate Meetings: Try Computer-Assisted
Notetaking Instead**
Self Help for Hard of H
7910 Woodmont Avenue   301-657-2248
Bethesda, MD 20814-3079   Fax: 301-913-9413
                                  TTY: 301-657-2249
                            e-mail: national@shhh.org
                                      www.shhh.org

Audio & Video

4728 ASL Poetry: Selected Works of Clayton Valli
DawnSignPress
6130 Nancy Ridge Drive   858-625-0600
San Diego, CA 92121-3223   800-549-5350
                                  Fax: 858-625-2336
                                  TTY: 858-625-0600
                       e-mail: comments@dawnsign.com
                                      www.dawnsign.com
Twenty one original Valli poems recited by a diversity of native
signers. Guided experience through the richness of poetry in an-
other language.
105 minutes
ISBN: 0-915035-23-5
Barry Howland, Marketing Director

4729 Basic Course in American Sign Language Vid eotape Package
TJ Publishers
2544 Tarpley Road   972-416-0800
Carrollton, TX 75006   800-999-1168
                                  Fax: 972-416-0944
                    e-mail: customerservice@tjpublishers.com
                              www.tjpublishers.com/index.html
The A Basic Course in American Sign Language Vocabulary Videotape features four Deaf models signing each vocabulary word
contained in all 22 lessons of the text plus the alphabet and numbers. The tape has captions and voice which can be turned off to
sharpen visual acuity. It is ideal for classroom reinforcement and
independent home study.
Angela K Thames, President
Jerald A Murphy, VP

4730 Beginning Reading and Sign Language Video
TJ Publishers

2544 Tarpley Road   972-416-0800
Carrollton, TX 75006   800-999-1168
                                  Fax: 972-416-0944
                    e-mail: customerservice@tjpublishers.com
                              www.tjpublishers.com/index.html
Learning sign improves reading, motor skills and visual percep-
tion and increases language acquisition abilities. For kids from 2 to
12, this video picture book features deaf actress Susan Bressler
signing over a hundred words at the zoo, at home and around the
community.
Video
Angela K Thames, President
Jerald A Murphy, VP

4731 Come Sign With Us
Gallaudet University
11030 S Langley Avenue
Chicago, IL 60628-3819   800-621-2736
                                  Fax: 800-621-8476
                                  TTY: 888-630-9347
                              www.gallaudet.edu/~gupress
Lessons including fingerspelling and signing are overviewed.
90 minutes
ISBN: 1-563680-50-5

4732 Deaf Children Signers
Harris Communications
15155 Technology Drive   952-906-1180
Eden Prairie, MN 55344   800-825-6758
                                  Fax: 952-906-1099
                                  TTY: 800-825-9187
                            e-mail: info@harriscomm.com
                                      www.harriscomm.com/
This 5-part collection of children signers is great for children,
teachers, parents and interpreters.
Robert Harris Ph.D, Founder/President/CEO

4733 Deaf Culture Autobiographies
Harris Communications
15155 Technology Drive   952-906-1180
Eden Prairie, MN 55344   800-825-6758
                                  Fax: 952-906-1099
                                  TTY: 800-825-9187
                            e-mail: info@harriscomm.com
                                      www.harriscomm.com/
Inspiring videotapes offer encouragement and enlightenment to
the hearing impaired. Total of eight videotapes.
Robert Harris Ph.D, Founder/President/CEO

4734 Deaf Culture Series
Harris Communications
15155 Technology Drive   952-906-1180
Eden Prairie, MN 55344   800-825-6758
                                  Fax: 952-906-1099
                                  TTY: 800-825-9187
                            e-mail: info@harriscomm.com
                                      www.harriscomm.com/
Each video in this 5-part series features a variety of Deaf talent. It
is an excellent resource for Deaf studies programs, Interpreter
Preparation programs and Sign Language programs.
Robert Harris Ph.D, Founder/President/CEO

4735 Deaf Mosaic Series
Harris Communications
15155 Technology Drive   952-906-1180
Eden Prairie, MN 55344   800-825-6758
                                  Fax: 952-906-1099
                                  TTY: 800-825-9187
                            e-mail: info@harriscomm.com
                                      www.harriscomm.com/
A national magazine show produced monthly by Gallaudet University, this show has been awarded nine Emmys. As the only nation-wide program about the Deaf community, these videotapes
are the best of the best from the shows programs.
Robert Harris Ph.D, Founder/President/CEO

4736 Diagnosis and Treatment of Unilateral Hearing Loss
American Academy of Otolaryngology

1 Prince Street
Alexandria, VA 22314-3357

703-836-4444
Fax: 703-683-5100
www.entnet.org

This CD-ROM focuses on evaluation and treatment of unilateral hearing loss arising from skull base lesion.

4737 Do You Hear That?
Alexander Graham Bell Association
3417 Volta Place NW
Washington, DC 20007-2737

202-337-5220
Fax: 202-337-8270
TTY: 202-337-5220

This video documents auditory-verbal therapy as it is practiced at North York General Hospital in Toronto, Canada.
1992 35 minutes

4738 Fantastic Series
Gallaudet University Bookstore
800 Florida Avenue NE
Washington, DC 20002-3660

800-451-1073
Fax: 800-621-8476
TTY: 888-630-9347
www.gallaudet.edu/~gupress

Tapes designed to encourage both deaf and hearing children to use their imaginations.
Ages 6-10

4739 Fingers that Tickle and Delight
National Association of the Deaf
8630 Fenton Street
Silver Spring, MD 20910

301-587-1788
Fax: 301-587-1791
TTY: 301-587-1789
www.nad.org

One's woman's experiences from childhood, school, marriage, her career as a teacher and interpreter trainer, and her life as an entertainer. Closed captioned.
13+ 32 minutes
Bill Stark, Project Director
Donna Morris, Publications Manager

4740 Fingerspelling and Numbers Software
American Sign Language (ASL) Productions
c/o Harris Communications
Eden Prairie, MN 55344

952-906-1180
800-767-4461
Fax: 952-906-1099
TTY: 800-767-4461
e-mail: ASLProductions@harriscomm.com
www.americansignlanguageproductions.com

Fingerspelling practice partner that allows you to control the speed and vocabulary level. Requires Windows 3.1 or greater.
Robert Harris Ph.D, Founder/President-Harris Communications
Jenna Cassell, Founder ASL Productions

4741 Getting in Touch
Research Press
2612 N Mattis Avenue
Champaign, IL 61822-1053

217-352-3273
800-519-2707
Fax: 217-352-1221
e-mail: rp@researchpress.com
www.researchpress.com

Shows how to create an individualized communications system based on the abilities and needs of the child. Illustrates seven basic communication procedures that involve the use of touch cues and object cues.

4742 Gospel of Luke
Gallaudet University Bookstore
800 Florida Avenue NE
Washington, DC 20002-3660

800-451-0173
Fax: 800-621-8476
TTY: 888-630-9347
www.gallaudet.edu/~gupress

A set of five videotapes of the Gospel of Luke told in ASL.
Set of five

4743 Granny Good's Sign of Christmas
Gallaudet University Bookstore

800 Florida Avenue NE
Washington, DC 20002-3660

800-451-1073
Fax: 800-621-8476
TTY: 888-630-9347
www.gallaudet.edu/~gupress

Twas The Night Before Christmas told in American Sign Language.

4744 Hearing Loss and Rehabilitation
American Academy of Otolaryngology
1 Prince Street
Alexandria, VA 22314-3357

703-836-4444
Fax: 703-683-5100
www.entnet.org

Slides.

4745 I Can Hear!
Alexander Graham Bell Association
3417 Volta Place NW
Washington, DC 20007-2737

202-337-5220
Fax: 202-337-8270
TTY: 202-337-5220

This inspirational video describes the auditory-verbal approach for developing speech and language for hearing impaired children and adults.
1992 23 minutes

4746 I Can Hear!: II
Alexander Graham Bell Association
3417 Volta Place NW
Washington, DC 20007-2737

202-337-5220
Fax: 202-337-8270
TTY: 202-337-5220

An exciting videotape that gives more examples of auditory-verbal therapy and a variety of kids who have been taught to speak using this method.
1996 19 minute video

4747 I See What You Say: Self Help Lip Reading Program
Alexander Graham Bell Association
3417 Volta Place NW
Washington, DC 20007-2737

202-337-5220
Fax: 202-337-8270
TTY: 202-337-5220

Easy to follow videotape and manual for consumers teaches visual recognition of speech sounds in single words and phrases.
1995 54 minutes

4748 Interpreters in Public Schools Kit
Sign Media
4020 Blackburn Lane
Burtonsville, MD 20866-1167

301-421-0268
800-475-4756
Fax: 301-421-0270
TTY: 301-421-4460
e-mail: signmedia@aol.com
www.signmedia.com

Videotapes individually specialized for administrators, classroom teachers and for interpreters. Provides practical insights to some of the most crucial issues and problems facing mainstreamed programs. Contains reproducible printed material.
Three videos
Barbara Olmert, Director Marketing

4749 Interview with Kirsten Gonzales
Alexander Graham Bell Association
3417 Volta Place NW
Washington, DC 20007-2737

202-337-5220
Fax: 202-337-8270
TTY: 202-337-5220

Interviews a longtime user and trainer of oral interpreters who offers techniques in articulation and natural gestures.
20 minutes

4750 It's Not Just Hearing AIDS: Deaf People and the Epidemic
National Association of the Deaf
8630 Fenton Street
Silver Spring, MD 20910

301-587-1788
Fax: 301-587-1791
TTY: 301-587-1789
www.nad.org

Straightforward and factual information on how AIDS is transmitted, who gets AIDS, procedures for an HIV test, and an interview with a person who actually has the AIDS virus.
9 - 13+ Video
Bill Stark, Project Director
Donna Morris, Publications Manager

4751 Joy of Signing
Gallaudet University Bookstore
800 Florida Avenue NE
Washington, DC 20002-3660

800-451-1073
Fax: 800-621-8476
TTY: 888-630-9347
www.gallaudet.edu/~gupress

Three tapes full of useful information to help increase skill and comfort with sign.
1 Videotape

4752 King Midas
Gallaudet University
11030 S Langley Avenue
Chicago, IL 60628-3819

800-621-2736
Fax: 800-621-8476
TTY: 888-630-9347
www.gallaudet.edu/~gupress

30 minutes
ISBN: 0-930323-71-8

4753 King Midas Videotape
Gallaudet University Bookstore
800 Florida Avenue NE
Washington, DC 20002-3660

800-451-1073
Fax: 800-621-8476
TTY: 888-630-9347
www.gallaudet.edu/~gupress

Story of King Midas told in American Sign Language.

4754 Learning to Communicate: The First Three Years Videotape
Alexander Graham Bell Association
3417 Volta Place NW
Washington, DC 20007-2737

202-337-5220
Fax: 202-337-8270
TTY: 202-337-5220

This video shows normal communication development in young children under three years of age. It discusses factors which can affect speech and language development, including anatomy and environment. Closed captioned.
11 minutes

4755 Let's Be Friends
Britannica Film Company
345 4th Street
San Francisco, CA 94107-1206

415-597-5555

The teacher left the room and asked Shelly, a hearing impaired child to be the mother. Margaret, an emotionally disturbed child, became frightened and verbally attacked Shelly. The teacher worked to get them to become friends and understand each other's problems.
Films

4756 Once Upon a Time - Children's Classics Ret old in American Sign Language
Harris Communications
15155 Technology Drive
Eden Prairie, MN 55344

952-906-1180
800-825-6758
Fax: 952-906-1099
TTY: 800-825-9187
e-mail: info@harriscomm.com
www.harriscomm.com/

Children's classics come alive on videotapes.
Robert Harris Ph.D, Founder/President/CEO

4757 Parent Sign Video Series
TJ Publishers
2544 Tarpley Road
Carrollton, TX 75006

972-416-0800
800-999-1168
Fax: 972-416-0944
e-mail: customerservice@tjpublishers.com
www.tjpublishers.com/index.html

Ten instructional videotapes specifically designed for parents of deaf children, present frequently used vocabulary and phrases. The tapes are perfect for home use and as a compliment to sign language and educational programs. Deaf and hearing parents, each having a deaf and a hearing child, reflect common communication needs of all families.
Video
Angela K Thames, President
Jerald A Murphy, VP

4758 People vs. Noise
Better Hearing Institute
5021B Backlick Road
Annandale, VA 22003-6043

703-684-3391
e-mail: mail@betterhearing.org
www.betterhearing.org

4759 Read My Lips
Alexander Graham Bell Association
3417 Volta Place NW
Washington, DC 20007-2737

202-337-5220
Fax: 202-337-8270
TTY: 202-337-5220

A six videotape series that takes adults from lip reading to basic words to complex phrases and sentences in a variety of real life situations.

4760 See What I'm Saying
Thomas Kaufman, author

Fanlight Productions
4196 Washington Street
Boston, MA 02131-1731

617-469-4999
800-937-4113
Fax: 617-469-3379
e-mail: fanlight@fanlight.com
www.fanlight.com

Follows Patricia, a deaf child from a hearing, Spanish speaking family, through her first year of elementary school. Illustrates how the acquisition of communication skills enhances a child's self-esteem, confidence and family relationships. Open captioned.
1992 31 Minutes
ISBN: 1-572950-90-0

4761 Seeing and Hearing Speech: Lessons in Lipreading and Listening
Hearing Loss Association of America
7910 Woodmont Avenue
Bethesda, MD 20814-3079

301-657-2248
Fax: 301-913-9413
TTY: 301-657-2249
e-mail: info@hearingloss.org
www.hearingloss.org

This CD-Rom helps people with hearing loss learn to combine what they see with what they hear to understand speech better in difficult situations. This interactive CD-ROM contains carefully planned lessons to improve speech understanding through lipreading.
CD-ROM
Jerry Portis, Executive Director
Brenda Battat, Assistant Executive Director

4762 Show & Tell: Explaining Hearing Loss to Teachers
Alexander Graham Bell Association
3417 Volta Place NW
Washington, DC 20007-2737

202-337-5220
Fax: 202-337-8270
TTY: 202-337-5220

This video introduces mainstreamed teachers to the challenges that hearing impairments impose on normal communication.
20 minutes

4763 Show 'N' Tell Stories
Modern Signs Press
PO Box 1181
Los Alamitos, CA 90720-1181

562-596-8548
800-572-7332
Fax: 562-795-6614
TTY: 562-493-4168
e-mail: modsigns@aol.com
www.modsigns.com

A bilingual storytelling series for Deaf children and their families, featuring both Signing Exact English (SEE) and American Sign Language (ASL).
Videotape

4764 Sign-Me-A-Story
DawnSignPress
6130 Nancy Ridge Drive
San Diego, CA 92121-3223

858-625-0600
800-549-5350
Fax: 858-625-2336
TTY: 858-625-0600
e-mail: info@dawnsign.com
www.dawnsign.com/

Linda Bove, the deaf actress from Sesame Street, introduces children to American Sign Language. Teaches simple signs and then

acts out fairy tales. Stories are voiced and closed captioned, accessible to all.
30 minutes
ISBN: 0-394892-32-1
Joe Dannis, Founder/Publisher/President

4765 Sleeping Beauty Videotape
Gallaudet University Bookstore
800 Florida Avenue NE
Washington, DC 20002-3660
800-451-1073
Fax: 800-621-8476
TTY: 888-630-9347
www.gallaudet.edu/~gupress
Presents the entire story of Sleeping Beauty told in American Sign Language.

4766 Sleeping Beauty: With Selected Sentences in ASL
Gallaudet University
11030 S Langley Avenue
Chicago, IL 60628-3819
800-621-2736
Fax: 800-621-8476
TTY: 888-630-9347
www.gallaudet.edu/~gupress
Features the full story in ASL and includes vocabulary and sentence structure focusing on adjectives, with a voice-over throughout.
30 minutes
ISBN: 0-930323-98-X

4767 Sound Hearing
Hearing Loss Association of America
7910 Woodmont Avenue
Bethesda, MD 20814-3079
301-657-2248
Fax: 301-913-9413
TTY: 301-657-2249
e-mail: info@hearingloss.org
www.hearingloss.org
Provides listening samples to illustrate sound, hearing, and hearing loss. Listeners will hear as people who have hearing loss might, listening to music, a story, etc.
CD-ROM, 26 mins
Jerry Portis, Executive Director
Brenda Battat, Assistant Executive Director

4768 Telecoil: Plugging Into Sound
Hearing Loss Association of America
7910 Woodmont Avenue
Bethesda, MD 20814-3079
301-657-2248
Fax: 301-913-9413
TTY: 301-657-2249
e-mail: info@hearingloss.org
www.hearingloss.org
In The Telecoil: Plugging Into Sound, members of SHHH give accounts of their experiences with using the telecoil, describing how the telecoil makes a noticeable difference in their social and professional lives.
Open Captioned
Jerry Portis, Executive Director
Brenda Battat, Assistant Executive Director

4769 Telecoil: Plugging into Sound
7910 Woodmont Avenue
Bethesda, MD 20814-3079
301-657-2248
Fax: 301-913-9413
TTY: 301-657-2249
e-mail: national@shhh.org
www.shhh.org
Guide for consumers concerning why they should include a telecoil in their hearing aid. SHHH members are featured, talking about their experiences. Includes 50 brochures. Open-captioned.
1996 10 minutes

4770 Telling Stories
Harris Communications
15155 Technology Drive
Eden Prairie, MN 55344
952-906-1180
800-825-6758
Fax: 952-906-1099
TTY: 800-825-9187
e-mail: info@harriscomm.com
www.harriscomm.com/

This international, award winning play, now on video, uses the symbols and myths drawn from the struggles between the world of the deaf and the world of the hearing.
Robert Harris Ph.D, Founder/President/CEO

4771 Treasure
Gallaudet University Bookstore
800 Florida Avenue NE
Washington, DC 20002-3660
773-568-1550
Fax: 800-621-8476
TTY: 888-630-9347
www.gallaudet.edu/~gupress
Ella Mae Lentz, a well-known deaf poet, signs some of her poems.

4772 Unheard Voices
Hearing Loss Association of America
7910 Woodmont Avenue
Bethesda, MD 20814-3079
301-657-2248
Fax: 301-913-9413
TTY: 301-657-2249
e-mail: info@hearingloss.org
www.hearingloss.org
Unheard Voices is a candid and compassionate portrayal of people coping with the life-changing impact of hearing loss. Open-captioned.
23 minutes
Jerry Portis, Executive Director
Brenda Battat, Assistant Executive Director

Web Sites

4773 Alexander Graham Bell Association
www.agbell.org
Information on pediatric hearing loss, and educational issues for hearing impaired children, promotes better public understanding of hearing loss in children and adults, provides scholarships and financial aid to families of children with hearing loss, and promotes early detection of hearing loss in infants.

4774 American Academy of Audiology
www.audiology.org
Provides professional development, education and research and provides increased public awareness of hearing disorders and audiologic services.

4775 American Academy of Otolaryngology
www.entnet.org
Advance the art and science of otalaryngology-head and neck surgury through state-of-the-art education, research, and learning; and to unite, serve, and represent the interests of its members and their patients to the public.

4776 American Society for Deaf Children
www.deafchildren.org
Provides support, encouragement, and current information about deafness to families with deaf and hard of hearing children.

4777 American Tinnitus Association
www.ata.org
Provides information about tinnitus and referrals to local contacts/support groups nationwide.

4778 Auditory-Verbal International
www.auditory-verbal.org
Promotes the Auditory-Verbal Therapy approach, which is based on the belief that the overwhelming majority of these children can hear and talk by using their residual hearing and hearing aids.

4779 Better Hearing Institute
www.betterhearing.org
Information programs on hearing loss and available medical, surgical, hearing aid, and rehabilitation assistance for millions with uncorrected hearing problems.

4780 Council on Education of the Deaf
www.deafed.net
Offers information and referral services to the hearing impaired.

4781 Deafness Research Foundation
www.drf.org
Committed to public awareness and support for basic and clinical research into deafness and hearing disabilities.

4782 EAR Foundation

www.earfoundation.org

Provides the general public support services promoting the integration of the hearing and balance impaired into mainstream society and to educate young people and adults about hearing preservation and early detection of hearing loss, enabling them to prevent at an early age hearing and balance disorders.

4783 Healing Well

www.healingwell.com

An online health resource guide to medical news, chat, information and articles, newsgroups and message boards, books, disease-related web sites, medical directories, and more for patients, friends, and family coping with disabling diseases, disorders, or chronic illnesses.

4784 Health Finder

www.healthfinder.gov

Searchable, carefully developed web site offering information on over 1000 topics. Developed by the US Department of Health and Human Services, the site can be used in both English and Spanish.

4785 Healthlink USA

www.healthlinkusa.com

Health information concerning treatment, cures, prevention, diagnosis, risk factors, research, support groups, email lists, personal stories and much more. Updated regularly.

4786 Hear Now

www.sotheworldmayhearnow.org

Committed to making technology accessible to deaf and hard of hearing individuals throughout the United States. Also raises funds to provide hearing aids, cochlear implants and related services to children and adults who have hearing losses but do not have financial resources to purchase their own devices.

4787 Hearing Education and Awareness for Rocker

www.hearnet.com

Educates the public about the real dangers of hearing loss resulting from repeated exposure to excessive noise levels.

4788 Helios Health

www.helioshealth.com

Online resource for your health information. Detailed information about specific health topics, access to expert advice from our Medical Advisory Board, and up-to-date health news.

4789 House Ear Institute

www.hei.org

A national non-profit otologic research and educational institute that provides information on hearing and balance disorders.

4790 John Tracy Clinic

www.johntracycyclinic.org

An educational facility for preschool age children who have hearing losses and their families. In addition to on-site services, worldwide correspondence courses in English and Spanish are offered to parents whose children are of preschool age and are hard of hearing, deaf, or deaf-blind.

4791 MedicineNet

www.medicinenet.com

An online resource for consumers providing easy-to-read, authoritative medical and health information.

4792 Medscape

www.medscape.com

Medscape offers specialists, primary care physicians, and other health professionals the Web's most robust and integrated medical information and educational tools.

4793 National Association of the Deaf

www.nad.org

Focus on advocacy, captioned media, deafness-related information/publications, legal assistance and more.

4794 National Captioning Institute

ncicap.org

Advocates captioned television for people who want to see, as well as hear, the dialogue of a television program. It not only enables deaf and hard-of-hearing people to understand all of a program's content, but it is also beneficial for new Americans learning English as a second language, as well as children learning to read.

4795 National Information Center on Deafness

www.gallaudet.edu

Provides information or referrals on questions about deafness, including general information, education, research, legislation, assistive devices and more. Offers a bibliography of readings available on 30 topics relating to deafness.

4796 National Information Clearinghouse on Children Who are Deaf-Blind

www.tr.wou.edu/dblink

Collects, organizes and disseminates information related to children and youth who are deaf-blind and connects consumers of deaf-blind information to sources of information about deaf-blindness, assistive technology and deaf-blind people.

4797 National Institute on Deafness and Other Communication Disorders

www.nih.gov/nidcd

A national resources center for information about hearing, balance, smell, taste, voice, speech and language.

4798 Registry of Interpreters for the Deaf

www.RID.org

Professional interpreters and translators, persons with deafness or hearing impairments and professionals in related fields.

4799 Self-Help for Hard of Hearing People

www.shhh.org/

Promotes awareness and information about hearing loss, communication, assistive devices, and alternative communication skills through publications, exhibits and presentations.

4800 USA Deaf Sports Federation

www.usadsf.org

Website published by a governing body for all deaf sports and recreation in the United States.

4801 WebMD

www.webmd.com

Information on deafness, including articles and resources.

Description

4802 # Heart Disease

There is a wide range of heart (cardiac) diseases that can be divided into several major categories: heart failure; problems in electrical conduction; heart rate and rhythm; and malfunction of the heart valves. Coronary disease relates to the arteries that supply oxygen to the heart muscle itself.

Heart failure is the general inability of the heart to function effectively as the pumping mechanism to distribute oxygenated blood and nutrients to the cells and tissues. As the heart's pumping action declines, blood does not get distributed properly and normal circulation gets disrupted. As a result, the fluid accumulates, or backs up, causing swelling (edema) in the body, often noticeable in the ankles, as well as within the lungs (pulmonary edema) causing difficulty in breathing. Numerous mechanisms are responsible for heart failure so treatment is aimed at the underlying causes, improving heart contractibility (and thus pump efficiency), and removal of excess fluid through the kidneys.

Problems in the electrical conduction that makes the heart contract result in irregular heart rate and rhythm, either slower, faster, or, in life-threatening situations, absence of heart beat or ineffective heart contractions. Specific medications and procedures are used in treatment, again depending on the underlying problem.

New diagnostic (angiography) and therapeutic catheter techniques have been developed to accurately identify the rhythm problem, and in some cases, cure it bydelivering radio frequency energy to the abnormal pathway.

Malfunctions of heart valves are also common, but surgical advances enable successful repair and replacement of defective or diseased valves.

The arteries that directly supply the heart (known as coronary arteries) can also be affected by disease processes. Deposits or fatty plaques may cause narrowing of the arteries, or the arteries can become blocked by a clot that originated somewhere else in the body. Either way, the heart may be deprived of oxygenated blood and the particular muscle that is fed by the artery is injured or dies. Angina is chest pain produced when the heart is not receiving enough oxygen but no direct damage occurs. A heart attack (or myocardial infarction) occurs when the heart is deprived of its blood for a significant amount of time. The outcome of a heart attack depends on the amount of damage sustained by the affected heart muscle and the speed with which treatment is started. Immediate medical intervention has a marked effect on long-term prognosis. Administration of agents that dissolve the clot (blood thinners, antithrombotics) significantly reduce heart attack deaths when given within 6 hours of the onset of chest pain. Catheter interventions (angioplasty) can include balloons and metallic stents that are placed in coronary arteries to push obstructions against the arterial walls thereby re-opening the vessel. The most recent advance is a stent that is coated with a drug that is coated to prevent reformation of the clot.

The symptoms of heart disease are varied, but may include chest pain, difficulty breathing, fatigue, palpitations, dizziness and fainting. See also *Congenital Heart Disease*.

National Agencies & Associations

4803 **American Heart Association**
7272 Greenville Avenue
Dallas, TX 75231   800-242-8721
www.americanheart.org
Supports research education and community service programs with the objective of reducing premature death and disability from cardiovascular diseases and stroke; coordinates the efforts of health professionals and other engaged in the fight against heart disease.
M Cass Wheeler, CEO

4804 **Canadian Adult Congenital Heart Network**
6835 Century Avenue
Mississauga, Ontario, L5N-2L2   e-mail: jtherrien@cachnet.org
www.cachnet.org
Was created to pool the knowledge and experience of congenital heart disease professionals in Canada to help strengthen their skills and knowledge of the discipline, and to create a community of individuals committed to caring for adults with congenital heart disease and their families.
Dr Erwin Oechslin, President

4805 **Children's Heart Society**
Box 52088 Garneau Postal Outlet   780-454-7665
Edmonton, Alberta, T6G-2T5   888-247-9404
Fax: 780-454-7665
e-mail: contact@childrensheart.org
www.childrensheart.org
Supports families of children with acquired and congenital heart disease.
Sue E North, President

4806 **National Heart, Lung and Blood Institute**
National Institutes of Health
31 Center Drive, Building 31   301-592-8573
Bethesda, MD 20892   Fax: 240-629-3246
TTY: 240-629-3255
e-mail: NHLBIinfo@nhlbi.nih.gov
www.nhlbi.nih.gov
Primary responsibility of this organization is the scientific investigation of heart, blood vessel, lung and blood disorders. Oversees research, demonstration, prevention, education, control and training activities in these fields and emphasizes the prevention and control of heart diseases.
Susan B Shurin MD, Director

4807 **Pulmonary Hypertension Association**
801 Roeder Road   301-565-3004
Silver Spring, MD 20910   800-748-7274
Fax: 301-565-3994
e-mail: pha@PHAssociation.org
www.PHAssociation.org
A nonprofit organization for pulmonary hypertension patients, families, caregivers and PH-treating medical professionals. The mission of the Pulmonary Hypertension Association (PHA) is to find ways to prevent and cure pulmonary hypertension, and to provide hope for the pulmonary hypertension community through support, education, advocacy and awareness.
Laura D'Anna, President

Research Centers

4808 Arizona Heart Institute
2632 N 20th Street
Phoenix, AZ 85006-1300 602-266-2200
800-345-4278
Fax: 602-604-5047
e-mail: information@azheart.com
www.azheart.com
Edward Diethrich, Medical Director and Founder

4809 Baylor College of Medicine: Debakey Heart Center
Texas Medical Center
1 Baylor Plaza 713-798-4951
Houston, TX 77030-3411 Fax: 713-798-6990
e-mail: research@bcm.edu
www.bcm.tmc.edu
Research activities have an emphasis on therapeutic intervention
and prevention of heart disease.
Steve Sigworth MD, Chief Medical Officer
Paul Klotman MD, President

4810 Baylor College of Medicine: General Clinical Research Center Adults
Baylor College of Medicine
1 Baylor Plaza 713-798-4951
Houston, TX 77030-3498 Fax: 713-798-6990
e-mail: asander1@bcm.edu
www.bcm.tmc.edu
Steve Sigworth MD, Chief Medical Officer
Paul Klotman MD, President

4811 Bees-Stealy Research Foundation
2001 4th Avenue 619-235-8744
San Diego, CA 92101-2303 Fax: 619-234-8190
Basic cardiac research.
HD Peabody Jr, Director

4812 Bockus Research Institute Graduate Hospital
Graduate Hospital
415 S 19th Street
Philadelphia, PA 19146-1464 215-893-2000
Offers research in cardiovascular diseases with emphasis on mus-
cle tissue studies.
Dr Robert Cox, Director

4813 Boston University, Whitaker Cardiovascular Institute
715 Albany Street 617-638-4887
Boston, MA 02118 Fax: 617-638-4066
www.bumc.bu.edu
Offers basic and clinical care research relating to cardiovascular
diseases.
Gary J Balady MD, Clinical Investigator

4814 CHASER Congenital Heart Disease Anomalies Anomalies Support, Education & Resources
2112 N Wilkins Road 419-825-5575
Swanton, OH 43558-9445 Fax: 419-825-2880
e-mail: myer106w@wonder.em.cdc.gov
www.csun.edu
An organization established to meet the emotional and educational
needs of parents and professionals who deal with congenital heart
disease in children. Offers resource materials and support for parent to parent networking.

4815 Cardiovascular Research and Training Center University of Alabama
THT Room 311 205-934-3624
Birmingham, AL 35294-6 Fax: 205-345-96
Robert C Bueourge, Director

4816 Children's Heart Institute of Texas
PO Box 3966 512-887-4505
Corpus Christi, TX 78463-3966 Fax: 512-887-0539
Offers research and statistical information on pediatric cardiology.
Laura Berlanga, Director

4817 Cleveland Clinic Foundation Research Institute
9500 Euclid Avenue 216-444-3900
Cleveland, OH 44195 Fax: 216-444-3279
www.lerner.ccf.org
Research institute focusing on diseases of the cardiovascular sys-
tem.
Clemencia Commenares PhD, Director
Paul E DiCorleto PhD, Staff/ Institute Chairman

4818 Columbia University Irving Center for Clinical Research Adult Unit
Presbyterian Hospital
116 Street and Broadway 212-854-1754
New York, NY 10027 Fax: 212-053-13
e-mail: askcuit@columbia.edu
www.columbia.edu
Research center focusing on pulmonary diseases.
Henry Ginsberg, Director

4819 Creighton University Cardiac Center
3006 Webster Street 402-280-4566
Omaha, NE 68131-2137 800-237-7828
Fax: 402-280-4938
thecardiaccenter.creighton.edu
Research into the clinical aspects of cardiology and heart disease.
Dennis J Esterbrooks MD, Chief of the Division of Cardiology
Michael G Del Core MD, Associate Professor of Medicine

4820 Duke University Pediatric Cardiac Catheterization Laboratory
PO Box 3352 DUMC 919-681-4080
Durham, NC 27710-0001 Fax: 919-681-2714
e-mail: john.rhodes@duke.edu
pediatrics.duke.edu
Research into pediatric cardiology.
Brenda E Armstrong MD, Director
John F Rhodes MD, Chief Clinical Cardiology

4821 Framingham Heart Study
73 Mount Wayte Avenue 508-935-3434
Framingham, MA 01702-5828 Fax: 508-626-1262
e-mail: levyD@nih.gov
www.framinghamheartstudy.org
Daniel Levy, Medical Director
Philip A Wolf, Principal Investigator

4822 General Clinical Research Center at Beth Israel Hospital
330 Brookline Avenue 617-735-2151
Boston, MA 02215-5400
Studies into cardiology pulmonary disorders and heart disease.
Lewis Landsb MD, Program Director

4823 General Clinical Research Center: University of California at LA
Center for Health Sciences
10833 Le Conte Avenue 310-825-7177
Los Angeles, CA 90095 Fax: 310-206-5012
e-mail: lshakerirwin@mednet.ucla.edu.
www.gcrc.medsch.ucla.edu
Cardiovascular and heart disease disorders and illness research.
Isidro Salus MD, Program Director
Gerald Levey, Principal Investigator

4824 Georgetown University Research Resources Facility
3800 Reservoir Road NW
Washington, DC 20007-2195 202-444-2000
www.georgetownuniversityhospital.org
Studies of medical sciences with particular emphasis on heart dis-
ease.
Linda Winger, Vice President of Professional Services
Joy Drass MD, President

4825 Hahnemann University Likoff Cardiovascular Institute
Broad & Vine Streets 215-854-8100
Philadelpia, PA 19102
Diseases of the heart and vessels.
William S Frankl MD, Director

4826 Harvard Throndike Laboratory Harvard Medical Center
Harvard Medical Center
330 Brookline Avenue 617-735-3020
Boston, MA 02215-5400 Fax: 617-735-4833
Dr James Morgan, Director

4827 Heart Disease Research Foundation
50 Court Street   718-649-6210
Brooklyn, NY 11201-4801
Robert A Teters, Director

4828 Heart Research Foundation of Sacramento
1007 39th Street   916-456-3365
Sacramento, CA 95816-5502   e-mail: rjfrink@pol.net
www.hrfsac.org

Dr Frink, Founder/Principal Investigator

4829 Hope Heart Institute
1380 112th Ave. NE   425-456-8700
Bellvue, WA 98004   Fax: 425-456-8701
e-mail: info@hopeheart.org
www.hopeheart.org

Heart and blood vessel research.
Dr Lester Sauvage MD, Founder & Medical Director Emeritus
Mark Nudelman, President & CEO

4830 John L McClellan Memorial Veterans' Hospital Research Office
4300 W 7th Street   501-257-1000
Little Rock, AR 72205-5446   Fax: 501-671-2510
www2.va.gov

Karl David Straub MD, Chief Staff

4831 Krannert Institute of Cardiology
1801 N Senate Boulevard   317-962-0500
Indianapolis, IN 46202-4832   800-843-2786
Fax: 317-962-0501
medicine.iupui.edu/krannert
The cardiovascular program at the Indiana University School of Medicine is recognized throughout the world for its commitment to excellence in patient care research and education. While we're known for our experience and ability to take care of the most complex cardiovascular problems we are equally focused on prevention and early detection.
Peng-Sheng C MD, Division Chief

4832 Loyola University of Chicago Cardiac Transplant Program
2160 S 1st Avenue   708-216-4977
Maywood, IL 60153-3304   Fax: 708-216-4918
www.luhs.org
Loyola University Health System is committed to excellence in patient care and the education of health professionals. They believe that our Catholic heritage and Jesuit traditions of ethical behavior academic distinction and scientific research lead to new knowledge and advance our healing mission in the communities we serve.
Dr Maria Rosa Costanzo-Nordin, Director

4833 Miami Heart Institute
4300 Alton Road   305-672-1111
Miami Beach, FL 33140-2997   Fax: 305-743-09
www.msmc.com

General cardiovascular research.
Steven D Sonenreich, President & Chief Executive Officer

4834 Miami Heart Research Institute
4770 Biscayne Boulevard   305-674-3020
Miami, FL 33137   Fax: 305-535-3642
e-mail: pak@floridaheart.org
www.miamiheartresearch.org
General cardiovascular research.
Paul Kurlansky, Director Research
Maria Terris MD, Medical Director

4835 Oklahoma Medical Research Foundation: Cardiovascular Research Program
825 NE 13th Street   405-271-6673
Oklahoma City, OK 73104-5097   800-522-0211
Fax: 405-271-3980
e-mail: contact@omrf.org
www.omrf.ouhsc.edu
The Cardiovascular Biology Research Program investigates fundamental mechanisms involved in blood coagulation inflammation and atherogenesis with special emphasis on the regulation of theses processes.
William G Thurman MD, President
Rodger P McEver, Member and Program Chair

4836 Pennsylvania State University Artificial Heart Research Project
Milton S Hershey Medical Center
500 University Drive   717-531-8407
Hershey, PA 17033-2391   Fax: 717-531-5011
www.psu.edu

William S Pierce MD, Director

4837 Preventive Medicine Research Institute
900 Bridgeway   415-332-2525
Sausalito, CA 94965-2158   Fax: 415-325-30
e-mail: dean.ornish@pmri.org
www.pmri.org
Nonprofit organization focusing on prevention and treatment of heart disease through modification of diet exercise and relaxation techniques.
Dean Ornish MD, President
Anne Ornish, Vice President

4838 Purdue University William A Hillenbrand Biomedical Engineering Center
AA Potter Engineering Center
206 S. Martin Jischke Drive   765-494-7015
W Lafayette, IN 47907-2032   877-598-4233
Fax: 765-494-6628
engineering.purdue.edu/BME
Cardiology and heart disease research.
George R Wodicka, Professor and Head

4839 Rockefeller University Laboratory of Cardiac Physiology
1230 York Avenue   212-327-8000
New York, NY 10065   Fax: 212-327-7974
www.rockefeller.edu
Causes of cardiac arrhythmias and prevention of heart disease.
Paul Nurse, Head

4840 San Francisco Heart Institute
1900 Sullivan Avenue   650-991-6601
Daly City, CA 94015-2200   800-82H-EART
Fax: 650-755-7315
e-mail: webmaster@sfhi.com
www.sfhi.com
At Seton Medical Center we are committed to providing a full range of high quality services and state-of-the-art cardiovascular treatments for our patients. Our medical nursing and social services staff provide quality care and compassion as a coordinated team focusing on the medical emotional and spiritual needs of patients and their families.
Colman Ryan, Executive Director
Louis Manila RN BA, Manager of Research and Operations

4841 Specialized Center of Research in Ischemic Heart Disease
1802 6th Avenue South   205-934-4011
Birmingham, AL 35294-0001   800-822-8816
www.health.uab.edu
Coronary artery disease.
Will Ferniany, CEO
Becky Armstrong, Program Manager

4842 Texas Heart Institute St Lukes Episcopal Hospital
St Lukes Episcopal Hospital
6770 Bertner Avenue   832-355-1000
Houston, TX 77225-0345   800-292-2221
Fax: 713-791-3089
e-mail: mmattsson@heart.thi.tmc.edu
www.texasheartinstitute.org

Denton A Cooley MD, President Emeritus
James T Willerson MD, President, Medical Director

4843 University of Alabama at Birmingham: Congenital Heart Disease Center
1201 University Blvd.   205-934-2344
Birmingham, AL 35233   Fax: 205-934-7514
www.uab.edu

Dr. Albert Pacifico, Director
Dr. Carol Garrison, President

4844 University of California San Diego General Clinical Research Center
UCSD Medical Center

200 W Arbor Drive
San Diego, CA 92103-1910
619-543-6014
Fax: 619-435-36
gcrc.ucsd.edu

General clinical research.
Michael G Zieglor, Program Director
Melinda Richards, Administrative Manager

4845 University of California: Cardiovascular Research Laboratory
Center for Health Sciences
UCLA Medical Center
Los Angeles, CA 90024
310-825-6824
Fax: 310-206-5777
Cellular and subcellular cardiac conditions.
Dr Glenn Langer, Director

4846 University of Cincinnati Department of Pathology & Laboratory Medicine
P.O. Box 670529
Cincinnati, OH 45267-0529
513-558-4500
Fax: 513-558-2289
e-mail: decourgm@ucmail.uc.edu
pathology.uc.edu

C Fenoglio Preiser, Director
Meifeng Xu PhD, Research Instructor

4847 University of Iowa: Iowa Cardiovascular Center
College of Medicine
200 Hawkins Drive
Iowa City, IA 52242
319-335-8588
Fax: 319-335-6969
www.int-med.uiowa.edu
The purpose is to coordinate the cardiovascular programs of the College into a more cohesive unit to permit us to 1) utilize our cardiovascular resources optimally 2) intensify expand and integrate basic and clinical research programs in areas related to cardiovascular research and 3) evaluate the role of new measures for prevention diagnosis and treatment of cardiovascular disease.
John B Stokes, Executive Vice Chair
Rebecca Hegeman, Vice Chair Clinical Programs

4848 University of Michigan Pulmonary and Critical Care Division
University Hospital
1500 E Medical Center Drive
Ann Arbor, MI 48109
734-936-4000
888-287-1082
Fax: 734-763-7390
www2.med.umich.edu
Ora Hirsch Pescovitz MD, Executive Vice President

4849 University of Michigan: Division of Cardiology
1500 E Medical Center Drive
Ann Arbor, MI 48109-0001
734-936-4000
www2.med.umich.edu
Focuses on the diagnosis, treatment and prevention of cardiovascular and heart diseases.
Ora Hirsch Pescovitz MD, Executive Vice President

4850 University of Missouri Columbia Division of Cardiothoracic Surgery
School of Medicine
1 Hospital Drive
Columbia, MO 65212
573-882-6955
Fax: 573-884-0437
e-mail: sissonwhitem@health.missouri.edu
www.missouri.edu
Cardiac surgery research.
Brady J Deaton, Chancellor

4851 University of Pennsylvania Pennsylvania Muscle Institute
School of Medicine
3600 Market Street
Philadelphia, PA 19104-2646
215-662-4000
Fax: 215-898-2653
e-mail: mafoster@mail.med.upenn.edu
www.med.upenn.edu
Studies in tissue science.
Aurther H Rubenstein, Dean
Michael Osta PhD, Associate Director

4852 University of Pittsburgh: Human Energy Research Laboratory
242 Trees Hall
Pittsburgh, PA 15261-0001
412-624-4387
www.pitt.edu
Focuses on exercise and cardiac rehabilitation.
Dr Robert Robertson, Director

4853 University of Rochester: Clinical Research Center
601 Elmwood Avenue
Rochester, NY 14642-0001
585-275-3676
Fax: 585-256-3805
e-mail: germaine_reinhardt@urmc.rochester.edu
www.urmc.rochester.edu
Studies of normal tissue functions pertaining to heart diseases.
John E Gerich MD, Director
David S Guzick MD, Principal Investigator

4854 University of Southern California: Coronary Care Research
1200 N State Street
Los Angeles, CA 90033-1029
213-226-7242
Dr. L Julian Haywood, Director

4855 University of Tennessee: Division of Cardiovascular Diseases
920 Madison Avenue
Memphis, TN 38163-0001
901-448-5750
Fax: 901-448-8084
www.utmem.edu\cardiology
Cardiovascular system disorders including heart disease prevention and treatment.
Karl T Weber MD, Director

4856 University of Texas Southwestern Medical Center at Dallas
University of Texas
5323 Harry Hines Boulevard
Dallas, TX 75390-7208
214-648-3111
Fax: 214-483-11
www.utsouthwestern.edu
Cardiology department research.
Francisco G. Cigarroa, M.D., Chancellor

4857 University of Utah: Artificial Heart Research Laboratory
803 N 300 W
Salt Lake City, UT 84103-1414
801-581-6991
Fax: 801-581-4044
healthsciences.utah.edu
Cardiac and blood vessel research.
Allen Stephens, Associate Director

4858 University of Utah: Cardiovascular Genetic Research Clinic
420 Chipeta Way
Salt Lake City, UT 84108-0001
801-581-3888
Fax: 801-581-6862
medicine.utah.edu
Cardiovascular genetics research.
Dr Roger Williams, Founder
Sara Frogley, Research Manager

4859 Urban Cardiology Research Center
2300 Garrison Boulevard
Baltimore, MD 21216-2308
410-945-8600
Causes diagnosis and treatment of cardiovascular diseases.
Arthur White MD, Director

4860 Warren Grant Magnuson Clinical Center
National Institute of Health
10 Center Drive
Bethesda, MD 20892
301-496-4000
800-411-1222
Fax: 301-480-9793
TTY: 866-411-1010
e-mail: prpl@mail.cc.nih.gov
www.clinicalcenter.nih.gov
Established in 1953 as the research hospital of the National Institutes of Health. Designed so that patient care facilities are close to research laboratories so new findings of basic and clinical scientists can be quickly applied to the treatment of patients. Upon referral by physicians, patients are admitted to NIH clinical studies.
John Gallin, Director
David Henderson, Deputy Director for Clinical Care

4861 Yeshiva University General Clinical Research Center
500 West 185th Street
New York, NY 10033
212-960-5400
www.yu.edu
Cardiovascular research.
Harriet S Gilbert MD, Program Director
Richard M Joel, President

Support Groups & Hotlines

4862   American Autoimmune Related Diseases Association
22100 Gratiot Avenue   586-776-3900
Eastpointe, MI 48021   800-598-4668
Fax: 586-776-3903
e-mail: aarda@aarda.org
www.aarda.org
Awareness, education, referrals for patients with any type of autoimmune disease.
Virginia T. Ladd, President/Executive Director

4863   Mended Hearts
7272 Greenville Avenue   214-706-1442
Dallas, TX 75231   888-432-7899
Fax: 214-706-5231
e-mail: dbonham@Heart.org
www.mendedhearts.org
Mutual support for persons who have heart disease, their families,
friends, and other interested persons.

4864   Mitral Valve Prolapse Program of Cincinnati Support Group
10525 Montgomery Road   513-745-9911
Cincinnati, OH 45242   e-mail: kscordo@wright.edu
www.nursing.wright.edu
Brings together persons frightened by their symptoms in order to
learn to better cope with MVP. Fosters use of non-drug therapies.
Supervised exercise sessions, diagnostic evaluations and specialized testing. Information and referrals, conferences, literature,
group meetings, MVP Hot Line, and assistance in starting groups.

4865   National Health Information Center
PO Box 1133   310-565-4167
Washington, DC 20013   800-336-4797
Fax: 301-984-4256
e-mail: info@nhic.org
www.health.gov/nhic
Offers a nationwide information referral service, produces directo-
ries and resource guides.

4866   National Society for MVP and Dysautonomia
880 Montclair Road   205-595-8229
Birmingham, AL 35213   866-595-8229
Fax: 205-595-8222
e-mail: nancysawyermd@bellsouth.net
Assists individuals suffering from mitral valve prolapse syndrome
and dysautonomia to find support and understanding. Education on
symptoms and treatment. Other areas of focus are Fibromyalgia
and Sjogren's Syndrome.
Nancy Sawyer, MD

4867   Pulmonary Hypertension Association
850 Sligo Avenue   301-565-3004
Silver Spring, MD 20907   800-748-7274
Fax: 301-565-3994
e-mail: pha@phassociation.org
www.phassociation.org
A nonprofit organization funded and for pulmonary hypertension
patients. Our mission is to seek a cure, provide hope, support, education and to promote awareness and advocate for the PH community.
Rind Alrrighetti, President

4868   Society of Mitral Valve Prolapse Syndrome
PO Box 431   630-250-9327
Itasca, IL 60143-0431   Fax: 630-773-0478
e-mail: bonnie0107@aol.com
www.mitralvalveprolapse.com/
Provides support and education to patients, families and friends
about mitral valve prolapse syndrome.
Phillip C Watkins, Director MVP Center
Cheryl Durante, Editor

Books

4869   Advances in Cardiac and Pulmonary Rehabilitation
Haworth Press

10 Alice Street   607-722-5857
Binghamton, NY 13904-1580   800-429-6784
Fax: 607-722-0012
www.haworthpress.com
Enhance your rehabilitation program with this authoritative vol-
ume.
74 pages Hardcover
ISBN: 0-866569-86-0

4870   Congenital Heart Disease
Northwestern University Press
625 Colfax Street   847-491-5313
Evanston, IL 60208-4210   800-621-2736
www.nupress.nwu.edu
1993 300 pages
ISBN: 1-880416-82-4

4871   Dr. Dean Ornish's Program for Reversing Heart Disease
Random House Trade Books
400 Hahn Road
Westminster, MD 21157-4663   800-733-3000
Fax: 800-659-2436

ISBN: 0-804110-38-7

**4872   Expert Guide to Beating Heart Disease: What You Absolutely
Must Know**
Dr. Harlan M. Krumholz, author
HarperCollins
10 E. 53rd Street   212-207-7000
New York, NY 10022-5299   e-mail: orders@harpercollins.com
www.harpercollins.com
Translates key medical data into clear guidelines capturing the
highest treatment standards for heart disease. Profiles care
alternatices from supplements to stress reduction as well as treatments on the horizon.
2005 288 pages
ISBN: 0-060578-34-3

4873   Heart Disease
Franklin Watts Grolier
90 Old Sherman Turnpike   203-797-3500
Danbury, CT 06816-0001   800-621-1115
Fax: 203-797-3197
www.grolier.com
Using diagrams, this book discusses strokes and other blood vessel
disorders, as well as their treatment and prevention.
112 pages Grades 7-12
ISBN: 0-531108-84-8

**4874   Heart of a Child: What Families Need to Know About Heart
Disorders: 2nd Edition**
Johnss Hopkins University Press
2715 N Charles Street   410-935-6900
Baltimore, MD 21218-4319   800-537-5487
Fax: 410-516-6998
www.press.jhu.edu
1993 352 pages Paperback
ISBN: 0-801866-36-7

4875   Living with Heart Disease
Franklin Watts Grolier
90 Old Sherman Turnpike   203-797-3500
Danbury, CT 06816-0001   800-621-1115
Fax: 203-797-3197
www.grolier.com
Shows how persons with heart disease can overcome their illness
and lead productive lives.
32 pages Grades 5-7
ISBN: 0-531108-45-7

4876   Mitral Valve Prolapse Syndrome/Dysautonomia Survival Guide
Society of Mitral Valve Prolapse Syndrome
PO Box 431   630-250-9327
Itasca, IL 60143-0431   Fax: 630-773-0478
e-mail: bonnie0107@aol.com
www.mitralvalveprolapse.com

Provides support and education to patients, families and friends about mitral valve prolapse syndrome.
175 pages
ISBN: 1-572243-03-1
Bonnie Durante, Vice President
Cheryl Durante, Editor

4877 What Every Woman Must Know About Heart Disease
Warner Books
1271 Avenue of the Americas   212-484-2900
New York, NY 10020-1300   Fax: 818-507-5596
e-mail: nylandimmunojobs@boxter.com
www.twbookmark.com

1996
ISBN: 0-446519-86-3

4878 Women Take Heart
Putnam Publishing Group
200 Madison Avenue   212-951-8400
New York, NY 10016-3903
1993 224 pages
ISBN: 0-399138-88-9

4879 Women and Heart Disease
Random House Trade Books
400 Hahn Road
Westminster, MD 21157-4663
800-733-3000
Fax: 800-659-2436

ISBN: 0-345386-20-5

Children's Books

4880 Village by the Sea
Franklin Watts Grolier
90 Old Sherman Turnpike   203-797-3500
Danbury, CT 06816-0001   Fax: 203-797-3197
www.grolier.com
This story focuses on the relationship between Emma and her father as he prepares to undergo bypass surgery.
Grades 5-8

Newsletters

4881 American Heart Association News
American Heart Association
7272 Greenville Avenue   214-706-1162
Dallas, TX 75231-5129   Fax: 214-696-5211
News reports and journal reports on the latest information concerning heart disease.

4882 And the Beat Goes On
Society of Mitral Valve Prolapse Syndrome
PO Box 431   630-250-9327
Itasca, IL 60143-0431   Fax: 630-773-0478
e-mail: bonnie0107@aol.com
www.mitralvalveprolapse.com
Bi-monthly newsletter. Provides support and education to patients, families and friends about mitral valve prolapse syndrome.
6 pages
Bonnie Durante, Vice President
Cheryl Durante, Editor

4883 Heartstyle
American Heart Association
7272 Greenville Avenue   214-706-1162
Dallas, TX 75231-5129   Fax: 214-696-5211
Reports on heart and blood vessel diseases and stroke.
Quarterly

4884 MVPS & Anxiety
Society of Mitral Valve Prolapse Syndrome

PO Box 431   630-250-9327
Itasca, IL 60143-0431   Fax: 630-773-0478
e-mail: bonnie0107@aol.com
www.mitralvalveprolapse.com
6 pages
Bonnie Durante, Vice President
Cheryl Durante, Editor

Pamphlets

4885 About High Blood Pressure
American Heart Association
7272 Greenville Avenue   214-706-1162
Dallas, TX 75231-5129   Fax: 214-696-5211
Offers information on what blood pressure is, risk factors and at risk persons.

4886 American Heart Association Diet
American Heart Association
7272 Greenville Avenue   214-706-1162
Dallas, TX 75231-5129   Fax: 214-696-5211
An eating plan for healthy americans.

4887 Cholesterol and Your Heart
American Heart Association
7272 Greenville Avenue   214-706-1162
Dallas, TX 75231-5129   Fax: 214-696-5211
Offers information on lowering blood cholesterol levels.

4888 Congenital Heart Defects
March of Dimes
233 Park Avenue South   212-353-8353
New York, NY 10003   Fax: 212-254-3518
e-mail: NY639@marchofdimes.com
www.marchofdimes.com

4889 E is for Exercise
American Heart Association
7272 Greenville Avenue   214-706-1162
Dallas, TX 75231-5129   Fax: 214-696-5211
Offers information on what kinds of exercise are the best and how to exercise properly.

4890 Easy Food Tips for Heart Healthy Eating
American Heart Association
7272 Greenville Avenue   214-706-1162
Dallas, TX 75231-5129   Fax: 214-696-5211
Offers food selection hints for fat-controlled meals.

4891 Eat Well, But Wisely
American Heart Association
7272 Greenville Avenue   214-706-1162
Dallas, TX 75231-5129   Fax: 214-696-5211
Offers information on good nutrition to reduce the risks of heat attacks.

4892 Exercise and Your Heart
American Heart Association
7272 Greenville Avenue   214-706-1162
Dallas, TX 75231-5129   Fax: 214-696-5211
Offers information on how to get enough exercise from daily activities, what the benefits of exercise are and what the risks of exercising are.

4893 Heart Defects
Association of Birth Defect Children
5400 Diplomat Circle
Orlando, FL 32810-5603   800-922-9234
Informational sheet on the causes, symptoms and statistics of heart defects and heart disease in children.

4894 How to Have Your Cake and Eat It Too
American Heart Association
7272 Greenville Avenue   214-706-1162
Dallas, TX 75231-5129   Fax: 214-696-5211
A guide to low-fat, low-cholesterol eating.

Web Sites

4895 American Heart Association

www.americanheart.org

Supports research, education and community service programs with the objective of reducing premature death and disability from cardiovascular diseases and stroke; coordinates the efforts of health professionals, and other engaged in the fight against heart and circulatory disease.

4896 Healing Well

www.healingwell.com

An online health resource guide to medical news, chat, information and articles, newsgroups and message boards, books, disease-related web sites, medical directories, and more for patients, friends, and family coping with disabling diseases, disorders, or chronic illnesses.

4897 Health Finder

www.healthfinder.gov

Searchable, carefully developed web site offering information on over 1000 topics. Developed by the US Department of Health and Human Services, the site can be used in both English and Spanish.

4898 Healthlink USA

www.healthlinkusa.com

Health information concerning treatment, cures, prevention, diagnosis, risk factors, research, support groups, email lists, personal stories and much more. Updated regularly.

4899 Helios Health

www.helioshealth.com

Online resource for your health information. Detailed information about specific health topics, access to expert advice from our Medical Advisory Board, and up-to-date health news.

4900 MedicineNet

www.medicinenet.com

An online resource for consumers providing easy-to-read, authoritative medical and health information.

4901 Medscape

www.medscape.com

Medscape offers specialists, primary care physicians, and other health professionals the Web's most robust and integrated medical information and educational tools.

4902 National Heart, Lung and Blood Institute

www.nhlbi.nih.gov

Primary responsibility of this organization is the scientific investigation of heart, blood vessel, lung and blood disorders. Oversees research, demonstration, prevention, education, control and training activities in these fields and emphasizes the prevention and control of heart diseases.

4903 WebMD

www.webmd.com

Information on Heart disease, including articles and resources.

Description

4904 **Hemophilia**

Hemophilia is a genetic disorder that disrupts the body's normal blood clotting function because there is a deficiency of specific proteins known as clotting factors—specifically, factor VIII and factor IX. About 20,000 Americans are affected with the disorder and, currently, there is no cure.

Hemophilia is linked to the X-chromosome because that is where both factor genes are located. As a result, hemophilia affects males almost exclusively, with females being carriers, whose sons have a 50 percent chance of having the disorder.

Hemophiliacs, like anyone else, will bleed if injured, but they will bleed longer and more profusely. They may also bleed in response to injuries that are inconsequential in other people. For instance, normal daily activities may cause bleeding within a joint, leading to severe pain and swelling, and over time destroying the joint.

The severity of hemophilia varies dramatically depending on the factor VIII and IX levels, thus, affecting a person's prognosis and need for therapy. Treatment is with transfusions of the appropriate factor, and usually has to be repeated frequently. Most hemophiliacs treated with plasma concentrate in the early 1980s are infected with HIV contracted from contaminated blood and transfusions. HIV is now responsible for over half of deaths among hemophiliacs.

Most hemophiliacs are now treated at comprehensive hemophilia centers, which offer not just factor replacement but multispecialty expertise, sophisticated laboratory testing, physical therapy and psychological support. New techniques allow for identification of carrier females in these families. This is important for genetic counseling and family planning.

National Agencies & Associations

4905 **American Red Cross Blood Services**
8550 Arlington Blvd.
Arlington, VA 22203
70- 58- 840
800-733-2767
e-mail: lkeefe@arlingtonredcross.org
www.redcross.org
Distributes a wide variety of plasma therapeutics to benefit people with hemophilia A and B, immune disorders and hypoalbuminemia.
Linda C Mathes, CEO

4906 **Baxter Hyland Division**
One Baxter Parkway
Deerfield, IL 60015-1900
847-948-4770
800-422-9837
Fax: 847-948-3642
www.baxter.com
Government affairs office that monitors and selectively lobbies on issues relating to Medicare Medicaid Orphan Drugs and other subjects relating to hemophilia.
Pam Koo, Programs Manager

4907 **Canadian Hemophilia Society**
400-1255 University Street
Montreal, Quebec, H3B-3B6
514-848-0503
800-668-2686
Fax: 514-848-9661
e-mail: chs@hemophilia.ca
www.hemophilia.ca
Strives to improve the health and quality of life for all people with inherited bleeding disorders and to find a cure.
Craig Upshaw, President
David Page, National Executive Director

4908 **Hemophilia Health Services**
201 Great Circle Road
Nashville, TN 37228
615-352-2500
800-800-6606
Fax: 615-261-6730
e-mail: info@hemophiliahealth.com
www.hemophiliahealth.com
Largest homecare company devoted solely to serving people with bleeding disorders.
Ken Trader, VP of Sales and Marketing

4909 **National Hemophilia Foundation**
116 W 32nd Street
New York, NY 10001
212-328-3700
800-424-2634
Fax: 212-328-3777
e-mail: info@hemophilia.org
www.hemophilia.org
Dedicated to the treatment and the cure of hemophilia, related bleeding disorders and complications of those disorders or their treatment, including HIV infection, as well as improving the quality of life of all those affected.
Val Bias, Chief Executive Officer
Neil Frick, Vice President

4910 **National Hemophilia Foundation's Information Center**
116 W 32nd Street
New York, NY 10001
212-328-3700
800-424-2634
Fax: 212-328-3777
e-mail: info@hemophilia.org
www.hemophilia.org
Offers various information articles resources books and more for the hemophilia and HIV/AIDS community.
Val Bias, CEO
Neil Frick, Vice President

4911 **World Federation of Hemophilia**
1425 Rene Levesque Boulevard W
Montreal, Quebec, H3G-1T7
514-875-7944
Fax: 514-875-8916
e-mail: wfh@wfh.org
www.wfh.org
An international not-for-profit organization to improving the lives of people with hemophilia and related bleeding disorders.
Claudia Black, CEO/Executive Director
Mark Skinner, President

State Agencies & Associations

Alabama

4912 **Alabama Chapter of the National Hemaphilia Foundation**
802 Midland Avenue
Muscle Shoals, AL 35661-1640
205-381-5925

Arkansas

4913 **Hemophilia Foundation of Arkansas**
351 Valley Oak Lane
Austin, AR 72007
501-941-3109
888-941-4366
e-mail: angieclark1315@sbcglobal.net
www.hemophilia.org

Angie Clark, President
John Little, VP

California

4914 Central California Chapter of the National Hemophilia Foundation
PO Box 163689
Sacramento, CA 95816
91- 2-6 90
Fax: 916-489-1569
e-mail: seanahubbert@yahoo.com
www.cchfsac.org
A very small and family-oriented chapter. Offers an active youth group, an annual summer camp, a men's and women's group and various family activities for persons living in the central California valley from its center in Sacramento to the borders of Nevada.
Sean Hubbert, President

4915 Hemophilia Association of San Diego County
3570 Camino Del Rio N
San Diego, CA 92108
619-325-3570
Fax: 619-325-4350
e-mail: web@hasdc.org
www.hasdc.org
Provides summer camp programs for young persons with hemophilia, sponsors educational programs for the general public, sponsors support groups for parents to help them deal with hemophilia, monitors legislation pertaining to hemophilia and related conditions.
Michael Brown, Board President

4916 Hemophilia Foundation of Northern California
6400 Hollis Street
Emeryville, CA 94608-3024
510-658-3324
Fax: 510-658-3384
e-mail: support@hemofoundation.org
www.hemofoundation.org
A volunteer, nonprofit organization serving the needs of people with hemophilia and other related bleeding disorders in 35 counties in Northern California. Provides hemophilia literature, scholarships, youth programs and annual summer camps.
Nancy Trunzo, Office Administrator
Merlin Wedepohl, Executive Director

4917 Hemophilia Foundation of Southern California
6720 Melrose Avenue
Hollywood, CA 90038
323-525-0440
800-371-4123
Fax: 323-525-0445
e-mail: hfsc@hemosocal.org
www.hemosocal.org

Helena Smith, Office Manager
Linda Corrente, Executive Director

Colorado

4918 Hemophilia Society of Colorado
P.O. Box 4943
Englewood, CO 80155
30- 6-2 75
88- 7-2 02
e-mail: hsc@cohemo.org
www.cohemo.org

Emily Davis, Executive Director
Diane Cadwell, Vice President

Florida

4919 Florida Chapter of the National Hemophilia Foundation
18001 Old Cutler Road
Palmetto Bay, FL 33157
813-367-0050
888-880-8330
Fax: 813-367-0051
e-mail: linda316@bellsouth.net
www.floridahemophilia.org
Janelle Espinosa, Secretary/Treasurer
Rhonda McNeil, President

Georgia

4920 Hemophilia Foundation of Georgia
8800 Roswelll Road
Atlanta, GA 30350
770-518-8272
Fax: 770-518-3310
e-mail: mail.@hog.org
www.hog.org
Established to help Georgia residents with hemophilia lead normal and productive lives. Because this organization is comprised of patients, their friends and families, it is especially motivated to provide the best in personalized and comprehensive services.
Patricia Dominic, CEO
Dave Fronk, Vice Chief Governance Officer

Hawaii

4921 Hemophilia Foundation of Hawaii Kapiolani Medical Center
Kapiolani Medical Center
1164 Bishop Street
Honolulu, HI 96813
808-638-2910
Fax: 808-638-2910
e-mail: hemophiliafoundation@hawaii.rr.com
http://www.kapiolani.org/women-and-child
Jeanine Keoh Kam, Executive Manager

Idaho

4922 Hemophilia Foundation of Idaho
1220 Vista Avenue
Boise, ID 83707-1622
208-344-4476
866-453-4476
Fax: 208-344-4476
e-mail: kmay@hemophilia.org
www.hemophilia.org
Janet Angell, Foundation Administrator
Kari May, Executive Director

Illinois

4923 Hemophilia Foundation of Illinois
210 S. DesPlaines St
Chicago, IL 60661
312-427-1495
Fax: 312-427-1602
e-mail: info@hfi-il.org
www.hemophiliaillinois.org
Serves as an information source referral service and advocate for persons with hemophilia and their families. The mission of this chapter is to provide counseling, educational information and support services to persons affected by hemophilia and related disorders.
Robert P Robinson, Executive Director
Lily Schwartz, Associate Director

Indiana

4924 Hemophilia Foundation of Indiana
5170 E 65th Street
Indianapolis, IN 46220
317-570-0039
800-241-2873
Fax: 317-570-0058
e-mail: cfeay@hoii.org
www.hemophiliaofindiana.org
Chad Feay, Executive Director
Debbie Ford, Office Manger

Kentucky

4925 Kentucky Hemophilia Foundation
1850 Taylor Avenue
Louisville, KY 40213
502-456-3233
800-582-2873
Fax: 502-456-3234
e-mail: info@kyhemo.org
www.kyhemo.org
Assists individuals with hemophilia and related inherited bleeding disorders through education, advocacy and support services. Services include quarterly newsletter, post secondary education scholarship, summer camp for children, seminars and support functions.
Quarterly
Ursela M Lacer, Executive Director

Louisiana

4926 Louisiana Chapter of the National Hemophilia Foundation
3636 S Sherwood Forest
Baton Rouge, LA 70816-2285
225-291-1675
800-749-1680
Fax: 225-291-1679
e-mail: lahemophilia@hipoint.net
http://www.lahemo.org/

Lori Keels, Executive Director
Edgar Guedry, President

Maryland

4927 Hemophilia Foundation of Maryland
13 Class Court   410-661-2307
Baltimore, MD 21234-2602   800-964-3131
                                                              Fax: 410-661-2308
                                                              www.hfmonline.org
The Hemophilia foundation of Maryland is a private not for profit organization which devotes its efforts to improving the quality of life for persons affected with bleeding disorders and their complications.

4928 Maryland Chapter of the National Hemophilia Foundation
PO Box 164   410-291-1675
Phoenix, MD 21131-0164   Fax: 410-285-3271

Massachusetts

4929 New England Hemophilia Association
347 Washington Street   781-326-7645
Dedham, MA 02026   Fax: 781-329-5122
                                                 e-mail: info@newenglandhemophilia.org
                                                              www.newenglandhemophilia.org
New England Hemophilia Association is dedicated to improving the quality of life for persons with bleeding disorders (hemophilia, von Willebrands, and other factor deficiencies) and their families through education, support and advocacy.
Kevin R Sorge, Executive Director
Lisa Schmitt, Program Director

Michigan

4930 Hemophilia Foundation of Michigan
1921 W Michigan Avenue   734-544-0015
Ypsilanti, MI 48197   800-482-3041
                                                              Fax: 734-544-0095
                                                              e-mail: hfm@hfmich.org
                                                              www.hfmich.org
Coordinates funding, professional education, and networking, with Hemophilia Treatment Centers in Michigan, Indiana, and Ohio. Provides educational services, including workshops, meetings, symposiums, and numerous publications.
Ivan C Harner, Executive Director
Jennifer Faunce, President

Minnesota

4931 Hemophilia Foundation of Minnesota and the Dakotas
750 S Plaza Drive   651-406-8655
Mendota Heights, MN 55120   Fax: 651-406-8656
                                                 e-mail: hemophiliafound@visi.com
                                                              www.hfmd.org
A nonprofit organization established to be a leader and a catalyst within the community to enable and inspire members to impact their own lives, with the ultimate aim of cures for both hemophilia and HIV/AIDS.
Aaron Reeves, President/Board of Directors
Bob Stone Jr, Vice President

Mississippi

4932 Mississippi Hemophilia Foundation
PO Box 13608   601-957-6483
Jackson, MS 39236   e-mail: haleyjones80@yahoo.com
                                                              www.hemophilia.org
Haley Jones, President
Patty Lyons, Treasurer

Missouri

4933 Gateway Hemophilia Association
4515 Olive Street   314-361-9500
Saint Louis, MO 63108   877-623-8300
                                                              Fax: 314-729-7033
                                                 e-mail: info@gatewayhemophilia.org
                                                              www.gatewayhemophilia.org
Daniel Kahmke, President
Bridget Tyrey, Vice-President

Nebraska

4934 Nebraska Chapter of the National Hemophilia Foundation
215 Centennial Mall S   402-742-5663
Lincoln, NE 68508   Fax: 402-742-5677
                                                 e-mail: office@nebraskanhf.org
                                                              www.nebraskanhf.org
The mission of this chapter is to provide support, education, communication and advocacy for men, women and children challenged by Hemophilia. Services provided include a toll free telephone hotline for persons seeking information on HIV and hemophilia.
Carl Clark, President
Jacob Wilke, Vice-President

Nevada

4935 Hemophilia Foundation of Nevada
7473 W. Lake Mead Blvd.   702-564-4368
Las Vegas, NV 89128   Fax: 702-446-8134
                                                 e-mail: Info@hfnv.org
                                                              www.hfnv.org
Ramona Alice RN, President Executive Committee
Paulette Shimaburkuro, Vice President Executive Committee

New Mexico

4936 Hemophilia Foundation of New Mexico
PO Box 51494   505-341-9321
Albuquerque, NM 87181   866-341-9321
                                                              Fax: 505-292-5818
                                                 e-mail: sangredeoro@comcast.net
                                                              www.hemophilia.org
Loretta Cordova, Executive Director
Johanna Chappelle, President

New York

4937 Hemophilia Center of Western New York
936 Delaware Ave   716-896-2470
Buffalo, NY 14215   800-669-2299
                                                              Fax: 716-898-5537
                                                 e-mail: info@hemophiliawny.com
                                                              www.hemophiliawny.com
Rosemary Holmberg, Executive Director
Thomas Long, President

4938 Mary M Gooley Hemophilia Center: A Chapter of the NHF
1415 Portland Avenue   585-922-5700
Rochester, NY 14621   Fax: 585-922-5775
                                                 e-mail: robert.fox@rochestergeneral.org
                                                              www.hemocenter.org
Robert Fox, CEO/ President
Peter Kouides, Medical & Research Director

North Carolina

4939 Hemophilia Foundation of North Carolina
260 Town Hall Dr.   919-319-0014
Cary, NC 27560   800-990-5557
                                                              Fax: 919-319-0016
                                                 e-mail: info@hemophilia-nc.org
                                                              www.hemophilia-nc.org
A nonprofit organization that serves as an information source for the hemophilia community of North Carolina. Supply the most up-to-date information concerning hemophilia and hemophilia related HIV/AIDS.
Richard Atwood, President
Leonard Poe, Vice President & Advocacy Chair

Ohio

4940 Central Ohio Chapter of the National Hemophilia Foundation
834 W Third Avenue   614-429-2120
Columbus, OH 43212-0345   800-847-0345
                                                              Fax: 614-429-2150
                                                 e-mail: ralexander@hemophilia.org
                                                              www.nhfcentralohio.org
Jim Wasserstrom, President
Rob Alexander, Executive Director

4941 **Greater Cincinnati/Northern Kentucky Chapter of the NHF**
1008 Marshall Avenue 513-961-4366
Cincinnati, OH 45225 Fax: 513-961-1740
e-mail: hemophilia@fuse.net
tristatebleedingdisorderfoundation.org

Lisa Raterman, Executive Director
Brad Sanders, President

4942 **Northern Ohio Chapter of the National Hemophilia Foundation**
One Independence Place
4807 Rockside Road 216-834-0051
Independence, OH 44131 800-554-4366
Fax: 216-834-0055
e-mail: lynnecapretto@nohf.org
www.nohf.org

Lynne Capretto, Executive Director
Marlene Piatek, President

4943 **Northwest Ohio Hemophilia Association**
P.O. Box 12606 41- 2-1 58
Toledo, OH 43606 Fax: 41- 4-9 32
e-mail: carla@nwohemophilia.org
http://www.hemophilia.org/NHFWeb/MainPgs

Carla Wells, Executive Director
Jim Knepp, President

4944 **Southwestern Ohio Chapter of the National Hemophilia Foundation**
3131 S Dixie Drive 937-298-8000
Moraine, OH 45439 Fax: 937-298-8080
e-mail: info@swohiohemophilia.org
www.swohiohemophilia.org
This chapter serves persons with hemophilia and blood clotting disorders in an 11 county area. It is dedicated to offering people with hemophilia and related blood disorders and their families educational opportunities about the diseases.
Sharon DiLorenzo, Executive Director
Dena M Shepard, President

Oklahoma

4945 **Oklahoma Chapter of the National Hemophilia Foundation**
720 W. Wilshire Blvd 40- 4-3 66
Oklahoma City, OK 73116 800-735-3855
e-mail: TAyers007@aol.com
www.okhemophilia.org

Nathan Holloway, President
Bob Goodley, Executive Director

Oregon

4946 **Hemophilia Foundation of Oregon**
5319 SW Westgate Drive 503-297-7207
Portland, OR 97221 Fax: 503-297-0127
e-mail: hfo@easystreet.com
www.hfo.info

Chris Leland, President
Dawn Johnson, Vice President

Pennsylvania

4947 **Delaware Valley Chapter of the National Hemophilia Foundation**
222 S Easton Road 215-885-6500
Glenside, PA 19038 Fax: 215-885-6074
e-mail: hemophilia@navpoint.com
www.hemophiliasupport.org

Ann Rogers, Executive Director
Clifford Cohn, President

4948 **Western Pennsylvania Chapter of the National Hemophilia Foundation**
20411 Rt. 19 724-741-6160
Pittsburgh, PA 16066 800-824-0016
Fax: 724-741-6167
e-mail: info@westpennhemophilia.org
www.westpennhemophilia.org
Brings together and serves as a focal point for those segments of the community most concerned with hemophilia. They include medical and social service providers, people with hemophilia and their families educators and the general public.
Kerry Fatula, Executive Director
Ida McFarren, President

Rhode Island

4949 **Rhode Island Hemophilia Foundation**
160 Plainfield Street 401-944-6950
Providence, RI 02909

South Carolina

4950 **Hemophilia Association of South Carolina**
PO Box 2386
Irmo, SC 29063 888-829-4849
e-mail: Factoreight@aol.com
http://www.hemophiliaofsouthcarolina.org

Tennessee

4951 **TN Hemo & Bleeding Disorders Foundation**
203 Jefferson Street 615-220-4868
Smyrna, TN 37167-5281 888-703-3269
Fax: 615-220-4889
e-mail: mary@thbdf.org
www.thbdf.org
Offers a hemophilia clinic, social workers and consultants, a state hemophilia program, blood donor programs, counseling programs, genetic counseling, literature and resources, summer camp, grants, and more for the hemophilia and HIV/AIDS community.
Mary Hord, Executive Director
Kent Russ, President

Texas

4952 **Lone Star Chapter of the National Hemophilia Foundation**
10500 NW Freeway 713-686-6100
Houston, TX 77092 888-LSC-NHF1
Fax: 713-686-6102
e-mail: Debbiedelariva@yahoo.com
www.lonestarhemophilia.org

Luis Ramirez, Executive Director
Brian Compton, President

4953 **Texas Central Chapter of the National Hemophilia Foundation**
3530 Forest Lane 214-351-4595
Dallas, TX 75234 Fax: 214-654-9954
e-mail: mail@texcen.org
www.texcen.org
A group of volunteers seeking solutions to the various aspects of the hemophilia problem. Supports blood drives sponsors a summer camp for hemophiliac children, conducts educational member meetings, arranges for genetic counseling and sponsors group support meetings.
Shanna Garcia, President
Shelley Embry, Secretary and Executive Director

Utah

4954 **Utah Chapter of the National Hemophilia Foundation**
772 E 3300 S 801-484-0325
Salt Lake City, UT 84106 877-463-6893
Fax: 801-484-4177
www.hemophiliautah.org
Offers educational information, pamphlets, fundraising events and more for persons and families affected by hemophilia.
Scott Muir, Executive Director
David Winslow, President

Virginia

4955 **Hemophilia Association of the Capital Area**
10560 Main Street 703-352-7641
Fairfax, VA 22030-1504 Fax: 703-352-2145
e-mail: hacacares@verizon.net
www.hacacares.org
A nonprofit organization serving persons with bleeding disorders and their families in northern Virginia Washington DC and Mont-

gomery and Prince George's Counties in Maryland. This chapter's mission is to improve the quality of life for persons with hemophilia.
Sandi Qualley, Executive Director
Miriam Goldstein, President

4956 United Virginia Chapter of the National Hemophilia Foundation
PO Box 188   804-748-7896
Midlothian, VA 23113-8824   800-266-8438
Fax: 800-266-8438
e-mail: vahemophiliaed@verizon.net
www.vahemophilia.org

Kelly Waters, Executive Director
Jeff Krecek, President

Washington

4957 Hemophilia Foundation of Washington
9639 Firdale Avenue   206-533-1660
Edmunds, WA 98020   Fax: 206-533-1686
e-mail: info@bdfwa.org
www.bdfwa.org

Regina Timmons, Executive Director
Reid Morgan, President

4958 Inland Empire Bleeding Disorders
1010 Riverside Drive   509-967-7417
W Richland, WA 99353   866-710-4323
e-mail: iebd4u@verizon.net
www.hemophilia.org

Debbie Campeau, President
Jill McCary, President

Wisconsin

4959 Great Lakes Hemophilia Foundation
638 N 18th Street   414-257-0200
Milwaukee, WI 53233   888-797-4543
Fax: 414-257-1225
e-mail: info@glhf.org
www.glhf.org
The only Wisconsin organization that addresses the physical, emotional social and financial needs of individuals affected by hemophilia. This chapter supports high-quality cost-effective programs for patient care, education, research and public awareness.
Michael Kohler, President
Brandon Young, VP

Foundations

4960 National Hemophilia Foundation
116 West 32nd Street   212-328-3700
New York, NY 10001   800-42H-ANDI
Fax: 212-328-3777
e-mail: handi@hemophilia.org
www.hemophilia.org
The National Hemophilia Foundation is dedicated to finding better treatments and cures for bleeding and clotting disorders and to preventing the complications of these disorders through education, advocacy and research.
Alan Kinniburgh, PhD, Chief Executive Officer

Research Centers

4961 Albert Einstein Medical Center Hemophilia Program
5501 Old York Road   215-456-3880
Philadelphia, PA 19141   Fax: 215-456-6179
www.einstein.edu
With humanity humility and honor to heal by providing exceptionally intelligent and responsive healthcare and education for as many as we can reach
Mehdi K Kajani MD

4962 American Red Cross Hemophilia Center
4860 Sheboygan Avenue   608-227-1303
Madison, WI 53705-0905   Fax: 608-233-8318
www.redcross.org
Greg Novinska, CEO

4963 Boston Hemophilia Center Fegan 5 Children's Hospital
Fegan 5 Children's Hospital
300 Longwood Avenue   617-355-6000
Boston, MA 02115   Fax: 617-730-0152
www.childrenshospital.org
The program offers comprehensive care to people with hemophilia and their families. Our services range from medical treatment counseling and support to discounts on clotting-factor replacement and other products that people with hemophilia require.
James Mandell, CEO
Sandra Fenwick, President

4964 Bowman Grey School of Medicine: Hemophilia Diagnostic Center
Wake Forest University
Department of Pediatrics   919-716-4324
Winston Salem, NC 27157-0001   Fax: 910-716-7100
Christine A Johnson MD

4965 Children's Hospital Hemophilia Treatment Center
3333 Burnet Avenue   513-636-4200
Cincinnati, OH 45229   800-344-2462
Fax: 513-636-5599
TTY: 513-636-4900
www.cincinnatichildrens.org
Cincinnati Children's will improve child health and transform delivery of care through fully integrated globally recognized research education and innovation.
Ralph Gruppo MD, Director
Michael Fisher, CEO

4966 Childrens Hospital of Philadelphia Hemophilia Program
Division of Hematology
34th Street and Civic Center Boulev   215-590-1000
Philadelphia, PA 19104   Fax: 215-903-92
www.chop.edu
The Children's Hospital of Philadelphia the oldest hospital in the United States dedicated exclusively to pediatrics strives to be the world leader in the advancement of healthcare for children by integrating excellent patient care innovative research and quality professional education into all of its programs.
Alan R Cohen MD, Medical Director

4967 Comprehensive Hemophilia Diagnostic and Treatment Center
University of North Carolina
101 Manning Drive   919-966-4131
Chapel Hill, NC 27514   Fax: 919-966-3036
e-mail: lccc@med.unc.edu
www.unchealthcare.org
Multidisciplinary clinics are dedicated to patients with hemophilia (through the Comprehensive Hemophilia Diagnostic and Treatment Center) sickle cell disease brain tumors late effects of anticancer therapy as well as general hematology/oncology.
William Roper, CEO
Dr.Richard Krasno, Chair

4968 Comprehensive Pediatric Hemophilia Center University of South Florida
University of South Florida
450 W Drive   813-974-2201
Tampa, FL 33612-4742
Sara Griggs RN

4969 Eastern Michigan Hemophilia Center St. Joseph Hospital
St. Joseph Hospital
302 Kensington Avenue   810-762-8656
Flint, MI 48503-2044
Leslie Kirschke

4970 Eau Claire Hemophilia Center
900 W Clairemont Avenue   715-839-4418
Eau Claire, WI 54701   Fax: 715-833-4976
Vicky Anders RN

4971 **Fairview-University Hemophilia & Thrombosis Center**
Harvard Street at E River Road
Minneapolis, MN 55455   612-626-6455
    800-688-5252
    Fax: 612-625-4955
Serves over 700 adults and children in Minnesota with inherited bleeding disorders. Offers access to current technologies and treatments. Special programs include patient support group family retreats and camps.
Linda Swanso RN, Program Manager

4972 **Great Plains Regional Hemophilia Center University of Iowa Hospitals**
University of Iowa Hospitals
200 Howkins Drive   319-384-8442
Iowa City, IA 52242   800-777-8442
    Fax: 319-567-59
    www.uiowa.edu

Donald E Macfarlane, Director

4973 **Greater Grand Rapids Pediatric Hemophilia Program**
DeVos at Spectrum Health Systems
100 Michigan NE   616-391-2033
Grand Rapids, MI 49503
James B Fahner MD

4974 **Gulf States Hemophilia Diagnostic and Treatment Center**
University of Texas Health Science Center Houston
6655 Travis Street   713-500-8360
Houston, TX 77030-3005   800-464-1440
    Fax: 713-500-8364
    www.livingwithhaemophilia.com
Marisela Trujillo, Financial Administer
W Hoots, Medical Director

4975 **Gundersen Clinic Comprehensive Hemophilia Treatment Center**
Gundersen Clinic
1900 S Avenue   608-782-7300
LaCrosse, WI 54601   800-362-9567
    Fax: 608-775-6692
    e-mail: info@GundLuth.org
    www.gundluth.com
Jeff Thompson, Chief Executive Officer
Joan Curran, Chief Government Relations and External

4976 **Hematology Treatment Center of the Great Lakes Hemophilia Foundation**
Milwaukee, WI 53201-2178   414-257-2424
    Fax: 414-257-1225
    e-mail: info@hemophilia.org
    www.hemophilia.org
Michael Kohler, President

4977 **Hemophilia Association of the Huntington Area**
Marshall University School of Medicine
1600 Medical Center Drive   304-691-1384
Huntington, WV 25703-1518   877-691-1600
    Fax: 304-691-1375

Andrew Tendleton, Medical Director

4978 **Hemophilia Association of the Huntington A Marshall University School of Medicine**
1600 Medical Center Drive   304-691-1700
Huntington, WV 25701   877-691-1600
    Fax: 304-691-1375
    musom.marshall.edu
Charles H McKowen, Dean, Vice President
Andrew Tendleton, Medical Director

4979 **Hemophilia Center of Central Pennsylvania Penn State Milton S Hershey Medical Cent**
Penn State Milton S Hershey Medical Center
500 University Drive   717-531-8521
Hershey, PA 17033   Fax: 717-310-4021
    www.hmc.psu.edu
Edward Junker, Chairman
Harold Paz, CEO, Director

4980 **Hemophilia Center of Rhode Island Rhode Island Hospital**
Rhode Island Hospital

593 Eddy Street   401-444-4000
Providence, RI 02903   Fax: 401-444-5914
    www.rirad.org
Lawrence Aubin, Chairman of the Board
Timothy Babineau, President, CEO

4981 **Hemophilia Center of West Virginia University Health Sciences Center**
University Health Sciences Center
Medical Center Drive   304-293-4229
Morgantown, WV 26506   Fax: 304-293-3793
John S Rogers II MD

4982 **Hemophilia Center of Western New York Erie County Medical Center**
Erie County Medical Center
462 Grider Street   716-896-2470
Buffalo, NY 14215-3021   Fax: 716-898-5537
    www.hemophiliawny.com
The center provides a variety of services to the hemophilia and HIV/AIDS community. Included among these services are diagnostics registration outpatient treatment home care programs home visits school visits dental services and counseling services. Offers an adult unit and a pediatric unit.
Rosemary Holmberg, Executive Director
Thomas Long, President

4983 **Hemophilia Center of the Huntington Hospital**
100 W California Boulevard
Pasadena, CA 91105-3023   626-397-5000
    www.huntingtonhospital.com
At Huntington our mission is to excel at the delivery of health care to our community.
Stephen Ralph, President and CEO
Jim Noble, Sr Vice President, CFO

4984 **Hemophilia Center of the New England Medical Center**
Tufts New England Medical Center
800 Washington Street   617-636-5000
Boston, MA 02111-1526   Fax: 617-636-7738
    www.tuftsmedicalcenter.org
Comprehensive care for pediatric and young adult individuals with bleeding and prothrombotic disorders.
Ellen Zane, President and Chief Executive Officer
David G Fairchild MD MP, Chief Medical Officer

4985 **Hemophilia Clinic: Childrens' Rehabilitation Service**
1870 Pleasant Avenue   334-479-8617
Mobile, AL 36617   800-879-8163
Nancy Woodall RN

4986 **Hemophilia Treatment Center at Children's National Medical Center**
Department of Hematology/Oncology
111 Michigan Avenue NW   202-884-3622
Washington, DC 20010   Fax: 202-884-2976
    www.livingwithhaemophilia.com
Gordon L Bray MD

4987 **Louisiana Comprehensive Hemophilia Care Center**
6823 Saint Charles Avenue   504-862-8000
New Orleans, LA 70118-2699   Fax: 504-883-08
    e-mail: cleissi@tulane.edu
    tulane.edu
Scott S Cowen, President

4988 **Maine Hemophilia Treatment Center**
19 Bramhall Street   207-885-7683
Portland, ME 04102   Fax: 207-885-7565
Nancy Roy RN

4989 **Mayo Comprehensive Hemophilia Center Mayo Clinic**
Mayo Clinic
200 1st Street SW   507-284-2021
Rochester, MN 55905-1   800-344-7726
    Fax: 507-284-8286
A World Federation of Hemophilia-designated International Hemophilia Training Center provides multidisciplinary assessment and care of persons with bleeding disorders. Offers consultation

with hemotologists specializing in the care of pediatric and adult patients a special consultation laboratory testing center and more.
Harlan Langstraat, Director

4990 Miami Comprehensive Hemophilia Center Jackson Medical Towers
Jackson Medical Towers
1500 NW
Miami, FL 33136-3609   305-243-4791
Susan Schmal ARNP   Fax: 305-324-9785

4991 Michigan State University Hemophilia Comprehensive Care Clinic
Michigan State University
2900 Hannah Boulevard
E Lansing, MI 48823   517-353-9385
                                    800-759-5595
                                    Fax: 517-353-9421

John Penner MD, Head Physician

4992 Missouri Illinois Regional Hemophilia Comprehensive Treatment Center
3635 Vista Avenue & Grand Boulevard
Saint Louis, MO 63104-1003   314-268-5275
Kathleen P Gioia RN   Fax: 314-268-5104

4993 Mountain State Regional Hemophilia Center University of Arizona Health Sciences Ce
University of Arizona Health Sciences Center
1501 N Campbell Avenue   520-626-1197
Tucson, AZ 85724-0001   Fax: 520-626-1460
                                    www.ahsc.arizona.edu

William Crist MD, Vice President

4994 Nadeene Brunini Comprehensive Hemophilia Care Center
St Michael s Medical Center
197 Route 18 South   732-249-6000
East Brunswick, NJ 08816-2011   Fax: 732-249-7999
                                    e-mail: hemnj@comcast.net
                                    www.hanj.org
Hemophilia and other bleeding disorder treatment center.
Louis Greene, Director

4995 North Dakota Comprehensive Hemophilia Center
Roger Maris Cancer Center
820 4th Street N   701-234-7544
Fargo, ND 58122-0001   800-437-4010
                                    Fax: 701-234-7592
A treatment center for diseases of hemotosis and thrombosis which includes a clinical research program in bleeding disorders. Hemotologists are available for consultation 24 hours a day.

4996 North Dakota Hemostasis and Thrombosis Treatment Center
Roger Maris Cancer Center
820 4th Street N   701-234-7544
Fargo, ND 58122-0001   800-437-4010
                                    Fax: 701-234-7577
                                    www.meritcare.com
A treatment center for diseases of hemotosis and thrombosis which includes a clinical research program in bleeding disorders. Hemotologists are available for consultation 24 hours a day.
Dr Nathan Kobrinsky MD, Hemophilia Treatment Director

4997 North Texas Comprehensive Adult Hemophilia Center
University of Texas Southwestern Medical Center
5323 Harry Hines Boulevard
Dallas, TX 75390-7208   214-648-3111
                                    www.utsouthwestern.edu
Daniel K Podolsky MD, President

4998 North Texas Comprehensive Pediatric Hemophilia Center
1935 Motor Street   214-456-2382
Dallas, TX 75235-7701   Fax: 214-456-6133
                                    www.hemophiliaregion6.org
Andrea Johns RN PNP

4999 Northwest Ohio Hemophilia Treatment Center
The Toledo Hospital

2142 N Cove Boulevard   419-471-2291
Toledo, OH 43606-3895   Fax: 412-916-01
                                    www.toledochildrens.org

Barbara Steele, President
Ann Gilbert, Director

5000 Oklahoma Comprehensive Hemophilia Diagnostic Treatment Center
940 NE 13th Street   405-271-3661
Oklahoma City, OK 73126-0307   800-688-5288
                                    Fax: 405-271-3756
Beverly Stev RN

5001 Orthopaedic Hospital's Hemophilia Treatment Center
2400 S Flower Street   213-742-1000
Los Angeles, CA 90007-2629   Fax: 213-742-1103
                                    e-mail: info@laoh.ucla.edu
                                    www.orthohospital.org

Carol K Kasper, Hematology
Richard W Cook, Chairman, CEO

5002 Puget Sound Blood Center
921 Terry Avenue   206-292-6500
Seattle, WA 98104-1256   e-mail: keithw@psbc.org
                                    www.psbc.org

James AuBuchon MD, Presidnent, CEO

5003 Regional Comprehensive Center for Hemophilia and VonWillebrand Disease
43 New Scotland Avenue   518-262-3125
Albany, NY 12208-3479   800-773-7080
                                    Fax: 518-262-6320
                                    e-mail: albanyhtc@mail.amc.edu
                                    www.amc.edu
Providing excellence in medical education biomedical research and patient care.ÿ
Joanne Porter, Medical Director
Christine Coonrad, Billing/ Grant Support

5004 Regional Hemophilia Treatment Center Children's Hospital of Michigan
Children's Hospital of Michigan
1921 W. Michigan Avenue   73- 54- 001
Ypsilanti, MI 48197-2196   800-482-3041
                                    Fax: 313-745-5237
                                    www.hfmich.org

Jennifer Faunce, President

5005 Richland Memorial Comprehensive Pediatric Hemophilia Center
Children's Hospital for Cancer & Blood Disorders
7 Richland Medical Park Drive   803-434-3533
Columbia, SC 29203   Fax: 803-434-4598
Robert S Etinger MD

5006 Riley Hemophilia & Hemophilia Center Riley Hospital for Children
Riley Hospital for Children
702 Barnhill Drive   317-274-2060
Indianapolis, IN 46202-5200   800-248-1199
                                    Fax: 317-278-0616
                                    e-mail: mheiny@iupui.edu
                                    rileychildrenshospital.com

Elaine South RN PNP, Nurse Coordinator
Daniel Fink, President, CEO

5007 South Texas Comprehensive Hemophilia Center: Santa Rosa Health Corporation
Children's Hospital
333 N Santa Rosa Street   210-704-2011
San Antonio, TX 78207-3108   Fax: 210-704-2396
                                    www.christussantarosa.org

John Drake RN
Patrick Carrier, President, CEO

5008 Southern Tier Hemophilia Center United Health Services-Wilson Hospital
United Health Services-Wilson Hospital
33-57 Harrison Street   607-763-6436
Johnson City, NY 13790   Fax: 607-763-5514
Doris Michal RN

5009 St. Joseph's Hemophilia Center
2927 N 7th Avenue 602-406-3770
Phoenix, AZ 85013-4102
Rachel Stuar RN

5010 Ted R Montoya Hemophilia Program University of New Mexico
University of New Mexico
2211 Lomas Boulevard NE 505-277-0111
Albuquerque, NM 87131-0001 Fax: 505-272-6845
www.unm.edu

Prasad Mathe MD, Director

5011 Thomas Jefferson University: Cardenza Foundation for Hematologic Research
1020 Walnut Street 215-955-6000
Philadelphia, PA 19107-5005 Fax: 215-955-2342
www.jefferson.edu

Robert L Barchi, President

5012 UCD Northern Central California Hemophilia Program
PO Box 163689 916-296-9066
Sacramento, CA 95816-2208 Fax: 916-489-1569
www.cchfsac.org
An all-volunteer nonprofit organization dedicated to helping people with bleeding disorders.
Charles F Abildgaard MD

5013 UCSD Comprehensive Hemophilia Treatment Center
9500 Gilman Drive, MC-0726 619-471-0336
La Jolla, CA 92093 Fax: 858-822-6444
e-mail: kdherbst@ucsd.edu
hem-onc.ucsd.edu

Sanford Shattil MD, Program Director
Kenneth D Herbst, Medical Director

5014 University Medical Center Hemophilia Program
1800 W Charleston Boulevard
Las Vegas, NV 89102-2329 702-383-2000
www.umcsn.com

Jack Lazerso MD
Kathleen Silver, CEO

5015 University Treatment Center of University Hospitals of Cleveland
11100 Euclid Avenue 216-844-1000
Cleveland, OH 44106 Fax: 216-844-5431
www.uhhospitals.org

Thomas S Zenty, CEO
Alex Y Huang, Director

5016 University of Cincinnati Adult Hemophilia Treatment Program
231 Bethesda Avenue 513-558-4233
Cincinnati, OH 45267-0001 Fax: 513-558-3878
Kathleen E Palascak MD

5017 University of Michigan Hemophilia Center
1500 E Medical Center Drive 734-647-5705
Ann Arbor, MI 48109 Fax: 734-635-15
www.umich.edu

Mary Sue Coleman, President

5018 University of Tennessee Hemophilia Clinic
203 Jefferson Street 901-220-4868
Smyrna, TN 37167 888-703-3269
Fax: 615-220-4889
www.thbdf.org

Mary Hord, Executive Director

5019 Vanderbilt Comprehensive Hemophilia Center
2200 Children's Way, 6105 DOT 615-936-1765
Nashville, TN 37232-9830 866-372-5663
Fax: 61- 93- 840
www.mc.vanderbilt.edu/vhtc
The mission of the Vanderbilt Hemostasis-Thrombosis Clinic is to provide the highest quality compassionate care for individuals with inherited disorders of bleeding or clotting. The team emphasizes the empowerment of patients in their own care while also providing opportunities to participate in scientific advances in the diagnosis and treatment of bleeding and clotting disorders.
Dr Robert L Janco, Director Hematologist
Dr Anne Neff, Co-Director Hematologist

5020 Vermont Regional Hemophilia Center
108 Cherry Street 80- 86- 720
Burlington, VT 05402 800-464-4343
Fax: 802-865-7754
e-mail: vtadap@vdh.state.vt.us
healthvermont.gov
Provides care to persons with types of bleeding disorders. We see people from Vermont and upstate New York.
Miriam Huste RN, Hemophilia Nurse Coordinator
Donald R Swartz, Medical Director

5021 West Central Ohio Hemophilia Center Childens Medical Center
Childens Medical Center
1 Childrens Plaza 937-641-3000
Dayton, OH 45404-1815 800-228-4055
Fax: 937-641-5878
www.childrensdayton.org
The center provides complete care for individuals and families with hemophilia and related bleeding disorders. Some of the services offered include a comprehensive clinic emergency treatment network consultations diagnostic coagulation laboratory home infusion programs HIV/AIDS education and counseling and more.
David Kinsaul, President, CEO
Emmett Broxson, Director Hemothology

Support Groups & Hotlines

5022 National Health Information Center
PO Box 1133 310-565-4167
Washington, DC 20013 800-336-4797
Fax: 301-984-4256
e-mail: info@nhic.org
www.health.gov/nhic
Offers a nationwide information referral service, produces directories and resource guides.

Books

5023 Avoiding Indecision and Hesitation with Hemophilia-Related Emergencies
American Health Consultants
3525 Piedmont Road NE
Atlanta, GA 30305 800-688-2421
Provides detailed information necessary for physicians, and ED staff to deal effectively and expeditiously with hemophilia emergencies.
12 pages

5024 Federal Medicaid Drug Program
1730 E Street NW 202-628-9292
Washington, DC 20006-5300
Discusses changes in government reimbursement and its effect on plasma derived products distributed by the American Red Cross. Includes law information, individual state billing procedures and Medicaid program coverage for the hemophilia community.

5025 Guide to Insurance Coverage for People with Hemophilia
Armour Pharmaceutical Company
500 Arcola Road 215-454-3720
Collegeville, PA 19426-3930
An educational guide designed to assist with health insurance concerns.

5026 Hemophilia Camp Directory
National Hemophilia Foundation
116 W 32nd Street 212-219-8180
New York, NY 10001-3212 800-424-2634
Fax: 212-328-3777
www.hemophilia.org
Lists camps in the United States for children with hemophilia and other coagulation disorders.
16 pages
Alan Kinniburgh, PhD, CEO

5027 Procedure Coding for Hemophilia Treatment
Armour Pharmaceutical Company
500 Arcola Road 215-454-3720
Collegeville, PA 19426-3930

Educational guide designed to facilitate the appropriate use of CPT codes for the hemophilia community.

Children's Books

5028 Adventures of Maxx
Nova Factor
1620 Century Centery Parkway   901-348-8129
Memphis, TN 38137   800-424-2634
                                       Fax: 901-385-3778
An activity book for children with hemophilia, this publication is intended to be both educational and entertaining.
15 pages

5029 Children's Hemophilia Book
Porton Products Limited
30401 Agoura Road   818-879-2200
Agoura Hills, CA 91301-2006
Coloring book that discusses what hemophilia is, bleeding episodes and treatment from a child's point of view.
25 pages

5030 Harold Talks About How He Inherited Hemophilia
Kentucky Hemophilia Foundation
982 Eastern Parkway   502-634-8161
Louisville, KY 40217-1571   800-582-2873
                                       Fax: 502-634-9995
                                   e-mail: info@kyhemo.org
                                          www.kyhemo.org
Children's brochure explaining hemophilia causes, symptoms and living a regular life.
Ursela M Lacer, Executive Director

5031 Harold's Secret: A Boy with Hemophilia
Bayer
400 Morgan Lane   203-937-2765
West Haven, CT 06516-4175
A comic book for youngsters pertaining to children with hemophilia and understanding of the illness among school friends.
16 pages

5032 Understanding Hemophilia: A Young Person's Guide
Armour Pharmaceuticals Company
500 Arcola Road
Collegeville, PA 19426-3930   800-424-2634
This publication is designed for young persons with hemophilia. Presented in very basic and accessible language, this text with colored illustrations points out what hemophilia is, how to cope and more.
91 pages

Magazines

5033 HEMALOG
Maleria Medica
101 W 23rd Street PMB 2246   212-725-5151
New York, NY 10011-2490   Fax: 212-725-2794
                                  e-mail: hemalog@hotmail.com
The purpose of Hemalog is to serve as a national forum for the hemophilia community, providing current news, information, opinion and contact with others in the community. The material contained in this journal reflects the experience and opinion of a wide range of people connected with hemophilia and encourages story and art contributions.
36 pages Quarterly
Barbara Robin Slonevsky, Publisher
Janet Spencer-King, Editor-in-Chief

5034 HemAware
National Hemophilia Foundation
116 W 32nd Street   888-463-6643
New York, NY 10001-3212   800-424-2634
                                       Fax: 212-328-3777
                                          www.hemophilia.org
NHF magazine that offers treatment news about bleeding disorders and provides comprehensive articles on the latest developments in treatment and research as well as highlighting new programs and new resources in the field.
Bi-Monthly
Alan Kinniburgh, PhD, CEO

5035 Human Factor
Hemophilia Health Services
6820 Charlotte Pike
Nashville, TN 37209-4206   800-800-6606
This journal is provided as a free service for the purpose of informing, educating and empowering the hemophilia community.
Quarterly

Newsletters

5036 Artery
Hemophilia Foundation of Michigan
230 1 Platt Road   734-761-2535
Ann Arbor, MI 48103-2973   800-482-3041
                                       Fax: 734-975-2889
                                          www.hfmich.org
Offers information on the chapter's activities and events, support groups and hotlines, technical and medical updates pertaining to the hemophilia and HIV/AIDS community.
Quarterly
Susan Lerch, Editor

5037 Big Red Factor
National Hemophilia Foundation: Nebraska
215 Centennial Mall South   402-742-5663
Lincoln, NE 68508   Fax: 402-742-5677
                                  e-mail: office@nebraskanhf.org
                                  www.nebraskanhf.org/chapter/
Chapter newsletter offering legislative and medical updates, technology, resources, assistive devices and more for persons affected by hemophilia and other blood disorders.

5038 Bloodlines
Hemophilia Association of San Diego County
3570 Camoni del Rio N   619-325-3570
San Diego, CA 92108   Fax: 619-325-4350
                                          www.hasdc.org
Updates membership on the newest techniques and technologies on the treatment of hemophilia.
Quarterly
Jessica Swann, Executive Director
Teresa Ramirez, Coordinator Member Services

5039 Concentrate
Hemophilia of North Carolina
2 Centerview Drive   919-852-4788
Greensboro, NC 27407-3708
Offers information on summer camps, resources, book reviews, parent information and articles pertaining to hemophilia.
Monthly

5040 Factor Nine News
Coalition for Hemophilia B
225 W 34th Street   212-628-3445
New York, NY 10122   Fax: 212-554-6906
                                  e-mail: cfb@web-depot.com
                                          www.boygenius.com/cfb
Offers information on FDA approvals, annual meetings and the latest in technology and information regarding hemophilia.
Kimberly Phelan, VP

5041 Hemophilia NewsBriefs
Great Lakes Hemophilia Foundation
638 North 18th Street   414-257-0200
Milwaukee, WI 53233   Fax: 414-257-1225
                                   e-mail: info@glhf.org
                                          www.glhf.org

5042 Infusion
Kentuckian Hemophilia Foundation

982 Eastern Parkway
Louisville, KY 40217-1571

510-634-8161
800-582-CURE
Fax: 510-568-6111
e-mail: officeinfo@HFNonline.org
www.hfnconline.org

Offers information on summer camps, association activities and events, national projects touching on hemophilia and HIV related disorders and articles on the newest breakthroughs and technology for fighting bleeding disorders.
Quarterly

5043 Initiatives
Quantum Health Resources
790 The City Drive S
Orange, CA 92868-4941

714-750-1610

Aimed at keeping patients and other interested individuals informed on important economic trends, legislation and medical issues.
Quarterly
Lynne Brightman

5044 Linking Factor
National Hemophila Foundation: Utah Chapter
340 E 400 S
Salt Lake City, UT 84111-2909

800-800-6606

A newsletter offering chapter association news and information.
BiMonthly
Charles Hand, Executive Director
Linda Aagard, Editor

5045 New England Hemophilia Association Newsletter
180 Rustcraft Road
Dedham, MA 02026-4558

781-326-7645
800-228-6342
e-mail: neha@world.std.com
www.newenglandhemophilia.org

New England Hemophilia Association is dedicated to improving the quality of life for persons with bleeding disorders (hemophilia, von Williebrands, and other factor deficiencies) and their families through education, support and advocacy. NEHA is a chapter of the National Hemophilia Foundation.
Quarterly
Catherine I Cornell, Executive Director

5046 TN Hemo & Bleeding Disorders Foundation Newsletter
TN Hemo & Bleedin Disorders Foundation
203 Jefferson Street
Smyrna, TN 37167-5281

615-220-4868
888-703-3269
Fax: 615-220-4889
e-mail: mary@thbdf.org
www.thbdf.org

3x/year
Mary Hord, Executive Director
H Kent Russ, President

5047 Ways & Means
Quantum Health Resources
790 The City Drive S
Orange, CA 92868-4941

714-750-1610

Features pertinent health care information for hemophilia patients and their families.
Quarterly
Lynne Brightman

5048 Infusion
Northern California Chapter of the NHF
7700 Edgewater Drive
Oakland, CA 94621-3023

650-568-NCHF

Informs members of medical, dental and orthopedic treatment advances and the latest research in the field. Helps to keep people with hemophilia and their families aware of relevant local and national meetings and includes important updates regarding research and treatment.
BiMonthly

Pamphlets

5049 Anyone Can Have a Bleeding Problem
Hemophilia Foundation of Michigan

411 Huronview Boulevard
Ann Arbor, MI 48103-2973

734-761-2535
800-482-3041

Offers information on Hemophilia and Von Willebrand's Disease. How persons can get it, prevention and causes of the illnesses.

5050 Article Reprint Exchange
HANDI-The National Hemophilia Foundation
116 W 32nd Street
New York, NY 10001-3212

212-219-8180
800-424-2634
Fax: 212-328-3777

Offers various reprinted articles concerning hemophilia and the newest medical technology.

5051 Basics of HIV Disease: Questions and Answers
National Hemophilia Foundation
116 W 32nd Street
New York, NY 10001-3212

888-463-6643
800-424-2634
Fax: 212-328-3777
www.hemophilia.org

This publication contains basic information about hemophilia and HIV disease.
1992 28 pages
Alan Kinniburgh, PhD, CEO

5052 Clotting Agents Are Lifesavers
Hemophilia Foundation of Michigan
411 Huronview Boulevard
Ann Arbor, MI 48103-2973

734-761-2535

Offers information on what hemophilia is, treatments, occurances, heredity, Von Willebrand's Disease, patient services and direct services for hemophiliacs and HIV/AIDS patients.

5053 Comprehensive Care
National Hemophilia Foundation
116 W 32nd Street
New York, NY 10001-3212

888-463-6643
800-424-2634
Fax: 212-328-3777
www.hemophilia.org

Discusses the nature of comprehensive care and its functions and defines the care team. Also touches upon essential resources, HIV, and the benefits of comprehensive care.
1991 12 pages
Alan Kinniburgh, PhD, CEO

5054 Comprehensive Services for Persons with Hemophilia
Hemophilia Foundation of Minnesota/Dakotas
2304 Park Avenue
Minneapolis, MN 55404-3712

612-871-3340
Fax: 612-871-1359

Offers information on what hemophilia is and information and resources for persons with hemophilia and other bleeding disorders.

5055 Consumer Bill of Rights and Responsibilities for Healthcare Service
National Hemophilia Foundation
116 W 32nd Street
New York, NY 10001-3212

888-463-6643
800-424-2634
Fax: 212-328-3777
www.hemophilia.org

Serves as a set of goals for both the provider and consumer in seeking, providing, and receiving high quality health care within a setting of honesty and respect.
1994
Alan Kinniburgh, PhD, CEO

5056 Countdown to a Cure
Louisiana Hemophilia Foundation
3636 S Sherwood Forest Boulevard
Baton Rouge, LA 70816-2285

225-291-1675
Fax: 225-291-1679
e-mail: lahemophilia@hipoint.net
www.louisianahemophilia.org/

Offers information on chapter resources and services for hemophiliacs and their families. Offers information and services to families/patients affected by bleeding disorders.
Lori Keels, Executive Director

5057 Fight Hemophilia with Facts Not Fiction
Great Lakes Hemophilia Foundation
638 North 18th Street
Milwaukee, WI 53233

414-257-0200
Fax: 414-257-1225
www.glhf.org

Offers information on what hemophilia is, research information and treatments.

5058 Get Real and Be Safe!
National Hemophilia Foundation
116 W 32nd Street 888-463-6643
New York, NY 10001-3212 800-424-2634
Fax: 212-328-3777
www.hemophilia.org
Comic book style, this pamphlet offers information to young adults on the hazards and precautions of sex. Offers an Ask The Doctor question and answer section to books and resources for young adults on safer sex and HIV/AIDS.
1991 14 pages
Alan Kinniburgh, PhD, CEO

5059 Guidelines for Finding Childcare
National Hemophilia Foundation
116 W 32nd Street 888-463-6643
New York, NY 10001-3212 800-424-2634
Fax: 212-328-3777
www.hemophilia.org
Information for parents on how to hire a good babysitter, information on daycare centers, how to tell daycare staff about hemophilia, cooperative childcare and suggested reading for parents.
1987 10 pages
Alan Kinniburgh, PhD, CEO

5060 HIV Disease in People with Hemophilia: Your Questions Answered
National Hemophilia Foundation
116 W 32nd Street 888-463-6643
New York, NY 10001-3212 800-424-2634
Fax: 212-328-3777
www.hemophilia.org
Discusses hemophilia and HIV disease, AIDS, management of HIV disease, risks to sexual partners, and issues for children with hemophilia.
1991 48 pages
Alan Kinniburgh, PhD, CEO

5061 HIV Infection and Hemophilia
Hemophilia Foundation of Illinois
332 S Michigan Avenue 312-427-1495
Chicago, IL 60604-4434
Offers information on HIV/AIDS relating to persons with hemophilia.

5062 Hemophilia: Current Medical Management
National Hemophilia Foundation
116 W 32nd Street 888-463-6643
New York, NY 10001-3212 800-424-2634
Fax: 212-328-3777
www.hemophilia.org
Provides an overview of all aspects of hemophilia treatment, including prophylaxis, home therapy, inhibitors, orthopedic solutions, surgery, and dental care.
1994 30 pages
Alan Kinniburgh, PhD, CEO

5063 How to Control Bleeds: Inspired by Vince, an 8-year-old Boy with Hemophilia
Bayer
400 Morgan Lane 203-937-2765
West Haven, CT 06516-4175
An educational comic book story by Vince about hemophilia and treatment for bleeds.
26 pages

5064 Living with HIV: Talking with Your Child
Bobbie Steinhart, author
National Hemophilia Foundation
116 W 32nd Street 888-463-6643
New York, NY 10001-3212 800-424-2634
Fax: 212-328-3777
www.hemophilia.org
A pamphlet directed at caregivers of young children living with hemophilia and HIV disease.
1990 8 pages
Alan Kinniburgh, PhD, CEO

5065 Mild Hemophilia
National Hemophilia Foundation
116 W 32nd Street 888-463-6643
New York, NY 10001-3212 800-424-2634
Fax: 212-328-3777
www.hemophilia.org
Defines mild hemophilia and details its discovery, diagnosis, inheritance, symptoms, treatment, and activity limitations.
1994 25 pages
Alan Kinniburgh, PhD, CEO

5066 Participating in a Clinical Trial: Your Life, Your Choice
National Hemophilia Foundation
116 W 32nd Street 888-463-6643
New York, NY 10001-3212 800-424-2634
Fax: 212-328-3777
www.hemophilia.org
This brochure explains what clinical trials are and what they are like for patients, describes what kinds of HIV therapies are being tested in clinical trials, and lists questions to ask before joining a trial. This publication is ideal for patients, their families, and/or healthcare personnel who counsel HIV-positive patients.
1994 6 pages
Alan Kinniburgh, PhD, CEO

5067 Physical Therapy in Hemophilia
Nationa Hemophilia Foundation
110 Greene Street 212-328-3700
New York, NY 10012-3832 800-424-2634
Fax: 212-328-3777
www.hemophilia.org
Targeted at physical therapy students or new therapists at comprehensive hemophilia care clinics. Also provides basic treatment care information for persons with hemophilia and their families.
1986 13 pages

5068 Simple & Complex: A Hemophilia Primer
Western Pennsylvania Chapter of the NHF
580 S Aiken Avenue 412-685-2231
Pittsburgh, PA 15232-1531 Fax: 412-683-2568
Offers information on what hemophilia is, explains AIDS and HIV infection, offers information on the treatments for hemophilia and what hemophilia care costs.

5069 Student with Hemophilia: A Resource for the Educator
National Hemophilia Foundation
116 W 32nd Street 888-463-6643
New York, NY 10001-3212 800-424-2634
Fax: 212-328-3777
www.hemophilia.org
Written for teachers, nurses, and other school personnel, this booklet aims to dispel the myths and fears surrounding hemophilia.
1995 16 pages
Alan Kinniburgh, PhD, CEO

5070 Treatment of Hemophilia: Current Orthopedic Management
Marvin Gilbert, Jerome Wiedel, author
National Hemophilia Foundation
116 W 32nd Street 888-463-6643
New York, NY 10001-3212 800-424-2634
Fax: 212-328-3777
www.hemophilia.org
Covers a wide range of orthopedic treatment issues, including hemophilic arthropathy, clinical considerations, diagnostic imaging, surgical and nonsurgical treatments, hemophilic synovitis, soft-tissue bleeding, the hemophilia pseudotumor, fracture care, other musculoskelatal problems, and HIV infections.
1995 25 pages
Alan Kinnibrugh, PhD, CEO

5071 Understanding Hepatitis
Leonard Seeff, Maribel Johnson, author
National Hemophilia Foundation
116 W 32nd Street 888-463-6643
New York, NY 10001-3212 800-424-2634
Fax: 212-328-3777
www.hemophilia.org
Provides comprehensive information about viral hepatitis for people with bleeding disorders, their caregivers, and families. Dis-

cusses the different hepatitis viruses, viral transmissions, how the liver is affected by hepatitis, blood product concerns, prevention, diagnosis, treatment, and psychosocial issues.
1997 24 pages
Alan Kinniburgh, PhD, CEO

5072   Von Willebrand Disease: A Guide for Patients and Families
Hemophilia Health Services
6820 Charlotte Pike
Nashville, TN 37209-4206   800-800-6606
Offers information on this disease, explains the causes, treatments, prevention and offers resources and books.

5073   What Is Hemophilia?
Hemophilia Foundation of Georgia
8800 Roswell Road   770-518-8272
Atlanta, GA 30328-1689   800-866-4366
                                            Fax: 770-518-3310
                                            e-mail: hog@america.net
                                            www.hog.org
Offers information on what hemophilia is, common factors in hemophilia, the cost and treatments offered to hemophiliacs and more.

5074   What Women Should Know About HIV Infection AIDS and Hemophilia
Hemophilia Foundation of Illinois
332 S Michigan Avenue   312-427-1495
Chicago, IL 60604-4434
For spouses/partners of men with hemophilia and women with bleeding disorders. Provides information about HIV/AIDS and how it affects women in the hemophilia community.
25 pages

5075   What You Should Know About Hemophilia
National Hemophilia Foundation
116 W 32nd Street   888-463-6643
New York, NY 10001-3212   800-424-2634
                                            Fax: 212-328-3777
                                            www.hemophilia.org
Defines hemophilia, explains its effects, and provides a historical overview of treatment and treatment complications.
1991 13 pages
Alan Kinniburgh, PhD, CEO

5076   Who Will Tell Them of Your Special Needs?
MedicAlert
2323 Colorado Avenue
Turlock, CA 95382-2018   800-432-5378
Offers information on MedicAlert bracelets, personal identification medical information needed for treatment in case of emergency.

Audio & Video

5077   Song of Superman
National Hemophilia Foundation
116 W 32nd Street   888-463-6643
New York, NY 10001-3212   800-424-2634
                                            Fax: 212-328-3777
                                            www.hemophilia.org
Designed to help young people with bleeding disorders come to terms with their HIV status, sexuality, and living with HIV. The video explores issues of disclosure in relationships and safer sex through dramatic scenes and frank testimonials by young people living with hemophilia and/or HIV. The companion workbook contains group exercises that follow each of the main topics of the video and serve as a bridge to discussion.
1993 49 pages
Alan Kinnibrugh, PhD, CEO

5078   Treat Yourself to a Brighter Future - It's Time to Hit the Freedom Trail
c/o Hemophilia Association of the Capital Area
10560 Main Street   703-352-7641
Fairfax, VA 22030-7182   Fax: 703-352-2145
                                            e-mail: info@hacacares.org
                                            www.hacacares.org/ed_publist.html

A booklet and videotape published by the American Red Cross providing a list of required supplies and equipment for self-infusion concentrates for persons with hemophilia A. It is an instructional piece for home self-infusion and concise text and illustrations depict seven steps for self-infusion.
20 pages Video & Booklet
Keith Bushey, President
Cliff Krug Jr, Vice President

Web Sites

5079   American Red Cross Blood Services
                                            www.redcross.org/services/biomed
Distributes a wide variety of plasma therapeutics to benefit people with hemophilia A and B, immune disorders and hypoalbuminemia.

5080   Healing Well
                                            www.healingwell.com
An online health resource guide to medical news, chat, information and articles, newsgroups and message boards, books, disease-related web sites, medical directories, and more for patients, friends, and family coping with disabling diseases, disorders, or chronic illnesses.

5081   Health Finder
                                            www.healthfinder.gov
Searchable, carefully developed web site offering information on over 1000 topics. Developed by the US Department of Health and Human Services, the site can be used in both English and Spanish.

5082   Healthlink USA
                                            www.healthlinkusa.com
Health information concerning treatment, cures, prevention, diagnosis, risk factors, research, support groups, email lists, personal stories and much more. Updated regularly.

5083   Helios Health
                                            www.helioshealth.com
Online resource for your health information. Detailed information about specific health topics, access to expert advice from our Medical Advisory Board, and up-to-date health news.

5084   MedicineNet
                                            www.medicinenet.com
An online resource for consumers providing easy-to-read, authoritative medical and health information.

5085   Medscape
                                            www.medscape.com
Medscape offers specialists, primary care physicians, and other health professionals the Web's most robust and integrated medical information and educational tools.

5086   National Hemophilia Foundation
                                            www.hemophilia.org
Information on the treatment and the cure of hemophilia, related bleeding disorders and complications of those disorders or their treatment, including HIV infection, as well as improving the quality of life of all those affected.

5087   WebMD
                                            www.webmd.com
Information on Hemophilia, including articles and resources.

Description

5088 Hepatitis

Hepatitis, or inflammation of the liver, has multiple causes and several stages. Hepatitis is usually caused by viruses or by excess alcohol consumption. Less common causes include prescription medications, accidental poisoning, and auto-immune diseases in which the body attacks its own liver.

The severity of the disease is highly variable. At an early stage, hepatitis may cause no symptoms, vague mild symptoms, or overwhelming disease. Early symptoms include vague abdominal pain, jaundice, fever, loss of appetite and nausea. If the disease becomes chronic, it may lead to irreversible scarring, or cirrhosis, which causes weakness, fatigue and weight loss. Late stage disease includes fluid accumulation in the abdominal cavity, gastrointestinal bleeding and mental changes. Abdominal pain and liver enlargement are generally present. Advanced cirrhosis is a risk factor for cancer of the liver.

There are four major kinds of viral hepatitis. Type A is very common world-wide, is spread by contaminated food and water, and generally causes a mild to moderately severe illness that runs its course over several weeks and disappears without further damage. Type B is also very common, and is spread by bodily fluids, generally through blood transfusion, sexual intercourse, sharing of needles or contaminated items like shaving razors and tattoo needles. The disease may resolve without further consequences, but frequently becomes chronic and may lead to cirrhosis as well as chronic infections. Hepatitis C is also spread through blood transfusion and needle sharing. Although it is not usually severe at onset, it can lead to the same serious consequences as type B. Finally, there is a type D, which is spread by blood products, and only infects people who already have Type B. Type D is associated with a more severe course.

Prevention of any of these forms of viral hepatitis depends on avoiding the usual routes of transmission. In addition, there is an effective vaccine available for hepatitis B. Close family contacts of persons with this disease should receive the vaccine if they have not yet received it as part of routine childhood immunization.

Treatment of hepatitis is largely supportive, but antiviral drugs and interferon are used in certain stages of Type B and Type C infection. End-stage or overwhelming infection may necessitate liver transplantation. See also *Liver Disease*.

National Agencies & Associations

5089 American Hepatitis Association
133 E 58th Street
New York, NY 10022
212-753-8068
Conducts educational and prevention programs concerning hepatitis provides screening and vaccines and offers support groups for individuals with hepatitis.

5090 Centers for Disease Control and Prevention Hepatitis Branch
1600 Clifton Road
Atlanta, GA 30333
404-639-2709
800-232-4636
www.cdc.gov/ncidod/diseases/hepatitis
Monitors the rates of viral hepatitis in the United States; provides epidemiologic assistance for outbreaks of viral hepatitis; coordinates and implements epidemiologic studies to define the risk factors for acute and chronic viral hepatitis; provides viral hepatitis reference/diagnostic services; serves as the World Health Organization Collaborating Center for Reference and Research on Viral Hepatitis.
Julie Louise Gerberding, MD, Director

5091 HIV/Hepatitis C in Prison (HIP) Committee
California Prison Focus
San Francisco, CA 94103
510-665-1935
e-mail: contact@prisons.org
www.prisons.org/hivin
The HIV/HCV in Prison Committee of California Prison Focus works on behalf of prisoners to fight for consistent access to quality medical care including access of all new HIV and hepatitis C medications, diagnostic testing and combination therapies.
Michelle Foy, Contact
Judy Greenspan, Contact

5092 Hepatitis B Coalition
1573 Selby Avenue
Saint Paul, MN 55104
651-647-9009
Fax: 651-647-9131
e-mail: admin@immunize.org
www.immunize.org
Works to prevent transmission of hepatitis B in high-risk groups; to promote HBsAG screening for all pregnant women; to achieve vaccination of all infants children and adolescents; and to promote education and treatment for the person who is chronically ill.
Deborah L Wexler MD, Executive Director
Diane C Peterson, Associate Director for Immunization

5093 Hepatitis Foundation International
504 Blick Drive
Silver Spring, MD 20904-2901
301-622-4200
800-891-0707
Fax: 301-622-4702
e-mail: hfi@comcast.net
www.hepfi.org
Grassroots support network for persons with viral hepatitis. Provides education about the prevention diagnosis and treatment of viral hepatitis as well as phone network support and various literature.
Thelma King Thiel, Chief Executive Officer
Karen Wirth MBA, Vice Chairwoman

5094 Immunization Action Coalition
1573 Selby Avenue
Saint Paul, MN 55104
651-647-9009
Fax: 651-647-9131
e-mail: admin@immunize.org
www.immunize.org
The mission of the Immunization Action Coalition is to boost immunization rates and prevent disease. The coalition promotes physician, community and family awareness of and responsibility for appropriate immunization of all children and adults against all diseases.
Deborah L Wexler MD, Executive Director
Diane C Peterson, Associate Director for Immunization

5095 Living Positive Resource Centre
#201-19232 Enterprise Way
Surrey, BC, V3S-6J9
604-576-5740
800-616-2437
Fax: 604-576-5790
e-mail: inbox@iprc.ca
www.iprc.ca
Through partnerships and collaboration, will work to reduce the incidence of new HIV/AIDS/HEP C and other blood borne pathogens and to improve the quality of life for those infected and affected.
Daryle Roberts, Executive Director
Sean Lang, President

5096 National Hepatitis C Coalition
PO Box 5058
Hemet, CA 92544
951-766-8238
e-mail: mail@nationalhepatitis-c.org
www.nationalhepatitis-c.org

The National Hepatitis C Coalition is a 501(c) (3) tax exempt organization that relies on private donations from good folks like you in order to continue helping others with hepatitis C.
Patty Krueger, Co-Founder/Board Chair/President

Foundations

5097 Hepatitis B Foundation
3805 Old Easton Road
Doylestown, PA 18902
215-489-4900
Fax: 215-489-4313
e-mail: info@hepb.org
www.hepb.org
We are dedicated to finding a cure and improving the quality of life for those affected by hepatitis B worldwide. Our commitment includes funding focused research, promoting disease awareness, supporting immunization and treatment initiatives, and serving as the primary source of information for patients and their families, the medical and scientific community, and the general public.

Molli Conti, Chair
Timothy Block, PhD, Founder/President

Libraries & Resource Centers

5098 Hepatitis Education Project
4603 Aurora Avenue N
Seattle, WA 98103
206-732-0311
Fax: 206-732-0312
e-mail: hep@scn.org
www.scn.org/hepatitis
The mission of the Hepatitis Education Project is to help raise awareness among patients, medical personnel and the public of the facts concerning hepatitis patients and the resources available to help those who live with the disease.
Steve Graham, President
Michael Ninburg, Executive Director

Support Groups & Hotlines

5099 Christ Hospital Hepatitis C Support Group
Christ Hospital
176 Palisade Avenue
Jersey City, NJ 07306
201-795-1230
e-mail: dkatz65717@aol.com
For anyone interested in becoming advocates for increasing awareness of this illness.

5100 Hepatitis Education Project
The Maritime Building
Seattle, WA 98104
206-732-0311
e-mail: hepinfo@hepeducation.org
www.hepeducation.org
Helps raise awareness among patients, medical personeel and the public of the facts concerning hepatitis patients and the resources available to help those who live with the disease
Steve Graham, President
Michael Ninburg, Executive Director

5101 National Health Information Center
PO Box 1133
Washington, DC 20013
310-565-4167
800-336-4797
Fax: 301-984-4256
e-mail: info@nhic.org
www.health.gov/nhic
Offers a nationwide information referral service, produces directories and resource guides.

Books

5102 Hepatitis B Prevention: A Resource Guide
National Digestive Diseases Info. Clearinghouse
2 Information Way
Bethesda, MD 20824
301-654-3810
800-891-5389
Fax: 301-907-8906
e-mail: nddic@info.niddk.uih.goc
www.niddk.nih.gov

Designed to assist health care and other professionals who work in planning or administering hepatitis B prevention programs.
252 pages

5103 Understanding Hepatitis
James L Achord, MD, author
University Press of Mississippi
3825 Ridgewood Road
Jackson, MS 39211-6492
601-432-6205
Fax: 601-432-6217
e-mail: kburgess@ihl.state.ms.us
www.upress.state.ms.us
For general readers a comprehensive discussion of the causes and of the treatments of hepatitis.
2002 152 pages Paperback
ISBN: 1-578064-36-8
Kathy Burgess, Advertising/Marketing Services Manager

5104 Viral Hepatitis: Scientific Basis and Clinical Management
Churchill Livingstone
PO Box 3188
Secaucus, NJ 07096-3188
201-319-9800
800-553-5426
Fax: 201-319-9659
www.harcourt-international.com/cl/
1997 800 pages Hardcover
ISBN: 0-443057-97-4

Magazines

5105 Hepatitis Magazine
Quality Publishing Services
523 N Sam Houston Parkway E
Houston, TX 77060
281-272-2744
800-310-7047
Fax: 281-847-5440
e-mail: info@hepatitismag.com
www.hepatitismag.com
Magazine for those with hepatitis. Price listed is for a one year subscription.
Quarterly
Barbara Veres, Publisher
Geoff Drushel, Editor

Newsletters

5106 American Liver Foundation: Progress Newsletter
75 Maiden Lane
New York, NY 10038-4826
212-668-1000
800-465-4837
Fax: 212-483-8179
e-mail: info@liverfoundation.org
www.liverfoundation.org
The American Liver Foundation is the nation's leading nonprofit organization promoting liver health and disease prevention. ALF provides research education and sdvocacy for those affected by liver-related diseases, including hepatitis
8 pages 2 per year
Sarah Wilson Brown, Manager Marketing/Communications

5107 B Connected
3805 Old Easton Road
Doylestown, PA 18902
215-489-4900
Fax: 215-489-4313
e-mail: info@hepb.org
www.hepb.org
Features practical health tips, frequently asked questions, and other useful information for patients and families to live well with chronic hepatitis B. Available in both print and online versions.
3x/year
Molli Conti, Chair
Timothy Block, PhD, Founder/President

5108 B-Informed Newsletter
Hepatitis B Foundation
3805 Old Easton Road
Doylestown, PA 18902
215-489-4900
Fax: 215-489-4920
e-mail: info@hepb.org
www.hepb.org

Includes a Drug Watch of approved and experimental therapies for Hepatitis B, reasearch updates, Foundation news and events, and feature articles on special topics. Available in print and online.
Molli C. Conti, Executive Director

5109 Hepatitis Alert
Hepatitis Foundation International (HFI)
30 Sunrise Terrace   973-239-1035
Cedar Grove, NJ 07009-1423   800-891-0707
                                         Fax: 973-875-5044
                                     e-mail: hfi@intac.com
                                              www.hepfi.org
Provides information for the public, patients, educators, and medical professionals about the diagnosis, treatment, and prevention of viral hepatitis.

5110 Hepatitis B Coalition News
Hepatitis B Coalition
1573 Selby Avenue   651-647-9009
Saint Paul, MN 55104-6328   Fax: 651-647-9131
                                  e-mail: admin@inmunize.org
Newsletter with brochures, articles, videotapes, audio-cassette tapes and manuals for different ethnic populations.

5111 NEEDLE TIPS & the Hepatitis B Coalition News
Hepatitis B Coalition
1573 Selby Avenue   651-647-9009
St. Paul, MN 55104-6328   Fax: 651-647-9131
                                  e-mail: admin@immunize.org
                                             www.immunize.org
Information on immunization for health professionals.
28 pages 2x Year
Deborah L Wexler

5112 VACCINATE ADULTS! Coalition News
Hepatitis B Coalition
1573 Selby Avenue   651-647-9009
St. Paul, MN 55104-6328   Fax: 651-647-9131
                                  e-mail: admin@immunize.org
                                             www.immunize.org
Information on immunization: adult medicine specialist.
12 pages 2x Year
Deborah L Wexler MD

Pamphlets

5113 Advice to Parents of Children with HBV
Hepatitis B Foundation
3805 Old Easton Road
Doylestown, PA 18902   215-489-4900
                                        Fax: 215-489-4920
                                      e-mail: info@hepb.org
                                               www.hepb.org
Provides information to people affected by hepatitis B and their loved ones. Current HBV research, telephone numbers, and a medical glossary.
Molli C. Conti, Executive Director

5114 Caring for Your Liver
Hepatitis Foundation International (HFI)
30 Sunrise Terrace   973-239-1035
Cedar Grove, NJ 07009-1423   800-891-0707
                                         Fax: 973-875-5044
                                     e-mail: hfi@intac.com
                                              www.hepfi.org
Information for the person with hepatitis.

5115 Caution! Treating Children with Acetaminophen
Hepatitis Foundation International (HFI)
30 Sunrise Terrace   973-239-1035
Cedar Grove, NJ 07009-1423   800-891-0707
                                         Fax: 973-875-5044
                                     e-mail: hfi@intac.com
                                              www.hepfi.org
Information on hepatitis.

5116 Chronic Viral Hepatitis Backgrounder
Schering Corporation

Kenilworth, NJ 07033
                                              908-298-4000
                                          www.sch-plough.com
Offers information and statistics on viral hepatitis.

5117 Cirrhosis: Many Causes
American Liver Foundation
1425 Pompton Avenue
Cedar Grove, NJ 07009-1000   800-223-0179
                                         Fax: 973-256-3214
                              e-mail: info@liverfoundation.org
                                        www.liverfoundation.org
Gives basic facts about cirrhosis including causes, signs, symptoms and treatments.
Rick Smith, President & CEO
Rebecca Frank, Chief Development Officer

5118 Diagnosis and Treatment
Hepatitis Foundation International (HFI)
30 Sunrise Terrace   973-239-1035
Cedar Grove, NJ 07009-1423   800-891-0707
                                         Fax: 973-875-5044
                                     e-mail: hfi@intac.com
                                              www.hepfi.org
Information for the person with hepatitis.

5119 Health Insurance
Hepatitis Foundation International (HFI)
30 Sunrise Terrace   973-239-1035
Cedar Grove, NJ 07009-1423   800-891-0707
                                         Fax: 973-875-5044
                                     e-mail: hfi@intac.com
                                              www.hepfi.org
Information on hepatitis and health insurance.

5120 Helpful Tips for Carriers of HBV
Hepatitis Foundation International (HFI)
30 Sunrise Terrace   973-239-1035
Cedar Grove, NJ 07009-1423   800-891-0707
                                         Fax: 973-875-5044
                                     e-mail: hfi@intac.com
                                              www.hepfi.org
Information for people with Hepatitis B.

5121 Hepatitis
National Institute of Allergy & Infectious Disease
31 Center Drive
Bethesda, MD 20892-0001   301-496-4000
                                www.niaid.nih.gov/default.htm
A pamphlet discussing the cause, symptoms, transmission, diagnosis, tests, prevention and the latest research on Hepatitis.

5122 Hepatitis A and B Vaccination
Hepatitis Foundation International (HFI)
30 Sunrise Terrace   973-239-1035
Cedar Grove, NJ 07009-1423   800-891-0707
                                         Fax: 973-875-5044
                                     e-mail: hfi@intac.com
                                              www.hepfi.org
Information on hepatitis vaccination.

5123 Hepatitis A, B & C
Hepatitis Foundation International (HFI)
30 Sunrise Terrace   973-239-1035
Cedar Grove, NJ 07009-1423   800-891-0707
                                         Fax: 973-875-5044
                                     e-mail: hfi@intac.com
                                              www.hepfi.org
Information for the person with hepatitis.

5124 Hepatitis A, B & C: Liver Disease You Should Know About
American Liver Foundation
1425 Pompton Avenue
Cedar Grove, NJ 07009   800-465-4837
                                         Fax: 973-256-3214
                              e-mail: info@liverfoundation.org
                                        www.liverfoundation.org
Explains viral hepatitis, transmission, symptoms, testing and acute chronic hepatitis.
Rick Smith, President & CEO
Rebecca Frank, Chief Development Officer

5125 Hepatitis B Prevention
National Center For Infectious Diseases
Hepatitis Branch   404-332-4555
Atlanta, GA 30333
Explains what hepatitis B is, what behaviors are risky and how to protect oneself against it.

5126 Hepatitis Fact Sheet
www.cdc.gov/ncidod/diseases/hepatitis/c
Offers information on the causes, symptoms, prevention and treatments for hepatitis.

5127 How Many Times a Day Do You Risk Being Infected with Hepatitis B?
American Liver Foundation
1425 Pompton Avenue
Cedar Grove, NJ 07009   800-465-4837
Fax: 973-256-3214
e-mail: info@liverfoundation.org
www.liverfoundation.org
A flyer emphasizing the importance of vaccination against hepatitis B.
Rick Smith, President & CEO
Rebecca Frank, Chief Development Officer

5128 Is Your Liver Giving You the Silent Treatment?
Hepatitis Foundation International (HFI)
30 Sunrise Terrace   973-239-1035
Cedar Grove, NJ 07009-1423   800-891-0707
Fax: 973-875-5044
e-mail: hfi@intac.com
www.hepfi.org
Provides information for patients with hepatitis.

5129 Living with Hepatitis C: Self Help Tips
Hepatitis Foundation International (HFI)
30 Sunrise Terrace   973-239-1035
Cedar Grove, NJ 07009-1423   800-891-0707
Fax: 973-875-5044
e-mail: hfi@intac.com
www.hepfi.org
Information for people with Hepatitis C.

5130 Protect Yourself and Those You Love Against HBV
Hepatitis B Foundation
3805 Old Easton Road   215-489-4900
Doylestown, PA 18902   Fax: 215-489-4920
e-mail: info@hepb.org
www.hepb.org
Provides information to people affected by hepatitis B and their loved ones.
Molli C. Conti, Executive Director

5131 Q and A: Hepatitis B Prevention
SmithKline Beecham Pharmaceuticals
1 Franklin Plaza   215-751-4000
Philadelphia, PA 19102-1282
Informational booklet written for healthcare personnel by the manufacturer of Engerix-B vaccine, reviews hepatitis B prevention.

5132 Someone You Know Has Hepatitis B
Hepatitis B Foundation
3805 Old Easton Road   215-489-4900
Doylestown, PA 18902   Fax: 215-489-4920
e-mail: info@hepb.org
www.hepb.org
Provides information to people affected by hepatitis B and their loved ones.
Molli C. Conti, Executive Director

5133 Tips on Coping with Chronic Hepatitis
Hepatitis Foundation International (HFI)
30 Sunrise Terrace   973-239-1035
Cedar Grove, NJ 07009-1423   800-891-0707
Fax: 973-875-5044
e-mail: hfi@intac.com
www.hepfi.org
Information for people with hepatitis.

5134 Viral Hepatitis: Everybody's Problem?
American Liver Foundation

1425 Pompton Avenue
Cedar Grove, NJ 07009-1000   800-223-0179
Fax: 973-256-3214
e-mail: info@liverfoundation.org
www.liverfoundation.org
Covering a broad range of topics including: a definition of the disease, descriptions of types of infections, transmission, symptoms, treatment options and prevention of hepatitis.
Rick Smith, President & CEO
Rebecca Frank, Chief Development Officer

5135 What Health Care Workers Should Know About Hepatitis B
Channing L Bete Company
200 State Road
South Deerfield, MA 01373   800-628-7733
Presents information in easy-to-read, simple English for health care workers about hepatitis B.
15 pages

Audio & Video

5136 Hepatitis B Video
Hepatitis B Foundation
3805 Old Easton Road   215-489-4900
Doylestown, PA 18902   Fax: 215-489-4920
e-mail: info@hepb.org
www.hepb.org
Provides information to people affected by hepatitis B and their loved ones.
Molli C. Conti, Executive Director

5137 Hepatitis C: A Viral Mystery
Terry Strauss, Stephen Steady, author

Fanlight Productions
4196 Washington Street   617-469-4999
Boston, MA 02131-1731   800-937-4113
Fax: 617-469-3379
e-mail: fanlight@fanlight.com
www.fanlight.com
This timely video is about living with a serious, chronic illness. In addition to discussing the medical treatments available, the video also explores alternatives which appear to help some people.
2000 30 Minutes
ISBN: 1-572953-08-X

Web Sites

5138 HIV/Hepatitis C in Prison (HIP) Committee
www.prisons.org/hivin.htm
Fighting for consistent access to quality medical care including access to all new HIV and Hepatitis C medications, diagnostic testing and combination therapies.

5139 Healing Well
www.healingwell.com
An online health resource guide to medical news, chat, information and articles, newsgroups and message boards, books, disease-related web sites, medical directories, and more for patients, friends, and family coping with disabling diseases, disorders, or chronic illnesses.

5140 Health Finder
www.healthfinder.gov
Searchable, carefully developed web site offering information on over 1000 topics. Developed by the US Department of Health and Human Services, the site can be used in both English and Spanish.

5141 Healthlink USA
www.healthlinkusa.com
Health information concerning treatment, cures, prevention, diagnosis, risk factors, research, support groups, email lists, personal stories and much more. Updated regularly.

5142 Healthy Lives
www.healthylives.com/hepatitis

5143 Helios Health
www.helioshealth.com

Online resource for your health information. Detailed information about specific health topics, access to expert advice from our Medical Advisory Board, and up-to-date health news.

5144   Hepatitis B Coalition

www.immunize.org

Works to prevent transmission of hepatitis B in high-risk groups; to promote HBsAG screening for all pregnant women; to achieve vaccination of all infants, children, and adolescents; and to promote education and treatment for the person who is chronically infected with hepatitis B.

5145   Hepatitis Information Network

www.hepnet.com

5146   MedicineNet

www.medicinenet.com

An online resource for consumers providing easy-to-read, authoritative medical and health information.

5147   Medscape

www.medscape.com

Medscape offers specialists, primary care physicians, and other health professionals the Web's most robust and integrated medical information and educational tools.

5148   WebMD

www.webmd.com

Information on hepatitis, including articles and resources.

Description

5149 Hydrocephalus

The normal brain and spinal cord are surrounded with a watery substance called cerebro-spinal fluid, CSF, which collects within the brain in several larger pools called ventricles, connected to one another through tiny channels. The CSF is formed in some of these ventricles, circulates widely and is eventually reabsorbed. If CFS production exceeds reabsorption, or if the fluid is blocked from circulating and it may build up pressure that expands the ventricles and presses on the normal brain tissue, causing hydrocephalus, or water on the brain.

Hydrocephalus can cause change in behavior, headache, visual loss, vomiting and weakness. Hydrocephalus may be congenital, that is, present from birth. If it occurs in a child whose skull bones have not yet fused together, it may cause the head to enlarge.

In adults whose brains are encased in the rigid skull, there is no room to expand and pressure builds up in the brain. Excess CSF may be in response to infection such as meningitis or to blockage of CSF movement by tumor. Treatment and outlook depend on the underlying cause. Medical therapy may cause limited temporary improvement. Surgical treatment may be able to correct the underlying cause. If it cannot, the surgeon may still give substantial relief by placing a shunt which allows extra CSF to drain from the ventricles to some other part of the body.

National Agencies & Associations

5150 Association of Hydrocephalus Education Advocacy & Discussion (AHEAD)
1730 Autumn Leaf Lane   215-355-4728
Huntingdon Valley, PA 19006-1515
Organized by young adults with hydrocephalus for the purpose of providing telephone support nationwide.
Lane Borden, NE Regional Contact

5151 Guardians of Hydrocephalus Research Foundation
2640 E 28 Street   718-743-9650
Brooklyn, NY 11235-2023   Fax: 718-743-9650
e-mail: ghrf2618@aol.com
ghrf.homestead.com/ghrf.html
Non-profit organization made up of concerned parents and dedicated volunteers. The goal is to wipe out this top ranking birth defect.
Michael Fischetti, Founder
Jamie Fischetti, Secretary

5152 Hydrocephalus Association Hydrocephalus Association
Hydrocephalus Association
870 Market Street   415-732-7040
San Francisco, CA 94102   888-598-3789
Fax: 415-732-7044
e-mail: info@hydroassoc.org
www.hydroassoc.org
The association provides support education and advocacy for families and professionals. The goal is to insure that families and individuals dealing with the complexities of hydrocephalus receive personal support, comprehensive educational materials and outreach.
Dory Kranz, Director of Research
Pip Marks, Director of Support & Education

5153 Hydrocephalus Foundation
910 Rear Broadway   781-942-1161
Saugus, MA 01906   e-mail: HyFII@netscape.net
www.hydrocephalus.org
Dedicated to providing support educational resources and networking opportunities to patients and families affected by hydrocephalus. The Foundation also promotes related research and facilitates the training of healthcare professionals to improve patient care.
Greg A Tocco MIR, Founder/Executive Director
Donna H West, Board of Directors Member

5154 Kidney Foundation
300-5165 Sherbrooke Street W   514-369-4806
Montreal, QC, H4A-1T6   800-361-7494
Fax: 514-369-2472
e-mail: webmaster@kidney.ca
www.kidney.ca
A national volunteer organization committed to reducing the burden of kidney disease through: funding and stimulating innovative research; providing education and support; promoting access to high quality healthcare; and increasing public awareness and commitment to advancing kidney health and organ donation.

5155 National Hydrocephalus Foundation
12413 Centralia Road   562-924-6666
Lakewood, CA 90715   888-857-3434
Fax: 562-924-6666
e-mail: nhf@earthlink.net
www.nhfonline.org
The foundation is a national organization with almost 30 years of history. We provide information and education along with peer-to-peer support a physician referral sheet along with patient and family comments and several different types of help sheets.
Debbi Fields, Executive Director
Michael Fields, President/Treasurer

5156 Spina Bifida & Hydrocephalus Association of Nova Scotia
PO Box 341   902-679-1124
Coldbrook, Nova Scotia, B4R-1B6   800-304-0450
Fax: 902-679-1433
e-mail: spina.bifida@ns.sympatico.ca
www3.ns.sympatico.ca
It is a non-profit, registered charitable organization affiliated with the Spina Bifida and Hydrocephalus Association of Canada, and currently has one chapter in Cape Breton.

5157 Spina Bifida & Hydrocephalus Association o f Ontario
PO Box 341   902-679-1124
Coldbrook Nova Scotia, B4R 1-3B1   800-304-0450
Fax: 902-679-1433
e-mail: spina.bifida@ns.sympatico.ca
www.sbhans.ca
It is a non-profit registered charitable organization affiliated with the Spina Bifida and Hydrocephalus Association of Canada and currently has one chapter in Cape Breton.

5158 World Hypertension League
Medical University of Ohio   419-383-5270
Toledo, OH 43614-5809   Fax: 419-383-3120
e-mail: gmonhollen@meduohio.edu
hsc.utoledo.edu
Devoted to the advancement of hypertension prevention and control through joint efforts of all national leagues and societies.
Lloyd A Jacobs MD, President

State Agencies & Associations

California

5159 Hydrocephalus Support Group of Southern California
870 Market Street   415-732-7040
San Francisco, CA 94102   888-598-3789
Fax: 415-732-7044
e-mail: info@hydroassoc.org
www.hydroassoc.org

Founded in 1976 this group was formed as a group of concerned families and patients with hydrocephalus to share information and experiences in dealing with this disease locally and nationwide.
Paul Gross, Chairman
Raymond Moser, Vice Chairman

Michigan

5160 Hydrocephalus Support Group of Michigan Children's Hospital of Michigan
Children's Hospital of Michigan
3901 Beaubien   313-745-5437
Detroit, MI 48201   Fax: 313-993-8744
Founded in 1992 this group provides information to families and gives them support.
Mary Smellie RN MSN, Clinical Nurse Specialist

Pennsylvania

5161 Hydrocephalus Association of Philadelphia
PO Box 2099   610-497-0375
Boothwyn, PA 19061-8099   Fax: 610-497-2836
Founded in 1992 the Association provides support information advocacy and telephone support to families in Pennsylvania New Jersey and Delaware.

Rhode Island

5162 Hydrocephalus Association of Rhode Island
PO Box 343   401-723-6065
Valley Falls, RI 02864-0343
Founded in 1993 the mission of this Association is to provide information support and advocacy for individuals with hydrocephalus and for friends and family members.
Gabriella Halmi, Director

Texas

5163 Hydrocephalus Association of North Texas
PO Box 670552
Dallas, TX 74637-0552   214-528-2877
http://nhfonline.org/treatment.php?id=or
Founded in 1987 the mission is to provide information and support to parents of children with hydrocephalus in the state of Texas and neighboring states.
Beverly Pike, President

Washington

5164 Hydrocephalus Support Group of Seattle
PO Box 1611   425-482-0479
Woodinville, WA 98072   e-mail: lpoliski@hydrosupport.org
www.hydrosupport.org
Founded in 1993 the group of Seattle provides support to individuals with hydrocephalus.
Diana Pozzi

Libraries & Resource Centers

5165 LINK Program
Emily Fudge, author

Hydrocephalus Association
870 Market Street   415-732-7040
San Francisco, CA 94102-2912   888-598-3789
Fax: 415-732-7044
e-mail: info@hydroassoc.org
www.hydroassoc.org
National network of 1300 individuals and families listed in directory format, giving our members direct access to others in similar circumstances.
Dory Kranz, Executive Director
Pip Marks, Director Outreach Services

Support Groups & Hotlines

5166 Cerebrospinal Fluid Shunt Systems for the Management of Hydrocephalus
Hydrocephalus Association
870 Market Street   415-732-7040
San Francisco, CA 94102-2912   888-598-3789
Fax: 415-732-7044
e-mail: info@hydroassoc.org
www.hydroassoc.org
Nonprofit organization that provides support, education and advocacy for all families, individuals and professionals affected by hydrocephalus.
Pip Marks, Director Outreach Services

5167 Hydrocephalus Parents Support Group
1325 Louis Street   908-722-4691
Manville, NJ 08835
Founded in 1993, the group provides support for parents of children with hydrocephalus.
Andrea Liptak, Founder

5168 National Health Information Center
PO Box 1133   310-565-4167
Washington, DC 20013   800-336-4797
Fax: 301-984-4256
e-mail: info@nhic.org
www.health.gov/nhic

Offers a nationwide information referral service, produces directories and resource guides.

Books

5169 Hydrocephalus: A Guide for Patients, Families, and Friends
O'Reilly and Associates
101 Morris Street
Sebastopol, CA 95472   800-998-9938
Fax: 707-829-0104
e-mail: order@oreilly.com
www.oreilly.com
Hydrocephalus: A Guide for Patients, Families, and Friends provides individuals and families with the guidance, information and support needed to make the right decisions at the right time.
350 pages Paperback
ISBN: 1-565924-10-X

5170 Spina Bifida Association of America: Insights into Spina Bifida
Spina Bifida Association of America
4590 MacArthur Boulevard NW   202-944-3285
Washington, DC 20007-4226   800-621-3141
Fax: 202-944-3295
e-mail: sbaa@sbaa.org
www.sbaa.org

News on medical, legislative and education topics relevant to individuals with spina bifida.
bi-monthly
Marybeth Leamyini, Communications Director

Children's Books

5171 Loving Ben
Delacorte
1540 Broadway
New York, NY 10036-4039   212-354-6500
This is a moving story of a sister who cares for her baby brother and tries to help him learn despite his birth defects and deteriorating health.
Grades 7-10

Newsletters

5172 Alliance of Genetic Support Groups
35 Wisconsin Circle   202-331-0942
Chevy Chase, MD 20815   800-336-4363

A coalition of voluntary genetic support groups, consumers and professionals addressing the needs of individuals and families affected by genetic disorders from a national perspective.

5173 Hydrocephalus Association Newsletter
Hydrocephalus Association
870 Market Street   415-732-7040
San Francisco, CA 94102-2912   888-598-3789
                                            Fax: 415-732-7044
                              e-mail: info@hydroassoc.org
                                        www.hydroassoc.org
Offers information on association news, conference articles, meetings, support and educational groups.
12 pages Quarterly
Dory Kranz, Executive Director
Pip Marks, Director Outreach Services

5174 Hydrocephalus Parents Support Group Newsletter
1325 Louis Street   908-722-4691
Manville, NJ 08835
Founded in 1993, the group provides support for parents of children with hydrocephalus.
Andrea Liptak, Founder

5175 Hydrocephalus Support Group Newsletter
PO Box 4236   636-532-8228
Chesterfield, MO 63005-4236   Fax: 314-995-4108
                              e-mail: hydrodb@earthlink.net
Founded in 1986, this group provides information, education and support to anyone dealing with hydrocephalus.
Debby Buffa, Founder/Chairman

5176 National Hydrocephalus Foundation Newsletter
12413 Centrailia Road   562-402-3523
Lakewood, CA 90715-1623   888-857-3434
                                            Fax: 562-924-6666
                            e-mail: hydrobrat@earthlink.net
                                                 nhfonline.org
Founded in 1979, the foundation is a national organization whose purpose is to provide information and education, along with peer support newsletter quarterly. Group meeting quarterly in Long Beach, CA. $35 a year.
Quarterly
Debbie Fields, Executive Director

5177 New York University Medical Center Auxiliary of Tisch Hospital
560 1st Avenue
New York, NY 10016   212-263-5040
                                        www.nyukidshealth.org
Conducts national symposiums on hydrocephalus.
Doris Farrelly, Contact

Pamphlets

5178 About Hydrocephalus: A Book for Families
Hydrocephalus Association
870 Market Street   415-732-7040
San Francisco, CA 94102-2912   888-598-3789
                                            Fax: 415-732-7044
                              e-mail: info@hydroassoc.org
                                        www.hydroassoc.org
A booklet in either English or Spanish, detailing all aspects of hydrocephalus from diagnosis and treatment to complications and follow-up care.
36 pages Paperback
Dory Kranz, Executive Director
Pip Marks, Director Outreach Services

5179 About Normal Pressure Hydrocephalus: A Book for Adults & Their Families
Hydrocephalus Association
870 Market Street   415-732-7040
San Francisco, CA 94102-2912   888-598-3789
                                            Fax: 415-732-7044
                              e-mail: info@hydroassoc.org
                                        www.hydroassoc.org

Booklet discusses the diagnosis and treatment of adult-onset normal pressure hydrocephalus.
24 pages Paperback
Dory Kranz, Executive Director
Pip Marks, Director Outreach Services

5180 Directory of Neurosurgeons Who Treat Adults
Hydrocephalus Association
870 Market Street   415-732-7040
San Francisco, CA 94102-2912   888-598-3789
                                            Fax: 415-732-7044
                              e-mail: info@hydroassoc.org
                                        www.hydroassoc.org
Names and addresses of neurosurgeons who treat adult-onset normal pressure hydrocephalus and adult-acquired hydrocephalus, listed alphabetically and geographically.
Dory Kranz, Executive Director
Pip Marks, Director Outreach Services

5181 Directory of Pediatric Neurosurgeons
Hydrocephalus Association
870 Market Street   415-732-7040
San Francisco, CA 94102-2912   888-598-3789
                                            Fax: 415-732-7044
                              e-mail: info@hydroassoc.org
                                        www.hydroassoc.org
Names and addresses of more than 200 neurosurgeons who specialize in pediatrics, listed alphabetically and geographically.
Dory Kranz, Executive Director
Pip Marks, Director Outreach Services

5182 Endoscopic Third Ventriculotomy
Hydrocephalus Association
870 Market Street   415-732-7040
San Francisco, CA 94102-2912   888-598-3789
                                            Fax: 415-732-7044
                              e-mail: info@hydroassoc.org
                                        www.hydroassoc.org
Series includes information on primary care, learning disabilities, eye problems, social skills development, headaches, endoscopic third ventriculostomy, shunts and more.
Dory Kranz, Executive Director
Pip Marks, Director Outreach Services

5183 Eye Problems Associated with Hydrocephalus in Children
Hydrocephalus Association
870 Market Street   415-732-7040
San Francisco, CA 94102-2912   888-598-3789
                                            Fax: 415-732-7044
                              e-mail: info@hydroassoc.org
                                        www.hydroassoc.org
Series includes information on primary care, learning disabilities, eye problems, social skills development, headaches, endoscopic third ventriculostomy, shunts and more.
Dory Kranz, Executive Director
Pip Marks, Director Outreach Services

5184 Fact Sheet: Hydrocephalus
Hydrocephalus Association
870 Market Street   415-732-7040
San Francisco, CA 94102-2912   888-598-3789
                                            Fax: 415-732-7044
                              e-mail: info@hydroassoc.org
                                        www.hydroassoc.org
Available in Spanish.
Dory Kranz, Executive Director
Pip Marks, Director Outreach Services

5185 Headaches and Hydrocephalus
Hydrocephalus Association
870 Market Street   415-732-7040
San Francisco, CA 94102-2912   888-598-3789
                                            Fax: 415-732-7044
                              e-mail: info@hydroassoc.org
                                        www.hydroassoc.org
Series includes information on primary care, learning disabilities, eye problems, social skills development, headaches, endoscopic third ventriculostomy, shunts and more.
Dory Kranz, Executive Director
Pip Marks, Director Outreach Services

5186 Hospitalization Tips
Hydrocephalus Association
870 Market Street
San Francisco, CA 94102-2912
415-732-7040
888-598-3789
Fax: 415-732-7044
e-mail: info@hydroassoc.org
www.hydroassoc.org

1997
Dory Kranz, Executive Director
Pip Marks, Director Outreach Services

5187 How to Be an Assertive Parent on the Treatment Team
Hydrocephalus Association
870 Market Street
San Francisco, CA 94102-2912
415-732-7040
888-598-3789
Fax: 415-732-7044
e-mail: info@hydroassoc.org
www.hydroassoc.org

Dory Kranz, Executive Director
Pip Marks, Director Outreach Services

5188 ID Card for Third Ventriculostomy Patients
Hydrocephalus Association
870 Market Street
San Francisco, CA 94102-2912
415-732-7040
888-598-3789
Fax: 415-732-7044
e-mail: info@hydroassoc.org
www.hydroassoc.org

Dory Kranz, Executive Director
Pip Marks, Director Outreach Services

5189 LINK Directory Information
Hydrocephalus Association
870 Market Street
San Francisco, CA 94102-2912
415-732-7040
888-598-3789
Fax: 415-732-7044
e-mail: info@hydroassoc.org
www.hydroassoc.org
A nationwide network of individuals listed in directory format giving members direct access to others in similar circumstances.
Dory Kranz, Executive Director
Pip Marks, Director Outreach Services

5190 Learning Disabilities in Children with Hydrocephalus
Hydrocephalus Association
870 Market Street
San Francisco, CA 94102-2912
415-732-7040
888-598-3789
Fax: 415-732-7044
e-mail: info@hydroassoc.org
www.hydroassoc.org
Available in Spanish.
Dory Kranz, Executive Director
Pip Marks, Director Outreach Services

5191 Nonverbal Learning Disorder Syndrome
Hydrocephalus Association
870 Market Street
San Francisco, CA 94102-2912
415-732-7040
888-598-3789
Fax: 415-732-7044
e-mail: info@hydroassoc.org
www.hydroassoc.org

1998
Dory Kranz, Executive Director
Pip Marks, Director Outreach Services

5192 Prenatal Hydrocephalus: A Book for Parents
Hydrocephalus Association
870 Market Street
San Francisco, CA 94102-2912
415-732-7040
888-598-3789
Fax: 415-732-7044
e-mail: info@hydroassoc.org
www.hydroassoc.org

Dory Kranz, Executive Director
Pip Marks, Director Outreach Services

5193 Resource Guide
Hydrocephalus Association
870 Market Street
San Francisco, CA 94102-2912
415-732-7040
888-598-3789
Fax: 415-732-7044
e-mail: info@hydroassoc.org
www.hydroassoc.org
A comprehensive listing of 450 articles on all aspects of hydrocephalus. Articles may be ordered from the association for a small fee.
Dory Kranz, Executive Director
Pip Marks, Director Outreach Services

5194 Resource Guide: Normal Pressure Hydrocephalus/Adult Onset
Hydrocephalus Association
870 Market Street
San Francisco, CA 94102-2912
415-732-7040
888-598-3789
Fax: 415-732-7044
e-mail: info@hydroassoc.org
www.hydroassoc.org

Dory Kranz, Executive Director
Pip Marks, Director Outreach Services

5195 Social Skills Development in Children with Hydrocephalus
Hydrocephalus Association
870 Market Street
San Francisco, CA 94102-2912
415-732-7040
888-598-3789
Fax: 415-732-7044
e-mail: info@hydroassoc.org
www.hydroassoc.org

Dory Kranz, Executive Director
Pip Marks, Director Outreach Services

5196 Survival Skills for the Family Unit
Hydrocephalus Association
870 Market Street
San Francisco, CA 94102-2912
415-732-7040
888-598-3789
Fax: 415-732-7044
e-mail: info@hydroassoc.org
www.hydroassoc.org

Dory Kranz, Executive Director
Pip Marks, Director Outreach Services

5197 Understanding Your Child's Education Needs/Individualized Education Program
Hydrocephalus Association
870 Market Street
San Francisco, CA 94102-2912
415-732-7040
888-598-3789
Fax: 415-732-7044
e-mail: info@hydroassoc.org
www.hydroassoc.org

Dory Kranz, Executive Director
Pip Marks, Director Outreach Services

Audio & Video

5198 Hydrocephalus: A Neglected Disease
Guardians of Hydrocephalus Research Foundation
2618 Avenue Z
Brooklyn, NY 11235-2023
718-743-4473
Fax: 718-743-1171
e-mail: ghrf2618@aol.com
www.homestead.com/ghrf.html

Marie Fischetti, Founder

Web Sites

5199 Healing Well
www.healingwell.com
An online health resource guide to medical news, chat, information and articles, newsgroups and message boards, books, disease-related web sites, medical directories, and more for patients, friends, and family coping with disabling diseases, disorders, or chronic illnesses.

5200 Health Finder
www.healthfinder.gov
Searchable, carefully developed web site offering information on over 1000 topics. Developed by the US Department of Health and Human Services, the site can be used in both English and Spanish.

5201 Healthlink USA

www.healthlinkusa.com

Health information concerning treatment, cures, prevention, diagnosis, risk factors, research, support groups, email lists, personal stories and much more. Updated regularly.

5202 Helios Health

www.helioshealth.com

Online resource for your health information. Detailed information about specific health topics, access to expert advice from our Medical Advisory Board, and up-to-date health news.

5203 Hydrocephalus Association

www.hydroassoc.org

Provides support, education and advocacy for families and professionals. The goal is to insure that families and individuals dealing with the complexities of hydrocephalus receive personal support, comprehensive educational materials and on-going medical care.

5204 Hydrocephalus Center

www.patientcenters.com/hydrocephalus

An online reference that was created especially as a resource for those with hydrocephalus and their families.

5205 MedicineNet

www.medicinenet.com

An online resource for consumers providing easy-to-read, authoritative medical and health information.

5206 Medscape

www.medscape.com

Medscape offers specialists, primary care physicians, and other health professionals the Web's most robust and integrated medical information and educational tools.

5207 Neurology Channel

www.neurologychannel.com

Find clearly explained, medically accurate information regarding conditions, including an overview, symptoms, causes, diagnostic procedures and treatment options. On this site it is possible to ask questions and get information from a neurologist and connect to people who have similar health interests.

5208 WebMD

www.webmd.com

Information on hydrocephalus, including articles and resources.

Description

5209 Hypertension

Hypertension is an abnormal elevation of blood pressure. Blood pressure is noted as a top number (systolic) over a bottom number (diastolic) with a reading of 120/80 being recognized as normal. Hypertension is defined as a systolic pressure greater than 140 and/or a diastolic pressure greater than 90. It is a common disorder that affects about 20 percent of the population. Primary, or essential, hypertension is the most common form, and it has no known cause. It is more prevalent in African-Americans, males, and those with a family history of high blood pressure. Other risk factors include obesity, diabetes, high levels of fat and cholesterol, smoking, sedentary lifestyle and psychological stress. It is a significant risk factor for coronary heart disease, heart failure, stroke, and kidney failure.

Patients with hypertension generally have no symptoms. Diagnosis is made by simple measurement with a blood pressure cuff. Several measurements are necessary at different times to establish the diagnosis.

Treatment of hypertension is done in a step-wise fashion beginning with lifestyle modifications (weight reduction, regular exercise, smoking cessation, a low salt, fat and cholesterol diet and improved stress reduction.) If medications are necessary, doctors can choose from a wide variety of effective and usually well-tolerated drugs. Therapy generally must be lifelong.

Occasionally the blood pressure may be refractory, or difficult to control with medicines. In this instance, screening is needed for unusual causes of hypertension, such as renovascular disease (narrowing of the arteries feeding the kidneys), hyperaldosteronism (a tumor or overgrowth of the adrenal gland which secretes hormones that raise the blood pressure), or aortic coarctation (a congenital malformation of the major blood vessels near the heart.) If no specifically treatable cause is identified, the patient will require combination therapy with high doses of drugs. Given a commitment to doing so, it is almost always possible to control the pressure.

National Agencies & Associations

5210 American Society of Hypertension
148 Madison Avenue
New York, NY 10016
212-696-9099
Fax: 212-696-0711
e-mail: ash@ash-us.org
www.ash-us.org
To organize and conduct educational seminars, materials and products in all aspects of hypertension and other cardiovascular diseases.
Torry Mark Sansone, Executive Director
Mary Trifault, Executive Associate

5211 Lifeclinic.Com
4032 Blackburn Lane
Burtonsville, MD 20866
301-476-9888
Fax: 301-476-9388
e-mail: salesteam@lifeclinic.com
www.lifeclinic.com

The lifeclinic.com web site was developed to provide an in-depth resource for information about prevalent, long-term health conditions and an online service to track your health over time. It also provides the information, resources and tools that can help patients and their families.
David Read, SVP
Shane Knee, VP-Business Development

5212 National Heart, Lung & Blood Institute
PO Box 30105
Bethesda, MD 20824-0105
301-592-8573
Fax: 240-629-3246
TTY: 240-629-3255
e-mail: nhlbiinfo@nhlbi.nih.gov
www.nhlbi.nih.gov
Primary responsibility of this organization is the scientific investigation of heart, blood vessel, lung and blood disorders. Oversee research, demonstration, prevention, education and training activities in these fields and emphasizes the control of stroke.
Elizabeth G Nabel, MD, Director

5213 National Hypertension Association
324 E 30th Street
New York, NY 10016
212-889-3557
Fax: 212-447-7032
e-mail: nathypertension@aol.com
www.nathypertension.org
Conducts research on the cause of hypertension through basic laboratory and clinical studies sponsors seminars and symposia to keep the medical profession and public abreast of services and advances in the treatment of hypertension.
William M Manger MD PhD, Chairman

5214 National Stroke Association
9707 E Easter Lane
Centennial, CO 80112-3747
303-649-9299
800-787-6537
Fax: 303-649-1328
e-mail: Info@stroke.org
www.stroke.org
A national organization whose sole purpose is to reduce the incidence and impact of stroke through prevention treatment rehabilitation and research and support for stroke survivors and their families. NSA produces a variety of education materials and other support services.
James Baranski, Chief Executive Officer
Mike Stefanski, Controller

5215 Pulmonary Hypertension Association
801 Roeder Road
Silver Spring, MD 20910
301-565-3004
800-748-7274
Fax: 301-565-3994
e-mail: pha@PHAssociation.org
www.PHAssociation.org
A nonprofit organization for pulmonary hypertension patients families caregivers and PH-treating medical professionals. The mission of the Pulmonary Hypertension Association (PHA) is to find ways to prevent and cure pulmonary hypertension.
Rino Aldrighetti, President
Carl Hicks, Chair

Research Centers

5216 Creighton University Midwest Hypertension Research Center
601 N 30th Street
Omaha, NE 68131-2137
402-280-4507
Fax: 402-280-4101
Dr William Pettinger, Director

5217 Hahnemann University: Division of Surgical Research
Broad & Vine Streets
Philadelphia, PA 19102
215-762-7000
Fax: 215-762-8109
www.hahnemannhospital.com
Studies hypertension and management of stress ulcers.
Teuro Matsum PhD, Director

5218 Henry Ford Hospital: Hypertension and Vascular Research Division
2799 W Grand Boulevard
Detroit, MI 48202-2689
313-972-1693
Fax: 313-876-1479
e-mail: ocarret1@hfhs.org
www.hypertensionresearch.org

Basic biomedical research seeks to understand: The role of vaso-constrictors and vasodilators (angiotensin II bradykinin nitric ox-ide natriuretic peptides) in the regulation of blood pressure development of hypertension and development of target organ damage (myocardial infarction heart failure vascular injury and renal disease); The generation of reactive oxygen species by blood vessels and kidney cells and how this contributes to target organ damage; and The mechanisms by which therape
Dr Oscar Carretero, Division Head
William H Beierwaltes, Scientist

5219 Indiana University: Hypertension Research Center
541 Clinical Drive   317-274-8153
Indianapolis, IN 46202-0001   800-274-4862
                             Fax: 317-278-0673
                             www.indiana.edu/medical
The mission of the Center is to conduct research in the causes diagnosis treatment and prevention of high blood pressure and its complications.
Dr Myron Weinberger, Director

5220 New York University General Clinical Research Center
NYU Medical Center
550 First Avenue   212-263-7900
New York, NY 10016   Fax: 212-263-8501
                             www.med.nyu.edu
Focuses in the areas of hypertension and studies into endocrinology.
Dr William Rom MPH, Director
Eric Schips, Divisional Administrator

5221 University of Michigan: Division of Hypertension
1500 E Medical Center   734-936-4000
Ann Arbor, MI 48109   800-914-8561
                             www.med.umich.edu
Excellence in medical education patient care and research.
Douglas L Strong, Director
Robert P Kelch, Executive Vice President for Medical Aff

5222 University of Minnesota: Hypertensive Research Group
611 Beacon Street SE   612-624-1438
Minneapolis, MN 55455
Research pertaining to hypertension and stress disorders.
Jack Stoulil, Study Coordinator

5223 University of Southern California: Division of Nephrology
2025 Zonal Avenue   213-226-7307
Los Angeles, CA 90033-1034   Fax: 213-226-3958
Research into hypertension and sleep disorders.
Dr. Shaul G Massry, Head

5224 University of Virginia: Hypertension and Atherosclerosis Unit
Medical Center   804-924-8470
Charlottesville, VA 22908-0001 Fax: 804-924-2581
Dr Carlos Ayers, Director

5225 Wake Forest University: Arteriosclerosis Research Center
Department of Comparative Medicine
300 S Hawthorne Road   336-764-3600
Winston-Salem, NC 27103-2732 Fax: 336-764-5818
Hypertension research.
Thomas Clark DVM, Director

Support Groups & Hotlines

5226 National Health Information Center
PO Box 1133   310-565-4167
Washington, DC 20013   800-336-4797
                             Fax: 301-984-4256
                             e-mail: info@nhic.org
                             www.health.gov/nhic
Offers a nationwide information referral service, produces directories and resource guides.

Books

5227 Courage: Poems & Positive Thoughts for Stroke Survivors
National Stroke Association

9707 E Easter Lane   303-649-9299
Englewood, CO 80112-3747   800-787-6537
                             Fax: 303-649-1328
                             www.stroke.org
Words of inspiration from survivors and caregivers.
83 pages
Colette Lafosse, Director Rehabilitation/Recovery Program

5228 Discovery Circles
National Stroke Association
9707 E Easter Lane   303-649-9299
Englewood, CO 80112-3747   800-787-6537
                             Fax: 303-649-1328
                             www.stroke.org
NSA's guide to organizing and facilitating stroke support groups. This detailed manual describes the support group structure and the facilitator's role.
213 pages
Colette Lafosse, Director Rehabilitation/Recovery Program

5229 Magic of Humor in Caregiving
National Stroke Association
9707 E Easter Lane   303-649-9299
Englewood, CO 80112-3747   800-787-6537
                             Fax: 303-649-1328
                             www.stroke.org
A dynamic researching tool focusing on the necessity of humor in daily caregiving interaction.
Colette Lafosse, Director Rehabilitation/Recovery Program

5230 Management of Hypertension
EMIS Medical Publishers
PO Box 1607   580-924-0643
Durant, OK 74702-1607   800-225-0694
                             Fax: 580-924-9414

ISBN: 0-929240-62-6

5231 November Days
National Stroke Association
9707 E Easter Lane   303-649-9299
Englewood, CO 80112-3747   800-787-6537
                             Fax: 303-649-1328
                             www.stroke.org
A caregiver's story of her struggle with a loved one's stroke.
225 pages

5232 Ted's Stroke: The Caregiver's Story
National Stroke Association
9707 E Easter Lane   303-649-9299
Englewood, CO 80112-3747   800-787-6537
                             Fax: 303-649-1328
                             www.stroke.org
Personal experiences, guidance and tips for caregivers.
175 pages
ISBN: 0-962487-61-9

5233 Women in Your Life: Protect Yourself, Protect Your Family
National Stroke Association
9707 E Easter Lane   303-649-9299
Englewood, CO 80112-3747   800-787-6537
                             Fax: 303-649-1328
                             www.stroke.org
Valuable information about the unique toll stroke takes on women.
Colette Lafosse, Director Rehabilitation/Recovery Program

Magazines

5234 American Journal of Hypertension
American Society of Hypertension
515 Madison Avenue   212-644-0650
New York, NY 10022   Fax: 212-644-0658
                             e-mail: ash@ash-us.org
                             www.ash-us.org

5235 Ethnicity & Disease
International Society on Hypertension in Blacks

2045 Manchester Street NE
Atlanta, GA 30324-4110

404-875-6263
Fax: 404-875-6334
e-mail: member@ishib.org
www.ishib.org

International journal on ethnic minority population differences in diease patterns. Provides a comprehensive source of information on the causal relationships in the etiology of common illnesses through the study of ethnic patterns of disease.
Quarterly
Christopher T Fitzpatrick, CEO
Melanie T Cockfield, Director Administration

5236 Ethnicity Disease
International Society on Hypertension in Blacks
2045 Manchester Street NE
Atlanta, GA 30324-4110

404-875-6263
Fax: 404-875-6334
e-mail: member@ishib.org
www.ishib.org

Determined to accomplish the overall mission to improving the health and life expectancy of ethnic minority populations around the world. Publishes a quarterly journal and holds an annual conference.
150 pages Quarterly
Christopher T Fitzpatrick, CEO
Melanie T Cockfield, Director Administration

5237 Magazine of the National Institute of Hypertension Studies
13217 Livernois Avenue
Detroit, MI 48238-3162

313-931-3427

Association news.

Newsletters

5238 News Report
National Hypertension Association
324 E 30th Street
New York, NY 10016-8329

212-889-3557
Fax: 212-447-7032
e-mail: nathypertension@aol.com
www.nathypertension.org

Offers information and medical updates regarding hypertension. Recent book publication: 100 Questions and Answers about Hypertension by WM Manger, MD, PhD, and RW Gifford, Jr, MT available through National Hypertension Association.
W.M. Manger MD, PhD, Chairman

Pamphlets

5239 African-Americans and Stroke
National Stroke Association
9707 E Easter Lane
Englewood, CO 80112-3747

303-649-9299
800-787-6537
Fax: 303-649-1328
www.stroke.org

Colette Lafosse, Director Rehabilitation/Recovery Program

5240 Aneurysm Answers
National Stroke Association
9707 E Easter Lane
Englewood, CO 80112-3747

303-649-9299
800-787-6537
Fax: 303-649-1328
www.stroke.org

Colette Lafosse, Director Rehabilitation/Recovery Program

5241 Check Your Pulse, America: Atrial Fibrillation
National Stroke Association
9707 E Easter Lane
Englewood, CO 80112-3747

303-649-9299
800-787-6537
Fax: 303-649-1328
www.stroke.org

Colette Lafosse, Director Rehabilitation/Recovery Program

5242 Cholesterol and Stroke
National Stroke Association
9707 E Easter Lane
Englewood, CO 80112-3747

303-649-9299
800-787-6537
Fax: 303-649-1328
www.stroke.org

Colette Lafosse, Director Rehabilitation/Recovery Program

5243 High Blood Pressure and Stroke
National Stroke Association
9707 E Easter Lane
Englewood, CO 80112-3747

303-649-9299
800-787-6537
Fax: 303-649-1328
www.stroke.org

Colette Lafosse, Director Rehabilitation/Recovery Program

5244 Mobility: Issues Facing Stroke Survivors and Their Families
National Stroke Association
9707 E Easter Lane
Englewood, CO 80112-3747

303-649-9299
800-787-6537
Fax: 303-649-1328
www.stroke.org

Colette Lafosse, Director Rehabilitation/Recovery Program

5245 Recurrent Stroke
National Stroke Association
9707 E Easter Lane
Englewood, CO 80112-3747

303-649-9299
800-787-6537
Fax: 303-649-1328
www.stroke.org

Colette Lafosse, Director Rehabilitation/Recovery Program

5246 Smoking Cessation: Be Smoke Free in 3 Minutes
National Stroke Association
9707 E Easter Lane
Englewood, CO 80112-3747

303-649-9299
800-787-6537
Fax: 303-649-1328
www.stroke.org

Colette Lafosse, Director Rehabilitation/Recovery Program

5247 Transient Ischemic Attack
National Stroke Association
9707 E Easter Lane
Englewood, CO 80112-3747

303-649-9299
800-787-6537
Fax: 303-649-1328
www.stroke.org

Colette Lafosse, Director Rehabilitation/Recovery Program

Audio & Video

5248 Stroke: Touching the Soul of Your Family
National Stroke Association
9707 E Easter Lane
Englewood, CO 80112-3747

303-649-9299
800-787-6537
Fax: 303-649-1328
www.stroke.org

Fifteen minute video chronicling three stroke survivors and their courageous struggle to overcome daily challenges and educate others about stroke.
Colette Lafosse, Director Rehabilitation/Recovery Program

Web Sites

5249 American Society of Hypertension

www.ash-us.org

To organize and conduct educational seminars, materials, and products in all aspects of hypertension and other cardiovascular diseases.

5250 Healing Well

www.healingwell.com

An online health resource guide to medical news, chat, information and articles, newsgroups and message boards, books, disease-related web sites, medical directories, and more for patients, friends, and family coping with disabling diseases, disorders, or chronic illnesses.

5251 Health Finder

www.healthfinder.gov

Searchable, carefully developed web site offering information on over 1000 topics. Developed by the US Department of Health and Human Services, the site can be used in both English and Spanish.

5252 Healthlink USA

www.healthlinkusa.com

Links to websites which may include treatment, cures, diagnosis, prevention, support groups, email lists, messageboards, personal stories, risk factors, statistics, research and more.

5253 Helios Health

www.helioshealth.com

Online resource for your health information. Detailed information about specific health topics, access to expert advice from our Medical Advisory Board, and up-to-date health news.

5254 Hypertension: Journal of the American Heart Association

hyper.ahajournals.org

Lists current issues of journals about hypertension and the American Heart Association.

5255 Inter-American Society of Hypertension

www.iashonline.org

Website hosted by IASH, a non-profit professional organization devoted to the understanding, prevention and control of hypertension and vascular diseases in the American population. Members from 20 different countries in the Americas as well as Europe, Australia and Asia. Stimulates research and the exchange of ideas in hypertension and vascular diseases amoung physicians and scientists. Promotes the detection, control and prevention of hypertension and other cardiovascular risk factors.

5256 Lifeclinic.Com

www.lifeclinic.com

Online information about blood pressure, hypertension, diabetes, cholesterol, stroke, heart failure and more. Maintains current, up-to-date and accurate information for patients to help them manage their conditions better and to improve communications between them and their doctors.

5257 Mayo Clinic Health Oasis

www.mayohealth.org

Mission is to empower people to manage their health, by providing useful and up-to-date information and tools that reflect the expertise and standard of excellence of the Mayo Clinic.

5258 MedicineNet

www.medicinenet.com

An online resource for consumers providing easy-to-read, authoritative medical and health information.

5259 Medscape

www.medscape.com

Medscape offers specialists, primary care physicians, and other health professionals the Web's most robust and integrated medical information and educational tools.

5260 National Heart, Lung & Blood Institute

www.nhlbi.nih.gov

Information on the scientific investigation of heart, blood vessel, lung and blood disorders. Oversee research, demonstration, prevention, education and training activities in these fields and emphasizes the control of stroke.

5261 WebMD

www.webmd.com

Information on hypertension, including articles and resources.

Description

5262 Impotence

Impotence, also called erectile dysfunction (ED), is defined as the inability of a male to achieve and maintain an erection of sufficient quality to allow sexual intercourse. ED is very common, affecting millions of American males. Although it may occur at any age, it becomes dramatically more common with advancing age. Impotence may be caused by diabetes, circulatory disturbance, genital injury, hormonal disorders, medication side effects, depression, surgery (for instance, prostate removal) and many less well-characterized physical and psychological states. Impotence may be situational, that is, involving place, time, partner and degree of self-esteem.

Few cases of impotence are completely cured, but several kinds of effective treatment exist, including correction, if possible, of underlying causes. Oral medications that increase blood flow to the penis have been effective in many instances. Psychological factors that accompany ED should be considered in every case, including behavioral therapy and counseling, as needed.

National Agencies & Associations

5263 Impotence Institute of America
119 S Ruth Street
Maryville, TN 37803
865-379-2154
800-669-1603
e-mail: iwatenn@aol.com
A non-profit organization dedicated to education about impotence. The IIA is a division of the Impotence World Association. Provides information on the causes, impact and treatments on this topic. Also publishes a quarterly newsletter on impotence topics.

5264 Impotence Resource Center of the Geddings Osbon Sr Foundation
PO Box 1593
Augusta, GA 30903
800-433-4215
Fax: 706-821-2782
e-mail: impotence@afud.org
www.impotence.org
Offers a free medical discussion where the consumer can obtain accurate unblessed information in a confidential understanding and thoughtful manner.

5265 National Kidney and Urologic Diseases Information Clearinghouse
Center Drive MSC 2560
Bethesda, MD 20892-2560
301-654-4415
800-891-5390
Fax: 301-907-8906
e-mail: nkudic@info.niddk.nih.gov
www.niddk.nih.gov
Provides information about diseases of the kidneys and urologic system to people with such afflictions and to their families, health care professionals and the public. Answers inquiries; develops, reviews and distributes publications.
Griffin P Rodgers, Director

5266 Sexual Function Health Council American Foundation for Urologic Disease
American Foundation for Urologic Disease
1000 Corporate Boulevard
Linthicum, MD 21090
410-689-3700
866-746-4282
Fax: 410-689-3800
e-mail: auafoundation@auafoundation.org
www.auafoundation.org
The American Foundation for Urologic Disease Inc. is a charitable organization established to raise funds for research lay education

and patient advocacy for the prevention detection management and cure of urologic disease.
John M Barry, President
Sandra Vassos, Executive Director

Research Centers

5267 CNY Male Sexual Dysfunction Center
357 Genesee Street
Oneida, NY 13421
315-363-8862
888-269-6732
Fax: 315-363-5477
www.cnymsdc.com

5268 Male Sexual Dysfunction Clinic
3401 N Central Avenue
Chicago, IL 60634
800-788-2873
800-788-2873
Fax: 847-231-4130
e-mail: info@msdclinic.com
www.msdclinic.com
Helping men overcome male sexual dysfunctions such as impotence since 1981.
Sheldon O Burman, Director

5269 New York Male Reproductive Center: Sexual Dysfunction Unit
161 Fort Washington Avenue
New York, NY 10032
212-305-0123
Fax: 212-305-0126
e-mail: rshabsigh@urology.columbia.edu
The New York Male Reproductive Center at Columbia-Presbyterian Medical Center offers state-of-the-art diagnosis and treatment for impotence. Treatments include surgical and non-surgical procedures.
Ridwan Shabs MD, Director

Support Groups & Hotlines

5270 Impotence Information Center
PO Box 9
Minneapolis, MN 55440
800-843-4315

5271 Impotents Anonymous
8630 Fenton Street
Silver Spring, MD 20910-3803
301-588-5777
Serves as an educational organization providing concerned individuals with information regarding impotence.
Bruce MacKenzie, Founder

5272 National Health Information Center
PO Box 1133
Washington, DC 20013
310-565-4167
800-336-4797
Fax: 301-984-4256
e-mail: info@nhic.org
www.health.gov/nhic
Offers a nationwide information referral service, produces directories and resource guides.

Books

5273 Impotence: How to Overcome It
HealthProInk Publishing
562 Wind Drift Lane
Spring Lake, MI 49456-2168
313-355-3686

5274 It's Not All in Your Head
Impotence Institute of America
8201 Corporate Drive
Landover, MD 20785-2230
301-577-0650
A couple's guide to overcoming impotence.

Newsletters

5275 Impotence Worldwide
8201 Corporate Drive
Landover, MD 20785-2230
301-577-0650
Provides information from professionals and lay persons concerning impotence plus manufactured product information.
Monthly

5276 Your Sexuality & Health
Impotence Resource Center
PO Box 1593
Augusta, GA 30903-1593   800-433-4215
                                e-mail: info@gdo.org
                                www.impotence.org
Quarterly newsletter that features articles by medical experts and highlights current research and tidbits of healthy living advice.
Quarterly

Pamphlets

5277 Answers to the Most Asked Questions About Impotence
Impotence World Services
8201 Corporate Drive   301-577-0650
Landover, MD 20785-2230

5278 Impotence Causes and Treatments
American Medical Systems
10700 Bren Road E   952-933-4666
Minnetonka, MN 55343   800-843-4315
                                 Fax: 952-930-6157
                                 www.visitams.com
Offers information on what impotence is, physical and emotional causes, treatments, questions and answers.

5279 Male Treatment Guide
Impotence Resource Center
PO Box 1593
Augusta, GA 30903-1593   800-433-4215
                                e-mail: info@gdo.org
                                www.impotence.org
Explains impotence - what it is, what causes it and how it is treated.
Free

5280 Woman's Perspective
Impotence Resource Center
PO Box 1593
Augusta, GA 30903-1593   800-433-4215
                                e-mail: info@gdo.org
                                www.impotence.org
Talking with your partner about impotence and choosing a treatment together.
Free

Audio & Video

5281 Impotence Treatment Options
Impotence Resource Center
PO Box 1593
Augusta, GA 30903-1593   800-433-4215
                                e-mail: info@gdo.org
                                www.impotence.org
Actual taping of a men's sexual health seminar - presented by Gary Leach, MD.

5282 Male Treatment Guide
Impotence Resource Center
PO Box 1593
Augusta, GA 30903-1593   800-433-4215
                                e-mail: info@gdo.org
                                www.impotence.org
Explains impotence - what it is, what causes it and how it is treated.
Audio Tape

5283 Medical Management of Impotence
Impotence Resource Center
PO Box 1593
Augusta, GA 30903-1593   800-433-4215
                                e-mail: info@gdo.org
                                www.impotence.org

5284 Woman's Perspective
Impotence Resource Center
PO Box 1593
Augusta, GA 30903-1593   800-433-4215
                                e-mail: info@gdo.org
                                www.impotence.org

Talking with your partner about impotence and choosing a treatment together.
Audio Tape

Web Sites

5285 American Foundation for Urologic Disease
                                www.impotence.org
Online information about impotence, provided by the Sexual Function Health Council of the American Foundation for Urologic Disease.

5286 Family Meds
                                www.familymeds.com
A site providing information on impotence and its various treatments, including over the counter, natural, and prescription medication choices.

5287 Healing Well
                                www.healingwell.com
An online health resource guide to medical news, chat, information and articles, newsgroups and message boards, books, disease-related web sites, medical directories, and more for patients, friends, and family coping with disabling diseases, disorders, or chronic illnesses.

5288 Health Finder
                                www.healthfinder.gov
Searchable, carefully developed web site offering information on over 1000 topics. Developed by the US Department of Health and Human Services, the site can be used in both English and Spanish.

5289 Healthlink USA
                                www.healthlinkusa.com
Health information concerning treatment, cures, prevention, diagnosis, risk factors, research, support groups, email lists, personal stories and much more. Updated regularly.

5290 Helios Health
                                www.helioshealth.com
Online resource for your health information. Detailed information about specific health topics, access to expert advice from our Medical Advisory Board, and up-to-date health news.

5291 Impotence Resource Center of the Geddings Osbon Sr Foundation
                                www.impotence.org
Offers a free medical discussion service where the consumer can obtain accurate, unblassed information in a confidential, understanding and thoughtful manner.

5292 Impotence Specialists.com
                                www.impotencespecialists.com
Offers information on physicians in your area, treatment options, online resources and more. A guide to the nation's impotence specialists.

5293 Impotence World Association
                                www.impotence.com
Informs and educates the public on the subject of impotence and its causes and treatments. Serving the impotence industry since 1983 by bringing total care to the treatment of impotence.

5294 MedicineNet
                                www.medicinenet.com
An online resource for consumers providing easy-to-read, authoritative medical and health information.

5295 Medscape
                                www.medscape.com
Medscape offers specialists, primary care physicians, and other health professionals the Web's most robust and integrated medical information and educational tools.

5296 WebMD
                                www.webmd.com
Information on impotence, including articles and resources.

Description

5297 Incontinence

Urinary incontinence is the involuntary leakage of urine, whether during waking or sleeping hours. One common type is urge incontinence, resulting from involuntary bladder contractions. The person feels a sudden urge to urinate, so intense that it may not be controlled long enough to reach the toilet. Common causes of urge incontinence are urinary tract infections, spinal cord injury, and kidney stones. Stress incontinence is the instantaneous leakage of urine without bladder contractions. It manifests as loss of urine during stress events, such as coughing, sneezing, laughing, or lifting. This may occur in women due to weak bladder tone from multiple pregnancies. In men, stress incontinence can occur after prostate removal or trauma to the bladder. Overflow incontinence, in which the bladder cannot control urine output, can be caused by nerve injury, alcoholism, and some diseases. Symptoms include urgency, and having to urinate more often (frequency) and at night (nocturia).

Treatment of incontinence focuses on therapy for the underlying causes. Infections are treated with the appropriate antibiotics. Stress incontinence in women can be treated with exercises to strengthen the bladder muscles. Other therapies include biofeedback and electrical stimulation. Severe cases may require surgical repair. Urinary incontinence remains largely a neglected problem, despite the fact that it can often be successfully treated.

National Agencies & Associations

5298 American Urological Association
1000 Corporate Boulevard
Linthicum, MD 21090

410-689-3700
866-746-4282
Fax: 410-689-3800
e-mail: auafoundation@auafoundation.org
www.urologyhealth.org

A charitable organization whose mission is the prevention and cure of urologic diseases through the expansion of research education and public awareness.
Sandra Vasso MPA, Executive Director
John M Barry MD, President

5299 International Foundation for Functional Gastrointestinal Disorders (IFFGD)
PO Box 170864
Milwaukee, WI 53217-8076

414-964-1799
888-964-2001
Fax: 414-964-7176
e-mail: iffgd@iffgd.org
www.iffgd.org

Nonprofit education, support and research organization devoted to increasing awareness and understanding of functional gastrointestinal disorders including irritable bowel syndrome (IBS), constipation, diarrhea, pain and incontinence.
Nancy J Norton, President

5300 Intestinal Disease Foundation
100 W Station Square Drive
Pittsburgh, PA 15219-1122

412-261-5888
877-587-9606
Fax: 412-471-2722
www.intestinalfoundation.org

Provides one-on-one telephone support, educational programs and materials and self-help groups for people with irritable bowel syndrome (IBS), diverticular disease, inflammatory bowel diseases

and short bowel syndrome; sponsors educational seminars; provides educational materials.
Harriet Gibb LPN, Client Services Manager

5301 National Association for Continence
PO Box 1019
Charleston, SC 29402-1019

843-377-0900
800-252-3337
Fax: 843-377-0905
e-mail: memberservices@nafc.org
www.nafc.org

Founded as Help for Incontinent People, NAFC is the foremost consumer advocacy organization dedicated to helping people who struggle with incontinence and related voiding dysfunction. Its mission is focused on public education, awareness and collaboration.
Nancy Muller, Executive Director
Pam Knox, Communications and Public Relations

5302 National Council on Aging
1901 L Street NW
Washington, DC 20036

202-479-1200
Fax: 202-479-0735
TTY: 202-479-6674
TDD: 202-479-6674
e-mail: info@ncoa.org
www.ncoa.org

Organizations and professionals promoting the dignity self-determination and well-being of older persons.
James P Firman EdD, President/CEO

5303 Simon Foundation for Continence
PO Box 815
Wilmette, IL 60091

847-864-3913
800-237-4666
Fax: 847-864-9758
e-mail: cbgartley@simonfoundation.org
www.simonfoundation.org

Seeks to bring the topic of incontinence out of the closet and remove the associated stigma; provides educational materials to patients their families and the health care professionals who provide patient care.
Cheryle B Gartley, President/Founder
Anita Saltmarche, Vice President

Support Groups & Hotlines

5304 Greater New York Pull-Thru Network
62 Edgewood Avenue
Wyckoff, NJ 07481

201-891-5977

National support network providing emotional support and information to patients and families of children who have had or will have a pull-thru type surgery to correct an imperforate anus or associated malformation, Hirschsprung's or other fecal incontinence problems. Support group meetings held quarterly.

5305 National Health Information Center
PO Box 1133
Washington, DC 20013

310-565-4167
800-336-4797
Fax: 301-984-4256
e-mail: info@nhic.org
www.health.gov/nhic

Offers a nationwide information referral service, produces directories and resource guides.

5306 Simon Foundation Helpline for Incontinence Information
Simon Foundation for Continence
PO Box 815
Wilmette, IL 60091

847-864-3913
800-237-4666
Fax: 847-864-9758
e-mail: cbgartley@simonfoundation.org
www.simonfoundation.org

Offers information and help to persons with incontinence problems and professionals who work with them.
Cheryle Gartley, Founder/President
Jasmine Schmidt, Director of Education

5307 University of California at San Francisco Women's Continence Center
2356 Sutter Street
San Francisco, CA 94115

415-885-7788
877-366-8325
coe.ucsf.edu/wcc

Offers a comprehensive array of clinical services for women with incontinence, urethal or bladder dysfuntion and pelvic support problems.
Jeanette S Brown MD, Director

Books

5308   Managing Incontinence: a Guide to Living with Loss of Bladder Control
Simon Foundation for Incontinence
PO Box 815   847-864-3913
Wilmette, IL 60091   800-237-4666
                                          Fax: 847-864-9768
                     e-mail: simoninfo@simonfoundation.org
                                    www.simonfoundation.org
Seeks to bring the topic of incontinence out of the closet and remove the associated stigma; provides information to patients, their families and the health care professionals who provide patient care.
Quarterly
Cheryle B Gartley, President

5309   Pocket Guide for Continence Care
National Association for Continence
PO Box 1019   843-377-0900
Charleston, SC 29402   800-252-3337
                                          Fax: 843-377-0905
                          e-mail: memberservices@nafc.org
                                              www.nafc.org
Condensed version of the Blueprint for Continence Care, this guide is designed for a first line supervisor or any health care professional in any eldercare environment to help address any issues related to bladder health. The guide is perfect for a quick referral because it can actually fit in the healthcare professional's pocket.
Nancy Muller, Executive Director
Caryn Antos, Publicity/Publications Associate

5310   Resource Guide: Products and Services for Incontinence
National Association for Continence
PO Box 1019   843-377-0900
Charleston, SC 29402   800-252-3337
                                          Fax: 843-377-0905
                          e-mail: memberservices@nafc.org
                                              www.nafc.org
Complete directory of products and services available. Categories include disposable products, reusable products, skin care products, deodorizing products, pelvic organ support devices, medications to treat incontinence and others. Also includes a listing of distributors and mail/phone order companies.
Nancy Muller, Executive Director
Caryn Antos, Publicity/Publications Associate

5311   Your Personal Guide to Bladder Health
National Association for Continence
PO Box 1019   843-377-0900
Charleston, SC 29402   800-252-3337
                                          Fax: 843-377-0905
                          e-mail: memberservices@nafc.org
                                              www.nafc.org
Designed for residents of assisted living environments, other older individuals living independently and their involved family members. It encompasses a wide variety of informative topics, including diet and daily habits, pelvic muscle exercises odor control and more.
48 pages
Nancy Muller, Executive Director
Caryn Antos, Publicity/Publications Associate

Magazines

5312   Digestive Health Matters
Intl. Foundation for Gastrointestinal Disorders
PO Box 170864   414-964-1799
Milwaukee, WI 53217-0864   888-964-2001
                                          Fax: 414-964-7176
                                  e-mail: iffgd@iffgd.org
                                              www.iffgd.org

Quarterly journal focuses on upper and lower gastrointestinal disorders in adults and children. Educational pamphlets and factsheets are available. Patient and professional membership.

Newsletters

5313   Discoveries
National Association for Continence
PO Box 1019   843-377-0900
Charleston, SC 29402   800-252-3337
                                          Fax: 843-377-0905
                          e-mail: memberservices@nafc.org
                                              www.nafc.org
Compendium comprised of the most recently released incontinence products and newly approved protocol. Includes editorial sections, authored by leading clinicians and researchers, describing new product technology and research in other medical advances related to continence care.
32 pages BiAnnual
Nancy Muller, Executive Director
Caryn Antos, Publicity/Publications Associate

5314   Informer
Simon Foundation for Incontinence
PO Box 815   847-864-3913
Wilmette, IL 60091   800-237-4666
                                          Fax: 847-864-9768
                     e-mail: simoninfo@simonfoundation.org
                                    www.simonfoundation.org
Seeks to bring the topic of incontinence out of the closet and remove the associated stigma; provides information to patients, their families, and the health care professionals who provide patient care.
Quarterly
Cheryle B Gartley, President

5315   Intestinal Fortitude
Intestinal Disease Foundation
One Station Square, Suite 525   412-261-5888
Pittsburgh, PA 15219   Fax: 412-471-2722
                                    www.intestinalfoundation.org
Newsletter, brochures and books for Intestinal Disease Foundation members.

5316   Participate
IFFGD
PO Box 17864   414-964-1799
Milwaukee, WI 53217-0864   888-964-2001
                                          Fax: 414-964-7176
                                  e-mail: iffgd@iffgd.org
                                    www.aboutincontinence.org
Provides information for people affected by the various forms of functional bowel disorders, including irritable bowel syndrome, constipation, diarrhea, pain and incontinence.
Quarterly

5317   Pull-Thru Network News
Greater New York Pull-Thru Network
62 Edgewood Avenue
Wyckoff, NJ 07481-3456   201-891-5977
                                    www.pullthrough.org/ptnn.html
Quarterly newsletter for patients and families who have had or will have a pull-thru type surgery to correct an imperforate anus or associated malformation, Hirschsprung's or other fecal incontinence problem.

5318   Quality Care
National Association for Continence
PO Box 1019   843-377-0900
Charleston, SC 29402   800-252-3337
                                          Fax: 843-377-0905
                          e-mail: memberservices@nafc.org
                                              www.nafc.org
Quarterly newsletter addressing causes, symptoms, management and treatment options for incontinence and related disorders.
Quarterly
Nancy Muller, Executive Director
Caryn Antos, Publicity/Publications Associate

Pamphlets

5319 Bladder Control for Women
National Kidney and Urologic Diseases Information
3 Information Way
Bethesda, MD 20892-3580   800-891-5390
                                Fax: 301-907-8906
                    e-mail: nkudic@info.nidkk.nih.gov
Comprehensive introduction to the causes, symptoms, and treatments for bladder control problems in women.

5320 Exercising Your Pelvic Muscles
National Kidney and Urologic Diseases Information
3 Information Way
Bethesda, MD 20892-3580   800-891-5390
                                Fax: 301-907-8906
                    e-mail: nkudic@info.nidkk.nih.gov
A description of exercises for the pelvic floor muscles, called Kegel exercises, and how they can help to restore or maintain bladder control.

5321 Menopause and Bladder Control
National Kidney and Urologic Diseases Information
3 Information Way
Bethesda, MD 20892-3580   800-891-5390
                                Fax: 301-907-8906
                    e-mail: nkudic@info.nidkk.nih.gov
An introduction to the changes to your body that occur during menopause, how these changes can result in loss of bladder control, and how your health care team can help you restore or maintain bladder control.

5322 NAFC Fact Sheets
National Association for Continence
PO Box 1019   843-377-0900
Charleston, SC 29402   800-252-3337
                                Fax: 843-377-0905
                    e-mail: memberservices@nafc.org
                                      www.nafc.org
Offering helpful tips and information on a variety of topics, the sheets provide consumers and professionals with the necessary information on managing incontinence. Some titles include medications, diet and daily habits, odor control, prostatectomy and many more.
Nancy Muller, Executive Director
Caryn Antos, Publicity/Publications Associate

5323 Pregnancy, Childbirth, and Bladder Control
National Kidney and Urologic Diseases Information
3 Information Way
Bethesda, MD 20892-3580   800-891-5390
                                Fax: 301-907-8906
                    e-mail: nkudic@info.nidkk.nih.gov
A look at the effects that pregnancy and childbearing can have on bladder control and ways you can counter those effects.

5324 Talking to Your Health Care Team About Bladder Control
National Kidney and Urologic Diseases Information
3 Information Way
Bethesda, MD 20892-3580   800-891-5390
                                Fax: 301-907-8906
                    e-mail: nkudic@info.nidkk.nih.gov
Tips for giving your health care provider the information needed to diagnose and treat your bladder control problem. Includes a questionnaire for you to fill out and take to your first appointment.

5325 Urinary Incontinence in Women
National Kidney and Urologic Diseases Information
3 Information Way
Bethesda, MD 20892-3580   800-891-5390
                                Fax: 301-907-8906
                    e-mail: nkudic@info.nidkk.nih.gov
An overview of the types, diagnosis, and treatment of urinary incontinence in women.

5326 What Your Female Patients Want to Know About Bladder Control
National Kidney and Urologic Diseases Information
3 Information Way
Bethesda, MD 20892-3580   800-891-5390
                                Fax: 301-907-8906
                    e-mail: nkudic@info.nidkk.nih.gov
Fact sheet with tips for health care providers on raising the issue of incontinence with female patients who may be reluctant to talk about their problem.

5327 Your Body's Design for Bladder Control
National Kidney and Urologic Diseases Information
3 Information Way
Bethesda, MD 20892-3580   800-891-5390
                                Fax: 301-907-8906
                    e-mail: nkudic@info.nidkk.nih.gov
An introduction to the female urinary system. Includes diagrams of the bladder and pelvic floor muscles.

5328 Your Daily Bladder Diary
National Kidney and Urologic Diseases Information
3 Information Way
Bethesda, MD 20892-3580   800-891-5390
                                Fax: 301-907-8906
                    e-mail: nkudic@info.nidkk.nih.gov
An easy-to-use form for patients to note liquid intake, trips to the bathroom, urine leaks, and other details that may help explain your incontinence.

5329 Your Medicines and Bladder Control
National Kidney and Urologic Diseases Information
3 Information Way
Bethesda, MD 20892-3580   800-891-5390
                                Fax: 301-907-8906
                    e-mail: nkudic@info.nidkk.nih.gov
Booklet describing the effects that your medications could have on bladder control, with a recommendation for discussing all your medicines with your doctor.

Audio & Video

5330 Solution Starts with You
Simon Foundation for Continence
PO Box 815   847-864-3913
Wilmette, IL 60091   800-237-4666
                                Fax: 847-864-9758
            e-mail: cbgartley@simonfoundation.org
                          www.simonfoundation.org
Seeks to bring the topic of incontinence out of the closet and remove the associated stigma; provides information to patients, their families, and the health care professionals who provide patient care.
Quarterly
Cheryle Gartley, Founder/President
Jasmine Schmidt, Director of Education

Web Sites

5331 American Foundation for Urologic Disease
                                    www.incontinence.org
Large website detailing information on incontinence, ranging from various treatment options to links and resources.

5332 Healing Well
                                      www.healingwell.com
An online health resource guide to medical news, chat, information and articles, newsgroups and message boards, books, disease-related web sites, medical directories, and more for patients, friends, and family coping with disabling diseases, disorders, or chronic illnesses.

5333 Health Finder
                                      www.healthfinder.gov
Searchable, carefully developed web site offering information on over 1000 topics. Developed by the US Department of Health and Human Services, the site can be used in both English and Spanish.

5334 Healthlink USA
                                      www.healthlinkusa.com

Health information concerning treatment, cures, prevention, diagnosis, risk factors, research, support groups, email lists, personal stories and much more. Updated regularly.

5335   Helios Health

www.helioshealth.com

Online resource for your health information. Detailed information about specific health topics, access to expert advice from our Medical Advisory Board, and up-to-date health news.

5336   MedicineNet

www.medicinenet.com

An online resource for consumers providing easy-to-read, authoritative medical and health information.

5337   Medscape

www.medscape.com

Medscape offers specialists, primary care physicians, and other health professionals the Web's most robust and integrated medical information and educational tools.

5338   National Association for Continence

www.nafc.org

Interactive website packed with useful information about diagnosis, treatment options and management solutions for incontinence. The site currentlyfeatures a specialist search engine of healthcare providers who have recieved specific training in the diagnosis and treatment of incontinence to assist consumers in locating a specialist in their area. Other features include archived Quality Care articles, a message board, online database of active support groups and much more.

5339   Simon Foundation for Continence

www.simonfoundation.org

Seeks to bring the topic of incontinence out of the closet and remove the associated stigma; provides educational materials to patients, their families, and the health care professionals who provide patient care.

5340   WebMD

www.webmd.com

Information on incontinence, including articles and resources.

Description

5341 Infertility

Infertility is defined as the failure to achieve conception by couples who have not used contraception for at least one year, and affects 1 in 5 couples in the United States.

Female causes of infertility include dysfunction of the ovaries (20 percent of couples), blockage of the tubes connecting the ovaries to the uterus (30 percent), and abnormal secretions (5 percent). Infertility in males is mostly related to sperm disorders (35 percent of couples), either insufficient production of sperm, ineffective sperm, or defective delivery of sperm. Unidentified factors account for the remaining 10 percent of couples.

A variety of tests are needed to determine the exact cause of infertility and then identify the appropriate treatment options. Failure to conceive can be both an emotional and financial burden on couples. Counseling and psychological support are important parts of treatment.

National Agencies & Associations

5342 Adopt-A-Special-Kid America
8201 Edgewater Drive
Oakland, CA 94621
510-553-1748
888-680-7349
Fax: 510-553-1747
e-mail: info@aask.org
www.adoptaspecialkid.org
Adopt-A-Special-Kid provides information on adoption of children with special needs.
Amirah Revels-Bey, President/Board of Directors
Vali Ebert, Executive Director

5343 American Fertility Association
666 5th Avenue
New York, NY 10103-0004
888-917-3777
Fax: 718-601-7722
e-mail: info@theafa.org
www.theafa.org
Purpose is to educate the public about reproductive disease and support families during struggles with infertility and adoption. Exists to serve the unique needs of men and women confronting infertility issues.
Ken Mosesian, Executive Director
Stuart Miller, Co-Chair of the Board

5344 American Society for Reproductive Medicine
1209 Montgomery Highway
Birmingham, AL 35216-2809
205-978-5000
Fax: 205-978-5005
e-mail: asrm@asrm.org
www.asrm.com
Purpose is to educate the public about reproductive disease and support families during struggles with infertility and adoption. Exists to serve the unique needs of men and women confronting infertility issues.
Robert W Rebar MD, Executive Director
Andrew LaBar PhD, Scientific Director

5345 Hysterectomy Educational Resources & Services (HERS) Foundation
422 Bryn Mawr Avenue
Bala Cynwyd, PA 19004
610-667-7757
888-750-4377
Fax: 610-677-8096
e-mail: hersfdn@earthlink.net
www.hersfoundation.com
A nonprofit foundation which provides information about the alternatives to hysterectomy the risks of the alternatives and the consequences of the surgery. HERS provides telephone counseling by appointment.

5346 International Council on Infertility Information Dissemination
PO Box 6836
Arlington, VA 22206
703-379-9178
Fax: 703-379-1593
e-mail: INCIIDinfo@inciid.org
www.inciid.org
Provides information on infertility pregnancy loss adoption high risk pregnancy and parenting after the above.
Gary S Berger MD FACOG, Member of Advisory Board
Mike Berkley LAc DA, Member of Advisory Board

5347 RESOLVE: The National Infertility
7910 Woodmont Avenue
Bethesda, MD 20814
301-652-8585
Fax: 301-652-9375
e-mail: info@resolve.org
www.resolve.org
A nationwide nonprofit consumer organization serving the unique needs of those striving to build a family. Provides compassionate and informed help to people who are experiencing the infertility crisis and strives to increase the visibility of infertility in the community.
Joseph C Isaacs CAE, President/CEO
Barbara Collura, Executive Director

State Agencies & Associations

Alabama

5348 RESOLVE of Alabama
1760 Old Meadow Road
McLean, VA 22102
703-556-7172
888-623-0744
Fax: 703-506-3266
e-mail: bcollura@resolve.org
www.resolve.org
Barbara Collura, Executive Director
Dawn Gannon, Professional Outreach Manager

Arizona

5349 RESOLVE of Valley of the Sun
PO Box 36252
Phoenix, AZ 85067-6252
602-995-3933
e-mail: resolveaz@hotmail.com
www.resolveaz.org
Tina Nelson, President
Denny Ceizyk, VP

Arkansas

5350 RESOLVE Affiliate of Northwest Arkansas
2230 Country Way
Fayetteville, AR 72703-4215
501-521-3763

California

5351 RESOLVE of Greater Los Angeles
PO Box 12529
Newport Beach, CA 92658
310-326-2630
866-888-7452
e-mail: socalresolve@gmail.com
www.southwest.resolve.org
Jennifer Munro, Los Angeles Local Area Affiliate Chair
Kirsten Hanson-Press, Adoption

5352 RESOLVE of Greater San Diego
PO Box 12529
Newport Beach, CA 92658-7385
310-326-2630
866-888-7452
e-mail: mariwaldron@yahoo.com
www.southwest.resolve.org
Mari Waldron, San Diego Chair
Jennifer Bolger, Speaker Coordinator

5353 RESOLVE of Northern California
312 Sutter Street
San Francisco, CA 94108
415-788-6772
Fax: 415-788-6774
e-mail: info@YourOpenPath.org
www.resolvenc.org
Volunteer-based organization that provides infertility education adoption information advocacy and support.
Roberta Rodriguez-Ha, Executive Director
Renee Cullinan, President

5354 RESOLVE of Orange County
1760 Old Meadow Road
McLean, VA 22102   877-203-7771
                    e-mail: pennyjf@sbcglobal.net
                    www.resolve.org/regions/southwest
Penny Joss Fletcher, Local Area Affiliate Chair

Colorado

5355 RESOLVE of Colorado
PO Box 260725   303-469-5261
Littleton, CO 80163-0725   866-469-5261
                    www.resolvecolorado.org

Connecticut

5356 RESOLVE of Fairfield County
PO Box 930   914-686-1490
S Norwalk, CT 06856-0930   Fax: 203-255-2561
                    e-mail: anncrane4@aol.com
                    northeast.resolve.org

Joan Gill, Volunteer Coordinator

5357 RESOLVE of Greater Hartford
PO Box 290964   860-523-8337
Wetherfield, CT 06129-0964 e-mail: info@resolveofgreaterhartford.org
                    www.resolveofgreaterhartford.org

Janice Falk, President
Gwen Hamil, Treasurer

District of Columbia

5358 RESOLVE of the Washington Metro Area
PO Box 3423   202-362-5555
Merrifield, VA 22116-3423   e-mail: mary.stern@erols.com
                    www.resolvedc.org

Mary Stern, Adoption Resource

Florida

5359 RESOLVE Affiliate of Central Florida
1050 W Morse Boulevard   407-637-0142
Winter Park, FL 32789   e-mail: admin@resolveofcentralflorida.org
                    www.resolveofcentralflorida.org

5360 RESOLVE of North Florida
1929 Logging Lane
Jacksonville, FL 32221-2071   904-737-0140
                    rushservices.com/resolve

5361 RESOLVE of South Florida
3342 SW 51 Street   954-749-9500
Ft Lauderdale, FL 33312   e-mail: elinder33134@gmail.com
                    southeast.resolve.org

Elise Linder, Coordinator

Georgia

5362 RESOLVE of Georgia
3904 N Druid Hills Road   404-233-8443
Decatur, GA 30333   e-mail: Katie9924@hotmail.com
                    southeast.resolve.org

Kate Badey, Coordinator
Renee Whitley, Advocacy Chair

Hawaii

5363 RESOLVE of Hawaii
PO Box 29193   808-528-8559
Honolulu, HI 96820   e-mail: info@resolveofhawaii.org
                    www.resolveofhawaii.org

Illinois

5364 RESOLVE of Illinois
PO Box 56   773-743-1623
Hinsdale, IL 60521   e-mail: info@resolveofillinios.org
                    greatlakes.resolve.org

Indiana

5365 RESOLVE of Indiana
5155 Sandy Court   317-329-9519
Pittsboro, IN 46167-9129   e-mail: resolveofindiana@hotmail.com
                    greatlakes.resolve.org

Robin Scott, President

Iowa

5366 RESOLVE Affiliate of Iowa
1348 Atlantic   319-557-2763
Dunuque, IA 52001

Kentucky

5367 RESOLVE of Kentucky
851 Van Dyke Mill Road   502-834-7568
Taylorsville, KY 40071-9502   e-mail: jannetteburns@msn.com
                    greatlakes.resolve.org

Louisiana

5368 RESOLVE of Louisiana
PO Box 55693   504-454-6987
Metairie, LA 70055-5693

Maryland

5369 RESOLVE of Maryland
PO Box 3423   202-362-5555
Merrifield, VA 22116   888-362-4414
                    e-mail: info@resolve.org
                    www.resolve.org

Holly Kortright, Support Services Coordinator
Jane Castanias, Co-Chair

5370 RESOLVE of West Virginia
PO Box 3423   202-362-5555
Merrifield, VA 22116   888-362-4414
                    e-mail: info@resolve.org
                    www.resolve.org

Joanne MacMillan, Co-Chair
Joann Mirgon, Professional Relations Coordinator

Massachusetts

5371 RESOLVE of the Bay State
395 Totten Pond Road   781-890-2225
Waltham, MA 02451-1553   Fax: 781-890-2249
                    e-mail: admin@resolveofthebaystate.org
                    www.resolveofthebaystate.org
Information on the Massachusetts chapter of a national, nonprofit
consumer based infertility support organization. Information and a
variety of services to answer your questions about infertility, treatments, coping techniquesand insurance issues.
1,000 Homes
Rebecca Lubens, Executive Director
Lisa Rothstein, Programming Coordinator

Michigan

5372 RESOLVE of Michigan
3601 W Thirteen Mile Road   248-975-8866
Royal Oak, MI 48068-9998   888-255-1399
                    e-mail: info@greatlakes.resolve.org
                    www.greatlakes.resolve.org

Kathy Rollinger, President
Heather Hall, Vice President

Minnesota

5373 RESOLVE: Minnesota Chapter
1161 E Wayzata Boulevard   651-659-0333
Wayzata, MN 55391   888-959-0333
                    e-mail: info@midwest.resolve.org
                    www.resolve.org

Missouri

5374 RESOLVE of St. Louis, Missouri
PO Box 411072
Saint Louis, MO 63141-3072   314-567-8788
e-mail: info@resolvestl.org
www.resolvestl.org

Jan DeMasters, MD, Media Contact

Nevada

5375 RESOLVE of Nevada Barbara Greenspun Women's Care Center
Barbara Greenspun Women's Care Center
8280 W Warm Springs Road
Las Vegas, NV 89074   702-616-4900
877-203-7778
e-mail: rpbooklover@cox.net
www.southwest.resolve.org

Robyn Isaacson, Local Area Affiliate Chair\Help Line
Suzanne Allen, Office Liaison/New Member Coordinator

New Hampshire

5376 RESOLVE of New Hampshire
131 Daniel Webster Highway
Nashua, NH 03060-5224   603-303-9144

New Jersey

5377 RESOLVE of New Jersey
1830 Front Street   908-322-9180
Scotch Plains, NJ 07076-0335   888-RNJ-2810
e-mail: info@resolvenj.org
www.resolvenj.org

Dr Lidia Abrams, Executive Director
Daria Venezia, Secretary

New Mexico

5378 RESOLVE of New Mexico
PO Box 93386   505-291-5066
Albuquerque, NM 87199   888-895-6055
e-mail: info@southcentral.resolve.org
www.resolve.org

New York

5379 RESOLVE of Long Island
PO Box 303   631-385-5026
Long Island, NY 11714-0303 e-mail: racchair@northeast.resolve.org
www.northeast.resolve.org

Arelys Soto-Lugo, President Advocacy Chair
April R Simanoff, VP Outreach Coordinator

5380 RESOLVE of New York City
178 Columbus Avenue   212-799-7400
New York, NY 10023   888-765-2810
e-mail: info@northeast.resolve.org
www.northeast.resolve.org

5381 RESOLVE of the Capital District
PO Box 14591   518-242-3848
Albany, NY 12212-4591

North Carolina

5382 RESOLVE of North Carolina
101 Gettysburg Drive   919-380-8497
Cary, NC 27513

Ohio

5383 RESOLVE of Ohio
3000 NW Boulevard   614-340-0905
Columbus, OH 43221   800-414-6446
Fax: 614-340-0916
e-mail: info@greatlakes.resolve.org
www.resolveofohio.org

Carole White, President
Kris Henniger, Secretary

Oklahoma

5384 RESOLVE of Oklahoma
PO Box 18151   405-949-8857
Oklahoma City, OK 73154-0151   888-895-6055
e-mail: info@southcentral.resolve.org
www.resolve.org

Oregon

5385 RESOLVE of Oregon
PO Box 175   503-762-0449
Scappoose, OR 97056 e-mail: resolve_oregon@yahoo.com
www.northpacific.resolve.org

Pennsylvania

5386 RESOLVE of Philadelphia
PO Box 2456   215-849-3920
Southeastern, PA 19399-2456   888-765-2810
e-mail: info@resolve.org
www.northeast.resolve.org

Marge McKeone, President and Conference Co-Chair
Jennifer Kaczur, Recording Secretary

5387 RESOLVE of Pittsburgh
PO Box 11203   703-861-2910
Pittsburgh, PA 15238-0203   888-255-1399
e-mail: CantrellMVHS@hotmail.com
www.greatlakes.resolve.org

5388 RESOLVE of Southcentral Pennsylvania
PO Box 402   717-234-8583
Camp Hill, PA 17001-0402

Rhode Island

5389 RESOLVE of the Ocean State
PO Box 28201   401-421-4695
Providence, RI 02908-0201

South Carolina

5390 RESOLVE of South Carolina
204 Fernbrook Circle   864-542-9092
Spartanburg, SC 29307-2966   888-867-7970
www.resolve.org

Tennessee

5391 RESOLVE of Tennessee
4770 Riverdale Road   615-244-5582
Memphis, TN 38141-8529   888-867-7970
www.resolve.org

Texas

5392 RESOLVE of Central Texas
PO Box 49783   512-453-2171
Austin, TX 78765 e-mail: resolvecentraltexas@gmail.com
www.resolvecentraltexas.org

Renaye Thornborrow

5393 RESOLVE of Dallas/Fort Worth
434 N Manus Drive
Dallas, TX 77244   888-563-6376

5394 RESOLVE of Houston
PO Box 441212   713-975-5324
Houston, TX 77244-1212   888-814-1119
e-mail: info@southcentral.resolve.org
www.southcentral.resolve.org

5395 RESOLVE of South Texas
PO Box 782061   210-967-6771
San Antonio, TX 78278 e-mail: info@southcentral.resolve.org
www.southcentral.resolve.org

Christie Goo APR, Contact

5396 RESOLVE of Utah
PO Box 57531   801-483-4024
Salt Lake City, UT 84157-0531   888-592-4449
e-mail: info@resolve.org
www.mountain.resolve.org

5397 RESOLVE of Vermont
PO Box 1094   802-657-2542
Williston, VT 05495-1094

5398 RESOLVE of Washington State
1760 Old Meadow Road   703-556-7172
McLean, VA 22102-1231   888-591-6663
Fax: 703-506-3266
e-mail: WAinfo@northpacific.resolve.org
www.resolvewa.org

5399 RESOLVE of Wisconsin
PO Box 13842   262-521-4590
Wauwatosa, WI 53213-0842   e-mail: info@resolvewi.org
www.resolvewi.org

Gary Dalton, Web Site Contact

5400 Society for the Study of Reproduction
1619 Monroe Street   608-256-2777
Madison, WI 53711-2063   Fax: 608-256-4610
e-mail: ssr@ssr.org
www.ssr.org
International scientific society promotes the study of reproductive biology by fostering interdisciplinary communication within the science by holding conferences and by publishing meritorious studies.
2,400 members
Judith Jansen, Executive Director
Asgerally T Fazleabas, President

Foundations

5401 Fertility Research Foundation
877 Park Avenue   212-744-5500
New York, NY 10021   Fax: 212-744-6536
e-mail: info@frfbaby.com
www.frfbaby.com
Offers information on treatment and the latest research on male and female infertility.
Masood Khatamee MD, Executive Director

Libraries & Resource Centers

5402 National Women's Health Resource Center
157 Broad Street, Suite 106
Red Bank, NJ 07701   877-986-9472
Fax: 732-530-3347
e-mail: info@healthywomen.org
www.healthywomen.org
NWHRC provides the most current women's health care information through website articles, online mini-courses, a monthly electronic newsletter, and periodic news releases.
Elizabeth Battaglino Cahill, RN, Executive Director
Maria Bushee, Director of Marketing & Communications

Research Centers

5403 Fertility Clinic at the Shepherd Spinal Center
Shepherd Spinal Center
2020 Peachtree Road NW
Atlanta, GA 30309-1465   404-352-2020
www.shepherd.org

This clinic makes it possible for paralyzed men to father children.
Gary Ulicny, Chief Executive Officer

5404 Fertility and Women's Health Care Center
130 Maple Street   413-781-8220
Springfield, MA 01103-2202   Fax: 413-732-9088
Conducts basic and clinical studies of male and female infertility.
Ronald K Burke MD, Head

5405 Melpomene Institute for Women's Health Research
550 Rice Street   651-789-0140
Saint Paul, MN 55103   Fax: 651-292-9417
e-mail: shawne@melpomene.org
www.melpomene.org
Focuses on women's health including fertility issues.
Judy Mahle Lutter, President

5406 Tufts University: Baystate Medical Center
759 Chestnut Street
Springfield, MA 01199-1001   413-784-5252
www.tufts.edu
Dr Donald Higby, Director

5407 University of California: UCLA Population Research Center
1124 W Carson Street   310-212-1867
Torrance, CA 90502-2006   Fax: 310-320-6515
Clinical investigations of overpopulation and infertility.
Dr Ronald Sweridloff, Director

5408 University of Michigan Reproductive Sciences Program
1301 E Catherine Street   734-764-0445
Ann Arbor, MI 48109   Fax: 734-368-20
e-mail: jenic@umich.edu
www.med.umich.edu
Research done into reproductive medicine and infertility treatments.
Larry Warren, Chief Executive Director
Jeffrey B Halter, Director

5409 Vand erbilt University: Center for Fertili
C-1100 MCN   615-322-6576
Nashville, TN 37232   Fax: 615-343-4902
Reproductive biology and fertility research.

5410 Vanderbilt University: Center for Fertility and Reproductive Research
C-1100 MCN   615-322-6576
Nashville, TN 37232-0001   Fax: 615-343-4902
Reproductive biology and fertility research.

5411 Wayne State University
4707 St Antoine   313-993-2666
Detroit, MI 48201   Fax: 313-745-0203
wsupg.med.wayne.edu
Reproductive endocrine infertility and gynecologic surgery research. The research spans the woman's life cycle. Reseach projects include: endometriosis polycystic ovary syndrome sexual dysfunction fibroids and menopause.
Michael Diam MD, Director

5412 Wayne State University: University Women's Care
26400 W 12 Mile Road   248-352-8200
Southfield, MI 48034   Fax: 248-356-8224
wayne.edu
Reproductive endocrine infertility and gynecologic surgery research. The research spans the woman's life cycle. Research projects include: endometriosis polycystic ovary syndrome sexual dysfunction fibroids and menopause. Additional studies pertaining to women's health and male infertility.
Elizabeth Pu MD, Associate Professor
Nancy Angel RN, Research Nurse Coordinator

Support Groups & Hotlines

5413 National Health Information Center
PO Box 1133   310-565-4167
Washington, DC 20013   800-336-4797
Fax: 301-984-4256
e-mail: info@nhic.org
www.health.gov/nhic

Offers a nationwide information referral service, produces directories and resource guides.

5414   National Infertility Network Exchange
PO Box 204   516-794-5772
East Meadow, NY 11554   Fax: 516-794-0008
                                      e-mail: info@nine-infertility.org
                                              www.nine-infertility.org/
The National Infertility Network Exchange (NINE) is a national, notfor profit organization for persons and couples with impaired fertility. NINE supportes the decision of legal and medical means to build families as well as the decision to remain childfree.

Books

5415   Adopt the Baby You Want
Simon & Schuster
1230 Avenue of the Americas   212-698-7000
New York, NY 10020-1586   800-223-2348
A how-to adoption book written by an attorney specializing in all areas of adoption.
272 pages

5416   Adopting After Infertility: The Decision, the Commitment, the Experience
American Society for Reproductive Medicine
1209 Montgomery Highway   205-978-5000
Birmingham, AL 35216-2809   Fax: 205-978-5018
Emphasizes the importance of communication between partners and offers several guidelines for maintaining a healthy relationship during such a stressful process.
318 pages

5417   Adoption Directory
American Society for Reproductive Medicine
1209 Montgomery Highway   205-978-5000
Birmingham, AL 35216-2809   Fax: 205-978-5018
An extensive reference text covering such specifics as state statutes, adoption agencies, exchanges and agencies.
515 pages

5418   Adoption Fact Book
American Society for Reproductive Medicine
1209 Montgomery Highway   205-978-5000
Birmingham, AL 35216-2809   Fax: 205-978-5018
A comprehensive source of statistics, regulations and facts on adoption.
277 pages

5419   Adoption Resource Book
Harper Collins
10 E 53rd Street   212-207-7000
New York, NY 10022-5299   800-242-7737
Explores and describes all types and styles of adoption and provides excellent resources for each path taken.
421 pages Third edition

5420   Baby of Your Own: New Ways to Overcome Infertility
Taylor Publishing Company
1550 W Mockingbird Lane   214-637-2800
Dallas, TX 75235-5007
Provides current information regarding the psychological aspects of infertility.
244 pages

5421   Conquering Infertility: A Guide for Couples
Prentice Hall Press
15 Columbus Circle   212-373-8000
New York, NY 10023-7707
Covers various aspects of infertility.

5422   Consumer's Guide to Insurance
American Society for Reproductive Medicine
1209 Montgomery Highway   205-978-5000
Birmingham, AL 35216-2809   Fax: 205-978-5018
A how-to book for infertile couples who are experiencing difficulty with insurance reimbursement.
106 pages

5423   Consumer's Legal Guide to Today's Health Care
American Society for Reproductive Medicine
1209 Montgomery Highway   205-978-5000
Birmingham, AL 35216-2809   Fax: 205-978-5018
Provides accurate and up-to-date information concerning patient rights and medical care.
384 pages

5424   Designs on Life
American Society for Reproductive Medicine
1209 Montgomery Highway   205-978-5000
Birmingham, AL 35216-2809   Fax: 205-978-5018
Provides real life stories regarding assisted reproductive technology.
276 pages

5425   Family Bonds: Adoption and the Politics of Parenting
American Society for Reproductive Medicine
1209 Montgomery Highway   205-978-5000
Birmingham, AL 35216-2809   Fax: 205-978-5050
A well organized book is written for people struggling with some of the issues encountered in their journey through infertility and ultimately adoption.
1993 273 pages

5426   Fertility and Pregnancy Guide for DES Daughters and Sons
American Society for Reproductive Medicine
1209 Montgomery Highway   205-978-5000
Birmingham, AL 35216-2809   Fax: 205-978-5018
Guide offering information related to the reproductive potential of individuals who have been exposed to DES in utero.
48 pages

5427   For Want of a Child: A Psychologist and His Wife Explore Infertility
Continuum Publishing Corporation
370 Lexington Avenue   212-532-3650
New York, NY 10017-6503
A psychologist and his wife go through the emotional effects and challenges of infertility.

5428   Getting Pregnant When You Thought You Couldn't
Warner Books
1271 Avenue of the Americas
New York, NY 10020   www.twbookmark.com
A concise guide to understanding infertility that covers issues from diagnosis to treatment and is useful for couples at any stage of infertility treatment.
1993 512 pages

5429   Guide for the Childless Couple
American Society for Reproductive Medicine
1209 Montgomery Highway   205-978-5000
Birmingham, AL 35216-2809   Fax: 205-978-5018
A short text which focuses on the emotional aspects of infertility, including its effects on marriage and self-esteem.
201 pages

5430   Guide to In Vitro Fertilization & Other Assisted Reproduction Methods
Pharos Books
200 Park Avenue   212-692-3700
New York, NY 10166-0005   800-221-4816
This book discusses assisted reproductive technologies from a laboratory and a patient's perspective.

5431   Having Your Baby By Donor Insemination
Houghton Mifflin Company
222 Berkeley Street
Boston, MA 02116   617-351-5000
                                                                www.hmco.com
A resource guide to donor insemination which discusses the experience, traditions and techniques of donor insemination, sperm freezing, and known vs. anonymous donors.
352 pages

5432   Healing the Infertile Family
University of California Press

1445 Lower Ferry Road
Ewing, NJ 08618

205-978-5000
800-777-4726
Fax: 800-999-1958
e-mail: orders@cpfs.pupress.princeton.edu

This well-written book is dedicated to the psychological concerns of the infertile couple.
335 pages
ISBN: 0-520211-80-4

5433　Hormones
American Society for Reproductive Medicine
1209 Montgomery Highway
Birmingham, AL 35216-2809

205-978-5000
Fax: 205-978-5018

Highly recommended text for patients who are suffering from reproductive disorders.
216 pages

5434　How Can I Help?: A Handbook for Practical Suggestions for Infertility
American Society for Reproductive Medicine
1209 Montgomery Highway
Birmingham, AL 35216-2809

205-978-5000
Fax: 205-978-5018

Designed to provide greater understanding of the infertility experience.
18 pages

5435　How to Be a Successful Fertility Patient
American Society for Reproductive Medicine
1209 Montgomery Highway
Birmingham, AL 35216-2809

205-978-5000
Fax: 205-978-5018

Offers extensive interviews with dozens of male and female infertility patients.
1993 447 pages

5436　In Pursuit of Fertility
American Society for Reproductive Medicine
1209 Montgomery Highway
Birmingham, AL 35216-2809

205-978-5000
Fax: 205-978-5018

A comprehensive text which can be used as a tool for couples who want to achieve an understanding of their problem as well as treatment options.
348 pages

5437　In Vitro Fertilization
Facts on File
11 Penn Plaza
New York, NY 10001

212-967-8800
800-322-8755
Fax: 800-678-3633

The A.R.T. of making babies. (Assisted Reproductive Technology) A complete and caring overview of the options available to infertile couples.
208 pages Hardcover
ISBN: 0-816032-69-6

5438　Infertility Book: A Comprehensive Medical & Emotional Guide
American Society for Reproductive Medicine
1209 Montgomery Highway
Birmingham, AL 35216-2809

205-978-5000
Fax: 205-978-5018

Enables the infertile couple to learn how to take control and educate themselves about the trials and tribulations of infertility treatment.
420 pages Softcover

5439　Infertility: A Comprehensive Text
Appleton & Lange
11 W 19th Street
New York, NY 10011-4209

203-838-4400
800-423-1359

A medical reference book.

5440　Issues in Reproductive Management
Thieme Med Publishers
381 Park Avenue S
New York, NY 10016-8806

212-683-5088
Fax: 212-779-9020
1993
ISBN: 0-865775-05-2

5441　Lethal Secrets: The Psychology of Donor Insemination
Warner Books
1271 Avenue of the Americas
New York, NY 10020

www.twbookmark.com

An interview of a cross-section of people who participated in donor insemination.
1993 277 pages
ISBN: 1-567430-20-1

5442　Lifeline: The Action Guide to Adoption Search
American Society for Reproductive Medicine
1209 Montgomery Highway
Birmingham, AL 35216-2809

205-978-5000
Fax: 205-978-5018

A very interesting text describing how an adoptee or adoptive parent may track down birth parents.
384 pages

5443　Long-Awaited Stork: A Guide to Parenting After Infertility
Jossey-Bass
350 Sansome Street
San Francisco, CA 94104

415-433-1740
Fax: 415-433-0499
e-mail: webperson@jbp.com
www.josseybass.com

An excellent resource for couples who are moving from being patients to being parents.
300 pages
ISBN: 0-787940-53-4

5444　Love Cycles: The Science of Intimacy
Random House
1540 Broadway
New York, NY 10036

212-782-9000
Fax: 212-302-7985

Book providing patients with refreshing, scientific concepts of rhythms and relationships between the sexes.
330 pages

5445　Loving Journeys Guide to Adoption
American Society for Reproductive Medicine
1209 Montgomery Highway
Birmingham, AL 35216-2809

205-978-5000
Fax: 205-978-5018

Describes the basic prerequisits agencies and social workers expectations of prospective adoptive parents. Part two offers a directory of state-by-state listings of public and private adoption agencies and adoption attorneys.
394 pages

5446　Male Body
Firestone Touchstone Paperbacks/Simon & Schuster
200 Old Tappan Road
Old Tappan, NJ 07675-7005

800-999-5479

An informative and reassuring reference written to meet increasing interest in male health issues. This book discusses varied aspects of health such as infections and injuries, vasectomies, the emotional aspects of sexual difficulties and preventive measures that can be taken against AIDS and other sexually transmitted diseases.
208 pages
ISBN: 0-671864-26-2

5447　Men, Women and Infertility
American Society for Reproductive Medicine
1209 Montgomery Highway
Birmingham, AL 35216-2809

205-978-5000
Fax: 205-978-5018

A helpful book offering suggestions for a positive self-image and high self-esteem through the trauma of infertility.
1993 256 pages

5448　Miscarriage Women: Sharing from the Heart
American Society for Reproductive Medicine
1209 Montgomery Highway
Birmingham, AL 35216-2809

205-978-5000
Fax: 205-978-5018

A well organized book offering help and information to benefit patients who have experienced pregnancy loss as well as professionals working with these couples.
1993 258 pages

5449　Missed Conceptions: Overcoming Infertility
McGraw-Hill
1221 Avenue of the Americas
New York, NY 10020

212-512-2000

Book about infertility and the emotional agony that goes along with it. Addresses all aspects surrounding infertility care and of-

fers in-depth discussions of the many fertility options now available.
377 pages

5450 Motherhood: A Feminist Perspective
American Society for Reproductive Medicine
1209 Montgomery Highway   205-978-5000
Birmingham, AL 35216-2809   Fax: 205-978-5018
A compilation of papers from conference proceedings designed to define motherhood. Offers information on infertility, emotional and financial difficulties and daily living.
234 pages

5451 Mothers of Thyme: Customs and Rituals of Infertility and Miscarriage
Lida Rose Press
PO Box 5076 book that offers details on rituals and misconceptions Ann Arbor, MI 48106 tility and miscarriage.
128 pages
ISBN: 0-962595-75-6

5452 Never to Be a Mother
Harper Collins Publishers
10 E 53rd Street   212-207-7000
New York, NY 10022-5299   800-242-7737
Offers childless women a plan for confronting their grief, anger and guilt, as well as offering alternative ways to mother and live.

5453 No-Hysterectomy Option
American Society for Reproductive Medicine
1209 Montgomery Highway   205-978-5000
Birmingham, AL 35216-2809   Fax: 205-978-5018
An excellent reference for women faced with decisions regarding hysterectomy.
265 pages

5454 One Women's Passionate Quest to Complete Her Family
Viking Penguin
375 Hudson Street   212-366-2000
New York, NY 10014-3658
The author presents a highly emotional account of the years of anguish, disappointment, and finally the joy she achieved in trying to complete her family.

5455 Overcoming Infertility
Doubleday
666 5th Avenue   212-765-6500
New York, NY 10103-0001   800-223-6834
Paints a clear picture of the medical and emotional aspects of infertility.

5456 Preventing Miscarriage: The Good News
American Society for Reproductive Medicine
1209 Montgomery Highway   205-978-5000
Birmingham, AL 35216-2809   Fax: 205-978-5018
Provides information on possible causes of miscarriages with information on infections, abnormalities and more.
240 pages Softcover

5457 Reproductive Hazards in the Workplace: Mending Jobs, Managing Pregnancies
Regina H Kenen, PhD, author
Haworth Press
10 Alice Street   607-722-5857
Binghamton, NY 13904-1580   800-429-6784
                                 Fax: 607-722-0012
                                 www.haworthpress.com
Offers information on the history and present of potential reproductive hazards. Includes pregnancy hazard hotlines, specific contact points where women can get information on working environments and more.
286 pages Hardcover
ISBN: 1-560241-54-3

5458 Resolving Infertility
RESOLVE: National Infertility Association

1310 Broadway   617-623-1156
Somerville, MA 02144-1779   888-623-0744
                                 Fax: 617-623-0252
                            e-mail: info@resolve.org
                                 www.resolve.org
Understanding the options and choosing solutions when you want to have a baby is a definitive resource to help you sort out the options and negative through the experience with confidence. This book tells you everything you need to know about infertility treatment and exploring other family building options.
370 pages
ISBN: 0-062735-22-5
Bonny Gilbert, Executive Director

5459 Science and Babies: Private Decisions, Public Dilemmas
American Society for Reproductive Medicine
1209 Montgomery Highway   205-978-5000
Birmingham, AL 35216-2809   Fax: 205-978-5018
Offers a superb summary of key reproductive issues ranging from conception to contraception.
250 pages

5460 Silent Sorrow
Delta-Dell Publishers
666 5th Avenue   212-765-6500
New York, NY 10103-0001   800-223-6834
A book dealing with the emotional and psychological aspects of losing a child.

5461 Surrogate Motherhood: The Legal and Human Issues
Harvard University Press
79 Garden Street   617-495-2600
Cambridge, MA 02138-1423
A discussion of the psychological, legal and policy questions raised by surrogacy.

5462 Surviving Infertility
Tapestry Books
PO Box 359   908-806-6695
Ringoes, NJ 08551-0359   800-765-2367
                                 Fax: 732-288-2999
A valuable source of support and practical advice for coping with the many intense feelings associated with being infertile.
389 pages

5463 Surviving Pregnancy Loss: A Complete Sourcebook for Women & Their Families
American Society for Reproductive Medicine
1209 Montgomery Highway   205-978-5000
Birmingham, AL 35216-2809   Fax: 205-978-5018
Contains practical approaches to coping with the emotional and psychological problems associated with pregnancy loss.
298 pages

5464 Sweet Grapes: How to Stop Being Infertile and Living Again
American Society for Reproductive Medicine
1209 Montgomery Highway   205-978-5000
Birmingham, AL 35216-2809   Fax: 205-978-5018
Recommended for couples nearing the end of their options or for those who are unsure if they wish to pursue infertility therapy.

5465 To Love a Child
Addison Wesley Publishing
Route 128   781-944-3700
Reading, MA 01867   800-447-2226
A thoughtful and informative overview of alternatives to bio/genetic parenting.

5466 Understanding and Infertility
Tapestry Books
PO Box 359   908-806-6695
Ringoes, NJ 08551-0359   800-765-2367
                                 Fax: 732-288-2999
Provides specific advice to the family on how to be supportive of members and/or friends who suffer from infertility.
28 pages

5467 WHO Laboratory Manual
American Society for Reproductive Medicine

1209 Montgomery Highway   205-978-5000
Birmingham, AL 35216-2809   Fax: 205-978-5018
Third edition

5468   **Waiting: A Diary of Loss and Hope in Pregnancy**
American Society for Reproductive Medicine
1209 Montgomery Highway   205-978-5000
Birmingham, AL 35216-2809   Fax: 205-978-5018
Provides clear insight into coping with the trials and tribulations of infertility.
121 pages

5469   **Without Child**
American Society for Reproductive Medicine
1209 Montgomery Highway   205-978-5000
Birmingham, AL 35216-2809   Fax: 205-978-5018
Covers topics including the doctor-patient relationship, religion and infertility, living child-free and the adoption process for persons without children investigating their options.
226 pages

5470   **Women Without Children**
Pharos Books
200 Park Avenue   212-692-3700
New York, NY 10166-0005   800-221-4816
Offers women without children support through their struggle and decision making.

Children's Books

5471   **Mommy, Did I Grow in Your Tummy? Where Some Babies Come From**
American Society for Reproductive Medicine
1209 Montgomery Highway   205-978-5000
Birmingham, AL 35216-2809   Fax: 205-978-5018
Illustrated book that helps parents explain the different ways children can come into the world, including IVF, surrogacy, game donation and adoption.
28 pages Ages 4-8

Magazines

5472   **American Society for Reproductive Medicine: Clinic Specific Annual Report**
1209 Montgomery Highway   205-978-5000
Birmingham, AL 35216-2809   Fax: 205-978-5005
     e-mail: asrm@asrm.com
     www.asrm.com
Gives the success rates of treatment for fertility centers around the country.

5473   **Biology of Reproduction**
1603 Monroe Street   608-256-2777
Madison, WI 53711-2021   Fax: 608-256-4610
     e-mail: bor@ssr.org
     www.biolreprod.org
A monthly, peer-reviewed journal.
250 pages Monthly

5474   **Family Building Magazine**
RESOLVE: National Infertility Association
1310 Broadway   617-623-1156
Somerville, MA 02144-1779   888-623-0744
     Fax: 617-623-0252
     e-mail: info@resolve.org
     www.resolve.org
Offers various information on the newest technology and advances in infertility treatments, support groups, helplines, centers and in depth articles written by professionals in the field.
15-18 pages Quarterly
Bonny Gilbert, Executive Director

5475   **Infertility and Adoption**
RESOLVE: National Infertility Association

1310 Broadway   617-623-1156
Somerville, MA 02144-1779   888-623-0744
     Fax: 617-623-0252
     e-mail: info@resolve.org
     www.resolve.org
Published by RESOLVE: The National Infertility Association.
Bonny Gilbert, Executive Director

5476   **Journal of Occupational & Environmental Medicine**
Williams & Wilkins
351 W Camden Street   301-528-4000
Baltimore, MD 21201-7912   800-638-0672

Newsletters

5477   **Hers Newsletter**
Hysterectomy Educational Resources & Services
422 Bryn Mawr Avenue   610-667-7757
Bala Cynwyd, PA 19004-2708   800-777-4377
     Fax: 610-667-8096
     e-mail: hersfdn@aol.com
     www.hersfoundation.com
Offers information and support for women who have had or are going through hysterectomies.
Quarterly
Nora W Coffey, President

5478   **RESOLVE of the Bay State**
PO Box 541553   781-647-1614
Waltham, MA 02454-1553   Fax: 781-899-7207
     e-mail: admin@resolveofthebaystate.org
     www.resolveofthebaystate.org
Information on the Massachusetts chapter of a national, nonprofit, consumer based infertility support organization. Information on a variety of services to answer your questions about infertility, treatments, coping techniques, insurance issues and family building options.

Pamphlets

5479   **ART-Assisted Reproductive Technologies**
Serono Symposia USA
100 Longwater Circle
Norwell, MA 02061-1616   800-283-8088

5480   **Abnormal Uterine Bleeding**
American Society for Reproductive Medicine
1209 Montgomery Highway   205-978-5000
Birmingham, AL 35216-2809   Fax: 205-978-5018
     e-mail: asrm@asrm.com
1996

5481   **Adoption**
American Society for Reproductive Medicine
1209 Montgomery Highway   205-978-5000
Birmingham, AL 35216-2809   Fax: 205-978-5018
     e-mail: asrm@asrm.com
1990

5482   **Affording Your Infertility**
Serono Symposia USA
100 Longwater Circle
Norwell, MA 02061-1616   800-283-8088

5483   **Age and Fertility**
American Society for Reproductive Medicine
1209 Montgomery Highway   205-978-5000
Birmingham, AL 35216-2809   Fax: 205-978-5018
     e-mail: asrm@asrm.com
1996

5484   **Bibliography**
RESOLVE: National Infertility Association
1310 Broadway   617-623-1156
Somerville, MA 02144-1779   888-623-0744
     Fax: 617-623-0252
     e-mail: info@resolve.org
     www.resolve.org

Annotated guide to books and articles on medical and emotional aspects of infertility.
Bonny Gilbert, Executive Director

5485 Birth Defects of the Female Reproductive System
American Society for Reproductive Medicine
1209 Montgomery Highway
Birmingham, AL 35216-2809
205-978-5000
Fax: 205-978-5018
e-mail: asrm@asrm.com
1993

5486 Coping with the Holidays
RESOLVE
1310 Broadway
Somerville, MA 02144-1779
781-643-0744

5487 Donor Insemination
American Society for Reproductive Medicine
1209 Montgomery Highway
Birmingham, AL 35216-2809
205-978-5000
Fax: 205-978-5018
e-mail: asrm@asrm.com
1995

5488 Early Menopause (Premature Ovarian Failure)
American Society for Reproductive Medicine
1209 Montgomery Highway
Birmingham, AL 35216-2809
205-978-5000
Fax: 205-978-5018
e-mail: asrm@asrm.com
1996

5489 Ectopic Pregnancy
American Society for Reproductive Medicine
1209 Montgomery Highway
Birmingham, AL 35216-2809
205-978-5000
Fax: 205-978-5018
e-mail: asrm@asrm.com
1996

5490 Emotional Aspects of Infertility
RESOLVE: National Infertility Association
1310 Broadway
Somerville, MA 02144-1779
617-623-1156
888-623-0744
Fax: 617-623-0252
e-mail: info@resolve.org
www.resolve.org
Published by RESOLVE: The National Infertility Association.
Bonny Gilbert, Executive Director

5491 Ending Infertility Treatment
RESOLVE: National Infertility Association
1310 Broadway
Somerville, MA 02144-1779
617-623-1156
888-623-0744
Fax: 617-623-0252
e-mail: info@resolve.org
www.resolve.org
Published by RESOLVE: The National Infertility Association.
Bonny Gilbert, Executive Director

5492 Endometriosis
American Society for Reproductive Medicine
1209 Montgomery Highway
Birmingham, AL 35216-2809
205-978-5000
Fax: 205-978-5018
e-mail: asrm@asrm.com
Available in Spanish.
1994

5493 Environmental Toxins and Fertility
RESOLVE: National Infertility Association
1310 Broadway
Somerville, MA 02144-1779
617-623-1156
888-623-0744
Fax: 617-623-0252
e-mail: info@resolve.org
www.resolve.org
Published by the National Infertility Association (RESOLVE).
Bonny Gilbert, Executive Director

5494 Fertility After Cancer Treatment
American Society for Reproductive Medicine
1209 Montgomery Highway
Birmingham, AL 35216-2809
205-978-5000
Fax: 205-978-5018
e-mail: asrm@asrm.com
1995

5495 Getting Started: How Do I Know If I'm Infertile?
RESOLVE
1310 Broadway
Somerville, MA 02144-1779
781-643-0744

5496 Hirsutism and Polycystic Ovarian Syndrome
American Society for Reproductive Medicine
1209 Montgomery Highway
Birmingham, AL 35216-2809
205-978-5000
Fax: 205-978-5018
e-mail: asrm@asrm.com
1995

5497 Husband Insemination
American Society for Reproductive Medicine
1209 Montgomery Highway
Birmingham, AL 35216-2809
205-978-5000
Fax: 205-978-5018
e-mail: asrm@asrm.com
1995

5498 IVF & GIFT: A Guide to Assisted Reproductive Technologies
American Society for Reproductive Medicine
1209 Montgomery Highway
Birmingham, AL 35216-2809
205-978-5000
Fax: 205-978-5018
e-mail: asrm@asrm.com
Available in Spanish.
1995

5499 If You are Having Trouble Conceiving
American Society for Reproductive Medicine
1209 Montgomery Highway
Birmingham, AL 35216-2809
205-978-5000
Fax: 205-978-5018

5500 Infertility Insurance
Serono Symposia USA
100 Longwater Circle
Norwell, MA 02061-1616
800-283-8088

5501 Infertility: An Overview
American Society for Reproductive Medicine
1209 Montgomery Highway
Birmingham, AL 35216-2809
205-978-5000
Fax: 205-978-5018
e-mail: asrm@asrm.com
Available in Spanish.
1994

5502 Infertility: Causes and Treatment
American College/Obstetricians and Gynecologists
409 12th Street SW
Washington, DC 20024
www.acog.com
To obtain a free copy of this publication, please send a self-addressed stamped #10 envelope and request by title. (#AP002)

5503 Infertility: Coping and Decision Making
American Society for Reproductive Medicine
1209 Montgomery Highway
Birmingham, AL 35216-2809
205-978-5000
Fax: 205-978-5018
e-mail: asrm@asrm.com
1995

5504 Infertility: The Emotional Roller Coaster
Serono Symposia USA
100 Longwater Circle
Norwell, MA 02061-1616
800-283-8088

5505 Insights Into Infertility
Serono Symposia USA
100 Longwater Circle
Norwell, MA 02061-1616
800-283-8088

5506 Introduction to Infertility: The First Steps
RESOLVE: National Infertility Association
1310 Broadway
Somerville, MA 02144-1779
617-623-1156
888-623-0744
Fax: 617-623-0252
e-mail: info@resolve.org
www.resolve.org
Published by RESOLVE: The National Infertility Association.
Bonny Gilbert, Executive Director

5507 Laparoscopy and Hysteroscopy
American Society for Reproductive Medicine

1209 Montgomery Highway
Birmingham, AL 35216-2809
1995

205-978-5000
Fax: 205-978-5018
e-mail: asrm@asrm.com

5508 Male Infertility
Serono Symposia USA
100 Longwater Circle
Norwell, MA 02061-1616

800-283-8088

5509 Male Infertility and Vasectomy Reversal
American Society for Reproductive Medicine
1209 Montgomery Highway
Birmingham, AL 35216-2809
1995

205-978-5000
Fax: 205-978-5018
e-mail: asrm@asrm.com

5510 Managing Family & Friends
RESOLVE
1310 Broadway
Somerville, MA 02144-1779

781-643-0744

5511 Miscarriage
American Society for Reproductive Medicine
1209 Montgomery Highway
Birmingham, AL 35216-2809
1995

205-978-5000
Fax: 205-978-5018
e-mail: asrm@asrm.com

5512 Myths & Facts
RESOLVE
1310 Broadway
Somerville, MA 02144-1779

781-643-0744

5513 Ovulation Detection
American Society for Reproductive Medicine
1209 Montgomery Highway
Birmingham, AL 35216-2809
1995

205-978-5000
Fax: 205-978-5018
e-mail: asrm@asrm.com

5514 Ovulation Drugs
American Society for Reproductive Medicine
1209 Montgomery Highway
Birmingham, AL 35216-2809
1995

205-978-5000
Fax: 205-978-5018
e-mail: asrm@asrm.com

5515 Patient Information Series Publications
American Society for Reproductive Medicine
1209 Montgomery Highway
Birmingham, AL 35216-2809

205-978-5000
Fax: 205-978-5018
e-mail: asrm@asrm.com

Offers a set of 20 various brochures ranging from artificial insemination to male infertility problems.

5516 Pelvic Pain
American Society for Reproductive Medicine
1209 Montgomery Highway
Birmingham, AL 35216-2809
1997

205-978-5000
Fax: 205-978-5018
e-mail: asrm@asrm.com

5517 Pregnancy After Infertility
American Society for Reproductive Medicine
1209 Montgomery Highway
Birmingham, AL 35216-2809
1997

205-978-5000
Fax: 205-978-5018
e-mail: asrm@asrm.com

5518 Premenstrual Syndrome (PMS)
American Society for Reproductive Medicine
1209 Montgomery Highway
Birmingham, AL 35216-2809
1997

205-978-5000
Fax: 205-978-5018
e-mail: asrm@asrm.com

5519 Third Party Reproduction (Donor Eggs, Donor Sperm, Donor Embryos, & Surrogacy)
American Society for Reproductive Medicine

1209 Montgomery Highway
Birmingham, AL 35216-2809
1996

205-978-5000
Fax: 205-978-5018
e-mail: asrm@asrm.com

5520 Tubal Factor Infertility
American Society for Reproductive Medicine
1209 Montgomery Highway
Birmingham, AL 35216-2809
1995

205-978-5000
Fax: 205-978-5018
e-mail: asrm@asrm.com

5521 Understanding: A Guide to Impaired Fertility for Family and Friends
American Society for Reproductive Medicine
1209 Montgomery Highway
Birmingham, AL 35216-2809

205-978-5000
Fax: 205-978-5018

A pamphlet designed for families of patients with infertility and for distribution to individuals who may want to become involved in the counseling and support of these couples.
28 pages

5522 Unexplained Infertility
American Society for Reproductive Medicine
1209 Montgomery Highway
Birmingham, AL 35216-2809
1997

205-978-5000
Fax: 205-978-5018
e-mail: asrm@asrm.com

5523 Uterine Fibroids
American Society for Reproductive Medicine
1209 Montgomery Highway
Birmingham, AL 35216-2809
1997

205-978-5000
Fax: 205-978-5018
e-mail: asrm@asrm.com

Audio & Video

5524 Candid Talk About Loss in Adoption
Mary Martin Mason
4505 York Avenue S
Minneapolis, MN 55410-1422

612-922-1136

Discusses losses incurred by the adopted persons and adoptive persons issues for children adopted into different race families.
Videotape

5525 Coping with Infertility
Distributed By UC Video
425 Ontario Street SE
Minneapolis, MN 55414-3002

612-627-4444

Features five couples talking about their infertility experiences.
Odessa Flores

5526 Infertility: Exploring the Male Factor
American Society for Reproductive Medicine
1209 Montgomery Highway
Birmingham, AL 35216-2809

205-978-5000
Fax: 205-978-5018

A well-orchestrated video discussing male factor infertility, including the infertility workup, physical exam, semen analysis, and surgical options available.
1993 47 minutes

5527 One, Two, Three, Zero: Infertility
Filmmaker's Library
133 E 58th Street
New York, NY 10022-1236
Videotape

212-355-6545

5528 Six Phases of Infertility Treatment: Medical & Emotional Aspects
RESOLVE of Maryland
PO Box 19049
Baltimore, MD 21284-9049

410-243-0235

Gives an overview of infertility treatment, addressing the medical and emotional aspects.
Videotape

5529 So You're Going to Adopt
Mary Martin Mason
4505 York Avenue S
Minneapolis, MN 55410-1422

612-922-1136

This video prepares adoptive parents for pre and post adoption issues.
Videotape

Web Sites

5530 Adopt-A-Special-Kid America

www.adoptaspecialkid.org
Adopt-A-Special-Kid provides information on adoption of children with special needs.

5531 American Society for Reproductive Medicine

www.asrm.com
Devoted to advancing the knowledge, understanding and expertise in all phases of reproductive medicine and biology. Offers patient education brochures, recommended readings and support.

5532 Center for Disease Control

www.cdc.gov
Reproductive health information source. Also a resource for the Society of Reproductive Technology. Invitro fertilization data reports and men's reproductive health. Interesting well balanced site.

5533 Fertilethoughts.com

www.fertilethoughts.com
A support sytem concerned with helping reach a goal of finding the perfect doctor, the diagnosis, as well as the treatment.

5534 Healing Well

www.healingwell.com
An online health resource guide to medical news, chat, information and articles, newsgroups and message boards, books, disease-related web sites, medical directories, and more for patients, friends, and family coping with disabling diseases, disorders, or chronic illnesses.

5535 Health Finder

www.healthfinder.gov
Searchable, carefully developed web site offering information on over 1000 topics. Developed by the US Department of Health and Human Services, the site can be used in both English and Spanish.

5536 Healthlink USA

www.healthlinkusa.com
Health information concerning treatment, cures, prevention, diagnosis, risk factors, research, support groups, email lists, personal stories and much more. Updated regularly.

5537 Helios Health

www.helioshealth.com
Online resource for your health information. Detailed information about specific health topics, access to expert advice from our Medical Advisory Board, and up-to-date health news.

5538 Infertility Books

www.infertilitybooks.com
Nonprofit site includes book titles regarding infertility and a short explanation of each book and how to get it.

5539 International Council on Infertility Information Dissemination

www.inciid.org
A nonprofit organization that helps individuals and couples explore their family-building options.

5540 Internet Health Resources

www.ihr.com/infertility
This web site provides extensive information about IVF, ICSI, infertility clinics, donor egg and surrogate services, sperm banks, pharmacies, infertility books and videotapes, sperm testing, infertility newsgroups and support organizations, and drugs and medications.

5541 Ivf.com

www.ivf.com
Goal is to provide the latest women's healthcare innovations to address infertility, polycystic ovaries, endometriosis, and pelvic pain treatment.

5542 MedicineNet

www.medicinenet.com
An online resource for consumers providing easy-to-read, authoritative medical and health information.

5543 Medscape

www.medscape.com
Medscape offers specialists, primary care physicians, and other health professionals the Web's most robust and integrated medical information and educational tools.

5544 National Institutes of Health

www.medlineplus.gov
Information regarding all aspects of infertility. Some of the topics include: Latest news, overview of anatomy and physiology, clinical trails, diagnoses and symptoms, treatment, genetics, plus lots of links to other sites. Type infertility into the search engine.

5545 RESOLVE

www.resolve.org
Provides help to people who are experiencing the infertility crisis and strives to increase the visibility of infertility issues via concerted advocacy and public education.

5546 Uterine Artery Embolization

www.uterinearteryembolization.com
Provides information on Uterine Artery Embolization, or Uterine Fibroid Embolization as an alternative to hysterectomy or myomectomy as a treatment for uterine fibroids.

5547 WebMD

www.webmd.com
Information on infertility, including articles and resources.

Description

5548 ## Kidney Disease

The diseases that affect the kidney can be divided into diseases of the kidney itself, such as nephritis, polycystic kidney disease, kidney infections and stones, and diseases of other body systems that cause damage to the kidneys, such as diabetes, high blood pressure and lupus. In either instance, disruption of kidney function results in failure to remove excess fluids and wastes from the blood. This may lead to end stage kidney, or renal, failure.

Symptoms of kidney disease and their severity, depend on the underlying cause. If there is damage or disease in the urinary tract, there can be pain when urinating, blood in the urine, or changes in frequency and urgency of urination. If excess fluid cannot be removed, there may be swelling around the eyes and ankles. When the kidney is damaged directly, back or flank tenderness may be present. In many cases, kidney disease causes no symptoms until the advanced stages, although it may be detected much earlier through tests of blood or urine.

Treatment is directed to the cause, and may include antibiotics for infections, removal of kidney stones by surgery or ultrasound waves, management of the systemic disease such as diabetes, dietary modification, especially of salt and protein intake, and close monitoring and correction of fluids and electrolytes. Treatment may also include control of high blood pressure, which can be caused by kidney disease and further damage the kidney. The most severe cases of kidney failure require either dialysis, in which the blood's toxins are mechanically filtered and removed, or a kidney transplant.

National Agencies & Associations

5549 **American Association of Kidney Patients**
3505 East Frontage Road
Tampa, FL 33607-1796
813-636-8100
800-749-2257
Fax: 813-636-8122
e-mail: info@aakp.org
www.aakp.org
Serves the needs and interests of all kidney patients and their families. Founded in 1969 by kidney patients, for kidney patients, the purpose of this association is to help patients and their families cope with the emotional, physical and social impact of kidney disease.
Kim Buettner, Executive Director

5550 **American Kidney Fund**
6110 Executive Boulevard
Rockville, MD 20852
301-881-3052
800-638-8299
Fax: 301-881-0898
e-mail: helpline@kidneyfund.org
www.akfinc.org
A nonprofit national health organization providing direct financial assistance to thousands of Americans who suffer from kidney disease.
Mike Hartness, Council Chair
Robert J Burnstein, Council Treasurer

5551 **National Institute of Diabetes & Digestive & Kidney Diseases**
National Institutes of Health
31 Center Drive MSC 2560
Bethesda, MD 20892-2560
301-496-4000
e-mail: NIHInfo@OD.NIH.GOV
www.diabetes.niddk.nih.gov

Conducts and supports research on many of the most serious diseases affecting public health. The Institute supports much of the clinical research on the diseases of internal medicine and related subspecialty fields as well as many basic science disciplines.
Dr Griffin Rodgers, Acting Director

5552 **National Kidney Foundation**
30 E 33rd Street
New York, NY 10016
212-889-2210
800-622-9010
Fax: 212-689-9261
e-mail: info@kidney.org
www.kidney.org
A major voluntary health organization dedicated to preventing kidney and urinary tract diseases improving the health and well-being of individuals and families affected by these diseases and increasing the availability of all organs for transplantation.
Allan J Collins MD, Immediate Past President
Bryan N Becker, President

5553 **National Kidney and Urologic Diseases Information Clearinghouse**
31 Center Drive MSC 2560
Bethesda, MD 20892-3580
301-496-3583
800-891-5390
Fax: 301-907-8906
e-mail: nkudic@info.niddk.nih.gov
www.niddk.nih.gov
Strives to increase knowledge and understanding about diseases of the kidneys and urologic system among people with these conditions their families health care professionals and the general public.
Griffin P Rodgers, Director

State Agencies & Associations

Alabama

5554 **Alabama Chapter of the American Association of Kidney Patients**
3404 Sheffield Drive
Birmingham, AL 35223-2238
205-967-4307
Lynn Royale

5555 **National Kidney Foundation of Alabama**
4150 Carmichael Court
Montgomery, AL 36106
334-396-9870
888-533-1981
Fax: 334-396-9872
e-mail: nkfal@kidney.org
www.nkfalabama.org

Barbara A Jackson, Regional Vice President
Renae White, Division Special Events Manager

Arizona

5556 **Arizona Kidney Foundation**
4203 E Indian School Road
Phoenix, AZ 85018
602-840-1644
Fax: 602-840-2360
www.azkidney.org

Jeffrey D Neff, Chief Executive Officer
Samuel H Rogers Jr, Chairman

5557 **Central Arizona Chapter of the American Association of Kidney Patients**
4401 W Hatcher Road
Glendale, AZ 85302-3821
602-939-7248
Dale A Ester, President

Arkansas

5558 **National Kidney Foundation of Arkansas**
1818 N Taylor Street
Little Rock, AR 72207
501-664-4343
800-282-0190
Fax: 816-221-7984
e-mail: nkfar@kidney.org
www.kidney.org

Nonprofit health organization. Our mission is to prevent kidney and urinary tract disease improve the health and well being of indi-

viduals and families affected by these diseases and increase the availability of all organs for transplantation.
R D Todd Baur, Member of the Board of Directors
Derek E Bruce, Member of the Board of Directors

California

5559 Harbor-South Bay Orange County Chapter of the American Assoc. of Kidney Patients
PO Box 8
Seal Beach, CA 90740
714-527-8009
e-mail: delrita@aol.com
www.aakp.org

Rita McQuire, President

5560 Los Angeles Chapter of the American Association of Kidney Patients
9854 National Boulevard
Los Angeles, CA 90034
310-364-1807
e-mail: aakpla@yahoo.com
www.aakp.org

Robin Siegal, President

5561 National Kidney Foundation of Northern California
131 Steuart Street
San Francisco, CA 94105
415-543-3303
Fax: 415-543-3331
e-mail: info@kidneynca.org
www.kidneynca.org
Work with kidney patients both pre ESRD dialysis and transplant. Financial assistance educational workshops scholarships children's and family camps transplant games information and referral.
Brad J Price, President
Pamela Evans, Vice President

5562 National Kidney Foundation of Southern California
15490 Ventura Boulevard
Sherman Oaks, CA 91403
818-783-8153
800-747-5527
Fax: 818-783-8160
e-mail: info@kidneysocal.org
www.kidneysocal.org

Linda D Small, Division President
Connie M Nieri, Division Director of Finance/Operations

5563 Redding Chapter of the American Association of Kidney Patients
790 Pioneer Drive
Redding, CA 96001-0258
530-241-6451
e-mail: teamward@c-zone.net
www.aakp.org

5564 Sacramento Valley Chapter of the American Association of Kidney Patients
565 Morrison Avenue
Sacramento, CA 95838
916-924-1996
Patricia Jones

Colorado

5565 Colorado Chapter of the American Association of Kidney Patients
PO Box 8442
Denver, CO 80201
303-758-8610
Lew Gaiter

5566 National Kidney Foundation of Colorado: Idaho, Montana, and Wyoming
30 East 33rd Street
New York, NY 10016
720-748-9991
800-263-4005
Fax: 720-748-1273
www.kidney.org

5567 Western Slope Chapter of the American Association of Kidney Patients
1539 Ptarmigan Ridge
Grand Junction, CO 81056
970-244-9196
Vicki Ladd

Connecticut

5568 National Kidney Foundation of Connecticut
2139 Silas Deane Highway
Rocky Hill, CT 06067
860-257-3770
800-441-1280
Fax: 860-257-3429
e-mail: info@kidneyct.org
www.kidneyct.org

Kimberly Hathaway, CEO
Donna Sciacca, Director of Patient Programs/Services

District of Columbia

5569 Georgetown University Center for Hypertension and Renal Disease Research
3800 Reservoir Road NW
Washington, DC 20007
202-687-9183
Fax: 202-687-7893
e-mail: wilcoxch@qunet.georgetown.edu
www.georgetown.edu/research/hrdrc
International institute for basic and clinical investigation education and clinical practice in hypertension and renal disease.
Christopher MD PhD, Chief

5570 National Kidney Foundation of the National Capital Area
5335 Wisconsin Avenue NW
Washington, DC 20015-2030
202-244-7900
Fax: 202-244-7405
e-mail: info@kidneywdc.org
www.kidneywdc.org

Preston A Englert, Jr. CAE, President/CEO

5571 National Kidney Foundation of the Texas
5335 Wisconsin Avenue NW
Washington, DC 20015
202-244-7900
Fax: 202-244-7405
e-mail: ncdc@kidney.org
www.kidneywdc.org

Preston A Englert, Division President/Government Relations
Lisa Taylor, Division Development Director

Florida

5572 National Kidney Foundation of Florida
1040 Woodcock Road
Orlando, FL 32803
407-894-7325
800-927-9659
Fax: 407-895-0051
e-mail: nkf@kidneyfla.org
www.kidneyfla.org

Stephanie Hutchinson, CEO
Richard Salick, Community Relations Director

5573 Palm Beach Chapter of the American Association of Kidney Patients
6801 Lake Worth Road
Lake Worth, FL 33467
561-434-4559
e-mail: jansym@bellsouth.net
www.aakp.org

Jan Symonette, President

5574 South Florida Chapter of the American Association of Kidney Patients
2375 NE 173rd Street
N Miami Beach, FL 33160
305-324-1727
e-mail: diazgray@aol.com
www.aakp.org

Robert Kirby, President

5575 Sunshine Chapter of the American Association of Kidney Patients
PO Box 4716
Hialeah, FL 33014-0716
305-821-4827
Elaine Kamsler

Georgia

5576 Atlanta Georgia Chapter of the American Association of Kidney Patients
6409 Lakeview Drive
Buford, GA 30518
404-932-1100
Pamela Printup

5577 National Kidney Foundation of Georgia
2951 Flowers Road S
Atlanta, GA 30341

770-452-1539
800-633-2339
Fax: 770-452-7564
e-mail: nkfga@kidney.org
www.kidneyga.org

Barbara Sachs, Division President
Tracy Jenny, Division Program Director

5578 Rome Georgia Chapter of the American Association of Kidney Patients
118 Woodcrest Drive
Rome, GA 30161

706-232-8989

Hazel McDowell, President

Hawaii

5579 National Kidney Foundation of Hawaii
1314 S King Street
Honolulu, HI 96814

808-593-1515
800-488-2277
Fax: 808-589-5993
e-mail: Glen@kidneyhi.org
www.kidneyhi.org

Hawaii's leading voluntary health agency to the education prevention and treatment of kidney and urinary tract diseases and increase the availability of all organs for transplantation in Hawaii.
Glen Hayashida, Chief Executive Officer
Diana Pinard, Director of Organization Planning

Idaho

5580 National Kidney Foundation of Colorado, Idaho, Montana, and Wyoming
3545 South Tamarac Drive
Denver, CO 80237

303-713-1523
800-263-4005
Fax: 303-713-0989
www.kidney.org

ML Hanson, CEO

Illinois

5581 Chicagoland Chapter of the American Association of Kidney Patients
70 Lincoln Oaks Drive
Chicago, IL 60514

708-325-3475

Gloria Combs, President

5582 National Kidney Foundation of Illinois
215 W Illinois
Chicago, IL 60610

312-321-1500
Fax: 312-321-1505
e-mail: kidney@nkfi.org
www.nkfi.org

Willa Iglitz Lang, Chief Executive Officer
Kate Grubbs O'Connor, Chief Operating Officer

Indiana

5583 National Kidney Foundation of Indiana
911 E 86th Street
Indianapolis, IN 46240-1840

317-722-5640
800-382-9971
Fax: 317-722-5650
e-mail: nkfi@kidneyindiana.org
www.kidneyindiana.org

The mission of the NKFI is to prevent kidney and urinary tract disease improve the health and well-being of individuals and family affected by these disease and increase the availability of all organs for transplantation.
Margie Fort, CEO
Marilyn Winn, Programs Director

Iowa

5584 Mississippi Valley, Iowa Chapter of the Association of Kidney Patients
2203 75th Place
Davenport, IA 52806-1107

319-391-1194

Dave King

5585 National Kidney Foundation of Iowa NKFI Mercy Medical Center
NKFI Mercy Medical Center
PO Box 1364
Cedar Rapids, IA 52406-1364

319-369-4474
800-369-3619
Fax: 800-724-8314
e-mail: info@kidneyia.org
www.kidneyia.org

Diane Hagarty, Executive Director
Lori Donald, Accounting Coordinator

Kansas

5586 National Kidney Foundation of Kansas and Western Missouri
6405 Metcalf Avenue
Overland Park, KS 66202

913-262-1551
800-444-8113
Fax: 913-722-4841
e-mail: nkfkswmo@kidney.org
www.kidneyksmo.org

Randy K Williams, Regional Vice President
Holly Hagman, Division Program Manager

Kentucky

5587 National Kidney Foundation of Kentucky
250 E Liberty Street
Louisville, KY 40202

502-585-5433
800-737-5433
Fax: 502-585-1445
e-mail: lallgood@nkfk.org
www.nkfk.org

Lisa Allgood, Program Director
Leann Wiley, Bookkeeper/Office Manager

Louisiana

5588 Bayou Area Chapter of the American Association of Kidney Patients
PO Box 400
Lockport, LA 70374

504-532-3542

Louisiana Barrios

5589 National Kidney Foundation of Louisiana
8200 Hampson Street
New Orleans, LA 70118

504-861-4500
800-462-3694
Fax: 504-861-1976
e-mail: info@kidneyla.org
www.kidneyla.org

Torie Kranze, Chief Executive Officer
Tracey Eldridge, Director of Special Events

Maine

5590 National Kidney Foundation of Maine
470 Forest Avenue
Portland, ME 04101

207-772-7270
800-639-7220
Fax: 207-772-4202
e-mail: nkfme@kidney.org
www.kidneyme.org

Tammy Atwood, Regional Vice President
Jaime Hanks, Regional Programs Assistant

Maryland

5591 National Kidney Foundation of Maryland
1107 Kenilworth Drive
Baltimore, MD 21204-2136

410-494-8545
800-671-5369
Fax: 410-494-8549
e-mail: rmcguire@kidneymd.org
www.kidneymd.org

Also covers the Harrisburg area of Pennsylvania and portions of Virginia and West Virginia.
Raquel McGuire, Executive Director
Brenda Falcone, Director of Community/Patient Services

Massachusetts

5592 National Kidney Foundation of MA/RI/NH/VT
11 Vanderbilt Avenue
Norwood, MA 02062
781-278-0222
800-542-4001
Fax: 781-278-0333
e-mail: asavisky@kidneyhealth.org
www.kidneyhealth.org
Andrea Savisky RN CNN, Director Patient Services

Michigan

5593 National Kidney Foundation of Michigan
1169 Oak Valley Drive
Ann Arbor, MI 48108
734-222-9800
800-482-1455
Fax: 734-222-9801
e-mail: info@nkfm.org
www.nkfm.org
Dan Carney, President and Chief Executive Officer
Maurie Ferriter, Director of Programs and Services

Minnesota

5594 National Kidney Foundation of Minnesota
1970 Oakcrest Avenue
Saint Paul, MN 55113
651-636-7300
800-596-7943
Fax: 651-636-9700
e-mail: nkfmndk@kidney.org
www.nkfmn.org
Also covers North Dakota and South Dakota.
Jill Evenocheck, Division President
Julie Iverson, Regional Vice President

Mississippi

5595 National Kidney Foundation of Mississippi
3000 Old Canton Road
Jackson, MS 39216
601-981-3611
800-232-1592
Fax: 601-981-3612
www.kidneyms.org
Gail G Sweat, Executive Director
Lynda Richards, Director of Patient Services

Missouri

5596 National Kidney Foundation of Eastern Missouri and Metro East
10803 Olive Boulevard
Saint Louis, MO 63141
314-961-2828
800-489-9585
Fax: 314-961-0888
e-mail: nkfemo@kidney.org
www.kidneyemo.org
Steve Engel, Division President
Anne Carpenter, Director of Program Services

Montana

5597 National Kidney Foundation of Colorado/Idaho/Montana/Wyoming
3151 South Vaughn Way
Aurora, CO 80014
720-748-9991
800-263-4005
Fax: 720-748-1273
www.kidneycimw.org

5598 National Kidney Foundation of Colorado,
3151 S Vaughn Way
Aurora, CO 80014
720-748-9991
Fax: 720-748-1273
e-mail: jnorman@kidneycimw.org
www.kidneycimw.org
Judy Norman, Executive Director
Tracey Nilson, Director of Development

Nebraska

5599 Nebraska Kidney Association
11725 Arbor Street
Omaha, NE 68144-2116
402-932-7200
800-642-1255
Fax: 402-933-0087
e-mail: nkfnoffice@kidneyne.org
www.kidneyne.org

Improve the lives of all Nebraskans through advocacy, education, early disease detection and patient services.
Tim Neal, Chief Executive Officer
Sherri Petersen, Development Director

Nevada

5600 National Kidney Foundation of Nevada
2550 E Desert Inn Road
Las Vegas, NV 89121-3611
702-735-9222
800-282-0190
Fax: 816-221-7984
e-mail: info@nkfnv.org
www.kidney.org

New Hampshire

5601 National Kidney Foundation of MA/RI/NH/VT
11 Vanderbilt Avenue
Norwood, MA 02062
781-278-0222
800-542-4001
Fax: 781-278-0333
e-mail: asavisky@kidneyhealth.org
www.kidneyhealth.org
Andrea Savisky RN CNN, Director Patient Services

New Jersey

5602 Garrett Mountain Chapter of the American Association of Kidney Patients
PO Box 8496
Haledon, NJ 07538
973-523-3959

5603 Meadowlands Chapter of the American Association of Kidney Patients
PO Box 3032
Clifton, NJ 07012-3032
201-471-5674
Howard Hurwitz, President

5604 Northern New Jersey Chapter of the American Association of Kidney Patients
1095 Stone Street
Rahway, NJ 07065-1913
732-382-1092

New Mexico

5605 National Kidney Foundation of New Mexico
3167 San Mateo Boulevard NE
Albuquerque, NM 87110
505-830-3542
800-282-0190
Fax: 816-221-7984
e-mail: nkfnm@kidney.org
www.kidney.org
Connie Burnett

New York

5606 Kidney & Urology Foundation of America
152 Madison Avenue
New York, NY 10016
212-629-9770
800-633-6628
Fax: 212-629-5652
e-mail: info@kidneyurology.org
www.kidneyurology.org
Sam Giarrusso, President
Shirley Baer, Executive Director

5607 Long Island Chapter of the American Association of Kidney Patients
2 Maplewood Avenue
Farmingdale, NY 11735
516-756-9126
Margie Ng Gencarelli, President

5608 National Kidney Foundation of Central New York
731 James Street
Syracuse, NY 13203
315-476-0311
877-8KI-DNEY
Fax: 315-476-3707
e-mail: info@cnykidney.org
www.cnykidney.org
Marion E Makhuli, Chief Executive Officer
Laura Squadrito, Director of Programs and Services

5609 National Kidney Foundation of Northeast New York
99 Troy Road   518-458-9697
E Greenbush, NY 12061   800-999-9697
                                                   Fax: 518-458-9690
                                            e-mail: info@nkfneny.org
                                                     www.nkfneny.org

Carol LaFleur, Executive Director
Alicia Jacobs, Director of Special Events

5610 National Kidney Foundation of Upstate New York
15 Prince Street   585-697-0874
Rochester, NY 14607   800-724-9421
                                                   Fax: 585-697-0895
                                           e-mail: infoupny@kidney.org
                                                    www.kidneynyup.org

Jan Miller MS Ed CFRE, Executive Director
Mary Jones, Division Development Director

5611 National Kidney Foundation of Western New York
3871 Harlem Road   716-835-1323
Buffalo, NY 14215   Fax: 716-835-2281
                                        e-mail: nkfofwny@hotmail.com
                                                       www.nkfwny.org

Nonprofit health organization.
Victoria Keidel, CEO
E Timothy Danahy III, Board President

**5612 New York Chapter of the American Association of Kidney
Patients**
450 Clarkson Avenue   718-270-1548
Brooklyn, NY 11203   e-mail: linda.cohen@downstate.edu
                                                          www.aakp.org

Linda Cohen, President

North Carolina

5613 National Kidney Foundation of North Carolina
5950 Fairview Road   704-552-1351
Charlotte, NC 28210   800-356-5362
                                                   Fax: 704-552-7870
                                                        www.nkfnc.org
Kenya Welch, Kidney Early Evaluation Program Contact

5614 National Kidney Foundation of North Texas
5950 Fairview Road   704-552-1351
Charlotte, NC 28210   Fax: 704-552-7870
                                             e-mail: info@nkfnc.org
                                                        www.nkfnc.org
Kenya Welch, Kidney Early Evaluation Program Contact

Ohio

**5615 Miami Valley Ohio Chapter of the American Association of
Kidney Patients**
4511 W State Route   513-698-5847
W Milton, OH 45383
Bob Felter, President

5616 National Kidney Foundation of Ohio
1373 Grandview Avenue   614-481-4030
Columbus, OH 43212-2804   800-242-2133
                                                   Fax: 614-481-4038
                                           e-mail: patti.gold@kidney.org
                                                     www.nkfofohio.org

Patti V B Gold, Division President
Danielle Estep, Division Program Director

Oklahoma

5617 American Association of Kidney Patients
911 N Woodland Drive   918-241-3969
Sand Springs, OK 74063   800-749-2257
                                       e-mail: jasonmikles@hotmail.com

Jason Mikles, President

5618 American Association of Kidney Patients: Tulsa Chapter
911 North Woodland Drive   918-241-3969
Sand Springs, OK 74063   800-749-2257
                                       e-mail: jasonmikles@hotmail.com

Jason Mikles, President

5619 National Kidney Foundation of Oklahoma
10600 S Pennsylvania Avenue   816-221-9559
Oklahoma City, OK 73170   800-282-0190
                                                   Fax: 816-221-7984
                                            e-mail: nkfok@kidney.org
                                                     www.kidneyok.org

Jeff Tallent, CEO

Oregon

5620 National Kidney Foundation of Oregon and Washington
465 NE 181st Avenue   503-963-5364
Portland, OR 97230   888-354-3639
                                                   Fax: 503-238-1754
                                           e-mail: nkforwa@kidney.org
                                                            www.kidney.org

Prevention treatment and cures for kidney diseases! Provides public education health screenings research funding and dialysis and
transplant patient services. Increases awareness for organ donation.
Susan Baumgardner, CEO
Glenda McClure, Operations Manager

Pennsylvania

**5621 Lehigh Valley Chapter of the American Association of Kidney
Patients**
1242 N 19th Street   610-776-1091
Allentown, PA 18104-3058   e-mail: info@aakp.org
                                                          www.aakp.org

Jill Davis, President

5622 National Kidney Foundation of Delaware Valley
111 S Independence Mall E   215-923-8611
Philadelphia, PA 19106   800-697-7007
                                                   Fax: 215-923-2199
                                             e-mail: nkfdv@kidney.org
                                                          www.nkfdv.org

Also covers Delaware and Southern New Jersey.
Joanne Spink, Division President
Mary Reilly, Development Director

5623 National Kidney Foundation of Western Pennsylvania
700 5th Avenue   412-261-4115
Pittsburgh, PA 15219   800-261-4115
                                                   Fax: 412-261-1405
                                            e-mail: nkfalg@kidney.org
                                                       www.kidneyall.org

Also covers Northern West Virginia.
Mary Grace Diana, Regional Program Director
Deborah A Hartman CFRE, Regional Vice President

Rhode Island

5624 National Kidney Foundation of MA/RI/NH/VT
85 Astor Avenue   781-278-0222
Norwood, MA 02062   800-542-4001
                                                   Fax: 781-278-0333
                                         e-mail: nkfmarinhvt@kidney.org
                                                     www.kidneyhealth.org

Andrea Savis RN CNN, Division Program Director
Linda Plazonja, Division President

South Carolina

5625 National Kidney Foundation of South Carolina
500 Taylor Street   803-798-3870
Columbia, SC 29201   800-488-2277
                                           e-mail: info@kidney-sc.org
                                                       www.kidney-sc.org

Beth Irick, CEO
Sheilah Derrick, Office Manager

South Dakota

5626 National Kidney Foundation of South Dakota
1000 East 21st Street   605-322-7025
Sioux Falls, SD 57105   Fax: 605-322-7029
Kori Baade, Executive Director

5627 National Kidney Foundation of Southeast
2601 S Minnesota Avenue   605-321-1668
Sioux Falls, SD 57105   Fax: 651-636-9700
                              e-mail: nkfmndk@kidney.org
                                        www.nkfdak.org

Jill Evenocheck, Division President
Julie Iverson, Regional Vice President

Tennessee

5628 National Kidney Foundation of East Tennessee
4450 Walker Boulevard   865-688-5481
Knoxville, TN 37917-1523   Fax: 865-688-5495
                              e-mail: nkfetn@kidney.org
                                        www.kidneyetn.org

The National Kidney Foundation of East Tennessee works to prevent kidney and urinary tract diseases improve the health and well-being of individuals and family members affected by these diseases and increase the availability of all organs for transplantation.
Helen Harb, President
Judy Roitman, Senior Program Manager

5629 National Kidney Foundation of West Tennessee
849 Mount Moriah Road   901-683-6185
Memphis, TN 38117   800-273-3869
                                            Fax: 901-683-6189
                              e-mail: nkf@bellsouth.net
                                        www.kidney.org

5630 National Kidney Foundation of West Texas
857 Mount Moriah Road   901-683-6185
Memphis, TN 38117   Fax: 901-683-6189
                              e-mail: info@nkfwtn.org
                                        www.nkfwtn.org

5631 Tennessee Kidney Foundation
2120 Crestmoor Road   615-383-3887
Nashville, TN 37215-2613   800-380-3887
                                            Fax: 615-383-2647
                       e-mail: info@tennesseekidneyfoundation.org
                             www.tennesseekidneyfoundation.org
Teresa Davidson, Executive Director

Texas

5632 American Association of Kidney Patients
PO Box 1012   903-537-7031
Mount Vernon, TX 75457   800-749-2257
                              e-mail: edwinhargraves@webtv.net
                                        www.aakp.org

Edwin Hargraves, President

5633 American Association of Kidney Patients: Piney Woods Chapter
PO Box 1012   903-537-7031
Mount Vernon, TX 75457   800-749-2257
                              e-mail: edwinhargraves@webtv.net
Edwin Hargraves, President

5634 Lone Star Chapter of the American Association of Kidney Patients
10042 Sugarloaf Drive
San Antonio, TX 78245
                                            210-523-1605
                                            www.aakp.org

Robert Wager, President

5635 National Kidney Foundation of North Texas
5429 Lyndon B Johnson Freeway   214-351-2393
Dallas, TX 75240   877-543-6397
                                            Fax: 214-351-3797
                              e-mail: nkfntx@kidney.org
                                        www.nkft.org

Public and professional education about kidney and urinary tract diseases. Peer mentoring medical emergency identification jewelry kidney early evaluation program Camp Reynal transplant games.
Mary Van Eaton, CEO
Cameron Hernholm, Director of Development

5636 National Kidney Foundation of South Texas
1919 Oakwell Farms Parkway   210-829-1299
San Antonio, TX 78218-1777   888-829-1299
                                            Fax: 210-829-1248
                              e-mail: nkfsctx@kidney.org
                                        www.kidneytx.org

5637 National Kidney Foundation of Southeast Texas
2400 Augusta Drive   713-952-5499
Houston, TX 77057   800-961-5683
                                            Fax: 713-952-5497
                       e-mail: customerservice@nkfset.org
                                        www.nkfset.org
Provides services for people who suffer with kidney and urinary tract diseases.

5638 National Kidney Foundation of West Texas
4601 50th Street   806-799-7753
Lubbock, TX 79414   Fax: 806-799-0277
                              e-mail: nkfwtx@kidney.org
                                        www.nkfwt.org

Amy Garms, Regional Vice President
Jennifer Ray, Regional Administrative Assistant

5639 National Kidney Foundation of the Texas Coastal Bend
PO Box 9172   361-884-5892
Corpus Christi, TX 78469   Fax: 361-884-2332
                 e-mail: info@coastalbendkidneyfoundation.org
                       www.coastalbendkidneyfoundation.org

Bess Stone, President
William Alle MD, Vice President

Utah

5640 National Kidney Foundation of Utah
3707 N Canyon Road   801-226-5111
Provo, UT 84604-4585   800-869-5277
                                            Fax: 801-226-8278
                              e-mail: NKFU@KidneyUT.org
                                        www.kidneyut.org

Serving kidney dialysis and transplant patients through out Utah providing patient service and support programs medical research and public and patient education regarding kidney disease and its treatment and prevention and the promotion of organ donations.
David C Trimble, President
Dean Vetterli, CEO

Vermont

5641 National Kidney Foundation of MA/RI/NH/VT
85 Astor Avenue   781-278-0222
Norwood, MA 02062   800-542-4001
                                            Fax: 781-278-0333
                              e-mail: nkfmarinhvt@kidney.org
                                        www.kidneyhealth.org

Andrea Savis RN CNN, Division Program Director
Linda Plazonja, Division President

Virginia

5642 National Kidney Foundation of Virginia
1742 E Parham Road   804-288-8342
Richmond, VA 23228   800-543-6398
                                            Fax: 804-282-7835
                              e-mail: welcome@kidneyva.org
                                        www.kidneyva.org

An affiliate of the National Kidney Foundation it serves kidney patients and their families in Virginia and portions of West Virginia. Mission includes professional and public education prevention and working to increase the availability of all organs for donation.
Lou Markwith, CEO
Betty Sloan, Executive Assistant

Washington

5643 **National Kidney Foundation of Oregon and Washington**
2142 NW Overton
Portland, OR 97210
503-963-5364
Fax: 503-238-1754
e-mail: help@kidneyorwa.org
www.kidneyorwa.org+R16

Susan Baumgardner, CEO
Glenda McClure, Operations Manager

Wisconsin

5644 **National Kidney Foundation of Wisconsin**
16655 W Bluemound Road
Brookfield, WI 53005-5935
262-821-0705
800-543-6393
Fax: 262-821-5641
e-mail: nkfw@kidneywi.org
www.kidneywi.org
Offers prevention detection and education programs for those at risk for kidney disease. The National Kidney Foundation of Wisconsin is making life's better through its programs and services. Brochures are offered at no charge.
Cindy Huberÿ, Chief Executive Officer
Kimberly Mueller, Director of Special Events

Wyoming

5645 **National Kidney Foundation of Colorado/Idaho/Montana/Wyoming**
3151 South Vaughn Way
Aurora, CO 80014
720-748-9991
800-263-4005
Fax: 720-748-1273
www.kidneycimw.org

5646 **National Kidney Foundation of Colorado,**
3151 S Vaughn Way
Aurora, CO 80014
720-748-9991
Fax: 720-748-1273
e-mail: jnorman@kidneycimw.org
www.kidneycimw.org

Judy Norman, Executive Director
Tracey Nilson, Director of Development

Research Centers

5647 **Associates in Nephrology**
210 S Desplaines Street
Chicago, IL 60611
312-654-2720
Fax: 312-654-0118
e-mail: charlotte.chapple@ainmd.com
www.associatesinnephrology.com
A medical group practicing nephrology in the Chicago metropolitan area and it suburbs. Includes 21 nephrologists with expertise in many areas in the field of nephrology including hypertension chronic and acute renal failure hemodialysis and peritoneal dialysis glomerulonephritis acid base disturbances fluid and electrolytes management. Provides personal high quality care to patients with kidney diseases.
Eduardo Cremer, Physician
Paul Crawford, Physician

5648 **Kantor Nephrology Consultants**
1750 E Desert Inn Road
Las Vegas, NV 89169
702-732-2438
Fax: 702-737-5043
www.kncvegas.com
Specializes in nephrology hypertension evaluation and treatment osteoporosis evaluation and treatment chronic in-center hemodialysis home dialysis programs transplantation nephrology nutritional support and more.
Gary L Kantor MD, Founder

5649 **Kidney Disease Institute Wadsworth Center for Laboratories and Re**
Wadsworth Center for Laboratories and Research
Empire State Plaza
Albany, NY 12201
518-474-7354
Fax: 518-737-71
www.nyhealth.gov
An information and referral organization for polycystic kidney disease autoimmune kidney disease and transplantation.
Lorraine Fla MD, Director

5650 **Kidney Disease Program of the University of Louisville**
615 S Preston Street
Louisville, KY 40202-0001
502-852-7350
Fax: 502-852-7643
e-mail: cbrown@kdp.louisville.edu
kdpnet.kdp.louisville.edu
Educates residents and patients regarding kidney diseases and offers a dialysis clinic for people afflicted with kidney disease.
George R Aronoff MD, Chief
Cynthia Brown, Program Coordinator

5651 **Lovelace Medical Foundation**
2425 Ridgecrest Drive SE
Albuquerque, NM 87108-5127
505-348-9400
Fax: 505-348-8541
e-mail: info@lrri.org
www.lrri.org

David J Ottensmeyer, President

5652 **PKD Foundation Polycystic Kidney Disease Foundation**
Polycystic Kidney Disease Foundation
9221 Ward Parkway
Kansas City, MO 64114-3367
816-931-2600
800-PKD-CURE
Fax: 816-931-8655
e-mail: pkdcure@pkdcure.org
www.pkdcure.org
The foundation exists to win the war with PKD. Their mission is to promote research into the treatment and cure of polycystic kidney disease by raising financial support for peer approved biomedical research projects and fostering public awareness among medical professionals patients and the general public.
Dave Switzer, National Director, Educational Programs

5653 **University of Kansas Kidney and Urology Research Center**
3901 Rainbow Boulevard
Kansas City, KS 66160
913-588-5000
Fax: 913-588-3995
TTY: 913-588-7963
www.kumc.edu

Jared J Grantham, Director
Tomas L Griebling, Vice Chair

5654 **University of Michigan Nephrology Division**
University of Michigan Health System
1500 E Medical Center Drive
Ann Arbor, MI 48109
734-936-5645
Fax: 734-763-4151
www.med.umich.edu/intmed/nephrology
Focuses on kidney research.
Frank Brosius, Chief
Joseph Messana, Professor/ Service Chief

5655 **University of Rochester: Nephrology Research Program**
601 Elmwood Avenue
Rochester, NY 14642-0001
585-275-3660
Fax: 716-442-9201
www.urmc.rochester.edu

Focuses on kidney disorders.
Rebeca Monk, Fellowship Director
Marilyn C Miran, Fellowship Coordinator

5656 **Warren Grant Magnuson Clinical Center**
National Institute of Health
9000 Rockville Pike
Bethesda, MD 20892
800-411-1222
Fax: 301-480-9793
TTY: 866-411-1010
e-mail: prpl@mail.cc.nih.gov
www.clinicalcenter.nih.gov
Established in 1953 as the research hospital of the National Institutes of Health. Designed so that patient care facilities are close to research laboratories so new findings of basic and clinical scientists can be quickly applied to the treatment of patients. Upon referral by physicians, patients are admitted to NIH clinical studies.
John Gallin, Director
David Henderson, Deputy Director for Clinical Care

5657 **Washington University Chromalloy American Kidney Center**
One Barnes-Jewish Hospital Plaza
Saint Louis, MO 63110-1036
314-362-7209
Fax: 314-747-3743
renal.wustl.edu

Offers a dialysis unit for people afflicted with kidney disease.
Dr Eduardo Slatopolsky, Director

Support Groups & Hotlines

5658 Kidneeds
Greater Cedar Rapids Community Foundation
200 First Street Southwest   319-366-2862
Cedar Rapids, IA 52404
                                    Fax: 319-386-0431
                    e-mail: kidneedsmpgn@yahoo.com
                    www.medicine.uiowa.edu/kidneeds/
Primary mission of kidneeds is to fund research on
membranoproliferative giomerulonephritis type 2 (MPON type 2,
aka, dense deposit disease). Phone support and annual newsletter
availiable. No computerized version availiable. No mailing list
availble.
Lynne Lanning RN/JD, President Board of Directors
Sean Tully, Vice President Board of Directors

5659 National Health Information Center
PO Box 1133   310-565-4167
Washington, DC 20013   800-336-4797
                                    Fax: 301-984-4256
                            e-mail: info@nhic.org
                            www.health.gov/nhic
Offers a nationwide information referral service, produces directo-
ries and resource guides.

Books

5660 Family and ADPKD: A Guide for Children and Parents
Polycystic Kidney Disease Foundation
9221 Ward Parkway   816-931-2600
Kansas City, MO 64114   800-753-2873
                                    Fax: 816-931-8655
                        e-mail: pkdcure@pkdcure.org
                        www.pkdcure.org
This book focuses on the questions most commonly asked by chil-
dren and parents about ADPKD. It is divided into two sections: one
for children and one for parents.
48 pages
ISBN: 0-961456-75-2
Dave Switzer, National Director, Educational Programs

**5661 Kidney Beginnings: A Patient's Guide to Li ving with Reduced
Kidney Function**
American Association of Kidney Patients
3505 E Frantage Road   813-636-8100
Tampa, FL 33607   800-749-2257
                                    Fax: 813-636-8122
                            e-mail: info@aakp.org
                            www.aakp.org
Provides patients with the information they need to take control of
their healthcare and do what is necessary to preserve and protect
their kidney function. The book addresses concerns of those at risk
for kidney disease and their family members; featuring information about the workings of the kidneys, common medications,
hypertention, testing, and answers to health, diet and lifestyle
questions.
62 pages
Kim Buettner, Executive Director

5662 Kidney Cooking
National Kidney Foundation of Georgia
1639 Tullie Circle NE   404-248-1315
Atlanta, GA 30329-2304
A unique cookbook with over one hundred recipes that have been
analyzed for sodium, potassium and protein content.

5663 Nutrition & the Kidney
Little Brown & Company
34 Beacon Street   617-227-0730
Boston, MA 02108-1415   Fax: 617-227-4633
1993 480 pages
ISBN: 0-316575-00-3

5664 PKD Patient's Manual
Polycystic Kidney Disease Foundation

9221 Ward Parkway   816-931-2600
Kansas City, MO 64114   800-753-2873
                                    Fax: 816-931-8655
                        e-mail: pkdcure@pkdcure.org
                        www.pkdcure.org
Covers everything from cysts to how persons can be active if they
have ARPKD.
Dave Switzer, National Director, Educational Programs

5665 Q&A on PKD
Polycystic Kidney Disease Foundation
9221 Ward Parkway   816-931-2600
Kansas City, MO 64114   800-753-2873
                                    Fax: 816-931-8655
                        e-mail: pkdcure@pkdcure.org
                        www.pkdcure.org
A goldmine of information for the PKD patient and physician. In-
cludes 88 pages of PKD questions and answers by the scientific ad-
visers of the PKR Foundation.
88 pages Paperback
ISBN: 0-961456-72-8
Dave Switzer, National Director, Educational Programs

5666 Real Lifestyles Manual
R&D Laboratories
4204 Glencoe Avenue
Marina Del Rey, CA 90292-5612   800-338-9066
A complete renal guide including diets for hemodialysis and
CAPD patients. Delicious menus, ADA exchange lists, gourmet
recipes with nutritional analysis for renal patients and exercises.

5667 Your Child, Your Family & ARPKD
Polycystic Kidney Disease Foundation
9221 Ward Parkway   816-931-2600
Kansas City, MO 64114   800-753-2873
                                    Fax: 816-931-8655
                        e-mail: pkdcure@pkdcure.org
                        www.pkdcure.org
This second edition book focuses on the questions most commonly
asked about ARPKD in order to help families understand more
about the disease.
Dave Switzer, National Director, Educational Programs

**5668 Your Child, Your Family and Autosomal Recessive Polycystic
Kidney Disease**
Polycystic Kidney Disease Foundation
9221 Ward Parkway   816-931-2600
Kansas City, MO 64114   800-753-2873
                                    Fax: 816-931-8655
                        e-mail: pkdcure@pkdcure.org
                        www.pkdcure.org
This secong edition book focuses on the questions most commonly
asked about autosomal recessive PKD in order to help families un-
derstand more about the disease.
26 pages Paperback
Dave Switzer, National Director, Educational Programs

Magazines

5669 Kindey Beginnings: The Magazine
American Association of Kidney Patients
3505 E Frantage Road   813-636-8100
Tampa, FL 33607   800-749-2257
                                    Fax: 813-636-8122
                            e-mail: info@aakp.org
                            www.aakp.org
This quarterly member magazine provides articles, news items and
information of interest to those at risk or recently diagnosed with
kidney disease, their famliy, and healthcare professionals.
Kmi Buettner, Executive Director

5670 aakpRENALIFE
American Association of Kidney Patients
35052 E Frantage Road   813-636-8100
Tampa, FL 33607   800-749-2257
                                    Fax: 813-636-8122
                            e-mail: info@aakp.org
                            www.aakp.org

The official publication for AAKP members, offering articles, news and health care information for kidney patients,and health care professionals.
BiMonthly
Kim Buettner, Executive Director

Newsletters

5671 Family Focus
National Kidney Foundation
30 E 33rd Street   212-889-2210
New York, NY 10016-5337   800-622-9010
                                                            Fax: 212-689-9261
                                                            www.kidney.org
A patient and family newspaper targeted toward dialysis populations.
Quarterly

5672 PKD Progress
PKD Foundation
4901 Main Street   816-931-2600
Kansas City, MO 64112-2634   800-753-2873
                                                            Fax: 816-931-8655
                                                  e-mail: pkdcure@pkdcure.org
                                                            www.pkdcure.org
Offers information and updated medical news for persons and professionals with an interest in kidney disorders.
Monthly
Dave Switzer, Marketing/Public Relations Director

5673 Renal Recipes Quarterly
R&D Laboratories
4204 Glencoe Avenue
Marina Del Rey, CA 90292-5612   800-338-9066
Features timely holiday and ethnic food menus and recipes, shopping and food tips, analysis of nutrients and calculation of food exchanges.
Quarterly

5674 Transplant Chronicles
National Kidney Foundation
30 E 33rd Street   212-889-2210
New York, NY 10016   800-622-9010
                                                            Fax: 212-689-9261
                                                            www.kidney.org
A patient and family newsletter targeted towards transplant recipients.
Quarterly

Pamphlets

5675 About Kidney Stones
National Kidney Foundation
30 E 33rd Street   212-889-2210
New York, NY 10016   800-622-9010
                                                            Fax: 212-689-9261
                                                            www.kidney.org
Discusses causes, treatment and prevention of kidney stones.

5676 Advance Directives: A Guide for Patients and Their Families
National Kidney Foundation
30 E 33rd Street   212-889-2210
New York, NY 10016-5337   800-622-9010
                                                            Fax: 212-689-9261
                                                            www.kidney.org
Everyone has the right to make an advance directive, which is a legal document stating how you want decisions made concerning your medical care when your no longer able to make them yourself. This booklet describes the different types of advance directives and the medical decisions they cover.
12 pages Package

5677 American Kidney Fund Helps When Nobody Else Will
American Kidney Fund

6110 Executive Boulevard   301-881-3052
Rockville, MD 20852-3915   800-638-8299
                                                            Fax: 301-881-0898
                                                  e-mail: helpline@AFINC.org
                                                            www.kidneyfund.org
Focuses on the services and programs offered by the American Kidney Fund.

5678 At Home with AAKP
American Association of Kidney Patients
3505 E Frantage Road   813-636-8100
Tampa, FL 33607   800-749-2257
                                                            Fax: 813-636-8122
                                                  e-mail: info@aakp.org
                                                            www.aakp.org
A free publication, this was developed to address the growing need for information about home dialysis treatment options.
Kim Buettner, Executive Director

5679 Children and Kidney Disease
American Kidney Fund
6110 Executive Boulevard   301-881-3052
Rockville, MD 20852-3915   800-638-8299
                                                            Fax: 301-881-0898
                                                            www.arbon.com/kidney/

5680 Choosing a Treatment for Kidney Failure
National Kidney Foundation
30 E 33rd Street   212-889-2210
New York, NY 10016   800-622-9010
                                                            Fax: 212-689-9261
                                                            www.kidney.org
Introduces treatment options for kidney failure and explains the pros and cons of each.
16 pages

5681 Diabetes and Kidney Disease
National Kidney Foundation
30 E 33rd Street   212-889-2210
New York, NY 10016-5337   800-622-9010
                                                            Fax: 212-689-9261
                                                            www.kidney.org
Explains the connection between diabetes and kidney disease covering prevention, recognition and treatments.
12 pages Pkg. of 100

5682 Dialysis Patient: An Informative Guide for the Dentist
American Kidney Fund
6110 Executive Boulevard   301-881-3052
Rockville, MD 20852-3915   800-638-8299
                                                            Fax: 301-881-0898
                                                            www.arbon.com/kidney/

5683 Diet Guide for the CAPD Patient
American Kidney Fund
6110 Executive Boulevard   301-881-3052
Rockville, MD 20852-3915   800-638-8299
                                                            Fax: 301-881-0898
                                                            www.arbon.com/kidney/

5684 Diet Guide for the Hemodialysis Patient
American Kidney Fund
6110 Executive Boulevard   301-881-3052
Rockville, MD 20852-3915   800-638-8299
                                                            Fax: 301-881-0898
                                                            www.arbon.com/kidney/

5685 Facts About Kidney Diseases and Their Treatment
American Kidney Fund
6110 Executive Boulevard   301-881-3052
Rockville, MD 20852-3915   800-638-8299
                                                            Fax: 301-881-0898
                                                            www.arbon.com/kidney/
Offers information about what kidneys are and their functions, diagnosis and treatment of kidney disease.

5686 Facts About Kidney Stones
American Kidney Fund

6110 Executive Boulevard
Rockville, MD 20852-3915

301-881-3052
800-638-8299
Fax: 301-881-0898
www.arbon.com/kidney/

5687 Glomerulonephritis
National Kidney Foundation
30 E 33rd Street
New York, NY 10016-5337

212-889-2210
800-622-9010
Fax: 212-689-9261
www.kidney.org

Defines the types of Glomerulonephritis, signs, causes and symptoms.
8 pages Pkg. of 100

5688 Hemodialysis
National Kidney Foundation
30 E 33rd Street
New York, NY 10016

212-889-2210
800-622-9010
Fax: 212-689-9261
www.kidney.org

Introduces and explains the hemodialysis treatment process.
12 pages Pkg. of 100

5689 High Blood Pressure and Your Kidneys
National Kidney Foundation
30 E 33rd Street
New York, NY 10016-5337

212-889-2210
800-622-9010
Fax: 212-689-9261
www.kidney.org

Offers a description of hypertension, including symptoms, detection, causes and effects. Also available in Spanish.
8 pages Pkg. of 100

5690 High Blood Pressure and its Effects on the Kidneys
American Kidney Fund
6110 Executive Boulevard
Rockville, MD 20852

301-881-3052
800-638-8299
Fax: 301-881-0898
www.arbon.com/kidney/

5691 Kid
American Kidney Fund
6110 Executive Boulevard
Rockville, MD 20852-3915

301-881-3052
800-638-8299
Fax: 301-881-0898
www.arbon.com/kidney/

5692 Kidney Disease: A Guide for Patients and Their Families
American Kidney Fund
6110 Executive Boulevard
Rockville, MD 20852

301-881-3052
800-638-8299
Fax: 301-881-0898
www.arbon.com/kidney/

Offers information on how the kidneys work, symptoms of kidney disease, kidney failure and treatment alternatives.

5693 Kidney Transplant: A New Lease on Life
National Kidney Foundation
30 E 33rd Street
New York, NY 10016

212-889-2210
800-622-9010
Fax: 212-689-9261
www.kidney.org

A brochure that answers common questions about transplants, such as patient expectations, drug therapy, complications including rejection and recovery.
10 pages Pkg. of 100

5694 Kidneys for Kids
American Kidney Fund
6110 Executive Boulevard
Rockville, MD 20852-3915

301-881-3052
800-638-8299
Fax: 301-881-0898
www.arbon.com/kidney/

5695 Nutrition and Changing Kidney Function
National Kidney Foundation
30 E 33rd Street
New York, NY 10016-5337

212-889-2210
800-622-9010
Fax: 212-689-9261
www.kidney.org

Explains how to slow the progression of kidney disease by controlling the intake of vitamins, minerals, fluids, calories and proteins.
12 pages Pkg. of 100

5696 Organ Donor Program
National Kidney Foundation
30 E 33rd Street
New York, NY 10016-5337

212-889-2210
800-622-9010
Fax: 212-689-9261
www.kidney.org

A comprehensive description of the organ donor program that explains organ and tissue donation, brain death, routine inquiry and becoming an organ donor.
12 pages Pkg. of 100

5697 Peritoneal Dialysis
National Kidney Foundation
30 E 33rd Street
New York, NY 10016

212-889-2210
800-622-9010
Fax: 212-689-9261
www.kidney.org

Introduces and explains the peritoneal dialysis treatment process
8 pages

5698 Understanding Nephrotic Syndrome
American Kidney Fund
6110 Executive Boulevard
Rockville, MD 20852-3915

301-881-3052
800-638-8299
Fax: 301-881-0898
www.arbon.com/kidney/

5699 Urinary Tract Infections
National Kidney Foundation
30 E 33rd Street
New York, NY 10016-5337

212-889-2210
800-622-9010
Fax: 212-689-9261
www.kidney.org

Defines urinary tract infections, its symptoms, causes and treatments.
10 pages Pkg. of 100

5700 Warning Signs of Kidney Disease
National Kidney Foundation
30 E 33rd Street
New York, NY 10016-5337

212-889-2210
800-622-9010
Fax: 212-689-9261
www.kidney.org

A one-panel leaflet that numbers and lists the six early warning signs of kidney disease.
Pkg. of 100

5701 Winning the Fight Against Silent Killers
National Kidney Foundation
30 E 33rd Street
New York, NY 10016-5337

212-889-2210
800-622-9010
Fax: 212-689-9261
www.kidney.org

Written for the African-American community, this brochure discusses the increased risk of high blood pressure and diabetes in this population.
12 pages Pkg. of 100

5702 Your Kidneys: Master Chemists of the Body
National Kidney Foundation
30 E 33rd Street
New York, NY 10016-5337

212-889-2210
800-622-9010
Fax: 212-689-9261
www.kidney.org

Offers an overview of kidneys and urinary system, describing the kidneys' filtering system, hereditary, congenital and acquired kidney diseases.
12 pages Pkg. of 100

Audio & Video

5703 It's Just Part of My Life
National Kidney Foundation

30 E 33rd Street
New York, NY 10016-5337

212-889-2210
800-622-9010
Fax: 212-689-9261
www.kidney.org

A 15-minute program for adolescent dialysis patients and their families.

5704 People Like Us
National Kidney Foundation
30 E 33rd Street
New York, NY 10016-5337

212-889-2210
800-622-9010
Fax: 212-689-9261
www.kidney.org

A seven-part video series targeted toward the newly-diagnosed chronic kidney disease patient.

Web Sites

5705 American Association of Kidney Patients

www.aakp.org

Serves the needs and interests of kidney patients, for kidney patients, the purpose of this Association is to help patients and their families cope with the emotional, physical and social impact of kidney disease.

5706 American Kidney Fund

www.akfinc.org/

A nonprofit, national health organization providing direct financial assistance to thousands of Americans who suffer from kidney disease.

5707 Healing Well

www.healingwell.com

An online health resource guide to medical news, chat, information and articles, newsgroups and message boards, books, disease-related web sites, medical directories, and more for patients, friends, and family coping with disabling diseases, disorders, or chronic illnesses.

5708 Health Finder

www.healthfinder.gov

Searchable, carefully developed web site offering information on over 1000 topics. Developed by the US Department of Health and Human Services, the site can be used in both English and Spanish.

5709 Healthlink USA

www.healthlinkusa.com

Links to websites which may include treatment, cures, diagnosis, prevention, support groups, email lists, messageboards, personal stories, risk factors, statistics, research and more.

5710 Helios Health

www.helioshealth.com

Online resource for your health information. Detailed information about specific health topics, access to expert advice from our Medical Advisory Board, and up-to-date health news.

5711 MedicineNet

www.medicinenet.com

An online resource for consumers providing easy-to-read, authoritative medical and health information.

5712 Medscape

www.medscape.com

Medscape offers specialists, primary care physicians, and other health professionals the Web's most robust and integrated medical information and educational tools.

5713 Polycystic Kidney Research Foundation

www.pkdcure.org

Provide information on research into the cause, treatment, and cure of polycystic kidney disease by raising financial support for peer approved biomedical research projects and fostering public awareness among medical professionals, patients and the general public.

5714 WebMD

www.webmd.com

Information on kidney disease, including articles and resources.

Description

5715 **Liver Disease**

Liver disease covers a wide range of disorders that can result in chronic liver damage, such as scarring (fibrosis) or the development of cirrhosis. An estimated 43,000 Americans die each year from liver disease.

Specific liver diseases that damage the liver include infection (e.g., viral hepatitis), chronic alcoholism or drug abuse, medications and certain systemic illnesses. Severe disease can permanently damage the liver, causing it to fail totally.

Common signs of liver damage are fatigue, loss of appetite, nausea and tea-colored urine. Yellowing of the skin and the whites of the eye (jaundice) is seen in 50 percent of cases. Other symptoms include liver enlargement and tenderness, and fluid collection in the abdominal cavity. A shriveling liver indicates more chronic and severe damage.

Treatment for liver disease depends on the underlying cause. In less severe injury, due to its remarkable capacity to heal itself, the liver can completely recover. Liver transplantation is accepted as appropriate treatment for end-stage liver dysfunction. See also *Hepatitis*.

National Agencies & Associations

5716 **(AASLD) American Association for the Study of Liver Diseases**
1729 King Street 703-299-9766
Alexandria, VA 22314 Fax: 703-299-9622
e-mail: aasld@aasld.org
www.aasld.org
Physicians, researchers, and allied hepatology health professionals.
Sherrie H. Cathcart, Executive Director

5717 **American Liver Foundation**
75 Maiden Lane 212-668-1000
New York, NY 10038 800-465-4837
Fax: 212-483-8179
e-mail: info@liverfoundation.org
www.liverfoundation.org
National, nonprofit organization dedicated to the prevention treatment and cure of hepatitis and other liver diseases through research and advocacy. The ALF offers information, physician referrals, a 24-hour, 7 day-a-week national helpline and support groups.
Rick Smith, President/CEO
Newton Guerin, COO

State Agencies & Associations

Arizona

5718 **American Liver Foundation Arizona Chapter**
4545 E Shea Boulevard 602-953-1800
Phoenix, AZ 85028 866-953-1800
Fax: 602-953-1806
e-mail: arizona@liverfoundation.org
www.liverfoundation.org
Melissa McCracken, Executive Director
Pamela White, Events Manager

California

5719 **American Liver Foundation Greater Los Angeles Chapter**
5777 Century Boulevard 310-670-4624
Los Angeles, CA 90045 Fax: 310-670-4672
e-mail: sfranklin@liverfoundation.org
www.liverfoundation.org
Taly Fantini, Executive Director
Jessica Goltermann, Event Coordinator

5720 **American Liver Foundation Northern CA Chapter**
870 Market Street 415-248-1060
San Francisco, CA 94102 800-292-9099
Fax: 415-248-1066
e-mail: northernca@liverfoundation.org
www.liverfoundation.org
Linden Young, Division Vice President
Michelle Flatley, Special Events Manager

5721 **American Liver Foundation San Diego Chapte r**
2515 Camino del Rio S 619-291-5483
San Diego, CA 92108 800-749-2630
Fax: 619-295-7181
e-mail: KFurrow@liverfoundation.org
www.liverfoundation.org
Kristina Furrow, Executive Director
Lisa A Haile JD PhD, President of the Board

Colorado

5722 **American Liver Foundation Rocky Mountain Division**
1660 S Albion Street 303-988-4388
Denver, CO 80222 Fax: 303-988-4398
e-mail: rminfo@liverfoundation.org
www.liverfoundation.org
Jeffrey Petrovic, Division VP
Cassie Thomas, Community Events Manager

Connecticut

5723 **American Liver Foundation: Connecticut Chapter**
127 Washington Avenue 203-234-2022
N Haven, CT 06473 Fax: 203-234-1386
e-mail: info@ctalf.org
www.ctalf.org
Offers support for patients and families provides educational meetings and conferences raising vital liver research dollars; encouraging the beautifully unselfish gift of organ donation and the medical miracle of organ transplantation.
12 pages Quarterly
JoAnn Thompson, Executive Director
Marla Hannah Sadler, Event Coordinator

Florida

5724 **American Liver Foundation Gulf Coast Chapter**
202 S 22nd Street 813-248-3337
Ybor City, FL 33605 Fax: 813-248-3340
e-mail: jbourgeois@liverfoundation.org
www.liverfoundation.org
Jennifer Bourgeois, Executive Director

Hawaii

5725 **American Liver Foundation Hawaii Chapter**
3660 Waialae Avenue 808-737-0400
Honolulu, HI 96816 Fax: 808-737-3230
e-mail: alfhawaii@liverfoundation.org
www.liverfoundation.org
Janice M Nillias, Executive Director

Illinois

5726 **American Liver Foundation Illinois Chapter**
180 N Michigan Avenue 312-377-9030
Chicago, IL 60601 Fax: 312-377-9035
e-mail: info@illinois-liver.org
www.illinois-liver.org
Kevin Gianotto, Executive Director
Emily Nuzzo MA LSW, Program Manager

Indiana

5727 American Liver Foundation Indiana Chapter
921 E 86th Street   317-635-5074
Indianapolis, IN 46240   877-548-3730
                                                         Fax: 317-635-5075
e-mail: dsparksunsworth@liverfoundation.org
www.liverfoundation.org

Natalie Sutton, Executive Director
Kristin Gray, Development Coordinator

Massachusetts

5728 American Liver Foundation New England Chapter
88 Winchester Street   617-527-5600
Newton, MA 02461   800-298-6766
                                                         Fax: 617-527-5636
e-mail: info@liverfoundation.org
www.liverfoundation.org

Kelly Leigh Beckett, Executive Director
Laura Dempsey, Director of Campaigns

Michigan

5729 American Liver Foundation Michigan Chapter
21886 Farmington Road   248-615-5768
Farmington, MI 48336   888-MYL-IVER
                                                         Fax: 248-615-5778
e-mail: michigan@liverfoundation.org
www.liverfoundation.org

Jennifer L Dale, Executive Director

Minnesota

5730 American Liver Foundation Minnesota Chapte r
2626 E 82nd Street   952-854-6181
Bloomington, MN 55425   Fax: 952-854-6956
e-mail: dstibbe@liverfoundation.org
www.liverfoundation.org

David Stibbe, Executive Director
Meghan Likes, Community Events Coordinator

Missouri

5731 American Liver Foundation Greater Kansas Greater kC Chapter
Greater kC Chapter
309 NE 88th Terrace   816-420-9446
Kansas City, MO 64155   Fax: 612-892-8442
e-mail: kcchapal@amail.com

Stan Adkins, Chapter Director

New York

5732 American Liver Foundation Greater New York Chapter
75 Maiden Lane   212-943-1059
New York, NY 10004   877-307-7507
                                                         Fax: 212-943-1314
e-mail: greaterny@liverfoundation.org
www.liverfoundation.org

Gina Parziale, Executive Director
Tracy Merlau, Programs Manager

5733 American Liver Foundation Western New York Chapter
25 Canterbury Road   585-271-2859
Rochester, NY 14607   Fax: 585-271-8642
e-mail: nkoris@liverfoundation.org
www.liverfoundation.org

Nancy Koris, Executive Director

Ohio

5734 American Liver Foundation Ohio Chapter
5755 Granger Road   216-635-2780
Independence, OH 44131-1455   Fax: 216-635-2781
e-mail: ohio@liverfoundation.org
www.liverfoundation.org

Susan S Rodwa MNO, Executive Director

Pennsylvania

5735 American Liver Foundation Delaware Valley Chapter
111 Presidential Boulevard   610-668-0152
Bala Cynwyd, PA 19004   Fax: 610-668-0155
e-mail: emurphy@liverfoundation.org
www.liverfoundation.org

Elizabeth Murphy, Executive Director

5736 American Liver Foundation Western Pennsylv ania
100 W Station Square Drive   412-434-7044
Pittsburgh, PA 15219   Fax: 412-434-7040
e-mail: spmasartis@liverfoundation.org
www.liverfoundation.org

Suzanna Masartis, Division Vice-President
Kara Hartner, Event Manager

Tennessee

5737 American Liver Foundation Midsouth Chapter
5050 Poplar Avenue   901-766-7668
Memphis, TN 38157   866-756-7668
                                                         Fax: 901-766-2061
e-mail: midsouth@liverfoundation.org
www.liverfoundation.org

Karen Viotti, Executive Director
Deri Whittaker, Community Events Coordinator

Texas

5738 American Liver Foundation South Texas Chap ter
2425 W Loop S   713-622-1318
Houston, TX 77027   Fax: 713-622-1376
e-mail: texas@liverfoundation.org
www.liverfoundation.org

Patricia Wittlif, Executive Director

Virginia

5739 American Liver Foundation National Capital
127 S Peyton Street   703-535-8880
Alexandria, VA 22314   Fax: 703-535-8890
e-mail: jjacobs@liverfoundation.org
www.liverfoundation.org

Jodie Campbe Jacobs, Community Events Coordinator

Washington

5740 American Liver Foundation Pacific Northwest Chapter
2033 6th Avenue   206-443-3805
Seattle, WA 98121   800-465-4837
                                                         Fax: 206-443-1511
www.liverfoundation.org

David de la Fuente, Executive Director
Molly Scott, Community Events Manager

Wisconsin

5741 American Liver Foundation Wisconsin Chapter
4927 N Lydell Avenue   414-961-4936
Glendale, WI 53217   Fax: 414-961-7288
e-mail: infowi@liverfoundation.org
www.liverfoundation.org

Dee Girard, Executive Director
Samantha Chartrau, Event/Program Coordinator

Research Centers

5742 Clinical Research Center: Pediatrics Children's Hospital Research Foundation
Children's Hospital Research Foundation
Elland & Bethesda Avenues   513-559-4412
Cincinnati, OH 45229   Fax: 513-559-7431
Studies of pediatric acquired diseases including liver disease and Reye's Syndrome.
Dr James Heubi, Director

5743 University of California Liver Research Unit
7601 E Imperial Highway
Downey, CA 90242
562-940-8961
Fax: 562-940-6628
Dr Allan G Redeker, Co-director

5744 University of Texas Southwestern Medical Center
5323 Harry Hines Boulevard
Dallas, TX 75390-9151
214-648-8311
www.utsouthwestern.edu
William M Lee MD Facp, Professor InteRNal Medicine / Director

5745 University of Texas Southwestern Medical
5323 Harry Hines Boulevard
Dallas, TX 75235
214-648-3404
Fax: 214-648-9119
e-mail: news@utsouthwestern.edu
www.utsouthwestern.edu
William M Lee MD Facp, Professor Internal Medicine / Director

5746 Yeshiva University Marion Bessin Liver Research Center
Albert Einstein College of Medicine
1300 Morris Park Avenue
Bronx, NY 10461-1975
718-430-2000
Fax: 718-918-0857
www.aecom.yu.edu
Liver disease research and therapy.
Dr David Shafritz, Director

Support Groups & Hotlines

5747 Children's Liver Association for Support S ervices
25379 Wayne Mills Place
Valencia, CA 91355
661-263-9099
877-679-8256
Fax: 661-263-9099
e-mail: Support Srv@aol.com
www.classkids.org
Dedicated to addressing the emotional, educational, and financial needs of families with children with liver disease or liver transplantation. Telephone hotline, newsletter, parent matching, literature and financial assistance. supports research and educates public about organ donations.
Diane Summer, President Board of Directors
Ann Whitehead RN/JD, Vice President Board of Directors

5748 National Gaucher Foundation (NGF)
2227 Idlewood Road
Tucker, GA 30084
800-504-3189
Fax: 770-934-2911
e-mail: rhonda@gaucherdisease.org
www.gaucherdisease.org/
The National Gaucher Foundation (NGF), established in 1984, supports and promotes research into the causes of, and a cure for Gaucher Disease. NGF provides information and assistance for those affected by Gaucher disease in addition to education and outreach to increase public awareness. NGF operates the Gaucher Disease Family Support Network.
Robin A Ely MD, President/Medical Director
Rhonda P Buyers, CEO/Executive Director

5749 National Health Information Center
PO Box 1133
Washington, DC 20013
310-565-4167
800-336-4797
Fax: 301-984-4256
e-mail: info@nhic.org
www.health.gov/nhic
Offers a nationwide information referral service, produces directories and resource guides.

5750 National Reye's Syndrome Foundation
PO Box 829
Bryan, OH 43506
419-636-2679
800-233-7393
Fax: 419-636-9897
e-mail: nrsf@reyessyndrome.org
www.reyessyndrome.org
Devoted to conquering Reye's syndrome, primarily a children's disease affecting the liver and brain, but can affect all ages. Provides support, information and referrals. Encourages research.
John Freudenberger, President
Larry Lasky, Vice President

5751 Wilson's Disease Association
1802 Brookside Drive
Wooster, OH 44691
330-264-1450
888-264-1450
Fax: 330-264-0974
e-mail: info@wilsonsdisease.org
www.wilsonsdisease.org
Serves as a communications support network for individuals affected by Wilson's disease; distributes information to professionals and the public; makes referrals; and holds meetings.
8 pages
Kimberly Symonds, Executive Director

Books

5752 Liver Cancer
Churchill Livingstone
PO Box 3188
Secaucus, NJ 07096-3188
201-319-9800
800-553-5426
Fax: 201-319-9659
www.churchillmed.com
1997 640 pages Hardcover
ISBN: 0-443054-81-9

5753 Liver Disease in Children
Mosby Year Book
11830 Westline Industrial Drive
Saint Louis, MO 63146-3313
314-872-8370
800-325-4177
1993 800 pages
ISBN: 1-556443-77-2

Magazines

5754 American Association for the Study of Liver Diseases
1729 King Street
Alexandria, VA 22314
703-299-9766
Fax: 703-299-9622
e-mail: aasld@aasld.org
www.aasld.org
Information for professionals interested in disease of the liver and biliary tract.
Sherrie H Cathcart, Executive Director

5755 Hepatology
American Assoc. for the Study of Liver Disease
1729 King Street
Alexandria, VA 22314
703-299-9766
Fax: 703-299-9622
e-mail: aasld@aasld.org
www.aasld.org
Information for professionals interested in disease of the liver and biliary tract.
Sherrie H Cathcart, Executive Director

Newsletters

5756 Children's Liver Association for Support S ervices Newsletter
25379 Wayne Mills Place
Valencia, CA 91355
661-263-9099
877-679-8256
Fax: 661-263-9099
e-mail: SupportSrv@aol.com
www.classkids.org
Dedicated to addressing the emotional, educational, and financial needs of families with children with liver disease or liver transplantation. Telephone hotline, newsletter, parent matching, literature and financial assistance. supports research and educates public about organ donations.
Yearly
Diane Summer, President Board of Directors
Ann Whitehead RN/JD, Vice President Board of Directors

5757 Liver Update
American Liver Foundation
1425 Pompton Avenue
Cedar Grove, NJ 07009-1000
800-465-4837
Fax: 973-256-3214
e-mail: info@liverfoundation.org
www.liverfoundation.org

Clinical newsletter for physicians.
BiAnnually
Rick Smith, President & CEO
Rebecca Frank, Chief Development Officer

5758 LiverLink
Alagille Syndrome Alliance
10630 SW Garden Park Place   503-639-6217
Tigard, OR 97223-3832
Newsletter for Alagille Syndrome.

5759 Progress
American Liver Foundation
1425 Pompton Avenue
Cedar Grove, NJ 07009-1000   800-465-4837
                                    Fax: 973-256-3214
                        e-mail: info@liverfoundation.org
                                www.liverfoundation.org

Newsletter about liver disease and ALF.
TriAnnually
Rick Smith, President & CEO
Rebecca Frank, Chief Development Officer

Pamphlets

5760 Alcohol and the Liver: Myth vs. Facts
American Liver Foundation
1425 Pompton Avenue   973-256-2550
Cedar Grove, NJ 07009-1000   800-223-0179
                        e-mail: info@liverfoundation.org
                                www.liverfoundation.org

Rick Smith, President & CEO
Rebecca Frank, Chief Development Officer

5761 Biliary Atresia
American Liver Foundation
1425 Pompton Avenue   973-857-2626
Cedar Grove, NJ 07009-1000   800-223-0179
                        e-mail: info@liverfoundation.org
                                www.liverfoundation.org

Rick Smith, President & CEO
Rebecca Frank, Chief Development Officer

5762 Diet and Your Liver
American Liver Foundation
1425 Pompton Avenue
Cedar Grove, NJ 07009-1000   800-223-0179
                                    Fax: 973-256-3214
                        e-mail: info@liverfoundation.org
                                www.liverfoundation.org

Rick Smith, President & CEO
Rebecca Frank, Chief Development Officer

5763 Facts on Liver Transplantation
American Liver Foundation
1425 Pompton Avenue
Cedar Grove, NJ 07009-1000   800-223-0179
                                    Fax: 973-256-3214
                        e-mail: info@liverfoundation.org
                                www.liverfoundation.org

Rick Smith, President & CEO
Rebecca Frank, Chief Development Officer

5764 Fatty Liver
American Liver Foundation
1425 Pompton Avenue
Cedar Grove, NJ 07009-1000   800-223-0179
                                    Fax: 987-256-3214
                        e-mail: info@liverfoundation.org
                                www.liverfoundation.org

Rick Smith, President & CEO
Rebecca Frank, Chief Development Officer

5765 Gallstones
American Liver Foundation

1425 Pompton Avenue
Cedar Grove, NJ 07009-1000   800-223-0179
                                    Fax: 973-256-3214
                        e-mail: info@liverfoundation.org
                                www.liverfoundation.org

Rick Smith, President & CEO
Rebecca Frank, Chief Development Officer

5766 Getting Help to Hepatitis
American Liver Foundation
1425 Pompton Avenue
Cedar Grove, NJ 07009-1000   800-223-0179
                                    Fax: 973-256-3214
                        e-mail: info@liverfoundation.org
                                www.liverfoundation.org

Rick Smith, President & CEO

5767 Hemochromatosis
American Liver Foundation
1425 Pompton Avenue
Cedar Grove, NJ 07009-1000   800-223-0179
                                    Fax: 973-256-3214
                        e-mail: info@liverfoundation.org
                                www.liverfoundation.org

Rick Smith, President & CEO

5768 Hepatitis A, B & C
American Liver Foundation
1425 Pompton Avenue
Cedar Grove, NJ 07009-1000   800-223-0179
                                    Fax: 973-256-3214
                        e-mail: info@liverfoundation.org
                                www.liverfoundation.org

Rick Smith, President & CEO

5769 Hepatitis B: Your Child at Risk
American Liver Foundation
1425 Pompton Avenue
Cedar Grove, NJ 07009-1000   800-223-0179
                                    Fax: 973-256-3214
                        e-mail: info@liverfoundation.org
                                www.liverfoundation.org

Rick Smith, President & CEO

5770 How Can You Love Me
American Liver Foundation
1425 Pompton Avenue   973-857-2626
Cedar Grove, NJ 07009-1000   800-223-0179
                                    Fax: 973-256-3214
                        e-mail: info@liverfoundation.org
                                www.liverfoundation.org

Rick Smith, President & CEO

5771 Liver Function Tests
American Liver Foundation
1425 Pompton Avenue   973-256-2550
Cedar Grove, NJ 07009-1000   800-223-0179
                                    Fax: 973-256-3214
                        e-mail: info@liverfoundation.org
                                www.liverfoundation.org

Rick Smith, President & CEO

5772 Liver Transplant Fund
American Liver Foundation
1425 Pompton Avenue   973-256-2550
Cedar Grove, NJ 07009-1000   800-223-0179
                                    Fax: 973-256-3214
                        e-mail: info@liverfoundation.org
                                www.liverfoundation.org

Rick Smith, President & CEO

5773 Liver Transplantation
American Liver Foundation
1425 Pompton Avenue   973-857-2626
Cedar Grove, NJ 07009-1000   800-223-0179
                                    Fax: 973-256-3214
                        e-mail: info@liverfoundation.org
                                www.liverfoundation.org

Rick Smith, President & CEO

5774 Viral Hepatitis
American Liver Foundation
1425 Pompton Avenue
Cedar Grove, NJ 07009-1000
973-256-2550
800-223-0179
Fax: 973-256-3214
e-mail: info@liverfoundation.org
www.liverfoundation.org

Rick Smith, President & CEO

5775 Your Liver Lets You Live
American Liver Foundation
1425 Pompton Avenue
Cedar Grove, NJ 07009-1000
973-256-2550
800-223-0179
Fax: 973-256-3214
e-mail: info@liverfoundation.org
www.liverfoundation.org

Rick Smith, President & CEO

Web Sites

5776 American Association for the Study of Liver Diseases
www.aasld.org/
Conducts symposia and educational courses for professionals interested in disease of the liver and biliary tract. The leading organization for advancing the science and practice of hepatology.

5777 Children's Liver Alliance
www.liverkids.org.au/
Empowering the hearts and minds of children with liver disease, their families and the medical professionals who care for them.

5778 Healing Well
www.healingwell.com
An online health resource guide to medical news, chat, information and articles, newsgroups and message boards, books, disease-related web sites, medical directories, and more for patients, friends, and family coping with disabling diseases, disorders, or chronic illnesses.

5779 Health Finder
www.healthfinder.gov
Searchable, carefully developed web site offering information on over 1000 topics. Developed by the US Department of Health and Human Services, the site can be used in both English and Spanish.

5780 Healthlink USA
www.healthlinkusa.com
Health information concerning treatment, cures, prevention, diagnosis, risk factors, research, support groups, email lists, personal stories and much more. Updated regularly.

5781 Helios Health
www.helioshealth.com
Online resource for your health information. Detailed information about specific health topics, access to expert advice from our Medical Advisory Board, and up-to-date health news.

5782 Liver Support
www.liversupport.com
Information about the world's safest, most powerful liver-protecting supplement, milk thistle. Specifically facts about the safe, yet highly potent, Phytosome form.

5783 MedicineNet
www.medicinenet.com
An online resource for consumers providing easy-to-read, authoritative medical and health information.

5784 Medscape
www.medscape.com
Medscape offers specialists, primary care physicians, and other health professionals the Web's most robust and integrated medical information and educational tools.

5785 WebMD
www.webmd.com
Information on liver disease, including articles and resources.

Description

5786 Lung Disease

The lungs are in intimate contact with a person's environment, so they may be damaged by scores of agents, including dusts, gases and micro-organisms. The majority of lung, or pulmonary, diseases are related to exposure to external irritants, such as cigarette smoke, asbestos, bacteria and viruses. The most common chronic lung diseases of this type are emphysema and chronic bronchitis; both are part of the class of diseases called Chronic Obstructive Pulmonary Disease, or COPD. Most cases are associated with tobacco usage. High-risk occupations for lung disease include mining, farming, building construction and certain types of manufacturing. Lung cancer may be primary (originating in the lung) or secondary (spread, or metastasized, from another area). Bronchogenic cancer accounts for more than 90 percent of all lung tumors; cigarette smoking is the principal cause. Lung cancer is usually seen in people with COPD, because the two conditions have similar causes. Other lung disorders are secondary to clots originating from other sites in the body, systemic illness, and skeletal abnormalities that interfere with chest expansion during breathing.

Symptoms of lung disease may include coughing, sputum production, breathlessness, and sometimes fever or chest pain. In advanced cases, breathlessness is constant, and cyanosis (a bluish discoloration of the lips and fingernails) may occur.

Diagnosis of pulmonary disorders depends on a very careful history, physical examination, chest x-ray and pulmonary function testing, or spirometry. These measures are also important in following disease progression and response to treatment. Other chest imaging techniques, such as computed tomography (CT) scans and MRIs, and examination of fluid in the lung and lung tissue help establish a diagnosis. Recent research indicates that PET (positron emission tomography) scans may be helpful in the earlier diagnosis and treatment of lung cancer. Treatment of lung disease depends on the underlying cause. Management of COPD includes avoiding tobacco or other environmental exposure, antibiotics to control heavy sputum production and drugs to open up the narrowed airways. In advanced cases, breathing oxygen directly by nasal prongs improves quality of life and survival. Lung transplantation has occasionally been attempted, usually when COPD is due to a genetic disorder. Early screening for lung cancer has been disappointing; quitting smoking early is the only meaningful way of reducing one's risk of dying of the disease. Treatment may include surgery, radiation, or chemotherapy; success depends on the stage of the tumor and its precise type as determined by tissue biopsy.

Severe Acute Respiratory Syndrome, known as SARS, is an infectious disease that first appeared in China in 2002. SARS is caused by a corona-virus, which is related to the virus behind the common cold. The symptoms of SARS are a fever, greater than 100.4 degrees, fatigue, headache and chills. It is also accompanied by a dry cough and difficulty breathing, owing to the inflamed lungs. Until effective treatment or a vaccine is developed, prevention in SARS-infected areas includes isolating patients, wearing protective surgical masks, and restricting travel.

National Agencies & Associations

5787 American Association for Respiratory Care

9425 N MacArthur Boulevard
Irving, TX 75063-4706

972-243-2272
Fax: 972-484-2720
e-mail: info@aarc.org
www.aarc.org

Committed to enhancing professionalism as a respiratory care practitioner improving your performance on the job and helping to broaden the scope essential for success.
Sam Giordano, Executive Director
Tim Goldsbury, Sales Director

5788 American Lung Association

1301 Pennsylvania Avenue NW
Washington, DC 20004

212-315-8700
800-LUN-GUSA
www.lungusa.org

The mission of the American Lung Association is to prevent lung disease and promote lung health. Founded in 1904 to fight tuberculosis the American Lung Association today fights disease in all its forms with special emphasis on asthma and tobacco control.
H James Gooden, Secretary
Stephen J Nolan, Chair

5789 Coalition for Pulmonary Fibrosis

1659 Branham Lane
San Jose, CA 95118

888-222-8541
Fax: 408-266-3289
e-mail: info@coalitionforpf.org
www.coalitionforpf.org

Founded to further education patient support and research efforts for pulmonary fibrosis specifically idiopathic pulmonary fibrosis.
Marvin Schwa MD, Chairman

5790 Lung Association

1750 Courtwood Crescent
Ottawa, K2C 2-2B5

613-569-6411
888-566-5864
Fax: 613-569-8860
e-mail: info@lung.ca
www.lung.ca

At the national provincial and community levels to improve and promote lung health.
Nora Sobolov, President/CEO
Mary-Pat Shaw, VP National Programs & Operations

5791 National Jewish Medical and Research Center

1400 Jackson Street
Denver, CO 80206

303-388-4461
800-222-5864
e-mail: allstetterw@njhealth.orgÿ
www.nationaljewish.org

Offers comprehensive diagnosis treatment and rehabilitation of people with chronic obstructive pulmonary disease asthma allergies and other respiratory and immune diseases.
William Allstetter, Media Contact
Pamela Meister, Patient Representative Office

5792 Public Information Center US Environmental Protection Agency

US Environmental Protection Agency
1200 Pennsylvania Avenue NW
Washington, DC 20460

202-272-0167
800-368-5888
TTY: 202-272-0165
www.epa.gov

Provides information on handling asbestos and explanation of legislation.
Lisa Jackson, Administrator

5793 Pulmonary Fibrosis Association
1332 N Halstead Street
Chicago, IL 60642-0004
312-587-9272
Fax: 312-587-9273
e-mail: pulmonaryfibrosisinfo@yahoo.com
www.pulmonaryfibrosis.org
Dedicated to finding a cure for and raising awareness of pulmonary fibrosis an often fatal lung disease.
Michael Rose PhD, President/CEO
Leanne Storch, Executive Director

5794 Pulmonary Fibrosis Foundation
1332 N Halsted Street
Chicago, IL 60642
312-587-9272
Fax: 312-587-9273
e-mail: pulmonaryfibrosisinfo@yahoo.com
www.pulmonaryfibrosis.org
A non-profitÿ corporation founded in the state of Colorado in 2000 by Albert Rose and Michael Rosenzweig, both of whom were diagnosed with Pulmonary Fibrosis (IPF).
Mike Rosenzweig, President/CEO
Leanne Storch, Executive Director

5795 Pulmonary Hypertension Association
801 Roeder Road
Silver Spring, MD 20910
301-565-3004
800-748-7274
Fax: 301-565-3994
e-mail: pha@PHAssociation.org
www.PHAssociation.org
A nonprofit organization for pulmonary hypertension patients, families, caregivers and PH-treating medical professionals. The mission of the Pulmonary Hypertension Association (PHA) is to find ways to prevent and cure pulmonary hypertension.
Rino Aldrighetti, President
Carl Hicks, Chair

5796 US Environmental Protection Agency: Indoor Environments Division
1200 Pennsylvania Avenue NW
Washington, DC 20460
202-343-9370
Fax: 202-343-2392
e-mail: iaqinfo@aol.com
www.epa.gov/iaq
Responsible for implementing EPA's Indoor Environments Program, a voluntary (non-regulatory) program to address indoor air pollution.

5797 White Lung Association
PO Box 1483
Baltimore, MD 21203-1483
410-243-5864
e-mail: jfite@whitelung.org
www.whitelung.org
A national nonprofit organization dedicated to the education of the public to the hazards of asbestos exposure. The association developed programs of public education and consults with victims of asbestos exposure, school boards, building owners and government representatives.
Jim Fite, Contact

State Agencies & Associations

Alabama

5798 American Lung Association of Alabama
3125 Independence Drive
Birmingham, AL 35209
205-933-8821
e-mail: kperry@alabamalung.org
www.alabamalung.org
Kim Perry, Director of Development

Alaska

5799 American Lung Association of Alaska
500 W International Airport Road
Anchorage, AK 99518-1105
907-276-5864
800-LUN-GUSA
Fax: 907-565-5587
e-mail: mlarson@aklung.org
www.aklung.org
Marge Larson, Steering Committee Member
Michelle Ferreira, Asthma Coalition Coordinator

Arizona

5800 American Lung Association of Arizona
102 W McDowell Road
Phoenix, AZ 85003-1299
602-258-7505
800-LUN-GUSA
Fax: 602-258-7507
e-mail: bpfeifer@lungaz.org
www.lungarizona.org
Through research education and advocacy the American Lung Association of Arizona works to prevent lung disease and promote lung health. Our areas of focus are asthma air quality and tobacco control.
Bill J Pfeifer, President/CEO

Arkansas

5801 American Lung Association of Arkansas
211 Natural Resources Drive
Little Rock, AR 72205-1539
501-224-5864
800-880-5864
Fax: 501-224-5654
e-mail: klackey@lungark.org
www.lungark.org
Karen S Lackey, CEO
Melinda Rogers, Data Entry Coordinator

California

5802 American Lung Association of California
424 Pendleton Way
Oakland, CA 94621-2189
510-638-5864
Fax: 510-638-8984
e-mail: contact@californialung.org
www.californialung.org
Ben Abate, President/CEO
Sylvia Goodin, Secretary

Colorado

5803 American Lung Association of Colorado
5600 Greenwood Plaza Boulevard
Greenwood Village, CO 80111
303-388-4327
800-LUN-GUSA
Fax: 303-377-1102
e-mail: chuber@lungcolorado.org
www.alacolo.org
Curt Huber, Executive Director
Connor Michael, Communications Manager

Connecticut

5804 American Lung Association of Connecticut
45 Ash Street
E Hartford, CT 06108-3272
860-289-5401
800-586-4872
Fax: 860-289-5405
e-mail: bcase@alact.org
www.alact.org
Part of the American Lung Association the oldest voluntary health agency dedicated to fighting a single disease. Highest priorities are asthma tobacco control and clean air.
Lisa Blumetti, Director Development/Special Events

Delaware

5805 American Lung Association of Delaware
1021 Gilpin Avenue
Wilmington, DE 19806-3280
302-655-7258
800-LUN-GUSA
Fax: 302-655-8546
e-mail: dbrown@alade.org
www.lunginfo.org
Deborah Brown, VP Community Outreach
Susan DeNardo, Development Director

District of Columbia

5806 American Lung Association of the District of Columbia
1725 K Street N.W.
Washington, DC 20001-2617
202-466-5864
e-mail: info@aladc.org
www.aladc.org
Resource for information and programs in the area of lung health, including asthma, tobacco control, air quality, sarcoidosis, and turberculosis.

5807 American Lung Association of the Northern
530 7th Street SE
Washington, DC 20003
202-546-5864
Fax: 202-546-5607
e-mail: info@aladc.org
www.aladc.org

Resource for information and programs in the area of lung health, including asthma, tobacco control, air quality, sarcoidosis, and tuberculosis.
David A McWilliams Sr, Chairman
Henry Yeager Jr MD, Vice Chairman

Florida

5808 American Lung Association of Florida
6852 Belfort Oaks Place
Jacksonville, FL 32216-5216
904-743-2933
800-940-2933
Fax: 904-743-2916
e-mail: alaf@lungfla.org
www.lungfla.org

Works for the prevention and control of lung disease through education, advocacy and research.
Denise Grimsley, President

5809 Goodwill Industries-Suncoast
Goodwill Industries-Suncoast
10596 Gandy Boulevard
St. Petersburg, FL 33702
727-523-1512
888-279-1988
Fax: 727-563-9300
e-mail: gw.marketing@goodwill-suncoast.com
www.goodwill-suncoast.org

A non-profit community based organization whose purpose is to improve the quality of life for people who are disabled, disadvantaged and/or aged. This mission is accomplished through a staff of over 1,200 employees providing independent living skills, affordable housing, career assessment and planning, job skills, training, placement, and job retention assistance with useful employment. Annually, Goodwill Industries-Suncoast serves over 30,000 people in Citrus, Hernando, Levy, Marion and more.
R Lee Waits, CEO
Martin W Gladysz, Chair

Georgia

5810 American Lung Association of Georgia
2452 Spring Road
Smyrna, GA 30080-3862
770-434-5864
Fax: 770-319-0349
e-mail: aburger@alase.org
www.alaga.org

Charles J White, Chief Executive Officer
June Deen, Vice President of Public Affairs

Hawaii

5811 American Lung Association of Hawaii
680 Iwilei Road
Honolulu, HI 96817
808-537-5966
Fax: 808-537-5971
e-mail: lung@ala-hawaii.org
www.ala-hawaii.org

Jean Evans, Executive Director
Karen J Lee, President

Idaho

5812 American Lung Association of Idaho
8030 Emerald Street
Boise, ID 83704
208-345-5864
800-LUN-GUSA
Fax: 208-345-5896
www.lungidaho.org

Illinois

5813 American Lung Association of Illinois
3000 Kelly Lane
Springfield, IL 62711
217-787-5864
800-LUN-GUSA
Fax: 217-787-5916
e-mail: info@lungil.org
www.lungil.org

Harold Wimmer, CEO
Kim Streib, Vice President Finance

Indiana

5814 American Lung Association of Indiana
115 W Washington Street
Indianapolis, IN 46204-1470
317-819-1181
800-LUN-GUSA
Fax: 317-819-1187
e-mail: info@lungin.org
www.lungin.org

Chris Brooks, Director Program Services
Melissa Henderson, Director Operations

Iowa

5815 American Lung Association of Iowa
2530 73rd Street
Des Moines, IA 50322-1800
515-278-5864
800-LUN-GUSA
Fax: 515-334-9564
e-mail: info@lungia.org
www.lungia.org

Harold Wimmer, President & CEO
Kim Streib, Manager/Controller

Kansas

5816 American Lung Association of Kansas
4300 SW Drury Lane
Topeka, KS 66604-2419
785-272-9290
800-LUN-GUSA
Fax: 785-272-9297
e-mail: jkeller@kslung.org
www.kslung.org

Judy Keller, Executive Officer
Kris Scothorn, Office Manager

Kentucky

5817 American Lung Association of Kentucky
4100 Churchman Avenue
Louisville, KY 40209-0067
502-363-2652
800-LUN-GUSA
Fax: 502-363-0222
e-mail: info@kylung.org
www.kylung.org

Ann Evans, Regional Director
Barry Gottschalk, Senior VP Operations

Louisiana

5818 American Lung Association of Louisiana
2325 Severn Avenue
Metairie, LA 70001-6918
504-828-5864
800-586-4872
Fax: 504-828-5867
e-mail: info@louisianalung.org
www.louisianalung.org

Aline Palmisano-Vita, Deputy Executive Director
Thomas P Lotz RRT MEd, Chief Executive Officer

Maine

5819 American Lung Association of Maine
122 State Street
Augusta, ME 04330
207-622-6394
888-241-6566
Fax: 207-626-2919
e-mail: info@lungme.org
www.lungme.org

Edward Miller, Executive Director
Norman Anderson, Regional Research Director

Maryland

5820 American Lung Association of Maryland
11350 McCormick Road
Hunt Valley, MD 21031
410-560-2120
800-LUN-GUSA
Fax: 410-560-0829
e-mail: info@marylandlung.org
www.marylandlung.org

Stephen J Nolan Esq, Chairman of the Board
Melina Davis-Martin, President and CEO

Massachusetts

5821 American Lung Association of Massachusetts
5 Mountain Road
Burlington, MA 01903   781-272-2866

Michigan

5822 American Lung Association of Michigan
25900 Greenfield Road   248-784-2000
Oak Park, MI 48237   800-543-LUNG
                                              Fax: 248-784-2008
                                              e-mail: alam@alam.org
                                              www.alam.org
Rose Adams, CEO
Nicole Crumpton, Executive Office Manager

Minnesota

5823 American Lung Association of Minnesota
490 Concordia Avenue   651-227-8014
Saint Paul, MN 55103-2441   800-LUN-GUSA
                                              Fax: 651-227-5459
                                              e-mail: info@alamn.org
                                              www.alamn.org
Jerry Orr, CEO

Mississippi

5824 American Lung Association of Mississippi
PO Box 2178   601-206-5810
Ridgeland, MS 39157

5825 American Lung Association of Missouri
731 Pear Orchard Road   601-206-5810
Ridgeland, MS 39157   Fax: 601-206-5813
                                              www.alams.org
Greg Wynne, Chairman
Tara Pierre Ellis, Vice-Chairman

Missouri

5826 American Lung Association of Eastern Missouri
1118 Hampton Avenue   314-645-5505
Saint Louis, MO 63139-3196   Fax: 314-645-7128
                              www.lungusa2.org/missouri/index.html

5827 American Lung Association: Kansas City Office
2400 Troost   816-842-5242
Kansas City, MO 64108   Fax: 816-842-5470
                                              e-mail: qnimrod@breathehealthy.org
                                              www.lungusa.org
National health association dedicated to promoting lung health and
preventing lung disease.

Montana

5828 American Lung Association of Northern Rockies
825 Helena Avenue   406-442-6556
Helena, MT 59601-3459   Fax: 406-442-2346
                                              e-mail: ala-nr@ala-nr.org
                                              www.lungusa.org

Nebraska

5829 American Lung Association of Nebraska
7101 Newport Avenue   402-572-3030
Omaha, NE 68152   800-LUN-GUSA
                                              e-mail: ala@lungnebraska.org
                                              www.lungnebraska.org

Nevada

5830 American Lung Association of Nevada
PO Box 7056   775-829-5864
Reno, NV 89510   800-LUN-GUSA
                                              Fax: 775-829-5850
                                              e-mail: dszabo@lungs.org
                                              www.lungusa.org

New Hampshire

5831 American Lung Association of New Hampshire
9 Cedarwood Drive   603-669-2411
Bedford, NH 03110   800-83L-UNGS
                                              Fax: 603-645-6220
                                              e-mail: dfortin@nhlung.org
                                              www.nhlung.org
Dan Fortin, President/CEO
Lois McKenna, Office Manager

New Jersey

5832 American Lung Association of New Jersey
1600 Route 22 E   908-687-9340
Union, NJ 07083-3410   Fax: 908-851-2625
                                              e-mail: info@alanewjersey.org
                                              www.alanewjersey.org
John A Rutkowski MBA RRT, President
Howard Hellman, First Vice President

New Mexico

5833 American Lung Association of New Mexico
7001 Menaul Boulevard NE   505-265-0732
Albuquerque, NM 87110   800-LUN-GUSA
                                              Fax: 505-260-1739
                                              e-mail: jdemaria@LungNewMexico.org
                                              www.lungnewmexico.org
Support group for adults with lung disease. Also offers lung health
education.
JoAnna DeMaria, Lung Health Coordinator
Lorrie Loomis, Office Coordinator

New York

5834 American Lung Association of New York State
155 Washington Avenue   518-465-2013
Albany, NY 12210-2804   Fax: 518-465-2926
                                              e-mail: info@alany.org
                                              www.alany.org
Deborah Carioto, President
Michael Seilback, Vice President of Public Policy

North Carolina

5835 American Lung Association of North Carolina
3801 Lake Boone Trail   919-832-8326
Raleigh, NC 27607   800-586-4872
                                              Fax: 919-856-8530
                                              e-mail: info@lungnc.org
                                              www.lungnc.org
Better breathing clubs for chronic lung disease patients.
Deborah Bryan, CEO
Susan King Cope, VP Programs/Advocacy

North Dakota

5836 American Lung Association of North Dakota
PO Box 5004   701-223-5613
Bismarck, ND 58501   800-252-6325
                                              Fax: 701-223-5727
                                              e-mail: lungnd@gcentral.com
A voluntary health agency whose objective is the conquest of lung
disease and the promotion of lung health. We sponsor Super
Asthma Saturday and open airways for schools events to educate
asthmatics and their families and Dakota Superkids Asthma Camp
for kids 8-15 with asthma. Smoking cessation classes for adults
and youth.

Ohio

5837 American Lung Association of Ohio
1950 Arlingate Lane   614-279-1700
Columbus, OH 43228-4102   800-LUN-GUSA
                                              Fax: 614-279-4940
                                              www.ohiolung.org
Tracy Ross, President/CEO

Oklahoma

5838 American Lung Association of Oklahoma
11212 N May Avenue
Oklahoma City, OK 73120
405-748-4674
800-LUN-GUSA
Fax: 405-748-6274
e-mail: ktodd@oklung.org
www.oklung.org

Kay Todd PhD CAE, CEO
Jimmy Beth, Member

Oregon

5839 American Lung Association of Oregon
7420 SW Bridgeport Road
Tigard, OR 97224-7790
503-924-4094
800-LUN-GUSA
Fax: 503-924-4120
e-mail: info@lungoregon.org
www.lungoregon.org

Dana Kaye, Executive Director
Jennifer Baldwin, Director of Development

Pennsylvania

5840 American Lung Association of Pennsylvania
3001 Old Gettysburg Road
Camp Hill, PA 17011
717-541-5864
800-932-0903
Fax: 717-541-8828
e-mail: info@lunginfo.org
www.lungusa.org
Provide education, research and information on lung disease and
lung health, including asthma, tobacco prevention and cessation,
chronic obstructive pulmonary disease, indoor and outdoor air
quality, children's summer camps, support groups and specialty
programs.

5841 American Respiratory Alliance of Western Pennsylvania
201 Smith Drive
Cranberry Township, PA 16066
724-772-1750
800-220-1990
Fax: 724-772-1180
www.healthylungs.org
Dedicated to the prevention and control of lung disease through education training, direct services, research funding and advocacy
since 1904.
Christine R Weaver, Executive Director
George B Miller, President

Rhode Island

5842 American Lung Association of Rhode Island
260 W Exchange Street
Providence, RI 02903-3700
401-421-6487
800-586-4872
Fax: 401-331-5266
e-mail: ALARI@lungri.org
www.lungne.org

Lucille Cavan, Director
Robert Petix, Chair/Executive Committee

South Carolina

5843 American Lung Association of South Carolina
1212 West Elkhorn Street
Columbia, SC 29201-2344
803-779-5864
800-849-5864
Fax: 803-254-2711
www.lungsc.org

South Dakota

5844 American Lung Association of South Dakota
1212 West Elkhorn
Sioux Falls, SD 57104-0233
605-336-7222
800-873-5864
Fax: 605-336-7227
e-mail: lung@americanlungsd.org

Linda Redder, Coordinator

Tennessee

5845 American Lung Association of Tennessee
1 Vantage Way
Nashville, TN 37228
615-329-1151
800-LUN-GUSA
Fax: 615-329-1723
e-mail: alastaff@alatn.org
www.lungtn.org
A statewide organization the oldest national health agency in the
US. Our mission is to prevent lung disease and to promote lung
health. Our program priorities include environmental health
asthma education tobacco control for children and finding a cure.

Texas

5846 American Lung Association of Texas
5926 Balcones Drive
Austin, TX 78731
512-467-6753
800-252-LUNG
Fax: 512-467-7621
e-mail: info@texaslung.org
www.texaslung.org

Lewis Brown MD, Chairman
Ted Balistreri, Member

Utah

5847 American Lung Association of Utah
1930 S 1100 E
Salt Lake City, UT 84106-2317
801-484-4456
800-548-8252
Fax: 801-484-5461
e-mail: info@utahlung.org
www.lungutah.org

Craig Cutright, Executive Director
Don Hooper, Development Director

Virginia

5848 American Lung Association of Virginia
9221 Forest Hill Avenue
Richmond, VA 23235
804-267-1900
800-345-5864
Fax: 804-267-5634
e-mail: info@lungac.org
www.lungva.org

Washington

5849 American Lung Association of Washington
2625 3rd Avenue
Seattle, WA 98121
206-441-5100
800-732-9339
Fax: 206-441-3277
e-mail: alaw@alaw.org
www.alaw.org

Marina Cofer-Wildsmi, CEO
Darlene Madenwald, President

West Virginia

5850 American Lung Association of West Virginia
415 Dickinson Street
Charleston, WV 25301
304-342-6600
800-LUN-GUSA
Fax: 304-342-6096
e-mail: sara@alawv.org
www.alawv.org

Sarah Crickenberger, Executive Director
Chantal Fields, Assistant Executive Director

Wisconsin

5851 American Lung Association of Wisconsin
13100 W Lisbon Road
Brookfield, WI 53005-2508
262-703-4200
800-LUN-GUSA
Fax: 262-781-5180
e-mail: amlung@lungwisconsin.org
www.lungwi.org

Susan Gloede Swan, Executive Director
Dona Wininsky, Director of Public Policy

Research Centers

5852 Enzymology Research Laboratory Dept. of Veterans Affairs Medical Center
Dept. of Veterans Affairs Medical Center
150 Muir Road   925-228-6800
Martinez, CA 94553
Studies affecting emphysema in mankind.
Michael C Geokas MD, Chief

5853 National Jewish Center for Immunology
1400 Jackson Street
Denver, CO 80206   303-388-4461
                                           www.nationaljewish.org
Offers basic and clinical research into the causes and treatments of various lung diseases and respiratory problems.
Lynn Gaussig, President

5854 University of Utah Rocky Mountain Center for Occupational & Environmental Health
University of Utah
391 Chipeta Way   801-581-4800
Salt Lake City, UT 84108   Fax: 801-817-24
                                 e-mail: rmoser@rmcoeh.utah.edu
                                           www.rmcoeh.utah.edu
Provides graduate and continuing education programs in occupational medicine occupational health nursing ergonomics and safety industrial hygiene and hazardous materials. Additionally provides clinical evaluations and consultations in the listed areas.
Royce Moser Jr MD, Deputy Director
Kurt Hedmann, Director

5855 Warren Grant Magnuson Clinical Center
National Institute of Health
9000 Rockville Pike
Bethesda, MD 20892   800-411-1222
                                      Fax: 301-480-9793
                                      TTY: 866-411-1010
                                 e-mail: prpl@mail.cc.nih.gov
                                      www.clinicalcenter.nih.gov
Established in 1953 as the research hospital of the National Institutes of Health. Designed so that patient care facilities are close to research laboratories so new findings of basic and clinical scientists can be quickly applied to the treatment of patients. Upon referral by physicians, patients are admitted to NIH clinical studies.
John Gallin, Director
David Henderson, Deputy Director for Clinical Care

Support Groups & Hotlines

5856 American Lung Association Help Line
American Lung Association
3000 Kelly Lane   217-787-5864
Springfield, IL 62711   800-586-4872
                                      Fax: 217-787-5916
                                           www.helpline.org
Provides information for the lung association of the state in which you make the call. Offers support group referrals.
Michael Mark, Lung Help Line Director

5857 Lung Facts
National Jewish Center for Immunology
1400 Jackson Street   303-388-4461
Denver, CO 80206   800-222-5864
                                      Fax: 303-270-2220
                                 e-mail: allstetterw@njc.org
                                           www.njc.org/
An automated information service with recorded health messages developed by Lung Line Information Service. The information provided on this system offers help and support, as well as medical updates for persons suffering from lung diseases.
Michael Salem MD, President/CEO
William Allstetter, Public Affairs/Media

5858 National Health Information Center
PO Box 1133   310-565-4167
Washington, DC 20013   800-336-4797
                                      Fax: 301-984-4256
                                      e-mail: info@nhic.org
                                           www.health.gov/nhic
Offers a nationwide information referral service, produces directories and resource guides.

Books

5859 American Lung Association Family Guide to Asthma and Allergies
American Lung Association
1740 Broadway   212-315-8700
New York, NY 10019-4315   e-mail: info@lungusa.org
                                           www.lungusa.org

5860 Health Consequences of Smoking: Cancer & Chronic Lung Disease in the Workplace
DIANE Publishing Company
330 Pusey Avenue, Unit #3 Rear   610-461-6200
Darby, PA 19023   800-782-3833
                                      Fax: 610-461-6130
                            e-mail: dianepublishing@gmail.com
                                           www.dianepublishing.net
Examines the relationship between cigarette smoking and occupational exposures. Establishes that in order to protect the workers fully, forces of labor, management, insurers and government must become as engaged in attempts to reduce the prevalence of cigarette smoking as they are in occupational exposure. Tables and figure. Extensive bibliography, index.
542 pages Paperback
ISBN: 0-788123-11-4
Herman Baron, Publisher

5861 Management of Acute Exacerbations of Chronic Obstructive Pulmonary Disease
DIANE Publishing Company
330 Pusey Avenue, Unit #3 Rear   610-461-6200
Darby, PA 19023   800-782-3833
                                      Fax: 610-461-6130
                            e-mail: dianepublishing@gmail.com
                                           www.dianepublishing.net
This report describes evidence about the clinical assessment and management of patients presenting with acute exacerbation of chronic obstructive pulmonary disease, a frequent cause of health care utilization, morality and decreased quality of life.
256 pages Paperback
ISBN: 0-756721-99-7
Herman Baron, Publisher

5862 Seven Steps to a Smoke-Free Life
American Lung Association
1740 Broadway   212-315-8700
New York, NY 10019-4315   e-mail: info@lungusa.org
                                           www.lungusa.org

Pamphlets

5863 Around the Clock with COPD
American Lung Association
1740 Broadway   212-315-8700
New York, NY 10019-4315   800-586-4872
                                 e-mail: info@lungusa.org
                                           www.lungusa.org
A booklet with non-medical helpful hints written by persons living with a chronic lung disease for others.

5864 Asbestos in Your Home
American Lung Association
1740 Broadway   212-315-8700
New York, NY 10019-4315   800-586-4872
Offers information on asbestos.

5865 Black Lung
National Jewish Center for Immunology

1400 Jackson Street 303-388-4461
Denver, CO 80206-2762 800-222-5864
Offers information on black lung and the respiratory system.

5866 Emphysema
American Lung Association of Connecticut
45 Ash Street 860-289-5401
East Hartford, CT 06108-3294 800-586-4872
Fax: 860-289-5405
www.alact.org
Offers information on who gets emphysema, how it attacks, causes, effects, prevention and treatment.
John E Zinn, President/CEO

5867 Exercise Guidelines for the Person with Lung Disease
American Lung Association of Connecticut
45 Ash Street 860-289-5401
East Hartford, CT 06108-3294 800-586-4872
Fax: 860-289-5405
www.alact.org
Offers exercise information and illustrations for persons with lung disease.
John E Zinn, President/CEO

5868 Facts About AAT Deficiency-Related Emphysema
American Lung Association
1740 Broadway 212-315-8700
New York, NY 10019-4315
Offers information on this type of emphysema, risk factors, development, symptoms and early detection.

5869 Facts About Asbestos
American Lung Association
1740 Broadway 212-315-8700
New York, NY 10019-4315
Offers information on lung hazards on the job and what employers can do to protect themselves and the people that work for them.

5870 Facts About Asthma
American Lung Association
1740 Broadway 212-315-8700
New York, NY 10019-4315 800-586-4872
Offers information on...

5871 Steps to a Better Understanding of Lung Cancer: A Patient and Family Guide
American Lung Association
1740 Broadway 212-315-8700
New York, NY 10019-4315 800-586-4872
e-mail: info@lungusa.org
www.lungusa.org
A booklet with non-medical helpful hints written by persons living with a chronic lung disease for others.

5872 Understanding Emphysema
National Jewish Center for Immunology
1400 Jackson Street 303-388-4461
Denver, CO 80206-2762 800-222-5864
Offers information on emphysema, causes, treatments, symptoms and prevention.

Audio & Video

5873 Keeping the Balance
Fanlight Productions
4196 Washington Street 617-469-4999
Boston, MA 02131-1731 800-937-4113
Fax: 617-469-3379
e-mail: fanlight@fanlight.com
www.fanlight.com
Siblings of children with serious lung disease share their experiences of being the normal child, exploring the frequent conflict between their feelings of love and concern and their resentment over the attention denied to them because of the sibling's illness. Offers advice on how parents can keep the balance between the needs of all of their children.
1993 23 Minutes
ISBN: 1-572950-89-7

5874 Sickle Cell Disease: Faces of Our Children
Fanlight Productions

4196 Washington Street 617-469-4999
Boston, MA 02131-1731 800-937-4113
Fax: 617-469-3379
e-mail: fanlight@fanlight.com
www.fanlight.com
This program examines the devastating impact of sickle cell disease on these young people and their families and caregivers. It will be an important tool for increasing awareness in the community and among healthcare and social service providers in community clinics, hospitals, and other settings.
1999 14 Minutes
ISBN: 1-572953-05-5

Web Sites

5875 American Lung Association
www.lungusa.org
Offers research, medical updates, fund-raising, educational materials and public awareness campaigns relating to lung disease causes.

5876 Healing Well
www.healingwell.com
An online health resource guide to medical news, chat, information and articles, newsgroups and message boards, books, disease-related web sites, medical directories, and more for patients, friends, and family coping with disabling diseases, disorders, or chronic illnesses.

5877 Health Central
www.healthcenter.com
Provides support group and diagnostic information regarding lung disease.

5878 Health Finder
www.healthfinder.gov
Searchable, carefully developed web site offering information on over 1000 topics. Developed by the US Department of Health and Human Services, the site can be used in both English and Spanish.

5879 Healthlink USA
www.healthlinkusa.com
Health information concerning treatment, cures, prevention, diagnosis, risk factors, research, support groups, email lists, personal stories and much more. Updated regularly.

5880 Helios Health
www.helioshealth.com
Online resource for your health information. Detailed information about specific health topics, access to expert advice from our Medical Advisory Board, and up-to-date health news.

5881 Lung Disease
www.lungusa.org
The American Lung Association's website, including information on diseases A to Z, living with lung disease, tobacco control, air quality, data, statistics, research, and more.

5882 MedicineNet
www.medicinenet.com
An online resource for consumers providing easy-to-read, authoritative medical and health information.

5883 Medscape
www.medscape.com
Medscape offers specialists, primary care physicians, and other health professionals the Web's most robust and integrated medical information and educational tools.

5884 National Heart, Lung & Blood Institute
www.nhlbi.nih.gov
A website maintained by the National Institute of Health offering general information regarding the heart, lungs, and blood.

5885 WebMD
www.webmd.com
Information on lung disease, including articles and resources.

431

Description

5886 Lupus Erythematosus

Lupus erythematosus refers to two distinct but overlapping conditions. Systemic lupus erythematosus, SLE, is a chronic multi-organ inflammatory illness that may involve the brain, skin, kidneys, joints, bowel, and eyes. Discoid lupus erythematosus, DLE, is a much less serious disease that is limited to the skin. In DLE, patches of skin may turn red and develop white scales, followed by thinning and scarring. About 10 percent of patients with DLE will go on to develop SLE; roughly 25 percent of patients with SLE also have the manifestations of DLE.

Of SLE cases, 90 percent are women, and the disease usually begins during the child-bearing years. Although the cause is unclear, SLE causes its damage through auto-immune mechanisms. The body's own immune system, designed to fight off invasion from micro-organisms, turns against its own tissues, evidence of which can be measured in the blood. Almost any organ system can be affected, and symptoms include fatigue, fever, loss of appetite, skin rash, sensitivity to light (photophobia), joint pain, headaches, personality change, eye irritation, and inflammation of the kidney.

In general, the course of SLE is chronic and relapsing, often with long periods (years) of remission. It may only be mild or progress towards more serious illness and death from infection, kidney failure, or neurologic damage. Survival has improved markedly in the past two decades because, for most patients with SLE, the disease can be controlled with large, prolonged doses of steroids, and other drugs that affect the immune system. Some of these therapies may be associated with long-term complications.

National Agencies & Associations

5887 American Juvenile Arthritis Organization (AJAO)
1330 West Peachtree Street   404-872-7100
Atlanta, GA 30309   800-283-7800
Fax: 440-872-9559
e-mail: help@arthritis.org
www.arthritis.org
A council of the Arthritis Foundation devoted to serving the special needs of children, teens and young adults with childhood rheumatic diseases (including systemic lupus erythematosus) and their families. Provides support groups, information, advocacy, research updates, and conferences.
Janet S Austin, PhD

5888 American Juvenile Arthritis Organization
1330 W Peachtree Street   404-872-7100
Atlanta, GA 30309   800-283-7800
Fax: 440-872-9559
e-mail: help@arthritis.org
www.arthritis.org
A council of the Arthritis Foundation devoted to serving the special needs of children teens and young adults with childhood rheumatic diseases (including systemic lupus erythematosus) and their families. Provides support groups, information and advocacy.
John H Klippel, President/CEO
Roberta K Byrum, Assistant Secretary

5889 Autoimmune Diseases Association
22100 Gratiot Avenue   586-776-3900
E Detroit, MI 48021   Fax: 586-776-3903
e-mail: aarda@aarda.org
www.aarda.org
Provides mutual support and education for patients with any type of autoimmune disease. Support includes advocacy referral to support groups literature and conferences.
Stanley M Finger PhD, Chairman of the Board
Noel R Rose MD PhD, Chairman Emeritus

5890 Lupus Foundation of America
2000 L Street NW   202-349-1155
Washington, DC 20036   800-558-0121
Fax: 202-349-1156
e-mail: info@lupus.org
www.lupus.org
The Lupus Foundation of America is the nation's leading non-profit voluntary health organization dedicated to finding the causes and cure for lupus. Our mission is to improve the diagnosis and treatment of lupus and support individuals and families affected by this disease.
Karen B Evans, Chair
Sandra C Raymond, President & CEO

5891 Lupus Network
230 Ranch Drive   203-372-5795
Bridgeport, CT 06606
Seeks to foster better understanding of the disease among patients and the general public educators and professionals through the distribution of educational materials.

State Agencies & Associations

Alabama

5892 Lupus Foundation of America: Alabama Chapter
4 Office Park Circle   205-870-0504
Birmingham, AL 35223

Alaska

5893 Lupus Foundation of America: Alaska Chapter
PO Box 240628   907-338-6332
Anchorage, AK 99524   800-307-5878
e-mail: LFA_Alaska@hotmail.com
www.geocities.com/lfa_alaska
Anna Tillman, Executive Director
Judy Powell, President

Arizona

5894 Lupus Foundation of America: Greater Arizona Chapter
2001 West Camelback Road   602-242-2213
Phoenix, AZ 85015-4908   e-mail: LupusAZ@aol.com
www.lupusarizona.org
Catherine Lamphier

5895 Lupus Foundation of America: Southern Arizona Chapter
2583 North 1st Avenue   520-622-9006
Tucson, AZ 85719
Sharon Smiley, Office Manager

Arkansas

5896 Lupus Foundation of America: Arkansas Chapter
220 Mockingbird   501-525-9380
Hot Springs, AR 71913   800-294-8878
e-mail: lupusarkhs@direclynx.net
www.lupus-arkansas.com

California

5897 Bay Area LE Foundation
2635 N 1st Street   408-954-8600
San Jose, CA 95134   800-523-3363
Chapter of the Lupus Foundation of America.

5898 **Lupus Foundation of America: San Diego/Imperial County Chapter**
PO Box 837 760-579-7744
El Cajon, CA 92022-0837

5899 **Lupus Foundation of America: Northern California Chapter**
2775 Cottage Way 916-973-0776
Sacramento, CA 95825 877-225-8787
Fax: 916-973-8124
e-mail: Saclupus@excite.com
www.saclupus.org

Cynthia L Holton, Executive Director Team
Stephanie Pringle-Fox, Executive Director Team

5900 **Lupus Foundation of America: Sacramento Chapter**
4200 Prospect Drive 916-973-0776
Carmichael, CA 95608-1941

5901 **Lupus Foundation of America: Southern California Chapter**
17985 Sky Park Circle 714-833-2121
Irvine, CA 92614 800-426-6026

Colorado

5902 **Lupus Foundation of Colorado**
1211 S Parker Road 303-597-4050
Denver, CO 80231 800-858-1292
Fax: 303-597-4054
e-mail: info@lupuscolorado.org
www.lupuscolorado.org
Chapter of the Lupus Foundation of America.
Skip Schlenk, CEO
Debbie Lynch, Director of Development

Connecticut

5903 **Lupus Foundation of America: Connecticut Chapter**
97 S Street 860-953-0387
W Hartford, CT 06110-2402 800-699-6967
e-mail: CTLFA@sbcglobal.net
www.lupusct.org
A non-profit organization and a National Health Agency established for the purpose of enlightening the public by focusing professional and public attention on Lupus Erythematosus promotes research by providing financial assistance and serves as the support bond for patients and their families.
Marilyn Sousa, Founder
Lisa Voglesong, President

Delaware

5904 **Lupus Foundation of America: Delaware Chapter**
PO Box 6391 302-622-8700
Wilmington, DE 19804 800-880-8686

Florida

5905 **Lupus Foundation of America: Northeast Florida Chapter**
PO Box 10486 904-645-8398
Jacksonville, FL 32247-0486 800-853-8398

5906 **Lupus Foundation of America: Northwest Florida Chapter**
PO Box 17841 904-444-7070
Pensacola, FL 32522-7841 800-458-8211
e-mail: info@lupus.pensacola.com
www.lupus.pensacola.com

Brenda Lee, President
Jon Kagan, Vice President

5907 **Lupus Foundation of America: Southeast Florida Chapter**
75 NE 6th Avenue 561-279-8606
Delray Beach, FL 33483 800-339-0586
Fax: 561-279-9772
e-mail: info@lupusfl.org
www.lupusfl.com

Claudia Kirk Barto, Executive Director
Kathleen Laca, Director of Operations

5908 **Lupus Foundation of America: Suncoast Chapter**
3637 4th Street N 727-447-7075
St Petersburg, FL 33704-7485 800-684-9276
Fax: 727-447-8925
e-mail: info@lupusflorida.org
www.lupusfl.com

Michael J Keefer, President/CEO
Maggi McQueen, Chairman

5909 **Lupus Foundation of America: Tampa Area Chapter**
Dibbs Plaza
4119-20A Gunn Highway 813-960-3992
Tampa, FL 33624 800-330-3992
www.milupus.org/southeast.htm

5910 **Lupus Foundation of Florida**
4406 Urban Court 727-447-7075
Orlando, FL 32810 800-684-9276
Fax: 727-447-7075
Chapter of the Lupus Foundation of America.

Georgia

5911 **Lupus Foundation of America: Columbus Chapter**
233 12th Street
Columbus, GA 31901 706-571-8950
www.milupus.org/southeast.htm

5912 **Lupus Foundation of America: Greater Atlanta Chapter**
340 Interstate North Parkway NW 404-952-3891
Atlanta, GA 30339-2203 800-800-4532

Hawaii

5913 **Hawaii Lupus Foundation**
1200 College Walk 808-538-1522
Honolulu, HI 96817 800-201-1522
Chapter of the Lupus Foundation of America.

Idaho

5914 **Lupus Foundation of America: Idaho Chapter**
4696 Overland Road
Boise, ID 83705-2864 208-343-4907
www.lupuswest.topcities.com

Illinois

5915 **Lupus Foundation of America: Illinois Chapter**
740 N Rush Street 312-542-0002
Chicago, IL 60611 800-258-7872
Fax: 312-255-8020
e-mail: charles@lupusil.org
www.lupusil.org
Offers support to individuals and families affected by Lupus, and looks to improve the diagnosis of and treatment of Lupus.
Charles Brummell, President & CEO
Mary Dollear, Vice President

Indiana

5916 **Lupus Foundation of America: Northeast Indiana Chapter**
5401 Keystone Drive 219-482-8205
Fort Wayne, IN 46825

5917 **Lupus Foundation of America: Northwest Indiana Lupus Chapter**
PO Box 2763 219-762-6575
Portage, IN 46368 800-948-8806
e-mail: lupusnwichapter@aol.com
www.lupusnwichapter.org

Tammie Largent, Director

5918 **Lupus Foundation of Indiana**
PO Box 51066
Indianapolis, IN 46251 317-858-9133
www.milupus.org/midwest.htm
Chapter of the Lupus Foundation of America.

Iowa

5919 Lupus Foundation of America: Iowa Chapter
PO Box 13174   515-279-3048
Des Moines, IA 50310-1044   888-279-3048
e-mail: info@lupusia.org
www.lupusia.org

Barb Hildebrandt, Executive Director
Braxton Pulley, Chair

Kansas

5920 Lupus Foundation of America: Kansas Chapter
PO Box 16094   316-262-6180
Wichita, KS 67216   e-mail: lupus@kansaslupus.org
www.kansaslupus.org

James Logue, President
Marilyn Rumsey, Treasurer

5921 Lupus Foundation of America: Kansas City
PO Box 12204   316-262-6180
Wichita, KS 67277   e-mail: lupus@kansaslupus.org
www.kansaslupus.org

Ruth Busch, President
Sandy Blaylock, Recording Secretary

Kentucky

5922 Lupus Foundation of Kentuckiana
1939 Goldsmith Lane   502-456-5265
Louisville, KY 40218   800-277-9681
www.milupus.org/southeast.htm
Chapter of the Lupus Foundation of America.

Louisiana

5923 Louisiana Lupus Foundation
7732 Goodwood Boulevard   225-927-8052
Baton Rouge, LA 70806   800-355-7473
www.milupus.org/southwest.htm
Chapter of the Lupus Foundation of America.

5924 Lupus Foundation of America: Cenla Chapter
PO Box 12565
Alexandria, LA 71315-2565   318-473-0125
www.lupus.org

5925 Lupus Foundation of America: Northeast Louisiana
102 Susan Drive   318-396-1333
West Monroe, LA 71291

5926 Lupus Foundation of America: Shreveport Chapter
6321 W Canal Boulevard
Shreveport, LA 71108   318-631-6531
www.lupus.org

Maine

5927 Lupus Group of Maine
PO Box 8168
Portland, ME 04104   207-878-8104
www.milupus.org/northeast.htm
Chapter of the Lupus Foundation of America.

Maryland

5928 Maryland Lupus Foundation
7400 York Road   410-337-9000
Baltimore, MD 21204   800-777-0934
Fax: 410-337-7406
e-mail: dwatson@lupusmd.org
www.lupusmd.org

Chapter of the Lupus Foundation of America.
Dick Watson, Executive Director
Jessica Gilbart, Health Education Coordinator

Massachusetts

5929 Lupus Foundation of America: Massachusetts Chapter
425 Watertown Street   617-332-9014
Newton, MA 02158   e-mail: info@lupusne.org
www.lupusmass.org

Elyse Smith, President
Lee McGraw, Board of Trustees Chair

Michigan

5930 Lupus Foundation of America: Michigan Lupus Foundation
26507 Harper Avenue   586-775-8310
Saint Clair Shores, MI 48081   800-705-6677
Fax: 586-775-8494
e-mail: info@milupus.org
www.milupus.org

Minnesota

5931 Lupus Foundation of America: Minnesota Chapter
2626 E 82nd Street   952-746-5151
Bloomington, MN 55425   800-645-1131
e-mail: info@lupusmn.org
www.lupusmn.org

Lynn Clarey, Chair
Chris McPartland, Chair Elect

Mississippi

5932 Lupus Foundation of America: Mississippi Chapter
PO Box 24292   601-366-5655
Jackson, MS 39225-4292   800-866-9606
www.milupus.org/southeast.htm

Missouri

5933 Lupus Foundation of America: Kansas City Chapter
6700 Troost   816-761-0850
Kansas City, MO 64131   866-761-0850
Fax: 816-361-0446
e-mail: info@lifewithlupus.org
www.lifewithlupus.org

5934 Lupus Foundation of America: Missouri Chapter
5701 Columbia Avenue   314-644-2222
Saint Louis, MO 63139   800-9LU-PUS6
e-mail: adminlupus@sbcglobal.net
www.lupusmo.org

Gina Banks, Chair
Necole Powell, Vice-Chair

5935 Lupus Foundation of America: Ozarks Chapter
3150 W Marty Street
Springfield, MO 65807   417-887-1560
www.lupus.org

Montana

5936 Lupus Foundation of America: Montana Chapter
29 1/2 Alderson
Billings, MT 59102   406-254-2082
www.lupus.org

Nebraska

5937 Lupus Foundation of America: Omaha Chapter
Community Health Plaza
7101 Newport Avenue
Omaha, NE 68152   402-572-3150
www.milupus.org/midwest.htm

5938 Lupus Foundation of America: Western Nebraska Chapter
HCR 72 Box 58   308-764-2474
Sutherland, NE 69165

Nevada

5939 Lupus Foundation of America: Las Vegas Chapter
1555 E Flamingo Suite 439
Las Vegas, NV 89119   702-369-0474
                                       www.lupus.org

5940 Lupus Foundation of America: Northern Nevada Chapter
1755 Vassar Street
Reno, NV 89502   702-323-2444
                                       www.lupus.org

New Hampshire

5941 New Hampshire Lupus Foundation
PO Box 444
Nashua, NH 03061-0444   603-424-0111
                                       www.milupus.org

Chapter of the Lupus Foundation of America.

New Jersey

5942 Lupus Foundation of America: New Jersey Chapter
150 Morris Avenue Suite 102   973-379-3226
Springfield, NJ 07081   800-322-5816
                                       Fax: 973-379-1053
                                       e-mail: info@lupusnj.org
                                       www.lupusnj.org

Dianna Beck-Clemens, Interim President and CEO
Adam Gold, Development Associate

5943 Lupus Foundation of America: South Jersey Chapter
One Greentree Center   856-988-5444
Marlton, NJ 08053   Fax: 856-596-8359
                                       e-mail: lupusinfo@sjlupus.org
                                       www.sjlupus.org

New Mexico

5944 Lupus Foundation of America: New Mexico Chapter
6001 Marble Avenue NE   505-881-9081
Albuquerque, NM 87110   800-843-9081
                                       e-mail: info@lupusnm.org
                                       www.lfanm.org

New York

5945 Lupus Alliance of America LIQ Affiliate
2255 Centre Avenue   516-783-3370
Bellmore, NY 11710   800-850-9000
                                       Fax: 516-826-2058
                                       e-mail: info@lupusliqueens.org
                                       www.lupusliqueens.org

JoAnn Quinn, Executive Director
Nancy Beder, Director of Resources

5946 Lupus Foundation of America: Bronx Chapter
PO Box 1117
Bronx, NY 10462   718-822-6542
                                       www.milupus.org/northeast.htm

5947 Lupus Foundation of America: Central New York Chapter
Pickard Office Building
5858 E Molloy Road   315-454-9886
Syracuse, NY 13211   e-mail: cnylupus@dreamscape.com
                                       www.milupus.org/northeast.htm

5948 Lupus Foundation of America: Genessee Valley Chapter
500 Helendale Road   585-288-2910
Rochester, NY 14609   Fax: 585-288-1608
                                       e-mail: lupusgvc@frontiernet.net
                                       www.lupusgvc.org

Eileen M Aman, President/CEO
Bob Stewart, Chairperson

5949 Lupus Foundation of America: Marguerite Curri Chapter
PO Box 139   315-829-4272
Utica, NY 13503   866-2LU-PUS4
                                       Fax: 315-829-4272
                                       e-mail: lupusmidny@aol.com
                                       www.nolupus.org

Kathleen A Arntsen, President/CEO
James E Mitchell Jr, Vice President

5950 Lupus Foundation of America: New York Southern Tier Chapter
PO Box 139   315-829-4272
Utica, NY 13503   866-2LU-PUS4
                                       Fax: 315-829-4272
                                       e-mail: lupusmidny@aol.com
                                       www.nolupus.org

Kathleen A Arntsen, President/CEO
James E Mitchell Jr, Vice President

5951 Lupus Foundation of America: Northeastern New York Chapter
1300 Piccard Drive   301-670-9292
Rockville, MD 20850-4303   800-558-0121
                                       Fax: 301-670-9486
                                       e-mail: nenylfa@aol.com
                                       nenylfa.tripod.com

5952 Lupus Foundation of America: Westchester
100 S Bedford Road   914-948-1032
Mt Kisco, NY 10549   888-57L-UPUS
                                       e-mail: pguidice@stellarishealth.org
                                       www.lupushudsonvalley.org

5953 Lupus Foundation of America: Western New York Chapter
3871 Harlem Road   716-835-7161
Cheektowaga, NY 14215   800-300-4198
                                       Fax: 716-835-7251
                                       e-mail: info@lupusupstateny.org
                                       www.lupusupstateny.org

5954 SLE Foundation
330 Seventh Avenue   212-685-4118
New York, NY 10001   800-74L-UPUS
                                       Fax: 212-545-1843
                                       e-mail: lupus@lupusny.org
                                       www.lupusny.org

Chapter of the Lupus Foundation of America.
Richard D DeScherer, President
Margaret G Dowd, Executive Director

North Carolina

5955 Lupus Foundation of America: Winston-Triad Lupus Chapter NCLF
2841 Foxwood Lane   910-768-1493
Winston Salem, NC 27103
Ruth Banbury, President

5956 Lupus Foundation of America: Charlotte Chapter
2540 Plantation Center Drive   704-849-8271
Matthews, NC 28105   877-849-8271
                                       Fax: 704-849-8272
                                       e-mail: info@lupuslinks.org
                                       www.lupuslinks.org

Christine M John, President/CEO
Ginger Dickerson, Chairman of the Board

5957 Lupus Foundation of America: Raleigh Chapter
5409 Belsay Drive
Raleigh, NC 27612   919-783-8288
                                       www.milupus.org/southeast.htm

Ohio

5958 Lupus Foundation of America: Akron Area Chapter
2769 Front Street   330-945-6767
Cuyahoga Falls, OH 44221   877-635-8787
                                       Fax: 330-945-5703
                                       www.lupus.org

Sharon Combs

5959 **Lupus Foundation of America: Columbus**
6119 E Main Street
Columbus, OH 43213   614-755-5077
Fax: 614-755-5066
e-mail: lupusoff@aol.com
www.lupusohio.org

Janice Washington, President
Melvyn Little, Chair of Public Relations

5960 **Lupus Foundation of America: Columbus, Marcy Zitron Chapter**
6161 Busch Boulevard   614-221-0811
Columbus, OH 43229

5961 **Lupus Foundation of America: Greater Cleveland Chapter**
12930 Chippewa Road   440-717-0183
Brecksville, OH 44141   Fax: 440-717-0186
e-mail: info@lupuscleveland.org
www.lupuscleveland.org

Suzanne Tierney, Executive Director
David Wonsetler, Counselor

5962 **Lupus Foundation of America: North Texas**
1800 N Blanchard Street   419-423-9313
Findlay, OH 45840   Fax: 419-423-5959
e-mail: info@lupusnwoh.org
www.lupus.org

Bob Scherger, President/CEO
Jackie Urbanski, VP Education & Volunteer Programs

5963 **Lupus Foundation of America: Northwest Ohio Lupus Chapter**
1710 Manor Hill Road   419-423-9313
Findlay, OH 45840   888-33L-UPUS
Fax: 419-423-5959
e-mail: info@lupusnwoh.org
www.lupusnwoh.org

Oklahoma

5964 **Oklahoma Lupus Association**
4100 N Lincoln Boulevard   405-427-8787
Oklahoma City, OK 73105   Fax: 405-427-8778
e-mail: oklupus@flash.net
www.oklupus.com

Chapter of the Lupus Foundation of America.
Katherine Scheirman, Vice Chairman
Janna D Hall, Chairman

Pennsylvania

5965 **Lupus Foundation of America: Central Pennsylvania Chapter**
Old Liberty Square
4813 Jonestown Road   717-671-9515
Harrisburg, PA 17109   e-mail: cplclfa@aol.com

5966 **Lupus Foundation of America: Northeast Pennsylvania Chapter**
615 Jefferson Avenue   570-558-2008
Scranton, PA 18510   888-995-8787
Fax: 570-558-2009
e-mail: neinfo@lupuspa.org
www.lupuspa.org

Beth Rundell MS, Branch Director
Cathy Wilcox, Patient Services Director

5967 **Lupus Foundation of America: Northwestern Pennsylvania Chapter**
PO Box 885   724-962-0368
Erie, PA 16512-0885   866-292-1472
Fax: 724-962-0368
e-mail: erieinfo@lupuspa.org
www.lupuspa.org

Jane Lippinc RN, Patient Services Consultant
Bill Trainor, Events Coordinator

5968 **Lupus Foundation of America: Philadelphia Tri-State Chapter**
500 Old York Road   215-517-5070
Jenkintown, PA 19046   866-517-5070
Fax: 215-517-8483
e-mail: info@lupustristate.org
www.lupustristate.org

Annette Myarick, CEO

5969 **Lupus Foundation of America: Western Pennsylvania Chapter**
Landmarks Building
100 West Station Square Drive   412-261-5886
Pittsburgh, PA 15219   800-800-5776
Fax: 412-261-5365
e-mail: info@lupuspa.org
www.lupuspa.org

Deborah Nigro, Executive Director
Barbara Hastings, RN, Patient Services Director

5970 **Lupus Foundation of Pennsylvania**
Landmarks Building
Pittsburgh, PA 15219   412-261-5886
Fax: 412-261-5365
e-mail: info@lupuspa.org
www.lupuspa.org

Deborah Nigro, Executive Director
Marian Belotti RN, Patient Services Director

5971 **Lupus Foundation of Philadelphia**
5415 Claridge Street   215-877-9061
Philadelphia, PA 19124
Chapter of the Lupus Foundation of America.

Rhode Island

5972 **Lupus Foundation of America: Rhode Island Chapter**
#8 Fallon Avenue
Providence, RI 02908   401-421-7227
www.milupus.org

South Carolina

5973 **Lupus Foundation of America: South Carolina Chapter**
L.E. Support Club
8039 Nova Court   843-764-1769
Charleston, SC 29420-8934   e-mail: hmeisic@awod.com
www.galaxymall.com/commerce/lupus

Tennessee

5974 **Lupus Foundation of America Memphis Area Chapter**
3181 Poplar Avenue   901-458-5320
Memphis, TN 38111   888-915-8787
Fax: 901-217-3193
e-mail: info@memphislupus.org
memphislupus.org

To educate and support those affected by lupus and to assist in finsing its cure. The goal is to unite and provide moral support and group strength for those individuals who are suspected of or diagnosed victims of Systemic Lupus Erythematosus and related disorders.
Yvonne D Nelson, Executive Director

5975 **Lupus Foundation of America: East Tennessee Chapter**
5612 Kingston Pike   615-584-5215
Knoxville, TN 37919   e-mail: lupustn@aol.com
www.lupus.org/chapters/southeastern.html

5976 **Lupus Foundation of America: Mid-South Area Chapter**
4004 Hillsboro Road   615-298-2273
Nashville, TN 37215   877-865-8787
Fax: 615-292-0520
e-mail: info@lupusmidsouth.org
www.lupustennessee.org

Sherry Hammond, Executive Director
Renee Levay Stewart, President

Texas

5977 **Lupus Foundation of America: North Texas Chapter**
15441 Knoll Trail   469-374-0590
Dallas, TX 75248   800-285-2369
Fax: 469-374-0794
e-mail: info@lupus-northtexas.org
www.lupus-northtexas.org

Tessie Holloway, President/CEO
Lisa Christensen, Development Director

5978 Lupus Foundation of America: South Central Texas Chapter
9330 Corporate Drive 210-651-9480
Selma, TX 78154 800-809-3953
e-mail: salupus@texas.net
www.milupus.org/southwest.htm

5979 Lupus Foundation of America: Texas Gulf Coast Chapter
3730 Kirby Drive 713-529-0126
Houston, TX 77098 800-458-7870
Fax: 713-529-0780
e-mail: info@lupustexas.org
www.lupustexas.org
Janice Gipson, President
Christine Smith, Vice President

5980 Lupus Foundation of America: West Texas Chapter
1717 Avenue K 806-744-6666
Lubbock, TX 79401 800-580-5878
e-mail: lfawesttx@juno.com
www.milupus.org/southwest.htm

Utah

5981 Lupus Foundation of America Utah Chapter
455 E 500 S 801-364-0366
Salt Lake City, UT 84111 800-657-6398
e-mail: info@utahlupus.org
www.utahlupus.org

Noelle Reymond, Executive Director
Katie Fillnow, President

Vermont

5982 Lupus Foundation of America: Vermont Chapter
57 S Main Street 802-244-5988
Waterbury, VT 05676 877-735-8787
e-mail: lupusvermont@myfairpoint.net
www.central-vt.com/web/lupus

Virginia

5983 Lupus Foundation of America: Central Virginia Chapter
PO Box 25418 804-262-9622
Richmond, VA 23260-5418

5984 Lupus Foundation of America: Eastern Virginia Chapter
Pembroke One
281 Independence Boulevard
Virginia Beach, VA 23462 757-490-2793
www.lupus.org

5985 Lupus Foundation of Greater Washington
2000 L Street NW 202-349-1167
Washington, DC 20036 888-349-1167
Fax: 202-223-1970
e-mail: info@lupusgw.org
www.lupusgw.org

Penelope C Fletcher, President
Sarah Guy, Executive Assistant

Washington

5986 Lupus Foundation of America: Pacific Northwest Chapter
1207 N 200th Street 206-546-6785
Shoreline, WA 98133 Fax: 206-546-8946
e-mail: lupus@lupuspnw.org
www.lupuspnw.org

Kathy Casey, Executive Director
Tonita Webb, President

Wisconsin

5987 Lupus Foundation of America: Wisconsin Chapter
1109 N Mayfair Road 414-443-6400
Milwaukee, WI 53226 866-LUP-USWI
Fax: 414-443-6400
e-mail: lupuswi@lupuswi.org
www.lupuswi.org

Sandra Hofstetter, Executive Director
Angela K Nelson, Chairman

Foundations

5988 SLE Lupus Foundation
330 Seventh Avenue 212-685-4118
New York, NY 10001 Fax: 212-545-1843
e-mail: lupus@lupusny.org
www.lupusny.org

The Foundation helps people with lupus, as well as their families and friends, cope with the anxieties and frustrations that often accompany daily living with a chronic illness. Sharing information and networking among patients and their families further helps dispel myths and provides daily support to those learning to live with lupus.
Richard K DeScherer, President
Margaret G Dowd, Executive Director

Research Centers

5989 Alliance for Lupus Research
28 W 44th Street 212-218-2840
New York, NY 10036 800-867-1743
e-mail: info@lupusresearch.org
www.lupusresearch.org
Research foundation dedicated to providing information about lupus.

5990 Hahnemann University Lupus Study Center Hahnemann University Medical Center
Hahnemann University Medical Center
Broad and Vine Street 215-762-7000
Philadelphia, PA 19102 Fax: 215-762-8109
www.hahnemannhospital.com
Raphael J Dehoratius, Director

5991 Terri Gotthelf Lupus Research Institute
3 Duke Place 800-828-87
S Norwalk, CT 06854 Fax: 203-852-9720
Founded to help millions of lupus victims in the world and to encourage coordinate and direct future progress in the etiology diagnosis and treatment of this disease.
Theodore Gotthelf, President

Support Groups & Hotlines

5992 National Health Information Center
PO Box 1133 310-565-4167
Washington, DC 20013 800-336-4797
Fax: 301-984-4256
e-mail: info@nhic.org
www.health.gov/nhic

Offers a nationwide information referral service, produces directories and resource guides.

Books

5993 Coping with Lupus
Lupus Foundation of America
1300 Piccard Drive 301-670-9292
Rockville, MD 20850-4303 800-558-0121
www.lupus.org

A practicing psychologist offers sound, meaningful and compassionate advice to individuals who must deal with lupus.
276 pages Paperback
ISBN: 0-895294-75-3

5994 Disability Workbook for Social Security Disability Applicants
Lupus Foundation of America
1300 Piccard Drive 301-670-9292
Rockville, MD 20850-4303 800-558-0121
www.lupus.org

Helps people get their disability benefits promptly, without unnecessary appeals. Tells what you have to prove and how to prove it.
137 pages

5995 Get to Sleep! How to Sleep Well...Despite Lupus
Lupus Foundation of America

1300 Piccard Drive 301-670-9292
Rockville, MD 20850-4303 800-558-0121
Written in a simple, straightforward style, this easy-to-follow action guide teaches you the most effective strategies for enabling you to get the sleep you want and need!
17 pages

5996 Lupus Book
Lupus Foundation of America
1300 Piccard Drive 301-670-9292
Rockville, MD 20850-4303 800-558-0121
Packed with useful, easy-to-understand information and practical guidance for people with lupus, their family members, friends and physicians. This hardcover book explains virtually every aspect of the disease and will help people better manage their day-to-day fight with lupus.

ISBN: 0-195084-43-8

5997 Lupus Erythematosus: A Handbook for Physicians, Patients & Families
Lupus Foundation of America
1300 Piccard Drive 301-670-9292
Rockville, MD 20850-4303 800-558-0121
www.lupus.org
Written for physicians, people with lupus, their families and friends, this is LFA's most popular publication. The handbook provides a brief, but detailed, overview of the disease and guide for living well with lupus.
60 pages

5998 Lupus: Everything You Need to Know
Lupus Foundation of America
1300 Piccard Drive 301-670-9292
Rockville, MD 20850-4303 800-558-0121
e-mail: lupusinfo@aol.com
www.lupus.org
Resource written for patients that want to learn more about lupus than what their doctors may or may not tell them.
236 pages

5999 Sick and Tired of Feeling Sick and Tired
Lupus Foundation of America
1300 Piccard Drive 301-670-9292
Rockville, MD 20850-4303 800-558-0121
www.lupus.org
Written in simple terms, the authors offer all readers- people with invisible chronic illness (ICI's), spouses, friends, family members, employers or health care providers, both understanding and practical guidance. This is a very useful resource for all those who live with ICI's and those who care for and about them.
288 pages

6000 We Are Not Alone: Learning to Live with Chronic Illness
Lupus Foundation of America
1300 Piccard Drive 301-670-9292
Rockville, MD 20850-4303 800-558-0121
www.lupus.org
Complete and comprehensive, this book is about redesigning your life... about how to live better, not just differently.
335 pages

Children's Books

6001 Embracing the Wolf: A Lupus Victim and Her Family Learn to Live
Cherokee Publishing Company
PO Box 1730 770-438-7366
Marietta, GA 30061-1730 800-653-3952
This book gives a very detailed account of the effects of the disease that include emotions and moods for the victim and the way in which these attributes affect loved ones.
192 pages Hardcover
ISBN: 0-877971-66-8
Kenneth W Boyd, Publisher

6002 In Search of the Sun: A Woman's Courageous Victory Over Lupus
Scribner

866 3rd Avenue 212-702-2000
New York, NY 10022-6221 800-257-5755
This book is a revision of Henrietta Aladjem's book, The Sun Is My Enemy. In this book, with Peter Schur she discusses her fight with this deadly and widespread disease.
Grades 10-12

6003 When Mom Gets Sick
Lupus Foundation of America
1300 Piccard Drive 301-670-9292
Rockville, MD 20850-4303 800-558-0121
www.lupus.org
Written and illustrated by a 9-year-old, this is a compelling story based on the experiences of a sensitive and insightful young girl who makes the best from what could be a devastating situation.
27 pages

Newsletters

6004 Heliogram
Lupus Network
230 Ranch Drive
Bridgeport, CT 06606-1747 203-372-5795
Includes book reviews, medical abstracts and resource listings of physicians.
Quarterly
ISBN: 0-887168-0 -
Linda Rosinsky, Editor

6005 Informer
Simon Foundation
PO Box 815 847-864-3913
Wilmette, IL 60091-0815 Fax: 847-864-9758
Offers information and the latest updates concerning incontinence treatments, cures, medical aspects, resources and more.
Quarterly

6006 Lupus Foundation of America Memphis Area Chapter Newsletter
Lupus Foundation of America Memphis Area Chapter
3181 Poplar Avenue 901-458-5320
Memphis, TN 38111 888-915-8787
Fax: 901-217-3193
e-mail: info@memphislupus.org
memphislupus.org

Monthly
Yvonne D Nelson, Executive Director

6007 Lupus News
Lupus Foundation of America
1300 Piccard Drive 301-670-9292
Rockville, MD 20850-4303 800-558-0121
Provides detailed news for physicians, patients, their families and friends on lupus.
Quarterly

6008 Pennsylvania Lupus News
Lupus Foundation of Pennsylvania
Landmarks Building 412-261-5886
Pittsburgh, PA 15219 Fax: 412-261-5365
e-mail: info@lupuspa.org
www.lupuspa.org

Deborah Nigro, Executive Director
Marian Belotti RN, Patient Services Director

6009 The Loop
SLE Lupus Foundation
330 Seventh Avenue 212-685-4118
New York, NY 10001 Fax: 212-545-1843
e-mail: lupus@lupusny.org
www.lupusny.org

Richard K DeScherer, President
Margaret G Dowd, Executive Director

Pamphlets

6010 Control Your Pain!
Lupus Foundation of America

1300 Piccard Drive
Rockville, MD 20850-4303
301-670-9292
800-558-0121
www.lupus.org

This easy to read booklet offers 144 concrete strategies for reducing and managing the pain of lupus.
48 pages

6011 Facts About Lupus

Lupus Foundation of America
1300 Piccard Drive
Rockville, MD 20850-4303
301-670-9292
800-558-0121

A series of brochures on a wide range of lupus-related topics including lab tests, medications, joint and muscle involvement, skin involvement, lupus and the kidneys, central nervous system involvement, lupus in men, pregnancy, well/coping, etc.
21 Brochures

6012 Handout on Health: Systemic Lupus Erythematosus

NAMSIC/National Institutes of Health
1 AMS Circle
Bethesda, MD 20892-0001
301-495-4484
877-226-4267
Fax: 301-718-6366
TTY: 301-565-2966
e-mail: niamsinfo@mail.nih.gov
www.nih.gov/niams

6013 Living Well, Despite Lupus!

Lupus Foundation of America
1300 Piccard Drive
Rockville, MD 20850
301-670-9292
800-558-0121

This booklet offers 204 sure-fire strategies for taking charge of your life to enable you to live well.
1996 50 pages
ISBN: 0-895294-75-3

6014 Lupus Eritematoso (Spanish Booklet)

Lupus Foundation of America
1300 Piccard Drive
Rockville, MD 20850-4303
301-670-9292
800-558-0121
www.lupus.org

Written for physicians, people with lupus, their families and friends, this is LFA's most popular publication. The handbook provides a brief, but detailed, overview of the disease and guide for living well with lupus.

6015 Lupus Erythematosus

Lupus Foundation of America
1300 Piccard Drive
Rockville, MD 20850-4303
301-670-9292
800-558-0121
www.lupus.org/lupus

This booklet is intended to help patients understand what lupus is, how it may affect their lives and what they can do to help themselves and their physician in the management of the illness.

6016 Lupus Information Package

NAMSIC/National Institutes of Health
1 AMS Circle
Bethesda, MD 20892-0001
301-495-4484
877-226-4267
Fax: 301-718-6366
TTY: 301-565-2966
e-mail: niamsinfo@mail.nih.gov
www.nih.gov/niams

6017 Many Shades of Lupus: Information for Multicultural Communities

NAMSIC/National Institutes of Health
1 AMS Circle
Bethesda, MD 20892-0001
301-495-4484
877-226-4267
Fax: 301-587-4352
TTY: 301-565-2966
e-mail: niamsinfo@mail.nih.gov
www.nih.gov/niams

Audio & Video

6018 For Life: More Stories of Lupus
Marcia Urbin Raymond, author

Fanlight Productions

4196 Washington Street
Boston, MA 02131
617-469-4999
800-937-4113
Fax: 617-469-3349
e-mail: fanlight@fanlight.com
www.fanlight.com

Three years after 'Stories of Lupus', the filmmaker revisits five people from the earlier film, to explore the day-to-day challenges and gifts that come to people living with a chronic illness as it evolves over time.
2002 53 Minutes
ISBN: 1-572954-17-5
Nicole Johnson, Publicity Coordinator

6019 Stories of Lupus

Fanlight Productions
4196 Washington Street
Boston, MA 02131
617-469-4999
800-937-4113
Fax: 617-469-3379
e-mail: fanlight@fanlight.com
www.fanlight.com

Recently diagnosed with lupus, the filmmakers go on the road to interview others enduring the precarious roller coaster of symptoms, treatment, flare-ups and recoveries which characterize this complex, mysterious, and often life-threatening disease.
1999 27 Minutes
ISBN: 1-572954-16-7
Nicole Johnson, Publicity Coordinator

Web Sites

6020 Healing Well

www.healingwell.com

An online health resource guide to medical news, chat, information and articles, newsgroups and message boards, books, disease-related web sites, medical directories, and more for patients, friends, and family coping with disabling diseases, disorders, or chronic illnesses.

6021 Health Finder

www.healthfinder.gov

Searchable, carefully developed web site offering information on over 1000 topics. Developed by the US Department of Health and Human Services, the site can be used in both English and Spanish.

6022 Healthlink USA

www.healthlinkusa.com

Health information concerning treatment, cures, prevention, diagnosis, risk factors, research, support groups, email lists, personal stories and much more. Updated regularly.

6023 Helios Health

www.helioshealth.com

Online resource for your health information. Detailed information about specific health topics, access to expert advice from our Medical Advisory Board, and up-to-date health news.

6024 Lupus Foundation of America

www.lupus.org

The LFA mission is to assist local chapters in their efforts to provide supportive services to individuals living with lupus, educate the public about lupus, and supports research into the cause and cure of lupus.

6025 MedicineNet

www.medicinenet.com

An online resource for consumers providing easy-to-read, authoritative medical and health information.

6026 Medscape

www.medscape.com

Medscape offers specialists, primary care physicians, and other health professionals the Web's most robust and integrated medical information and educational tools.

6027 WebMD

www.webmd.com

Information on Lupus Erythematosus, including articles and resources.

Description

6028 Mental Illness/General

Mental illness includes disorders of mood, thinking and behavior, with psychiatry being the branch of medicine responsible for their study, diagnosis, treatment, and prevention. Mental illness may be determined by genetic, physical, chemical, psychological, and social factors. Mental or emotional illness includes such conditions as major depression, schizophrenia, bipolar disorder (i.e., manic depression), panic and other anxiety disorders, substance abuse and dependence, and dementia and other cognitive disorders.

Psychiatric diagnoses generally are based on criteria outlined in *Diagnostic and Statistical Manual of Mental Disorders* (DSM-IV), published by the American Psychiatric Association. DSM-V, due out in May 2013, is thought by many to be one of the most anticipated events in the mental health field. Depending on the specific diagnosis, treatment can include medication, counseling, behavior modification, psychotherapy, and modification of the patient's environment. See also *Mental Illness/Depression* and *Mental Illness/Schizophrenia*.

National Agencies & Associations

6029 Action Autonomie
1260 Ste-Cataherine E #208
Montreal, Quebec, H2L-2H2   514-525-5060
                           Fax: 514-525-5580
e-mail: lecollectif@actionautonomie.qc.ca
www.actionautonomie.qc.ca
Community organization set up by people living or having lived with mental health problems who believed in the necessity of uniting their efforts collectively in order to defend their rights.

6030 American Academy of Child & Adolescent Psychiatry
3615 Wisconsin Avenue NW   202-966-7300
Washington, DC 20016   Fax: 202-966-2891
e-mail: communications@aacap.org
www.aacap.org
A professional organization that represents 7 500 child and adolescent psychiatrists that actively research diagnose and treat psychiatric and mental illness disorders in children and adolescents.
Robert Hendren, President

6031 American Association of Children's Residential Centers
11700 W Lake Park Drive   877-332-2272
Milwaukee, WI 53224   Fax: 877-36A-ACRC
e-mail: info@aacrc-dc.org
www.aacrc-dc.org
Brings professionals together to advance the frontiers of knowledge pertaining to the spectrum of therapeutic living environments for adolescents with behavioral health disorders.
Steven Elson, President
Richard Altman, Secretary

6032 American Association on Mental Retardation
444 N Capitol Street NW   202-387-1968
Washington, DC 20001-1512   800-424-3688
                           Fax: 202-387-2193
www.aamr.org
Promotes progressive policies sound research effective practices and universal human rights for people with intellectual and developmental disabilities.
Steve M Eidelman, President
Doreen M Croser, Executive Director

6033 American Psychiatric Association
1000 Wilson Boulevard   703-907-7300
Arlington, VA 22209-3901   888-357-7924
e-mail: apa@psych.org
www.psych.org
Works to promote the best interest of patients and those actually or potentially making use of psychiatric services.

6034 American Psychological Association
750 1st Street NE   202-336-5500
Washington, DC 20002-4242   800-374-2721
TTY: 202-336-6123
e-mail: practice@apa.org
www.apa.org
A scientific and professional organization the represents psychology in the United States. The largest association of psychologists worldwide.
James H Bray, President

6035 Calgary Association of Self Help
1019-7th Avenue SW   403-266-8711
Calgary, Alberta, T2P-1A8   Fax: 403-266-2478
e-mail: info@calgaryselfhelp.com
www.calgaryselfhelp.com
Calgary Association of Self Help have been assisting people with a mental illness to live full lives within our community since 1973.
Marion McGrath, CEO
Anneisa Lauchlan, COO

6036 Canadian Federation of Mental Health Nurse s
1185 Eglinton Avenue E   416-426-7029
Toronto, Ontario, M3C-3C6   Fax: 416-426-7280
e-mail: info@cfmhn.ca
www.cfmhn.ca
A national voice for psychiatric and mental health (PMH) nursing.
Chris Davis, President

6037 Canadian Mental Health Association
180 Dundas Street W   416-484-7750
Toronto, Ontario, M5G-1Z8   Fax: 416-484-4617
e-mail: info@cmha.ca
www.cmha.ca
Promotes the mental health of all and supports the resilience and recovery of people experiencing mental illness.
Glenn Thompson, CEO
Christine Saracino, Director Finance

6038 Center for Mental Health Services: Knowledge Exchange Network
PO Box 42557
Washington, DC 20015   800-789-2647
                           Fax: 240-221-4295
                           TTY: 866-889-2647
                           TDD: 866-889-2647
e-mail: ken@mentalhealth.org
www.mentalhealth.org
Goal is to provide the treatment and support services needed by adults with mental disorders and children with serious emotional problems.
A Kathryn Power MEd, Director
Jeffrey A Buck PhD, Branch Chief

6039 Coalition of Voluntary Mental Health Agencies
90 Broad Street   212-742-1600
New York, NY 10014   Fax: 212-742-2080
e-mail: mailbox@cvmha.org
www.coalitionny.org
An umbrella advocacy organization of New York's mental health community representing over 100 non-profit community health agencies that serve more than 300 000 clients in the five boroughs of New York City and its environs.
Peter Campan PsyD, Past President
Donna Colonna, Vice President

6040 Community Access
666 Broadway   212-780-1400
New York, NY 10012   Fax: 212-780-1412
e-mail: info@communityaccess.org
www.cairn.org

A nonprofit agency providing housing and advocacy for people with psychiatric disabilities.
Stephen Chase, President
Karen Roth, Vice President

6041 Federation of Families for Children's Mental Health
1101 King Street   703-684-7710
Alexandria, VA 22314   Fax: 703-836-1040
e-mail: ffcmh@ffchm.org
www.ffcmh.org
Provides leadership to develop and sustain a nationwide network of family-run organizations.
Sandra Spencer, Executive Director
Marion Mealing, Administrative Assistant

6042 Mental Health America
2000 N Beauregard Street   703-684-7722
Alexandria, VA 22311   800-969-6642
Fax: 703-684-5968
TTY: 800-433-5959
e-mail: infoctr@mentalhealthamerica.net
www.mentalhealthamerica.net
Mental Health America (formerly National Mental Health Association) is dedicated to helping all people live mentally healthier lives. With our more than 320 affiliates nationwide, we represent a growing movement of Americans who promote mental health.
340+ Members
David L Shern PhD, President/CEO
Eileen Sexton, Vice President Communications

6043 Mental Health America (formerly NMHA) Resource Center
2000 North Beauregard Street   703-684-7722
Alexandria, VA 22311   800-969-6642
Fax: 703-684-5968
TTY: 800-433-5959
e-mail: www.mentalhealthamerica.net/help/index.c
www.nmha.org
The NMHA publishes pamphlets and booklets on many aspects of mental health and mental illnesses. Topics include children and families, recovery, doctor/patient communication, mental health policy, culturally competent services, teen suicide, coping, schizphrenia, stress, depression and many others.
340+ Members

6044 National Alliance for the Mentally Ill
Colonial Place Three
2107 Wilson Boulevard   703-524-7600
Arlington, VA 22201-3042   800-950-6264
Fax: 703-524-9094
TDD: 703-516-7227
e-mail: bbc@naimi.org
www.nami.org
The leading self-help organization for families and friends of those suffering from serious mental illnesses and those persons themselves. Over 900 affiliate groups nationwide offer support to members, advocate better lives for their loved ones, support research efforts and educate the public to reduce the stigma attached to serious mental illnesses.
Bob Carolla, Director Communications

6045 National Association of State Mental Health Program Directors
66 Canal Center Plaza   703-739-9333
Alexandria, VA 22314   Fax: 703-548-9517
e-mail: webmaster@nasmhpd.org
www.nasmhpd.org
Offers referrals to state mental health programs services and physicians for persons with mental illness.
Virginia Tro Betts, President
James S Reinhard, Vice President

6046 National Association of Therapeutic Wilderness Camps
437 William Avenue Suite 5
Davis, WV 26260   e-mail: natwc@gcol.net
www.natwc.org
Represents nearly fifty therapeutic wilderness camps located all over the US. We believe therapeutic wilderness camps represent the most effective method to help troubled young people change the way they deal with their parents, school and other authorities.
Rick McClintock, Executive Director

6047 National Council for Community Behavior Healthcare
12300 Twinbrook Parkway   301-984-6200
Rockville, MD 20852   Fax: 301-881-7159
e-mail: lindar@thenationalcouncil.org
www.thenationalcouncil.org
Represents community mental health centers working on Capitol Hill to ensure funding for community mental health services. Offers technical support and guidance and serves as a liaison with state organizations and other mental health related organizations.
Linda Rosenb MSW CSW, President/ CEO
Jeannie Campbell, Executive Vice President

6048 National Hispanic Coalition of Health and Human Service Organizations
1501 16th Street NW   202-387-5000
Washington, DC 20036   Fax: 202-265-8027
e-mail: alliance@hispanichealth.org
www.hispanichealth.org
Members are Spanish-speaking mental health professionals and patients and those interested in the special emotional needs of Hispanics.
Jane L Delgado PhD, President
Adolph Falcon, Vice President for Science and Policy

6049 National Institute of Mental Health
6001 Executive Boulevard   301-443-4513
Bethesda, MD 20892-9663   866-615-6464
Fax: 301-443-4279
TTY: 301-443-8431
e-mail: nimhinfo@nih.gov
www.nimh.nih.gov
A federal agency that supports research nationwide on mental illness and mental health. The Institute provides research, demonstrations and technical assistance concerning the housing and service needs of the homeless mentally ill population.
Thomas R Insel MD, Director
Aleisha S James, Grants Management Specialist (AFP)

6050 National Mental Health Services Knowledge Exchange Network
PO Box 42557
Washington, DC 20015   800-789-2647
Fax: 240-747-5470
TTY: 866-889-2647
TDD: 866-889-2647
e-mail: nmhic-info@samhsa.hhs.gov
www.mentalhealth.org
The National Mental Health Information Center was developed for users of mental health services and their families, the general public, policy makers, providers and the media.
A Kathryn Power MEd, Director
Edward B Searle, Deputy Director

6051 National Network for Mental Health (NNMH) s
55 King Street   905-682-2423
St. Catharines, Ontario, L2R-3H5   888-406-4663
Fax: 905-682-7469
e-mail: info@nnmh.ca
www.nnmh.ca
Network with Canadian consumer/survivors and family and friends of consumer/survivors to provide opportunities for resource sharing, information distribution and education on mental health issues.
Roy Muise, President
Joan Edwards-Karmazyn, VP

6052 Obsessive Compulsive Information Center Dean Foundation
Dean Foundation
7617 Mineral Point Road   608-827-2470
Madison, WI 53717-1914   Fax: 608-827-2479
e-mail: mim@miminc.org
www.miminc.org
Provides access to published literature on obsessive compulsive disorder certain obsessive compulsive spectrum disorders and their treatments.

6053 Option Istitute Learning and Training Center
2080 S. Undermountain Road 413-229-2100
Sheffield, MA 01257 800-714-2779
Fax: 413-229-8931
e-mail: happiness@option.org
www.option.org
As the worldwide teaching center for the Option Process(R). The Option Institute offers empowering personal growth programs and seminars using life-changing experiential learning techniques that help people overcome adversity, maximize their success and happiness and greatly improve their health, career, relationships and quality of life.
Zoe

6054 Texas Mining and Reclamation Association
100 Congress Avenue 512-236-2325
Austin, TX 78701 Fax: 512-236-2002
e-mail: information@tmra.com
www.tmra.com
Serves as a unified voice for mental health patients in consumer social and political affairs. Helps members to live outside a hospital setting by providing assistance in the areas of resocialization, employment and housing.
Mark Pelizza, Chairman
Mike Kezar, Vice Chair

6055 World Federation for Mental Health
12940 Harbor Drive 703-494-6515
Woodbridge, VA 22192 Fax: 703-494-6518
e-mail: info@wfmh.com
www.wfmh.com
WFMH is an international membership organization founded in 1948 to advance among all peoples and nations the prevention of mental and emotional disorders the proper treatment and care of those with such disorders and the promotion of mental health.
Tony Fowke, President
Dr Vijay Ganju, CEO

State Agencies & Associations

Alabama

6056 National Alliance on Mental Illness of Alabama: NAMI Alabama
4122 Wall Street 334-396-4797
Montgomery, AL 36106-1902 800-626-4199
Fax: 334-396-4794
e-mail: Terri@NAMIAlabama.org
www.namialabama.org
James Walsh, President
Terri Beasley, Executive Director

Alaska

6057 National Alliance on Mental Illness of Alaska
144 W 15th Avenue 907-277-1300
Anchorage, AK 99501-5106 Fax: 907-277-1400
e-mail: trishmcd@nami.org
www.nami.org/sites/alaska
Trish McDonald, Program/Education Director
Beth LaCrosse, Treasurer

Arizona

6058 Mentally Ill Kids In Distress
2642 E Thomas Road 602-253-1240
Phoenix, AZ 85016-2723 800-35M-IKID
Fax: 602-253-1250
e-mail: Phoenix@MIKID.org
www.mikid.org
Vicki Johnso MA, Executive Director
Steve Carter, President

6059 Mentally Ill Kids in Distress Sue Gilbertson
Sue Gilbertson

2642 E Thomas Road 602-253-1240
Phoenix, AZ 85016 800-35M-IKID
Fax: 602-253-1250
e-mail: Phoenix@MIKID.org
www.mikid.org
Vicki Johnso MA, Executive Director
Steve Carter, President

6060 National Alliance on Mental Illness of Arizona
2210 N 7th Street 602-244-8166
Phoenix, AZ 85006-1604 Fax: 602-244-9264
e-mail: namiaz@namiaz.org
www.namiaz.org
Provides emotional support education and advocacy to persons of all ages who are affected by serious mental illnesses. Supports research to find a cure.
Robert Hess, Executive Director
Cheryl Fanning, President

6061 Navaho Nation K'E Project: Tuba City Children & Families Advocacy Corp
PO Box 3937 520-283-5415
Tuba City, AZ 86045 Fax: 520-283-5413
Rueben McCabe

6062 Navaho Nation K'E Project: Winslow Children & Families Advocacy Corp
HC 63 Box E 520-657-3234
Winslow, AZ 86047 Fax: 520-657-3207
Jayne Clark

Arkansas

6063 Arkansas FFCMH Jane Burgan
Jane Burgan
PO Box 56667 501-374-7218
Little Rock, AR 72215-4023 Fax: 501-374-2711
e-mail: pammarshall7218@sbcglobal.net
www.ffcmh.org

6064 NAMI Arkansas
1012 Autumn Road 501-661-1548
Little Rock, AR 72211-2222 800-844-0381
Fax: 501-312-7540
e-mail: karnold@nami.org
www.nami.org
Grassroots organization that focuses on improving mental health services. The mission is three prong: Support, Education, and Advocacy. Support Group meetings are held at 11 locations across the state.
Rick Owen, President
Kim Arnold, Executive Director

California

6065 NAMI California
1010 Hurley Way 916-567-0163
Sacramento, CA 95825-3218 Fax: 916-567-1757
e-mail: support@namicalifornia.org
www.namicalifornia.org
Brenda Scott, First Vice President
Karen H Henry, President

6066 United Advocates for Children of California
2035 Hurley Way 916-643-1530
Sacramento, CA 95825 866-643-1530
Fax: 916-643-1592
e-mail: sduval@uacf4hope.org
www.uacf4hope.org
Oscar Wright, Chief Executive Officer
Poppy Johal, Chief Officer of Strategic Planning

Colorado

6067 **Colorado FFCMH**
2950 Tennyson Street 303-572-0302
Denver, CO 80212 888-569-7500
Fax: 303-433-1605
e-mail: tdillingham@coloradofederation.org
www.coloradofederation.org

Tom Dillingham, Executive Director
Margie Grimsley, Technical Assistance Coordinator

6068 **FFCMH: Denver/Aurora Chapter**
12485 E 13th Avenue 303-343-1019
Aurora, CO 80011 Fax: 720-859-9367
e-mail: **ffcmhda@comcast.net

Carmen Held
Debra White

6069 **National Alliance for the Mentally Ill of Colorado**
1100 Fillmore Street 303-321-3104
Denver, CO 80206-3334 888-566-6264
Fax: 303-321-0912
e-mail: nami-co@nami.org
www.namicolorado.org

The National Alliance for the Mentally Ill Of Colorado is a state-wide, grassroots, nonprofit organization whose mission is; To give strength and hope to individuals with mental illness and their families.

Henry Mohr, President
Carol Reynolds, Executive Director

6070 **No. Colorado FFCMH**
1400 White Peak Court 970-223-3036
Fort Collins, CO 80525 Fax: 303-377-0245
e-mail: thefeds@attbi.com
www.ffcmh.org

Connecticut

6071 **Families United For CMH, Inc.**
PO Box 151 860-537-6125
New London, CT 06320 Fax: 860-537-6130
e-mail: **ctfamiliesunited@sbcglobal.net
www.familiesunited.org

Morgan Meltz

6072 **National Alliance for the Mentally Ill of Connecticut**
30 Jordan Lane 860-882-0236
Wethersfield, CT 06109 800-215-3021
Fax: 860-882-0240
e-mail: namicted@namict.org
www.namict.org

Robert Correll, President
Sheila King, Executive Director

Delaware

6073 **Alliance for the Mentally Ill in Delaware (AMID)**
2400 W 4th Street 302-427-0787
Wilmington, DE 19805-3306 888-427-2643
Fax: 302-427-2075
e-mail: namide@namide.org
www.namide.org

Julius Meisel, President
Ken Singleton, Executive Director

6074 **Delaware FFMCH**
19 Baltusrol Court 302-730-0325
Dover, DE 19904 866-994-0000
Fax: 302-730-8952
e-mail: marags1@aol.com
www.ffcmh.org

Earline Jackson, Executive Director

6075 **Mental Health Association of Delaware**
100 W 10th Street 302-654-6833
Wilmington, DE 19801 800-287-6423
Fax: 302-654-6838
e-mail: information@mhainde.org
www.mhainde.org

Laurie McArthur, Director Development/Communications

District of Columbia

6076 **DC Threshold Alliance for the Mentally Ill**
422 8th Street SE 202-546-0646
Washington, DC 20003-2832 Fax: 202-546-6817
e-mail: namidc@juno.com
www.nami.org

Adrian Green, President

6077 **Family Advocacy and Support Association**
PO Box 74884 202-234-2325
Washington, DC 20056 Fax: 202-576-7154
Lynne M Smith

Florida

6078 **Career Assessment & Planning Services Goodwill Industries-Suncoast**
Goodwill Industries-Suncoast
10596 Gandy Boulevard 727-523-1512
St Petersburg, FL 33702 888-279-1988
Fax: 727-579-0850
e-mail: gw.marketing@goodwill-suncoast.com
www.goodwill-suncoast.org

Provides a comprehensive assessment, which can predict current and future employment and potential adjustment factors for physically, emotionally or developmentally disabled persons who may be unemployed or underemployed.

Martin W Gladysz, Chair
R Lee Waits, President

6079 **Florida Alliance for the Mentally Ill**
316 E Park Avenue 850-671-4445
Tallahassee, FL 32301-2646 877-626-4352
Fax: 850-671-5272
e-mail: namifl@namifl.org
www.nami.org

Marcia Mathes, President
Judith Evans, Executive Director

6080 **Florida FFCMH: Tampa Chapter**
13301 Bruce B Downs Boulevard 813-974-7930
Tampa, FL 33612 Fax: 813-974-7712
e-mail: ffcmh@earthlink.net
www.federationoffamilies.org

Linda M Callejas, Board of Director
Albert J Duchnowski, Board of Director

6081 **Suncoast Residential Training Center/Developmental Services Program**
Goodwill Industries-Suncoast
10596 Gandy Boulevard 727-523-1512
St. Petersburg, FL 33733 888-279-1988
Fax: 727-577-2749
e-mail: gw.marketing@goodwill-suncoast.com
www.goodwill-suncoast.org

A large group home which serves individuals diagnosed as mentally retarded with a secondary diagnosed of psychiatric difficulties as evidenced by problem behavior. Providing residential, behavioral and instructional support and services that will promote the development of adaptive, socially appropriate behavior, each individual is assessed to determine strecths and needs in such skill areas as self-care, daily living, human growth and development, socialization, basic academics and recreation.

Martin W Gladysz, Chair
R Lee Waits, President/CEO

Georgia

6082 **Georgia Alliance for the Mentally Ill**
3050 Presidential Drive 770-234-0855
Atlanta, GA 30340-3916 800-728-1052
Fax: 770-234-0237
e-mail: nami-ga@nami.org
www.namiga.org

Nora Haynes, President
Eric Spencer, Executive Director

Hawaii

6083 NAMI: The Local Affiliate of the National Alliance for the Mentally Ill
85-175 Farrington Highway   808-591-1297
Waianae, HI 96792-2025   Fax: 808-591-2058
e-mail: namihawaii@hawaiiantel.net
namihawaii.org
Members include consumers families health professionals and interested persons/organizations. Programs include advocacy support and education and are free and open to the public. Office has lending library of books and videos. Newsletter is published.
6 pages Quarterly
Marion Poirier, Executive Director
Mike Durant, President

Idaho

6084 FFCMH: Idaho Chapter
1509 S Robert Street   208-433-8845
Boise, ID 83705   800-905-3436
Fax: 208-433-8337
e-mail: info@idahofederation.org
www.idahofederation.org
Courtney Lester, Administrative Director
Lacey Sinn, Development Director

6085 Idaho Alliance for the Mentally Ill
362 W Street   208-673-6672
Albion, ID 83311-0068   800-572-9940
Fax: 208-673-6685
e-mail: namiid@atcnet.ne
www.nami.org
President, President
Lee Woodland, Executive Director

Illinois

6086 Illinois Alliance for the Mentally Ill
218 W Lawrence Avenue   217-522-1403
Springfield, IL 62704-2612   800-346-4572
Fax: 217-522-3598
e-mail: namiil@sbcglobal.net
il.nami.org
Doug Call, President
Lora Thomas, Executive Director

6087 Illinois Federation of Families
PO Box 413   847-265-0500
McHenry, IL 60051   800-871-8400
Fax: 847-265-0501
e-mail: iffcmh@msn.com
www.iffcmh.net
Cynthia Sheppard, Executive Director

Indiana

6088 FFCMH: Indiana Chapter
2205 Costello Drive   765-643-4357
Anderson, IN 46011   Fax: 765-643-4357
e-mail: Indianafedfam@insightbb.com
www.ffcmh.org
Brenda Hamilton

6089 Family Action Network
214 W 2nd Street   765-643-4357
Anderson, IN 46016-2206
Brenda Hamilton

6090 NAMI Indiana
PO Box 22697   317-925-9399
Indianapolis, IN 46222-0697   800-677-6442
Fax: 317-925-9398
e-mail: NAMI-IN@nami.org
www.nami.org
Grass roots advocacy support and educational group for families affected by severe and persistent mental illnesses.
Pamela McConey, Executive Director
Teresa Hatten, President

Iowa

6091 FFCMH: Iowa Chapter
106 S Booth   319-462-2187
Anamosa, IA 52205   888-400-6302
Fax: 319-462-6789
e-mail: help@iffcmh.org
www.iffcmh.org
Lori Reynolds

6092 NAMI Iowa: National Alliance on Mental Illness
5911 Meredith Drive   515-254-0417
Des Moines, IA 50322-1903   800-417-0417
Fax: 515-254-1103
e-mail: info@namiiowa.com
www.namiiowa.com
Dawn Olson, President
Margaret Stout, Executive Director

Kansas

6093 Keys for Networking: Kansas FFCMH
211 W 33rd Street   785-233-8732
Topeka, KS 66611   800-499-8732
Fax: 785-235-8732
e-mail: jadams@keys.org
www.keys.org
Jane Adams

6094 NAMI Kansas: Kansas' Voice on Mental Illness
112 SW 6th Avenue   785-233-0755
Topeka, KS 66601-0675   800-539-2660
Fax: 785-233-4804
e-mail: namikansas@nami.org
www.nami.org
Sharon Manson, President
Richard Cagan, Executive Director

Kentucky

6095 KY Partnership For Families and Children
207 Holmes Street   502-875-1320
Frankfort, KY 40601   Fax: 502-875-1399
e-mail: kpfc@kypartnership.org
www.kypartnership.org
Carol W Cecil, Executive Director
Kate Tilton, Program Coordinator

6096 Kentucky Alliance for the Mentally Ill
10510 Lagrange Road   502-245-5284
Louisville, KY 40223-1277   800-257-5081
Fax: 502-245-6390
e-mail: namiky@nami.org
www.nami.org
Bob McFadden, President
Carol Carrithers, Executive Director

Louisiana

6097 Louisiana Alliance for the Mentally Ill
5700 Florida Boulevard   225-926-8770
Baton Rouge, LA 70806-2398   866-851-6264
Fax: 225-926-8773
e-mail: namilouisiana@bellsouth.net
www.namilouisiana.org
Roselynn Nobles, President
Jennifer N Jantz, Executive Director

Maine

6098 Maine Alliance for the Mentally Ill
1 Bangor Street   207-622-5767
Augusta, ME 04330-4701   800-464-5767
Fax: 207-621-8430
e-mail: info@namimaine.org
www.nami.org
Julie O'Brien, President
Carol Carothers, Executive Director

6099 United Families for Children's Mental Health
PO Box 2107   207-622-3309
Augusta, ME 04338-2107   Fax: 207-622-1661
Pat Hunt

Maryland

6100 National Alliance for the Mentally Ill: Maryland
804 Landmark Drive   410-863-0470
Glen Burnie, MD 21061-4486   800-467-0075
                                                   Fax: 410-863-0474
                                              e-mail: amimd@aol.com
                                                        md.nami.org

Barbara Bellack, Executive Director
Dana Lefko

6101 Parents Supporting Parents of MD
PO Box 30
Kensington, MD 20895-0030   800-498-5551
                              e-mail: Marge_Samels@umail.umd.edu
Marge Samels, Executive Director

Massachusetts

6102 Massachusetts Alliance for the Mentally Ill
400 W Cummings Park   781-938-4048
Woburn, MA 01801-6528   800-370-9085
                                                   Fax: 781-938-4069
                                       e-mail: helpline@namimass.org
                                                    www.namimass.org

Rita Sagalyn, President
Toby Fisher, Director of Public Policy

Michigan

6103 Association for Children's Mental Health
6017 W Street Joseph Highway   517-372-4016
Lansing, MI 48917   888-226-4543
                                                   Fax: 517-372-4032
                                          e-mail: ajwinans@aol.com
                                                     www.acmh-mi.org

Amy J Winans, Executive Director
Mary Porter, Business Manager

6104 JIMHO Affiliated Centers (Justice in Mental Health Organization)
421 Seymour Street   517-371-2266
Lansing, MI 48933   800-831-8035
                                                   Fax: 517-371-5770
                                        e-mail: brwellwood@aol.com
                                             members.aol.com/jimhofw/
JIMHO advocates for the rights and dignity that all people suffering from mental or emotional illness deserve.

6105 Michigan Alliance for the Mentally Ill
921 N Washington Avenue   517-485-4049
Lansing, MI 48906-5137   800-331-4264
                                                   Fax: 517-485-2333
                                     e-mail: namimichigan@acd.net
                                                        mi.nami.org

Hubert Huebl, President
Sharon Solomon, Executive Director

Minnesota

6106 Minnesota Alliance for the Mentally Ill
800 Transfer Road   651-645-2948
Saint Paul, MN 55114-1146   888-NAM-IHEL
                                                   Fax: 651-645-7379
                                        e-mail: nami-mn@nami.org
                                                    www.namihelps.org

Karen Lloyd, President
Sue Abderholden, Executive Director

6107 Minnesota Association for Children's Mental Health
165 Western Avenue   651-644-7333
Saint Paul, MN 55102   800-528-4511
                                                   Fax: 651-644-7391
                                        e-mail: dsaxhaug@macmh.org
                                                      www.macmh.org

Deborah Saxhaug, Executive Director
Michele Willert, President

Mississippi

6108 Mississippi Alliance for the Mentally Ill
411 Briarwood Drive   601-899-9058
Jackson, MS 39206-3058   800-357-0388
                                                   Fax: 601-956-6380
                                        e-mail: namimiss1@aol.com
                                                        www.nami.org

Annette Giessner, President
Wendy Mahoney, Executive Director

6109 Mississippi Families as Allies
5166 Keele Street   601-981-1618
Jackson, MS 39206   800-833-9671
                                                   Fax: 601-981-1696
                                        e-mail: info@msfaacmh.org
                                                     www.msfaacmh.org

Tessie Bruni LMSW, Executive Director
Tressa Knuts LMSW, Family Support Coordinator

Missouri

6110 MO-SPAN
440 Rue Saint Francois   314-972-0600
Florissant, MO 63031   Fax: 314-972-0606
                                                     www.mo-span.org

Donna Dittrich, Executive Director
Tina VarVera, Administrative Assistant

6111 Missouri Coalition Alliance for the Mentally Ill
230 W Dunklin Street   573-634-7727
Jefferson City, MO 65101-3260   800-374-2138
                                                   Fax: 573-761-5636
                                           e-mail: Keele@aol.com

6112 NAMI of Missouri
1001 SW Boulevard   573-634-7727
Jefferson City, MO 65109-2501   800-374-2138
                                                   Fax: 573-761-5636
                                    e-mail: namimosjf@yahoo.com
                                                        mo.nami.org
A nonprofit education adudcacy, referal and support organization serving people with mental illness and their families.
12 pages newsletter
Cindi Keele, Executive Director
Karren Jones, President

Montana

6113 Family Support Network
1002 10th Street W   406-256-7783
Billings, MT 59102   877-376-4850
                                                   Fax: 406-256-9879
                                     e-mail: admin@mtfamilysupport.org
                                                  www.mtfamilysupport.org

Barbara Sample, Executive Director

6114 Montana Alliance for the Mentally Ill Mihelish's Residence
Mihelish's Residence
616 Helena Avenue   406-443-7871
Helena, MT 59624-6946   888-280-6264
                                                   Fax: 406-862-6352
                                        e-mail: mattkuntz@msn.com
                                                        www.namimt.org

Gary Milhelish, President
Matt Kuntz, Executive Director

Nebraska

6115 National Alliance for the Mentally Ill: Nebraska (NAMI)
1941 South 42nd Street   402-345-8101
Omaha, NE 68105-2986   877-463-6264
Fax: 402-346-4070
e-mail: nami.nebraska@nami.org
www.nami.org/sites/ne
NAMI is a nonprofit organization dedicated to providing support,
education and advocacy to and for anyone whose life has been
touched by a mental illness.
Colleen Wuebben, Executive Director
Carole Denton, President

Nevada

6116 Nevada Alliance for the Mentally Ill
2251 N Rampart Boulevard   702-310-5764
Las Vegas, NV 89128   Fax: 775-329-1618
e-mail: joetyler@sdi.net
www.nami-nevada.org

Joe Tyler, President
Mark Burchell, Vice President

New Hampshire

6117 Granite State FFCMH
940 Mammoth Road   603-296-0692
Manchester, NH 03104   e-mail: gsffcmh@aol.com
www.ffcmh.org

Kathleen Abate

6118 National Alliance for the Mentally Ill
15 Green Street   603-225-5359
Concord, NH 03301   800-242-6264
Fax: 603-228-8848
e-mail: info@naminh.org
www.naminh.org
Family support and advocacy for consumers and family members.
Michael Cohen, Executive Director
Win Saltmarsh, Development Director

6119 National Alliance for the Mentally Ill: New Hampshire
15 Green Street   603-225-5359
Concord, NH 03301-4020   800-242-6264
Fax: 603-228-8848
e-mail: naminh@naminh.org
www.naminh.org
Family support and advocacy for consumers and family members.
Michael Cohen, Executive Director
Mary Ann Aldrich, President

New Jersey

6120 Association for Advancement of Mental Health
Information
819 Alexander Road   609-452-2088
Princeton, NJ 08540   Fax: 609-452-0627
e-mail: info@aamh.org
www.aamh.org
This organization was founded to create a permanent community
support system for mentally ill and developmentally disabled
adults and their families living in the Greater Mercer County area
of New Jersey.
Lisa Lynch, Director of Development
Marc Helberg, President

6121 Community Mental Health Foundation
610 Industrial Avenue   201-986-5070
Paramus, NJ 07652   Fax: 201-265-3543
e-mail: staff@cmhf.org
www.cmhf.org

6122 New Jersey Alliance for the Mentally Ill
1562 US Highway 130   732-940-0991
N Brunswick, NJ 08902-3004   Fax: 732-940-0355
e-mail: info@naminj.org
www.naminj.org

Mark Perrin, President
Sylvia Axelrod, Executive Director

New Mexico

6123 Navaho Nation K'E Project Children and Families Advocacy Corp
PO Box 309   505-733-2474
Tohatchi, NM 87325   Fax: 505-733-2444
Vera Kieyoomia

6124 Navajo Nation K'E Project: Shiprock Children & Families Advocacy Corp
PO Box 1240   505-368-4479
Shiprock, NM 87420   Fax: 505-368-5582
Evelyn Balwin

6125 New Mexico Alliance for the Mentally Ill
6001 Marble NE Suite 8   505-260-0154
Albuquerque, NM 87190-3086   Fax: 505-260-0342
e-mail: naminm@aol.com
www.nami.org

Becky Beckett, President
Elaine Jones, Executive Director

New York

6126 Children's Mental Health Coalition of WNY, Inc.
814 Kenmore Avenue   716-871-8997
Buffalo, NY 14216   Fax: 716-871-8656
e-mail: mtskorupa@aol.com
www.raisingminds.org

Mary Skorupa, Executive Director

6127 Families Together in New York State
737 Madison Avenue   518-432-0333
Albany, NY 12208   888-326-8644
Fax: 518-434-6478
e-mail: info@ftnys.org
www.ftnys.org

Paige Pierce, Executive Director
Joan Cullen, Program Director/Family Specialist

6128 New York Alliance for the Mentally Ill
260 Washington Avenue   518-462-2000
Albany, NY 12210   800-950-3228
Fax: 518-462-3811
e-mail: info@naminys.org
www.naminys.org

Trix Niernberger, Executive Director
Jeff Keller, Deputy Director

6129 Parents United Network: Parsons Child Family Center
60 Academy Road   518-426-2600
Albany, NY 12208   Fax: 518-447-5234
e-mail: info@parsonscenter.org
www.parsonscenter.org

Rose Mary Bailly, Executive Director
Thomas Luzzi, Chief Financial Officer

North Dakota

6130 North Dakota Alliance for the Mentally Ill
PO Box 3215   701-852-8202
Minot, ND 58702-6016   Fax: 701-725-4334
e-mail: naminwnd@min.midco.net
www.nami.org

Janet Sabol, President

6131 North Dakota FFCMH
PO Box 3061   701-222-1223
Bismarck, ND 58502-3061   Fax: 701-250-8835
e-mail: carlottamccleary@bis.midco.nrt
www.ffcmh.org

Ohio

6132 1st Capital FFCMH
394 Chestnut Street   740-775-2674
Chillicothe, OH 45601   Fax: 740-775-7834
e-mail: rmh1@adelphia.net

Rosemary Hill

6133 **Ohio Alliance for the Mentally Ill**
747 E Broad Street
Columbus, OH 43205
614-224-2700
800-686-2646
Fax: 614-224-5400
TTY: 866-924-1478
e-mail: amiohio@amiohio.org
www.namiohio.org

Harvey Snider, President
Jim Mauro, Executive Director

Oklahoma

6134 **Oklahoma Alliance for the Mentally Ill**
500 N Broadway Avenue
Oklahoma City, OK 73102-6200
405-230-1900
800-583-1264
Fax: 405-230-1903
e-mail: nami-OK@swbell.net
www.nami.org

Barney Allen, President
Karina Forrest, Executive Director

6135 **Tulsa Unified FFCMH**
1022 N Howard
Tulsa, OK 74115
918-838-8033
e-mail: sherryscoobydoo@aol.com
www.ffcmh.org

Sherry Hamby

Oregon

6136 **NAMI-Oregon**
3550 SE Woodward Street
Portland, OR 97202-1552
503-230-8009
800-343-6264
Fax: 503-230-2751
e-mail: namioregon@qwest.net
www.nami.org

Providing support education and advocacy for people with biological mental illness and their families. The in-state 800 phone number is Oregon's NAMI-Line. Callers to this line are provided with information about mental illnesses and referrals to support and treatment services.
Molly Gorger, Education Program Director
Cora Palazzolo, Communications Coordinator

6137 **Oregon Family Support Network**
PO Box 324
Marylhurst, OR 97036
503-675-2294
800-323-8521
Fax: 503-675-6932
e-mail: ofsn@ofsn.org
www.ofsn.org

Jammie Farish, Executive Director
Sandy Bumpus, President

Pennsylvania

6138 **Parents Involved Network**
1211 Chestnut Street
Philadelphia, PA 19107
215-751-1800
800-688-4226
e-mail: pin@pinofpa.org
www.pinofpa.org

Janet Lonsdale

6139 **Pennsylvania Alliance for the Mentally Ill**
2149 N 2nd Street
Harrisburg, PA 17110-1005
717-238-1514
800-223-0500
Fax: 717-238-4390
TTY: 800-890-6093
e-mail: nami-pa@nami.org
namipa.nami.org

James W Jordan Jr, Executive Director
Jyoti Shah, President

Rhode Island

6140 **National Alliance for the Mentally Ill**
154 Waterman Street
Providence, RI 02906
401-331-3060
800-749-3197
Fax: 401-274-3020
e-mail: chaznami@cox.net
www.namirhodeisland.org

Fred Sneesby, President
Charles Gross, Executive Director

6141 **National Alliance for the Mentally Ill of Rhode Island (NAMI)**
82 Pitman Street
Providence, RI 02906-4312
401-331-3060
800-749-3197
Fax: 401-274-3020
e-mail: nicknami@aol.com
www.namiri.org

Henry Saccoccia, President
Nicki Sahlin, Executive Director

South Carolina

6142 **NAMI-SC: National Alliance on Mental Illness: South Carolina**
PO BOX 1267
Columbia, SC 29202-1267
803-733-9592
800-788-5131
Fax: 803-733-9593
e-mail: namisc@namisc.org
www.namisc.org

Advocacy, Education and Support
Bill Lindsey, Executive Director

South Dakota

6143 **NAMI South Dakota**
3920 S Western Avenue
Sioux Falls, SD 57109-1204
605-271-1871
800-551-2531
Fax: 605-271-1871
e-mail: namisd@midconetwork.com
www.nami.org/sites/NAMISouthDakota

Shelly Fuller, President
Robin Deming

Tennessee

6144 **Tennessee Alliance for the Mentally Ill**
1101 Kermit Drive
Nashville, TN 37217-2126
615-361-6608
800-467-3589
Fax: 615-361-6698
e-mail: sdiehl@namitn.org
www.namitn.org

Tod Jablonski, President
Sita Diehl, Executive Director

Texas

6145 **Central Texas FFCMH**
6814 Orange Blossom
Austin, TX 78744
512-282-7126
Fax: 512-282-5817
e-mail: mattie_dixon@hotmail.com

Mattie Dixon

6146 **North Texas FFCMH**
722 E Summitt
Sherman, TX 75090
e-mail: patoadv@msn.com
Pat Owens

6147 **San Antonio Bexar County FFCMH**
2516 Bandara
San Antonio, TX 78238
210-523-2351
Fax: 210-523-2352
e-mail: ideasjn@aol.com

Joseph Nazaroff

6148 **Texas Alliance for the Mentally Ill**
Foundtain Park Plaza III
Austin, TX 78704
512-693-2000
800-633-3760
Fax: 512-693-8000
e-mail: rpeyson@namitexas.org
www.namitexas.org

Robin Peyson, Executive Director
Donna Fisher, President

6149 **Texas FFCMH**
7800 Shoal Creek Road   512-407-8844
Austin, TX 78752   866-893-3264
Fax: 512-407-8266
e-mail: PattiDerr@txffcmh.org
www.txffcmh.org

Patti Derr, Executive Director

Utah

6150 **Utah Alliance for the Mentally Ill**
450 S 900 E   801-323-9900
Salt Lake City, UT 84102-1701   Fax: 801-323-9799
e-mail: Education@namiut.org
www.namiut.org

Don Muller, President
Sherri Wittwer, Executive Director

Vermont

6151 **Vermont Alliance for the Mentally Ill**
162 S Main Street   802-244-1396
Waterbury, VT 05676-1519   800-639-6480
Fax: 802-244-1405
e-mail: info@namivt.org
www.nami.org

Fran Levine, President
Larry Lewack, Executive Director

6152 **Vermont FFCMH**
95 Main Street   802-244-1955
Waterbury, VT 05676-0607   800-639-6071
Fax: 802-329-2135
e-mail: vffcmh@vffcmh.org
www.vffcmh.org

Kathy Holsopple, Executive Director
Ted Tighe, President

Virginia

6153 **Virginia Alliance for the Mentally Ill**
PO Box 8260   804-225-8264
Richmond, VA 23226-1903   888-486-8264
Fax: 80 -85 -464
e-mail: namiva@comcast.net
www.nami.org

Bill Farrington, President
Mira Signer, Executive Director

Washington

6154 **NAMI Washington (National Alliance for the Mentally Ill of Washington)**
4305 Lacey Boulevard SE   360-584-9622
Lacey, WA 98503-5580   800-782-9264
e-mail: office@namiwa.comcastbiz.net
www.nami.org
Advocacy, support and education for the mentally ill, their families and friends.
Barbara Bate, President
Bill Waters, Vice President

6155 **Washington FFCMH**
801 E 141 Street   253-537-2145
Tacoma, WA 98445-2768   Fax: 253-537-2162
e-mail: acvmarge@comcast.net
www.ffcmh.org/

Marge Critchlow

West Virginia

6156 **Mountain State/Parents/Children/ Adolescents Network**
1201 Garfield Street   304-233-5399
McMechen, WV 26040   800-CHI-LD35
Fax: 304-233-3847
e-mail: ttoothman@mcpcan.org
www.mspcan.org

Hope Coleman, President
Terrie Isaly, Fast Track Program Director

6157 **NAMI West Virginia**
PO Box 2706   304-342-0497
Charleston, WV 25330-2706   800-598-5653
Fax: 304-342-0499
e-mail: namiwv@aol.com
www.namiwv.org
Educational advocacy and support for families consumers and friends of people with mental illnesses.
Randal Johnson, President
Michael W Ross, Executive Director

Wisconsin

6158 **Wisconsin Alliance for the Mentally Ill**
4233 W Beltline Highway   608-268-6000
Madison, WI 53711-3814   800-236-2988
Fax: 608-268-6004
e-mail: namiwisc@choiceonemail.com
www.namiwisconsin.org

Pat Rutkowski, Co-President
Terence Schnapp, Interim Executive Director

6159 **Wisconsin Family Ties**
16 N Carroll Street   608-267-6888
Madison, WI 53703   800-422-7145
Fax: 608-267-6801
e-mail: info@wifamilyties.org
www.wifamilyties.org

Hugh Davis, Executive Director
Ginger Fobart, Statewide Family Network Coordinator

Wyoming

6160 **Wyoming Alliance for the Mentally Ill**
133 W 6th Street   307-265-2573
Casper, WY 82601-3124   888-882-4968
Fax: 307-234-0440
e-mail: nami-wyo@qwestoffice.net
www.nami.org/sites/namiwyoming

Jane Johnson, President
Deion Hagemeister, Vice-President

Libraries & Resource Centers

6161 **Alta Bates Summit Medical Center**
2001 Dwight Way
Berkeley, CA 94704-2608   510-204-4444
www.altabatesherrick.org
Alta Bates Summit Medical Center has made community healthcare a priority. We are proud of our many areas of clinical excellence including cardiovascular, behavioral health, women and infants, orthopedics, rehabilitation, and oncology care.
Carolyn Kemp, Director Public Relations

6162 **Central Louisiana State Hospital Medical and Professional Library**
242 West Shamrock Street   318-484-6363
Pineville, LA 71360   Fax: 318-484-6284
e-mail: bentonmcgee@hotmail.com
www.clmlc.org

The Consortium was established to increase and better utilize the health information resources of Central Louisiana. Information offered on psychiatry, psychology and mental health.
Carol McGee, Medical Librarian

6163 **National Mental Health Consumer's Self-Help Clearinghouse**
1211 Chestnut Street   215-751-1810
Philadelphia, PA 19107   800-553-4539
Fax: 215-735-0275
e-mail: info@mhselfhelp.org
www.mhselfhelp.org

The National Mental Health Consumers' Self-Help Clearinghouse, the nation's first national consumer technical assistance center, has played a major role in the development of the mental health consumer movement. The consumer movement strives for dignity, respect, and opportunity for those with mental illnesses.
Joseph Rogers, Director

6164 National Mental Health Consumers' Self- Help Clearinghouse
1211 Chestnut Street   215-751-1810
Philadelphia, PA 19107   800-553-4539
                                          Fax: 215-636-6312
                                   e-mail: info@mhselfhelp.org
                                          www.mhselfhelp.org
The National Mental Health Consumers' Self-Help Clearinghouse, the nation's first national consumer technical assistance center, has played a major role in the development of the mental health consumer movement. The consumer movement strives for dignity, respect, and opportunity for those with mental illnesses. Consumers—those who receive or have received mental health services—continue to reject the label of 'those who cannot help themselves.'
Joseph Rogers, Director

Research Centers

6165 Anxiety Disorders Center University of Wisconsin
University of Wisconsin
Department of Psychiatry   608-263-1530
Madison, WI 53792-0001
Provides evaluation and treatment for individuals suffering from anxiety disorders as well as training and education for clinicians.

6166 Institute of Psychiatry and Human Behavior: University of Maryland
701 Weat Pratt Street   410-328-6735
Baltimore, MD 21201-1542   Fax: 410-328-3693
                             e-mail: alehman@psych.umaryland.edu
                                  www.medschool.umaryland.edu
Studies in psychiatric disorders.
Anthony Lehm MD, Director

6167 Langley Porter Psychiatric Institute University of California
University of California
401 Parnassus Avenue
San Francisco, CA 94143-9911   415-476-7365
                                www.universityofcalifornia.edu
Conducts clinical studies of psychiatric disorders.
Samuel Barno MD, Director
Craig Vantyke, Chief Executive Officer

6168 Medical College of Pennsylvania: Eastern Psychiatric Institute
3200 Henry Avenue   215-842-6990
Philadelphia, PA 19129-1137
Offers research into all aspects of mental illness.
Michael Faucher, Director

6169 Menninger Clinic: Department of Research
PO Box 829   785-350-5000
Topeka, KS 66601-0829   Fax: 785-350-5392
Focuses research on mental illness and mental health issues.
Dr Herbert Spohn, Director

6170 Mental Illness Research and Education Institute
Eastern State Hospital
PO Box 800   509-299-3121
Medical Lake, WA 99022-800   Fax: 509-997-15
Governmental organization focusing on mental illness research.
Harold Wilson, Director

6171 State University of New York At Stony Brook: Mental Health Research
450 Clarkson Avenue   718-270-1270
Brooklyn, NY 11203-2056
Oliver David, Director

6172 Thresholds Psychiatric Rehabilitation
2700 N Ravenswood Avenue   773-281-3800
Chicago, IL 60614-1894   Fax: 773-818-90
                               e-mail: thresholds@thresholds.org
                                               www.luc.edu
A psychosocial rehabilitation agency serving persons with severe and persistent mental illness.
Tom Kinley, Director
Ellen Rodman, Assistant Director

6173 University of California Los Angeles Program on Psychosocial Adaptation
Neuropsychiatric Institute
760 Westwood Plaza   310-825-0511
Los Angeles, CA 90024   800-825-9989
                                            www.semel.ucla.edu
Studies behavior disorders and psychosocial adaptation and the future.
Roderic GoRN MD, Director
Peter Whybrow, Director

6174 University of Michigan: Mental Health Research Institute
205 Washtenaw Place   734-763-2462
Ann Arbor, MI 48109   e-mail: UMresearch@umich.edu
                                               www.umich.edu
Focuses on the diagnosis treatment and prevention of mental illnesses and disorders.
Dr Bernard Agranoff, Director

6175 University of Minnesota Department of Psychiatry
420 Delaware Street SE   612-624-2430
Minneapolis, MN 55455-374   Fax: 612-265-91
                                               www.umn.edu
Behavior and mental illness research.
S Charles Schulz, Chair of Psychiatry

6176 University of Missouri: Columbia Missouri Institute of Mental Health
5247 Fyler Avenue   573-634-8787
Saint Louis, MO 63139-1300   Fax: 314-644-8834
Mental health policy and ethics studies.
Danny Weddin PhD, Director

6177 University of Pittsburgh: Western Psychiatric Institute & Clinic
3811 Ohara Street   412-246-6356
Pittsburgh, PA 15213-2593   Fax: 412-246-6350
                                 e-mail: reitzpm@msx.upmc.edu
                                               www.pitt.edu
Advancement of basic and clinical knowledge in mental health and psychiatric care.
Thomas Detre MD, Director

6178 Vanderbilt University John F Kennedy Center for Research/Human Development
Vanderbilt University
230 Appleton Place   615-322-8240
Nashville, TN 37203-5701   Fax: 615-228-36
                                    e-mail: kc@vanderbilt.edu
                                           www.kc.vanderbilt.edu
Mental health research.
Stephen Camarata, Acting Director

6179 Veterans Medical Center: Mental Health Clinical Research Center
3801 Miranda Avenue
Palo Alto, CA 94304-1207   650-858-3941
                                               www.va.gov
Jerome Yesavage, Director Advanced Psychiatry
Ruth O'Hara, Co-Director Advanced Psychology

6180 Warren Grant Magnuson Clinical Center National Institute of Health
National Institute of Health
9000 Rockville Pike   301-496-4000
Bethesda, MD 20892   800-411-1222
                                          Fax: 301-480-9793
                                          TTY: 866-411-1010
                                  e-mail: prpl@mail.cc.nih.gov
                                               www.cc.nih.gov
Established in 1953 as the research hospital of the National Institutes of Health. Designed so that patient care facilities are close to research laboratories so new findings of basic and clinical scientists can be quickly applied to the treatment of patients. Upon referral by physicians patients are admitted to NIH clinical studies.
John I Gallin, Director
David Henderson, Deputy Director for Clinical Care

6181 Yeshiva University: Soundview-Throgs Neck Community Mental Health Center
2527 Glebe Avenue   718-904-4400
Bronx, NY 10461-3109   Fax: 718-931-7307
Mental health mental illness and recovery from mental illness research.
Dr Itamar Salamon, Director

Support Groups & Hotlines

6182 National Health Information Center
PO Box 1133
Washington, DC 20013   310-565-4167
                                     800-336-4797
                                     Fax: 301-984-4256
                                     e-mail: info@nhic.org
                                     www.health.gov/nhic
Offers a nationwide information referral service, produces directories and resource guides.

Alabama

6183 Alabama Education of Homeless Children and Youth Program
Alabama State Department of Education
5348 Gordon Persons Building
Montgomery, AL 36130-3901   334-242-8199
                                     Fax: 334-420-9633
                                     e-mail: mrivers@alsde.edu
                                     www.alsde.edu/html/home.asp
The major responsibilities of the Federal Programs Section are to administer all federally funded education programs and to provide technical assistance to local education agencies and schools. These responsibilities include promoting, supervising, and coordinating statewide educational programs with federal programs in addition to assisting schools in developing, revising, and implementing their school wide plans.
Maggie Rivers, Federal Program Coordinator

Alaska

6184 National Alliance for the Mentally Ill (NA MI) Alaska
144 West 15th Avenue   907-227-1300
Anchorage, AK 99501-5106   800-478-4462
                                     Fax: 907-227-1400
                                     e-mail: info@nami-alaska.org
                                     www.nami.org/sites/alaska
NAMI Alaska is a grassroots, 501(c)(3) nonprofit, support, educational and advocacy organization of consumers, families, and friends of people with severe brain disorders such as schizophrenia, schizo-affective disorder, bipolar disorder, major depressive disorder, obsessive-compulsive disorder, panic and anxiety disorders, and attention deficit/hyperactivity disorder. In addition, NAMI provides information and referral services and works with local media on stories about mental illness.
Trish McDonald, Program/Education Director
Augusta Reimer, Leadership Project Coordinator

Arizona

6185 Navajo Nation Office Special Education & R ehabilitation Services
IHS PO Box 1337   505-722-1454
Gallup, NM 87301   Fax: 505-722-1554
                                     e-mail: osers@navajo.org
                                     www.osers.navajo.org/
Navajo OSERS is a program within the Division of DINE Education, which offers vocational rehabilitation to people with disabilities. Vocational Rehabilitation includes an array of services, which are funded by a grant to the Navajo Nation from the U.S. Department of Education. The goal of vocational rehabilitation is to assist people with disabilities to obtain or maintain employment.
Rosemary Smith, Parent Training Coordinator

6186 Navajo Nation Office of Special Education & Rehabilitation Services (OSERS)
PO Box 1420   928-871-6338
Window Rock, AZ 86515   866-341-9918
                                     Fax: 928-871-7865
                                     e-mail: osers@navajo.org
                                     www.osers.navajo.org/

Navajo OSERS is a program within the Division of DINE Education, which offers vocational rehabilitation to people with disabilities. Vocational Rehabilitation includes an array of services, which are funded by a grant to the Navajo Nation from the U.S. Department of Education. The goal of vocational rehabilitation is to assist people with disabilities to obtain or maintain employment.
Treva M Roanhorse, Director
Paula S Seanez, Assistant Director

Colorado

6187 Laradon Services for Children and Adults w ith Developmental Disabilities
5100 Lincoln Street   303-296-2400
Denver, CO 80216   Fax: 303-296-4012
                                     TDD: 7209746821
                                     www.laradon.org/Index.shtml#
Laradon specializes in services to children and adults with developmental disabilities, operating 15 programs that are designed to help each individual develop to his or her fullest potential and maximize self-sufficiency.
Annie Green, Deputy Director

Florida

6188 Florida Institute for Family Involvement (FIFI)
3927 Spring Creek Highway   305-293-7626
Crawfordville, FL 32327   877-926-3514
                                     Fax: 863-582-9358
                                     e-mail: HewFLMOM@aol.com
                                     www.fifionline.org
Florida Institute for Family Involvement (FIFI), an affiliate of Federation of Families for Children's Mental Health (FFCMH), enhances, facilitates, and supports family and consumer involvement in the development of responsive, family centered, and community based systems of care. FIFI works in collaboration with state, federal, and private programs to develop a resource and training information center to enable individuals to advocate for appropriate services and make wise service choices.
Connie Wells, Executive Director
Lindsay Phillips, Business Manager

6189 Parent Education Network (PEN) Project Health
Family Network on Disabilities of Florida
2735 Whitney Road   727-523-1130
Clearwater, FL 33760   800-825-5736
                                     Fax: 727-523-8687
                                     e-mail: wilbur@fndfl.org
                                     www.fndfl.org/PEN/index.htm
The PEN Project provides: information on specific disabilities; individual assistance by telephone, email, and in-person; referrals to local, state, and national resources; opportunities for youths with disabilities to be involved in training to parents and students; and, collaboration with Family Network on Disabilities Heart and Hope annual statewide conference for families.
Wilbur Hawke, Co-Director
Tara Bremer, Co-Director

Georgia

6190 Georgia Parent Support Network (GPSN)
1381 Metropolitan Parkway   404-758-4500
Atlanta, GA 30310   Fax: 404-758-6833
                                     e-mail: rheba.smith@gpsn.org
                                     www.gpsn.org/
Georgia Parent Support Network (GPNS) provides support, education, and advocacy for children and youth with mental illness, emotional disturbances, and behavioral differences and their families.
Sue L Smith, Co-Chief Executive Officer
Anna M McLaughlin, Co-Chief Executive Officer

Hawaii

6191 Hawaii Families As Allies (HFAA)
99-209 Moanalua Road   808-487-8785
Aiea, HI 96701   866-361-8825
                                     Fax: 808-487-0514
                                     e-mail: hfaa@hfaa.net
                                     www.hfaa.net/

Hawaii Families as Allies (HFAA) is a statewide parent-controlled family network organization that provides support, services and information for families of children and adolescents with emotional and/or behavioral challenges. HFAA is the Hawaii state chapter of the Federation of Families for Children's Mental Health, a national organization that advocates for service system change so that families are valued and treated as true partners.

Susan Cooper, Executive Director
Shanelle Lum, Public Policy Information Specialist

Illinois

6192 CANDU Parent Group
24W 681 Woodcrest Drive   630-983-9027
Naperville, IL 60540
Cathy Bozett

6193 KALEIDOSCOPE
1279 N Milwaukee Avenue   773-278-7200
Chicago, IL 60622   Fax: 773-278-5663
                                 TTY: 773-292-4086
e-mail: information@kaleidoscope4kids.org
                                 www.kaleidoscope4kids.org
Karl Dennis

6194 Parents Information Network FFCMH
1926 1700th Avenue   217-735-1662
Lincoln, IL 62656
Bridget Schneider

Indiana

6195 Bloomington: NAMI Bloomington
NAMI Indiana
PO Box 22697   812-334-8117
Indianapolis, IN 46222-0697   800-677-6442
                                 Fax: 317-925-9398
e-mail: lev@bloomington.in.us
                                 www.namiindiana.org
Meets on the first and third Thursday at 7:00 p.m., at the First United Methodist Church on 219 E 4th Street, room 307.
Paul Van Gogh, President

6196 Elkhart: NAMI Elkhart County
NAMI Indiana
PO Box 22697
Indianapolis, IN 46222-0697   800-677-6442
                                 Fax: 317-925-9398
e-mail: hsgjan@aol.com
                                 www.namiindiana.org
Meets on the second and fourth Thursday at 7:30 p.m., at the St. Paul Methodist Church.
Harold Grieb, President

6197 Evansville NAMI Evansville
NAMI Indiana
PO Box 22697   317-925-9399
Indianapolis, IN 46222-697   800-677-6442
                                 Fax: 317-925-9398
e-mail: daRNeson4051@insightbb.com
                                 www.namiindiana.org
Meets on the second and fourth Tuesday, 6:45 p.m., at Southwestern Indiana CMHC.
Diane Arneson, President
Jo Vanable, President Nami Indiana

6198 Fort Wayne: NAMI Fort Wayne
NAMI Indiana
PO Box 22697   260-447-8990
Indianapolis, IN 46222-0697   800-677-6442
                                 Fax: 317-925-9398
e-mail: tahat10@aol.com
                                 www.namiindiana.org
Meets every Tuesday, 6:45 p.m., at Carriage House, 3327 Lake Avenue.
Teresa Hatten, President

6199 Indianapolis: NAMI Indianapolis
NAMI Indiana

PO Box 22697   317-767-7653
Indianapolis, IN 46222-0697   800-677-6442
                                 Fax: 317-925-9398
                                 www.namiindiana.org
For information please call our voice mail information line (317-767-7653) or write P.O. Box 40866, Indianapolis, IN 46240-0866. We have central, east, north, south and west support groups.
Don Fearrin, President

6200 Jeffersonville: NAMI Sunnyside
NAMI Indiana
PO Box 22697   812-282-6494
Indianapolis, IN 46222-0697   800-677-6442
                                 Fax: 317-925-9398
                                 www.namiindiana.org
Consumers meet on the second Monday of each month, 6:00 p.m., and family members meet on the second Tuesday of each month at 7:00 p.m. at Clark Memorial Hospital. Please call for directions.
Charlotte Davis, Contact Person

6201 Kendallville NAMI Northeast
NAMI Indiana
PO Box 22697   260-347-2291
Indianapolis, IN 46222-697   800-677-6442
                                 Fax: 317-925-9398
                                 www.namiindiana.org
Meets on the first Thursday of each month, 7:00 p.m., at the Kendallville Public Library.
Mary Smith, President

6202 Kokomo NAMI Kokomo
NAMI Indiana
128 Grant   765-628-7920
Green town, IN 46936-697   800-677-6442
                                 Fax: 317-925-9398
e-mail: vkharris1010@aol.com
                                 www.namiindiana.org
Meets on the first Tuesday of every month, 7:00 p.m., at the First Christian Church.
Alice Harris, President
Verl Harris, Treasurer

6203 Lafayette: NAMI West Central
NAMI Indiana
PO Box 22697   765-423-6939
Indianapolis, IN 46222-0697   800-677-6442
                                 Fax: 317-925-9398
                                 www.namiindiana.org
Meets on the second and fourth Monday of each month, at St. Elizabeth School of Nursing, room 4-901.
Cecilia Weber, Executive Director

6204 Lake County: NAMI Lake County
NAMI Indiana
PO Box 22697   219-374-5408
Indianapolis, IN 46222-0697   800-677-6442
                                 Fax: 317-925-9398
                                 www.namiindiana.org
Meets on the second and fourth Friday, 7:00 p.m., at the Southlake Mental Health Center.
Debbie Ganns, President

6205 Lawrenceburg: NAMI Southeast
NAMI Indiana
PO Box 22697   812-926-0199
Indianapolis, IN 46222-0697   800-677-6442
                                 Fax: 317-925-9398
                                 www.namiindiana.org
Meets on the first Tuesday of each month at the Dearborn County Mental Health Clinic, Dearborn Shopping Plaza. Call for meeting time.
Nancy McDaniel, President

6206 Logansport: NAMI Cass County
NAMI Indiana
PO Box 22697   574-753-6667
Indianapolis, IN 46222-0697   800-677-6442
                                 Fax: 317-925-9398
                                 www.namiindiana.org

451

Meets on the second Monday, 6:00 p.m., at the Four County Counseling Center. Call for more information.
Karen Menzie, President

6207   Marion NAMI Grant Blackford Counties
NAMI Indiana
PO Box 22697   765-664-0227
Indianapolis, IN 46222-697   800-677-6442
                                      Fax: 317-925-9398
                                      www.namiindiana.org
Meets on the first Wednesday, 7:00 p.m. Please call details.
Sandy Westafer, President

6208   Muncie: NAMI Delaware County
NAMI Indiana
PO Box 22697
Indianapolis, IN 46222-0697   800-677-6442
                                      Fax: 317-925-9398
                                      www.namiindiana.org
Please call the state office for details.

6209   NAMI Highland
NAMI
PO Box 22697   317-925-9399
Indianapolis, IN 46222-697   800-677-6442
                                      Fax: 317-925-9398
                                      e-mail: namiin@nami.org
                                      www.namiindiana.org
Pamela Mcconey, Executive Director
Leslie Gay, Office Coordinator

6210   NAMI Indiana - National Alliance on Mental Illness
PO Box 22697   317-925-9399
Indianapolis, IN 46222-0697   800-677-6442
                                      Fax: 317-925-9398
                                      e-mail: nami-in@nami.org
                                      www.namiindiana.org
NAMI Indiana is a non-profit grassroots organization dedicated to improving the lives of people afflicted by serious and persistent mental illness. NAMI Indiana consists of families, consumers, and professionals that are dedicated to helping families through a network of support, education, advocacy, and promotion of research. NAMI Indiana is affiliated with the National Alliance on Mental Illness (NAMI), which is located in Arlington, Virginia.
Pamela McConey, Executive Director
B Kellie Meyer, Development Director

6211   NAMI South Central Indiana
National Alliance for the Mentally Ill
1916 Central Avenue   812-376-0020
Columbus, IN 47201   Fax: 317-925-9398
                      e-mail: dweeks@seidata.com OR nami-in@nami.org
                                      www.namiindiana.org
NAMI Indiana is a non-profit grassroots organization dedicated to improving the lives of people afflicted by serious and persistent mental illness. NAMI Indiana consists of families, consumers, and professionals that are dedicated to helping families through a network of support, education, advocacy, and promotion of research. NAMI Indiana is affiliated with the National Alliance on Mental Illness (NAMI), which is located in Arlington, Virginia.
Dee Weeks, Executive Director

6212   Richmond: NAMI East Central
NAMI Indiana
PO Box 22697   765-458-6758
Indianapolis, IN 46222-0697   800-677-6442
                                      Fax: 317-925-9398
                                      e-mail: nami@dunncenter.org
                                      www.namiindiana.org
Meets on the first Tuesday of each month, 7:00 p.m., at 831 Dillon Drive, room 231.
Bernice Issac, Contact Person

6213   South Bend: NAMI St. Joseph County
NAMI Indiana
PO Box 22697   574-272-8580
Indianapolis, IN 46222-0697   800-677-6442
                                      Fax: 317-925-9398
                                      e-mail: Gary.E.Herr.1@nd.edu
                                      www.namiindiana.org

Please call for our schedule.
Patricia Herr, President

6214   Terre Haute: NAMI Wabash Valley
NAMI Indiana
PO Box 22697   812-877-9950
Indianapolis, IN 46222-0697   800-677-6442
                                      Fax: 317-925-9398
                                      www.namiindiana.org
Currently meeting on the second Wednesday of each month, 7:00 p.m., at the Hamilton Center. Please call for directions and more information.
Betty Porter, Contact Person

6215   Warsaw NAMI Warsaw
NAMI Indiana
NAMI Indiana   317-925-9399
Indianapolis, IN 46222-697   800-677-6442
                                      Fax: 317-925-9398
                                      e-mail: toddataeq@earthlink.com
                                      www.namiindiana.org
Meets every Tuesday from 7:00 to 9:00 p.m. at the First United Methodist Church.
Todd Biller, President
Joseph Vanable, President Nami Indiana

Iowa

6216   Iowa Federaion of Families for Children's Mental Health (FFCMH)
106 South Boothtreet   319-462-2187
Anamosa, IA 52205   888-400-6302
                                      Fax: 319-462-6789
                                      e-mail: lori@iffcmh.org
                                      www.iffcmh.org
The mission of Iowa Federation of Families for Children's Mental Health is to link families to community, county and state partners for needed supports and services; and to promote systems change that will enable families to live in a safe, stable and respectful environment.
Lori Reynolds, Executive Director

Kentucky

6217   Kentucky IMPACT
275 E Main Street   502-564-7610
Frankfort, KY 40621
Sandra Noble Canon

Massachusetts

6218   Parent Professional Advocacy League
59 Temple Place   617-542-7860
Boston, MA 2111   866-815-8122
                                      Fax: 617-542-7832
                                      e-mail: info@ppal.net
                                      www.ppal.net
Donna Welles, Executive Director

6219   Windhorse Associates
Windhorse Associates
31 Trumbull Road   413-586-0207
Northampton, MA 01060-2328   Fax: 413-585-1521
                                      e-mail: info@windhorseassociates.org
                                      www.windhorseassociates.org
Creating therapeutic environments to promote recovery from mental illness.
Molly Fortuna, Director Nursing/Admissions

Minnesota

6220   Emotional Health Anonymous
PO Box 4245   651-647-9712
St Paul, MN 55104-0245   Fax: 651-647-1593
                      e-mail: infodf3498fjsd@enotionsanonymous.org
                                      www.emotionsanonymous.org
A twelve-step organization, similar to Alcoholics Anonymous. Compsed of people who come together in weekly meetings for the purpose of working toward recovery from emotional difficulties.

6221 **PACER Center**
8161 Normandale Boulevard
Minneapolis, MN 55437-1044
952-838-9000
800-537-2237
Fax: 952-838-0199
TTY: 952-838-0190
e-mail: pacer@pacer.org
www.pacer.org

Dixie Jordan, Advocate
Paula Goldberg, Executive Director

Missouri

6222 **MO-SPAN Southwest Region**
210 W Vine Street
Butler, MO 64730
660-679-5767
Eldonna Carroll

6223 **MOSPAN Northwest Region**
440 Rue Street François
Jefferson City, MO 63031
314-972-0600
Fax: 314-720-06
e-mail: mospan2@fid.net.com
www.mospan.org

Donna Dittrich, Executive Director
Tina Vervara, Administrative Assistant

Nevada

6224 **Nevada PEP**
2355 Red Rock Street
Las Vegas, NV 89146
702-388-8899
800-216-5188
Fax: 702-388-2966
e-mail: pepinfo@nvpep.org
www.nvpep.org
A statewide non-profit helping families who have children with disabilities, and the professionals who work with them. Support groups, training, workshops, lending resource library. Services are provided at no cost.
Karen Taycher, Executive Director

New Hampshire

6225 **National Alliance for the Mentally Ill: New Hampshire**
15 Green Street
Concord, NH 03301
603-225-5359
800-242-6264
Fax: 603-228-8848
e-mail: info@naminh.org
www.naminh.org
Family support and advocacy for consumers and family members.
Michael Cohen, Executive Director

New York

6226 **Family Ties of Orange County**
Mental Health Association of Orange County
20 Walker Street
Goshen, NY 10924-1906
845-294-7411
800-832-1200
Fax: 845-294-7348
e-mail: mha@mhaorangeny.com
www.mhaorangeny.com/
Mental Health Association of Orange County/MHA is a private, not-for-profit organization seeking to promote the mental health and emotional well being of Orange County residents. Under the leadership of a volunteer Board of Directors, MHA's staff members, consultants and volunteers provide free mental health services to thousands of Orange County residents each year. Several volunteers answer several hotlines, provide companionship, public education, direct services and assist with fundraisers.
Nadia Allen, Executive Director

6227 **Mental Health Association in Dutchess Coun ty**
510 Haight Avenue
Poughkeepsie, NY 12603
845-473-2500
Fax: 845-473-4870
e-mail: mhadc@hvc.rr.com
www.mhadc.com/
The Mental Health Association in Dutchess County promotes mental well-being and advances the recovery from mental illness, pro-

vides rehabilitation programs and support services for adults with a history of mental illness and their families.
Jacki Brownstein MPS, Executive Director
Emily Robisch, Director Finance and Operations

North Dakota

6228 **ND FFCMH Region II**
PO Box 3061
Bismarck, ND 58502-3061
701-222-1223
Fax: 701-250-8835
e-mail: carlottamccleary@bis.midco.nrt
www.ffcmh.org

Carlotta McCleary

6229 **ND Region V FFCMH Chapter-Federation of Fa milies for Children's Mental Health**
1104 2nd Avenue South
Fargo, ND 58103
701-235-9923
Fax: 701-235-9923
e-mail: ndffrgv@nbinternet.com
www.ffcmh.org/who_chapters.php
The FFCMH, a national family-run organization serves to: provide advocacy at the national level for the rights of children and youth with emotional, behavioral and mental health challenges and their families; provide leadership and technical assistance to a nation-wide network of family run organizations; and, collaborate with family run and other child serving organizations to transform mental health care in America.
Deborah Jendro, Executive Director

6230 **ND Region VII FFCMH-Federation of Families for Children's Mental Health**
2252 La Corte Loop
Bismarck, ND 58503
701-258-1628
Fax: 701-258-1628
e-mail: ndffrg7@btinet.net
www.ffcmh.org/who_chapters.php
The FFCMH, a national family-run organization serves to: provide advocacy at the national level for the rights of children and youth with emotional, behavioral and mental health challenges and their families; provide leadership and technical assistance to a nation-wide network of family run organizations; and, collaborate with family run and other child serving organizations to transform mental health care in America.
Becky Sevart, Executive Director

Ohio

6231 **Child & Adolescent Service Center (CASC)**
919 2nd Street NE
Canton, OH 44704
330-454-7917
Fax: 330-454-1476
e-mail: bsnyder@casrv.org
www.casrv.org/
The Child and Adolescent Service Center (CASC) was founded and incorporated in 1976 by a standing committee of the Stark County Mental Health Foundation. CASC provides dynamic leadership through innovative service, training and evaluation and is committed to providing culturally-sensitive programs and services throughout the community.
Bobbi L Beale Psy.D, Group Programs Director
David J Coleman Ph.D, Director of Psychological Services

6232 **First Ohio Chapter: FFCMH**
4505 Quaker Court
Canfield, OH 44406-9131
330-726-9570
Fax: 330-726-9031
e-mail: xuparents@aol.com OR ffcmh@ffcmh.org
www.ffcmh.org/who_chapters.php
The Federation of Families for Children's Mental Health (FFCMH) is a national organization dedicated exclusively to helping children with mental health needs and their families achieve a better quality of life.
Chrysanne Mitzel, Director First Ohio Chapter
Sandra Spencer, Executive Director Corporate Office (MD)

Rhode Island

6233 Parent Support Network
400 Warwick Avenue Suite 12   401-467-6855
Warwick, RI 2888   800-483-8844
                                     Fax: 401-467-6903
                                     e-mail: psnosri@aol.com
                                     www.psnri.org

Cathy Cianon, Executive Director
Brenda Alego, Assistant Director

6234 Parent Support Network of Rhode Island
400 Warwick Avenue   401-467-6855
Warwick, RI 2888   800-483-8844
                                     Fax: 401-467-6903
                                     e-mail: psnori@aol.com
                                     www.psnori.org
Family-run organization whose mission is to provide support, education and advocacy to parents of children at risk for or who have emotional, behavioral, and/or mental health challenges.
Cathy Cianon, Executive Director

South Carolina

6235 FFCMH: South Carolina Chapter
PO Box 1266   803-779-0402
Columbia, SC 29201   866-779-0402
                                     Fax: 803-779-0450
                                     e-mail: diane.flashnick@fedfamsc.org
                                     www.fedfamsc.org/
The Federation of Families of South Carolina (FFCMH) is a nonprofit organization established to serve the families of children with any degree of emotional, behavioral or psychiatric disorder. Through support networks, educational materials, publications, conferences/workshops and other activities, the Federation provides many avenues of support for families of children with emotional, behavioral or psychiatric disorders.
Dianne Flashnick, Executive Director
Phoebe Malloy, Board of Directors President

6236 Family Support Network/SC AMI
PO Box 2538   803-779-7849
Columbia, SC 29202   800-788-5131
                                     Fax: 803-779-2655

Diane Flashnick

6237 Federation of Families of South Carolina
PO Box 1266   803-779-0402
Columbia, SC 29202-2344   866-779-0402
                                     Fax: 803-779-0450
                                     e-mail: FedFamSC@yahoo.com
                                     www.midnet.sc.edu/ffsc

Cookie Cloyd

Tennessee

6238 Tennessee Voices for Children
1315 8th Avenue S   615-269-7751
Nashville, TN 37203   800-670-9882
                                     Fax: 615-269-8914
                                     e-mail: tvc@tnvoices.org
                                     www.tnvoices.org

Charlotte Bryson, Director

Texas

6239 Harris County FFCMH
431 Breeze Park Drive   713-455-8962
Houston, TX 77015   e-mail: annn@flash.net
Elizabeth Neimeyer

Utah

6240 Allies with Families
450 East 1000   801-292-2515
North Salt Lake, UT 84054-2979   877-477-0764
                                     Fax: 801-292-2680
                                     e-mail: Allies@AlliesWithFamilies.org
                                     www.allieswithfamilies.org

Allies with Families was created in 1991 to offer practical support and resources for parents and their children and youth who face serious emotional, behavioral and mental health challenges. It was created to support all families in the state of Utah.
Lori Cerar, Executive Director
Karen Greenwell, Community Education Coordinator

Vermont

6241 Vermont FFCMH
PO Box 607   802-434-6757
Montpelier, VT 05676-0507   800-639-6071
                                     Fax: 802-434-6741
                        e-mail: vffcmh@together.net OR ffcmh@ffcmh.org
                                     www.ffcmh.org/who_chapters.php
The Federation of Families for Children's Mental Health (FFCMH) is a national organization dedicated exclusively to helping children with mental health needs and their families achieve a better quality of life.
Kathleen Holsopple, Executive Director
Sandra Spencer, Executive Director Corporate Office (MD)

Virginia

6242 PACCT
8032 Mechanicsville Turnpike   804-559-6833
Mechanicsville, VA 23111   Fax: 804-559-6835
Joyce Kube

6243 PACCT of Roanoke Valley
PO Box 21112   703-989-5042
Roanoke, VA 24018   Fax: 703-989-5675
                                     e-mail: scheibe.p@worldnet.att.net

Sue Scheibe

Washington

6244 Common Voice for Pierce County Parents
801 East 141st Street   253-537-2145
Tacoma, WA 98445-2768   Fax: 253-537-2162
                        e-mail: acvmarge@comcast.net OR ffcmh@ffcmh.org
                                     www.ffcmh.org/who_chapters.php
A Common Voice for Pierce County Parents is affiliated with the Federation of Families for Children's Mental Health (FFCMH), a national organization dedicated exclusively to helping children with mental health needs and their families achieve a better quality of life.
Marge Critchlow, Director
Sandra Spencer, Executive Director Corporate Office (MD)

Wisconsin

6245 We Are the Children's Hope/Support Group
First Love Outreach Ministries
PO Box 06204   414-263-1323
Milwaukee, WI 53206   Fax: 414-263-1148
                                     e-mail: zelodius@aol.com
                                     www.firstlovelifecoaching.com

Pr Zelodius Morton, CEO

Wyoming

6246 Concerned Parent Coalition
1125 Sioux Avenue   307-682-6684
Gillette, WY 82718-6529
Michelle Gerlosky

6247 Uplift
200 W 17th Street   307-778-8686
Cheyenne, WY 82003   888-875-4383
                                     Fax: 307-778-8681
                                     e-mail: uplift@upliftwy.org
                                     www.upliftwy.org

Peggy Nikkel, Executive Director
Carla Schroeder, Deputy Director

Books

6248   **Anatomy of a Psychiatric Illness**
American Psychiatric Press
1400 K Street NW   202-682-6268
Washington, DC 20005-2403   Fax: 202-789-2648
Answers questions, provides clinical anecdotes, explains what medical science does and does not know about mental illnesses and discusses compassion and hard scientific facts surrounding the psychiatric profession.
230 pages
ISBN: 0-880485-21-3

6249   **Assessing Psychopathology and Behavior Problems: Mentally Ill Persons**
National Clearinghouse for Alcohol and Drug Abuse
PO Box 2345
Rockville, MD 20857-0001   800-729-6686
    www.health.org
239 pages

6250   **Caring for People with Severe Mental Disorders: A National Plan**
Superintendent of Documents
PO Box 371954   202-512-2250
Pittsburgh, PA 15250-7954
This report offers, from three panels of expert consultants, recommendations for strengthening both services research and research resources that should lead to improvement of the standard and provision of care for persons who have severe mental disorders.
80 pages

6251   **Complete Mental Health Directory**
Grey House Publishing
4919 Route 22   518-789-8700
Amenia, NY 12501   800-562-2139
    Fax: 518-789-0545
    e-mail: books@greyhouse.com
    www.greyhouse.com
Offers critical and comprehensive information on disorders, support groups, clinical management, government agencies, professional conferences, research centers and training.
687 pages
ISBN: 1-930956-06-1
Leslie Mackenzie, Publisher

6252   **Creating New Options**
Bazelon Center for Mental Health Law
1101 15th Street NW   202-467-5730
Washington, DC 20005-5002   Fax: 202-223-0409
    TDD: 202-467-4342
    e-mail: pubs@bazelon.org
    www.bazelon.org
Training for corrections administrators and staff on access to federal benefits for people with mental illnesses who are leacing jail or prison. Available as a manual ($7.50), a PowerPoint presentation on CD ($5), or both ($11).
2008
Lee Carly, Communications Director

6253   **Creating a Circle of Learning: The Church and the Mentally Ill**
National Alliance for the Mentally Ill
PO Box 753   301-524-7600
Waldorf, MD 20604-0753   Fax: 301-843-0159
    www.NAMI.org
A curriculum designed to sensitize adults in the church to the plight of people with severe mental illnesses and their families. Leaders can teach the study as 12 one-hour lessons or six two-hour lessons. The teaching sessions build on a Biblical-based theological reflection calling congregations to minister to their brothers and sisters with mental illnesses.
1997

6254   **Culture and the Restructuring of Community Mental Health**
William A Vega, author
Greenwood Publishing Group, Inc.
PO Box 6926
Portsmouth, NH 03802-6926   800-225-5800
    Fax: 877-231-6980
    e-mail: service@greenwood.com
    www.greenwood.com
Examines treatment, organizational planning and research issues and offers a critique of the theoretical and programmatic aspects of providing mental health services to traditionally undeserved populations.
168 pages
ISBN: 0-313268-87-8

6255   **Dealing with Mental Incapacity**
Center for Public Representation
PO Box 260049   608-251-4008
Madison, WI 53726-0049   800-369-0388
    Fax: 608-251-1263
This manual contains a comprehensive introduction to the problem of guardianship as well as chapters of financial and health care planning tools, guardianship under Wisconsin law, protective placement and Watts reviews.
Training Manual

6256   **Design of Rehabilitation Services in Psychiatric Hospital Settings**
American Occupational Therapy Association
PO Box 1725   301-948-9626
Rockville, MD 20849-1725   800-729-2082
Presents a design for constructing a rehabilitation system that will ensure the delivery of quality services to patients in a psychiatric hospital setting.
130 pages
Jeanette Bair, Executive Director

6257   **Dimensions of State Mental Health Policy**
Greenwood Publishing Group, Inc/Praeger Publishers
PO Box 6926
Portsmouth, NH 03802-6926   800-225-5800
    Fax: 877-231-6980
    e-mail: service@greenwood.com
    www.greenwood.com
Introduces students to the emerging field of state mental health policy.
320 pages
ISBN: 0-275932-52-4

6258   **Dual Diagnosis of Major Mental Illness and Substance Disorder**
National Alliance for the Mentally Ill
PO Box 753   703-524-7600
Waldorf, MD 20604-0753   Fax: 703-524-9094
    www.NAMI.org
Written for professionals, readable for families including descriptions of model programs.

6259   **Educating Patients and Families About Mental Illness: A Practical Guide**
Aspen Publishers
7201 McKinney Circle
Frederick, MD 21704-8356   800-638-8437
Introducing the manual to specifically address educating your patients and their families about mental illness.
496 pages

6260   **Elderly with Chronic Mental Illness**
Springer Publishing Company
536 Broadway   212-431-4370
New York, NY 10012-3955   877-687-7476
    Fax: 212-941-7842
    e-mail: marketing@springerpub.com
    www.springerpub.com
384 pages Hardcover
ISBN: 0-826172-80-6
Annette Imperati, Marketing Director

6261   **Elders Assert Their Rights**
Bazelon Center for Mental Health Law
1101 15th Street NW   202-467-5730
Washington, DC 20005-5002   Fax: 202-223-0409
    TDD: 202-467-4342
    e-mail: pubs@bazelon.org
    www.bazelon.org

A guide for residents, family members and advocates to the legal rights of elderly people with mental disabilities in nursing homes.
Paperback
Lee Carly, Communications Director

6262 Encyclopedia of Mental Health
Facts on File
11 Penn Plaza
New York, NY 10001
212-967-8800
800-322-8755
Fax: 800-678-3633
Here, readers will find inciseve definitions of theories, syndromes, symptons, treatments, and contemporary issues in easy-to-understand language.
480 pages Hardcover

6263 Encyclopedia of Phobias, Fears, and Anxieties
Facts on File
11 Penn Plaza
New York, NY 10001
212-967-8800
800-322-8755
Fax: 800-678-3633
500 pages Hardcover

6264 Evaluation and Treatment of the Psychogeriatric Patient
Diane Gibson, MS, author
Haworth Press
10 Alice Street
Binghamton, NY 13904-1580
607-722-5857
800-429-6784
Fax: 607-722-0012
www.haworthpress.com
This pertinent book assists occupational therapists and other health care providers in developing up-to-date psychogeriatric programs.
111 pages Hardcover
ISBN: 1-560240-52-1

6265 Family Caregiving in Mental Illness
National Alliance for the Mentally Ill
PO Box 753
Waldorf, MD 20604-0753
301-524-7600
Fax: 301-843-0159
www.NAMI.org
Examines patients' rights and treatment needs from the point of view of all those involved. Focuses on family burden and research and theoretical perspectives that influence mental health professionals.
1996

6266 Federal Law of the Mentally Handicapped
William Hein & Company
1285 Main Street
Buffalo, NY 14209-1987
716-882-2600
Chronological compilation of all relevant federal laws dealing with the mentally handicapped along with supporting documentation necessary to create a complete legislative history.
42 volumes/set

6267 Focal Group Psychotherapy for Mental Health Professionals
New Harbinger Publications
5674 Shattuck Avenue
Oakland, CA 94609-1662
800-748-6273
Fax: 510-652-5472
www.newharbinger.com
Definitive guide to leading brief, theme-based groups. This book offers an extensive week-by-week description of the basic concepts and interventions for 14 theme or focal groups.
544 pages

6268 Handbook of Mental Health and Mental Disor der Among Black Americans
Greenwood Publishing Group, Inc.
PO Box 6926
Portsmouth, NH 03802-6926
800-225-5800
Fax: 877-231-6980
e-mail: service@greenwood.com
www.greenwood.com
In addition to providing a wealth of new data on the mental health status of black communities, this handbook presents analyses of specific social, structural, and cultural conditions that affect the lives of individual black Americans.
352 pages
ISBN: 0-313263-30-2

6269 How to Live with a Mentally Ill Person: A Handbook of Day-to-Day Strategies
National Alliance for the Mentally Ill
PO Box 753
Waldorf, MD 20604-0753
301-524-7600
Fax: 301-843-0159
www.NAMI.org
Offers self-help-styled advice to caregivers. Includes personal experiences, education, stigma, coping, and the mental health system.
1996

6270 Last in Line
Bazelon Center for Mental Health Law
1101 15th Street NW
Washington, DC 20005-5002
202-467-5730
Fax: 202-223-0409
TDD: 202-467-4342
e-mail: pubs@bazelon.org
www.bazelon.org
discusses barriers to community integration of older adults with mental illnesses, and recommendations for change.
2006 72 pages
Lee Carly, Communications Director

6271 Living with Mental Handicaps
Jessica Kingsley Publishers
118 Pentonville Road
London, England,
071-833-2307
Fax: 071-837-2917
The focus of this book lies in its insistence that mentally handicapped people make transitions like the rest of us from youth to old age.
176 pages

6272 Madness in the Streets
Free Press
866 3rd Avenue
New York, NY 10022-6221
800-323-7445
Fax: 800-943-9831
www.simonsays.com
How psychiatry and the law abandoned the mentally ill.
436 pages
ISBN: 0-029153-80-8

6273 Making Child Welfare Work
Bazelon Center for Mental Health Law
1101 15th Street NW
Washington, DC 20005-5002
202-467-5730
Fax: 202-223-0409
TDD: 202-467-4342
e-mail: pubs@bazelon.org
www.bazelon.org
How the RC lawsuit forged new partnership to protect children and sustain families. The story of systems reform from the bottom up and the rededication of a burocracy to focus on the children and families it is meant to serve.
1998 126 pages
Lee Carly, Communications Director

6274 Managed Mental Health Care
American Psychiatric Press
1400 K Street NW
Washington, DC 20005-2403
202-682-6268
Fax: 202-789-2648
This text presents the collective wisdom of 40 experts experienced in clinical and managerial issues in managed care.
425 pages Hardcover
ISBN: 0-880483-55-5

6275 Managing Managed Care: A Mental Health Practitioner's Survival Guide
American Psychiatric Press
1400 K Street NW
Washington, DC 20005-2403
202-682-6268
Fax: 202-789-2648
Provides an easy-to-learn system for communicating with external reviewers and documenting quality of care.
200 pages Hardcover
ISBN: 0-880483-69-5

6276 Manic Depressive Illness
National Alliance for the Mentally Ill
PO Box 753
Waldorf, MD 20604-0753
703-524-7600
Fax: 703-524-9094
www.NAMI.org

A definitive overview of bipolar disorder.

6277 Medicare Rx Consumer Workbook
Mental Health America
2000 North Beauragard Street 703-684-7722
Alexandria, VA 22311 800-969-6642
Fax: 703-684-5968
TTY: 800-433-5959
www.mentalhealthamerica.net
This workbook is designed to help you as a mental health consumer to get educated about and get enrolled in the new Medicare prescription drug program. Designed as a pocket folder, the workbook includes basic language explanations, tips for enrollment preparation, questions you should ask regarding plan options, worksheets, and definitions.

6278 Membership Directory
Natl. Council for Community Behavioral Healthcare
12300 Twinbrook Parkway 301-984-6200
Rockville, MD 20852

6279 Mental Disability Law: A Primer
Commission on The Mentally Disabled
1800 M Street NW 202-331-2240
Washington, DC 20036-5802
An updated and expanded version of the 1984 edition. Addresses the considerations involved in representing clients with mental disabilities.

6280 Mental Health Care in Prisons and Jails
Vance Bibliographies
PO Box 229 217-762-3831
Monticello, IL 61856-0229
A bibliography regarding health care in prisons.
30 pages
ISBN: 0-792006-94-1

6281 Mental Health Concepts and Techniques for the Occupational Therapy Assistant
Raven Press
1185 Avenue of the Americas 212-930-9500
New York, NY 10036-2601 800-777-2295
This text offers clear and easily understood explanations of the various theoretical and practice health models. Second edition.
344 pages
ISBN: 0-781700-74-4

6282 Mental Health Law Reporter
Business Publishers, Inc.
PO Box 17592
Baltimore, MD 21297
800-274-6737
e-mail: custserv@bpinews.com
www.bpinews.com
Brings you the most timely, focused and thorough information on the legal issues that concern you in mental health litigation.
monthly
Leonard Eiserer, Publisher

6283 Mental Health: Counseling Services
Vance Bibliographies
PO Box 229 217-762-3831
Monticello, IL 61856-0229
Selected annotated bibliography on counseling services for the mentally handicapped from a black perspective.
23 pages
ISBN: 1-555903-76-2

6284 Mental Illness-Opposing Viewpoints Series
Greenhaven Press
Thomson Gale
Farmington Hills, MI 48333-9187 800-877-4253
Fax: 800-414-5043
e-mail: gale.customerservice@thomson.com
www.gale.com/greenhaven
In-depth overview of the topic written for upper elementary and junior/senior high school students.
2006
ISBN: 1-560061-68-5

6285 Mental and Physical Disability Law Report
American Bar Association

1800 M Street NW 202-331-2240
Washington, DC 20036-5802
Covers case law, legislative and regulatory developments that affect persons with mental or physical disabilities.

6286 Mentally Ill Individuals
Mainstream
1030 5th Street NW 202-898-1400
Washington, DC 20001-2504
Mainstreaming mentally ill individuals into the workplace.
12 pages

6287 Mood Apart: Depression, Mania, and Other Afflictions of the Self
National Alliance for the Mentally Ill
PO Box 753 301-524-7600
Waldorf, MD 20604-0753 Fax: 301-843-0159
www.NAMI.org
Discussion of depression and mania includes the symptoms, human costs, biological underpinnings, and therapies. Uses case histories, appendices, and historical references.
1997

6288 National Plan for Research on Child and Adolescent Mental Disorders
Superintendent of Documents
PO Box 371954 202-512-2250
Pittsburgh, PA 15250-7954
Summarizes the current knowledge about the prevalence and causes of mental disorders among children, identifies the possible treatments and prevention strategies and notes promising areas of research.
64 pages

6289 Occupational Therapy Practice Guidelines for Adults with Mood Disorders
American Occupational Therapy Association
4720 Montgomery Lane 301-652-2682
Bethesda, MD 20824-1220 Fax: 301-652-7711
TDD: 800-377-8555
www.aota.org
27 pages
ISBN: 1-569001-10-3

6290 Playing Cure
Jason Aronson
PO Box 15100
York, PA 17405-7100 800-782-0015
www.aronson.com
400 pages Hardcover
ISBN: 0-765700-21-2

6291 Protection and Advocacy Program for the Mentally Ill
US Department of Health and Human Services
5600 Fishers Lane 301-443-3667
Rockville, MD 20857-0001
Federal formula grant program to protect and advocate the rights of people with mental illnesses who are in residential facilities and to investigate abuse and neglect in such facilities.
Natalie Reatia, Chief

6292 Somatization Disorder in the Medical Setting
Superintendent of Documents
PO Box 371954 202-512-2250
Pittsburgh, PA 15250-7954
Somatization is a process in which psychological distress is expressed in multiple physical symptoms that have no discernible medical cause.
98 pages

6293 Strengthening the Role of Families in States' Early Intervention Systems
CEC, Department K00757 703-471-9543
Herdon, VA 22091
Policy guide for procedural safeguards for infants and toddlers under Part H of the Individuals with Disabilities Education Act.
213 pages Report

6294 Surviving Mental Illness
National Alliance for the Mentally Ill

PO Box 753
Waldorf, MD 20604-0753
703-524-7600
Fax: 703-524-9094
www.NAMI.org
The subjective experiences of people with multiple diagnoses including schizophrenia, bipolar disorder and manic depression.

6295 Teaching Adults with Mental Handicaps
Sunday School Board of the Southern Baptists
127 9th Avenue N
Nashville, TN 37234-0001
800-458-BSSB
Offers guidelines in methods of teaching adults with mental handicaps, their needs, outreach ideas, curriculum resources, adaptation procedures, and ministry suggestions.

6296 Troubled Journey
National Alliance for the Mentally Ill
PO Box 753
Waldorf, MD 20604-0753
301-524-7600
Fax: 301-843-0159
www.NAMI.org
Long associated with NAMI's former Siblings and Adult Children Network, the authors use their years of listening to stories - plus Marsh's professional experience - to provide a book that offers support to siblings and a caring and heartfelt approach to healing.
1997

6297 Turning Point
American Psychiatric Press
1400 K Street NW
Washington, DC 20005-2403
202-682-6268
Fax: 202-789-2648
The first comprehensive chronicle of the contributions made by conscientious objectors who volunteered for service in America's mental hospitals and state institutions for the developmentally disabled.
314 pages Hardcover
ISBN: 0-880485-60-4

6298 Understanding Depression
Patricia Ainsworth, MD, author
University Press of Mississippi
3825 Ridgewood Road
Jackson, MS 39211-6492
601-432-6205
Fax: 601-432-6217
e-mail: kburgess@ihl.state.ms.us
www.upress.state.ms.us
A clear explanation for those who know the illness personally and for those who want to understand them.
2000 120 pages Paperback
ISBN: 1-578061-69-5
Kathy Burgess, Advertising/Marketing Services Manager

6299 Understanding Mental Retardation
Patricia Ainsworth, MD; Pamela C Baker, PhD, author
University Press of Mississippi
3825 Ridgewood Road
Jackson, MS 39211-6492
601-432-6205
Fax: 601-432-6217
e-mail: kburgess@ihl.state.ms.us
www.upress.state.ms.us
A resource for parents, caregivers, and counselors.
2004 192 pages Paperback
ISBN: 1-578066-47-6
Kathy Burgess, Advertising/Marketing Services Manager

6300 Understanding Panic and Other Anxiety Disorders
Benjamin Root, MD, author
University Press of Mississippi
3825 Ridgewood Road
Jackson, MS 39211-6492
601-432-6205
Fax: 601-432-6217
e-mail: kburgess@ihl.state.ms.us
www.upress.state.ms.us
A patients guide to panic disorders, panic attacks, and other stress-related maladies.
2000 128 pages Paperback
ISBN: 1-578062-45-4
Kathy Burgess, Advertising/Marketing Services Manager

6301 Victims of Dementia
Haworth Press

10 Alice Street
Binghamton, NY 13904-1580
607-722-5857
800-429-6784
Fax: 607-722-0012
www.haworthpress.com
Provides an in-depth look at the concept, construction and operation of Wesley Hall, a special living area at the Chelsea United Methodist retirement home in Michigan.
1993 155 pages Hardcover
ISBN: 1-560242-64-0

6302 Way to Go: School Success for Children with Mental Health Care Needs
Bazelon Center for Mental Health Law
1101 15th Street NW
Washington, DC 20005-5002
202-467-5730
Fax: 202-223-0409
TDD: 202-467-4342
e-mail: pubs@bazelon.org
www.bazelon.org
A report and fact sheets that document how states and school districts have successfully combined school-wide positive behavior support (PBS) with effective mental health services to foster a school environment that is conducive to learning, and improves children's lives. Order book and fact sheets sheets seperately or together. Pricing according to volume begins at $25 per book, $10 per fact sheet, or $29 for the combination.
1998
Lee Carly, Communications Director

6303 What

6304 What Fair Housing Means for People with Disabilities
Bazelon Center for Mental Health Law
1101 15th Street NW
Washington, DC 20005-5002
202-467-5730
Fax: 202-223-0409
TDD: 202-467-4342
e-mail: pubs@bazelon.org
www.bazelon.org
Explains in plain language how three federal laws protect the housing rights of people with mental or physical disabilities. 2003 edition available as pdf download.
2006 56 pages
Lee Carly, Communications Director

6305 When Madness Comes Home
National Alliance for the Mentally Ill
PO Box 753
Waldorf, MD 20604-0753
301-524-7600
Fax: 301-843-0159
www.NAMI.org
Personal accounts offer first-hand, day-to-day experiences with mental illness of a sibling (mostly) and partner/spouse (briefly) and discuss the effects of growing up in a family whose energies are focused on an ill family member.
1997

6306 When Someone You Love Has a Mental Illness
National Alliance for the Mentally Ill
PO Box 753
Waldorf, MD 20604-0753
703-524-7600
Fax: 703-524-9094
www.NAMI.org
Excellent for families recently stricken with severe mental illness.

Children's Books

6307 Compassion Books, Inc.
7036 State Highway 80 South
Burnsville, NC 28714-7569
828-675-5909
800-970-4220
Fax: 828-675-9687
e-mail: orders@compassionbooks.com
www.compassionbooks.com
Hand picked resources to help people through loss, grief and changes of all kinds. Carry over 400 books and videos on death and dying, bereavement and change, comfort and healing, hope and much more.
Bruce Greene, VP

Magazines

6308 AJMR
American Association on Mental Retardation
444 N Capitol Street NW   202-387-1968
Washington, DC 20001-1508   800-424-3688
                                  Fax: 202-387-2193
                    e-mail: AAMR@access.digex.net
                                      www.aamr.org
Provides information on the latest program advances, current research, and information on products and services in the developmental disabilities field.
BiMonthly

6309 American Journal of Psychiatry
American Psychiatric Association
1400 K Street NW   202-682-6220
Washington, DC 20005-2492
Professional papers on topics in psychiatry.
Monthly
Public Affairs, Division

6310 American Psychologist
American Psychological Association
750 First Street NE   202-336-5510
Washington, DC 20002-4242   800-374-2721
                                  Fax: 202-336-5502
                                  TDD: 202-336-6123
                             e-mail: books@apa.org
                                       www.apa.org
Articles on current issues in psychology as well as empirical, theoretical and practical articles on broad aspects of psychology.
9x a year

6311 Journal of Clinical Psychology
Clinical Psychology Publishing Company
4 Conant Square   802-247-6877
Brandon, VT 05733-1018
Scholarly research reports in the field of psychology.

6312 Mental Retardation
American Association on Mental Retardation
444 N Capitol Street NW   202-387-1968
Washington, DC 20001-1508   800-424-3688
                                  Fax: 202-387-2193
                    e-mail: AAMR@access.digex.net
                                      www.aamr.org
Provides information on the latest program advances, current research, and information on products and services in the developmental disabilities field.
BiMonthly

6313 Psychopharmacology Bulletin
Superintendent of Documents/NIMH Journal
PO Box 371954   202-512-2250
Pittsburgh, PA 15250-7954
Emphasizes rapid, informal dissemination of recent research findings that have not previously appeared in the more formal literature.
Quarterly

6314 Psychosocial Rehabilitation Journal
Int'l Assoc. of Psychosocial Rehab. Services
730 Commonwealth Avenue   617-353-3549
Boston, MA 02215-1209
Discusses issues, programs and research on psychiatric rehabilitation.

Newsletters

6315 ACMH Newsletter
Association for Children's Mental Health
1705 Coolidge Road   517-336-7222
East Lansing, MI 48823-1735   800-782-0883
Offers the latest information, including unmet needs and notices of relevant agency and legislative activities, hearings, public meet-

ings and other opportunities for promoting children's mental health.
Quarterly
Gail Allen, Director
Marla Holle, Parent Advocate

6316 Advocate
National Alliance for the Mentally Ill
200 N Glebe Road   703-524-7600
Arlington, VA 22203-3754   Fax: 703-524-9094
Offers reviews of books, medical information, legislative information and Alliance activities for persons with mental illness, their families and professionals who work with them.
Quarterly

6317 Mental Health Law News
Interwood Publications
PO Box 20241   513-221-3715
Cincinnati, OH 45220-0241
Mental health case law summaries.
6 pages Monthly
ISBN: 0-889017-0 -
Frank J Bardack, Editor

6318 News & Notes
American Association on Mental Retardation
444 N Capitol Street NW   202-387-1968
Washington, DC 20001-1508   800-424-3688
                                  Fax: 202-387-2193
                    e-mail: AAMR@access.digex.net
                                      www.aamr.org
Covers legislative, program, and research developments of interest to the field, as well as international news, Association activities, job ads and other classifieds, and upcoming events.
BiMonthly

Pamphlets

6319 14 Worst Myths About Recovered Mental Patients
National Institutes of Health
5600 Fishers Lane   301-496-4000
Rockville, MD 20857-0001   e-mail: NIHInfo@nih.gov
                                       www.nih.gov
Refutes false beliefs that stigmatize recovered mental patients and suggests ways that the public can help advance the truth.

6320 Bipolar Disorder
National Institutes of Health
5600 Fishers Lane   301-443-3706
Rockville, MD 20857-0001   Fax: 301-443-6349
A short booklet offering a concise description of this disorder, which is also called manic-depressive illness.

6321 Coping with Mental Illness in the Family
National Alliance for the Mentally Ill
PO Box 753   703-524-7600
Waldorf, MD 20604-0753   Fax: 703-524-9094
                                      www.NAMI.org
A handbook for families.

6322 Dual Diagnosis: Substance Abuse and Mental Illness
National Alliance for the Mentally Ill
PO Box 753   703-524-7600
Waldorf, MD 20604-0753   Fax: 703-524-9094
                                      www.NAMI.org
A booklet for families and consumers.

6323 Helping Families Understand PTSD
National Veterans Services Fund
PO Box 2465   203-656-0003
Darien, CT 06820-0465   Fax: 203-656-1957
                         e-mail: NatVetSvc@aol.com

Pamphlet

6324 Let's Talk Facts About Childhood Disorders
American Psychiatric Association
1400 K Street NW   202-682-6220
Washington, DC 20005-2492

Offers information on depression and depressive disorders including the causes, symptoms, treatments, anxiety, and various other phobias.
Public Affairs, Division

6325 Mental Health Problems of Vietnam Veterans
National Veterans Services Fund
PO Box 2465
Darien, CT 06820-0465
203-656-0003
Fax: 203-656-1957
e-mail: NatVetSvc@aol.com
Pamphlet

6326 Minority Advocacy Notebook
Bazelon Center for Mental Health Law
1101 15th Street NW
Washington, DC 20005-5002
202-467-5730
Fax: 202-223-0409
TDD: 202-467-4342
e-mail: pubs@bazelon.org
www.bazelon.org
Selected materials and models from our manual on outreach and advocacy for African Americans and Latinos with mental disabilities; includes Impediments to Services and Advocacy for Black and Hispanic People with Mental Illness.
1998
Lee Carly, Communications Director

6327 New Challenge: Responding to Families
Federation for Children with Special Needs
95 Berkeley Street
Boston, MA 02116-6230
617-482-2915
800-331-0688
Addresses the needs of children with emotional, behavioral and mental disorders and their families.

6328 PTSD and the Family: Secondary Traumatization
National Veterans Services Fund
PO Box 2465
Darien, CT 06820-0465
203-656-0003
Fax: 203-656-1957
e-mail: NatVetSvc@aol.com
Pamphlet

6329 Plain Talk About...Dealing with the Angry Child
Superintendent of Documents
PO Box 371954
Pittsburgh, PA 15250-7954
202-512-2250
A flyer that offers suggestions for helping children cope with their anger in a healthy and constructive way.

6330 Plain Talk About...Handling Stress
Superintendent of Documents
PO Box 371954
Pittsburgh, PA 15250-7954
202-512-2250
Information on stress and how you can make it work for you rather than against you.

6331 Psychotherapy with Traumatized Vietnam Combatants
National Veterans Services Fund
PO Box 2465
Darien, CT 06820-0465
203-656-0003
Fax: 203-656-1957
e-mail: NatVetSvc@aol.com
Pamphlet

6332 Triumph Over Fear
National Alliance for the Mentally Ill
PO Box 753
Waldorf, MD 20604-0753
703-524-7600
Fax: 703-524-9094
www.NAMI.org
Step-by-step treatment plans for the many faces of phobias, panic disorder, obsessive-compulsive disorder, and post-traumatic stress. Includes case histories.
1994 Softcover

Audio & Video

6333 And After Tomorrow
G. Allan Roeher Institute
4700 Keele Street
Downsview, ON, M3J 1P3,
416-661-9611

A film about lives of people with a mental handicap and their families, in which parents and friends speak candidly about their personal experiences.
Films

6334 With a Little Help from My Friends
L'institut Roeher Institute
York University, 4700 Keele Street
North York, ON, M3J 1P3,
416-661-9611
Fax: 416-661-5701
This three-part video provides insight into inclusive education for people with mental handicaps.

Web Sites

6335 American Psychological Association
www.apa.org
Mission is to advance psychology as a science and professional organization that represents psychology in the United States.

6336 Coalition of Voluntary Mental Health Agencies
www.cvmha.org/
An umbrella advocacy organization of New York's mental health community, representing over 100 non-profit community based mental health agencies that serve more than 300,000 clients in the five boroughs of New York City and its environs.

6337 Community Access
www.cairn.org/
A nonprofit agency providing housing and advocacy for people with psychiatric disabilities.

6338 Federation of Families for Children's Mental Health
www.ffcmh.org/
Providing leadership to develop and sustain a nationwide network of family-run organizations.

6339 Healing Well
www.healingwell.com
An online health resource guide to medical news, chat, information and articles, newsgroups and message boards, books, disease-related web sites, medical directories, and more for patients, friends, and family coping with disabling diseases, disorders, or chronic illnesses.

6340 Health Finder
www.healthfinder.gov
Searchable, carefully developed web site offering information on over 1000 topics. Developed by the US Department of Health and Human Services, the site can be used in both English and Spanish.

6341 Healthlink USA
www.healthlinkusa.com
Health information concerning treatment, cures, prevention, diagnosis, risk factors, research, support groups, email lists, personal stories and much more. Updated regularly.

6342 Helios Health
www.helioshealth.com
Online resource for your health information. Detailed information about specific health topics, access to expert advice from our Medical Advisory Board, and up-to-date health news.

6343 Internet Mental Health
www.mentalhealth.com
A site whose goal is to improve understanding, diagnosis, and treatment of mental illness throughout the world. Includes information on specific disorders, medications, diagnosis, research, news, and other internet links.

6344 MedicineNet
www.medicinenet.com
An online resource for consumers providing easy-to-read, authoritative medical and health information.

6345 Medscape
www.medscape.com
Medscape offers specialists, primary care physicians, and other health professionals the Web's most robust and integrated medical information and educational tools.

6346   Mental Health America (formerly NMHA) Information Center
www.mentalhealthamerica.net
Provides informational materials, lobbies for Federal mental health legislation, stimulates funding of research on the causes and treatment of mental illnesses.

6347   National Alliance for the Mentally Ill
www.nami.org
Over 900 affiliate groups nationwide offer support to members, advocate better lives for their loved ones, support research efforts and educate the public to reduce the stigma attached to serious mental illnesses.

6348   National Mental Health Services Knowledge Exchange Network
www.mentalhealth.org
Leading the national system that delivers mental health services. Provides the treatment and support services neede by adults with mental disorders and children with serious emotional problems.

6349   WebMD
www.webmd.com
Information on mental illness, including articles and resources.

6350   World Federation for Mental Health
www.wfmh.com
Mission is to promote, among all people and nations, the highest possible level of mental health in its broadest biological, medical, educational, and social aspects.

Description

6351 Mental Illness/Depression

Depression is a mood disorder that can cause marked impairment of physical and social function and work capacity. It differs from normal grief which occurs in response to a significant separation or loss. It affects twice as many women as men and is more common in people with a family history of depression.

Research is gathering evidence of the relationship between depression and chemical imbalances in the brain. Clinical depression can also be associated with medication or other physical illnesses.

Common symptoms associated with depression include irritability, sleeping problems, changes in appetite, sadness, apathy, loss of interest in previously enjoyed activities and anxiety. Depression frequently disrupts a person's relationship with friends, family members and colleagues. It is also associated with alcohol and substance abuse. Suicide is the cause of death in approximately 15 percent of untreated patients.

Treatment must be tailored to the individual and can include talk therapy and/or medication. Newer groups of antidepressant medications have markedly improved the success of treatment. Patient and family education can play a crucial role. See also *Mental Illness/General and Mental Illness/Schizophrenia.*

National Agencies & Associations

6352 American Counseling Association
5999 Stevenson Avenue
Alexandria, VA 22304
800-347-6647
Fax: 800-473-2329
www.counseling.org
The American Counseling Association is a non-profit professional and educational organization that is dedicated to the growth and enhancement of the counseling profession. Founded in 1952 ACA is the world's largest such association.
Colleen R Logan, President
Richard Yep, Executive Director

6353 American Psychiatric Association
1000 Wilson Boulevard
Arlington, VA 22209-3901
703-907-7300
888-357-7924
e-mail: apa@psych.org
www.psych.org
The American Psychiatric Association is a medical specialty society recognized world wide. Its over 35,000 U.S. and international member physicians work together to ensure humane care and effective treatment for all persons with mental disorders.

6354 Anxiety Disorders Association of America
8730 Georgia Avenue
Silver Spring, MD 20910
240-485-1001
Fax: 240-485-1035
e-mail: information@adaa.org
www.adaa.org
The Anxiety Disorders Association (ADAA) is a non profit organization whose mission is to promote the prevention treatment and cure of anxiety disorders and to improve the lives of all people who suffer from them.
Abby J Fyer, Treasurer
Jerilyn Ross, President & CEO

6355 NARSAD: Mental Health Research Association
60 Cutter Miller Road
Great Neck, NY 11021-3104
516-829-0091
800-829-8289
Fax: 516-487-6930
e-mail: info@narsad.org
www.narsad.org
NARSAD Information and helpline staff is available to answer basic questions about the symptoms, causes and treatments of psychiatric illnesses. Information on support groups and other mental health organizations can also be provided.
Joel Gurin, Acting President
Louis Innamorato, Vice President Finance/CFO

6356 National Alliance for the Mentally Ill
2107 Wilson Boulevard
Arlington, VA 22201
703-524-7600
800-950-6264
Fax: 703-524-9097
TDD: 703-516-7227
www.nami.org
Membership organization with over 858 affiliates in 50 states, offers newsletters, a mail-order bookstore and many programs, conferences, symposia and groups meetings for family members and patients.
Liz Smith, Regional Director

6357 National Anxiety Foundation
3135 Custer Drive
Lexington, KY 40517-4001
606-272-7166
www.lexington-on-line.com/naf.html
Offers information and help to persons with panic disorders manic and depressive disorders and mental illness.
Stephen Cox, President & Medical Director
Linda Vermon Blair, Vice President

6358 National Foundation for Depressive Illness
PO Box 2257
New York, NY 10116-2257
800-239-1265
www.depression.org
Founded in 1983 to correct the myths and misconceptions surrounding the illness and help reverse the devastating effects depression has on the individual and our society. NAFDI's purpose is to educate the public and primary health care providers.
Jim Estepp, President/CEO
Joe Conoscenti, Vice President of Global Customers

6359 National Mental Health Association
2000 N Beauregard Street
Alexandria, VA 22311
703-684-7722
800-969-6642
Fax: 703-684-5968
TTY: 800-433-5959
e-mail: infoctr@nmha.org
www.mentalhealthamerica.net
Serves over 700 affiliates nationally providing information publications and other services.
David L Shern PhD, President & CEO
Eileen Sexton, Vice President Communications

6360 National Mental Health Information Center
PO Box 42557
Washington, DC 20015
800-789-2647
Fax: 240-747-5470
TTY: 866-889-2647
TDD: 866-889-2647
e-mail: nmhic-info@samhsa.hhs.gov
www.mentalhealth.samhsa.gov
The Center for Mental Health Services (CMHS) is charged with leading the national system that delivers mental health services. The goal of this system is to provide the treatment and support services needed by adults and children with mental disorders.
A Kathryn Power, Director
Edward B Searle, Deputy Director

6361 Option Institute
2080 S Undermountain Road
Sheffield, MA 01257
413-229-2100
800-714-2779
Fax: 413-229-8931
e-mail: participantsupport@option.org
www.option.org
Self-defeating beliefs, along with attitudes and judgments can lead to depression and a host of physical and psychological challenges.

The Option Institute offers programs designed to help uproot self-defeating beliefs and remove roadblocks to happiness.
Barry Kaufman, Co-Founder
Samahria Lyt Kaufman, Co-Founder

6362   Screening For Mental Health
Screening For Mental Health
One Washington Street   781-239-0071
Wellesley Hills, MA 02481   Fax: 781-431-7447
                    e-mail: smhinfo@mentalhealthscreening.org
                    www.mentalhealthscreening.org
Screening for Mental Health (SHM) is the non-profit organization that first introduced the concept of large-scale mental health screenings with its flagship program National Depression Screening Day in 1991. SHM programs now include both in-person and online.
Douglas G Jacobs, President/CEO
James Henry Scully Jr, Medical Director

Research Centers

6363   University of Pennsylvania: Depression Research Unit
School of Medicine
Department of Psychiatry   215-662-3462
Philadelphia, PA 19104   Fax: 215-662-6443
Focuses on mental health and depression.
Jay D Amsterdam MD, Director

6364   University of Texas Mental Health Clinical Research Center
University of Texas
5323 Harry Hines Boulevard   214-648-5555
Dallas, TX 75390   Fax: 214-485-99
                    e-mail: news@utsouthwester.edu
                    www.utsouthwesteRN.edu
Research activity of major and atypical depression.
Eric Nestler MD, Chairman
Alex Cabrera, Clinic Manager

6365   Yale University: Behavioral Medicine Clinic
Yale School of Medicine
333 Cedar Street   203-785-4184
New Haven, CT 06510
Focuses on mental disorders including schizophrenia and depression.
Hoyle Leigh MD, Director

6366   Yale University: Ribicoff Research Facilities/CT Mental Health Center
34 Park Street   203-789-7300
New Haven, CT 06511   Fax: 203-562-7079
Clinical research in the areas of schizophrenia depression and mental disorders.
George Henin MD, Director

Support Groups & Hotlines

6367   Depression and Bipolar Support Alliance
730 N Franklin Street   312-642-0049
Chicago, IL 60654   800-826-3632
                                           Fax: 312-642-7243
                                           www.dbsalliance.org
Consists of approximately 900 patient groups providing support and direct services to persons with clinical depression and/or bipolar disorder.
Peter Ashenden, President

6368   National Health Information Center
PO Box 1133   310-565-4167
Washington, DC 20013   800-336-4797
                                           Fax: 301-984-4256
                                           e-mail: info@nhic.org
                                           www.health.gov/nhic
Offers a nationwide information referral service, produces directories and resource guides.

Books

6369   Columbia University Complete Home Guide to Mental Health
Henry Holt & Company
115 W 18th Street   212-886-9200
New York, NY 10011-4113   Fax: 212-633-0748
A compendium of information on all aspects of mental health; written primarily for the lay reader.
476 pages

6370   Coping with Depression and Mood Disorders
Rosen Publishing Group
29 E 21st Street   212-777-3017
New York, NY 10010   800-237-9932
                                           Fax: 888-436-4643
                    e-mail: customerservice@rosenpub.com
                    www.rosenpublishing.com
With an emphasis on life's myriad difficulties, the authors help teens find practical ways to cope with depression.

ISBN: 0-823929-73-6
Lawrence Clayton PhD, Author
Sharon Carter, Author

6371   Depression Sourcebook
Brian P. Quinn, author
McGraw-Hill Companies
Returns Department
Dubuque, IA 52002   877-833-5524
                                           Fax: 614-759-3749
            e-mail: pbg.ecommerce_custserv@mcgrw-hill.com
                    www.mcgraw-hill.com
Everything anyone afflicted with a depressive disorder - or the people who care about them - need to know about unipolar and bipolar depression.
2000 288 pages
ISBN: 0-737303-79-4

6372   Depression and its Treatment
Warner Books
1271 Avenue of the Americas   212-522-7200
New York, NY 10020-1300
A layman's guide to help one understand and cope with America's #1 mental health problem.
157 pages

6373   Depressive Illnesses: Treatments Bring New Hope
Superintendent of Documents
PO Box 371954   202-512-2250
Pittsburgh, PA 15250-7954
Offers the general public an overview of the various depressive illnesses. Topics include causes, symptoms and types of depression, clinical evaluation and treatment, helpful suggestions for family and friends, and other sources of information.
28 pages

6374   Encyclopedia of Depression
Facts on File
11 Penn Plaza   212-967-8800
New York, NY 10001   800-322-8755
                                           Fax: 800-678-3633
This volume defines and explains all terms and topics relating to depression.
170 pages Hardcover

6375   Essential Guide to Psychiatric Drugs
St. Martin's Press
175 5th Avenue   212-674-5151
New York, NY 10010-7848   800-221-7945
                                           Fax: 212-420-9314
Basic information on 123 drugs used for depression, anxiety and bipolar illness.

6376   Everything You Need to Know About Depression
Rosen Publishing Group

29 E 21st Street
New York, NY 10010

212-777-3017
800-237-9932
Fax: 888-436-4643
e-mail: customerservice@rosenpub.com
www.rosenpublishing.com

An important resource for teens who are looking for help with depression.
Grades 7-12
ISBN: 0-823934-39-X
Elanor H Ayer, Author

6377 Inside Manic Depression
Sunnyside Press
PO Box 1717
San Marcos, CA 92079-1717

619-424-3348

The true story of one victim's triumph over despair. A first person account.
176 pages

6378 Medical Management of Depression
EMIS Medical Publishers
PO Box 1607
Durant, OK 74702-1607

580-924-0643
800-225-0694
Fax: 580-924-9414

ISBN: 0-929240-62-6

6379 Mood Apart
Basic Books
10 E 53rd Street
New York, NY 10022-5244

212-207-7057

An overview of the depression and manic depression and the available treatments for them.
363 pages

6380 Overcoming Depression
Harper & Row
10 E 53rd Street
New York, NY 10022-5299

212-207-7000

318 pages Paperback

6381 Panic Disorder in the Medical Setting
Superintendent of Documents
PO Box 371954
Pittsburgh, PA 15250-7954

202-512-2250

This book serves the primary care physicians as a helpful guide in recognizing and treating panic disorder in patients and in identifying those who need psychiatric consultation or rerferrals.
1993 135 pages

6382 Pastoral Care of Depression
The Haworth Press
10 Alice Street
Binghamton, NY 13904-1580

607-722-5857
800-429-6784
Fax: 607-895-0582
e-mail: getinfo@haworth.com
www.haworth.com

Helps caregivers by overcoming the simplistic myths about depressive disorders and probing the real issues.
Paperback
ISBN: 0-789002-65-5

6383 Prozac Nation: Young & Depressed in America: A Memoir
Houghton Mifflin Company
Wayside Road
Burlington, MA 01803

800-225-3362

Struck with depression at 11, now 27, Wurtzel chronicles her struggle with the illness. Witty, terrifying and sometimes funny, it tells the story of a young life almost destroyed by depression.
317 pages

6384 Psychotherapy of Severe and Mild Depression
Jason Aronson
PO Box 15100
York, PA 17405-7100

800-782-0015
Fax: 201-840-7242
www.aronson.com

464 pages Softcover
ISBN: 1-568211-46-5

6385 Questions & Answers About Depression & Its Treatment
Ivan K Goldberg, MD, author
Charles Press Publishers
PO Box 15715
Philadelphia, PA 19103-0715

215-561-2786
Fax: 215-561-0191
e-mail: mailbox@charlespresspub.com
www.charlespresspub.com

All the questions you'd like to ask, asked and answered.
139 pages
ISBN: 0-914783-68-8

6386 Report of the Secretary's Task Force on Youth Suicide, Volume 1
Superintendent of Documents
PO Box 371954
Pittsburgh, PA 15250-7954

202-512-2250

A comprehensive review of information about youth suicide. The task force recommendations are presented in Volume 1.
110 pages

6387 Touched with Fire:- Manic Depressive Illness & the Artistic Temperment
Free Press
866 3rd Avenue
New York, NY 10022-6221

Fax: 800-943-9831
www.simonsays.com

Describing and discussing the markedly increased rates of severe mood disorders and suicides among the artistically creative and the reasons why.
370 pages

6388 Winter Blues
Norman E Rosenthal, author
Guilford Press
72 Spring Street
New York, NY 10012-4019

800-265-7006
Fax: 212-966-6708
e-mail: info@guilford.com
www.guilford.com

Complete information about Seasonal Affective Disorder and its treatment.
2005
ISBN: 1-593852-14-2

6389 Women and Depression
Springer Publishing Company
536 Broadway
New York, NY 10012-3955

212-431-4370
877-687-7476
Fax: 212-941-7842
e-mail: marketing@springerpub.com
www.springerpub.com

This volume examines depression in women within a developmental context. It ranges from issues in childhood and adolescence through premenstrual syndrome and postpartum depression to issues of menopause and aging.
328 pages Hardcover
ISBN: 0-826151-40-X
Annette Imperati, Marketing Director

6390 Yesterday's Tomorrow
Hazelden
15251 Pleasant Valley Road
Center City, MN 55012-9640

651-257-4010
800-328-9000
Fax: 651-213-4426
www.hazelden.org

A meditation book that shows why and how recovery works, from the author's own experiences.
432 pages Paperback
ISBN: 1-568381-60-3

Children's Books

6391 Compassion Books, Inc.
7036 State Highway 80 South
Burnsville, NC 28714-7569

828-675-5909
800-970-4220
Fax: 828-675-9687
e-mail: orders@compassionbooks.com
www.compassionbooks.com

Hand picked resources to help people through loss, grief and changes of all kinds. Carry over 400 books and videos on death and dying, bereavement and change, comfort and healing, hope and much more.
Bruce Greene, VP

Newsletters

6392 **NFDI Newsletter**
National Foundation for Depressive Illness
PO Box 2257   212-268-4260
New York, NY 10116-2257   800-248-4344
                                         Fax: 212-268-4434
                                         e-mail: pross@att.net
                                         www.depression.org
To correct the myths and misconceptions surrounding the illness and help reverse the devastating effects depression has on the individual and our society and to inform the public, primary health care providers, other healthcare professionals and corporations about depression and manic depression and to provide the information about correct diagnosis and treatment and the availability of qualified doctors and support groups.
4 pages Quarterly

Pamphlets

6393 **Depression is a Treatable Illness: A Patients Guide**
Department of Health & Human Services
2101 E Jefferson Street   301-217-1245
Rockville, MD 20852-4908
Tells about major depressive disorder, which is only one form of depressive illness. This booklet answers important questions regarding this disorder and gives information on where to go for more help.

6394 **If You're Over 65 and Feeling Depressed...**
National Institutes on Mental Health
5600 Fishers Lane   301-443-3706
Rockville, MD 20857-0001   Fax: 301-443-6349
Many older people believe that their age alone is responsible for feelings of exhaustion, helplessness and worthlessness. This brochure discusses the causes of depression in the older years, symptoms, types of treatment and where to go for help.
12 pages

6395 **Let's Talk About Depression**
Superintendent of Documents
PO Box 371954   202-512-2250
Pittsburgh, PA 15250-7954
Targeted especially for inner-city youth. The colorful design will capture attention and focus on depression in a way that young people will understand and identify with.

6396 **Lithium and Manic Depression**
Lithium Info. Center-Dean Foundation for Health
8000 Excelsior Drive   608-836-8070
Madison, WI 53717-1972
A guidebook about lithium and its effects on bipolar affective disorders and manic depression.
1992 32 pages

6397 **Living Without Depression & Manic Depression: A Workbook**
National Alliance for the Mentally Ill
PO Box 753
Waldorf, MD 20604-0753   703-524-7600
                                         www.NAMI.org
Workbook offering checklists and helpful advice targeted for individuals whose depressive illness is stabilized.
1994

6398 **Panic Disorder**
National Institutes of Health
5600 Fishers Lane   301-443-3706
Rockville, MD 20857-0001   Fax: 301-443-6349
Written for the lay public, this pamphlet contains a description of panic disorder, gives the symptoms, describes treatment methods, and encourages the person who has the symptoms to seek treatment.

6399 **Plain Talk About Depression**
Superintendent of Documents
PO Box 371954   202-512-2250
Pittsburgh, PA 15250-7954
A flyer discussing types of depression, major depression, symptoms and causes.

6400 **Understanding Panic Disorder**
National Institutes of Health
5600 Fishers Lane   301-443-3706
Rockville, MD 20857-0001   Fax: 301-443-6349
Offers information on what an panic disorder is, symptoms, causes, treatment, medications and therapy.

6401 **Useful Information on Phobias and Panic**
Superintendent of Documents
PO Box 371954   202-512-2250
Pittsburgh, PA 15250-7954
This booklet provides information on both phobias and panic. Symptoms, causes and treatments of these disorders are referred to. If you know someone who is excessively fearful, this booklet will be of great help to them in understanding their problem.
40 pages 50 copies

6402 **What to Do When a Friend is Depressed: Guide for Students**
Superintendent of Documents
PO Box 371954   202-512-2250
Pittsburgh, PA 15250-7954
Offers information on depression and its symptoms and suggests things a young person can do to guide a depressed friend in finding help.

6403 **What to Do When an Employee is Depressed: A Guide for Supervisors**
Superintendent of Documents
PO Box 371954   202-512-2250
Pittsburgh, PA 15250-7954
A D/ART program brochure that will enable an employer to recognize the symptoms of depression in an employee and offers suggestions on what to say to the employee to encourage him or her to seek help.

Audio & Video

6404 **Four Lives: A Portrait of Manic Depression**
Fanlight Productions
4196 Washington Street   617-469-4999
Boston, MA 02131-1731   800-937-4113
                                         Fax: 617-469-3379
                                         e-mail: fanlight@fanlight.com
                                         www.fanlight.com
Four patients, families and psychiatrists share their perspectives on living with manic depression.
1987 60 Minutes
ISBN: 1-572950-29-3

6405 **Taking Control of Depression**
                                         800-228-2495
Dramatic program offering new hope in the understanding and treatment of depression, with actor Ed Asner and Alan Xenakis, M.D.

6406 **When Someone You Love Suffers from Depression**
Medcom/Trainex
                                         800-320-1444
Helping family and friends identify depression in a loved one - offers ways to help stop the suffering and get appropriate treatment.

Web Sites

6407 **Healing Well**
                                         www.healingwell.com
An online health resource guide to medical news, chat, information and articles, newsgroups and message boards, books, disease-related web sites, medical directories, and more for patients, friends,

and family coping with disabling diseases, disorders, or chronic illnesses.

6408 Health Finder

www.healthfinder.gov

Searchable, carefully developed web site offering information on over 1000 topics. Developed by the US Department of Health and Human Services, the site can be used in both English and Spanish.

6409 Healthlink USA

www.healthlinkusa.com

Health information concerning treatment, cures, prevention, diagnosis, risk factors, research, support groups, email lists, personal stories and much more. Updated regularly.

6410 Helios Health

www.helioshealth.com

Online resource for your health information. Detailed information about specific health topics, access to expert advice from our Medical Advisory Board, and up-to-date health news.

6411 MedicineNet

www.medicinenet.com

An online resource for consumers providing easy-to-read, authoritative medical and health information.

6412 Medscape

www.medscape.com

Medscape offers specialists, primary care physicians, and other health professionals the Web's most robust and integrated medical information and educational tools.

6413 National Anxiety Foundation

www.lexington-on-line.com/naf.html

Offers information and help to persons with panic disorders, manic and depressive disorders and mental illness.

6414 National Foundation for Depressive Illness

www.depression.org

Provide the information about correct diagnosis and treatment and the availability of qualified doctors and support groups.

6415 WebMD

www.webmd.com

Information on depression, including articles and resources.

Description

6416 # Mental Illness/Schizophrenia

Schizophrenia is a chronic mental illness that is characterized by disturbances of thinking, feeling, and behavior. It usually begins in late adolescence or early adult life, with a lifetime prevalence between 0.2 to 1 percent. Despite its literal translation of split mind, schizophrenia is not the same as split personality. Although its specific cause is unknown, most cases of schizophrenia are believed to result from a complex interaction between biologic, inherited and environmental factors.

Symptoms of schizophrenia vary in type and severity and may include delusions and auditory hallucinations (hearing voices), incoherent thought patterns, catatonic behavior, and a flat or grossly inappropriate emotional state.

Drug treatment is the cornerstone of managing schizophrenia. When treated early, patients tend to respond quickly and more fully. Effective drugs have been available for several decades, and have revolutionized treatment of the disease. However, these drug treatments may be limited by side effects (especially movement disorders resembling Parkinsons disease) and by the patient's failure or refusal to stay on treatment. Patient non-compliance is sometimes addressed with long-acting injectable medications. A new class of drugs, lacking the Parkinson-like side effects, and sometimes dramatically more effective than previously used drugs, became available during the 1990s. Their use is limited by high costs and the threat of serious blood-related side effects. Treatment includes counseling, social support, rehabilitation, and skills retraining. Poor outcome frequently leads to extensive and long-term disability. Psychological and educational interventions can reduce the rate of relapse. People close to persons with schizophrenia are often very affected by the disease and can be helped by support and advocacy groups. See also *Mental Illness/General and Mental Illness/Depression*.

National Agencies & Associations

6417 **International Society for the Study of Dissociation**
8400 Westpark Drive
McLean, VA 22102
703-610-9037
Fax: 703-610-0234
e-mail: info@isst-d.org
www.issd.org
A nonprofit professional association that promotes research and training in the identification of treatment of multiple personality, provides professional and public education about multiple personality and initiates international communication among clinicians.
Kathy Steele, President
Paul F Dell PhD, President-Elect

6418 **NARSAD: Mental Health Research Association**
60 Cutter Miller Road
Great Neck, NY 11021-3104
516-829-0091
800-829-8289
Fax: 516-487-6930
e-mail: info@narsad.org
www.narsad.org
NARSAD Information and helpline staff is available to answer basic questions about the symptoms, causes and treatments of psychi-

atric illnesses. Information on support groups and other mental health organizations can also be provided.
Joel Gurin, Acting President
Louis Innamorato, Vice President Finance/CFO

6419 **National Alliance for the Mentally Ill**
Colonial Place Three
2107 Wilson Boulevard
Arlington, VA 22201-3042
703-524-7600
800-950-6264
Fax: 703-524-9094
TDD: 703-516-7227
e-mail: membership@naminyc.org
www.nami-nyc-metro.org
Nonprofit, self-help, volunteer organization that offers practical support, useful education, advocacy, comfort and understanding to those in the greater New York area who suffer or have family members suffering from mental illnesses. Chapter of the National Alliance for the Mentally Ill and the New York State Alliance for the Mentally Ill.
Charolette Moses Fischman, President
Karen Gormandy, Vice President

Research Centers

6420 **Huxley Insititue-American Schizophrenic Association**
86-B Dorchester Drive
Lakewood, NJ 08701
www.schizohprenia.org
The ASA works to bring effective, low-cost treatment to patients woth schizophrenia and help them in a cooperative effort to cope with the disorder.
Abram Hoffer, MD PhD, President
Elizabeth Plante, Director, Huxley Institute

6421 **Maryland Psychiatric Research Center**
Box 21247
Baltimore, MD 21228
410-402-7666
Fax: 410-788-3837
www.umaryland.edu/mprc
Providing treatment to patients with schizophrenia and related disorders educating professionals and consumers about schizophrenia and conducting basic and translational research into the manifestations causes and treatment of schizophrenia.
Dr William Carpenter Jr, Director
Vito J Seskunas, Deputy Director for Administration

6422 **National Alliance for Research on Schizophrenia and Depression**
Grants Office
60 Cutter Mill Road
Great Neck, NY 11021
516-829-0091
800-829-8289
Fax: 516-487-6930
e-mail: info@narsad.org
www.narsad.org
Research focusing on varieties of mental illness and mental disorders.
Steve Lieber, Chairman of the Board & Treasurer
Joel Gurin, Acting President

6423 **Schizophrenia Research Branch: Division of Clinical and Treatment Research**
5600 Fisher Lane, Parklawn Building
Rockville, MD 20857
301-443-4707
Fax: 301-443-6000
Plans, supports, and conducts programs of research, research training, and resource development of schizophrenia and related disorders. Reviews and evaluates research developments in the field and recommends new program directors. Collaborates with organizations in and outside of the National Institue of Mental Health (NIMH) to stimulate work in the field through conferences and workshops.

6424 **Schizophrenia Research Branch: Division of**
5600 Fisher Lane Parklawn Building
Rockville, MD 20857
301-443-4707
Fax: 301-443-6000
Plans supports and conducts programs of research research training and resource development of schizophrenia and related disorders. Reviews and evaluates research developments in the field and recommends new program directors. Collaborates with organizations in and outside of the National Institute of Mental Health (NIMH) to stimulate work in the field through conferences and workshops.

6425 **Tennessee Neuropsychiatric Institute Middle Tennessee Mental Health Institute**
Middle Tennessee Mental Health Institute
221 Stewarts Ferry Pike
Nashville, TN 37217   615-902-7535
Michael Eber MD, Director

6426 **University of Iowa Mental Health Clinical Research Center**
University of Iowa Hospitals & Clinics
200 Hawkins Drive   319-356-1553
Iowa City, IA 52242   877-575-2864
Fax: 319-353-8300
www.iowa-mhcrc.psychiatry.uiowa.edu
Schizophrenia studies and other cognitive disorder research.
Nancy C Andreassen MD, Director

Support Groups & Hotlines

6427 **National Health Information Center**
PO Box 1133   310-565-4167
Washington, DC 20013   800-336-4797
Fax: 301-984-4256
e-mail: info@nhic.org
www.health.gov/nhic
Offers a nationwide information referral service, produces directories and resource guides.

Books

6428 **Encyclopedia of Schizophrenia and the Psychotic Disorders**
Facts on File
11 Penn Plaza   212-967-8800
New York, NY 10001   800-322-8755
Fax: 800-678-3633
This volume details recent theories and research findings on schizophrenia and psychotic disorders, together with a complete overview of the field's history.
368 pages Hardcover

6429 **Experiences of Schizophrenia**
Guilford Press
72 Spring Street
New York, NY 10012   800-365-7006
Fax: 212-966-6708
e-mail: info@guilford.com
www.guilford.com
This authoritative book presents new information on seasonal affective disorder. It includes remedies such as recent advances in light box therapy, research on the effectiveness of antidepressants, and new recipes to counterbalance unhealthy winter food cravings. This book also helps distinguish various degrees of the disorder ranging from winter blues to full blown SAD, and provides a self test that readers can use to evalutate their own seasonal mood changes.
2005 372 pages
ISBN: 1-593852-14-2

6430 **Occupational Therapy Practice Guidelines for Adults with Schizophrenia**
American Occupational Therapy Association
4720 Montgomery Lane   301-652-2682
Bethesda, MD 20824-1220   Fax: 301-652-7711
TDD: 800-377-8555
www.aota.org
24 pages
ISBN: 1-569001-53-7

6431 **Return from Madness**
Jason Aronson
PO Box 15100
York, PA 17405-7100   800-783-0015
www.aronson.com
256 pages Hardcover
ISBN: 1-568216-25-4

6432 **Schizophrenia and Primitive Mental States**
Jason Aronson

PO Box 15100
York, PA 17405-7100   800-782-0015
Fax: 201-840-7242
www.aronson.com
288 pages Softcover
ISBN: 0-765700-27-1

6433 **Schizophrenia: From Mind to Molecule**
American Psychiatric Press
1400 K Street NW   202-682-6268
Washington, DC 20005-2403   Fax: 202-789-2648
Presents a change in the scientific understanding and outlook regarding the devastating disorder of schizophrenia. It provides a thorough, up-to-date look at schizophrenia that includes neural behavioral studies, technologies and medical treatments.
274 pages Hardcover
ISBN: 0-880489-50-2

Children's Books

6434 **Year it Rained**
MacMillan Publishing Company
866 3rd Avenue
New York, NY 10022-6221   212-702-2000
www.mcp.com
The story of a girl traumatized by an alcoholic father and her desire to commit suicide. Hospitalized for schizophrenia, Elizabeth reaches a catharsis and, with the help of a poet, discovers that her talent and therapy may be in writing.
Grades 7-10

Magazines

6435 **Dissociation**
ISSMP&D
5700 Old Orchard Road   847-966-4322
Skokie, IL 60077-1036   Fax: 847-966-9418
A professional journal offering the latest information about the issues and research into multiple personalities and related disorders.

6436 **Schizophrenia Bulletin**
Superintendent of Documents/NIMH Journal
PO Box 371954   202-512-2250
Pittsburgh, PA 15250-7954
Serves as a forum for multidisciplinary exchange of information about schizophrenia and is exclusively devoted to the exploration of this severe disorder.
Quarterly

Newsletters

6437 **ISSD News**
Int'l Society for the Study of Dissociation
60 Revere Drive   847-480-0899
Northbrook, IL 60062   Fax: 847-480-9282
e-mail: issd@issd.org
www.issd.org
Includes current news from other onzations of interest to members, information about recent articles and books, news from US and international affiliates and the latest issues concerning multiple personality/dissociative states.
17 pages 6 times a year
Julie A Theander, Administrative Director
Richard Koepke, Executive Director

Pamphlets

6438 **Schizophrenia**
National Alliance for the Mentally Ill
200 N Glebe Road   703-524-7600
Arlington, VA 22203-3754   Fax: 703-524-9094
Part of the NAMI medical information series offering information on the causes, symptoms and treatments of Schizophrenia.

Web Sites

6439   Healing Well

www.healingwell.com

An online health resource guide to medical news, chat, information and articles, newsgroups and message boards, books, disease-related web sites, medical directories, and more for patients, friends, and family coping with disabling diseases, disorders, or chronic illnesses.

6440   Health Finder

www.healthfinder.gov

Searchable, carefully developed web site offering information on over 1000 topics. Developed by the US Department of Health and Human Services, the site can be used in both English and Spanish.

6441   Healthlink USA

www.healthlinkusa.com

Health information concerning treatment, cures, prevention, diagnosis, risk factors, research, support groups, email lists, personal stories and much more. Updated regularly.

6442   Helios Health

www.helioshealth.com

Online resource for your health information. Detailed information about specific health topics, access to expert advice from our Medical Advisory Board, and up-to-date health news.

6443   International Society for the Study of Dissociation

www.issd.org

Association that promotes research and training in the identification of treatment of multiple personality.

6444   MedicineNet

www.medicinenet.com

An online resource for consumers providing easy-to-read, authoritative medical and health information.

6445   Medscape

www.medscape.com

Medscape offers specialists, primary care physicians, and other health professionals the Web's most robust and integrated medical information and educational tools.

6446   National Alliance for the Mentally Ill

www.nami-nyc-metro.org

Organization that offers practical support, useful education, advocacy, comfort, and understanding to those in the greater New York area who suffer or have family members suffering from neurobiologically based disorders.

6447   Schizophrenia Therapy Online Resource Center

www.schizophreniatherapy.com

A website which provides effective and lasting alternatives to traditional treatment for individuals suffering with schizophrenia. Offers an effective and full continium of services ranging from psychopharmacology to individual and group psychotherapy to social rehabilitation, supported work experience, assertive community training and supported housing.

6448   WebMD

www.webmd.com

Information on schizophrenia, including articles and resources.

Description

6449 Migraine

Roughly 45 million Americans suffer from chronic headaches, the most disabling of which is migraine. Classified as a vascular headache, migraine headaches are caused by intracranial vasospasm, that is, alternating swelling and constricting of blood vessels on the surface of the brain. The swelling phase brings on intense pain and nausea, while the constricting phase may cause neurologic symptoms such as focal loss of vision or numbness involving one side of the body. Another theory is that migraines are due to a different dysfunction of the neurovascular system that results in the release of a substance that leads to migraine. More than 50 percent of patients have a family history of migraine. They also appear to have a hormonal component, being more common in women and often affected by menstrual cycles or pregnancy.

Management of migraine begins with careful observation for triggering agents like foods, alcohol, or irregular sleep patterns. Acute treatment to stop a migraine involves a class of drugs which antagonize the action of the 5-HT that aggravates the migraine process. They block inflammation and can abort migraine in about 70 percent of patients. Sumatriptan, the prototype, is available in oral and subcutaneous injection forms. Ergot drugs, also available in oral and injectable forms, work by helping the swollen blood vessels constrict down to normal size. If headaches become very frequent, doctors may recommend preventive therapy, which requires daily drug administration. Drugs used in this way include beta-blockers and calcium-channel blockers, which were originally developed for hypertension and heart disease, and certain medicines ordinarily used for depression or seizures.

Pain medication should be used sparingly. Nonsteroidal anti-inflammatory drugs, such as ibuprofen are best for mild to moderate headaches. Narcotic medications should be avoided except under special circumstances and with strict guidelines. Most migraine sufferers can be satisfactorily managed by their primary care physician or a neurologist, but in refractory cases a multi-disciplinary headache center may be of help.

Tension is the other common cause of disabling headaches. They are not migraine and are not considered vascular headache, but are mentioned here because they are so common. Some of the resources listed in this section may be helpful for persons with tension headache.

National Agencies & Associations

6450 American Academy of Neurology
1080 Montreal Avenue
Saint Paul, MN 55116-2311
651-695-2717
800-879-1960
Fax: 651-695-2791
e-mail: memberservices@aan.com
www.aan.com

A professional organization representing neurologists worldwide.
Catherine Rydell, Executive Director & CEO
Stephen M Sergay, President

6451 American Council for Headache Education
19 Mantua Road
Mount Royal, NJ 08061
856-423-0258
800-255-2243
Fax: 856-423-0082
e-mail: achehq@talley.com
www.achenet.org

A not-for-profit alliance of headache sufferers and physicians who are working together to improve the quality of care and the quality of information available to people with chronic or severe headache conditions.
Jan Lewis Brandes MD, President

6452 American Headache Society
19 Mantua Road
Mount Royal, NJ 08061
856-423-0043
Fax: 856-423-0082
e-mail: ahshq@talley.com
www.ahsnet.org

Professional society of health care providers who study and treat headache and face pain. AHS brings physicians from various fields and specialties together to share concepts and developments about headache and related conditions.
Linda McGillicuddy, Executive Director
Fred Sheftell, President

6453 Help for Headaches
515 Richmond Street
London, Ontario, N6A-5M3
519-434-0008
e-mail: brent@helpforheadaches.org
www.headache-help.org

A non-profit organization, and a registered Canadian charity that is committed to educational services for those suffering from and treating headaches.
G Brent Lucas BA, Director

6454 Migraine Association of Canada
356 Bloor Street E
Toronto Ontario, M4W
416-920-4916
800-663-3557
Fax: 416-920-3677
www.migraine.ca

A registered charity funded through memberships. Activities include a 24 hour telephone information access line the development of materials and assistance for those who start community self-help groups, workplace seminars and awareness programs.

6455 Migraine Awareness Group: A National Understanding for Migraineurs
100 N Union Street
Alexandria, VA 22314
703-349-1929
Fax: 703-739-2432
e-mail: comments@migraines.org
www.migraines.org

Works to bring public awareness utilizing the electronic print and artistic mediums to the fact that migraine is a true organic neurological disease.
Michael J Coleman, President
Terri Miller Burchfield, Exec VP & Legislative Director

6456 National Headache Foundation
820 N Orleans
Chicago, IL 60610-3132
312-640-5399
888-643-5552
Fax: 312-640-9049
e-mail: nhf1970@headaches.org
www.headaches.org

A nonprofit organization established in 1970 dedicated to serve as an information resource to headache sufferers, their families and the healthcare providers who treat them. Promotes research into potential headache causes and treatments.
Arthur HE Elkind MD, President
Roger K Cady M D, Vice President

Research Centers

6457 Baltimore Headache Institute
11 E Chase Street
Baltimore, MD 21202
410-547-0200
Brian E Mondell MD, Medical Director

6458 **San Francisco Clinical Research Center**
909 Hyde Street
San Francisco, CA 94109

415-673-4600
Fax: 415-673-9352
e-mail: SFHACLIN@aol.com
www.sfcrc.com

This research center also specializes in diagnosis of Alzheimer's related dementia in addition to migraine headaches.
Jerome Goldstein, Director

Support Groups & Hotlines

6459 **National Health Information Center**
PO Box 1133
Washington, DC 20013

310-565-4167
800-336-4797
Fax: 301-984-4256
e-mail: info@nhic.org
www.health.gov/nhic

Offers a nationwide information referral service, produces directories and resource guides.

Books

6460 **Conquering Headache**
Alan Rapoport, MD, author
B.C Decker, Inc.
50 King Street E, Floor 2 PO Box620
Ontario, Canada L8N 3K7,

905-522-7017
800-568-7281
Fax: 905-522-7839
e-mail: info@bcdecker.com
www.bcdecker.com

2003 128 pages Paperback
ISBN: 1-550092-33-2

6461 **Freedom from Headaches**
Simon & Schuster Order Department
200 Old Tappan Road
Old Tappan, NJ 07675-7095

800-999-5479

ISBN: 0-671254-04-9

6462 **Handbook of Headache Disorders**
Essential Medical Information Systems
PO Box 1607
Durant, OK 74702-1607

580-924-0643
800-225-0694
Fax: 580-924-9414

1993 Paperback
ISBN: 0-929240-62-6

6463 **Handbook of Headache Management: A Practic al Guide to Diagnosis & Treatment**
Williams & Wilkins
351 W Camden Street
Baltimore, MD 21201-7912

301-528-4000
800-638-0672
www.wwilkins.com

1993 224 pages
ISBN: 0-683058-01-0

6464 **Migraine and Other Headaches: Vascular Mechanisms**
Raven Press
1185 Avenue of the Americas
New York, NY 10036-2601

212-930-9500
800-777-2295
www.raven.com

Leading international experts present new concepts on the mechanisms of migraine and other vascular headaches and detail the latest strategies for diagnosis and treatment of migraine with and without aura, tension-type headaches, cluster headaches and other vascular disorders.
368 pages
ISBN: 0-881677-95-7

6465 **Migraine: The Complete Guide**
American Council for Headache Education
19 Mantua Road
Mount Royal, NJ 08061

856-423-0258
800-255-2243
Fax: 856-423-0082
e-mail: achehq@talley.com
www.achenet.org

A comprehensive resource book for people with migraine, their families and physicians (updated in 1999) by Lynne M Constantine, Suzanne Scott and ACHE.

6466 **Overcoming Headaches & Migraines**
Longmeadow Press
PO Box 10218
Stamford, CT 06904-1469

203-352-2110

1993 128 pages Paperback
ISBN: 0-681417-92-7

6467 **Understanding Migrain and Other Headaches**
Stewart J Tepper, MD, author
University Press of Mississippi
3825 Ridgewood Road
Jackson, MS 39211-6492

601-432-6205
Fax: 601-432-6217
e-mail: kburgess@ihl.state.ms.us
www.upress.state.ms.us

A comprehensive overview of causes, diagnoses, and treatments.
2004 112 pages Paperback
ISBN: 1-578065-92-5
Kathy Burgess, Advertising/Marketing Services Manager

6468 **Wolff's Headaches & Other Head Pain**
Oxford University Press
2001 Evans Road
Cary, NC 27513-2010

212-726-6000
800-451-7556
Fax: 919-677-1303
www.oup-usa.org

1993
ISBN: 0-195082-50-8

Newsletters

6469 **Headache**
American Council for Headache Education
19 Mantua Road
Mount Royal, NJ 08061

856-423-0258
800-255-2243
Fax: 856-423-0082
e-mail: achehq@talley.com
www.achenet.org

The ACHE 12 page quarterly newsletter provides valuable and current information on new treatments, as well as time proven headache management strategies. All articles are written or reviewed by headache experts from the American Headache Society (AHS). Recent issues have included articles by headache experts on drug and nondrug treatment options and information on new treatments and research is regularly included.
Quarterly

6470 **NHF Head Lines**
National Headache Foundation
820 N Orleans
Chicago, IL 60610-3132

312-640-5399
888-643-5552
Fax: 312-640-9049
e-mail: nhf1970@headaches.org
www.headaches.org

Offers the latest information on headaches, causes and treatments. Contains news on drugs and medical forums, in depth discussions of headaches and preventions and a question and answer section in which physicians respond to reader inquiries and support group information.
16 pages Quarterly

Pamphlets

6471 **52 Proven Stress Reducers**
National Headache Foundation
820 N Orleans
Chicago, IL 60610

888-643-5552
Fax: 312-640-9049
e-mail: nhf1970@headaches.org
www.headaches.org

Members only.
Suzanne Simons, Executive Director

6472 About Headaches
National Headache Foundation
820 N Orleans
Chicago, IL 60610
888-643-5552
Fax: 312-640-9049
e-mail: nhf1970@headaches.org
www.headaches.org
Contains an in depth look at headaches, tips on when to seek medical advice, methods of treatment and more.
16 pages
Suzanne Simons, Executive Director

6473 Analgesic Rebound Headaches: Fact Sheet
National Headache Foundation
820 N Orleans
Chicago, IL 60610
888-643-5552
Fax: 312-640-9049
e-mail: nhf1970@headaches.org
www.headaches.org
Offers information on analgesic agents or drugs used to control pain including migraine and other types of headaches.
Suzanne Simons, Executive Director

6474 Cluster Headache: Fact Sheet
National Headache Foundation
820 N Orleans
Chicago, IL 60610
888-643-5552
Fax: 312-640-9049
e-mail: nhf1970@headaches.org
www.headaches.org
Offers information on cluster headaches and the treatment available for them. This information sheet can be downloaded from the web site.
Suzanne Simons, Executive Director

6475 Diet and Headache: Fact Sheet
National Headache Foundation
820 N Orleans
Chicago, IL 60610
888-643-5552
Fax: 312-640-9049
e-mail: nhf1970@headaches.org
www.headaches.org
Offers information on what foods should be avoided and what foods trigger headaches in all migraine sufferers. This information sheet can be dowloaded from the web site.
Suzanne Simons, Executive Director

6476 Headache Facts: What Everyone Should Know
American Council for Headache Education
19 Mantua Road
Mount Royal, NJ 08061
856-423-0258
800-255-2243
Fax: 856-423-0082
e-mail: achehq@talley.com
www.achenet.org

6477 Headache Handbook
National Headache Foundation
820 N Orleans
Chicago, IL 60610
888-643-5552
Fax: 312-640-9049
e-mail: nhf1970@headaches.org
www.headaches.org
Gives information on causes and types of headaches as well as treatments available.
8 pages

6478 Headache in Children: Fact Sheet
National Headache Foundation
820 N Orleans
Chicago, IL 60610
888-643-5552
Fax: 312-640-9049
e-mail: nhf1970@headaches.org
www.headaches.org
Offers information on vascular headaches, tension-type headaches, traction and inflammatory headaches and treatment. This information sheet can be downloaded from the web site.
Suzanne Simons, Executive Director

6479 Hormones and Migraines: Fact Sheet
National Headache Foundation
820 N Orleans
Chicago, IL 60610
888-643-5552
Fax: 312-640-9049
e-mail: nhf1970@headaches.org
www.headaches.org
Offers information on the link between hormones and migraines.
Suzanne Simons, Executive Director

6480 How to Talk to Your Doctor About Headaches
National Headache Foundation
820 N Orleans
Chicago, IL 60610
888-643-5552
Fax: 312-640-9049
e-mail: nhf1970@headaches.org
www.headaches.org
Learn how to keep a headache diary to pinpoint symptoms and effective diagnosis.
Suzanne Simons, Executive Director

6481 Impact of Migraine: A Disabling and Costly Condition
American Council for Headache Education
19 Mantua Road
Mount Royal, NJ 08061
856-423-0258
800-255-2243
Fax: 856-423-0082
e-mail: achehq@talley.com
www.achenet.org

6482 Migraine and Coexisting Conditions: Other Illnesses That May Affect Migraine
American Council for Headache Education
19 Mantua Road
Mount Royal, NJ 08061
856-423-0258
800-255-2243
Fax: 856-423-0082
e-mail: achehq@talley.com
www.achenet.org

6483 Migraine: Fact Sheet
National Headache Foundation
820 N Orleans
Chicago, IL 60610
888-643-5552
Fax: 312-640-9049
e-mail: nhf1970@headaches.org
www.headaches.org
Offers information on migraines and treatments.
Suzanne Simons, Executive Director

6484 Tap the Best Resource
National Headache Foundation
820 N Orleans
Chicago, IL 60610
888-643-5552
Fax: 312-640-9049
e-mail: nhf1970@headaches.org
www.headaches.org
Informational brochure offering facts and statistics on headaches. Everything from muscle contraction, vascular headaches, sinus headaches, TMJ and much more.
Suzanne Simons, Executive Director

6485 Tension-Type Headache: Fact Sheet
National Headache Foundation
820 N Orleans
Chicago, IL 60610
888-643-5552
Fax: 312-640-9049
e-mail: nhf1970@headaches.org
www.headaches.org
Offers information on the least known type of headache, chronic tension-type headaches. This information sheet can be downloaded from the web site.

6486 What's the Best Medicine for My Headaches?
American Council for Headache Education
19 Mantua Road
Mount Royal, NJ 08061
856-423-0258
800-255-2243
Fax: 856-423-0082
e-mail: achehq@talley.com
www.achenet.org

Audio & Video

6487 Relaxation Tape
National Headache Foundation
820 N Orleans
Chicago, IL 60610   888-643-5552
                                  Fax: 312-640-9049
                        e-mail: nhf1970@headaches.org
                                      www.headaches.org

Contains techniques to assist the listener in experiencing greater self control and relaxation.
Audio Tape
Suzanne Simons, Executive Director

6488 Stretch and Relax Tape
National Headache Foundation
820 N Orleans
Chicago, IL 60610   888-643-5552
                                  Fax: 312-640-9049
                        e-mail: nhf1970@headaches.org
                                      www.headaches.org

Based on a series of progressive relaxation techniques which involve the tightening and relaxing of specific muscle groups.
Audio Tape
Suzanne Simons, Executive Director

Web Sites

6489 American Academy of Neurology
                                        www.aan.com/
A professional organization representing neurologists worldwide.

6490 American Council for Headache Education (ACHE)
                                      www.achenet.org
The ACHE website offers an extensive library of headache information, including a searchable database of past articles from our newsletter, discussion forums that provide virtual contact with leading headache specialists and fellow headache sufferers, a searchable database of physicians to find a specialist in your area and more.

6491 American Headache Society
                                      www.ahsnet.org
The AHS website offers clinically oriented information on headache, as well as information on AHS programs and activities.

6492 American Medical Association
Journal of the American Medical Association
                                    www.ama-assn.org/
An organized web site focusing on treatment options, education and support available to those suffering from migraine headaches.

6493 Cluster Headaches
                                www.clusterheadaches.com
A web site devoted completely and exclusively to those that suffer from cluster headaches.

6494 Healing Well
                                    www.healingwell.com
An online health resource guide to medical news, chat, information and articles, newsgroups and message boards, books, disease-related web sites, medical directories, and more for patients, friends, and family coping with disabling diseases, disorders, or chronic illnesses.

6495 Health Finder
                                    www.healthfinder.gov
Searchable, carefully developed web site offering information on over 1000 topics. Developed by the US Department of Health and Human Services, the site can be used in both English and Spanish.

6496 Healthlink USA
                                  www.healthlinkusa.com
Health information concerning treatment, cures, prevention, diagnosis, risk factors, research, support groups, email lists, personal stories and much more. Updated regularly.

6497 Helios Health
                                    www.helioshealth.com

Online resource for your health information. Detailed information about specific health topics, access to expert advice from our Medical Advisory Board, and up-to-date health news.

6498 MedicineNet
                                    www.medicinenet.com
An online resource for consumers providing easy-to-read, authoritative medical and health information.

6499 Medscape
                                    www.medscape.com
Medscape offers specialists, primary care physicians, and other health professionals the Web's most robust and integrated medical information and educational tools.

6500 Medsupport
                                    www.medsupport.com
An up-to-date website dedicated towards giving the headache sufferer some important insights through the eyes of those who treat headache disorders.

6501 Migraine Awareness Group: A National Understanding for Migraineurs
                                    www.migraines.org/
Works to bring public awareness, utilizing the electronic, print, and artistic mediums, to the fact that migraine is a true organic neurological disease.

6502 National Headache Foundation
                                      www.headaches.org
Information for headache sufferers, their families, and the physicians who treat them.

6503 Neurology Channel
                                www.neurologychannel.com
Find clearly explained, medically accurate information regarding conditions, including an overview, symptoms, causes, diagnostic procedures and treatment options. On this site it is possible to ask questions and get information from a neurologist and connect to people who have similar health interests.

6504 WebMD
                                        www.webmd.com

Information on migraine, including articles and resources.

Description

6505 ## Multiple Sclerosis

Multiple sclerosis, MS, is a chronic disease that affects the central nervous system and impairs many of its functions. Over 300,000 Americans have MS. Although its cause is unknown, an immunologic abnormality is suspected. There also appear to be both genetic and environmental factors involved. Interestingly, the incidence of MS increases the further one lives from the equator.

Age of onset is typically between 20 and 40 years, and women are affected somewhat more than men. MS destroys the protective myelin sheath that surrounds nerve fibers. This special sheath normally allows passage of electrical signals through the brain, spinal cord, and nerves of the body. The disease is characterized by remissions and recurring exacerbations. The clinical signs vary depending on the area of demyelination and can include: generalized or focal weakness; difficulty walking; clumsiness; slurred speech; easy fatigability; numbness and tingling; visual loss; incontinence (loss of bladder and bowel control); loss of sexual function; and problems with short-term memory, judgment, or reason.

Significant strides are being made in both treating and understanding MS. Currently there is no curative treatment, but corticosteroids, interferon and other new medications may shorten or prevent relapses.

Supportive treatment includes medications to control muscle spasticity, fatigue and pain. Maintaining a normal lifestyle is recommended, avoiding fatigue and exposure to excessive heat. Physical therapy may also be helpful. Because of the debilitating nature of MS, counseling, psychiatric support, and antidepressant medication may be warranted.

National Agencies & Associations

6506 **Multiple Sclerosis Association of America**
706 Haddonfield Road
Cherry Hill, NJ 08002-2652
856-488-4500
800-532-7667
Fax: 856-661-9797
e-mail: webmaster@msassociation.org
www.msassociation.org
A national nonprofit organization dedicated to enriching the quality of life for everyone affected by multiple sclerosis.

6507 **Multiple Sclerosis Foundation**
6350 N Andrews Avenue
Fort Lauderdale, FL 33309
954-776-6805
888-MSF-OCUS
Fax: 954-938-8708
e-mail: admin@msfocus.org
www.msfocus.org
Dedicated to helping create a brighter tomorrow for those with MS the foundation offers a wide array of free services including: national toll-free support, educational programs, homecare, support groups, assistive technology and publications.
Toni Somma, Public Relations Coordinator

6508 **National Institute of Neurological Disorders and Stroke**
NIH Neurological Institute
Bethesda, MD 20824
301-496-5751
800-352-9424
Fax: 301-402-2186
TTY: 301-468-5981
www.ninds.nih.gov

The mission of NINDS is to reduce the burden of neurological disease - a burden borne by every age group, by every segment of society, by people all over the world.
Story Landis PhD, Director
Walter J Koroshetz, Deputy Director

6509 **National Multiple Sclerosis Society**
733 3rd Avenue
New York, NY 10017-3288
212-986-3240
800-344-4867
Fax: 212-986-7981
e-mail: nat@nmss.org
www.nmss.org
Serves persons with MS, their families, health professionals and the interested public. The Society provides funding for research, public and professional education, advocacy and the design of rehabilitative and psychosocial programs. Direct services to MS persons are provided through local chapters and branches. Among the services offered are counseling, referral, equipment loan and other support activities.
Joyce Nelson, President & CEO

6510 **Toronto Parents of Multiple Births Associa tion**
790 Bay Street
Toronto, Ontario, M5G-1N9
416-760-3944
e-mail: info@tpomba.org
www.tpomba.org
A not-for-profit self-help and support organization in Canada for parents of twins, triplets, and more.
Laura Dallal, President

State Agencies & Associations

Alabama

6511 **National Multiple Sclerosis Society: Alabama Chapter**
3840 Ridgeway Drive
Birmingham, AL 35209
205-879-8881
800-FIG-HTMS
e-mail: alc@nmss.org
www.nationalmssociety.org/alc
Dedicated to serving people with MS and their families by providing programs and services designed to enhance quality of life.
Melissa Daniel, Chapter President
Taylor Lander, Development Manager

6512 **National Mutiple Sclerosis Society: Alabama Chapter**
3840 Ridgeway Drive
Birmingham, AL 35209
205-879-8881
800-344-4867
Fax: 205-879-8869
e-mail: alc@nmss.org
www.nationalmssociety.org
Serving people with MS and their families through education and emotional support.
Melissa Dani Patterson, Chapter President
Hillary Ball Ryan, Development Manager

Alaska

6513 **National Multiple Sclerosis Society: Alaska Chapter**
511 W 41st Avenue
Anchorage, AK 99503-6643
907-563-1115
800-344-4867
Fax: 907-562-6673
e-mail: aka@nmss.org
www.nationalmssociety.org/aka
Nonprofit organization providing equipment loan, information and referral, leading library, self-help groups, advocacy, education, training, newsletter, educational programs, volunteer opportunities, exercise/aquatics, newly diagnosed support and educational material.
Gary Wells, Regional Development Manager
Pam McElrath, President, All American Chapter

Arizona

6514 **Desert Southwest Chapter 1 National Multiple Sclerosis Society**
National Multiple Sclerosis Society
315 S 48th Street
Tempe, AZ 85281-2343
602-968-2488
Fax: 602-966-4049
e-mail: info@dsw.nmss.org
www.dsw.nmss.org
Serves Central and Northern Arizona.

6515 Desert Southwest Chapter 2 National Multiple Sclerosis Society
National Multiple Sclerosis Society
3003 S Country Club Road 520-322-6601
Tucson, AZ 85713 Fax: 520-322-6739
Serves Southern Arizona.

Arkansas

6516 National Multiple Sclerosis Society: Arkansas Chapter
Evergreen Place
1100 N University Avenue 501-663-6767
Little Rock, AR 72207-6367 Fax: 501-666-4355
e-mail: arr@nmss.org
www.nationalmssociety.org/arr

Rick Selig, Division Manager

California

6517 Central California Chapter National Multiple Sclerosis Society
National Multiple Sclerosis Society
334 Shaw Avenue 209-325-9293
Clovis, CA 93612-3839 Fax: 209-325-9295
Dan Dietrich, Development Director
Karen Nunn, Service Director

6518 National Multiple Sclerosis Society: Southern California Chapter
2440 S Sepulveda Boulevard 310-479-4456
Los Angeles, CA 90064 800-344-4867
Fax: 310-479-4436
e-mail: cal@nmss.org
www.cal.nmss.org

Leon A LeBuffe, President

6519 National Multiple Sclerosis Society Channel Islands Chapter
14 W Valerio Street 805-682-8783
Santa Barbara, CA 93101 Fax: 805-563-1489
e-mail: cat@nmss.org
nationalmssociety.org

Joan Young, Chapter President

6520 National Multiple Sclerosis Society: Silicon Valley Chapter
2589 Scott Boulevard 408-988-7557
Santa Clara, CA 95050-2508 800-344-4867
Fax: 408-988-1816
e-mail: cau@nmss.org
www.nmss.org

Funds, researches and supports people with MS and their families to end the devastating effects of multiple sclerosis.
Carla Hines, Chapter President
Michelle Spam-Allen, Program Director

6521 Northern California Chapter National Multiple Sclerosis Society
National Multiple Sclerosis Society
1700 Owens Street 415-230-6678
San Francisco, CA 94158 800-344-4867
Fax: 510-268-0575
e-mail: info@msconnection.org
www.nationalmssociety.org

David Hartman, Chapter President
Denise Casey, Director of Chapter Programs

6522 Orange County Chapter National Multiple Sclerosis Society
National Multiple Sclerosis Society
5950 La Place Court 760-448-8400
Carlsbad, CA 92008-5677 800-344-4867
Fax: 949-833-3104
e-mail: msinfo@mspacific.org
www.nmssoc.org

Richard V Israel, Chapter President
Karen Hooper, Vice President Programs & Services

6523 San Diego Area Chapter National Multiple Sclerosis Society
National Multiple Sclerosis Society
8840 Complex Drive 619-974-8640
San Diego, CA 92123-1498 Fax: 619-974-8646
e-mail: mswalksd@aol.com
www.nmssoc.org

Allan Shaw, Chapter President
Karen Barton, Service Director

Colorado

6524 National MS Society: Colorado Chapter
900 S Broadway 303-698-7400
Denver, CO 80209-3442 800-344-4867
Fax: 303-698-7421
e-mail: COCRECEPTIONIST@NMSS.ORG
www.nationalmssociety.org/chapters/COC/i
Carrie Nolan, President
Mary Ann Peters, Executive Assistant

Connecticut

6525 National MS Society: Greater Connecticut Chapter
659 Tower Avenue 860-714-2300
Hartford, CT 06112 Fax: 860-714-2301
e-mail: info@ctfightsMS.org
www.nationalmssociety.org/chapters/CTN/i
Lisa Gerrol, President and Chief Professional Officer
Cheryl Donati, Executive Vice President

6526 National MS Society: Western Connecticut Chapter
1 Selleck Street 203-831-2971
Norwalk, CT 06855-1120 Fax: 203-831-2973
www.nationalmssociety.org/chapters/CTN/i

Delaware

6527 National MS Society: Delaware Chapter
2 Mill Road 302-655-5610
Wilmington, DE 19806-2175 Fax: 302-655-0993
e-mail: KATE.COWPERTHWAIT@DED.NMSS.ORG
www.nationalmssociety.org/chapters/DED/i
Provides the encouragement, materials and skills needed to achieve and maintain a productive lifestyle with multiple sclerosis. The organization is a voluntary, nonprofit entity.
1100 members
Kate Cowperthwait, Chapter President
Helen Serbu, Director of Finance

District of Columbia

6528 National MS Society: National Capital Chapter
1800 M Street 202-296-5363
Washington, DC 20036-1003 Fax: 202-296-3425
e-mail: INFORMATION@MSandYOU.ORG
www.nationalmssociety.org/chapters/DCW/i
J Christophe Broullire, Chapter President
Kevin Dougherty, Vice President Programs and Services

Florida

6529 Central Florida Chapter
2701 Maitland Center Parkway 407-478-8880
Orlando, FL 32751-6726 Fax: 407-478-8893
e-mail: INFO@FLC.NMSS.ORG
www.nationalmssociety.org/chapters/FLC/i

Tami Caesar, President
Ryan Bumgardner, Bike MS Manager

6530 Florida Gulf Coast Chapter National Multiple Sclerosis Society
National Multiple Sclerosis Society
4919 Memorial Highway 813-889-8303
Tampa, FL 33634-3540 800-344-4867
Fax: 813-889-8313
www.nationalmssociety.org/chapters/FLC/i
Judy Wilkinson, Service Director
Tim Hanke, Chairman

6531 Goodwill Industries-Suncoast
Goodwill Industries-Suncoast
10596 Gandy Boulevard 727-523-1512
St. Petersburg, FL 33733 Fax: 727-577-2749
www.goodwill-suncoast.org
A nonprofit community based organization whose purpose is to improve the quality of life for people who are disabled, disadvantaged and/or aged. This mission is accomplished through a staff of over 1,200 employees providing independent living skills, affordable housing, career assessment and planning, job skills, training, placement, and job retention assistance with useful employment.

Annually, Goodwill Industries-Suncoast serves over 30,000 people in Citrus, Hernando, Levy, Marion and more.
Jay Mc Cloe, Director Resource Development

6532 Mid Florida Chapter National Multiple Sclerosis Society
National Multiple Sclerosis Society
733 Third Avenue   212-463-7787
New York, NY 10017   Fax: 212-986-7981
                              e-mail: INFO@MSNYC.ORG
                        www.nationalmssociety.org/chapters/NYN/i
Ruth Brenner, President
Robin Einbinder, Executive Vice President Programs

6533 National Multiple Sclerosis Society: North Florida Chapter
9550 Regency Square Boulevard   904-725-6800
Jacksonville, FL 32225-8171   800-344-4867
                                 Fax: 904-725-0500
                                  TDD: 800-955-8770
                            e-mail: msnorfla@fln.nmss.org
                          www.nationalmssociety.org/fln

Jennifer Lee, Chapter President
Sabrah Witkamp, Client Program Director

6534 South Florida Chapter National Multiple Sclerosis Society
National Multiple Sclerosis Society
3201 W Commercial Boulevard   954-731-4224
Fort Lauderdale, FL 33309-6350   800-344-4867
                                 Fax: 954-739-1398
                                 e-mail: fls@nmss.org
                                 fls.nationalmssociety.org

Karen Dresbach, Chapter President
Fred Zuckerman, Chairman

Georgia

6535 National MS Society: Georgia Chapter
1117 Perimeter Center W   678-672-1000
Atlanta, GA 30338-3097   800-822-3379
                                 Fax: 678-672-1015
                             e-mail: mailbox@nmssga.org
                         www.nationalmssociety.org/chapters/GAA/i
Roy A Rangel, Chapter President
Nicole Hill, Director of Finance & Administrative

Hawaii

6536 National MS Society: Hawaii Chapter
418 Kuwili Street   808-532-0806
Honolulu, HI 96817   Fax: 808-532-0814
                               e-mail: HIH@NMSS.ORG
                        www.nationalmssociety.org/chapters/HIH/i
Jeffrey D Peier, Chairman
Pam McElrath, President

Idaho

6537 National MS Society: Idaho Division
6901 W Emerald Street   208-388-4253
Boise, ID 83704   800-344-4867
                                 Fax: 208-388-1907
                                 e-mail: idi@nmss.org
                        www.nationalmssociety.org/chapters/IDI/i
Pam McElrath, Chapter President
Suzanne Bland, Executive Vice President

Illinois

6538 National MS Society: Chicago, Greater Illinois Chapter
600 S Federal Street   312-922-8000
Chicago, IL 60605-3814   Fax: 312-922-2752
The Greater Illnois Chapter is comprised of all the Illinoisans whohave chosen to fight MS and the work that they do through the National Multiple Sclerosis Society Volunteers, staff, healthcare workers, researchers, donors, advocated, and partners together represent the Greater Illinoisans Chapter, and all the many ways it's possible to join the fight against multiple sclerosis.
Steven Pratapous, Chapter President

Indiana

6539 National MS Society: Indiana State Chapter
7301 Georgetown Road   317-870-2500
Indianapolis, IN 46268   800-344-4867
                                 Fax: 317-870-2520
                              e-mail: Indiana@NMSS.org
                        www.nationalmssociety.org/chapters/INI/i
Tiffany Bogard, Chapter President
Lisa Coffman, Director of Chapter Programs

Iowa

6540 National MS Society: Iowa Chapter
8187 University Boulevard   515-270-6337
Clive, IA 50325   800-798-6677
                                 Fax: 515-270-0337
                            e-mail: mark.davis@nmss.org
                        www.nationalmssociety.org/chapters/NTH/a
Brett Ridge, Chapter President
Mark Davis, Area Director

Kansas

6541 National MS Society: Mid-America Chapter
7611 State Line   913-432-3926
Kansas City, KS 64114-2915   800-745-3148
                                 Fax: 913-432-6912
                              e-mail: info@nmsskc.org
                        www.nationalmssociety.org/chapters/KSG/i
The National Multiple Sclerosis Society is a not-for-profit organization serving people with MS in every state. The Mid-America Chapter serves the 25,000 people who are affected by MS in eastern Kansas and western Missouri.
Kay Julian, Chapter President
Amy Goldstein, Program Director

6542 National MS Society: South Central & West Kansas Division
9415 E Harry Street   316-264-7043
Wichita, KS 67211-1515   800-344-4867
                                 Fax: 316-264-5436
                              e-mail: KSS@NMSS.ORG
                        www.nationalmssociety.org/chapters/KSS/i
Cammy Mathews, Donor Relations Coordinator
Becky Kimbell, Regional Programs and Services Manager

Kentucky

6543 National MS Society: Kentucky Chapter
11700 Commonwealth Drive   502-451-0014
Louisville, KY 40299   e-mail: KYW@NMSS.ORG
                                www.nationalmssociety.org

Jeff Hamilton, Chairman
Stacy Funk, Chapter President

Louisiana

6544 National Multiple Sclerosis Society
4613 Fairfield Street   504-832-4013
Metairie, LA 70006   800-344-4867
                                 Fax: 504-831-7188
                       e-mail: louisianachapter@lam.nmss.org
                        www.nationalmssociety.org/chapters/LAM/i
Brian Berrigon, Chapter President
Crystal Smith, Director of Programs and Services

6545 National Multiple Sclerosis Society: Louisiana Chapter 3
3616 S I 10 Service Road W   504-832-4013
Metairie, LA 70001-1874   800-344-4867
                                 Fax: 504-831-7188
                       e-mail: louisianachapter@lam.nmss.org
                                www.nationalmssociety.org
Brian Berrigon, Chapter President
Crystal Smith, Director Chapter Programs

Maine

6546 National MS Society: Maine Chapter
170 US Route One   800-344-4867
Falmouth, ME 04105   Fax: 207-781-7961
e-mail: info@msmaine.org
www.nationalmssociety.org/chapters/MEM/i
The National Multiple Sclerosis Societ is dedicated to enind the
devastating the devastating effects of multiple sciersis, a chronic,
disease of the central nervous system often diagnosed in young
adults
Robin Doughty, Director of Finance & Operations
Denise Clavette, Chapter President

Maryland

**6547 National MS Society: Maryland Chapter Hunt Valley Business
Center**
Hunt Valley Business Center
11403 Cronhill Drive   443-641-1200
Owings Mills, MD 21117   Fax: 443-641-1201
e-mail: INFO@NMSS-MD.ORG
www.nationalmssociety.org/chapters/MDM/i
Mark Roeder, Chapter President
Nicole Weedon, Executive Assistant/Office Manager

Massachusetts

6548 National MS Society: Central New England Chapter
101A 1st Avenue   781-890-4990
Waltham, MA 02451-1160   800-493-9255
Fax: 781-890-2089
e-mail: COMMUNICATIONS@MAM.NMSS.ORG
www.nationalmssociety.org/chapters/MAM/i
Linda Guiod, Executive Vice President
Arlyn White, Chapter President & CEO

6549 National MS Society: Massachusetts Chapter
101A 1st Avenue   781-890-4990
Waltham, MA 02451-1160   Fax: 781-890-2089
e-mail: COMMUNICATIONS@MAM.NMSS.ORG
www.nationalmssociety.org/chapters/MAM/i
Linda Guiod, Executive Vice President
Arlyn White, Chapter President & CEO

Michigan

6550 National MS Society: Michigan Chapter
21311 Civic Center Drive   248-350-0020
Southfield, MI 48076   800-344-4867
Fax: 248-350-0029
e-mail: info@mig.nmss.org
www.nationalmssociety.org/mig
Offer a variety of programs and services benefiting people with
multiple sclerosis and their family members. Programs include educational seminars, information and referrals, peer support, advocacy, free legal clinic, financial assistance for medical equipment,
medical transportation, home care, technical assistance and much
more
Elana Sullivan, Chapter President
Melissa Ryan, Executive Administrative Assistant

Minnesota

6551 National MS Society: Minnesota Chapter
200 12th Avenue S   612-335-7900
Minneapolis, MN 55415   800-582-5296
Fax: 612-335-7997
e-mail: INFO@MSSOCIETY.ORG
www.nationalmssociety.org/chapters/MNM/i

Mississippi

**6552 National Multiple Sclerosis Society: Alaba ma-Mississippi
Chapter**
145 Executive Drive   601-856-5831
Madison, MS 39110-9198   800-344-4867
Fax: 601-856-7173
e-mail: alc@nmss.org
www.nationalmssociety.org/alc
Angie Jackson, Area Director
Andi Agnew, Programs and Services Coordinator

Missouri

6553 National MS Society: Gateway Area Chapter
1867 Lackland Hill Parkway   314-781-9020
Saint Louis, MO 63146-3545   800-344-4867
Fax: 314-781-1440
e-mail: info@mos.nmss.org
www.nationalmssociety.org/chapters/MOS/i
Sponsors research and offers educational programs, counseling,
lending library, referral services, independent living aids, legislative advocacy and therapeutic recreation for people with MS.
Phyllis Robsham, Chapter President
Kathi Taylor, Executive Assistant

Montana

6554 National MS Society: Montana Division
1629 Avenue D   406-252-5927
Billings, MT 59102   800-344-4867
Fax: 406-252-5956
e-mail: MTT@NMSS.ORG
www.nationalmssociety.org/chapters/MTT/i
Rebecca Wiehe, Regional Programs and Services Manager
Heather Ohs, Regional Developmentÿ Manager

Nebraska

**6555 National MS Society: Midlands Chapter Community Health
Plaza**
Community Health Plaza
328 S 72nd Street   402-505-4000
Omaha, NE 68114-2153   Fax: 402-572-3002
e-mail: NEN@NMSS.ORG
www.nationalmssociety.org/chapters/NEN/i
Lisa Brink, Chapter President
Milton Trabal, Director of Finance

Nevada

6556 Desert Southwest Chapter 3 National Multiple Sclerosis Society
National Multiple Sclerosis Society
6000 S Eastern Avenue   702-736-1478
Las Vegas, NV 89119-3157   800-344-4867
Fax: 702-736-2487
e-mail: NVL@NMSS.ORG
www.nationalmssociety.org/chapters/NVL/i
Serves southern Nevada & northwest Arizona.
Nicole Rainey, Development Coordinator Special Events
Linda Nowell, Programs and Services Coordinator

6557 National MS Society: Great Basin Sierra Chapter
4600 Keitzke Lane   702-329-7180
Reno, NV 89502   800-344-4867
Fax: 775-827-3167
e-mail: nvn@nvn.nmss.org
www.nationalmssociety.org/chapters/NVN/i
Linda Lott, Regional Development Manager
Danielle Lutzow, Programs and Services Coordinator

New Hampshire

6558 National MS Society: Central New England Chapter
101A First Avenue   781-890-4990
Waltham, MA 02451-1115   800-493-9255
Fax: 781-490-2089
e-mail: COMMUNICATIONS@MAM.NMSS.ORG
www.msnewengland.org

Serving people with MS in Massachusetts and New Hampshire.
Judy Cotton, Director Chapter Services
Arlyn White, Chapter President & CEO

New Jersey

6559 National MS Society: Greater North Jersey Chapter
1 Kalisa Way   201-967-5599
Paramus, NJ 07652-3550   Fax: 201-967-7085
e-mail: INFO@NJM.NMSS.ORG
www.nationalmssociety.org/chapters/NJM/i
Michael Elkow, Chapter President
Marianne Maddocks, Vice President of Operations

6560 National MS Society: Mid-Jersey Chapter
246 Monmouth Road   732-660-1005
Oakhurst, NJ 07755   800-344-4867
Fax: 732-660-1388
e-mail: INFO@NJM.NMSS.ORG
www.nationalmssociety.org/chapters/NJM/i
The National Multiple Sclerosis Society is the only voluntary
health agency that supports an international program of scientific
research designed to cure, prevent and treat MS.
Michael Elkow, Chapter President
Marianne Maddocks, Vice President of Operations

New Mexico

6561 National MS Society: Rio Grande Division
4125-A Carlisle Boulevard NE   505-243-2792
Albuquerque, NM 87107   800-344-4867
Fax: 505-244-0629
e-mail: NMX@NMSS.ORG
www.nationalmssociety.org/chapters/NMX/i
Maggie Schold, Development Coordinator Special Events
Sheri Wharton, Programs and Services Coordinator

New York

6562 National MS Society: Long Island Chapter
40 Marcus Drive   631-864-8337
Melville, NY 11747   Fax: 631-864-8342
e-mail: PMASTROTA@NMSSLI.ORG
www.nationalmssociety.org/chapters/NYH/i
The National Multiple Sclerosis Society, Long Island Chapter, is
dedicated to helping people with MS and their families live useful
and fulfilling lives by opening their minds to opportunities and
providing the tools to live with dignity.
Pamela Jones Mastrota, President & CEO
Barbara Travis, Vice President of Donor Development

6563 National MS Society: New York City Chapter
733 Third Avenue   212-463-7787
New York, NY 10017-2098   800-344-4867
Fax: 212-989-4362
e-mail: INFO@MSNYC.ORG
www.nationalmssociety.org/chapters/NYN/i
Committed to providing comprehensive support services to help
people with MS and their families cope with the consequences of
the disease. The goal is to empower people with MS and their loved
ones so that they can better control their lives.
Ruth Brenner, Chapter President
Robin Einbinder, Executive Vice President Programs

6564 National MS Society: Northeastern New York Chapter
421 New Karner Road   518-464-0630
Albany, NY 12205-5156   800-344-4867
Fax: 518-464-1232
e-mail: chapter@msupstateny.org
www.nationalmssociety.org/chapters/NYR/i
Barbara R Milano, Chapter President
Elliey Kiale-Ingalsb, Chapter Chair

6565 National MS Society: Southern New York Chapter
2 Gannett Drive   914-694-1655
White Plains, NY 10604-2145   800-344-4867
Fax: 914-345-3504
e-mail: NYV@NMSS.ORG
www.nationalmssociety.org/chapters/NYV/i

The mission of the National MS Society is to end the devastating
effects of multiple sclerosis. The Southern NY Chapter is committed to helping people with MS to live independently.
Andrea Maloney, Interim Chapter President
Christina Szeliga, Administrative Coordinator

6566 National MS Society: Upstate New York Chapter
457 State Street   607-724-5464
Binghamton, NY 13901-2341   800-344-4867
Fax: 607-722-1485
e-mail: chapter@msupstateny.org
www.nationalmssociety.org/chapters/NYR/i
James Ahearn, Chapter President
Jonathan Smith, Program Coordinator

**6567 National MS Society: Western New York/ Northwestern
Pennsylvania Chapter**
4245 Union Road   716-634-2261
Buffalo, NY 14225-5040   800-344-4867
Fax: 716-634-2979
e-mail: chapter@msupstateny.org
www.nationalmssociety.org/chapters/NYR/i
Arthur V Cardella, Chapter President
Betsy Farkas, Director Chapter Programs

6568 National Multiple Sclerosis: Upstate New York Chapter
National Multiple Sclerosis Society
1650 S Avenue   716-271-0801
Rochester, NY 14620-3901   877-869-6677
Fax: 716-442-2817
e-mail: CHAPTER@MSUPSTATENY.ORG
www.nationalmssociety.org/chapters/NYR/i
Randal A Simonetti, Presidentÿ& CEO
Stephanie Mincer, Senior Vice President of Programs

North Carolina

6569 National MS Society: Central North Carolina Chapter
2211 W Meadowview Road   336-299-4136
Greensboro, NC 27407-3400   Fax: 336-855-3039
e-mail: NCC@NMSS.ORG
www.nationalmssociety.org/chapters/NCC/i
Elizabeth Green, Chapter President
Davishia Baldwin, Volunteer Coordinator

6570 National MS Society: Eastern North Carolina Chapter
3101 Industrial Drive   919-781-0676
Raleigh, NC 27609-7577   Fax: 919-781-1042
e-mail: NCT@NMSS.ORG
www.nationalmssociety.org/chapters/NCT/i
Craig Robertson, Interim Chapter President
Debbie Hoffman, Vice President Operations

6571 National Multiple Sclerosis Society
9801-I Southern Pine Boulevard   704-525-2955
Charlotte, NC 28273-5561   800-344-4867
Fax: 704-527-0406
e-mail: mac@nmss.org
www.nationalmssociety.org/mac
The Mid-Atlantic chapter of the National MS Society serves
80,000 people with multiple sclerosis in South Carolina and western North Carolina. The Chapter is dedicated to helping people
with MS learn to manage and understand their disease and to
achieve maximum independence.
Allison Mertens, Chair Board of Trustees
Jennifer Lee, Chapter President

North Dakota

6572 National MS Society: Dakota Chapter
5990 14th Street S   701-235-2678
Fargo, ND 58104   Fax: 701-235-6358
www.nationalmssociety.org/chapters/NTH/i
Kelly Boeddeker, Senior Development Manager
Amanda Noce, Programs Manager

Ohio

6573 Columbus Center of the National Multiple Sclerosis Society
National Multiple Sclerosis Society

651 G Lakeview Plaza Boulevard
Worthington, OH 43229-3626

614-880-2290
800-667-7131
Fax: 614-880-2296
www.nationalmssociety.org

Stacey Wilko LSW, Program Coordinator
Tony Bernard LSW, Program Coordinator

6574 National MS Soceity: Western Ohio Chapter The Woolpert Building
The Woolpert Building
409 E Monument Avenue
Dayton, OH 45402-1261

937-461-5232
800-344-4867
Fax: 937-461-3500
e-mail: donnasimpson@ohm.nmss.org
www.nationalmssociety.org

Providing accurate, up-to-date information to individuals with MS, their families and healthcare providers is central to our mission.
12 pages
Karen Joseph, Program Director
Judy LaMusga, Chapter Chair

6575 National MS Society: Southwestern Ohio/Northern Kentucky
4460 Lake Forest Drive
Cincinnati, OH 45242-3755

513-281-5200
Fax: 513-769-6019

Tena Bunnell, Chapter President
Becky Wiehe, Service Director

6576 National MS Society: Northeast Ohio Chapter
The Hanna Building
6155 Rockside Road
Independence, OH 44131-1901

216-696-8220
800-667-7131
Fax: 216-696-2817
e-mail: WEBMASTER@NMSSOHA.ORG
www.nationalmssociety.org

Janet Kramer, Chapter President
Greg Kovach, Director of Services

6577 National MS Society: Northwest Ohio Chapter
401 Tomahawk Drive
Maumee, OH 43537-1633

419-897-9533
800-368-7459
Fax: 419-897-9733
e-mail: NWOHIO@AMPLEX.NET
www.nationalmssociety.org/chapters/OHO/i

Jacque Pratt, Chapter Program Coordinator
Tonya Scherf, Program Director

Oklahoma

6578 National MS Society: Oklahoma Chapter
4604 E 67th Street
Tulsa, OK 74136-4946

918-488-0882
800-777-7814
Fax: 918-488-0913
e-mail: LISA.GRAY@OKE.NMSS.ORG
www.nationalmssociety.org/chapters/OKE/i

Paula Cortner, Chapter President
Denise Allen, Finance/HR Manager

Oregon

6579 National MS Society: Oregon Chapter
104 SW Clay Street
Portland, OR 97201

503-223-9511
800-344-4867
Fax: 503-223-2912
e-mail: INFO@DEFEATMS.COM
www.nationalmssociety.org/chapters/ORC/i

The Pregon Chapter is aggressively pursuing the mission to end the devastating effects of MS by providing programs designed to enhance the families throughout Oregon and Clark County, Washington.
Wendy Allison, Office Coordinator
Sally Alworth, Director of Finance

Pennsylvania

6580 National MS Society: Central Pennsylvania Chapter
2040 Linglestown Road
Harrisburg, PA 17110-1095

717-652-2108
Fax: 717-652-2590
e-mail: PAC@NMSS.ORG
www.nationalmssociety.org/chapters/PAC/i

Margie Adelmann, President
Debbie Rios, Executive Vice President

6581 National MS Society: Greater Delaware Valley Chapter
1 Reed Street
Philadelphia, PA 19147-5519

215-271-1500
800-548-4611
Fax: 215-271-6122
e-mail: PAE@NMSS.ORG
www.nationalmssociety.org/chapters/PAE/i

John H Scott, President
Randee Forstein, VP Programs & Community Outreach

Rhode Island

6582 National MS Society: Rhode Island Chapter
205 Hallene Road
Warwick, RI 02886-2452

401-738-8383
800-344-4867
Fax: 401-738-8469
e-mail: CATIE.DUSSAULT@RIR.NMSS.ORG
www.nationalmssociety.org/chapters/RIR/i

Provides local programs and services to people with MS and their families. These services include information and referral, equipment loans, purchase assistance, programs for the newly diagnosed and education and support groups.
3M Members
Kathy Mechnig, Chapter President
Catie Dussault, Director of Special Events

South Carolina

6583 National MS Society: South Carolina Branch
2711 Middleburg Drive
Columbia, SC 29204-2413

803-799-7848
800-922-7591
www.nationalmssociety.org/chapters/NCP/i

Tennessee

6584 National MS Society: Sutheast Tennessee/North Georgia Chapter
5720 Uptain Road
Chattanooga, TN 37411-5642

423-954-9700
Fax: 423-855-9667
e-mail: questions@msmidsouth.org
www.nationalmssociety.org

Jeanne Brice, Services Manager

6585 National MS Society: Mid-South Chapter
3100 Walnut Grove Road
Memphis, TN 38111-3530

901-324-9610
Fax: 901-324-9668

The mission of the National Multiple Sclerosis Society is to end the devastating effects of MS.
Dee Blake, Chapter President
Sherree Wilson, Services Director

6586 National MS Society: Mid-South Chapter, Nashville Office
4219 Hillsboro Road
Nashville, TN 37215-3332

615-269-9055
800-269-9055
Fax: 615-269-9470
e-mail: TNS@NMSS.ORG
www.nationalmssociety.org/chapters/TNS/i

Jim Ward, Chapter President
Beth Smith, Vice President of Client Programs

Texas

6587 National MS Society: North Central Texas Chapter
4086 Sandshell Drive
Fort Worth, TX 76137

817-306-7003
Fax: 817-877-1205
www.nationalmssociety.org/chapters/TXH/i

Educational programs, self-help groups, and information and referral for persons and families diagnosed with multiple sclerosis.
12 pages Quarterly
Justin Martin, Coordinator Development
Lynette Jarvis-Barre, Senior Manager Programs & Services

6588 National MS Society: Panhandle Chapter
6222 Canyon Drive   806-468-8005
Amarillo, TX 79109-6730   800-344-4867
                                        Fax: 806-468-8022
                               e-mail: TXP@NMSS.ORG
                   www.nationalmssociety.org/chapters/TXP/i
Gail Lindsey, Programs and Services Coordinator
April Brownlee, Development Coordinator Special Events

6589 National MS Society: Southern Texas
8111 N Stadium Drive   713-526-8967
Houston, TX 77054   Fax: 713-394-7422
                               e-mail: TXH@NMSS.ORG
                   www.nationalmssociety.org/chapters/TXH/i
Mark Neagli, Chapter President
Deborah Pope, VP - Operations

6590 National MS Society: West Texas Division
1031 Andrews Highway   432-522-2143
Midland, TX 79701-4636   Fax: 432-694-7970
                               e-mail: TXQ@NMSS.ORG
                   www.nationalmssociety.org/chapters/TXQ/i
Sharon Rader, Regional Development Manager
Rona Bowerman, Regional Programs and Services Manager

6591 National MS Socisty: Southeast Texas Chapter
8111 N Stadium Drive   713-526-8967
Houston, TX 77054-4051   Fax: 281-526-4049
                                www.nationalmssociety.org
Mark Neagli, Chapter President
Jim Tidwell, Chairman

Utah

6592 National MS Society: Utah State Chapter
6364 S Highland Drive   801-493-0113
Salt Lake City, UT 84121-3537   800-527-8116
                                        Fax: 801-493-0122
                               e-mail: infoutah@nmss.org
                                    www.fightmsutah.org
Our mission is to end the devastating effects of MS. Serving indi-
viduals with MS and their families through programs, research,
awareness and education.
Annette Royle, Chapter President
Dee Dee Fox, Director of Client Programs and Services

Vermont

6593 National MS Society: Vermont Division
75 Talcott Road   802-864-6356
Williston, VT 05495   800-344-4867
                                        Fax: 802-864-6509
                               e-mail: VTN@NMSS.ORG
                   www.nationalmssociety.org/chapters/VTN/i
Committed to ending the devastating effects of MS.
Christine Newberr, Programs and Services Coordinator
Lindsay Going, Development Coordinator Special Events

Virginia

6594 National MS Society: Blue Ridge Chapter
One Morton Drive   804-971-8010
Charlottesville, VA 22903   Fax: 804-979-4475
                               e-mail: VAB@NMSS.ORG
                   www.nationalmssociety.org/chapters/VAB/i
Faith Painter, Chapter President
Delton Hanson, Operations Director

6595 National MS Society: Central Virginia Chapter
2112 W Laburnum Avenue   804-353-5008
Richmond, VA 23227   Fax: 804-353-5595
                       e-mail: JUDY.GRIFFIN@NMSS.ORG
                   www.nationalmssociety.org/chapters/VAR/i
Sherri Ellis, Chapter President
Andy Page, Director of Community Development

6596 National MS Society: Hampton Roads Chapter
760 Lynnhaven Parkway   757-490-9627
Virginia Beach, VA 23452-6311   Fax: 757-490-1617
                               e-mail: info@fightms.com
                   www.nationalmssociety.org/chapters/VAX/i
Sharon Grossman, Chapter President
Michelle Derr, Vice President Finance/Administration

Washington

6597 National MS Society: Greater Washington Chapter
192 Nickerson Street   206-284-4236
Seattle, WA 98109   800-800-7047
                                        Fax: 206-284-4972
                   e-mail: GREATERWAINFO@NMSSWAS.ORG
                   www.nationalmssociety.org/chapters/WAS/i
Patricia Shepherd-Ba, Chapter President
Erin Poznanski, Vice President Chapter Programs

6598 National MS Society: Inland Northwest Chapter
818 E Sharp Avenue   509-482-2022
Spokane, WA 99202-1935   Fax: 509-483-1077
                               e-mail: WAI@NMSS.ORG
                   www.nationalmssociety.org/chapters/WAI/i
Robert Hansen, Chapter President
Patty Mathias, Office Manager

West Virginia

6599 National MS Society: West Virginia Chapter
1 Morton Drive   434-971-8010
Charlottesville, VA 22903   800-344-4867
                                        Fax: 434-979-4475
                               e-mail: VAB@NMSS.ORG
                   www.nationalmssociety.org/chapters/VAB/i
The National MS Society is committed to building a movement by
and for people with MS that will move us closer to a world free of
this disease.
Fay Painter, Chapter President
Delton Hanson, Operations Director

Wisconsin

6600 National MS Society: Wisconsin Chapter
1120 James Drive   262-369-4400
Hartland, WI 53029   Fax: 262-369-4410
                               e-mail: info@wisms.org
                   www.nationalmssociety.org/chapters/WIG/i
Colleen Kalt, President & CEO
Melissa Palfery, Executive Assistant

Wyoming

6601 National MS Society: Wyoming Chapter
525 Randall Avenue   307-433-9590
Cheyenne, WY 82001-1627   Fax: 307-433-8657
                               e-mail: WYY@NMSS.ORG
                   www.nationalmssociety.org/chapters/WYY/i
Cheryl Seaberg, Programs and Services Coordinator
Stephanie Batson, Development Coordinator Special Events

Libraries & Resource Centers

6602 Information Resource Center and Library
National Multiple Sclerosis Society
733 Third Avenue
New York, NY 10017   800-344-4867
                                www.nationalmssociety.org
The primary venue for educating the community about multiple
sclerosis.Offers the latest information about MS information and
provides referrals to local MS care centers, physicians and service
providers.
Weyman T Johnson, Jr, Chairman
Joyce M Nelson, President/CEO

6603 St. Agnes Hospital Medical: Health Science Library
305 North Street 914-681-4500
White Plains, NY 10605 Fax: 914-328-6408
Labe C Scheinberg MD, Director

Research Centers

6604 Brigham and Women's Hospital: Center for Neurologic Diseases
LMRC Building
75 Francis Street 617-732-5500
Boston, MA 02115 800-294-9999
TTY: 617-732-6458
www.brighamandwomens.org
Offers research relating to Multiple Sclerosis and other autoimmune diseases.
Dr Howard Weiner, Coordinator

6605 Center for Neuroimmunology: University of Alabama at Birmingham
1720 7th Ave S 205-934-0683
Birmingham, AL 35294 Fax: 205-996-4039
www.main.uab.edu/neurology
Evaluate and treat acute and chronic neurological and neuromuscular diseases which are caused by autoimmune mechanisms or linked to presumed abnormalities affecting the immune system.
Khurram Bashir, Director

6606 Jimmie Heuga Center
27 Main Street 970-926-1290
Edwards, CO 81632 800-367-3101
Fax: 970-926-1295
e-mail: Info@heuga.org
www.heuga.org
Conducts research and studies on multiple sclerosis patients.
Kim Lennox Sharkey, Chief Executive Officer
Carrie Van Beek, Office Coordinator

6607 Neuromuscular Treatment Center: Univ. of Texas Southwestern Medical Center
Department of Neurology
Dallas, TX 75390 214-648-3111
www.utsouthwestern.edu
Basic and clinical studies of myasthenia gravis.
Dr Ralph Greenlee, Director

6608 Rush University Multiple Sclerosis Center
1725 W Harrison Street 312-942-8011
Chicago, IL 60612 888-352-RUSH
TTY: 312-942-2207
e-mail: contact_rush@rush.edu
www.rush.edu
The Multiple Sclerosis Center combines comprehensive treatment with clinical and laboratory research to provide the highest quality patient care.
Floyd A Davis, Director

Support Groups & Hotlines

6609 MS Toll-Free Information Line
National Multiple Sclerosis Society
733 3rd Avenue
New York, NY 10017-3288 800-344-4867
Offers public and professional information, brochures and referrals to MS patients, their families and health care professionals.

6610 MSWorld
1943 Morrill Street 415-701-1117
Sarasota, FL 34236 877-710-0302
e-mail: msworld@msworld.org
www.msworld.org/
MSWorld is for people with multiple sclerosis their families and friends, offer support via chat, e-mail, message boards, magazines.
Kathleen Wilson, Founder/President

6611 Multiple Sclerosis Action Group
National Multiple Sclerosis Society

733 3rd Avenue 409-883-2282
New York, NY 10017 800-344-4867
e-mail: msag@erasems.com
www.nmss.org
Richard J Mengel, Treasurer
Fred J Lublin, Director

6612 National Health Information Center
PO Box 1133 310-565-4167
Washington, DC 20013 800-336-4797
Fax: 301-984-4256
e-mail: info@nhic.org
www.health.gov/nhic
Offers a nationwide information referral service, produces directories and resource guides.

6613 Traditional Tibetan Healing
13 Harrison Street 617-666-8635
Sommerville, MA 2143-6504 866-628-6504
e-mail: Kelob@gte.net
www.tibetanherbalhealing.com/
To rid mankind from chronic illnesses using alternative methods.
Keyzon Bhutti, Chief Physician

Books

6614 300 Tips for Making Life with Multiple Sclerosis Easier
Demos Medical Publishing
386 Park Avenue S 212-683-0072
New York, NY 10016 Fax: 212-683-0118
e-mail: orderdept@demospub.com
www.demosmedpub.com
Techniques for better living.
109 pages
ISBN: 1-888799-23-4
Dr. Diana M Schneider

6615 Alternative Medicine and Multiple Sclerosis
Demos Medical Publishing
386 Park Avenue S 212-683-0072
New York, NY 10016 Fax: 212-683-0118
e-mail: orderdept@demospub.com
www.demosmedpub.com
272 pages
ISBN: 1-888799-52-8
Dr. Diana M Schneider

6616 Fall Down Seven Times Get Up Eight
Miramar Communications
PO Box 8987
Malibu, CA 90265-8987 800-543-4116
The second in Dr. Wolf's series on MS management: including chapters on stress and fatigue, planning for serious disability and lots more.
211 pages

6617 Living with Multiple Sclerosis
Demos Medical Publishing
386 Park Avenue S 212-683-0072
New York, NY 10016 Fax: 212-683-0118
e-mail: orderdept@demospub.com
www.demosmedpub.com
ISBN: 1-888799-26-9
Dr. Diana M Schneider

6618 Living with Multiple Sclerosis: A Wellness Approach
Demos Vermande
386 Park Avenue S 212-683-0072
New York, NY 10016-8804 800-532-8663
112 pages
ISBN: 1-888799-00-5

6619 Meeting the Challenge of Progressive Multiple Sclerosis
Demos Medical Publishing

386 Park Avenue S
New York, NY 10016

212-683-0072
Fax: 212-683-0118
e-mail: orderdept@demospub.com
www.demosmedpub.com

128 pages
ISBN: 1-888799-46-3
Dr. Diana M Schneider

6620 Multiple Sclerosis
Demos Medical Publishing
386 Park Avenue S
New York, NY 10016

212-683-0072
800-532-8663
Fax: 212-683-0118
e-mail: orderdept@demospub.com
www.demosmedpub.com

A consistent bestseller in multiple sclerosis management.
224 pages
ISBN: 1-888799-54-4
Dr. Diana M Schneider

6621 Multiple Sclerosis, The Questions you Have Answers You Need
Demos Medical Publishing
386 Park Avenue S
New York, NY 10016

212-683-0072
Fax: 212-683-0118
e-mail: orderdept@demospub.com
www.demosmedpub.com

592 pages
ISBN: 1-888799-43-9
Dr. Diana M Schneider

6622 Multiple Sclerosis: A Guide for Families
Demos Medical Publishing
386 Park Avenue S
New York, NY 10016-8804

212-683-0072
800-532-8663
Fax: 212-683-0118
e-mail: orderdept@demospub.com
www.demosmedpub.com

With its complex and unpredictable course, MS affects every area of family life. This book covers a broad range of medical, psychological, social, vocational, economic and legal problems.
1997 207 pages Paperback
ISBN: 1-888799-14-5
Dr. Diana M Schneider, President

6623 Multiple Sclerosis: A Guide for Patients and Their Families
Raven Press
1185 Avenue of the Americas
New York, NY 10036-2601

212-930-9500
800-777-2295

Second edition.
288 pages Paperback
ISBN: 0-881672-55-6

6624 Multiple Sclerosis: A Personal Exploration
Demos Vermande
386 Park Avenue S
New York, NY 10016-8804

212-683-0072
800-532-8663
Fax: 212-683-0118

1993 192 pages
ISBN: 0-285650-18-1

6625 Multiple Sclerosis: Your Legal Rights
Demos Medical Publishing
386 Park Avenue S
New York, NY 10016

212-683-0072
Fax: 212-683-0118
e-mail: orderdept@demospub.com
www.demosmedpub.com

156 pages
ISBN: 1-888799-31-5
Dr. Diana M Schneider

6626 The Comfort of Home Multiple Sclerosis Edi tion: A Guide for Caregivers
Marie M. Meyer and Paula Derr, RN, author
CareTrust Publications
PO Box 10283
Portland, OR 97296-0283

800-565-1533
Fax: 415-673-2005
e-mail: sales@comfortofhome.com
www.comfortofhome.com

Reviews caregiving options and discusses the financial and legal decisions you may encounterr. Readers will learn how to set up a safe and comfortable home for the person whose needs are changing and abilities declining. Comfort offers guidance through every caregiving stage and most decisions one will face in daily living, as well as in avoiding caregiver burnout. Valuable for the caregiver and the patient.
324 pages
ISBN: 0-966476-76-X

6627 Understanding Multiple Sclerosis
Melissa Stauffer, author
University Press of Mississippi
3825 Ridgewood Road
Jackson, MS 39211-6492

601-432-6205
Fax: 601-432-6217
e-mail: kburgess@ihl.state.ms.us
www.upress.state.ms.us

For patients and companions, an overview of all aspects of MS.
2006 144 pages Paperback
ISBN: 1-578068-03-7
Kathy Burgess, Advertising/Marketing Services Manager

Magazines

6628 Inside MS
National Multiple Sclerosis Society
733 3rd Avenue
New York, NY 10017-3288

212-986-3240
800-344-4867
Fax: 212-986-7981
www.nmss.org

Full color quarterly magazine on living well with mutiple sclerosis. Articles by people with MS; daily living, achievments, news, treatments, research, advocacy, humor, travel, helpful resources, large type. The magazine is a benefit of membership.
64 pages 4x Year

Newsletters

6629 Inside MS Bulletin
National Multiple Sclerosis Society
733 3rd Avenue
New York, NY 10017-3288

212-986-3240
800-344-4867
Fax: 212-986-7981

Newsletter offering information on the organization activities. Profiles of donors, and reports on MS research programs.

6630 MS Connection
National Multiple Sclerosis Society
9801-I Southern Pine Boulevard
Charlotte, NC 28273

704-525-2955
Fax: 704-527-0406
e-mail: mac@nmss.org
www.nationalmssociety.org/mac

Provides education, support and information about Chapter activities for people living with multiple sclerosis in South Carolina and western North Carolina.
Quarterly
Allison Mertens, Chair, Board of Trustees
Jennifer Lee, Chapter President

6631 Motivator
Multiple Sclerosis Foundation
6350 N Andrews Avenue
Fort Lauderdale, FL 33309-2130

954-776-6805
800-441-7055
e-mail: msfacts@icanect.net
www.msfacts.org

Reports on the latest advancements regarding medical treatments/therapies for MS, inspirational feature stories, coping skills, correspondence from readers, and ongoing MSAA programs, services, and activities.
BiMonthly

6632 Multiple Sclerosis Quarterly Report
Demos Vermande
386 Park Avenue S
New York, NY 10016-8804

212-683-0072
800-532-8663
Fax: 212-683-0118

This is the definitive newsletter for everyone who has MS, with feature articles, research updates, book reviews, and more. It is developed with the sponsorship of the Eastern Paralyzed Veterans of America and the National Multiple Sclerosis Society. The MSQR will keep you informed of new developments in the management of MS and strategies for living successfully with the disease.
1997 Quarterly

6633 National Multiple Sclerosis Society: Allegheny District Chapter
1040 5th Avenue — 412-261-6347
Pittsburgh, PA 15219-6220 — 800-544-5250
Fax: 412-232-1461
e-mail: pa@nmss.org
www.nmss-pgh.org

12 pages 4 per year
Colleen McGuire, Chapter President

Pamphlets

6634 ADA and People with MS
National Multiple Sclerosis Society
733 3rd Avenue — 212-986-3240
New York, NY 10017-3288 — 800-344-4867
Fax: 212-986-7981
What the Americans with Disabilities Act means in employment, public accommodations, transportation, and telecommunications.
24 pages

6635 At Home with MS: Adapting Your Environment
National Multiple Sclerosis Society
733 3rd Avenue — 212-986-3240
New York, NY 10017-3288 — 800-344-4867
Fax: 212-986-7981
Modify a house or apartment to save energy, compensate for reduced vision or mobility, and live comfortably. Many do-it-yourself changes.
28 pages

6636 At Our House
National Multiple Sclerosis Society
733 3rd Avenue — 212-986-3240
New York, NY 10017-3288 — 800-344-4867
Fax: 212-986-7981
A coloring book for children, ages 5-8, about a Mama Bear with MS. contains some very basic facts with an afterword for parents on how to talk to young children about MS.
20 pages

6637 Chapter Services at a Glance
National Multiple Sclerosis Society
733 3rd Avenue — 212-986-3240
New York, NY 10017-3288 — 800-344-4867
Fax: 212-986-7981
A summary of services offerred by local chapters. Contains membership form.

6638 Check Your Multiple Sclerosis Facts
National Multiple Sclerosis Society
733 3rd Avenue — 212-986-3240
New York, NY 10017-3288 — 800-344-4867
Fax: 212-986-7981
A brief checklist of MS basics - definition, symptoms, and outlook.

6639 Choosing a Pharmacy Service
National Multiple Sclerosis Society
733 3rd Avenue — 212-986-3240
New York, NY 10017-3288 — 800-344-4867
Fax: 212-986-7981
What to look for when choosing a prescription drug provider.
20 pages

6640 Clear Thinking About Alternative Therapies
National Multiple Sclerosis Society
733 3rd Avenue — 212-986-3240
New York, NY 10017-3288 — 800-344-4867
Fax: 212-986-7981
Highlights facts and common misconceptions, compares alternative and conventional medicine, and suggests ways to evaluate benefits and risks.

6641 Controlling Spasticity
National Multiple Sclerosis Society
733 3rd Avenue — 212-986-3240
New York, NY 10017-3288 — 800-344-4867
Fax: 212-986-7981
An overview of ways to control this common and sometimes disabling MS symptpom. Includes roles of self-help, medications, physical therapists, nurses, and physicians.

6642 Food for Thought: MS and Nutrition
National Multiple Sclerosis Society
733 3rd Avenue — 212-986-3240
New York, NY 10017-3288 — 800-344-4867
Fax: 212-986-7981
A guide to healthy eating and coping with symptoms that may affect eating habits.
20 pages

6643 Getting a Grip on Gait
National Multiple Sclerosis Society
733 3rd Avenue — 212-986-3240
New York, NY 10017-3288 — 800-344-4867
Fax: 212-986-7981
Walking problems and how they can be addressed.

6644 Hiring Help at Home?
National Multiple Sclerosis Society
733 3rd Avenue — 212-986-3240
New York, NY 10017-3288 — 800-344-4867
Fax: 212-986-7981
Checklists and worksheets for people who need help at home. Forms for needs assessment, job description, and employment contract.

6645 Insight Into Eyesight
National Multiple Sclerosis Society
733 3rd Avenue — 212-986-3240
New York, NY 10017-3288 — 800-344-4867
Fax: 212-986-7981
Current therapy for MS-related eye disorders. Discusses low-vision aids.

6646 Living with MS
National Multiple Sclerosis Society
733 3rd Avenue — 212-986-3240
New York, NY 10017-3288 — 800-344-4867
Fax: 212-986-7981
Answers to 28 questions most often asked when the diagnosis is MS - from possible causes to advice on coping.
20 pages

6647 Moving with Multiple Sclerosis
National Multiple Sclerosis Society
733 3rd Avenue — 212-986-3240
New York, NY 10017-3288 — 800-344-4867
Fax: 212-986-7981
Step-by-step illustrations of passive and active stretching, balance, and conditioning exercises.
30 pages

6648 Multiple Sclerosis and Your Emotions
National Multiple Sclerosis Society
733 3rd Avenue — 212-986-3240
New York, NY 10017-3288 — 800-344-4867
Fax: 212-986-7981
How to manage some of the emotional challenges created by MS.
32 pages

6649 On the Question of Pregnancy
National Multiple Sclerosis Society
733 3rd Avenue — 212-986-3240
New York, NY 10017-3288 — 800-344-4867
Fax: 212-986-7981
Reassuring answers on pregnancy, delivery, and nursing.

6650 On: Alternative Therapies
National Multiple Sclerosis Society
733 3rd Avenue — 212-986-3240
New York, NY 10017-3288 — 800-344-4867
Fax: 212-986-7981
Checklist for people who are considering an alternative treatment.

6651 On: Diagnosis...Putting the Pieces Together
National Multiple Sclerosis Society
733 3rd Avenue   212-986-3240
New York, NY 10017-3288   800-344-4867
                                Fax: 212-986-7981
Explains usual steps and tests. Includes how to prepare for an MRI.

6652 On: Energy Management
National Multiple Sclerosis Society
733 3rd Avenue   212-986-3240
New York, NY 10017-3288   800-344-4867
                                Fax: 212-986-7981
Guidelines for budgeting your energy when it's limited by fatigue through prioritizing, delegating, and simplifying tasks.

6653 On: Fatigue
National Multiple Sclerosis Society
733 3rd Avenue   212-986-3240
New York, NY 10017-3288   800-344-4867
                                Fax: 212-986-7981
The mystery of MS fatigue, practical tips for coping, and the medications sometimes prescribed.

6654 On: Genes
National Multiple Sclerosis Society
733 3rd Avenue   212-986-3240
New York, NY 10017-3288   800-344-4867
                                Fax: 212-986-7981
Recent information on MS and heredity.

6655 On: Pain
National Multiple Sclerosis Society
733 3rd Avenue   212-986-3240
New York, NY 10017-3288   800-344-4867
                                Fax: 212-986-7981
Myths and facts about MS pain. Covers types of pain and possible treatment.

6656 Plaintalk: A Booklet About MS for Families
National Multiple Sclerosis Society
733 3rd Avenue   212-986-3240
New York, NY 10017-3288   800-344-4867
                                Fax: 212-986-7981
Discusses some of the more difficult physical and emotional problems families may face.
32 pages

6657 Rehab Outlook
National Multiple Sclerosis Society
733 3rd Avenue   212-986-3240
New York, NY 10017-3288   800-344-4867
                                Fax: 212-986-7981
What rehabilitation can do for mobility, fatigue, driving, speech, memory, bowel or bladder problems, sexuality, and more.
24 pages

6658 Research Directions in Multiple Sclerosis
National Multiple Sclerosis Society
733 3rd Avenue   212-986-3240
New York, NY 10017-3288   800-344-4867
                                Fax: 212-986-7981
An overview of current research on key areas of immunology, genetics, virology, and cell biology explained for nonscientists.
16 pages

6659 Sexual Problems Your Doctor Didn't Mention
National Multiple Sclerosis Society
733 3rd Avenue   212-986-3240
New York, NY 10017-3288   800-344-4867
                                Fax: 212-986-7981
How MS may affect sexuality and what can be done.

6660 Solving Cognitive Problems
National Multiple Sclerosis Society
733 3rd Avenue   212-986-3240
New York, NY 10017-3288   800-344-4867
                                Fax: 212-986-7981
Mental functions most likely to be affected by MS. Suggestions for self-help and information about cognitive rehabiitation.
20 pages

6661 Someone You Know Has MS: A Book for Families
National Multiple Sclerosis Society
733 3rd Avenue   212-986-3240
New York, NY 10017-3288   800-344-4867
                                Fax: 212-986-7981
For children ages 6-12 who have a parent with MS. Provides facts and explores children's fears and concerns.
32 pages

6662 Taking Care: A Guide for Well Partners
National Multiple Sclerosis Society
733 3rd Avenue   212-986-3240
New York, NY 10017-3288   800-344-4867
                                Fax: 212-986-7981
Introduces the concept of carepartnering to balance both partners' needs. Includes practical suggestions about getting and giving help.
16 pages

6663 Taming Stress in Multiple Sclerosis
National Multiple Sclerosis Society
733 3rd Avenue   212-986-3240
New York, NY 10017-3288   800-344-4867
                                Fax: 212-986-7981
Stress and depression, and how both relate to MS. Tips on simplifying daily life. Instructions on muscle relaxation, deep breathing, and visualization relaxation.
36 pages

6664 Things I Wish Someone Had Told Me
National Multiple Sclerosis Society
733 3rd Avenue   212-986-3240
New York, NY 10017-3288   800-344-4867
                                Fax: 212-986-7981
First-person story. A positive and practical approach to adjusting to life with MS.
20 pages

6665 Understanding Bladder Problems in Multiple Sclerosis
National Multiple Sclerosis Society
733 3rd Avenue   212-986-3240
New York, NY 10017-3288   800-344-4867
                                Fax: 212-986-7981
The three main types of bladder dysfunction explained. Guidelines for management.
12 pages

6666 Understanding Bowel Problems in MS
National Multiple Sclerosis Society
733 3rd Avenue   212-986-3240
New York, NY 10017-3288   800-344-4867
                                Fax: 212-986-7981
An exploration of ways to manage bowel problems in MS.
24 pages

6667 What Everyone Should Know About Multiple Sclerosis
National Multiple Sclerosis Society
733 3rd Avenue   212-986-3240
New York, NY 10017-3288   800-344-4867
                                Fax: 212-986-7981
Overview of MS, suitable for the whole family.
16 pages

6668 What Is Multiple Sclerosis?
National Multiple Sclerosis Society
733 3rd Avenue   212-986-3240
New York, NY 10017-3288   800-344-4867
                                Fax: 212-986-7981
For the newly diagnosed and others who need an overview of symptoms, disease patterns, diagnosis, prognosis, treatment, and research efforts.

6669 When a Parent Has MS: A Teenager's Guide
National Multiple Sclerosis Society
733 3rd Avenue   212-986-3240
New York, NY 10017-3288   800-344-4867
                                Fax: 212-986-7981
For older children and teenagers who have a parent with MS. Discusses issues brought up by real kids.
24 pages

6670 **Win-Win Approach to Reasonable Accommodations**
National Multiple Sclerosis Society
733 3rd Avenue   212-986-3240
New York, NY 10017-3288   800-344-4867
                                  Fax: 212-986-7981
A practical guide to obtaining workplace accommodations.
20 pages

Audio & Video

6671 **Aqua Exercises for Multiple Sclerosis**
National Multiple Sclerosis Society
733 3rd Avenue   212-986-3240
New York, NY 10017-3288   800-344-4867
                                  Fax: 212-986-7981
A workout that cools and supports the body, with exercises to reduce spasticity, build muscles, and improve posture. With waterproof chart.
20 minutes

6672 **Clinical Trials in Multiple Sclerosis: Searching for New Therapies**
National Multiple Sclerosis Society
733 3rd Avenue   212-986-3240
New York, NY 10017   800-344-4867
                                  Fax: 212-986-7981
Describes studies to determine the safety and efficacy of new drugs to treat MS. Why studies are essential, how they are conducted, and the role of participants.
20 minutes

6673 **Now, More Than Ever: Progress in Multiple Sclerosis Research**
National Multiple Sclerosis Society
733 3rd Avenue   212-986-3240
New York, NY 10017-3288   800-344-4867
                                  Fax: 212-986-7981
Traces the National Multiple Sclerosis Society's historic role in propelling MS research and explains current approaches for nonscientists.
10 minutes

Web Sites

6674 **Healing Well**
                                  www.healingwell.com
An online health resource guide to medical news, chat, information and articles, newsgroups and message boards, books, disease-related web sites, medical directories, and more for patients, friends, and family coping with disabling diseases, disorders, or chronic illnesses.

6675 **Health Finder**
                                  www.healthfinder.gov
Searchable, carefully developed web site offering information on over 1000 topics. Developed by the US Department of Health and Human Services, the site can be used in both English and Spanish.

6676 **Healthlink USA**
                                  www.healthlinkusa.com
Health information concerning treatment, cures, prevention, diagnosis, risk factors, research, support groups, email lists, personal stories and much more. Updated regularly.

6677 **Helios Health**
                                  www.helioshealth.com
Online resource for your health information. Detailed information about specific health topics, access to expert advice from our Medical Advisory Board, and up-to-date health news.

6678 **MedicineNet**
                                  www.medicinenet.com
An online resource for consumers providing easy-to-read, authoritative medical and health information.

6679 **Medscape**
                                  www.medscape.com
Medscape offers specialists, primary care physicians, and other health professionals the Web's most robust and integrated medical information and educational tools.

6680 **Multiple Sclerosis Foundation**
                                  www.msfocus.org
Dedicated to helping create a brighter tomorrow for those with MS, the foundation offers a wide array of free services including: national toll-free support, educational programs, homecare, support groups, assitive technology, publications, a comprehensive website and more to improve the quality of life for those affected by MS.

6681 **National Multiple Sclerosis Society**
                                  www.nmss.org
Provides research, public and professional education, advocacy and the design of rehabilitative and psychosocial programs.

6682 **Neurology Channel**
                                  www.neurologychannel.com
Find clearly explained, medically accurate information regarding conditions, including an overview, symptoms, causes, diagnostic procedures and treatment options. On this site it is possible to ask questions and get information from a neurologist and connect to people who have similar health interests.

6683 **WebMD**
                                  www.webmd.com
Information on Multiple Sclerosis, including articles and resources.

Description

6684 Muscular Dystrophy

Muscular dystrophy is a group of genetic disorders marked by progressive weakness and degeneration of the skeletal, or voluntary, muscles that control movement. The muscles of the heart and other involuntary muscles may also affected in some forms of muscular dystrophy, and a few forms of the disease involve other organs as well.

Muscular dystrophy can affect people of all ages. The most common form, Duchenne, appears in childhood, but others may not appear until middle age or later.

Duchenne muscular dystrophy affects males almost exclusively. By age five, those with Duchenne experience progressive weakness and difficulty in climbing, jumping and hopping. By ages eight to ten, leg braces are often required, and eventually walking is impossible. Duchenne is also associated with heart problems, although without symptoms, and intellectual impairment that affects verbal ability more than performance. Death usually occurs in the third decade of life, often as a result of pneumonia.

No specific treatment exists. Daily prednisone provides significant benefit but owing to the medication's numerous side effects, it should be reserved for patients with major functional decline. Other treatment includes physical therapy, which can help minimize the shortening of the muscles that occurs around joints; assistive devices; and avoidance of prolonged immobility. There are now techniques available to detect female carriers of the defective gene, enabling genetic counseling for families and couples considering conception.

Other forms of muscular dystrophy are myotonic, Becker, limb-girdle and facioscapulohumeral. Information about when and where muscle weakness first occurred, and its severity, is very helpful in classifying the type of muscular dystrophy. Studying a small piece of muscle tissue can indicate whether the disorder is muscular dystrophy and which form of the disease it is.

National Agencies & Associations

6685 Muscular Dystrophy Association
3300 E Sunrise Drive
Tucson, AZ 85718-3299
520-529-2000
800-572-1717
e-mail: mda@mdausa.org
www.mda.org

Primary objective of MDA is the support of scientific investigators seeking the causes of and effective treatments for muscular dystrophy and related neuromuscular disorders. The worldwide research program supports over 400 scientific investigations annually.
Robert Ross, President/CEO

6686 Muscular Dystrophy Canada
2345 Yonge Street
Toronto, Ontario, M4P-2E5
866-687-2538
Fax: 416-488-7523
e-mail: info@muscle.ca
www.muscle.ca

Since 1954, Muscular Dystrophy Canada has been committed to improving the quality of life for the tens of thousands of Canadians with neuromuscular disorders and funding leading research for the discovery of therapies and cures for neuromuscular disorders.

6687 Parent Project: Muscular Dystrophy
1012 N University Boulevard
Middletown, OH 45042
513-424-0696
800-714-5437
Fax: 513-425-9907
e-mail: pat@parentprojectmd.org
www.parentprojectmd.org

Organization of families around the world who have children diagnosed with DMD/BMD. Our goal is to invest significant amounts of money raised into medical research with clinical application.
Patricia Furlong, President
Kimberly Galberaith, Executive Vice President

6688 Society for Muscular Dystrophy Information International
PO Box 7490
Bridgewater, Nova Scotia, B4V-2X6
902-685-3961
Fax: 902-685-3962
e-mail: smdi@auracom.com
users.auracom.com

A registered Canadian charity founded in 1983 by us, to provide a non-technical worldwide information links via publications and now this web site, for neuromuscular disorders.

Research Centers

6689 Baylor College of Medicine: Jerry Lewis Neuromuscular Disease Research
Methodist Neurological Institute
Department of Neurology
Houston, TX 77030
713-798-5971
Fax: 713-798-3854
e-mail: neurons@bcm.edu
www.bcm.edu/neurology

Offers research into biochemistry molecular genetics and neuromuscular disorders.
Stanley Appe MD, Director

6690 Columbia Presbyterian Medical Center Neurological Institute
Columbia University
710 W 168th Street
New York, NY 10032
212-305-2700
Fax: 212-058-98
www.cumc.columbia.edu

Neuromuscular clinical research center.
Hiroshi Mits MD, Division Head Neuromuscular Division

6691 Columbia University Clinical Research Center for Muscular Dystrophy
College of Physicians & Surgeons
630 W 168th Street
New York, NY 10032
212-305-3806
Fax: 212-305-1343
www.columbia.edu

Salvatore DiMauro, Co Director

6692 Hospital of the University of Pennsylvania University of Pennsylvania
University of Pennsylvania
3400 Spruce Street
Philadelphia, PA 19104
215-662-4000
800-789-PENN
Fax: 215-903-09
e-mail: pleasure@email.chop.edu
www.pennhealth.com

Research program centering its efforts on finding better ways to prevent and treat neuromuscular disorders.
David E Pleasure MD, Director

6693 Mayo Clinic and Foundation Mayo Foundation
Mayo Foundation
201 W Center Street
Rochester, MN 55905
507-284-2511
Fax: 507-284-0161
TTY: 507-284-9786
www.mayo.edu

Neuromuscular clinical research center with a primary research interest in neuropathies.
Peter J Dyck MD, Director Nerve Studies
Andrew G Engel MD, Director Muscle Studies

6694 **Muscular Dystrophy Association**
3300 E Sunrise Drive
Tucson, AZ 85718-3299
520-529-2000
800-572-1717
Fax: 520-529-5300
e-mail: mda@mdausa.org
www.MDausa.org
Fights neuromuscular disease including all muscular dystrophies. Conducts extensive programs of research services and public education including 230 clinics.
Robert Ross, President/CEO

6695 **University of Utah Utah Genome Depot University of Utah**
University of Utah
20 S 2030 E
Salt Lake City, UT 84112
801-585-7606
Fax: 801-857-7177
e-mail: bob.weiss@genetics.utah.edu
www.genome.utah.edu
Focuses research on human muscular dystrophies.
Robert Weiss, Principal Investigator
Jackie Tyce, Program Coordinator

Support Groups & Hotlines

6696 **Facioscapulohumeral Muscular Dystrophy Soc iety (FSH Society)**
3 Westwood Road
Lexington, MA 02420
781-860-0501
Fax: 781-860-0599
e-mail: solvefshd@fshsociety.org
www.fshsociety.org
The Facioscapulohumeral Muscular Dystrophy Society (FSH Society) serves as a resource for individuals and families with FSHD, representing them and advocating on their behalf. Purposes of the organization are to accumulate, disseminate and encourage the exchange of information about FSHD, including educating the general public, relevant governmental bodies, and the medical and scientific professions about the existence, diagnosis and treatment of FSHD.
Daniel Paul Perez, President/CEO
Carol A Perez, Executive Director

6697 **National Health Information Center**
PO Box 1133
Washington, DC 20013
310-565-4167
800-336-4797
Fax: 301-984-4256
e-mail: info@nhic.org
www.health.gov/nhic
Offers a nationwide information referral service, produces directories and resource guides.

Books

6698 **Clinical Evaluation and Diagnostic Tests for Neuromuscular Disorders**
Butterworth-Heinemann Medical
200 Wheeler Road
Burlington, MA 01803
781-221-2212
Fax: 781-221-1615
e-mail: custserv.bh@elsevier.com
www.bh.com
Expert advice from leading authorities on how and when to use the numerous evaluation tests now available for diagnosis and management of neuromuscular disorders.
2002

6699 **Everyday Life with ALS: A Practical Guide**
Muscular Dystrophy Association
3300 E Sunrise Drive
Tucson, AZ 85718-3299
520-529-2000
800-572-1717
Fax: 520-529-5383
e-mail: publications@mdausa.org
www.mda.org
Advice and information addressing degrees of affliction of those with ALS. Ways to conserve energy, to modifying your home space, to medical devices and equipment. Consider using the Guide with your care team.
2005
Christina Medvescek, Director of Editorial Services

6700 **Journey of Love: Parent's Guide to Duchenne Muscular Dystrophy**
Muscular Dystrophy Association
3300 E Sunrise Drive
Tucson, AZ 85718-3299
520-529-2000
800-572-1717
Fax: 520-529-5383
e-mail: publications@mdausa.org
www.mda.org
Complete guide for parents with children diagnosed with DMD. Information includes explanation of the disease, treatments, research, services provided by MDA, guides to finding assistance and more.
170 pages Paperback
Bob Mackle, Director Public Information
Christina Medvescek, Director of Editorial Services

6701 **MDA ALS Caregiver's Guide**
Muscular Dystrophy Association
3300 E Sunrise Drive
Tucson, AZ 85718-3299
520-529-2000
800-572-1717
e-mail: publication@mdusa.org
www.mda.org
A comprehensive guide to caring for a person with ALS at home. Covers everything from physical care to psychological and emotional concerns to getting financial assistance. Companion to Everyday Life with ALS: A Practical Guide.
2008 58 pages Paperback
Bob Mackle, Director Public Information
Christina Medvescek, Director of Editorial Services

6702 **Moonrise: One Family, Genetic Identity, & Muscular Dystrophy**
St. Martin's Press
175 5th Avenue
New York, NY 10010
212-674-5151
Fax: 212-420-9314
www.stmartins.com
A mother writes about her teen-age son who has Duchenne muscular dystrophy, the life he leads, and the one he can look forward to.
2003

6703 **Muscular Dystrophy & Other Neuromuscular Diseases: Psychological Issues**
Leon Charash, Robert Lovelace, author
Haworth Press
10 Alice Street
Binghamton, NY 13904
607-722-5857
800-429-6784
Fax: 607-722-0012
www.haworthpress.com
Thoughtful book from professionals who assist people with neuromuscular disorders to help them adapt to lifestyle changes accompanying these disorders.
250 pages Hardcover
ISBN: 1-560240-77-0

6704 **Muscular Dystrophy in Children: Guide for Families**
Demos Medical Publishing
386 Park Avenue S
New York, NY 10015
800-532-8663
Fax: 212-683-0118
e-mail: orderdept@demospub.com
www.demosmedpub.com
Addresses emotional as well as physical challenges that families and caregivers will have to face and gives readers information on muscular dystrophy, how to adapt to a child's needs, and present research being conducted. In addition, it gives parents and caregivers sources for additional support and suggestions for further reading.
1999

6705 **Neuromuscular Dis. of Infancy, Childhood & Adolesesce: A Clinician's Approach**
Butterworth-Heinemann Medical
200 Wheeler Road
Burlington, MA 01803
781-221-2212
Fax: 781-221-1615
e-mail: custserv.bh@elsevier.com
www.bh.com
Explains how childhood neuromuscular diseases differ from those in adult patients, and provides clinicians with all the knowledge they need to successfully diagnose and treat pediatric patients.
2003

6706 Noninvasive Mechanical Ventilation
John Bach, MD, author
Elsevier
Book Customer Service Department
St. Louis, MO 63146
Fax: 800-545-2522
Fax: 800-535-9935
e-mail: usbkinfo@elsevier.com
www.elsevier.com

Describes the use of inspiratory and expiratory muscle aids to prevent the pulmonary complications of lung disease and conditions with muscle weakness. It also describes treatment and rehabilitation interventions specific for patients with these conditions. This book is unique in presenting the use of entirely noninvasive management alternatives to eliminate respiratory morbidity and avoid the need to resort to tracheostomy for the majority of patients with lung or neuromuscular disease.
2002 348 pages Paperback
ISBN: 1-560535-49-0

6707 Physical Medicine & Rehabilitation
WB Saunders/Elsevier Science/Harcourt
200 Wheeler Road
Burlington, MA 01803
781-221-2212
Fax: 781-221-1615
e-mail: custserv.bh@elsevier.com
www.us.elsevierhealth.com

Current aspects of physical medicine and rehabilitation in a single, readable volume. Completely updated and revised edition includes all the latest advances and techniques.
2001

Children's Books

6708 Abby & the South Seas Adventure Series
Tyndale House Publishers
PO Box 80
Wheaton, IL 60189
630-668-8300
Fax: 630-668-3245
www.tyndalecatalog.com

Delightful new series, focusing on the travels of Abby Kendall, who has muscular dystrophy, is a sure-fire hit for 8 to 12 year old girls. Lots of surprises will keep them coming back for each new Abby title.
2000

6709 Heartsongs, Journey Through Heartsongs, Hope Through Heartsongs, Celebrate
Hyperion Books
1344 Crossman Avenue
Sunnyvale, CA 94089
408-744-9500
Fax: 408-744-0400
www.hyperion.com

By the 2002-2003 National Goodwill Ambassador for the Muscular Dystrophy Association. The first two books of inspiring poems were both on the New York Times bestseller list. Mattie's struggle with muscular dystrophy has never kept him from feeling deep love for his family, friends, country and faith — heartfelt emotions that are reflected throughout these pages by a precociously brilliant boy.
2001-2003
Carol Sowell, Director Publications

6710 Muscular Dystrophy
Enslow Publishers
40 Industrial Road
Berkeley Heights, NJ 07922-0398
800-398-2504
Fax: 908-771-0925
e-mail: info@enslow.com
www.enslow.com

Written for children, this book follows two families with muscular dystrophy and describes various forms of the disease, who gets it, and how to learn to live with it.
2000

Magazines

6711 Quest Magazine
Muscular Dystrophy Association

3300 E Sunrise Drive
Tucson, AZ 85718-3299
520-529-2000
800-572-1717
Fax: 520-529-5300
e-mail: publications@mdusa.org
www.mda.org

Quarterly magazine. Contains stories about vital concerns of people with meuromuscular diseases and their community. Find tips, hobbies, resources, treatments, findings, and products. Available online.
30 pages Paperback
Bob Mackle, Director Public Information
Christina Medvescek, Director of Editorial Services

Pamphlets

6712 Breathe Easy: Respiratory Care with Muscular Dystrophy
Muscular Dystrophy Association
3300 E Sunrise Drive
Tucson, AZ 85718-3299
520-529-2000
800-572-1717
Fax: 520-529-5383
e-mail: publications@mda.org
www.mda.org

Members of a respiratory care team describe how muscular dystrophy can affect breathing, maintaining respiratory health and types of therapies. Also available in Spanish.
2006
Christina Medvescek, Director of Editorial Services

6713 Everybody's Different Nobody's Perfect
Muscular Dystrophy Association
3300 E Sunrise Drive
Tucson, AZ 85718-3299
520-529-2000
800-572-1717
Fax: 520-529-5300
e-mail: publications@mdusa.org
www.mda.org

Children's Book. Explains how muscular dystrophy affects children and describes how people are different from each other in many ways. Emphasizing fun, friendship and caring, this booklet is ideal for heightening awareness and encouraging understanding of persons with disabilities. Also available in Spanish.
1999 11 pages Paperback
Bob Mackle, Director Public Information
Christina Medvescek, Director of Editorial Services

6714 Facts About Charcot-Marie-Tooth Disease
Muscular Dystrophy Association
3300 E Sunrise Drive
Tucson, AZ 85718-3299
520-529-2000
800-572-1717
Fax: 520-529-5383
e-mail: publications@mdausa.org
www.mda.org

Covers the forms of the disease and outlines the characteristics and genetic patterns of the CMTs. Research efforts aimed at finding the causes, treatments and cures are also described. Also available in Spanish.
15 pages
Christina Medvescek, Director of Editorial Services

6715 Facts About Duchenne & Becker Muscular Dystrophies
Muscular Dystrophy Association
3300 E Sunrise Drive
Tucson, AZ 85718-3299
520-529-2000
800-572-1717
Fax: 520-529-5383
e-mail: publications@mdausa.org
www.mda.org

Introductory booklet describes the two disorders, testing, inheritance and treatments. Also available in Spanish.
Christina Medvescek, Director of Editorial Services

6716 Facts About Facioscapulohumeral Muscular Dystrophy
Muscular Dystrophy Association
3300 E Sunrise Drive
Tucson, AZ 85718-3299
520-529-2000
800-572-1717
Fax: 520-529-5383
e-mail: publications@mdausa.org
www.mda.org

Introductory booklet describes FSHD in easy-to-understand terms and answers commonly asked questions about the disease. Also available in Spanish.

Christina Medvescek, Director of Editorial Services

6717 Facts About Friedreich's Ataxia
Muscular Dystrophy Association
3300 E Sunrise Drive   520-529-2000
Tucson, AZ 85718-3299   800-572-1717
                                        Fax: 520-529-5300
                  e-mail: publications@mdausa.org
                                               www.mda.org
Explains Friedreich's ataxia in layman's terms and answers commonly asked questions about the disease. Also available in Spanish.
15 pages Paperback
Bob Mackle, Director Public Information
Christina Medvescek, Director of Editorial Services

6718 Facts About Limb-Girdle Muscular Dystrophy
Muscular Dystrophy Association
3300 E Sunrise Drive   520-529-2000
Tucson, AZ 85718-3299   800-572-1717
                                        Fax: 520-529-5383
                  e-mail: publications@mdausa.org
                                               www.mda.org
Introductory booklet provides basic facts about LGMD and contains information regarding the many forms, diagnostic tests and current treatments. Also available in Spanish.
Christina Medvescek, Director of Editorial Services

6719 Facts About Metabolic Diseases of Muscle
Muscular Dystrophy Association
3300 E Sunrise Drive   520-529-2000
Tucson, AZ 85718-3299   800-572-1717
                                        Fax: 520-529-5300
                  e-mail: publications@mdausa.org
                                               www.mda.org
Provides an overview of the 11 inheritable metabolic diseases of muscle encompassed by MDA's program. Addresses commonly asked questions and highlights MDA's research efforts aimed at finding the causes of and effective treatments for these disorders. Also available in Spanish.
20 pages Paperback
Bob Mackle, Director Public Information
Christina Medvescek, Director of Editorial Services

6720 Facts About Mitochondrial Myopathies
Muscular Dystrophy Association
3300 E Sunrise Drive   520-529-2000
Tucson, AZ 85718-3299   800-572-1717
                                        Fax: 520-529-5300
                  e-mail: publications@mdausa.org
                                               www.mda.org
Explains mitochondrial myopathies in layman's terms and answers the most frequently asked questions about this disease. Also available in Spanish.
24 pages Paperback
Bob Mackle, Director Public Information
Christina Medvescek, Director of Editorial Services

6721 Facts About Myasthenia Gravis
Muscular Dystrophy Association
3300 E Sunrise Drive   520-529-2000
Tucson, AZ 85718-3299   800-572-1717
                                        Fax: 520-529-5300
                  e-mail: publications@mdausa.org
                                               www.mda.org
Explains myasthenia gravis and Lambert-Eaton syndrome in layman's terms and answers the most frequently asked questions about these diseases. Also available in Spanish.
19 pages Paperback
Bob Mackle, Director Public Information
Carol Sowall, Director Publications

6722 Facts About Myopathies
Muscular Dystrophy Association

3300 E Sunrise Drive   520-529-2000
Tucson, AZ 85718-3299   800-572-1717
                                        Fax: 520-529-5300
                  e-mail: publications@mdusa.org
                                               www.mda.org
Overview of the myopathies encompassed by MDA's program. Addresses commonly asked questions and highlights MDA's research efforts aimed at finding the causes of and effective treatments for these disorders. Also available in Spanish.
18 pages Paperback
Bob Mackle, Director Public Information
Christina Medvescek, Director of Editorial Services

6723 Facts About Myotonic Muscular Dystrophy
Muscular Dystrophy Association
3300 E Sunrise Drive   520-529-2000
Tucson, AZ 85718-3299   800-572-1717
                                        Fax: 520-529-5383
                  e-mail: publications@mdausa.org
                                               www.mda.org
Introductory booklet provides basic facts about the disorder and explains the causes and effects, as well as tests used to diagnose and MDA's search for treatments and cures. Also available in Spanish.
Christina Medvescek, Director of Editorial Services

6724 Facts About Plasmapheresis
Muscular Dystrophy Association
3300 E Sunrise Drive   520-529-2000
Tucson, AZ 85718-3299   800-572-1717
                                        Fax: 520-529-5300
                  e-mail: publications@mdusa.org
                                               www.mda.org

Describes plasmapheresis, a plasma exchange procedure often utilized as a treatment for autoimmune disease such as myasthenia gravis and Lambert-Eaton syndrome.
Paperback
Bob Mackle, Director Public Information
Christina Medvescek, Director of Editorial Services

6725 Facts About Polymyostis/Dermatomyositis
Muscular Dystrophy Association
3300 E Sunrise Drive   520-529-2000
Tucson, AZ 85718-3299   800-572-1717
                                        Fax: 520-529-5300
                  e-mail: publications@mdusa.org
                                               www.mda.org
Outlines these two front forms of inflammatory myopathy. Current approaches to treatment and MDA's efforts in continued research are described. Also available in Spanish.
13 pages Paperback
Bob Mackle, Director Public Information
Christina Medvescek, Director of Editorial Services

6726 Facts About Rare Muscular Dsytrophies
Muscular Dystrophy Association
3300 E Sunrise Drive   520-529-2000
Tucson, AZ 85718-3299   800-572-1717
                                        Fax: 520-529-5300
                  e-mail: publications@mdusa.org
                                               www.mda.org
This brochure gives basic facts about four forms of muscular dystrophy (Congenital, Distal, Emery-Dreifuss and Oculopharyngeal) and addresses commonly asked questions. Also available in Spanish.
28 pages Paperback
Bob Mackle, Director Public Information
Christina Medvescek, Director of Editorial Services

6727 Facts About Spinal Muscular Atrophy
Muscular Dystrophy Association
3300 E Sunrise Drive   520-529-2000
Tucson, AZ 85718-3299   800-572-1717
                                        Fax: 520-529-5300
                  e-mail: publications@mdusa.org
                                               www.mda.org
Covers the four forms of the disease and outlines the characteristics and genetic patterns of the SMAs. Research efforts aimed at

finding the causes, treatments and cures are also described. Also available in Spanish.
15 pages Paperback
Bob Mackle, Director Public Information
Christina Medvescek, Director of Editorial Services

6728 Genetics and Neuromuscular Diseases
Muscular Dystrophy Association
3300 E Sunrise Drive   520-529-2000
Tucson, AZ 85718-3299   800-572-1717
                                        Fax: 520-529-5383
                        e-mail: publications@mdausa.org
                                            www.mda.org
Booklet describes what a genetic disorder is and explains how genetic testing and counseling can help people understand how disorders that may affect them or their children are inherited. Also available in Spanish.
Christina Medvescek, Director of Editorial Services

6729 Hey, I'm Here Too
Muscular Dystrophy Association
3300 E Sunrise Drive   520-529-2000
Tucson, AZ 85718-3299   800-572-1717
                                        Fax: 520-529-5383
                        e-mail: publications@mdausa.org
                                            www.mda.org
Help for siblings of boys with Duchenne muscular dystrophy. Explores how they feel about themselves, their brothers and their families. Also provides specific answers to some questions that siblings may wonder about. Also available in Spanish.
28 pages
Bob Mackle, Director Public Information
Christina Medvescek, Director of Editorial Services

6730 Learning to Live with Neuromuscular Desease: A Message to Parents
Muscular Dystrophy Association
3300 E Sunrise Drive   520-529-2000
Tucson, AZ 85718-3299   800-572-1717
                                        Fax: 520-529-5383
                        e-mail: publications@mdausa.org
                                            www.mda.org
Helps parents and families cope with the fact that their child has a neuromuscular disease and with the impact the disease will have on everyday life. Also available in Spanish.
Christina Medvescek, Director of Editorial Services

6731 MDA Camp: A Special Place
Muscular Dystrophy Association
3300 E Sunrise Drive   520-529-2000
Tucson, AZ 85718-3299   800-572-1717
                                        Fax: 520-529-5300
                        e-mail: publications@mdusa.org
                                            www.mdusa.org
Highlights the activities of MDA dummer camps for youngsters diagnosed with one of the more than 40 diseases in MDA's program. Shares camper and volunteer reactions. Also available in Spanish.
Paperback
Bob Mackle, Director Public Information
Carol Sowall, Director Publications

6732 MDA Fact Sheet
Muscular Dystrophy Association
3300 E Sunrise Drive   520-529-2000
Tucson, AZ 85718-3299   800-572-1717
                                        Fax: 520-529-5383
                        e-mail: publications@mdausa.org
                                            www.mda.org
Basic information on MDA's origins and purposes; the more than 40 neuromuscular diseases in MDA's program, and brief symptom descriptions by category. Also available in Spanish.
Christina Medvescek, Director of Editorial Services

6733 MDA Services for the Individual, Family and Community
Muscular Dystrophy Association
3300 E Sunrise Drive   520-529-2000
Tucson, AZ 85718-3299   800-572-1717
                                        Fax: 520-529-5383
                        e-mail: publications@mdausa.org
                                            www.mda.org

Lists the diseases covered by MDA as well as eligibility criteria for MDA's services program, a list of MDA-sponsored clinics nationwide, and the services available through local MDA offices. Also available in Spanish.
Christina Medvescek, Director of Editorial Services

6734 Teacher's Guide to Neuromuscular Disease
Muscular Dystrophy Association
3300 E Sunrise Drive   520-529-2000
Tucson, AZ 85718-3299   Fax: 520-529-5383
                        e-mail: publications@mdausa.org
                                            www.mda.org
This publication provides a source of guidance and information to teachers, giving details about neuromuscular diseases, how they affect school participation, and ways that teachers can help meet the needs of students affected by these disorders.
2005
Christina Medvescek, Director of Editorial Services

6735 Travis, I Got Lots of Neat Stuff Children Living with Muscular Dystrophy
Muscular Dystrophy Association
3300 E Sunrise Drive   520-529-2000
Tucson, AZ 85718-3299   800-572-1717
                                        Fax: 520-529-5383
                        e-mail: publications@mdausa.org
                                            www.mda.org
Booklet illustrates that a child with muscular dystrophy can do many things. Adapted for MDA's Hop-a-Thon program, the booklet heightens awareness and understanding of people with disabilities. It's suitable for youngsters in elementary school. Also available in Spanish.
24 pages
Christina Medvescek, Director of Editorial Services

Audio & Video

6736 Muscular Dystrophy
Films for the Humanities & Sciences
Box 2053   609-419-8000
Princeton, NJ 08543-2053   800-257-5126
                                        Fax: 609-275-3767
Video deals with how Muscular Dystrophy sufferers deal with the disease that has no cure. Three life stories dealing with surgery, medicine, therapy and bracing as a means to survive. Dr. Betty Banke discusses the need to find a cure while Richard Nordgren from the Dartmouth-Hitchcock Medical Center discusses treatment.
20 Minutes

Web Sites

6737 Healing Well
                                    www.healingwell.com
An online health resource guide to medical news, chat, information and articles, newsgroups and message boards, books, disease-related web sites, medical directories, and more for patients, friends, and family coping with disabling diseases, disorders, or chronic illnesses.

6738 Health Finder
                                        www.healthfinder.gov
Searchable, carefully developed web site offering information on over 1000 topics. Developed by the US Department of Health and Human Services, the site can be used in both English and Spanish.

6739 Healthlink USA
                                    www.healthlinkusa.com
Health information concerning treatment, cures, prevention, diagnosis, risk factors, research, support groups, email lists, personal stories and much more. Updated regularly.

6740 Helios Health
                                    www.helioshealth.com
Online resource for your health information. Detailed information about specific health topics, access to expert advice from our Medical Advisory Board, and up-to-date health news.

6741   MedicineNet

www.medicinenet.com

An online resource for consumers providing easy-to-read, authoritative medical and health information.

6742   Medscape

www.medscape.com

Medscape offers specialists, primary care physicians, and other health professionals the Web's most robust and integrated medical information and educational tools.

6743   Muscular Dystrophy Association

www.mdausa.org

Information on effective treatments for muscular dystrophy, related neuromuscular disorders and research programs. In addition, MDA offers a comprehensive program of patient and community services, with access to over 230 MDA-supported clinics nationwide.

6744   Parent Project: Muscular Dystrophy

www.parentdmd.org

Organization of families around the world who have children diagnosed with DMD/BMD. Our goal is to invest significant amounts of money raised into medical research with clinical application.

6745   WebMD

www.webmd.com

Information on Muscular Dystrophy, including articles and resources.

Description

6746 ## Myasthenia Gravis

Myasthenia gravis is a disease of the neuromuscular junction - the structure which carries the nerve's chemical signal that tells the muscle to contract. Circulating antibodies attack this junction, leading to weakness of voluntary muscles and muscle fatigue after exercise. Any muscle may be involved, but muscles in the face and throat are especially susceptible. The disease therefore especially affects chewing, swallowing, coughing and facial expressions. These manifestations fluctuate in intensity over hours to days.

Because this disease is caused by an overactive immune system, most treatments target this system. These include corticosteroids, immunosuppressive drugs such as azathioprine, plasmapheresis (filtration of the blood with retention of the cells and removal of the plasma), intravenous immunoglobulins and surgical removal of the thymus gland. In addition, anticholinesterase drugs like pyridostigmine increase the level of the messenger chemical at the neuromuscular junction, thereby increasing muscle strength.

Because of the progressive weakness associated with this disease, physical therapy and assistive devices are generally required.

National Agencies & Associations

6747 **Myasthenia Gravis Association of BC**
2805 Kingsway
Vancouver, BC, V5R-5H9
640-451-5511
e-mail: mgabc@centreforability.bc.ca
www.myastheniagravis.ca
Informs members about new treatment thods and research concerning myasthenia gravis.

6748 **Myasthenia Gravis Foundation**
1821 University Avenue W
St Paul, MN 55104
651-917-6256
800-541-5454
Fax: 651-917-1835
e-mail: mgfa@myasthenia.org
www.myasthenia.org
The mission of the Foundation is to facilitate the timely diagnosis end optimal care of individuals affected by myasthenia gravis and closely related disorders and to improve their lives through programs of patient services, public information and medical reports.
Marcia Lorimer, Executive Committee
Sam Schulhof, Chair

6749 **Myasthenia Gravis Foundation of America**
5841 Cedar Lake Road
Minneapolis, MN 55416
43- 29- 986
800-541-5454
Fax: 952-646-2028
e-mail: mgfa@myasthenia.org
www.myasthenia.org
Dedicated to the conquest of the disease through research education information and patient services. Offers over 34 chapters and over 100 support groups across the country as well as 8 international chapters.
Tor Holtan, CEO
Jennifer Heidelberge, Chapter Relations Manager

State Agencies & Associations

Alabama

6750 **Alabama Chapter of the Myasthenia Gravis Foundation of America**
PO Box 530623
Birmingham, AL 35253
205-868-1210
866-749-0844
Fax: 205-868-1211
e-mail: alabama@myasthenia.org
www.myasthenia.org

Michael Greene, President
Joyce Wood, Vice President

Arizona

6751 **Jim L Walker: Arizona Chapter of the Myasthenia Gravis Foundation of America**
PO Box 34173
Phoenix, AZ 85067-1136
480-451-3060
877-347-7905
Fax: 480-767-7029
e-mail: azmgfa@mystheniagravisfoundation.phxcox
www.azmgfa.org

Wayne Magee, CEO/ President
Edward C Kaps, Chairman

Arkansas

6752 **Arkansas Chapter of the Myasthenia Gravis Foundation of America**
5204 Crystal Hill Road
N Little Rock, AR 72118
501-753-5974
877-455-4442
Fax: 501-753-5978
e-mail: mgfoundationar@sbcglobal.net
www.myasthenia.org

Connecticut

6753 **Connecticut Chapter of the Myasthenia Gravis Foundation of America**
33 Patmar Drive
Monroe, CT 06468-4511
203-926-9910
866-329-8784
e-mail: conn@myasthenia.org
www.myasthenia.org

Irving Beck ED

Delaware

6754 **MD/DC/Delaware Chapter of Myasthenia Gravis Foundation of America**
PO Box 186
Pasedena, MD 21123-0186
866-437-2881
e-mail: lhwaltz@aol.com

District of Columbia

6755 **MD/DC/Delaware Chapter of Myasthenia Gravis Foundation of America**
PO Box 186
Pasedena, MD 21113-0186
866-437-2881
e-mail: lhwaltz@aol.com

Florida

6756 **East Central Florida Chapter of the Myasthenia Gravis Foundation of America**
14502 87 Avenue N
Seminole, FL 33776-0623
727-596-1491
877-596-1491
Fax: 727-596-1491
e-mail: wcflorida@myasthenia.org
www.myasthenia.org

6757 **South Florida Gold Coast Chapter of the Myasthenia Gravis Foundation of America**
6185 Winding Brook Way
Delray Beach, FL 33484
561-638-2636
e-mail: oldjack@gateway.net
www.4-mga.org/orgsNEW.html

Jack Moore, Chairman
Loise Cororan, Vice Chairman

6758 West Central Florida Chapter of the Myasthenia Gravis Foundation of America
13540 Andova Drive
Largo, FL 33774-4633
727-596-1491
e-mail: mpeters@aol.com
www.4-mga.org/orgsNEW.html

Marie Peters, Chairman

Georgia

6759 Georgia Chapter of the Myasthenia Gravis Foundation of America
PO Box 93604
Atlanta, GA 30318
770-973-3269
800-743-4339
Fax: 770-973-3269
e-mail: gachapter_mgfa@hotmail.com
www.ga-mgfa.or

Indiana

6760 Greater Indianapolis Chapter of the Myasthenia Gravis Foundation of America
8922 Haverstick Road
Indianapolis, IN 46240
317-846-1462
e-mail: Spknke@aol.com
www.4-mga.org/orgsNEW.html

Earl Zimmerman, Chair

Kentucky

6761 Kentucky Chapter of the Myasthenia Gravis Foundation of America
2628 Rush Trail
Owensboro, KY 42303
270-684-4555
Fax: 270-926-2234
e-mail: shlane@bellsouth.net
www.myasthenia.org

Maryland

6762 MD/DC/Delaware Chapter of Myasthenia Gravis Foundation of America
PO Box 186
Pasadena, MD 21123-0186
410-432-6193
866-437-2881
e-mail: maryland@myasthenia.org
www.myasthenia.org

Massachusetts

6763 Mass./New Hampshire Chapter of the Myasthenia Gravis Foundation of America
5 Alcott Drive
Northboro, MA 01532
978-562-4570
e-mail: djemery@juno.com

6764 Massachusetts Chapter of the MG Foundation
5 Alcott Drive
Northboro, MA 01532
508-393-1403
Fax: 508-393-1403
e-mail: djemery@juno.com
www.4-mga.org/orgsNEW.html

6765 Myasthenia Gravis: Massachusetts Chapter
28 Bayview Road
Wellesley, MA 02181
508-851-3218
www.4-mga.org/orgsNEW.html

Michelle Ronchetti

Michigan

6766 Great Lakes Chapter of the Myasthenia Gravis Foundation of America
2680 Horizon Drive SE
Grand Rapids, MI 49546
616-956-0622
800-224-9180
Fax: 616-956-9234
e-mail: myasthenia.info@gmail.com
www.myasthenia-mi.org

Autoimmune, neuromuscular disease manifest in weakness of voluntary muscles; arms, legs, eyes, facial expressions, severe cases of breathing.
Susan Richards, Executive Director
Paulus Heule, President

6767 Myasthenia Gravis Association
17117 W Nine Mile Road
Southfield, MI 48075
248-423-9700
Fax: 248-423-9705
e-mail: mgadetroit1@hotmail.com
www.mgadetroit-easternmi.org

Agnes Wisner, Executive Director
Taylor Bleibtrey, Board Member

Minnesota

6768 Minnesota State Chapter of the Myasthenia Gravis Foundation of America
29234 Piney Way
Breezy Point, MN 56472-1715
218-562-4594
e-mail: minnesota@myasthenia.org
www.myasthenia.org

Missouri

6769 Myasthenia Gravis Foundation: Greater St. Louis Chapter
PO Box 58785
Renton, WA 98058
425-235-1435
877-252-0677
Fax: 425-204-2070
e-mail: washington@myasthenia.org
www.myasthenia.org

Babette Figler, President

New Hampshire

6770 Mass./New Hampshire Chapter of the Myasthenia Gravis Foundation of America
460 S River Street
Marshfield, MA 02050
508-435-3808
e-mail: massachusetts@myasthenia.org
www.ma-nhmgfa.org

Marilyn Buckner, Chair
Marc Weinberg, Treasurer

New Jersey

6771 Garden State Chapter of the Myasthenia Gravis Foundation of America
PO Box 4258
Wayne, NJ 07474-1362
973-633-6900
800-437-4949
Fax: 973-633-6908
e-mail: gsmg@webspan.net
www.mgnj.org

New Mexico

6772 New Mexico Chapter of the Myasthenia Gravis Foundation of America
PO Box 34173
Phoenix, AZ 85067-6873
480-451-3060
877-347-7905
Fax: 623-321-9032
e-mail: azmgfa@myastheniagravisfoundation.phxcox
www.azmgfa.org

Wayne Magee, CEO/President
Edward C Kaps, Chairman

New York

6773 Metro New York Chapter of Myasthenia Gravis Foundation of America
PO Box 40
Stony Brook, NY 11790
516-538-0738
800-667-9807
e-mail: MetroNY@myasthenia.org
www.metronymgfa.org

Cindie Killeen, Chairperson
Debbie Thompsen, Vice Chairperson

6774 Myasthenia Gravis Support Group: Long Island
N Shore University Hospital
Manhasset, NY
516-785-7538
e-mail: KARKENN@SPEC.NET
www.members.tripod.com/LIMGer/limgsuppor

Carol

6775 Upstate NY Chapter of the Myasthenia Gravis Foundation of America
14 Summit Road
Delmar, NY 12054
518-439-5377
800-581-5377
Fax: 518-439-8783
e-mail: upstatenewyork@myasthenia.org
www.myasthenia-gravis.com
Barry Levine, President/Chair

North Carolina

6776 Carolinas Chapter of the Myasthenia Gravis Foundation of America
506 E Forest Hills Boulevard
Durham, NC 27707-1801
919-490-2937
800-842-8711
Fax: 919-489-7564
e-mail: tvassar56@aol.com
www.med.unc.edu/mgfa/mgnc-hom.htm

Ohio

6777 Mahoning-Shenango Chapter of the Myasthenia Gravis Foundation of America
PO Box 282
Girard, OH 44420-0282
330-539-5582

6778 Ohio Chapter of the Myasthenia Gravis Foundation of America
2907 B Lincoln Way E
Massillon, OH 44646
330-834-9066
Fax: 330-834-9067
e-mail: ohiochaptermgf@att.net
www.ohiochaptermgf.org
Jackie Held, Executive Director

Oklahoma

6779 Oklahoma Chapter of the Myasthenia Gravis Foundation of America
6465 S Yale Avenue
Tulsa, OK 74136
918-494-4951
Fax: 918-494-4951
e-mail: oklahoma@myasthenia.org
www.myasthenia.org
Peggy Foust, Executive Director
Margret Feller, Vice-President/Treasurer

Pennsylvania

6780 Myasthenia Gravis Association of Western Pennsylvania
490 EN Avenue
Pittsburgh, PA 15212
412-566-1545
Fax: 412-566-1550
e-mail: mgaoffice@mgawpa.org
www.mgawpa.org
A neuromuscular disorder with no known cause or cure. The mission is to provide access to superior medical treatment and medications at reasonable cost providing those patients and their families adequate social and psychological support and education.
Barbara Lefler, Executive Director

6781 Pennsylvania Chapter of the Myasthenia Gravis Foundation of America
2665 Pinewood Road
Lancaster, PA 17601
717-581-1271
e-mail: PennaMGFA@aol.com
www.pamgfa.org

Rhode Island

6782 Rhode Island 'Hope' Chapter
33 Patmar Drive
Monroe, CT 06468
203-926-9910
866-329-8784
e-mail: conn@myasthenia.org
www.myasthenia.org

South Carolina

6783 Carolinas Chapter of the Myasthenia Gravis Foundation of America
506 E Forest Hills Boulevard
Durham, NC 27707-1801
919-490-2937
800-842-8711
Fax: 919-489-7564
e-mail: tvassar56@aol.com
www.med.unc.edu/mgfa/mgnc-hom.htm

Texas

6784 Greater South Texas Chapter of the Myasthenia Gravis Foundation of America
10592 Fuqua Street #A
Houston, TX 77089-1402
281-987-9393
Fax: 281-328-2430
e-mail: gowens@accesscomm.net

6785 Northwest Texas Chapter of the Myasthenia Gravis Foundation of America
3406 Manioca Road
Lubbock, TX 79403
806-749-3126
Fax: 915-554-7044
e-mail: nwtexas@myasthenia.org
www.nwtcmg.org
Lowell McBroom, Vice-Chairperson

Utah

6786 Utah State Intermountain Chapter of the Myasthenia Gravis Foundation of America
8717 S 910 E
Sandy, UT 84094-1831
801-816-2204
Fax: 801-572-1787
e-mail: dawnascheib@waterfordschool.org
www.myasthenia.org

Virginia

6787 Virginia Chapter of the Myasthenia Gravis Foundation of America
PO Box 71193
Richmond, VA 23255
804-308-1674
800-728-4405
Fax: 804-308-1674
e-mail: va-wvchapmgfa@comcast.net
www.myasthenia-va.org
Georgiann C Davis, President
Anita Steele, VP

Washington

6788 Pacific Northwest Chapter of the Myasthenia Gravis Foundation of America
PO Box 58785
Renton, WA 98058-6562
425-235-1435
877-252-0677
Fax: 425-204-2070
e-mail: washington@myasthenia.org
www.myasthenia.org

Wisconsin

6789 Wisconsin Chapter of the Myasthenia Gravis Foundation of America
2474 S 96 Street
W Allis, WI 53227
262-938-9800
800-541-5454
Fax: 262-789-3363
e-mail: wisconsin@myasthenia.org
www.myasthenia.org
The Myasthenia Gravis Foundation of America is the only national volunteer health agency dedicated solely to fight against myasthenoia gravis.
Patricia Lamp, Chairperson
Ellie Burbach, Vice-Chairperson

Support Groups & Hotlines

6790 Myasthenia Gravis Association of Colorado
PO Box 18567
Denver, CO 80218
303-360-7080
Fax: 303-360-7080
e-mail: 4mga@4-mga.org
Sharon Leahy, Chairperson

6791 Myasthenia Gravis Support Group
6465 S Yale Ave
Tulsa, OK 74136-7808
918-494-4951
Fax: 918-494-4951
e-mail: oklahoma@myasthenia.org
www.myasthenia.rg
Provides education and patient services to improve the lives of all people affected by MG and to promote awareness of the disease myasthenia gravis.
Peggy Foust, Executive Director/President

6792 Myasthenia Gravis Support Group East Central Illinois
Myasthenia Gravis Foundation of Illinois
310 W Lake Street   630-835-0153
Elmhurst, IL 60126   800-888-6208
e-mail: myastheniaill@aol.org
www.myastheniagravis.org
To facilitate the timely diagnosis and optimal care of individuals affected by myasthenia gravis and to improve their lives through programs of patient services, public awareness, medical research, professional education, advocacy and patient care

6793 Myasthenia Gravis Support Group of Wiscons in
2474 S 96 Street   262-938-9800
West Allis, WI 53227-2204   Fax: 262-789-3363
e-mail: wisconsin@myasthenia.org
www.myasthenia.org
Serves patients and their families throughout the state of Wisconsin. The goal is to help achieve the conquest of Myasthenia Gravis through research, education, public awareness, anf fundraising.

6794 Myasthenia Gravis Support Group: Virginia/ West Virginia
PO Box 71193   804-308-1674
Richmond, VA 23255   Fax: 804-308-1647
e-mail: va-wvchapmgfa@comcast.net
www.myasthenia-va.org
To facilitate the timely diagnosis and optimal care of individuals affected by MG and closely related disorders and to improve their lives with programs of patient services, public information, medical research, professional education, advocacy and patient care.
Georgiann Davis, President

6795 National Health Information Center
US Department of Health and Human Services
PO Box 1133   301-565-4167
Washington, DC 20013-1133   800-336-4797
Fax: 301-984-4256
e-mail: info@nhic.org
www.health.gov/nhic
Offers a nationwide referral service, produces directories and resource guides.

Books

6796 Myasthenia Gravis
CRC Press
2000 NW Corporate Boulevard   561-994-0555
Boca Raton, FL 33431-7385   Fax: 561-994-3625
1993
ISBN: 0-849363-43-8

Newsletters

6797 Alabama Chapter of the Myasthenia Gravis Foundation of America
Alabama Chapter of the Myasthenia Gravis Found
300 Office Park Drive   205-868-1210
Birmingham, AL 35223   Fax: 205-868-1211
e-mail: alchaptermgfa@aol.com
Three to four newsletters per year. Support Group Information, articles about MG and it's treatment, information about chapters operations.

6798 Connecticut Nutmeg
Myasthenia Gravis Foundation
113 Folly Brook Boulevard   860-529-8784
Wetherfield, CT 06109   Fax: 860-529-8784

6799 Conquer
Myasthenia Gravis Foundation of Illinois
2411 New Street   708-385-3888
Blue Island, IL 60406-2328   800-888-6208
Fax: 708-385-0447
e-mail: myastheniaill@aol.com
myastheniagravis.org
A quarterly newsletter containing articles and stories relating to myasthenia gravis.
16 pages Quarterly
Gerald Tarka, Executive Director

6800 East Central Florida Chapter of the Myasthenia Gravis Foundation of America
PO Box 623   904-672-2635
Ormond Beach, FL 32175-0623
Published bi-monthly, and contains information about latest research. area meetings, and topics of concern for our readers.

6801 Facts About Myasthenia Gravis for Patients and Families
Myasthenia Gravis Foundation of America
5841 Cedar Lake Road   952-545-9438
Minneapolis, MN 55416   800-541-5454
Fax: 952-646-2028
e-mail: myastheniagravis@msn.com
www.myasthenia.org
Offers information on the history, clinical symptoms and features, causes, diagnosis, treatment and prognosis of Myasthenia Gravis.
16 pages 4 per year
Debora K Boelz, CEO
Jennifer Heidelberger, Chapter Relations Manager

6802 MG Communicator
Great Lakes Chapter of the Myasthenia Gravis Found
2680 Horizon Drive SE   616-956-0622
Grand Rapids, MI 49546   800-224-9180
Fax: 616-956-9234
e-mail: myasthenia.info@gmail.com
www.myasthenia-mi.org
3x/year
Susan Richards, Executive Director
Paulus Heule, President

6803 Myasthenia Gravis Association
2300 E Meyer Boulevard   816-276-4585
Kansas City, MO 64132-1199   Fax: 816-276-4569
e-mail: mga@planetkc.org
A nonprofit, United Way agency offering a variety of programs. The programs include; individualized education and advocacy, specialized outpatient clinics, patient support group meetings and newsletters.
Carole Bowe Thompson, Executive Director
Danna Garabedian, Administrative Assistant

6804 Myasthenia Gravis Association: Detroit Chapter
17117 W Nine Mile Road   248-423-9700
Southfield, MI 48075
A quarterly newslatter containing medical articles, personal stories relating to myasthenia gravis.

6805 Myasthenia Gravis Foundation: Geater South Texas
10592-A Fuqua   281-987-9393
Houston, TX 77089-1402   Fax: 281-328-2430
e-mail: gowens@accesscomm.net
Six issues per year. Support Group Information, articles about MG and it's treatment, information about Chapter operations.
Gary Owens, Chair

6806 Myasthenia Gravis Foundation: Northwest Texas Chapter
281 County Road 135
Ovalo, TX 79541   e-mail: nwtxmg@hotmail.com
A quarterly newsletter containing articles and stories relating myasthenia gravis.
Jenne McVicker, Editor

6807 Myasthenia Gravis Foundation: Ohio Chapter
PO Box 6392   330-477-7727
Canton, OH 44706   e-mail: ohiochaptermgf@nci2000,net

6808 Puget Sound Chapter Newsletter
PO Box 587853   206-235-1435
Renton, WA 98058-1785   Fax: 206-204-2070
A quarterly newsletter containing the latest articles and stories relating to myasthenia gravis.

Web Sites

6809 Healing Well
www.healingwell.com
An online health resource guide to medical news, chat, information and articles, newsgroups and message boards, books, disease-re-

lated web sites, medical directories, and more for patients, friends, and family coping with disabling diseases, disorders, or chronic illnesses.

6810 Health Finder

www.healthfinder.gov

Searchable, carefully developed web site offering information on over 1000 topics. Developed by the US Department of Health and Human Services, the site can be used in both English and Spanish.

6811 Healthlink USA

www.healthlinkusa.com

Health information concerning treatment, cures, prevention, diagnosis, risk factors, research, support groups, email lists, personal stories and much more. Updated regularly.

6812 Helios Health

www.helioshealth.com

Online resource for your health information. Detailed information about specific health topics, access to expert advice from our Medical Advisory Board, and up-to-date health news.

6813 MedicineNet

www.medicinenet.com

An online resource for consumers providing easy-to-read, authoritative medical and health information.

6814 Medscape

www.medscape.com

Medscape offers specialists, primary care physicians, and other health professionals the Web's most robust and integrated medical information and educational tools.

6815 Myasthenia Gravis Foundation of America

www.myasthenia.org

Dedicated to the conquest of the disease through research, education, information and patient services. Offers over 54 chapters and over 100 support groups across the country as well as 8 international chapters.

6816 Neurology Channel

www.neurologychannel.com

Find clearly explained, medically accurate information regarding conditions, including an overview, symptoms, causes, diagnostic procedures and treatment options. On this site it is possible to ask questions and get information from a neurologist and connect to people who have similar health interests.

6817 WebMD

www.webmd.com

Information on Myasthenia Gravis, including articles and resources.

Description

6818 Neurofibromatosis

Neurofibromatosis, or von Recklinghausen disease, named after a German pathologist, is an inherited genetic disorder. The more common form occurs once in 4,000 births. The skin and the nervous system are the primary target organs. Characteristic skin lesions are large, flat brown freckles, called cafe au lait spots, owing to their light coffee color. They are apparent at birth or in infancy in more than 90 percent of patients. Flesh-colored tumors appear in late childhood. Abnormal growths may be detectable in the brain, perhaps accounting for the seizures and learning difficulties commonly seen in this syndrome. Tumors may appear on the nerves from the eyes or the ears, sometimes causing hearing loss or visual disturbance.

There is no specific therapy for this condition, but tumors that produce severe symptoms can be surgically removed or irradiated. Genetic counseling is important for the entire family.

National Agencies & Associations

6819 Association for the Neurologically Disable d of Canada
59 Clement Road
Etobicoke, Ontario, M9R-1Y5
416-244-1992
Fax: 416-244-4099
e-mail: info@and.ca
www.and.ca
Provides functional rehabilitation programs to individuals with neurological disabilities.
Basil Ziv, Executive Director
Dr John Unruh, Director of Rehabilitation

6820 BC Centre for Ability
2805 Kingsway
Vancouver, BC, V5R-5H9
604-451-5511
Fax: 604-451-5651
e-mail: home@centreforability.bc.ca
www.centreforability.bc.ca
Founded in 1969 by families who desired alternatives to hospital or institutional-based services. The centre provides education and promotes the rights of individuals with disabilities to participate as valued members of their communities.
Angie Kwok, Executive Director
Moses Gabriel, Director of Resource Development

6821 Children's Tumor Foundation
95 Pine Street
New York, NY 10005
212-344-6633
800-323-7938
Fax: 212-747-0004
e-mail: info@ctf.org
www.ctf.org
Dedicated to health and well being of individuals and families affected by the neurofibromatoses (NF).
Allison Walsh, Communications Officer
John Risner, President

6822 NF Canada
800-1010 Sherbrooke Street W
Montreal, Quebec, H3A-2R7
888-986-3876
e-mail: infocanada@nfcanada.ca
www.nfcanada.ca
To ensure that all Canadians living with neurofibromatosis benefit from support, understanding, appropriate medical treatment and the hope that a cure is on the horizon.

6823 Neurofibromatosis
Po Box 18246
Minneapolis, MN 55418
651-225-1720
800-942-6825
Fax: 301-918-0009
e-mail: info@nfinc.org
www.nfinc.org

A national nonprofit organization with independent and regional chapters that provides support and services to NF families. Simulates funds and encourages participation in NF research. Works closely with clinical and research professionals.
Miguel Lessing, President
Rosemary Anderson, Vice President

6824 Neurofibromatosis Society of Ontario
180 Circle Lake Road
North Bay, Ontario, P1A-3T2
705-685-1409
Fax: 705-685-1409
e-mail: info@nfon.ca
www.nfon.ca
Support individuals and families affected by NF, to educate its members, professionals, and the general public about NF, and support NF research.
Lynne Leyland, Director
Gladys Hamilton, Director

6825 Neurological Science Federation
7015 Macleod Trail SW
Calgary, AB, T2H-2K6
403-229-9544
Fax: 403-229-1661
e-mail: info@cnsfederation.org
www.ccns.org

To promote and encourage all aspects of neurology, including research, education, assessment and accreditation.

State Agencies & Associations

Alabama

6826 NNFF Alabama Affiliate
1205 Branchwater Lane
Birmingham, AL 35216
205-529-8006
e-mail: jeffalb@charter.net
www.ctf.org

Jeff Albright, Chairperson

Arizona

6827 Neurofibromatosis Association of Arizona
Po Box 2718
Chandler, AZ 85244
480-945-9650
Fax: 480-945-9650
e-mail: info@nfaz.org
www.nfaz.org

Nicole Hicks, Executive Director
Michael Sheedy, President

Arkansas

6828 NNFF Arkansas Affilaite
139 Rainbow Lne
Bigelow, AR 72016
501-759-2710
e-mail: lesleyo@arbbs.net
www.ctf.org

Lesley Oslica, Information and Support

Colorado

6829 NNFF Colorado Chapter
70 N Ranch Road
Littleton, CO 80127
303-734-9942
e-mail: mark.ebel@eyeris.com
www.ctf.org

Mark Ebel, Chapter President

Connecticut

6830 NNFF Connecticut Chapter
8 S Barn Hill Road
Bloomfield, CT 06002-1622
860-286-2705
Fax: 860-286-2705
TTY: 860-286-2705
TDD: 860-286-2705
e-mail: StevenSand@aol.com

Steve Sandler, Chapter President

Florida

6831 NF Center: North Broward Medical Center Neurofibromatosis
Neurofibromatosis
201 E Sample Road
Pompano Beach, FL 33064-3502
954-786-7346
www.nfinc.org

6832 NNFF Florida Chapter
PO Box 410684
Melbourne, FL 32941
321-253-1622
800-540-5721
e-mail: NNFFflorida@aol.com
www.ctf.org

Suzanne Earle, Chapter President

Georgia

6833 NNFF Georgia Affiliate
5 Ardmore Circle
Cartersville, GA 30120
678-428-9711
e-mail: ctfgeorgia@bellsouth.net
www.ctf.org

Randy Watkins, Chairman

Idaho

6834 NNFF Idaho Chapter
4419 E Linden Street
Caldwell, ID 83605-8037
208-459-6022
Suzy Crici, Chapter President

Illinois

6835 Illinois Midwest Neurofibromatosis
Neurofibromatosis
Po Box 1923
Lombard, IL 60148
630-932-8111
800-322-6363
Fax: 630-932-8119
e-mail: info@nfmidwest.org
nfmidwest.org

6836 NNFF Illinois Chapter: Chicago Area
5604 W Henderson 3 W
Chicago, IL 60634
e-mail: ilnfchapter@hotmail.com
www.ctf.org

Debbi Callahan, Vice President

6837 NNFF Illinois Chapter: Silvis Area
513 16th Street
Silvis, IL 61282
309-792-4195
e-mail: nfquadcities@juno.com
Sue Rockwell, Patient Information and Support

6838 NNFF Illinois Chapter: Springfield Area
5 Twilight Lane
Springfield, IL 62712
217-529-0834
e-mail: ma.miller@InsightBB.com
www.ctf.org

Marcia Miller, Treasurer

6839 NNFF Illinois Chapter:Peoria Region
PO Box 213
Emden, IL 62635
217-732-8568
e-mail: beachph@cs.com
www.ctf.org

Paul Beach, President

Indiana

6840 NNFF Indiana Chapter
1173 Hague Court
Franklinolis, IN 46131
317-736-7577
e-mail: pdavis@athensmed.org
www.ctf.org

Dottie Whitehurst, Chapter President

Iowa

6841 NNFF Iowa Chapter
321 Glenview Drive
De Moines, IA 50312
515-277-8494
e-mail: drev@aol.com
www.ctf.org

Sheila Drevyanko, Chapter President

Kansas

6842 NNFF Kansas Affiliate
12606 E 49th Terrace
Independence, MO 64055
816-737-8378
e-mail: annette_novak@yahoo.com
www.ctf.org

Annette Novak, Chairperson

6843 Neurofibromatosis Kansas and Central Plains
Neurofibromatosis
PO Box 1792
Hutchinson, KS 67504-1792
620-669-8453
800-942-6825
e-mail: nprieb@sbcglobal.net
www.nfinc.org

Louisiana

6844 NNFF Louisiana Chapter
PO Box 499
Baton Rouge, LA 70821
225-665-3547
e-mail: nflouisiana1@cox.net
www.ctf.org

Debbie Bouy, Chairperson

Maryland

6845 Neurofibromatosis: Mid-Atlantic
Neurofibromatosis
8855 Annapolis Road
Lanham, MD 20706-2924
301-577-8984
800-942-6825
Fax: 301-577-0016
e-mail: info@nfmidatlantic.org
www.nfmidatlantic.org

Mid-Atlantic Chapter serves the following states: Maryland Virginia District of Columbia Delaware New Jersey Pennsylvania West Virginia and North Carolina.
Barbra Levin, Executive Director
Beverly B Dobson, President

Massachusetts

6846 Neurofibromatosis: New England
Neurofibromatosis
9 Bedford Street
Burlington, MA 01803-3702
781-272-9936
Fax: 781-272-9937
e-mail: info@nfincne.org
www.nfincne.org

Karen Peluso, Executive Director
Dr Paul Epstein, President

Minnesota

6847 Neurofibromatosis: Minnesota
Neurofibromatosis
PO Box 18246
Minneapolis, MN 55418
651-225-1720
e-mail: JohnE@cipmn.org
www.nfincmn.org

John Everett, President
Steven Schutts, Vice-President

Nevada

6848 NNFF Nevada Affiliate: Reno Area
8065 White Falls Drive
Reno, NV 89506
775-972-1882
e-mail: daverenorice@yahoo.com
www.ctf.org

David Rice, Chairperson

New Hampshire

6849 NNFF Northern New England Chapter
75 McNeil Way
Dedham, MA 02026
508-879-5638
888-585-5316
Fax: 781-326-4940
e-mail: nfe.ed@verizon.net
www.ctf.org

The Northern New England Chapter serves these states: Maine, New Hampshire, Vermont, Connecticut, Massachusetts, and Rhode Island.
Michelle M Braden, Vice President

New York

6850 **Tri-State Region: New York, New Jersey, An d Connecticut**
Tri-State Development

212-344-6633
800-323-7938
e-mail: jradziejewski@ctf.org
www.ctf.org

John Radziejewski, Vice President

North Dakota

6851 **NNFF Northern Plains Chapter: North Dakota South Dakota, And Nebraska**
The Childrens Tumor Foundation

310-216-9570
888-314-6633
e-mail: csilberstein@ctf.org
www.ctf.org

Cathy Silberstein, Director Training and Development
Kelly McGowan, Chapter and Affiliate Coordinator

Oregon

6852 **NNFF Oregon Affiliate Kaiser Permanente Northwest**
Kaiser Permanente Northwest
2806 SW Troy
Portland, OR 97227

503-331-6325
Fax: 503-331-6320
e-mail: crowkas@pop.mts.kpnw.org
www.ctf.org

Katie Crow, Genetic Counselor

South Carolina

6853 **NNFF South Carolina Chapter**
111 Oakview Drive
Darlington, SC 29532

843-393-9672
e-mail: pmschrisley@aol.com
www.ctf.org

Pat Chrisely, Chairperson

Virginia

6854 **NNFF Mid-Atlantic Region Affiliate: Virgin a, District Of Columbia, And Maryland**
The Childrens Tumor Foundation

800-323-7938
e-mail: csilberstein@ctf.org
www.ctf.org

Cathy Silberstein, Director Training and Development

Wisconsin

6855 **NNFF Wisconsin Chapter**
6562 W Glenbrook Road
Brown Deer, WI 53223

414-362-0211
e-mail: epankownf@aol.com
www.ctf.org

Elaine Pankow, President

Support Groups & Hotlines

6856 **Children's Tumor Foundation**
95 Pine Street
New York, NY 10005

212-344-6633
800-323-7938
Fax: 212-747-0004
e-mail: info@ctf.org
www.ctf.org

Sponsors critical research, public awareness and patient support services.
Allison Walsh, Communications Officer

6857 **NF Support Group of West Michigan**
Spectrum Health
230 Michigan Street NE
Grand Rapids, MI 49503

616-451-3699
e-mail: nfwestmich@aol.com
www.nfsupport.org

Rose Mary Anderson, Patient Advocate

6858 **National Health Information Center**
PO Box 1133
Washington, DC 20013

310-565-4167
800-336-4797
Fax: 301-984-4256
e-mail: info@nhic.org
www.health.gov/nhic

Offers a nationwide information referral service, produces directories and resource guides.

6859 **Neurofibromatosis**
9320 Annapolis Road
Lanham, MD 20706-3123

301-918-4600
800-942-6825
Fax: 301-918-0009
e-mail: nfinfo@nfinc.com
www.nfinc.org

Dedicated to individuals and families affected by the neurofibromatosis through educational, support, clinical and research programs.
Miguell Lessing, President
Rosemary Anderson, Vice President

6860 **Neurofibromatosis Foundation: Colorado**
2280 S Columbine Street
Denver, CO 80210

303-460-8313
800-323-7938
e-mail: UsRKids@aol.com
www.unitedwaydenver.org

Offers a support group to persons affected by neurofibromatosis. Offers panel discussion, sharing, fundraising, and fun activities. Also provides new patient information.
Charles Taylor
Jane Cahn

6861 **Neurofibromatosis Support Network**
Parents Helping Parents
3041 Olcott Street
Santa Clara, CA 95054

408-727-5775
Fax: 408-727-0182
www.php.com

Helping children with special needs receive the resources, love, hope, respect, health care, education and other services they need to achieve their full potential by providing them with strong families and dedicated professionals to serve them.
Sheri Sobrato, MA/MFC

6862 **Neuroscience Institute at Mercy Hospital**
4120N W Memorial Road
Oklahoma City, OK 73120

800-996-3729
Fax: 405-752-3977
www.okmercy.net

Mike Patt, Chief Executive Officer

6863 **Texas Neurofibromatosis Foundation**
415 Travis Street
Dallas, TX 75205

214-528-5557
www.texasnf.org

Newsletters

6864 **Neurofibromatosis**
9320 Annapolis Road
Lanham, MD 20706-3123

301-918-4600
800-942-6825
Fax: 301-918-0009
e-mail: nfinfo@nfinc.org
www.nfinc.org

Provides a variety of resources for NF families, professionals and researchers.
SemiAnnual
Gwen Charest, Executive Director

Pamphlets

6865 **Child with Neurofibromatosis 1**
Children's Tumor Foundation
95 Pine Street
New York, NY 10005-1703

212-344-NNFF
800-323-7938
e-mail: info@ctf.org
www.ctf.org

Offers information on the prognosis, management, complications, genetic implications, and sources of support for children with neurofibromatosis 1.
Allison Walsh, Communications Officer

6866 Guide for Teens
Children's Tumor Foundation
95 Pine Street
New York, NY 10005-1703
212-344-NNFF
800-323-7938
e-mail: info@ctf.org
www.ctf.org
Offers information for teenagers on how to face neurofibromatosis on a daily basis.
Allison Walsh, Communications Officer

6867 How NF-1 Affects the Body
Neurofibromatosis
9320 Annapolis Road
Lanham, MD 20706-3123
301-918-4600
800-942-6825
Fax: 301-918-0009
e-mail: nfinfo@nfinc.org
www.nfinc.org
A graphic showing the parts of the body where symptoms of NF-1 can occur.
Gwen Charest, Executive Director

6868 How NF-2 Affects the Body
Neurofibromatosis
9320 Annapolis Road
Lanham, MD 20706-3123
301-918-4600
800-942-6825
Fax: 301-918-0009
e-mail: nfinfo@nfinc.org
www.nfinc.org
A graphic showing the parts of the body where symptoms of NF-2 can occur.
Gwen Charest, Executive Director

6869 National NF Medical Resource Listing
Neurofibromatosis
9320 Annapolis Road
Lanham, MD 20706-3123
301-918-4600
800-942-6825
Fax: 301-918-0009
e-mail: nfinfo@nfinc.org
www.nfinc.org
A listing of medical centers in the US where geneticists and NF experts are located.
Gwen Charest, Executive Director

6870 Neurofibromatosis
March of Dimes
233 Park Avenue South
New York, NY 10003
212-353-8353
Fax: 212-254-3518
e-mail: NY639@marchofdimes.com
www.marchofdimes.com
Located on the website.

6871 Neurofibromatosis Type 2: Information for Patients and Families
Children's Tumor Foundation
95 Pine Street
New York, NY 10005-1703
212-344-6633
800-323-7938
e-mail: info@ctf.org
www.ctf.org
Offers extensive information on what NF2 is and answers the most asked about questions regarding the illness.
Allison Walsh, Communications Officer

6872 Understanding Neurofibromatosis
9320 Annapolis Road
Lanham, MD 20706-3123
301-918-4600
800-942-6825
Fax: 301-918-0009
e-mail: nfinfo@nfinc.org
www.nfinc.org
A handbook specifically designed for the newly diagnosed NF families.
Gwen Charest, Executive Director

Web Sites

6873 Healing Well
www.healingwell.com
An online health resource guide to medical news, chat, information and articles, newsgroups and message boards, books, disease-related web sites, medical directories, and more for patients, friends, and family coping with disabling diseases, disorders, or chronic illnesses.

6874 Health Finder
www.healthfinder.gov
Searchable, carefully developed web site offering information on over 1000 topics. Developed by the US Department of Health and Human Services, the site can be used in both English and Spanish.

6875 Healthlink USA
www.healthlinkusa.com
Health information concerning treatment, cures, prevention, diagnosis, risk factors, research, support groups, email lists, personal stories and much more. Updated regularly.

6876 Helios Health
www.helioshealth.com
Online resource for your health information. Detailed information about specific health topics, access to expert advice from our Medical Advisory Board, and up-to-date health news.

6877 MGH Neurology
www.mgh.harvard.edu
Provides both unmonderated message boards and chat rooms for specific neurological disorders including: amyloidosis, arachnoiditis, cerebellar ataxia, congenital fiber type disproportion, CFS leak, DeMorsiers syndrome, erythromealgia, Lewy body disease, meningitis, meralgia paresthetic, Norrie disease, periodic paralysis, phantom limb pain, Romberg disorder, Syndenhams chorea, tethered cord syndrome, and thoracic outlet syndrome.

6878 MedicineNet
www.medicinenet.com
An online resource for consumers providing easy-to-read, authoritative medical and health information.

6879 Medscape
www.medscape.com
Medscape offers specialists, primary care physicians, and other health professionals the Web's most robust and integrated medical information and educational tools.

6880 Neurology Channel
www.neurologychannel.com
Find clearly explained, medically accurate information regarding conditions, including an overview, symptoms, causes, diagnostic procedures and treatment options. On this site it is possible to ask questions and get information from a neurologist and connect to people who have similar health interests.

6881 WebMD
www.webmd.com
Information on Neurofibromatosis, including articles and resources.

Description

6882 Obesity

Obesity refers to a condition in which there is an excessive accumulation of fat in subcutaneous and other tissues of the body. Being obese and being overweight are not necessarily synonymous, as people who are overweight may have increased body size as a result of increased muscle or skeletal tissue mass. Obesity may develop at any age, but peak development periods occur during the first 12 months of life, between the ages of five and six years, and during the adolescent years in children. In adults, obesity may develop at any time, but many people may find that weight gain progresses through the 3rd-6th decade. It is clear from numerous medial, public health and sociologic studies that obesity in the United States occurs in a staggering proportion of the population and many consider it to be an epidemic.

Obesity may result from an increase in the actual number of fat cells or from an increase in the size of the individual fat cells. Researchers believe that fat cells increase in number in proportion to caloric intake increase and that this increase is particularly evident in the first 12 months of life. As children grow, increases in fat cell populations continue at a slower rate. Because the number of fat cells cannot be decreased, except surgically, later weight loss must result from the reduction of fat in individual cells.

Obesity usually results when caloric intake exceeds the energy demands of the body, thus increasing the storage of body fat. Fat accumulation is usually a progressive process, resulting from repeated episodes of food intake exceeding the body's demand for energy (calories). Many factors may influence appetite or obesity. Such factors may include environmental influences; psychosocial disturbances that may be induced by stress or emotional upset or trauma; brain lesions that may involve certain area of the brain such as the hypothalamus or the pituitary gland (both essential to hormone production); an overabundance of insulin in the body (hyperinsulinism); and genetic influences. In addition, in rare instances, obesity may be a feature of certain genetic disorders (see *Prader-Willi syndrome*). the most common cause in North America however, is the excessive intake of calories, particularly those from fats and sugars, and the concomitant lack of physical exercise and activity that uses calories.

Complications of obesity in the child and the adult may include respiratory difficulties such as shortness of breath and increased cardiovascular risk factors such as high blood pressure, elevated total cholesterol levels as well as increased bad or LDL cholesterol and decreased good or HDL cholesterol, and increased levels of fatty acid and glycerol compounds (triglycerides). These are risk factors for the development of coronary artery disease, one of the leading causes of morbidity and the mortality in North America. In addition, obesity may be associated with a resistance to the hormone insulin that aids in the metabolism of glucose, fats, carbohydrates, and proteins. This resistance may lead to excessive levels of circulating insulin in the body (hyperinsulinism); however, the body is not able to appropriately use insulin and high blood sugar (hyperglycemia) may occur. This condition is known as Type II Diabetes Mellitus and its incidence in the population is also increasing dramatically in both children and adults. The diagnosis of obesity in children, adolescents and adults is usually determined through the use of certain screening methods such as measurement of the body mass index (BMI) as well as the triceps skinfold thickness.

Patterns of behavior that may lead to obesity may be established as early as infancy. For example, if parents or caregivers persistently use a bottle to pacify a crying baby, the baby may learn that food is equivalent to relief of stress. Treatment for obesity should include the cooperation and support of the entire family and may be directed toward psychological considerations, as well as proper exercise and nutrition to psychological and emotional needs may include behavior modification, as well as individual and family counseling. See also *Eating Disorders*.

National Agencies & Associations

6883 Active Healthy Kids Canada
1185 Eglinton Avenue E
Toronto, Ontario, M3C-3C6
416-426-7120
888-446-7432
Fax: 416-426-7373
e-mail: info@activehealthykids.ca
www.activehealthykids.ca
Established in 1994 to advocate the importance of quality, accessible, and enjoyable physical activity participation experiences for children and youth.
Elio Antunes, Executive Director
Jennifer Crowie-Bonne, Director of Development/Programs

6884 American Obesity Association
1250 24th Street NW
Washington, DC 20037
202-776-7711
Fax: 202-776-7712
e-mail: executive@obesity.org
obesity1.tempdomainname.com
AOA provides obesity awareness and prevention information.
Morgan Downey, Executive Director
Richard L Atkinson, President

6885 Canadian Obesity Network
237 Barton Street E
Hamilton, Ontario, L8L-2X2
905-527-4322
Fax: 905-528-7114
e-mail: info@obesitynetwork.ca
www.obesitynetwork.ca
Focuses the expertise and deciation of more than 1,000 member researchers, clinicans, allied health care providers and other professionals with an interest in obesity in a unified effort to reduce the mental, physical and economic burden of obesity in Canadians.
Alice Bradbury, Manager

6886 National Association to Advance Fat Acceptance
PO Box 22510
Oakland, CA 94609
916-558-6880
Fax: 916-558-6881
e-mail: naafa@naafa.org
www.naafa.org
NAAFA provides educational information a newsletter and hosts a national conference.
Carole Cullum, Co-Chair
Kara Brewer Allen, Co-Chair

6887 Overeaters Anonymous World Service Office
World Service Office

PO Box 44020
Rio Rancho, NM 87174-4020

505-891-2664
Fax: 505-891-4320
e-mail: info@oa.org
www.oa.org

A fellowship of men and women from all walks of life who meet in order to help solve a common problem - compulsive overeating.
Naomi, Managing Director, Board Administrator

6888 Research Chair on Obesity
2725 Chemin Sainte-Foy
Quebec, Canada, G1V

418-656-8711
Fax: 418-656-4929
e-mail: obesite.chair@crhl.ulaval.ca
http://obesity.chair.ulaval.ca

Provides understanding of the pathophysiology of obesity. Promotes communication and interaction among basic scientists and clinicians, involved in nutrition, energy metabolism, obesity, lipid metabolism and cardiovascular research., Provides continuing education about the best possible knowledge on obesity to health professionals, physicians and to the public at large regarding the causes, the complications and the treatment of obesity.
Paul Boisvert, Coordinator

Libraries & Resource Centers

6889 Weight-control Information Network
1 WIN Way
Bethesda, MD 20892-3665

202-828-1025
877-946-4627
Fax: 202-828-1028
e-mail: win@info.niddk.nih.gov
http://win.niddk.nih.gov/

WIN addresses the health information needs of individuals through the production and dissemination of educational materials. In addition, WIN is developing communication strategies for a pilot program to encourage at-risk individuals to achieve and maintain a healthy weight by making changes in their lifestyle.

Research Centers

6890 Harvard Clinical Nutrition Research Center
Harvard Medical School
Boston, MA 02215

617-998-8803
Fax: 617-998-8804
e-mail: allan_walker@hms.harvard.edu
nutrition.med.harvard.edu

Mission is to derive the benefit of continuity in assessing the effectiveness of the Center from year to year while still allowing flexibility for new insights as the Center's activities evolve.
W Allan Walker, Director
George Blackburn, Associate Director

6891 Minnesota Obesity Center
1334 Eckles Avenue
St Paul, MN 55108

763-807-0559
e-mail: mnoc@tc.umn.edu
www1.umn.edu/mnoc

Mission is to find ways to prevent weight gain obesity and its complications. The Center incorporates 46 Participating Investigators who are studying the causes and treatments of obesity. Provides the general public with a source of information on the happenings of the Center and on the current developments in the field of obesity.
Catherine C Welch, Program Coordinator

6892 New York Obesity/Nutrition Research Center
31 Center Drive MSC 2560
Bethesda, MD 20892-2560

301-496-3583
www.niddk.nih.gov/fund/other/centers.htm
Griffin P Rodgers, Director

6893 Obesity Research Center St. Luke's-Roosevelt Hospital
St. Luke's-Roosevelt Hospital
1090 Amsterdam Avenue
New York, NY 10025

212-523-4196
Fax: 212-523-3416
e-mail: dg108@columbia.edu
www.nyorc.org

The mission of the New York Obesity Research Center is to help reduce the incidence of obesity and related diseases through leadership in basic research clinical research epidemiology and public health patient care lib public education.
Dr Xavier Pi-Sunyer, Director
Janet Crane, Dietitians

Support Groups & Hotlines

6894 Greater New York Metro Intergroup of Overeaters Anonymous
Madison Square Station
New York, NY 10159-1235

212-946-4599
e-mail: office@oanyc.org
www.oanyc.org

6895 Office of Chronic Disease Prevention and Nutrition Services
Obesity Prevention Program
150 N. 18th Avenue
Phoenix, AZ 85007

602-542-1886
Fax: 602-542-1890
www.azdhs.gov/phs/oncdps/opp

Mission is to improve the health and quality of life of Arizona residents by reducing the incidence and severity of chronic disease and obesity through physical activity and nutrition interventions.
Renae Cunnien, Program Manager

Books

6896 An Atlas of Obesity and Weight Control
George A. Bray, author

212-216-7800
Fax: 212-564-7854
www.taylorandfrancisgroup.com

This informative guide is a clearly written, beautifully illustrated color atlas on obesity, including its etiology, development and treatment. Contains nearly 150 clinical pictures of obesity and its related conditions, as well as many pertinent clinical guidelines and up-to-the-minute data on assessment and treatment.
135 pages

6897 Dietary Guidelines for Americans 2005
U.S. Government Printing Office
200 Independence Avenue, S.W.
Washington, DC 20201

202-619-0257
877-696-6775
www.health.gov/dietaryguidelines

80 pages
Tommy G. Thompson, HHS-Secretary
Ann M. Veneman, USDA-Secretary

6898 Encyclopedia of Obesity and Eating Disorders
Facts on File
11 Penn Plaza
New York, NY 10001

212-967-8800
800-322-8755
Fax: 800-678-3633

From abdominoplasty to Zung Rating Scale, this volume defines and explains these disorders, along with medical and other problems associated with them.
272 pages Hardcover

6899 Handbook of Obesity Treatment
Guilford Press
72 Spring Street
New York, NY 10012

800-365-7006
Fax: 212-966-6708
e-mail: info@guilford.com
www.guilford.com

This comprehensive handbook guides mental, medical, and allied health professionals through the process of planning and delivering individualized treatment services for those seeking help for Obesity.
2001 624 pages Hardcover
ISBN: 1-572307-22-6

6900 Obesity
National Academies Press
500 Fifth Street, NW
Washington, DC 20055

202-334-3313
888-624-8373
Fax: 202-334-2451
www.nap.edu

A ground breaking report on childhood obesity providing indepth background and instructive case studies that illustrate just how serious and widespread the problem is; gives honest, authorative, based advice that consitute our best weapons in this critical battle.
280 pages

6901 Overeaters Anonymous
World Service Office

117 W 26th Street
New York, NY 10001-6807
505-891-2664
Fax: 505-891-4320
www.overeatersanonymous.org
World Service Office offers literature, provides information or meetings world wide.
204 pages Hardcover

6902 Preventing Childhood Obesity: Health in the Balance
National Academies Press
500 Fifth Street NW
Washington, DC 20055
202-334-3313
888-624-8373
Fax: 202-334-2451
www.nap.edu
Provides a broad-based examination of the nature, extent, and consequences of obesity. Also explores the underlying causes of this serious health problem and the actions needed to initiate support, and sustain the societal and lifestyle changes that can reverse the trend among our children and youth.
436 pages
ISBN: 0-309091-96-9

6903 Shape Up America!
6707 Democracy Boulevard
Bethesda, MD 20817
www.shapeup.org
A high profile national initiative to promote healthy weight and increased physical activity in America. Involves a broad based coalition of industry, medical/health, nutrition, physical fitness, and related organizations and experts.
C. Everett Koop, Founder
Barbara J. Moore, President And CEO

6904 Understanding Childhood Obesity
J Clinton Smith, MD, author
University Press of Mississippi
3825 Ridgewood Road
Jackson, MS 39211-6492
601-432-6205
Fax: 601-432-6217
e-mail: press@ihl.state.ms.us
www.upress.state.ms.us
A clear explanation of causes, diagnosis, and treatment of childhood obesity.
1999 120 pages Paperback
ISBN: 1-578061-34-2
Kathy Burgess, Advertising/Marketing Services Manager

6905 Understanding Obesity: The Five Medical Causes
Lance Levy, author
Firefly Books Ltd
66 Leek Crescent
Richmond Hill, Ontario, L4B-1H1
416-499-8412
Fax: 416-499-1142
www.fireflybooks.com
An authoritative book that focuses on the causes of, and the treatment for, obesity. Obesity is usually related to other health problems and treatment for them is the first step.
200 pages

Children's Books

6906 I Was a Fifteen-Year-Old Blimp
Harper & Row
10 E 53rd Street
New York, NY 10022-5299
212-207-7000
This story focuses on Gabby, a teenage girl who overhears others discuss her weight and takes radical steps to become popular.
Grades 6-9

Magazines

6907 CheckUp
Medical University of South Carolina
135 Cannon Street
Charleston, SC 29425
843-792-1414
800-424-6872
www.muschealth.com/weight

Provides health information about screenings, treatments, medical advances and services available through MUSC, as well as advice about nutrition and prevention.
Susan Kammeraad-Campbell, Managing Editor
Damon Simmons, Art Director

6908 Official Journal of NAASO
NAASO
Boston Med. Center, 650 Albany St.
Boston, MA 02118
617-638-7107
Fax: 617-638-6630
e-mail: teffk!niddk.nih.gov
www.naaso.org
Promotes research, education and advocacy to better understand, prevent and treat obesity and improve the lives of those affected.
Barbara E. Corkey, Editor-In-Chief
Deborah Moskowitz, Managing Editor

6909 Progress Notes
Medical University of South Carolina
135 Cannon Street
Charleston, SC 29425
843-792-2200
800-922-5250
www.muschealth.com/weight
Designed to inform the medical community developments at the Medical University of South Carolina and as a continuing medical education resource for practicing physicians and faculty.
Susan Kammeraad-Campbell, Managing Editor
Lynne Barber Associate Editor, Alex Sargent, Associate Editor

Newsletters

6910 Trim & Fit
Obesity Foundation
5600 S Quebec Street
Englewood, CO 80111-2202
303-850-0328
Offers nutrition facts and articles, low-fat recipes, medical information on heart disease and cancer relating to nutrition and more.
James F Merker CAE, Editor

Pamphlets

6911 About Overeaters Anonymous
Metro Intergroup of Overeaters Anonymous
117 W 26th Street
New York, NY 10001-6807
212-206-8621

6912 An Inside View
Metro Intergroup of Overeaters Anonymous
117 W 26th Street
New York, NY 10001-6807
212-206-8621

6913 Anonymity
Metro Intergroup of Overeaters Anonymous
117 W 26th Street
New York, NY 10001-6807
212-206-8621

6914 Before You Take That First...
Metro Intergroup of Overeaters Anonymous
117 W 26th Street
New York, NY 10001-6807
212-206-8621

6915 Compulsive Overeaters in the Military
Metro Intergroup of Overeaters Anonymous
117 W 26th Street
New York, NY 10001-6807
212-206-8621

6916 Compulsive Overeating & Overaters Anonymous
Metro Intergroup of Overeaters Anonymous
117 W 26th Street
New York, NY 10001-6807
212-206-8621

6917 For the Obese Employee
Metro Intergroup of Overeaters Anonymous
117 W 26th Street
New York, NY 10001-6807
212-206-8621

6918 Guide to the 12 Steps for You
Metro Intergroup of Overeaters Anonymous
117 W 26th Street
New York, NY 10001-6807
212-206-8621

6919 **Hazelden Step Pamphlets for Overeaters**
Hazelden
15251 Pleasant Valley Road   651-257-4010
Center City, MN 55012-9640   800-328-9000
                                                    Fax: 651-213-4426
                                                    www.hazelden.org
A 12 pamphlet collection that offers one person's interpretation of
the Twelve Steps for overeaters.

6920 **If God Spoke to Overeaters Anonymous**
Metro Intergroup of Overeaters Anonymous
117 W 26th Street   212-206-8621
New York, NY 10001-6807

6921 **Many Symptoms, One Disease**
Metro Intergroup of Overeaters Anonymous
117 W 26th Street   212-206-8621
New York, NY 10001-6807

6922 **Members in Relapse**
Metro Intergroup of Overeaters Anonymous
117 W 26th Street   212-206-8621
New York, NY 10001-6807

6923 **One Day at a Time**
Metro Intergroup of Overeaters Anonymous
117 W 26th Street   212-206-8621
New York, NY 10001-6807

6924 **Overeaters Anonymous Cares**
Metro Intergroup of Overeaters Anonymous
117 W 26th Street   212-206-8621
New York, NY 10001-6807

6925 **Overeaters Anonymous is Not a Diet Club**
Metro Intergroup of Overeaters Anonymous
117 W 26th Street   212-206-8621
New York, NY 10001-6807

6926 **Person to Person**
Metro Intergroup of Overeaters Anonymous
117 W 26th Street   212-206-8621
New York, NY 10001-6807

6927 **Program of Recovery**
Metro Intergroup of Overeaters Anonymous
117 W 26th Street   212-206-8621
New York, NY 10001-6807

6928 **Questions and Answers**
Metro Intergroup of Overeaters Anonymous
117 W 26th Street   212-206-8621
New York, NY 10001-6807

6929 **So You've Reached Goal Weight**
Metro Intergroup of Overeaters Anonymous
117 W 26th Street   212-206-8621
New York, NY 10001-6807

6930 **Think First...**
Metro Intergroup of Overeaters Anonymous
117 W 26th Street   212-206-8621
New York, NY 10001-6807

6931 **To the Family**
Metro Intergroup of Overeaters Anonymous
117 W 26th Street   212-206-8621
New York, NY 10001-6807

6932 **To the Man**
Metro Intergroup of Overeaters Anonymous
117 W 26th Street   212-206-8621
New York, NY 10001-6807

6933 **To the Newcomer**
Metro Intergroup of Overeaters Anonymous
117 W 26th Street   212-206-8621
New York, NY 10001-6807

6934 **To the Teen**
Metro Intergroup of Overeaters Anonymous
117 W 26th Street   212-206-8621
New York, NY 10001-6807

6935 **Tools of Recovery**
Metro Intergroup of Overeaters Anonymous
117 W 26th Street   212-206-8621
New York, NY 10001-6807

6936 **Twelve Traditions of Overeaters Anonymous**
Metro Intergroup of Overeaters Anonymous
117 W 26th Street   212-206-8621
New York, NY 10001-6807

6937 **Welcome Back**
Metro Intergroup of Overeaters Anonymous
117 W 26th Street   212-206-8621
New York, NY 10001-6807

Audio & Video

6938 **Obesity Online**
NAASO
                                                    301-563-6526
Educational resource for clinicians, researchers and educators
with an interest in obesity and its related disorders.
Samuel Klein, Editor
Christie M. Ballantyne, Editor

Web Sites

6939 **Boston Obesity Nutrition Research Center (BONRC)**
                                                    www.bmc.org
Provides resources and support for studies in the area of obesity
and nutrition. Comprised of four research cores located within the
Boston area. In the areas of adipocytes, epidemiology and statistics, body composition, energy expenditure and genetic analyses,
and transgenic animal models.

6940 **Center for Human Nutrition**
                                                    www.uchsc.edu/nutrition
A interdisciplinary team encompassing basic and clinical research,
post-graduate training and career development of nutrition professionals, and commuity outreach. The research conducted at the
CHN focuses on obesity prevention and treatment, nutrient metabolism, and micronutrient status in children. Activities conducted
aim to improve the quallity of life by promoting physical activity
and nutritional awareness.

6941 **Clinical Nutrition Research Unit (CNRU)**
                                                    http://depts.washington.edu/uwcnru
Promotes and enhances the interdisciplinary nutrition research and
education at the Univeristy of Washington. By providing a number
of Core Facilities, the CNRU attempts to integrate and coordinate
the abundant ongoing activities with the goals of fostering new
interdiscilinary research collaborations, stimulating new research
activities, improving nutrition education at multiple levels, and facilitating the nutritional management of patients.

6942 **MedicineNet**
                                                    www.medicinenet.com
An online resource for consumers providing easy-to-read, authoritative medical and health information.

6943 **New York Obesity/Nutrition Research Center (ONRC)**
                                                    www.niddk.nih.gov/fund/other/centers.htm
Funded by the National Institute of Diabetes and Digestive and
Kidney Diseases (NIDDK). A combined effort of Columbia ane
Cornell Universities. Provides participating investigators of
funded projects relevant to obesity research with valuable laboratory, technical, and educational services that otherwise would not
be available to them, thereby improving the productivity an efficiency of their operations.

6944 **North American Association for the Study of Obesity**
                                                    www.naaso.org
The leading scientific society dedicated to the study of obesity.
Committed to encouraging research on the causes and treatment of
obesity, and to keeping the medical community and public informed of new advances.

6945 **Research Chair on Obesity**
2725 Chemin Sainte Foy   418-656-8711
Quebec,Canada,   e-mail: obesite.chair@crhl.ulaval.ca
                           http://obesity.chair.ulaval.ca
Expand our understanding of the pathophysiology of obesity, through scientific research program, to promote communication and interaction among basic scientists and clinicians, involved in nutrition, energy metabolism, obesity, lipid metabolism and cardiovascular research, and to provide continuing education about the best possible knowledge on obesity to health professionals, physicians and to the public at large regarding the causes, the complications and the treatment of obesity.

6946 **University of Pittsburgh Obesity/Nutrition Research Center**
www.pitt.edu/~onrc
Goal is to develop more effective interventions for the prevention and treatment of obesity. Exists to support research functions for investigators studying the broad areas of obesity and nutrition. Focuses on behavioral aspects of obesity and behavioral treatment of this disease.

6947 **Vanderbilt Clinical Nutrition Research Unit (CNRU)**
www.vanderbilt.edu/nutrition/index.html
A core center grant funded by the National Institute of Diabetes and Digestive and Kidney Diseases (NIDDK). Nutrition research is carried out by faculty members i most academic departments and extends from basic laboratory research to clinical and applied research. Maintains service facilities to support both basic and clinical research. Supports research cores that bring nutrition investigators together to discuss their work.

6948 **Weight-control Information Network**
www.niddk.nih.gov/health/nutrit/win.htm
WIN addresses the health information needs of individuals through the production and dissemination of educational materials. In addition, WIN is developing communication strategies for a pilot program to encourage at-risk individuals to achieve and maintain a healthy weight by making changes in their lifestyle.

Description

6949 Osteogenesis Imperfecta

Osteogenesis imperfecta, OI, often called "brittle bone" disease, is actually is a group of serious genetic disorders that are characterized by abnormally fragile bones that break or fracture easily. There are at least four distinct forms of the disorder, with neonatal (congenital) being the most severe. A person with OI has either less collagen, the major protein of the connective tissue, including bone, or a poorer quality collagen. Infants born with OI may have multiple bone fractures and hearing loss, and routine vaginal delivery may lead to significant bone fracture, hemorrhage into the brain and other major problems. Survivors develop shortened extremities and other bony abnormalities. If no injury to the brain occurs then mental and intellectual function should be unaffected. Hearing loss may occur.

At present, there is no effective treatment for this disorder. Careful handling of these infants is essential. Gentle exercise and physical therapy are directed at preventing fractures and increasing function. Surgical implants can provide stability to the skeletal structure. Genetic counseling is also important.

National Agencies & Associations

6950 NIH Osteoporosis and Related Bone Diseases - National Resource Center
2 AMS Circle
Bethesda, MD 20892-3676
202-223-0344
800-624-2663
Fax: 202-293-2356
TTY: 202-466-4315
e-mail: niamsboneinfo@mail.nih.gov
www.osteo.org
Provides patients, health professionals and the public with an important link to resources and information on osteoporosis, Paget's disease of bone, osteogenesis imperfecta, and other metabolic bone diseases. The National Resource Center's mission is to expand awareness and enhance knowledge and understanding of the prevention, early detection, and treatment of these diseases.

6951 NIH Osteoporosis and Related Bone Disease
2 AMS Circle
Bethesda, MD 20892
202-223-0344
800-624-2663
Fax: 202-293-2356
TTY: 202-466-4315
e-mail: nihboneinfo@email.nih.gov
www.bones.nih.gov
Provides patients, health professionals and the public with an important link to resources and information on osteoporosis, Paget's disease of bone, osteogenesis imperfecta and other metabolic bone diseases.
Stephen I Katz, Director
John O'Shea, Scientific Director

6952 National Institute of Child Health and Human Development
National Institutes of Health
31 Center Drive
Bethesda, MD 20892-0001
301-496-5133
Fax: 301-496-7107
Supports several basic and clinical research projects on osteogenesis imperfecta.
Duane Alexander, Director

6953 Osteogenesis Imperfecta Foundation
804 W Diamond Avenue
Gaithersburg, MD 20878-1414
301-947-0083
800-981-2663
Fax: 301-947-0456
TTY: 202-466-4315
TDD: 202-466-4315
e-mail: BoneLink@oif.org
www.oif.org
Support and resources for families and medical professionals dealing with osteogeneis imperfecta.
Mary Beth Huber, Information/Resource Director
Tracy Smith Hart, CEO

Libraries & Resource Centers

6954 NIH Osteoporosis and Related Bone Diseases - National Resource Center
2 AMS Circle
Bethesda, MD 20892-3676
202-223-0344
800-624-2663
Fax: 202-293-2356
TTY: 202-466-4315
e-mail: niamsboneinfo@mail.nih.gov
www.osteo.org
Provides patients, health professionals and the public with an important link to resources and information on osteoporosis, Paget's disease of bone, osteogenesis imperfecta, and other metabolic bone diseases. The National Resource Center's mission is to expand awareness and enhance knowledge and understanding of the prevention, early detection, and treatment of these diseases.

Research Centers

6955 American Society for Bone and Mineral Research
2025 M Street NW
Washington, DC 20036-3309
202-367-1161
Fax: 202-672-2161
e-mail: asbmr@asbmr.org
www.asbmr.org
The mission of the ASBMR is to be the premier society in the field of bone and mineral metabolism through promoting excellence in bone and mineral research fostering integration of clinical and basic science and facilitating the translation of that science to health care and clinical practice.
Ann Elderkin, Executive Director
Douglas Fesler, Associate Executive Director

6956 Children's Brittle Bone Foundation
7701 95th Street
Pleasant Pride, WI 53158
847-433-4981
866-694-2223
Fax: 262-947-0724
e-mail: info@cbbf.org
www.cbbf.org
The mission of the Children's Brittle Bone Foundation is to provide for research into the causes diagnosis treatment prevention a eventual cure for Osteogenesis Imperfecta (OI) while supporting programs which improve the quality of life for people afflicted.

Support Groups & Hotlines

6957 National Health Information Center
PO Box 1133
Washington, DC 20013
310-565-4167
800-336-4797
Fax: 301-984-4256
e-mail: info@nhic.org
www.health.gov/nhic
Offers a nationwide information referral service, produces directories and resource guides.

6958 Osteogenesis Imperfecta Foundation
804 W Diamond Avenue
Gaithersburg, MD 20878
301-947-0083
800-981-2663
Fax: 301-947-0456
TDD: 202-466-4315
e-mail: BoneLink@oif.org
www.oif.org

Support and resources for families and medical professional dealing with osteogeneis imperfecta.

Marybeth Huber, Information Resource Director
Bill Bradner, Director Communication/Events

Books

6959 Children with Ostegogenesis Imperfecta: St raties to Enhance Performance
Holly Lea Cintas, Lynn Gerber, author
Osteogenesis Imperfecta Foundation
804 W Diamond Avenue   301-947-0083
Gaithersburg, MD 20878   800-981-2663
                                    Fax: 301-947-0456
                              e-mail: BoneLink@oif.org
                                         www.oif.org

This guide covers the same issues, but has been written especially for elementary school readers.
252 pages Paperback
ISBN: 0-964218-95-X
Mary Beth Huber, Information/Resource Director

6960 Growing Up with OI: A Guide for Children
Ellen Painter Dollar, author
Osteogenesis Imperfecta Foundation
804 W Diamond Avenue   301-947-0083
Gaithersburg, MD 20878   800-981-2663
                                    Fax: 301-947-0456
                              e-mail: bonelink@oif.org
                                         www.oif.org

This guide covers the same issues as the adult book, Growing Up with OI: A Guide for Families and Caregivers, but has been written especially for elementary school readers.
122 pages Paperback
ISBN: 0-964218-92-5
Mary Beth Huber, Information/Resource Director

6961 Growing Up with OI: A Guide for Families a nd Caregivers
Ellen Painter Dollar, author
Osteogenesis Imperfecta Foundation
804 W Diamond Avenue   301-947-0083
Gaithersburg, MD 20878-1414   800-981-2663
                                    Fax: 301-947-0456
                              e-mail: BoneLink@oif.org
                                         www.oif.org

This guide covers common questions parents, family members and caregivers have about raising a child with OI. The focus is onmaximizing abilities and proactive problem solving. Chapters cover medical, financial, emotional and school related issues.
295 pages Paperback
ISBN: 0-964218-91-7
Mary Beth Huber, Information/Resource Director

6962 Managing Osteogenesis Imperfecta: A Medical Manual
Priscilla Wacaster, MD, author
Osteogenesis Imperfecta Foundation
804 W Diamond Avenue   301-947-0083
Gaithersburg, MD 20878-1414   800-981-2663
                                    Fax: 301-947-0456
                              e-mail: BoneLink@oif.org
                                         www.oif.org

The manual is designed for physicians, physical and occupational therapists, orthopedic technologists, early intervention providers and others who come in contact with persons with OI. It covers a broad range of topics including genetics, diagnosis, pregnancy, arthritis, osteoperosis and rodding.
Mary Beth Huber, Information/Resource Director

6963 Therapeutic Strategies: A Guide for Occupational & Physical Therapists
Ellen Painter Dollar, author
Osteogenesis Imperfecta Foundation

804 W Diamond Avenue   301-947-0083
Gaithersburg, MD 20878-1414   800-981-2663
                                    Fax: 301-947-0456
                              e-mail: BoneLink@oif.org
                                         www.oif.org

This booklet is intended for medical professionals, or for families to use as a resource while working with a medical professional.
14 pages
Mary Beth Huber, Information/Resource Director

Newsletters

6964 Breakthrough
Osteogenesis Imperfecta Foundation
804 W Diamond Avenue   301-947-0083
Gaithersburg, MD 20878-1414   800-981-2663
                                    Fax: 301-947-0456
                              e-mail: BoneLink@oif.org
                                         www.oif.org

Newsletter of the Osteogenesis Imperfecta Foundation that provides information on current research and OIF fundraising activities as well as support features.
15 pages Quarterly
Mary Beth Huber, Information/Resource Director

Pamphlets

6965 Caring for Infants and Children with Osteogenesis Imperfecta
Osteogenesis Imperfecta Foundation
804 W Diamond Avenue   301-947-0083
Gaithersburg, MD 20878-1414   800-981-2663
                                    Fax: 301-947-0456
                              e-mail: BoneLink@oif.org
                                         www.oif.org

A companion to the videotape You Are Not Alone. Presents some basic information and unique tips on caring for a baby with OI. Available in Spanish.
24 pages
Mary Beth Huber, Information/Resource Director

6966 Osteogenesis Imperfecta: A Guide for Medic al Professionals, Individuals & Families
Osteogenesis Imperfecta Foundation
804 W Diamond Avenue   301-947-0083
Gaithersburg, MD 20878-1414   800-981-2663
                                    Fax: 301-947-0456
                              e-mail: BoneLink@oif.org
                                         www.oif.org

This pamphlet contains basic information about the types of OI, inheritance factors, diagnosis and treatment.
10 pages Paperback
Mary Beth Huber, Information/Resource Director

Audio & Video

6967 Going Places and Plan for Success: An Educ ator's Guide to Students with OI
Osteogenesis Imperfecta Foundation
804 W Diamond Avenue   301-947-0083
Gaithersburg, MD 20878-1414   800-981-2663
                                    Fax: 301-947-0456
                              e-mail: BoneLink@oif.org
                                         www.oif.org

A 15-minute video with booklet that guides educators and parents through planning steps that will help children with OI fully participate in school activities.
Mary Beth Huber, Information/Resource Director

6968 Within Reach
Osteogenesis Imperfecta Foundation
804 W Diamond Avenue   301-947-0083
Gaithersburg, MD 20878-1414   800-981-2663
                                    Fax: 301-947-0456
                                    TDD: 202-466-4315
                              e-mail: BoneLink@oif.org
                                         www.oif.org

This 50-minute video features in-depth interviews with adults living with OI. They talk candidly about how they have achieved independent and satisfying lives, addressing such issues as travel, career, marriage and family.

VHS/DVD

Mary Beth Huber, Information/Resource Director

6969 You Are Not Alone

Osteogenesis Imperfecta Foundation

804 W Diamond Avenue   301-947-0083
Gaithersburg, MD 20878-1414   800-981-2663
Fax: 301-947-0456
TDD: 202-466-4315
e-mail: BoneLink@oif.org
www.oif.org

Explores the emotional turmoil of dealing with the diagnosis of OI and offers practical and uplifting solutions for caring for infants with Type II to severe Type III OI. Also valuable for new families with the more mild forms of OI. Available open captioned or with Spanish subtitles (specify if needed). Add $5.00 per video for Canadian orders and $11.00 per video for overseas orders.

Mary Beth Huber, Information/Resource Director

Web Sites

6970 Healing Well

www.healingwell.com

An online health resource guide to medical news, chat, information and articles, newsgroups and message boards, books, disease-related web sites, medical directories, and more for patients, friends, and family coping with disabling diseases, disorders, or chronic illnesses.

6971 Health Finder

www.healthfinder.gov

Searchable, carefully developed web site offering information on over 1000 topics. Developed by the US Department of Health and Human Services, the site can be used in both English and Spanish.

6972 Healthlink USA

www.healthlinkusa.com

Health information concerning treatment, cures, prevention, diagnosis, risk factors, research, support groups, email lists, personal stories and much more. Updated regularly.

6973 Helios Health

www.helioshealth.com

Online resource for your health information. Detailed information about specific health topics, access to expert advice from our Medical Advisory Board, and up-to-date health news.

6974 MedicineNet

www.medicinenet.com

An online resource for consumers providing easy-to-read, authoritative medical and health information.

6975 Medscape

www.medscape.com

Medscape offers specialists, primary care physicians, and other health professionals the Web's most robust and integrated medical information and educational tools.

6976 Osteogenesis Imperfecta Foundation

www.oif.org

A website for those who want to learn more about Osteogenesis Imperfecta, the OI Foundation, and what they do.

6977 Osteoporosis and Related Bone Diseases: National Resource Center (NIGH)

www.osteo.org

Provides patients, health professionals and the public with an important link to resources and information on osteoporosis and other metabolic bone diseases.

6978 WebMD

www.webmd.com

Information on Osteogenesis Imperfecta, including articles and resources.

Description

6979 Osteoporosis

Osteoporosis is a general term for many conditions which result in a reduction in bone mass. Most cases occur in post-menopausal women because estrogen loss is associated with decreased bone mass. These women are at risk for fractures of the wrist, spine and hip. Post-menopausal osteoporosis may also cause marked reduction in a woman's height, as multiple vertebral bodies in the spine compress downwards over the years. Risk factors for osteoporosis include white race, cigarette smoking, thin body build and early menopause. Men can develop a similar condition, but it is generally much less severe. Excessive activity of the adrenal glands (Cushing's syndrome), the thyroid gland (thyrotoxicosis), the parathyroid glands (hyperparathyroidism), and the pituitary gland (hyperprolactinemia) cause bones to thin, as does underactivity of the testes or ovaries. Anorexia nervosa and prolonged administration of cortisone or heparin will also thin the bones.

Treatment is in part nonspecific, and can include surgery or other immobilization to treat fractures of the hip or wrist, control of pain with medications and physical therapy to encourage return to pre-fracture function. Specific therapy includes calcium and Vitamin D supplementation and weight-bearing exercises. Biphosphonates, such as alendronate, have been approved for osteoporosis and other new therapies are being developed.

National Agencies & Associations

6980 National Osteoporosis Foundation
1232 22nd Street NW 202-223-2226
Washington, DC 20037-1292 800-223-9994
Fax: 202-223-2237
e-mail: communications@nof.org
www.nof.org
The nation's leading resource for people seeking up-to-date medically sound information on the causes prevention detection and treatment of osteoporosis.
Leo Schargorodski, Executive Director
Ethel Siris, President

6981 Osteoporosis Canada
1090 Don Mills Road 416-696-2663
Toronto, Ontario, M3C-3R6 800-463-6842
Fax: 416-696-2673
e-mail: info@osteoporosis.ca
www.osteoporosis.ca
A registered charity, is the only national organization serving people who have, or are at risk for, osteoporosis.
Dr. Famida Jiwa, MHSc, DC, BSc, President/CEO

Libraries & Resource Centers

6982 NIH Osteoporosis and Related Bone Diseases - National Resource Center
2 AMS Circle 202-223-0344
Bethesda, MD 20892-3676 800-624-2663
Fax: 202-293-2356
TTY: 202-466-4315
e-mail: niamsboneinfo@mail.nih.gov
www.osteo.org

Provides patients, health professionals and the public with an important link to resources and information on osteoporosis, Paget's disease of bone, osteogenesis imperfecta, and other metabolic bone diseases. The National Resource Center's mission is to expand awareness and enhance knowledge and understanding of the prevention, early detection, and treatment of these diseases.

Research Centers

6983 Medical College of Pennsylvania Center for the Mature Woman
3300 Henry Avenue 215-842-6000
Philadelphia, PA 19129
our purpose is to provide consumers information to help them get high quality services and products at the best possible prices.
Jon Schneider,MD, Director

6984 Osteoporosis Center Memorial Hospital/Advanced Medical Diagn
Memorial Hospital/Advanced Medical Diagnostic
1700 Coffee Road
Modesto, CA 95355 209-526-4500
www.memorialmedicalcenter.org
Memorial Medical Center is part of Memorial Hospitals Association a not-for-profit organization that exists to maintain and improve the health status of citizens in the greater Stanislaus County.
David Benn, Director
Bev Finley, Director

6985 Regional Bone Center Helen Hayes Hospital
Helen Hayes Hospital
51-55 Route 9W 845-786-4839
W Haverstraw, NY 10993 Fax: 845-947-3000
e-mail: info@helenhayeshospital.org
www.helenhayeshospital.org
The mission of the Regional Bone conduct a broad-based research program focused on the elucidation of cellular mechanisms underlying metabolic bone disease and the development of new treatments for bone disease.
David W Dempster PhD, Director
Adrienne Tewksbury, Grants Administrator

6986 University of Connecticut Osteoporosis Center
263 Farmington Avenue 860-679-7692
Farmington, CT 06030 800-535-6232
Fax: 860-679-1258
www.uchc.edu

Jay R Lieberman, Director

6987 University of Connecticut: Exercise Research Laboratory
Health Center
263 Farmington Avenue 860-679-1000
Farmington, CT 06032
Studies the effects of hormone treatment and exercise on osteoporosis in women.
Gail Dalsky PhD, Director

Support Groups & Hotlines

6988 National Health Information Center
PO Box 1133 310-565-4167
Washington, DC 20013 800-336-4797
Fax: 301-984-4256
e-mail: info@nhic.org
www.health.gov/nhic
Offers a nationwide information referral service, produces directories and resource guides.

6989 National Osteoporosis Foundation (NOF)
1232 22nd Street NW 202-223-2226
Washington, DC 20037-1292 Fax: 202-223-2237
e-mail: webmaster@nof.org
www.nof.org
Dedicated to reducing the widespread prevalence of osteoporosis through programs of research, education and advocacy. Provides referrals to existing support groups, as well as free resources, training and materials to assist people to start groups.
Leo Schargorodski, Executive Director
Daniel A Mica, Chairman of the Board

Books

6990 One-Hundred-Fifty Most Asked Questions About Osteoporosis
Hearst Books
1350 Avenue of the Americas   212-261-6500
New York, NY 10016   Fax: 212-261-6595
1993
ISBN: 0-688123-34-1

6991 Preventing & Reversing Osteoporosis: Every Woman's Guide
Prima Publishing
PO Box 1260
Rocklin, CA 95677-1260   916-624-5718
                                     www.primapub.com
1993 275 pages
ISBN: 1-559582-98-7

6992 Preventing and Managing Osteoporosis
Springer Publishing Company
536 Broadway   212-431-4370
New York, NY 10012-3955   877-687-7476
                                     Fax: 212-941-7842
e-mail: springer@springerpub.com
www.springerpub.com
This book will raise awareness and inform health professionals about this often preventable and treatable disease. Written by a team of authors from medicine, nursing, nutrition, exercise physiology, and physical therapy, the book provides an overview of the disease process.
216 pages Hardcover
ISBN: 0-826113-18-4
M Susan Burke MD, Editor
Helen Wright PhD, Editor

Newsletters

6993 Osteoporosis Report
National Osteoporosis Foundation
1232 22nd Street NW   202-223-2226
Washington, DC 20037-1292   800-223-9994
                                     Fax: 202-223-2237
e-mail: communications@nof.org
www.nof.org
A benefit to members of the National Osteoporosis Foundation (NOF), the Osteoporosis Report includes updates on recent research, strategies for bone health and other information. NOF is the only nonprofit, voluntary health organization dedicated to reducing the widespread prevalence of osteoporosis through programs of research, education and advocacy. Contact the foundation for membership information.
Quarterly

Pamphlets

6994 Boning Up on Osteoporosis
National Osteoporosis Foundation
1232 22nd Street NW   202-223-2226
Washington, DC 20037-1292   800-223-9994
                                     Fax: 202-223-2237
e-mail: communications@nof.org
www.nof.org
Risk factor card.

6995 How Strong Are Your Bones?
1232 22nd Street NW   202-223-2226
Washington, DC 20037-1292   800-223-9994
                                     Fax: 202-223-2237
e-mail: communications@nof.org
www.nof.org
Describes the various methods for determining bone mass, including types of equipment and how bone density testing is used in the diagnosis and treatment of osteoporosis.
12 pages

6996 Living with Osteoporosis
1232 22nd Street NW   202-223-2226
Washington, DC 20037-1292   800-223-9994
                                     Fax: 202-223-2237
e-mail: communications@nof.org
www.nof.org
A guide to preventing falls in the home and to protecting yourself from injury during your daily routine.

6997 Medications and Bone Loss
1232 22nd Street NW   202-223-2226
Washington, DC 20037-1292   800-223-9994
                                     Fax: 202-223-2237
e-mail: communications@nof.org
www.nof.org
Designed for women dealing with menopause, this brochure provides information of estrogen replacement therapy and its relationship to bone health and osteoporosis prevention and treatment.

6998 Men with Osteoporosis: In Their Own Words
1232 22nd Street NW   202-223-2226
Washington, DC 20037-1292   800-223-9994
                                     Fax: 202-223-2237
e-mail: communications@nof.org
www.nof.org

6999 Official Prevention Month Poster
1232 22nd Street NW   202-223-2226
Washington, DC 20037-1292   800-223-9994
                                     Fax: 202-223-2237
e-mail: communications@nof.org
www.nof.org
Poster promotes public awareness about osteoporosis. It can be used as a compliment to the education kit, or by itself for exhibits, health fairs or community programs.

7000 Official Prevention Week Poster
1232 22nd Street NW   202-223-2226
Washington, DC 20037-1292   800-223-9994
                                     Fax: 202-223-2237
e-mail: communications@nof.org
www.nof.org
Poster promotes public awareness about osteoporosis. It can be used as a compliment to the education kit, or by itself for exhibits, health fairs or community programs.

7001 Osteoporosis Education Kit
1232 22nd Street NW   202-223-2226
Washington, DC 20037-1292   800-223-9994
                                     Fax: 202-223-2237
e-mail: communications@nof.org
www.nof.org
This kit is designed for preparing public and patient education programs. Updated annually and includes age-targeted materials, nutrition information and osteoporosis fact sheets that are easily duplicated.

7002 Osteoporosis Education Poster
1232 22nd Street NW   202-223-2226
Washington, DC 20037-1292   800-223-9994
                                     Fax: 202-223-2237
e-mail: communications@nof.org
www.nof.org
Ideal for health care settings, the poster clearly illustrates the effect of osteoporosis on bone tissue and common fracture sites.

7003 Osteoporosis Information Package
NAMSIC/National Institutes of Health
1 AMS Circle   301-495-4484
Bethesda, MD 20892-0001   877-226-4267
                                     Fax: 301-718-6366
                                     TTY: 301-565-2966
e-mail: niamsinfo@mail.nih.gov
www.nih.gov/niams
19 pages

7004 Osteoporosis International
1232 22nd Street NW
Washington, DC 20037-1292

202-223-2226
800-223-9994
Fax: 202-223-2237
e-mail: communications@nof.org
www.nof.org

An international multidisciplinary, clinically oriented journal for the exchange of ideas concerning osteoporosis.

7005 Osteoporosis in Men Information Package
NAMSIC/National Institutes of Health
1 AMS Circle
Bethesda, MD 20892-0001

301-495-4484
877-226-4267
Fax: 301-715-6366
TTY: 301-565-2966
e-mail: niamsinfo@mail.nih.gov
www.nih.gov/niams

19 pages

7006 Osteoporosis: Clinical Updates
1232 22nd Street NW
Washington, DC 20037-1292

202-223-2226
800-223-9994
Fax: 202-223-2237
e-mail: communications@nof.org
www.nof.org

NOF's health profession newsletter provides an in depth focus on varying clinical topics.

7007 Osteoporosis: The Silent Disease-Slide Lecture Presentation
1232 22nd Street NW
Washington, DC 20037-1292

202-223-2226
800-223-9994
Fax: 202-223-2237
e-mail: communications@nof.org
www.nof.org

This 42-slide presentation is ideal for community, patient and worksite education progams. It covers basic bone biology, osteoporosis risk factors, diagnosis, prevention and treatment and concludes with a patient case history. A question and answer document is also provided to assist the presenter with audience questions.
Slide set

7008 Patient Education Sample Pack
1232 22nd Street NW
Washington, DC 20037-1292

202-223-2226
800-223-9994
Fax: 202-223-2237
e-mail: communications@nof.org
www.nof.org

This pack contains one of each of NOF's patient education brochures and a catalog; health professionals can select the brochures appropriate for their audience.
Ten brochures

7009 Risk Factor Card: Can It Happen to You?
National Osteoporosis Foundation
1232 22nd Street NW
Washington, DC 20037-1292

202-223-2226
800-223-9994
Fax: 202-223-2237
e-mail: communications@nof.org
www.nof.org

Explains osteoporosis, the causes, symptoms and preventions and high risk persons.

7010 Stand Up to Osteoporosis
National Osteoporosis Foundation
1232 22nd Street NW
Washington, DC 20037-1292

202-223-2226
800-223-9994
Fax: 202-223-2237
e-mail: communications@nof.org
www.nof.org

One of 25 educational brochures on all aspects of this chronic and debilitating disease. The National Osteoporosis Foundation (NOF) is the nation's only private, nonprofit organization dedicated to education, advocacy and public services. Memberships are available to health professionals and public. Quarterly newsletter and physician's guide.

7011 Strategies for People with Osteoporosis
1232 22nd Street NW
Washington, DC 20037-1292

202-223-2226
800-223-9994
Fax: 202-223-2237
e-mail: communications@nof.org
www.nof.org

This series of articles from NOF's newsletter helps patients learn how to cope with osteoporosis. Articles cover hip, vertebrae and wrist fracture recovery, fall-proofing your home, finding the right doctor, what to do after you've been diagnosed and more.

Audio & Video

7012 Be BoneWise: Exercise
National Osteoperosis Foundation
1232 22nd Street NW
Washington, DC 20037-1292

202-223-2226
800-223-9994
Fax: 202-223-2237
e-mail: communications@nof.org
www.nof.org

Take steps toward better bones, health, flexibility and balance with the offical weight bearing and strength training exercise video.

7013 Osteoperosis: The Silent Disease
National Osteoperosis Foundation
1232 22nd Street NW
Washington, DC 20037-1292

202-223-2226
800-223-9994
Fax: 202-223-2237
e-mail: communications@nof.org
www.nof.org

A scripted, visual presentation covers basic bone biology, osteoperosis risk factors, diagnosis, prevention and treatment. Available as a slide presentation or power point CD Rom.

7014 Patient Education Video
National Osteoporosis Foundation
1232 22nd Street NW
Washington, DC 20037-1292

202-223-2226
800-223-9994
Fax: 202-223-2237
e-mail: communications@nof.org
www.nof.org

Discusses treatment, exercise, nutrition and coping strategies for those already diagnoses with osteoporosis.
15 minutes

Web Sites

7015 Healing Well

www.healingwell.com

An online health resource guide to medical news, chat, information and articles, newsgroups and message boards, books, disease-related web sites, medical directories, and more for patients, friends, and family coping with disabling diseases, disorders, or chronic illnesses.

7016 Health Finder

www.healthfinder.gov

Searchable, carefully developed web site offering information on over 1000 topics. Developed by the US Department of Health and Human Services, the site can be used in both English and Spanish.

7017 Healthlink USA

www.healthlinkusa.com

Health information concerning treatment, cures, prevention, diagnosis, risk factors, research, support groups, email lists, personal stories and much more. Updated regularly.

7018 Helios Health

www.helioshealth.com

Online resource for your health information. Detailed information about specific health topics, access to expert advice from our Medical Advisory Board, and up-to-date health news.

7019 MedicineNet

www.medicinenet.com

An online resource for consumers providing easy-to-read, authoritative medical and health information.

7020 Medscape

www.medscape.com

Medscape offers specialists, primary care physicians, and other health professionals the Web's most robust and integrated medical information and educational tools.

7021 NIH Osteoporosis and Related Bone Disease

www.osteo.org

Information on prevention, early detection, and treatment of these diseases is also available. The Resource Center is operated by the National Osteoporosis Foundation, in collaboration with The Paget Foundation and the Osteogenesis Imperfecta Foundation.

7022 National Osteoporosis Foundation

www.nof.org

The nation's leading resource for people seeking up-to-date, medically sound information on the causes, prevention, detection and treatment of osteoporosis.

7023 WebMD

www.webmd.com

Information on osteoporosis, including articles and resources.

Description

7024 ## Paget's Disease

Paget's disease is a disorder of the bone, which typically results in enlarged and deformed bones in one or more regions of the skeleton. Excessive bone breakdown and formation cause new bone to be dense but fragile. Paget's disease occurs most frequently in the spine, skull, pelvis, and legs.

Early symptoms of Paget's disease include bone and joint pain and fatigability, as well as headaches and hearing loss, when the skull is affected. Deformities of bone such as enlargement of the forehead, bowing of a limb, and curvature of the spine may occur as the disease progresses.

The cause of Paget's disease is unknown. It is sometimes familial, but a specific genetic pattern is unclear.

The course of the disease varies greatly and may range from complete stability to rapid progression. Generally, symptoms progress slowly in affected bones with usually no spread to normal ones.

Although there is no cure for Paget's disease at the present, treatments include drugs that suppress disease activity. Orthopedic surgery for joint replacement or stabilization may also be beneficial.

National Agencies & Associations

7025 **Arthritis Foundation**
1330 W Peachtree Street
Atlanta, GA 30309
404-872-7100
800-283-7800
Fax: 404-872-0457
e-mail: help@arthritis.org
www.arthritis.org

A nonprofit organization that depends on volunteers to provide services to help people with arthritis. Supports research to find ways to cure and prevent arthritis and provides services to improve the quality of life for those affected by arthritis.
Cecile Perich, Chair
John H Klippel MD, President and CEO

7026 **Paget Foundation for Paget's Disease of Bone & Related Disorders**
120 Wall Street
New York, NY 10005-4001
212-509-5335
800-237-2438
Fax: 212-509-8492
e-mail: PagetFdn@aol.com
www.paget.org

Private voluntary health agency that provides information to patients and health professionals on several bone disorders including: Paget's disease of bone, primary hyperparathyroidism, fibrous dysplasia, osteoporosis (not osteoporosis) and complications of these conditions.
Charlene Waldman, Executive Director
Christal Sumpter, Administrator & Web Manager

Support Groups & Hotlines

7027 **National Health Information Center**
PO Box 1133
Washington, DC 20013
310-565-4167
800-336-4797
Fax: 301-984-4256
e-mail: info@nhic.org
www.health.gov/nhic

Offers a nationwide information referral service, produces directories and resource guides.

Newsletters

7028 **Update**
Paget Foundation
120 Wall Street
New York, NY 10005-4001
212-509-5335
800-237-2438
Fax: 212-509-8492
e-mail: PagetFdn@aol.com
www.paget.org

Provides information for consumers and health professionals on the following disorders: paget's disease of bone, primary hyperparathyroidism, fibrous dysplasia, osteopetrosis (not osteoporosis) and the complications of breast and prostate cancer metastic to the bone.
3 per year
Charlene Waldman, Executive Director

Pamphlets

7029 **Questions & Answers About Paget's Disease of Bone**
Paget Foundation
120 Wall Street
New York, NY 10005-4001
212-509-5335
800-237-2438
Fax: 212-509-8492
e-mail: pagetfdn@aol.com
www.paget.org

The Paget Foundation provides this and other question and answer booklets and fact sheets on Paget's disease of bone, primary hyperparathyroidism,, fibrous dysplasia, osteopetrosis (not osteoporosis) and breast and prostate cancer metastic to bone. These publications are available on the foundation websit and in print.
Charlene Waldman, Executive Director

Web Sites

7030 **Healing Well**
www.healingwell.com

An online health resource guide to medical news, chat, information and articles, newsgroups and message boards, books, disease-related web sites, medical directories, and more for patients, friends, and family coping with disabling diseases, disorders, or chronic illnesses.

7031 **Health Finder**
www.healthfinder.gov

Searchable, carefully developed web site offering information on over 1000 topics. Developed by the US Department of Health and Human Services, the site can be used in both English and Spanish.

7032 **Healthlink USA**
www.healthlinkusa.com

Health information concerning treatment, cures, prevention, diagnosis, risk factors, research, support groups, email lists, personal stories and much more. Updated regularly.

7033 **Helios Health**
www.helioshealth.com

Online resource for your health information. Detailed information about specific health topics, access to expert advice from our Medical Advisory Board, and up-to-date health news.

7034 **MedicineNet**
www.medicinenet.com

An online resource for consumers providing easy-to-read, authoritative medical and health information.

7035 **Medscape**
www.medscape.com

Medscape offers specialists, primary care physicians, and other health professionals the Web's most robust and integrated medical information and educational tools.

513

7036 **Paget Foundation for Paget's Disease of Bone & Related Disorders**

www.paget.org

Includes information for patients and health professionals on Paget's disease of bone, primary hyperparathyroidism, fibrous dysplasia, osteopetrosis (not osteoporosis) and the complications of certain cancers on the skeleton.

7037 **WebMD**

www.webmd.com

Information on Paget's disease, including articles and resources.

Description

7038 Parkinson Disease

Parkinson disease is a neurological condition characterized by slow and decreased movement. It affects about 1 percent of those over age 65. The cause of Parkinson disease is unknown, but both genetic and environmental factors may play a role. In a minority of cases, Parkinson disease develops after repeated head trauma, carbon monoxide poisoning, drug use, or viral infections that affect the brain.

In about 50 percent to 80 percent of patients, Parkinson disease begins with a slight tremor in the hands, resembling "pill-rolling." With fatigue and stress, the tremor becomes more pronounced. As the disease progresses, voluntary movements, such as walking and eating, become more and more difficult. Rigidity and postural instability (difficulty standing up) develop. Dementia affects approximately one third of patients with advanced Parkinson disease.

Because Parkinson disease is characterized by reduced levels of neurotransmitter chemicals, notably dopamine, in certain parts of the brain, therapy has focused on restoring these levels to normal. Monoamine oxidase type B inhibitors given early in the disease, may protect the cells that secrete these chemicals, and thus delay the need for other therapy. When it is necessary to directly manipulate the chemical levels because of progression of the disease, levodopa, related to dopamine, is the mainstay of treatment and is associated with improvement of all Parkinson symptoms. Anticholinergic medications are especially helpful in treating tremor.

Parkinson disease is the subject of intense research, and experimental surgical or drug treatments are frequently available to patients whose response to standard therapy has been unsatisfactory. General supportive care should not be neglected, and includes physical therapy and an exercise program to help optimize mobility.

National Agencies & Associations

7039 American Parkinson Disease Association

135 Parkinson Avenue   718-981-8001
Staten Island, NY 10305-1943   800-223-2732
Fax: 718-981-4399
e-mail: apda@apdaparkinson.org
www.apdaparkinson.org

Funds research towards finding the cause(s) and cure for Parkinson's Disease, patient education, information, support groups nationwide.
Joel A Miele, President
Joel Gerste, Executive Director

7040 Michael J. Fox Foundation for Parkinson's Research

Grand Central Station
New York, NY 10163
800-708-7644
www.michaeljfox.org

The Michael J. Fox Foundation is dedicated to ensuring the development of a cure for Parkinson's disease within this lifetime through an aggressively funded research center.
Deborah W Brooks, Co-Founder
Katie Hood, CEO

7041 National Institute of Neurological Disorders and Stroke

NIH Neurological Institute   301-496-5751
Bethesda, MD 20824   800-352-9424
Fax: 301-402-2186
TTY: 301-468-5981
www.ninds.nih.gov

The mission of NINDS is to reduce the burden of neurological disease - a burden borne by every age group, by every segment of society, by people all over the world.
Story C Landis PhD, Director
Walter J Koroshetz, Deputy Director

7042 National Parkinson Foundation

1501 NW 9th Avenue   305-243-6666
Miami, FL 33136-1407   800-327-4545
Fax: 305-243-6824
e-mail: contact@parkinson.org
www.parkinson.org

A nonprofit organization dedicated to research, diagnosis, treatment and care for men and women suffering from Parkinson's and other related neurological diseases. The Foundation also supports the Bob Hope research and rehabilitation center.
Nathan Slewett, Chairman
Joyce A Oberdorf, President and Chief Executive Officer

7043 Parkinson Society Canada

4211 Yonge Street   416-227-9700
Toronto, Ontario, M2P-2A9   800-565-3000
Fax: 416-227-9600
e-mail: info@parkinson.ca
www.parkinson.ca

A not-for-profit, national charitable organization. The Society raises money through corporate sponsorships, public donations, and planned gifts. Finding the cause and cure for Parkinson's disease remains our mission.
Joyce Gordon, President/CEO
Beverly Crandell, National Director, Resource Development

7044 Parkinson's Action Network (PAN)

1025 Vermont Avenue NW   202-638-4101
Washington, DC 20005   800-850-4726
Fax: 202-638-7257
e-mail: info@parkinsonaction.org
www.parkinsonsaction.org

The Parkinson's Action Network is the unified voice of the Parkinson's disease community-advocating for more than one million Americans and their families.
Amy Comstock Rick, Chief Executive Officer
Michelle Duelley, Executive Assistant to the CEO

7045 Parkinson's Institute

675 Almanor Avenue   408-734-2800
Sunnyvale, CA 94085-1605   800-655-2273
Fax: 408-734-8522
e-mail: info@thepi.org
www.thepi.org

The mission of the Parkinson's Institute is to find the cause(s) and a cure for Parkinson's Disease and provide the best possible treatment to those afflicted with the disease.
J William Langston, Founder/CEO/Chief Scientific Officer
Melanie M Brandabur, Clinic Director

7046 WE MOVE

204 W 84th Street   212-875-8312
New York, NY 10024   e-mail: wemove@wemove.org
www.wemove.org

WE MOVE's mission is to raise awareness of neurologic movement disorder among healthcare professionals, patients and families and the public.
Susan B Bressman, President
Mo Moadeli, Vice President

State Agencies & Associations

Arizona

7047 Arizona Chapter of the National Parkinson Foundation
20280 N 59th Avenue   480-607-1960
Glendale, AZ 85308-6182   866-637-8772
                                    Fax: 480-607-1957
                                 e-mail: info@aznpf.org
                                          www.aznpf.org
Affiliate chapter of The National Parkinson Foundation Inc.
Alan Marks, President
Kenneth Larkin, Vice President

California

7048 Los Angeles Alliance Against Parkinson's Disease
3251 Oakley Drive   323-851-3230
Los Angeles, CA 90068-1315   e-mail: Millard@millardtipp.com
                                 www.parkinson.org/chapters.htm#
Affiliate of the National Parkinson Foundation.

7049 National Parkinson Foundation: California Office
4929 Wilshire Boulevard   323-442-8434
Los Angeles, CA 90010-3899

7050 National Parkinson Foundation: Orange County Chapter
PO Box 2207   949-764-6998
Newport Beach, CA 92659   Fax: 949-548-4624
                                 e-mail: info@yahoo.com
                                          www.npfocc.org
Affiliate of The National Parkinson Foundation.
Mignone M Trenary, President
Laurie Gerberding, Office Manager

7051 Northstate Parkinson's Chapter
1003 Yuba Street
Redding, CA 96001
                                            530-229-0878
                                          www.parkinson.org
Affiliate of The National Parkinson Foundation, Inc.
Craig Boyer

7052 Parkinson Association of the Sacramento Valley
900 Fulton Avenue   916-489-0226
Sacramento, CA 96825-4502   Fax: 916-489-0241
                              e-mail: parkanc@sbcglobal.net
                                 www.parkinsonsacramento.org
Bernardine Ford, President
George Johnston, 2nd Vice President

7053 Parkinson Network of Mount Diablo
Po Box 3127   925-284-2189
Walnut Creek, CA 94598-0127 e-mail: mmhansell@hotmail.com
                                          www.parkinson.org
Affiliate of the National Parkinson Foundation.
Mary Hansell

7054 Parkinson's Action Network (PAN) Parkinson's Action Network
Parkinson's Action Network
1025 Vermont Avenue NW   202-638-4101
Washington, DC 20005   800-850-4726
                                    Fax: 202-638-7257
                              e-mail: info@parkinsonsaction.org
                                 www.parkinsonsaction.org
Amy Comstock Rick, Chief Executive Officer
Anne Udall, Chair/Founding Chair

Colorado

7055 Colorado Parkinson Foundation
1155 Kelly Johnson Boulevard   719-884-0103
Colorado Springs, FL 90920-1494   800-327-4545
                                    Fax: 719-495-909
                                 e-mail: rpfarrer@msn.com
                                 colorado.parkinson.org
The mission of the National Parkinson Foundation if to find the
cause of the cure for Parkinson disease through research. To improve the quality if life for persons with Parkinson and their caregivers. To also educate persons with Parkinson their carecar
Ric Pfarrer, Chairperson

Florida

7056 Alzheimer/Parkinson Association of Indian River County
2501 27th Avenue   772-563-0505
Vero Beach, FL 32960   e-mail: alzsupport@fastmail.fm
                                          www.parkinson.org
Toni Teresi, Chairperson

7057 Goodwill Industries-Suncoast
Goodwill Industries-Suncoast
10596 Gandy Boulevard   727-523-1512
St. Petersburg, FL 37023   888-279-1988
                                    Fax: 727-563-9300
                      e-mail: gw.marketing@goodwill-suncoast.org
                                 www.goodwill-suncoast.org
A nonprofit community based organization whose purpose is to improve the quality of life for people who are disabled, disadvantaged and/or aged. This mission is accomplished through a staff of
over 1,200 employees providing independent living skills, affordable housing, career assessment and planning, job skills, training,
placement, and job retention assistance with useful employment.
Annually, Goodwill Industries-Suncoast serves over 30,000 people in Citrus, Hernando, Levy, Marion and more.
R Lee Waits, President/CEO
Martin W Gladysz, Chair

7058 Parkinson Association of Greater Daytona Beach
111 North Frederick Avenue   386-252-8959
Daytona Beach, FL 32114   e-mail: goatie@cfl.rr.com
                                          www.parkinson.org
Nancy Dawson, Chairperson

7059 Parkinson Association of Greater Kansas
111 N Frederick Avenue
Daytona Beach, FL 32114   386-252-8959
                                          www.parkinson.org
Nancy Dawson, Chairperson

7060 Parkinson Association of Southwest Florida
6226 Trail Boulevard   239-254-7791
Naples, FL 34108   Fax: 239-254-9421
                                 e-mail: pasfi@aol.com
                                          www.pasfi.org
Affiliate of the National Parkinson Foundation.
Jacqueline Urso, Executive Director
Ellen Chaney, Secretary

7061 South Palm Beach County Chapter of NFP
PO Box 880145
Boca Raton, FL 33433-0145   561-482-2867
                                          www.parkinson.org
Irving Layton, Chairperson

7062 Southeast Parkinson Disease Association
6530 Metrowest Boulevard   407-489-4124
Orlando, FL 32835-6520   e-mail: srh_pres@sepda.org
                                          www.sepda.org
Steve Hochberger, Chairperson

Georgia

7063 Northwest Georgia Parkinson Disease Association
708 Glen Milner Boulevard   706-235-3164
Rome, GA 30161   e-mail: webmaster@gaparkinsons.org
                                 www.gaparkinsons.org
James Trussel, Chairperson

Hawaii

7064 Hawaii Parkinson Association Gwendolyn A Montibon President
Gwendolyn A Montibon, President
347 N Kuakini Street   808-528-0935
Honolulu, HI 96817   Fax: 808-528-1897
                                 e-mail: kekim@hawaii.edu
                                          www.parkinson.org
Affiliate of The National Parkinson Foundation.

Kansas

7065 Northeast Kansas Parkinson Association
PO Box 251
Topeka, KS 66601   785-228-1337
                                        www.parkinson.org

Mary Hatke, Chairperson

7066 Parkinson Association of Greater Kansas City
8900 State Line Road   913-341-8828
Leawood, KS 66206   Fax: 913-341-8885
                          e-mail: meg@parkinsonheartland.org
                                        www.parkinsonheartland.org
Affiliate of The National Parkinson Foundation.
Meg Duggan, Executive Director
Katie Fuchs, Program Coordinator

Louisiana

7067 Eljay Foundation for Parkinson Syndrome Awareness
715 Ryan Street   337-310-0083
Lake Charles, LA 70601   e-mail: info@eljayfd.org
                                        www.eljayfd.org

Eligha Guillory, Chairperson

Massachusetts

7068 Cape Cod Chapter National Parkinson Foundation
33 Ships Way   508-385-2333
Buzzards Bay, MA 02532-0584   e-mail: meacapecod@yahoo.com
                                        www.parkinson.org
Affiliate of The National Parkinson Foundation.
Joseph Wimbrow, President

7069 National Parkinson Foundation:Cape Cod Chapter
33 Ships Way   508-385-2333
Buzzards Bay, MA 02532-0584   e-mail: meacapecod@yahoo.com
                                        www.parkinson.org

Garland Smith, Chairperson

7070 Northeast Parkinson's and Caregivers
27 Sutcliffe Road   508-756-7721
Brimfield, MA 01010   e-mail: rstake@northeastparkinsons.com
                                        www.northeastparkinsons.com

Richard Stake, Chairperson

Minnesota

7071 Parkinson Association of Minnesota
2205 Zealand Avenue N   763-545-1272
Golden Valley, MN 55427-4602   800-327-4545
                          e-mail: info@parkinsonmn.org
                                        www.parkinsonmn.org
Affiliate of The National Parkinson Foundation.
Paul Blom, President

New Jersey

7072 Parkinson Alliance
PO Box 308   609-688-0870
Kingston, NJ 08540   800-579-8440
                                        Fax: 609-688-0875
                      e-mail: admin@parkinsonalliance.net
                                        www.parkinsonalliance.net
The Princeton-New Jersey based Parkinson Alliance is a National
nonprofit organization dedicated to raising funds to help finance
the most promising research to find the cause and curefor Parkin-
son's disease.
Carol Walton, Executive Director

New York

7073 National Parkinson Foundation: New York Office
122 E 42nd Street
New York, NY 10017-5622   800-457-6676

7074 Parkinsons Wellness Group of Western New York
222 Seabert Avenue   716-684-0650
Depew, NY 14043   e-mail: coach71395@aol.com
                                        www.parkinsonswny.com

Richard Lipka, Chairperson

Oklahoma

7075 Parkinson Foundation of the Heartland Oklahoma Branch
1000 W Wilshire   405-810-0695
Oklahoma City, OK 73116   e-mail: jimk@parkinsonheartland.org
                                        www.parkinson.org
Satellite office of the Kansas Chapter
Jim Keating, Chairperson

Oregon

7076 Parkinsons Resources of Oregon
3975 Mercantile Drive   503-594-0901
Lake Oswego, OR 97035   800-426-6806
                                        Fax: 503-594-0547
                       e-mail: info@parkinsonsresources.org
                                        www.parkinsonsresources.org

Holly Chaimov, Executive Director

Pennsylvania

7077 Parkinson Chapter of Greater Pittsburgh
6507 Wilkins Avenue   412-365-2086
Pittsburgh, PA 15217   e-mail: info@pfwpa.org.
                                        www.parkinsonpittsburgh.org

Doreen Grasso, Chairperson
Maggie Schmidt, Executive Director

7078 Parkinson Council
111 Presidential Boulevard   610-668-4292
Bala Cynwyd, PA 19004   Fax: 610-668-4275
                       e-mail: info@theparkinsoncouncil.org
                                        www.theparkinsoncouncil.org
The Parkinson Council is dedicated to promoting research initiat-
ing to find the causes and cure for Parkinson Disease educating patients their caregivers healthcare professionals and the general
public about Parkinson's and improving the quality of lif
Mark Vernon, Chairperson
Sally J Bellet, Executive Director

South Dakota

7079 Parkinson Association of South Dakota
PO Box 87952   605-328-4227
Sioux Falls, SD 57109-9938   Fax: 605-328-7150
                          e-mail: info@parkinsonsd.org
                                        www.parkinsonsd.org
Affiliate of The National Parkinson Foundation.
Elaine Spader, President
Lori Jones, Vice President

Virginia

7080 Parkinson Foundation of the National Capitol Area
8300 Greensboro Drive   703-287-8729
McLean, VA 22102-4201   Fax: 703-918-4847
                       e-mail: pfnca@parkinsonfoundation.org
                                        www.parkinsonfoundation.org

Susan D Hamburger, Chairperson

Washington

7081 Parkinson Educational Society of Puget Sound
Evergreen Nursing And Rehabilitation
1501 NW 9th Avenue   305-243-6666
Miami, FL 33136-1494   800-327-4545
                                        Fax: 305-243-6824
                          e-mail: contact@parkinson.org
                                        www.parkinson.org
The National Parkinson Foundation is the largest organization in
the world serving persons affected by Parkinson disease. The

Foundation supports research for a cure and programs dedicated to improving care and quality of life.
Bernard J Fogel, Chairman

Wisconsin

7082 Wisconsin Parkinson Association
945 N 12th Street   414-219-7061
Milwaukee, WI 53233   800-972-5455
Fax: 414-219-6564
www.wiparkinson.org
Chapter of The National Parkinson Foundation.
Keith Brewer, President

Foundations

7083 Parkinsons Disease Foundation
1359 Broadway   212-923-4700
New York, NY 10018   800-457-6676
Fax: 212-923-4778
e-mail: info@pdf.org
www.pdf.org
The foundation has been one of teh leaders in subsidizing research into Parkinson's Disease. Offers many services including The Summer Fellowship Program, The Postdoctoral Fellowship Program, support groups nationwide, grants for clinical and laboratory studies, public awareness and government promotion of the disease.
Lewis P Rowland, MD, President
Robin A Elliott, Executive Director

Libraries & Resource Centers

7084 Parkinson's Resource Organization
74090 El Paseo   760-773-5628
Palm Desert, CA 92260-4135   877-775-4111
Fax: 760-773-9803
e-mail: info@parkinsonsresource.org
www.parkinsonsresource.org
Our mission is to help families affected by Parkinson's forge through the journey of the disease's progression with as much quality as life can provide. Working so no one is isolated because of Parkinson's
Jo Rosen, Visionary, President, Founder
Bonnie Shoemaker, Programs Director

Research Centers

7085 California Institute for Medical Research
2260 Clove Drive   408-998-4554
San Jose, CA 95128   Fax: 408-998-2723
e-mail: admin@clmr.org
www.cimr.org
Medical research including infectious diseases stroke and cancer specializing in Parkinson's Disease related studies.
David A Stevens, Researcher Infectious Diseases
J William Langston, Researcher Parkinson's Disease

7086 Texas Tech University Tarbox Parkinson's Disease Institute
3601 4th Street
Lubbock, TX 79430   806-743-1000
www.ttuhsc.edu
The current objectives of the Tarbox Institute are to provide services for Parkinson's disease patients and their families in the underserved West Texas area; to maintain a Parkinson's Disease Information and Referral Center to enable both healthcare professionals and affected families to obtain the latest information on services available new developments in research support groups and educational literature.
Joseph Green, Chairman

7087 University of Alabama at Birmingham Parkinsons Disease Center
1720 7th Avenue S   205-934-9100
Birmingham, AL 35294   Fax: 205-346-78
e-mail: apda@uab.edu
www.uab.edu
Offers educational emotional and political support to Parkinson disease patients and their families.
Ray Watts, Interim CEO
David G Standaert, Director

7088 William T Gossett Parkinson's Disease Center
Henry Ford Hospital
Department of Neurology   313-972-1693
Detroit, MI 48202
Jay M Gorell MD, Director

Support Groups & Hotlines

7089 National Health Information Center
PO Box 1133   310-565-4167
Washington, DC 20013   800-336-4797
Fax: 301-984-4256
e-mail: info@nhic.org
www.health.gov/nhic
Offers a nationwide information referral service, produces directories and resource guides.

California

7090 Parkinson's Disease Association of San Die go (PDASD)
8555 Areo Drive   858-273-6763
San Diego, CA 92123-1746   877-737-7576
Fax: 858-273-6764
e-mail: info@pdasd.org
www.pdasd.org
Information and referral research center for Parkinson's disease patients and their families.
Ronald C Hendrix, Executive Director
Kathleen Wescott, Program Director

Florida

7091 Greater Daytona Area Parkinson Support Group
Bishop's Glen Retirement Center   904-322-4748
Daytona, FL   e-mail: boba@n-jcenter.com
www.parkinson.org/shell/areacode.pl
Affiliate of the National Parkinson Foundation.

7092 National Parkinson Foundation Hotline
National Parkinson Foundation
1501 NW 9th Avenue Bob Hope Road   305-243-6666
Miami, FL 33136   800-327-4545
Fax: 305-243-5595
www.parkinson.org
Offers support and emergency information for persons with Parkinson's and their families.
Jose Garcia Pebrosa, Director

7093 Pembroke Pines Parkinson Support Group
Century Village, Club House
Pembroke Pines, FL 33027   954-433-0947
www.parkinson.org/shell/areacode.pl
Affiliate of the National Parkinson Foundation.

Hawaii

7094 Kuakini Parkinson Disease (PD) Information & Referral
Kuakini Medical Center
347 North Kuakini Street   808-528-0935
Honolulu, HI 96817   800-570-1101
Fax: 808-528-1897
e-mail: pr@kuakini.org
www.kuakini.org/SiteMap.asp
The Kuakini Parkinson Disease (PD) Information & Referral Office provides referrals to neurologists and other special services for Parkinson disease patients; provides information about community services to assist PD patients and their caregivers in finding

optimal care; distributes educational materials; conducts educational conferences and other activities; and assists with support groups for PD patients and caregivers.
Gary K Kajiwara, President/Chief Executive Officer
Gregg Oishi, SVP/Chief Operating Officer

Illinois

7095 Rockford Parkinson's Support Group
5415 Watson Road
Rockford, IL 61108
815-654-0614
800-972-5455
Affiliate of The National Parkinson Foundation, Inc.

Maryland

7096 Parkinson Support Groups of America
11376 Cherry Hill Road
Beltsville, MD 20705
301-937-1545
Offers support networks and groups for persons with Parkinson's disease, families, friends and professionals.

Mississippi

7097 APDA Center for Advanced Parkinson Disease Research
Washington University School of Medicine
660 South Euclid
St Louis, MO 63110
314-362-6909
Fax: 314-362-0168
e-mail: joel@npg.wustl.edu
www.neuro.wustl.edu/parkinson/
Information and referral research center for Parkinson's disease patients and their families.
Joel Perlmutter, Director

Missouri

7098 Ozarks Parkinson Support Group
Po Box 50595
Springfield, MO 65805
417-885-9595
www.parkinson.org/shell/areacode.pl
Affiliate of the National Parkinson Foundation.
Monty Montgomery, Contact

New Jersey

7099 New Jersey Parkinson's Disease Information Center
Robert Wood Johnson University Hospital
One Robert Wood Johnson Place
New Brunswick, NJ 08901
732-745-7520
Fax: 732-745-3114
e-mail: elizabeth.schaaf@rwjuh.edu
www.rwjuh.edu/medical_services/
The New Jersey Parkinson's Disease Information and Referral Center reaches out to persons affected by Parkinson's disease, including patients, families and healthcare professionals. This Information and Referral Center is committed to providing community education and information as well as support groups for caregivers and persons with Parkinson's disease.
Elizabeth Schaaf, Parkinson's Disease Center Coordinator

New York

7100 American Parkinson Disease Association Hotline
1250 Hylan Boulevard
Staten Island, NY 10305
800-908-2732
Fax: 718-981-4399
www.attaparkinson.org
Offers information and physician referrals to patients and their families.
Joel Gerstel, Director

7101 New York College of Osteopathic Medicine
PO Box 8000
Old Westbury, NY 11568-8000
516-686-7516
800-345-6948
Fax: 516-686-7613
e-mail: Barbara
www.iris.nyit.edu/nycom/
Information and referral research center for Parkinson's disease patients and their families.
Rosslee Vice President

7102 Parkinson's Support Group of Upstate New York
PO Box 23204
Rochester, NY 14692-3204
716-377-6718
www.parkinson.org/upstate.htm
Affiliate of The National Parkinson Foundation, Inc.
David Look, President

7103 St. John's Episcopal Hospital
Rt 25A
Smithtown, NY 11787
631-361-4100
Information and referral research center for Parkinson's disease patients and their families.

7104 University of Rochester
500 Wilson Boulevard
Rochester, NY 14627
585-275-2121
www.rochester.edu/
Information and referral research center for Parkinson's disease patients and their families.

Oregon

7105 Oregon Health Sciences University
3181 SW Sam Jackson Park Road
Portland, OR 97201
503-494-5285
888-222-6478
Information and referral research center for Parkinson's disease patients and their families.

Pennsylvania

7106 University of Pittsburgh
Forbes Avenue
Pittsburgh, PA 15260
412-624-4141
e-mail: helpdesk+@pitt.edu
www.pitt.edu
Information and referral research center for Parkinson's disease patients and their families.
Mark Nordenberg, Counselor

Texas

7107 Presbyterian Hospital of Dallas
8200 Walnut Hill Lane
Dallas, TX 75231
214-345-6789
www.texashealth.org
Information and referral research center for Parkinson's disease patients and their families.
Mark H Merril

7108 University of Texas HSC at San Antonio
7703 Floyd Curl Drive
San Antonio, TX 78229-3900
512-567-6688
www.uthscsa.edu/
Information and referral research center for Parkinson's disease patients and their families.

Washington

7109 University of Washington
Box 355840
Seattle, WA 98195-5840
206-543-5369
e-mail: uwvic@u.washington.edu
www.washington.edu/
Information and referral research center for Parkinson's disease patients and their families.

Books

7110 Coping with Parkinson's Disease
American Parkinson's Disease Association
1250 Hylan Boulevard
Staten Island, NY 10305-1944
800-223-2732
88 pages

7111 Living with Parkinson's Disease
Demos Medical Publishing
386 Park Avenue S
New York, NY 10016-8804
212-683-0072
800-532-8663
Fax: 212-683-0118
e-mail: orderdept@demospub.com
www.demospub.com

Written specifically for anyone who has been diagnosed with Parkinson's disease, as well as family members and friends.
1996 150 pages
ISBN: 1-888799-10-2
Dr. Diana M Schneider, President

7112 Parkinson's - A Personal Story of Acceptance
Branden Publishing Company
17 Station Street Box 843   617-734-2045
Brookline Village, MA 02147   Fax: 617-734-2046
www.branden.com
1993 162 pages Paperback
ISBN: 0-828319-49-9

7113 Parkinson's Disease & Movement Disorders
Williams & Wilkins
351 W Camden Street   301-528-4000
Baltimore, MD 21201-7912   800-638-0672
1993 640 pages
ISBN: 0-683043-80-3

7114 Parkinson's Disease Handbook
National Parkinson Foundation
1501 NW 9th Avenue   305-547-6666
Miami, FL 33136-1407   800-327-4545
Fax: 305-548-4403
www.parkinson.org
A guide for patients and their families regarding the illness of Parkinson's.
Paperback

7115 Parkinson's Disease: A Guide for Patient and Family
Raven Press
1185 Avenue of the Americas   212-930-9500
New York, NY 10036-2601   800-777-2295
Recommended by patients, the medical community and the leading medical journals, this guide offers information on the most recent medical advances in the field of Parkinson's disease and answers the patients most frequently asked questions about the illness.
224 pages Hardcover
ISBN: 0-781703-12-3

7116 Parkinsonian Syndromes
John H Dekker & Sons
2941 Clydon Avenue SW   616-538-5160
Grand Rapids, MI 49509-2403   Fax: 616-538-0720
1993 584 pages
ISBN: 0-824788-38-9

7117 The Comfort of Home for Parkinson Disease: A Guide for Caregivers
Marie Meyer & Paula Derr, RN with Susa Imke, RN/MS, author

CareTrust Publications
PO Box 10283
Portland, OR 97296-0283   800-565-1533
Fax: 415-673-2005
e-mail: sales@comfortofhome.com
www.comfortofhome.com
Comfort will help caregivers be equipped with information about everything from the importance of and noticing wearing off signs to making difficult decisions to travel, equipment options, therapies and dietary guidelines. It offers caregivers mental and emotional support in coping with their challenging role, as well.
2007 298 pages
ISBN: 0-966476-77-8

Children's Books

7118 Journey to Almost There
Clarion Books
215 Park Avenue S
New York, NY 10003-1603   212-420-5800
An interesting tale that surrounds the relationship of Alison and her Granfather O'Brien when Alison's mother feels that he should enter an elderly home.
Grades 6-9

Newsletters

7119 APDA Newsletter
American Parkinson Disease Association
135 Parkinson Avenue   718-981-8001
Staten Island, NY 10305-1943   800-223-2732
Fax: 718-981-4399
e-mail: apda@apdaparkinson.org
www.apdaparkinson.org
Current information on matters of interest for PD patients and families.
Joel A Miele, President
Joel Gerste, Executive Director

7120 American Parkinson Disease Association Newsletter
60 Bay Street   718-981-8001
Staten Island, NY 10301-2514   800-223-2732
Offers information on the association activities and events, convention and legislative information, medical updates and research reports for the Parkinson's patient and their families.
Quarterly

7121 News & Review
Parkinsons Disease Foundation
1359 Broadway   212-923-4700
New York, NY 10018   800-457-6676
Fax: 212-923-4778
e-mail: info@pdf.org
www.pdf.org
In each issue we include reports on scientific research and discoveries, treatments and therapies, commentary from physicians and insight from Parkinson's specialists. We also provide practical suggestions, tips and articles from people who live with the disease and wish to share their experiences.
Quarterly
Lewis P Rowland, MD, President
Robin A Elliott, Executive Director

7122 Parkinson Report
National Parkinson Foundation
1501 NW 9th Avenue   305-547-6666
Miami, FL 33136-1407   800-327-4545
Fax: 305-548-4403
www.parkinson.org
Offers association news and events, conference and symposia news, legislative and medical updates, research reports and more for the Parkinson's patient, their families and the general public.
Quarterly

7123 Parkinson's Disease Foundation Newsletter
Parkinson's Disease Foundation
650 W 168th Street   212-923-4700
New York, NY 10032-3702   800-457-6676
Provides information on Parkinson's Disease Foundation events, news stories of research findings, and technical advances in the field of patient care.

Pamphlets

7124 A One-Stop Shop for Parkinson's Informatio n
Parkinsons Disease Foundation
1359 Broadway   212-923-4700
New York, NY 10018   800-457-6676
Fax: 212-923-4778
e-mail: info@pdf.org
www.pdf.org
An explanation of PDF's services and resources that are available to answer your most important questions about Parkinson's disease. These services include a toll-free helpline, our Ask the Expert web service and print/video materials.
Lewis P Rowland, MD, President
Robin A Elliott, Executive Director

7125 Adjustment, Adaptation and Accomodation: Psychological Approaches
National Parkinson Foundation

1501 NW 9th Avenue
Miami, FL 33136-1407

305-547-6666
800-327-4545
Fax: 305-548-4403
www.parkinson.org

Coping strategies for Parkinson's disease.

7126 Akathisia in Parkinson's Disease
Parkinson United Foundation
833 W Washington Boulevard   312-733-1893
Chicago, IL 60607
1990

7127 Answering Your Questions About PROPATH
525 Middlefield Road
Menlo Park, CA 94025-3447   800-776-7284
This brochure explains and offers an introduction to PROPATH, a
program for Parkinson's disease patients.

7128 Autonomic Failure and Parkinson's Disease
United Parkinson Foundation
833 W Washington Boulevard   312-733-1893
Chicago, IL 60607-2316
1990

7129 Balance Disturbances and Parkinson's Disease
United Parkinson Foundation
833 W Washington Boulevard   312-733-1893
Chicago, IL 60607-2316
1990

7130 Basic Information About Parkinson's Disease
American Parkinson's Disease Association
1250 Hylan Boulevard
Staten Island, NY 10305-1944   800-223-2732
Offers information on the illness, incidence, treatments, education
and support for both patients and professionals.

7131 Deep Brain Stimulation for Parkinson's Disease
Parkinsons Disease Foundation
1359 Broadway   212-923-4700
New York, NY 10018   800-457-6676
Fax: 212-923-4778
e-mail: info@pdf.org
www.pdf.org
This booklet addresses the newest area of surgical options in the
treatment of PD symptoms _ deep brain stimulation (or DBS) sur-
gery _ while also describing older surgical approaches used to treat
PD.
Lewis P Rowland, MD, President
Robin A Elliott, Executive Director

7132 Dental Care for the Patient with Parkinson's Disease
United Parkinson Foundation
833 W Washington Boulevard   312-733-1893
Chicago, IL 60607-2316
1987

7133 Depression and Dementia in Parkinson's Disease
United Parkinson Foundation
833 W Washington Boulevard   312-733-1893
Chicago, IL 60607-2316
1993

7134 Diagnosis Parkinson's Disease: You Are Not Alone
Parkinsons Disease Foundation
1359 Broadway   212-923-4700
New York, NY 10018   800-457-6676
Fax: 212-923-4778
e-mail: info@pdf.org
www.pdf.org
Designed for the person newly diagnosed with Parkinson's, this informational booklet serves as a reference for the many questions
that may arise. It shares resources, medical expert testimony and
the experiences of people who have dealt with the diagnosis of Parkinson's disease.
Booklet
Lewis P Rowland, MD, President
Robin A Elliott, Executive Director

7135 Dietary Considerations for Parkinson's Disease Patients
United Parkinson Foundation

833 W Washington Boulevard   312-733-1893
Chicago, IL 60607-2316

7136 Differential Diagnosis of Parkinsonism
United Parkinson Foundation
833 W Washington Boulevard   312-733-1893
Chicago, IL 60607-2316
1984

**7137 Driving and the Parkinson's Disease Patient: Some
Considerations**
United Parkinson Foundation
833 W Washington Boulevard   312-733-1893
Chicago, IL 60607-2316
1994

7138 Efficacy of Antiparkinson Medications
United Parkinson Foundation
833 W Washington Boulevard   312-733-1893
Chicago, IL 60607-2316
1983

7139 Equipment and Suggestions for Persons with Parkinson's Disease
American Parkinson's Disease Association
1250 Hylan Boulevard
Staten Island, NY 10305-1944   800-223-2732
19 pages

7140 Eyes and Parkinson's Disease
United Parkinson Foundation
833 W Washington Boulevard   312-733-1893
Chicago, IL 60607-2316
1986

7141 Fighting Back Against PD: One Women's Story
National Parkinson Foundation
1501 NW 9th Avenue   305-547-6666
Miami, FL 33136-1407   800-327-4545
Fax: 305-548-4403
www.parkinson.org
One woman's battle against Parkinson's disease.

**7142 Fulfilling the Hope: Our Commitment to the Parkinson's
Community**
Parkinsons Disease Foundation
1359 Broadway   212-923-4700
New York, NY 10018   800-457-6676
Fax: 212-923-4778
e-mail: info@pdf.org
www.pdf.org
This brochure provides an overview of Parkinsons Disease Foun-
dations services and programs.
Lewis P Rowland, MD, President
Robin A Elliott, Executive Director

7143 Good Nutrition in Parkinson's Disease
American Parkinson Disease Association
60 Bay Street
Staten Island, NY 10301-2514   800-223-2732
Offers information on diet, nutrients, proteins and recipes for peo-
ple with Parkinson's disease.

7144 How to Start a Parkinson's Disease Support Group
American Parkinson's Disease Association
1250 Hylan Boulevard
Staten Island, NY 10305-1944   800-223-2732
42 pages

7145 MR Imaging in Parkinson's Disease
United Parkinson Foundation
833 W Washington Boulevard   312-733-1893
Chicago, IL 60607-2316
1990

7146 Micrographia
United Parkinson Foundation
833 W Washington Boulevard   312-733-1893
Chicago, IL 60607-2316
1991

7147 Neuropsychology and Parkinson's Disease
United Parkinson Foundation

833 W Washington Boulevard
Chicago, IL 60607-2316   312-733-1893
1992

7148 Neurotrophic Factors in Parkinson's Disease
United Parkinson Foundation
833 W Washington Boulevard   312-733-1893
Chicago, IL 60607-2316
1992

7149 One Step at a Time Brochure
United Parkinson Foundationon
833 W Washington Boulevard   312-733-1893
Chicago, IL 60607-2316
An exercise manual for the Parkinsonian patient.
1985

7150 Pain Syndromes and Parkinson's Disease
United Parkinson Foundation
833 W Washington Boulevard   312-733-1893
Chicago, IL 60607-2316
1990

7151 Parkinson Handbook: A Guide for Patients and Their Families
National Parkinson Foundation
1501 NW 9th Avenue   305-547-6666
Miami, FL 33136-1407   800-327-4545
Fax: 305-548-4403
www.parkinson.org
Offers informative, up-to-date information on exercises, hobbies, treatments, speech impairments and psychological aspects.

7152 Parkinson's Advocacy: The Keys to Empowerment
Parkinsons Disease Foundation
1359 Broadway   212-923-4700
New York, NY 10018   800-457-6676
Fax: 212-923-4778
e-mail: info@pdf.org
www.pdf.org
Use this informational brochure to learn how to harness your power as a person living with Parkinson's and join the fight for a cure.
Lewis P Rowland, MD, President
Robin A Elliott, Executive Director

7153 Parkinson's Disease Handbook
American Parkinson's Disease Association
1250 Hylan Boulevard
Staten Island, NY 10305-1944
800-223-2732
40 pages

7154 Parkinson's Disease Q&A: A Guide for Patients
Parkinsons Disease Foundation
1359 Broadway   212-923-4700
New York, NY 10018   800-457-6676
Fax: 212-923-4778
e-mail: info@pdf.org
www.pdf.org
This booklet answers the most frequently asked questions about Parkinson's disease. Movement disorder specialists from the Columbia University Medical Center address topics ranging from signs of Parkinson's to treatment options to daily living issues.
Booklet
Lewis P Rowland, MD, President
Robin A Elliott, Executive Director

7155 Parkinson's Disease and the Menstrual Cycle
United Parkinson Foundation
833 W Washington Boulevard   312-733-1893
Chicago, IL 60607-2316
1990

7156 Parkinson's Disease: The Patient Experience
United Parkinson Foundation
833 W Washington Boulevard   312-733-1893
Chicago, IL 60607-2316
Booklet designed for patients with Parkinson's disease and their families to explain medical terminology and offer suggestions on how to deal with the disease more easily.
1986

7157 Parkinson's Patient: What You and Your Family Should Know
National Parkinson Foundation
1501 NW 9th Avenue   305-547-6666
Miami, FL 33136-1407   800-327-4545
Fax: 305-548-4403
www.parkinson.org
Offers a brief overview of Parkinson's Disease causes, symptoms and treatments as well as offering an insight into statistical information on the illness.

7158 Patient Perspectives on Parkinson's
National Parkinson Foundation
1501 NW 9th Avenue   305-547-6666
Miami, FL 33136-1407   800-327-4545
Fax: 305-548-4403
www.parkinson.org
Offers a brief overview of Parkinson's disease, the onset of the illness, depression, sexuality, exercise, sleep and nutrition information for daily living.
45 pages

7159 Perioperative Management of Parkinson's Disease
United Parkinson Foundation
833 W Washington Boulevard   312-733-1893
Chicago, IL 60607-2316
1989

7160 Pet Scans: A New Look at Parkinson's Disease
United Parkinson Foundation
833 W Washington Boulevard   312-733-1893
Chicago, IL 60607-2316
1989

7161 Podiatry and Parkinson's Disease
United Parkinson Foundation
833 W Washington Boulevard   312-733-1893
Chicago, IL 60607-2316
1983

7162 Postural Hypotension
United Parkinson Foundation
833 W Washington Boulevard   312-733-1893
Chicago, IL 60607-2316
1988

7163 Practical Pointers for Parkinson Patients
National Parkinson Foundation
1501 NW 9th Avenue   305-547-6666
Miami, FL 33136-1407   800-327-4545
Fax: 305-548-4403
www.parkinson.org

7164 Role of Physical Therapy in Parkinson's Disease
United Parkinson Foundation
833 W Washington Boulevard   312-733-1893
Chicago, IL 60607-2316
1985

7165 Sexual and Bladder Difficulties in Parkinson's Disease
United Parkinson Foundation
833 W Washington Boulevard   312-733-1893
Chicago, IL 60607-2316
1988

7166 Sleep Problems with Parkinson's Disease
United Parkinson Foundation
833 W Washington Boulevard   312-733-1893
Chicago, IL 60607-2316
1992

7167 Speech & Swallowing Problems for Parkinsonians
National Parkinson Foundation
1501 NW 9th Avenue   305-547-6666
Miami, FL 33136-1407   800-327-4545
Fax: 305-548-4403
www.parkinson.org

7168 Speech Problems & Swallowing Problems in Parkinson's Disease
American Parkinson Disease Association
60 Bay Street
Staten Island, NY 10301-2514
800-223-2732

Offers information on speech problems, swallowing problems, hearing impairments and facial mobility for the person with Parkinson's.

7169   Speech and Voice Impairment
United Parkinson Foundation
833 W Washington Boulevard   312-733-1893
Chicago, IL 60607-2316
1983

7170   Stages of Parkinson's Disease
United Parkinson Foundation
833 W Washington Boulevard   312-733-1893
Chicago, IL 60607-2316
1983

7171   Suggested Exercise Program for People with Parkinson's Disease
American Parkinson Disease Association
60 Bay Street
Staten Island, NY 10301-2514   800-223-2732
Exercise program pamphlet with full illustrations explaining each exercise.
23 pages

7172   Treatment of Parkinson's Disease with Carbidopa-Levodopa
National Parkinson Foundation
1501 NW 9th Avenue   305-547-6666
Miami, FL 33136-1407   800-327-4545
Fax: 305-548-4403
www.parkinson.org
Offers information on treating Parkinson's Disease.

Audio & Video

7173   Diagnosis Parkinson's Disease: You Are Not Alone
Parkinsons Disease Foundation
1359 Broadway   212-923-4700
New York, NY 10018   800-457-6676
Fax: 212-923-4778
e-mail: info@pdf.org
www.pdf.org

Designed for the person newly diagnosed with Parkinson's, this informational booklet and video serve as a reference for the many questions that may arise. It shares resources, medical expert testimony and the experiences of people who have dealt with the diagnosis of Parkinson's disease.
Video & Booklet
Lewis P Rowland, MD, President
Robin A Elliott, Executive Director

7174   Motivating Moves for People with Parkinson's
Parkinsons Disease Foundation
1359 Broadway   212-923-4700
New York, NY 10018   800-457-6676
Fax: 212-923-4778
e-mail: info@pdf.org
www.pdf.org

Motivating Moves is a unique program of 24 seated exercises designed especially for people with Parkinson's. Exercises address typical Parkinson's symptoms such as stability, flexibility, posture, vocal range and facial expressivity. The video is divided into three sections, How to Do Motivating Moves (45 minutes), The Exercise Class (36 minutes) and Practical Tips for Daily Living (4 minutes).
Video
Lewis P Rowland, MD, President
Robin A Elliott, Executive Director

7175   PDF Exercise Program
Parkinsons Disease Foundation
1359 Broadway   212-923-4700
New York, NY 10018   800-457-6676
Fax: 212-923-4778
e-mail: info@pdf.org
www.pdf.org

This program consists of three sets of exercises specifically designed for PD patients. Each exercise is clearly illustrated in a

3-ring binder with flip-chart pages and includes two cassette tapes, which provide verbal cues and music for timing.
Cassettes
Lewis P Rowland, MD, President
Robin A Elliott, Executive Director

7176   Parkingson's: Lynda's Story
David Tucker, author
Fanlight Productions
4196 Washington Street   617-469-4999
Boston, MA 02131   800-937-4113
Fax: 617-469-3379
e-mail: fanlight@fanlight.com
www.fanlight.com

Parkinson's disease is robbing Lynda McKenzie of normal coordination and movement. She's prepared to participate in a clinical study of surgery to transplant fetal cells directly into her brain, but she will have to live for a year not knowing whether she has received the actual cells or a placebo.
1999 46 Minutes
ISBN: 1-572954-22-1
Nicole Johnson, Publicity Coordinator

Web Sites

7177   Healing Well
www.healingwell.com
An online health resource guide to medical news, chat, information and articles, newsgroups and message boards, books, disease-related web sites, medical directories, and more for patients, friends, and family coping with disabling diseases, disorders, or chronic illnesses.

7178   Health Finder
www.healthfinder.gov
Searchable, carefully developed web site offering information on over 1000 topics. Developed by the US Department of Health and Human Services, the site can be used in both English and Spanish.

7179   Healthlink USA
www.healthlinkusa.com
Health information concerning treatment, cures, prevention, diagnosis, risk factors, research, support groups, email lists, personal stories and much more. Updated regularly.

7180   Helios Health
www.helioshealth.com
Online resource for your health information. Detailed information about specific health topics, access to expert advice from our Medical Advisory Board, and up-to-date health news.

7181   MedicineNet
www.medicinenet.com
An online resource for consumers providing easy-to-read, authoritative medical and health information.

7182   Medscape
www.medscape.com
Medscape offers specialists, primary care physicians, and other health professionals the Web's most robust and integrated medical information and educational tools.

7183   National Parkinson Foundation
www.parkinson.org
Information on research, diagnosis, treatment and care for men and women suffering from parkinson's and other related neurological diseases.

7184   Neurology Channel
www.neurologychannel.com
Find clearly explained, medically accurate information regarding conditions, including an overview, symptoms, causes, diagnostic procedures and treatment options. On this site it is possible to ask questions and get information from a neurologist and connect to people who have similar health interests.

7185   WebMD
www.webmd.com

Description

7186 ## Post-Polio Syndrome

Post-Polio syndrome, PPS, also known as the late effects of polio or post polio sequelae, is characterized by new symptoms that occur in people with a history of polio after a long period of stability during which whatever strength they had recovered remained unchanged. PPS affects approximately 60 percent of polio survivors, 20 to 40 years after the initial episode. The hallmark of PPS is new weakness. Other symptoms include fatigue, pain, difficulty breathing and swallowing, intolerance to cold, and new muscle atrophy.

While the cause of PPS is not clearly understood, two theories exist. One suggests that it is caused by normal muscle loss that accompanies aging. The other is that PPS is caused by the repeated over use of muscle groups. In both cases, muscle groups not previously known to have been affected by polio are weakened, and it is this weakness that is the major indicator of PPS. A polio survivor with an affected leg may find that his or her arms are newly affected. Whether the arm problems are a result of undetected muscle damage that occurred at the time of the original polio or newer damage resulting from the over use of the remaining good muscles, or a combination of the two, is not clearly understood.

PPS is frequently emotionally difficult for polio survivors. Many feel they have triumphed over their initial polio, or have come to terms with their resulting disabilities. To think that the polio is coming back is often terrifying. These emotional issues are frequently made more difficult by the fact that PPS is often mis-diagnosed as other conditions or normal aging. Also, patients are often given misinformation about PPS.

Post-polio syndrome, like most diseases classified as syndromes, does not have a specific diagnostic test, but a diagnosis of exclusion. This means that other medical conditions that may present with symptoms similar to those found in PPS should be considered and excluded, if possible. Once diagnosis of PPS is determined, treatment is individualized by primary symptoms and may include medications, supervised therapy, injections and, in some cases, surgery.

National Agencies & Associations

7187 **Post Polio Awareness and Support Society o f British Columbia**
#2-2630 Ross Lane   250-477-8244
Victoria, BC, V8T-5L5   Fax: 250-477-8287
                                        e-mail: ppass@ppass.bc.ca
                                                www.ppass.bc.ca
A non-profit society that links area groups, through our board and our provincial office in Victoria.
Joan Toone, President

Support Groups & Hotlines

7188 **PostPolio Health International**
4207 Lindell Boulevard   314-534-0475
Saint Louis, MO 63108-2915   Fax: 314-534-5070
                                        e-mail: info@postpolio.org
                                                www.post-polio.org/
Post-Polio Health International's mission is to enhance the lives and independence of polio survivors and home ventilator users through education, advocacy, research and networking.
Joan L Headley, Executive Director
Sheryl Rudy, Webmaster

Books

7189 **Managing Post-Polio: A Guide for Polio Survivors and Their Families**
Yale University Press
PO Box 209040   203-732-0960
New Haven, CT 06520-9040   Fax: 203-432-0948
Diagnosis and management of polio-related health problems . Essential resources for polio survivors, their families and health care providers.

7190 **Managing Post-Polio: A Guide to Living Well with Post-Polio Syndrome**
ABI Professional Publications
PO Box 5243   703-525-5488
Arlington, VA 22205   Fax: 703-524-4105
Practical information resulting from a combination of professional knowledge and personal experience. A comprehensive array of topics are addressed: the diagnostic process, finding expert medical care, energy conservation, psychosocial aspects of disability, support groups, vocational strategies, managed care concerns, Social Security benefits, and internet resources.
256 pages

Newsletters

7191 **Polio Network News**
Post-Polio Health International
4207 Lindell Boulevard   314-534-0475
St. Louis, MO 63108-2915   Fax: 314-534-5070
                                        e-mail: ventinfo@post-polio.org
                                                www.post-polio.org/IVUN
Joan Headley, Executive Director

7192 **Post-Polio Health**
Post-Polio Health International
4207 Lindell Boulevard   314-534-0475
Saint Louis, MO 63108-2915   Fax: 314-534-5070
                                        e-mail: ventinfo@post-polio.org
                                                www.post-polio.org/IVUN
12 pages Quarterly
Joan Headley, Executive Director

7193 **Post-Polio Health International**
Joan L Headley, author
4207 Lindell Boulevard   314-534-0475
St. Louis, MO 63108-2915   Fax: 314-534-5070
                                        e-mail: info@post-polio.org
                                                www.post-polio.org
Provides educational materials, advocacy, networking and support research to enhance the lives and independence of polio survivors and users of home mechanical ventilators. Minimum $25.00 with membership.
12 pages
Joan Headley, Executive Director

7194 **Ventilator-Assisted Living**
Joan L Headley, author
4207 Lindell Boulevard   314-534-0475
St. Louis, MO 63108-2915   Fax: 314-534-5070
                                        e-mail: info@post-polio.org
                                                www.post-polio.org

Provides educational materials, advocacy, networking and support research to enhance the lives and independence of polio survivors and users of home mechanical ventilators. Minimum $25.00 with membership.
12 pages
Joan Headley, Executive Director

7195 Ventilator: Assisted Living
Post-Polio Health International
4207 Lindell Boulevard   314-534-0475
St. Louis, MO 63108-2915   Fax: 314-534-5070
                                  e-mail: ventinfo@post-polio.org
                                       www.post-polio.org/IVUN
The newsletter of the International Ventilator Users Network, an affiliate of Post-Polio Health International.
12 pages Newsletter
Joan Headley, Executive Director

Pamphlets

7196 Guidelines for People Who Have Had Polio
March of Dimes
PO Box 1657   717-820-8104
Wilkes-Barre, PA 18703   800-367-6630
                                     Fax: 570-825-1987
Located on website as a PDF file. Information based on March of Dimes International Conference on Post-Polio Syndrome.

7197 Post-Polio Syndrome: Identifying Best Practices in Diagnosis and Care
March of Dimes
233 Park Avenue South   212-353-8353
New York, NY 10003   Fax: 212-254-3518
                          e-mail: NY639@marchofdimes.com
                                       www.marchofdimes.com
Located on website as PDF file.

Web Sites

7198 EMedicine
                       www.emedicine.com/pmr/topic110.htm
EMedicine was launched in 1996 and is the largest and most current clinical knowledge base available to physicians and health professionals.

7199 International Rehabilitation Center for Polio
                                          www.polioclinic.org
International Rehabilitation Center for Polio (IRCP) at Spaulding Rehabilitation HOspital website offers information about PPS and resources for polio survivors and others with an interest in post-polio syndrome.

7200 MedicineNet
                                          www.medicinenet.com
An online resource for consumers providing easy-to-read, authoritative medical and health information.

7201 Polio Experience Network
                                          www.polionet.org
The Polio Experience Network offers information, inspiration, ideas and resources for polio survivors and those seeking information on post-polio syndrome.

7202 Social Security Administration
                                          www.ssa.gov/disability
The Social Security Administration website on disability benefits includes information about how to apply for benefits.

Description

7203 Prader-Willi Syndrome

Prader-Willi syndrome, PWS, is a group of abnormalities first described by Drs. Prader, Labart, and Willi in 1956. This uncommon condition occurs in about one in every 20,000 births. In about 50 percent of PWS patients, there is a missing piece (deletion) of part of chromosome 15.

PWS is characterized by obesity, short stature, small penis and testicles (hypogonadism), small hands and feet, mental retardation and decreased muscle tone. During the toddler years, many patients begin to overeat. Some persons with PWS may show signs of obsessive-compulsive disorder, apart from their obsessions with food. In addition to insatiable hunger, other behavioral features include emotional highs and lows, poor motor skills and cognitive impairment. Sexual development is halted, and facial and skeletal abnormalities develop.

Therapies for PWS are aimed at symptoms with an emphasis on specialized diets and customized exercise programs and support.

National Agencies & Associations

7204 National Institute of Child Health and Human Development
31 Center Drive
Bethesda, MD 20892
301-496-5133
Fax: 301-496-7101
www.nih.gov
Offers reprints, articles and various information on Prader-Willi Syndrome in children and adults.
Duane Alexander, Director

7205 Prader-Willi Syndrome Association (USA) Prader-Willi Syndrome Association
Prader-Willi Syndrome Association (USA)
8588 Potter Park Drive
Sarasota, FL 34238
941-312-0400
800-926-4797
Fax: 941-312-0142
e-mail: webmaster1@pwsausa.org
www.pwsausa.org
Provides to parents and professionals a national and international network of information, support services and research endeavors to expressly meet the needs of affected children and adults and their families. Offers 31 state chapters and published materials.
Janalee Heinemann, Executive Director

State Agencies & Associations

Arizona

7206 Prader-Willi Syndrome Arizona Association: Phoenix Area
Prader-Willi Syndrome Association
3920 East Bronco Trail
Phoenix, AZ 85044
480-598-0966
e-mail: shemc@netzero.net
www.pwsausa.org
Sheila McMahon, President

7207 Prader-Willi Syndrome Arizona Association Prader-Willi Syndrome Association
Prader-Willi Syndrome Association
13839 N Bentwater Drive
Tucson, AZ 85737
520-297-7025
e-mail: p.penta@comcast.net
www.pwsausa.org
Tammie Penta, President

Arkansas

7208 Prader-Willi Arkansas Association Prader-Willi Syndrome Association
Prader-Willi Syndrome Association
2504 S Drive
N Little Rock, AR 72118-4245
501-753-8715
e-mail: jpattpnlr@msn.com
www.pwsausa.org
Jim Patton, President

California

7209 Prader-Willi California Foundation
514 N Prospect Avenue
Redondo Beach, CA 90277
310-372-5053
800-400-9994
Fax: 310-372-4329
e-mail: PWCF1@aol.com
www.pwsausa.org
Lisa Graziano, Executive Director

7210 Prader-Willi California Foundation: Newport Area
419 Fullerton Avenue
Newport Beach, CA 92663
949-642-9772
e-mail: olsonbb@adelphia.net
www.pwsausa.org
Robert J Olsen, President

Colorado

7211 Prader-Willi Colorado Association Prader-Willi Syndrome Association
Prader-Willi Syndrome Association
8290 S Yukon Way
Littleton, CO 80128
303-973-4780
e-mail: hosler@dynamicsolutions.com
www.pwsausa.org
Lynette Hosler, President

Connecticut

7212 Prader-Willi Connecticut Association Prader-Willi Syndrome Association
Prader-Willi Syndrome Association
35 Ansonia Drive
N Haven, CT 06473-3306
203-239-9902
e-mail: pwsactchapter@yahoo.com
www.pwsausa.org
Vicki Knoph, President

Delaware

7213 Prader-Willi Delaware Association Prader-Willi Syndrome Association
Prader-Willi Syndrome Association
300 Bethel Circle Millwood
Middletown, DE 19709
302-378-7385
e-mail: swede455@aol.com
www.pwsausa.org
Karen Swanson, President

Florida

7214 Prader-Willi Florida Assocition Prader-Willi Syndrome Association
Prader-Willi Syndrome Association
17777 S W 285 Street
Homestead, FL 33030
305-245-6484
e-mail: pwfa2000@aol.com
www.pwsausa.org
Debbie Stallings, Co-President
John Stallings, Co-President

Georgia

7215 PWSA of Georgia Prader-Willi Syndrome Association
Prader-Willi Syndrome Association
562 Lakeland Plaza
Cumming, GA 30040
770-886-2334
877-866-2334
Fax: 770-886-2335
e-mail: pwsaga@earthlink.net
www.pwsausa.org
Debbie Lang, Executive Director

Hawaii

7216 Prader-Willi Northwest Association
Prader-Willi Syndrome Association
269 Kaha Street
Hailua, HI 96734   808-263-8177
                                    e-mail: susanlundh@yahoo.com
                                    www.pwsausa.org

Susan Lundh, President

Idaho

7217 Prader-Willi Northwest Association
Prader-Willi Syndrome Association
550 Lodgepole Road
Athol, ID 83801   208-683-2993
                                    e-mail: idaho4ts@aol.com
                                    www.pwsausa.org

Susan Lundh, President
Gene Todhunter, Local Contact

Illinois

7218 PWSA Illinois Prader-Willi Syndrome Association
Prader-Willi Syndrome Association
2128 N Sedgwick Street
Chicago, IL 60614   773-281-9170
                                    e-mail: illinois@pwsausa.org
                                    www.pwsausa.org

Jeffrey Fender, President

Indiana

7219 PWSA of Indiana Prader-Willi Syndrome Association
Prader-Willi Syndrome Association
7536 Moonbeam Drive
Indianapolis, IN 46259   317-527-9173
                                    e-mail: pwsain@yahoo.com
                                    www.pwsausa.org

Jacque McGuire, President

Iowa

7220 PWSA of Iowa Prader-Willi Syndrome Association
Prader-Willi Syndrome Association
15130 Holcomb Avenue
Clive, IA 50325-9695   515-987-0288
                                    e-mail: ktcaedav@netins.net
                                    www.pwsausa.org

Tammi Davis, President
Edie Bogaczyk, President

Kansas

7221 PWSA of Kansas Prader-Willi Syndrome Association
Prader-Willi Syndrome Association
14 NE Bayview Drive
Lees Summit, MO 64064-1624   816-350-1375
                                    e-mail: national@pwsausa.org
                                    www.pwsausa.org

Terri Douglas, Prader-Willi Syndrome Advocate
Barry Douglas, Prader-Willi Syndrome Advocate

Kentucky

7222 Prader-Willi Kentucky Association Prader-Willi Syndrome Association
Prader-Willi Syndrome Association
9213 Reigate Court
Louisville, KY 40222   502-339-7872
                                    e-mail: national@pwsausa.org
                                    www.pwsausa.org

Frank Beckles, President
Rick Settles

Maine

7223 Prader-Willi New England Association
Andover, MA 01757   978-475-5570
                                    e-mail: pwsane@aol.com
                                    www.pwsausa.org

Eileen Rullo, President

Massachusetts

7224 Prader-Willi New England Association Prader-Willi Syndrome Association
Prader-Willi Syndrome Association
Andover, MA 01757   978-475-5570
                                    e-mail: pwsane@aol.com
                                    www.pwsausa.org

Eileen Rullo, President

7225 Prader-Willi Syndrome of Western Massachusetts
Prader-Willi Syndrome Association
10 Cottage Avenue
Holyoke, MA 01040   413-533-8335
                                    e-mail: national@pwsausa.org
                                    www.pwsausa.org

Violet Gingras, President

Michigan

7226 Prader-Willi Syndrome Association of Michigan
10756 Woodbushe   616-642-0017
Lowell, MI 49331   e-mail: chrishendrick@cablespeed.com
                                    www.pwsausa.org

Jon Hendrick, Co-Chairperson
Chris Hendrick, Co-Chairperson

Minnesota

7227 PWSA of Minnesota Prader-Willi Syndrome Association
Prader-Willi Syndrome Association
7209 Oaklawn Avenue
Woodbury, MN 55105   952-893-9318
                                    e-mail: national@pwsausa.org
                                    www.pwsausa.org

Jey Behnken, President

Missouri

7228 PWSA Missouri Chapter Prader-Willi Syndrome Association
Prader-Willi Syndrome Association
1465 S Grand Boulevard Missouri Str 314-268-4027
Louis, MO 63104   Fax: 314-935-7461
                                    e-mail: national@pwsausa.org
                                    www.pwsausa.org

Barbara Whitman, President

Montana

7229 Prader-Willi Northwest Association
3706 29th Avenue W   206-285-7679
Seattle, WA 98199   e-mail: susanlundh@yahoo.com
                                    www.pwsausa.org

This association covers Washington, Oregon, Idaho, Montana, Alaska, and Hawaii.
Susan Lundh, President

Nebraska

7230 PWSA Nebraska Chapter Prader-Willi Syndrome Association
Prader-Willi Syndrome Association
302 S 49th Avenue
Omaha, NE 68132   402-551-9168
                                    e-mail: national@pwsausa.org
                                    www.pwsausa.org

Jennifer Varner, Local Contact

New Jersey

7231 Prader-Willi New Jersey Association Prader-Willi Syndrome Association
Prader-Willi Syndrome Association
514 Gatewod Road
Cherry Hill, NJ 08003   856-795-4229
                                    e-mail: national@pwsausa.org
                                    www.pwsausa.org

Sybil Cohen, President
Judy Livny, Vice-President

7232 Prader-Willi Alliance of New York Prader-Willi Syndrome Association
Prader-Willi Syndrome Association
PO Box 1114
Niagara Falls, NY 14304
716-276-2211
800-442-1655
e-mail: alliance@prader-willi.org
www.prader-willi.org

Barbara McManus, President

North Carolina

7233 Prader-Willi Syndrome Association of North Carolina
Prader-Willi Syndrome Association
1404 Sutton Drive
Kinston, NC 28501
252-527-1813
e-mail: national@pwsausa.org
www.pwsausa.org

Sally St John, President

North Dakota

7234 PWSA Fargo Chapter Prader-Willi Syndrome Association
Prader-Willi Syndrome Association
2902 S University Drive
Fargo, ND 58103-6032
701-232-3301
Fax: 701-237-5775
e-mail: fraser@fraserltd.org
www.fraserltd.org

Ohio

7235 PWSA Ohio Chapter Prader-Willi Syndrome Association
Prader-Willi Syndrome Association
4075 W 226 Street
Fairview Park, OH 44126
440-716-0552
e-mail: pwsaohio@aol.com
www.pwsausa.org

Jennifer Bolander, President

Oklahoma

7236 PWSA Oklahoma Chapter Prader-Willi Syndrome Association
Prader-Willi Syndrome Association
3816 SE 89th Street
Oklahoma City, OK 74135-6222
405-677-8089
e-mail: national@pwsausa.org
www.pwsausa.org

Daphne Mosley, President

7237 Prader-Willi Association: Tulsa Area
4444 S Columbia Avenue
Tulsa, OK 74105-5221
918-747-7848
e-mail: marishack@aol.om
www.pwsausa.org

Curt Shacklett, Chairman

Oregon

7238 PWSA Oregon Chapter Prader-Willi Syndrome Association
Prader-Willi Syndrome Association
303 E Historic Columbia
Troutdale, OR 97060
503-669-7191
e-mail: national@pwsausa.org
www.pwsausa.org

Cory Eliason, President

Pennsylvania

7239 PWSA Pennsylvania Chapter Prader-Willi Syndrome Association
Prader-Willi Syndrome Association
104 Persimmon Place
Cranberry Township, PA 16066
724-779-4415
e-mail: national@pwsausa.org
www.pwsausa.org

Debbie Fabio, President

South Carolina

7240 PWSA South Carolina Chapter Prader-Willi Syndrome Association
Prader-Willi Syndrome Association
912 Lake Spur Lane
Chapin, SC 29036
803-345-1379
e-mail: national@pwsausa.org
www.pwsausa.org

Rhett Eleazer, Local Contact

Tennessee

7241 PWSA Tennessee Chapter Prader-Willi Syndrome Association
Prader-Willi Syndrome Association
105 Foxwood Lane
Franklin, TN 37065
615-790-6659
e-mail: national@pwsausa.org
www.pwsausa.org

Terry Bolander, Local Contact

Texas

7242 PWSA Texas Chapter Prader-Willi Syndrome Association
Prader-Willi Syndrome Association
14427 Perchin Drive
San Antonio, TX 78247
210-946-6789
e-mail: national@pwsausa.org
www.pwsausa.org

Susan Carvajal, Local Contact

Utah

7243 Prader-Willi Utah Association Prader-Willi Syndrome Association
Prader-Willi Syndrome Association
2652 Nottingham Way
Salt Lake City, UT 84108
801-582-0998
Fax: 801-768-3924
e-mail: national@pwsausa.org
www.pwsausa.org

Lisa Thornton, President

Virginia

7244 PWSA of Maryland, Virginia & DC
Prader-Willi Syndrome Association
2601 Chriswell Place
Hernson, VA 20171-2940
410-822-3752
e-mail: pwsausa@pwsausa.org
www.pwsausa.org

Linda Keder, President
Susie Wood, Maryland Contact

Washington

7245 Prader-Willi Northwest Association Prader-Willi Syndrome Association
Prader-Willi Syndrome Association
16208 SE 46th Place
Bellevue, WA 98006
206-285-7679
e-mail: jlubderwood@juno.com
www.pwsausa.org

Joanne Underwood, Co-President
Susan Lundh, Co-President

Wisconsin

7246 PWSA of Wisconsin Prader-Willi Syndrome Association
Prader-Willi Syndrome Association
2701 N Alexander Street
Appleton, WI 54911-2512
920-882-6371
866-797-2947
e-mail: wisconsion@pwsausa.org
www.pwsausa.org

Mary Lynn Larson, Program Director
Mike Larson, President

Support Groups & Hotlines

7247 National Health Information Center
PO Box 1133
Washington, DC 20013
310-565-4167
800-336-4797
Fax: 301-984-4256
e-mail: info@nhic.org
www.health.gov/nhic

Offers a nationwide information referral service, produces directories and resource guides.

7248 PraderWilli Syndrome Association
PraderWilli Syndrome Association
5700 Midnight Pass Road   941-312-0400
Sarasota, FL 34242   800-926-4797
                                  Fax: 941-312-0142
                            e-mail: pwsuasa@aol.com
                                    www.pwsausa.org

Jenalee Heinemann, Executive Director
Steve Dudrow, Business Manager

Books

7249 Child with Prader-Willi Syndrome: Birth to Three
Prader-Willi Syndrome Association (USA)
8588 Potter Park Drive   941-312-0400
Sarasota, FL 34238   800-926-4797
                                  Fax: 941-312-0142
                            e-mail: info@pwsausa.com
                                    www.pwsausa.org
Discusses the common concerns of the first three years and offers specific recommendations for early intervention strategies. A helpful and positive resource for families, physicians, early intervention workers and other care providers. Booklet
2004 34 pages
Craig Pulhemus, Executive Director

7250 Early Years
Prader-Willi Syndrome Association (USA)
8588 Potter Park Drive   941-312-0400
Sarasota, FL 34238   800-926-4797
                                  Fax: 941-312-0142
                            e-mail: info@pwsausa.com
                                    www.pwsausa.org
Collection of articles regarding young children with PWS — many from a parent's perspective.
1998 37 pages
Craig Polhemus, Executive Director

7251 Growing Up with Prader-Willi Syndrome: Personal Reflections of a Mother
Prader-Willi Syndrome Association (USA)
8588 Potter Park Drive   941-312-0400
Sarasota, FL 34238   800-926-4797
                                  Fax: 941-312-0142
                            e-mail: info@pwsausa.com
                                    www.pwsausa.org
Collection of 15 articles. Tips for managing family life on a practical level. Booklet
2003 37 pages
Craig Polhemus, Executive Director

7252 Growth Hormone & Prader-Willi Syndrome: A Reference for Familes & Care Providers
Linda S. Keder, author
Prader-Willi Syndrome Association (USA)
8588 Potter Park Drive   941-312-0400
Sarasota, FL 34238   800-926-4797
                                  Fax: 941-312-0142
                            e-mail: info@pwsausa.com
                                    www.pwsausa.org
Reference for families and care providers.
2001 52 pages
Craig Polhemus, Executive Director

7253 Handbook for Parents
Shirley Neason, author
Prader-Willi Syndrome Association (USA)
8588 Potter Park Drive   941-312-0400
Sarasota, FL 34238   800-926-4797
                                  Fax: 941-312-0142
                            e-mail: info@pwsausa.com
                                    www.pwsausa.org
Parent-to-Parent handbook for understanding and managing issues related to PWS, from birth to adulthood.
1999 75 pages
Craig Polhemus, Executive Director

7254 Nutrition Care for Children with PWS: Infants and Toddlers
J. Hovasi & D. Doorlag, with J. Loker & C. Loker, author
Prader-Willi Syndrome Association (USA)
8588 Potter Park Drive   941-312-0400
Sarasota, FL 34238   800-926-4797
                                  Fax: 941-312-0142
                            e-mail: info@pwsausa.com
                                    www.pwsausa.org
Provides answers to frequently asked questions about nutrition and feeding infants and toddlers with PWS.
2004 62 pages
Craig Polhemus, Executive Director

7255 Sometimes I'm Mad, Sometimes I'm Glad - A Sibling Booklet
Sarah Heinemann, author
Prader-Willi Syndrome Association (USA)
8588 Potter Park Drive   941-312-0400
Sarasota, FL 34238   800-926-4797
                                  Fax: 941-312-0142
                            e-mail: info@pwsausa.com
                                    www.pwsausa.org
Explains sibling relationships and how they are affected by Prader-Willi syndrome. Written in the voice of a sibling of someone with PWS. Ages 5-13
32 pages
Craig Polhemus, Executive Director

7256 Supporting Adults with Prader-Willi Syndro me in a Residential Setting
B.J. Goff, Ed.D, author
Prader-Willi Syndrome Association (USA)
8588 Potter Pass Drive   941-312-0400
Sarasota, FL 34238   800-926-4797
                                  Fax: 941-312-0142
                            e-mail: info@pwsausa.com
                                    www.pwsausa.org
Filling a large gap for care givers of those with Prader-Willi Sydrome, this is an extensive manual covering residential care issues; including management strategies, specifics for phase of life, and a number of additional ideas.
2002 121 pages
Craig Polhemus, Executive Director

Newsletters

7257 Gathered View
Prader-Willi Syndrome Association (USA)
8588 Potter Park Drive   941-312-0400
Sarasota, FL 34238   800-926-4797
                                  Fax: 941-312-0142
                            e-mail: info@pwsausa.com
                                    www.pwsausa.org
The official newsletter of PWSA, mailed 6 time/year to members. Offers current research findings, behavior and weight management techniques, educational news, articles and more.
BiMonthly
Craig Polhemus, Executive Director

Pamphlets

7258 An Early Prader-Willi Syndrome Diagnosis & How to Make it Easier on Parents
Prader-Willi Foundation
40 Holly Lane   516-944-8136
Roslyn Hts, NY 11577-1533   800-253-7993
                                  Fax: 516-944-3173
                 e-mail: foundation@prader-willi.inter.net
                                    www.prader-willi.org
A parent of a child with PWS and an advocate for others with the afflication speaks.

7259 Behavior Management: Collection of Articless
Prader-Willi Syndrome Association (USA)

8588 Potter Park Drive
Sarasota, FL 34238

941-312-0400
800-926-4797
Fax: 941-312-0142
e-mail: info@pwsausa.com
www.pwsausa.org

Includes general articles of behavior concerns, use of psychotropic medications, skin picking and teaching social skills.
2003 49 pages
Craig Polhemus, Executive Director

7260 Educational Choices for Children with PWS
Prader-Willi Foundation
40 Holly Lane
Roslyn Hts, NY 11577-1533

516-944-8136
800-253-7993
Fax: 516-944-3173
e-mail: foundation@prader-willi.inter.net
www.prader-willi.org

Parents of young children with Prader-Willi syndrome discuss their individual philosophies of educational choice - inclusion vs. specialized setting.

7261 Nutrition Care for Adolescents and Adults with PWS
Karenn H. Borgie, MA, RD, author

Prader-Willi Syndrome Association (USA)
8588 Potter Park Drive
Sarasota, FL 34238

941-312-0400
800-926-4797
Fax: 941-312-0142
e-mail: info@pwsausa.com
www.pwsausa.org

covers essential diet information for families, caregivers, and residential service providers.
Craig Polhemus, Executive Director

7262 Nutrition Care for Children with PWS, Ages 3-9
Karen H. Borgie, MA, RD, author

Prader-Willi Syndrome Association (USA)
8588 Potter Park Drive
Sarasota, FL 34238

941-312-0400
800-926-4797
Fax: 941-312-0142
e-mail: info@pwsausa.com
www.pwsausa.org

Discusses calorie needs, supplements, diet planning, food management, and exchange lists. Softvcover.
Craig Polhemus, Executive Director

7263 What Educators Should Know About Prader-Willi Syndrome
Prader-Willi Syndrome Association (USA)
8588 Potter Park Drive
Sarasota, FL 34238

941-312-0400
800-926-4797
Fax: 941-312-0142
e-mail: info@pwsausa.com
www.pwsausa.org

Offers guidelines and strategies for helping the student with PWS stay focused, develop skills and knowledge, and minimize problems associated with the syndrome in the school setting.
Craig Polhemus, Executive Director

Audio & Video

7264 Prader-Willi Syndrome: An Overview for Health Professionals
Prader-Willi Syndrome Association
5700 Midnight Pass Road
Sarasota, FL 34242-3000

941-312-0400
800-926-4797
Fax: 941-312-0142
e-mail: national@pwsausa.org
www.pwsausa.org

Essential viewing for all health care professionals who are not experts on prader-willi syndrome. It deals with all major genetics and health care issues of the child with PWS.
2002

7265 Prader-Willi Syndrome: the Early Years
Prader-Willi Syndrome Association
5700 Midnight Pass Road
Sarasota, FL 34242-3000

941-312-0400
800-926-4797
Fax: 941-312-0142
e-mail: national@pwsausa.org
www.pwsausa.org

Offers help and practical suggestions for those families with a young child newly diagnosed with PWS. Genetics, medical, early intervention and family issues are presented, personalized with family interviews. Although focusing on young children, this video is a wonderful resource for schools and families with children of all ages.
2002

Web Sites

7266 Healthlink USA

www.healthlinkusa.com

Health information concerning treatment, cures, prevention, diagnosis, risk factors, research, support groups, email lists, personal stories and much more. Updated regularly.

7267 MedicineNet

www.medicinenet.com

An online resource for consumers providing easy-to-read, authoritative medical and health information.

7268 Medscape

www.medscape.com

Medscape offers specialists, primary care physicians, and other health professionals the Web's most robust and integrated medical information and educational tools.

Description

7269 Raynaud's Disease

Raynaud's disease is the spasm of blood vessels to fingers and toes, resulting in restricted blood supply in response to cold or emotional upset. Symptoms include tingling and numbness. During an episode, which can last from minutes to hours, the arteries contract briefly and the skin, deprived of oxygen, turns pale and then blue. As arteries relax and blood begins to flow, reddening, tingling, or swelling may occur. While hands and feet are most commonly affected, the nose and ears can also be subject to Raynaud's.

Raynaud's most commonly affects women under 40, accounting for perhaps 90 percent of all cases. When the classic symptoms are present, without other complaints, the condition is referred to as Raynaud's disease (primary Raynaud's), and generally results in no serious consequences. The second form, Raynaud's phenomenon (secondary Raynaud's), is the result of other underlying medical conditions, including scleroderma, vascular disease, rheumatoid arthritis and lupus.

Certain drugs can also trigger Raynaud's, including ergotamine and a number of beta-blocking drugs that are used in the treatment of heart disease. About 10 percent of Raynaud's cases are related to specific repetitive stress activities such as the operation of pneumatic drills and other hand-held vibrating machinery. In most Raynaud's cases, symptoms are discomforting but not serious. In extreme cases, Raynaud's can result in tissue atrophy and gangrene. Preventative measures include protection from cold, even when taking food out of the refrigerator or freezer, and avoiding behavior that disrupts bloodflow, for instance, smoking cigarettes.

Medical treatment of Raynaud's is directed toward improving blood flow to the extremities. In many cases, simple exercises are prescribed, and relaxation techniques, such as biofeedback, teach the body to ignore trivial or transient signals of cold. In other cases, vasodilator drugs which are designed to relax and open blood vessels to improve blood flow are prescribed. In the most extreme cases, surgery may be performed to cut nerves that may be inappropriately triggering the contraction of arteries, although relief may last only 1 to 2 years. Herbal remedies have been used in the treatment of Raynaud's and other circulatory conditions, especially the Chinese herb Dong quai. There is also evidence that foods rich in vitamin E, and fish oils, may help to reduce or moderate the vascular spasms that produce Raynaud's symptoms.

National Agencies & Associations

7270 Arthritis Foundation
1330 W Peachtree Street
Atlanta, GA 30309
404-872-7100
800-283-7800
Fax: 404-872-0457
e-mail: help@arthritis.org
www.arthritis.org

A nonprofit organization that depends on volunteers to provide services to help people with arthritis. Supports research to find ways to cure and prevent arthritis and provides services to improve the quality of life for those affected by arthritis.
Cecile Perich, Chair
John H Klippel MD, President and CEO

7271 Raynaud's Foundation
PO Box 346176
Chicago, IL 60634-6176
773-622-9220
Fax: 773-622-9221
members.aol.com/raynauds/index.ht

The Raynaud's Foundation is a non-profit dedicated to the promotion of education and research Raynaud's Phenomenon and related diseases, both autoimmune and non-autoimmune.
Ida Therese Jablanovec, Executive Director

7272 United Scleroderma Foundation
300 Rosewood Drive
Danvers, MA 01923-0350
978-463-5843
800-722-4673
Fax: 978-463-5809
www.scleroderma.org

Offers materials and referrals conducts workshops and support groups for those with Raynaud's and their families.
Mary Ann Berman, Office Assistant
Liz Dorsett, Communications Manager

Libraries & Resource Centers

7273 Arizona Telemedicine Program
University of Arizona, Health Science Center
PO Box 245105
Tucson, AZ 85724-5105
520-626-4785
Fax: 520-626-1027
e-mail: kerps@email.arizona.edu
www.telemedicine.arizona.edu/index.html

The Arizona Telemedicine Program is a large, multidisciplinary, university-based program that provides telemedicine services, distance learning, informatics training, and telemedicine technology assessment capabilities to communities throughout Arizona, the sixth largest state in the United States, in square miles.
Ronald S Weinstein, MD, Director
Richard A McNeeley, Co-Director

Support Groups & Hotlines

7274 National Health Information Center
PO Box 1133
Washington, DC 20013
310-565-4167
800-336-4797
Fax: 301-984-4256
e-mail: info@nhic.org
www.health.gov/nhic

Offers a nationwide information referral service, produces directories and resource guides.

Books

7275 Raynaud's Phenomenon
Oxford University Press
This is a detailed and technical work on the physiology finger circulation, and on diagnosis and treatment of Raynaud's Phenomenon and Raynaud's Disease. Includes a chapter on Acrocyanosis and Livedo reticularis.
186 pages
ISBN: 0-195057-56-2

Pamphlets

7276 Raynaud's Phenomenon
Arthritis Foundation
PO Box 7669
Atlanta, GA 30357-0669
404-872-7100
800-283-7800
Fax: 404-872-0457

Web Sites

7277 Health Finder

www.healthfinder.gov

Searchable, carefully developed web site offering information on over 1000 topics. Developed by the US Department of Health and Human Services, the site can be used in both English and Spanish.

7278 MedicineNet

www.medicinenet.com

An online resource for consumers providing easy-to-read, authoritative medical and health information.

7279 United Scleroderma Foundation

www.scleroderma.org

Offers materials and referrals, conducts workshops and support groups for those with Raynaud's and their families.

Description

7280 Sarcoidosis

Sarcoidosis is a chronic disease that can affect almost any part of the body. It is characterized by the deposit of small masses of tissue (granulomas) in multiple organs. The cause is unknown, although it is speculated to be related to an immunologic defect or infection. Incidence varies widely between countries. In the United States, sarcoidosis is 10- to 18-fold higher in African Americans than in whites. Most cases start between the ages of 30 and 50 years.

Clinical features vary considerably, depending on the site and extent of involvement. Systemic symptoms may include fatigue, weight loss, loss of appetite and fever. Local symptoms may involve any organ, but the most commonly affected are the lungs, skin, eyes and lymph nodes. If the disease becomes severe and life-threatening, it is usually because of lung involvement. Patients develop cough, wheeze, chest pain and difficulty breathing.

Both the severity and the long-term outlook are extremely variable. In most patients, the disease regresses within 2 years and does not recur. In approximately 25 percent of patients, the disease progresses and causes serious disability. If progressive symptoms require treatment, corticosteroids are usually given. If these are not effective or tolerated, immuno suppressive drugs such as methotrexate or azathioprine may be tried. Approximately 5 percent of patients die of respiratory failure.

National Agencies & Associations

7281 National Sarcoidosis Family Aid and Research Foundation
268 Martin Luther King Boulevard 973-624-4703
Newark, NJ 07102 800-223-6429
Fax: 973-877-2850
www.php.com
Provides information on a rare disease involving inflammation in lymph nodes and other body tissues, usually in young adults.
Mary Ellen Peterson, Executive Director
Melissa King, Program Coordinator

7282 National Sarcoidosis Resource Center
PO Box 1593 732-699-0733
Piscataway, NJ 08855-1593 Fax: 732-699-0882
www.nsrc-global.net
The center provides a national computer database with statistical information and studies, telephone support for patients, subscriptions to national magazines and newsletters and public information provided by mail.
Sandra Conroy, President

7283 Sarcoidosis Networking Program National Sarcoidosis Resource Center
National Sarcoidosis Resource Center
437 Rivercrest Drive 732-699-0733
Piscataway, NJ 08855-1593 800-223-6429
Fax: 732-699-0882
A program meant to educate give encouragement and build public awareness of the illness. Also provides information to encourage the formation of self-help groups and to eliminate the isolation that is often felt by the Sarcoidosis sufferer.

Research Centers

7284 Sarcoidosis Center
6005 Park Avenue 901-761-5877
Memphis, TN 38119 866-727-2643
Fax: 901-761-2280
e-mail: sarcoid@sarcoidcenter.com
www.sarcoidcenter.com
A nonprofit tax exempt organization dedicated to increasing knowledge of the disease sarcoidosis. This broad goal encompasses three main areas: Disseminating information to professionals who assist with treatment of the disease obtaining and dispersing funds to assist with investigation into the cause and treatment of the disease and providing support for individuals afflicted with the disease.

7285 Sarcoidosis Treatment and Research Center Thomas Jefferson University Hospital
Thomas Jefferson University Hospital
111 S 11th Street 215-955-6590
Philadelphia, PA 19107-5092

Support Groups & Hotlines

7286 Better Breather's Clubs
American Lung Association of Virginia
9221 Forest Hill Avenue 804-267-1900
Richmond, VA 23235 800-586-4872
Fax: 804-267-5634
e-mail: chamm@lungva.org
www.lungusa.org
Support Groups for those suffering from chronic obstructive pulmonary disease (COPD) such as emphysema, chronic bronchitis and asthma. In these meetings members give and receive support, and learn more about chronic lung disease from health care professionals who share trends in therapy, medication and other topics, or simply answer members' questions.
Catherine G Hamm, President/Chief Executive Officer
Michelle LaRose, Development Director

7287 Let's Breathe Sarcoidosis Support Group
2225 Foster Street 708-328-9410
Evanston, IL 60201-3353 e-mail: bharris354@aol.com
Brenda Harris, Facilitator

7288 Middle Tennessee Sarcoidosis Support Group
PO Box 1342
Cookesville, TN 38503 931-528-7826
www.tennesseesarcoidosisawareness.org
Becky Robertson, Group Leader

7289 Mount Sinai Sarcoidosis Support Group
One Gustave L. Levy Place
New York, NY 10029 212-241-8733
www.mountsinai.org

7290 National Health Information Center
PO Box 1133 310-565-4167
Washington, DC 20013 800-336-4797
Fax: 301-984-4256
e-mail: info@nhic.org
www.health.gov/nhic
Offers a nationwide information referral service, produces directories and resource guides.

7291 Pacific NW Support Group
Providence Hospital
Casey Room 500 17th Avenue 206-784-9365
Seattle, WA 98107
Ed Girvan, Facilitator

7292 Sarcoidosis HelpNet
PO Box 022642 718-802-1970
Brooklyn, NY 11202 Fax: 212-241-8733
Soneni B Smith, Contact

7293 Sarcoidosis Research Institute (SRI)
3475 Central Avenue
Memphis, TN 38111
901-766-6951
Fax: 901-774-7294
e-mail: sarcoid@sarcoidcenter.com
www.sarcoidcenter.com/saradd.htm
The Sarcoidosis Research Institute is a non-profit, tax-exempt organization dedicated to increasing knowledge of the disease sarcoidosis. This broad goal encompasses three main areas: Disseminating information to professionals who assist with treatment of the disease; Obtaining and dispersing funds to assist with investigation into the cause and treatment of the disease; and, providing support for individuals afflicted with the disease.
Paula Yette Polite, Board of Directors President
Wayne Crook, Vice President Board of Directors

7294 Sarcoidosis Self-Help Group: New York
Nassau County Medical Center
2201 Hempstead Turnpike
East Meadow, NY 11554
516-483-2666
Robert Schoenfeld, Facilitator

7295 Sarcoidosis Self-Help Group: Virginia
American Lung Association of Northern Virginia
9735 Main Street
Fairfax, VA 22031
703-591-4131
Carolyn Thomas, Facilitator

7296 Sarcoidosis Support Group Delaware
American Lung Association of Delaware
1021 Gilpin Avenue
Wilmington, DE 19806
302-655-7258
800-586-4872
Fax: 302-655-8546
e-mail: dbrown@alade.org
www.alade.org
Peter Shanley, Chairman
Martha Bogdan, President/CEO

7297 Sarcoidosis Support Group: New Jersey
268 Dr. ML King Boulevard
Newark, NJ 07106
201-374-7570
Jean Curlin-Miller, Facilitator

7298 Sarcoidosis Support Group: Washington DC
110 Irving Street
Washington, DC 20010
202-877-6286
Fax: 202-877-5779
Carol Bartlett

7299 Triangle Area Sarcoidosis Support Group
Soapstone UM Church
12837 Norwood Road
Raleigh, NC 27613
919-676-6498
e-mail: fairleyl@bellsouth.net
Priscilla Fairley, Facilitator

7300 Understanding Sarcoidosis Self-Help Group
2112 Highland Avenue
New Castle, PA 16105
412-652-6089
Della Emmanuel

7301 University of North Carolina Sarcoidosis Support Group
UNC Chapel Hill Healthcare
130 Mason Farm Road
Chapel Hill, NC 27599
919-966-2531
e-mail: sharikia_burt@med.unc.edu
Sharikia Burt, Clinical Coordinator

7302 West Tennessee Sarcoidosis Support Group
1670 McLemoresville Road
Huntington, TN 38344
731-986-9832
www.tennesseesarcoidosisawareness.org
Patricia Coleman, Group Leader

Books

7303 Sarcoidosis Resource Guide and Directory
PC Publications
PO Box 1593
Piscataway, NJ 08855-1593
732-699-0733
Fax: 732-699-0882
1993 304 pages Paperback
ISBN: 0-963122-25-8

Newsletters

7304 Online Sarcoidosis Newsletter
National Sarcoidosis Resource Center
PO Box 1593
Piscataway, NJ 08855-1593
732-699-0733
Fax: 732-699-0882
Offers information on the center's activities and events, medical and legislative updates for the patients and their families.
Quarterly

Pamphlets

7305 Anemia of Sarcoidosis
PC Publications
PO Box 1593
Piscataway, NJ 08855-1593
732-699-0733
800-223-6429
Fax: 732-699-0882

7306 Bronchoalveolar Lymphocytes in Sarcoidosis
PC Publications
PO Box 1593
Piscataway, NJ 08855-1593
732-699-0733
800-223-6429
Fax: 732-699-0882

7307 Case Report: MR Imaging of Myocardial Sarcoidosis
PC Publications
PO Box 1593
Piscataway, NJ 08855-1593
732-699-0733
800-223-6429
Fax: 732-699-0882

7308 Case Report: Osseous Sarcoidosis and Chronic Polyarthritis
PC Publications
PO Box 1593
Piscataway, NJ 08855-1593
732-699-0733
800-223-6429
Fax: 732-699-0882

7309 Case Report: Overlap of Granulomatous Vasculitis and Sarcoidosis
PC Publications
PO Box 1593
Piscataway, NJ 08855-1593
732-699-0733
800-223-6429
Fax: 732-699-0882

7310 Case Report: Rapidly Dev. Confusion, Impaired Memory and Unsteady Gait
PC Publications
PO Box 1593
Piscataway, NJ 08855-1593
732-699-0733
800-223-6429
Fax: 732-699-0882

7311 Coping with Sarcoidosis
National Sarcoidosis Resource Center
PO Box 1593
Piscataway, NJ 08855-1593
732-699-0733
800-223-6429
Fax: 732-699-0882
A pamphlet offering information on how to manage and live with sarcoidosis.

7312 Disability Law: A Legal Primer
PC Publications
PO Box 1593
Piscataway, NJ 08855-1593
732-699-0733
800-223-6429
Fax: 732-699-0882

7313 Drugs That Have Been Used for the Treatment of Sarcoidosis
PC Publications
PO Box 1593
Piscataway, NJ 08855-1593
732-699-0733
800-223-6429
Fax: 732-699-0882

7314 Effect of Corticosteroid or Methotrexate Therapy on Lung Lymphocytes
PC Publications
PO Box 1593
Piscataway, NJ 08855-1593
732-699-0733
800-223-6429
Fax: 732-699-0882

7315 Effects of Sarcoid and Steroids on Angiotensin-Converting Enzyme
PC Publications

PO Box 1593   732-699-0733
Piscataway, NJ 08855-1593   800-223-6429
    Fax: 732-699-0882

7316 Evaluation of the Efficacy and Toxicity of the Cyclosporine
PC Publications
PO Box 1593   732-699-0733
Piscataway, NJ 08855-1593   800-223-6429
    Fax: 732-699-0882

7317 Gastrointestinal Presentation of Churg Strauss Syndrome
PC Publications
PO Box 1593   732-699-0733
Piscataway, NJ 08855-1593   800-223-6429
    Fax: 732-699-0882

7318 Governor New Jersey Proclamation: Sarcoidosis Awareness Day
PC Publications
PO Box 1593   732-699-0733
Piscataway, NJ 08855-1593   800-223-6429
    Fax: 732-699-0882

7319 How to Get the Most Out of Your Doctor: A Neurologist's Perspective
PC Publications
PO Box 1593   732-699-0733
Piscataway, NJ 08855-1593   800-223-6429
    Fax: 732-699-0882

7320 Ideas and Considerations for Starting a Self-Help Mutual Aid Group
PC Publications
PO Box 1593   732-699-0733
Piscataway, NJ 08855-1593   800-223-6429
    Fax: 732-699-0882

7321 Masqueraders of Sarcoidosis
PC Publications
PO Box 1593   732-699-0733
Piscataway, NJ 08855-1593   800-223-6429
    Fax: 732-699-0882

7322 Mayor Piscataway, NJ Proclamation: Sarcoidosis Awareness Day
PC Publications
PO Box 1593   732-699-0733
Piscataway, NJ 08855-1593   800-223-6429
    Fax: 732-699-0882

7323 Multidisciplinary Clinico-Pathologic Conference
PC Publications
PO Box 1593   732-699-0733
Piscataway, NJ 08855-1593   800-223-6429
    Fax: 732-699-0882

7324 National Sarcoidosis Resource Center
PC Publications
PO Box 1593   732-699-0733
Piscataway, NJ 08855-1593   Fax: 732-699-0882
    www.nsrc-global.net
A booklet offering a brief introduction to the illness and offers information on the role of the Center in finding a cure and educating the public on Sarcoidosis.

7325 Neurosarcoidosis
PC Publications
PO Box 1593   732-699-0733
Piscataway, NJ 08855-1593   800-223-6429
    Fax: 732-699-0882

7326 Neurosarcoidosis or Multiple Sclerosis?
National Sarcoidosis Resource Center
PO Box 1593   732-699-0733
Piscataway, NJ 08855-1593   800-223-6429
    Fax: 732-699-0882

7327 Paranoid Psychosis Due to Neurosarcoidosis
PC Publications
PO Box 1593   732-699-0733
Piscataway, NJ 08855-1593   800-223-6429
    Fax: 732-699-0882

7328 Patient Information Package
National Sarcoidosis Resource Center

PO Box 1593   732-699-0733
Piscataway, NJ 08855-1593   800-223-6429
    Fax: 732-699-0882
Contains various brochures and pamphlets offering information about Sarcoidosis.

7329 Physician Listings
PC Publications
PO Box 1593   732-699-0733
Piscataway, NJ 08855-1593   800-223-6429
    Fax: 732-699-0882

7330 Possible Association of Rheumatoid Arthritis & Sarcoidosis
PC Publications
PO Box 1593   732-699-0733
Piscataway, NJ 08855-1593   800-223-6429
    Fax: 732-699-0882

7331 Presidential Proclamation - National Sarcoidosis Awareness Day
PC Publications
PO Box 1593   732-699-0733
Piscataway, NJ 08855-1593   800-223-6429
    Fax: 732-699-0882

7332 Psychological Factors in Sarcoidosis
PC Publications
PO Box 1593   732-699-0733
Piscataway, NJ 08855-1593   800-223-6429
    Fax: 732-699-0882

7333 Public Law 102-94
PC Publications
PO Box 1593   732-699-0733
Piscataway, NJ 08855-1593   800-223-6429
    Fax: 732-699-0882

7334 Pulmonary Sarcoidosis: Evaluation with High Resolution
PC Publications
PO Box 1593   732-699-0733
Piscataway, NJ 08855-1593   800-223-6429
    Fax: 732-699-0882

7335 Pulmonary Sarcoidosis: What We Are Learning
PC Publications
PO Box 1593   732-699-0733
Piscataway, NJ 08855-1593   800-223-6429
    Fax: 732-699-0882

7336 Questionnaire Responses for Demographics and Symptoms from 1000 Patients
PC Publications
PO Box 1593   732-699-0733
Piscataway, NJ 08855-1593   800-223-6429
    Fax: 732-699-0882

7337 Right & Left Ventricular Function at Rest in Patients with Sarcoidosis
PC Publications
PO Box 1593   732-699-0733
Piscataway, NJ 08855-1593   800-223-6429
    Fax: 732-699-0882

7338 Role of Magnetic Resonance Imaging in Neurosarcoidosis
PC Publications
PO Box 1593   732-699-0733
Piscataway, NJ 08855-1593   800-223-6429
    Fax: 732-699-0882

7339 Sarcoidosis
PC Publications
PO Box 1593   732-699-0733
Piscataway, NJ 08855-1593   800-223-6429
    Fax: 732-699-0882
Offers information on the illness, causes, symptoms and treatments.

7340 Sarcoidosis Diagnosed in a Patient with Known HIV Infection
PC Publications
PO Box 1593   732-699-0733
Piscataway, NJ 08855-1593   800-223-6429
    Fax: 732-699-0882

7341   Sarcoidosis Patient Questionnaire
PC Publications
PO Box 1593   732-699-0733
Piscataway, NJ 08855-1593   800-223-6429
Fax: 732-699-0882

7342   Sarcoidosis Questionnaire: Demographics and Symptomatology-The Patients Respond
PC Publications
PO Box 1593   732-699-0733
Piscataway, NJ 08855-1593   800-223-6429
Fax: 732-699-0882

7343   Sarcoidosis and Pregnancy: Clinical Observation
PC Publications
PO Box 1593   732-699-0733
Piscataway, NJ 08855-1593   800-223-6429
Fax: 732-699-0882

7344   Sarcoidosis and You: A Listing of Possible Symptoms
PC Publications
PO Box 1593   732-699-0733
Piscataway, NJ 08855-1593   800-223-6429
Fax: 732-699-0882

7345   Sarcoidosis in India: A Review of 125 Biopsy-Proven Cases from India
PC Publications
PO Box 1593   732-699-0733
Piscataway, NJ 08855-1593   800-223-6429
Fax: 732-699-0882

7346   Sarcoidosis of the Liver
PC Publications
PO Box 1593   732-699-0733
Piscataway, NJ 08855-1593   800-223-6429
Fax: 732-699-0882

7347   Sarcoidosis: A Multisystem Disease
PC Publications
PO Box 1593   732-699-0733
Piscataway, NJ 08855-1593   800-223-6429
Fax: 732-699-0882
Explains the effects of the illness on the lungs and joints.

7348   Sarcoidosis: International Review
PC Publications
PO Box 1593   732-699-0733
Piscataway, NJ 08855-1593   800-223-6429
Fax: 732-699-0882

7349   Sarcoidosis: Pleural Involvement Mimicking a Coin Lesson
PC Publications
PO Box 1593   732-699-0733
Piscataway, NJ 08855-1593   800-223-6429
Fax: 732-699-0882

7350   Sarcoidosis: Usual and Unusual Manifestations
PC Publications
PO Box 1593   732-699-0733
Piscataway, NJ 08855-1593   800-223-6429
Fax: 732-699-0882

7351   Seasonal Clustering of Sarcoidosis
National Sarcoidosis Resource Center
PO Box 1593   732-699-0733
Piscataway, NJ 08855-1593   800-223-6429
Fax: 732-699-0882

7352   Successful Treatment of Myocardial Sarcoidosis with Steriods
PC Publications
PO Box 1593   732-699-0733
Piscataway, NJ 08855-1593   800-223-6429
Fax: 732-699-0882

7353   Support Group Listing
PC Publications
PO Box 1593   732-699-0733
Piscataway, NJ 08855-1593   800-223-6429
Fax: 732-699-0882

7354   Use of Low Dose Methotrexate in Refractory Sarcoidosis
PC Publications
PO Box 1593   732-699-0733
Piscataway, NJ 08855-1593   800-223-6429
Fax: 732-699-0882

7355   World Association Sarcoidosi Other Granulatomous
PC Publications
PO Box 1593   732-699-0733
Piscataway, NJ 08855-1593   800-223-6429
Fax: 732-699-0882

Audio & Video

7356   Dialogue with Doris
PC Publications
PO Box 1593   732-699-0733
Piscataway, NJ 08855-1593   800-223-6429
Fax: 732-699-0882

7357   Help with a Hidden Disease Update
PC Publications
PO Box 1593   732-699-0733
Piscataway, NJ 08855-1593   800-223-6429
Fax: 732-699-0882

7358   Of Their Own: Person to Person Show
PC Publications
PO Box 1593   732-699-0733
Piscataway, NJ 08855-1593   800-223-6429
Fax: 732-699-0882

7359   Sarcoidosis Conference 2
PC Publications
PO Box 1593   732-699-0733
Piscataway, NJ 08855-1593   800-223-6429
Fax: 732-699-0882

7360   Sarcoidosis Conference 3
PC Publications
PO Box 1593   732-699-0733
Piscataway, NJ 08855-1593   800-223-6429
Fax: 732-699-0882

7361   Sarcoidosis and Lyme Disease
PC Publications
PO Box 1593   732-699-0733
Piscataway, NJ 08855-1593   800-223-6429
Fax: 732-699-0882

7362   Sarcoidosis: What's That?
PC Publications
PO Box 1593   732-699-0733
Piscataway, NJ 08855-1593   800-223-6429
Fax: 732-699-0882

7363   XIV International World Conference on Sarcoidosis: Patient Symposium
PC Publications
PO Box 1593   732-699-0733
Piscataway, NJ 08855-1593   800-223-6429
Fax: 732-699-0882
Cassette.

Web Sites

7364   Healing Well
www.healingwell.com
An online health resource guide to medical news, chat, information and articles, newsgroups and message boards, books, disease-related web sites, medical directories, and more for patients, friends, and family coping with disabling diseases, disorders, or chronic illnesses.

7365   Health Finder
www.healthfinder.gov
Searchable, carefully developed web site offering information on over 1000 topics. Developed by the US Department of Health and Human Services, the site can be used in both English and Spanish.

7366 Healthlink USA

www.healthlinkusa.com

Health information concerning treatment, cures, prevention, diagnosis, risk factors, research, support groups, email lists, personal stories and much more. Updated regularly.

7367 Helios Health

www.helioshealth.com

Online resource for your health information. Detailed information about specific health topics, access to expert advice from our Medical Advisory Board, and up-to-date health news.

7368 MedicineNet

www.medicinenet.com

An online resource for consumers providing easy-to-read, authoritative medical and health information.

7369 Medscape

www.medscape.com

Medscape offers specialists, primary care physicians, and other health professionals the Web's most robust and integrated medical information and educational tools.

7370 National Sarcoidosis Resource Center

www.nsrc-global.net

Provides the general public with sarcoidosis information, for patients to obtain medical and emotional help and to provide government officials with the information they need.

7371 WebMD

www.webmd.com

Information on sarcoidosis, including articles and resources.

Description

7372 Scleroderma

Scleroderma, literally "hard skin", is a form of systemic sclerosis, a generalized disturbance of connective and vascular tissue which leads to scarring (sclerosis). Scleroderma is a rare disease, with about 5,000 new cases in the United States each year. Women are 3 or 4 times as likely as men to get the disease, which typically begins between the ages of 30 and 50 years. It is comparatively rare in children. The cause of the disease is unknown.

Since almost any organ may be involved, the list of possible symptoms is extensive. Important ones include weakness, fatigue, stiffness, weight loss, shortness of breath, abdominal bloating and pain, diarrhea and irritation of the eyes. Kidney involvement usually causes abrupt acceleration of high blood pressure. A very characteristic symptom, although not unique to this disease, is Raynaud's phenomenon. On exposure to cold, the arteries of the patient's hands and feet contract, causing the skin color to change from red, to white (blanch), to blue (cyanosis), accompanied by pain and numbness.

If the disease is limited to the skin the outlook is good, but involvement of lung and kidney in the systemic form may be fatal. Use of the ACE inhibitor class of anti-hypertensive drugs has helped preserve kidney function. Many immunosuppressive drugs have been tried without clear success. Clinical trials of new agents are often available to patients. When end-stage kidney disease cannot be prevented, dialysis and transplant can be used, although the death rate remains high.

National Agencies & Associations

7373 Canadian Dermatology Association
1385 Bank Street 613-738-1748
Ottawa, Ontario, K1H-8N4 800-267-3376
Fax: 613-738-4695
e-mail: contact.cda@dermatology.ca
www.dermatology.ca
Ensure the Canadian public has equal access to timely and exemplary dermatologic care, by advocating on dermatologic issues, providing leadership in continuing medical and public education, and promoting and disseminating dermatologic knowledge and research.
Dr Louis Weatherhead, President of the Board
Dr Laurence Warshawski, President of the Board

7374 Scleroderma Foundation
300 Rosewood Drive 978-463-5843
Danvers, MA 01923 800-722-4673
Fax: 978-463-5809
e-mail: sfinfo@scleroderma.org
www.scleroderma.org
A national nonprofit organization serving the interests of persons with Scleroderma. The Foundation's 26 chapters and 135 support groups nationwide help to carry out its three-fold mission of support, education and research.
Joseph Camerino, Chair
Carol Feghali-Bostwi, Vice Chair

7375 Scleroderma Society of Ontario
393 University Avenue 800-321-1433
Toronto, Ontario, M5G-1E6 Fax: 416-979-8366
www.sclerodermaontario.ca

Committed to promoting increased public awareness, advancing patient wellness and supporting research in scleroderma.
Carroll Vapsva, Scleroderma Society Canada Liaison
Peter Woolcott, President of the Board

State Agencies & Associations

Arizona

7376 Scleroderma Foundation: Arizona Chapter
18402 N 19th Avenue 623-847-3757
Phoenix, AZ 85023 e-mail: carolnader@cox.net
Local chapter of the national Scleroderma Foundation in Byfield, Massachusetts. Please contact this group for information on area support groups.
Carol Nader, President

California

7377 Scleroderma Foundation: Greater San Diego Chapter
8748 Cherry Hills Road 619-448-6301
Santee, CA 92071 e-mail: GSDchapter@scleroderma.org
www.scleroderma.org
Local chapter of the national Scleroderma Foundation in Byfield, Massachusetts. Please contact this group for information on area support groups.
Fletcher Diehl, President
Carol Ireland, Vice President

7378 Scleroderma Foundation: Northern California Chapter
PO Box 601313 916-832-1102
Sacramento, CA 95860-1313 e-mail: NoCAchapter@scleroderma.org
www.scleroderma.org
Local chapter of the national Scleroderma Foundation in Byfield, Massachusetts. Please contact this group for information on area support groups.
Cathy Eddy, President
Cheryl George, Vice President

7379 Scleroderma Foundation: Southern California Chapter (& LA Area)
11704 Wilshire Boulevard 310-477-8225
Los Angeles, CA 90025 877-443-5755
Fax: 310-477-8774
e-mail: SoCAchapter@scleroderma.org
www.scleroderma.org
Local chapter of the national Scleroderma Foundation in Byfield, Massachusetts. Please contact this group for information on area support groups.
Brian Ross Adams, Executive Director
Dan Furst, President

Colorado

7380 Scleroderma Foundation: Colorado Chapter
2280 S Albion Street 303-806-6686
Denver, CO 80222-0940 e-mail: COchapter@scleroderma.org
www.scleroderma.org
Local chapter of the national Scleroderma Foundation in Danvers, Massachusetts. Please contact this group for information on area support groups.
Rita Miller, President
Fran Penk, Vice President

Connecticut

7381 Scleroderma Foundation: Tri-State Chapter
Binghamton, NY 201-837-9826
800-867-0885
e-mail: sdtristate@aol.com
Local chapter of the national Scleroderma Foundation in Byfield, Massachusetts. Please contact this group for information on area support groups.
Rosemary Markoff, President

Delaware

7382 Scleroderma Foundation: Delaware Valley Chapter
385 Kings Highway N
Cherry Hill, NJ 08034
732-449-7001
866-675-5545
e-mail: DVchapter@scleroderma.org
www.scleroderma.org
Local chapter of the national Scleroderma Foundation in Byfield, Massachusetts. Please contact this group for information on area support groups.
Melissa Kuscher, Executive Director
Colleen Ferara, Administrative Assistant

District of Columbia

7383 Scleroderma Foundation: Greater Washington DC Chapter
2010 Corporate Ridge
McLean, VA 22102
888-233-4779
e-mail: carolsod@att.net
Local chapter of the national Scleroderma Foundation in Byfield, Massachusetts. Please contact this group for information on area support groups.
Carol Sodetz, President

Florida

7384 Scleroderma Foundation: Southeast Florida Chapter
6145 NW 123rd Lane
Coral Springs, FL 33076-3913
954-255-8335
Fax: 954-255-8081
e-mail: SEFLchapter@scleroderma.org
www.scleroderma.org
Local chapter of the national Scleroderma Foundation in Byfield, Massachusetts. Please contact this group for information on area support groups.
Berna Falkoff, President
Ruth Greenspan, Vice - Chair

Georgia

7385 Scleroderma Foundation: Georgia Chapter Scleroderma Foundation
Scleroderma Foundation

800-722-4673
e-mail: swright@cleroderma.org
www.scleroderma.org
Local chapter of the national Scleroderma Foundation in Byfield, Massachusetts. Call the national office for contact information on the Georgia Chapter. Please contact this group for information on area support groups.
Stacy Wright, Contact
Mary Haulk, Contact

Illinois

7386 Scleroderma Foundation: Greater Chicago Chapter
203 N Wabash Street
Chicago, IL 60601
312-660-1131
Fax: 312-660-1133
e-mail: GCchapter@scleroderma.org
www.scleroderma.org
Local chapter of the national Scleroderma Foundation. Please contact group for information on area support groups.
Mike Robbins, President

Maine

7387 Scleroderma Foundation: New England Chapter
462 Boston Street
Topsfield, MA 01983
888-525-0658
e-mail: sclfndne@aol.com
Local chapter of the national Scleroderma Foundation in Byfield, Massachusetts. Please contact this group for information on area support groups. Includes MA, ME, NH, VT, & RI.
Marie Coyle, President

Maryland

7388 Scleroderma Foundation: Greater Washington DC Chapter
2010 Corporate Ridge
McLean, VA 22102
888-233-4779
e-mail: carolsod@att.net
Local chapter of the national Scleroderma Foundation in Byfield, Massachusetts. Please contact this group for information on area support groups.
Carol Sodetz, President

Massachusetts

7389 Scleroderma Foundation: New England Chapter
462 Boston Street
Topsfield, MA 01983
888-525-0658
e-mail: sclfndne@aol.com
Local chapter of the national Scleroderma Foundation in Byfield, Massachusetts. Please contact this group for information on area support groups.
Marie Coyle, President

Michigan

7390 Scleroderma Foundation: Michigan Chapter
23999 Telegraph
Southfield, MI 48033
800-716-6554
e-mail: MIchapter@scleroderma.org
www.scleroderma.org/chapters/michigan
Local chapter of the national Scleroderma Foundation in Danvers, Massachusetts. Please contact this group for information on area support groups, medical referrals, conference dates and fund raising activities.
Laura Dyas, Executive Director
Janus Landrum, Executive Assistant

Minnesota

7391 Scleroderma Foundation: Minnesota Chapter
5775 Wayzata Boulevard
Saint Louis Park, MN 55416
952-525-2273
877-794-0347
e-mail: MNChapter@scleroderma.org
www.scleroderma.org
Local chapter of the national Scleroderma Foundation in Byfield, Massachusetts. Please contact this group for information on area support groups.
Lee Roy Jones, President
Chris Woo, Executive Director

Missouri

7392 Scleroderma Foundation: Missouri Chapter
Springfield, MO 65808
417-887-3269
e-mail: MOchapter@scleroderma.org
www.scleroderma.org
Local chapter of the national Scleroderma Foundation in Byfield, Massachusetts. Please contact this group for information on area support groups.
Mary Blades, President
Ben Blades, Vice President

Nevada

7393 Scleroderma Foundation: Nevada Chapter
6760 Surrey Street
Las Vegas, NV 89119
702-368-1572
e-mail: NVchapter@scleroderma.org
www.scleroderma.org
Local chapter of the national Scleroderma Foundation in Byfield, Massachusetts. Please contact this group for information on area support groups.
Barbara Dempsey, President
Sheila Gray, VP Support Group

New Hampshire

7394 Scleroderma Foundation: New England Chapter
462 Boston Street
Topsfield, MA 01983
888-525-0658
e-mail: sclfndne@aol.com

Local chapter of the national Scleroderma Foundation in Byfield, Massachusetts. Please contact this group for information on area support groups.
Marie Coyle, President

New Jersey

7395 Scleroderma Foundation: Tri-State Chapter
59 Front Street
Binghamton, NY 13905
607-723-2239
800-867-0885
Fax: 607-723-2039
e-mail: chribar@scleroderma.org
www.scleroderma.org
Local chapter of the national Scleroderma Foundation in Byfield, Massachusetts. Please contact this group for information on area support groups.
Jeff Mace, President
Corey Hribar, Executive Director

New York

7396 Scleroderma Foundation: Central New York Chapter
59 Front Street
Binghamton, NY 13905
607-723-2239
e-mail: chribar@scleroderma.org
www.scleroderma.org
Local chapter of the national Scleroderma Foundation in Byfield, Massachusetts. Please contact this group for information on area support groups.
Corey Hribar, Executive Director
Tom Knapp, Office Manage

7397 Scleroderma Foundation: Tri-State Chapter
59 Front Street
Binghamton, NY 13905
607-723-2239
800-867-0885
Fax: 607-723-2039
e-mail: chribar@scleroderma.org
www.scleroderma.org
Local chapter of the national Scleroderma Foundation in Byfield, Massachusetts. Please contact this group for information on area support groups.
Jeff Mace, President
Corey Hribar, Executive Director

7398 Scleroderma Foundation: Western New York Chapter
PO Box 708
Hamburg, NY 14075
716-627-2283
877-969-2478
e-mail: wnychpt@aol.com
www.scleroderma.org
Local chapter of the national Scleroderma Foundation in Byfield, Massachusetts. Please contact this group for information on area support groups.
Laura Henry, Co-President

Ohio

7399 Scleroderma Foundation: Ohio Chapter
PO Box 846
Hilliard, OH 43026-0846
614-334-0846
866-849-9030
e-mail: OHchapter@scleroderma.org
www.scleroderma.org
Local chapter of the national Scleroderma Foundation in Byfield, Massachusetts. Please contact this group for information on area support groups.
Mariann Boyanowski, President
Amelia Yaussy, Past President

Oregon

7400 Scleroderma Foundation: Oregon Chapter
PO Box 19296
Portland, OR 97280-0296
503-246-0235
e-mail: ORchapter@scleroderma.org
www.scleroderma.org
Local chapter of the national Scleroderma Foundation in Byfield, Massachusetts. Please contact this group for information on area support groups.
Liz Orem-Bedel, Vice President
Richard Bates, President

Pennsylvania

7401 Scleroderma Foundation: Delaware Valley Chapter
385 Kings Highway N
Cherry Hill, NJ 08034
732-449-7001
866-675-5545
e-mail: DVchapter@scleroderma.org
www.scleroderma.org
Local chapter of the national Scleroderma Foundation in Byfield, Massachusetts. Please contact this group for information on area support groups.
Melissa Kuscher, Executive Director
Colleen Ferara, Administrative Assistant

7402 Scleroderma Foundation: Western Pennsylvania Chapter
3500 Terrace Street
Pittsburgh, PA 15261
724-869-2515
800-722-4673
e-mail: WPAchapter@scleroderma.org
www.scleroderma.org
Local chapter of the national Scleroderma Foundation in Byfield, Massachusetts. Please contact this group for information on area support groups.
Betty Aquino, President
Thomas A Medsger Jr, Treasurer

Rhode Island

7403 Scleroderma Foundation: New England Chapter
462 Boston Street
Topsfield, MA 01983
888-525-0658
e-mail: sclfndne@aol.com
Local chapter of the national Scleroderma Foundation in Byfield, Massachusetts. Please contact this group for information on area support groups.
Marie Coyle, President

South Carolina

7404 Scleroderma Foundation: South Carolina Chapter
1027 S Pendleton Street
Easley, SC 29642
843-832-9486
866-557-3729
e-mail: SCchapter@scleroderma.org
www.scleroderma.org
Local chapter of the national Scleroderma Foundation in Byfield. Massachusetts. Please contact this group for information on area support groups.
Amy Parrish, President
Dolores Collins, Vice President

Tennessee

7405 Scleroderma Foundation: Tennessee Chapter
PO Box 2844
Hendersonville, TN 37077
615-792-4610
800-497-5193
Fax: 615-792-4610
e-mail: TNchapter@scleroderma.org
www.scleroderma.org
Local chapter of the national Scleroderma Foundation in Byfield, Massachusetts. Please contact this group for information on area support groups.
April Simpkins, President
Charles Cowell, Vice President

Texas

7406 Scleroderma Foundation: Bluebonnet Chapter
PO Box 1836
Allen, TX 75013-1894
972-396-9400
866-532-7673
Fax: 972-649-7910
e-mail: TXchapter@scleroderma.org
www.scleroderma.org
Local chapter of the national Scleroderma Foundation in Byfield, Massachusetts. Please contact this group for information on area support groups.
Cindi Brannum, President
Peggy Brown, Vice President

Vermont

7407 Scleroderma Foundation: New England Chapter
462 Boston Street
Topsfield, MA 01983
978-887-0658
888-525-0658
Fax: 978-887-0659
e-mail: sclfndne@aol.com
www.scleroderma.org
Local chapter of the national Scleroderma Foundation in Byfield, Massachusetts. Please contact this group for information on area support groups.
Marie Coyle, President
Tom Curran, Executive Director

Virginia

7408 Scleroderma Foundation: Greater Washington DC Chapter
2010 Corporate Ridge
McLean, VA 22102
703-938-2191
888-233-4779
e-mail: GWDCchapter@scleroderma.org
www.scleroderma.org
Local chapter of the national Scleroderma Foundation in Byfield, Massachusetts. Please contact this group for information on area support groups.
Carol Sodetz, President
Fi Fi J Lin, Vice President

Washington

7409 Scleroderma Foundation: Evergreen Chapter
PO Box 84506
Seattle, WA 98124-5806
206-285-9822
e-mail: WAchapter@scleroderma.org
www.scleroderma.org
Local chapter of the national Scleroderma Foundation in Byfield, Massachusetts. Please contact this group for information on area support groups.
Bunny Garthe, President
Nic Evans, Vice President

Foundations

7410 Juvenile Scleroderma Network
1204 W 13th Street
San Pedro, CA 90731
310-519-9511
866-338-5892
e-mail: OutreachJSDN@jsdn.org
www.jsdn.org
Organization that is working to provide educational programs about JSD, and to help children and their families to gain a better understanding.
Jerry Gaither, Chairman
Kathy Gaither, President

Research Centers

7411 Boston University University Medical Center
University Medical Center
One Boston Medical Center Place
Boston, MA 02118
617-638-8000
Fax: 617-385-26
www.bmc.org
Ongoing clinical trials and studies in scleroderma. Office hours by appointment.
Melynn Nuite RN, Clinical Trails Contact
Elaine Ullian, President/CEO

7412 Center for Rheumatology
1367 Washington Avenue
Albany, NY 12206
518-489-4471
e-mail: cbarr@joint-docs.com
www.joint-docs.com
This is a committed research facility as well as a medical practice. Our research practice is made up of seven physicians a certified physician's assistant and four research coordinators. We may have as many as 20 ongoing trails at a time in various indications within the study of rheumatology. Investigational treatment of interstitial lung disease associated with systemic sclerosis.
Norman R Romanoff, Practitioner
Joel M Kremer, Practitioner

7413 Georgetown University Hospital: Department of Rheumatology
3800 Reservoir Road NW
Washington, DC 20007
202-444-8233
Fax: 202-444-8579
www.medicine.georgetown.edu
Research is based on clinical trials and special interest in scleroderma and kidney pulmonary hypertension pregnancy epidemiology and natural history of scleroderma subsets.
Thomas R Cupps, Division Chief
James N Baraniuk, Associate Professor

7414 Johns Hopkins University: Scleroderma Center
Johns Hopkins Bayview Medical Center
5501 Hopkins Bayview Circle
Baltimore, MD 21224
410-550-7715
Fax: 410-550-1363
www.scleroderma.jhmi.edu
Specializes in the management of systemic sclerosis (scleroderma) Raynaud's phenomenon and related disorders. In addition to patient care the center is involved in both basic and clinical research projects.
Frederick M Wigley MD, Director
Barbara Whit MD, Director

7415 Mayo Clinic Scottsdale Center for Scleroderma Care & Research
Mayo Clinic
13400 E Shea Boulevard
Scottsdale, AZ 85259
480-301-8000
Fax: 480-301-7006
www.mayoclinic.org/rheumatology
Integrates multiple medical as well as surgical specialties under the direction of the Division of Rheumatology to provide coordinated and comprehensive evaluations and treatment. New clinical trails are in development.
Lester Mertz MD, Assistant Professor of Medicine
April Chang-Miller, Assistant Professor of Medicine

7416 Medical University of South Carolina Medical University of South Carolina
Medical University of South Carolina
96 Johnathan Lucas Street
Charleston, SC 29403
843-792-2300
800-424-MUSC
Fax: 843-792-2601
e-mail: wickman@musc.edu
www.musc.edu
Actively engaged in basic and clinical research of scleroderma.
Richard M Silver, Director of Rheumatology and Immunology
W Stuart Smith, Vice President for Clinical Operations a

7417 Scleroderma Clinical & Research Center State University of New York at Stonybro
State University of New York at Stonybrook
26 Research Way
E Setauket, NY 01173-9260
631-444-6345
Fax: 631-444-0562
Ongoing research of scleroderma.

7418 Scleroderma Research Foundation
220 Montgomery Street
San Francisco, CA 94104
415-834-9444
800-637-4005
Fax: 415-834-9177
e-mail: info@sclerodermaresearch.org
www.srfcure.org
Mission is to find a cure for scleroderma a life threatening and degenerative illness by funding and facilitating the most promising highest quality research and placing the disease and its need for a cure in the public eye.
Luke Evnin PhD, Chairman
Nancy Bechtle, Member of Board of Directors

7419 Thomas Jefferson University Hospital
111 S 11th Street
Philadelphia, PA 19107
215-955-6000
Fax: 215-923-5828
www.jeffersonhospital.org
Provides diagnostic evaluations treatment and access to the latest research studies for more than one thousand patients with scleroderma and related diseases.
Oscar Irigoyen, Director Division of Rheumatology
Sergio Jimen MD, Professor

7420 University of Alabama Birmingham
6th Avenue S
Birmingham, AL 35294
205-934-4011
Fax: 205-755-54
www.uab.edu

Located in the Clinical Immunology and Rheumatology department Oral Type 1 Collagen in Scleroderma is studied.
Carol Garrison, President
William Ferniany, CEO

7421 University of Chicago Center for Advanced Medicine Duchossis Center
University of Chicago hospital
5841 S Maryland Avenue
Chicago, IL 60637
773-702-1000
888-UCH-0200
Fax: 773-028-02
e-mail: orogers@medicine.bsd.uchicago.edu
www.uchospitals.com
Scleroderma clinic.
Michael Ellm MD, Clinic Contact
Ornery Rogers, Clinic Contact

7422 University of Illinois at Chicago Medical Center Outpatient Clinical Center
University of Illinois
600 S Hoyne Avenue
Chicago, IL 60612
312-996-7000
800-UIC-1002
Fax: 312-633-3434
TTY: 312-413-0123
e-mail: info@iMDc.org
www.uic.edu
Scleroderma clinic held on the first and third Thursdays of every month.
Sylvia Manning, Chancellor
Michael R Tanner, Provost and Vice Chancellor for Academic

7423 University of Pittsburgh
3500 Terrance Street
Pittsburgh, PA 15261
412-624-4141
Fax: 412-383-2264
www.pitt.edu
Clinic and research of scleroderma.
Carol Blair RN, Clinic Contact

7424 University of Tennessee Medical Group
956 Court Avenue
Memphis, TN 38103
901-448-5775
Fax: 901-448-7265
www.utmedicalgroup.com
Ongoing research protocols.
Arnold E Postlewaite MD, Research Contact

7425 University of Texas Health Science Center
7000 Fannin
Houston, TX 77030
713-500-4472
Fax: 713-500-3026
e-mail: sclerodermaregister@uth.tmc.edu
www.uthouston.edu
Clinic research and clinical trials concerning scleroderma.
Maureen Mayes, Research Contact

Support Groups & Hotlines

7426 National Health Information Center
PO Box 1133
Washington, DC 20013
310-565-4167
800-336-4797
Fax: 301-984-4256
e-mail: info@nhic.org
www.health.gov/nhic
Offers a nationwide information referral service, produces directories and resource guides.

7427 Rhode Island Scleroderma Support Group
18 Talbot Manor
Cranston, RI 02905
401-781-5013
e-mail: scleroderma@hotmail.com
www.angelfire.com/ri/scleroderma
Meets on the fourth Wednsday of every month at Roger Williams Hospital.
Carole Cowell, President

7428 Scleroderma Support Groups
Scleroderma Foundation
12 Kent Way
Byfield, MA 01922
978-463-5843
800-722-4633
Fax: 978-463-5809
e-mail: sfinfo@scleroderma.org
www.scleroderma.org

Please contact the Scleroderma Foundation or visit our web site for a listing of support groups in your area.

Books

7429 Best of the Beacon
Scleroderma Foundation
12 Kent Way
Byfield, MA 01922
978-463-5843
800-722-4673
Fax: 978-463-5809
e-mail: sfinfo@scleroderma.org
www.scleroderma.org/store.html#books
Interesting, readable and highly practical collection of articles of particular interest to those living with scleroderma. This mini encyclopedia includes 11 medical articles, 358 most frequently asked questions, 34 sharing stories, 62 articles of special interest on a variety of useful topics and a glossary that defines 240 words you may encounter when reading about scleroderma.
Marie Coyle, Editor

7430 Handout on Health: Scleroderma
NAMSIC/National Institutes of Health
1 AMS Circle
Bethesda, MD 20892-0001
301-495-4484
877-226-4267
Fax: 301-718-6366
TTY: 301-565-2966
e-mail: niamsinfo@mail.nih.gov
www.nih.gov/niams
143 pages

7431 Helpful Hints for Living with Scleroderma
Scleroderma Foundation
12 Kent Way
Byfield, MA 01922
978-463-5843
800-722-4673
Fax: 978-463-5809
e-mail: sfinfo@scleroderma.org
www.scleroderma.org/store.html#books
Booklet of helpful suggestions from our chapters and members, for the comfort and convienience of others who share the same challenges.
57 pages

7432 Perspectives on Living with Scleroderma
Scleroderma Foundation
12 Kent Way
Byfield, MA 01922
978-463-5843
800-722-4673
Fax: 978-463-5809
e-mail: sfinfo@scleroderma.org
www.scleroderma.org/store.html#books
Insightful articles on coping with scleroderma come from not only from Dr. Flapan's counseling and volunteer work, but also from his personal experience as a scleroderma patient.
233 pages

7433 Scleroderma Book
Scleroderma Foundation
12 Kent Way
Byfield, MA 01922
978-463-5843
800-722-4673
Fax: 978-463-5809
e-mail: sfinfo@scleroderma.org
www.scleroderma.org/store.html#books
Definitive guide to scleroderma for patients and their families, with easy to understand explanations.
182 pages

7434 Scleroderma: Surviving a Seventeen-Year Itch
Scleroderma Foundation
978-463-5809
800-722-4673
Fax: 978-463-5809
e-mail: sfinfo@scleroderma.org
www.scleroderma.org
Self-help manual including history, diagnosis, daily routines and exercise programs for persons with scleroderma.

7435 Scleroderma: a New Role for Patients and Families
Scleroderma Foundation

12 Kent Way
Byfield, MA 01922

978-463-5843
800-722-4673
Fax: 978-463-5809
e-mail: sfinfo@scleroderma.org
www.scleroderma.org/store.html#books

Provides an overview of key issues and offers resources that enable patients and their families to find more resources on thier own.
168 pages

7436 Understanding & Managing Scleroderma
Scleroderma Foundation
12 Kent Way
Byfield, MA 01923

978-463-5843
800-722-4633
Fax: 978-463-5809
e-mail: sfinfo@scleroderma.org
www.scleroderma.org

Booklet intended to help persons with scleroderma, their families and others interested in scleroderma to better understand what scleroderma is, what effects it may have, and what those with scleroderma can do to help themselves and their physicians manage the disease. It answers some of the most frequently asked questions about scleroderma.

Magazines

7437 Scleroderma Voice
Scleroderma Foundation
12 Kent Way
Byfield, MA 01922

978-463-5843
800-722-4673
Fax: 978-463-5809
e-mail: sfinfo@scleroderma.org
www.scleroderma.org

Feautures the latest information available on scleroderma treatments and research. Subscription to the Voice includes a one-year membership in the Scleroderma Foundation.
Quarterly

Pamphlets

7438 If You Have Scleroderma You Need Not Feel Alone
Scleroderma Foundation
12 Kent Way
Byfield, MA 01922

978-463-5843
800-722-4673
Fax: 978-463-5809
e-mail: sfinfo@scleroderma.org
www.scleroderma.org/store.html#brochures

Scleroderma Foundation's membership brochure. Free of charge, also available in Spanish.

7439 Scleroderma: an Overview
Scleroderma Foundation
12 Kent Way
Byfield, MA 01922

978-463-5843
Fax: 978-463-5809
e-mail: sfinfo@scleroderma.org
www.scleroderma.org/store.html#brochures

Concise genral overview of sytemic scleroderma. Also available in Spanish, and downloadable in Portugese.

7440 What Causes Scleroderma?
Scleroderma Foundation
12 Kent Way
Byfield, MA 01922

978-463-5843
800-722-4673
Fax: 978-463-5809
e-mail: sfinfo@scleroderma.org
www.scleroderma.org/store.html#brochures

Discusses the puzzling nature of scleroderma. Also available in Spanish, and downloadable in Portugese.

Web Sites

7441 Healing Well

www.healingwell.com

An online health resource guide to medical news, chat, information and articles, newsgroups and message boards, books, disease-related web sites, medical directories, and more for patients, friends, and family coping with disabling diseases, disorders, or chronic illnesses.

7442 Health Finder

www.healthfinder.gov

Searchable, carefully developed web site offering information on over 1000 topics. Developed by the US Department of Health and Human Services, the site can be used in both English and Spanish.

7443 Healthlink USA

www.healthlinkusa.com

Health information concerning treatment, cures, prevention, diagnosis, risk factors, research, support groups, email lists, personal stories and much more. Updated regularly.

7444 Helios Health

www.helioshealth.com

Online resource for your health information. Detailed information about specific health topics, access to expert advice from our Medical Advisory Board, and up-to-date health news.

7445 MedicineNet

www.medicinenet.com

An online resource for consumers providing easy-to-read, authoritative medical and health information.

7446 Medscape

www.medscape.com

Medscape offers specialists, primary care physicians, and other health professionals the Web's most robust and integrated medical information and educational tools.

7447 Scleroderma Foundation

www.scleroderma.org

501 (c)3 national nonprofit organization serving the interests of persons with scleroderma. The Foundation's 26 chapters and 135 support groups nationwide help to carry out its three-fold mission of support, education and research. The Scleroderma Foundation is a leading nonprofit supporter of scleroderma research — funding over $1 million of new grants each year to find the cause and cure of scleroderma.

7448 WebMD

www.webmd.com

Information on scleroderma, including articles and resources.

Description

7449 **Scoliosis**

Scoliosis is a lateral curvature of the spine, with 60 to 80 percent of the cases occurring in girls. It may first be suspected when one of the teenager's shoulders appears higher than the other or clothes don't hang straight. The spinal curve is more pronounced when the adolescent bends forward. More than 80 percent of scoliosis is idiopathic, that is, there is no known cause.

Symptoms include prominent shoulder blades, uneven hip levels, and fatigue in the lower back after sitting or standing for prolonged periods of time. In many cases there are no symptoms unless the scoliosis is severe.

The prognosis depends on the site and severity of the curve, and the age of onset of symptoms. Early detection through school screening provides more treatment options, and prompt referral to an orthopedist is indicated. The majority of cases require only observation for progression. Approximately 20 percent of those with scoliosis will require an orthopedic brace or spinal fusion surgery.

National Agencies & Associations

7450 **American Academy of Orthopaedic Surgeons**
6300 N River Road
Rosemont, IL 60018-4238
847-823-7186
800-346-2267
Fax: 847-823-8125
e-mail: custserv@aaos.org
www.aaos.org
The American Academy of Orthopaedic Surgeons provides education and practice management services for orthopaedic surgeons and allied health professionals. The Academy also serves as an advocate for improved patient care and informs the public.
Karen L Hackett FACHE CAE, CEO
Richard J Stewart, Chief Financial Officer

7451 **International Federation of Spine Associations**
Howard M Shulman
9908 Cape Scott Court
Raleigh, NC 27614-9025
919-846-2204
www.scoliosisrx.com
IFOSA is a federation of various national Spine Associations from countries in North America Europe and Australia. These organizations principally represent the spine patients and their families.

7452 **National Scoliosis Foundation**
5 Cabot Place
Stoughton, MA 02072
781-341-6333
800-673-6922
Fax: 781-341-8333
e-mail: NSF@scoliosis.org
www.scoliosis.org
Promotes school screening offers public awareness materials to promote public education maintains a resource center for professional information conducts scoliosis conferences and offers support groups to people affected by the disease.
Joseph P O'Brien, President/CEO
Dennis J Fusco, Treasurer

7453 **Scoliosis Association**
PO Box 811705
Boca Raton, FL 33481-1705
561-994-4435
800-800-0669
Fax: 561-994-2455
e-mail: normlipin@aol.com
www.scoliosis-assoc.org
Sponsors and encourages spinal screening programs. Disseminates information throughout the country and raises funds for scoliosis research. Membership fee includes subscription to newsletter. Videos and printed information available.

7454 **Spinal Connection National Scoliosis Foundation**
National Scoliosis Foundation
5 Cabot Place
Stoughton, MA 02072
781-341-6333
800-673-6922
Fax: 781-341-8333
e-mail: NSF@scoliosis.org
www.scoliosis.org
Offers updated information and the latest medical advances in the area of spinal cord injury and spina bifida. Includes resources reviews support group and meeting information.
Joseph P O'Brien, President/CEO
Dennis J Fusco, Treasurer

Research Centers

7455 **Scoliosis Research Society**
555 E Wells Street
Milwaukee, WI 53202
414-289-9107
Fax: 414-276-3349
e-mail: info@srs.org
www.srs.org
This society provides an international forum for those interested in the management of spinal deformities. It holds a yearly meeting at which health professionals meet to share observations and results and to explore new avenues of research.
Tressa Goulding, Executive Director
Kathryn Agard, Administrative Assistant

7456 **Shriners Hospital for Crippled Children Chicago Unit**
Chicago Unit
2211 N Oak Park Avenue
Chicago, IL 60707
773-622-5400
Fax: 773-855-88
www.shrinersplural2hopitals.org
A 60-bed orthopedic hospital providing comprehensive spinal cord injury care to children. Provides care for spinal deformities Cerebral Palsy Osteoeneisis Imperfecta and Scoliosis as well as others.
Chara Jones, Administrator
Diether Sturm, Chief of Staff

Support Groups & Hotlines

7457 **National Health Information Center**
PO Box 1133
Washington, DC 20013
310-565-4167
800-336-4797
Fax: 301-984-4256
e-mail: info@nhic.org
www.health.gov/nhic
Offers a nationwide information referral service, produces directories and resource guides.

Books

7458 **Adult Scoliosis Surgery...It Can Be Done**
St. Luke's Spine Center
11311 Shaker Boulevard
Cleveland, OH 44104-3805
216-368-7000
Describes various types of surgery and procedures used in adult scoliosis patients.
21 pages

7459 **Coalition Index**
American School Health Association
PO Box 708
Kent, OH 44240
330-678-1601
800-445-2742
Fax: 330-678-4526
e-mail: asha@ashaweb.org
www.ashaweb.org
A professional membership organization dedicated to promoting the health and well being of children and youth through coordinated school health programs.
Susan Wooley, Executive Director

7460 Getting Ready, Getting Well
National Scoliosis Foundation
5 Cabot Place   781-341-6333
Stoughton, MA 02072   800-673-6922
                                                               Fax: 781-341-8333
                                               e-mail: NSF@scoliosis.org
                                                        www.scoliosis.org
Guide for those anticipating surgery. Divided into three sections:
Making up Your Mind, Taking Charge, and Home Again.
73 pages
Joseph P O'Brien, President/CEO

7461 Handbook of Scoliosis
Scoliosis Research Society
555 East Wells Street   414-289-9107
Milwaukee, WI 53202   Fax: 414-276-3349
                                                               www.srs.org

Tressa Goulding, Executive Director

7462 Stopping Scoliosis
National Scoliosis Foundation
5 Cabot Place   781-341-6333
Stoughton, MA 02072   800-673-6922
                                                               Fax: 781-341-8333
                                               e-mail: NSF@scoliosis.org
                                                        www.scoliosis.org
Filled with accurate, currently researched information for adults
concerned with their condition or that of a young person.
Joseph P O'Brien, President/CEO

7463 Twenty Years at Hull House
New American Library
375 Hudson Street   212-366-2000
New York, NY 10014
Book dealing with Scoliosis.
Grades 7-12

Children's Books

7464 Deenie
Bradbury Press
866 3rd Avenue   212-702-2000
New York, NY 10022-6221   800-257-5755
Deenie, a beautiful thirteen-year-old girl, had a mother who was
pushing her to become a model. The agency representatives told
Deenie she had the looks but walked differently. Deenie's main
wish was to become a cheerleader. Her close friend, Janet, made
the cheerleading squad but Deenie didn't make the finalist list. After this her gym teacher noticed her posture and called her family.
After seeing therapists, the diagnosis of adolescent idiopathic
scoliosis was made.
159 pages Hardcover
ISBN: 0-027110-20-6

7465 Tina's Story...Scoliosis and Me
Alfred I DuPont Institute
PO Box 269   302-651-4000
Wilmington, DE 19801
Suggested for parents of children anticipating surgery. This out-
standing book, written as an eighth grade project by a gifted thir-
teen year old writer and scoliosis patient, relates her experiences
and emotions while wearing a brace for three years prior to surgery.

7466 What Young People and Parents Need to Know about Scoliosis
American Physical Therapy Association
1111 N Fairfax Street   703-684-2782
Alexandria, VA 22314
A physical therapist's perspective.

Newsletters

7467 Backtalk
Scoliosis Association
PO Box 811705   561-994-4435
Boca Raton, FL 33481-1705   800-800-0669
                                                               Fax: 561-994-2455
                                               e-mail: scolioassn@aol.com
                                                        www.scoliosis.org

Information for families, patients and health care professionals.

Pamphlets

7468 1 in Every 10 Persons Has Scoliosis
National Scoliosis Foundation
5 Cabot Place   781-341-6333
Stoughton, MA 02072   800-673-6922
                                                               Fax: 781-341-8333
                                               e-mail: NSF@scoliosis.org
                                                        www.scoliosis.org
Explains what scoliosis is and illustrates how to screen for it. It
also contains facts about the Foundation.
Joseph P O'Brien, President/CEO

7469 Adolescent Idiopathic Scoliosis: Prevelance, Natural History, Treatments
National Scoliosis Foundation
5 Cabot Place   781-341-6333
Stoughton, MA 02072   800-673-6922
                                                               Fax: 781-341-8333
                                               e-mail: NSF@scoliosis.org
                                                        www.scoliosis.org
Expert overview of a condition that affects many young people.
Joseph P O'Brien, President/CEO

7470 Boston Bracing System for Idiopathic Scoliosis
National Scoliosis Foundation
5 Cabot Place   781-341-6333
Stoughton, MA 02072   800-673-6922
                                                               Fax: 781-341-8333
                                               e-mail: NSF@scoliosis.org
                                                        www.scoliosis.org
Explaination of an available option.
Joseph P O'Brien, President/CEO

7471 Brace & Her Brace is No Handicap
National Scoliosis Foundation
5 Cabot Place   781-341-6333
Stoughton, MA 02072   800-673-6922
                                                               Fax: 781-341-8333
                                               e-mail: NSF@scoliosis.org
                                                        www.scoliosis.org
Contains two illustrated short stories, each about a teenage girl
coping successfully with scoliosis.
Joseph P O'Brien, President/CEO

7472 Getting a Second Opinion
National Scoliosis Foundation
5 Cabot Place   781-341-6333
Stoughton, MA 02072   800-673-6922
                                                               Fax: 781-341-8333
                                               e-mail: NSF@scoliosis.org
                                                        www.scoliosis.org
Reprinted from Health Tips.
Joseph P O'Brien, President/CEO

7473 Going Home
University Hospital Spine Center
2074 Abington Road   216-844-1616
Cleveland, OH 44106
Instructions for pediatric and adult patients who have had a spinal
fusion.

7474 Medical Update Column
National Scoliosis Foundation
5 Cabot Place   781-341-6333
Stoughton, MA 02072   800-673-6922
                                                               Fax: 781-341-8333
                                               e-mail: NSF@scoliosis.org
                                                        www.scoliosis.org
Reprints from past issues of the Spinal Connections Medical Up-
date Column available on various topics.
Joseph P O'Brien, President/CEO

7475 NSF Packets
National Scoliosis Foundation

5 Cabot Place
Stoughton, MA 02072
781-341-6333
800-673-6922
Fax: 781-341-8333
e-mail: NSF@scoliosis.org
www.scoliosis.org

Packet contains information for parents and young people, adults, and healthcare professionals.
Joseph P O'Brien, President/CEO

7476 Patient with Scoliosis
Educational Services, Division of AJV Company
555 W 57th Street
New York, NY 10019-2925
212-996-6473

A reprint from the American Journal of nursin.

7477 Postural Screening Program
National Scoliosis Foundation
5 Cabot Place
Stoughton, MA 02072
781-341-6333
800-673-6922
Fax: 781-341-8333
e-mail: NSF@scoliosis.org
www.scoliosis.org

Guidelines for physicians and school nurses.
Joseph P O'Brien, President/CEO

7478 Questions Most Often Asked the NSF
National Scoliosis Foundation
5 Cabot Place
Stoughton, MA 02072
781-341-6333
800-673-6922
Fax: 781-341-8333
e-mail: NSF@scoliosis.org
www.scoliosis.org

Answers the most frequently asked questions about scoliosis and the foundation in general.
Joseph P O'Brien, President/CEO

7479 Scoliosis
Scoliosis Research Society
611 E Wells Street
Milwaukee, WI 53202
414-289-9107
Fax: 414-276-3349
www.srs.org

Brochure describing scoliosis, kyphosis, lordosis; causes, prevention, treatment and adult scoliosis.
Tressa Goulding, Executive Director

7480 Scoliosis Patient Becomes a Model
National Scoliosis Foundation
5 Cabot Place
Stoughton, MA 02072
781-341-6333
800-673-6922
Fax: 781-341-8333
e-mail: NSF@scoliosis.org
www.scoliosis.org

Reprinted from Children's Today.
Joesph P O'Brien, President/CEO

7481 Scoliosis Road Map
University Hospital Spine Center
2074 Abington Road
Cleveland, OH 44106
216-844-1616

Written for teenagers affected by this illness.

7482 Scoliosis Screening: The Carlsbad Program
National Scoliosis Foundation
5 Cabot Place
Stoughton, MA 02072
781-341-6333
800-673-6922
Fax: 781-341-8333
e-mail: NSF@scoliosis.org
www.scoliosis.org

Exceptional scoliosis screening program.
Joseph P O'Brien, President/CEO

7483 Scoliosis Surgery, What's It All About?
University Hospital Spine Center
2074 Abington Road
Cleveland, OH 44106
216-844-1616

This pamphlet answers many of the questions patients ask before having surgery.

7484 Scoliosis and Kyphosis
Scoliosis Research Society

555 East Wells Street
Milwaukee, WI 53202
414-289-9107
Fax: 414-276-3349
www.srs.org

Information and advice from parents.
Tressa Goulding, Executive Director

7485 Scoliosis, Me?
North Dallas Scoliosis Center
1910 N Collins Boulevard
Richardson, TX 75080-3525
972-644-1930

Detailed answers to questions most asked by parents and teens.

7486 Scoliosis... Now it Can Be Treated in Adults as Well as Children
National Scoliosis Foundation
5 Cabot Place
Stoughton, MA 02072
781-341-6333
800-673-6922
Fax: 781-341-8333
e-mail: NSF@scoliosis.org
www.scoliosis.org

Reprinted from Cleveland Magazine.
Joseph P O'Brien, President/CEO

7487 Scoliosis: Handbook for Patients
National Scoliosis Foundation
5 Cabot Place
Stoughton, MA 02072
781-341-6333
800-673-6922
Fax: 781-341-8333
e-mail: NSF@scoliosis.org
www.scoliosis.org

Information on detection and treatment of adolescent scoliosis, kyphosis and lordosis and adult scoliosis.
Joseph P O'Brien, President/CEO

7488 Screening Procedure Guidelines for Spinal Deformity
Scoliosis Research Society
555 East Wells Street
Milwaukee, WI 53202
414-289-9107
Fax: 414-276-3349
www.srs.org

Seven page brochure covers reasons, organizations and procedures for spinal screening. Signs of spinal deformity, as seen in both standing and forward bending positions are illustrated and discussed. Includes sample screening form.
7 pages
Tressa Goulding, Executive Director

7489 Spinal Deformity: Congenital Scoliosis and Kyphosis
Scoliosis Research Society
555 East Wells Street
Milwaukee, WI 53202
414-289-9107
Fax: 414-276-3349
www.srs.org

Discusses signs and causes of congenital spinal deformities, associated conditions, treatment options and a glossary of terms.
12 pages
Tressa Goulding, Executive Director

7490 Spinal Deformity: Scoliosis and Kyphosis
Scoliosis Research Society
555 East Wells Street
Milwaukee, WI 53202
414-289-9107
Fax: 414-276-3349
www.srs.org

Twelve page brochure discusses signs and causes of scoliosis and kyphosis, indications for treatment, treatment options, commonly asked questions and a glossary of terms.
12 pages
Tressa Goulding, Executive Director

7491 What Young People & Their Parents Need to Know About Scoliosis
American Physical Therapy Association
1111 N Fairfax Street
Alexandria, VA 22314-1488
703-684-2782

A physical therapists' perspective.

7492 What if You Need an Operation for Scoliosis?
St. Luke's Spine Center
11311 Shaker Boulevard
Cleveland, OH 44104-3805
216-368-7000

7493 When the Spine Curves
National Scoliosis Foundation

5 Cabot Place
Stoughton, MA 02072

781-341-6333
800-673-6922
Fax: 781-341-8333
e-mail: NSF@scoliosis.org
www.scoliosis.org

Joseph P O'Brien, President/CEO

7494 You and Your Brace
University Hospital Spine Center
2074 Abington Road
Cleveland, OH 44106

216-844-1616

Audio & Video

7495 Cutting Edge Medical Report
National Scoliosis Foundation
5 Cabot Place
Stoughton, MA 02072

781-341-6333
800-673-6922
Fax: 781-341-8333
e-mail: NSF@scoliosis.org
www.scoliosis.org

As seen on the Discovery Channel, this video is an indepth examination of the latest developments in the diagnosis and treatment of scoliosis.
Joseph P O'Brien, President/CEO

7496 Growing Straighter and Stronger
National Scoliosis Foundation
5 Cabot Place
Stoughton, MA 02072

781-341-6333
800-673-6922
Fax: 781-341-8333
e-mail: NSF@scoliosis.org
www.scoliosis.org

Fifteen-minute presentation available in VHS video format, for the pre-screening education of students in grades 5 through 7.
Videotape
Joseph P O'Brien, President/CEO

7497 Preparing Yourself for Spinal Surgery for Teenagers with Severe Scoliosis
National Scoliosis Foundation
5 Cabot Place
Stoughton, MA 02072

781-341-6333
800-673-6922
Fax: 781-341-8333
e-mail: NSF@scoliosis.org
www.scoliosis.org

Patient education video helping to reduce anxiety for teenagers facing surgery by giving a sense of what to expect before, during, and after surgery.
Joseph P O'Brien, President/CEO

7498 School Screening with Dr. Robert Keller
National Scoliosis Foundation
5 Cabot Place
Stoughton, MA 02072

781-341-6333
800-673-6922
Fax: 781-341-8333
e-mail: NSF@scoliosis.org
www.scoliosis.org

Training video that teaches the proper technique for doing spinal screening. Defines scoliosis and kyphosis. Four teenagers, three with curves and one without, are examined and the findings explained.
Videotape
Joseph P O'Brien, President/CEO

7499 Scoliosis: An Adult Perspective
National Scoliosis Foundation
5 Cabot Place
Stoughton, MA 02072

781-341-6333
800-673-6922
Fax: 781-341-8333
e-mail: NSF@scoliosis.org
www.scoliosis.org

Dr. Blackman and five women patients provide an overall perspective of what scoliosis is, who gets it, the types of devices, myths about the disorder, and options for treatment.
Joseph P O'Brien, President/CEO

7500 Sharing Scoliosis: You're Not Alone
National Scoliosis Foundation

5 Cabot Place
Stoughton, MA 02072

781-341-6333
800-673-6922
Fax: 781-341-8333
e-mail: NSF@scoliosis.org
www.scoliosis.org

The Missouri chapter of the NSF, shares their experience with scoliosis including diagnosis, wearing a brace, surgery, and recovery. It is a good source of support for patients of all ages and their families.
Joseph P O'Brien, President/CEO

7501 Spinal Screening Program
Scoliosis Research Society
555 East Wells Street
Milwaukee, WI 53202

414-289-9107
Fax: 414-276-3349
www.srs.com

Twenty minute videotape designed to instruct screeners in the spinal screening program. It demonstrates methods of screening, showing adolescents with normal and abnormal spines. Includes sample screening form.
VHS Video Tape
Tressa Goulding, Executive Director

7502 Taking the Mystery Out of Spinal Deformities
Children's Hospital of LA, Div. of Orthopaedics
4650 Sunset Boulevard
Los Angeles, CA 90027

213-660-2450
800-841-7439
e-mail: RWETZEL@chla.usc.edu

Answers questions most often asked by screeners, patients and parents.
Videotape

7503 Understanding Scoliosis
National Scoliosis Foundation
5 Cabot Place
Stoughton, MA 02072

781-341-6333
800-673-6922
Fax: 781-341-8333
e-mail: NSF@scoliosis.org
www.scoliosis.org

Kaiser Permanente's educational video clearly and positively addresses the patient community. In this video four teenagers at various stages of treatment talk about their life with scoliosis.
Joseph P O'Brien, President/CEO

7504 What's This Thing Called Scoliosis
National Scoliosis Foundation
5 Cabot Place
Stoughton, MA 02072

781-341-6333
800-673-6922
Fax: 781-341-8333
e-mail: NSF@scoliosis.org
www.scoliosis.org

Comprehensive overview of scoliosis using the latest computer technology. The anatomical spine and animated model work together to truly show the 3D aspects of scoliosis and the corresponding impact on the patient.
Joseph P O'Brien, President/CEO

7505 You Are Not Alone
Minnesota Spine Center
606 24th Avenue S
Minneapolis, MN 55454-1438

612-332-3843

A video presenting two women's experiences with surgery. Personal life, concerns, hospital experience, recovery and improved lifestyle are openly discussed.
Videotape

Web Sites

7506 American Association of Neurological Surgeons
www.neurosurgery.org/

Official web site of the American Association of Neurological Surgeons and Congress of Neurological Surgeons. Whether you are a patient, physician, health care professional, or member of the media, this site is your online resource for neurosurgical information.

7507 British Scoliosis Research Society
www.ndos.ox.ac.uk/pzs/

This site contains: background to the meeting, Scoliosis Research Society review papers on the aetiology of idiopathic scoliosis, a list of participants, abstracts classified by discussion group and the chairman's conclusions for each group.

7508 Healing Well

www.healingwell.com

An online health resource guide to medical news, chat, information and articles, newsgroups and message boards, books, disease-related web sites, medical directories, and more for patients, friends, and family coping with disabling diseases, disorders, or chronic illnesses.

7509 Health Finder

www.healthfinder.gov

Searchable, carefully developed web site offering information on over 1000 topics. Developed by the US Department of Health and Human Services, the site can be used in both English and Spanish.

7510 Healthlink USA

www.healthlinkusa.com

Health information concerning treatment, cures, prevention, diagnosis, risk factors, research, support groups, email lists, personal stories and much more. Updated regularly.

7511 Helios Health

www.helioshealth.com

Online resource for your health information. Detailed information about specific health topics, access to expert advice from our Medical Advisory Board, and up-to-date health news.

7512 MedicineNet

www.medicinenet.com

An online resource for consumers providing easy-to-read, authoritative medical and health information.

7513 Medscape

www.medscape.com

Medscape offers specialists, primary care physicians, and other health professionals the Web's most robust and integrated medical information and educational tools.

7514 Patients Rate Their Scoliosis Doctors

This web site is a free internet service for communicating subjective impressions of medical doctor (MD) reputations among scoliosis patients. Please use this system to learn some of the subjective impressions of the treatment other patients have received from their doctors.

7515 Scoliosis Association

www.sauk.org.uk/

The Scoliosis Association (UK) was founded in 1981. It is the only independent support group for scoliosis in the UK. SAUK aims to provide information about scoliosis, eliminate fear and stigma, and offer contacts for shared experiences.

7516 WebMD

www.webmd.com

Information on scoliosis, including articles and resources.

Description

7517 # Seizure Disorders

There are two types of seizure disorders: an isolated, nonrecurring attack, such as may occur with high fevers in children, head trauma, or from other diseases (metabolic abnormalities or brain tumor) and epilepsy, which is characterized by recurrent, sudden, rapid changes in brain function caused by abnormalities in the electrical activity of the brain. Roughly 2 million Americans suffer from epilepsy, with half of the cases found in children and adolescents.

Seizures can be classified as generalized, affecting the whole brain at once, or partial, affecting a part of the brain. Absence (petit mal) attacks are generalized seizures in which there is only a brief (10-30 second) loss of consciousness, with eye and muscle fluttering but no loss of muscle tone. A generalized tonic-clonic seizure (grand mal) usually lasts 1-2 minutes, and includes loss of consciousness, falling, and involuntary contractions of the arms and legs. Some patients report that they see flashing lights and experience a heightened sense of taste and smell (known as an aura) that indicates they are about to have a seizure.

In many cases there is no apparent cause of the disorder, and it is therefore called idiopathic epilepsy.

Treatment aims primarily to control seizures. Causative or precipitating factors should be eliminated. Drug treatment is the mainstay of therapy for most types of seizures. In order to limit toxic effects, an attempt is made to use only a single drug. Some patients may need to take more than one drug. In most cases, acceptable control can be achieved with medications alone. Rarely, seizures will not respond to drugs, and surgery on the brain will be recommended. In this procedure, the surgeon tries to identify and destroy the part of the brain that is triggering the seizures.

National Agencies & Associations

7518 **American Epilepsy Society**
342 N Main Street   860-586-7505
W Hartford, CT 06117-2500   Fax: 860-568-7550
e-mail: ctubby@aesnet.org
www.aesnet.org
Fosters treatment of epilepsy in its biological clinical and social phases.
M Suzanne C Berry, Executive Director
Cheryl-Ann Tubby, Assistant Executive Director

7519 **Epilepsy Foundation**
8301 Professional Place   301-459-3700
Landover, MD 20785   800-332-1000
Fax: 301-577-2684
e-mail: postmaster@efa.org
www.epilepsyfoundation.org
A national charitable nonprofit volunteer agency in the US dedicated to the welfare of people with epilepsy. Its goals are the prevention and cure of seizure disorders, the alleviation of their effects and the promotion of independence.
Steven T Sabatini, Chair of the Board of Directors
Eric R Hargis, President & CEO

7520 **National Association of Epilepsy Centers**
5775 Wayzata Boulevard   612-525-4526
Minneapolis, MN 55416-1222   888-525-6232
Fax: 612-525-1560
e-mail: info@naec-epilepsy.org
www.naec-epilepsy.org
A nonprofit organization that encourages and supports professional and technical education in the treatment of epilepsy. Over 50 centers nationwide are members of the trade association which will make referrals to its member centers.
Robert J Gumnit MD, President
Gregory L Barkley, VP

7521 **National Institute of Neurological Disorders and Stroke**
NIH Neurological Institute   301-496-5751
Bethesda, MD 20824   800-352-9424
Fax: 301-402-2186
TTY: 301-468-5981
www.ninds.nih.gov
The mission of NINDS is to reduce the burden of neurological disease - a burden borne by every age group, by every segment of society, by people all over the world.
Story C Landis PhD, Director
Walter J Koroshetz, Deputy Director

State Agencies & Associations

California

7522 **Epilepsy Foundation of Northern California**
5700 Stoneridge Mall Road   925-224-7760
Pleasanton, CA 94588-2824   800-632-3532
Fax: 925-224-7770
e-mail: efnca@epilepsynorcal.org
www.epilepsynorcal.org
Nonprofit organization serving families affected by epilepsy.
Neva Hirschkorn, Executive Director
Bill Stack, Associate Director

Florida

7523 **Epilepsy Association of Big Bend**
1215 Lee Avenue   850-222-1777
Tallahassee, FL 32303-2651   Fax: 850-222-7440
e-mail: epilepsyassoc@embarqmail.com
www.epilepsyassoc.org
Services include: Case management, prevention education, counseling and advocacy, information and referral.

7524 **Epilepsy Foundation of South Florida**
7300 N Kendall Drive   305-670-4949
Miami, FL 33156-7840   Fax: 305-670-0904
e-mail: information@epilepsysofla.org
www.epilepsyfound.org
A twenty five year old nonprofit community based organization dedicated to enhancing the personal and social adjustments of individuals with seizure disorders and their families.
Karen Basha Egozi, Executive Director
Ana Alfonso, Executive Administrator

7525 **Epilepsy Services Foundation**
4618 N Armenia Avenue   813-870-3414
Tampa, FL 33603-2706   Fax: 813-870-1321
e-mail: info@epilepsysf.org
www.epilepsysf.org
Information on medical and supportive services for persons affected by epilepsy living in West Central Florida. Raise funds to provide medical and supportive services and to build an endowment to make a difference in the lives of generations to come.
Thomas Orth, Executive Director

7526 **Epilepsy Services of North Central Florida**
11200 NW 8th Avenue   352-392-6449
Gainesville, FL 32601-4946   800-330-9746
Fax: 352-392-5792
e-mail: jlyons@college.med.ufl.edu
www.floridaepilepsy.org/northcentral.htm

Jim Lyons, Program Director
Mike Dorsey, PE Coordinator

7527 Epilepsy Services of Northeast Florida
5209 San Jose Boulevard 904-731-3751
Jacksonville, FL 32207-2267 e-mail: epilepsy@bellsouth.net
Services include: Program case management, program prevention
and education, employment services, children's summer camp,
counseling and advocacy, and information and referrals.

7528 Epilepsy Services of Southwest Florida
1900 Main Street 941-953-5988
Sarasota, FL 34236 Fax: 941-366-5890
www.epilepsyservicesofswfl.org
Dedicated to providing case management and medical services for
individuals with seizure disorders who meet eligibility criteria.
Provides employment education for individuals and families affected by seizure disorders and prevention education to the com
Thomas Garrity, Executive Director

7529 Manattee County Office Epilepsy Services of Southwest Florida
1701 14th Street W 941-746-6488
Bradenton, FL 34205-7132 Fax: 941-746-8382
e-mail: bardentonep@aol.com

Brian Larocque, Social Worker

New Jersey

7530 Epilepsy Foundation of New Jersey
429 River View Plaza 609-392-4900
Trenton, NJ 08611-3420 800-336-5843
Fax: 609-392-5621
TTY: 800-852-7899
TDD: 800-852-7899
e-mail: efnj@efnj.com
www.efnj.com

Eric M Joice, Executive Director
Liza Gundell, Deputy Director

New York

7531 Epilepsy Foundation of Long Island
506 Stewart Avenue 516-739-7733
Garden City, NY 11530-4700 888-672-7154
Fax: 516-794-2180
e-mail: info@epil.org
www.efli.org

Robert A Karson, President
John Savarese, Vice President

Pennsylvania

7532 Epilepsy Foundation of Western Pennsylvania
1323 Forbes Avenue 412-261-5880
Pittsburgh, PA 15219-4725 Fax: 412-261-5361
e-mail: staff@efwp.org
www.efwp.org

Washington

7533 Epilepsy Foundation of North West Washington
2311 N 45th Street 206-547-4551
Seattle, WA 98103 800-752-3509
Fax: 206-547-4557
e-mail: mail@epilepsynw.org
www.epilepsyfoundation.org

Brent Herrmann, President/CEO
Alta C Hancock, Associate Director

Research Centers

7534 Baylor College of Medicine: Epilepsy Research Center
Texas Medical Center
6550 Fannin 713-798-8259
Houston, TX 77030 Fax: 713-798-7533
e-mail: neurochair@bcm.edu
www.bcm.edu/neurology
The clinical program at Baylor College of Medicine for the comprehensive evaluation of those with epilepsy or those suspected of
having seizures or epilepsy.
Eli Mizrahi MD, Director

7535 Duke University Center for the Advanced Study of Epilepsy
Duke Neuroscience Clinic
200 Trent Drive 919-668-7600
Durham, NC 27710 888-ASK-DUKE
www.dukehealth.org
Clinical and research unit that experiments in limbic epilepsy.
James McNama MD, Director
William B Gallentine

7536 Duke University Epilepsy Research Center
Trent Drive 919-684-8111
Durham, NC 27710 888-275-3853
www.mc.duke.edu

Dr James McNamara, Director

7537 Neurology Research Center Helen Hayes Hospital
Helen Hayes Hospital
53-55 Route 9W 845-786-4535
W Haverstraw, NY 10993 888-70R-EHAB
Fax: 845-947-3097
e-mail: info@helenhayeshospital.org
www.helenhayeshospital.org
Robert Linds MD, Chief Internal medicine
Jason P Greenberg, Assistant Clinical Professor of Neurolog

7538 University of Illinois at Chicago Consultation Clinic for Epilepsy
912 S Wood Street 312-996-6906
Chicago, IL 60612-7330 Fax: 312-996-4169
e-mail: neu50@uic.edu
www.uic.edu

Dr. John R Hughes, Director

7539 University of Tennessee: Center for Neuroscience
875 Monroe Avenue 901-448-5960
Memphis, TN 38163-0001 Fax: 901-448-4685
www.utmem.edu/neuroscience

Epilepsy research and studies.
William E Armstrong, Director
Anton J Reiner, Co-Director

7540 University of Wisconsin Madison Neurophysiology Laboratory
UW Hospital and Clinics
600 Highland Avenue 608-263-6400
Madison, WI 53792 800-323-8942
Fax: 608-265-5512
www.uwhealth.org

Epilepsy research.
Thomas P Sutula, Chairman of Neurology
Paul A Rutecki, Vice Chairman of Neurology

Support Groups & Hotlines

7541 Epilepsy Foundation of America Helpline
Epilepsy Foundation of America
4351 Garden City Drive 301-459-3700
Landover, MD 20785-7223 800-332-1000
Fax: 301-577-4941
e-mail: postmaster@esa.org
www.epilepsyfoundation.org
A toll free information and referral service staffed by specially
trained people who will answer questions and discuss concerns
about seizure disorders and their treatment. Staff will direct callers
to local affiliates of the EFA and tell about a broad range of medical
services that respond to the needs of people with seizure disorders.
Eric Hargis, Chief Executive Officer

7542 National Health Information Center
PO Box 1133 310-565-4167
Washington, DC 20013 800-336-4797
Fax: 301-984-4256
e-mail: info@nhic.org
www.health.gov/nhic

Offers a nationwide information referral service, produces directories and resource guides.

Books

7543 Americans with Disabilities Act
Epilepsy Foundation of America
4351 Garden City Drive   301-459-3700
Landover, MD 20785-2267   800-332-1000
                                    Fax: 301-577-9056
Learn how the Americans With Disabilities Act of 1990 can benifit you. Excellent comprehensive resource for individuals with seizure disorders.
46 pages Softcover
ISBN: 0-802774-65-2

7544 Bomb in the Brain: A Heroic Tale of Science, Surgery and Survival
MacMillan Publishing Company
866 3rd Avenue   212-702-2000
New York, NY 10022
The autobiographical account of this author's struggle with epilepsy and the debilitating effects it has on health, emotions, and mental stability.
Grades 10-12

7545 Brainstorms: Epilepsy in Our Words
4351 Garden City Drive   301-459-3700
Landover, MD 20785-2267   800-332-1000
                                    Fax: 301-577-9056
Patients describe their experiences with seizures. Sixty-eight in-depth personal accounts of actual seizures are followed by a short section on how epilepsy affects the lives of the patients.
197 pages Paperback
ISBN: 0-802774-65-2

7546 Children with Epilepsy
Epilepsy Foundation of America
4351 Garden City Drive   301-459-3700
Landover, MD 20785-2267   800-332-1000
                                    Fax: 301-577-9056
Offers direction and support to parents of a child with epilepsy, by first educating them about epilepsy and then helping them cope with the effects this disorder will have on their child and family.
314 pages Paperback
ISBN: 0-933149-19-0

7547 Does Your Child Have Epilepsy?
4351 Garden City Drive   301-459-3700
Landover, MD 20785-2267   800-332-1000
                                    Fax: 301-577-9056
This book establishes Ten Basic Rules for parents of children with epilepsy.
201 pages Softcover

7548 Embrace the Dawn
Epilepsy Foundation of America
4351 Garden City Drive   301-459-3700
Landover, MD 20785-2267   800-332-1000
                                    Fax: 301-577-9056
A moving biographical account of one person's lifelong experience with epilepsy.
127 pages Softcover

7549 Epilepsy A to Z
4351 Garden City Drive   301-459-3700
Landover, MD 20785-2267   800-332-1000
                                    Fax: 301-577-9056
This book is designed to give health-care personnel a convenient way to find brief answers to questions about epilepsy. It includes definitions of terms, ranging all the way from abdominal epilepsy to Zonisimide.
322 pages Softcover

7550 Epilepsy Diet Treatment: An Introduction to the Ketogenic Diet
Epilepsy Foundation of America
4351 Garden City Drive   301-459-3700
Landover, MD 20785-2267   800-332-1000
                                    Fax: 301-577-9056
The only book devoted exclusively to the ketogenic diet - a rigid, mathematically calculated, doctor-supervised diet that is high in fat and low in carbohydrate and protein with strictly limited calories and liquid intake. Gives all the facts about the diet, plus quotes

from parents showing what the experience is really like and 30 sample recipes.
1996 200 pages
ISBN: 0-939957-86-8

7551 Epilepsy Surgery
Raven Press
1185 Avenue of the Americas   212-930-9500
New York, NY 10036-2601
The most complete and current references on surgical treatments of the epilepsies.
880 pages
ISBN: 0-881678-21-0

7552 Epilepsy and the Family: A New Guide
Harvard University Press
79 Garden Street
Cambridge, MA 02138   800-448-2242
                    www.hup.harvard.edu/catalog/LECEPF.html

ISBN: 0-674258-97-5

7553 Epilepsy: 199 Answers
Demos Medical Publishing
386 Park Avenue S   212-683-0072
New York, NY 10016-8804   800-532-8663
                                    Fax: 212-683-0118
                    e-mail: orderdept@demosmed.com
                                    www.demosmedpub.com
Addresses the needs of everyone with epilepsy. A helpful guide to the most common questions asked by people with epilepsy and will help the reader to work with his physician and take charge of the epilepsy.
1996 152 pages
ISBN: 1-888799-09-9
Dr. Diana M Schneider, President

7554 Epilepsy: A Behavior Medicine Approach to Assessment & Treatment in Children
Hogrefe & Huber Publications
PO Box 51   716-282-1610
Lewiston, NY 14092-0051   Fax: 716-484-4200
1993 200 pages
ISBN: 0-889371-06-7

7555 Epilepsy: Current Approaches to Diagnosis and Treatment
Raven Press
1185 Avenue of the Americas   212-930-9500
New York, NY 10036-2601
288 pages
ISBN: 0-881676-15-2

7556 Epilepsy: I Can Live with That
4351 Garden City Drive   301-459-3700
Landover, MD 20785-2267   800-332-1000
                                    Fax: 301-577-9056
The experience of epilepsy as recorded by a group of ordinary men and women living in Australia. Each story focuses on personal growth, triumph over disability and emphasizes individual courage and hope.
Softcover
ISBN: 0-802774-65-2

7557 Epilepsy: Models, Mechanisms & Concepts
Cambridge University Press
40 W 20th Street   212-924-3900
New York, NY 10011-4211   800-221-4512
                                    Fax: 212-691-3239
                    e-mail: customerservice@cup.org
                                    www.cup.org

1993 400 pages
ISBN: 0-521392-98-5
Alice Ra, Assistant Marketing Manager

7558 Epilepsy: Patient and Family Guide
O Devinsky, MD, author
FA Davis Company

1915 Arch Street
Philadelphia, PA 19103

215-568-2172
800-523-4049
Fax: 215-568-5065
e-mail: mrt@fadavis.com
www.fadavis.com

Epilepsy expert Dr. Orrin Devinsky provides an easy-to-read guide to understanding the disease so that patients can achieve — and maintain — a higher quality of life. This book will educate recently-diagnosed patients, as well as those who have been living with epilepsy for years.
434 pages Paperback
ISBN: 0-803604-98-X
Michael Torso, Marketing Manager

7559 Equal Partners
Epilepsy Foundation of America
4351 Garden City Drive
Landover, MD 20785-2267

301-459-3700
800-332-1000
Fax: 301-577-9056

This book tells the story of a young Harvard-trained doctor whose experiences with seizures, brain surgery and subsequent epilepsy turns her from physician to patient.
257 pages Hardcover
ISBN: 0-802774-65-2

7560 Guide to Understanding and Living with Epilepsy
4351 Garden City Drive
Landover, MD 20785-2267

301-459-3700
800-332-1000
Fax: 301-577-9056

Easy-to-understand resource for people with epilepsy and their families. Covers a wide range of medical, social and legal issues. Topics include expanation of seizures and epilepsy; information about medication, side effects and risks; and getting the best medical care.

7561 Ketogenic Diet: A Treatment for Epilepsy
Demos Medical Publishing
386 Park Avenue S
New York, NY 10016

212-683-0072
Fax: 212-683-0118
e-mail: orderdept@demopub.com
www.demosmedpub.com

256 pages
ISBN: 1-888799-39-0
Dr. Diana M Schneider

7562 Living Well with Epilepsy
Epilepsy Foundation of America
4351 Garden City Drive
Landover, MD 20785-2267

301-459-3700
800-332-1000
Fax: 301-577-9056

Designed to help both health-care professionals and patients to understand all aspects of diagnosis and of pharmacologic and surgical management; to enable patients to participate more knowledgeably in interactions with their health care team and to help steer them toward a more normal, fulfilling life.
166 pages Softcover
ISBN: 1-888799-11-0

7563 Managing Seizure Disorder
Epilepsy Foundation of America
4351 Garden City Drive
Landover, MD 20785-2267

301-459-3700
800-332-1000
Fax: 301-577-9056

Provides health professionals with detailed information, on a variety of subjects, designed to help them help people with epilepsy live the kind of life they desire.
276 pages Softcover
ISBN: 0-802774-65-2

7564 Miles to Go Before I Sleep
Epilepsy Foundation of America
4351 Garden City Drive
Landover, MD 20785-2267

301-459-3700
800-332-1000
Fax: 301-577-9056

This book tells the story of a hijacking in which the author sustained a severe brain injury that, among other things, affected her vision, her memory, and left her with epilepsy.
230 pages Hardcover
ISBN: 0-802774-65-2

7565 Students with Seizures: A Manual for School Nurses
Epilepsy Foundation of America
4351 Garden City Drive
Landover, MD 20785-2267

301-459-3700
800-332-1000
Fax: 301-577-9056

A professional text with the sole purpose of creating a more accepting and understanding school environment for children with seizure disorders.
131 pages Paperback

Children's Books

7566 Dotty the Dalmatian has Epilepsy
Epilepsy Foundation of America
4351 Garden City Drive
Landover, MD 20785-2267

301-459-3700
800-332-1000
Fax: 301-577-9056

This is the story of Dotty the Dalmatian who discovers she has epilepsy.
16 pages Softcover
ISBN: 0-802774-65-2

7567 Epilepsy
Franklin Watts Grolier
90 Old Sherman Tpke
Danbury, CT 06816-0001

203-797-3500
800-621-1115
Fax: 203-797-3197
www.grolier.com

This book explains what epilepsy is, causes of epileptic seizures, diagnosis and treatments.
96 pages Grades 7-12
ISBN: 0-531108-07-4

7568 Lee the Rabbit with Epilepsy
4351 Garden City Drive
Landover, MD 20785-2267

301-459-3700
800-332-1000
Fax: 301-577-9056

Written for children ages 3-6, this illustrated picture book follows the adventures of a small rabbit who has seizures during a fishing trip with her Grandpa.
23 pages Hardcover

7569 Season of Secrets
Little, Brown & Company
3 Center Plz
Boston, MA 02108

617-227-0730
800-759-0190
Fax: 800-286-9471

Grades 4-6

Newsletters

7570 Epilepsia: Journal of the International League Against Epilepsy
Blackwell Publishing, Inc.
Commerce Place
Malden, MA 02148

781-388-8200
800-862-6657
Fax: 781-388-8210
www.blackwellpublishing.com

The leading international journal on the epilepsies for more than 30 years, Epilepsia provides comprehensive coverage of current clinical and research results.

7571 Epilepsy Services Foundation Newsletter
4618 N Armenia Avenue
Tampa, FL 33603-2706

813-870-3414
Fax: 813-870-1321
e-mail: eswcf@epilepsyservices.com
www.epilepsyservices.com

Information on medical and supportive services for persons affected by epilepsy living in West Central Florida. Raise funds to provide medical and supportive services to build and endowment to make a difference in the lives of generations to come.
2 pages 2-3 x/year
Thomas Orth, Executive Director

Pamphlets

7572 Child with Epilepsy at Camp
Epilepsy Foundation of America
4351 Garden City Drive 301-459-3700
Landover, MD 20785-2267 800-332-1000
Fax: 301-577-9056
Helps to explain why the child with epilepsy should be included in the camping experience.
14 pages Pamphlet

7573 Children and Seizures: Information for Babysitters
Epilepsy Foundation of America
4351 Garden City Drive 301-459-3700
Landover, MD 20785-2267 800-332-1000
Fax: 301-577-9056
Explains seizures, routine and special care, emergency aid and first aid to babysitters. Also offers a graph to write down important information about the child with seizure disorders for a quick reference.

7574 Epilepsy Medicines and Dental Care
Epilepsy Foundation of America
4351 Garden City Drive 301-459-3700
Landover, MD 20785-2267 800-332-1000
Fax: 301-577-9056
Explains dental care and includes instructions for brushing and flossing.

7575 Epilepsy: Legal Rights, Legal Issues
Epilepsy Foundation of America
4351 Garden City Drive 301-459-3700
Landover, MD 20785-2267 800-332-1000
Fax: 301-577-9056
Offers persons diagnosed with epilepsy information on their legal rights in employment, education, insurance and general disability benefits.
9 pages

7576 Epilepsy: Part of Your Life Series
Epilepsy Foundation of America
4351 Garden City Drive 301-459-3700
Landover, MD 20785-2267 800-332-1000
Fax: 301-577-9056
Provides information for staying healthy, describes various tests and diagnostic procedures, includes information for parents of children with epilepsy and provides general answers to questions about epilepsy.
Series of 4

7577 Epilepsy: You and Your Child, a Guide for Parents
Epilepsy Foundation of America
4351 Garden City Drive 301-459-3700
Landover, MD 20785-2267 800-332-1000
Fax: 301-577-9056
This instructional booklet offers information on emotional aspects of epilepsy, how to handle seizures, medication, diet and nutrition, and offers referral organizations for parents.

7578 Epilepsy: You and Your Treatment
Epilepsy Foundation of America
4351 Garden City Drive 301-459-3700
Landover, MD 20785-2267 800-332-1000
Fax: 301-577-9056
Reviews medical tests and diagnostic procedures used by physicians in diagnosing epilepsy.

7579 Facts About Epilepsy
Epilepsy Foundation of America
4351 Garden City Drive 301-459-3700
Landover, MD 20785-2267 800-332-1000
Fax: 301-577-9056
Designed for use by physicians and other health professionals with an interest in or who deal with the problems of people with epilepsy.
16 pages Softcover

7580 Finding Out About Seizures: A Guide to Medical Tests
Epilepsy Foundation of America

4351 Garden City Drive 301-459-3700
Landover, MD 20785-2267 800-332-1000
Fax: 301-577-9056
Introduces adults and children with epilepsy to the types of tests they may have to undergo.

7581 Kits for Adults with Epilepsy
Epilepsy Foundation of America
4351 Garden City Drive 301-459-3700
Landover, MD 20785-2267 800-332-1000
Fax: 301-577-9056
A variety of informative pamphlets for persons with epilepsy or seizure disorders.

7582 Management by Common Sense
Epilepsy Foundation of America
4351 Garden City Drive 301-459-3700
Landover, MD 20785-2267 800-332-1000
Fax: 301-577-9056
Promotes the employability of people with seizure disorders. Provides employers with information about epilepsy, customer/client reactions, workers' compensation issues, side effects of medication and other information relevant to employing a person with epilepsy.
46 pages Paperback
ISBN: 0-802774-65-2

7583 Me and My World Packet for Children
Epilepsy Foundation of America
4351 Garden City Drive 301-459-3700
Landover, MD 20785-2267 800-332-1000
Fax: 301-577-9056
Collection of pamphlets designed for children with epilepsy.

7584 Medicines for Epilepsy
Epilepsy Foundation of America
4351 Garden City Drive 301-459-3700
Landover, MD 20785-2267 800-332-1000
Fax: 301-577-9056
Offers information on medication and treatments, generic drugs, side effects, drug abuse and more. Contains a color chart with picyures of the most common medications for epilepsy.

7585 Mom I Have a Staring Problem
Epilepsy Foundation of America
4351 Garden City Drive 301-459-3700
Landover, MD 20785-2267 800-332-1000
Fax: 301-577-9056
Tiffany, a seven-year-old, describes her experience with petit mal seizures; her feelings, wishes and fears. Written to help adults recognize a hidden problem that could be occuring with a child who has learning problems.
24 pages Softcover
ISBN: 0-802774-65-2

7586 My Brother Matthew
Woodbine House
4351 Garden City Drive 301-459-3700
Landover, MD 20785-2267 800-332-1000
Fax: 301-577-9056
A picture and text book for children who have a brother or sister with developmental delay.
25 pages Harcoverr
ISBN: 0-802774-65-2

7587 My Friend Emily
Epilepsy Foundation of America
4351 Garden City Drive 301-459-3700
Landover, MD 20785-2267 800-332-1000
Fax: 301-577-9056
A story about Emily and her best friend Katy. Emily, a self confident child who enjoys life, shows that kids with epilepsy are just like other kids.
35 pages Softcover
ISBN: 0-802774-65-2

7588 Patient's Guide to Everyday Life
Epilepsy Foundation of America
4351 Garden City Drive 301-459-3700
Landover, MD 20785-2267 800-332-1000
Fax: 301-577-9056

Provides information for the newly diagnosed individual with epilepsy.

7589 Preventing Epilepsy
Epilepsy Foundation of America
4351 Garden City Drive   301-459-3700
Landover, MD 20785-2267   800-332-1000
                                         Fax: 301-577-9056
Examines some known causes of seizures and suggests precautionary measures which may prevent the occurrence of epilepsy.
16 pages

7590 Recognizing the Signs of Childhood Seizures
Epilepsy Foundation of America
4351 Garden City Drive   301-459-3700
Landover, MD 20785-2267   800-332-1000
                                         Fax: 301-577-9056
Explains what seizures are and what to look for in your child.

7591 Seizure Recognition and First Aid
Epilepsy Foundation of America
4351 Garden City Drive   301-459-3700
Landover, MD 20785-2267   800-332-1000
                                         Fax: 301-577-9056
Helps you recognize a seizure when it happens and give basic first aid.

7592 Surgery for Epilepsy
Epilepsy Foundation of America
4351 Garden City Drive   301-459-3700
Landover, MD 20785-2267   800-332-1000
                                         Fax: 301-577-9056
Describes current surgical treatment and the testing that precedes it.
12 pages

7593 Talking to Your Doctor About Seizure Disorders
Epilepsy Foundation of America
4351 Garden City Drive   301-459-3700
Landover, MD 20785-2267   800-332-1000
                                         Fax: 301-577-9056
Designed to help the patient talk with medical personnel about treatment of epilepsy.
Pamphlet

7594 Teacher's Role, A Guide for School Personnel
Epilepsy Foundation of America
4351 Garden City Drive   301-459-3700
Landover, MD 20785-2267   800-332-1000
                                         Fax: 301-577-9056
Provides tips on recognizing seizures and handling a seizure in the classroom.
14 pages

Audio & Video

7595 Comprehensive Clinical Management of the Epilepsies
Epilepsy Foundation of America
4351 Garden City Drive   301-459-3700
Landover, MD 20785-2267   800-332-1000
                                         Fax: 301-577-9056
Excellent reference on the treatment of epilepsy.
17 minutes

7596 How to Recognize and Classify Seizures
Epilepsy Foundation of America
4351 Garden City Drive   301-459-3700
Landover, MD 20785-2267   800-332-1000
                                         Fax: 301-577-9056
Discusses the classification of seizures and epileptic syndromes.
25 minutes

7597 Just Like You and Me
TASH
1025 Vermont Avenue   202-263-5600
Washington, DC 20005   Fax: 202-637-0138
                                    e-mail: btrader@tash.org
                                    www.tash.org/index.html

A video/print package on successful living with epilepsy.
Lu Zeph, Executive of Board Operating Committee
Barbara A Trader, Human Resources Director

7598 Meeting the Challenge: Employment Issues and Epilepsy
Epilepsy Foundation of America
4351 Garden City Drive   301-459-3700
Landover, MD 20785-2267   800-332-1000
                                         Fax: 301-577-2684
This video answers the fquestions most often asked by emloyers. It covers issues such as driving, absenteeism, productivity, accidents and first aid, and emphasized that most people with epilepsy can be gainfully employed.
9 minutes

7599 Rest of the Family
Epilepsy Foundation of America
4351 Garden City Drive   301-459-3700
Landover, MD 20785-2267   800-332-1000
                                         Fax: 301-577-9056
Presents the feelings and concerns of other family members including siblings, of children with epilepsy.
Video cassette

7600 Seizure First Aid
Epilepsy Foundation of America
4351 Garden City Drive   301-459-3700
Landover, MD 20785-2267   800-332-1000
                                         Fax: 301-577-9056
This video combines footage of real seizures with reenactments to demonstrate proper first aid procedures. In addition, people with epilepsy talk about how they feel when they have a seizure, discuss how they would like friends, family and the general public to react when a seizure occurs.
10 minutes

7601 Understanding Seizure Disorders
Epilepsy Foundation of America
4351 Garden City Drive   301-459-3700
Landover, MD 20785-2267   800-332-1000
                                         Fax: 301-577-9056
Provides an explanation of seizure disorders in everyday language and dispels many misconceptions about epilepsy with medically accurate information.
Video cassette

7602 Voices from the Workplace
Epilepsy Foundation of America
Epilepsy Foundation of America   301-459-3700
4351 Garden City Drive, MD 20785   800-332-1000
                                         Fax: 301-577-2684
Inspirational tape to help people with epilepsy cope with employment challenges. Individuals with epilepsy describe personal and social challenges in the workplace. They explain how they cope with their seizures and the reactions of co-workers and the public.

Web Sites

7603 American Epilepsy Society
                                         www.aesnet.org
Fosters treatment of epilepsy in its biological, clinical and social phases.

7604 Epilepsy Foundation of America
                                         www.efa.org
Information on the prevention and cure of seizure disorders, the alleviation of their effects, and the promotion of independence and optimal quality of life for people who have these disorders.

7605 Healing Well
                                         www.healingwell.com
An online health resource guide to medical news, chat, information and articles, newsgroups and message boards, books, disease-related web sites, medical directories, and more for patients, friends, and family coping with disabling diseases, disorders, or chronic illnesses.

7606 Health Finder
                                         www.healthfinder.gov

Searchable, carefully developed web site offering information on over 1000 topics. Developed by the US Department of Health and Human Services, the site can be used in both English and Spanish.

7607   Healthlink USA

www.healthlinkusa.com

Health information concerning treatment, cures, prevention, diagnosis, risk factors, research, support groups, email lists, personal stories and much more. Updated regularly.

7608   Helios Health

www.helioshealth.com

Online resource for your health information. Detailed information about specific health topics, access to expert advice from our Medical Advisory Board, and up-to-date health news.

7609   MedicineNet

www.medicinenet.com

An online resource for consumers providing easy-to-read, authoritative medical and health information.

7610   Medscape

www.medscape.com

Medscape offers specialists, primary care physicians, and other health professionals the Web's most robust and integrated medical information and educational tools.

7611   National Institute of Neurological Disorders and Stroke

www.ninds.nih.gov

The mission of NINDS is to reduce the burden of neurological disease - a burden borne by every age group, by every segment of society, by people all over the world.

7612   Neurology Channel

www.neurologychannel.com

Find clearly explained, medically accurate information regarding conditions, including an overview, symptoms, causes, diagnostic procedures and treatment options. On this site it is possible to ask questions and get information from a neurologist and connect to people who have similar health interests.

7613   WebMD

www.webmd.com

Information on seizure disorders, including articles and resources.

Description

7614 # Sexually Transmitted Diseases

Sexually transmitted diseases, STDs, are among the most common infectious diseases in the U.S. More than 20 STDs have been identified, and roughly 13 million persons are affected. Fortunately, most STDs are curable with prompt treatment, and do not become chronic. These include bacterial vaginosis, gonorrhea, syphilis, trichomoniasis and chlamydia. People who suffer from these diseases over long periods almost always do so because of re-infection rather than treatment failure. HIV and hepatitis B are commonly transmitted through sexual intercourse; see also *AIDS* and *Hepatitis*.

Fortunately, behavioral changes in sexual practices can drastically reduce the risk of STDs. Abstinence from intercourse or having a long-term mutually faithful monogamous relationship with an uninfected partner give essentially complete protection. Risk rises with multiple partners, unprotected intercourse between males, anonymous sex and contact with high-risk individuals, such as prostitutes. Barrier methods, notably condoms, give significant but not complete protection.

Until recently, no vaccines were available for any common STD except hepatitis B. However, researchers developed a vaccine for human papilloma virus (HPV) that is, amazingly, 100 percent effective. The vaccine is such a critical discovery because one specific type of HPV causes cervical cancer. Common STDs which may become chronic despite treatment are described below.

Genital herpes is a virus of the herpes family characterized by blisters (vesicles) in the genital area. The appearance of the blisters is often preceded by low-grade fever and by burning pain in the affected area. The first episode is often the most painful. Specific anti-viral therapy will shorten the duration and intensity of an attack. Herpes infections are self-limited but recurrent because the virus chronically infects nerves that radiate from the spinal column. Under certain conditions, such as febrile illness and physical or emotional stress, the virus reactivates and causes another outbreak. People with frequent recurrences can lower the risk of repeat attacks by taking a low dose of the anti-viral medication every day.

Genital warts are caused by the human papilloma virus (HPV.) There are roughly 750,000 new cases each year in the United States. The warts may appear anywhere in the genital and rectal area, making transmission difficult to prevent with a condom. Genital warts in the male, unless quite large, are often just a cosmetic nuisance, although a wart inside the urinary passage may cause discomfort. Women with genital warts not only need to have the warts removed, but to be observed for pre-cancerous changes in the cervix. Warts are generally destroyed by application of chemicals, but doctors have also used laser beams, freezing and electrical currents to destroy them. Recurrence after treatment is common, even in the absence of re-infection.

Pelvic inflammatory disease (PID) is not always sexually transmitted, but it is included here because chlamydia and gonorrhea, which are sexually transmitted, are commonly the cause of PID. In this condition, the sensitive pelvic reproductive organs are attacked, leading to fever and lower abdominal pain and occasionally collection of pus in a pelvic abscess. Even after the attack is treated with high doses of antibiotics, residual scarring may lead to chronic pelvic pain, pain with intercourse, infertility and ectopic pregnancy, in which the fertilized egg implants in other pelvic structures outside the uterus. Prompt recognition and vigorous treatment of the acute attack of PID are important.

National Agencies & Associations

7615 **American Foundation for the Prevention of Venereal Disease**
799 Broadway
New York, NY 10003   212-759-2069
www.chclibrary.org
Encourages every individual to assume responsible sexual relations and proper personal hygiene.
Mary O'Connell, Secretary

7616 **American Social Health Association**
PO Box 13827   919-361-8400
Research Triangle Park, NC 27709-3827   800-227-8922
Fax: 919-361-8425
www.ashastd.org
Provides resources to local communities to improve STD control programs through citizen action.
Lynn Barclay, President CEO
Deborah Arrindell, Vice President Health Policy

7617 **American Venereal Disease Association**
PO Box 1753
Baltimore, MD 21203-1753   301-955-3150
www.alternativemedicine.com
Primary interest of this organization is in the reduction of the prevalence of the diseases.
Edward Hook III MD, Secretary

7618 **Centers for Disease Control and Prevention**
1600 Clifton Road   404-639-3111
Atlanta, GA 30333   800-232-4636
TTY: 888-232-6348
e-mail: cdcinfo@cdc.gov
www.cdc.gov
Offers reprints reports public awareness and educational materials and research on sexually transmitted diseases.
Richard E Besser, Director

7619 **Citizens Alliance for VD Awareness**
5002 W Madison   773-379-1000
Chicago, IL 60644   Fax: 773-379-1342
e-mail: info@cfhcn.org
www.circlefamilycare.org
Seeks to increase commitment of health professionals to venereal disease and AIDS control.
Bruce Peoples, President/CEO
Patrick C Nwaezeigwe, CFO

7620 **Herpes Resource Center**
PO Box 13827   919-361-8400
Research Triangle Park, NC 27709-3827   800-227-8922
Fax: 919-361-8425
www.ashastd.org
Gives emotional support to individuals and provides information to the public about herpes.
Carolyn Mabry, Coordinator
Lynn Barclay, President CEO

7621 National Institute of Allergy and Infectious Diseases
6610 Rockledge Drive
Bethesda, MD 20892-6612   301-496-5717
www.niaid.nih.gov

Research Centers

7622 Herpes Resource Center
PO Box 13827   919-361-8400
Research Triangle Park, NC 27709   800-227-8922
Fax: 919-361-8425
www.ashastd.org
Offers information and referrals for persons affected by herpes and other sexually transmitted disease prevention.
Lynn Barclay, President and Chief Executive Officer
Deborah Arrindell, Vice President Health Policy

7623 International Union Against Venereal Diseases
New York Hospital - Cornell Medical Center
1153 York Avenue   212-746-1200
New York, NY 10021   Fax: 212-746-1202
e-mail: ajacobso@myp.org
Encourages campaigns medical and social against venereal disease.
Lewis Drusin MD, Director

7624 University of Chicago Committee on Virology
Marjorie B Kovler Viral Oncology Laboratories
910 E 58th Street   773-702-1898
Chicago, IL 60637   Fax: 773-702-1631
mgcb.bsd.uchicago.edu
Focuses research into the area of sexually transmitted disease.
Bernard Roizman, Chairman
Olaf Schneewind, Professor and Chairman

Support Groups & Hotlines

7625 National Health Information Center
PO Box 1133   310-565-4167
Washington, DC 20013   800-336-4797
Fax: 301-984-4256
e-mail: info@nhic.org
www.health.gov/nhic
Offers a nationwide information referral service, produces directories and resource guides.

7626 STI Resource Center Hotline
919-361-8488
800-227-8922
www.ashastd.org
Provides information, materials and referrals to anyone concerned about sexually transmitted infections.
Lynn Barclay, President/CEO
Deborah Arrindell, VP Health Policy

Books

7627 Herpes and Papilloma Viruses Volume I & II
Raven Press
1185 Avenue of the Americas   212-930-9500
New York, NY 10036-2601
382 pages
ISBN: 0-881671-95-9

7628 Sexually Transmitted Diseases
Raven Press
1185 Avenue of the Americas   212-930-9500
New York, NY 10036-2601
Focuses on the clinically important subject of the immune response to sexually transmitted diseases.
350 pages
ISBN: 0-881678-82-1

7629 Understanding Helps
University Press of Mississippi

3825 Ridgewood Road   601-432-6205
Jackson, MS 39211-6492   800-737-7788
Fax: 601-432-6217
e-mail: press@ihl.state.ms.us
www.upress.state.ms.us
This book is for people who wish to learn about herpes simplex viruses, two remarkably complex microbes capable of causing a wide variety of infections. These include genital herpes, a very common chronic sexually transmitted disease.
120 pages Hardcover
ISBN: 1-578060-40-0
Kathy Burgess, Advertising Manager/Marketing Assistant

7630 Understanding Herpes: Revised Second Edition
Lawrence R Stanberry, MD; PhD, author
University Press of Mississippi
3825 Ridgewood Road   601-432-6205
Jackson, MS 39211-6492   Fax: 601-432-6217
e-mail: kburgess@ihl.state.ms.us
www.upress.state.ms.us
A concise overview of advances and resources.
2006 144 pages Paperback
ISBN: 1-578068-68-1
Kathy Burgess, Advertising/Marketing Services Manager

7631 Women at Risk
Bristol Publishing
PO Box 1737   415-895-4461
San Leandro, CA 94577-0811   Fax: 415-895-4459
1993 159 pages
ISBN: 0-917851-62-5

Children's Books

7632 Teen Guide to Safe Sex
Franklin Watts Grolier
90 Old Sherman Tpke   203-797-3500
Danbury, CT 06816-0001   800-621-1115
Fax: 203-797-3197
www.grolier.com
A basic book about sexually transmitted diseases. Describes what they are, what causes them, how to recognize them and how teenagers can protect against them.
64 pages Grades 9-12
ISBN: 0-531105-92-0

Newsletters

7633 Sexually Transmitted Diseases: Journal
Julius Schachter, PhD, author
Lippincott Wiliiams & Wilkins
PO Box 1600
Hagerstown, MD 21741-1600   800-638-3030
Fax: 301-223-2400
e-mail: orders@lww.com
www.lww.com
This timely, scholarly journal publishes original, peer-reviewed articles on clinical, laboratory, immunologic, epidemiologic, sociologic, and historical topics pertaining to sexually transmitted diseases and related fields.
Monthly

7634 Step Perspective
Seattle Treatment Education Project
127 Broadway E   206-329-4857
Seattle, WA 98102-5711   800-869-7837
A publication of the Seattle Treatment Education Project. Published three times a year.
Michael Auch, Executive Director

Pamphlets

7635 AIDS...What We Need To Know Pamphlet
March of Dimes

233 Park Avenue South
New York, NY 10003
212-353-8353
Fax: 212-254-3518
e-mail: NY639@marchofdimes.com
www.marchofdimes.com

Discusses the facts about HIVÆinfection and AIDS and how you can reduce your risk.
Pkg of 50
ISBN: 0-923500- -

7636 Chlamydial Infection
National Institute of Allergy/Infectious Diseases
National Institutes of Health   301-496-5717
Bethesda, MD 20892-0001
Offers information on diagnosis, treatment, effects, prevention and research.

7637 Genital Herpes
National Institute of Allergy/Infectious Diseases
National Institutes of Health   301-496-5717
Bethesda, MD 20892-0001
Offers information on symptoms, causes, diagnosis and reccurences.

7638 Genital Herpes Fact Sheet
March of Dimes
233 Park Avenue South
New York, NY 10003
212-353-8353
Fax: 212-254-3518
e-mail: NY639@marchofdimes.com
www.marchofdimes.com

Fact Sheets: one to two page review written for the general public. Also available electronically from our website www.marchofdimes.com

7639 Gonorrhea
National Institute of Allergy/Infectious Diseases
National Institutes of Health   301-496-5717
Bethesda, MD 20892-0001
Offers information on the symptoms, diagnosis, treatment, complications, prevention and research.

7640 Human Papillomavirus and Genital Warts
National Institute of Allergy/Infectious Diseases
National Institutes of Health   301-496-5717
Bethesda, MD 20892-0001
Offers information on diagnosis, treatment, complications and prevention of the diseases.

7641 Introduction to Sexually Transmitted Diseases
National Institute of Allergy/Infectious Diseases
National Institutes of Health   301-496-5717
Bethesda, MD 20892-0001
Offers information on STDs, various types and symptoms, research, and referral services.

7642 Other Important STD's
National Institute of Allergy/Infectious Diseases
National Institutes of Health   301-496-5717
Bethesda, MD 20892-0001
Lists over ten of the most common sexually transmitted diseases. Offers information on what they are, the causes and treatments, research being done in these areas and referral numbers of where to call for more information on the diseases.

7643 Pelvic Inflammatory Disease
National Institute of Allergy/Infectious Diseases
National Institutes of Health   301-496-5717
Bethesda, MD 20892-0001
Offers information on the causes, symptoms, risk factors, diagnosis, treatment, and prevention.

7644 Syphilis
National Institute of Allergy/Infectious Diseases
National Institutes of Health   301-496-5717
Bethesda, MD 20892-0001
Offers information on what syphilis is, the symptoms, complications, diagnosis, prevention and treatment methods available.

7645 Vaginal Infections
National Institute of Allergy/Infectious Diseases
National Institutes of Health   301-496-5717
Bethesda, MD 20892-0001

Lists three specific types of vaginitis, with information on their symptoms, prevention, complications and treatments.

Web Sites

7646 American Social Health Association
sunsite.unc.edu/asha
Provides resources to local communities to improve STD control programs through citizen action.

7647 Centers for Disease Control
www.cdc.gov
Offers reprints, reports, public awareness and educational materials and research on sexually transmitted diseases.

7648 Healing Well
www.healingwell.com
An online health resource guide to medical news, chat, information and articles, newsgroups and message boards, books, disease-related web sites, medical directories, and more for patients, friends, and family coping with disabling diseases, disorders, or chronic illnesses.

7649 Health Finder
www.healthfinder.gov
Searchable, carefully developed web site offering information on over 1000 topics. Developed by the US Department of Health and Human Services, the site can be used in both English and Spanish.

7650 Healthlink USA
www.healthlinkusa.com
Health information concerning treatment, cures, prevention, diagnosis, risk factors, research, support groups, email lists, personal stories and much more. Updated regularly.

7651 Helios Health
www.helioshealth.com
Online resource for your health information. Detailed information about specific health topics, access to expert advice from our Medical Advisory Board, and up-to-date health news.

7652 MedicineNet
www.medicinenet.com
An online resource for consumers providing easy-to-read, authoritative medical and health information.

7653 Medscape
www.medscape.com
Medscape offers specialists, primary care physicians, and other health professionals the Web's most robust and integrated medical information and educational tools.

7654 WebMD
www.webmd.com
Information on sexually transmitted diseases, including articles and resources.

Description

7655 Sickle Cell Disease

Sickle cell disease (also called sickle cell anemia) is an inherited defect of hemoglobin, the oxygen-carrying element in the blood. Under some circumstances, the normally disc-shaped red blood cell takes on a crescent or sickle shape. It then becomes lodged in small capillaries and prevents normal oxygen flow to the tissues. This oxygen deprivation can cause sickle cell crises, with symptoms of severe pain in the back, joints, hands, and feet, and may even include neurologic changes. Severe abdominal pain and vomiting may also occur.

Sickle cell anemia occurs almost exclusively in African Americans. There are approximately 55,000 people in the United States with this condition. These children have sickle cell trait, occurring when one receives a copy of the sickle cell gene from only one parent. Only if a child receives a copy of the defective gene from both parents will the full-blown disease develop.

Therapy for sickle cell disease is aimed at preventing and treating infections, maintaining an adequate diet and fluid intake, and managing acute attacks with painkillers, oxygen, antibiotics and blood transfusion. Hydroxyurea has been shown to reduce the number of attacks by 50 percent as well as the need for transfusion. In the past, death typically occurred because of overwhelming infection or from organ destruction brought about by multiple sickling crises. Modern therapy has improved life expectancy dramatically, but some level of disability is common. Geneticcounseling is important for the patient and all family members.

National Agencies & Associations

7656 American Sickle Cell Anemia
10300 Carnegie Avenue
Cleveland, OH 44106-0171
216-229-8600
Fax: 216-229-4500
e-mail: irabragg@ascaa.org
www.ascaa.org
Provides education testing counseling and supportive services for sickle cell anemia and its hemoglobinopathy variants.
Ira Bragg-Grant, Executive Director
Leslie Carter, Newborn Screening Coordinator

7657 Comprehensive Sickle Cell Center
80 Jesse Hill Jr Drive SE
Atlanta, GA 30303
404-616-3572
Fax: 404-616-5998
e-mail: aplatt@emory.edu
www.scinfo.org
The mission of Sickle Cell Information Center is to provide sickle cell patient and professional education, news, research updates and world wide sickle cell resources, as well as world class compassionate care.
James R Eckman, Medical Director
Lewis Hsu, Interim Director

7658 Sickle Cell Anemia Foundation
503 S Center Street
Statesville, NC 28687
704-878-0732
This program is designed to provide information about sickle cell disease symptoms available treatments and service facilities by distributing literature and dispatching foundation members to address organizations church or school groups.
Priscilla Dudley

7659 Sickle Cell Association of Ontario
3199 Bathurst Street
Toronto, Ontario, M6A-2B2
416-789-2855
Fax: 416-789-1903
e-mail: sicklecell@look.ca
www.sicklecellontario.com
A voluntary, non-profit, charitable organization which is funded by donations from individuals, organizations and employee charitable funds.
Dotty Nicholas RN, President

7660 Sickle Cell Disease Association of America
231 E Baltimore Street
Baltimore, MD 21202
410-528-1555
800-421-8453
Fax: 410-528-1495
e-mail: scdaa@sicklecelldisease.org
www.sicklecelldisease.org
Purpose is to promote leadership on a national level in order to create awareness in all circles of the impact of sickle cell disease on emotional and economic well-being of families and the individual.
Willarda V Edwards, President/COO
Jeannine Knight, Executive Assistant to the President/COO

7661 Sickle Cell Information Center Grady Memorial Hospital
Grady Memorial Hospital
80 Jesse Hill Jr Drive SE
Atlanta, GA 30303
404-616-3572
Fax: 404-616-5998
e-mail: aplatt@emory.edu
www.SCInfo.org
Our mission is to provide sickle cell patient and professional education news research updates and world wide sickle cell resources. It is the mission of our organizations to provide world class compassionate care.
James R Eckman, Medical Director
Lewis Hsu, Interim Director

Foundations

7662 James R Clark Memorial Sickle Cell Foundation
1420 Gregg Street
Columbia, SC 29201
803-765-9916
800-506-1273
Fax: 803-799-6471
e-mail: sicklecell@sc.rr.com
Genetic Blood Disorder Disease.
Melodie A Hunnicutt, Executive Director
Saundra Kidwell, Director Finance

7663 Northeast Louisiana Sickle Cell Anemia Foundation
1604 Winnsboro Road
Monroe, LA 71202
318-322-0896
Fax: 318-387-4740
e-mail: sickle@bayou.com
The Foundation is a community-based non-profit, tax-exempt organization whose purpose is to provide services to sickle cell patients and their families, as well as be a resource in the communities we serve (12 northeast parishes) We provide education, trait counseling, patient assistance and social services. Our services are free.
Lasandre R Starks, Executive Director
Cheryl Minor, Registered Social Worker

7664 Sickle Cell Foundation of Georgia
2391 Benjamin E Mays Drive
Atlanta, GA 30311
404-755-1641
800-326-5287
Fax: 404-755-7955
e-mail: n_nichols@sicklecellatlaga.org
www.sicklecellatlaga.org
Our mission is dedicated to providing education, screening and counseling programs for Sickle Cell and other abnormal hemoglobin.
D Jean Brannan, President
Nesby Gibson, Project Director

7665 Sickle Cell Foundation of Greater Montgomery
3180 US Highway 8 West
Montgomery, AL 36108
334-286-9122
800-742-5534
e-mail: sicklec2@aol.com
www.scfgm.org
The main objectives of the Foundation are to give accurate information about sickle cell disease and related hemoglobinopathies, to provide testing and diagnostic services to interested persons, to

counsel individuals with positive test results so they can make informed decisions about their lives and to provide supportive services for clients and their family members.
Willie Owens, Executive Director

Research Centers

7666 Boston Sickle Cell Center Boston Medical Center
Boston Medical Center
88 E Newton Street   617-414-1020
Boston, MA 02118-2999   Fax: 617-414-1021
                                          e-mail: mhsteinb@bu.edu
                                                www.bu.edu/sicklecel
The treatment facility of choice for Boston-area patients with sickle cell disease. The Center also promotes interactive basic and clinical research and patient and professional educational activities.
Martin Steinberg, Director
Shawn H Eung, Program Manager

7667 Columbia University: Comprehensive Sickle Cell Center
Harlem Hospital
506 Lenox Avenue
New York, NY 10037-1000   212-939-1426
                          www.nyc.gov/html/hhc/html/facilities/har
Research into sickle cell disease.
Dr Jeanne Smith, Director

7668 Comprehensive Sickle Cell Center Children's Hospital Research Foundation
Children's Hospital Research Foundation
3333 Burnet Avenue   513-636-4541
Cincinnati, OH 5229—3039   800-344-2462
                                          Fax: 513-636-5562
                                         e-mail: blood@cchmc.org
                                       www.cincinnatichildrens.org
Offers research and statistical information in the area of sickle cell disease.
Clinton Joiner, Director
Karen Kalinyak, Clinical Director

7669 Howard University Center for Sickle Cell Disease
1840 7th Street NW   202-865-8292
Washington, DC 20001   Fax: 202-232-6719
                                      e-mail: sicklecell@howard.edu
                                         www.sicklecell.howard.edu

Victor R Gordeuk, Director
Catherine Nwokolo, Clinical Staff Member

7670 Medical College of Georgia: Sickle Cell Center
1521 Pope Avenue   706-721-2171
Augusta, GA 30912-0002   Fax: 706-721-4575
                                      www.mcg.edu/centers/sicklecel
Offers research into sickle cell disease.
Abdullah Kutlar, Director
Kavita Natarajan

7671 Philadelphia Biomedical Research Institute
100 Ross and Royal Road   610-962-0615
King of Prussia, PA 19406   Fax: 610-254-9332
                                       e-mail: stohmishi@aol.com
                               members.aol.com/stohinishi/phila_biomed
Study on the management of sickle cell anemia through nutrition.
S Tsuyoshi Ohinishi PhD, Director

7672 SUNY Health Science Center at Brooklyn Sickle Cell Center
450 Clarkson Avenue   718-270-1000
Brooklyn, NY 11203   Fax: 718-270-7592
                                            www.hscbklyn.edu

John C LaRosa, President
Paul J Davis, Interim Chief Financial Officer

7673 Sickle Cell Anemia Research Foundation
2625 3rd Street   318-487-8019
Alexandria, LA 71309   877-722-7370
                                          Fax: 318-487-9990
                               e-mail: scarf@sicklecelldisease.org
                                                www.kumc.edu

The Sickle Cell Anemia Research Foundation provides a comprehensive program on Sickle Cell Disease. We offer education training counseling and help with prescriptions.

7674 Sickle Cell Association of the Texas Gulf Coast
2626 S Loop W   713-666-0300
Houston, TX 77054-2649   Fax: 713-660-17
Rebecca Jasso, Executive Director

7675 University of California Northern Comprehensive Sickle Cell Center
Childrens Hospital Research Center
747 50 2nd Street   510-428-3651
Oakland, OK 94609-3594
Sickle cell disease research.
Elliot Vichinsky, Director

7676 University of Southern California: Comprehensive Sickle Cell Center
2025 Zonal Avenue   213-342-1259
Los Angeles, CA 90033-1034
Dr Cage S Johnson, Director

7677 University of Texas Southwestern Medical Center/Sickle Cell Management
Southwestern Medical Center
1935 Medical District Drive   214-456-7000
Dallas, TX 75235-7701   Fax: 214-648-3122
                              e-mail: jsquires@childmed.dallas.tx.us
                                              www.childrens.com
Focuses on the prevention of disease complications and management using the newest treatment strategies including hydroxyurea chronic transfusions stem cell (bone marrow) transplantation and state-of-the-art approaches to infection prevention pain management and treatment of specific organ-related complications (chest syndrome priapism avascular necrosis of the femoral head etc.).
George Bucha MD, Director
James F Amatruda

7678 Wayne State University: Comprehensive Sickle Cell Center
Curricular Affairs Office
Scott Hall   313-577-1546
Detroit, MI 48201   Fax: 313-577-8777
                                                wayne.edu

Charles F Whitten MD, President

Support Groups & Hotlines

7679 Keon Paschal Perry Sickle Cell Anemia Disease Awareness
7510 Granby Street, Perry Building
Norfolk, VA 23505   888-406-5111
                                        e-mail: keon4u@aol.com
International Sickle Cell Anemia Disease Awareness Campaign.
Roy L Perry-Bey, CEO/Executive Director

7680 Lehigh Valley Sickle Cell Support Group
PO Box 1711   610-706-0636
Allentown, PA 18105-1711   e-mail: SororW@aol.com
                              www.members.aol.com/SororW/index.html
Anyone affected/effected by Sickle Cell and all interested persons. Our mission is to educate the local community about Sickle Cell.

7681 National Health Information Center
PO Box 1133   310-565-4167
Washington, DC 20013   800-336-4797
                                          Fax: 301-984-4256
                                         e-mail: info@nhic.org
                                            www.health.gov/nhic
Offers a nationwide information referral service, produces directories and resource guides.

7682 Sickle Cell Anemia Association of Austin: Marc Thomas Chapter
PO Box 201092   512-335-2306
Austin, TX 78720-1092   e-mail: llthomas@austin.cc.tx.us
                                            www.tdh.state.tx.us
To raise awareness, resources and support for clients with sickle cell disease.
Linda L Thomas

7683 Sickle Cell Disease Association of America Philadelphia/Delaware Valley Chapter
4601 Market Street   215-471-8686
Philadelphia, PA 19139   Fax: 215-471-7441
e-mail: scdaa.pdvc@verizon.net
www.sicklecelldisorder.com
The Philadelphia/Delaware Valley Chapter of the Sickle Cell Disease Association of America (SCDAA/PDVC) assists the sickle cell community by serving as a vehicle and resource center for the psycho-social and social service needs of those individuals affected by the disease through the following services: case management; counseling; hospital/clinic visits; advocacy; career/vocational assistance; newborn screening follow-up; transportation; and outreach/community education.
Stanley A Simpkins, Executive Director
Karin Darius, Program Director

Pamphlets

7684 Sickle Cell Disease
March of Dimes
233 Park Avenue South   212-353-8353
New York, NY 10003   Fax: 212-254-3518
e-mail: NY639@marchofdimes.com
www.marchofdimes.com
Fact Sheets: one to two page review written for the general public. Also available electronically from the website www.marchofdimes.com

Web Sites

7685 American Sickle Cell Anemia
www.ascaa.org
Provides education, testing, counseling and supportive services for sickle cell anemia and its hemoglobinopathies variants.

7686 Healing Well
www.healingwell.com
An online health resource guide to medical news, chat, information and articles, newsgroups and message boards, books, disease-related web sites, medical directories, and more for patients, friends, and family coping with disabling diseases, disorders, or chronic illnesses.

7687 Health Finder
www.healthfinder.gov
Searchable, carefully developed web site offering information on over 1000 topics. Developed by the US Department of Health and Human Services, the site can be used in both English and Spanish.

7688 Healthlink USA
www.healthlinkusa.com
Health information concerning treatment, cures, prevention, diagnosis, risk factors, research, support groups, email lists, personal stories and much more. Updated regularly.

7689 Helios Health
www.helioshealth.com
Online resource for your health information. Detailed information about specific health topics, access to expert advice from our Medical Advisory Board, and up-to-date health news.

7690 MedicineNet
www.medicinenet.com
An online resource for consumers providing easy-to-read, authoritative medical and health information.

7691 Medscape
www.medscape.com
Medscape offers specialists, primary care physicians, and other health professionals the Web's most robust and integrated medical information and educational tools.

7692 Sickle Cell Disease Association of America
sicklecelldisease.org
Purpose is to promote leadership on a national level in order to create awareness in all circles of the impact of sickle cell disease on emotional and economic well-being of families and the individual.

7693 WebMD
www.webmd.com
Information on Sickle Cell disease, including articles and resources.

Description

7694 ## Sjogren's Syndrome

Sjogren's syndrome (also called sicca syndrome) is an autoimmune disorder characterized by dryness of the mouth, eyes and mucous membranes. Variable enlargement of the lacrimal (tear) or salivary gland can occur. The disorder has no known cause, but many researchers believe that it has a genetic basis. Sjogren's syndrome is divided into primary (affecting only the eyes and mouth) and secondary (generalized) forms which may be associated with connective tissue diseases such as rheumatoid arthritis, systemic lupus erythematosus, polymyositis or scleroderma.

Patients who suffer from Sjogren's syndrome often complain initially of a gritty sensation in the eyes or severe dryness of the mouth. Patients may develop kidney, skin, neurologic, pulmonary or joint problems.

Treatment for Sjogren's is mainly symptomatic in the form of artificial tears, sipping fluids throughout the day, chewing gum and using special mouthwash. Pilocarpine may be used to stimulate saliva production. Severe cases, especially if they affect parts of the body outside of the glands, may require corticosteroid therapy. Dental caries (cavities) are a complication of dry mouth, so close dental follow-up is important.

National Agencies & Associations

7695 **National Sjogren's Syndrome Foundation NSSA**
NSSA
5815 N Blk Canyon Highway
Phoenix, AZ 85015-2200

602-433-9844
800-395-6772
Fax: 602-433-9838
e-mail: NSSA@aol.com
www.sjogrens.org

Provides educational materials to members about medical developments and research concerning SS nationally and internationally. Membership also includes assorted discounts on additional materials and events.
Steven Taylor, National Executive Director
Sheriese DeFruscio, Vice President of Development

7696 **Sjogren's Syndrome Foundation**
6707 Democracy Boulevard
Bethesda, MD 20817-2025

301-530-4420
800-475-6473
Fax: 301-530-4415
e-mail: tms@sjogrens.org
www.sjogrens.org

A non-profit voluntary health organization whose purposes are to educate patients and their families about Sjogren's syndrome and help them cope with the problems and frustrations of living with Sjogren's syndrome and to increase public and medical awareness.
Philip C Fox, President
Steven Taylor, CEO

Support Groups & Hotlines

7697 **National Health Information Center**
PO Box 1133
Washington, DC 20013

310-565-4167
800-336-4797
Fax: 301-984-4256
e-mail: info@nhic.org
www.health.gov/nhic

Offers a nationwide information referral service, produces directories and resource guides.

Books

7698 **New Sjogren's Syndrome Handbook**
Sjogren's Syndrome Foundation
366 N Broadway
Jericho, NY 11753-2025

516-933-6365
800-475-4736
Fax: 516-933-6368
www.sjogrens.org

An authoritative guide for patients and health care providers on the many aspects of Sjogren's syndrome written by renowned experts, plus practical suggestions for living more comfortably with this chronic illness.
Hardcover
ISBN: 0-195117-24-7
Steven Carsons MD, Editor
Elaine K Harris, Editor

Newsletters

7699 **Moisture Seekers Newsletter**
Sjogren's Syndrome Foundation
366 N Broadway
Jericho, NY 11753-2025

516-933-6365
800-475-4736
Fax: 516-933-6368
www.sjogrens.org

Contains up-to-date information on Sjogren's syndrome including new treatments, new products, and clinical trails; also features articles on the ways members cope with this chronic disease.
9x Year
Linda Saslow, Editor

Pamphlets

7700 **Dry Eyes? Dry Mouth? Dry Nose? Arthritis? If Two or More: Sjogren's Syndrome**
Sjogren's Syndrome Foundation
382 Main Street
Port Washington, NY 11050-3136

516-767-2866
Fax: 516-767-7156

Offers a brief overview of what the illness is, a history, statistical information, causes, symptoms and treatments.

7701 **Sjogren's Syndrome**
NAMSIC/National Institutes of Health
1 AMS Circle
Bethesda, MD 20892-0001

301-495-4484
Fax: 301-587-4352
TTY: 301-565-2966
www.nih.gov/niams/

14 pages

Audio & Video

7702 **SjoGren's Syndrome Survival Guide**
6707 Democracy Boulevard
Bethesda, MD 20817

301-530-4420
800-475-6473
Fax: 301-530-4415
e-mail: staylor@sjogrens.org
www.sjogrens.org

A complete resource for Sjogren's sufferers providing the newest medical information, research results, and treatment methods available, as well as the most effective and practical self-help strategies. Sjogren's syndrome is an autoimmune disease in which the body's immune system mistakenly attacks its own moisture producing glands.
Steven Taylor, Chief Executive Officer
Sheriese DeFruscio, Vice President of Development

Web Sites

7703 **Healing Well**

www.healingwell.com

An online health resource guide to medical news, chat, information and articles, newsgroups and message boards, books, disease-related web sites, medical directories, and more for patients, friends, and family coping with disabling diseases, disorders, or chronic illnesses.

7704 Health Finder

www.healthfinder.gov

Searchable, carefully developed web site offering information on over 1000 topics. Developed by the US Department of Health and Human Services, the site can be used in both English and Spanish.

7705 Healthlink USA

www.healthlinkusa.com

Health information concerning treatment, cures, prevention, diagnosis, risk factors, research, support groups, email lists, personal stories and much more. Updated regularly.

7706 Helios Health

www.helioshealth.com

Online resource for your health information. Detailed information about specific health topics, access to expert advice from our Medical Advisory Board, and up-to-date health news.

7707 MedicineNet

www.medicinenet.com

An online resource for consumers providing easy-to-read, authoritative medical and health information.

7708 Medscape

www.medscape.com

Medscape offers specialists, primary care physicians, and other health professionals the Web's most robust and integrated medical information and educational tools.

7709 National Sjogren's Syndrome Association

www.sjogrens.org

Provides educational materials to members about medical developments and research concerning SS nationally and internationally. Membership also includes assorted discounts on additional materials and events.

7710 Sjogren's Syndrome Foundation

www.sjogrens.org

Information on Sjogren's Syndrome, the SS Foundation, and links to other related sites.

7711 WebMD

www.webmd.com

Information on Sjogren's Syndrome, including articles and resources.

Description

7712 Skin Disorders

The three most common chronic skin disorders are acne, psoriasis and eczema. Although these conditions do not shorten one's life, or cause significant disability, they can have a profound effect on one's quality of life and self-esteem.

Acne is probably the most common skin disorder, and can affect all age groups. It typically occurs in adolescents and young adults. Acne involves the sebaceous glands - glands that produce sebum, a substance that preserves the skin's natural oiliness. In acne, the glands' pores become plugged, trapping the sebum and bacteria. Inflammation follows, resulting in small red tender bumps with a corresponding blackhead or whitehead. These lesions can become pus-filled or even cystic ranging from 1 mm to 5 mm. Acne is seen most commonly on the face, neck, back and shoulders. Treatment starts with keeping affected areas clean. Locally-applied creams include retinoic acid, benzoyl peroxide and various antibiotics. Oral antibiotics (tetracycline) are especially effective for large, deep pimples. Oral tretinoin (Accutane) is very affective, but causes birth defects and other side effects and should be used only as a last resort and in consultation with a dermatologist. Oral contraceptives are often helpful in young women.

Psoriasis usually begins in early adult life, and affects 2 to 4 percent of the white population. A family history is common. The disease is characterized by scaly patches, some as small rain drop, others a few inches in diameer. Typical locations are the scalp, knees and elbows, but any part of the body may be affected. The patches are extremely itchy, and compulsive scratching may further damage the skin. In roughly 10 percent there is an associated arthritis. Milder cases are treated with steroid creams applied to skin and tar preparations or oral psoralen drugs, is effective in more severe cases. The most severe cases may require immunomodulating drugs like methotrexate or cyclosporine.

Eczema is a catchall term for many diseases which involve skin inflammation in response to some irritant. The irritant may be a direct one, such as contact dermatitis from the metal in a belt buckle, or an indirect one, as in atopic dermatitis triggered by various environmental agents (inhalants) and factors (certain foods). Atopic dermatitis is frequently associated with a personal or family history of allergic disorders (hay fever, asthma). For either situation, treatment consists of identifying and eliminating the offending agent(if possible) and local application of corticosteroid creams or nonspecific soothing and hydrating substances. Topical tacrolimus, approved by the FDA in 2000, is an immunosuppressive ointment effective for severe eczema without damaging the skin in the way that long-term topical steroids sometimes do.

National Agencies & Associations

7713 American Academy of Dermatology
PO Box 4014   847-330-0230
Schaumburg, IL 60168-4014   866-503-7546
                                    Fax: 847-240-1859
                              e-mail: volunteer@aad.org
                                          www.aad.org
The largest, most influential dermatologic association in the world. The Academy is committed to the highest quality standards in continuing medical education and plays a major role in formulating socioeconomic solutions.
Cyndi Del Boccio, Board of Director
Barbara Greenan, Advisory Board

7714 American Board of Dermatology American Society for Dermatologic Surger
American Society for Dermatologic Surgery
5550 Meadowbrook Drive   847-956-0900
Rolling Meadows, IL 60008   Fax: 847-956-0999
                              e-mail: info@asds.net
                                          www.asds-net.org
Sole mission is to ensure competence for patients with cutaneous diseases through board representation.
Katherine J Svedman, Executive Director
Debra Kennedy, Associate Executive Director

7715 American Dermatological Association University of Iowa Hospital and Clinics
University of Iowa Hospital and Clinics
Department of Dermatology   319-356-2274
Iowa City, IA 52242   Fax: 319-356-8317
Professional society of physicians specializing in dermatology. Promotes teaching, practice, public education and research into dermatology.
John S Strauss MD, Secretary

7716 American Society for Dermatologic Surgery
5550 Meadowbrook Drive   847-956-0900
Rolling Meadows, IL 60008-2005   Fax: 847-956-0999
                              e-mail: info@asds.net
                                          www.asds.net
Seeks to improve the quality of abnormal skin conditions especially the structural changes produced by skin cancer and other disease.
Katherine J Svedman, Executive Director
Robert A Weiss, President

7717 American Society of Plastic and Reconstructive Surgeons
444 E Algonquin Road   847-228-9900
Arlington Heights, IL 60005-4654   800-475-2784
                        e-mail: media@plasticsurgery.org
                                     www.plasticsurgery.org
This Society sends free information about various surgical procedures and also provides the names of board certified plastic surgeons in a patient's area.

7718 Dermatology Foundation
1560 Sherman Avenue   847-328-2256
Evanston, IL 60201-4808   Fax: 847-328-0509
                  e-mail: dfgen@dermatologyfoundation.org
                                          www.dermfnd.org
Raises funds for the control of skin diseases through research improved education and better patient care. Supports basic clinical investigations.

7719 Eczema Association for Science and Education
4460 Redwood Highway   415-499-3474
San Rafael, CA 94903   800-818-7546
                                    Fax: 415-472-5345
                          e-mail: info@nationaleczema.org
                                     www.nationaleczema.org
Offers research and information to persons with eczema and other skin disorders.
Donald S Young, Chair
John [Jack] R Crossen, CFO

7720 International Society of Dermatology
2323 N State Street
Bunnell, FL 32110-0001
386-437-4405
Fax: 386-437-4427
e-mail: info@intsocderm.org
www.intsocderm.org
Promotes interest education and research in dermatology.
Sigfrid A Muller MD, President
Luitgard Wie MD, Executive Vice President

7721 National Arthritis and Musculoskeletal & Skin Diseases Information Clearinghouse
National Institutes of Health
31 Center Drive - MSC 2350
Bethesda, MD 20892-2350
301-496-8190
Fax: 301-480-2814
e-mail: niamsinfo@mail.nih.gov
www.niams.nih.gov
Our mission is to support research into the causes, treatment and prevention of arthritis and musculoskeletal and skin diseases, the training of basic and clinical scientists to carry out this research and the dissemination of information on research.
Stephen I Katz MD PhD, Director

7722 National Institute of Arthritis and Musculoskeletal and Skin Disease (NIAMS)
1 AMS Circle
Bethesda, MD 20892
301-495-4484
877-226-4267
Fax: 301-718-6366
TTY: 301-565-2966
e-mail: niamsinfo@mail.nih.gov
www.niams.nih.gov
The NIAMS Information Clearinghouse provides free information about various forms of arthritis and rheumatic disease and bone, muscle and skin diseases. It distributes patient and professional education materials and refers people to other sources of information.
Stephen I Katz MD PhD, Director

Foundations

7723 National Psoriasis Foundation
6600 SW 92nd Avenue
Portland, OR 97223-7195
503-244-7404
800-723-9166
Fax: 503-245-0626
e-mail: getinfo@psoriasis.org
www.psoriasis.org
Misson: To find a cure for psoriasis arthritis and to eliminate their devastating effects through research, advocacy, and education. Provides: patient services; public and professional education; community services; government affairs; research.
Randy Beranek, President/CEO
Catie Coman, Director Communications

Research Centers

7724 Agromedicine Program Medical University of South Carolina
Medical University of South Carolina
295 Calhoun Street
Charleston, SC 29425-0100
843-792-2281
Fax: 843-792-1798
www.musc.edu
Does research into the effects of pesticides on humans including epidemiology and skin diseases.
Dr Stanley Schuman, Director
W Stuart Smith, Vice President for Clinical Operations a

7725 Duke University Plastic Surgery Research Laboratories
Medical Center
Box 3974
Durham, NC 27710-1
919-681-8555
e-mail: elizabeth.yundt@duke.edu
plastic.surgery.duke.edu
Conducts studies on skin cancer and aging skin.
L Scott Levin, Chief Division of Plastic and Reconstru
Detlev Erdmann, Associate Professor of Surgery

7726 Laboratory of Dermatology Research Memorial Sloane-Kettering Cancer Center
Memorial Sloane-Kettering Cancer Center
1275 York Avenue
New York, NY 10065-6007
212-639-2000
Fax: 212-717-3363
www.mskcc.org/mskcc
Specific studies on the identification of skin disorders and dermatology.
Allan C Halpern, Chief Dermatology Service

7727 Massachusetts General Hospital: Harvard Cutaneous Biology Research Center
Massachusetts General Hospital
55 Fruit Street
Boston, MA 02114
617-726-5254
Fax: 617-726-1875
TTY: 617-724-8800
www.massgeneral.org
Dermatology research.
Dr John Parrish, Director

7728 Orentreich Foundation for the Advancement of Science
855 Route 301
Cold Spring, NY 10516-4155
212-606-0836
Fax: 845-265-4210
e-mail: ofas@orentreich.org
Conducts biomedical research on dermatology.
Norman Orentreich, Founder and Co-Director
David S Orentreich, Co-Director

7729 Psoriasis Research Institute
600 Town & Country Center
Palo Alto, CA 94301
650-326-1848
Fax: 650-326-1262
Studies the causes symptoms and treatments of psoriasis.

7730 Rockefeller University Laboratory for Investigative Dermatology
Rockefeller University
1230 York Avenue
New York, NY 10021-6399
212-327-7458
Fax: 212-708-32
www.rockefeller.edu
Research into skin disorders and the whole specialty of dermatology in general.

7731 Rockefeller University, Laboratory for Investigative Dermatology
1230 York Avenue
New York, NY 10021-6399
212-327-7458
Fax: 212-570-8232
D Martin Carter MD, PhD, Head

7732 Scripps Clinic and Research Foundation: Autoimmune Disease Center
10550 N Torrey Pines Road
La Jolla, CA 92037-1092
858-784-1000
Fax: 619-554-6805
www.scripps.edu
Research into dermatomyositis and polymyositis.
Eng Tan, Professor Emeritus

7733 Sulzberger Institute for Dermatologic Education
PO Box 94020
Palatine, IL 60094-4020
847-330-0230
Fax: 847-330-0050
A nonprofit research center whose sole goal is to enhance patient care through the development and promotion of quality educational programs on the care and disorders of the skin, hair, nails and mucous membranes.

7734 Sulzberger Institute for Dermatologic Educ
PO Box 94020
Palatine, IL 60094
847-330-0230
Fax: 847-330-0050
A nonprofit research center whose sole goal is to enhance patient care through the development and promotion of quality educational programs on the care and disorders of the skin hair nails and mucous membranes.

7735 University of California: San Francisco Dermatology Drug Research
515 Spruce
San Francisco, CA 94143-0001
415-476-2001
Fax: 415-221-4751
www.ucsf.edu
Conducts clinical testing of new or existing pharmalogic agents used in the treatment of skin disorders.
John Koo MD, Director

7736 University of Texas: Southwestern Medical Center at Dallas, Immunodermatology
5323 Harry Hines Boulevard
Dallas, TX 75390-7208
214-648-3111
Fax: 214-688-8275
www.utsouthwestern.edu

Provides a focus for research into the causes prevention and management of diseases such as immune deficiencies and infections. Studies are aimed at increasing basic-level understanding of immunologic skin diseases.
Paul Bergtresser, Chair in Dermatology
Kiyoshi Ariizumi, Associate Professor

Support Groups & Hotlines

7737 National Health Information Center
PO Box 1133   310-565-4167
Washington, DC 20013   800-336-4797
                                        Fax: 301-984-4256
                                    e-mail: info@nhic.org
                                    www.health.gov/nhic
Offers a nationwide information referral service, produces directories and resource guides.

Books

7738 Managing Your Psoriasis
MasterMedia
33 Beecker Street   212-260-5600
New York, NY 10012   800-334-8232
1993 Paperback
ISBN: 0-942361-83-0

7739 Psoriasis and Psoriatic Arthritis Pocket Guide
National Psoriasis Foundation
6600 SW 92nd Avenue   503-244-7404
Portland, OR 97223-7195   800-723-9166
                                        Fax: 503-245-0626
                                    e-mail: getinfo@psoriasis.org
                                    www.psoriasis.org
The Pocket Guide includes algorithms for therapy including combination and biologic treatments based on patient types. This second edition was revised to provide guidance for managing patients with severe psoriasis and to put the roll of new biologics into perspective.
2005 79 pages

7740 Q&A's About Psoriasis
NAMSIC/National Institutes of Health
1 AMS Circle   301-495-4484
Bethesda, MD 20892-0001   877-226-4267
                                        Fax: 301-718-6366
                                        TTY: 301-565-2966
                                    e-mail: niamsinfo@mail.nih.gov
                                    www.nih.gov/niams
Offers various information for the psoriasis patient and their family regarding treatments, risks, nutrition and more.
24 pages

7741 Therapy of Moderate-to-Severe Psoriasis
National Psoriasis Foundation
6600 SW 92nd Avenue   503-244-7404
Portland, OR 97223-7195   800-723-9166
                                        Fax: 503-245-0626
                                    e-mail: getinfo@psoriasis.org
                                    www.psoriasis.org
Edited by Gerald D. Weinstein, MD, and Alice Gottlieb, MD, PhD, this book includes information on state-of-the-art clinical management through contributions from national experts on psoriasis.
2002
Gail M Zimmerman, President/CEO
Paula Fasano, Director Marketing/Communications

7742 Treatment Guide for the Health Insurance Industry
National Psoriasis Foundation
6600 SW 92nd Avenue   503-244-7404
Portland, OR 97223-7195   800-723-9166
                                        Fax: 503-245-0626
                                    e-mail: getinfo@psoriasis.org
                                    www.psoriasis.org
This easy-to-read general overview is a valuable tool for the insurer or any health professional interested in detailed information

about psoriasis and psoriatic arthritis, patient quality of life issues, and many available treatments.
Gail M Zimmerman, President/CEO
Paula Fasano, Director Marketing/Communications

Magazines

7743 International Journal of Dermatology
International Society of Dermatology
200 1st Street SW   507-284-3736
Rochester, MN 55905-0001
Focuses on information for dermatologists and the whole specialty of dermatology research and education.
10x Year

7744 Journal of Dermatologic Surgery and Oncology
International Society for Dermatologic Surgery
930 N Meachan Road   847-330-9830
Schaumburg, IL 60173   Fax: 847-330-1135
Focuses on medical updates and information on dermatology.
Monthly

7745 Journal of the Academy of Dermatology
American Academy of Dermatology
PO Box 94020   847-330-0230
Palatine, IL 60094-4020   Fax: 847-330-0050
A scientific publication serving the clinical needs of the specialty and provides a wide selection of articles on various topics important to continuing medical education of Academy members and the international dermatologic community.
Monthly

7746 Psoriasis Advance
National Psoriasis Foundation
6600 SW 92nd Avenue   503-244-7404
Portland, OR 97223-7195   800-723-9166
                                        Fax: 503-245-0626
                                    e-mail: getinfo@npfusa.org
                                    www.psoriasis.org
Written especially for the psoriatis community four times a year. Provides current articles to keep you up to date with treatmetnt and research information, pave the way to empowerment, and connect you with others.
40 pages BiMonthly
Sheri Decker, Director Communication

7747 Psoriasis Forum
National Psoriasis Foundation
6600 SW 92nd Avenue   503-244-7404
Portland, OR 97223-7195   800-723-9166
                                        Fax: 503-245-0626
                                    e-mail: getinfo@psoriasis.org
                                    www.psoriasis.org
Dedicated to providing up-to-date and practical information to health care providers on the frontline of psoriasis treatment. Professional Members only.
Quarterly
Gail M Zimmerman, President/CEO
Paula Fasano, Director Marketing/Communications

Newsletters

7748 Dermatology Focus
Dermatology Foundation
1560 Sherman Avenue   847-328-2256
Evanston, IL 60201-4808   Fax: 847-328-0509
                                    e-mail: dfgen@dermatologyfoundation.org
                                    www.dermfnd.org
Designed to communicate to practitioners the latest advances in medical and surgical dermatology. The publication also serves as the Foundation's newsletter, recognizing the accomplishments and activities of the many dermatologists who give not only their monetary support, but countless hours to develop the research and teaching careers of future leaders throughout the specialty.
Quarterly
Sandra Rahn Benz, Executive Director

7749 Dermatology Focus
Dermatology Foundation
1560 Sherman Avenue — 847-328-2256
Evanston, IL 60201-4808 — Fax: 847-328-0509
e-mail: dfgen@dermatologyfoundation.org
www.dermfnd.org
Designed to communicate to practitioners the latest advances in medical and surgical dermatology. The publication also serves as the Foundation's newsletter recognizing the accomplishments and activities of the many dermatologists who give not only their monetary support, but countless hours to develop the research and teaching careers of future leaders throughout the specialty.
Quarterly
Sandra Rahn Benz, Executive Director

7750 Dermatology World
American Academy of Dermatology
PO Box 94020 — 847-330-0230
Palatine, IL 60094-4020 — Fax: 847-330-0050
Offers Academy members information outside the clinical realm. It carries news of government actions, reports of socioeconomic issues, societal trends and other events which impinge on the practice of dermatology.
Monthly

7751 Progress in Dermatology
Dermatology Foundation
1560 Sherman Avenue — 847-328-2256
Evanston, IL 60201-4808 — Fax: 847-328-0509
e-mail: dfgen@dermatologyfoundation.org
www.dermfnd.org
The journal provides in-depth coverage of clinically relevant topics as well as basic scientific advances affecting all of dermatology. Distributed exclusively to members of the Foundation.
Quarterly
Sandra Rahn Benz, Executive Director

7752 Psoriasis Newsletter
Psoriasis Research Institute
600 Town & Country Center — 650-326-1848
Palo Alto, CA 94301 — Fax: 650-326-1262
e-mail: emfpri@aol.com
Offers information and medical updates on the disease of psoriasis, events, fundraising and more.
4 pages Quarterly

Pamphlets

7753 Acne
American Academy of Dermatology
PO Box 4014 — 847-330-0230
Schaumburg, IL 60168-4014 — Fax: 847-330-0050
Explains the causes of acne. Treatments are explored, including diet, medications, antibiotics, and sun exposure. Available in Spanish.
1996

7754 Allergic Contact Rashes
American Academy of Dermatology
PO Box 4014 — 847-330-0230
Schaumburg, IL 60168-4014 — Fax: 847-330-0050
Lists the common causes of skin rashes, including jewelry and hidden ingredients in fabrics and household products.
1997

7755 Athlete's Foot
American Academy of Dermatology
PO Box 4014 — 847-330-0230
Schaumburg, IL 60168-4014 — Fax: 847-330-0050
This common fungal infection is not only a problem for athletics. Discusses what causes it and how to treat it.
1994

7756 Black Skin
American Academy of Dermatology
PO Box 4014 — 847-330-0230
Schaumburg, IL 60168-4014 — Fax: 847-330-0050
Explains the skin diseases common with black skin and how they are diagnosed and treated.
1996

7757 Conception, Pregnancy & Psoriasis
National Psoriasis Foundation
6600 SW 92nd Avenue — 503-244-7404
Portland, OR 97223-7195 — 800-723-9166
Fax: 503-245-0626
e-mail: getinfo@npfusa.org
www.psoriasis.org
Explains pregnancy factors for persons with psoriasis.

7758 Cosmetics & Skin Care
American Academy of Dermatology
PO Box 4014 — 847-330-0230
Schaumburg, IL 60168-4014 — Fax: 847-330-0050
Discusses skin reactions to fragrances, makeup, and bath and body care products.
1994

7759 Darker Side of Tanning
American Academy of Dermatology
PO Box 4014 — 847-330-0230
Schaumburg, IL 60168-4014 — Fax: 847-330-0050
Discusses the dangers of ultraviolet radiation from the sun, tanning beds, and sun lamps. Includes descriptions of the different skin types and tips to help minimize the sun's damage to the skin and eyes.
1996

7760 Eczema/Atopic Dermatitis
American Academy of Dermatology
PO Box 4014 — 847-330-0230
Schaumburg, IL 60168-4014 — Fax: 847-330-0050
Explains how to recognize and treat dermatitis.
1995

7761 For Parents
National Psoriasis Foundation
6600 SW 92nd Avenue — 503-244-7404
Portland, OR 97223-7195 — 800-723-9166
Fax: 503-245-0626
e-mail: getinfo@npfusa.org
www.psoriasis.org
Offers advice and resources on how to educate yourself about psoriasis and your child, as well as treatment information and summer camps.

7762 Genital Psoriasis
National Psoriasis Foundation
6600 SW 92nd Avenue — 503-244-7404
Portland, OR 97223-7195 — 800-723-9166
Fax: 503-245-0626
e-mail: getinfo@npfusa.org
www.psoriasis.org
Introduces the reader to the basics of genital psoriasis, and treatment options.

7763 Hand Eczema
American Academy of Dermatology
PO Box 4014 — 847-330-0230
Schaumburg, IL 60168-4014 — Fax: 847-330-0050
Shows examples of hand rashes, explains causes, lists protective measures and treatments.
1993

7764 Hives
American Academy of Allergy, Asthma and Immunology
611 E Wells Street — 414-272-6071
Milwaukee, WI 53202-3889 — 800-822-2762
Fax: 414-272-6070
www.aaaai.org
This brochure offers information on what causes hives, what is Angioedema, and how hives can be treated.

7765 Home Phototherapy
National Psoriasis Foundation

6600 SW 92nd Avenue
Portland, OR 97223-7195

503-244-7404
800-723-9166
Fax: 503-245-0626
e-mail: getinfo@npfusa.org
www.psoriasis.org

Talks about the use of a home UVB unit to treat psoriasis.

7766 Methotrexate (MTX)
National Psoriasis Foundation
6600 SW 92nd Avenue
Portland, OR 97223-7195

503-244-7404
800-723-9166
Fax: 503-245-0626
e-mail: getinfo@npfusa.org
www.psoriasis.org

An introductions to MTX treatment.

7767 Oral Retinoid Therapy (Soriatane)
National Psoriasis Foundation
6600 SW 92nd Avenue
Portland, OR 97223-7195

503-244-7404
800-723-9166
Fax: 503-245-0626
e-mail: getinfo@npfusa.org
www.psoriasis.org

Explains Soriatane treatment options.

7768 PUVA (Psoralen Plus Ultraviolet Light A)
National Psoriasis Foundation
6600 SW 92nd Avenue
Portland, OR 97223-7195

503-244-7404
800-723-9166
Fax: 503-245-0626
e-mail: getinfo@npfusa.org
www.psoriasis.org

Explains PUVA treatment options, pros, cons, and potential side-effects.

7769 Pityriasis Rosea
American Academy of Dermatology
PO Box 4014
Schaumburg, IL 60168-4014

847-330-0230
Fax: 847-330-0050

Discusses the appearance, symptoms, and causes of this common rash. Diagnosis and treatment are also explained.
1996

7770 Psoriasis on Specific Skin Sites
National Psoriasis Foundation
6600 SW 92nd Avenue
Portland, OR 97223-7195

503-244-7404
800-723-9166
Fax: 503-245-0626
e-mail: getinfo@npfusa.org
www.psoriasis.org

Including nails, ears, eyelids, face, mouth and lips, hands and feet.

7771 Psoriasis: How It Makes You Feel
National Psoriasis Foundation
6600 SW 92nd Avenue
Portland, OR 97223-7195

503-244-7404
800-723-9166
Fax: 503-245-0626
e-mail: getinfo@npfusa.org
www.psoriasis.org

7772 Psoriatic Arthritis
National Psoriasis Foundation
6600 SW 92nd Avenue
Portland, OR 97223-7195

503-244-7404
800-723-9166
Fax: 503-245-0626
e-mail: getinfo@npfusa.org
www.psoriasis.org

7773 Rosacea
American Academy of Dermatology
PO Box 4014
Schaumburg, IL 60168-4014

847-330-0230
Fax: 847-330-0050

The condition, do's and don'ts for rosacea patients, and treatment are explained.
1995

7774 Scabies
American Academy of Dermatology
PO Box 4014
Schaumburg, IL 60168-4014

847-330-0230
Fax: 847-330-0050

Explains the nature of the scabies parasite, symptoms, at-risk groups, individual and large group treatments. Available in Spanish.
1997

7775 Scalp Psoriasis
National Psoriasis Foundation
6600 SW 92nd Avenue
Portland, OR 97223-7195

503-244-7404
800-723-9166
Fax: 503-245-0626
e-mail: getinfo@npfusa.org
www.psoriasis.org

7776 Seborrheic Dermatitis
American Academy of Dermatology
PO Box 4014
Schaumburg, IL 60168-4014

847-330-0230
Fax: 847-330-0050

Answers the most frequently asked questions about this common, easily treatable skin condition.
1995

7777 Seborrheic Keratoses
American Academy of Dermatology
PO Box 4014
Schaumburg, IL 60168-4014

847-330-0230
Fax: 847-330-0050

Describes seborrheic keratosis growths, causes, and treatments.
1997

7778 Skin Cancer
American Academy of Dermatology
PO Box 4014
Schaumburg, IL 60168-4014

847-330-0230
Fax: 847-330-0050

Warning signs and how to perform self-examinations are discussed.
1994

7779 Skin Conditions Related to AIDS
American Academy of Dermatology
PO Box 4014
Schaumburg, IL 60168-4014

847-330-0230
Fax: 847-330-0050

What AIDS is, who's at risk, and other important information about this major health problem are discussed.
1997

7780 Specific Forms of Psoriasis
National Psoriasis Foundation
6600 SW 92nd Avenue
Portland, OR 97223-7195

503-244-7404
800-723-9166
Fax: 503-245-0626
e-mail: getinfo@npfusa.org
www.psoriasis.org

Pustular, Guttate, Inverse, and Erythrodermic.

7781 Spider Veins, Varicose Vein Therapy
American Academy of Dermatology
PO Box 4014
Schaumburg, IL 60168-4014

847-330-0230
Fax: 847-330-0050

Discusses the latest methods for removing unsightly and unwanted blood vessels that appear mostly on the legs.
1995

7782 Sun & Water Therapy
National Psoriasis Foundation
6600 SW 92nd Avenue
Portland, OR 97223-7195

503-244-7404
800-723-9166
Fax: 503-245-0626
e-mail: getinfo@npfusa.org
www.psoriasis.org

7783 Sun Protection for Children
American Academy of Dermatology
PO Box 4014
Schaumburg, IL 60168-4014

847-330-0230
Fax: 847-330-0050

Teaches parents how to protect their children from the sun's harmful rays.
1996

7784 Sun and Your Skin
American Academy of Dermatology
PO Box 4014
Schaumburg, IL 60168-4014

847-330-0230
Fax: 847-330-0050

Information on acute sunburn, premature aging of the skin, allergies, and skin cancer. Tips on how to be sun smart.
1994

7785 Sunlight, Ultraviolet Radiation and the Skin
National Cancer Institute
Building 31
Bethesda, MD 20892-0001   800-422-6237

7786 Tinea Versicolor
American Academy of Dermatology
PO Box 4014   847-330-0230
Schaumburg, IL 60168-4014   Fax: 847-330-0050
Discusses the symptoms, diagnosis, and treatment of this often misunderstood fungal infection.
1995

7787 Treatment Overview
National Psoriasis Foundation
6600 SW 92nd Avenue   503-244-7404
Portland, OR 97223-7195   800-723-9166
                                 Fax: 503-245-0626
                                 e-mail: getinfo@npfusa.org
                                 www.psoriasis.org
Discusses a number of available psoriasis treatments, what is considered by the doctor when developing a treatment plan, and treatment resources.

7788 Vascular Birthmarks
American Academy of Dermatology
PO Box 4014   847-330-0230
Schaumburg, IL 60168-4014   Fax: 847-330-0050
Includes descriptions and treatments for most common types of vascular birthmarks - macular stains, hemangiomas, and port-wine stains.
1997

7789 Vitiligo
American Academy of Dermatology
PO Box 4014   847-330-0230
Schaumburg, IL 60168-4014   Fax: 847-330-0050
Discusses lost skin pigmentation and what can be done about it, including repigmentation therapy.
1994

7790 Young People and Psoriasis
National Psoriasis Foundation
6600 SW 92nd Avenue   503-244-7404
Portland, OR 97223-7195   800-723-9166
                                 Fax: 503-245-0626
                                 e-mail: getinfo@npfusa.org
                                 www.psoriasis.org
Infancy through adolescence.

7791 Your Diet & Psoriasis
National Psoriasis Foundation
6600 SW 92nd Avenue   503-244-7404
Portland, OR 97223-7195   800-723-9166
                                 Fax: 503-245-0626
                                 e-mail: getinfo@npfusa.org
                                 www.psoriasis.org
A discussion of particular diets, foods and supplements and the effect they have on psoriasis.

7792 Your Skin and Your Dermatologist
American Academy of Dermatology
PO Box 4014   847-330-0230
Schaumburg, IL 60168-4014   Fax: 847-330-0050
Explains why a dermatologist is the appropriate specialist for the care of diseases of the skin, hair, nails, and mucous membranes.
1997

Audio & Video

7793 Allergic Skin Reactions
American Academy of Allergy, Asthma and Immunology
611 E Wells Street   414-272-6071
Milwaukee, WI 53202-3889   800-822-2762
                                 Fax: 414-272-6070
                                 www.aaaai.org

In some people, allergy symptoms include itching redness, rashes, or hives. This video describes the symptoms, triggers, and treatment for common skin reactions such as dermatitis, hives and angioedema.
10-13 minutes

7794 Basic Science Series
American Academy of Dermatology
PO Box 4014   847-330-0230
Schaumburg, IL 60168-4014   Fax: 847-330-0050
Combines high-quality 35mm slides and accompanying narration on audiocassette and features topics that underline and support clinical dermatology. The series is useful for residents in training as well as practicing dermatologists.
Slides

7795 CME Video Library
American Academy of Dermatology
PO Box 4014   847-330-0230
Schaumburg, IL 60168-4014   Fax: 847-330-0050
A series of video programs developed by AAD experts recognized for their continued efforts in dermatologic advancement.
Videotapes

7796 Facts About Acne
American Academy of Dermatology
PO Box 4014   847-330-0230
Schaumburg, IL 60168-4014   Fax: 847-330-0050
The etiology of acne and treatment choices are explained by consultants, with patient encounters.
13 minutes

7797 Mystery of Contact Dermatitis
American Academy of Dermatology
PO Box 4014   847-330-0230
Schaumburg, IL 60168-4014   Fax: 847-330-0050
The causes and treatment of some common forms of contact dermatitis are shown with consultation and commentary.
10 minutes

7798 National Library of Dermatologic Teaching Slides
American Academy Of Dermatology
PO Box 94020   847-330-0230
Palatine, IL 60094-4020   Fax: 847-330-0050
A collection of dermatologic teaching slides offering the most comprehensive series ever assembled. Each set offers a realistic presentation of classic clinical skin conditions encountered by the dermatologist.

7799 Skin Cancer: The Undeclared Epidemic
American Academy of Dermatology
PO Box 4014   847-330-0230
Schaumburg, IL 60168-4014   Fax: 847-330-0050
Examples of skin cancer lesions, interviews with patients at screenings, and comments from Academy members.
9 minutes

7800 Skin Care Under the Sun
American Academy of Dermatology
PO Box 4014   847-330-0230
Schaumburg, IL 60168-4014   Fax: 847-330-0050
Dramatization of the dangers of overexposure to the sun, providing explanations of the effects of ultraviolet radiation on the skin.
7 minutes

Web Sites

7801 American Academy of Dermatology
                                 www.aad.org
Promotes and advances the science and art of medicine and surgery related to the skin, promotes the highest possible standards in clinical practice, education and research.

7802 American Society of Plastic and Reconstructive Surgeons
                                 www.plasticsurgery.org
This Society sends free information about various surgical procedures and also provides the names of board certified plastic surgeons in a patient's area.

7803 Derma Doctor

www.dermadoctor.com
The most informative skin care site on the Web. An extensive library of newsletters to help answer your questions.

7804 Dermatology Foundation

www.dermfnd.org
Raises funds for the control of skin diseases through research, improved education and better patient care. Supports basic clinical investigations.

7805 Healing Well

www.healingwell.com
An online health resource guide to medical news, chat, information and articles, newsgroups and message boards, books, disease-related web sites, medical directories, and more for patients, friends, and family coping with disabling diseases, disorders, or chronic illnesses.

7806 Health Finder

www.healthfinder.gov
Searchable, carefully developed web site offering information on over 1000 topics. Developed by the US Department of Health and Human Services, the site can be used in both English and Spanish.

7807 Healthlink USA

www.healthlinkusa.com
Health information concerning treatment, cures, prevention, diagnosis, risk factors, research, support groups, email lists, personal stories and much more. Updated regularly.

7808 Helios Health

www.helioshealth.com
Online resource for your health information. Detailed information about specific health topics, access to expert advice from our Medical Advisory Board, and up-to-date health news.

7809 MedicineNet

www.medicinenet.com
An online resource for consumers providing easy-to-read, authoritative medical and health information.

7810 Medscape

www.medscape.com
Medscape offers specialists, primary care physicians, and other health professionals the Web's most robust and integrated medical information and educational tools.

7811 Nat'l Arthritis and Musculoskeletal Skin

www.niams.nih.gov
Supports and provides clinical and public information and research to increase understanding of the many skin diseases and related disorders. Also provides lists and order forms for their resources and materials.

7812 Nat'l Institute of Arthritis

www.nih.gov
Handles inquiries on the following - arthritis, bone diseases and skin diseases. Consumer and professional education materials are available.

7813 National Psoriasis Foundation

www.psoriasis.org
Offers information, support and referrals for victims of psoriasis and their families.

7814 Skin Store

www.skinstore.com
Carries over 500 of the finest skincare products, available at the lowest prices, delivered immediately to your home.

7815 WebMD

www.webmd.com
Information on skin disorders, including articles and resources.

Description

7816 Sleep Disorders

Sleep disorders are defined as disturbances that affect the ability to fall or stay asleep, that involve sleeping too much, or that result in abnormal sleep-related behavior. They can be categorized into primary sleep disorders; sleep disorders related to another mental disorder or a general medical condition; and substance induced sleep disorder. The two conditions discussed here, narcolepsy and obstructive sleep apnea, are both primary sleep disorders.

Narcolepsy is a rare disorder of abnormal and irresistible daytime drowsiness. Excessive daytime sleepiness with involuntary daytime sleep episodes, disturbed nighttime sleep, and cataplexy (sudden weakness or loss of muscle tone, often triggered by emotion), are the most common symptoms of narcolepsy. Generally, symptoms appear between the onset of puberty and age 25, and worsen as the patient ages. There are 100,000 people in the US with this condition.

Although the exact cause of narcolepsy is unknown, there appears to be a genetic link.

Oral medication, including stimulant agents, as well as specific sleep schedules and other forms of behavioral therapy are also prescribed.

Obstructive sleep apnea is a serious and common sleep disorder that features heavy snoring and breathing irregularities. It is chronic and relapsing, and varies in severity from mild to lethal. Almost 90 percent of the estimated 12 million sleep apnea sufferers are male. Obstructive sleep apnea is biomechanical and usually occurs when tissues in the back of the throat collapse and close the breathing passage. Sufferers experience heavy snoring, periods during sleep when breathing halts for 10 seconds or more, and many short awakenings which they do not remember. In the worst cases, sufferers may cease breathing for more than half of total sleeping time, which can result in daytime fatigue, oxygen deprivation and hypertension.

Signs of sleep apnea or a related sleeping disorder include loud, habitual snoring, fatigue on waking, daytime sleepiness, and choking, gasping or holding one's breath while asleep. Overweight persons and smokers are more prone to develop this disorder. Heavy eating, late-night snacking, sedative use, and alcohol consumption are often contributing factors.

The diagnosis of sleep apnea often requires a polysomnography, or sleep study, which monitors brain waves, muscle tension, eye movement, respiration and blood-oxygen levels. Obviously, a partner can easily help to confirm these symptoms; single people can arrange for sleep observation in a hospital or clinic setting. Behavior modification is frequently sufficient to reduce or eliminate many snoring problems, as is sleeping on one's side and/or without a pillow. In addition to behavioral changes, mild cases are often responsive to oral devices that help to keep airways open by bringing the jaw forward, elevating the soft palate, or repositioning the tongue. More severe cases can be treated with a C-PAP (continuous positive airway pressure) machine, or a Bi-Level (Bi-PAP) machine, both of which blow air into the patient's airways in a regulated manner. Surgery is sometimes indicated, when facial or oral irregularities, such as jaw irregularities, small throat openings, enlarged tonsils, a large tongue or other tissue in front of the airway, or a deviated septum, impede proper airflow.

National Agencies & Associations

7817 American Narcolepsy Association
PO Box 26230
San Francisco, CA 94126-6230   800-222-6085
Offers help and information to persons with narcolepsy and their families.

7818 American Sleep Apnea Association
6856 E Avenue   202-293-3650
Washington, DC 20012   Fax: 202-293-3656
e-mail: asaa@sleepapnea.org
www.sleepapnea.org
Offers help and information to persons with sleep apnea and their families.
Michael P Coppola MD, President and Chief Medical Officer
Nancy Rothstein, Secretary

7819 Association of Professional Sleep Societies
One Westbrook Corporate Center   708-492-0930
Westchester, IL 60154   Fax: 708-273-9354
www.apss.org
Works to facilitate the research and development of sleep disorders medically by encouraging exchange of information among members.
Jerome A Barrett, Executive Director
Jennifer Markkanen, Assistant Executive Director

7820 Lung Association
Station S   780-488-6819
Edmonton, AB, T6E-6K2   Fax: 780-488-7195
e-mail: lasa@sleep-apnea.ab.ca
www.sleep-apnea-ab.ca
The Lung Association - Sleep Apnea (LASA) is a patient and professional coalition providing support through improved care for patients with respiratory disorders of sleep.

7821 NIH/National Institute of Neurological Disorders and Stroke
PO Box 5801   301-496-5751
Bethesda, MD 20824   800-352-9424
TTY: 301-468-5981
www.ninds.nih.gov
Mission is to reduce the burden of neurological disease, a burden borne by every age group, by every segment of society, by people all over the world.
Story C Landis, Director
Walter J Koroshetz, Deputy Director

7822 Narcolepsy Institute/Montefiore Medical Center
111 E 210th Street   718-920-6799
Bronx, NY 10467-2490   Fax: 718-654-9580
e-mail: MGoswami@aol.com
www.montefiore.org
Offers services such as screening, information on narcolepsy, counseling and referrals for individuals and their families with problems arising as a consequence of narcolepsy, and adult and teenage support groups to help individuals develop positive self-images.
Dr Meeta Goswami, Director

7823 Narcolepsy Network
PO Box 294
Pleasantville, NY 10570

410-667-2523
888-292-6522
Fax: 401-633-6567
e-mail: narnet@aol.com
www.narcolepsynetwork.org

Nonprofit organization consisting of memberships by people who have narcolepsy (or related sleep disorders), their families and friends and professionals involved in treatment, research and public education.
Eveline Honig, Executive Director
Collen A Rettig, Office Manager

7824 National Sleep Foundation
1522 K Street NW
Washington, DC 20005-1253

202-347-3471
Fax: 202-347-3472
e-mail: nsf@sleepfoundation.org
www.sleepfoundation.org

The National Sleep Foundation (NSF) is an independent nonprofit organization dedicated to improving public health and safety by achieving understanding of sleep and sleep disorders and by supporting education sleep-related research and advocacy.
Meir H Kryger, Chairman
Thomas J Balkin, Vice Chairman

7825 Sleep Research Society American Academy of Sleep Medicine
American Academy of Sleep Medicine
One Westbrook Corporate Center
Westchester, IL 60154

708-492-1093
Fax: 708-492-0943
e-mail: ncekosh@srsnet.org
www.sleepresearchsociety.org

Facilitates communication among research workers in this field but does not sponsor research investigations on its own.
Michael V Vitiello, President
Ronald Szymusiak, Secretary/Treasurer

Research Centers

7826 Baylor College of Medicine: Sleep Disorder and Research Center
10019 S Main Street
Houston, TX 77025-3498

713-798-3300
Fax: 713-796-9718
www.baylorclinic.com

Internal unit of the College that focuses on research into sleep and sexual dysfunction in males.
Shyam Subramanian, Medical Director
Charlie Lan, Assistant Professor of Medicine

7827 Capital Regional Sleep-Wake Disorders Center
St. Peter's Hospital and Albany Medical Center
25 Hackett Boulevard
Albany, NY 12208-3420

518-436-9253

Cheryl Carlu MD

7828 Center for Narcolepsy Research at the University of Illinois at Chicago
University of Illinois
845 S Damen Avenue
Chicago, IL 60612-7350

312-996-5176
Fax: 312-99-700
e-mail: julielaw@uic.edu
www.uic.edu/depts/cnr

Provides information to health professionals and people with sleep disorders regarding diagnosis and treatment. Maintain national network with sleep professionals throughout the US.
6-8 pages 2 per year
David W Carley, Director
Julie Law, Center Administrator

7829 Center for Research in Sleep Disorders Affiliated with Mercy Hospital
Mercy Hospital of Hamilton/Fairfield
1275 E Kemper Road
Cincinnati, OH 45246

513-671-3101

Martin Schar PhD

7830 Center for Sleep & Wake Disorders: Miami Valley Hospital
One Wyoming Street
Dayton, OH 45409-2722

513-220-2515
www.miamivalleyhospital.org

Offering the largest variety of sleep disorder testing available in the area it also offers comprehensive sleep care and care of related issues with a sleep lab clinical treatment pulmonary treatment and behavioral treatment in the same facility.
Kevin Huban, Director
Amy Cline, Administrative Director of Respiratory C

7831 Center for Sleep Medicine of the Mount Sinai Medical Center
1176 Fifth Avenue
New York, NY 10029-6500

212-241-5098
Fax: 212-875-84
www.mountsinai.org

The Center for Sleep Medicine at The Mount Sinai Medical Center is a comprehensive program dedicated to the diagnosis and treatment of all aspects of sleep pathology including breathing related sleep disorders periodic limb movements in sleep insomnia and narcolepsy. Mechanical (CPAP BiPAP ventilator) surgical dental and pharmacologic therapies are available.
E Neil Schachter, Professor
Gwen S Skloot, Associates Professor

7832 Geisinger Wyoming Valley Medical Center: Sleep Disorders Center
1000 E Mountain Drive
Wilkes-Barre, PA 18711

570-819-5770
www.geisinger.org

Our dedicated sleep team operates service sleep centers and laboratories to diagnose and treat a broad range of sleep disorders.ÿ Geisinger sleep centers are conveniently located in Danville Bloomsburg Shamokin Wilkes-Barre and Mt. Pocono.
Andrew Paul Matragrano, Director
Stephanie Schaefer, Nurse Practitioner

7833 Johns Hopkins University: Sleep Disorders Francis Scott Key Medical Center
Francis Scott Key Medical Center
601 N Caroline Street
Baltimore, MD 21287

410-550-0545
www.hopkinshospital.org

The Johns Hopkins University Sleep Disorders Center is a tertiary care center for patients with sleep/wake disorders and medical disorders associated with sleep.
Phillip L Smith, Director

7834 Knollwoodpark Hospital Sleep Disorders Center
5600 Girby Road
Mobile, AL 36693-3398

334-660-5757
Fax: 334-660-5254
e-mail: 71054.2530@compuserve.com

7835 Knollwoodpark Hospital Sleep Disorders Cen
5600 Girby Road
Mobile, AL 36693

334-660-5757
Fax: 334-660-5254
e-mail: 71054.2530@compuserve.com
www.southalabama.edu/usakph

7836 Loma Linda University Sleep Disorders Clinic
VA Hospital Medical Services Center
11201 Benton Street
Loma Linda, CA 92357-1

909-825-7084
800-741-8387
Fax: 909-963-64
www.lom.med.va.gov

Ralph Downey III MD, Director

7837 Methodist Hospital Sleep Center Winona Memorial Hospital
Rehab Centers
3232 N Meridian Street
Indianapolis, IN 46208-8126

317-927-2100
Fax: 317-927-2914
Kenneth Wies MD

7838 MidWest Medical Center: Sleep Disorders Center
Winona Memorial Hospital
3232 N Meridian Street
Indianapolis, IN 46208-4688

317-927-2100
Fax: 317-927-2914
Kenneth Wiesert MD

7839 Northwest Ohio Sleep Disorders Center Toledo Hospital
Toledo Hospital
2142 N Cove Boulevard
Toledo, OH 43606-3896

419-471-5629

Frank O Horton III MD, Director

7840 Ohio Sleep Medicine Institute
4975 Bradenton Avenue   614-766-0773
Dublin, OH 43017-3521   Fax: 614-766-2599
e-mail: info@sleepmedicine.com
www.sleepmedicine.com
A comprehensive accredited sleep disorders center that is dedicated to excellence in sleep medicine care. Offer evaluation, diagnosis and treatment for adults and children with sleep apnea, insomnia, restless legs syndrome, narcolepsy, parasomnias, circadian rhythms disorders, shift work, fatigue and other sleep problems.
Betty Palmer, Director

7841 Penn Center for Sleep Disorders: Hospital of the University of Pennsylvania
3400 Spruce Street   215-662-7772
Philadelphia, PA 19104-4204   Fax: 215-349-8038
Joanne Getsy MD, Director

7842 Presbyterian-University Hospital: Pulmonary Sleep Evaluation Center
DeSoto At O'Hara Street   412-647-3475
Pittsburgh, PA 15213
Mark Sanders MD, Director

7843 Scripps Clinic Sleep Disorders Center Scripps Clinic
Scripps Clinic
10666 N Torrey Pines Road   858-455-9100
La Jolla, CA 92037-1027   Fax: 858-828-64
e-mail: malcoRN@scrippsclinic.com
www.scripps.org
The Scripps Clinic Sleep Center provides evaluation diagnosis and treatment of a full range of sleep disorders such as Circadian rhythm disorders Insomnia Narcolepsy Night terror Nightmares Restless legs syndrome Sleep apnea Sleepwalking and Snoring.
Dan Dworsky MD, Medical Director
Merrill M Mitler MD, Scientific Director

7844 Sleep Alertness Center: Lafayette Home Hospital
2400 S Street   765-447-6811
Lafayette, IN 47904-3027   e-mail: glenda.eberhard@glhsi.org
Frederick Ro MD

7845 Sleep Center: Community General Hospital
4900 Broad Road
Syracuse, NY 13215-5100   315-492-5877
www.cgh.org
The Sleep Center at Community General Hospital is a specialized facility providing accurate diagnosis and recommending treatment of sleep-related problems.
Robert Westl MD, Medical Director
Antonio Cule MD, Neurology Consultant

7846 Sleep Disorders Center Bethesda Oak Hospital
619 Oak Street
Cincinnati, OH 45206-1613   513-569-6320
www.trihealth.com
Milton Krame MD

7847 Sleep Disorders Center Columbia Presbyterian Medical Center
The University Hospital of Columbia & Cornell
161 Fort Washington Avenue   212-305-1860
New York, NY 10032   Fax: 212-305-5496
e-mail: inquire@sleepNYP.com
www.sleepnyp.com
A Highly specialized outpatient facility for the evaluation and treatment of patients with problems related to sleep and wakefulness.
Neil B Kavey, Medical Director
Andrew Tucker, Director

7848 Sleep Disorders Center Dartmouth Hitchcock Medical Center
Darthmouth Hitchcock medical Center
One Medical Center Drive   603-650-7534
Lebanon, NH 03756-1   866-346-2362
Fax: 603-650-7820
e-mail: Joanne.MacQuarrie@dartmouth.edu
dms.dartmouth.edu
Provides consultation and testing for all varieties of sleep-related disturbances including snoring sleep apnea narcolepsy restless legs syndrome periodic limb movement disorder insomnia parasomnias and circadian rhythm disorders.
Glen Greenough, Fellowship Director
Michael Sate MD, Director

7849 Sleep Disorders Center Lankenau Hospital
100 E Lancaster Avenue   610-645-3400
Wynnewood, PA 19096-3498   Fax: 610-645-2291

7850 Sleep Disorders Center Ohio State University Medical Center
1492 E Broad Street   614-257-2500
Columbus, OH 43205-1228   800-293-5123
Fax: 614-257-2551
medicalcenter.osu.edu
Ulysses J Magalang MD, Medical Director

7851 Sleep Disorders Center at California: Pacific Medical Center
2340 Clay Street   415-923-3336
San Francisco, CA 94115-1932   Fax: 415-923-3584
e-mail: 76307.2221@compuserve.com

7852 Sleep Disorders Center at California: Paci
2340 Clay Street   415-923-3336
San Francisco, CA 94115   Fax: 415-923-3584
e-mail: 76307.2221@compuserve.com

7853 Sleep Disorders Center of Metropolitan Toronto
2888 Bathurst Street   416-785-1128
Toronto Ontario, M6B-4H6   Fax: 416-782-2740
e-mail: sleep@compuserve.com
www.sdc.ca
Jeffrey Lips MD, Director

7854 Sleep Disorders Center of Rochester: St. Mary's Hospital
2110 Clinton Avenue S   716-442-4141
Rochester, NY 14618-2616
Donald Green MD

7855 Sleep Disorders Center of Western New York Millard Fillmore Hospital
3 Gates Circle   716-887-5337
Buffalo, NY 14209-1120   Fax: 716-887-5332
gates.kaleidahealth.org
Daniel Rifkin, Director

7856 Sleep Disorders Center: Cleveland Clinic Foundation
9500 Euclid Avenue   216-636-5860
Cleveland, OH 44195-0001   800-588-2264
Fax: 216-445-1022
my.clevelandclinic.org
Accredited by the American Academy of Sleep Medicine the Cleveland Clinic Sleep Disorders Center is staffed by physicians specializing in sleep disorders from a variety of disciplines including adult and child neurology pulmonary and critical care medicine psychology psychiatry otolaryngology and dentistry.
Nancy Foldva Schaefer DO, Director
Petra Podmor RPSGT, Laboratory Manager

7857 Sleep Disorders Center: Community Medical Center
1822 Mulberry Street   717-969-8931
Scranton, PA 18510-2375
John Goodnow, Director

7858 Sleep Disorders Center: Crozer-Chester Medical Center
Sleep Disorders Center
175 E Chester Pike
Ridley Park, PA 19078-3975   610-447-2689
www.crozer.org
A multidisciplinary facility for the investigation and treatment of sleep problems
Calvin Staff MD, Medical Director

7859 Sleep Disorders Center: Good Samaritan Medical Center
1020 Franklin Street   814-533-1661
Johnstown, PA 15905-4109
Richard Parc DO, Director

7860 Sleep Disorders Center: Kettering Medical Center
3935 Southern Boulevard
Kettering, OH 45439-1295 · 937-395-8805
Fax: 937-395-8821
www.kmcnetwork.org

Donna Arand PhD, Clinical Director
George G Burton MD, Medical Director

7861 Sleep Disorders Center: Medical College of Pennsylvania
3200 Henry Avenue · 215-842-4250
Philadelphia, PA 19129-1137
June M Fry MD PhD, Director

7862 Sleep Disorders Center: Newark Beth Israel Medical Center
201 Lyons Avenue at Osborne Terrace
Newark, NJ 07112-2027 · 973-926-2973
www.sbhcs.com

Evaluates a wide range of disorders including sleep apnea snoring insomnia narcolepsy sleep-wake schedule disorders and male impotency. The center also provides board-certified consultants in sleep medicine neurology urology endocrinology psychiatry cardiology and ear nose and throat surgery in addition to certified sleep technologists.
Monroe S Karetzky MD

7863 Sleep Disorders Center: Rhode Island Hospital
70 Catamore Boulevard · 401-431-5420
E Providence, RI 02914 · Fax: 401-431-5429
www.lifespan.org

Richard Mill MD, Director

7864 Sleep Disorders Center: St. Vincent Medical Center
2213 Cherry Street · 419-321-4980
Toledo, OH 43608-2691
Joseph Schaf PhD, Director

7865 Sleep Disorders Center: University Hospital, SUNY at Stony Brook
240 Middle Country Road · 631-444-2500
Smithtown, NY 11787-0001 · Fax: 631-444-2580
uhmc-xweb1.uhmc.sunysb.edu/sleepdisorder
Wallace Mend MD

7866 Sleep Disorders Center: Winthrop, University Hospital
222 Station Plaza N
Mineola, NY 11501-3808 · 516-663-3907
www.winthrop.org

Steven H Feinsilver MD

7867 Sleep Disorders Unit Beth Israel Deaconess Medical Center
330 Brookline Avenue
Boston, MA 02215-5400 · 617-667-3237
www.bidmc.org

Jean K Matheson MD

7868 Sleep Laboratory St Joseph's Hospital
St Joseph's Hospital
945 E Genesee Street · 315-475-3379
Syracuse, NY 13210 · Fax: 315-755-77
www.sjhsyr.org

The Sleep Lab focuses on diagnosing and treating Obstructive Sleep Apnea and sleep-related breathing disorders and has the largest number of sleep-credentialed physicians and registered sleep technologists of any sleep lab in the area.
Edward T Downing, Director

7869 Sleep Laboratory, Maine Medical Center
22 Bramhall Street · 207-871-2279
Portland, ME 04102-3134
George E Bokinsky Jr

7870 Sleep Medicine Associates of Texas
5477 Glen Lakes Drive · 214-750-7776
Dallas, TX 13210-4353 · Fax: 214-750-4621
e-mail: smat@sleepmed.com
www.sleepmed.com

First largest and longest standing accredited sleep center in North Texas.
Philipp Becker, President and Founding Partner
Andrew O Jamieson MD, Chairman of the Board and Founding Partn

7871 Sleep Research Foundation
170 Morton Street · 617-522-9270
Boston, MA 02130-3735
Ernest Hartm MD, Director

7872 Sleep Wake Disorders Center Montefiore Sleep Disorders Center
111 E 210th Street · 718-920-4841
Bronx, NY 10467-2401 · Fax: 718-798-4352
www.montefiore.org

Provide outstanding clinical care for patients with disorders that affect the sleep-wake cycle and are committed to performing high quality research and to making outstanding contributions to the areas of clinical research that includes the entire spectrum of sleep medicine.
Michael J Thorpy MD, Director
Karen Ballab MD, Associate Director

7873 Sleep and Chronobiology Center: Western Psychiatric Institute and Clinic
3811 Ohara Street · 412-624-2246
Pittsburgh, PA 15213-2593
Charles F Reynolds III MD, Director

7874 Sleep-Wake Disorders Center: New York Hospital-Cornell Medical Center
520 E 70th Street · 212-746-2623
New York, NY 10021-1504 · Fax: 212-746-5509
www.weillcornell.org

Charles Poll MD, Director

7875 Sleep/Wake Disorders Center: Community Hospitals of Indianapolis
1500 N Ritter Avenue · 317-355-4275
Indianapolis, IN 46219-3027 · Fax: 317-351-2785
e-mail: mevollmer@pol.net
Marvin E Vollmer MD

7876 Sleep/Wake Disorders Center: Hampstead Hospital
E Road · 603-329-5311
Hampstead, NH 03841
Deborah Sewi PhD

7877 Stanford University Center for Narcolepsy Dept of Psychiatry & Behavioral Sciences
450 Broadway Street · 650-725-6517
Redwood City, CA 94063-5102 · Fax: 650-498-7761
e-mail: jck@stanford.edu
med.stanford.edu

Dr Emanuel Mignot, Director
Marlene Iry, Admin Associate

7878 Thomas Jefferson University: Sleep Disorders Center
Jefferson Medical College
211 S Ninth Street · 215-955-6175
Philadelphia, PA 19107-5083 · 800-JEF-FNOW
Fax: 215-955-9783
www.jefferson.edu

A comprehensive clinical research and educational program in sleep and sleep disorders medicine.
Karl Doghram MD, Medical Director

7879 University of Texas Sleep/Wake Disorders Center
Southwestern Medical Center
5323 Harry Hines Boulevard · 214-648-7350
Dallas, TX 75390-9070 · Fax: 214-487-59

Studies sleep/wake disorders including insomnia apnea and narcolepsy.
Howard Roffw MD, Director

Support Groups & Hotlines

7880 Narcolepsy Institute/Montefiore Medical Center
111 E 210th Street · 718-920-6799
Bronx, NY 10467-2490 · Fax: 718-654-9580
e-mail: MGoswami@aol.com
www.narcolepsyinstitute.org

The Narcolepsy Institute provides psychosocial support services for narcolepsy.
Dr. Meeta Goswami, Director

7881 Narcolepsy Network
110 Ripple Lane
North Kingstown, RI 02852
401-667-2523
888-292-6522
Fax: 401-633-6567
e-mail: narnet@narcolepsynetwork.org
www.narcolepsynetwork.org
Provides advocacy and education, supports research. Newsletter, conferences, phone support and group development guidelines.
Patricia Higgins, President
Eveline V. Honig, Md, MPh, Executive Director

7882 National Health Information Center
PO Box 1133
Washington, DC 20013
310-565-4167
800-336-4797
Fax: 301-984-4256
e-mail: info@nhic.org
www.health.gov/nhic
Offers a nationwide information referral service, produces directories and resource guides.

Books

7883 ABC of ZZZs
National Sleep Foundation
1522 K Street NW
Washington, DC 20005-1235
202-347-3471
Fax: 202-347-3472
www.sleepfoundation.org
A primer on sleep basics, including getting enough sleep, why sleep is important, and ' sleep stealers.'
Emerson Darbonne, Communications Coordinator

7884 Doctor, I Can't Sleep: Insomnia Training Manual
Narcolepsy Network
PO Box 42460
Cincinnati, OH 45242-0460
513-891-3522
Fax: 513-891-9936
e-mail: narnet@aol.com
Comprehensive course manual for primary care physicians and the public. Outlines basic facts about epidemiology, sleep hygiene, relaxation techniques, diagnosis, and treatment.
100+ pages

7885 International Classification of Sleep Disorders
American Academy of Sleep Medicine
One Westbrook Corporate Center
Westchester, IL 60154
708-492-0930
Fax: 708-492-0943
www.aasmnet.org
A comprehensive manual for physicians and other healthcare professionals containing information on 84 sleep disorders. The extensive text describes the diagnostic features of each disorder and includes specific diagnostic and severity criteria for each disorder.
396 pages Paperback

7886 Living with Narcolepsy
National Sleep Foundation
1522 K Street
Washington, DC 20005-1235
202-347-3471
Fax: 202-347-3472
www.sleepfoundation.org
Defines and describes narcolepsy and what can be expected after diagnosis, including effects on education, career, social and family life.
Emerson Darbonne, Communications Coordinator

7887 Melatonin: The Basic Facts
National Sleep Foundation
1522 K Street
Washington, DC 20005-1235
202-347-3471
Fax: 202-347-3472
www.sleepfoundation.org
If you're curious about melatonin, it's not suprising. There has been a lot of attention paid to the hormone in popular magazines and books, scholarly journals, and advertisements. You may habe heard claims that malatonin cures everything from jet lag to insomnia to aging.
Emerson Darbonne, Communications Coordinator

7888 Narcolepsy Primer
Meeta Goswami, Michael Thorpy, author
Narcolepsy Institute/Montefiore Medical Center

111 E 210th Street
Bronx, NY 10467-2401
718-920-6799
Fax: 718-654-9580
e-mail: MGsowami@aol.com
narcolepsyinstitute.org
A guide for physicians, patients and their families on the affects, causes and prevention of narcolepsy.
Dr. Meeta Goswami, Director

7889 Narcolepsy Primer Package
Meeta Goswami, Michael Thorpy, author
Narcolepsy Institute/Montefiore Medical Center
111 E 210th Street
Bronx, NY 10467-2401
718-920-6799
Fax: 718-654-9580
e-mail: MGsowami@aol.com
narcolepsyinstitute.org
The package includes: Narcolepsy Primer; Manuel on Narcolepsy and A Counseling Service for Narcolepsy: A Sociomedical Model.
Dr. Meeta Goswami, Director

7890 Pain and Sleep
National Sleep Foundation
1522 K Street NW
Washington, DC 20005-1235
202-347-3471
Fax: 202-347-3472
www.sleepfoundation.org
Whether pain results from headache, backache, arthritis, or other conditions, it frequently occurs with sleep difficulty. This overview of the pain and sleep connection describes behavioral and pharmacological approaches to pain management.
Emerson Darbonne, Communications Coordinator

7891 Sleep Aids: Everything You Wanted To Know But Were Too Tired To Ask
National Sleep Foundation
1522 K Street NW
Washington, DC 20005-1235
202-347-3471
Fax: 202-347-3472
www.sleepfoundation.org
If you have trouble falling or staying asleep, or you wake up feeling unrefreshed, you may be suffering from insomnia. Insomnia is a symptom. It may be caused by stress, anxiety, depression, disease, pain, medications, sleep disorders or poor sleep habits.
Emerson Darbonne, Communications Coordinator

7892 Sleep Apnea
National Sleep Foundation
1522 K Street, NW
Washington, DC 20005-1235
202-347-3471
Fax: 202-347-3472
www.sleepfoundation.org
A brochure about sleep apnea, a breathing disorder characterized by brief interruptions of breathing during sleep. Brochure explains what it is, who gets it, and how it is diagnosed and treated.
Emerson Darbonne, Communications Coordinator

7893 Snoring and Sleep Apnea
Demos Medical Publishing
386 Park Avenue S
New York, NY 10016
212-683-0072
Fax: 212-683-0118
e-mail: orderdept@demopub.com
www.demosmedpub.com
A straightforward, jargon-free approach to dealing with snoring and sleep problems.
222 pages
ISBN: 1-888799-29-3
Dr. Diana M Schneider, President

7894 You Don't LOOK Sick!: Living Well with Invisible Chronic Illness
Joy Selak, Steven Overman, author
Haworth Press
10 Alice Street
Binghamton, NY 13904-1580
607-722-5857
800-429-6784
Fax: 607-722-0012
www.haworthpress.com
Chronicles a patient's true-life stories and her physician's compassionate commentary as they take a journey through the three stages of chronic illness - Getting Sick, Being Sick, and Living Well. Hardcover $29.95 (ISBN): 978-0-7890-2488-0, Paperback $14.95 (ISBN): 978-0-7890-2499-7.
145 pages Hrdcover/Ppbck

Magazines

7895 **SleepMatters**
National Sleep Foundation
1522 K Street NW   202-347-3471
Washington, DC 20005-1235   Fax: 202-347-3472
                                   www.sleepfoundation.org
Covering hot sleep news, profiles, advice from experts and much more!
Quarterly
Cameron Darbonne, Communications Coordinator

Newsletters

7896 **Eye Opener**
American Narcolepsy Association
425 California Street, Suite 201   415-788-4793
San Francisco, CA 94126-6230
Offers information on sleep disorders including a question and answer column for persons suffering from disorders.

7897 **Narcolepsy Institute/Montefiore Medical Center**
Meeta Goswami, author

Narcolepsy Institute
111 E 210th Street   718-920-6799
Bronx, NY 10467-2490   Fax: 718-654-9580
                                   e-mail: MGsowami@aol.com
                                   narcolepsyinstitute.org
The Narcolepsy Institute provides psychosocial support services for narcolepsy and has a newsletter, a video, and a primer on narcolepsy.
8 pages Bi-Annual
Dr. Meeta Goswami, Director

7898 **Sleep Medicine Alert**
Nationa Sleep Foundation
1522 K Street NW   202-347-3471
Washington, DC 20005-1235   Fax: 202-347-3472
                                   www.sleepfoundation.org
This quearterly newsletter is for healthcare professionals. It offers updates on sleep research and its clinical implications, information on diagnosing and treating a variety of sleep disorders.

7899 **Wake-Up Call**
American Sleep Apnea Association
6856 E Avenue   202-293-3650
Washington, DC 20012   Fax: 202-293-3656
                                   e-mail: asaa@sleepapnea.org
                                   www.sleepapnea.org
Contains information of interest to APNEA patients and their families.
Quarterly
Michael P Coppola MD, President and Chief Medical Officer
Nancy Rothstein, Secretary

Pamphlets

7900 **Get the Facts About Sleep Apnea**
American Sleep Apnea Association
1424 K Street NW   202-293-3650
Washington, DC 20005   Fax: 202-293-3656
                                   e-mail: asaa@sleepapnea.org
                                   www.sleepapnea.org

7901 **Helping Yourself to a Good Night's Sleep**
Nantional Sleep Foundation
1522 K Street NW   202-347-3471
Washington, DC 20005-1253   Fax: 202-347-3472
                                   www.sleepfoundation.org
About half of Americans report sleep difficulty at least occasionally, according to National Sleep Foundation surveys. These woes-called insomnia by doctors-have far reaching effects. This brochure details the many things you can do to improve your sleep.

7902 **Narcolepsy**
American Academy of Sleep Medicine

One Westbrook Corporate Center   708-492-0930
Westchester, IL 60154   Fax: 708-492-0943
                                   www.aasmnet.org
Describes the causes, symptoms and treatments of a disorder characterized by excessive sleepiness.
Lot of 50

7903 **Sleep Diary**
National Sleep Foundation
1522 K Street, NW   202-347-3471
Washington, DC 20005-1235   Fax: 202-347-3472
                                   www.sleepfoundation.org
It includes sections on sleep schedules, quality and quantity of sleep, sleep disturbances, sleep hygiene and daytime sleepiness. It enables people to identify their sleep and health habits and note any sleep problems they may have.
Emerson Darbonne, Communications Coordinator

7904 **Sleep Strategies for Shift Workers**
National Sleep Foundation
1522 K Street NN   202-347-3471
Washington, DC 20005-1235   Fax: 202-347-3472
                                   www.sleepfoundation.org
This brochure outlines the common effects of shift work on health, workplace alertness and productivity and offers tips about diet, sleep environment, medications, light therapy and sleep hygiene.
Cameron Darbonne, Communications Coordinator

7905 **Wake Up! Brochure**
National Sleep Foundation
1522 K Street NW   202-347-3471
Washington, DC 20005-1235   Fax: 202-347-3472
                                   www.sleepfoundation.org
A blooklet dedicated to the drowsy driving problem, including the risks, the myths, the danger signals and recommendations.
Cameron Darbonne, Communications Coordinator

7906 **When You Can't Sleep**
Narcolepsy Network
Po Box 294   401-667-2523
Pleasantville, NY 10570-0460   888-292-6522
                                   Fax: 401-633-6567
                                   e-mail: narnet@aol.com
A primer on sleep basics, including getting enough sleep, why sleep is important, and sleep stealers. Plus a sleep quotient quiz.

7907 **Women and Sleep**
National Sleep Foundation
1522 K Street NW   202-347-3471
Washington, DC 20005-1235   Fax: 202-347-3472
                                   www.sleepfoundation.org
A brochure dealing with the effects of sleep on women which explores reasons for tiredness, increased accidents, problems concentrating, and poor performance on the job and in school, and possible increased sickness.
Cameron Darbonne, Communications Coordinator

Audio & Video

7908 **Narcolepsy**
American Academy of Sleep Medicine
One Westbrook Corporate Center   708-492-0930
Westchester, IL 60154   Fax: 708-492-0943
                                   www.aasmnet.org
Addresses the etiology, pathophysiology, diagnosis and management of narcolepsy.
58 slides

7909 **Narcolepsy: Fanlight Productions**
Jason Margolis, author

Fanlight Productions
4196 Washington Street   617-469-4999
Boston, MA 02131-1731   800-937-4113
                                   Fax: 617-469-3379
                                   e-mail: fanlight@fanlight.com
                                   www.fanlight.com

This remarkable film presents the experiences of three individuals whose lives and relationships have been disrupted by narcolepsy.
2000 25 Minutes
ISBN: 1-572953-23-2

7910 Video on Narcolepsy
Narcolepsy Institute/Montefiore Medical Center
111 E 210th Street   718-920-6799
Bronx, NY 10467   Fax: 718-654-9580
                                    e-mail: MGsowami@aol.com
                                    www.narcolepsyinstitute.org
Clinical symptoms, genetics, diagnosis, effects of Narcolepsy, support groups.
Dr. Meeta Goswami, Director

Web Sites

7911 American Sleep Apnea Association
                                    www.sleeppapnea.org
The ASAA is a 501(c)(3) organization dedicated to reducing injury, disability, and depth from sleep apnea and to enhancing the well-being of those affected by this common disorder. The ASAA promotes education and awareness, the ASAA A.W.A.K.E. network of voluntary mutual support groups, research, and continuous improvement of care.

7912 American Sleep Disorders Association
Provides full diagnostic and treatment services to improve the quality of care for patients with all types of sleep disorders.

7913 Healing Well
                                    www.healingwell.com
An online health resource guide to medical news, chat, information and articles, newsgroups and message boards, books, disease-related web sites, medical directories, and more for patients, friends, and family coping with disabling diseases, disorders, or chronic illnesses.

7914 Health Finder
                                    www.healthfinder.gov
Searchable, carefully developed web site offering information on over 1000 topics. Developed by the US Department of Health and Human Services, the site can be used in both English and Spanish.

7915 Healthlink USA
                                    www.healthlinkusa.com
Health information concerning treatment, cures, prevention, diagnosis, risk factors, research, support groups, email lists, personal stories and much more. Updated regularly.

7916 Helios Health
                                    www.helioshealth.com
Online resource for your health information. Detailed information about specific health topics, access to expert advice from our Medical Advisory Board, and up-to-date health news.

7917 MGH Neurology WebForums
Online. Provides both unmoderated message boards and chat rooms for specific neurological disorders.

7918 MedicineNet
                                    www.medicinenet.com
An online resource for consumers providing easy-to-read, authoritative medical and health information.

7919 Medscape
                                    www.medscape.com
Medscape offers specialists, primary care physicians, and other health professionals the Web's most robust and integrated medical information and educational tools.

7920 National Sleep Foundation
                                    www.sleepfoundation.org
Information for millions of Americans who suffer from sleep disorders, and to prevent the catastrophic accidents that are related to poor or disordered sleep through research, education and the dissemination of information.

7921 Neurology Channel
                                    www.neurologychannel.com

Find clearly explained, medically accurate information regarding conditions, including an overview, symptoms, causes, diagnostic procedures and treatment options. On this site it is possible to ask questions and get information from a neurologist and connect to people who have similar health interests.

7922 Sleep Research Society
                                    www.sleepresearchsociety.org
Facilitates communication among research workers in this field, but does not sponsor research investigations on its own.

7923 WebMD
                                    www.webmd.com
Information on Narcolepsy, including articles and resources.

Description

7924 **Spina Bifida**

Spina bifida refers to conditions which result in an incomplete closure of the spinal column during fetal development. It is the most serious of a group of disorders called neural tube defects. The severity of spina bifida ranges from mild to severe.

Spina bifida occulta is an opening in one or more vertebrae without damage to the spinal cord. Meningocele is when the protective covering around the spinal cord (meninges) has protruded into the vertebrae, with little, if any, damage. Myelomeningocele, the most severe form of spina bifida, is when part of the actual spinal cord pushes through the back and exposes nerves and tissues.

The effects of spina bifida, in its most extreme state, are serious. They can include paralysis, loss of bowel and bladder control and hydrocephalus. Other inherited abnormalities may be present. Open spina bifida can be diagnosed in utero by finding elevations of a specific protein in maternal amniotic fluid. Prevention involves supplementation with folic acid. Treatments for spina bifida require a united effort by a team of specialists, and depend on the severity of the defects. With proper care, many children with spina bifida live fairly normal lives. See also *Birth Defects*.

National Agencies & Associations

7925 **Canadian & American Spinal Research Organi zation**
120 Newkirk Road
Richmond Hill, ON, L4C-9S7
905-508-4000
Fax: 905-508-4002
e-mail: info@csro.com
www.csro.com
Dedicated to the improvement of the physical quality of life for persons with a spinal cord injury and those with related neurological deficits, through targeted medical and scientific research.
Barry Munro, Chair
Dave Lostchuk, Treasurer

7926 **Easter Seals**
230 W Monroe Street
Chicago, IL 60606-4703
312-726-6200
800-221-6827
Fax: 312-726-1494
TTY: 312-726-4258
e-mail: info@easter-seals.org
www.easter-seals.org
Provides serves to children and adults with disabilities as well as support to their families.
Reenie Kavalar, VP Medical/Rehabilitation Services

7927 **March of Dimes Birth Defects Foundation**
1275 Mamaroneck Avenue
White Plains, NY 10605
914-949-7166
www.marchofdimes.com
Our mission is to improve the health of babies by preventing birth defects premature birth and infant mortality. The March of Dimes carries out this mission through programs of research community services education and advocacy to save babies' lives.

7928 **Spina Bifida Association of America**
4590 Macarthur Boulevard NW
Washington, DC 20007-4226
202-944-3285
800-621-3141
Fax: 202-944-3295
e-mail: sbaa@sbaa.org
www.sbaa.org

The association works for people with spina bifida and their families through education advocacy research and service. There is also an annual conference and publications available.
Cindy Brownstein, CEO
Maya House, Resource Center Manager

7929 **Spina Bifida and Hydrocephalus Association of Canada**
#977-167 Lombard Avenue
Winnipeg, Manitoba, R3B-0V3
204-925-3650
Fax: 204-925-3654
e-mail: spinab@mts.net
www.sbhac.ca

To improve the quality of life of all individuals with spina bifida and/or hydrocephalus and their families, through awareness, education, research, and advocacy, and to reduce the incidence of neural tube defects.
Lorelei Fletcher, President
Gene Layton, VP

State Agencies & Associations

Alabama

7930 **Spina Bifida Association of Alabama**
PO Box 13254
Birmingham, AL 35202-0538
256-617-1414
e-mail: info@sbaofal.org
www.sbaofal.org
Lori Turner, President
David Little, Executive Director

Arizona

7931 **Spina Bifida Association of Arizona**
1001 E Fairmount Avenue
Phoenix, AZ 85014-4806
602-274-3323
Fax: 602-274-7632
e-mail: office@sbglobal.net
www.sbaaz.org
Benjaman D Scanlan, President
Ron Whiteside, Treasurer

Arkansas

7932 **Spina Bifida Association of Arkansas**
PO Box 24663
Little Rock, AR 72221-4663
501-978-7222
Fax: 501-320-6805
e-mail: sigmondr@sbglobal.net
www.sbaa.org
James Rucker, President

California

7933 **Spina Bifida Association of Greater San Diego**
PO Box 232272
San Diego, CA 92193-2272
619-491-9018
Fax: 619-275-3361
e-mail: sbaofgsd@hotmail.com
www.sbaa.org
Erika Jorquera, President

Colorado

7934 **Spina Bifida Association of Colorado**
PO Box 22994
Denver, CO 80222-0994
303-797-7870
Fax: 303-730-8032
e-mail: sbacolorado@gmail.com
www.coloradospinabifida.org
Marge Hayes, Equipment Swap
Marie Arroyo, President

Connecticut

7935 **Spina Bifida Association of Connecticut**
PO Box 2545
Hartford, CT 06146-2545
860-832-8905
800-574-6274
Fax: 860-832-6260
e-mail: sbac@sbac.org
www.sbac.org
Mary Attardo, President
Kiley J Carlson, Executive Director

Delaware

7936 Spina Bifida Association of Delaware
PO Box 807
Wilmington, DE 19899-0807

302-478-4805
e-mail: kbasar@aol.com
www.angelfire.com/de/sbaofde/

Blake Heath, Vice President
Andy Anderso Jr, Treasurer

Florida

7937 Spina Bifida Association of Florida Space Coast
3685 Starlight Avenue
Merrit Island, FL 32953-2549

321-454-9737
Fax: 321-454-9737
e-mail: sbafscearthlink.com
www.sbaa.org

Robin Reinarts, President

7938 Spina Bifida Association of Jacksonville
807 Childrens Way
Jacksonville, FL 32207-8426

904-390-3686
800-722-6355
Fax: 904-390-3466
e-mail: sbaj@sbaj.org
www.sbaj.org

Michael Erhard, Chairperson

7939 Spina Bifida Association of Tampa
PO Box 151038
Tampa, FL 33684-1038

813-933-4827
Fax: 813-872-9845
e-mail: sbatampabay@aol.com
www.sbaj.org

Dianne Gore, President

Georgia

7940 Spina Bifida Association of Georgia
1448 Mclendon Drive
Decatur, GA 30033

770-939-1044
Fax: 770-939-1049
e-mail: info@spinabifidaga.org
www.spinabifidaofgeorgia.org

Provides referrals, evaluation, treatment and therapeutic activities for children and teens afflicted with spina bifida. The goal of this center is to help children or teenagers prepare for life.
William Turnispeed, President
Judy Thibadeau, Vice President

Illinois

7941 Illinois Spina Bifida Association
8765 W Higgins Road
Chicago, IL 60631-1693

773-444-0305
800-969-4722
Fax: 630-637-1066
e-mail: sbail@sbail.org
www.sbail.org

Dedicated to improving the quality of life of people with spina bifida through direct services, information and referral and public awareness. Direct services include a residential summer camp for children with spina bifida over the age of seven.
Scott J Munkvold, President
Amy Maggio, CEO

Indiana

7942 Spina Bifida Association of Central Indiana
PO Box 19814
Indianapolis, IN 46279-0814

317-592-1630
Fax: 317-351-2010
e-mail: pres@sbaci.org
www.sbaci.org

James Zetzl, President

Iowa

7943 Spina Bifida Association of Iowa
PO Box 1456
Des Moines, IA 50305-1456

515-964-8810
e-mail: spinabifidaiowa@yahoo.com
www.spinabifidaia.com

Rod Tressel, President

Kentucky

7944 Spina Bifida Association of Kentucky Kosair Charities Center
Kosair Charities Center
982 Eastern Parkway
Louisville, KY 40217-1568

502-637-7363
866-340-7225
Fax: 502-637-1010
e-mail: sbak@sbak.org
www.sbak.org

Angela Cosby, President
Patty Dissell, Executive Director

Louisiana

7945 Spina Bifida Association of Greater New Orleans
PO Box 1346
Kenner, LA 70063-1346

504-737-5181
Fax: 504-538-9046
e-mail: sbagno@sbagno.com
www.sbagno.org

Al Hitt, President
Judy Otto, Vice-President

Maryland

7946 Spina Bifida Association of Maryland
2416 Lampost Lane
Baltimore, MD 21234-1460

410-665-1543
Fax: 410-833-1700
e-mail: sbamaryland@comcast.net ÿÿ
www.home.comcast.net/~sbamaryland

7947 Spina Bifida Association of the Eastern Shore
316 Prospect Avenue
Easton, MD 21601-4046

410-822-8609
Fax: 410-822-5455
www.spinabifidaassociation.org

Massachusetts

7948 Spina Bifida Association of Massachusetts
321 Fortune Boulevard
Milford, MA 01757-2741

617-742-2574
888-479-1900
Fax: 978-649-8725
e-mail: bsullivan@sbaMass.org
www.msbaweb.org

Brendan Sullivan, President
Cara Packard, Vice President

Michigan

7949 Spina Bifida Association of Grand Rapids
235 Wealthy Street SE
Grand Rapids, MI 49503-5299

616-240-9672
Fax: 616-222-1541
e-mail: WMiSBA@hotmail.comÿ
www.spinabifidaassociation.org

Carol Carpenter, President

7950 Spina Bifida Association of Upper Peninsula Michigan
1220 N 3rd Street
Ishpeming, MI 44849-1108

906-485-5127
Fax: 906-225-7230
e-mail: cbengson@chartermi.net
www.sba-up.8m.com

Lois Bengson, President

7951 Spina Bifida and Hydrocephalus Association of Southwestern Michigan
PO Box 212
Mattawan, MI 49071-0212

269-385-3959
Fax: 269-392-9765
e-mail: marenhorkness@yahoo.com

Richard Benthnin, President

7952 Spina Bifida and Hydrocephalus Association
PO Box 212
Mattawan, MI 49071

269-385-3959
Fax: 269-392-9765
e-mail: marenharkness@yahoo.com
www.spinabifidasupport.com

Richard Benthnin, President

Minnesota

7953 Spina Bifida Association of Minnesota
PO Box 29323
Minneapolis, MN 55429-0212

651-222-6395
Fax: 952-591-0246
e-mail: sbamn@hotmail.com
www.sbamn.com

Wendy Swanson, President
Jim Thayer, Executive Director

Missouri

7954 Spina Bifida Association of Greater St. Louis
8050 Watson Road
Saint Louis, MO 63119-2000

314-843-2244
800-784-0983
Fax: 314-353-1446
e-mail: sbastl@charter.net
www.sbstl.com

Mark Abbott, President

Nebraska

7955 Spina Bifida Association of Nebraska
7612 Maple Street
Omaha, NE 68134-2153

402-932-5826
Fax: 402-572-3002
www.spinabifidanebraska.org

LeAnn Karman, President

New Jersey

7956 Spina Bifida Association of the Tri-State Region
84 Park Avenue
Flemington, NJ 08822-1174

908-782-7475
877-722-8774
Fax: 908-782-6102
e-mail: info@thesbrn.org
www.sbatsr.org

Serves New Jersey, New York Metro Area and Southern Connecticut.
Jane Horowitz, Executive Director and President
K David Holmes, Chairman of the Board

New Mexico

7957 Spina Bifida Association of New Mexico
1127 University Boulevard NE
Albuquerque, NM 87102-1740

505-242-1184
www.sbanm.com

Rey Garduno, Executive Director
Ann Beddingfield, Interim Treasurer

New York

7958 Spina Bifida Association of Albany/Capital District
100 Spring
Scotia, NY 12302-3312

518-399-9151
e-mail: sbaalbany102@aol.com
www.abaalbany.org

Kevin Chamberlain, Co-President
Vanessa Chamberlain, Co-President

7959 Spina Bifida Association of Greater Rochester
PO Box 3
Fairport, NY 14450-0003

585-381-5471
Fax: 585-264-9547
e-mail: jarmst4459@aol.com

JoAnn Armstrong, President

7960 Spina Bifida Association of Nassau County
12 Hampton Road
Sound Beach, NY 11789

631-821-9028
e-mail: kid3418@optonline.net
www.spinabifidaassociation.org

Leslieann Sussman, President

North Carolina

7961 Spina Bifida Association of North Carolina
3915 Grace Court
Indian Trail, NC 28079

704-882-0988
800-847-2262
Fax: 704-882-0988
e-mail: sbanc@mindspring.com
www.spinabifidaassociation.org

Julie Yindra, President
Kin Gates, Executive Director

Ohio

7962 Spina Bifida Association of Canton
S Cherokee Trail
Malvern, OH 44644

330-863-2531
Fax: 330-863-1172
e-mail: cmgriffin@nero.rr.com
www.spinabifidasupport.com

Connie Griffin, President

7963 Spina Bifida Association of Central Ohio
7239 Upper Cambridge Way
Westerville, OH 43082

614-818-3840
e-mail: sbaco@sbaco.net
www.sbaco.net

Laurie Schulze, Treasurer
Chrissy Zepfel, President

7964 Spina Bifida Association of Cincinnati
3245 Deborah Lane
Cincinnati, OH 45239-0152

513-923-1378
e-mail: sbacincy@sbacincy.org
www.sbacincy.org

Brady Sellet, President
Diane Burns, Executive Director

7965 Spina Bifida Association of Greater Dayton
4801 Springfield Street
Dayton, OH 45431

937-236-1122
Fax: 937-434-4899
e-mail: mvspinabifida@yahoo.com
www.sbadayton.org

David Skinner, President
Lisa Maas, Vice President

7966 Spina Bifida Association of Northwest Ohio
2211 River Road
Maumee, OH 43537

419-794-0561
Fax: 419-533-3952
e-mail: sba@sbaofnorthwestohio.org
www.sbaofnorthwestohio.org

Ginnette Clark, President
Julie Harley, Vice President

Pennsylvania

7967 Spina Bifida Association of Central Pennsylvania
209 E State Street
Quarryville, PA 17566-1242

717-786-9280
888-770-SBPA
Fax: 717-786-8821
e-mail: SBAofPA@aol.com
www.geocities.com/sbaofgpa

Patricia Fulvio, President
Amy Graver, Chairman

7968 Spina Bifida Association of Delaware Valley
PO Box 859
Worcester, PA 19490-0289

610-584-5530
Fax: 215-412-9396
e-mail: info@sbadv.org
www.sbadv.org

Marilyn Lieb, President
Keri Mascaro, Executive Director

7969 Spina Bifida Association of Greater Pennsylvania
209 E State Street
Quarryville, PA 17566-9614

717-786-9280
Fax: 717-786-8821
e-mail: sbaofpa@aol.com
www.spinabifidasupport.com

Amy Graver, President
Patricia Fulvio, Executive Director

Rhode Island

7970 **Spina Bifida Association of Rhode Island**
PO Box 6948
Warwick, RI 02887-6948
401-732-7862
Fax: 401-732-7862
www.spinabifidaassociation.org

Tennessee

7971 **Spina Bifida Association of Tennessee**
PO Box 23056
Nashville, TN 37202-5529
615-791-8117
Fax: 615-791-1518
e-mail: lynnhess56@comcast.net
www.spinabifidasupport.com

Lynn Cook, President

Texas

7972 **Spina Bifida Association of Austin**
9301 Bradner Drive
Austin, TX 78748
512-292-6317
Fax: 512-479-3845
e-mail: austinspinabifida@yahoo.com
www.spinabifidasupport.com

Kelley Hively, President

7973 **Spina Bifida Association of Dallas**
705 W Avenue B
Garland, TX 75040
972-238-8755
Fax: 972-414-3772
e-mail: sbdal@aol.com
www.sbdallas.org

Robin Leeÿ, President
Ryan McCoy, Vice President

7974 **Spina Bifida Association of Texas, Gulf Coast**
440 Benmar
Houston, TX 77060-2460
281-493-4349
Fax: 281-997-2278
e-mail: Yvonne.Horner@sbahgc.org
www.sbahgc.org

Yvonne Horner, President
Donnis Collier, Vice President

Washington

7975 **Spina Bifida Association of Evergreen**
2128 N Pines Road
Spokane, WA 99208
253-589-3700
888-289-3700
Fax: 775-766-1654
e-mail: patti_logan04@yahoo.com
www.evergreenspinabifida.org

Patti Logan, Secretary
Ed Kennedy, President

Wisconsin

7976 **Spina Bifida Association of Northern Wisconsin**
PO Box 421
Schofield, WI 54476-0421
715-798-3944
e-mail: dtackley@chegnet.net
David Blanchard, President

7977 **Spina Bifida Association of Northwest Ohio**
PO Box 421
Schofield, WI 54476
715-359-9674
e-mail: thutton@cheqnet.net
www.spinabifidasupport.com

Teresa Vullings, President

7978 **Spina Bifida Association of Southeastern Wisconsin**
830 N 109th Street
Wauwatosa, WI 53226
414-607-9061
Fax: 414-607-9602
e-mail: sbawi@sbawi.org
www.sbawi.org

Karen Drzewiecki, President
Heather Lynn Flohr, Executive Director

7979 **Spina Bifida Association of the Greater Fox Valley**
325 N John Street
Kimberly, WI 54136
920-687-0801
e-mail: fus1234@athenet.net
www.spinabifidasupport.com

Kelly Richard, President

Support Groups & Hotlines

7980 **National Health Information Center**
PO Box 1133
Washington, DC 20013
310-565-4167
800-336-4797
Fax: 301-984-4256
e-mail: info@nhic.org
www.health.gov/nhic

Offers a nationwide information referral service, produces directories and resource guides.

Books

7981 **Answering Your Questions About Spina Bifida**
Spina Bifida Association of America
4590 Macarthur Boulevard NW
Washington, DC 20007-4226
202-944-3285
800-621-3141
Fax: 202-944-3295
e-mail: sbaa@sbaa.org
www.sbaa.org

Provides information to help people understand the basic medical, educational and social issues which commonly affect people with Spina Bifida.

7982 **Bowel Continence and Spina Bifida**
Spina Bifida Association of America
4590 Macarthur Boulevard NW
Washington, DC 20007-4226
202-944-3285
800-621-3141
Fax: 202-944-3295
e-mail: sbaa@sbaa.org
www.sbaa.org

An excellent book aimed at anyone (infant or adult) trying to attain bowel continence. Focuses on continence programs, bowel management development and techniques.

7983 **Clinic Directory**
Spina Bifida Association of America
4590 Macarthur Boulevard NW
Washington, DC 20007-4226
202-944-3285
800-621-3141
Fax: 202-944-3295
e-mail: sbaa@sbaa.org
www.sbaa.org

A directory of health care clinics throughout the United States for children and adults with spina bifida.
200 pages 3-Ring Binder

7984 **Complete IEP Guide: How to Advocate for Your Special Ed Child**
Spina Bifida Association
4590 Macarthur Boulevard NW
Washington, DC 20007-4226
202-944-3285
800-621-3141
e-mail: sbaa@sbaa.org
www.sbaa.org

This all-in-one guide will help you understand special education law, identify your child's needs, prepare for meetings, develop the IEP and resolve disputes.

7985 **Confronting the Challenges of Spina Bifida**
Spina Bifida Association of America
4590 Macarthur Boulevard NW
Washington, DC 20007-4226
202-944-3285
800-621-3141
Fax: 202-944-3295
e-mail: sbaa@sbaa.org
www.sbaa.org

A group curriculum addressing self-care, self-esteem, and social skills in 8 to 13 year olds.

7986 **Healthcare Guidelines**
Spina Bifida Association of America
4590 Macarthur Boulevard NW
Washington, DC 20007-4226
202-944-3285
800-621-3141
Fax: 202-944-3295
e-mail: sbaa@sbaa.org
www.sbaa.org

7987 **Learning Disabilities and the Person with Spina Bifida**
Spina Bifida Association of America

4590 Macarthur Boulevard NW   202-944-3285
Washington, DC 20007-4226   800-621-3141
Fax: 202-944-3295
e-mail: sbaa@sbaa.org
www.sbaa.org

7988   **Negotiating the Special Education Maze: A Guide for Parents and Teachers**
Spina Bifida Association
4590 Macarthur Boulevard NW   202-944-3285
Washington, DC 20007-4226   800-621-3141
e-mail: sbaa@sbaa.org
www.sbaa.org
An excellent aid for the development of an effective special education program.

7989   **New Language of Toys: Teaching Communication Skills to Children...**
Spina Bifida Association
4590 Macarthur Boulevard NW   202-944-3285
Washington, DC 20007-4226   800-621-3141
e-mail: sbaa@sbaa.org
www.sbaa.org
A guide for parents and teachers, this reader-friendly resource guide provides a wealth of information on how play activities affect a child's language development (with a focus on special needs) and where to get the toys and materials to use in these activities.

7990   **Nick Joins In**
Spina Bifida Association
4590 Macarthur Boulevard NW   202-944-3285
Washington, DC 20007-4226   800-621-3141
e-mail: sbaa@sbaa.org
www.sbaa.org
When Nick, who is in a wheelchair, enters a regular classroom, for the first time he realizes that he has much to contribute.

7991   **Princess Pooh**
Spina Bifida Association
4590 Macarthur Boulevard NW   202-944-3285
Washington, DC 20007-4226   800-621-3141
e-mail: sbaa@sbaa.org
www.sbaa.org
Jealous of her disabled sister's royal treatment as she sits on her throne with wheels, Patty Jean borrows it and discovers that life in a wheelchair isn't so easy.

7992   **SBAA General Information Packet**
Spina Bifida Association of America
4590 Macarthur Boulevard NW   202-944-3285
Washington, DC 20007-4226   800-621-3141
Fax: 202-944-3295
e-mail: sbaa@sbaa.org
www.sbaa.org

7993   **Sexuality and the Person with Spina Bifida**
Spina Bifida Association of America
4590 Macarthur Boulevard NW   202-944-3285
Washington, DC 20007-4226   800-621-3141
Fax: 202-944-3295
e-mail: sbaa@sbaa.org
www.sbaa.org
Focuses on sexuality, sexual development, sexual activity, and other important issues.

7994   **Social Development and the Person with Spina Bifida**
Spina Bifida Association of America
4590 Macarthur Boulevard NW   202-944-3285
Washington, DC 20007-4226   800-621-3141
Fax: 202-944-3295
e-mail: sbaa@sbaa.org
www.sbaa.org

7995   **Steps to Independence: Teaching Everyday Skills to Children with Special Needs**
Spina Bifida Association
4590 Macarthur Boulevard NW   202-944-3285
Washington, DC 20007-4226   800-621-3141
e-mail: sbaa@sbaa.org
www.sbaa.org
A guide to help parents teach life skills to their disabled child.

7996   **Taking Charge**
Spina Bifida Association of America
4590 Macarthur Boulevard NW   202-944-3285
Washington, DC 20007-4226   800-621-3141
Fax: 202-944-3295
e-mail: sbaa@sbaa.org
www.sbaa.org
Teenagers talk about life and physical disabilities.

7997   **Unlocking Potential: College and Other Choices for People with LD and AD/HD**
Spina Bifida Association
4590 Macarthur Boulevard NW   202-944-3285
Washington, DC 20007-4226   800-621-3141
e-mail: sbaa@sbaa.org
www.sbaa.org
An indispensible tool for high school students with learning disabilities and AD/HD. Includes a comprehensive listing of resources.

Children's Books

7998   **Margaret's Moves**
Dutton Children's Books
375 Hudson Street   212-366-2000
New York, NY 10014-3658
This story deals with all the nuances and impairments that children afflicted with spina bifida must encounter and succeed in overcoming.
Grades 4-6

7999   **Rolling Along with Goldilocks and the Three Bears**
Spina Bifida Association
4590 Macarthur Boulevard NW   202-944-3285
Washington, DC 20007-4226   800-621-3141
e-mail: sbaa@sbaa.org
www.sbaa.org
The familiar folktale with a special-needs twist.

8000   **Views from Our Shoes: Growing Up with a Brother or Sister with Special Needs**
Spina Bifida Association
4590 Macarthur Boulevard NW   202-944-3285
Washington, DC 20007-4226   800-621-3141
e-mail: sbaa@sbaa.org
www.sbaa.org
A balanced view of the positives and negatives of living with a disabled sibling. Written for siblings ages nine and up.

Newsletters

8001   **Insights Into Spina Bifida**
Spina Bifida Association of America
4590 Macarthur Boulevard NW   202-944-3285
Washington, DC 20007-4226   800-621-3141
Fax: 202-944-3295
e-mail: sbaa@sbaa.org
www.sbaa.org
Includes articles on the latest research, the latest up-dates on legislation, features and emotional aspects specific to Spina Bifida, educational information and information on the Association's national conference.
BiMonthly

8002   **NASS News**
222 S Prospect Avenue   847-698-1628
Park Ridge, IL 60068-4037
Association activities newsletter.

Pamphlets

8003   **Educational Issues Among Children with Spina Bifida**
Spina Bifida Association of America

4590 Macarthur Boulevard NW
Washington, DC 20007-4226

202-944-3285
800-621-3141
Fax: 202-944-3295
e-mail: sbaa@sbaa.org
www.sbaa.org

1995

8004 Learning Among Children with Spina Bifida
Spina Bifida Association of America
4590 Macarthur Boulevard NW
Washington, DC 20007-4226

202-944-3285
800-621-3141
Fax: 202-944-3295
e-mail: sbaa@sbaa.org
www.sbaa.org

1995

8005 Monetary Allowance, Health Care and Vocational Training
National Veterans Services Fund
PO Box 2465
Darien, CT 06820-0465

203-656-0003
Fax: 203-656-1957
e-mail: NatVetSvc@aol.com

Monetary allowance, health care and vocational training and rehabilitation for Vietnam Veterans' children with spine bifida.
Pamphlet

8006 Sexual Issues in Spina Bifida
Spina Bifida Association of America
4590 Macarthur Boulevard NW
Washington, DC 20007-4226

202-944-3285
800-621-3141
Fax: 202-944-3295
e-mail: sbaa@sbaa.org
www.sbaa.org

1993

8007 Urologic Care of the Child with Spina Bifida
Spina Bifida Association of America
4590 Macarthur Boulevard NW
Washington, DC 20007-4226

202-944-3285
800-621-3141
Fax: 202-944-3295
e-mail: sbaa@sbaa.org
www.sbaa.org

1994

Audio & Video

8008 Protecting Against Latex Allergy
Spina Bifida Association of America
4590 Macarthur Boulevard NW
Washington, DC 20007-4226

202-944-3285
800-621-3141
Fax: 202-944-3295
e-mail: sbaa@sbaa.org
www.sbaa.org

Audio-visual resource focusing on the awareness of latex aller-
gies.
Audio-Visual
Cindy Brownstein, Chief Executive Officer
Caroline Alston, Program Director

8009 Raising a Child with Spina Bifida: An Introduction
Ajn Company
New York, NY 10019

212-582-8820
800-226-6256
Fax: 212-586-5462

Offers information parents need when their child is born with spina
bifida. Uses clear explanations to define spina bifida and discuss
its implications for the child. Covers procedures the child may
face, such as a ventricular shunt. Emphasizes the importance of
early intervention and contains footage of happy and healthy children and interviews with parents.
29 minutes

8010 The Challenge
Spina Bifida Association of America
4590 Macarthur Boulevard NW
Washington, DC 20007-4226

202-944-3285
800-621-3141
Fax: 202-944-3295
e-mail: sbaa@sbaa.org
www.sbaa.org

A human look of how people come to grips with and overcome the
challenges related to living with Spina Bifida.
14 minutes
Cindy Brownstein, Chief Executive Officer
Caroline Alston, Program Director

Web Sites

8011 Healing Well

www.healingwell.com

An online health resource guide to medical news, chat, information
and articles, newsgroups and message boards, books, disease-related web sites, medical directories, and more for patients, friends,
and family coping with disabling diseases, disorders, or chronic
illnesses.

8012 Health Finder

www.healthfinder.gov

Searchable, carefully developed web site offering information on
over 1000 topics. Developed by the US Department of Health and
Human Services, the site can be used in both English and Spanish.

8013 Healthlink USA

www.healthlinkusa.com

Health information concerning treatment, cures, prevention, diagnosis, risk factors, research, support groups, email lists, personal
stories and much more. Updated regularly.

8014 Helios Health

www.helioshealth.com

Online resource for your health information. Detailed information
about specific health topics, access to expert advice from our Medical Advisory Board, and up-to-date health news.

8015 March of Dimes Birth Defects Foundation

www.modimes.org

Information on the treatment and prevention of birth defects, including spina bifida.

8016 MedicineNet

www.medicinenet.com

An online resource for consumers providing easy-to-read, authoritative medical and health information.

8017 Medscape

www.medscape.com

Medscape offers specialists, primary care physicians, and other
health professionals the Web's most robust and integrated medical
information and educational tools.

8018 Spina Bifida Association of America

www.sbaa.org

Represents approximately 60 chapters of parents and other members of families having children born with spina bifida, individuals
with spina bifida, and health professionals who work with them.

8019 WebMD

www.webmd.com

Information on Spina Bifida, including articles and resources.

Description

8020 # Spinal Cord Injuries

Spinal cord injury results from trauma to or disease of the spinal cord. Depending on where the spinal cord was injured, paraplegia (paralysis affecting the legs and lower part of the body) or quadriplegia (paralysis affecting all muscles below the neck and therefore all four limbs), may occur. Bladder and/or sexual function may be damaged. Each year, 12,000 people, mostly teenage males, sustain a spinal cord injury as a result of motor vehicle or sports-related accidents, or violent crimes.

Modern medical and surgical care has dramatically increased both long-term survival and quality of life in victims of spinal cord injury. This improvement reflects intensive medical care and appropriate surgical stabilization at the time of the injury, and in later years, attention to preventing the complications, such as skin breakdown, bladder infection and lung dysfunction. One of the greatest challenges is helping persons with spinal cord injuries to live as productive and independent a life as possible. Rehabilitation should begin as soon as possible after the injury. It usually starts with several weeks at a specialized inpatient facility, then transitions to family-assisted or independent living, depending on the extent of the disability. The multidisciplinary team provides education, emotional support, physical and occupational therapy, assistive devices, braces, and beds, and helps arrange special vans or modifications to the patient's home. Many voluntary societies and government agencies can help with the transition to life in the community.

National Agencies & Associations

8021 **American Association of Spinal Cord Injury Nurses**
801 18th Street NW   202-416-7704
Washington, DC 20006   Fax: 202-416-7641
e-mail: aascin@pva.org
www.aascin.org
Comprised of nurses who specialize in spinal cord research nursing and education.
Sara Lerman MPH, Program Manager
Maurice L Jordan, Acting Executive Director

8022 **American Paraplegic Society**
801 18th Street NW   202-416-7704
Washington, DC 20006-1131   Fax: 202-416-7641
e-mail: aps@pva.org
www.apssci.org
A professional membership organization for physicians scientists and allied health care professionals.
Maurice L Jordan, Acting Executive Director
Brenda Finkel, Administrative Assistant

8023 **American Spinal Cord Injury Association**
2020 Peachtree Road NW   404-355-9772
Atlanta, GA 30309   Fax: 404-355-1826
e-mail: ASIA_Office@shepherd.org
www.asia-spinalinjury.org
Provides a forum for doctors, nurses, rehabilitation professionals and others to exchange information through seminars and workshops. Scientific conferences include workshops on chronic SCI problems, neurophysiology, bioengineering and outpatient care.
Lesley M Hudson, Executive Director
Patricia Duncan, Administrative Coordinator

8024 **American Spinal Injury Association (ASIA)**
2020 Peachtree Road NW   404-355-9772
Atlanta, GA 30309   Fax: 404-355-1826
e-mail: ASIA_Office@shepherd.org
www.asia-spinalinjury.org
Professional association for physicians and other clinicians working in the field of spinal cord injury research prevention and care delivery.
Lesley Hudson, Director Meetings/Publications
Patricia Duncan, Administrative Coordinator

8025 **Association of Spinal Cord Injury Psychologists and Social Workers**
801 18th Street NW   202-416-7704
Washington, DC 20006-1131   Fax: 202-416-7641
e-mail: aascipsw@epua.org
www.aascipsw.org
Formed in 1986 to provide a forum for the exchange of ideas and information with assistance of the Eastern Paralyzed Veterans Association.
Maurice L Jordan, Acting Executive Director
Brenda Finkel, Administrative Assistant

8026 **Christopher & Dana Reeve Foundation Paralysis Resource Center**
636 Morris Turnpike   973-467-8270
Short Hills, NJ 07078   800-225-0292
e-mail: info@paralysis.org
www.paralysis.org
The Paralysis Resource Center is a national clearinghouse of information referral and educational materials on paralysis. Services include a free lending library of books and videos and quality of life grants to qualifying non-profit organizations.
Paul Daversa, CEO
John McConnell, Senior Vice President of Programming

8027 **Eastern Paralyzed Veterans Association of America**
7520 Astoria Boulevard   718-803-3782
E Elmhurst, NY 11370-1177   800-444-0120
Fax: 718-803-0414
Dedicated to serving veterans with a spinal cord injury or disease in New York New Jersey Connecticut or Pennsylvania. Based in New York City EPVA is the leader in funding SCI research and care.
Angela Wu, Director of Library Information

8028 **FES Information Center WO Walker Industrial Rehabilitation Cent**
WO Walker Industrial Rehabilitation Center
11000 Cedar Avenue
Cleveland, OH 44106-3052   800-666-2353
FES offers technology to persons with neuromuscular disorders resulting from spinal cord injury, head injury or stroke. The most widely known use of FES in the spinal community is for exercise.

8029 **International Medical Society of Paralegia: US Office**
T Giles
1333 Moursend Avenue   713-797-5910
Houston, TX 77030   Fax: 713-799-7017
National non-profit organization offers information resources and research for people with spinal cord injury or dysfunction. Professional organization for physicians.

8030 **International Spinal Cord Regeneration Center**
Po Box 451   619-463-5350
Bonita, CA 91908   Fax: 619-460-2699
e-mail: spinal@mailutopia.net
spinal.siteutopia.net
Specializes in spinal cord regeneration as well as Embryonic Cell Transplant Therapy.
Fernando C Ramirez del Rio, Medical Director
Wolfram W Kuhnau, Associate

8031 **Kent Waldrep National Paralysis Foundation Main Office**
Main Office
16415 Addison Road   972-248-7100
Addison, TX 75001   800-925-2873
Fax: 972-248-7313

National non-profit organization offers information referral resources and research for people with spinal cord injury their family members or service providers.

8032 National Spinal Cord Injury Association: Metropolitan Washington Chapter
6701 Democracy Boulevard 301-214-4006
Bethesdae, MD 20817 800-962-9629
Fax: 301-881-9817
e-mail: stevetowle@cs.com
The mission of the National Spinal Cord Injury A ssociation is to enable people with spinal cord injury and disease to achieve their highest level of indepedence, health, and personal fulfillment by providing resources, services, and peer support.
Harley Thomas, President

8033 National Spinal Cord Injury Statistical Center
University of Alabama, Dept. of Physical Medicine
619 19th Street S 205-934-3283
Birmingham, AL 35249 Fax: 205-975-4691
e-mail: sciweb@uab.edu
www.spinalcord.uab.edu
Supervises and directs the collection management and analysis of an extensive spinal cord injury database.
Amie Jackson, Project Director & Medical Director
Pam Mott, Director Research Services

8034 Paralysis Society of America
801 Eighteenth Street NW 202-973-8420
Washington, DC 20006-3517 888-772-1711
Fax: 202-973-8421
TTY: 2029738422
e-mail: info@psa.org
www.psa.org
Membership organization for people who have sustained a spinal cord injury or who have contracted a spinal cord disease; provides information services and advocacy.
Randy L Pleva, National President
Gene A Crayton, National Senior Vice President

8035 Paralyzed Veterans of America
801 18th Street NW 202-872-1300
Washington, DC 20006-3517 800-424-8200
Fax: 202-785-4452
e-mail: info@pva.org
www.pva.org
A congressionally chartered veterans service organization founded in 1946 has developed a unique expertise in a wide variety of issues involving the special needs of members - veterans of the armed forces who have experienced spinal cord injury or dysfunction.
Randy L Pleva, National President
Gene A Crayton, National Senior Vice President

8036 Rick Hansen Foundation
520 W 6th Avenue 604-876-6800
Vancouver, BC, V5Z-1A1 800-213-2131
Fax: 604-876-6666
e-mail: info@rickhanse.com
www.rickhansen.com
To inspire others to share in the achievement of big dreams that accelerate improvements in the quality of life of people with spinal cord injury.

8037 Spinal Cord Injury Network International
3911 Princeton Drive 707-577-8796
Santa Rosa, CA 95405-7013 800-548-2673
Fax: 707-577-0605
e-mail: spinal@sonic.net
www.spinalcordinjury.org
Provides information and referral for spinal cord injured individuals and their families. Video lending library with information about spinal cord injuries. Provides answers to many questions about disability and spinal cord injury and disease.
Lennice Ambrose, Executive Director
Sharon E Hunt, Medical Librarian

8038 Spinal Cord Society
19051 County Highway 1 218-739-5252
Fergus Falls, MN 56537 Fax: 218-739-5262
www.scsus.org

Funds research for spinal cord injuries and provides physician referrals.

State Agencies & Associations

Arizona

8039 Arizona United Spinal Cord Association Samaritan Rehab Institute R-2
Samaritan Rehab Institute R-2
901E Willetta Street 602-239-5929
Phoenix, AZ 85006 877-778-6588
Fax: 602-239-6268
e-mail: info@azspinal.org
www.azspinal.org
Organization dedicated to improving the quality of life for persons with spinal cord injuries and related disorders and their families. Seeks to fulfill this mission by raising awareness about spinal cord injury through education and injury prevention.
Paul Mortensen, Executive Director
Vangie Mortenson, Office Manager

California

8040 National Spinal Cord Injury Association: San Diego County Chapter
6645 Alvarado Road 619-229-7001
San Diego, CA 92120 e-mail: rehabdsg@gte.net
Organization dedicated to improving the quality of life for persons with spinal cord injury and related disorders and their families. Seeks to fufill this mission by raising awareness about spinal cord injury through education, injury prevention, improvement of medical, rehabilitative and supportive services, research and public policy formulation.
Royce Hamrick

8041 National Spinal Cord Injury Association: Los Angeles Chapter
311 Robertson Boulevard 310-553-4833
Beverly Hills, CA 90211 Fax: 310-230-0999
spinalcord.org
Organization dedicated to improving the quality of life for persons with spinal cord injury and related disorders and their families. Seeks to fufill this mission by raising awareness about spinal cord injury through education, injury prevention, improvement of medical, rehabilitative and supportive services, research and public policy formulation.
Paul Berns MD, President

Connecticut

8042 National Spinal Cord Injury Association: Connecticut Chapter
PO Box 400 203-284-1045
Wallingford, CT 06492 e-mail: nscia@sciact.org
www.sciat.org
Organization dedicated to improving the quality of life for persons with spinal cord injury and related disorders and their families. Seeks to fufill this mission by raising awareness about spinal cord injury through education, injury prevention, improvement of medical, rehabilitative and supportive services, research and public policy formulation.
Bill Mancini, President

Florida

8043 Goodwill Industries-Suncoast
Goodwill Industries-Suncoast
10596 Gandy Boulevard 727-523-1512
Saint Petersburg, FL 33702 888-279-1988
Fax: 727-579-0850
TTY: 727-579-1068
e-mail: gw.marketing@goodwill-suncoast.com
www.goodwill-suncoast.org
A nonprofit community based organization whose purpose is to improve the quality of life for people who are disabled, disadvantaged and/or aged. This mission is accomplished through a staff of over 1,200 employees providing independent living skills.
R Lee Waits, President/Chief Executive Officer
Chris Ward, Marketing and Media Relations Manager

Georgia

8044 **Shepherd Spinal Center**
2020 Peachtree Road NW
Atlanta, GA 30309

404-352-2020
e-mail: webmaster@shepherd.org
www.shepherd.org

A nationally recognized facility in the United States dedicated exclusively to the care of patients with paralyzing spinal cord injuries and neuromuscular diseases.
David F Apple Jr, Medical Director Emeritus
Brock K Bowman, Assistant Medical Director

Illinois

8045 **Spinal Cord Injury Association of Illinois**
1032 S LaGrange Road
LaGrange, IL 60525

708-352-6223
877-373-0301
Fax: 708-352-9065
e-mail: sciinjury@aol.com
www.sci-illinois.org

Organization dedicated to improving the quality of life for persons with spinal cord injury and related disorders and their families. Seeks to fulfill this mission by raising awareness about spinal cord injury through education and injury prevention.
Mercedes Rauen, Executive Director

Indiana

8046 **National Spinal Cord Injury Association: Central Indiana Chapter**
2109 Cleveland Street
Garyanapolis, IN 46404

219-944-8037
Fax: 317-329-2530
e-mail: rjackson@ci.gary.in.us

Organization dedicated to improving the quality of life for persons with spinal cord injury and related disorders and their families. Seeks to fulfill this mission by raising awareness about spinal cord injury through education, injury prevention, improvement of medical, rehabilitative and supportive services, research and public policy formulation.
Lucille Hightower

Kentucky

8047 **National Spinal Cord Injury Association: Derby City Area Chapter**
Center for Accessible Living
1518 Herr Lane
Louisville, KY 40222

502-589-6620
e-mail: dallgood@calky.org

Organization dedicated to improving the quality of life for persons with spinal cord injury and related disorders and their families. Seeks to fufill this mission by raising awareness about spinal cord injury through education, injury prevention, improvement of medical, rehabilitative and supportive services, research and public policy formulation.
David Allgood, President

Louisiana

8048 **National Spinal Cord Injury Association: Louisiana Chapter**
3650 18th Street
Metairie, LA 70002

504-455-1178
Fax: 504-455-7315

Organization dedicated to improving the quality of life for persons with spinal cord injury and related disorders and their families. Seeks to fufill this mission by raising awareness about spinal cord injury through education, injury prevention, improvement of medical, rehabilitative and supportive services, research and public policy formulation.
Yadi Mark

Maryland

8049 **National Spinal Cord Injury Association**
6701 Democracy Blvd.
Bethesda, MD 20817

301-214-4006
800-962-9629
Fax: 301-990-0445
e-mail: nscia2@aol.com
www.spinalcord.org

The missionof The National Spimal Cord Injury Association is to enable people with spinal cord injury and diesease to achieve their highest level of independence, health, and peronal fulfillment by providing resourcees, services, and peer support.
Steven A Towle, Contact

Massachusetts

8050 **National Spinal Cord Injury Association**
545 Concord Avenue
Cambridge, MA 02138-1173

301-588-6959
800-962-9629
Fax: 301-588-9414
e-mail: nscia2@aol.com
www.spinalcord.org

Organization dedicated to improving the quality of life for persons with spinal cord injury and related disorders and their families. Seeks to fufill this mission by raising awareness about spinal cord injury through education, injury prevention, improvement of medical, rehabilitative and supportive services, research and public policy formulation.

8051 **National Spinal Cord Injury Association: Greater Boston Chapter**
New England Rehabilitation Hospital
Two Rehabilitation Way
Woburn, MA 01801

781-933-8666
Fax: 781-933-0043
e-mail: sciboston@aol.com
www.sciboston.com

Organization dedicated to improving the quality of life for persons with spinal cord injury and related disorders and their families. Seeks to fufill this mission by raising awareness about spinal cord injury through education and injury prevention.
Kevin Gibson, Coordinator
Dave Estrada, Director

New Hampshire

8052 **New Hampshire Chapter NSCIA**
Northeast Rehabilitation Hospital
PO Box 197 North Salem
Salem, NH 03079-3974

603-479-0560
Fax: 928-438-9607
www.nhspinal.org

Lisa Thompson, President

New York

8053 **Greater Rochester Area Chapter NSCIA**
PO Box 20516
Rochester, NY 14602-0076

716-275-6345
e-mail: ascaram4@frontier.net

Karen Genet, Contact

Pennsylvania

8054 **Philadelphia Unit of Shriners Hospital**
3551 N Broad Street
Philadelphia, PA 19140

215-430-4000
800-281-4050
Fax: 215-430-4079
www.shrinershq.org

Studies and research done on children with spinal cord injuries.
Richard B Gallier, Chairman
Randal R Betz, Chief of Staff and Medical Director

8055 **Spinal Cord Injury Program at Harmarville Rehabilitation Center**
PO Box 11460
Pittsburgh, PA 15238

412-828-1300
800-624-4673

Most comprehensive center for the treatment of spinal cord injury and disease.

Texas

8056 **Rio Grande Chapter: NSCIA Rio Vista Rehabilitation Hospital**
Rio Vista Rehabilitation Hospital
1395 George Dieter
El Paso, TX 79936-2901

915-532-3004
www.spinalcord.org

Sukie Armendariz, Contact
Ron Prieto, Contact

8057 Old Dominion Area Chapter: NSCIA
5206 Markel Road
Richmond, VA 23226
804-726-4990
Fax: 888-752-7857
e-mail: info@odcnscia.org
www.odcnscia.org
Steve Fetrow, President
Craig Fabian, Vice President

8058 West Virginia Mountaineer Chapter: NSCIA
PO Box 1004
Institute, WV 25112-1004
304-766-4751
Fax: 304-766-4849
www.spinalcord.org
Steve Hill, President

8059 Greater Milwaukee Area Chapter: NSCIA Sacred Heart Rehabilitation Hospital
Sacred Heart Rehabilitation Hospital
1545 S Layton Boulevard
Milwaukee, WI 53215-1993
414-384-4022
Fax: 414-384-7820
e-mail: someone@example.com
www.nsciagmac.org
John Dzicwa, President

Research Centers

8060 Miami Project to Cure Paralysis
1095 NW 14th Terrace
Miami, FL 33136
305-243-6001
800-STA-NDUP
Fax: 205-243-6017
e-mail: miamiproject@med.miami.edu
www.miamiproject.miami.edu
The Project which began in 1985 is on the leading edge of basic science and clinical research to restore function after spinal cord injury. The Project is divided into three areas. The primary emphasis is on basic science research under the direction of Dr. Richard Bunge an eminent researcher. The second area is under the direction of Barth Green M.D. a neurosurgeon. The third area is rehabilitation research.
Suzie M Fayfie, Executive Director
Marc A Buoniconti, President

8061 Paralysis Project
PO Box 56141
Sherman Oaks, CA 91413-1141
818-785-5555
www.venturablvd.com
Funds scientific research and clinical studies that focus on spinal nerve repair and regeneration. The Project distributes current research data regarding paralysis and scientific projects public awareness and community information referral and support services for paralyzed individuals.

8062 Pushin On: RRTC on Secondary Conditions of Spinal
UAB Office of Research Services
619 19th Street S
Birmingham, AL 35249-7330
205-934-3283
Fax: 205-975-4691
e-mail: rtc@sun.rehabm.uab.edu
www.spinalcord.uab.edu
A federally funded rehabilitation research and training center.
8 pages 2 per year
Phil Klebine, Project Coordinator/Editor
Pamela Mott, Director Research Services

8063 RRTC on Aging with a Disability Los Amigos Research and Education Instit
Los Amigos Research and Education Institute
800 W Annex
Downey, CA 90242-3456
562-401-7402
Fax: 562-401-7011
e-mail: lcarrothers@agingwithdisability.org
www.agingwithdisability.org
A federally funded rehabilitation research and training center.
Leanne Carro Pt PhD, Training Director
Bryan Kemp PhD, Director

Support Groups & Hotlines

8064 Georgia National Spinal Cord Injury Association Support Group Network
PO Box 2645
Columbus, GA 31920
800-422-3352
Support group dedicated to improving the quality of life for persons with spinal cord injury and related disorders and their families. Seeks to fufill this mission by raising awareness about spinal cord injury through rehabilitative and supportive services, research and public policy formulation.
Andy Harp

8065 HEALTHSOUTH Capital Rehabilitation Hospital
1675 Riggins Road
Tallahassee, FL 32308
850-656-4800
Fax: 850-656-4809
www.healthsouth.com
Support group dedicated to improving the quality of life for persons with spinal cord injury and related disorders and their families. Seeks to fufill this mission by raising awareness about spinal cord injury through rehabilitative and supportive services, research and public policy formulation.
Lynn Streetman, Chief Executive Officer

8066 Maryland National Spinal Cord Injury Association Support Group Network
Kerman Hospital
2200 Kerman Drive
Baltimore, MD 21207
410-448-6307
800-962-9629
Support group dedicated to improving the quality of life for persons with spinal cord injury and related disorders and their families. Seeks to fufill this mission by raising awareness about spinal cord injury through rehabilitative and supportive services, research and public policy formulation.
Jessica Richard

8067 National Health Information Center
PO Box 1133
Washington, DC 20013
310-565-4167
800-336-4797
Fax: 301-984-4256
e-mail: info@nhic.org
www.health.gov/nhic
Offers a nationwide information referral service, produces directories and resource guides.

8068 National Spinal Cord Injury Hotline
2200 Kerman Drive
Baltimore, MD 21207
410-448-6824
800-492-5538
Fax: 410-448-6825
www.kernanhospital.com/pain
Provides information and referral services and peer support for people affected by a traumatic paralyzing injury.

8069 National Spinal Cord Injury Support Goups
Florida Rehabilitation and Sports Medicine
5165 Adanson Street
Orlando, FL 32804
407-895-7991
Support group dedicated to improving the quality of life for persons with spinal cord injury and related disorders and their families. Seeks to fufill this mission by raising awareness about spinal cord injury through rehabilitative and supportive services, research and public policy formulation.
Robin Kohn

8070 VIVA!
Health Enhancement Learning Programs
PO Box 543065
Dallas, TX 75354-3065
972-986-2977
800-334-4403
A computer-based patient education system on spinal cord injury.

8071 National Spinal Cord Injury Support Groups
Healthsouth Central Georgia Rehab Hospital
3351 Northside Drive
Macon, GA 31210
478-201-6500
800-491-3550
Fax: 478-633-5134
e-mail: tamboli.sara@mccg.org
www.centralgarehab.com/
Support group dedicated to improving the quality of life for persons with spinal cord injury and related disorders and their families. Seeks to fufill this mission by raising awareness about spinal

cord injury through rehabilitative and supportive services, research and public policy formulation.

Kathy Parks Combs RN, SCI Support Group Coordinator

8072 **National Spinal Cord Injury Support Groups**
HEALTHSOUTH, Sea Pines Rehabilitation Hospital
101 E Florida Avenue   407-984-4600
Melbourne, FL 32901
Support group dedicated to improving the quality of life for persons with spinal cord injury and related disorders and their families. Seeks to fulfill this mission by raising awareness about spinal cord injury through rehabilitative and supportive services, research and public policy formulation.

Dorn Williamson

8073 **National Spinal Cord Injury Support Groups**
115 Alpine Street   334-456-1768
Chickasaw, AL 36611
Support group dedicated to improving the quality of life for persons with spinal cord injury and related disorders and their families. Seeks to fulfill this mission by raising awareness about spinal cord injury through rehabilitative and supportive services, research and public policy formulation.

Marilyn McPherson

Books

8074 **Body Silent: An Anthropologist Embarks into the World of the Disabled**
WW Norton Publishing
500 Fifth Avenue   212-354-5500
New York, NY 10110   Fax: 212-869-0856
                                         www.wwnorton.com
Diagnosed at midlife in the early 1980s with an inoperable (and, at the time, untreatable) ependymona of the spine, an anthropologist frankly discusses his progressive disability.

ISBN: 0-393307-02-6
RF Murphy

8075 **Climbing Back**
Miramar Communications
PO Box 8987
Malibu, CA 90265-8987   800-543-4116
The author broke his back after a climbing fall. With his sights at the top of the mountain he climbs back in this inspiring story.
256 pages Hardcover

8076 **Occupational Therapy Practice Guidelines for Adults with Spinal Cord Injury**
American Occupational Therapy Association
4720 Montgomery Lane   301-652-2682
Bethesda, MD 20824-1220   Fax: 301-652-7711
                                      TDD: 800-377-8555
                                         www.aota.org

31 pages
ISBN: 1-569001-54-5

8077 **Options: Spinal Cord Injury and the Future**
National Spinal Cord Injury Association
8300 Colesville Road   301-588-6959
Silver Spring, MD 20910-3243   800-962-9629
                                      Fax: 301-588-9414
                                   e-mail: nscia2@aol.com
                                      www.spinalcord.org
A collection of conversations with people who have had spinal cord injuries who share some of their experiences and emotions.
150 pages

8078 **Spinal Cord Injury Home Care Manual**
Santa Clara Valley Medical Center
751 S Bascom Avenue
San Jose, CA 95128-2699   408-885-5000
                                         www.scvmed.org
Provides people with spinal cord injury, their families and professionals with information about physical care, independent living, psychosocial issues, attendant care and supplies.

8079 **Spinal Network**
Miramar Communications
PO Box 8987
Malibu, CA 90265   800-543-4116
Total wheelchair resource book.

Children's Books

8080 **Follow Your Dreams**
National Spinal Cord Injury Association
8300 Colesville Road   301-588-6959
Silver Spring, MD 20910-3243   800-962-9629
                                      Fax: 301-588-9414
                                   e-mail: nscia2@aol.com
                                      www.spinalcord.org
JT, born with spina bifida, goes on an adventure. Written for and by children with SCI, for children ages 9-12.
30 pages

8081 **Tell it Like it is**
National Spinal Cord Injury Association
8300 Colesville Road   301-588-6959
Silver Spring, MD 20910-3243   800-962-9629
                                      Fax: 301-588-9414
                                   e-mail: nscia2@aol.com
                                      www.spinalcord.org
Written by teenagers with SCI for teenagers with SCI.

Magazines

8082 **SCI Life**
National Spinal Cord Injury Association
8300 Colesville Road   301-588-6959
Silver Spring, MD 20910-3243   800-962-9629
                                      Fax: 301-588-9414
                                   e-mail: nscia2@aol.com
                                      www.spinalcord.org
Official magazine of NSCIA. Updates on topics such as research, medical issues, prevention, new products, books, and Association activities.
Quarterly

8083 **Spinal Column**
Shepherd Spinal Center
2020 Peachtree Road NW   404-352-2020
Atlanta, GA 30309-1465
This quarterly magazine from the spinal center offers information on the newest treatments, therapies, referral centers, assistive devices and much more for persons living with spina bifida, multiple sclerosis and other chronic physical ailments.
Quarterly

Newsletters

8084 **Progress in Research**
American Paralysis Association
500 Morris Avenue   973-379-2690
Springfield, NJ 07081-1020   800-225-0292
                                      Fax: 973-912-9433
Offers information on the association, news, reviews, books, and information on the latest medical and technological advances in spinal cord injury research.
Quarterly
Susan P Howley, Research Director
Mitchell R Stoller, President/CEO

8085 **Pushing on: University of Alabama**
Christopher Reeve Association
500 Morris Avenue   973-379-2690
Springfield, NJ 07081   800-225-0292
                                      Fax: 973-912-9433
A research newsletter regarding spinal cord injuries.
Quarterly
Mitchell R Stoller, President/CEO

8086 Spinal Cord Society Newsletter
Spinal Cord Society
19051 County Highway 1
Fergus Falls, MN 56537

218-739-5252
Fax: 218-739-5262
www.members.aol.com/scsweb

Offers medical reports, articles, convention news, chapter news and more for persons with spinal cord injury.
Monthly

8087 Walking Tomorrow: University of Alabama
Christopher Reeve Association
500 Morris Avenue
Springfield, NJ 07081-1020

973-379-2690
800-225-0292
Fax: 973-912-9433

A research newsletter regarding spinal cord injuries.
Quarterly
Mitchell R Stoller, President/CEO

Pamphlets

8088 Autonomic Dysreflexia
National Spinal Cord Injury Association
8300 Colesville Road
Silver Spring, MD 20910-3243

301-588-6959
800-962-9629
Fax: 301-588-9414
e-mail: nscia2@aol.com
www.spinalcord.org

8089 Choosing A Spinal Cord Injury Rehabilitation Program
National Spinal Cord Injury Association
8300 Colesville Road
Silver Spring, MD 20910-3243

301-588-6959
800-962-9629
Fax: 301-588-9414
e-mail: nscia2@aol.com
www.spinalcord.org

Includes a listing of programs accredited by CARF & Model Centers designated by NIDRR.

8090 Fun and Games
National Spinal Cord Injury Association
8300 Colesville Road
Silver Spring, MD 20910-3243

301-588-6959
800-962-9629
Fax: 301-588-9414
e-mail: nscia2@aol.com
www.spinalcord.org

8091 Functional Electrical Stimulation: Clinical Applications
National Spinal Cord Injury Association
8300 Colesville Road
Silver Spring, MD 20910-3243

301-588-6959
800-962-9629
Fax: 301-588-9414
e-mail: nscia2@aol.com
www.spinalcord.org

8092 Importance of Basic Science in Research
National Spinal Cord Injury Association
8300 Colesville Road
Silver Spring, MD 20910-3243

301-588-6959
800-962-9629
Fax: 301-588-9414
e-mail: nscia2@aol.com
www.spinalcord.org

8093 Male Reproductive Function After Spinal Cord Injury
National Spinal Cord Injury Association
8300 Colesville Road
Silver Spring, MD 20910-3243

301-588-6959
800-962-9629
Fax: 301-588-9414
e-mail: nscia2@aol.com
www.spinalcord.org

8094 Medical Facilities and Resources for Ventilator Users
National Spinal Cord Injury Association
8300 Colesville Road
Silver Spring, MD 20910-3243

301-588-6959
800-962-9629
Fax: 301-588-9414
e-mail: nscia2@aol.com
www.spinalcord.org

8095 Reading Resources on Spinal Cord Injury
National Spinal Cord Injury Association

8300 Colesville Road
Silver Spring, MD 20910-3243

301-588-6959
800-962-9629
Fax: 301-588-9414
e-mail: nscia2@aol.com
www.spinalcord.org

8096 Sexuality After Spinal Cord Injury
National Spinal Cord Injury Association
8300 Colesville Road
Silver Spring, MD 20910-3243

301-588-6959
800-962-9629
Fax: 301-588-9414
e-mail: nscia2@aol.com
www.spinalcord.org

8097 Spinal Cord Injury Awareness
National Spinal Cord Injury Association
8300 Colesville Road
Silver Spring, MD 20910-3243

301-588-6959
800-962-9629
Fax: 301-588-9414
e-mail: nscia2@aol.com
www.spinalcord.org

Understanding the importance of language and images.

8098 Spinal Cord Injury: Statistical Information
National Spinal Cord Injury Association
8300 Colesville Road
Silver Spring, MD 20910-3243

301-588-6959
800-962-9629
Fax: 301-588-9414
e-mail: nscia2@aol.com
www.spinalcord.org

8099 Starting a Support Group
National Spinal Cord Injury Association
8300 Colesville Road
Silver Spring, MD 20910-3243

301-588-6959
800-962-9629
Fax: 301-588-9414
e-mail: nscia2@aol.com
www.spinalcord.org

8100 Tendon Transfer Surgery
National Spinal Cord Injury Association
8300 Colesville Road
Silver Spring, MD 20910-3243

301-588-6959
800-962-9629
Fax: 301-588-9414
e-mail: nscia2@aol.com
www.spinalcord.org

8101 Travel After Spinal Cord Injury
National Spinal Cord Injury Association
8300 Colesville Road
Silver Spring, MD 20910-3243

301-588-6959
800-962-9629
Fax: 301-588-9414
e-mail: nscia2@aol.com
www.spinalcord.org

8102 Understanding Spinal Muscular Atrophy
Families of Spinal Muscular Atrophy
PO Box 196
Libertyville, IL 60048-0196

847-367-7620
800-886-1762
Fax: 847-367-7623
e-mail: info@fsma.org
www.curesma.com

Offers a brief overview of Spinal Muscular Atrophy, causes, treatments, symptoms and unknowns.
Kenneth Hobby, Executive Director

8103 What is Spinal Cord Injury?
National Spinal Cord Injury Association
8300 Colesville Road
Silver Spring, MD 20910-3243

301-588-6959
800-962-9629
Fax: 301-588-9414
e-mail: nscia2@aol.com
www.spinalcord.org

8104 What is a Physiatrist?
National Spinal Cord Injury Association
8300 Colesville Road
Silver Spring, MD 20910-3243

301-588-6959
800-962-9629
Fax: 301-588-9414
e-mail: nscia2@aol.com
www.spinalcord.org

8105 What's New in Spinal Cord Injury Research?
National Spinal Cord Injury Association
8300 Colesville Road 301-588-6959
Silver Spring, MD 20910-3243 800-962-9629
Fax: 301-588-9414
e-mail: nscia2@aol.com
www.spinalcord.org

Audio & Video

8106 Living with Spinal Cord Injury
Barry Corbet, author

Fanlight Productions
4196 Washington Street 617-469-4999
Boston, MA 02131-1731 800-937-4113
Fax: 617-469-3379
e-mail: fanlight@fanlight.com
www.fanlight.com

A series of three videos produced by an individual who has experienced spinal cord injury himself. Changes is about coming to terms with spinal cord injury and beginning rehabilitation. Outside looks at the life-long process by which some injured people have created active and rewarding lives. Survivors explores the problems of growing old with a disability.
1973 84 Minutes

8107 SCI and Lower Extremity Orthoses
Health Enhancement Learning Programs
PO Box 543065 214-902-8277
Dallas, TX 75354-3065 800-334-4403

A video presenting an overview of indications and use of HKAFO, KAFO and AFO. Perfect resource for medical presentations and professional workshops.

8108 Spinal Cord Injury Video Access
Spinal Cord Injury Access International
39111 Princeton Drive
Santa Rosa, CA 95405 800-548-2673
Offers informational videotapes on spinal cord injury.

8109 Spinal Injury Slide Series
Health Enhancement Learning Programs
PO Box 543065 214-902-8277
Dallas, TX 75354-3065 800-334-4403

A slide series based on the VIVA program, a patient education system on spinal cord injury.

Web Sites

8110 American Association of Spinal Cord Injury Nurses
www.aascin.org
Comprised of nurses who specialize in spinal cord research, nursing and education.

8111 American Paraplegic Society
www.apssci.org
A professional membership organization for physicians, scientists and allied health care professionals.

8112 Christopher Reeve Paralysis Foundation
www.apacure.com
Dedicated to finding a cure for paralysis caused by spinal cord injury, head injury and stroke. A network of chapters across the country formed to provide comfort to the paralyzed but primarily to help raise funds to find a paralysis cure.

8113 Healing Well
www.healingwell.com
An online health resource guide to medical news, chat, information and articles, newsgroups and message boards, books, disease-related web sites, medical directories, and more for patients, friends, and family coping with disabling diseases, disorders, or chronic illnesses.

8114 Health Finder
www.healthfinder.gov

Searchable, carefully developed web site offering information on over 1000 topics. Developed by the US Department of Health and Human Services, the site can be used in both English and Spanish.

8115 Healthlink USA
www.healthlinkusa.com
Health information concerning treatment, cures, prevention, diagnosis, risk factors, research, support groups, email lists, personal stories and much more. Updated regularly.

8116 Helios Health
www.helioshealth.com
Online resource for your health information. Detailed information about specific health topics, access to expert advice from our Medical Advisory Board, and up-to-date health news.

8117 MedicineNet
www.medicinenet.com
An online resource for consumers providing easy-to-read, authoritative medical and health information.

8118 Medscape
www.medscape.com
Medscape offers specialists, primary care physicians, and other health professionals the Web's most robust and integrated medical information and educational tools.

8119 Miami Project to Cure Paralysis
www.miamiproject.miami.edu
Science and clinical research to restore function after spinal cord injury. The primary emphasis is on basic science research, under the direction of Dr. Richard Bunge, an eminent researcher.

8120 Sexual Health Network
www.sexualhealth.com
Informative site dealing with disability, sexuality and fertility.

8121 Spinal Cord Injury Information Network Center
www.spinalcord.uab.edu
Supervises and directs the collection, management and analysis of an extensive spinal cord injury database.

8122 Spinal Cord Injury Network International
www.sonic.net/~spinal
A non-profit organization that provides information and referral services and lends videos.

8123 University of Alabama, (UAB)
www.spinalcord.uab.edu
Up-to-date statistical information as well as extensive fact sheets on many aspects of Spinal Cord Injury.

8124 WebMD
www.webmd.com
Information on spinal cord injuries, including articles and resources.

Description

8125 Stroke

Strokes are caused by an interruption of blood flow in the brain, and usually — 80 percent of cases — are the result of a blocked blood vessel. The incidence increases with age, is higher in men than in women, and is higher in blacks than in whites. Depending on the severity and location of the damage, symptoms of stroke may include sudden weakness or paralysis (especially on one side of the body), blurred vision, difficulty speaking, slurred speech, dizziness and falling, extreme headache, stiff neck, altered level of alertness, and loss of bladder control. High blood pressure, atherosclerosis (fatty deposits), heart disease, diabetes, cigarette smoking, and heavy alcohol use are the major risk factors predisposing someone to stroke.

Preventive therapy is aimed at treatment of high blood pressure, heart disease, and diabetes. If someone has had a stroke they may be treated with blood thinning agents and/or other medication to prevent brain swelling. Research has shown that patients who are given one of these agents within three hours of stroke symptoms may have some or total restoration of neurologic function. To that end, the Golden Hour program was developed in which emergency medical personnel can initiate therapy in certain patients on the way to the hospital. Rehabilitation after the stroke involves physical and occupational therapy. Many stroke survivors experience depression and difficulty regaining independence, so it is important to provide emotional supportfor both survivors and their families.

National Agencies & Associations

8126 American Heart Association
7272 Greenville Avenue
Dallas, TX 75231
214-373-6300
800-242-8721
www.americanheart.org
A national organization whose primary concern is the reduction of death and disability due to cardiovascular diseases and stroke.
M Cass Wheeler, CEO

8127 American Stroke Association
7272 Greenville Avenue
Dallas, TX 75231
888-478-7653
www.strokeassociation.org
The American Stroke Association is a division of the American Heart Association that focuses on reducing risk, disability and death from stroke through research, education, fund raising and advocacy.

8128 Heart and Stroke Foundation of Canada
222 Queen Street
Ottawa, Ontario, K1P-5V9
613-569-4361
Fax: 613-569-3278
ww2.heartlandstroke.ca
Volunteer-based health charity, leads in eliminating heart disease and stroke and reducing their impact through the advancement of research and its application, the promotion of healthy living and advocacy.

8129 National Heart, Lung & Blood Institute
PO Box 301051
Bethesda, MD 20824
301-592-8573
Fax: 240-629-3296
TTY: 240-629-3255
e-mail: nhlbiinfo@nhlbi.nih.gov
www.nhlbi.nih.gov

Primary responsibility of this organization is the scientific investigation of heart, blood vessel, lung and blood disorders. Oversee research, demonstration, prevention, education and training activities in these fields and emphasizes the control of stroke.
Elizabeth G Nabel, Director

8130 National Institute of Neurological Disorders and Stroke
NIH Neurological Institute
Bethesda, MD 20824
301-496-5751
800-352-9424
Fax: 301-402-2186
TTY: 301-468-5981
www.ninds.nih.gov
The mission of NINDS is to reduce the burden of neurological disease - a burden borne by every age group, by every segment of society, by people all over the world.
Story C Landis PhD, Director
Walter J Koroshetz, Deputy Director

8131 National Stroke Association
9707 E Easter Lane
Centennial, CO 80112-3747
303-649-9299
800-787-6537
Fax: 303-649-1328
e-mail: Info@stroke.org
www.stroke.org
A national organization whose sole purpose is to reduce the incidence and impact of stroke through prevention treatment rehabilitation and research and support for stroke survivors and their families.
James Baranski, Chief Executive Officer
Mike Stefanski, Controller

8132 Neurology Institute
P O Box 5801
Bethesda, MD 20824
301-496-5751
Fax: 301-402-2186
TTY: 301-468-5981
www.ninds.nih.gov
Offers information support and resources for persons with neurological disorders heart disease and stroke victims.
Story Landis, Director
Walter J Koroshetz, Deputy Director

8133 Stroke Recovery Canada
10 Overlea Boulevard
Toronto, Ontario, M4H-1A4
888-540-6666
Fax: 416-425-1920
e-mail: info@strokerecoverycanada.com
www.strokerecoverycanada.com
National service offering post-recovery support, education and programs for stroke survivors, their families and health care providers.

Foundations

8134 American Stroke Foundation
5960 Dearborn
Mission, KS 66202
913-649-1776
866-549-1776
Fax: 913-649-6661
www.americanstroke.org
The American Stroke Foundation helps those who can't help themseles. They offer compassionate-but practical-knowledge and service in a comfortable,home-like environment. Stroke survivors get the continued assistance and suppoort they need to reach their full potential.
Rita Griffith, Executive Director
Mark Bertrand, Director Development

Research Centers

8135 Bowman Gray School of Medicine
Medical Center Boulevard
Winston Salem, NC 27157-0001
919-716-7461
Fax: 919-716-5639
www.web.bgsm.edu

James Toole MD, Professor

8136 Cerebral Blood Flow Laboratories Veterans Administration Medical Center
Veterans Administration Medical Center
2002 Holcombe Boulevard
Houston, TX 77030-4211
713-795-5807
Fax: 713-957-01

Offers research in cerebrovascular disorders and risk factors for stroke.
John S Meyer MD, Director

8137 Comprehensive Stroke Center of Oregon University of Oregon Health Sciences Cen
University of Oregon Health Sciences Center
3181 SW Sam Jackson Park Road
Portland, OR 97239-3098   503-949-8311
                                www.ohsu.edu

Provide comprehensive treatment and prevention services to adults who have had a stroke or at risk of stroke.
Bruce Coull MD, Professor

8138 Departments of Neurology & Neurosurgery: University of California, San Francisco
UCSF Medical Center
505 Parnassus Avenue   415-353-1668
San Francisco, CA 94143   Fax: 415-353-8593
                e-mail: bill.dillon@radiology.ucsf.edu
                www.neurorad.ucsf.edu

Suzie M Fayfie, Professor

8139 Hospital of the University of Pennsylvania
3400 Spruce Street   215-662-4000
Philadelphia, PA 19104   800-789-PENN
                              Fax: 215-903-09
                e-mail: pleasure@email.chop.edu
                www.pennhealth.com

Research program centering its efforts on finding better ways to prevent and treat neuromuscular disorders.
David E Pleasure MD, Director

8140 Massachusetts General Departments of Neurology and Neurosurgery
Massachusetts General Hospital
55 Fruit Street
Boston, MA 02114   617-726-2000
                              www.massgeneral.org

Peter Slavin, Director

8141 Stroke Research and Treatment Center UAB Medical Center
Medical Center
1813 6th Avenue S   205-975-8569
Birmingham, AL 35294-7   800-822-6478
                              Fax: 205-975-6785
                              main.uab.edu/neurology

An interdisciplinary program specializing in the prevention diagnosis and treatment of stroke and stroke-related disorders. The CSRC integrates the latest in medical technology with a multi-faceted approach.
Andrei V Alexandrov MD, Director and Professor
James D Halsey Jr MD, Director Stroke Residency Program

8142 University of Iowa College of Medicine
200 CMAB   319-335-6707
Iowa City, IA 52242 e-mail: webmaster@mail.medicine.uiowa.edu
                     www.medicine.uiowa.edu

Donald D Heistad MD, Professor

8143 University of Maryland Center for Studies of Cerebrovascular Disease & Stroke
16 S Utah Street   410-328-4323
Baltimore, MD 21201   Fax: 410-328-1149

Thomas R Price MD, Principal Investor

8144 University of Miami School of Medicine Department of Neurology
1120 NW 14th Street   305-243-6732
Miami, FL 33136   877-243-4340
                              Fax: 305-243-1632
                e-mail: RSacco@med.miami.edu
                www.med.miami.edu

Myron D Ginsberg MD, Professor
Ralph L Sacco MD, Chairman Department of Neurology

8145 Wake Forest University: Cerebrovascular Research Center
Department of Neurology
300 S Hawthorne Road   336-748-2338
Winston-Salem, NC 27103-2732 Fax: 336-748-5477

Cerebrovascular research.
Dr James Toole, Director

8146 Washington University School of Medicine
660 S Euclid Avenue   314-362-5000
Saint Louis, MO 63110-1016   e-mail: web@medicine.wustl.edu
                             www.medicine.wustl.edu

Marcus Raich MD

Support Groups & Hotlines

8147 National Health Information Center
PO Box 1133   310-565-4167
Washington, DC 20013   800-336-4797
                              Fax: 301-984-4256
                              e-mail: info@nhic.org
                              www.health.gov/nhic

Offers a nationwide information referral service, produces directories and resource guides.

8148 Stroke Clubs International
805 12th Street   409-762-1022
Galveston, TX 77550   e-mail: strokeclubs@earthlink.net
                      www.ninds.nih.gov

Organization of persons who have experienced strokes, their families and friends for the purpose of mutual support, education, social and recreational activities. Provides information and assistance to Stroke Clubs (which are usually sponsored by local organizations).
Ellis Williamson

Books

8149 Alzheimer's, Stroke and 29 Other Neurological Disorders Sourcebook
Omnigraphics
615 Griswold Street   313-961-1340
Detroit, MI 48226-3993   800-234-1340
                              Fax: 800-875-1340
                              www.omnigraphics.com

Provides vital information for the nontechnical reader focusing on Alzheimer's disease, stroke and various neurological disorders. Answers thousands of questions related to afflications of the central nervous system with each chapter reviwing a particular disorder and offers in-depth discussions.

8150 Courage: Poems & Positive Thoughts for Stroke Survivors
National Stroke Association
9707 E Easter Lane   303-649-9299
Englewood, CO 80112-3747   800-787-6537
                              Fax: 303-649-1328
                              www.stroke.org

Words of inspiration from survivors and caregivers.
83 pages
Colette Lafosse, Director Rehabilitation/Recovery Program

8151 Discovery Circles
National Stroke Association
9707 E Easter Lane   303-649-9299
Englewood, CO 80112-3747   800-787-6537
                              Fax: 303-649-1328
                              www.stroke.org

NSA's guide to organizing and facilitating stroke support groups. This detailed manual describes the support group structure and the facilitator's role.
213 pages
Colette Lafosse, Director Rehabilitation/Recovery Program

8152 Magic of Humor in Caregiving
National Stroke Association
9707 E Easter Lane   303-649-9299
Englewood, CO 80112-3747   800-787-6537
                              Fax: 303-649-1328
                              www.stroke.org

A dynamic researching tool focusing on the necessity of humor in daily caregiving interaction.
Colette Lafosse, Director Rehabilitation/Recovery Program

8153   November Days
National Stroke Association
9707 E Easter Lane   303-649-9299
Englewood, CO 80112-3747   800-787-6537
                                 Fax: 303-649-1328
                                     www.stroke.org
A caregiver's story of her struggle with a loved one's stroke.
225 pages

8154   Occupational Therapy Practice Guidelines for Adults with Stroke
American Occupational Therapy Association
4720 Montgomery Lane   301-652-2682
Bethesda, MD 20824-1220   Fax: 301-652-7711
                                TDD: 800-377-8555
                                     www.aota.org
15 pages
ISBN: 1-569001-55-3

8155   Stroke Book
William Morrow & Company
1350 Avenue of the Americas   212-261-6500
New York, NY 10019-4702
1993
ISBN: 0-688090-55-9

8156   Stroke: A Clinical Approach
Butterworth-Heinemann
225 Wildwood Avenue   617-928-2500
Woburn, MA 01801-2079   800-366-2665
1993 584 pages
ISBN: 0-750691-81-6

8157   Stroke: A Guide for Patient and Family
Raven Press
1185 Avenue of the Americas   212-930-9500
New York, NY 10036-2601
224 pages
ISBN: 0-881672-79-3

8158   Stroke: Your Complete Exercise Guide
Human Kinetics Publishers
PO Box 5076   217-351-1549
Champaign, IL 61825-5076   800-747-4457
                                 Fax: 217-351-5076
Part of the Cooper Clinic and Research Institute Fitness Series providing exercise rehabilitation for persons suffering from strokes.
126 pages Paperback
ISBN: 0-873224-28-0

8159   Ted's Stroke: The Caregiver's Story
National Stroke Association
9707 E Easter Lane   303-649-9299
Englewood, CO 80112-3747   800-787-6537
                                 Fax: 303-649-1328
                                     www.stroke.org
Personal experiences, guidance and tips for caregivers.
175 pages
ISBN: 0-962487-61-9

8160   The Comfort of Home for Stroke: A Guide fo r Caregivers
Marie Meyer & Paula Derr, RN with Jon Caswell, author
CareTrust Publications
PO Box 10283
Portland, OR 97296-0283   800-565-1533
                                 Fax: 415-673-2005
                    e-mail: sales@comfortofhome.com
                             www.comfortofhome.com
Comfort guides readers through every caregiving stage, from understanding personality changes, preparing the home, equipment, the healthcare team, and the activities of daily living. It helps take the fear out of home care and assists caregivers in maintaining peace of mind.
2007 344 pages
ISBN: 0-966476-78-6

8161   Women in Your Life: Protect Yourself, Protect Your Family
National Stroke Association

9707 E Easter Lane   303-649-9299
Englewood, CO 80112-3747   800-787-6537
                                 Fax: 303-649-1328
                                     www.stroke.org
Valuable information about the unique toll stroke takes on women.
Colette Lafosse, Director Rehabilitation/Recovery Program

Magazines

8162   Stroke Connection
American Stroke Foundation
8700 Lamar   913-649-1776
Overland Park, KS 66207   Fax: 913-649-6661
                             www.americanstroke.org
Official magazine of the American Stroke Foundation. Supports stroke survivors, their families, caregivers and friends by providing resources, services, education and information that improves the quality of life.

Pamphlets

8163   African-Americans and Stroke
National Stroke Association
9707 E Easter Lane   303-649-9299
Englewood, CO 80112-3747   800-787-6537
                                 Fax: 303-649-1328
                                     www.stroke.org
Colette Lafosse, Director Rehabilitation/Recovery Program

8164   Aneurysm Answers
National Stroke Association
9707 E Easter Lane   303-649-9299
Englewood, CO 80112-3747   800-787-6537
                                 Fax: 303-649-1328
                                     www.stroke.org
Colette Lafosse, Director Rehabilitation/Recovery Program

8165   Check Your Pulse, America: Atrial Fibrillation
National Stroke Association
9707 E Easter Lane   303-649-9299
Englewood, CO 80112-3747   800-787-6537
                                 Fax: 303-649-1328
                                     www.stroke.org
Colette Lafosse, Director Rehabilitation/Recovery Program

8166   Cholesterol and Stroke
National Stroke Association
9707 E Easter Lane   303-649-9299
Englewood, CO 80112-3747   800-787-6537
                                 Fax: 303-649-1328
                                     www.stroke.org
Colette Lafosse, Director Rehabilitation/Recovery Program

8167   Facts on Heart Disease, Heart Attack, Stroke and Risk Factors
American Heart Association
7272 Greenville Avenue   214-373-6300
Dallas, TX 75231-5129   Fax: 214-706-1341
Offers information on how to recognize a heart attack or stroke, recovery and rehabilitation techniques and risk factors.

8168   High Blood Pressure and Stroke
National Stroke Association
9707 E Easter Lane   303-649-9299
Englewood, CO 80112-3747   800-787-6537
                                 Fax: 303-649-1328
                                     www.stroke.org
Colette Lafosse, Director Rehabilitation/Recovery Program

8169   Mobility: Issues Facing Stroke Survivors and Their Families
National Stroke Association
9707 E Easter Lane   303-649-9299
Englewood, CO 80112-3747   800-787-6537
                                 Fax: 303-649-1328
                                     www.stroke.org
Colette Lafosse, Director Rehabilitation/Recovery Program

8170   Recurrent Stroke
National Stroke Association

9707 E Easter Lane
Englewood, CO 80112-3747

303-649-9299
800-787-6537
Fax: 303-649-1328
www.stroke.org

Colette Lafosse, Director Rehabilitation/Recovery Program

8171 **Smoking Cessation: Be Smoke Free in 3 Minutes**
National Stroke Association
9707 E Easter Lane
Englewood, CO 80112-3747

303-649-9299
800-787-6537
Fax: 303-649-1328
www.stroke.org

Colette Lafosse, Director Rehabilitation/Recovery Program

8172 **Stroke: Hope Through Research**
Office of Scientific & Health Reports
Building 31
Bethesda, MD 20892-0001

301-496-5751
800-352-9424

Offers information on stroke, research and advances in treatments and rehabilitation programs to help patients.

8173 **Transient Ischemic Attack**
National Stroke Association
9707 E Easter Lane
Englewood, CO 80112-3747

303-649-9299
800-787-6537
Fax: 303-649-1328
www.stroke.org

Colette Lafosse, Director Rehabilitation/Recovery Program

Audio & Video

8174 **Secret Life of the Brain**
PBS Home Video
PO Box 751089
Charlotte, NC 28275

877-727-7467
Fax: 703-739-8131
www.pbs.org/wnet/brain/about.html

Reveals the facinating processes involved in brain development across a lifetime. The five-part series informs viewers of exciting new information in the brain sciences, introduces the foremost researchers in the field, and utilizes dynamic visual imagry and compelling human stories to help a general audience understand otherwise difficult scientific concepts.
5 Tapes
Paula Kerger, President/CEO
Wayne Godwin, Chief Operating Officer

8175 **Stroke: Touching the Soul of Your Family**
National Stroke Association
9707 E Easter Lane
Englewood, CO 80112-3747

303-649-9299
800-787-6537
Fax: 303-649-1328
www.stroke.org

Fifteen minute video chronicling three stroke survivors and their courageous struggle to overcome daily challenges and educate others about stroke.
Colette Lafosse, Director Rehabilitation/Recovery Program

Web Sites

8176 **American Heart Association**

www.americanheart.org
A national organization whose primary concern is the reduction of death and disability due to cardiovascular diseases and stroke.

8177 **Healing Well**

www.healingwell.com
An online health resource guide to medical news, chat, information and articles, newsgroups and message boards, books, disease-related web sites, medical directories, and more for patients, friends, and family coping with disabling diseases, disorders, or chronic illnesses.

8178 **Health Finder**

www.healthfinder.gov
Searchable, carefully developed web site offering information on over 1000 topics. Developed by the US Department of Health and Human Services, the site can be used in both English and Spanish.

8179 **Healthlink USA**

www.healthlinkusa.com
Health information concerning treatment, cures, prevention, diagnosis, risk factors, research, support groups, email lists, personal stories and much more. Updated regularly.

8180 **Helios Health**

www.helioshealth.com
Online resource for your health information. Detailed information about specific health topics, access to expert advice from our Medical Advisory Board, and up-to-date health news.

8181 **MedicineNet**

www.medicinenet.com
An online resource for consumers providing easy-to-read, authoritative medical and health information.

8182 **Medscape**

www.medscape.com
Medscape offers specialists, primary care physicians, and other health professionals the Web's most robust and integrated medical information and educational tools.

8183 **National Heart, Lung & Blood Institute**

www.nhlbi.nih.gov/nhlbi/nhlbi.htm
Primary responsibility of this organization is the scientific investigation of heart, blood vessel, lung and blood disorders. Oversee research, demonstration, prevention, education and training activities in these fields and emphasizes the control of stroke.

8184 **National Institute of Neurological Disorders and Stroke**

www.ninds.nih.gov
The mission of NINDS is to reduce the burden of neurological disease - a burden borne by every age group, by every segment of society, by people all over the world.

8185 **National Stroke Association**

www.stroke.org
A national organization whose sole purpose is to reduce the incidence and impact of stroke through prevention, treatment, rehabilitation and research, and support for stroke survivors and their families. Educational resources on all aspects of stroke available on website.

8186 **Neurology Channel**

www.neurologychannel.com
Find clearly explained, medically accurate information regarding conditions, including an overview, symptoms, causes, diagnostic procedures and treatment options. On this site it is possible to ask questions and get information from a neurologist and connect to people who have similar health interests.

8187 **WebMD**

www.webmd.com
Information on stroke, including articles and resources.

Description

8188 ## Substance Abuse

Substance abuse is a broad term that refers to any illegal, dangerous or destructive use of some substance. This use may be legal (binge drinking by an adult) or illegal (smoking marijuana). Abused substances include alcohol, nicotine, marijuana, heroin, prescription painkillers and tranquilizers, stimulants such as amphetamines and cocaine, and hallucinogens such as LSD. The abuse may be a danger to the user, family members, business associates, close friends or even total strangers. Substance dependence refers to a state of strong compulsion to use the substance, in many cases accompanied by physical withdrawal symptoms if the substance is not regularly available.

The cause of substance abuse is very complex, and involves an interplay between the individual's behavioral choices, their genetic background and past and present social environment. Some substance abusers also have a definable psychiatric disorder such as depression or schizophrenia; treatment of these dual-disorder patients is especially challenging.

The consequences of substance abuse are well-known, and include job loss, arrest, family breakup, automobile and other accidents, birth defects (fetal alcohol syndrome), direct toxic effects (cirrhosis of the liver from alcohol or lung cancer from smoking), and infections (HIV or hepatitis B from sharing needles). Substance abuse, unless it occurs in extremely isolated persons, greatly affects family members and loved ones. Family members often deny the reality of the abuse, and may help, or enable, the abuser to cover up the problem and avoid its consequences.

There is no quick and universally effective treatment for substance abuse. Options range from inexpensive peer-based organizations such as Alcoholics Anonymous to very expensive long-term inpatient programs. Some peer-based programs appeal to a niche defined by sex, race, age or religious affiliation. Treatment is much more likely to succeed if it is freely chosen by the individual rather than mandated by a court. Dropout during treatment and relapse after initial success are common, but many people do achieve life-long cures with abstinence from further substance abuse. Family members should look for education and support through groups like Al-Anon, which bring them together with people facing similar situations.

National Agencies & Associations

8189 **AAA Foundation for Traffic Safety**
607 14th Street NW
Washington, DC 20005-6001
202-638-5944
Fax: 202-638-5943
e-mail: info@aaafoundation.org
www.aaafoundation.org
This national organization publishes drinking and traffic safety programs for K-6 and junior high students. Courses offered are taught by school district teachers who have participated in two-hour in-service training seminars.
J Peter Kissinger, President
Kristin Backstrom, Senior Manager Development

8190 **African American Family Services**
2616 Nicollet Avenue
Minneapolis, MN 55408
612-871-7878
Fax: 612-871-2567
e-mail: contact@aafs.net
www.aafs.net
This institute provides training and technical assistance to programs that want to serve African-American/black clients and others of color more effectively.
Terry J Ticey, Chairman of the Board
Robert S Bradley, Treasurer

8191 **Al-Anon Family Group Headquarters**
1600 Corporate Landing Parkway
Virginia Beach, VA 23454-5617
757-563-1600
888-425-2666
Fax: 757-563-1655
e-mail: wso@al-anon.org
www.al-anon.alateen.org
A fellowship of relatives and friends of alcoholics who believe their lives have been affected by someone else's drinking and a mutual support group recovery program based on the 12 steps of Alcoholics Anonymous.
Robert Schneider, Director of Communications

8192 **Alateen Al-Anon Family Group Headquarters**
Al-Anon Family Group Headquarters
1600 Corporate Landing Parkway
Virginia Beach, VA 23454-5617
757-563-1600
800-425-2666
Fax: 757-563-1655
e-mail: wso@al-anon.org
www.al-anon.alateen.org
A part of the Al-Anon program Alateen is for teenagers who have been affected by someone else's drinking whether it be a family member or a friend.
Robert Schneider, Director Communications

8193 **Alcoholics Anonymous General Service Office/Grand Central Sta**
General Service Office/Grand Central Station
PO Box 459
New York, NY 10163-0459
212-870-3400
Fax: 212-870-3003
e-mail: www.aa.org
www.aa.org
Founded in 1935 Alcoholics Anonymous is a world-wide fellowship of men and women who have found solutions to their drinking problems. The only requirement for A.A. membership is a desire to stop drinking. There are no dues.

8194 **American Council for Drug Education**
50 Jay Street
Brooklyn, NY 11201-2301
718-222-6641
800-488-3784
Fax: 212-595-2553
e-mail: acde@phoenixhouse.org
www.acde.org
This organization provides information on drug use publishes books and offers films and curriculum materials for prevention.
J David Hawkins, Director
George E Woody, Chief of Staff

8195 **American Council on Alcohol Problems**
1000 E Indian School Road
Phoenix, AZ 85014
602-264-7897
800-527-5344
Fax: 602-264-7403
e-mail: info@aca-usa.org
www.aca-usa.org
Provides the forum and the mechanism through which concerned people can find common ground on alcohol and other drug problems and address these issues with a united voice.
Lloyd Vocovsky, Executive Director
Percy Menzies, Acting Chairman

8196 **American Dental Association Department of Library Services**
Department of Library Services
211 E Chicago Avenue
Chicago, IL 60611-2637
312-440-2500
Fax: 312-440-2822
e-mail: kittelson@ada.org
www.ada.org

Referrals to Chemical Dependency Support Groups that offer intervention services, referrals to dentists for treatment centers and doctors' support groups and assists with state licensing boards questions.
Linda Kittel MS RN, Manager
Brandon R Maddox, Representative

8197 Associate Administrator for Alcohol Prevention and Treatment Policy
Substance Abuse & Mental Health Services Offices
200 Independance Avenue   301-443-8956
Washington, DC 20201-0001   e-mail: info@samhsa.gov
www.samhsa.gov
Promotes monitors evaluates and coordinates programs for the prevention and treatment of alcoholism and alcohol abuse.

8198 Association of Halfway House Alcoholism Programs of North America
401 E Sangamon Avenue   217-523-0527
Springfield, IL 62702   Fax: 217-698-8234
e-mail: president@ahhap.org
www.ahhap.org
Acts as a clearinghouse of the latest literature on alcoholism assists chemical dependency counselors in placing post treatment individuals in halfway houses and helps in setting up halfway houses.
Olivia Howard, President
David Logan, Vice President

8199 BACCHUS of the US
PO Box 100430   303-871-0901
Denver, CO 80250   Fax: 303-871-0907
e-mail: admin@bacchusnetwork.org
www.bacchusgamma.org
Boosts alcohol consciousness concerning the health of university students.
Drew Hunter, President
Janet Cox, Vice President/COO

8200 CSAP State Liason Program CSAP Division of Communications Programs
CSAP Division of Communications Programs
7200 Wisconsin Avenue
Bethesda, MD 20857-0001   301-941-8500
www.covesoft.com/csap.html
This program is designed to support alcohol and other drug abuse prevention efforts in the States.

8201 Center for Substance Abuse Prevention
Substance Abuse and Mental Health Services Admin.
PO Box 2345
Rockville, MD 20847-2345   800-279-6686
TTY: 800-487-4886
TDD: 800-487-4886
e-mail: info@health.org.
ncadi.samhsa.gov
This organization's goal is to connect people and resources with innovative ideas strategies and programs designed to encourage creative and effective efforts aimed at reducing and eliminating alcohol tobacco and other drug problems in our society.

8202 Chemical People Project Public Television Outreach Alliance
Public Television Outreach Alliance
4802 5th Avenue   412-391-0900
Pittsburgh, PA 15213-2957
The project supplies information in the form of tapes literature and seminars.

8203 Cocaine Anonymous: World Service Office
3740 Overland Avenue   310-559-5833
Los Angeles, CA 90034-6337   800-999-9951
Fax: 310-559-2554
e-mail: cawso@ca.org
www.ca.org
A support group based on the twelve steps of Alcoholics Anonymous that focuses specifically on problems of cocaine addiction.

8204 Drug Abuse Resistance Education of America
PO Box 512090   310-215-0575
Los Angeles, CA 90051-0090   800-223-3273
www.dare.com

Provides information, resources, tips, warning signs and other information for parents and kids to help keep children off drugs.
Herb Kleber, Chairman
Carol J Boyd, Director

8205 Drugs Anonymous
PO Box 473   212-874-0700
New York, NY 10023
A twelve-step program that holds more than 30 meetings for drug addicts in the Greater New York Area including several in hospitals and institutions.

8206 Families Anonymous
PO Box 3475   310-313-5800
Culver City, CA 90231-3475   800-736-9805
Fax: 310-815-9682
e-mail: famanon@familiesanonymous.org
www.familiesanonymous.org
Addresses the needs of families who are concerned about a relative with a drug problem and with related behavioral problems. Offers informational packets meetings and support networks for these families.

8207 Families in Action National Drug Information Center
2957 Clairmont Road NE   404-248-9676
Atlanta, GA 30329   Fax: 404-248-1312
e-mail: nfia@nationalfamilies.org
www.nationalfamilies.org
Offers news and information for persons interested in drug abuse prevention.
Sue Rusche, President
Paula Kemp, Executive Vice President

8208 Hazelden
PO Box 11   651-213-4200
Center City, MN 55012-0011   800-257-7810
Fax: 651-213-4411
e-mail: info@hazeldon.org
www.hazelden.com
A nonprofit organization dedicated to providing quality rehabilitation education and professional services for chemical dependency and related addictive behaviors. Services offered include assessment and rehabilitation and family services.
Ellen Breyer, President

8209 Indian Health Service
801 Thompson Avenue
Rockville, MD 20852-1627   605-226-7456
www.ihs.gov
Charged with providing a comprehensive program of alcoholism and substance abuse prevention and treatment for Native Americans and Alaskan natives.

8210 Lawyers Concerned for Lawyers
2550 University Avenue W   651-646-5590
Saint Paul, MN 55114-4127   866-525-6466
Fax: 651-646-2364
e-mail: lcl.org@aol.com
www.mnlcl.org
A nonprofit organization of recovering lawyers and judges and concerned others. Educates lawyers and judges about the disease of chemical dependency assists in assessments and arranging interventions and offers lawyer-only AA meetings.
Joan Bibelhausen, Executive Director
Ellen Murphy-Fritsch, Case Manager

8211 Marijuana Anonymous: World Services
Marijuana Anonymous World Services
PO Box 2912
Van Nuys, CA 91404-2318   800-766-6779
e-mail: office@marijuana-anonymous.org
www.marijuana-anonymous.org
A fellowship of men and women who share our experience strength and hope with each other that we may solve our common problem and help others to recover from marijuana addiction.

8212 Mothers Against Drunk Driving (MADD)
511 E John Carpenter Freeway   214-744-6233
Irving, TX 75062   800-438-6233
Fax: 972-869-2206
www.madd.org

Founded by a small group of mothers and has turned into one of the largest crime victims organizations in the world.
Paul D Folkemer, Chairman of the Board
Charles A (Chuck) Hurley, Chief Executive Officer

8213 Narcotics Anonymous World Service Office
World Service Office
PO Box 9999 818-773-9999
Van Nuys, CA 91409-9099 Fax: 818-700-0700
e-mail: fsmail@na.org
www.na.org
Similar to Alcoholics Anonymous this program is a fellowship of men and women who meet to help one another with their drug dependency problems.

8214 National Association for Children of Alcoholics
11426 Rockville Pike 301-468-0985
Rockville, MD 20852-3007 888-554-2627
Fax: 301-468-0987
e-mail: nacoa@nacoa.org
www.nacoa.org
Advocates for all children and families affected by alcohol and other drug dependencies.
Sis Wenger, President/CEO
Judy Galloway, Coordinator-Affiliate Services

8215 National Association for Native American Children of Alcoholics
Seattle Indian Health Board
1402 Third Avenue 206-467-7686
Seattle, WA 98114-3364 800-322-5601
Fax: 206-467-7689
e-mail: nanacoa@aol.com
Formed to facilitate positive change in individuals and communities in order to break the intergenerational cycle of addiction among Native Americans.

8216 National Association of Alcoholism and Drug Abuse Counselors
1001 N Fairfax Street 703-741-7686
Alexandria, VA 22314 Fax: 800-377-1136
e-mail: naadac@naadac.org
www.naadac.org
Largest membership organization serving addiction counselors educators and other addiction-focused health care professionals who specialize in addiction prevention treatment and education.
Patricia M Greer, President
Sharon DeEsch, Secretary

8217 National Association on Drug Abuse Problems
Director of Corporate and Community Services
355 Lexington Avenue 212-986-1170
New York, NY 10017 Fax: 212-697-2939
e-mail: info@nadap.org
www.nadap.org
Provides skills evaluation job training and job placement to recovering drug addicts in the metropolitan New York area.
John A Darin, President & CEO
Gary Stankowski, Senior Vice President

8218 National Clearinghouse for Alcohol and Drug Information
11420 Rockville Pike Suite 200 301-468-2600
Rockville, MD 20847-2345 800-729-6686
Fax: 240-221-4292
TTY: 800-487-4889
TDD: 800-487-4889
e-mail: webmaster@health.org
www.health.org
Nation's one-stop resource for information about substance abuse prevention and addiction treatment.

8219 National Council on Alcoholism and Drug Dependence
244 E 58th Street 212-269-7797
New York, NY 10022-3128 800-622-2255
Fax: 212-269-7510
e-mail: national@ncadd.org
www.ncadd.org
The National Council on Alcoholism and Drug Dependence, Inc and it's Affiliate Network is a voluntary health organization dedicated to fighting the Nation's #1 health problem-alcholism, drug addiction and the devestating consequences of alcohol and other drugs on individuals, families and communities.
Robert Lindsey, President
Leah Brock, Director of Affiliate Relations

8220 National Crime Prevention Council
2345 Crystal Drive 202-466-6272
Arlington, VA 22202 Fax: 212-269-7510
www.ncpc.org
This organization works to prevent crime and drug use in many ways including developing materials for parents and children.
Alfonso E Lenhardt, President/CEO
David A Dean, Executive Committee Chair

8221 National Families in Action
2957 Clairmont Road NE 404-248-9676
Atlanta, GA 30329 Fax: 404-248-1312
e-mail: nfia@nationalfmailies.org
www.nationalfamilies.org
Mission is to help families and communities prevent drug use among children by promoting policies based on science.
Joseph A Califano Jr, Chairman and President
Susan P Brown, Vice President/Director of Finance

8222 National Organization on Fetal Alcohol Syndrome
900 17th Street NW 202-785-4585
Washington, DC 20006 800-666-6327
Fax: 202-466-6456
e-mail: information@nofas.org
www.nofas.org
Dedicated to eliminating birth defects caused by alcohol consumption during pregnancy and to improving the quality of life for those affected individuals and families.
Terry Lierman, Chairperson
Tom Donaldson, President

8223 National Parents Resources Institute for Drug Education
4 W Oak Street 231-924-1662
Fermont, MI 49412 800-668-9277
Fax: 231-924-5663
e-mail: info@prideyouthprograms.org
www.prideyouthprograms.org
A provider of prevention services in the area of alcohol and other drugs. Mission is to build a drug-free America.
Jay Dewispelaere, President/CEO
Lou Anne Wheater, Membership Coordinator

8224 Office of Applied Studies Substance Abuse & Mental Health Services
Substance Abuse & Mental Health Services Offices
5600 Fishers Lane
Rockville, MD 20857-0001 301-443-8956
www.oas.samhsa.gov
Provides the leadership needed for collecting data on mental illness and substance abuse including incidence and prevalence studies.

8225 Office of Substance Abuse Prevention
5600 Fishers Lane
Rockville, MD 20857-0001 301-443-0373
www.samhsa.gov
Reviews the government's alcohol and drug abuse policy operates a grant program supports development of model programs and conducts prevention workshops.

8226 Office of Women's Services Substance Abuse & Mental Health Services
Substance Abuse & Mental Health Services Offices
5600 Fishers Lane 301-443-8956
Rockville, MD 20857-0001
Provides leadership and guidance in creating and maintaining an agency-wide focus for addressing the substance abuse and mental health needs of women.

8227 Office on Smoking and Health: CDCP
Centers for Disease Control And Prevention
1600 Clifton Road 404-639-3311
Atlanta, GA 30333 TTY: 888-232-6348
e-mail: tobaccoinfo@cdc.gov
www.cdc.gov/tobacco

Offers reference services to researchers through the Technical Information Center. Publishes and distributes a number of titles in the field of smoking and health.

8228 Partnership for a Drug-Free America
405 Lexington Avenue   212-922-1560
New York, NY 10174-0002   Fax: 212-922-1570
www.drugfreeamerica.org
Non-profit coalition of communication health medical and educational professionals working to reduce illicit drug use and help people live health drug-free lives.
Stephen J Pasierb, President & CEO
Roy J Bostock, Chairman

8229 Remove Intoxicated Drivers (RID-USA)
PO Box 520   518-372-0034
Schenectady, NY 12301   Fax: 518-310-4917
e-mail: dwi@rid-usa.org
rid-usa.org
Volunteers working to deter impaired driving, to help its victims obtain justice, restitution and peace of mind when faced with the maze of criminal justice systems, and to curb the alcohol abuse which leads to drunken driving.
Doris Aiken, Founder/President
Bill Aiken, VP/Manager

8230 Safe Homes
4 Mann Street   508-366-4305
Worcester, MA 01602-0702   Fax: 508-836-5560
e-mail: safehomes@thebridgecm.org
www.safehomesma.org
This national organization encourages parents to sign a contract stipulating that when parties are held in one another's homes they will adhere to a strict no-alcohol/no-drug-use rule.

8231 Students Against Destructive Decisions
255 Main Street   508-481-3568
Marlborough, MA 01752   877-723-3462
Fax: 508-481-5759
e-mail: info@sadd.org
www.sadd.org
Offers materials to improve students' knowledge of and attitudes toward alcohol and other drugs and to help them plan their behavior so they can reduce the chances of becoming involved in drunk driving situations.
Penelope Wells, President and Executive Director
Stephen Wallace, Chairman and Chief Executive Officer

8232 Substance Abuse and Mental Health Services Administration
P O Box 2345   877-726-4727
Rockville, MD 20847-0001   877-696-6775
TTY: 800-487-4889
www.samhsa.gov
The goal of this organization is to reduce incidence and prevalence of mental disorders and substance abuse and improve treatment outcomes for persons suffering from addictive and mental health problems and disorders.

8233 Workplace Program CSAP Division of Communication Programs
CSAP Division of Communication Programs
5600 Fishers Lane   301-443-9936
Rockville, MD 20857-0001
This program sets standards for drug testing in workplace settings.

State Agencies & Associations

Alabama

8234 Division of Mental Illness and Substance Abuse Community Programs
Department of Mental Health
100 N Union Street   334-242-3456
Montgomery, AL 36130-1410   800-832-0952
Fax: 334-242-0759
e-mail: DMHMR@MH.Alabama.GOV
www.mh.alabama.gov
Kent Hunt, Associate Commissioner Substance Abuse
Susan P Chambers, Associate Commissioner Mental Illness

Alaska

8235 Office of Alcohol and Substance Abuse Department of Health and Social Services
Department of Health and Social Services
PO Box 110620   907-465-3370
Juneau, AK 99811   800-465-4828
Fax: 907-465-2668
e-mail: Stacy.Toner@Alaska.gov
www.hss.state.ak.us
Stacy Toner, Deputy Director
Cheryl Lowenstein, Administrative Operations Manager II

Arizona

8236 Alcoholism and Drug Abuse: Office of Community Behavioral Health
Department of Health Services
150 N 18th Avenue   602-364-4558
Phoenix, AZ 85007-3228   Fax: 602-364-4570
e-mail: cancerlr@azdhs.gov
www.azdhs.gov
January Contreras, Acting Director

Arkansas

8237 Office of Alcohol and Drug Abuse Prevention
4313 West Markham   501-686-9866
Little Rock, AR 72205   Fax: 501-686-9035
e-mail: linda.baker@arkansas.gov
www.state.ar.us

California

8238 California Women's Commission on Alcohol and Drug Dependencies
14622 Victory Boulevard   818-376-0470
Van Nuys, CA 91411
Dedicated to improving the quality and increasing the quantity of services to women with alcohol-related problems.

8239 Department of Alcohol and Drug Programs
1700 K Street   916-445-0834
Sacramento, CA 95811-4037   800-879-2772
Fax: 916-323-1270
e-mail: resourcecenter@adp.state.ca.us
www.adp.state.ca.us
Kathryn P Jett, Director

Colorado

8240 Alcohol and Drug Abuse Division Department of Human Services
Department of Human Services
4055 S Lowell Boulevard   303-866-7480
Denver, CO 80236-3120   Fax: 303-866-7481
e-mail: jaqueline.enriques@state.co.us
www.cdhs.state.co.us
Janet Wood, Director
Mary McCann, Acting Manager

Connecticut

8241 Connecticut Alcohol and Drug Abuse Commission
410 Capitol Avenue   860-418-7000
Hartford, CT 06134   800-446-7348
Fax: 860-418-6780
TTY: 860-418-6707
e-mail: ronna.keil@pa.state.ct.us
www.dmhas.state.ct.us
Thomas A Kirk Jr, Commissioner
Pat Rehmer, Deputy Commissioner

Delaware

8242 Delaware Division of Alcoholism, Drug Abuse and Mental Health
Alcohol And Drug Services

1901 North DuPont Highway
New Castle, DE 19720

303-255-9399
Fax: 302-255-4428
e-mail: DHSSInfor@state.de.us
www.dhss.delaware.gov

Renata J. Henry, Director

District of Columbia

8243   Health Planning and Development
825 N Capitol Street NE
Washington, DC 20002

202-422-5875
Fax: 202-442-4827
www.dchealth.dc.gov

Florida

8244   Alcohol and Drug Abuse Program Department Of Children And Families
Department Of Children And Families
1317 Winewood Boulevard
Tallahassee, FL 32399-6570

850-487-2920
Fax: 850-414-7474
www.dcf.state.fl.us/mentalhealth/sa

Cynthea Panzarino, Director

Georgia

8245   Alcohol and Drug Services Addictive Diseases Program
Addictive Diseases Program
Two Peachtree Street NW
Atlanta, GA 30303-3171

404-657-2331
Fax: 404-657-2160
www.mhddad.dhr.georgia.gov

Hawaii

8246   Alcohol and Drug Abuse Division Department of Health
Department of Health
601 Kamokila Boulevard
Kapoleiu, HI 96707

808-692-7506
Fax: 808-692-7521
e-mail: ATRINFO@doh.hawaii.gov
www.hawaii.gov/health

Chiyome Fukino, Director
Bernie Strand, Program Director

Idaho

8247   Department of Health and Welfare Department Of Health And Welfare
Department Of Health And Welfare
1720 Westgate Drive
Boise, ID 83704-0036

208-334-6747
800-926-2588
Fax: 208-334-6738
e-mail: rossil@dhw.idaho.gov
www.healthandwelfare.idaho.gov

Landis Rossi, Regional Director
Richard Armstrong, Director

Illinois

8248   Department of Alcoholism and Substance Abuse
Department Of Human Services
100 W Randolph Street
Chicago, IL 60601

312-814-3840
800-843-6154
Fax: 312-814-2419
TTY: 800-447-6404
e-mail: dhsas16@dhs.state.il.us
www.dhs.state.il.us

Theodora Binion-Tayl, Director

8249   Illinois Church Action on Alcohol Problems
1132 W Jefferson Street
Springfields, IL 62702

217-546-6871
Fax: 217-546-2814
e-mail: mail@ilcaaap.org
www.ilcaaap.org

An interdenominational Christian agency representing church groups in Illinois. Works to prevent alcohol and other drug-related problems through education legislative action and public awareness.

8250   Parkside Medical Services Corporation
205 W Touhy Avenue
Park Ridge, IL 60068-4256

847-698-9866
800-727-5723

This establishment offers treatment and hope for the alcoholic/substance abuser. A resource center that provides information books and resources pertaining to substance abuse and offers treatment facilities in various states across the country.

Indiana

8251   Division of Addiction Services Department of Mental Health
Department of Mental Health
402 W Washington Street
Indianapolis, IN 46204-3614

317-232-7800
800-662-4357
Fax: 317-233-3472
www.in.gov/fssa

Gina Eckart, Director
Alma Burrus, Operations Manager

Iowa

8252   Department of Public Health: Division of Substance Abuse and Health
Lucas State Office Building
321 E 12th Street
Des Moines, IA 50319-0075

515-281-7689
866-227-9878
Fax: 515-281-4535
e-mail: jzwick@idphstate.ia.us
www.idph.state.ia.us

Kathy Stone, Director

Kansas

8253   Alcohol and Drug Abuse Services
915 Harrison Street
Topeka, KS 66612

785-296-3959
800-586-3690
Fax: 785-296-7275
TTY: 785-296-1491
e-mail: dxmd@srskansas.org
www.srskansas.org

Don Jordan, Secretary
Laura Howard, Deputy Secretary and CFO

Kentucky

8254   Division of Substance Abuse: Department of Mental Health
Department For MH/MR Services
100 Fair Oaks Lane
Frankfort, KY 40621

502-564-2880
Fax: 502-564-7152
TTY: 502-564-5777
www.mhmr.ky.gov

Louisiana

8255   Office of Human Services: Division of Alcohol and Drug Abuse
628 N 4th Street
Baton Rouge, LA 70821-2790

225-342-6717
877-664-2248
Fax: 225-342-3875
e-mail: jbordeln@dhh.la.gov
www.dhh.louisiana.gov

Maine

8256   Office of Alcohol and Drug Abuse Prevention
Ofice Of Substance Abuse
AMHI Complex, Marquardt Building
Augusta, ME 04333-0159

207-289-2595
Fax: 207-287-4334
e-mail: osa.ircosa@state.me.us
www.maine.gove

Kimberly A. Johnson, Director

Maryland

8257   Maryland State Alcohol and Drug Abuse Administration
55 Wade Avenue
Catonsville, MD 21228

410-402-8600
Fax: 410-402-8601
e-mail: adaainfo@dhmh.state.md.us
www.maryland-adaa.org

Kathleen Rebbert-Fra, Acting Director
Steve Bocian, Acting Deputy Director

Massachusetts

8258 Division of Substance Abuse
250 Washington Street
Boston, MA 02108-4619

617-624-5111
800-327-5050
Fax: 617-624-5185
TTY: 617-536-5872
e-mail: bsas.questions@state.ma.us
www.mass.gov

Michael Botticelli, Director

Michigan

8259 Office of Substance Abuse Services Department of Public Health
Department of Public Health
320 S Walnut Street
Lansing, MI 48913

517-373-4700
888-736-0253
Fax: 517-335-2121
TTY: 517-373-3573
www.michigan.gov

Yvonne Blackmond, Director

Minnesota

8260 Chemical Dependency Program Division Department of Human Services
Department of Human Services
444 Lafayette Road
Saint Paul, MN 55155-3899

651-431-2460
800-627-3529
Fax: 651-582-1865
e-mail: DHS.ADAD@state.mn.us
www.dhs.state.mn.us

8261 Dentists Concerned for Dentists
450 N Syndicate
Saint Paul, MN 55104

651-641-0730
www.medhelp.org/amshc/amshc53.htm
A nonprofit organization for chemically dependent Minnesota dentists and concerned others.

Mississippi

8262 Division of Alcohol & Drug Abuse: Mississippi
Department of Mental Health
Robert E Lee State Office Building
Jackson, MS 39201

601-359-1288
Fax: 601-359-6295
www.dmh.state.ms.us

8263 Division of Alcohol & Drug Abuse: South Department of Mental Health
1101 Robert E Lee Building
Jackson, MS 39201

601-359-1288
Fax: 601-359-6295
TTY: 601-359-6230
www.dmh.state.ms.us

Edwin C LeGrand III, Executive Director

Missouri

8264 Missouri Division of Alcohol and Drug Abuse
Department of Mental Health
1706 E Elm Street
Jefferson City, MO 65102

573-751-4122
800-364-9687
Fax: 573-751-8224
TTY: 573-526-1201
e-mail: dmhmail@dmh.mo.gov
www.dmh.missouri.gov

Mark G Stringer, Director
Heidi DiBiaso, Administrative Assistant

Montana

8265 Department of Institutions, Alcohol and Drug Abuse Division
PO Box 202905nue
Helena, MT 59620-2905

406-444-3964
Fax: 406-444-9389
e-mail: jcassidy@mt. gov
www.dphhs.st.mt.us

Nebraska

8266 Department of Public Instruction: Division of Alcoholism and Drug Abuse
Division Of Behavioral Health
PO Box 98925
Lincoln, NE 68509-8925

402-471-7818
800-648-4444
Fax: 402-479-5162
e-mail: richard.deliberty@hhss.ne.gov
www.hhs.state.ne.us

Scot Adams, Director
GibsonBlaine Shaffer, CEO

Nevada

8267 Alcohol and Drug Abuse Bureau: Department of Human Resources
4126 Technology Way
Carson City, NV 89706

775-684-4190
Fax: 775-684-4185
e-mail: mcanfiel@nvhd.state.nv.us
www.mhds.nv.gov

Maria Canfield, Chief

New Hampshire

8268 Office of Alcohol and Drug Abuse Prevention
State Office Park South
105 Pleasant Street
Concord, NH 03301-3852

800-804-0909
Fax: 603-271-6105
e-mail: rosemary.shannon@dhhs.sate.nh.us
www.dhhs.state.nh.us

8269 Office of Alcohol and Drug Abuse Programs State Office Park South
105 Pleasant Street
Concord, NH 03301

603-271-6100
Fax: 603-271-6105
TTY: 800-735-2964
e-mail: rosemary.shannon@dhhs.sate.nh.us
www.dhhs.state.nh.us

New Jersey

8270 Department of Health
120 S Stockton Street
Trenton, NJ 08625-0362

609-292-7837
800-367-6543
Fax: 609-292-3816
e-mail: georgene.rhodunda@dhs.state.nj.us
www.state.nj.us

Heather Howard, Commissioner
Mary E O'Dowd, Chief of Staff

8271 Division of Narcotic and Drug Abuse Control
120 S Stockton Street
Trenton, NJ 08625-0362

609-292-5760
800-238-2333
Fax: 609-292-3816
www.state.nj.us/humanservices

Jeffers, Director

New Mexico

8272 Substance Abuse Bureau
1190 Saint Francis Drive
Santa Fe, NM 87502

505-827-2601
800-362-2013
Fax: 505-827-0097
www.nmcares.org

New York

8273 Division of Substance Abuse Services Substance Abuse Services
Substance Abuse Services
1450 Western Avenue
Albany, NY 12203-3526

518-473-3460
Fax: 518-457-5474
e-mail: communications@oasas.state.ny.us
www.oasas.state.ny.us

Karen M Carpenter-Palumbo, Commissioner
Kathleen Caggiano-Si, Executive Deputy Commissioner

North Carolina

8274 Alcohol and Drug Abuse Section Division of Mental Health & Mental Retar
Division of Mental Health & Mental Retardation
3001 Mail Service Center   919-733-7011
Raleigh, NC 27699-3007   800-662-7030
                                            Fax: 919-508-0951
                                            www.dhhs.state.nc.us

Leza Wainwright, Director
Michael S Lancaster, Director

North Dakota

8275 Division of Alcoholism & Drug Abuse: Department of Human Services
Department Of Human Services
1237 W Divide Avenue   701-328-8920
Bismarck, ND 58501   800-755-2719
                                            Fax: 701-328-8969
                                            e-mail: dhsmhsas@state.nd.us
                                            www.state.nd.us

Ohio

8276 Bureau on Alcohol Abuse and Recovery Ohio Department of Health
Ohio Department of Health
280 N Hight Street   614-466-3445
Columbus, OH 43215-2550   Fax: 614-752-8645
                                            e-mail: INFO@ada.ohio.gov
                                            www.odadas.state.oh.us

Angela Corne Dawson, Director
Jewel Neely, Deputy Director

8277 Bureau on Drug Abuse: Ohio Department of Health
Ohio Department of Health
280 N High Street   614-466-3445
Columbus, OH 43215   Fax: 614-752-8645
                                            e-mail: INFO@ada.ohio.gov
                                            www.odadas.state.oh.us

Angela Corne Dawson, Director
Jewel Neely, Deputy Director

Oklahoma

8278 Oklahoma Department of Mental Health and Substance Abuse Services
Substance Abuse Program
1200 NE 13th Street   405-522-3908
Oklahoma City, OK 73152-3277   800-522-9054
                                            Fax: 405-522-3650
                                            TTY: 405-522-3851
                                            e-mail: jglover@odmhsas.org
                                            www.odmhsas.org

Terri White, Commissioner

Oregon

8279 Office of Alcohol and Drug Abuse Programs
500 Summer Street NE   503-945-5763
Salem, OR 97301-1118   Fax: 503-378-8467
                                            TTY: 800-375-2863
                                            e-mail: omhas.web@state.or.us
                                            www.oregon.gov

Pennsylvania

8280 Drug and Alcohol Programs Department Of Health
Department Of Health
02 Kline Plaza   717-783-8200
Harrisburg, PA 17104-0090   877-724-3258
                                            Fax: 717-787-6285
                                            e-mail: rkauffman@state.pa.us
                                            www.dsf.health.state.pa.us

Rhode Island

8281 Division of Substance Abuse: Department of Mental Health and Hospitals
Department Of Mental Health And Retardation
14 Harrington Road   401-462-4680
Cranston, RI 02920-0944   800-622-7422
                                            Fax: 401-462-6078
                                            www.mhrh.state.ri.us

Craig S Stenning, Executive Director

South Carolina

8282 South Carolina Commission on Alcohol and Drug Abuse
Department Of Alcohol And Drug Abuse Services
101 Executive Center Drive   803-896-5555
Columbia, SC 29210-9498   Fax: 803-896-5557
                                            www.daodas.org

W Lee Catoe, Director
Lillian Roberson, Manager of Operation Division

South Dakota

8283 Division of Alcohol & Drug Abuse: South Dakota
Department Of Human Services
3800 E Highway 34   605-773-5990
Pierre, SD 57501-5070   800-265-9684
                                            Fax: 605-773-5483
                                            TTY: 605-773-6412
                                            e-mail: infodhs@state.sd.us
                                            www.dhs.sd.gov

Gilbert Sudbeck, Director

Tennessee

8284 Department of Mental Health and Mental Retardation, Alcohol & Drug Service
Bureau Of Alcohol And Drug Abuse Services
425 Fifth Avenue N   615-532-6500
Nashville, TN 37243-4401   800-560-5767
                                            Fax: 615-532-2419
                                            e-mail: oca.mhdd@tn.gov
                                            www.state.tn.us

Virginia Tro Betts, Commissioner

Texas

8285 Texas Commission on Alcohol and Drug Abuse Department Of State Health
Department Of State Health
PO Box 149347   512-206-5000
Austin, TX 78714   866-378-8440
                                            Fax: 512-458-7477
                                            TTY: 800-735-2989
                                            e-mail: contact@dshs.state.tx.us
                                            www.tcada.state.tx.us

Utah

8286 Department of Social Services: Division of Substance Abuse
Department Of Human Services
120 N 200 W Street   801-538-3939
Salt Lake City, UT 84103   Fax: 801-538-9892
                                            e-mail: dsamhwebmaster@utah.gov
                                            www.hsdsa.utah.gov

Paula Bell, Chairperson
Darryl Wagner, Vice Chairman

Vermont

8287 Alcohol and Drug Abuse Programs of Vermont Department Of Health
Department Of Health
108 Cherry Street   802-651-1550
Burlington, VT 05402-1531   Fax: 802-651-1573
                                            e-mail: vtadap@vdh.state.vt.us
                                            www.healthvermont.gov

Virginia

8288 Substance Abuse Services Office of Virginia
Department of Mental Health & Mental Retardation
PO Box 1797　　　　　　　　　　　804-786-3921
Richmond, VA 23218-1797　　　　　800-451-5544
　　　　　　　　　　　　　　Fax: 804-371-6638
　　　　　　　　　　　　　　TTY: 804-371-8977
　　　e-mail: wglover@co.dmhmrsas.virginia.gov
　　　　　　　　　　www.dmhmrsas.virginia.gov

James Reinhard, Commissioner
Heidi Dix, Deputy Commissioner

Washington

8289 Washington Department of Social and Health Services, Alcohol and Drug Prog.
Department Of Social And Health Services
PO Box 45130　　　　　　　　　　877-301-4557
Olympia, WA 98504-5330　　　　　800-562-1240
　　　　　　　　　　　　　　Fax: 360-438-8078
　　　　　　　　　　　　　　TTY: 877-301-4557
　　　　　e-mail: starkkd@dshs.wa.gov
　　　　　　　　　　www1.dshs.wa.gov

West Virginia

8290 West Virginia Division of Alcohol & Drug Abuse
Department Of Health And Human Resources
350 Capitol Street　　　　　　　　304-558-2276
Charleston, WV 25301-3702　　　Fax: 304-558-1008
　　　　　　　　　　　e-mail: obhs@wvdhhr.org
　　　　　　　　　　　　　　www.wvdhhr.org

Eugenie Taylor, Acting Commissioner

Wisconsin

8291 Office of Alcohol and Other Drug Abuse
1 W Wilson Street　　　　　　　　608-266-1865
Madison, WI 53703-7851　　　　Fax: 608-266-1533
　　　　　　　　　　　　　　TTY: 608-267-7371
　　　e-mail: DHSwebmaster@wisconsin.gov
　　　　　　　　　　www.dhfs.state.wi.us

John Easterday, Administrator
Susan Gadacz, Contact

Wyoming

8292 Alcohol & Drug Abuse Programs of Wyoming Department Of Health
Department Of Health
6101 Yellowestone Road　　　　　307-777-6494
Cheyenne, WY 82002-0480　　　　800-535-4006
　　　　　　　　　　　　　　Fax: 307-777-5849
　　　　　　　　　　e-mail: aburde@state.wy.us
　　　　　　　　　　　　　　wdh.state.wy.us

Korin Schmidt, Administrator
Rodger McDaniel, Deputy Director

Libraries & Resource Centers

8293 National Clearinghouse for Alcohol and Drug Information
PO Box 2345　　　　　　　　　　240-221-4019
Rockville, MD 20847-2345　　　　800-729-6686
　　　　　　　　　　　　　　Fax: 240-221-4292
　　　　　　　　　　　　　　TDD: 800-487-4889
　　　　　　　　　　　e-mail: info@health.org
　　　　　　　　　　www.ncadi.samhsa.gov
A resource for alcohol and other drug information. It carries a wide variety of publications dealing with alcohol and other drug abuse.
John Noble, Director

8294 Parents Resource Institute for Drug Education
160 Vanderbilt Court
Bowling Green, KY 42103　　　　800-279-6361
　　　　　　　　　　　　　　Fax: 270-746-9598
　　　e-mail: janie.pitcock@pridesurveys.com
　　　　　　　　　　www.pridesurveys.com

Offers national information and educational materials pertaining to alcohol and drug dependency.
Thomas J Gleaton, EdD, President
Janie Pitcock, Director Operations

Research Centers

8295 Alcohol Disease Foundation
33 Eglantine Avenue　　　　　　609-737-0088
Pennington, NJ 08534-2308
Founded in 1988 to promote research on testing systems that could diagnose the metabolic aspects of alcoholism. Seeks to educate the public on the validity of the disease concept of alcoholism.

8296 Alcohol Research Group Public Health Institute
Public Health Institute
6475 Christie Avenue　　　　　　510-597-3440
Emeryville, CA 94608-1324　　　Fax: 510-985-6459
　　　　　　　　　　　　e-mail: info@arg.org
　　　　　　　　　　　　　　www.arg.org
One of ten national research centers funded by the National Institute on Alcohol Abuse and Alcoholism. Its alcoholism library carries 5 500 books 130 journals 150 newsletters and 60 000 other materials.
Dominique La MPH, Executive Director
Debbie Gill, Manager Administrative Services

8297 Boston University Laboratory of Neuropsychology
Dept of Behavioral Neuroscience
80 E Concord Street M9　　　　　617-638-4803
Boston, MA 02118　　　　　　　Fax: 617-638-4806
　　　　　　　　　　　　　　www.bu.edu
Offers research and studies into the effects of Alcoholism pertaining to aphasia apraxia dementia memory disorders and various other neurological malfunctions.
Marlene Osca Berman PhD, Director

8298 Center for Alcohol & Addiction Studies Brown University
Brown University
Box G-S121-5　　　　　　　　　401-863-6600
Providence, RI 02912-0001　　　Fax: 401-863-6697
　　　　　　　　　　e-mail: CAAS@brown.edu
　　　　　　　　　　www.caas.brown.edu
The Center for Alcohol and Addiction Studies through its affiliation with the Brown Medical School occupies a unique position within the University. The Center brings together more that 90 faculty and professional staff members from 11 University departments and eight affiliated hospitals to promote the identification prevention and effective treatment of alcohol and other substance abuse.
Peter M Monti PhD, Center Director
Damaris Rohs PhD, Associate Director

8299 Cornerstone Medical Arts Center Hospital
Medical Arts Center Hospital
159-05 Union Turnpike　　　　　718-906-6700
Fresh Meadows, NY 11366-2802　　800-233-9999
　　　　　　　　　　　　　　Fax: 718-906-6840
　　　　　　　　　　www.cornerstoneny.com
Offers a complete integrated program for alcohol assessment alcohol and drug rehabilitation continuing care community education and comprehensive family recovery.

8300 Do it Now Foundation
PO Box 27658　　　　　　　　　480-736-0599
Tempe, AZ 85285-7658　　　　　Fax: 480-736-0599
　　　　　　　　　　e-mail: info@dci-dcitnaw.com
　　　　　　　　　　　　www.doitnow.org
An information clearinghouse for service providers that publishes well-written pamphlets booklets and materials on chemical dependency and recovery.

8301 Dorothea Dix Hospital Clinical Research Unit
809 Ruggles Drive　　　　　　　919-733-5227
Raleigh, NC 27603　　　　　　　866-349-5627
　　　　　　　　　　　　　　Fax: 919-733-5351
　　　　　　　　　　　　www.med.unc.edu

Researches the biological risk factors of alcoholism using young adults without the disease but with history of familial alcoholism.
Terry Spell, Director

8302 **Ernest Gallo Clinic and Research Center**
5858 Horton Street
Emeryville, CA 94608
510-985-3100
Fax: 510-985-3101
e-mail: ngreen@gallo.ucsf.edu
www.galloresearch.org
Alcoholism studies with a special emphasis on genetics.
Raymond L White PhD, Director
William R Sawyers JD, Chief Administrative Officer

8303 **Families in Action National Drug Abuse Center**
National Drug Abuse Center
PO Box 3553
Wilson, NC 27895
252-237-1242
Fax: 252-237-6544
e-mail: wfapmooring@simflex.com
www.familiesinaction.org
Publish prevention materials and serves as an information clearinghouse for families with a member suffering from a drug or alcohol addiction.
Phillip A Mooring, Executive Director
Elizabeth Bunn, Coordinator

8304 **Friends Medical Science Research Center**
11075 Santa Monica Boulevard
Los Angeles, CA 90025
310-479-9330
Fax: 310-477-9601
Studies narcotic addictions.
Meta P Barton, President

8305 **Hahnemann University Laboratory of Human Pharmacology**
Department of Pharmacology
Broad and Vine
Philadelphia, PA 19102
215-854-8100
Fax: 215-762-8109
www.hahnemannhospital.com
Benjamin Cal MD, Director

8306 **Harvard Cocaine Recovery Project**
1493 Cambridge Street
Cambridge, MA 02139-1099
617-498-1000
Fax: 617-642-58
Six-year study of relapse and recovery in cocaine addicts.
William McAu MD, Principal Investigator

8307 **Interdisciplinary Program in Cell and Molecular Pharmacology**
Medical University of South Carolina
173 Ashley Avenue BSB 358
Charleston, SC 29425
843-792-2471
Fax: 843-792-2475
www.musc.edu/pharm
Research into pharmacology and toxicology.
Kenneth D Tew, Professor and Chairman
Belinda Andersen, Administrative Coordinator

8308 **Johns Hopkins University: Behavioral Pharmacology Research Unit**
John Hopkins Bay View Campus
5510 Nathan Shock Drive
Baltimore, MD 21224-2735
410-550-1686
Fax: 410-550-0030
e-mail: bigelow@jhmi.edu
www.hopkinsmedicine.org
An internationally recognized center of excellence in research on psychoactive drugs. As the name implies BPRU's orientation is behavioral and pharmacological emphasizing a behavioral analysis of drug action.
George E Bigelow PhD, Scientific Director
Eric C Strain MD, Medical Director

8309 **Kettering-Scott Magnetic Resonance Laboratory**
Wright State University, School of Medicine
PO Box 927
Dayton, OH 45401-0927
937-296-7839
www.med.wright.edu
No information found on the website.
Joseph Manti MD, Director

8310 **Marin Institute**
24 Belvedere Street
San Rafael, CA 94901-4817
415-456-5692
Fax: 415-456-0491
www.marinInstitute.org
The mission of this Institute is to reduce the toll of alcohol and other drug problems on Marin County and society in general. The

Institute fulfills this mission by developing implementing evaluating and disseminating innovative approaches to prevention locally nationally and internationally.
Bruce Lee Livingston MPP, Executive Director
Michele Simo JD MPH, Research & Policy Director

8311 **Narcotic and Drug Research**
11 Beach Street
New York, NY 10013-2429
212-966-8700
Fax: 212-334-8058
Nonprofit organization that is devoted to drug abuse education treatment and prevention.
Douglas S Lipton PhD, Director

8312 **National Center on Addiction and Substance Abuse**
Columbia University
633 3rd Avenue
New York, NY 10017-6706
212-841-5200
800-622-4357
Fax: 212-956-8020
www.casacolumbia.org
The only nation-wide organization that brings together under one roof all the professional disciplines needed to study and combat abuse of all substances - alcohol nicotine as well as illegal prescription and performance enhancing drugs - in all sectors of society.
Susan Brown, Vice President
Joseph A Califano Jr, Chairman and President

8313 **National Prevention Resource Center CSAP Division of Communications Programs**
CSAP Division of Communications Programs
5600 Fishers Lane
Rockville, MD 20857-0001
301-443-9936
Supports an array of prevention program evaluation approaches including individual grantee evaluations program evaluations and a National Evaluation Project. Also offers a National Data Base to provide information on programs for prevention of substance abuse.

8314 **National Treatment Consortium for Alcohol and Other Drugs**
PO Box 1294
Washington, DC 20013
202-434-4780
www.ntc-usa.org

8315 **National Volunteer Training Center for Substance Abuse Prevention**
CSAP Division of Communications Programs
5600 Fishers Lane
Rockville, MD 20857
301-443-9936
Volunteers are always on hand to provide answers, information, referrals and resources pertaining to alcohol, drugs and substance abuse.

8316 **National Volunteer Training Center for Sub CSAP Division of Communications Programs**
5600 Fishers Lane
Rockville, MD 20857
301-443-9936
Volunteers are always on hand to provide answers information referrals and resources pertaining to alcohol drugs and substance abuse.

8317 **Ohio State University Clinical Pharmacology Division**
College of Medicine
333 Western 9th Avenue
Columbus, OH 43210-1239
614-292-8600
800-252-3636
Fax: 614-292-4293
www.medicine.osu.edu
Substance abuse and alcohol related research.

Glen Apsloss, Director

8318 **Ohio State University Clinical Pharmacolog College of Medicine**
333 Western 9th Avenue
Columbus, OH 43210
614-292-6908
800-252-3636
Fax: 614-292-4293
www.medicine.osu.edu
Substance abuse and alcohol related research.

Glen Apsloss, Director

8319 **RADAR Network National Clearinghouse for Alcohol & Dru**
National Clearinghouse for Alcohol & Drug Info

PO Box 2345
Rockville, MD 20847-2345

301-468-2600
877-SAM-HSA7
Fax: 240-221-4292
TTY: 800-487-4889
ncadi.samhsa.gov

Consists of state clearinghouses specialized information centers of national organizations and the Department of Education Regional Training Centers. Each RADAR member can offer the public a variety of information services.
John Noble, Director

8320 Research Institute on Alcoholism State University of New York at Buffalo
State University of New York at Buffalo
1021 Main Street
Buffalo, NY 14203

716-887-2566
Fax: 716-872-52
e-mail: connors@ria.buffalo.edu
www.ria.buffalo.edu

Integral part of the New York State Division of Alcoholism and Alcohol Abuse.
Gerard Conno MD, Director
Kimberly S Walitzer, Deputy Director

8321 Rockefeller University Laboratory of Biology
1230 York Avenue
New York, NY 10021

212-327-7458
Fax: 212-277-54
www.rockefeller.edu

Vincent P Doyle, Head

8322 Rutgers University Center of Alcohol Studies
Busch Campus
607 Allison Road
Piscataway, NJ 08854

732-445-2190
Fax: 732-445-5300
e-mail: alclib@rci.rutgers.edu
alcoholstudies.rutgers.edu

Causes and treatment of alcoholism.
Robert Pandi PhD, Director
Marsha E Bates PhD, Research Professor I of Psychology

8323 Rutgers University: Controlled Drug- Delivery Research Center
College of Pharmacy
PO Box 789
Piscataway, NJ 08855-0789

732-932-3834
Fax: 732-932-5767

Yie W Chien, Director

8324 Ruth E Golding Clinical Pharmacokinetics Laboratory
College of Pharmacy
1703 E Mabel
Tucson, AZ 85721-1427 e-mail: webmaster@pharmacy.arizona.edu

520-626-1938
www.pharmacy.arizona.edu

Conducts studies of drugs in humans and animals.
Michael Maye MD, Head

8325 Southern California Research Institute
7065 Hayvenhurst Avenue
Van Nuys, CA 91406

310-390-8481
Fax: 310-390-8482
www.scri.org

Effects of alcohol and drugs on behavior studies.
Dary Fiorent PhD, Executive Director
Bergetta Die BA, Research Associate

8326 Stanford Center for Research in Disease Prevention
Stanford University School of Medicine
1070 Arastradero Road
Palo Alto, CA 94304

650-725-6906
Fax: 650-723-6254
prevention.stanford.edu

Prevention and control of alcohol and drug abuse related disorders.
John W Farquhar MD, Director

8327 State University of New York at Buffalo Toxicology Research Center
3435 Main Street
Buffalo, NY 14214

716-831-2125
Fax: 716-829-2806
www.smbs.buffalo.edu

Toxicology-related research and services including the development of tests to evaluate toxins chemicals and drugs.
Paul Kostyni PhD, Director
Dr James R Olson, Assistant Director

8328 University of California: Los Angeles Alcohol Research Center
760 Westwood Plaza
Los Angeles, CA 90095-8353

310-825-1891
Fax: 310-206-7309
www.ucla.edu

Causes of alcoholism including genetics.
Dr Ernest Noble, Director

8329 University of Michigan: Alcohol Research Center
400 E Eisenhower Parkway
Ann Arbor, MI 48108-3318

734-763-7952
Fax: 734-998-7994
www.umich.edu

Alcohol abuse studies among the elderly including the relationship between alcohol and aged disorders.
Robert A Zucker PhD, Contact

8330 University of Michigan: Psychiatric Center
1500 E Medical Center Drive
Ann Arbor, MI 48109-0001

734-936-4960
Fax: 734-936-9761
www.umich.edu

Psychiatric disease research pertaining to the effects of alcoholism and drug abuse.
John F Greden, Chairman

8331 University of Minnesota: Program on Alcohol/Drug Control
Stadium Gate 27
Minneapolis, MN 55455

612-624-6861

Alcohol tobacco and drug research.
Dr James Schaefer, Director

8332 University of Missouri: Kansas City Drug Information Service
2464 Charlotte
Kansas City, MO 64108-2640

816-235-5490
Fax: 816-235-5491
dic.umkc.edu

Literature research and evaluation of clinical drug problems and questions.
Pat Bryant PhD, Director
Heather A Pace PhD, Assistant Director

8333 University of Tennessee Drug Information Center
875 Monroe Avenue
Memphis, TN 38163-1

901-528-5555
Fax: 901-448-5419
e-mail: utdic@utmem.edu
dop.utmem.edu/dic

Katie Suda, Director
Camille Thornton, Assistant Professor

8334 University of Texas Health Science Center Neurophysiology Research Center
Speech & Hearing Institute
1343 Moursund Street
Houston, TX 77030-3405

713-792-4542
Fax: 713-792-4513

Conducts clinical and animal studies aimed at combating alcohol drug and tobacco dependence.
Malcolm Skol PhD, Director

8335 University of Texas at Austin: Drug Synamics Institute
1 University Station
Austin, TX 78712

512-475-9746
Fax: 512-471-2746
www.utexas.edu

Pharmaceutical and drug research.
Janet C Walkow PhD, Director
Carla Van Den Berg PhD, Associate Professor

8336 University of Utah: Center for Human Toxicology
417 Wakara Way
Salt Lake City, UT 84112-1210

801-581-5117
Fax: 801-581-5034
e-mail: dwilkins@alanine.pharm.utah.edu
www.pharmacy.utah.edu

Clinical forensic and toxicology research.
Douglas Roll MD, Associate Director
Dennis Crouch, Director

8337 University of Wisconsin Milwaukee Medicinal Chemistry Group
University of Wisconsin
PO Box 413
Milwaukee, WI 53201-413

414-229-1122
www4.uwm.edu

Research on drugs including studies of valium receptors.
Carlos Santiago, Chancellor

Support Groups & Hotlines

8338 Al-Anon Alateen Family Group Hotline
1600 Corporate Landing Parkway
Virginia Beach, VA 10018-970

757-563-1600
888-425-2666
Fax: 757-563-1655
e-mail: wso@alanon.org
www.al-anon.alateen.org

A mutual peer-to-peer support program with groups meeting worldwide to provide hope and help to the families of alcoholics. Although a seperate entity from Alcoholics Anonymous, our program is based upon the Twelve Steps.
Ric Buchanan, Executive Director

8339 Alcohol Drug Treatment Referral
1316 South Coast Highway
Laguna Beach, CA 92651-3118

800-454-8966
Fax: 949-281-1933

National Help and Referral Network, a nonprofit organization available 24 hours a day to assist people troubled by drug or alcohol abuse. Here to provide information on addiction treatment and support services and to help save lives and mend broken dreams.
Mike Cohan, Director

8340 Alcoholics Anonymous World Services
PO Box 459
New York, NY 10163-4059

212-870-3400
Fax: 212-870-3003
www.aa.org

Alcoholics Anonymous is a fellowship of men and women who share their experience, strength and hope with each other that they may solve their common problem and help others to recover from alcoholism. The only requirement for membership is a desire to stop drinking. There are no dues or fees for AA membership; they are self-supporting through their own contributions.
Greg M, General Manager

8341 Drug Free Workplace Hotline
Division of Workplace Programs
Samhsa Diagonal CSAP 1 Choke Cherry
Rockville, MD 20857

240-276-2612
800-967-5752
Fax: 240-276-1210
www.drugfreeworkplace.gov

A hotline for businesses to obtain information on a wide range of drug abuse related problems, issues and services.
Robert Stephenson II, Director

8342 Friday Night Live
California Dept of Drug & Alcohol Programs
1700 K Street
Sacramento, CA 95814

916-445-7456
Fax: 916-230-59
e-mail: laura@tcoe.org
www.communitycounseling.org/fnl

These groups, located in California, are all run by students with a faculty adviser. They arrange local alcohol and drug free events, from dances and movies to visiting hospitalized children. Students not only have fun but they learn to have fun sober.
Jim Kooler, Administrator
Laura Purcellabuzo, Project Coordinator

8343 Images Within: A Child's View of Parental Alcoholism
Children of Alcoholics Foundation
PO Box 4185
New York, NY 10163-4185

212-595-5810
800-359-2623
e-mail: coaf@phoenixhouse.org
www.coaf.org

An innovative program designed to teach all children about family alcoholism. Middle-school-aged children learn how to get help for themselves or give help to their friends.

8344 International Lawyers in Alcoholics Anonymous
39 Smith Neck Road
Old Lyme, CT 6371

860-529-7474
e-mail: bert@bertwitehead.com
www.ilaa.org

Provides 40 independent local groups.

8345 National Health Information Center
PO Box 1133
Washington, DC 20013

310-565-4167
800-336-4797
Fax: 301-984-4256
e-mail: info@nhic.org
www.health.gov/nhic

Offers a nationwide information referral service, produces directories and resource guides.

8346 ToughLove International
PO Box 1069
Doylestown, PA 18901-0019

215-348-7090
800-333-1069
www.toughlove.org

This national self-help group for parents, children and communities emphasizes cooperation, personal initiative and action. Publishes books, brochures and promotional information and holds workshops and seminars across the country.

8347 WFS' New Life Program
Women for Sobriety
PO Box 618
Quakertown, PA 18951-0618

215-536-8026
Fax: 215-538-9026
e-mail: newlife@nni.com
www.womenforsobriety.org

A self-help program for women that can be used independent from AA or with AA. Groups are in many states in the United States. Donations suggested.
Rebecca M Fenner, Director

Books

8348 AA Comes of Age
Alcoholics Anonymous
PO Box 459
New York, NY 10163-0459

212-870-3400
Fax: 212-870-3137

Tells how AA was started, how the Steps and Traditions evolved and how the AA Fellowship grew and spread overseas.

8349 AA in Prison: Inmate to Inmate
Alcoholics Anonymous
PO Box 459
New York, NY 10163-0459

212-870-3400
Fax: 212-870-3137

Thirty-two stories that share the experience of men and women who found AA while in prison.
128 pages

8350 Accepting Ourselves & Others
Hazelden
15251 Pleasant Valley Road
Center City, MN 55012-9640

651-257-4010
800-328-9000
Fax: 651-213-4426
www.hazelden.org

Fully revised and expanded second edition. Examines recovery as it affects the gay, lesbian, and bisexual community, as well as their friends, family, and therapists. Addresses the relationship between substance abuse and being a sexual minority, and discusses the impact of other issues such as anxiety, depression, sexual abuse, and learning disabilities.
379 pages Paperback
ISBN: 1-568381-20-4

8351 Addiction and Responsibility
The Crossroad Publishing Company
370 Lexington Avenue
New York, NY 10017-6503

212-532-3650
800-395-0690
Fax: 212-532-4922

Anyone who has wrestled with such basic questions about addiction such as: Is drug addiction a behavior disorder or a character flaw? Is it genetic or learned? What is it like to be addicted? will find welcome answers in this groundbreaking philosophical inquiry into the addictive mind. The author helps readers understand addiction.
192 pages
ISBN: 0-824513-65-7

8352 Addictions Counseling
The Crossroad Publishing Company

370 Lexington Avenue
New York, NY 10017-6503

212-532-3650
800-395-0690
Fax: 212-532-4922

A practical guide to counseling people with chemical and other addictions.
144 pages Paperback
ISBN: 0-824513-86-0

8353 Addictive Personality
Hazelden
15251 Pleasant Valley Road
Center City, MN 55012-9640

651-257-4010
800-328-9000
Fax: 651-213-4426
www.hazelden.org

Understanding how an individual becomes an addict through examination of addiction's causes, stages of development, and consequences. Second edition further refines these ideas and includes the most recent information on the addictive process, cultural influences on addictive behaviors, recovery, genetic factors in addiction, mental health issues, and new research findings.
130 pages Paperback
ISBN: 1-568381-29-8

8354 Addictive Thinking Understanding Self-Deception
Hazelden
15251 Pleasant Valley Road
Center City, MN 55012-9640

651-257-4010
800-328-9000
Fax: 651-213-4426
www.hazelden.org

Illustrates the irrational perspective and complicated, contradictory thinking patterns of addictive thinking, and demonstrates how they lead to low self-esteen, addiction, and relapse. Revised edition includes expanded information on depression and affective disorders, the relationship between addictive thinking and relapse, and the new research related to the origins of addictive thinking.
140 pages Paperback
ISBN: 1-568381-38-7

8355 Adult Children of Alcoholics
Hazelden
15251 Pleasant Valley Road
Center City, MN 55012-9640

651-257-4010
800-328-9000
Fax: 651-213-4426
www.hazelden.org

Written to and for adult children of dysfunctional families.
138 pages Paperback

8356 Al-Anon Family Groups
Al-Anon Family Group Headquarters
1600 Corporate Landing Parkway
Virginia Beach, VA 23454-5617

757-563-1600
800-425-2666
Fax: 757-563-1655
e-mail: wso@al-anon.org
www.al-anon.alateen.org

Basic book that explains the purpose of fellowship, how it works and how it is held in unity. Includes real life stories by husbands, wives, parents and children of those who suffer from alcoholism.
177 pages
ISBN: 0-910034-54-0
Caryn Johnson, Director Communications

8357 Al-Anon's Twelve Steps and Twelve Traditions
Al-Anon Family Group Headquarters
1600 Corporate Landing Parkway
Virginia Beach, VA 23454-5617

757-563-1600
800-425-2666
Fax: 757-563-1655
e-mail: wso@al-anon.org
www.al-anon.alateen.org

Written for people whose lives have been affected by alcoholism.
142 pages Hardcover
ISBN: 0-910034-24-9
Caryn Johnson, Director Communications

8358 Alateen: A Day at a Time
Al-Anon Family Group Headquarters
1600 Corporate Landing Parkway
Virginia Beach, VA 23454-5617

757-563-1600
800-425-2666
Fax: 757-563-1655
e-mail: wso@al-anon.org
www.al-anon.alateen.org

A collection of positive, daily sharings written by teenagers around the world.
384 pages
ISBN: 0-910034-53-2
Caryn Johnson, Director Communications

8359 Alateen: Hope for Children of Alcoholics
Al-Anon Family Group Headquarters
1600 Corporate Landing Parkway
Virginia Beach, VA 23454-5617

757-563-1600
800-425-2666
Fax: 757-563-1655
e-mail: wso@al-anon.org
www.al-anon.alateen.org

A gold mine of information written by Alateens themselves. It covers the history of Alateen, understanding alcoholism and personal stories.
115 pages
ISBN: 0-910034-20-6
Caryn Johnson, Director Communications

8360 Alcohol and Other Drug Services: Dir. of California's Community Services
Department of Alcohol and Drug Programs
1700 K Street
Sacramento, CA 95814-4022

916-445-0834

A directory listing agencies, alcohol and drug providers, county 504 coordinators and county program administrators for the state of California.
136 pages

8361 Alcohol, Drug and Other Addictions: A Directory of Treatment Centers
Oryx Press
4041 N Central Avenue
Phoenix, AZ 85012-3397

602-265-2651
800-279-4663

Lists 18,000 federal, state and local addiction treatment regimens that include public and private centers.

8362 Alcohol, Tobacco and Other Drugs May Harm the Unborn
National Clearinghouse for Alcohol and Drug Info.
PO Box 2345
Rockville, MD 20847-2345

800-729-6686

Presents the most recent findings of basic research and clinical studies conducted on the effects of alcohol, drugs and tobacco on the unborn.

8363 Alcoholics Anonymous
Alcoholics Anonymous
PO Box 459
New York, NY 10163-0459

212-870-3400
Fax: 212-870-3137

Third edition of the Big Book, basic text of AA. Chapters describe the AA recovery program and personal histories have been added.

8364 Alcoholics Anonymous: The Big Book
Hazelden
15251 Pleasant Valley Road
Center City, MN 55012-9640

651-257-4010
800-328-9000
Fax: 651-213-4426
www.hazelden.org

Classic text that guides Alcoholics Anonymous programs and describes how millions of men and women have recovered from alcoholism.
575 pages Paperback

8365 American Academy of Psychiatrists in Alcoholism and Addiction Directory
Box 376
Greenbelt, MD 20768

301-220-0951
Fax: 301-220-0941

Lists 900 member professionals who are concerned with drug and alcohol abuse.

8366 An Annotated Bibliography of Recent Empirical Research In Methadone
National Clearinghouse for Alcohol and Drug Info.
PO Box 2345
Rockville, MD 20847-2345

800-729-6686

Provides guidelines and suggestions to investigators engaged in the demanding and essential task of followup research on intravenous drug users who have contracted AIDS.
97 pages

8367 As Bill Sees It
Alcoholics Anonymous
PO Box 459
New York, NY 10163-0459   212-870-3400
                                         Fax: 212-870-3137
This collection of Bill W's writings offers a daily source of comfort and inspiration.

8368 As We Understood...
Al-Anon Family Group Headquarters
1600 Corporate Landing Parkway   757-563-1600
Virginia Beach, VA 23454-5617   800-425-2666
                                         Fax: 757-563-1655
                                         e-mail: wso@al-anon.org
                                         www.al-anon.alateen.org
Al-Anon members share their understanding of a higher power, fellowship, spiritual awakening, prayer, meditation and letting go.
269 pages
ISBN: 0-910034-56-7
Caryn Johnson, Director Communications

8369 Black, Beautiful and Recovering
African American Family Services
2616 Nicollet Avenue S   612-871-7878
Minneapolis, MN 55408
A helpful guide for Black people who are in the process of recovering from alcohol or other substance abuse problems.
10 pages

8370 Body, Mind, and Spirit
Hazelden
15251 Pleasant Valley Road   651-257-4010
Center City, MN 55012-9640   800-328-9000
                                         Fax: 651-213-4426
                                         www.hazelden.org
Addressing such issues as self-esteem, fear, anger, and spirituality, these 366 daily meditations and affirmations integrate the physical, mental, and spiritual aspects of healing from addiction.
410 pages Paperback
ISBN: 1-568380-77-1

8371 Came to Believe
Alcoholics Anonymous
PO Box 459   212-870-3400
New York, NY 10163-0459   Fax: 212-870-3137
A collection of stories by AA members who write about what the phrase spiritual awakening means to them.
120 pages

8372 Chemically Dependent Older Adults
Hazelden
15251 Pleasant Valley Road   651-257-4010
Center City, MN 55012-9640   800-328-9000
                                         Fax: 651-213-4426
                                         www.hazelden.org
Reviews the importance of considering the older adult's health, living conditions and social and economic resources when developing treatment and aftercare plans.
136 pages Paperback

8373 Childhood and Adolescent Drug Abuse: A Physician's Guide
American Council on Drug Education
204 Monroe Street
Rockville, MD 20850-4425   800-488-3784
A scientific monograph which educates and sensitizes doctors to the dimensions of drug problems.
68 pages

8374 Circle of Hope
Hazelden
15251 Pleasant Valley Road   651-257-4010
Center City, MN 55012-9640   800-328-9000
                                         Fax: 651-213-4426
                                         www.hazelden.org
Spirituality, acceptance, and living one day at a time are show through personal stories of individuals living with HIV and AIDS and dealing with adiction and recovery.
364 pages Paperback
ISBN: 0-894866-10-9

8375 Citizen's Alcohol and Other Drug Prevention Directory
National Clearinghouse for Alcohol and Drug Info.
PO Box 2345
Rockville, MD 20847-2345   800-729-6686
National directory of over 3,000 state, local and government agencies dealing with alcohol and other drug-related topics.
276 pages

8376 Cocaine Today
American Council on Drug Education
204 Monroe Street
Rockville, MD 20850-4425   800-488-3784
A recent revision of this popular book. Cocaine Today takes a new look at cocaine and its derivative, crack.

8377 Codependent No More
Hazelden
15251 Pleasant Valley Road   651-257-4010
Center City, MN 55012-9640   800-328-9000
                                         Fax: 651-213-4426
                                         www.hazelden.org
Explains codependent behaviors in clear, simple terms.
208 pages Paperback

8378 Color of Light
Hazelden
15251 Pleasant Valley Road   651-257-4010
Center City, MN 55012-9640   800-328-9000
                                         Fax: 651-213-4426
                                         www.hazelden.org
These 366 meditations speak to both the practical and spiritual journey of living with HIV/AIDS, and demonstrate how to integrate personal values with those offered in chemical dependency recovery and the Twelve Steps.
400 pages Paperback
ISBN: 0-894865-11-0

8379 Confusion is a State of Grace
Hazelden
15251 Pleasant Valley Road   651-257-4010
Center City, MN 55012   800-328-9000
                                         Fax: 651-213-4426
                                         www.hazelden.org
Compilation of quotes that captures the wisdom, humor, and healing found in Al-Anon and other Twelve Step groups.
153 pages Paperback
ISBN: 1-568380-89-5

8380 Courage to Be Me: Living with Alcoholism
Al-Anon Family Group Headquarters
1600 Corporate Landing Parkway   757-563-1600
Virginia Beach, VA 23454-5617   800-425-2666
                                         Fax: 757-563-1655
                                         e-mail: wso@al-anon.org
                                         www.al-anon.alateen.org
Written for and by Alateens of all ages who will treasure the honesty and strength of recovery shown.
326 pages
ISBN: 0-910034-30-3
Caryn Johnson, Director Communications

8381 Daily Reflections: A Book of Reflections by AA Members for AA Members
Alcoholics Anonymous
PO Box 459   212-870-3400
New York, NY 10163-0459   Fax: 212-870-3137
AAs reflect on favorite quotations from A.A. literature. A reading for each day of the year.

8382 Day at a Time: Daily Reflections for Recovering People
Hazelden
15251 Pleasant Valley Road   651-257-4010
Center City, MN 55012-9640   800-328-9000
                                         Fax: 651-213-4426
                                         www.hazelden.org
Offers inspiration and hope for people recovering from chemical dependency or other addictions. Each daily passage reinforces the message of Twelve Step recovery.
384 pages Paperback
ISBN: 1-568380-36-4

8383 Day by Day
Hazelden
15251 Pleasant Valley Road   651-257-4010
Center City, MN 55012   800-328-9000
                                         Fax: 651-213-4426
                                         www.hazelden.org
A book of daily meditations for recovering addicts that reinforce Narcotics Anonymous principles and objectives.
400 pages Paperback

8384 Days of Healing, Days of Joy
Hazelden
15251 Pleasant Valley Road   651-257-4010
Center City, MN 55012-9640   800-328-9000
                                         Fax: 651-213-4426
                                         www.hazelden.org
Three hundred and sixty-six daily quotes, meditations and affirmations to help adult children in their search for serenity.
400 pages Paperback

8385 Developing Chemical Dependency Services for Black People
African American Family Services
2616 Nicollet Avenue S   612-871-7878
Minneapolis, MN 55408
This manual has been developed to address many of the questions asked by new or expanding programs as they establish new culturally specific initiatives for African-American clients.
78 pages

8386 Dilemma of the Alcoholic Marriage
Al-Anon Family Group Headquarters
1600 Corporate Landing Parkway   757-563-1600
Virginia Beach, VA 23454-5617   800-425-2666
                                         Fax: 757-563-1655
                                 e-mail: wso@al-anon.org
                                 www.al-anon.alateen.org
This book explores the problem of alcoholism in marriage and includes questions for applying the twelve steps to relationships.
100 pages
ISBN: 0-910034-18-4
Caryn Johnson, Director Communications

8387 Dr. Bob and the Good Oldtimers
Alcoholics Anonymous
PO Box 459   212-870-3400
New York, NY 10163-0459   Fax: 212-870-3137
The life story of the fellowship's co-founder, interwoven wth recollections of early AA in the Midwest.

8388 Drug Abuse and Addiction Information/Treatment Programs
American Business Directories
5711 S 86th Circle   402-593-4600
Omaha, NE 68127-4146   Fax: 402-331-1505
Number of entries is 9,425.

8389 Drug Use Among American High School Seniors, College Students & Youth
National Clearinghouse for Alcohol and Drug Info.
PO Box 2345
Rockville, MD 20847-2345   800-729-6686
Comprehensive reports presenting the results of the 16th national survey of the drug use and related attitudes of American high school seniors.
199 pages Volumes I & II

8390 Drugs and Pregnancy: It's Not Worth the Risk
American Council on Drug Education
204 Monroe Street
Rockville, MD 20850   800-488-3784
A scientific monograph for health care providers which teaches them to identify alcohol and drug problems in their patients.
48 pages

8391 Dual Diagnosis
Hazelden
15251 Pleasant Valley Road   651-257-4010
Center City, MN 55012-9640   800-328-9000
                                         Fax: 651-213-4426
                                         www.hazelden.org

Focuses on the issues surrounding the treatment of clients with co-existing chemical dependency and psychiatric conditions.
191 pages Paperback

8392 Dual Disorders
Hazelden
15251 Pleasant Valley Road   651-257-4010
Center City, MN 55012-9640   800-328-9000
                                         Fax: 651-213-4426
                                         www.hazelden.org
Presents case histories and analyses of psychiatric disorders.
140 pages Paperback

8393 Dual Disorders Recovery Book
Hazelden
15251 Pleasant Valley Road   651-257-4010
Center City, MN 55012-9640   800-328-9000
                                         Fax: 651-213-4426
                                         www.hazelden.org
Helps individuals with dual disorders develop a plan for daily living through a specially-designed Twelve-Step program.
242 pages Paperback
ISBN: 1-568380-34-8

8394 Each Day a New Beginning
Hazelden
15251 Pleasant Valley Road   651-257-4010
Center City, MN 55012-9640   800-328-9000
                                         Fax: 651-213-4426
                                         www.hazelden.org
Promotes the development of a significant spiritual core for recovery that can be enhanced throughout the rest of life.
400 pages Paperback

8395 Elephant in the Living Room: A Leader's Guide
Hazelden
15251 Pleasant Valley Road   651-257-4010
Center City, MN 55012-9640   800-328-9000
                                         Fax: 651-213-4426
                                         www.hazelden.org
The adult companion to the classic children's book. Caretakers learn how to explain addiction and its effect on the family to small children who's parents or siblings are chemically dependent.
129 pages Paperback
ISBN: 1-568380-34-8

8396 Encyclopedia of Drug Abuse
Facts on File
11 Penn Plaza   212-967-8800
New York, NY 10001   800-322-8755
                                         Fax: 800-678-3633
More that 500 entries explore: specific drugs, countries, organizations, treatment programs, laws, medical terms, and psychosocial concepts.
496 pages Hardcover

8397 Ethics for Addiction Professionals
Hazelden
15251 Pleasant Valley Road   651-257-4010
Center City, MN 55012-9640   800-328-9000
                                         Fax: 651-213-4426
                                         www.hazelden.org
Probes crucial, complex ethical issues including counselor relapse, paid referrals and discrimination.
60 pages

8398 Extent and Adequacy of Insurance Coverage for Substance Abuse I & II
National Clearinghouse for Alcohol and Drug Info.
PO Box 2345
Rockville, MD 20847-2345   800-729-6686
These volumes examine the extent to which the cost of alcohol and other drug treatments is covered by private insurance, public financing and other sources.

8399 Eye Opener
Hazelden
15251 Pleasant Valley Road   651-257-4010
Center City, MN 55012-9640   800-328-9000
                                         Fax: 651-213-4426
                                         www.hazelden.org

Daily meditations about understanding the Alcoholics Anonymous program, writen by a favorite early AA member and author.
380 pages Cloth
ISBN: 0-894860-23-2

8400   Fact Is...Hispanic Parents Can Help Their Children Avoid Alcohol/Drugs
National Clearinghouse for Alcohol and Drug Info.
PO Box 2345
Rockville, MD 20847-2345   800-729-6686

8401   Feeding the Hungry Heart, the Experience of Compulsive Eating
Gurze Books
PO Box 2238
Carlsbad, CA 92018-2238   800-756-7533
                                          Fax: 760-434-5476
                                          e-mail: gzcatl@aol.com
                                          www.bulimia.com
This is a widely respected, extremely readable book from Ms. Roth and the many participants of early breaking free workshops. It is an intimate, vulnerable sharing of experiences which continues to touch and change lives.
212 pages Paperback

8402   Food for Thought: Daily Meditations for Overeaters
Hazelden
15251 Pleasant Valley Road   651-257-4010
Center City, MN 55012-9640   800-328-9000
                                          Fax: 651-213-4426
                                          www.hazelden.org
Offers guidance in the early days of living a Twelve Step program.
400 pages Paperback
ISBN: 0-894860-90-9

8403   Forum Favorites: Volumes 1, 2, 3 & 4
Al-Anon Family Group Headquarters
1600 Corporate Landing Parkway   757-563-1600
Virginia Beach, VA 23454-5617   800-425-2666
                                          Fax: 757-563-1655
                                          e-mail: wso@al-anon.org
                                          www.al-anon.alateen.org
Personal sharings show how the fundamentals of the Al-Anon programs are applied to everyday situations.
428 pages Set of 4
ISBN: 0-910034-51-6
Caryn Johnson, Director Communications

8404   Freedom from Smoking at Work Program
American Lung Association
1740 Broadway
New York, NY 10017   212-315-8700
                                          www.lungusa.org
ALA program for organizations interested in creating a healthier workplace environment through a comprehensive, multicomponent smoking education, cessation and policy development program designed for the workplace.

8405   Future by Design/A Community Framework
National Clearinghouse for Alcohol and Drug Info.
PO Box 2345
Rockville, MD 20847-2345   800-729-6686
Provides communities with a manageable framework for getting involved in alcohol and other drug prevention.
234 pages

8406   Gentle Path Through the Twelve Steps
Hazelden
15251 Pleasant Valley Road   651-257-4010
Center City, MN 55012-9640   800-328-9000
                                          Fax: 651-213-4426
                                          www.hazelden.org
This workbook provides a unique set of structured forms and exercises to help recoving people integrate the Twelve Steps in all aspects of their lives.
224 pages Paperback
ISBN: 1-568380-58-5

8407   Getting Started in AA
Hazelden

15251 Pleasant Valley Road   651-257-4010
Center City, MN 55012-9640   800-328-9000
                                          Fax: 651-213-4426
                                          www.hazelden.org
Practical suggestions for staying sober, summaries of AA principles, concepts, and slogans, and a historical overview to help the reader understand the spirit of the program.
211 pages Paperback
ISBN: 1-568380-91-7

8408   Getting Tough on Gateway Drugs: A Guide for the Family
American Council On Drug Education
204 Monroe Street
Rockville, MD 20850-4425   800-488-3784
Gateway drugs including marijuana, alcohol and tobacco are those which open doors into all drug abuse. This family survival guide helps parents understand the consequences of drug dependence and suggests actions the family can take to prevent and solve drug problems.
332 pages

8409   Getting it Together: Promoting Drug Free Communities
National Clearinghouse for Alcohol and Drug Info.
PO Box 2345
Rockville, MD 20847   800-729-6686
Provides resources and step-by-step information on how local communities and organizations can work effectively with young people who are committed to preventing alcohol and other drug abuse.
71 pages

8410   God Grant Me the Laughter: A Treasury of Twelve Step Humor
Hazelden
15251 Pleasant Valley Road   651-257-4010
Center City, MN 55012-9640   800-328-9000
                                          Fax: 651-213-4426
                                          www.hazelden.org
Hearty cartoons and humorous anecdotes clearly demonstrate how readers' lives today contrast with their drinking and drug using in the past.
200 pages Paperback
ISBN: 1-568380-38-0

8411   Good First Step
Hazelden
15251 Pleasant Valley Road   651-257-4010
Center City, MN 55012-9640   800-328-9000
                                          Fax: 651-213-4426
                                          www.hazelden.org
Features a structured format and emphasis on the meaning of the First Step to help build a solid foundation for recovery.
60 pages Paperback
ISBN: 1-568381-13-1

8412   Goodbye Hangovers, Hello Life
Women for Sobriety
PO Box 618   215-536-8026
Quakertown, PA 18951-0618   Fax: 215-536-8026
                                          e-mail: NewLife@nni.com
                                          www.womenforsobriety.org
A book about recovery - how it happens, what problems arise and how to overcome these problems.
250 pages Paperback

8413   Grateful to Have Been There
Hazelden
15251 Pleasant Valley Road   651-257-4010
Center City, MN 55012   800-328-9000
                                          Fax: 651-213-4426
                                          www.hazelden.org
Aide and executive secretary to AA's co-founder Bill W. for 20 years, Wing shares her memories and impressions of 42 years of involvement with the Fellowship.
150 pages Paperback
ISBN: 0-942421-44-2

8414   Growing Up Drug Free: A Parent's Guide to Prevention
National Clearinghouse for Alcohol and Drug Info.
PO Box 2345
Rockville, MD 20852   800-729-6686

Offers information on what parents can do to prevent their child from becoming a substance abuser/alcoholic. Focuses on counseling, peer pressure issues, education, school-parent cooperation and offers an introduction to each drug, symptoms and how to spot the warning signs of drug addiction.
47 pages

8415 Handle with Care
Hazelden
15251 Pleasant Valley Road
Center City, MN 55012-9640
651-257-4010
800-328-9000
Fax: 651-213-4426
www.hazelden.org

A comprehensive look at how parents, teachers and other care givers of children ages 10 and younger can identify and meet their special needs.

8416 Help for Helpers: Daily Meditations for Counselors
Hazelden
15251 Pleasant Valley Road
Center City, MN 55012-9640
651-257-4010
800-328-9000
Fax: 651-213-4426
www.hazelden.org

Written by addiction treatment center staff members from across the country, these daily meditations encourage, comfort, and challenge helpers to understand others and themselves.
400 pages Paperback
ISBN: 1-568380-61-5

8417 Helping Homeless People with Alcohol and Other Drug Problems
National Clearinghouse for Alcohol and Drug Info.
PO Box 2345
Rockville, MD 20847
800-729-6686

Developed by professionals who work directly with homeless people, this manual provides basic information about homeless people with AOD problems.
50 pages

8418 Helping Your Students Say No Teacher's Guide
National Clearinghouse for Alcohol and Drug Info.
PO Box 2345
Rockville, MD 20847-2345
800-729-6686

Explains the effects of alcohol on the body, why children start to drink, how teachers can help their students refuse alcohol and deal with the first signs of drinking.
13 pages

8419 How to Manage Your Drug-Free Workplace Programs
American Council on Drug Education
204 Monroe Street
Rockville, MD 20850-4425
800-488-3784

Step-by-step process for introducing and managing a drug awareness program that includes a variety of additional tips to complement messages in the drug awareness pamphlet series.
48 pages

8420 I'm Black and I'm Sober
Hazelden
15251 Pleasant Valley Road
Center City, MN 55012-9640
651-257-4010
800-328-9000
Fax: 651-213-4426
www.hazelden.org

An autobiography written by a recovering African American woman who discusses the impact of discrimination and the obstacles faced through the journey back to sobriety.
279 pages Paperback
ISBN: 1-568380-71-2

8421 If Only I Could Quit
Hazelden
15251 Pleasant Valley Road
Center City, MN 55012-9640
651-257-4010
800-328-9000
Fax: 651-213-4426
www.hazelden.org

Promotes the Twelve Step process for recovery from nicotine addiction.
320 pages Paperback

8422 In God's Care
Hazelden

15251 Pleasant Valley Road
Center City, MN 55012-9640
651-257-4010
800-328-9000
Fax: 651-213-4426
www.hazelden.org

Excellent relaxation and education tool for clients working on their Second and Third Steps.
400 pages Paperback

8423 Keep Quit
Hazelden
15251 Pleasant Valley Road
Center City, MN 55012-9640
651-257-4010
800-328-9000
Fax: 651-213-4426
www.hazelden.org

Daily motivational guide to help the new nonsmoker understand the craving for nicotine and learn how to break the rituals and patterns associated with relapse.
300 pages Paperback
ISBN: 1-568381-04-2

8424 Keep it Simple
Hazelden
15251 Pleasant Valley Road
Center City, MN 55012-9640
651-257-4010
800-328-9000
Fax: 651-213-4426
www.hazelden.org

Daily prayers that help clients learn to ask for help and to turn their self-will over to a Higher Power.
400 pages Paperback

8425 Learning to Live Drug Free: A Curriculum Model for Prevention
National Clearinghouse for Alcohol and Drug Info.
PO Box 2345
Rockville, MD 20847-2345
800-729-6686

Provides a flexible framework for classroom-based prevention efforts for kindergarten through grade 12.
52 pages

8426 Let's Talk About Alcohol Abuse
Rosen Publishing Group's PowerKids Press
29 E 21st Street
New York, NY 10010
212-777-3017
800-237-9932
Fax: 888-436-4643
e-mail: customerservice@rosenpub.com
www.rosenpublishing.com

In gentle and sensitive terms this book talks about when a parent drinks and what alcohol can do to the body. Kids are told about the illegality of drinking as minors. Recommended for grade K-4.

ISBN: 0-823923-03-7
Marianne Johnston, Author

8427 Life of My Own: Daily Meditations on Hope and Acceptance
Hazelden
15251 Pleasant Valley Road
Center City, MN 55012-9640
651-257-4010
800-328-9000
Fax: 651-213-4426
www.hazelden.org

Offers daily access to strength, serenity, and insight in our relationships with chemically dependent people.
400 pages Paperback
ISBN: 0-894868-63-2

8428 Little Red Book
Hazelden
15251 Pleasant Valley Road
Center City, MN 55012-9640
651-257-4010
800-328-9000
Fax: 651-213-4426
www.hazelden.org

A primer for members of Alcoholics Anonymous. Each page acts as a study guide to the Big Book and its teachings.
164 pages Paperback
ISBN: 0-894869-85-X

8429 Living Sober
Hazelden
15251 Pleasant Valley Road
Center City, MN 55012-9640
651-257-4010
800-328-9000
Fax: 651-213-4426
www.hazelden.org

Offers clients sound advice about how to stay sober.
88 pages Paperback

8430 Lois Remembers
Al-Anon Family Group Headquarters
1600 Corporate Landing Parkway   757-563-1600
Virginia Beach, VA 23454-5617   800-425-2666
                                        Fax: 757-563-1655
                                        e-mail: wso@al-anon.org
                                        www.al-anon.alateen.org
The memoirs of a co-founder of Al-Anon. Lois tells her personal story and recalls the eventful years before and after the founding of AA and Al-Anon.
204 pages
ISBN: 0-910034-23-0
Caryn Johnson, Director Communications

8431 Marijuana
Branden Publishing Company
17 Station Street   617-734-2045
Brookline Village, MA 02147   Fax: 617-734-2046
                                        www.branden.com
Paperback
ISBN: 0-828319-49-9

8432 Marijuana Smoking Prevention Program for Schools
American Lung Association
1740 Broadway   212-315-8700
New York, NY 10017
Cast of the TV show FAME enlivens highly motivational program to inform parents about the dangers of pot and discourages 9-11 year olds from using it.

8433 Marijuana Today
American Council on Drug Education
204 Monroe Street
Rockville, MD 20850-4425   800-488-3784
A revision of the long time bestseller, this book examines the history of marijuana, its use, the risks associated with use and the short and long-term effects of use.

8434 Marijuana and Reproduction
American Council on Drug Education
204 Monroe Street
Rockville, MD 20850-4425   800-488-3784
A scientific monograph for physicians which describes marijuana, profiles the users and discusses the effects on the reproductive system.
30 pages

8435 Marketing Booze to Blacks
African American Family Services
2616 Nicollet Avenue S   612-871-7878
Minneapolis, MN 55408
This controversial book details how liquor industries target the black population with its advertising.
55 pages

8436 Mistaken Beliefs About Relapse
Hazelden
15251 Pleasant Valley Road   651-257-4010
Center City, MN 55012-9640   800-328-9000
                                        Fax: 651-213-4426
                                        www.hazelden.org
Examines mistaken beliefs people have about relapse.
30 pages Paperback

8437 My Mind is Out to Get Me: Humor and Wisdom in Recovery
Hazelden
15251 Pleasant Valley Road   651-257-4010
Center City, MN 55012   800-328-9000
                                        Fax: 651-213-4426
                                        www.hazelden.org
Five hundred inspirational sayings and slogans that reflect both the lighter side of living a sober life and the profound wisdom offered in recovery. Each quote has been drawn from the wisdom of Alcoholics Anonymous.
180 pages Paperback
ISBN: 1-568380-10-0

8438 Narcotics Anonymous
Hazelden
15251 Pleasant Valley Road   651-257-4010
Center City, MN 55012-9640   800-328-9000
                                        Fax: 651-213-4426
                                        www.hazelden.org
Men and women describe the N.A. program and how it works.
289 pages Paperback

8439 National Conference on Drug Abuse Researcg & Practice
National Clearinghouse for Alcohol and Drug Info.
PO Box 2345
Rockville, MD 20847   800-729-6686
Offers summaries of workshops, forums, dinner speeches and sessions presented at the National Conference on Drug Abuse Research and Practice.
275 pages

8440 National Directory of Drug Abuse and Alcoholism Treatment and Programs
US National Institute On Drug Abuse
5600 Fishers Lane
Rockville, MD 20857   202-625-8400
                                        www.nida.nih.gov
Eleven thousand listings of agencies that administer treatment and services on the federal, state and local levels.

8441 Night Light: A Book of Nighttime Meditations
Hazelden
15251 Pleasant Valley Road   651-257-4010
Center City, MN 55012-9640   800-328-9000
                                        Fax: 651-213-4426
                                        www.hazelden.org
Three hundred and sixty-six meditations designed to help relax and encourage prayer. Reminds readers to look to their Higher Power for strength, reassurance, comfort, and guidance.
400 pages Paperback
ISBN: 0-894863-81-9

8442 Not God: A History of Alcoholics Anonymous
Hazelden
15251 Pleasant Valley Road   651-257-4010
Center City, MN 55012-9640   800-328-9000
                                        Fax: 651-213-4426
                                        www.hazelden.org
Documenting AA's philosophical and social development within the larger context of American culture, this book follows the remarkable story of the evolution of a small group of Depression-era alcoholics into a worldwide movement.
436 pages Paperback
ISBN: 0-894860-65-8

8443 Occupational Therapy Practice Guidelines for Adults with Substance Use Disorders
American Occupational Therapy Association
4720 Montgomery Lane   301-652-2682
Bethesda, MD 20824-1220   Fax: 301-652-7711
                                        TDD: 800-377-8555
                                        www.aota.org
22 pages
ISBN: 1-569001-60-X

8444 Of Course You're Angry
Hazelden
15251 Pleasant Valley Road   651-257-4010
Center City, MN 55012-9640   800-328-9000
                                        Fax: 651-213-4426
                                        www.hazelden.org
Revised edition dealing with the nature and resolution of anger. Demonstrates how to make anger work in a positive and effective way that can ease, rather than exacerbate, the challenges of early recovery.
120 pages Paperback
ISBN: 1-568381-41-7

8445 One Day at a Time in Al-Anon
Al-Anon Family Group Headquarters

1600 Corporate Landing Parkway
Virginia Beach, VA 23454-5617

757-563-1600
800-425-2666
Fax: 757-563-1655
e-mail: wso@al-anon.org
www.al-anon.alateen.org

Inspirational daily readings cover various aspects of the Al-Anon philosopha and relate it to everyday situations.
376 pages
ISBN: 0-910034-21-4
Caryn Johnson, Director Communications

8446   Operation PAR
National Clearinghouse for Alcohol and Drug Info.
PO Box 2345
Rockville, MD 20847-2345   800-729-6686
Describes successful community alcohol and other drug abuse prevention and treatment programs.
40 pages

8447   Parent Training is Prevention
National Clearinghouse for Alcohol and Drug Info.
PO Box 2345
Rockville, MD 20847-2345   800-729-6686
Contains information to help communities identify and carry out programs on parenting.
184 pages

8448   Pass it On
Alcoholics Anonymous
World Services   212-870-3400
New York, NY 10163   Fax: 212-870-3137
The story of Bill Wilson, the co-founder of AA and the development of the Fellowship.

8449   Passages Through Recovery
Hazelden
15251 Pleasant Valley Road   651-257-4010
Center City, MN 55012-9640   800-328-9000
Fax: 651-213-4426
www.hazelden.org
Guides clients through the six stages of recovery.
130 pages Paperback

8450   Peer Pressure Reversal
Human Resource Development Press
22 Amherst Road   413-253-3488
Amherst, MA 01002-9730

8451   Pregnancy and Exposure to Alcohol and Other Drug Use
National Clearinghouse for Alcohol and Drug Info.
PO Box 2345
Rockville, MD 20847-2345   800-729-6686
www.health.org
This report is for health care professionals presenting the state-of-the-art information about preventing ATOD use among women of childbearing age.

8452   Preparing for the Drug-Free Years: A Family Activity Book
Developmental Research and Programs
130 Nickerson Street   206-286-1805
Seattle, WA 98145-1746   800-736-2630
Fax: 206-286-1462
www.drp.org

8453   Presence at the Center
Hazelden
15251 Pleasant Valley Road   651-257-4010
Center City, MN 55012-9640   800-328-9000
Fax: 651-213-4426
www.hazelden.org
About a new way of life that addresses transformation, change, the presence of a Higher Power, letting go of reluctance and fear, and the freedom commitment can bring.
76 pages Paperback
ISBN: 1-568380-01-1

8454   Prevention Plus II: Tools for Creating & Sustaining a Drug-Free Community
National Clearinghouse for Alcohol and Drug Info.

PO Box 2345
Rockville, MD 20847-2345   800-729-6686
www.health.org
Provides a framework for organizing or expanding community alcohol and other drug problem prevention activities for youth into a coordinated, complimentary system.
541 pages

8455   Prevention Plus III: Assessing Alcohol & Other Prevention Programs
National Clearinghouse for Alcohol and Drug Info.
PO Box 2345
Rockville, MD 20847-2345   800-729-6686
www.health.org
Provides tools and techniques for alcohol and other drug prevention, planning and implementation.
470 pages

8456   Prevention Resource Guide: Alcohol and Other Drug Related Periodicals
National Clearinghouse for Alcohol and Drug Info.
PO Box 2345
Rockville, MD 20847-2345   800-729-6686
www.health.org
Provides a concise annotated bibliography of journals, newsletters and other publications related to the AOD prevention field.
12 pages

8457   Prevention Resource Guide: American Indian/Native Alaskans
National Clearinghouse for Alcohol and Drug Info.
PO Box 2345
Rockville, MD 20847-2345   800-729-6686
www.health.org
This resource guide is a survey of current data on alcohol abuse among American Indians and Native Alaskans.
24 pages

8458   Prevention Resource Guide: Asian and Pacific Islander Americans
National Clearinghouse for Alcohol and Drug Info.
PO Box 2345
Rockville, MD 20847-2345   800-729-6686
www.health.org
Contains facts and figures about Asian and Pacific Islander Americans and alcohol and other drug prevention.
13 pages

8459   Prevention Resource Guide: Elementary Youth
National Clearinghouse for Alcohol and Drug Info.
PO Box 2345
Rockville, MD 20847-2345   800-729-6686
www.health.org
This resource guide includes materials specifically developed for youth that may be used in an elementary school setting.
23 pages

8460   Prevention Resource Guide: Pregnant Postpartum Women and Their Infants
National Clearinghouse for Alcohol and Drug Info.
PO Box 2345
Rockville, MD 20847-2345   800-729-6686
www.health.org
This resource guide targets health care providers, prevention program planners and counselors of pregnant and postpartum women between the ages of 15 and 44.
30 pages

8461   Prevention Resource Guide: Secondary School Students
National Clearinghouse for Alcohol and Drug Info.
PO Box 2345
Rockville, MD 20847-2345   800-729-6686
www.health.org
This resource guide targets teachers, administrators and program leaders who come in contact with secondary school youth.
27 pages

8462   Prevention Resource Guide: Women
National Clearinghouse for Alcohol and Drug Info.

PO Box 2345
Rockville, MD 20847-2345   800-729-6686
                                            www.health.org
This resource guide provides the latest information about the effects of drugs and alcohol on women.
32 pages

8463 Prevention in Action
National Clearinghouse for Alcohol and Drug Info.
PO Box 2345
Rockville, MD 20847-2345   800-729-6686
Provides descriptions selected by representatives of national organizations and State alcohol and drug agency representatives.
20 pages

8464 Program for You
Hazelden
15251 Pleasant Valley Road   651-257-4010
Center City, MN 55012-9640   800-328-9000
                                            Fax: 651-213-4426
                                            www.hazelden.org
Study guide interpreting the original AA program as described in Alcoholics Anonymous and helps apply the wisdom to everyday life.
183 pages Paperback
ISBN: 0-894867-41-5

8465 Promise of a New Day: A Book of Daily Meditations
Hazelden
15251 Pleasant Valley Road   651-257-4010
Center City, MN 55012-9640   800-328-9000
                                            Fax: 651-213-4426
                                            www.hazelden.org
Simple, inspiring wisdom about creating and maintaining inner peace. Each of the 366 daily meditations expresses the essence of Twelve Step spirituality without the program jargon.
400 pages Paperback
ISBN: 0-894862-03-0

8466 Quit & Stay Quit: A Personal Program to Stop Smoking
Hazelden
15251 Pleasant Valley Road   651-257-4010
Center City, MN 55012-9640   800-328-9000
                                            Fax: 651-213-4426
                                            www.hazelden.org
Guide to nicotine recovery offering an effective long-term program to quit by showing readers how smoking has subtly shaped their values, attitudes, and lives.
196 pages Paperback
ISBN: 1-568381-09-3

8467 Quit Smoking Manual
American Lung Association
1740 Broadway   212-315-8700
New York, NY 10019-4315
Original self-help smoking cessation manual showing the public how to quit smoking in 20 days.
64 pages

8468 Recovery Journal for Exploring Who I Am
Hazelden
15251 Pleasant Valley Road   651-257-4010
Center City, MN 55012-9640   800-328-9000
                                            Fax: 651-213-4426
                                            www.hazelden.org
Introduces clients to journal writing as an effective therapeutic adjunct for addiction recovery.
48 pages

8469 School Answers Back: Responding to Student Drug Use
American Council on Drug Education
204 Monroe Street
Rockville, MD 20850   800-488-3784
Provides teachers, counselors, administrators and parents with a model for schools to use in confronting drug and alcohol abuse.
145 pages

8470 Search for Serenity
Hazelden

15251 Pleasant Valley Road   651-257-4010
Center City, MN 55012-9640   800-328-9000
                                            Fax: 651-213-4426
                                            www.hazelden.org
Provides clients with practical inspiration to change their feelings toward people and situations.
152 pages Paperback

8471 Shame Faced
Hazelden
15251 Pleasant Valley Road   651-257-4010
Center City, MN 55012-9640   800-328-9000
                                            Fax: 651-213-4426
                                            www.hazelden.org
Discusses the relationship between shame and chemical dependency.
28 pages

8472 Skeptic's Guide to the 12 Steps
Hazelden
15251 Pleasant Valley Road   651-257-4010
Center City, MN 55012-9640   800-328-9000
                                            Fax: 651-213-4426
                                            www.hazelden.org
Investigates each of the 12 steps to gain a deeper understanding of a Higher Power.
241 pages Paperback

8473 Smoking and Pregnancy Kit for Health Care Providers
American Lung Association
1740 Broadway   212-315-8700
New York, NY 10019-4315
A program kit for health care providers designed to educate pregnant women not to smoke and to help them kick the habit.

8474 Smoking, Drinking & Illicit Drug Use
National Clearinghouse for Alcohol and Drug Info.
PO Box 2345
Rockville, MD 20847-2345   800-729-6686
Comprehensive reports representing the results of the 12th national survey on drug use and analyzing data collected from young Americans from 1975-1991.

8475 Sober But Stuck
Hazelden
15251 Pleasant Valley Road   651-257-4010
Center City, MN 55012-9640   800-328-9000
                                            Fax: 651-213-4426
                                            www.hazelden.org
Collection of personal stories by men and women who are long-time members of Alcoholics Anonymous. Each story shares the anecdotes and resources which helped members break through the barriers that limited their enjoyment of a sober life.
215 pages Paperback
ISBN: 1-568380-78-X

8476 Social Policy Prevention Handbook
African American Family Services
2616 Nicollet Avenue S   612-871-7878
Minneapolis, MN 55408
A manual that details IBCA's community based approach to the development of alcohol and drug abuse prevention strategies.
24 pages

8477 Staying Clean
Hazelden
15251 Pleasant Valley Road   651-257-4010
Center City, MN 55012-9640   800-328-9000
                                            Fax: 651-213-4426
                                            www.hazelden.org
Each section focuses on one of 33 proven ideas for staying drug-free, such as professional help, prayer, support groups and meditation.
76 pages Paperback

8478 Staying Sober
Hazelden
15251 Pleasant Valley Road   651-257-4010
Center City, MN 55012-9640   800-328-9000
                                            Fax: 651-213-4426
                                            www.hazelden.org

Discusses addictive diseases and its physical, psychological and social effects.
228 pages Paperback

8479   Step Zero: Getting to Recovery
Hazelden
15251 Pleasant Valley Road   651-257-4010
Center City, MN 55012-9640   800-328-9000
                                        Fax: 651-213-4426
                                        www.hazelden.org
Explains the concepts of Step Zero, when clients drop their defenses, begin to face themselves and start to assess their behavior and the reasons for it.
170 pages Paperback

8480   Stools and Bottles
Hazelden
15251 Pleasant Valley Road   651-257-4010
Center City, MN 55012-9640   800-328-9000
                                        Fax: 651-213-4426
                                        www.hazelden.org
Depicts the first Three steps using a three-legged stool and eight whiskey bottles representing character defects revealed when working Step Four.
160 pages Hardcover

8481   Substance Abuse and Physical Disability
Allen Heinemann, PhD, author
Haworth Press
10 Alice Street   607-722-5857
Binghamton, NY 13904-1580   800-429-6784
                                        Fax: 607-722-0012
                                        www.haworthpress.com
This book offers information on alcohol and drug abuse being a contributing factor in traumatic and disabling injuries.
1993 289 pages Hardcover
ISBN: 1-560242-89-3

8482   Success Stories from Drug-Free Schools
National Clearinghouse for Alcohol and Drug Info.
PO Box 2345
Rockville, MD 20847-2345   800-729-6686
                                        www.health.org
Salutes the 107 schools honored by the US Department of Education's Drug-Free Recognition Program.
59 pages

8483   Tackling Alcohol Problems on Campus: Tools for Media Advocacy
National Clearinghouse for Alcohol and Drug Info.
PO Box 2345
Rockville, MD 20847-2345   800-729-6686
Reviews the role of alcohol on campus and shows how to use the media to get attention and support.
38 pages

8484   Team Up for Drug Prevention with America's Young Athletes
Drug Enforcement Administration, Demand Reduction
1405 I Street NW
Washington, DC 20537-0001   202-307-5550
                                        www.usdoj.gov/dea/programs/demand.htm

8485   Ten Steps to Help Your Child Say No: A Parent's Guide
National Clearinghouse for Alcohol and Drug Info.
PO Box 2345
Rockville, MD 20847-2345   800-729-6686

8486   Things My Sponsors Taught Me
Hazelden
15251 Pleasant Valley Road   651-257-4010
Center City, MN 55012-9640   800-328-9000
                                        Fax: 651-213-4426
                                        www.hazelden.org
Features AA philosophy, quotes, slogans and refreshing reminders.
76 pages Paperback

8487   Today I Will Do One Thing: Daily Readings for Awareness & Hope
Hazelden

15251 Pleasant Valley Road   651-257-4010
Center City, MN 55012-9640   800-328-9000
                                        Fax: 651-213-4426
                                        www.hazelden.org
Specially designed to integrate recovery from addiction with the treatment of emotional or psychiatric illness. Each meditation focuses on a task or goal to be completed each day.
400 pages Paperback
ISBN: 1-568380-83-6

8488   Today's Gift
Hazelden
15251 Pleasant Valley Road   651-257-4010
Center City, MN 55012-9640   800-328-9000
                                        Fax: 651-213-4426
                                        www.hazelden.org
Inspiring meditations bringing families together and strengthening family bonds.
400 pages Paperback

8489   Touchstones
Hazelden
15251 Pleasant Valley Road   651-257-4010
Center City, MN 55012-9640   800-328-9000
                                        Fax: 651-213-4426
                                        www.hazelden.org
A book of daily meditations for men in the Twelve-Step program.
400 pages Paperback

8490   Turnabout
Women for Sobriety
PO Box 618   215-536-8026
Quakertown, PA 18951-0618   Fax: 215-536-8026
                                        e-mail: WFSobriey@aol.com
                                        www.mediapulse.com/wfs/
This is the story of the founder of Women for Sobriety and her struggle to quit drinking.
183 pages

8491   Turning Awareness Into Action: What Your Community Can Do About Drug Use
National Clearinghouse for Alcohol and Drug Info.
PO Box 2345
Rockville, MD 20847-2345   800-729-6686
                                        www.health.org
This bilingual booklet is designed to show leaders at the grassroots level how to make the most of their talents and their community's resources.
73 pages

8492   Twelve Step Sponsorship: How it Works
Hazelden
15251 Pleasant Valley Road   651-257-4010
Center City, MN 55012-9640   800-328-9000
                                        Fax: 651-213-4426
                                        www.hazelden.org
Complete handbook for working with a newcomer. Based on Twelve Step traditions and knowledge passed orally through the generations, this working manual defines the sponsorship role and guides sponsors through the rewards and pitfalls of reaching out to help new program members.
260 pages Paperback
ISBN: 1-568381-22-0

8493   Twelve Steps and Traditions
Hazelden
15251 Pleasant Valley Road   651-257-4010
Center City, MN 55012-9640   800-328-9000
                                        Fax: 651-213-4426
                                        www.hazelden.org
Outlines the core principles by which AA members recover and by which the fellowship functions.
192 pages Paperback

8494   Twelve Steps and Twelve Traditions
Alcoholics Anonymous
PO Box 459   212-870-3400
New York, NY 10163-0459   Fax: 212-870-3137
Twenty-four essays on the Steps and Traditions that discuss the principles of individual recovery and group unity.

8495 Twelve Steps and Twelve Traditions for Alateen
Al-Anon Family Group Headquarters
1600 Corporate Landing Parkway   757-563-1600
Virginia Beach, VA 23454-5617   800-425-2666
    Fax: 757-563-1655
    e-mail: wso@al-anon.org
    www.al-anon.alateen.org
Questions, discussions and personal reflections of Alateen members.
60 pages
Caryn Johnson, Director Communications

8496 Twelve Steps for Everyone...Who Really Wants Them
Hazelden
15251 Pleasant Valley Road   651-257-4010
Center City, MN 55012-9640   800-328-9000
    Fax: 651-213-4426
    www.hazelden.org
A basic primer outlining how spiritual and emotional health can be found by working and living the Twelve Steps. Emphasizes that the Twelve Steps are for anyone who wants to change.
208 pages Paperback
ISBN: 1-568380-47-X

8497 Twelve Steps of Alcoholics Anonymous
Hazelden
15251 Pleasant Valley Road   651-257-4010
Center City, MN 55012-9640   800-328-9000
    Fax: 651-213-4426
    www.hazelden.org
A series of short discussions that interpret each of the Twelve Steps, from admission of individual powerlessness outlined in Step One to the moral inventory of Step Four and the spiritual awakening of Step Twelve.
130 pages Paperback
ISBN: 0-894869-04-3

8498 Twenty Four Hours a Day
Hazelden
15251 Pleasant Valley Road   651-257-4010
Center City, MN 55012-9640   800-328-9000
    Fax: 651-213-4426
    www.hazelden.org
Offers a resource that serves as a solid foundation in a spiritual program. Simple, yet effective resource that helps clients relate to the Twelve-Step program.
400 pages Paperback

8499 Walk in Dry Places
Hazelden
15251 Pleasant Valley Road   651-257-4010
Center City, MN 55012-9640   800-328-9000
    Fax: 651-213-4426
    www.hazelden.org
Core-recovery book filled with practical spiritual advice and time-honored Twelve Step philosophy. Insightful explorations of the deeper issues of living in recovery address the daily concerns of those new to life without alcoholism, as well as those with long-term sobriety.
400 pages Paperback
ISBN: 1-568381-27-1

8500 Wasted Tales of a Gen X Drunk
Hazelden
15251 Pleasant Valley Road   651-257-4010
Center City, MN 55012-9640   800-328-9000
    Fax: 651-213-4426
    www.hazelden.org
Cynicism and black humor underscore this hard-edged memoir of a young journalist's alcoholism and subsequent recovery. Captures the ethos of a generation often suspicious and alienated by the Twelve-Step approach.
250 pages Cloth
ISBN: 1-568381-42-5

8501 What Works: Schools Without Drugs
National Clearinghouse for Alcohol and Drug Info.
PO Box 2345
Rockville, MD 20847-2345   800-729-6686

8502 What You Can Do About Drug Use in America
National Clearinghouse for Alcohol and Drug Info.
PO Box 2345   301-468-2600
Rockville, MD 20847-2345   800-729-6686
    www.health.org
Offers information on what parents and professionals can do to prevent drug use in America.

8503 Why Am I Afraid to Tell You Who I Am?
Hazelden
15251 Pleasant Valley Road   651-257-4010
Center City, MN 55012-9640   800-328-9000
    Fax: 651-213-4426
    www.hazelden.org
Outlines types of interpersonal relationships.

8504 Woman's Way Through the Twelve Steps
Hazelden
15251 Pleasant Valley Road   651-257-4010
Center City, MN 55012-9640   800-328-9000
    Fax: 651-213-4426
    www.hazelden.org
How women understnad and work the Twelve Steps of AA, including reflections of spirituality, powerlessness, and the emergence of a sense of the feminine soul.
228 pages Paperback
ISBN: 0-894869-93-0

8505 Young Teens: Who They Are and How to Talk to Them About Alcohol & Drugs
National Clearinghouse for Alcohol and Drug Info.
PO Box 2345
Rockville, MD 20847-2345   800-729-6686
Offers information on how parents, educators and concerned citizens can work together to help youngsters avoid alcohol and other drugs by understanding the risks and dangers.
57 pages

Children's Books

8506 Alcoholism
Franklin Watts Grolier
90 Old Sherman Tpke   203-797-3500
Danbury, CT 06816-0001   800-621-1115
    Fax: 203-797-3197
    www.grolier.com
This comprehensive overview describes the different types of alcoholism, the addictive personality and the warning signs.
112 pages Grades 7-12
ISBN: 0-531108-79-1

8507 Alcoholism and the Family
Franklin Watts Grolier
90 Old Sherman Tpke   203-797-3500
Danbury, CT 06816-0001   800-621-1115
    Fax: 203-797-3197
    www.grolier.com
This book, after discussing what alcoholism is, its effects on health and behavior modifications through alcohol, starts addressing one of the most important aspects of alcoholism, the effects on the family.
32 pages Grades 3-5
ISBN: 0-531125-48-3

8508 America's War on Drugs
Franklin Watts Grolier
90 Old Sherman Tpke   203-797-3500
Danbury, CT 06816   800-621-1115
    Fax: 203-797-3197
    www.grolier.com
An overview of the United States' attempts to combat illegal drugs on the supply side, from stopping the supply of drugs into the country.
160 pages Grades 7-12
ISBN: 0-531109-54-2

8509 Buzzy's Rebound
National Clearinghouse for Alcohol and Drug Info.

PO Box 2345
Rockville, MD 20847-2345   800-729-6686
A Fat Albert comic book that describes the pressure on a new kid in
town to drink.
18 pages

8510   Caffeine and Nicotine
Hazelden
15251 Pleasant Valley Road   651-257-4010
Center City, MN 55012-9640   800-328-9000
                                       Fax: 651-213-4426
                                          www.hazelden.org
Simple, clear, and accurate presentation of nicotine and caffeine
dependency. How to avoid these addictions, and why teens ought to
do so.
64 pages Paperback
ISBN: 1-568381-68-9

8511   Christy's Chance
Crestridge Corporate Center
10155 York Road   410-628-0390
Hunt Valley, MD 21030   Fax: 410-628-0398
                          e-mail: cboyce@networkpub.com
                                         www.networkpub.com
A story geared to younger teens that allows the reader to make a
nonuse decision about marijuana.

8512   Cocaine
Hazelden
15251 Pleasant Valley Road   651-257-4010
Center City, MN 55012-9640   800-328-9000
                                       Fax: 651-213-4426
                                          www.hazelden.org
The information that teens need to stay drug-free, promoting un-
derstanding of the ramifications, both social and personal.
64 pages Paperback
ISBN: 1-568381-64-6

8513   Coping with Codependency
Hazelden
15251 Pleasant Valley Road   651-257-4010
Center City, MN 55012-9640   800-328-9000
                                       Fax: 651-213-4426
                                          www.hazelden.org
Explains the cycle of codependency, describes its destructive effects on all involved, and suggests ways to break free and live in
more healthy relationships.
64 pages Paperback
ISBN: 1-568381-85-9

8514   Coping with Depression
Hazelden
15251 Pleasant Valley Road   651-257-4010
Center City, MN 55012-9640   800-328-9000
                                       Fax: 651-213-4426
                                          www.hazelden.org
Practical ways to cope with depression. Provides clear suggestions
for handling life's downers, and encourages readers to seek professional help when they feel they can't deal with problems themselves.
64 pages Paperback
ISBN: 1-568381-79-4

8515   Coping with Drinking and Driving
Hazelden
15251 Pleasant Valley Road   651-257-4010
Center City, MN 55012-9640   800-328-9000
                                       Fax: 651-213-4426
                                          www.hazelden.org
Addressing teens' illusion of invulnerability, the author describes
exactly how alcohol affects the body and one's driving skills, emphasizing that teens are not immune to alcohol's effects.
64 pages Paperback
ISBN: 1-568381-80-8

8516   Coping with Peer Pressure
Hazelden

15251 Pleasant Valley Road   651-257-4010
Center City, MN 55012-9640   800-328-9000
                                       Fax: 651-213-4426
                                          www.hazelden.org
Discussion of the positive and negative effects that members of a
peer group can have on each other and explores ways teens can handle the pressure they face.
64 pages Paperback
ISBN: 1-568381-83-2

8517   Coping with Stress
Hazelden
15251 Pleasant Valley Road   651-257-4010
Center City, MN 55012-9640   800-328-9000
                                       Fax: 651-213-4426
                                          www.hazelden.org
Outlines positive strategies to help teens learn to cope more effectively with stress, rather than turning to destructive outlets such as
drugs and even suicide.
64 pages Paperback
ISBN: 1-568381-76-X

8518   Coping with a Drug-Abusing Parent
Hazelden
15251 Pleasant Valley Road   651-257-4010
Center City, MN 55012-9640   800-328-9000
                                       Fax: 651-213-4426
                                          www.hazelden.org
Describes steps that teens, powerless to stop a drug-abusing parent
from continuing on that destructive path, can take to to learn to take
better care of themselves. Includes coping strategies and who to
call for help.
64 pages Paperback
ISBN: 1-568381-78-6

8519   Crack Down on Drugs
National Clearinghouse for Alcohol and Drug Info.
PO Box 2345
Rockville, MD 20847   800-729-6686
Coloring book for children featuring McGruff, the crime dog, that
teaches young children the importance of refusing alcohol and
drug abuse.
Ages 5-8

**8520   Different Like Me: A Book for Teens Who Worry About Their
Parents' Using**
Johnson Institute
Ohms Lane   612-831-1630
Edina, MN
Provides support and information for teens who are concerned,
confused, scared and angry because their parents abuse alcohol
and other drugs.
110 pages

8521   Drug Abuse: The Impact on Society
Franklin Watts Grolier
90 Old Sherman Tpke   203-797-3500
Danbury, CT 06816   800-621-1115
                                       Fax: 203-797-3197
                                          www.grolier.com
Discusses all major aspects of illegal drug usage and the health and
personality effects they cause.
144 pages Grades 7-12
ISBN: 0-531105-79-2

8522   Drugs and AIDS
Hazelden
15251 Pleasant Valley Road   651-257-4010
Center City, MN 55012-9640   800-328-9000
                                       Fax: 651-213-4426
                                          www.hazelden.org
Covers many topics through case studies, including the effects of
the disease on the body, transmission, homosexuality, condom use,
drug treatment, and peer pressure.
64 pages Paperback
ISBN: 1-568381-72-7

8523   Drugs and Anger
Hazelden

15251 Pleasant Valley Road
Center City, MN 55012-9640

651-257-4010
800-328-9000
Fax: 651-213-4426
www.hazelden.org

True-to-life scenarios and practical techniques found here can help teens cope constructively with their anger.
64 pages Paperback
ISBN: 1-568381-73-5

8524 Drugs and Depression
Hazelden
15251 Pleasant Valley Road
Center City, MN 55012-9640

651-257-4010
800-328-9000
Fax: 651-213-4426
www.hazelden.org

Describes positive ways of handling depression, as well as suggesting resources for receiving assistance.
64 pages Paperback
ISBN: 1-568381-74-3

8525 Drugs and Domestic Violence
Hazelden
15251 Pleasant Valley Road
Center City, MN 55012-9640

651-257-4010
800-328-9000
Fax: 651-213-4426
www.hazelden.org

Describes valuable coping tactics that can help teens stay safe in situations involving domestic violence and drug use.
64 pages Paperback
ISBN: 1-568381-75-1

8526 Drugs and Your Friends
Hazelden
15251 Pleasant Valley Road
Center City, MN 55012-9640

651-257-4010
800-328-9000
Fax: 651-213-4426
www.hazelden.org

Helps teens make sound decisions on vital choices and provides many suggestions for resisting peer pressure.
64 pages Paperback
ISBN: 1-568381-70-0

8527 Drugs and Your Parents
Hazelden
15251 Pleasant Valley Road
Center City, MN 55012-9640

651-257-4010
800-328-9000
Fax: 651-213-4426
www.hazelden.org

Practical advice for teenage children of parents addicted to alcohol or other drugs. How to cope initially with the situation as well as long-term survival strategies.
64 pages Paperback
ISBN: 1-568381-71-9

8528 Drugs in the Body: Effects of Abuse
Franklin Watts Grolier
90 Old Sherman Tpke
Danbury, CT 06816

203-797-3500
800-621-1115
Fax: 203-797-3197
www.grolier.com

Traces the effects of cocaine and crack, opium, morphine, heroine, marijuana and hashish, LSD and PCP in a person's system. Special emphasis is placed on long-term adverse effects in the body.
144 pages Grades 7-12
ISBN: 0-531125-07-6

8529 Elephant in the Living Room: The Children's Book
Hazelden
15251 Pleasant Valley Road
Center City, MN 55012-9640

651-257-4010
800-328-9000
Fax: 651-213-4426
www.hazelden.org

An activity book to help children understand and cope with the problem of chemical dependency in the family.
88 pages Paperback
ISBN: 1-568380-35-6

8530 Facts on Alcohol
Franklin Watts Grolier

90 Old Sherman Tpke
Danbury, CT 06816

203-797-3500
800-621-1115
Fax: 203-797-3197
www.grolier.com

Offers various information on alcohol so young children can have an opportunity to form their own opinions and the ability to make their own decisions when it comes to alcoholism.
32 pages Grades 5-7
ISBN: 0-531108-21-0

8531 Facts on the Crack and Cocaine Epidemic
Franklin Watts Grolier
90 Old Sherman Tpke
Danbury, CT 06816

203-797-3500
800-621-1115
Fax: 203-797-3197
www.grolier.com

Offers young children information on these deadly drugs to help them become informed.
32 pages Grades 5-7
ISBN: 0-531108-22-8

8532 Feed Your Head
Hazelden
15251 Pleasant Valley Road
Center City, MN 55012-9640

651-257-4010
800-328-9000
Fax: 651-213-4426
www.hazelden.org

Offers practical guidance for young people.
137 pages Paperback

8533 Gangs and Drugs
Hazelden
15251 Pleasant Valley Road
Center City, MN 55012-9640

651-257-4010
800-328-9000
Fax: 651-213-4426
www.hazelden.org

Encouraging and helpful message that goes beyond Just say no.
240 pages Paperback
ISBN: 1-568381-35-2

8534 How to Say No and Keep Your Friends
Hazelden
15251 Pleasant Valley Road
Center City, MN 55012-9640

651-257-4010
800-328-9000
Fax: 651-213-4426
www.hazelden.org

Ideas to help teens deal with negative peer pressure.
112 pages

8535 I Can Talk About What Hurts
Hazelden
15251 Pleasant Valley Road
Center City, MN 55012-9640

651-257-4010
800-328-9000
Fax: 651-213-4426
www.hazelden.org

Written and illustrated for children whose lives have been affected by someone else's chemical dependency.
56 pages Paperback

8536 I Wish Daddy Didn't Drink So Much
Judith Vigna, author

Albert Whitman & Company
6340 Oakton Street
Morton Grove, IL 60053-2723

847-581-0033
800-255-7675
Fax: 847-581-0039
e-mail: mail@awhitmanco.com
www.albertwhitman.com

A young girl shres her feelings and frustrations about her alcoholic father's behavior.
1993 32 pages Grades P-3
ISBN: 0-807535-23-0
Pat McPartland, Sales
Joe Campbell, Customer Service

8537 If Drugs Are So Bad, Why Do So Many People Use Them?
Hazelden
15251 Pleasant Valley Road
Center City, MN 55012-9640

651-257-4010
800-328-9000
Fax: 651-213-4426
www.hazelden.org

Uses direct language to explain drugs and their effects.
29 pages Grades 5-9

8538 In a Perfect World
Hazelden
15251 Pleasant Valley Road   651-257-4010
Center City, MN 55012-9640   800-328-9000
                                    Fax: 651-213-4426
                                    www.hazelden.org
Kevin thinks his world will be perfect when his father stops drinking, but Kevin is in for a few surprises.
160 pages Softcover

8539 Inhalants
Hazelden
15251 Pleasant Valley Road   651-257-4010
Center City, MN 55012-9640   800-328-9000
                                    Fax: 651-213-4426
                                    www.hazelden.org
Clear, straightforward explanation of the dangers and consequences of using seemingly harmless chemicals, such as model airplane glue, hair spray, whipping cream, and cleaning and lighter fluids, as well as sources of help for those who need it.
64 pages Paperback
ISBN: 1-568381-69-7

8540 Inside Out
Hazelden
15251 Pleasant Valley Road   651-257-4010
Center City, MN 55012-9640   800-328-9000
                                    Fax: 651-213-4426
                                    www.hazelden.org
Offers open-ended sentences for readers to fill in their responses.
97 pages Paperback

8541 Kids and Alcohol: Get High on Life
Health Communications
1721 Blount Road   954-360-0909
Pompano Beach, FL 33069
A workbook designed to help children make important decisions in their lives and feel good about themselves.
Ages 11-14

8542 Let's Talk About Drug Abuse
Rosen Publishing Group's PowerKids Press
29 E 21st Street   212-777-3017
New York, NY 10010   800-237-9932
                                    Fax: 888-436-4643
                                    e-mail: customerservice@rosenpub.com
                                    www.rosenpublishing.com
A first step in a child's education about the dangers of drugs. Recommended for grade K-4.

ISBN: 0-823923-02-9
Anna Kreiner, Author

8543 McGruff's Surprise Party
National Clearinghouse for Alcohol and Drug Info.
PO Box 2345
Rockville, MD 20847-2345   800-729-6686
A comic book that helps children understand the importance of refusing alcohol and other drugs.
14 pages Ages 8-10

8544 My Body is My House
Hazelden
15251 Pleasant Valley Road   651-257-4010
Center City, MN 55012   800-328-9000
                                    Fax: 651-213-4426
                                    www.hazelden.org
A coloring book about alcohol, drugs and health.
16 pages

8545 Sad Story of Mary Wanna or How Marijuana Harms You
Woodmere Press
PO Box 20
New York, NY 10025-0020
A comic book for children that contains pictures of the damage that marijuana does to the body.
40 pages Grades 1-4

8546 Should Drugs Be Legalized?
Franklin Watts Grolier

90 Old Sherman Tpke   203-797-3500
Danbury, CT 06816-0001   800-621-1115
                                    Fax: 203-797-3197
                                    www.grolier.com
Presents a discussion of this controversial subject.
160 pages Grades 7-12

8547 Smoking-At Issues Series
Greenhaven Press
Thomson Gale
Farmington Hills, MI 48333-9187   800-877-4253
                                    Fax: 800-414-5043
             e-mail: gale.customerservice@thomson.com
                                    www.gale.com/greenhaven
Written in a straightforward manner, this book answers questions most young adults are asking regarding smoking and health.

ISBN: 0-737701-57-9

8548 Stand Strong
African American Family Services
2616 Nicollet Avenue S   612-871-7878
Minneapolis, MN 55408
Comic book prevention for young adults. Profiles two African-American teens as they go through the hazards and risks of drug use and sexual behavior.
16 pages

8549 Summer of Sassy Jo
Houghton Mifflin
Wayside Road
Burlington, MA 01803   800-225-3362
A story of a thirteen-year-old girl faced with reconciliation with her recovered alcoholic mother after eight years of abandonment.
192 pages Grades 7+
ISBN: 0-395669-56-1

8550 Teen Alcoholism-Teen Issues
Lucent Books
Thomson Gale
San Diego, CA 48333-9187   800-877-4253
                                    Fax: 800-414-5043
             e-mail: gale.customerservice@thomson.com
                                    www.gale.com/lucent
Offers readable interviews for reports and answers the most frequently asked questions about alcohol.

ISBN: 1-590185-01-3

8551 Teen Guide to Pregnancy, Drugs and Smoking
Franklin Watts Grolier
90 Old Sherman Tpke   203-797-3500
Danbury, CT 06816-0001   800-621-1115
                                    Fax: 203-797-3197
                                    www.grolier.com
Outlines the risks of smoking and drug taking while pregnant and answers teenagers' questions about the use of legal, illegal and prescription drugs.
64 pages Grades 9-12
ISBN: 0-531108-35-0

8552 Understanding Drugs
Franklin Watts Grolier
90 Old Sherman Tpke   203-797-3500
Danbury, CT 06816-0001   800-621-1115
                                    Fax: 203-797-3197
                                    www.grolier.com
This series of books explains the current drug phenomenon at a high-interest, low-vocabulary level. Gives in-depth information about all aspects of commonly abused substances, including their negative mental, physical and social effects. Each book features photographs, diagrams, a glossary, an index and list of addresses for futher information and help. Set of seven volumes.
Grades 5-7

8553 Violence and Drugs
Franklin Watts Grolier

90 Old Sherman Tpke
Danbury, CT 06816-0001

203-797-3500
800-621-1115
Fax: 203-797-3197
www.grolier.com

This informative book studies the fascinating link between drug use and violent behavior.
112 pages Grades 9-12
ISBN: 0-531108-18-0

8554 What's Drunk Mama?
Al-Anon Family Group Headquarters
1600 Corporate Landing Parkway
Virginia Beach, VA 23454-5617

757-563-1600
800-425-2666
Fax: 757-563-1655
e-mail: wso@al-anon.org
www.al-anon.alateen.org

Large print illustrated booklet for use as a shared reading experience to help younger children understand alcoholism.
32 pages
Caryn Johnson, Director Communications

8555 Whiskers Says No to Drugs
Weekly Reader Skills Books
245 Long Hill Road
Middletown, CT 06457-4063

860-346-7157
www.weeklyreader.com

This book contains stories and follow-up activities for students to provide information and form attitudes before they face peer pressure to experiment.
Grades 2-3

8556 Why Do People Drink Alcohol?
Franklin Watts Grolier
90 Old Sherman Tpke
Danbury, CT 06816-0001

203-797-3500
800-621-1115
Fax: 203-797-3197
www.grolier.com

Answers young children's questions about alcoholism.
32 pages Grades 3-5
ISBN: 0-531171-34-5

8557 Why Do People Smoke?
Franklin Watts Grolier
90 Old Sherman Tpke
Danbury, CT 06816-0001

203-797-3500
800-621-1115
Fax: 203-797-3197
www.grolier.com

Raises and answers questions of specific interest to seven-to-ten year olds about smoking.
32 pages Grades 3-5
ISBN: 0-531171-92-2

8558 Why Do People Take Drugs?
Franklin Watts Grolier
90 Old Sherman Tpke
Danbury, CT 06816-0001

203-797-3500
800-621-1115
Fax: 203-797-3197
www.grolier.com

Raises important questions and offers some answers for young children on the aspects and everyday living with a drug addiction.
32 pages Grades 3-5
ISBN: 0-531171-13-2

8559 Winning the Battle Against Drugs: Rehabilitation Programs
Franklin Watts Grolier
90 Old Sherman Tpke
Danbury, CT 06816-0001

203-797-3500
800-621-1115
Fax: 203-797-3197
www.grolier.com

Programs contained in this book will help adolescents see that drug and alcohol addiction can be successfully treated.
160 pages Grades 7-12
ISBN: 0-531110-63-0

8560 Young Person's Guide to the Twelve Steps
Hazelden
15251 Pleasant Valley Road
Center City, MN 55012-9640

651-257-4010
800-328-9000
Fax: 651-213-4426
www.hazelden.org

Explains the Twelve Steps in the best way young people can understand: in their own language.
168 pages Paperback

8561 Young, Sober & Free
Hazelden
15251 Pleasant Valley Road
Center City, MN 55012-9640

651-257-4010
800-328-9000
Fax: 651-213-4426
www.hazelden.org

Features young peoples' personal experiences of living with addiction.
137 pages Paperback

Magazines

8562 ACAP Recap
American Council on Alcohol Problems
3426 Bridgeland Drive
Bridgeton, MO 63044-2603

314-739-5944
Fax: 314-739-0848

Offers information on organization activities and events, updates on resources and publications and legislative information for affiliate executives.
Monthly

8563 American Issue
American Council on Alcohol Problems
3426 Bridgeland Drive
Bridgeton, MO 63044-2603

314-739-5944
Fax: 314-739-0848

Offered to contributors of the organization.
Monthly

8564 Drug Abuse Update
2296 Henderson Mill Road
Atlanta, GA 30345-2739

770-934-6364

A journal of news and information for persons interested in drug prevention.
Quarterly

8565 Forum Magazine
Al-Anon Alateen Family Group Headquarters
1600 Corporate Landing Parkway
Virginia Beach, VA 10018-970

757-563-1600
888-425-2666
Fax: 757-563-1655
e-mail: wso@alanon.org
www.al-anon.alateen.org

Contains many personal stories of inspiration, some of which are maade available each month on the Internet by authorization of Al-Anon Family Group Headquarters, Inc.
Ric Buchanan, Executive Director

8566 Lead Line
Grapevine
PO Box 1980
New York, NY 10163-1980

212-870-3400
Fax: 212-870-3301

AA members all over the world communicate with each other through the pages of this magazine. It contains: insight into how AAs stay sober; readers' views; old-timers corner, beginners meeting, youth enjoying sobriety, and spotlight on service.
Monthly

Newsletters

8567 ADPA Professional
Alcohol/Drug Problems Association of North America
307 N Main Street
St. Charles, MO 63301

314-589-6702
Fax: 314-940-2358

Offers information to members on events, conferences and activities, reviews the newest resources and technology pertaining to alcoholism and drug addiction.

8568 Drug-Free Workplace Educator
American Council on Drug Education
204 Monroe Street
Rockville, MD 20850-4425

800-488-3784

Offers continuing education for employers and their supervisors responsible for substance abuse prevention. Practical articles fea-

ture information to help employers design, implement and maintain a drug-free workplace.
BiMonthly

8569 Just Say Notes
Just Say No International
2101 Webster Street   510-451-6666
Oakland, CA 94612-3065   800-258-2766
Offers information on the organizations, activities, programs, conferences and events.
BiMonthly

8570 RID-USA Newsletter
Remove Intoxicated Drivers (RID-USA)
PO Box 520   518-393-4357
Schenectady, NY 12301-0520   Fax: 518-370-4917
Membership news.
3x Year
Doris Aiken, President & CEO

8571 Sobering Thoughts
Women for Sobriety
PO Box 618   215-536-8026
Quakertown, PA 18951-0618   800-333-1606
Fax: 215-536-8026
e-mail: NewLife@nni.comcom
wwww.womenforsobriety.com
A monthly membership newsletter for women with an addiction problem who wish for recovery and start a new life.
16 pages Monthly
Rebecca Fenner, Director

8572 Substance Abuse Funding News
CD Publications
8204 Fenton Street   301-588-6380
Silver Spring, MD 20910-4571   800-666-6380
Fax: 301-588-6385
e-mail: chf@cdpublications.com
www.cdpublications.com
Detailed coverage of private and federal funding opportunities for alcohol, tobacco and drug abuse programs. Plus advice on successful grantseeking strategies and news affecting your programs.
18 pages BiWeekly
Mike Gerecht, Publisher
Amy Bernstein, Editor

Pamphlets

8573 AA Member: Medications and Other Drugs
Alcoholics Anonymous
PO Box 459   212-870-3400
New York, NY 10163-0459   Fax: 212-870-3137
Report from a group of doctors in Alcoholics Anonymous.

8574 AA Service Manual: Twelve Concepts for World Service
Alcoholics Anonymous
PO Box 459   212-870-3400
New York, NY 10163-0459   Fax: 212-870-3137
This manual opens with a history of AA services.

8575 AA and the Armed Services
Alcoholics Anonymous
PO Box 459   212-870-3400
New York, NY 10163-0459   Fax: 212-870-3137
Personal stories tell how men and women in the military can beat a drinking problem.

8576 AA and the Gay/Lesbian Alcoholic
Alcoholics Anonymous
PO Box 459   212-870-3400
New York, NY 10163-0459   Fax: 212-870-3137
Excerpts from experience, strength and hope of sober gay and lesbian alcoholics.

8577 AA as a Resource for Health Care Professionals
Alcoholics Anonymous
PO Box 459   212-870-3400
New York, NY 10163-0459   Fax: 212-870-3137

Information about the Fellowship and describes some approaches that health care professionals use in referring problem drinkers to AA.

8578 AA for the Native North American
Alcoholics Anonymous
PO Box 459   212-870-3400
New York, NY 10163-0459   Fax: 212-870-3137
Addressed to and contains stories by Native American AA members.

8579 AA for the Woman
Alcoholics Anonymous
PO Box 459   212-870-3400
New York, NY 10163-0459   Fax: 212-870-3137
Relates the experiences of alcoholic women, all ages and from all walks of life.

8580 AA in Correctional Facilities
Alcoholics Anonymous
PO Box 459   212-870-3400
New York, NY 10163-0459   Fax: 212-870-3137
Experience based on the functioning of AA groups in prisons, with institutional opinions recommending AA as a helpful ally.

8581 AA in Treatment Facilities
Alcoholics Anonymous
PO Box 459   212-870-3400
New York, NY 10163-0459   Fax: 212-870-3137
Shares experiences of treatment facility administrators and of AA's who have carried the message into these facilities.

8582 Acceptance
Hazelden
15251 Pleasant Valley Road   651-257-4010
Center City, MN 55012-9640   800-328-9000
Fax: 651-213-4426
www.hazelden.org
Addresses issues such as facing life, the kindness of God, suffering and contentment.

8583 Adult Children of Alcoholics Newcomer Packet
Al-Anon Family Group Headquarters
1600 Corporate Landing Parkway   757-563-1600
Virginia Beach, VA 23454-5617   800-425-2666
Fax: 757-563-1655
e-mail: wso@al-anon.org
www.al-anon.alateen.org
For those who have grown up with parental alcoholism, this is a loving introduction to Al-Anon and the twelve steps.
9 pieces
Caryn Johnson, Director Communications

8584 African Americans in Treatment
Hazelden
15251 Pleasant Valley Road   651-257-4010
Center City, MN 55012   800-328-9000
Fax: 651-213-4426
www.hazelden.org
Helps African American clients understand treatment from a cultural standpoint.
23 pages

8585 Al-Anon Newcomers Packet
Al-Anon Family Group Headquarters
1600 Corporate Landing Parkway   757-563-1600
Virginia Beach, VA 23454-5617   800-425-2666
Fax: 757-563-1655
e-mail: wso@al-anon.org
www.al-anon.alateen.org
Material specifically for the newcomer to Al-Anon packed in a handsome sleeve.
8 pieces
Caryn Johnson, Director Communications

8586 Al-Anon Spoken Here
Al-Anon Family Group Headquarters

1600 Corporate Landing Parkway
Virginia Beach, VA 23454-5617

757-563-1600
800-425-2666
Fax: 757-563-1655
e-mail: wso@al-anon.org
www.al-anon.alateen.org

Why are Al-Anon meetings the way they are? Questions and answers that lead to a better understanding of the importance of keeping Al-Anon principles.
8 pages
Caryn Johnson, Director Communications

8587   Al-Anon is for Men
Al-Anon Family Group Headquarters
1600 Corporate Landing Parkway
Virginia Beach, VA 23454-5617

757-563-1600
800-425-2666
Fax: 757-563-1655
e-mail: wso@al-anon.org
www.al-anon.alateen.org

Straight forward questions to help men identify their reactions to alcoholism in another person.
6 pages
Caryn Johnson, Director Communications

8588   Al-Anon, You and the Alcoholic
Al-Anon Family Group Headquarters
1600 Corporate Landing Parkway
Virginia Beach, VA 23454-5617

757-563-1600
800-425-2666
Fax: 757-563-1655
e-mail: wso@al-anon.org
www.al-anon.alateen.org

Answers the most frequently asked questions about Al-Anon and how it helps families deal with problems brought about by alcoholism.
12 pages
Caryn Johnson, Director Communications

8589   Alateen Newcomer Packet
Al-Anon Family Group Headquarters
1600 Corporate Landing Parkway
Virginia Beach, VA 23454-5617

757-563-1600
800-425-2666
Fax: 757-563-1655
e-mail: wso@al-anon.org
www.al-anon.alateen.org

Helpful leaflets assembled in a sleeve ready to give to the new young member.
13 pieces
Caryn Johnson, Director Communications

8590   Alateen Talk
Al-Anon Family Group Headquarters
1600 Corporate Landing Parkway
Virginia Beach, VA 23454-5617

757-563-1600
800-425-2666
Fax: 757-563-1655
e-mail: wso@al-anon.org
www.al-anon.alateen.org

Robert Schneider, Director Communications

8591   Alcohol Alert #11: Estimating the Cost of Alcohol Abuse
National Clearinghouse for Alcohol and Drug Info.
PO Box 2345
Rockville, MD 20847-2345

800-729-6686
www.health.org

Discusses the various problems of estimating the cost of alcohol abuse.

8592   Alcohol Alert #15: Alcohol and AIDS
National Clearinghouse for Alcohol and Drug Info.
PO Box 2345
Rockville, MD 20847-2345

800-729-6686
www.health.org

Discusses the relationship between alcohol consumption and HIV infection and AIDS.

8593   Alcohol Alert #16: Moderate Drinking
National Clearinghouse for Alcohol and Drug Info.
PO Box 2345
Rockville, MD 20847-2345

800-729-6686
www.health.org

Defines moderate drinking and explores the benefits and risks associated with moderate drinking.

8594   Alcohol Alert #17: Treatment Outcome Research
National Clearinghouse for Alcohol and Drug Info.
PO Box 2345
Rockville, MD 20847-2345

800-729-6686
www.health.org

Discusses purpose, methodology, randomization, blinding, followup and what treatment outcome research reveals.

8595   Alcohol Alert #18: The Genetics of Alcoholism
National Clearinghouse for Alcohol and Drug Info.
PO Box 2345
Rockville, MD 20847-2345

800-729-6686
www.health.org

Presents the results of studies that investigate the role of genes and the environment in the development of alcoholism.

8596   Alcohol Alert #21: Alcohol and Cancer
National Clearinghouse for Alcohol and Drug Info.
PO Box 2345
Rockville, MD 20847-2345

800-729-6686
www.health.org

8597   Alcohol Alert #23: Alcohol and Minorities
National Clearinghouse for Alcohol and Drug Info.
PO Box 2345
Rockville, MD 20847-2345

800-729-6686
www.health.org

8598   Alcohol Alert #24: Animal Models in Alcohol Research
National Clearinghouse for Alcohol and Drug Info.
PO Box 2345
Rockville, MD 20847-2345

800-729-6686
www.health.org

8599   Alcohol Alert #25: Alcohol-Related Impairment
National Clearinghouse for Alcohol and Drug Info.
PO Box 2345
Rockville, MD 20847-2345

800-729-6686
www.health.org

8600   Alcohol Alert #26: Alcohol and Hormones
National Clearinghouse for Alcohol and Drug Info.
PO Box 2345
Rockville, MD 20847-2345

800-729-6686
www.health.org

8601   Alcohol Alert #27: Alcohol Medication Interactions
National Clearinghouse for Alcohol and Drug Info.
PO Box 2345
Rockville, MD 20847-2345

800-729-6686
www.health.org

8602   Alcohol and Drug Abuse in Black America: A Guide for Community Action
African American Family Services
2616 Nicollet Avenue S
Minneapolis, MN 55408

612-871-7878

A booklet giving a description of the history and the current manifestations of alcohol and drug problems in Black America with a discussion of strategies for fundamental change.
24 pages

8603   Alcohol and Pregnancy
March of Dimes
233 Park Avenue South
New York, NY 10003

212-353-8353
Fax: 212-254-3518
e-mail: NY639@marchofdimes.com
www.marchofdimes.com

8604   Alcoholics Anonymous and Employee Assistance Program
Alcoholics Anonymous
PO Box 459
New York, NY 10163-0459

212-870-3400
Fax: 212-870-3137

Of interest to management and union officials, this pamphlet gives concise descriptions of the help AA can offer to the alcoholic employee.

8605   Alcoholism Tends to Run in Families
National Clearinghouse for Alcohol and Drug Info.
PO Box 2345
Rockville, MD 20847-2345

800-729-6686
www.health.org

Provides answers and questions about how to help children of alcoholics and where to find resources for additional information.

8606 Alcoholism: A Merry-Go-Round Named Denial
Al-Anon Family Group Headquarters
1600 Corporate Landing Parkway   757-563-1600
Virginia Beach, VA 23454-5617   800-425-2666
                                   Fax: 757-563-1655
                               e-mail: wso@al-anon.org
                               www.al-anon.alateen.org
Dramatic explanations that help family members and friends see the roles they play in the problems of alcoholism.
18 pages
Caryn Johnson, Director Communications

8607 Alcoholism: The Family Disease
Al-Anon Family Group Headquarters
1600 Corporate Landing Parkway   757-563-1600
Virginia Beach, VA 23454-5617   800-425-2666
                                   Fax: 757-563-1655
                               e-mail: wso@al-anon.org
                               www.al-anon.alateen.org
A treasury of information and inspiration with the purpose of the Al-Anon program, actual stories of people who found serenity in Al-Anon, questions/answers, slogans, evaluations and thoughts to live by.
48 pages
Caryn Johnson, Director Communications

8608 Anabolic Steroids: A Threat to Body and Mind
National Clearinghouse for Alcohol and Drug Info.
PO Box 2345
Rockville, MD 20847   800-729-6686
Summarizes the findings of recent studies on the use of anabolic steroids in the United States.
11 pages

8609 Anonymity
Al-Anon Family Group Headquarters
1600 Corporate Landing Parkway   757-563-1600
Virginia Beach, VA 23454-5617   800-425-2666
                                   Fax: 757-563-1655
                               e-mail: wso@al-anon.org
                               www.al-anon.alateen.org
Offers information on Al-Anon and Alateen traditions and what a big factor anonymity plays for members.
6 pages
Caryn Johnson, Director Communications

8610 Are You Concerned About Someone's Drinking
Al-Anon Family Group Headquarters
1600 Corporate Landing Parkway   757-563-1600
Virginia Beach, VA 23454-5617   800-425-2666
                                   Fax: 757-563-1655
                               e-mail: wso@al-anon.org
                               www.al-anon.alateen.org
12 pages
Caryn Johnson, Director Communications

8611 Be Kind to Nonsmokers
American Lung Association
1740 Broadway   212-315-8700
New York, NY 10019-4315
Explains why smoke hurts nonsmokers.

8612 Best of Public Outreach
Al-Anon Family Group Headquarters
1600 Corporate Landing Parkway   757-563-1600
Virginia Beach, VA 23454-5617   800-425-2666
                                   Fax: 757-563-1655
                               e-mail: wso@al-anon.org
                               www.al-anon.alateen.org
Helps groups, committees and individuals carry out their PI institutions and CPC activities; includes suggested activities and open letters to various professionals.
24 pages
Caryn Johnson, Director Communications

8613 Black, Beautiful and Recovering
Hazelden

15251 Pleasant Valley Road   651-257-4010
Center City, MN 55012-9640   800-328-9000
                                   Fax: 651-213-4426
                               www.hazelden.org
20 pages

8614 Chemical Dependency and the African American
Hazelden
15251 Pleasant Valley Road   651-257-4010
Center City, MN 55012-9640   800-328-9000
                                   Fax: 651-213-4426
                               www.hazelden.org
Reviews the impact alcohol and other drug abuse has on African American communities.
66 pages

8615 Chemical Dependency: An Acceptable Disease
Hazelden
15251 Pleasant Valley Road   651-257-4010
Center City, MN 55012-9640   800-328-9000
                                   Fax: 651-213-4426
                               www.hazelden.org
Help persons identify and acknowledge their chemical dependency.
14 pages

8616 Chew or Snuff is Real Bad Stuff
National Cancer Institute
Building 31   301-496-4000
Bethesda, MD 20892
A pamphlet describing the hazards of using smokeless tobacco.
8 pages

8617 Cigarette Smoking
American Lung Association
1740 Broadway   212-315-8700
New York, NY 10019-4315
Leaflet presenting the facts about how cigarette smoke is related to lung disease.

8618 Communication Skills
Hazelden
15251 Pleasant Valley Road   651-257-4010
Center City, MN 55012-9640   800-328-9000
                                   Fax: 651-213-4426
                               www.hazelden.org
Helps clients discover how to become better listeners.

8619 Community Campaign Brochure
National Clearinghouse for Alcohol and Drug Info.
PO Box 2345
Rockville, MD 20847-2345   800-729-6686
Information and promotional brochure discusses key prevention concepts and messages and details how to plan campaign events.

8620 Crack
Hazelden
15251 Pleasant Valley Road   651-257-4010
Center City, MN 55012-9640   800-328-9000
                                   Fax: 651-213-4426
                               www.hazelden.org
Explains history, use and effects of crack cocaine.

8621 Crack Cocaine: The Big Lie
National Clearinghouse for Alcohol and Drug Info.
PO Box 2345
Rockville, MD 20847-2345   800-729-6686
                               www.health.org
Offers information on what crack and cocaine are, how strong the addictions are from these drugs, how they affect the body and other risks in taking cocaine and crack.

8622 Crossing the Line Between Social Drinking and Alcoholism
Hazelden
15251 Pleasant Valley Road   651-257-4010
Center City, MN 55012-9640   800-328-9000
                                   Fax: 651-213-4426
                               www.hazelden.org
20 pages

8623 Denial
Hazelden
15251 Pleasant Valley Road   651-257-4010
Center City, MN 55012-9640   800-328-9000
Fax: 651-213-4426
www.hazelden.org
Describes denial and its role in the five-stage acceptance process.

8624 Depression and Recovery from Chemical Dependency
Hazelden
15251 Pleasant Valley Road   651-257-4010
Center City, MN 55012-9640   800-328-9000
Fax: 651-213-4426
www.hazelden.org
Outlines depression's warning signs.

8625 Detaching with Love
Hazelden
15251 Pleasant Valley Road   651-257-4010
Center City, MN 55012-9640   800-328-9000
Fax: 651-213-4426
www.hazelden.org
Addresses the essential recovery tools clients need to cope with addiction and detach from the problem.

8626 Detachment
Al-Anon Family Group Headquarters
1600 Corporate Landing Parkway   757-563-1600
Virginia Beach, VA 23454-5617   800-425-2666
Fax: 757-563-1655
e-mail: wso@al-anon.org
www.al-anon.alateen.org
Everything you always wanted to know about detachment in an easy-to-use leaflet.
Caryn Johnson, Director Communications

8627 Did You Grow Up with a Problem Drinker?
Al-Anon Family Group Headquarters
1600 Corporate Landing Parkway   757-563-1600
Virginia Beach, VA 23454-5617   800-425-2666
Fax: 757-563-1655
e-mail: wso@al-anon.org
www.al-anon.alateen.org
Twenty personal questions help individuals decide if they can benefit from Al-Anon.
Caryn Johnson, Director Communications

8628 Do You Think You're Different?
Alcoholics Anonymous
PO Box 459   212-870-3400
New York, NY 10163-0459   Fax: 212-870-3137
Speaks to newcomers who may wonder how AA can work for someone different.

8629 Don't Let Your Dreams Go Up in Smoke
American Lung Association
1740 Broadway   212-315-8700
New York, NY 10019-4315
Photos, testimonials and clear language to deliver the message that everyone can and should stop smoking.

8630 Don't Lose a Friend to Drugs
National Crime Prevention Council
1000 Connecticut Avenue NW   202-466-6272
Washington, DC 20036-3802   Fax: 202-296-1356
www.ncpc.org
Offers practical advice to teenagers on how to say no to drugs, how to help a friend who uses drugs and how to initiate community efforts to prevent drug use.

8631 Drinking Alcohol During Pregnancy
March of Dimes
233 Park Avenue South   212-353-8353
New York, NY 10003   Fax: 212-254-3518
e-mail: NY639@marchofdimes.com
www.marchofdimes.com
Fact Sheets: one to two page review written for the general public. Also available electronically from the website www.marchofdimes.com

8632 Drug Free Zones: A Manual
African American Family Services
2616 Nicollet Avenue S   612-871-7878
Minneapolis, MN 55408
This booklet describes a variety of strategies concerned citizens are using to reclaim their neighborhoods from rampant drug abuse and dealing.
24 pages

8633 Drugs and Pregnancy
March of Dimes
233 Park Avenue South   212-353-8353
New York, NY 10003   Fax: 212-254-3518
e-mail: NY639@marchofdimes.com
www.marchofdimes.com
Brochures: 3 panel color brochures written for the general public.
pkg 50

8634 Employer's Guide to Dealing with Substance Abuse
National Clearinghouse for Alcohol and Drug Info.
PO Box 2345
Rockville, MD 20847-2345   800-729-6686
www.health.org
Instructs employers in setting up comprehensive alcohol and other drug programs in the workplace.
18 pages

8635 Enabling
Hazelden
15251 Pleasant Valley Road   651-257-4010
Center City, MN 55012-9640   800-328-9000
Fax: 651-213-4426
www.hazelden.org
Describes problems families encounter when they focus their lives on their chemically dependent family member.

8636 Facts About Alateen
Al-Anon Family Group Headquarters
1600 Corporate Landing Parkway   757-563-1600
Virginia Beach, VA 23454-5617   800-425-2666
Fax: 757-563-1655
e-mail: wso@al-anon.org
www.al-anon.alateen.org
Offers information on Alateen member services.
4 pages
Caryn Johnson, Director Communications

8637 Facts About Alcohol Abuse
Medical Arts Center Hospital
57 W 57th Street   212-838-2169
New York, NY 10019-2802   Fax: 212-755-0200
A question and answer pamphlet that offers information on alcohol abuse and the effects the abuse has on the family unit.

8638 Family Denial
Hazelden
15251 Pleasant Valley Road   651-257-4010
Center City, MN 55012-9640   800-328-9000
Fax: 651-213-4426
www.hazelden.org
Describes ways for families to recognize denial, examine common fears that cause denial and develop methods for overcoming it.

8639 Fetal Alcohol Syndrome
Hazelden
15251 Pleasant Valley Road   651-257-4010
Center City, MN 55012-9640   800-328-9000
Fax: 651-213-4426
www.hazelden.org
A source of information about the effects of drinking while pregnant.

8640 Fight Drug Abuse at Home, Work, School and in the Community
American Council for Drug Education
204 Monroe Street
Rockville, MD 20850-4425   800-488-3784
A catalog of print and video materials pertaining to substance abuse, alcoholism and drugs.

8641 For a Strong and Healthy Baby
National Clearinghouse for Alcohol and Drug Info.

PO Box 2345
Rockville, MD 20847-2345   800-729-6686
                                  www.health.org
Recommends that women not drink or use other drugs if pregnant or planning to become pregnant.

8642 Free to Care
Hazelden
15251 Pleasant Valley Road   651-257-4010
Center City, MN 55012-9640   800-328-9000
                                  Fax: 651-213-4426
                                  www.hazelden.org
Explores today's definition of family and new attitudes about gender, technology, single-parents, relatives and friends.

8643 Freedom from Despair
Al-Anon Family Group Headquarters
1600 Corporate Landing Parkway   757-563-1600
Virginia Beach, VA 23454-5617   800-425-2666
                                  Fax: 757-563-1655
                                  e-mail: wso@al-anon.org
                                  www.al-anon.alateen.org
A message of hope for those faced with a problem they can't solve alone.
4 pages
Caryn Johnson, Director Communications

8644 Freedom from Smoking Flyer
American Lung Association
1740 Broadway   212-315-8700
New York, NY 10019-4315
4 color flyer describing all FFS programs.

8645 Getting in Touch with Al-Anon/Alateen
Al-Anon Family Group Headquarters
1600 Corporate Landing Parkway   757-563-1600
Virginia Beach, VA 23454-5617   800-425-2666
                                  Fax: 757-563-1655
                                  e-mail: wso@al-anon.org
                                  www.al-anon.alateen.org
A listing of Al-Anon information services throughout the world. Helps members, the public and professionals located nearby Al-Anon or Alateen groups.
Caryn Johnson, Director Communications

8646 Grieving
Hazelden
15251 Pleasant Valley Road   651-257-4010
Center City, MN 55012-9640   800-328-9000
                                  Fax: 651-213-4426
                                  www.hazelden.org
Outlines the five-phase grieving process for clients and the significance of each.

8647 Guidance on Our Journeys
Hazelden
15251 Pleasant Valley Road   651-257-4010
Center City, MN 55012-9640   800-328-9000
                                  Fax: 651-213-4426
                                  www.hazelden.org
Examines the relationship between the recovering person and his or her sponsor.

8648 Guide for the Family of the Alcoholic
Al-Anon Family Group Headquarters
1600 Corporate Landing Parkway   757-563-1600
Virginia Beach, VA 23454-5617   800-425-2666
                                  Fax: 757-563-1655
                                  e-mail: wso@al-anon.org
                                  www.al-anon.alateen.org
A clear and realistic look at alcoholism, problems encountered by those close to the alcoholic and choices available to the family.
16 pages
Caryn Johnson, Director Communications

8649 Have Fun! Figure Out the Smoking Puzzle
American Lung Association
1740 Broadway   212-315-8700
New York, NY 10019-4315
Crossword puzzles make stimulating points on the effects of smoking.

8650 Healthy Beginning, Promotional Flyers
American Lung Association
1740 Broadway   212-315-8700
New York, NY 10019-4315
Flyer offers tips to help protect newborn and young children from the harmful effects of passive smoking.

8651 Help a Friend to Stop Smoking
American Lung Association
1740 Broadway   212-315-8700
New York, NY 10019-4315
This original guide to helping family members and friends support a smoker who is trying to quit smoking.
12 pages

8652 Helping Smokers Get Ready to Quit
American Lung Association
1740 Broadway   212-315-8700
New York, NY 10019-4315
Offers suggestions on how to get smokers to think about quitting and how to open up a dialogue on the issue.

8653 Helping Your Child Say No: A Parent's Guide
National Clearinghouse for Alcohol and Drug Info.
PO Box 2345
Rockville, MD 20847-2345   800-729-6686
Explains to parents how alcohol affects the body, how to tell if your child has been drinking and why children start to drink.

8654 Homeward Bound
Al-Anon Family Group Headquarters
1600 Corporate Landing Parkway   757-563-1600
Virginia Beach, VA 23454-5617   800-425-2666
                                  Fax: 757-563-1655
                                  e-mail: wso@al-anon.org
                                  www.al-anon.alateen.org
A booklet designed to help beginners make the transition from the family treatment setting to Al-Anon. Contains forty members' personal sharings, a basic glossary of Al-Anon terms, brief explanations of Al-Anon slogans and helpful suggestions for newcomers.
48 pages
Caryn Johnson, Director Communications

8655 How Can I Help My Children?
Al-Anon Family Group Headquarters
1600 Corporate Landing Parkway   757-563-1600
Virginia Beach, VA 23454-5617   800-425-2666
                                  Fax: 757-563-1655
                                  e-mail: wso@al-anon.org
                                  www.al-anon.alateen.org
Parents can help their children achieve a healthier attitude. Improving our own attitudes and behavior will help the entire family.
20 pages
Caryn Johnson, Director Communications

8656 How Drug Abuse Takes Profit Out of Business
National Clearinghouse for Alcohol and Drug Info.
PO Box 2345
Rockville, MD 20847-2345   800-729-6686
Answers employers questions about substance abuse in the workplace.

8657 How to Get the Most Out of Group Therapy
Hazelden
15251 Pleasant Valley Road   651-257-4010
Center City, MN 55012-9640   800-328-9000
                                  Fax: 651-213-4426
                                  www.hazelden.org
Answers clients' questions about going to and getting help from group therapy.

8658 How to Help a Friend Quit Smoking
American Lung Association
1740 Broadway   212-315-8700
New York, NY 10019-4315
Discusses how friends, family and co-workers can assist smokers with their concerns about quitting smoking.

8659 How to Take Care of Your Baby Before Birth
National Clearinghouse for Alcohol and Drug Info.

625

PO Box 2345
Rockville, MD 20847-2345 800-729-6686
www.health.org
A low-literacy brochure aimed at pregnant women that describes what they should and should not do during pregnancy.

8660 I Can't Be Addicted Because...
Hazelden
15251 Pleasant Valley Road 651-257-4010
Center City, MN 55012-9640 800-328-9000
Fax: 651-213-4426
www.hazelden.org
Focuses on denial and elaborates on its most common forms.

8661 Ice Storm
Hazelden
15251 Pleasant Valley Road 651-257-4010
Center City, MN 55012-9640 800-328-9000
Fax: 651-213-4426
www.hazelden.org
Prepares treatment professionals for the complications of one of the most recently synthesized drugs - ice.

8662 If Someone Close to You Has a Problem with Alcohol or Other Drugs
National Clearinghouse for Alcohol and Drug Info.
PO Box 2345
Rockville, MD 20847-2345 800-729-6686
www.health.org
This booklet is aimed at the general public and gives support and suggestions on coping with someone close who has an alcohol or drug problem.

8663 If You Are a Professional, AA Wants to Work with You
Alcoholics Anonymous
PO Box 459 212-870-3400
New York, NY 10163-0459 Fax: 212-870-3137
Directed at professionals of all types who deal with alcoholics.

8664 If Your Parents Drink Too Much
Al-Anon Family Group Headquarters
1600 Corporate Landing Parkway 757-563-1600
Virginia Beach, VA 23454-5617 800-425-2666
Fax: 757-563-1655
e-mail: wso@al-anon.org
www.al-anon.alateen.org
Alateen's cartoon booklet.
24 pages
Caryn Johnson, Director Communications

8665 Illicit Drug Use During Pregnancy
March of Dimes
233 Park Avenue South 212-353-8353
New York, NY 10003 Fax: 212-254-3518
e-mail: NY639@marchofdimes.com
www.marchofdimes.com
Fact Sheets: one to two page review for the general public. Also available electronically from the website www.marchofdimes.com

8666 Index to Alcoholics Anonymous
Hazelden
15251 Pleasant Valley Road 651-257-4010
Center City, MN 55012-9640 800-328-9000
Fax: 651-213-4426
Features page and line references to the topics discussed in Alcoholics Anonymous, the Big Book.

8667 Is AA for Me?
Alcoholics Anonymous
PO Box 459 212-870-3400
New York, NY 10163-0459 Fax: 212-870-3137
An illustrated easy to read version of the 12 questions in Is AA for You? pamphlet.
32 pages

8668 Is AA for You?
Alcoholics Anonymous
PO Box 459 212-870-3400
New York, NY 10163-0459 Fax: 212-870-3137

Symptoms of alcoholism are summed up in 12 questions most AA's had answered to identify themselves as alcoholics.

8669 Is There a Safe Tobacco?
American Lung Association
1740 Broadway 212-315-8700
New York, NY 10019-4315
Offers information on the health risks of cigarette smoking, pipes and cigars.

8670 Is There an Alcoholic in Your Life?
Alcoholics Anonymous
PO Box 459 212-870-3400
New York, NY 10163-0459 Fax: 212-870-3137
Explains the AA program as it affects anyone close to an alcoholic.

8671 It Happened to Alice
Alcoholics Anonymous
PO Box 459 212-870-3400
New York, NY 10163-0459 Fax: 212-870-3137
Easy to read comic-book style format for women alcoholics.

8672 It Sure Beats Sitting in a Cell
Alcoholics Anonymous
PO Box 459 212-870-3400
New York, NY 10163-0459 Fax: 212-870-3137
An illustrated pamphlet which presents the experience of seven inmates who found AA while in prison. It also offers suggested dos and don'ts for staying sober after release.

8673 Kids and Drugs: A Handbook for Parents & Professionals
PANDAA Press
4111 Watkins Trl 703-750-9285
Annandale, VA 22003-2051

8674 Let's Solve the Smokeword Puzzle
American Lung Association
1740 Broadway 212-315-8700
New York, NY 10019-4315
Fifth graders will love getting an antismoking message through solving a crossword puzzle.

8675 Let's Talk
Hazelden
15251 Pleasant Valley Road 651-257-4010
Center City, MN 55012-9640 800-328-9000
Fax: 651-213-4426
www.hazelden.org
Offers 12 guidelines to promote effective communication between parent and child.

8676 Letter to a Woman Alcoholic
Alcoholics Anonymous
PO Box 459 212-870-3400
New York, NY 10163-0459 Fax: 212-870-3137
Describes with sensitive understanding the problem of the alcoholic woman.

8677 Letting Go of the Need to Control
Hazelden
15251 Pleasant Valley Road 651-257-4010
Center City, MN 55012-9640 800-328-9000
Fax: 651-213-4426
www.hazelden.org
Discusses how control issues are common among chemically dependent people.

8678 Lifetime of Freedom from Smoking: Maintenance Manual
American Lung Association
1740 Broadway 212-315-8700
New York, NY 10019-4315
Companion manual helps persons stay quit once they have stopped smoking.
28 pages

8679 Little More About Alcohol
Alcohol Research Information Service
1120 E Oakland Avenue 517-485-9900
Lansing, MI 48906-5513 Fax: 517-485-1928
e-mail: alcoholisadrugtoo@yoyoger.net

A cartoon character explains the facts about alcohol and its effects on the body.

8680 Living Sober
Alcoholics Anonymous
PO Box 459   212-870-3400
New York, NY 10163-0459   Fax: 212-870-3137
Practical book demonstrating through simple examples, how AA members throughout the world live and stay sober one day at a time.
88 pages

8681 Living in a Shelter?
Al-Anon Family Group Headquarters
1600 Corporate Landing Parkway   757-563-1600
Virginia Beach, VA 23454-5617   800-425-2666
                                                      Fax: 757-563-1655
                                        e-mail: wso@al-anon.org
                                        www.al-anon.alateen.org
100 pieces
Caryn Johnson, Director Communications

8682 Look at Cross-Addiction
Hazelden
15251 Pleasant Valley Road   651-257-4010
Center City, MN 55012-9640   800-328-9000
                                                      Fax: 651-213-4426
Discusses cross-addiction, denial, coping skills and avoidance.

8683 Look at Relapse
Hazelden
15251 Pleasant Valley Road   651-257-4010
Center City, MN 55012-9640   800-328-9000
                                                      Fax: 651-213-4426
Addresses emotional consequences of relapse, such as decreased feelings of self-esteem and self-confidence.

8684 Managing Cocaine Cravings
Hazelden
15251 Pleasant Valley Road   651-257-4010
Center City, MN 55012-9640   800-328-9000
                                                      Fax: 651-213-4426
                                             www.hazelden.org
Offers clients hands-on plan to help them stay away from cocaine.

8685 Marijuana
Hazelden
15251 Pleasant Valley Road   651-257-4010
Center City, MN 55012-9640   800-328-9000
                                                      Fax: 651-213-4426
                                             www.hazelden.org
Outlines the physical and psychological effects of marijuana unique to episodic and chronic use.
65 pages

8686 Media Kit
Al-Anon Family Group Headquarters
1600 Corporate Landing Parkway   757-563-1600
Virginia Beach, VA 23454-5617   800-425-2666
                                                      Fax: 757-563-1655
                                        e-mail: wso@al-anon.org
                                        www.al-anon.alateen.org
An attractive silver folder containing information necessary to work with radio and TV stations.
Caryn Johnson, Director Communications

8687 Member's Eye View of Alcoholics Anonymous
Alcoholics Anonymous
PO Box 459   212-870-3400
New York, NY 10163-0459   Fax: 212-870-3137
Designed to explain to people in the helping professionals how AA works.
30 pages

8688 Members of the Clergy Ask About Alcoholics Anonymous
Alcoholics Anonymous
PO Box 459   212-870-3400
New York, NY 10163-0459   Fax: 212-870-3137
Introduction to AA for members of the clergy unfamiliar with the Fellowship.

8689 Memo to an Inmate Who May Be an Alcoholic
Alcoholics Anonymous
PO Box 459   212-870-3400
New York, NY 10163-0459   Fax: 212-870-3137
A message from AA's who have themselves been inmates. Their personal stories offer a new outlook to inmate alcholics who want to know who AA can help.

8690 Men Newcomer Packet
Al-Anon Family Group Headquarters
1600 Corporate Landing Parkway   757-563-1600
Virginia Beach, VA 23454-5617   800-425-2666
                                                      Fax: 757-563-1655
                                        e-mail: wso@al-anon.org
                                        www.al-anon.alateen.org
For men who are not sure Al-Anon is for them, this collection offers a realistic look at alcoholism and straight forward answers to frequently asked questions.
8 pieces
Caryn Johnson, Director Communications

8691 Message to Correctional Facilities Administrators
Alcoholics Anonymous
PO Box 459   212-870-3400
New York, NY 10163-0459   Fax: 212-870-3137
Information about what AA is and can do, and how groups function in correctional facilities.

8692 Message to Teenagers
Alcoholics Anonymous
PO Box 459   212-870-3400
New York, NY 10163-0459   Fax: 212-870-3137
This brochure offers a simple, 12-question quiz designed to help teenagers decide when drinking is becoming a problem in their lives.

8693 Military Packet
Al-Anon Family Group Headquarters
1600 Corporate Landing Parkway   757-563-1600
Virginia Beach, VA 23454-5617   800-425-2666
                                                      Fax: 757-563-1655
                                        e-mail: wso@al-anon.org
                                        www.al-anon.alateen.org
For those in the armed services with loved ones or colleagues who are alcoholic, here's a collection that says, Al-Anon can help.
7 pieces
Caryn Johnson, Director Communications

8694 Moment to Reflect on Codependency
Hazelden
15251 Pleasant Valley Road   651-257-4010
Center City, MN 55012-9640   800-328-9000
                                                      Fax: 651-213-4426
A collection of four booklets offering meditations that emphasize and reinforce self-esteem for young people recovering from addiction.

8695 Moment to Reflect on Self-Esteem
Hazelden
15251 Pleasant Valley Road   651-257-4010
Center City, MN 55012-9640   800-328-9000
                                                      Fax: 651-213-4426
Focuses on the fundamental recovery issue of self-esteem.
4 Booklets

8696 Moving On! From Alateen to Al-Anon
Al-Anon Family Group Headquarters
1600 Corporate Landing Parkway   757-563-1600
Virginia Beach, VA 23454-5617   800-425-2666
                                                      Fax: 757-563-1655
                                        e-mail: wso@al-anon.org
                                        www.al-anon.alateen.org
Former Alateen members experience the joy of continued recovery in Al-Anon.
12 pages
Caryn Johnson, Director Communications

8697 NIDA Capsules
National Clearinghouse for Alcohol and Drug Info.

PO Box 2345
Rockville, MD 20847-2345 800-729-6686
www.health.org

8698 Newcomer Asks
Alcoholics Anonymous
PO Box 459 212-870-3400
New York, NY 10163-0459 Fax: 212-870-3137
Gives straightforward answers on 15 points that once puzzled many of us.

8699 Nicotine Addiction and Cigarettes
American Lung Association
1740 Broadway 212-315-8700
New York, NY 10019-4315
Offers information on nicotine and cigarette smoking.

8700 No Smoking Coloring Book
American Lung Association
1740 Broadway 212-315-8700
New York, NY 10019-4315
Preschool and primary grade children will enjoy drawing and coloring while getting an antismoking message.

8701 No Smoking: Lungs At Work
American Lung Association
1740 Broadway 212-315-8700
New York, NY 10019-4315
Describes how lungs work and how they are affected by smoking.

8702 Now What Do I Do for Fun?
Hazelden
15251 Pleasant Valley Road 651-257-4010
Center City, MN 55012-9640 800-328-9000
Fax: 651-213-4426
www.hazelden.org
Explores the dilemma of finding new interests in recovery after completing treatment.

8703 Older Adults After Treatment
Hazelden
15251 Pleasant Valley Road 651-257-4010
Center City, MN 55012-9640 800-328-9000
Fax: 651-213-4426
www.hazelden.org
Discusses aftercare issues, such as family relations, health, medication and relapse.

8704 Older Adults in Treatment
Hazelden
15251 Pleasant Valley Road 651-257-4010
Center City, MN 55012-9640 800-328-9000
Fax: 651-213-4426
www.hazelden.org
Examines past beliefs about addiction and defines chemical dependency as a disease.

8705 On the Air: A Guide to Creating A Smoke-Free Workplace
American Lung Association
1740 Broadway 212-315-8700
New York, NY 10019-4315
A step-by-step guide for organizations interested in developing and implementing a successful workplace smoking control policy.
24 pages

8706 Parents Newcomer Packet
Al-Anon Family Group Headquarters
1600 Corporate Landing Parkway 757-563-1600
Virginia Beach, VA 23454-5617 800-425-2666
Fax: 757-563-1655
e-mail: wso@al-anon.org
www.al-anon.alateen.org
For parents who realize their child is an alcoholic, this is a compassionate and reassuring welcome to Al-Anon.
9 pieces
Caryn Johnson, Director Communications

8707 Points for Parents Perplexed About Drugs
Hazelden

15251 Pleasant Valley Road 651-257-4010
Center City, MN 55012-9640 800-328-9000
Fax: 651-213-4426
www.hazelden.org
Clear guidelines to help adults recognize, evaluate and deal with adolescent drug abuse.
16 pages

8708 Preventing Relapse
Hazelden
15251 Pleasant Valley Road 651-257-4010
Center City, MN 55012-9640 800-328-9000
Fax: 651-213-4426
www.hazelden.org
Offers practical information and personal stories to help clients better understand the relapse process.
28 pages

8709 Program Booklet
Women for Sobriety
PO Box 618 215-536-8026
Quakertown, PA 18951-0618 Fax: 215-536-8026
e-mail: WFSobriety@aol.com
www.womenforsobriety.org
Purse size booklet that explains the Thirteen Statements of Dr. Kirkpatrick's New Life program, statement by statement.

8710 Put on the Brakes Bulletin: Take a Look at College Drinking
National Clearinghouse for Alcohol and Drug Info.
PO Box 2345
Rockville, MD 20847-2345 800-729-6686
www.health.org
This second edition continues CSAP's campaign to raise awareness about the problems of college drinking.

8711 Q&A About Smoking and Health
American Lung Association
1740 Broadway 212-315-8700
New York, NY 10019-4315
Gives fact-crammed answers to questions on smoking and health.

8712 Quick List to Build Pride in Your Communities
National Clearinghouse for Alcohol and Drug Info.
PO Box 2345
Rockville, MD 20847-2345 800-729-6686
This parent guide is an adaptation of CSAP's Be Smart! Quick List: 10 Steps to Help Your Child Say No.

8713 Reducing the Health Risks of Secondhand Smoke
American Lung Association
1740 Broadway 212-315-8700
New York, NY 10019-4315
What a person can do at home, work and in public places to reduce the health risks of secondhand smoke.

8714 Relapse and the Addict
Hazelden
15251 Pleasant Valley Road 651-257-4010
Center City, MN 55012-9640 800-328-9000
Fax: 651-213-4426
www.hazelden.org
Identifies specific stages and triggers of relapse.

8715 Releasing Anger
Hazelden
15251 Pleasant Valley Road 651-257-4010
Center City, MN 55012-9640 800-328-9000
Fax: 651-213-4426
www.hazelden.org
Discusses anger as a normal feeling and how anger can endanger recovery.

8716 Research on Drugs and the Workplace
National Clearinghouse for Alcohol and Drug Info.
PO Box 2345
Rockville, MD 20847-2345 800-729-6686
Discusses prevalence and costs to society of drug use in the workplace, along with information on employee assistance programs, drug testing, grants and additional resources.

8717 Secondhand Smoke
American Lung Association
1740 Broadway   212-315-8700
New York, NY 10019-4315
Documents the effects of tobacco smoke on nonsmokers.

8718 Seven Reasons Not to Use Drugs and Alcohol
American Council On Drug Education
204 Monroe Street
Rockville, MD 20850-4425   800-488-3784
A series of five pamphlets offering information on the hazards of
alcohol, crack, cocaine, steroids and tobacco products.
Grades 4-6

8719 Sexual Intimacy and the Alcoholic Relationship
Al-Anon Family Group Headquarters
1600 Corporate Landing Parkway   757-563-1600
Virginia Beach, VA 23454-5617   800-425-2666
                        Fax: 757-563-1655
                        e-mail: wso@al-anon.org
                        www.al-anon.alateen.org
Sex and alcohol? Al-Anon members face this personal problem
when they apply to the Al-Anon program indexed.
48 pages
Caryn Johnson, Director Communications

8720 Should Tobacco Advertising and Promotion Be Banned?
American Lung Association
1740 Broadway   212-315-8700
New York, NY 10019-4315
Answers many questions about tobacco advertising and promo-
tion, and explains how ads are targeted to vulnerable populations.

8721 Smoke Free Family Promotional Leaflet
American Lung Association
1740 Broadway   212-315-8700
New York, NY 10019-4315
Leaflet and order form describe an entire range of ALA's smok-
ing-related materials.

8722 Smokeless Tobacco: No Way
American Lung Association
1740 Broadway   212-315-8700
New York, NY 10019-4315
Written for junior and senior high school students, this booklet
presents the facts about health risks of smokeless tobacco use.

8723 Smoking and Pregnancy
American Lung Association
1740 Broadway   212-315-8700
New York, NY 10019-4315
Written in a question/answer format, this pamphlet discusses many
issues relating to smoking and pregnancy.

8724 Stop Smoking, Stay Trim
American Lung Association
1740 Broadway   212-315-8700
New York, NY 10019-4315
Outlines how to avoid gaining weight while quitting smoking.

8725 Stop Smoking: A Guide to Your Options
American Lung Association
1740 Broadway   212-315-8700
New York, NY 10019-4315
Describes a variety of approaches to smoking cessation. Offers
guidance on how to choose a program.

8726 Straight Back Home
Hazelden
15251 Pleasant Valley Road   651-257-4010
Center City, MN 55012-9640   800-328-9000
                        Fax: 651-213-4426
                        www.hazelden.org
Written for adolescents completing inpatient treatment and return-
ing home.

8727 Stress in Recovery
Hazelden

15251 Pleasant Valley Road   651-257-4010
Center City, MN 55012-9640   800-328-9000
                        Fax: 651-213-4426
                        www.hazelden.org
Outlines methods for clients to overcome stress in their daily lives.

8728 This Is AA
Alcoholics Anonymous
PO Box 459   212-870-3400
New York, NY 10163-0459   Fax: 212-870-3137
A pamphlet offering an introduction to the AA recovery program.

8729 Three Talks to Medical Societies
Alcoholics Anonymous
PO Box 459   212-870-3400
New York, NY 10163-0459   Fax: 212-870-3137
Contains Bill Wilson's, the co-founder of AA, principles borrowed
from medicine and religion and a summary of AA's first 23 years.

8730 Time to Start Living
Alcoholics Anonymous
PO Box 459   212-870-3400
New York, NY 10163-0459   Fax: 212-870-3137
Addresses the older alcoholic, with nine stories of men and women
who came to AA after the age of 60 (large print edition is also avail-
able).

**8731 Too Many Young People Drink and Know Too Little About the
Consequences**
National Clearinghouse for Alcohol and Drug Info.
PO Box 2345
Rockville, MD 20847-2345   800-729-6686
Provides up-to-date resources and statistics on the widespread use
of alcohol by youth under 21 years of age.

8732 Too Young?
Alcoholics Anonymous
PO Box 459   212-870-3400
New York, NY 10163-0459   Fax: 212-870-3137
This cartoon pamphlet speaks to teenagers in their own language,
telling the varied drinking stories of six youn people (13 to 18).

8733 Treating Nicotine Addiction
Hazelden
15251 Pleasant Valley Road   651-257-4010
Center City, MN 55012-9640   800-328-9000
                        Fax: 651-213-4426
                        www.hazelden.org
Describes the success of one chemical dependency treatment cen-
ter that began treating nicotine as an addiction.

8734 Twelve Steps Illustrated
Alcoholics Anonymous
PO Box 459   212-870-3400
New York, NY 10163-0459   Fax: 212-870-3137
An easy-to-read version of AA's twelve steps.

8735 Twelve Steps for Tobacco Users
Hazelden
15251 Pleasant Valley Road   651-257-4010
Center City, MN 55012-9640   800-328-9000
                        Fax: 651-213-4426
                        www.hazelden.org
Presents the Surgeon General's findings that classify nicotine as an
addictive substance.
25 pages

8736 Understanding Depression and Addiction
Hazelden
15251 Pleasant Valley Road   651-257-4010
Center City, MN 55012-9640   800-328-9000
                        Fax: 651-213-4426
                        www.hazelden.org
29 pages

8737 Understanding Major Anxiety Disorders and Addiction
Hazelden

15251 Pleasant Valley Road
Center City, MN 55012-9640
651-257-4010
800-328-9000
Fax: 651-213-4426
www.hazelden.org
36 pages

8738 Understanding Ourselves and Alcoholism
Al-Anon Family Group Headquarters
1600 Corporate Landing Parkway
Virginia Beach, VA 23454-5617
757-563-1600
800-425-2666
Fax: 757-563-1655
e-mail: wso@al-anon.org
www.al-anon.alateen.org
Explains how compulsion, obsession and denial affect those close to an alcoholic as well as the alcoholic.
6 pages
Caryn Johnson, Director Communications

8739 Understanding Personality Problems and Addiction
Hazelden
15251 Pleasant Valley Road
Center City, MN 55012-9640
651-257-4010
800-328-9000
Fax: 651-213-4426
www.hazelden.org
Describes common features of personality problems, such as self-centeredness and setting boundaries.
28 pages

8740 Understanding Post-Traumatic Stress Disorder and Addiction
Hazelden
15251 Pleasant Valley Road
Center City, MN 55012-9640
651-257-4010
800-328-9000
Fax: 651-213-4426
www.hazelden.org
17 pages

8741 Unpuffables Promotional Brochure
American Lung Association
1740 Broadway
New York, NY 10019-4315
212-315-8700
Describes the ALA Unpuffables program.

8742 What Are the Signs of Alcoholism?
Hazelden
15251 Pleasant Valley Road
Center City, MN 55012-9640
651-257-4010
800-328-9000
Fax: 651-213-4426
www.hazelden.org
Self-test for clients to review the role of alcohol in their lives.

8743 What Happened to Joe?
Alcoholics Anonymous
PO Box 459
New York, NY 10163-0459
212-870-3400
Fax: 212-870-3137
Dramatic story of a young construction worker and his drinking problem, told in brightly colored comic book style.

8744 What Happens After Treatment?
Al-Anon Family Group Headquarters
1600 Corporate Landing Parkway
Virginia Beach, VA 23454-5617
757-563-1600
800-425-2666
Fax: 757-563-1655
e-mail: wso@al-anon.org
www.al-anon.alateen.org
100 pieces
Caryn Johnson, Director Communications

8745 What is AA?
Hazelden
15251 Pleasant Valley Road
Center City, MN 55012-9640
651-257-4010
800-328-9000
Fax: 651-213-4426
www.hazelden.org
Answers the basic questions about Alcoholics Anonymous.

8746 What is NA?
Hazelden
15251 Pleasant Valley Road
Center City, MN 55012-9640
651-257-4010
800-328-9000
Fax: 651-213-4426
www.hazelden.org
Helps clients evaluate their addiction to narcotics and answers their questions about N.A.

8747 What's Your Cigarette Smoking IQ?
American Lung Association
1740 Broadway
New York, NY 10019-4315
212-315-8700
Brief true-or-false quiz that tests a person's knowledge of the effects of smoking.

8748 When You Go Back to Work
Hazelden
15251 Pleasant Valley Road
Center City, MN 55012-9640
651-257-4010
800-328-9000
Fax: 651-213-4426
www.hazelden.org
Stories demonstrating co-workers' attitudes clients may face upon their return to work.

8749 When Your Teen is in Treatment
Hazelden
15251 Pleasant Valley Road
Center City, MN 55012-9640
651-257-4010
800-328-9000
Fax: 651-213-4426
www.hazelden.org
A guide for parents.

8750 Where Do I Go from Here?
Alcoholics Anonymous
PO Box 459
New York, NY 10163-0459
212-870-3400
Fax: 212-870-3137
For people leaving treatment facilities, single-sheet flyer tells of continuing help offered by outside AAs.

8751 Why Anonymity in Al-Anon?
Al-Anon Family Group Headquarters
1600 Corporate Landing Parkway
Virginia Beach, VA 23454-5617
757-563-1600
800-425-2666
Fax: 757-563-1655
e-mail: wso@al-anon.org
www.al-anon.alateen.org
12 pages
Caryn Johnson, Director Communications

8752 Workers at Risk: Drugs and Alcohol on the Job
National Clearinghouse for Alcohol and Drug Info.
PO Box 2345
Rockville, MD 20847-2345
800-729-6686
Gives facts about drugs in the workplace and suggests appropriate behavior for employees who are confronted with a coworker's use of alcohol or other drugs.

8753 You Can Help Your Community Get Rid of Drugs
National Clearinghouse for Alcohol and Drug Info.
PO Box 2345
Rockville, MD 20847-2345
800-729-6686
Supports drug abuse treatment and explains how drug use can create problems for your community.

8754 Young Children and Drugs: What Parents Can Do
Wisconsin Clearinghouse
1964 E. Washington Avenue
Madison, WI 53704-5275

8755 Youth and the Alcoholic Parent
Al-Anon Family Group Headquarters
1600 Corporate Landing Parkway
Virginia Beach, VA 23454-5617
757-563-1600
800-425-2666
Fax: 757-563-1655
e-mail: wso@al-anon.org
www.al-anon.alateen.org
Questions and suggestions to help young people improve their own lives.
12 pages
Caryn Johnson, Director Communications

Audio & Video

8756 AA: Rap with Us
Alcoholics Anonymous

PO Box 459
New York, NY 10163-0459
212-870-3400
Fax: 212-870-3137
Features four anonymous young AA members. Rap music and lyrics bridge these four young people's stories of alcoholic despair and A.A. recovery.
16 minutes

8757 Al-Anon Video
Al-Anon Family Group Headquarters
1600 Corporate Landing Parkway
Virginia Beach, VA 23454-5617
757-563-1600
800-425-2666
Fax: 757-563-1655
e-mail: wso@al-anon.org
www.al-anon.alateen.org
12 pages
Caryn Johnson, Director Communications

8758 Al-Anon is for African Americans...and All People of Color
Al-Anon Family Group Headquarters
1600 Corporate Landing Parkway
Virginia Beach, VA 23454-5617
757-563-1600
800-425-2666
Fax: 757-563-1655
e-mail: wso@al-anon.org
www.al-anon.alateen.org
12 pages
Caryn Johnson, Director Communications

8759 Al-Anon's Path to Recovery: Al-Anon is for Americans/Aboriginals
Al-Anon Family Group Headquarters
1600 Corporate Landing Parkway
Virginia Beach, VA 23454-5617
757-563-1600
800-425-2666
Fax: 757-563-1655
e-mail: wso@al-anon.org
www.al-anon.alateen.org
12 pages
Caryn Johnson, Director Communications

8760 Alcoholics Anonymous: An Inside View
Alcoholics Anonymous
PO Box 459
New York, NY 10163-0459
212-870-3400
Fax: 212-870-3137
Depicts alcoholics, recovering in A.A., going about their daily lives, attending A.A. meetings, and other gatherings.
28 minutes

8761 Art of Living with Change: Turning Your Good Intentions Into Progress...
Hazelden
15251 Pleasant Valley Road
Center City, MN 55012-9640
651-213-4030
800-328-0094
Fax: 651-213-4426
www.hazelden.org
45 minutes
ISBN: 0-894868-40-3

8762 Bill Discusses the Twelve Traditions
Alcoholics Anonymous
PO Box 459
New York, NY 10163-0459
212-870-3400
Fax: 212-870-3137
Bill W. tells how the principles safe-guarding A.A. unity developed.
60 minutes

8763 Bill's Own Story
Alcoholics Anonymous
PO Box 459
New York, NY 10163-0459
212-870-3400
Fax: 212-870-3137
Co-founder Bill W. tells of his drinking and recovery.
60 minutes

8764 Caring for Ourselves: Hope for Healthy Relationships
Hazelden
15251 Pleasant Valley Road
Center City, MN 55012-9640
651-213-4030
800-328-0094
Fax: 651-213-4426
www.hazelden.org
50 minutes
ISBN: 0-894866-38-9

8765 Hope: Alcoholics Anonymous
Alcoholics Anonymous
PO Box 459
New York, NY 10163-0459
212-870-3400
Fax: 212-870-3137
Explains the principles of AA: what it is, steps, traditions, sponsorship, and basic recovery tools.
15 minutes

8766 It Sure Beats Sitting in a Cell
Alcoholics Anonymous
PO Box 459
New York, NY 10163-0459
212-870-3400
Fax: 212-870-3137
Filmed inside correctional facilities in the United States and Canada, this film tells the story of four young AA's who were in prison as a result of drinking, yet today are sober.
17 minutes

8767 Markings on the Journey
Alcoholics Anonymous
PO Box 459
New York, NY 10163-0459
212-870-3400
Fax: 212-870-3137
Videocassette depicts 45 years of AA history, using rare materials from our archives.
35 minutes

8768 Men's Work: How to Stop the Violence that Tears Our Lives Apart
Hazelden
15251 Pleasant Valley Road
Center City, MN 55012-9640
651-213-4030
800-328-0094
Fax: 651-213-4426
www.hazelden.org
50 minutes
ISBN: 0-894868-28-4

8769 Secret to a Satisfied Life: The Way You Encounter Life Can Bring Happiness...
Hazelden
15251 Pleasant Valley Road
Center City, MN 55012-9640
651-213-4030
800-328-0094
Fax: 651-213-4426
www.hazelden.org
45 minutes
ISBN: 0-894868-17-9

8770 Women: Coming Out of the Shadows
Elyse A Williams, author
Fanlight Productions
4196 Washington Street
Boston, MA 02131-1731
617-469-4999
800-937-4113
Fax: 617-469-3379
e-mail: fanlight@fanlight.com
www.fanlight.com
Ten women share their personal stories of addiction and recovery.
1991 27 Minutes
ISBN: 1-572950-84-6

8771 Young People and AA
Alcoholics Anonymous
PO Box 459
New York, NY 10163-0459
212-870-3400
Fax: 212-870-3137
Four young AA members describe what it is like drinking, what happened to bring them to AA, and what their lives are like sober today.
28 minutes

Web Sites

8772 AAA Foundation for Traffic Safety
www.aaafts.org
This national organization publishes drinking and traffic safety programs for K-6 and junior high students.

8773 Al-Anon
www.al-anon.alateen.org
The single purpose of this organization is to help families and friends of alcoholics, whether the alcoholic is still drinking or not.

8774 Alateen

A part of the Al-Anon program, Alateen is for teenagers who have been affected by someone else's drinking, whether it be a family member or a friend.

8775 American Council for Drug Education

www.acde.org/

This organization provides information on drug use, publishes books and offers films and curriculum materials for prevention.

8776 CSAP State Liason Program

www.samhsa.gov/centers/csap/csap.html

This program is designed to support alcohol and other drug abuse prevention efforts in the States.

8777 Center for Substance Abuse Prevention

www.samhsa.gov/centers/csap/csap.html

This organization's goal is to connect people and resources with innovative ideas, strategies and programs designed to encourage creative and effective efforts aimed at reducing and eliminating alcohol, tobacco and other drug problems in our society.

8778 Cocaine Anonymous

www.ca.org

A support group based on the twelve steps of Alcoholics Anonymous that focuses specifically on problems of cocaine addiction.

8779 Dentists Concerned for Dentists

www.medhelp.org/amshc/amshc53.htm

A nonprofit organization for chemically dependent Minnesota dentists and concerned others.

8780 Families Anonymous

www.familiesanonymous.org/

Addresses the needs of families who are concerned about a relative with a drug problem and with related behavioral problems.

8781 Hazelden

www.hazelden.com

Organization dedicated to providing quality rehabilitation, education and professional services for chemical dependency and related addictive behaviors.

8782 Healing Well

www.healingwell.com

An online health resource guide to medical news, chat, information and articles, newsgroups and message boards, books, disease-related web sites, medical directories, and more for patients, friends, and family coping with disabling diseases, disorders, or chronic illnesses.

8783 Health Finder

www.healthfinder.gov

Searchable, carefully developed web site offering information on over 1000 topics. Developed by the US Department of Health and Human Services, the site can be used in both English and Spanish.

8784 Healthlink USA

www.healthlinkusa.com

Health information concerning treatment, cures, prevention, diagnosis, risk factors, research, support groups, email lists, personal stories and much more. Updated regularly.

8785 Helios Health

www.helioshealth.com

Online resource for your health information. Detailed information about specific health topics, access to expert advice from our Medical Advisory Board, and up-to-date health news.

8786 Indian Health Service

www.ihs.gov

Charged with providing a comprehensive program of alcoholism and substance abuse prevention and treatment for Native Americans and Alaskan natives.

8787 Lawyers Concerned for Lawyers

www.mnlcl.org/

Organization of recovering lawyers and judges and concerned others. Educates lawyers and judges about the disease of chemical dependency, assists in assessments and arranging interventions and offers lawyer-only AA meetings.

8788 MedicineNet

www.medicinenet.com

An online resource for consumers providing easy-to-read, authoritative medical and health information.

8789 Medscape

www.medscape.com

Medscape offers specialists, primary care physicians, and other health professionals the Web's most robust and integrated medical information and educational tools.

8790 National Clearinghouse for Alcohol and Drug Information

www.health.org

8791 National Council on Alcoholism and Drug Dependence

www.ncadd.org

Provides education, information, help and hope in the fight against addictions. Nationwide network of affiliates, advocates prevention, intervention and treatment, and is committed to ridding the disease of its stigma and its sufferers of their denial and shame.

8792 National Crime Prevention Council

www.ncpc.org

This organization works to prevent crime and drug use in many ways, including developing materials for parents and children.

8793 Office on Smoking and Health

www.cdc.gov/tobacco/

Offers reference services to researchers through the Technical Information Center. Publishes and distributes a number of titles in the field of smoking and health.

8794 Safe Homes

www.yescap.org/safehomes/safehomes.htm

This national organization encourages parents to sign a contract stipulating that when parties are held in one another's homes they will adhere to a strict no-alcohol/no-drug-use rule.

8795 Substance Abuse and Mental Health Services Administration

www.samhsa.gov

The goal of this organization is to reduce incidence and prevalence of mental disorders and substance abuse and improve treatment outcomes for persons suffering from addictive and mental health problems and disorders.

8796 WebMD

www.webmd.com

Information on substance abuse, including articles and resources.

Description

8797 **Sudden Infant Death Syndrome**

Sudden Infant Death Syndrome, SIDS, is the sudden death of an infant or young child that is unexpected and for which there is no demonstrable cause. It is the most common cause of death in children between 1 and 12 months of age, with a peak incidence between the second and fourth month of life. Almost all SIDS deaths occur when the infant is thought to be sleeping.

Despite extensive research, no cause for SIDS has been found, although evidence suggests that it may be related to malfunction of the mechanisms that control the heart function and breathing process. The diagnosis cannot be made without an adequate investigation of the infant after its death. The incidence of SIDS is greater in babies born to mothers who are young, unwed, smoke, have had many births, did not complete high school and have had poor prenatal care. Other possible factors include exposure to cigarette smoke, cold months, soft bedding (lamb's wool), waterbed mattresses, an overheated environment, and being a sibling of a SIDS victim.

Recent studies have indicated that having babies sleep on their backs reduces the risks of SIDS. The American Academy of Pediatrics recommends that infants be placed on their back for sleep. It further advises to avoid overwrapping the infant, remove soft bedding, and avoid smoking during and after pregnancy. In 1994, the Back to Sleep Campaign was launched, a national campaign that encourages that infants be placed to sleep on their backs. Between 1992 and 1996,the rate of SIDS dropped 38 percent and has continued to decrease since then.

Parents who lose a child to SIDS are grief-stricken and, because no definitive cause can be found for their seemingly healthy baby's death, usually have excessive guilt feelings. Bereavement support is necessary not only during the days immediately following the infant's death, but also for at least several months.

National Agencies & Associations

8798 **American SIDS Institute**
509 Augusta Drive
Marietta, GA 30067-8657
770-426-8746
800-232-7437
Fax: 770-426-1369
e-mail: prevent@sids.org
www.sids.org
Dedicated to the prevention of sudden infant death and the promotion of infant health through research clinical services education and family support.
Betty McEnti PhD, Executive Director
Marc Peterzell, Chairman

8799 **Center for Research for Mothers & Children**
National Institute of Child Health & Development
PO Box 3006
Rockville, MD 20847
800-370-2943
800-370-2943
Fax: 301-984-1477
TTY: 888-320-6942
e-mail: NICHDinformationresourcecenter@mail.nih
www.nichd.nih.gov
Mission is to ensure that every person is born healthy and wanted, that women suffer no harmful effects from reproductive processes,

and that all children have the chance to achieve their full potential for healthy and productive lives free from disease.
Duane F Alexander, Director
Christine Ma Banks, Secretary

8800 **Compassionate Friends**
PO Box 3696
Oak Brook, IL 60522
630-990-0010
877-969-0010
Fax: 630-990-0246
e-mail: nationaloffice@compassionatefriends.org
www.compassionatefriends.org
A national organization that offers 600 local chapters that give support to parents and siblings who have experienced the death of a child. Offers monthly support meetings to get through the difficult times and learn how to cope.
Patricia Loder, Executive Director

8801 **National Center for Education in Maternal and Child Health**
Georgetown University
Box 571272
Washington, DC 20057-1272
202-784-9770
Fax: 202-784-9777
e-mail: mchlibrary@ncemch.org
www.ncemch.org
Provides national leadership to the maternal and child health community in three key areas—program development education and state-of-the-art knowledge—to improve the health and well-being of the nation's children and families.
Rochelle Mayer, Director

8802 **National Organization for Rare Disorders (NORD)**
55 Kenosia Avenue
Danbury, CT 06813-1968
203-744-0100
800-999-6673
Fax: 203-798-2291
TDD: 203-797-9590
e-mail: orphan@rarediseases.org
www.rarediseases.org
The NORD is a unique federation of voluntary health organizations dedicated to helping people with rare orphan diseases and assisting the organizations that serve them.
Frank Sasinowski, Chair
Carolyn Asbury, PhD, Vice Chair

8803 **Parent Care**
9041 Colgate Street
Indianapolis, IN 46268-1210
Fax: 317-872-5464
This organization was formed in 1982 to improve the neonatal intensive care experience for families and care providers. Provides leadership to promote the development of effective parent support services at the local level.
Sarah Killion, Administrative Director

8804 **Share Pregnancy and Infant Loss Support, Inc.**
The National Share Office
402 Jackson Street
St. Charles, MO 63301
636-947-6164
800-821-6819
Fax: 636-947-7486
www.nationalshare.org
Offers support, resources and education on miscarriage, stillborn and newborn death.
Cathi Lammert, Executive Director
Rose Carlson, Program Director

8805 **Sudden Infant Death Syndrome (SIDS) Network**
PO Box 520
Ledyard, CT 06339
86- 89- 704
Fax: 860-887-7309
e-mail: sidsnet1@sids-network.org
www.sids-network.org
Dedicated to eliminate Sudden Infant Death Syndrome through the support of SIDS research projects. Provides support for those who have been touched by the tragedy of Sudden Infant Death Syndrome and to raise public awareness of this event.
Chuck Mihalko, Co-founder and President

8806 **Sudden Infant Death Syndrome Alliance**
1314 Bedford Avenue
Baltimore, MD 21208-6605
410-653-8226
800-221-7437
Fax: 410-653-8709
e-mail: info@firstcandle.org
www.sidsalliance.org

The purpose of the Alliance is to help parents educate the community about SIDS and to support SIDS research. The Alliance assists parents to organize local chapters and provides services including a newsletter and other literature.

Marian Sokol, President
Deborah Boyd, Executive Director

State Agencies & Associations

Alabama

8807 Bureau of Family Health Services: Alabama Department of Public Health
19 South Jackson Street
201 Monroe Street   334-206-5300
Montgomery, AL 36104   800-ALA-1818
                                            Fax: 334-269-5200
                                        e-mail: llee@aap.net
                                                www.adph.org

Linda P Lee, Executive Director

Alaska

8808 SIDS Information and Counseling Program: Alaska Department of Health
550 W 8th Street   907-296-3900
Anchorage, AK 99501-3553   Fax: 907-296-3901
                            e-mail: william.hogan@alaska.gov
                                           www.hss.state.ak.us

Joel Bill Hogan, Commissioner
Jay Butler, Chief Medical Officer

Arizona

8809 Arizona SIDS Founation
PO Box 1111   520-297-6013
Phoenix, AZ 85001   800-597-7437
                                      e-mail: info@azsidf.org
                                                www.azsidf.org

Vanessa Seaney, President

8810 Office of Womens And Childrens Health: Alabama Department of Health
State Dapartment of Healths Services
150 N 18th Avenue   602-542-1000
Phoenix, AZ 85007-2602   Fax: 602-542-0883
                                   e-mail: newbers@azdhs.gov
                                                www.azdhs.gov

Susan Newber RN, Manager

Arkansas

8811 Arkansas Department of Health: SIDS Information & Counseling Program
4815 W Markham Street
Little Rock, AR 72205-3866   501-280-4560
                                    www.healthyarkansas.com

Jackie Whitfield, Program Coordinator
Dawn Graziani

California

8812 California SIDS Program
11344 Coloma Road   916-851-7437
Gold River, CA 95670-6052   800-369-7437
                                             Fax: 916-851-5937
                             e-mail: info@californiasids.com
                                         www.californiasids.com

Gwen Edelstein, Program Director
Cheryl McBride, Program Manager

8813 Region IX Office Program Consultants for Maternal and Child Health
90 7th Street   415-437-7873
San Francisco, CA 94103   Fax: 415-437-8336
                            e-mail: reginald.louie@acf.hhs.gov
                                           www.mchoralhealth.org

Reginald Lou DDS MPH, Oral Health Consultant

8814 SIDS Alliance Of Northern California
1547 Palos Verdes Mall   925-274-1109
Walnut Creek, CA 94597   877-938-7437
                                     e-mail: info@sidsnc.org
                                                www.sidsnc.org

Lorie Gehrke, President

8815 SIDS Foundation of Southern California
10811 Washington Boulevard   310-558-4511
Culver City, CA 90232   Fax: 310-558-7075
                                    e-mail: sidsfsc@aol.com
                          sidsfoundationofsoutherncalifornia.org

Margot Stern Bennett, Executive Director

Colorado

8816 Colorado SIDS Program
425 S Cherry Street   303-320-7771
Denver, CO 80224   888-285-7437
                                             Fax: 303-320-7827
                                    e-mail: rlouie@hrsa.gov
                                           www.coloradosids.org

Tena Saltzman, Executive Director

8817 Colordao Department of Health and Environment
4300 Cherry Creek Drive S   303-692-2000
Denver, CO 80246-1530   800-886-7689
                                             Fax: 303-782-5576
                                             TTY: 303-691-7700
                         e-mail: cdphe.information@state.co.us
                                           www.cdphe.state.co.us

Bill Letson, Director

8818 Region VIII Office Program Consultants for Maternal and Child Health
1961 Stout Street   303-844-1482
Denver, CO 80294-1961   Fax: 303-844-3642
                          e-mail: valeri.orlando@acf.hhs.gov
                                           www.mchoralhealth.org

Valerie Orla RDH BS, Oral Health Consultant

Connecticut

8819 Connecticut SIDS Alliance
PO Box 486   860-626-1542
Torrington, CT 06790   866-574-7437
                                             Fax: 860-496-9919
                                     e-mail: ctsids@aol.com
                                                www.ctsids.org

Shannon Strandberg, Secretary

8820 SIDS Program: Connecticut Department of Health
410 Capitol Avenue   860-509-8074
Hartford, CT 06134   Fax: 860-509-7720
                          e-mail: marilyn.binns@po.state.ct.us
                                           www.sidsalliance.org

Marilyn Binns, Program Coordinator

Delaware

8821 Delaware SIDS Alliance
PO Box 5449   302-996-9464
Wilmington, DE 19808   Fax: 302-255-2273
                                           www.sidsalliance.org

Linda Hawthorne, President

8822 SIDS Information & Counseling: Division of Public Health
1901 N DuPont Highway   302-255-9040
New Castle, DE 19720   Fax: 302-255-4429
                                 e-mail: dhssinfo@state/de/us
                                           www.dhss.delaware.gov

Elaine Marke LCSW BCD, Program Coordinator

District of Columbia

8823 DC Department of Health Maternal and Family Health Administration
Maternal And Family Health Administration

825 N Capitol Street NE
Washington, DC 20002
202-442-5955
Fax: 202-645-6491
e-mail: drena.reaves@dc.gov
www.dchealth.dc.gov

Pierre Vigilance, Director
Rosie McLaren, Program Manager

Florida

8824   Children's Medical Services Program: Florida SIDS Program
4052 Bald Cypress Way
Tallahassee, FL 32399
850-245-4444
Fax: 904-488-2341
e-mail: Health@doh.state.fl.us
www.doh.state.fl.us

Susan Potts

8825   Florida Department of Health
4052 Bald Cypress Way
Tallahassee, FL 32399
850-245-4444
Fax: 850-245-4047
e-mail: Health@doh.state.fl.us
www.doh.state.fl.us

Susan Potts, Coordinator

8826   Florida SIDS Alliance
4185 W Lake Mary Boulevard
Lake Mary, FL 32746
305-232-1640
800-SID-SFLA
e-mail: flasidsalliance@yahoo.com
www.flasids.com

Steve Bonwit, Officer
Roy Bagley, President

Georgia

8827   Georgia Department of Human Resources: Center for Family Resource Planning
2 Peach Tree Street NW
Atlanta, GA 30319
404-651-7371
Fax: 404-463-6729
e-mail: kotto@dhr.state.ga.us
Provides grief support for parents.
Katherine Ottoel, Coordinator

8828   Georgia Department of Human Resources: Inf ant and Child Health
2 Peach Tree Street NW
Atlanta, GA 30303
404-651-7371
Fax: 404-463-6729
e-mail: kotto@dhr.state.ga.us

Katherine Otto, Coordinator

8829   Georgia SIDS Project
4112-2 E Ponce De Leon Avenue
Clarkston, GA 30021
678-342-3360
Fax: 404-296-7211
e-mail: gasids@mindspring.com
www.sidsga.org
Sudden Infant Death Syndrome is the sudden death of an infant under one year of age which remains unexplained after a thorough case investigation.
Diane Manheim, Director

8830   Region IV Office Program Consultants for Maternal and Child Health
61 Forsyth Street SW
Atlanta, GA 30303-8909
404-562-2935
Fax: 404-562-2984
e-mail: ejalderman@comcast.net
www.mchoralhealth.org

E Joseph Alderman DDS MPH, Oral Health Consultant

Hawaii

8831   Hawaii Department of Health: Family Health Division
Child Wellness Program   r
1250 Punchbowl Street
Honolulu, HI 96813
808-586-4400
Fax: 808-733-9032
e-mail: gwen.palmer@fshd.health.state.hi.us
ww.hawaii.gov/health

Gwen Palmer, Coordinator

Idaho

8832   Child Health Improvement Program: Idaho Department of Health
450 W State Street
Boise, ID 83720
208-334-5507
www.healthandwelfare.idao.gov
Simonne deGl MS PNP, SIDS Coordinator

8833   Idaho Department of Health and Welfare
590 W Washington Street
Boise, ID 83720
208-334-4000
800-632-8000
Fax: 208-334-4015
e-mail: gainord@idhw.state.id.us
www.healthandwelfare.idaho.gov

Richard F Hudson PhD, Bureau Chief

Illinois

8834   SIDS of Illinois
710 E Ogden Avenue
Naperville, IL 60563
630-305-7300
Fax: 630-305-4773
e-mail: pam@sidsillinois.org
www.sidsillinois.org

Pam Borchardt, Facilitator

8835   Statewide SIDS Program: Illinois Department of Public Health
500 E Monroe Street
Springfield, IL 62761
217-557-2931
Fax: 217-524-2831
e-mail: bbreiden@idph.state.il.us
Babara Breidenbaugh, Program Specialist

Indiana

8836   Indiana State Board of Health: SIDS Project
2 N Meridian Street
Indianapolis, IN 46204-2829
317-233-1325
800-457-8283
e-mail: hpb6@hpb.in.gov.in.us
www.in.gov/hpb

Jayma Ellerbrook, Project Director

8837   Indiana State Department of Health Maternal And Child Health Services
Maternal And Child Health Services
2 N Meridian Street
Indianapolis, IN 46204
317-233-1325
800-457-8283
Fax: 317-233-1300
e-mail: bmjohnso@isdh.state.in.us
www.in.gov/hpb

Beth Johnson, Nurse Consultant

8838   SIDS Center of Indiana
1810 Broad Ripple Avenue
Indianapolis, IN 46220
317-484-1500
e-mail: sidscenter@insids.org
John Schutt, Chairperson

Iowa

8839   Iowa Department of Public Health Center for Congenital and Inherited Disorders
Center For Congenital And Inherited Disorders
321 E 12th Street
Des Moines, IA 50319
515-281-7689
Fax: 515-242-6384
e-mail: kipper@idph.state.ia.us
www.idph.state.ia.us

Patricia Young, Prevention Coordinator
Rob Walker, Surveillance Officer

8840   Iowa SIDS Alliance
406 SW School Street
Ankeny, IA 50023
515-965-7655
866-480-4741
Fax: 515-964-7506
e-mail: info@iowasids.org
www.iowasids.org

Patty Keeley, Executive Director
Jennifer Atzen, President

8841   Iowa SIDS Program Iowa Department of Public Health
Iowa Department of Public Health

321 E 12th Street
Des Moines, IA 50319-0075

515-281-7689
866-227-9878
www.idph.state.ia.us

Jane Borst, Bureau Chief
Sally Clausen

Kansas

8842   Kansas Department of Health & Environment Bureau of Family Health
Bureau Of Children, Youth And Families
1000 SW Jackson Street
Topeka, KS 66612-1274

785-291-3368
800-332-6262
Fax: 785-296-6553
e-mail: info@kdheks.gov
www.kdheks.gov

Linda kenney, Director
Kobi Gomel, Administrative Specialist

8843   SIDS Network of Kansas
1148 S Hillside
Wichita, KS 67211

316-682-1301
866-399-7437
Fax: 316-682-1274
e-mail: info@sidsks.org
www.sidsks.org

Christy Schunn, Executive Director

Kentucky

8844   Department of Public Health: Adult and Child Health Division
275 E Main Street
Frankfort, KY 40621

502-564-3236
800-372-2973
Fax: 502-564-8389
TTY: 800-627-4702
e-mail: marcia.burkow@ky.gov

Marcia Burkow, SIDS Coordinator

8845   SIDS Network of Kentucky
PO Box 186
Caneyville, KY 42721-3555

800-928-7437
Fax: 859-245-0717
e-mail: info@sidsky.org
www.sidsky.org

Adrienne Grizzell, Executive Director

Louisiana

8846   Office of Public Health
628 N 4th Street
Baton Rouge, LA 70802

225-342-9500
Fax: 225-342-5568
e-mail: hhwebadmin@la.gov
www.dhh.louisiana.gov/offices/?ID=79

Tracy Hubbard, Coordinator

8847   Public Health Services of Louisiana
628 N 4th Street
Baton Rouge, LA 70802-0629

225-342-9500
Fax: 225-342-5568
e-mail: dhhwebadmin@la.gov
www.dhh.state.la.us/

Jamie Roques RNC, SIDS Coordinator

Maine

8848   Department of Human Services
221 State Street
Augusta, ME 04333-0001

207-287-3707
Fax: 207-287-3005
TTY: 800-606-0215
www.state.me.us/dhs/

Brenda Harvey, Commissioner

8849   Maine SIDS Foundation
14 Charlonate Drive
Gray, ME 04039

207-657-2220
Fax: 207-657-3737
e-mail: roybagley@aol.com
www.sidsalliance.org

Roy Bagley, Chairperson

8850   Maine SIDS Program Department Of Human Services
Department Of Human Services

200 Main Street
Lewiston, ME 04240

207-795-4450
Fax: 207-795-4445
e-mail: luanne.crinion@maine.gov

Luanne Crinion, Program Coordinator

Maryland

8851   Maryland SIDS Information & Counseling Program
22 S Green Street
Baltimore, MD 21201

410-328-8667
800-492-5538
TTY: 410-328-9600
TDD: 410-328-9600
e-mail: webmaster@umm.edu
www.marylandsids.com

Jeffrey A Rivest, President and Chief Executive Officer
R Keith Allen, Senior Vice President

Massachusetts

8852   Massachusetts Chapter of SIDS Alliance Boston Medical Center
Boston Medical Center
PO Box 520
Ledyard, CT 06339-2908

617-414-SIDS
800-641-7437
Fax: 617-534-5555
e-mail: sidsnet1@sids-network.org
www.sids-network.org

State chapter offering educational resources and information on SIDS, parent groups, support networks, monthly meetings and workshops to the community.
Frederick Mandell, Co Director
Michael Corwin, Co Director

8853   Region I Office Program: Consultants for Maternal and Child Health
John F Kennedy Building
Boston, MA 02203

617-899-1355
Fax: 202-833-8288
e-mail: Mary.Foley@mcphs.edu
www.mchoralhealth.org

Mary Foley RDH MPH, Oral Health Consultant

Michigan

8854   Apnea Identification Program Children's Hospital of Michigan
Children's Hospital of Michigan
3901 Beaubien Street
Detroit, MI 48201-2196

313-745-5437
888-DMC-2500
www.childrensdmc.org

Karen Branif RN MSW, Nurse Specialist

8855   Genesee County Health Department
630 S Saignaw Street
Flint, MI 48502-3915

810-257-3612
Fax: 810-257-3147
e-mail: gchd-info@gchd.us
www.gchd.us

John Northrup, Chairperson
Michael Boucree, Vice-Chairperson

8856   Kent County Health Department
300 Monroe Avenue NE
Grand Rapids, MI 49503-1996

616-632-7590
www.accesskent.com

Colleen Jill RN, SIDs Coordinator
David Kraker

8857   Michigan Department of Community Health
3423 MLK Boulevard
Lansing, MI 48909

517-373-1820
Fax: 517-373-2129
e-mail: lauberc@michigan.gov
www.michigan.gov

Cheryl Lauber, Coordinator

8858 Oakland County Health Division: SIDS Project
1200 N Telegraph   248-858-1280
Pontiac, MI 48341-0482   800-774-4542
                                        Fax: 248-858-0178
                                        TTY: 248-452-2247
                                        TDD: 248-452-2247
                         e-mail: oakllbph@oakland.lib.mi.us
                                         www.oakgov.com

David Conklin, Librarian
George J Miller Jr MA, Director

8859 SIDS LEAD: Children's Special Health Care Services
Michigan Department of Public Health
201 Townsend Street   517-373-3740
Lansing, MI 48913-2934   TTY: 517-373-3573
                                        TDD: 517-373-3573
                            e-mail: norris@michigan.gov
                                  www.michigan.gov/mdch

Janet Olszewski, Director
Ed Dore, Chief Deputy Director

Minnesota

8860 Minnesota Sudden Infant Death Center Minneapolis Children's Medical Center
Minneapolis Children's Medical Center
2525 Chicago Avenue   612-813-6000
Minneapolis, MN 55404-4518   Fax: 612-813-7344
              e-mail: kathleen.fernbach@childreansHC.org
                www.childrensmn.org/Communities/SIDs.asp
Sara Schumacher, Project Coordinator

8861 STOP-SIDS Minnesota
2873 Upper 138th Street
Rosemont, MN 55068   Fax: 651-310-2106
                                       www.sidsalliance.org

Trish LaVictoire, President

Mississippi

8862 Mississippi SIDS Alliance
PO Box 2170
Madison, MS 39130-2170   877-471-7437
                             e-mail: mssids@jam.rr.com
                                       www.sidsalliance.org

Cathy Files, Chairperson

8863 Mississippi State Department of Health and Child Health Services
570 E Woodrow Wilson   601-576-7400
Jackson, MS 39216   866-458-4948
                                        Fax: 601-576-7498
                     e-mail: Linda.Proctor@msdh.state.ms.us
                                       www.msdh.state.ms.us

Linda Proctor, Coordinator

Missouri

8864 Region VII Office Program: Consultants for Maternal and Child Health
Federal Building
10031 Perry Drive   913-888-1377
Overland Park, KS 66212-2826   Fax: 816-426-3633
                             e-mail: lwalker17@kc.rr.com
                                     www.mchoralhealth.org
Lawrence Wal DDS MPH, Oral Health Consultant

8865 SIDS Resources
1120 S Sixth Street   314-822-2323
Saint Louis, MO 63104   800-421-3511
                                        Fax: 314-822-2098
                          e-mail: lahrens@sidsresources.org
                                     www.sidsresources.org

Lori Behrens, Executive Director
Teresa Buehler, Program Coordinator

8866 Western Region SIDS Resources
5700 Broadmoor   913-671-1818
Mission, MO 66202   Fax: 816-753-6906
                            e-mail: slogan@sidsresources.org
                                     www.sidsalliance.org

Shay Logan, Program Coordinator

Montana

8867 Department of Public Health and Human Services
1400 Broadway   406-444-3565
Helena, MT 59620   800-232-4636
                                        Fax: 406-444-2606
                             e-mail: WMcGraw@state.mt.us
                                        www.dphhs.mt.gov

Brad Pickhardt, Chairperson
Peggy Baker, Administrative Aide

8868 Montana Department of Health & Environmental Sciences
Health Plannin Program
PO Box 200901   406-444-4473
Helena, MT 59620-0901
Charles Aagenes

Nebraska

8869 Nebraska Department of Health Perinatal Child and Adolescent Health
301 Centennial Mall South   402-471-0165
Lincoln, NE 68509   Fax: 402-471-7049
                       e-mail: jan.heusinkvelt@hhss.ne.gov
Jan Heusinkvelt, RN, BSN, Community Health Nurse

8870 Nebraska SIDS Foundation University of Nebraska Medical Center
University of Nebraska Medical Center
PO Box 460905   402-431-8076
Papillion, NE 68046   e-mail: board@nesids.org
                                          www.nesids.com

Tammy Dawdy

Nevada

8871 Nevada State Health Division Bureau of Family Health Services
Bureau Of Family Health Services
3427 Goni Road   775-684-4285
Carson City, NV 89706   Fax: 775-684-4245
                          e-mail: chuth@nvhd.state.nv.us
                                    www.health2k.state.nv.us

Cynthia Huthht, Health Program Specialist

New Hampshire

8872 New Hampshire SIDS Alliance
13 Drew Road   617-828-4996
Derry, NH 03038   e-mail: declan4204@comcast.net
                                       www.sidsalliance.org

Charlie Foote, Chairperson

8873 New Hampshire SIDS Program
New Hampshire Division of Public Health Services
29 Hazen Drive   603-271-4536
Concord, NH 03301   Fax: 603-271-4519
                          e-mail: sidsnet1@sids-network.org
                                     www.sids-network.org

Audrey Knigh MSN CPNP, SIDS Coordinator

New Jersey

8874 New Jersey Department of Health: Child Health Program
PO Box 360   609-292-7837
Trenton, NJ 08625   800-367-6543
                        e-mail: lindajones@doh.state.nj.us
                                     www.state.nj.us/health

Linda Jones Hicks, Director
Shirley White-Walker, Chair

8875 New Jersey SIDS Alliance
15 Meadowbrook Road
Boonton Township, NJ 07005   973-299-6523
                                    e-mail: njsids@yahoo.com
                                    www.sidsalliance.org
Genny Elias-Warren, Chairperson

8876 SIDS Center of New Jersey
1 Robert Wood Johnson Place   732-249-2160
New Brunswick, NJ 08903-1766   800-704-7437
                                     Fax: 732-235-6609
                                     e-mail: hegyith@umdnj.edu
                                     www2.umdnj.edu/sids
Thomas Hegyi MD, Co-Medical Director
Barbara Ostf PhD, Program Director

8877 SIDS Center of New Jersey: Northern Site
Hackensack Medical Center
30 Prospect Avenue   201-996-5328
Hackensack, NJ 07601   800-704-7437
                                     Fax: 201-996-0754
                                     e-mail: rhinnen@humed.com
                                     www2.umdnj.edu/sids
Barbara Ostf PhD, Program Director
Thomas Hegyi MD, Co-Medical Director

New Mexico

8878 New Mexico SIDS Information and Counseling Program
University of New Mexico School of Medicine
2500 Marble NE   505-277-3053
Albuquerque, NM 87131   Fax: 505-272-3601
                                     e-mail: sidsnet1@sids-network.org
                                     www.sids-network.org
Beverly Whit RN MS, Director

New York

8879 NYS Center for SIDS
990 7th N Street   315-634-2191
Liverpool, NY 13088-6148   Fax: 315-634-1118
                                     e-mail: csquillace@hospice-pca.org
                                     www.sidsprojectimpact.com
Cynthia Squillace, Chairperson

8880 NYS Center for Sudden Infant Death: Eastern Satellite Office
Albany Medical College
47 New Scotland Avenue   518-262-5918
Albany, NY 12208   Fax: 518-262-7237
                                     e-mail: whittrm@mail.amc.edu
Mary Whittredge, Regional Coordinator

8881 New York City Center for SIDS
New York City Satellite Office
520 1st Avenue   212-686-8854
New York, NY 10016   800-522-5006
                                     Fax: 212-532-6564
                                     e-mail: evelyne.longchamp@sids1.ssw.sunysb.edu
Judith Gaine CSW PhD, SIDS Program Director

8882 New York State Center for SIDS: School of Social Welfare
Stony Brook University
Health Sciences Center Level 2
Stony Brook, NY 11794-0001   631-444-1441
                                     800-336-7437
                                     Fax: 631-444-6475
                                     e-mail: marie.chandick@stonybrook.edu
                                     www.hsc.stonybrook.edu
Marie Chandi CSW, Associate Project Director

8883 Region II Office Program: Consultants for Maternal and Child Health
345 E 24th Street   212-998-9654
New York, NY 10010-0004   Fax: 212-995-4364
                                     e-mail: ngh1@nyu.edu
                                     www.mchoralhealth.org
Neal Herman DDS, Oral Health Consultant

8884 WNYS Center for SIDS
3580 Harlem Road   716-837-5189
Buffalo, NY 14215   Fax: 716-836-1578
                                     e-mail: jwalkden@palliativecare.org
                                     www.sidsalliance.org
Jan Walkden, Family Service Coordinator

North Carolina

8885 Department of Health and Human Services
200 Independence Avenue SW   919-715-8430
Washington, DC 20201   Fax: 919-715-3410
                                     e-mail: april.ellis@ncmail.net
                                     www.hhs.gov
April Ellis, SIDS Program Manager

8886 SIDS Alliance of the Carolinas
306 Lucas Park Drive   336-545-3348
Greensboro, NC 27455   e-mail: sandylkennedy@hotmail.com
                                     www.sidsalliance.org
Sandy Kennedy, Chairperson

North Dakota

8887 North Dakota SIDS Alliance
128 Apollo Avenue   701-530-2507
Bismarck, ND 58503   Fax: 701-223-0440
                                     e-mail: ndsids@btinet.net
                                     www.sidsalliance.org
Barb Delvo, Chairperson

8888 North Dakota SIDS Management Program
Division of Maternal and Child Health
600 E Boulevard Avenue   701-328-2493
Bismarck, ND 58505-0200   800-472-2286
                                     Fax: 701-328-1412
                                     e-mail: kchintz@nd.gov
                                     www.ndhealth.gov
Provides support education and follow-up to parents/caregivers
family and childcare providers suffering a sudden infant death
Kjersti Hintz, Program Director

Ohio

8889 District Board of Health: Mahoning County
50 Westchester Drive   330-270-2855
Youngstown, OH 44515   800-873-MCHD
                                     Fax: 330-270-2860
                                     e-mail: mchealth@cboss.com
                                     www.mahoning-health.org
Lisa Weiss MD, Forum Health
Bev Fisher, Manager

8890 Ohio Department of Health
Child Fatality Review
246 N High Street   614-728-0773
Columbus, OH 43215   866-634-7654
                                     Fax: 614-564-2433
                                     e-mail: SmkInfo@odh.ohio.govÿ
                                     www.odh.ohio.gov
Alvin D Jackson, Director

8891 SIDS Network of Ohio
421 Graham Road
Cuyahoga Falls, OH 44221   Fax: 330-929-0593
                                     e-mail: SIDNetwork@sidsohio.org
                                     www.sidsohio.org
Pat Marquis, Chairperson

Oklahoma

8892 Oklahoma State Department of Health: Maternal and Child Health Services
1000 NE 10th Street   405-271-5600
Oklahoma City, OK 73117-1207   800-522-0203
                                     Fax: 405-271-9202
                                     e-mail: paulaw@health.ok.gov
                                     www.ok.gov
Paula Wood, Executive Assistant
Suzanna Dooley

Oregon

8893 Oregon Department of Human Services
500 Summer Street NE
Salem, OR 97301
503-945-5944
Fax: 503-378-2897
TTY: 503-945-6214
e-mail: dhs.info@state.or.us
www.oregon.gov

Joyce Edmonds, Public Nurse Consultant

Pennsylvania

8894 Pennsylvania Department of Health Bureau of Family Health
Bureau of Family Health
7th & Forster Streets
Harrisburg, PA 17120
717-772-2762
877-PAH-EALT
Fax: 717-772-0323
e-mail: bcaboot@state.pa.us
www.dsf.health.state.pa.us

Robert Torres, Deputy Secretary for Administration

8895 Region III Office Program: Consultants for Maternal and Child Health
Public Ledger Building
2115 Wisconsin Avenue NW
Washington, DC 20007-3309
202-784-9771
Fax: 202-784-9777
www.mchoralhealth.org

Jolene Bertness, Health Education Specialist
Katrina Holt, Director

8896 SIDS of Pennsylvania
810 River Avenue
Pittsburgh, PA 15212
412-322-5680
800-721-7437
Fax: 412-481-5968
e-mail: sidspa@aol.com
www.sids-pa.org

Judy Bannon, Executive Director
Joseph Dominick, Chairman

Rhode Island

8897 Rhode Island Department of Health
3 Capitol Hill
Providence, RI 02908
401-222-4606
800-942-7434
Fax: 401-222-6548
TTY: 711
e-mail: DOH@health.ri.gov
www.health.state.ri.us

David R Gifford MD MPH, Director
Donald L Carcieri, Governor

8898 Rhode Island Department of Health: National SIDS Foundation
29 Hannah Drive
Warwick, RI 02888
401-461-2162
e-mail: wilksme@aol.com
www.sidsalliance.org

Mary Wilks, Area Contact

South Carolina

8899 Division of Perinatal Systems Mills Jarret Complex
Mills Jarret Complex
Box 101106
Columbia, SC 29211
803-898-0734
Fax: 803-898-2065
e-mail: swansokm@dhec.sc.gov

Kathy Swanson, State FIMR Director

South Dakota

8900 South Dakota Department of Health
Health Building
600 E Capitol Avenue
Pierre, SD 57501
605-773-3361
800-738-2301
Fax: 605-773-5509
e-mail: DOH.info@state.sd.us
www.doh.sd.gov

Nancy Shoup, Program Coordinator

Tennessee

8901 Tennessee Department of Health
Division of Maternal & Child Health
425 5th Avenue N
Nashville, TN 37243-4701
615-741-3111
Fax: 615-741-1063
e-mail: tn.health@tn.gov
health.state.tn.us

Susan R Cooper MSN RN, Commissioner

8902 Tennessee SIDS Alliance
7603 Moon Crest Court
Powell, TN 37849
423-947-6669
e-mail: lisasids@cs.com
ww.sidsalliance.org

Lisa Hunt, Chairperson

Texas

8903 Department of State Health Offices
Title V And Health Resources
PO Box 149347
Austin, TX 78714
512-458-7111
888-963-7111
Fax: 512-458-7650
e-mail: chan.mcdermott@dshs.state.tx.us
www.dshs.state.tx.us

Mary Chan Mcdermott, Prenatal Coordinator

8904 Greater Houston Chapter SIDS Alliance
916 Satsuma Street
Pasadena, TX 77506
713-924-1419
Fax: 281-541-5340
e-mail: anita.carmona@us.rhodia.com
www.sidsalliance.org

Anita Carmona, Chairperson

8905 Harris County Public Health and Environmental Services
2223 W Lop S
Houston, TX 77027
713-439-6000
e-mail: publicinfo@hd.co.harris.tx.us
www.hcphes.org

Herminia Palacio, Executive Director

8906 Region VI Office Program Consultants for Maternal and Child Health
1301 Young Street
Dallas, TX 75202-4325
214-767-3003
Fax: 214-767-3038
e-mail: geurink@zeecon.com
www.mchoralhealth.org

Kathy Geurin RDH BS MA, Oral Health Consultant

8907 Southwest SIDS Research Institute
Brazosport Memorial Hospital
100 Medical Drive
Lake Jackson, TX 77566
409-297-4411
www.swsids.com

ISBN: 9-792992-81-4
CF Hogan, President
Loretta Washington, Vice-President

Utah

8908 Utah Department of Health
Child Adolescent & School Health Program
288 N 1460 W
Salt Lake City, UT 84114-3231
801-538-6870
Fax: 801-538-6200
www.health.utah.gov

David Sundwa MD, Executive Director
A Richard Melton, Deputy Director

8909 Utah SIDS Alliance
1760 American Park Circle
W Valley City, UT 84119
801-487-7800
Fax: 801-487-4477
e-mail: lisa.hughes@fnwmail.com
www.sidsalliance.org

Lisa Hughes, President
Troy Hughes, Co-President

Vermont

8910 Vermont Department of Health: SIDS Information and Counseling Program
108 Cherry Street
Burlington, VT 05402
802-652-2000
Fax: 802-652-2005
TTY: 800-253-0191
e-mail: kkelehe@vdh.state.vt.us
healthvermont.gov

Kathy Keleher, Assistant Director Public Health

Virginia

8911 SIDS Mid-Atlantic
PO Box 799
Haymarket, VA 20168
703-955-6899
Fax: 703-933-9101
e-mail: bconnal@aol.com
www.sidsma.org

Betty Connal, Executive Director

8912 Virginia SIDS Alliance
PO Box 752
Mechanicsville, VA 23111
Fax: 757-548-7074
e-mail: mail@vasids.org
www.vasids.org

Terri Newman, President
Mark Ferraro, Vice President

8913 Virginia SIDS Program: Virginia Department of Health
Virginia Department of Health
109 Governor Street
Richmond, VA 23219
804-846-7772
Fax: 804-973-9498
e-mail: WomensAndInfantsHealth@vdh.virginia.gov
www.vdh.virginia.gov

Robert Stroube, Commissioner
Rosanne Kolesar, Deputy Commissioner Public Health

Washington

8914 Region X Office Program Consultants for Maternal and Child Health
2201 Sixth Avenue
Seattle, WA 98121-1857
206-615-2518
Fax: 206-615-2500
e-mail: rslayton@acf.hhs.gov
www.mchoralhealth.org

Rebecca Slay DDS PhD, Oral Health Consultant

8915 SIDS Foundation of Washington
4649 Sunnyside Avenue N
Seattle, WA 98103
206-548-9290
800-533-0376
Fax: 206-548-9445
e-mail: execdirector@sidsofwa.org
www.nisa-sids.org

Inga Paige, Executive Director
Lindsey Hulet, Office Administrator

8916 SIDS Northwest Regional Center
Washington Department of Health
111 Israel Rd SE
Olympia, WA 98501-7880
360-236-3502
800-533-0376
Fax: 360-236-2323
e-mail: mch.support@doh.wa.gov
www.doh.wa.gov

Lorrie Grevstad

8917 Washington State Department of Health Maternal & Child Health Office
111 Israel Rd SE
Olympia, WA 98501
360-236-3502
Fax: 360-236-2323
e-mail: mch.support@doh.wa.gov
www.doh.wa.gov

Shumei Yun, Manager Maternal and Child Health
Riley Peters, Director

West Virginia

8918 Office of Maternal, Child & Family Health
Bureau For Public Health

350 Capitol Street
Charelston, WV 25301
304-558-7997
Fax: 304-558-3510
e-mail: annmunson@wvdhhr.org

Ann Munson, SIDS Coordinator

Wisconsin

8919 Counseling and Research Center for SIDS
9000 W Wisconsin Avenue
Wauwatosa, WI 53226
414-266-2746
Fax: 414-266-3338
e-mail: aharvieux@chw.org
www.idcw.org

Anne Harvieux, Program Administrator

8920 Infant Death Center of Wisconsin Childrens Hospital Of Wisconsin
Childrens Hospital Of Wisconsin
PO Box 1997
Milwaukee, WI 53201
414-266-2746
Fax: 414-266-3140
e-mail: aharvieux@chw.org
www.idcw.org

Anne Harvieux, Program Administrator

Wyoming

8921 Wyoming Department of Health
Community & Family Health Section
6101 Yellowstone Road
Cheyenne, WY 82002
307-777-6326
Fax: 307-777-7215
e-mail: mirandie.peterson@health.wyo.gov
wdh.state.wy.us

Molly M Bruner MSN RNC, Administrator

Research Centers

8922 Massachusetts Sudden Infant Death Syndrome Boston City Hospital
Boston City Hospital
1 Boston Medical Center Place
Boston, MA 02118
617-534-7434
Fax: 617-534-5555
www.bmc.org

A joint program of Boston City Hospital and Children's Hospital. Services provided include around-the-clock availability for consultation to health professionals and families counseling of families parent group meetings and supportive home visits.

8923 Pediatric Pulmonary Unit Massachusetts General Hospital
Massachusetts General Hospital
55 Fruit Street
Boston, MA 02114
617-726-0336
Fax: 617-242-03
www.massgeneral.org

Sudden infant death syndrome and childhood disorders research.
T Bernard Kinane MD, Head Physician

8924 Sudden Infant Death Syndrome Institute of the University of Maryland
22 S Green Street
Baltimore, MD 21201
410-538-3363
800-492-5538
www.umm.edu

Dr M John O'Brien MB, Director

8925 USC: Neonatology Research Units
1240 Mission Road
Los Angeles, CA 90033
213-226-3408
Fax: 213-226-3440

Focuses on clinical problems of the newborn and premature infant.
Paul YK Wu MD, Director

Support Groups & Hotlines

8926 National Center for the Prevention of SIDS
1314 Bedford Avenue
Baltimore, MD 21208-6605
800-638-7437

Offers medical updates and information on prevention of SIDS and other disorders to parents and professionals.

8927   National Health Information Center
PO Box 1133   310-565-4167
Washington, DC 20013   800-336-4797
                                                  Fax: 301-984-4256
                                                  e-mail: info@nhic.org
                                                  www.health.gov/nhic
Offers a nationwide information referral service, produces directories and resource guides.

8928   Parents Helping Parents A Family Resource Center
3041 Olcott Street   408-727-5775
Santa Clara, CA 95054   866-747-4040
                                                  Fax: 408-727-0182
                                                  www.php.com
A group of parents and professionals committed to alleviating some of the problems, hardships and concerns of families with children having special needs.
Mary Ellen Peterson, Director

8929   SIDS Information and Referral Hotline
SIDS Alliance
1314 Bedford Avenue   410-653-8226
Baltimore, MD 21208   800-221-7437
                                                  Fax: 410-653-8709
                                                  www.firstcandle.org
Twenty-four hour information and referral line for parents who wish to discuss their concerns with a SIDS counselor, request additional information about SIDS and to receive referrals to the local SIDS affiliate in their area.
Deborah Boyd, Director

8930   SIDS Support Group
Massachusetts Center for SIDS
Boston Medical Center   617-414-SIDS
Boston, MA 02118   800-641-7437
                                                  www.bmc.org
Aids in the resolution of the early trauma of grief experienced by parents following the sudden unexpected death of their infant. The purposes are to provide a safe environemnt for parents to express their feelings, to provide contact with others who share their grief and are at various stages of resolution, to provide a reliable source of information about SIDS and to provide the opportunity to go on to help others.

Books

8931   Apparent Life-Threatening Event and Sudden Infant Death Syndrome
National Maternal and Child Health Clearinghouse
2070 Chain Bridge Road   703-442-9051
Vienna, VA 22182-2588   888-275-4772
                                                  Fax: 703-821-2098
                                                  e-mail: ask@hrsa.gov
                                                  www.ask.hrsa.gov
Provides information about ALTE and its relationship to SIDS.

8932   Hospice Care for Children
Oxford University Press
2001 Evans Road   212-726-6000
Cary, NC 27513-2010   800-451-7556
                                                  Fax: 919-677-1303
                                                  www.oup-usa.org
A comprehensive book offering the most inclusive and up-to-date information about caring for terminally ill children and their families.
304 pages
ISBN: 0-195073-12-6
Ann Armstrong-Dailey, Editor

8933   Professional's Role in Sudden Infant Death Syndrome
National Maternal and Child Health Clearinghouse
2070 Chain Bridge Road   703-442-9051
Vienna, VA 22182-2588   888-275-4772
                                                  Fax: 703-821-2098
                                                  e-mail: ask@hrsa.gov
                                                  www.ask.hrsa.gov
Contains abstracts of articles on the role of professionals in SIDS.

8934   Smoking and Sudden Infant Death Syndrome
National Maternal and Child Health Clearinghouse
2070 Chain Bridge Road   703-442-9051
Vienna, VA 22182-2588   888-275-4772
                                                  Fax: 703-821-2098
                                                  e-mail: ask@hrsa.gov
                                                  www.ask.hrsa.gov
Contains abstracts of materials about tobacco use, its relationship to SIDS and the dangers to the unborn and the newly born from passive and secondary smoking.

Newsletters

8935   Newsletter: SIDS
Massachusetts Center For SIDS
1 Boston Medical Center Place
Boston, MA 02118-2905   617-414-8504
                                                  www.bmc.org/program/sids/
Offers information on SIDS, articles pertaining to the latest information available on the mystery condition, latest research and fund-raising news and professional resources available.
Monthly

8936   Parent Care News Brief
Parent Care
303 Watts Branch Parkway   301-294-9338
Rockville, MD 20850-1210   Fax: 301-294-8848
                                                  e-mail: drscott@parentcare.com
                                                  www.parentcare.com
Features articles and medical updates pertaining to the care of the critically ill child.
Quarterly

Pamphlets

8937   Crib Death: The Sudden Infant Death Syndrome
US Department Of Health & Human Services
202 Independence Avenue SW   202-619-0257
Washington, DC 20201-0001   877-696-6775
                                                  e-mail: hhsmail@os.dhhs.gov
                                                  www.os.dhhs.gov
Offers information on the most frequently asked questions pertaining to SIDS and crib death.
Kristen Brett
Kathy McKnight

8938   Developmental Delays and Developmental Disorders
National Maternal and Child Health Clearinghouse
2070 Chain Bridge Road   703-442-9051
Vienna, VA 22182-2588   888-275-4772
                                                  Fax: 703-821-2098
                                                  e-mail: ask@hrsa.gov
                                                  www.ask.hrsa.gov
Contains abstracts of selected articles on developmental delays and developmental disorders and the relationship to SIDS.
1997

8939   Facts About SIDS
Sudden Infant Death Syndrome Alliance
1314 Bedford Avenue   410-653-8226
Baltimore, MD 21208-6605   800-221-7437
                                                  Fax: 410-653-8709
Offers information on basic facts, answers to the most frequently asked questions about SIDS and information on numbers to call and referral centers for more help.

8940   Grief of Children After the Loss of a Sibling or Friend
National Maternal and Child Health Clearinghouse
2070 Chain Bridge Road   703-442-9051
Vienna, VA 22182-2588   888-275-4772
                                                  Fax: 703-821-2098
                                                  e-mail: ask@hrsa.gov
                                                  www.ask.hrsa.gov
Discusses some of the common expressions of childrens grief and offers ways adults can help during the grieving process.
1995

8941   Infant Positioning and Sudden Infant Death Syndrome
National Maternal and Child Health Clearinghouse
2070 Chain Bridge Road   703-442-9051
Vienna, VA 22182-2588   888-275-4772
                                          Fax: 703-821-2098
                                     e-mail: ask@hrsa.gov
                                          www.ask.hrsa.gov
Contains abstracts of selected articles on the topic of sleep position and SIDS.
1994

8942   Nationwide Survey of Sudden Infant Death Syndrome (SIDS) Service
National Maternal and Child Health Clearinghouse
2070 Chain Bridge Road   703-442-9051
Vienna, VA 22182-2588   888-275-4772
                                          Fax: 703-821-2098
                                     e-mail: ask@hrsa.gov
                                          www.ask.hrsa.gov
Analysis of availability of SIDS services.
1994

8943   Parents and the Grieving Process
National Maternal and Child Health Clearinghouse
2070 Chain Bridge Road   703-442-9051
Vienna, VA 22182-2588   888-275-4772
                                          Fax: 703-821-2098
                                     e-mail: ask@hrsa.gov
                                          www.ask.hrsa.gov
Defines grief, presents common reactions and emotions expressed by the bereaved.
1992

8944   SIDS Information for the EMT
National Maternal and Child Health Clearinghouse
2070 Chain Bridge Road   703-442-9051
Vienna, VA 22182-2588   888-275-4772
                                          Fax: 703-821-2098
                                     e-mail: ask@hrsa.gov
                                          www.ask.hrsa.gov
Provides suggestions for first response of emergency medical technicians and others at the time of sudden infant death.
1983

8945   SIDS Research: An Analysis in Three Parts
National Maternal and Child Health Clearinghouse
2070 Chain Bridge Road   703-442-9051
Vienna, VA 22182-2588   888-275-4772
                                          Fax: 703-821-2098
                                     e-mail: ask@hrsa.gov
                                          www.ask.hrsa.gov
Contains articles from a three part series on SIDS research.
1993

8946   SIDS: Toward Prevention and Improved Infant Health
American SIDS Institute
2480 Windy Hill Road SE   770-612-1030
Marietta, GA 30067-8657   800-232-7437
                                          Fax: 770-612-8277
                                     e-mail: prevent@sids.org
                                          www.sids.org
A practical guide for those planning a pregnancy, for parents to be and for new parents.
Betty McEntire PhD, Executive Director

8947   Selected Book on Sudden Infant Death Syndrome
National Maternal and Child Health Clearinghouse
2070 Chain Bridge Road   703-442-9051
Vienna, VA 22182-2588   888-275-4772
                                          Fax: 703-821-2098
                                     e-mail: ask@hrsa.gov
                                          www.ask.hrsa.gov
Provides a list of selected titles on SIDS covering topics such as research, support information and the professionals role.
1993

8948   Selected Resources for Children Grieving the Loss of Another Child
National Maternal and Child Health Clearinghouse
2070 Chain Bridge Road   703-442-9051
Vienna, VA 22182-2588   888-275-4772
                                          Fax: 703-821-2098
                                     e-mail: ask@hrsa.gov
                                          www.ask.hrsa.gov
Provides a list of materials suitable for grieving children and teenagers.
1995

8949   Sudden Infant Death Syndrome and Risk Reduction
National Maternal and Child Health Clearinghouse
2070 Chain Bridge Road   703-442-9051
Vienna, VA 22182-2588   888-275-4772
                                          Fax: 703-821-2098
                                     e-mail: ask@hrsa.gov
                                          www.ask.hrsa.gov
Contains abstracts of selected articles on risk reduction.
1997

8950   What Every Parent Should Know About SIDS
SIDS Alliance
1314 Bedford Avenue   410-653-8226
Baltimore, MD 21208-6605   800-221-7437
                                          Fax: 410-653-8709
Pamphlet offering information on what SIDS is, causes, prevention techniques and what parents can do.

8951   What is SIDS?
National Maternal and Child Health Clearinghouse
2070 Chain Bridge Road   703-442-9051
Vienna, VA 22182-2588   888-275-4772
                                          Fax: 703-821-2098
                                     e-mail: ask@hrsa.gov
                                          www.ask.hrsa.gov
Provides basic facts about SIDS and answers some of the most commonly asked questions.
1993

8952   When Sudden Infant Death Syndrome Occurs in Childcare Settings
National Maternal and Child Health Clearinghouse
2070 Chain Bridge Road   703-442-9051
Vienna, VA 22182-2588   888-275-4772
                                          Fax: 703-821-2098
                                     e-mail: ask@hrsa.gov
                                          www.ask.hrsa.gov
Presents information about SIDS for child care providers.
1993

Web Sites

8953   American SIDS Institute
                                               sids.org/
Dedicated to the prevention of sudden infant death and the promotion of infant health through research, clinical services, education and family support.

8954   Center for Research for Mothers & Children
                                          cdrwww.who.ch/
Mission is to make sure everyone is born healthy and wanted, that women suffer no harmful effects from reproductive processes, and that all children have the chance to achieve their full potential for healthy and productive lives, free from disease or disability, and to ensure the health, productivity, independence, and well-being of all people through optimal rehabilitation.

8955   Compassionate Friends
                                     www.compassionatefriends.org
A national organization that offers 600 local chapters that give support to parents and siblings who have experienced the death of a child.

8956   Healing Well
                                          www.healingwell.com
An online health resource guide to medical news, chat, information and articles, newsgroups and message boards, books, disease-related web sites, medical directories, and more for patients, friends, and family coping with disabling diseases, disorders, or chronic illnesses.

8957   Healthlink USA

www.healthlinkusa.com

Health information concerning treatment, cures, prevention, diagnosis, risk factors, research, support groups, email lists, personal stories and much more. Updated regularly.

8958   Helios Health

www.helioshealth.com

Online resource for your health information. Detailed information about specific health topics, access to expert advice from our Medical Advisory Board, and up-to-date health news.

8959   MedicineNet

www.medicinenet.com

An online resource for consumers providing easy-to-read, authoritative medical and health information.

8960   Medscape

www.medscape.com

Medscape offers specialists, primary care physicians, and other health professionals the Web's most robust and integrated medical information and educational tools.

8961   National Center for Education in Maternal and Child Health

www.ncemch.org

The National Center for Education in Maternal and Child Health provides national leadership to the maternal and child health community in three key areas - program development, policy analysis and education, and state-of-the-art knowledge to improve the health and well-being of the nation's children and families.

8962   WebMD

www.webmd.com

Information on Sudden Infant Death Syndrome, including articles and resources.

Description

8963 ## Tay-Sachs Disease

Tay-Sachs disease results from an absence of an enzyme (hexosaminidase A) which leads to an accumulation of fat (lipid) in the specific brain tissues (cerebral neurons). The disease is genetic and is autosomal recessive; if two carriers have children, the disease would have a 1 in 4 chance of being passed on. The disease is most prevalent in those of Jewish families, particularly those of Eastern European (Ashkenazi) background.

Symptoms usually present between 3-6 months of age. Early symptoms include mild muscle weakness, muscle spasms, and feeding difficulties. As the disease progresses, the patient may experience vision loss, seizures and eventually paralysis. Death usually occurs by the age of 4 years.

Treatment for Tay-Sachs disease is supportive and there is no cure. Genetic and premarital counseling is important to those at high risk.

National Agencies & Associations

8964 **National Foundation for Jewish Genetic Diseases**
Fifth Avenue at 100th Street   212-659-6774
New York, NY 10029   Fax: 212-241-6947
                                      www.mssm.edu/jewish_genetics
Offers information and support for persons suffering from Tay-Sachs Disease as well as their families and professionals working with them. The Foundation supports research into all areas of genetic disorders.
R J Desnick PhD MD, Center Director

8965 **National Institute of Child Health and Human Development**
31 Center Drive   301-496-5133
Bethesda, MD 20892   800-370-2943
                                      Fax: 866-760-5947
                                      TTY: 888-320-6942
                                      e-mail: mcgrathj@mail.nih.gov
                                      www.nichd.nih.gov
Offers reprints, articles and various information on Tay-Sachs Disease for patients and professionals.
Duane Alexan MD, Director
John McGrath, Coordinator

8966 **National Institute of Neurological Disorders and Stroke**
NIH Neurological Institute   301-496-5751
Bethesda, MD 20824   800-352-9424
                                      Fax: 301-402-2186
                                      TTY: 301-468-5981
                                      www.ninds.nih.gov
The mission of NINDS is to reduce the burden of neurological disease - a burden borne by every age group, by every segment of society, by people all over the world.
Story C Landis PhD, Director
Walter J Koroshetz, Deputy Director

8967 **National Organization for Rare Disorders**
55 Kenosia Avenue   203-744-0100
Danbury, CT 06813-1968   800-999-6673
                                      Fax: 203-798-2291
                                      TDD: 203-797-9590
                                      e-mail: orphan@rarediseases.org
                                      www.rarediseases.org
Serves as a clearinghouse for information about rare disorders and brings together families with similar disorders for mutual support; fosters communication among rare disease voluntary agencies, Government agencies, industry scientific researchers and academia.
Frank Sasinowski, Chair
Carolyn Asbury, PhD, Vice Chair

8968 **National Tay-Sachs and Allied Diseases Association (NTSAD)**
2001 Beacon Street
Brighton, MA 02135   800-906-8723
                                      Fax: 617-277-0134
                                      e-mail: info@ntsad.org
                                      www.ntstad.org
Offers programs of public and professional education prevention services testing research and family services and promotion of TSD genetic screening programs nationally.
Fran Berkwits, Director
Bradley L Campbell, President

Foundations

8969 **National Tay-Sachs and Allied Diseases Association (NTSAD)**
2001 Beacon Street
Brighton, MA 02135   800-906-8723
                                      Fax: 617-277-0134
                                      e-mail: info@ntsad.org
                                      www.ntsad.org
Dedicated to the treatment and preventin of Tay Sachs, Canavan, and related diseases, and to provide information and support services to individuals and families affected by these diseases, as well as the public at large.
John F Crowley MBA, JD, President

Support Groups & Hotlines

8970 **National Health Information Center**
PO Box 1133   310-565-4167
Washington, DC 20013   800-336-4797
                                      Fax: 301-984-4256
                                      e-mail: info@nhic.org
                                      www.health.gov/nhic
Offers a nationwide information referral service, produces directories and resource guides.

8971 **National Tay-Sachs Association: Delaware Valley (NTSAD-DV)**
720 Greenwood Avenue   215-887-0877
Jenkintown, PA 19046   877-599-9293
                                      Fax: 215-887-1931
                                      e-mail: NTSAD@aol.com
                                      www.tay-sachs.org

Rebecca Tantala, Executive Director

8972 **National TaySachs & Allied Diseases**
2001 Beacon Street   617-277-4463
Boston, MA 2135   800-906-8723
                                      Fax: 617-277-0134
                                      e-mail: info@ntsad.org
                                      www.ntsad.org
A mutual support group coordinated by staff and volunteers who are parents of affected children or affected adults. One of several programs supported and sponsored by the association.
Kim Crawford, Member Services Coordinator

Books

8973 **Home Care Book**
National Tay-Sachs and Allied Diseases Association
2001 Beacon Street
Brighton, MA 02135   800-906-8723
                                      Fax: 617-277-0134
                                      e-mail: info@ntsad.org
                                      www.ntsad.org
Written by parents for parents and professionals, the Home Care Book is a guide to caring for children with progressive neurological disorders at home.
John F Crowley MBA, JD, President

8974 Home-Care Book
National Tay-Sachs and Allied Diseases Association
2001 Beacon Street
Brookline, MA 02146   800-906-8723
A guide for caring for children with progressive neurological diseases.

8975 Late Onset Tay-Sachs Disease Medical Bibliography
National Tay-Sachs and Allied Diseases Association
2001 Beacon Street
Brookline, MA 02146   800-906-8723

8976 Lifting of Canavan's Carrier Testing Facilities
National Tay-Sachs and Allied Diseases Association
2001 Beacon Street
Brookline, MA 02146   800-906-8723

8977 Monograph on Canavan's Disease
National Tay-Sachs and Allied Diseases Association
2001 Beacon Street
Brookline, MA 02146   800-906-8723

8978 Tay-Sachs Carrier Testing Directory
National Tay-Sachs and Allied Diseases Association
2001 Beacon Street
Brookline, MA 02146   800-906-8723

8979 Tay-Sachs: The Dreaded Inheritance
National Tay-Sachs and Allied Diseases Assocation
2001 Beacon Street
Brighton, MA 02135   800-906-8723
                                             Fax: 617-277-0134
                          e-mail: NTSAD-Boston@worldnet.att.net
                                                www.ntsad.org
Descriptive narrative on caring for a child with Tay-Sachs Disease.

8980 There is Only One Child
National Tay-Sachs and Allied Diseases Association
2001 Beacon Street
Brookline, MA 02146   800-906-8723

8981 What Every Family Should Know Sixth Edition
National Tay-Sachs & Allied Diseases Association
2001 Beacon Street
Brighton, MA 02135   800-906-8723
                                             Fax: 617-277-0134
                                       e-mail: info@ntsad.org
                                                www.ntsad.org
Detailing lysosomal storage and leukodystrophy disorders, with
sections on Tay-Sachs, Sandhoff, Niemann-Pick, Gaucher,
Canavan, Fabry, Pompe, therapeutic approaches and unique disease table.
50 pages
John F Crowley MBA. JD, President

Newsletters

8982 Breakthrough
National Tay-Sachs and Allied Diseases Association
2001 Beacon Street
Boston, MA 02135   800-906-8723
                                             Fax: 617-277-0134
                                       e-mail: info@ntsad.org
                                                www.ntsad.org
Each year NTSAD publishes a newsletter for friends and supporters that focuses on the latest advances in research, profiles of families and individuals helped by NTSAD and disease profiles.
Annual
John F Crowley MBA, JD, President

8983 Late Onset Community Newsletter
National Tay-Sachs and Allied Diseases Association
2001 Beacon Street
Brighton, MA 02135   800-906-8723
                                             Fax: 617-277-0134
                                       e-mail: info@ntsad.org
                                                www.ntsad.org
PSG members dealing with chronic forms of the allied diseases receive this newsletter focused specifically on the issues and per-

spectives unique to adults struggling with long-term disability issues. Public editions of the newsletter are also available.
Bi-Monthly
John F Crowley MBA, JD, President

8984 Lifeline
National Tay-Sachs and Allied Diseases Association
2001 Beacon Street
Brighton, MA 02135   800-906-8723
                                             Fax: 617-277-0134
                                       e-mail: info@ntsad.org
                                                www.ntsad.org
The editorial content is wide ranging: symptom management and home health care; new product reviews; guidance in benefits and services advocacy for families and affected individuals of all ages; science and medical research updates; coverage of NTSAD events, fundraising, programs and administrative activities. Members only.
Quarterly
John F Crowley MBA, JD, President

Pamphlets

8985 Late Onset Tay-Sachs Fact Sheet
National Tay-Sachs and Allied Diseases Association
2001 Beacon Street
Brighton, MA 02135   800-906-8723
                                             Fax: 617-277-0134
                                       e-mail: info@ntsad.org
                                                www.ntsad.org
This quick reference information sheet on the chronic or late onset form of Tay-Sachs is available for no charge.
John F Crowley MBA, JD, President

8986 Services to Families
National Tay-Sachs and Allied Diseases Association
2001 Beacon Street
Brookline, MA 02146   800-906-8723
Offers information on the Association parent peer groups, referrals and advocacy services to families and patients.

8987 Tay-Sachs Information Sheet
March of Dimes
233 Park Avenue South   212-353-8353
New York, NY 10003   Fax: 212-254-3518
                        e-mail: NY639@marchofdimes.com
                                         www.marchofdimes.com
Offers a brief overview of the illness, causes, symptoms and treatments are covered. Availabe electronically on the website:
www.marchofdimes.com

8988 Tay-Sachs is
National Tay-Sachs and Allied Diseases Association
2001 Beacon Street
Brookline, MA 02146   800-906-8723
Information on the history of the disease, what a victim of the disease should know and what they can do as far as resources and referrals.

8989 Understanding Lysosomal Storage Diseases
National Tay-Sachs and Allied Diseases Association
2001 Beacon Street
Brookline, MA 02146   800-906-8723

8990 What is Canavan Disease?
National Tay-Sachs and Allied Diseases Association
2001 Beacon Street
Brighton, MA 02135   800-906-8723
                                             Fax: 617-277-0134
                                       e-mail: info@ntsad.org
                                                www.ntsad.org
The educational pamphlet describing Canavan Disease.
John F Crowley MBA, JD, President

8991 What is Tay-Sachs? Russian Translation
National Tay-Sachs and Allied Diseases Association

2001 Beacon Street
Brighton, MA 02135

800-906-8723
Fax: 617-277-0134
e-mail: info@ntsad.org
www.ntsad.org

This informative educational pamphlet describing Infantile Tay-Sachs, its inheritance and prevention is available for no charge.

John F Crowley MBA, JD, President

Audio & Video

8992　For My Sister, Elyssa
National Tay-Sachs & Allied Diseases Assocation
2001 Beacon Street
Brighton, MA 02135

800-906-8723
Fax: 617-277-0134
e-mail: NTSAD-Boston@worldnet.att.net
www.ntsad.org

Moving and informative 15 minute presentation told by a teenager who baby siter died from Tay-Sachs Disease. Contains information on Tay-Sachs Disease and simple steps each individual can take to prevent the tragedy of Tay-Sachs.

Web Sites

8993　Healing Well

www.healingwell.com

An online health resource guide to medical news, chat, information and articles, newsgroups and message boards, books, disease-related web sites, medical directories, and more for patients, friends, and family coping with disabling diseases, disorders, or chronic illnesses.

8994　Health Finder

www.healthfinder.gov

Searchable, carefully developed web site offering information on over 1000 topics. Developed by the US Department of Health and Human Services, the site can be used in both English and Spanish.

8995　Healthlink USA

www.healthlinkusa.com

Health information concerning treatment, cures, prevention, diagnosis, risk factors, research, support groups, email lists, personal stories and much more. Updated regularly.

8996　Helios Health

www.helioshealth.com

Online resource for your health information. Detailed information about specific health topics, access to expert advice from our Medical Advisory Board, and up-to-date health news.

8997　MedicineNet

www.medicinenet.com

An online resource for consumers providing easy-to-read, authoritative medical and health information.

8998　Medscape

www.medscape.com

Medscape offers specialists, primary care physicians, and other health professionals the Web's most robust and integrated medical information and educational tools.

8999　WebMD

www.webmd.com

Information on Tay-Sachs disease, including articles and resources.

Description

9000 **Thyroid Disease**

Thyroid Disease refers to a number of conditions that affect the thyroid, a small, butterfly-shaped gland located in the middle of the lower neck. Hormones T3 and T4, produced by the thyroid, deliver energy to cells of the body, thus controlling the body's metabolism. Conditions that result from an imbalance of these hormones are Hypothyroidism — not enough hormones that results in the body using energy slower than it should, and Hyperthyroidism — too much hormones that results in the body using energy faser than it should. These conditions can be caused by an inflammation of the thyroid gland, too much or too little iodine (used to produce thyroid hormones), or autoimmune disease, in which antibodies gradually either destroy the thyroid gland or speed up its function. Other thyroid conditions are Goiter — an enlarged thyroid; Thyroid Nodules — cysts, lumps, bumps and tumors that can be cancerous or benign; and Thyroiditis — inflammation of the thyroid gland. More than 20 million Americans have thyroid disease, and it affects many more women than men. Treatment includes synthetic hormone medication to replace missing hormones, radioactive iodine to deactivate the thyroid, and surgery for some goiters and cancerous nodules. Early diagnosis is often the key in prescribing treatment even before the onset of symptoms. Although thyroid disease is a chronic condition, careful disease management allows affected individuals to live healthy, normal lives.

National Agencies & Associations

9001 **American Thyroid Association**
6066 Leesburg Pike   703-998-8890
Falls Church, VA 22041   800-479-7634
                               Fax: 703-998-8893
                          e-mail: thyroid@thyroid.org
                               www.thyroid.org
Promotes excellence and innovation in clinical care research education and public policy.
Barbara R. Smith, CAE, Executive Director

9002 **National Women's Health Resource Center**
157 Broad Street   877-986-9472
Red Bank, NJ 07701   877-986-9472
                               Fax: 732-530-3347
                        e-mail: snelson@healthwomen.org
                              www.healthywomen.org
NWHRC develops and distributes up-to-date and objective women's health information based on the latest advances in medical research and practice.
Patricia Gurne, Chairman
Elizabeth Ba Cahill, Executive Director

9003 **Thyroid Federation International**
797 Princess Street   613-544-8364
Kingston, Ontario, K7L-1G1   Fax: 613-544-9731
                          e-mail: tfi@on.aibn.com
                              www.thyroid-fed.org
Aims to work for the benefit of those affected by thyroid disorders throughout the world.
Yvonne Andersson, President, Board of Directors
Peter Lakwijk, VP, Board of Directors

9004 **Thyroid Foundation of Canada**
797 Princess Street   613-544-8364
Kingston, Ontario, K7L-1G1   800-267-8822
                               Fax: 613-544-9731
                               www.thyroid.ca
Thyroid Foundation of Canada is a registered charity.
Katherine Keen, National Office Coordinator

Books

9005 **Autoimmune Connection: Essential Informati on for Women on Diagnosis, Treatment**
National Women's Health Resource Center
157 Broad Street   877-986-9472
Red Bank, NJ 07701   Fax: 732-530-3347
                          e-mail: info@healthywomen.org
                              www.healthywomen.org
Readers learn about the recent groundbreaking discovery of the links between the different autoimmune diseases and why women are more likely to develop them.
Elizabeth Battaglino Cahill, Executive Director

9006 **The Thyroid Gland**
Joel I Hamburger MD & Michael M Kaplan, author
Thyroid Foundation of Canada
797 Princess Street   613-544-8364
Kingston, Ontario, K7L-1G1   800-267-8822
                               Fax: 613-544-9731
                               www.thyroid.ca
Provides material for the patient to study at home, and to review at subsequent visits to the physician.

9007 **Thyroid Balance**
National Women's Health Resource Center
157 Broad Street   877-986-9472
Red Bank, NJ 07701   Fax: 732-530-3347
                          e-mail: info@healthywomen.org
                              www.healthywomen.org
An authoritative guide to treating thyroid issues-using both traditional and alternative methods.
Elizabeth Battaglino Cahill, Executive Director

9008 **Thyroid Disease: The Facts**
RIS Bayliss & WMG Tunbridge MD, author
Thyroid Foundation of Canada
797 Princess Street   613-544-8364
Kingston, Ontario, K7L-1G1   800-267-8822
                               Fax: 613-544-9731
                               www.thyroid.ca
Provides patients, their friends, and relatives with an up-to-date, readable account of disorders of the thyroid and the treatments which are now available.

9009 **Thyroid Power: Ten Steps to Total Health**
Richard Shames & Karilee H Shames, author
National Women's Health Resource Center
157 Broad Street   877-986-9472
Red Bank, NJ 07701   Fax: 732-530-3347
                          e-mail: snelson@healthwomen.org
                              www.healthywomen.org
Discusses the labyrinth of diagnostic and treatment issues a patient must endure.

9010 **Thyroid Solution: A Mind-Body Program for Beating Depression and Regaining Health**
National Women's Health Resource Center
157 Broad Street   877-986-9472
Red Bank, NJ 07701   Fax: 732-530-3347
                          e-mail: info@healthywomen.org
                              www.healthywomen.org
This book explains the link between stress and thyroid imbalance; how thyroid imbalance affects your emotions, sex life, and relationships; and how to cope with the effects of this imbalance.
Elizabeth Battaglino Cahill, Executive Director

9011 **Thyroid Sourcebook**
Thyroid Foundation of Canada

797 Princess Street
Kingston, Ontario, K7L-1G1

613-544-8364
800-267-8822
Fax: 613-544-9731
www.thyroid.ca

Provides the guidance, reassurance, and important information you need to manage your health and make informed decisions.

9012 Your Thyroid: A Home Reference
Lawrence Wood MD & David S Cooper MD, author
Thyroid Foundation of Canada
797 Princess Street
Kingston, Ontario, K7L-1G1

613-544-8364
800-267-8822
Fax: 613-544-9731
www.thyroid.ca

Explains the latest scientific advances can mean to you.

Magazines

9013 Clinical Thyroidology
American Thyroid Association
6066 Leesburg Pike
Falls Church, VA 12041

703-998-8890
800-849-7634
Fax: 703-998-8893
e-mail: editorclinthy@thyroid.org
www.thyroid.org

An online publication, available monthly, this is a broad-ranging look at clinical and preclinical thyroid literature. The Editor searches the world literature for excellent thyroid studies and then summarizes them along side his expert commentary.
Ernest L. Mazzaferri, MD, Editor

9014 THYROID
American Thyroid Association
6066 Leesburg Pike
Falls Church, VA 12041

703-998-8890
800-849-7643
Fax: 703-998-8893
e-mail: thyroideditor@umassmed.edu
www.thyroid.org

The Associations monthly journal that touches on topics from the molecular biology of the thyroid gland to clinical management of thyroid disorders. All Association members receive a suvscription, and it is available to non-members.

9015 Clinical Thyroidology for Patients
American Thyroid Association
6066 Leesburg Pike
Falls Church, VA 12041

703-998-8890
800-849-7634
Fax: 703-998-8893
e-mail: editorclinthy@thyroid.org
www.thyroid.org

A collection of summaries of recently published articles fromt the medical literature that covers the broad spectrum of thryroid disorders. Notes descxribing published research studies were prepared by THYROID Editor, Ernest Mazzaferri, MD.

Newsletters

9016 SIGNAL
American Thyroid Association
6066 Leesburg Pike
Falls Church, VA 12041

703-998-8890
800-849-7643
Fax: 703-998-8893
e-mail: thyroid@thyroid.org
www.thyroid.org

Covers Association news, meetings, policies, leaders, and important thyroid-related issues.

Pamphlets

9017 Hypothyroidism Web Booklet
American Thyroid Association
6066 Leesburg Pike
Falls Church, VA 12041

703-998-8890
800-489-7643
Fax: 703-998-8893
e-mail: thyroid@thyroid.org
www.thyroid.org

This online booklet introduces the thryroid and hypothyroidism to the reader, explains symptoms, treatments, causes, who's at risk, and more.
2003 25 pages

Web Sites

9018 American Thyroid Association

www.thyroid.com

Promotes excellence and innovation in clinical care, research, education, and public policy.
David S Cooper MD, President
Gregory A Brent MD, Secretary

9019 MedicineNet

www.medicinenet.com

An online resource for consumers providing easy-to-read, authoritative medical and health information.

9020 National Women's Health Resource Center

www.healthywomen.org

NWHRC developes and distributes up-to-date and objective women's health information based on the latest advances in medical research and practice.
Elizabeth Battaglino Cahill, RN, Executive Director
Maria Bushee, Director of Marketing & Communications

9021 Thyroid Federation International

www.thyroid-fed.org

Aims to work for the benefit of those affected by thyroid disorders throughout the world.

9022 Thyroid Foundation of Canada

www.thyroid.ca

Thyroid Foundation of Canada is a registered charity.

Description

9023 Tick-Borne Disease

Ticks transmit disease to humans by being carriers for a variety of microorganismns. The most common tick-borne illness is Lyme disease, first recognized and so named in 1975 because of a cluster of cases found in Lyme, Connecticut. It is a bacterial infection spread by the bite of an infected deer tick. The disease in its earliest stages causes an expanding red rash in at least 75 percent of patients. Flu-like symptoms—headaches, fever, fatigue—are common. The rash may be followed by progressive joint pain and swelling. Dysfunction of the heart (8 percent) and nervous system (15 percent) develop weeks to months later. Further progression causes arthritis and more serious neurologic problems.

Although only one third of patients remember a tick bite, greater than 60 percent do develop the tell-tale rash. Diagnosis requires a blood test to confirm the physical symptoms.

Oral antibiotics may be sufficient for the disease caught in the early stages. Long-standing, disseminated disease responds best to intravenous antibiotics.

Rocky Mountain spotted fever, also known as tick fever, is transmitted by a bite from either a dog tick or wood tick, depending on the part of the country. Like Lyme disease, it begin with flu-like symptoms — chills, fever and loss of appetite. A rash of small, reddish bumps, which gives the disease its name, begins on the wrist and ankle and spreads to the rest of the body. Aggressive antibotic treatment should begin as early as possible. If left untreated, Rocky Mountain spotted fever has a mortality rate of 10 to 80 percent.

Prevention of tick-borne disease requires avoidance of tick bites, by using insect repellants and protective clothing, plus daily checks for ticks during periods of exposure. A vaccine may provide partial protection from Lyme disease for those regularly engaged in high-risk activities (i.e. property maintenance), although other conditions may complicate this treatment.

National Agencies & Associations

9024 Lyme Disease Foundation
PO Box332
Tolland, CT 06084-0332
860-870-0070
800-886-5963
Fax: 860-870-0080
e-mail: info@lyme.org
www.lyme.org
Provides a wide range of services including information and referral network on Lyme Disease, distribution of educational videos to state libraries, educational materials for public and professionals, national public forums and training for community education.
John F Anderson, Board of Director
Willy Burgdorfer, Board of Director

Libraries & Resource Centers

9025 California Lyme Disease Association
PO Box 707
Weaverville, CA 96093
e-mail: info@lymedisease.org
www.lymedisease.org
The California Lyme Disease Association (CALDA) is an affiliate of the Lyme Disease Association, Inc. CALDA, a non-profit organization, was originally founded in 1990 as The Lyme Disease Resource Center (LDRC). We provide services for Lyme disease patients, their families and friends; provide a forum for physicians and health professionals for the exchange of ideas and information about symptoms, diagnosis, and treatment of Lyme disease.
Marilynn Barkley, Board of Directors
Barbara Barsoschinni, Board of Directors

Research Centers

9026 Ball State University Public Health Entomology Laboratory
2000 University Avenue
Muncie, IN 47306
765-289-1241
800-382-8540
www.bsu.edu
Offers information on mosquitoes and mosquito-born diseases specializing in Lyme Disease.
Bob Pinger, Director
Jeffrey Clark, Department Chair and Professor

9027 Centers for Disease Control Division of Vector Borne Infectious Diseases
US Public Health Service
PO Box 2087
Fort Collins, CO 80521
970-221-6400
Fax: 970-216-76
www.cdc.gov
Research done into lyme disease tularemia bubonic plague and all vector-borne infectious diseases — including west nile virus.
Lyle Petersen, Director

Support Groups & Hotlines

9028 Advocates 4 Health: Tick-borne Disease Self-Help Group
PALS
PO Box 1271
San Luis Obispo, CA 93406
805-544-0984
e-mail: advocates4heatlh@yahoo.com
Advocacy and support group increasing awareness, education and understanding of tick-borne disorders and other zoonotic diseases. This group fosters a supportive network between human/animal sufferers, caregivers, health care professionals and the general community.
Sheryl Glidden

9029 American Lyme Disease Foundation
PO Box 466
Lyme, CT 06371
e-mail: Inquire@aldf.com
www.aldf.com
Supports research and plays a key role in providing reliable and scientifically accurate information to the public and health care providers.
David L Weld, Executive Director
Jeffery Black, Partner

9030 Lyme Alliance
PO Box 454
Concord, MI 49237
517-563-3582
www.lymealliance.org
Lyme Alliance volunteers will address your questions concerning the newsletter, website, or questions about doctor referrals, medical treatment options, or information about Lyme disease.

9031 Lyme Disease Network
1613 Hewitt Avenue
St. Paul, MN 55104
651-644-7239
e-mail: olivierlynn@switchboardmail.com
Lynn M Olivier

9032 Lyme Disease Network Support Group of Alabama: Mobile Chapter
Mobile, AL 35758 256-772-6482
e-mail: alabamalyme@usa.com
www.lymnet.org/supportgroups
Support information, and referrals for victims of Lyme disease and their families.
Kara Tyson

9033 Lyme Disease Network of New Jersey
43 Winton Road
East Brunswick, NJ 08816 e-mail: carol@lymenet.org
www.lymenet.org
Support information, and referrals for victims of Lyme disease and their families. Maintains comuter information system.
Bill Stolow, President

9034 Lyme Disease Network of South Carolina
Po Box 6634 803-798-5963
Columbia, SC 29260-6634 e-mail: lyme@sc-lyme.org
www.sc-lyme.org
Sue Fox

9035 National Health Information Center
PO Box 1133 310-565-4167
Washington, DC 20013 800-336-4797
Fax: 301-984-4256
e-mail: info@nhic.org
www.health.gov/nhic
Offers a nationwide information referral service, produces directories and resource guides.

Books

9036 Coping with Lyme Disease: A Practical Guide
Henry Holt & Company
115 W 18th Street 212-886-9200
New York, NY 10011-4113 Fax: 212-633-0748
1993 288 pages Paperback
ISBN: 0-805026-50-9

9037 Ecology & Environment Management of Lyme Disease
Rutgers University Press
109 Church Street 201-932-7762
New Brunswick, NJ 08901-1242
1993 224 pages
ISBN: 0-813519-28-4

9038 Everything You Need to Know About Lyme Disease
John Wiley & Sons Publishing
605 3rd Avenue 212-850-6000
New York, NY 10158-0012 800-225-5945
Fax: 212-850-6088
www.wiley.com
237 pages
ISBN: 0-471160-61-X

9039 Let's Talk About Having Lyme Disease
Rosen Publishing Group's PowerKids Press
29 E 21st Street 212-777-3017
New York, NY 10010 800-237-9932
Fax: 888-436-4643
e-mail: customerservice@rosenpub.com
www.rosenpublishing.com
Kids are taught to take precautions when walking in the woods and how to inspect themselves for ticks. The illness and recovery are also explained.
Grades K-4
ISBN: 0-823950-29-8
Elizabeth Weitzman, Author

Children's Books

9040 Lyme Disease
Franklin Watts Grolier

90 Old Sherman Tpke 203-797-3500
Danbury, CT 06816-0001 800-621-1115
Fax: 203-797-3197
www.grolier.com
This book discusses the symptoms, prevention, treatments and the role of the tick. This source will not only help readers become aware of Lyme Disease, it will help them become informed.
64 pages Grades 5-7
ISBN: 0-531109-31-3

9041 Lyme Disease and Other Pest-Borne Illnesses
Franklin Watts Grolier
90 Old Sherman Turnpike 203-797-3500
Danbury, CT 06816-0001 800-621-1115
Fax: 203-797-3197
www.grolier.com
Scientific, without being technical, this book explains what Lyme Disease is, symptoms, causes and what a person can do if they contract it.
112 pages Grades 7-12
ISBN: 0-531125-23-8

Magazines

9042 Vector Borne & Zoonotic Diseases
Mary Ann Liebert
Two Madison Avenue 914-834-3100
Larchmont, NY 10538-1961 800-654-3238
Fax: 914-834-1388
www.liebertpub.com/vbz
Essential multidisiplinary journal dedicated to all aspects of human diseases that occur as zoonoses or are transmitted by invertibrate vectors.
Quarterly

Newsletters

9043 Lymelight Newsletter
Lyme Disease Foundation
1 Financial Plaza 860-525-2000
Hartford, CT 06103-2608 800-886-5963
Fax: 860-525-8425
Newsletter offering up to date information on Lyme Disease and related disorders, Foundation activities, conference and fund-raising information and resources.
4x Year

Pamphlets

9044 Frequently Asked Questions
Lyme Disease Foundation
1 Financial Plaza 860-525-2000
Hartford, CT 06103-2608 800-886-5963
Fax: 860-525-8425
Overview of testing, treatment, transmission, and pregnancy.

9045 Guide to Lyme Disease
Lyme Disease Foundation
1 Financial Plaza 860-525-2000
Hartford, CT 06103-2608 800-886-5963
Fax: 860-525-8425
Detailed information about Lyme disease and the LDF.

9046 Guide to Tick Spread Diseases
Lyme Disease Foundation
1 Financial Plaza 860-525-2000
Hartford, CT 06103-2608 800-886-5963
Fax: 860-525-8425
www.lyme.org
Symptoms, diagnosis and treatment for a variety of diseases.
16 pages

9047 Guide to Tick-Borne Disorders
Lyme Disease Foundation

1 Financial Plaza   860-525-2000
Hartford, CT 06103-2608   800-886-5963
    Fax: 860-525-8425
Symptoms, diagnosis, and treatment for a variety of diseases.

9048   **LD Alert Card**
Lyme Disease Foundation
1 Financial Plaza   860-525-2000
Hartford, CT 06103-2608   800-886-5963
    Fax: 860-525-8425
LD symptoms and prevention information.

9049   **LD Awareness Packet**
Lyme Disease Foundation
1 Financial Plaza   860-525-2000
Hartford, CT 06103-2608   800-886-5963
    Fax: 860-525-8425
Educational letter-size posters, brochures listed above, case counts, Spanish information, insurance problem information, General Diagnostic poster, & more.

9050   **Lyme Disease & Pets**
Lyme Disease Foundation
1 Financial Plaza   860-525-2000
Hartford, CT 06103-2608   800-886-5963
    Fax: 860-525-8425
    e-mail: lymefna@aol.com
    www.lyme.org
Offers information on Lyme Disease and other tick-borne disorders, through pets and animal transmission.
T Forchaser, Executive Director

9051   **Quick Guide to Lyme Disease**
American Lyme Disease Foundation
293 Route 100   914-277-6970
Somers, NY 10589   Fax: 914-277-6974
    e-mail: inquire@aldf.com
    www.aldf.com
Epidemiology, the cause of the disease, recognizing the symptoms, what to do if you are bitten, treatment, vaccine and other tick-borne diseases are all covered. One free copy, quantity prices vary.

9052   **Self-Help (S-H) Program**
Lyme Disease Foundation
1 Financial Plaza   860-525-2000
Hartford, CT 06103-2608   800-886-5963
    Fax: 860-525-8425
How to establish and conduct a S-H Group. Video, instruction manual, brochure masters, posters, and more.
28 minutes

9053   **Understanding Lyme Disease: Entendiendo Lyme Disease**
American Lyme Disease Foundation
293 Route 100   914-277-6970
Somers, NY 10589   Fax: 914-277-6974
    e-mail: inquire@aldf.com
    www.aldf.com
Only available in Spanish, this brochure is for children ages 10-15 years old. Includes a basic desription of Lyme disease, symptoms, diagnosis, prevention and proper tick removal. One free copy, quantity prices vary.

9054   **Understanding Ticks and Lyme Disease**
American Lyme Disease Foundation
293 Route 100   914-277-6970
Somers, NY 10589   Fax: 914-277-6974
    e-mail: inquire@aldf.com
    www.aldf.com
For children 10-15 years old, basic description of Lyme disease, symptoms, diagnosis, prevention and proper tick removal. One free copy, quantity prices vary.

Audio & Video

9055   **Case of the Great Imitator**
American Lyme Disease Foundation

293 Route 100   914-277-6970
Somers, NY 10589   Fax: 914-277-6974
    e-mail: inquire@aldf.com
    www.aldf.com
For children ages 9-14 years old. Educational video made in cooperation with the Centers for Disease Control and Prevention.

9056   **LD: Diagnosis & Treatment**
Lyme Disease Foundation
1 Financial Plaza   860-525-2000
Hartford, CT 06103-2608   800-886-5963
    Fax: 860-525-8425
Physicians discuss the challenges of diagnosing and treating LD.
60 minutes

9057   **LD: Facts for Kids**
Lyme Disease Foundation
1 Financial Plaza   860-525-2000
Hartford, CT 06103-2608   800-886-5963
    Fax: 860-525-8425
Targeted toward kindergarten to fourth grade children, these videos educate youngsters about Lyme Disease and ticks.

9058   **Lyme Disease: What You Should Know**
Lyme Disease Foundation
1 Financial Plaza   860-525-2000
Hartford, CT 06103-2608   800-886-5963
    Fax: 860-525-8425
Diagnosis, treatment, transmission, prevention, and research. Interviews with patients, doctors, school officials, researchers, and health department officials.
60 minutes

9059   **Tick Talk**
American Lyme Disease Foundation
293 Route 100   914-277-6970
Somers, NY 10589   Fax: 914-277-6974
    e-mail: inquire@aldf.com
    www.aldf.com
For children ages 5-8 years old. Educational video made in cooperation with the Centers for Disease Control and Prevention.

Web Sites

9060   **America's Doctor Online Consulting**
    www.americasdoctor.com
Provides pharmaceutical and biotech companies and contract research organizations an exclusive source for conducting phase II-IV clinical research.

9061   **American Lyme Disease Foundation**
    www.aldf.com
Provides a wide range of information, both in English and in Spanish, on the diagnosis, treatment, prevention and control of lyme disease and other tick-borne infections.

9062   **CDC Intro to Lyme Disease**
    www.cdc.gov/ncidod/dvbid/lyme/incex.htm
Accurate, evidence based information on symptoms, diagnosis, treatment and prevention of Lyme disease and other tick-borne illnesses. Includes vaccine information, late-braking news, frequently asked questions and related links.

9063   **Healing Well**
    www.healingwell.com
An online health resource guide to medical news, chat, information and articles, newsgroups and message boards, books, disease-related web sites, medical directories, and more for patients, friends, and family coping with disabling diseases, disorders, or chronic illnesses.

9064   **Health Finder**
    www.healthfinder.gov
Searchable, carefully developed web site offering information on over 1000 topics. Developed by the US Department of Health and Human Services, the site can be used in both English and Spanish.

9065   **Healthlink USA**
    www.healthlinkusa.com

Health information concerning treatment, cures, prevention, diagnosis, risk factors, research, support groups, email lists, personal stories and much more. Updated regularly.

9066 Helios Health

www.helioshealth.com

Online resource for your health information. Detailed information about specific health topics, access to expert advice from our Medical Advisory Board, and up-to-date health news.

9067 Lyme Disease Foundation

www.lyme.org

Provides a wide range of services including information and referral network on Lyme disease.

9068 MGH Neurology WebForums

Provides both unmoderated message board and chat rooms for specific neurological disorders including: amyloidosis, asachnoiditis, cerebellar ataxia, congenital fiber type disproportion, CFS leak, DeMorsiers syndrome, erythomelalgia, Lewy body disease, meningitis, meralgia paresthetic, Norrie disease, periodic paralysis, phantom limb pain, Romber disorder, Syndenhams chorea, tethered cord syndrome, and thoracic outlet syndrome.

9069 MedicineNet

www.medicinenet.com

An online resource for consumers providing easy-to-read, authoritative medical and health information.

9070 Medscape

www.medscape.com

Medscape offers specialists, primary care physicians, and other health professionals the Web's most robust and integrated medical information and educational tools.

9071 Neurology Channel

www.neurologychannel.com

Find clearly explained, medically accurate information regarding conditions, including an overview, symptoms, causes, diagnostic procedures and treatment options. On this site it is possible to ask questions and get information from a neurologist and connect to people who have similar health interests.

9072 Pubmed

www.ncbi.nlm.nih.gov/PubMed

National institutes of Health search engine for published medical and scientific research.

9073 University of Rhode Island Tick Research Laboratory

www.riaes.org/resources/ticklab

Pictures of ticks and tick-borne disease information.

9074 WebMD

www.webmd.com

Information on Lyme disease, including articles and resources.

Description

9075 ## Tourette Syndrome

Tourette syndrome, TS, is a neurological disorder characterized by tics - involuntary, rapid, sudden movements or vocalizations that occur repeatedly in the same way. Onset of the disorder occurs before 18 years of age, and usually before the age of 12. Roughly one person in 2000 will demonstrate this behavior at some time in his life. Boys are 3 or 4 times as likely as girls to develop TS.

Multiple motor and vocal tics can appear separately or simultaneously as part of the syndrome. Tics may occur many times daily, or intermittently, with periodic changes in their number, frequency, type and location. Sometimes they may disappear for weeks.

Over time, symptoms can range from hand jerking and throat clearing in the syndrome's early stages to jumping and vocalizing socially unacceptable phrases. Movements may also occur in combination with each other.

Although the cause of TS is unknown, researchers have identified factors which may be involved in producing the disease. Persons with TS may show subtle abnormalities in the structure of certain parts of the brain. The disease may reflect abnormal metabolism of a neurotransmitter (a chemical that brain cells use to signal one another) called dopamine; drugs affecting dopamine levels may reduce symptoms. Relatives of affected persons have an increased risk of disease, suggesting a genetic component. Finally, in some cases the brain's function may be affected by antibodies triggered by infection with a bacterium called Group A Strep. Children who are not bothered by their tics should not be treated with drugs. Medications are reserved for those whose tics lead to symptoms which impair behavioral, physiologic or social function. Simple tics respond to benzodiazepines (tranquilizers). For more severe cases, haloperidol, an antipsychotic, may be used, but should be started slowly. Unfortunately, it sometimes causes other movement disorders after prolonged use. Whether drug treatment is used or not, patients and their families may need counseling to deal with the disease's secondary effects, which may include bullying at school or conflict within the family. Fortunately, the condition often becomes much less severe, without any treatment, after 10 or 15 years.

National Agencies & Associations

9076 **American Academy of Neurology: Tourette Syndrome**
1080 Montreal Avenue   651-695-2717
Saint Paul, MN 55116-2311   800-879-1960
                          Fax: 651-695-2791
                   e-mail: memberservices@aan.com
                             www.aan.com
A medical specialty society established to advance the art and science of neurology and thereby promote the best possible care for patients wit neurological disorders.
Catherine Rydell, Executive Director

9077 **National Institute of Neurological Disorders and Stroke**
NIH Neurological Institute   301-496-5751
Bethesda, MD 20824   800-352-9424
                          Fax: 301-402-2186
                          TTY: 301-468-5981
                             www.ninds.nih.gov
The mission of NINDS is to reduce the burden of neurological disease - a burden borne by every age group, by every segment of society, by people all over the world.
Story C Landis PhD, Director
Walter J Koroshetz, Deputy Director

9078 **Tourette Syndrome Association**
42-40 Bell Boulevard   718-224-2999
Bayside, NY 11361   888-486-8738
                          Fax: 718-279-9596
                 e-mail: grantadministrator@tsa-usa.org
                             www.tsa-usa.org
The only national organization exclusively devoted to the research, diagnosis, education and treatments for persons with Tourette Syndrome.
Judit Ungar, President
Sue Levi-Pearl, VP Meical & Scientific Programs

9079 **Tourette Syndrome Foundation of Canada**
#206 194 Jarvis Street   800-361-3120
Toronto, Ontario, M5B-2B7   Fax: 416-861-2472
                          e-mail: tsfc@tourette.ca
                             www.tourette.ca

National voluntary organization dedicated to improving the quality of life for those with or affected by Tourette Syndrome through programs of education, advocacy, self-help and the promotion of research.
Rosie Wartecker, Executive Director

Research Centers

9080 **Tourette Syndrome Clinic Yale Child Study Center**
Yale Child Study Center
230 S Frontage Road
New Haven, CT 06520   203-785-5880
                             www.medicine.yale.edu
Clinical care center offering research solely into the causes symptoms and treatments for persons with Tourette Syndrome.
Diane B Findley, Associate Research Scientist and Clinic
Robert King, Medical Director

Support Groups & Hotlines

9081 **National Health Information Center**
PO Box 1133   310-565-4167
Washington, DC 20013   800-336-4797
                          Fax: 301-984-4256
                          e-mail: info@nhic.org
                             www.health.gov/nhic
Offers a nationwide information referral service, produces directories and resource guides.

Books

9082 **Children with Tourette Syndrome**
Woodbine House
6510 Bells Mill Road
Bethesda, MD 20817-1636   800-843-7323
This book offers parents information on Tourette Syndrome, causes, symptoms and medications, as well as the other disorders which are commonly linked with it. Other chapters include information on family life, education, advocacy and legal rights.
340 pages Paperback
ISBN: 0-933149-44-1

9083 **Children with Tourette Syndrome: A Parent's Guide**
Adam Ward Seligman, Echolalia Press
35158 Annapolis Road   707-886-1972
Annapolis, CA 95412-9713   e-mail: seligman@sonic.net
                          www.sonic.net/echolaliapress/

9084 Living with Tourette Syndrome
Simon & Schuster
611 W Bay Street
Tampa, FL 33606-2703   800-999-5479
Provides valuable advice for children and adults with TS, their families, co-workers, teachers and friends. Describes the symptoms and related disorders, exposes many myths surrounding the disease, and advises adults on business and personal relationships.
256 pages
ISBN: 0-684811-60-0

9085 Ryan: A Mother's Story of her TS/ADHD Child
Adam Ward Seligman, Echolalia Press
35158 Annapolis Road
Annapolis, CA 95412-9713   707-886-1972
Available in hardcover.
Softcover

9086 Teaching the Tiger: An Educator's Guide to TS/OCD/ADHD
Adam Ward Seligman, Echolalia Press
35158 Annapolis Road
Annapolis, CA 95412-9713   707-886-1972
Workbook

9087 Tourette Syndrome and Human Behavior
Adam Ward Seligman, Echolalia Press
35158 Annapolis Road
Annapolis, CA 95412-9713   707-886-1972
Available in hardcover.
Softcover

9088 Tourette Syndrome: Advances in Neurology
Tourette Syndrome Association
42-40 Bell Boulevard   718-224-2999
Bayside, NY 11361-2861   888-480-8737
                                        Fax: 718-279-9596
In this single-volume reference, more than 90 of the foremost research and clinical leaders in the field review the current state of knowledge about this disorder.
400 pages
Thomas N Chase MD, Editor
Arnold J Friedhoff MD, Editor

9089 What Makes Ryan Tic?
Adam Ward Seligman, Echolalia Press
35158 Annapolis Road
Annapolis, CA 95412-9713   707-886-1972
Softcover

Children's Books

9090 Adam and the Magic Marble
Adam Ward Seligman, Echolalia Press
35158 Annapolis Road
Annapolis, CA 95412-9713   707-886-1972

9091 Hi! I'm Adam!
Adam Ward Seligman, Echolalia Press
35158 Annapolis Road
Annapolis, CA 95412-9713   707-886-1972

9092 Matthew and the Tics
Tourette Syndrome Association
42-40 Bell Boulevard   718-224-2999
Bayside, NY 11361-2861   888-480-8738
                                        Fax: 718-279-9596
A story for young children with TS and their peers.
2 pages

Newsletters

9093 Tourette Syndrome Association Newsletter
42-40 Bell Boulevard   718-224-2999
Bayside, NY 11361   888-480-8738
                                        Fax: 718-279-9596
                                        e-mail: ts@tsa-usa.org
                                        www.tsa-usa.org/

Offers information, articles and news on the latest technology and advancements for persons with Tourette Syndrome.
Quarterly

Pamphlets

9094 Commentary on Alternative Therapies for TS
Tourette Syndrome Association
42-40 Bell Boulevard   718-224-2999
Bayside, NY 11361-2861   888-480-8738
                                        Fax: 718-279-9596
Summarizes physician/patient reports of symptom management through non-pharmacological interventions.
2 pages

9095 Consumer's Guide to TS Medications
Tourette Syndrome Association
42-40 Bell Boulevard   718-224-2999
Bayside, NY 11361-2861   888-480-8738
                                        Fax: 718-279-9596
Covers common medications used for the control of TS motor and vocal ties as well as those traditionally prescribed for associated behaviors.
1992 12 pages

9096 Coping with TS in the Classroom
Tourette Syndrome Association
42-40 Bell Boulevard   718-224-2999
Bayside, NY 11361-2820   Fax: 718-279-9596
Includes practical guidelines for education developed from a study about cognitive effects on learning.
18 pages

9097 Coping with TS, A Parent's Viewpoint
Tourette Syndrome Association
42-40 Bell Boulevard   718-224-2999
Bayside, NY 11361-2861   888-480-8738
                                        Fax: 718-279-9596
An accalaimed medical writer and mother of three children with TS, the author sensitively addresses common concerns and feelings of parents.
1994 23 pages

9098 Coping with Tourette Syndrome in Early Adulthood
Tourette Syndrome Association
42-40 Bell Boulevard   718-224-2999
Bayside, NY 11361-2861   888-480-8738
                                        Fax: 718-279-9596
Focuses on two fundamental challenges facing adults with TS: employment and interpersonal relationships. Provides specific techniques for overcoming barriers.

9099 Current Pharmacology of TS
Tourette Syndrome Association
42-40 Bell Boulevard   718-224-2999
Bayside, NY 11361-2861   888-480-8738
                                        Fax: 718-279-9596
Covers all current medications used to treat TS with specific information about clinical evaluations and diagnosis.
12 pages

9100 Dental Treatment of Patients with Gilles de la Tourette Syndrome
Tourette Syndrome Association
42-40 Bell Boulevard   718-224-2999
Bayside, NY 11361-2861   888-480-8738
                                        Fax: 718-279-9596
Discusses TS movements and possible adverse interactions of dentistry and TS medications.
5 pages

9101 Development of Behavioral and Emotional Problems in TS
Tourette Syndrome Association
42-40 Bell Boulevard   718-224-2999
Bayside, NY 11361-2861   888-480-8738
                                        Fax: 718-279-9596
Using the Child Behavior Checklist, 78 male children were assessed for a variety of behavioral problems. Relation to tic severity covered.
1989 3 pages

9102 Discipline and the Child with TS
Tourette Syndrome Association
42-40 Bell Boulevard   718-224-2999
Bayside, NY 11361   888-480-8738
                                          Fax: 718-279-9596

Helps children redirect impulses and compulsions through teaching cause and effect relationships.
15 pages

9103 Educator's Guide to Tourette Syndrome
Tourette Syndrome Association
42-40 Bell Boulevard   718-224-2999
Bayside, NY 11361-2861   888-480-8738
                                          Fax: 718-279-9596

Covers symptoms, treatments and techniques for classroom management, attentional, writing and language problems.
16 pages

9104 Genetics of Tourette's Syndrome: Who it Affects and How it Occurs in Families
Tourette Syndrome Association
42-40 Bell Boulevard   718-224-2999
Bayside, NY 11361-2861   888-480-8738
                                          Fax: 718-279-9596

10 pages

9105 Getting Into College: Strategies for the Student with TS
Tourette Syndrome Association
42-40 Bell Boulevard   718-224-2999
Bayside, NY 11361   888-480-8738
                                          Fax: 718-279-9596

10 pages

9106 Gift of Hope
Tourette Syndrome Association
42-40 Bell Boulevard   718-224-2999
Bayside, NY 11361-2861   888-480-8738
                                          Fax: 718-279-9596

TSA Brain Bank Program registration information. Includes donor cards.

9107 Grandparents Club
Tourette Syndrome Association
42-40 Bell Boulevard   718-224-2999
Bayside, NY 11361-2861   888-480-8738
                                          Fax: 718-279-9596

A flyer describing how to join with other grandparents to support TS research to benefit future generations.

9108 Guide to Diagnosis & Treatment
Tourette Syndrome Association
42-40 Bell Boulevard   718-224-2999
Bayside, NY 11361-2861   888-480-8738
                                          Fax: 718-279-9596

Covers symptoms, pharmacology and clinical assessments.
30 pages

9109 Guide to Housing for Adults with TS
Tourette Syndrome Association
42-40 Bell Boulevard   718-224-2999
Bayside, NY 11361-2861   888-480-8738
                                          Fax: 718-279-9596

A guide to finding housing, housing laws that help people with TS and ways to maximize living environments.
1991 16 pages

9110 Health Insurance & Tourette Syndrome
Tourette Syndrome Association
42-40 Bell Boulevard   718-224-2999
Bayside, NY 11361-2861   888-480-8738
                                          Fax: 718-279-9596

Detailed, up-to-date packet of medical information for obtaining health insurance as well as information for submission to insurance carriers.

9111 Helpful Techniques to Aid the Student with TS
Tourette Syndrome Association
42-40 Bell Boulevard   718-224-2999
Bayside, NY 11361-2861   888-480-8738
                                          Fax: 718-279-9596

Helpful hints for teacher with specific suggestions for test taking, math computation, and note taking.
1 pages

9112 Learning Problems & the Child with TS
Tourette Syndrome Association
42-40 Bell Boulevard   718-224-2999
Bayside, NY 11361-2861   888-480-8738
                                          Fax: 718-279-9596

Report on learning problems identified through a study of 200 children with TS.
1 pages

9113 Need to Know
Tourette Syndrome Association
42-40 Bell Boulevard   718-224-2999
Bayside, NY 11361-2861   888-480-8738
                                          Fax: 718-279-9596

Recollections of a young woman who was diagnosed with TS in her 20s.
4 pages

9114 Neuropsychological Performance in Adults with TS
Tourette Syndrome Association
42-40 Bell Boulevard   718-224-2999
Bayside, NY 11361-2861   888-480-8738
                                          Fax: 718-279-9596

Describes clinical and neuropsychological testing on learning and memory with TS adults.
7 pages

9115 Peer Problems in Tourette's Disorder
Tourette Syndrome Association
42-40 Bell Boulevard   718-224-2999
Bayside, NY 11361-2861   888-480-8738
                                          Fax: 718-279-9596

Detailed research findings of peer problems in children with TS. Includes statistical results obtained from these studies.
1991 7 pages

9116 Pharmacotherapy of TS and Associated Disorders
Tourette Syndrome Association
42-40 Bell Boulevard   718-224-2999
Bayside, NY 11361-2861   888-480-8738
                                          Fax: 718-279-9596

Overview with emphasis on the complexities of prescribing TS medications.
19 pages

9117 Problem Behaviors & TS
Tourette Syndrome Association
42-40 Bell Boulevard   718-224-2999
Bayside, NY 11361-2861   888-480-8738
                                          Fax: 718-279-9596

Describes recent research and what is now known about the relationship of a variety of behaviors and TS.
21 pages

9118 Recognizing TS in the Classroom
Tourette Syndrome Association
42-40 Bell Boulevard   718-224-2999
Bayside, NY 11361-2861   888-480-8738
                                          Fax: 718-279-9596

Provides an overview offering detailed symptoms checklist, post-diagnosis advice and covers special education needs.
4 pages

9119 Risperidone as a Treatment for TS
Tourette Syndrome Association
42-40 Bell Boulevard   718-224-2999
Bayside, NY 11361-2861   888-480-8738
                                          Fax: 718-279-9596

6 pages

9120 Specific Classroom Strategies and Techniques for Students with TS
Tourette Syndrome Association
42-40 Bell Boulevard   718-224-2999
Bayside, NY 11361-2861   888-480-8738
                                          Fax: 718-279-9596

An educator with TS spells out concrete methods for managing students with TS. She outlines many valuable classroom interventions to help youngsters deal with tic symptons, ADHD, visual motor and fine motor integration, and behavioral difficulties.
1994 2 pages

9121   TS and Other Tic Disorders
Tourette Syndrome Association
42-40 Bell Boulevard   718-224-2999
Bayside, NY 11361-2861   888-480-8738
                                        Fax: 718-279-9596
Comprehensive overview of the complexities of TS. Includes tic syndrome classifications, epidemiology, genetics, behavioral aspects, and summary.
17 pages

9122   TS and the School Nurse
Tourette Syndrome Association
42-40 Bell Boulevard   718-224-2999
Bayside, NY 11361-2861   888-480-8738
                                        Fax: 718-279-9596
Comprehensive professional guide to educational, social and medical implications.
19 pages

9123   TS and the School Psychologist
Tourette Syndrome Association
42-40 Bell Boulevard   718-224-2999
Bayside, NY 11361-2861   888-480-8738
                                        Fax: 718-279-9596
The role of the school psychologist is covered including testing procedures, counseling strategies and social implications.
1993 (rev.) 14 pages

9124   TS: A Look at the Interface Between TS & the Law
Tourette Syndrome Association
42-40 Bell Boulevard   718-224-2999
Bayside, NY 11361-2861   888-480-8738
                                        Fax: 718-279-9596
Summarizes important legislation protecting the rights of students with TS. Also covers resources and hints about how to prepare for dealing successfully with educators and school systems.
1 pages

9125   TSA Medical Letters
Tourette Syndrome Association
42-40 Bell Boulevard   718-224-2999
Bayside, NY 11361-2861   888-480-8738
                                        Fax: 718-279-9596
Annual publication of TSA's Medical Committe covering recent, significant findings from scientific articles.
16 pages

9126   Teens and Tourette Syndrome
Tourette Syndrome Association
42-40 Bell Boulevard   718-224-2999
Bayside, NY 11361-2820   Fax: 718-279-9596
                                       e-mail: ts@tsa-usa.org
                                        www.tsa-usa.org/
Covers self esteem, friends, dating, drugs and alcohol, stress, depression, academic and vocational planning, sibling relationships and medication.
16 pages

9127   Tourette Syndrome and the School Nurse
Tourette Syndrome Association
42-40 Bell Boulevard   718-224-2999
Bayside, NY 11361-2820   Fax: 718-279-9596
                                       e-mail: ts@tsa-usa.org
                                        http://tsa-usa.org
Includes symptoms, epidemiology, associated beviors, developmental consequences, causes, treatments, role of the school nurse and additional resources.
20 pages

9128   Tourette: The Man and His Times
Tourette Syndrome Association
42-40 Bell Boulevard   718-224-2999
Bayside, NY 11361-2861   888-480-8738
                                        Fax: 718-279-9596

Rare historical biography of the famous French neurologist G. Gilles De La Tourette.
9 pages

9129   What School Bus Drivers Need to Know About Students with Tourette Syndrome
Tourette Syndrome Association
42-40 Bell Boulevard   718-224-2999
Bayside, NY 11361-2820   Fax: 718-279-9596
                                       e-mail: ts@tsa-usa.org
                                        http://tsa-usa.org
Includes a description of the disorder, as well as related disorders and suggestions as to what school bus drivers can do for students with TS.
1 pages

Audio & Video

9130   A Regular Kid That's Me: Inservice Film for Educators
Tourette Syndrome Association
42-40 Bell Boulevard   718-224-2999
Bayside, NY 11361   888-480-8738
                                        Fax: 718-279-9596
                                       e-mail: ts@tsa-usa.org
                                        http://tsa-usa.org
Nineteen students with TS (ages 7-17) along with several educators are seen interacting in classroom settings. Includes the basic criteria for diagnosis, discussions of common associated behaviors, e.g. ADD with or without hyperactivity, obsessive compulsive symptoms and specific learning disabilities. Professionals describe the impact of having TS on educational placement and specific classroom strategies are presented. 45 minutes. May be purchased as part of a curriculum or separately. #AV-2
VHS 1/2 inch

9131   After the Diagnosis...the Next Steps
42-40 Bell Boulevard   718-224-2999
Bayside, NY 11361   888-480-8738
                                        Fax: 718-279-9596
                                       e-mail: ts@tsa-usa.org
                                        http://tsa-usa.org
When the diagnosis is Tourette Syndrome, what do you do first? How do you sort out the complexities of the disorder? Whose advice do you follow? What steps do you take to lead a normal life? Six people with TS—as different as any six people can be—relate the sometimes difficult, but finally triumphant path each took to lead the rich, fulfilling life they now enjoy. Narrated by Academy Award-winning actor, Richard Dreyfuss, the stories are blends of poignancy, fact and inspiration.

9132   Clinical Counseling: Towards a Better Understanding of TS
Tourette Syndrome Association
42-40 Bell Boulevard   718-224-2999
Bayside, NY 11361   888-480-8738
                                        Fax: 718-279-9596
                                       e-mail: ts@tsa-usa.org
                                        http://tsa-usa.org
Targeted to counselors, social workers, educators, psychologists and families, this video features expert physicians, allied professionals and several families summarizing key issues that can arise when counseling families with TS. 15 minutes. #AV-10A

9133   Complexities of TS Treatment: A Physician's Round Table
Tourette Syndrome Association
42-40 Bell Boulevard   718-224-2999
Bayside, NY 11361   888-480-8738
                                        Fax: 718-279-9596
                                       e-mail: ts@tsa-usa.org
                                        http://tsa-usa.org
Three internationally recognized TS experts provide colleagues with valuable information about the complexities of treating and advising families with TS. Emphasis is on different clinical approaches to patients with a broad range of symptom severity. Co-morbid and associated conditions are covered. 15 minutes. #AV-10

9134   Educator's In-Service Program
Tourette Syndrome Association

42-40 Bell Boulevard
Bayside, NY 11361

718-224-2999
888-480-8738
Fax: 718-279-9596

A curriculum designed to train educators to recognize and understand TS and guide students with TS and associated disorders in a classroom setting. Developed by the Tourette Syndrome Association for the training of all educational personnel. Includes 2 videos, a particpant's guide, a set of 20 transparencies, 2 scripted curriculum modules and a comprehensive teacher's guide. Discounted for members.

9135 Gift of Hope
Tourette Syndrome Association
42-40 Bell Boulevard
Bayside, NY 11361

718-224-2999
888-480-8738
Fax: 718-279-9596
e-mail: ts@tsa-usa.org
http://tsa-usa.org

The cause of TS lies in the brain. Because their are no animal models to study this disorder, human brain tissue is of vital importance for progress in research. Increased brain bank registration is a prime objective of the TSA. VHS 1/2 inch. 14 minutes. Available for shipping cost only. #AV- 7

9136 Guide to Diagnosis
Tourette Syndrome Association
42-40 Bell Boulevard
Bayside, NY 11361-2861

718-224-2999
888-480-8738
Fax: 718-279-9596

A video and companion guide for interested medical professionals who have not seen a substantial number of TS patients.
30 minutes

9137 I'm a Person Too
Tourette Syndrome Association
42-40 Bell Boulevard
Bayside, NY 11361

718-224-2999
888-480-8738
Fax: 718-279-9596
e-mail: ts@tsa-usa.org
http://tsa-usa.org

Narrated by Cliff Robertson, this video features 5 people with TS; 2 elementary school students and 3 adults from diverse social backgrounds. They talk about a broad variety of symptoms and their personal experiences living with the disorder. VHS 1/2 inch. 22 minutes. #AV1

9138 Panel of Experts
Tourette Syndrome Association
42-40 Bell Boulevard
Bayside, NY 11361-2861

718-224-2999
888-480-8738
Fax: 718-279-9596

Five leading authorities bring their in-depth knowledge and experience to bear in a wide-ranging discussion that covers current strategies in TS diagnosis, and medication.
30 minutes

9139 Parent's Perspective: Diplomacy in Action
Tourette Syndrome Association
42-40 Bell Boulevard
Bayside, NY 11361-2861

718-224-2999
888-480-8738
Fax: 718-279-9596

The child with TS faces a set of special problems in school. The level of achievement reached in large measure is dependent on the attitude of teachers and administrators. Therefore, educating the educators becomes a high priority with the parent.
45 minutes

9140 Stop It!... I Can't!
Tourette Syndrome Association
42-40 Bell Boulevard
Bayside, NY 11361

718-224-2999
888-480-8738
Fax: 718-279-9596
e-mail: ts@tsa-usa.org
http://tsa-usa.org

Narrated by William Shatner, this video promotes sensitivity, education, acceptance and confidence for children with TS. Produced in the 1970's, but provides a valuable and classic message. VHS 1/2 inch. 13 minutes.

9141 TS-The Parent's Perspective: Diplomacy in Action
Tourette Syndrome Association

42-40 Bell Boulevard
Bayside, NY 11361

718-224-2999
888-480-8738
Fax: 718-279-9596
e-mail: ts@tsa-usa.org
http://ts-usa.org

The child with TS faces a set of special problems in school. The level of achievement reached in large measure is dependent on the attitude of teachers and administrators. Therefore educating the educators becomes a high priority for the parent. Special education professionals provide firm guidance to famillies on school advocacy issues. Concrete suggestions are offered to smooth the road to success in school for the student with TS. VHS 1/2 inch. 45 minutes. #AV-6

9142 TS: A Panel of Experts
Tourette Syndrome Association
42-40 Bell Boulevard
Bayside, NY 11361

718-224-2999
888-480-8738
Fax: 718-279-9596
e-mail: ts@tsa-usa.org
http://tsa-usa.org

Five leading authorities bring their in-depth knowledge and experience to bear in a wide-ranging discussion that covers current strategies in TS diagnosis and medication, behavioral problems, predicted course and other aspects of this disorder. VHS 1/2 inch. 30 minutes. # AV-5

9143 Talking About Tourette Syndrome
Tourette Syndrome Association
42-40 Bell Boulevard
Bayside, NY 11361

718-224-2999
888-480-8738
Fax: 718-279-9596
e-mail: ts@tsa-usa.org
http://tsa-usa.org

When the professional is also the patient, a unique perspective emerges. A psychiatrist leads a candid probing discussion with a brother and sister- all have Tourette syndrome. This free-wheeling exchange brings to the viewer many instructive and often surprising observations about TS and obsessive compulsive symptoms. VHS 1/2 inch. 45 minutes. #AV-8

9144 Tourette Syndrome: Guide to Diagnosis
Tourette Syndrome Association
42-40 Bell Boulevard
Bayside, NY 11361

718-224-2999
888-480-8738
Fax: 718-279-9596
e-mail: ts@tsa-usa.org
http://tsa-usa.org

Video for interested medical professionals who have not seen substantial numbers of TS patients. Presents 7 patients with TS who exhibit the full range of movements, vocalizations and behavioral patterns associated with the disorder. Descriptions and demonstrations of other movement disorders are also presented for the purpose of differential diagnosis. VHS 1/2 inch. 30 minutes. A 29 page companion piece by Drs. Ruth Brunn, Donald Cohen and James Leckman is available at $6.00/3.50 shipping.#AV4

9145 Family Life with Tourette Syndrome... Personal Stories: Professor Peter
Tourette Syndrome Association
42-40 Bell Boulevard
Bayside, NY 11361

718-224-2999
888-480-8738
Fax: 718-279-9596
e-mail: ts@tsa-usa.org
tsa-usa.org

Now a world class scientific research expert and a professor of biology at Harvard and Purdue, Professor Hollenbeck talks about growing up positively with TS, never hesitating to have children, and offering good advice for newly diagnosed families. 7 minutes, 27 seconds. If purchased together, the six videos in this series are $50.00. #AV-11A

9146 Family Life with Tourette Syndrome... Personal Stories: Reverend Mike
Tourette Syndrome Association
42-40 Bell Boulevard
Bayside, NY 11361

718-224-2999
888-480-8738
Fax: 718-279-9596
e-mail: ts@tsa-usa.org
tsa-usa.org

Mike Higgins did not receive a diagnosis of TS until he was in the army! Mike overcame significant symptoms and childhood teasing. Reverend Mike talks about the value of strong family life, faith, support groups and acceptance of the person, and not the disorder as a good way to live positively with TS. If purchased together, the six videos in this series are $50.00. #AV-11B

9147   Family Life with Tourette Syndrome... Personal Stories: Rachel
Tourette Syndrome Association
42-40 Bell Boulevard   718-224-2999
Bayside, NY 11361   888-480-8738
                                                    Fax: 718-279-9596
                                                e-mail: ts@tsa-usa.org
                                                    http://tsa-usa.org
Challenged by TS, ADHD and OCD Rachel and her family endured difficult reactions, behavioral episodes, and at times, a great loss of hope. Now seventeen years old, Rachel and family overcame stresses and strains by sticking together through the highs and lows to find Rachel today a confident and happy teen. 10 minutes. If purchased together, the six videos in this series are $50.00. #AV-11C

9148   Family Life with Tourette Syndrome... Personal Stories: The Turners
Tourette Syndrome Association
42-40 Bell Boulevard   718-224-2999
Bayside, NY 11361   888-480-8738
                                                    Fax: 718-279-9596
                                                e-mail: ts@tsa-usa.org
                                                    http://tsa-usa.org
Three of the four Turner daughters have TS in varying degrees. The family wondered how their symptoms came to be, how to dispense attention fairly, what to say to teachers and friends. They learned how to deal with sibling issues and low self esteem among the sisters. This determined family never gave up! 12 minutes. If purchased together, the six videos in this series are $50.00. #AV-11D

9149   Family Life with Tourette Syndrome... Personal Stories: Ryan
Tourette Syndrome Association
42-40 Bell Boulevard   718-224-2999
Bayside, NY 11361   888-480-8738
                                                    Fax: 718-279-9596
                                                e-mail: ts@tsa-usa.org
                                                    http://tsa-usa.org
Ryan's family first thought his behavior was a deliberate way to get attention. A school principal was harshly critical. The family soon learned to educate themselves and others about Ryan's TS. Things turned around as a result. A good teacher took a great interest, friends began to seek him out and Ryan grew into a young man with a positive outlook. 11 minutes, 28 seconds. If purchased together, the six videos in this series are $50.00. #AV-11E

9150   Family Life with Tourette Syndrome... Personal Stories: Dakota
Tourette Syndrome Association
42-40 Bell Boulevard   718-224-2999
Bayside, NY 11361   888-480-8738
                                                    Fax: 718-279-9596
                                                e-mail: ts@tsa-usa.org
                                                    http://tsa-usa.org
A happy 11 year old baseball playing, video game whiz, Dakota was initially diagnosed as having a brain tumor! He was actually affected by TS and AHD. This is a story of a child who developed a strong confidence and a good attitude, learning to believe in himself. He says the love of his grandparents was a special help! 7 minutes, 12 seconds. If purchased together, the 6 videos in this series are $50.00. #AV-11F

Web Sites

9151   American Academy of Neurology: Tourette Syndrome
                                                        www.aan.com
The American Academy of Neurology (AAN) is a worldwide professional association of more than 17,000 neurologists and neuroscience professionals dedicating to providing the best possible care for patients with neurological disorders.

9152   Healing Well
                                                    www.healingwell.com
An online health resource guide to medical news, chat, information and articles, newsgroups and message boards, books, disease-re-

lated web sites, medical directories, and more for patients, friends, and family coping with disabling diseases, disorders, or chronic illnesses.

9153   Health Finder
                                                    www.healthfinder.gov
Searchable, carefully developed web site offering information on over 1000 topics. Developed by the US Department of Health and Human Services, the site can be used in both English and Spanish.

9154   Healthlink USA
                                                    www.healthlinkusa.com
Health information concerning treatment, cures, prevention, diagnosis, risk factors, research, support groups, email lists, personal stories and much more. Updated regularly.

9155   Helios Health
                                                    www.helioshealth.com
Online resource for your health information. Detailed information about specific health topics, access to expert advice from our Medical Advisory Board, and up-to-date health news.

9156   MedicineNet
                                                    www.medicinenet.com
An online resource for consumers providing easy-to-read, authoritative medical and health information.

9157   Medscape
                                                        www.medscape.com
Medscape offers specialists, primary care physicians, and other health professionals the Web's most robust and integrated medical information and educational tools.

9158   National Institute of Neurological Disorders and Stroke
                                                        www.ninds.nih.gov
The mission of NINDS is to reduce the burden of neurological disease - a burden borne by every age group, by every segment of society, by people all over the world.

9159   WebMD
                                                            www.webmd.com
Information on Tourette Syndrome, including articles and resources.

Description

9160 Transplant-Related Conditions

In recent decades, transplantation of solid organs (heart, liver, lung, kidney), bone marrow and stem cells has become an established part of medical care for advanced diseases in many patients who otherwise face end-organ failure and poor prognosis. While on one hand, transplantation may serve to cure the underlying disease it nonetheless often entails chronic medical therapy that will likely include the use of immunosuppressants, complications from chronic medications, frequent and long-term medical follow-up and diagnostic testing which may be invasive.

A number of clinical management protocols are utilized in the care of post-transplantation patient, and these vary depending on the type of transplant undertaken, the extent of the tissue match between donor and recipient, and the experience of the given transplantation center. In general however, most patients who receive a transplanted organ or cells will require some chronic therapy (short or long-term) with immunosuppressive medications. These can be several or many and are given in an effort to control the patient's own immunologic response to receiving an organ or cells from another person. The body's natural response after recognizing such an exposure is to "fight" these cells and tissues with its own defense cells, which are designed to attack and kill foreign material. The immunosuppressive medications help modulate this response so that the transplanted organ is not damaged, injured or "rejected" by the recipient who needs the organ or cells to function in a healthier manner. Immunosuppressive therapy and protection of the transplanted organ must be balanced against the adverse creation of an immunocompromised state in the patient placing him at greater risk for contracting infections that can be serious and even life threatening. Given these circumstances, transplant patients require close working relationships with their medical team along with a true commitment to be compliant with these potentially difficult and complicated medical regimens.

In addition to the medical therapy for patients who have received transplants, one must also consider the significant psychological and social aspects of having undergone such procedures. Strong social support systems and close attention to a healthy emotional and psychological status are important for successful management of these patients. Many transplant centers have extensive support services available to patients from which they and their families can benefit.

National Agencies & Associations

9161 American Society of Transplantation (AST)
15000 Commerce Parkway 856-439-9986
Mount Laurel, NJ 08054 Fax: 856-439-9982
e-mail: ast@ahint.com
www.a-s-t.org
The American Society of Transplantation is an international organization of transplant professionals dedicated to advancing the field of transplantation through the promotion of research education advocacy and organ donation to improve patient care.
Barbara Murphy, President
Susan J Nelson, Executive Vice President

9162 Association of Organ Procurement Organizations (AOPO)
1364 Beverly Road 703-556-4242
McLean, VA 22101 Fax: 703-556-4852
e-mail: aopo@aopo.org
www.aopo.org
Organization involved in helping people find and obtain the organs they need for transplantation.
Bruce A Wilson, Executive Director
Sue Dunn, President/CEO

9163 Children's Organ Transplant Association (COTA)
2501 COTA Drive 700-366-2682
Bloomington, IN 47403 800-366-2682
Fax: 812-336-8885
e-mail: cota@cota.org
www.cota.org
Not-for-profit national chairty dedicated to helping families and communities raise the necessary funds for transplant expenses.
Rick Lofgren, President/CEO
Lisa Fulkerson, VP/CFO

9164 Donate Life America
700 N Fourth Street 804-782-4920
Richmond, VA 23219 Fax: 804-782-4643
e-mail: coalition@donatelife.net
www.donatelife.net
A not-for-profit alliance of national organizations and local coalitions across the United States that have joined forces to educate the public about organ, eye and tissue donation, correcting misconceptions about donation and creating a greater willingness to donate.
Sara Pace Jones, Chairwoman
Bruce Wilson, Director of Organ Procurement

9165 Health Resources and Services Administration (HRSA)
5600 Fishers Lane 301-443-7577
Rockville, MD 20857 e-mail: comments@hrsa.gov
www.hrsa.gov
Envisions optimal health for all, supported by a health care system that assures access to comprehensive, culturally competant, quality care. Provides national leadership, program resources and services needed to improve access to culturally competant, quality health care.
Elizabeth M Duke PhD, Administrator
Dennis P Williams PhD MA, Deputy Administrator

9166 Jewish Hospital Transplant Center
200 Abraham Flexner Way
Louisville, KY 40202 502-587-4011
www.jewishhospital.com
An elite group approved to perform five solid organ transplants and has been named a Federally Designated Medicare Heart Lung Kidney Liver and Pancreas Transplant Center.
Robert L Shircliff, President/CEO
Barbara Mackovic, Senior Manager

9167 National Foundation for Transplants
5350 Poplar Avenue 901-684-1697
Memphis, TN 38119 800-489-3863
Fax: 901-684-1128
e-mail: info@transplants.org
www.transplants.org
Mission is to reach out to help those who seek a new life through transplantation by providing healthcare and financial support services and patient advocacy for transplant candidates families nationwide.
Jackie D Hancock, President
Connie Gonitzke, Vice President

9168 National Institute of Allergy and Infectious Diseases (NIAID)
6610 Rockledge Drive
Bethesda, MD 20892-6612 301-496-2263
www.niaid.nih.gov
Conducts and supports basic and applied research to better understand, treat, and ultimately prevent infectious, immunologic and allergic diseases. Research has led to new therapies, vaccines, di-

agnostic tests, and other technologies that have improved the health of millions of people in the United States and around the world.
Anthony S. Fauci, Director

9169 National Transplant Assistance Fund (NTAF)
150 N Radnor Chester Road 610-353-9684
Radnor, PA 19087 800-642-8399
Fax: 610-353-1616
e-mail: ntaf@transplantfund.org
www.transplantfund.org
Helps to raise funds for transplant and catastrophic injury patients by providing compassionate support education and expertise to them their families and communities.
Lynne Coughl Samson, Executive Director
Judy B Diner, Managing Director

9170 Organ Procurement and Transplantation Network (OPTN)
700 N 4th Street 804-782-4800
Richmond, VA 23219 888-TXI-NFO1
Fax: 804-782-4994
www.optn.org
A unified transplant network established by the United States Congress under the National Organ Transplant Act (NOTA) of 1984. A unique public-private partnership that links all of the professionals involved in the donation and transplantation system.
Robert S Higgins, President
James Wynn, Vice President

9171 United Network for Organ Sharing (UNOS)
700 N 4th Street 804-782-4800
Richmond, VA 23218 Fax: 804-782-4817
www.unos.org
Non-profit scientific and educational organization that administers the nation's only Organ Procurement and Transplantation Network (OPTN). Mission is to advance organ availability and transplantation by uniting and supporting our communities.
Walter K Graham, Executive Director
Marcia D Manning, Director of Community Affairs

9172 United Organ Transplant Association (UOTA)
3405 Arlington Avenue
Riverside, CA 92506 e-mail: pres@uota.org
www.uota.org
Non-profit charitable corporation dedicated to providing educational emotional and financial support to pre- and post- transplant patients.

State Agencies & Associations

Alabama

9173 Alabama Organ Center
500 S 22 Street S 205-731-9200
Birmingham, AL 35233 800-252-3677
Fax: 205-731-9250
e-mail: Rebecca.davis@ccc.uab.edu
alabamaorgancenter.org
A non-profit, independent organ procurement organization (OPO) serving the population of the Southeastern United States.
Demosthenes Lalisan I MBA CPTC, Director
R Alan Hicks MPH CPTC, Associate Director

Arizona

9174 Donor Network of Arizona
201 W Coolidge 602-222-2200
Phoenix, AR 85013 800-94D-ONOR
Fax: 602-222-2202
e-mail: Contact.Us@dnaz.org
www.dnaz.org
Participates in the equitable distribution of organs, tissues, and corneas for transplant. Also offers donor family support services, community and health care education, and presentations.
Sara Pace Jones, Public Education Contact

Arkansas

9175 Arkansas Regional Organ Recovery Agency
1701 Aldersgate Road 501-907-9150
Little Rock, AR 72205 800-727-6726
Fax: 501-372-6279
e-mail: info@arora.org
www.arora.org
Makes every effort to provide organs and tissues for life-saving and life-enhancing transplantation. Goal will be accomplished through continuous hospital involvement which includes hospital training community involvement andpublic education.
Audrey Brown, Director of Community Education
Boyd Ward, Executive Director

California

9176 California Transplant Donor Network
1000 Broadway 510-444-8500
Oakland, CA 94607 888-570-9400
Fax: 510-444-8501
e-mail: info@ctdn.org
www.ctdn.org
Helps patients in Northern and Central California and Northern Nevada receive organ and tissue transplants. Recovers organs from donors and matches them with the more than 6 000 people who are currently waiting for transplants in this region.
Cindy Siljestrom, Chief Executive Officer
Sonia Salloum, Community Outreach Coordinator

9177 Golden State Donor Services
1760 Creekside Oaks Drive 916-567-1600
Sacramento, CA 95833 Fax: 916-567-8300
e-mail: info@gsds.org
www.gsds.org
Support, enhance, and provide for the recovery and allocation of anatomical gifts. Also work to educate the public regarding the critical need for organ and tissue doors.
Katherine Doolittle, Senior Public Education Coordinator
Helen Nelson, Executive Director

9178 LifeSharing Community Organ & Tissue Donation
3465 Camino Del Rio S 619-521-1983
San Diego, CA 92108 Fax: 619-521-2833
e-mail: info@lifesharing.org
www.lifesharing.org
Non-profit unique and creative organ procurement organization that has centers at the University of California at San Diego Medical Center, Green Hospital of Scripps Clinic, Sharp Hospital.
Sharie Shipley, Public Education Contact
Bill Dawson, Chairman of Volunteer Action Committee

9179 One Legacy Transplant Donor Network
221 S Figueroa Street 213-229-5600
Los Angeles, CA 90012 800-786-4077
Fax: 213-229-5601
e-mail: tmone@onelegacy.org
www.onelegacy.org
One Legacy is dedicaated to achieving the donation of life saving and life enhancing organs and tissues for those in need of transplants and to providing a sense of purpose and comfort to those families we serve.
Stephanie Collazo, Director Clinical Education
Thomas Mone, Chief Executive Officer/EVP

Colorado

9180 Donor Alliance
720 S Colorado Boulevard 303-329-4747
Denver, CO 80246 888-868-4747
Fax: 303-321-0366
www.donoralliance.org
In cooperation with others Donor Alliance facilitates the donation and recovery of organs and tissues for people needing transplantation. Donor Alliance is one of 58 not-for-profit organ recovery organizations federally designated by the U.S..
Jennifer Moe, Director of Community Relations/PR
Nancy Williams, Chairman

Connecticut

9181 New England Organ Bank Connecticut
One Gateway Center   203-785-4237
Newton, MA 02158   800-446-NEOB
                                      Fax: 617-244-8755
                                      e-mail: info@neob.com
                                      www.neob.org
Non-profit organ procurement organization that the geographical
areas covered are New Haven Connecticut Area, Maine, Eastern
Massachusetts, New Hampshire, Rhode Island, and Vermont.
Sean Fitzpatrick, Public Education Director

Delaware

9182 Gift of Life Donor Program Delaware
401 N. 3rd St.   215-557-8090
Philadelphia, PA 19123   888-366-6771
                                      Fax: 215-963-0587
                                      e-mail: info@donors1.org
                                      www.donors1.org
Formerly (Delaware Valley Transplant Program) is the region's
nonprofit organ and tissue donor program serving eastern half of
Pennsylvania, southern New Jersey and the state of Delaware.
Also, considered a model program in the United States.
John Green, Director of Community Relations

District of Columbia

9183 Washington Regional Transplant Consortium
7619 Little River Turnpike   703-641-0100
Annandale, VA 22003   866-232-3666
                                      Fax: 703-658-0711
                                      e-mail: contactwrtc@wrtc.org
                                      www.wrtc.org
WRTC is the official link between organ and tissue donors and the
patients who are waiting for transplants.
Sara Idler, Public Education Contact

Florida

9184 LifeLink of Florida
409 Bayshore Boulevard   813-253-2640
Tampa, FL 33606   800-262-5775
                                      Fax: 813-348-0634
                                      e-mail: info@lifelinkfound.org
                                      www.lifelinkfound.org
Independent, nonprofit community service organization dedicated
to the recovery and transplantation of organs and tissues. Operates
under the authority of the Social Security Act, and in accordance
with the National Organ Transplant Act passed by Congress.
Dennis F Heinrichs, President
Dana L Shires Jr, Chairman of the Board

9185 LifeLink of Southwest Florida
409 Bayshore Boulevard   813-253-2640
Tampa, FL 33906   800-262-5775
                                      Fax: 813-348-0634
                                      e-mail: info@lifelinkfound.org
                                      www.lifelinkfound.org
LifeLink of Southwest Florida and Florida Gulf Coast University
joined forces to develop a survey instrument to assss student attitudes and opinions about donation. Worked to conduct and evaluate the impact of the multifaceted education campaign.
Dennis F Heinrichs, President
Dana L Shires Jr, Chairman of the Board

9186 TransLife/Florida Hospital
1560 Orange Avenue   407-644-3770
Winter Park, FL 32789   800-443-6667
                                      Fax: 407-303-2473
                                      www.translife.org
Works closely with hospitals and donor families to coordinate the
gift of life in Central Florida. Also a critical link between donors
and possible recipients.
Carol Rumsey, Public Education Contact

Georgia

9187 LifeLink of Georgia
2875 Northwoods Parkway   770-225-5465
Norcross, GA 30071   800-544-6667
                                      e-mail: info@lifelinkfound.org
                                      www.lifelinkfound.org/georgia/ga.html
The Foundation atempts to work in a sensitive diligent and com-
passionate manner with donor families to facilitate the donation of
desperately needed organs and tissues for waiting patients.
Dennis F Heinrichs, President
Dana L Shires, Chairman of the Board

Hawaii

9188 Organ Donor Center of Hawaii
1149 Bethel Street   808-599-7630
Honolulu, HI 96813   877-855-0603
                                      Fax: 808-599-7631
                                      e-mail: info@organdonorhawaii.com
                                      www.organdonorhawaii.com
Non-profit organ procurement organization.
Stephen A Kula, Executive Director
Christine L Bogee, Administrative Services Director

Illinois

9189 Regional Organ Bank of Illinois, Inc.
800 S. Wells   312-431-3600
Chicago, IL 60607   888-307-3668
                                      Fax: 312-803-7643
                                      e-mail: info@robi.org
                                      www.robi.org
ROBI'S mission is to save and enhance the lives of as many people
as possible through organ and tissue donation.
Kim McCullough, Public Education Contact

Indiana

9190 Indiana Organ Procurement Organization,
3760 Guion Road   317-685-0389
Indianapolis, IN 46222-1816   888-275-4676
                                      Fax: 317-685-1687
                                      e-mail: info@iopo.org
                                      www.iopo.org
Non-profit organ procurement organization designed to recover
and distribute organ and tissues for transplantation.
Sam Davis, Director of Professional Services
Lynn Driver, President and CEO

Iowa

9191 Iowa Donor Network
550 Madison Avenue   319-665-3787
N Liberty, IA 52317   800-831-4131
                                      Fax: 319-665-3788
                                      www.iowadonornetwork.org
Iowa Donor Network is dedicated to serving donow families
potentialdonors and candidates doe transplantation through identifying potential donorssupporting and respecting donation decisions and maximizing the recovery of transplantable organs and
tissues.
Kelly Sorensen, Public Education Contact

Kansas

9192 Midwest Transplant Network & Organ Bank
1900 W 47th Place   913-262-1668
Westwood, KS 66205   Fax: 913-262-5130
                                      e-mail: info@mwob.org
                                      www.mwtn.org
Provides quality transplantation related services that will maximize the availability of organs and tissues to the comunities we
serve. Provides procurement services for organ and tissue and laboratory services for HLA.
Ray Gable, Public Education Contact
Marcia Schoenfeld, Public Education Contact

Kentucky

9193 Kentucky Organ Donor Affiliates
106 E Broadway
Louisville, KY 40202
502-581-9511
800-525-3456
Fax: 502-589-5157
e-mail: info@kyorgandonor.org
www.kyorgandonor.org
Non-profit organ donor center that retrieves and distributes organs to qualified recipients.

Louisiana

9194 Louisiana Organ Procurement Agency
4441 N I-10 Service Road
Metairie, LA 70006-3626
504-837-3355
800-521-GIVE
Fax: 504-837-3587
e-mail: info@lopa.org
www.lopa.org
Non-profit organ procurement organization federally-designated to increase the number of transplantable organs by providing families an opportunity to donate organs and tissues to support these families regardless of their decision.
John Egan, Public Education Contact

Maine

9195 New England Organ Bank Maine
One Gateway Center
Newton, MA 02158
800-870-5230
800-446-NEOB
Fax: 617-244-8755
e-mail: info@neob.org
www.neob.org
Independent, not-for-profit agency whose mission is to recover, peerve, and distribute human organs and tissues for transplantation. The New England Organ Bank is a federally-designated organ procurement organization for all parts of the six New England states, it serves 177 acute care hospitals and 14 transplant centers.
Sean Fitzpatrick, Public Education Contact

Maryland

9196 Transplant Resource Center of Maryland
1730 Twin Springs Road
Baltimore, MD 21227
410-242-7000
800-641-HERO
Fax: 410-242-1871
e-mail: communications@TheLLF.org
www.mdtransplant.org
Provides organ and tissue donation and recovery services hospital donor program development and community education to 42 hospitals and the citizens living in Maryland.
Ann Bromery, Chief Financial Officer
Charles Alexander, President & Chief Executive Officer

9197 Washington Regional Transplant Consortium
7619 Little River Turnpike
Annandale, VA 22003
703-641-0100
866-232-3666
Fax: 703-658-0711
e-mail: contactwrtc@wrtc.org
www.wrtc.org
Recently partnered with fellow Mid-Atlantic Coalition on Donation members and a company called Sports America to sponsor the second annual DeMatha Invitational. WRTC is the official link between organ and tissue donors and the patients who are waiting for transplant.
Sara Idler, Public Education Contact

Massachusetts

9198 New England Organ Bank Massachusetts
One Gateway Center
Newton, MA 02158
800-446-NEOB
Fax: 617-244-8755
e-mail: info@neob.com
www.neob.org
Independent, not-for-profit agency whose mission is to recover, preserve, and distribute human organs and tissues for transplantation. A federally-designated organ procurement organization for all or part of the six New England states, it serves 177 acute care hospitals and 14 transplant centers.
Sean Fitzpatrick, Public Education Contact

9199 NorthEast Organ Procurement Organization
80 Seymour Street
Hartford, CT 06102-5037
800-874-5215
Fax: 860-545-4143
www.harthosp.org/NEOPO/index.html
Assures that comprehensive organ and tissue donation services are provided to the community in an efficient and professional manner.
Ginger Van Nostrand, Public Education Contact

Michigan

9200 Transplantation Society of Michigan
3861 Research Park Drive
Ann Arbor, MI 48108
734-973-1577
800-482-4881
Fax: 734-973-3133
e-mail: info@giftoflifemichigan.org
www.giftoflifemichigan.org
Nonprofit independent corporation certified by Medicare and designated by the Centers for Medicare and Medicaid Services as an organ recovery organization for Michigan.
Tammie Harvermahl, Public Education Contact

Minnesota

9201 LifeSource, Upper Midwest Organ Procurement Organization, Inc.
2550 University Avenue West
St. Paul, MN 55114-1904
651-603-7800
Fax: 651-603-7801
e-mail: info@life-source.org
www.life-source.org
Nonprofit, federally-designated organ procurement organization for the Upper Midwest, managing all organ donation activities in Minnesota.
Jill Halimi, Donor Family Services

Mississippi

9202 Mississippi Organ Recovery
12 River Bend Place
Flowood, MS 39232
601-933-1000
800-690-8878
Fax: 601-933-1006
www.msora.org
Not-for-profit organization coordinates the recovery of human organs for transplantation by working with and providing education to medical professionals donor families and the people of Mississippi.
Kelly Nations, Community Education Coordinator
Kevin Stump, Chief Executive Officer

Missouri

9203 Mid-America Transplant Services
1110 Highlands Plaza Drive E
Saint Louis, MO 63110-3205
314-735-8200
Fax: 314-991-2805
e-mail: info@mts-stl.org
www.mts-stl.org
Community based not-for-profit organ procurement organization dedicated to enhancing the quality of human life. Coordinates the procurement of vital organs tissues and eyes in hospitals throughout its service area.
Diane Brockmeier, COO
Dean F Kappel, President and CEO

Nebraska

9204 Nebraska Organ Retrieval System
8502 W Center Road
Omaha, NE 68124
402-733-1800
877-633-1800
Fax: 402-733-9312
www.NEdonation.org
Responsible for retrieving the proper organs and distrbuting them to the recipients.
Stephanie Lochmiller, Public Relations Coordinator
Karen Risk, Executive Director

Nevada

9205 Nevada Donor Network
2085 E Sahara Avenue
Las Vegas, NV 89104
702-796-9600
Fax: 702-796-4225
e-mail: ksatcher@nvdonor.org
www.nvdonor.org
Improving the quality of human life through the recovery of all
available organs and tissues for transplantation education and research while maintaining the dignity of the donors and their families.
Liliana Arredondo, Public Education Coordinator
Ken Richardson, Executive Director

New Hampshire

9206 New England Organ Bank New Hampshire
One Gateway Center
Newton, MA 02158
800-446-NEOB
Fax: 617-244-8755
e-mail: info@neob.com
www.neob.org
Non-profit organ procurement organization that the geographical
areas covered are New Haven Connecticut Area, Maine, Eastern
Massachusetts, New Hampshire, Rhode Island, and Vermont.
Sean Fitzpatrick, Public Education Director

New Jersey

9207 Gift of Life Donor Program New Jersey
2000 Hamilton Street
Philadelphia, PA 19103-3813
215-557-8090
888-366-6771
Fax: 215-963-0587
e-mail: info@donors1.org
www.donors1.org
Formerly (Delaware Valley Transplant Program) is the region's
nonprofit organ and tissue donor program serving eastern half of
Pennsylvania, southern New Jersey and the state of Delaware.
Also, considered a model program in the United States.
John Green, Director of Community Relations

9208 Sharing Network Organ Tissue Donation Services
841 Mountain Avenue
Springfield, NJ 07081
973-379-4535
800-742-7365
Fax: 973-379-5113
e-mail: tsn@sharenj.org
www.sharenj.org
Federally certified state-approved organ procurement organization responsible for recovering organ and tissue for New Jersey
residents currently awaiting transplants.
Melissa Honohan, Director of External Relations
Joseph Roth, President and Chief Executive Officer

New Mexico

9209 New Mexico Donor Services
2715 Broadbent Parkway NE
Albuquerque, NM 87107
505-843-7672
800-843-7672
Fax: 505-343-1828
e-mail: info@donatelifenm.org
www.donatelifenm.org
Transplant centers in the service area are: University of New Mexico Hospitals Presbyterian Hospital.
Maria Sanders, Community Services
Patricia Niles, Executive Director

New York

9210 Center for Donation & Transplantation
218 Great Oaks Boulevard
Albany, NY 12203
518-262-5606
800-256-7811
Fax: 518-262-5427
e-mail: dfloeser@cdtny.org
www.cdtny.org
Dedicated to increasing organ and tissue donation by following
procurement and equitable distribution of medically suitable organs and tissue for transplantation.
Antonio Di Carlo, Assistant Medical Director
David Conti, Board Chairman/Medical Director

9211 Finger Lakes Donor Recovery Network
Corporate Woods of Brighton
Rochester, NY 14623
585-272-4930
800-810-5494
Fax: 585-272-4956
e-mail: info@donorrecovery.org
www.donorrecovery.org
Nonprofit organization that covers the Finger Lakes Region Cen-
tral and Upstate New York for transplant centers.
Richard Padula, Operations Manager
Rob Kochik, Executive Director

9212 New York Organ Donor Network, Inc
132 West 31st Street
New York, NY 10001
646-291-4444
Fax: 646-291-4600
www.nyodn.org
The New York Organ Donor Network is dedicated to the recovery
of organs and tissues for people in need of life-saving and
life-improvving transplants.
Elaine Berg, President/CEO

9213 Upstate New York Transplant Services, Inc.
110 Broadway
Buffalo, NY 14203
716-853-6667
800-227-4771
Fax: 716-853-6674
e-mail: info@unyts.org
www.unyts.org
An independent nonprofit organization that encourages and coordinates the donation of human organs and tissue for transplantation.
Sallyann Ieraci, Vice President of Community Relations
Mark J Simon, President/CEO

North Carolina

9214 Life Share of the Carolinas
5000 D Airport Center Parkway
Charlotte, NC 28208
704-512-3303
800-932-4483
Fax: 704-512-3056
e-mail: lifeshare@carolinas.org
www.lifesharecarolinas.org
Mission is to improve the quality of human life through the provision of organs and tissues for transplantation and to serve our hospitals and their respective communities by rpoviding educational
support services which enhance the donation process.
Debbie Gibbs, Public Relations Manager
Bill Faircloth, Executive Director

Ohio

9215 Life Connection of Ohio
3661 Briarfield Boulevard
Maumee, OH 43537
419-893-1618
800-262-5443
Fax: 419-893-1827
e-mail: ksteele@lcotro.org
www.lifeconnectionofohio.org
Life Connection of Ohio is committed to serving humanity by ending the wait for organ and tissue transplants in a manner that is beneficial to patients, donor families, health care professionals and the
public.
Kara Steele, Director of Community Relations (Toledo)
Cathi Arends, Director of Community Relations (Dayton)

9216 LifeBanc
20600 Chaggrin Boulevard
Cleveland, OH 44122-5343
216-752-5433
888-558-LIFE
Fax: 216-751-4204
e-mail: info@lifebanc.org
www.lifebanc.org
Non-profit organization that covers all of Northeast Ohio.
Monica Morgan, Public Education Contact

9217 Lifeline of Ohio Organ Procurement Agency, Inc.
770 Kinnear Road
Columbus, OH 43212
614-291-5667
800-525-5667
Fax: 614-291-0660
www.lifelineofohio.org

Lifeline of Ohio (LOOP) is an independent non-profit organization whose purpose is to promote and coordinate the donation of human organs and tissue dor transplantation.
Roger L Walker, Vice-Chair Governing Board of Directors
Marilyn Tomasi, Chair Governing Board of Directors

9218 Ohio Valley LifeCenter
2925 Vernon Place
Cincinnati, OH 45219-2430
513-558-5555
800-981-5433
Fax: 513-558-5556
e-mail: info@lifepassiton.org
www.lifecnt.org
Encourages amd coordinates the donation of human organs and tissues in the Greater Cincinnati area. Provides educational and motivational progams to healthcare professionals regarding their important role in the donation of organs and tissues for transplant.
Mark Sommerville, Public Education Contact
Michael Edwards, Chairman

Oklahoma

9219 Oklahoma Organ Sharing Network
5801 N Broadway
Oklahoma City, OK 73118
888-580-5680
Fax: 405-840-9748
e-mail: philvs@oosn.org ÿ
www.oosn.org
LifeShare Transplant Donor Services of Oklahoma is committed to providing a better quality of life for those people who require organ or tissue transplantation while respecting and honoring those families who share the gift of life.
Harlan Wright, President

Oregon

9220 Pacific NW Transplant Bank
2611 SW 3rd Avenue
Portland, OR 97201-4952
503-494-5560
800-344-8916
Fax: 503-494-4725
e-mail: pntb@ohsu.edu
www.pntb.org
Federally designated nonprofit organ procurement organization serving Oregon southwest Washington and western Idaho.
Jean Shepard, Public Education Contact
Barbara Thompson, Clinical Director

Pennsylvania

9221 Center for Organ Recovery & Education
RIDC Park
Pittsburgh, PA 15238
800-366-6777
Fax: 412-963-3563
e-mail: hbulvony@core.org
www.core.org
Continues its efforts to lead the procurement field by becoming a full-service OPO.
Susan A Stuart, President & CEO
Joseph P Weber, Vice President Finance

9222 Gift of Life Donor Program Pennsylvania
2000 Hamilton Street
Philadelphia, PA 19103-3813
215-557-8090
888-366-6771
Fax: 215-963-0587
e-mail: info@donors1.org
www.donors1.org
Formerly (Delaware Valley Transplant Program) is the region's nonprofit organ and tissue donor program serving eastern half of Pennsylvania, southern New Jersey and the state of Delaware. Also, considered a model program in the United States.
John Green, Director of Community Relations

Rhode Island

9223 New England Organ Bank Rhode Island
One Gateway Center
Newton, MA 02158
800-446-NEOB
Fax: 617-244-8755
e-mail: info@neob.com
www.neob.org

Independent, not-for-profit agency whose mission is to recover, preserve, and distribute human organs and tissues for transplantation. A federally-designated organ procurement organization for all or part of the six New England states, it serves 177 acute care hospitals and 14 transplant centers.
Sean Fitzpatrick, Public Education Contact

South Carolina

9224 LifePoint
4200 Faber Place Drive
Charleston, SC 29405-5711
843-763-7755
800-462-0755
Fax: 843-763-6393
e-mail: info@lifepoint-sc.org
www.lifepoint-sc.org
Dedicated to saving and improving lives by providing organ recovery services to hospitals treating potential organ donors and to support donor families.
Peggy Drake, VP Organ Recovery Services
Nancy A Kay, President & CEO

Tennessee

9225 Mid-South Transplant Foundation, Inc. Tennessee
910 Madison Avenue
Memphis, TN 38103
901-328-4438
877-228-LIFE
Fax: 901-448-8126
www.midsouthtransplant.org
Mission is to provide the option of donation to all families of potential organ donors and to protect their rights and interest throughout the donation process.
Lisa Peoples, Public Education Contact

9226 Tennessee Donor Services
110 KLM Drive
Gray, TN 37615
423-915-0808
888-562-3774
Fax: 901-448-8126
e-mail: info@donatelifetn.org
donatelifetn.org
Mission is to represent the interests of the people of our service area in the formulation of policies procedures and regulations concerning organ donation and transplantation.
Lisa Peoples, Public Education Contact
Jennifer Jenks, Contact

Utah

9227 Intermountain Donor Services
230 S 500 E
Salt Lake City, UT 84102
801-521-1755
800-833-6667
Fax: 801-364-8815
e-mail: debbie@idslife.org
www.idslife.org
Provides high quality organ and tissue procurement services to the medical and public communities. Educating medical professionals and the poublic sector on the benefits of organ and tissue donation.
Alex McDonald, Public Education Director
Tracy C Schmidt, Executive Director

Vermont

9228 New England Organ Bank Vermont
One Gateway Center
Newton, MA 02158
802-656-8454
800-446-NEOB
Fax: 617-244-8755
e-mail: info@neob.com
www.neob.org
Independent, not-for-profit agency whose mission is to recover, preserve, and distribute human organs and tissues for transplantation. A federally-designated organ procurement organization for all or part of the six New England states, it serves 177 acute care hospitals and 14 transplant centers.
Sean Fitzpatrick, Public Education Contact

Virginia

9229 LifeNet
1864 Concert Drive
Virginia Beach, VA 23453

ÿ75- 46- 476
800-847-7831
Fax: 757-301-6582
e-mail: lifenet@trans.org
www.lifenet.org

An organ procurement agency and the largest full-service tissue bank in the United States providing musculoskeletal and cardiovascular tissues for transplant on a national and international basis.
Becky Lawson, Public Education Contact

Washington

9230 LifeCenter Northwest
11245 SE 6th Street
Bellevue, WA 98004

425-201-6563
877-275-5269
Fax: 425-688-7641
e-mail: info@lcnw.org
www.lcnw.org

LifeCenter Northwest Organ Donation Network is a nonprofit organization that facilitates organ donation for a population of over 7.5 million people throughout Washington Montana Alasks and Nothern Idaho. Our mission is to fund education and outreach programs.
Megan Erwin, Vice President Community Relations
Diana Clark, President & CEO

Wisconsin

9231 University of Wisconsin Organ Procurement Organization
University of Wisconsin Hospital and Clinics
450 Science Drive
Madison, WI 53711-1735

608-265-0356
Fax: 608-262-9099
e-mail: uwhcopo@uwhealth.org
www.uwhcopo.org

Located within a major academic center and is recognized as one of the most successful organ procurement programs in the nation.
Jill Ellefson, Public Education Contact

9232 Wisonsin Donor Network
9200 W Chester Street
Milwaukee, WI 53214

414-805-2024
800-432-5405
Fax: 414-259-8059
e-mail: cjastroc@fmlh.edu
www.wisdonornetwork.org

Recovers organs for transplant as well as provides public and professional education about the tremendous need for organ and tissue donors.
Judy Suchman, Director
Colleen McCarthy, Assistant Director

Wyoming

9233 Donor Alliance
720 S Colorado Boulevard
Denver, CO 80246

303-329-4747
888-868-4747
Fax: 303-321-0366
www.donoralliance.org

Jennifer Moe, Director of Community Relations/PR
Nancy Williams, Chairman

International

9234 Lifelink of Puerto Rico
Digital Plaza, Suite 402
Guaynabo, PR 00968

787-277-0900
800-558-0977
Fax: 787-277-0876
e-mail: lifelink@PPTC.Net
www.lifelinkfound.org

An independent, nonprofit community service organization dedicated to the recovery and transplantation of organs and tissues.
Ruth Duncan Bell, Public Education Contact

Foundations

9235 Musculoskeletal Transplant Foundation
125 May Street
Edison, NJ 08837

732-661-0202
Fax: 732-661-2298
e-mail: information@mtf.org
www.mtf.org

Non-profit service organization dedicated to providing quality tissue through a commitment to excellence in education, research, recovery and care for recipients, donors, and their families.
Bruce W Stroever, President/CEO
George A Oram, EVP Sales/Marketing

Research Centers

9236 Georgetown University Hospital Transplant Institute
3800 Reservoir Road, NW
Washington, DC 20007

202-444-2000
www.georgetownuniversityhospital.org

Founded to promote health through education, research, and patient care.

Books

9237 History of Organ and Cell Transplantation
Imperial College Press
57 Shelton St., Convent Garden
United Kingdom,

e-mail: edit@icpress.co.uk
www.icpress.co.uk

Covers the areas of modern medical literature.
464 pages Hardcover
ISBN: 1-860942-09-1

9238 Legal and Ethical Aspects of Organ Transplantation
David P T Price, author

Cambridge University Press
40 West 20th Street
New York, NY 10011-4221

212-924-3900
Fax: 212-691-3239
www.cambridge.org/us

A comprehensive analysis of existing laws and policies governing transplantation practices around the world. Examines the meaning of death, cadaver organ procurement policies, use of living donors, trading in human organs, experimental transplant procedures and xenotransplantation.
507 pages Hardcover
ISBN: 0-521651-64-6

9239 Organ Procurement and Transplantation:
Intitute of Medicine, author

National Academies Press
500 Fifth Street NW
Washington, DC 20055

202-334-3313
888-624-8373
Fax: 202-334-2451
www.nap.edu

This book assesses the potential impact of the Final Rule on organ transplantation. Prensents new, original data, and assesses medical practices, social and economic observations, and other information.
232 pages Hardcover

9240 Organ Transplants from Executed Prisoners:
Louis J Palmer, author

McFarland & Company
960 NC Hwy 88W
Jefferson, NC 28640

336-246-4460
Fax: 336-246-5018
e-mail: info@mcfarlandpub.com
www.mcfarlandpub.com

A study of the utilitarian creation of death sentence organ removal statutes that would make legal the harvesting of transplantable organs from the cadavers of executed capital murders.
156 pages
ISBN: 0-786406-73-9

9241 Transplantation Ethics
Robert M. Veatch, author

Georgetown University Press
3240 Prospect Street, NW
Washington, DC 20007   202-687-5889
    Fax: 202-687-6340
    e-mail: gupress@georgetown.edu
    www.press.georgetown.edu

The first complete and systematic account of the ethical and policy controversies surrounding organ transplants.
2000 448 pages Paperback
ISBN: 0-878408-12-2

9242 Twice Dead: Organ Transplants and the Reinvention of Death
Margaret Lock, author

University of California Press
1445 Lower Ferry Road
Ewing, NJ 08618   800-UCB-OOKS
    Fax: 800-999-1958
    www.ucpress.edu/index.html

Raises critically important questions about life and death in the modern world.
429 pages Paperback
ISBN: 0-520228-14-6

9243 US Organ Procurement System: A Prescription for Reform
David L. Kaserman, A.H. Barnett, author

American Enterprise Institute
1150 Seventeenth St, NW
Washington, DC 20036   202-862-5800
    Fax: 202-862-7177
    www.aei.org

Isolates the procurement issue from others to make a compelling and persuasive case for markets in cadaveric organs.
177 pages Paperback
ISBN: 0-844741-71-X

Magazines

9244 Encore: Another Chance for Life
Chronimed Pharmacy
Po Box 59032
Minneapolis, MN 55459-9686   800-888-5753
Published exclusively for transplant patients, their families, and friends, this publication provides a broad look at many issues surrounding transplantation and encourages personal stories and feedback from readers.
Quarterly

9245 Renalife
The American Association of Kidney Patients
100 S. Ashley Drive
Tampa, FL 33260   800-749-2257
    e-mail: aakpaz@enet.net
Provides articles, news items, and information of interest to kindey patients and their families, individuals, and organizations in the renal health care field.
3 Year

9246 Stadtlanders LifeTIMES
Stadtlanders Pharmacy
600 Penn Center Boulevard
Pittsburgh, PA 15235-5810   800-238-7828
    www.statlander.com/transplant/#resource
Designed to be an educational, informative and supportive, focusing on a variety of health-care issues of concern to patients (including transplant patients).

Newsletters

9247 Advocate
National Foundation for Transplants
1102 Brookfield Road
Memphis, TN 38119   901-684-1697
    800-489-3863
    Fax: 901-684-1128
    e-mail: info@transplants.org
    www.transplants.org
Judy Strickland, Patient Services Coordinator

9248 Children's Organ Transplant Association (COTA)
2501 COTA Drive
Bloomington, IN 47403   800-366-2682
    Fax: 812-336-8885
    e-mail: cota@cota.org
    www.cota.org
Provides fundraising assistance to children and young adults needing life-saving transplants and promotes organ, marrow and tissue donation.
Rick Lofgren, President/CEO
Lisa Fulkerson, VP/CFO

9249 New Start News
National Transplant Assistance Fund (NTAF)
3475 West Chester Pike
Newtown Square, PA 19073   610-353-9684
    800-642-8399
    Fax: 610-353-1616
    e-mail: ntaf@transplantfund.org
    www.transplantfund.org

Sidney P. Constien, Editor
Judy Walker, Editor

Web Sites

9250 American Society of Transplantation (AST)
    www.a-s-t.org
An organization of transplant professionals dedicated to research, education, advocacy and patient care in transplantation science and medicine.

9251 Association of Organ Procurement Organizations (AOPO)
    www.aopo.org
Organization involved in helping people find and obtain the organs they may need for transplantation.

9252 Children's Organ Transplant Association (COTA)
    www.cota.org
Not-for-profit national chairty dedicated to helping families and communities raise the necessary funds for transplant expenses.

9253 Donate Life America
    www.donatelife.net
A not-for-profit alliance of national organizations and local coalitions across the United States that have joined forces to educate the public about organ, eye and tissue donation, correcting misconceptions about donation and creating a greater willingness to donate.

9254 Georgetown University Hospital Transplant Institute
    www.georgetownuniversityhospital.org
Founded to promote health through education, research, and patient care.

9255 Health Resources and Services Administration (HRSA)
    www.hrsa.gov
Envisions optimal health for all, supported by a health care system that assures access to comprehensive, culturally competant, quality care. Provides national leadership, program resources and services needed to improve access to culturally competant, quality health care.

9256 Jewish Hospital Transplant Center
    www.jewishhospital.com
An elite group approved to perform five solid organ transplants and has been named a Federally Designated Medicare Heart, Lung, Kidney, Liver and Pancreas Transplant Center.

9257 MedicineNet
    www.medicinenet.com
An online resource for consumers providing easy-to-read, authoritative medical and health information.

9258 National Foundation for Transplants
    www.transplants.org
Mission is to reach out to help those who seek a new life through transplantation, by providing healthcare and financial support services and patient advocacy for transplant candidates families nationwide.

9259 National Transplant Assistance Fund (NTAF)
    www.transplantfund.org

Helps to raise funds for transplant and catastrophic injury patients by providing compassionate support, education and expertise to them, their families and communities.

9260   Organ Procurement and Transplantation Network (OPTN)

www.optn.org

A unified transplant network established by the United States Congress under the National Organ Transplant Act (NOTA) of 1984. A unique public-prvate partnership that links all of the professionals nvolved in the donation and transplantation system.

9261   Transweb: All About Transplantation and Donation

www.transweb.org

Non-profit educational website serving the world transplant community. Features news and events, real peoples experinces, the top 10 myths about donation, a donation quiz, and a large collection of questions and answers, as well as a reference area with everything from articles to videos.

9262   United Network for Organ Sharing (UNOS)

www.unos.org

Mon-profit, scientific and educational organization that administers the nation's only Organ Procurement and Transplantation Network(OPTN). Mission is to advance organ availability and transplantation by uniting and supporting our communities for the benefit of patients through education, technology and policy development.

9263   United Organ Transplant Association (UOTA)

www.uota.org

Non-profit charitable Corporation dedicated to providing educational, emotional and financial support to pre- and post- transplant patients.

Description

9264 Tuberculosis

Tuberculosis, TB, is an infectious disease caused by mycobacteria. It is spread through the air and normally affects the lungs (pulmonary tuberculosis). Extremely common in the United States early in the twentieth century, tuberculosis declined dramatically after 1950. This trend reversed itself after about 1985, due to immigration, the HIV epidemic, and the development of drug resistance by the germ responsible for the disease.

The usual symptoms of TB infection of the lungs include persistent cough, chest pain and coughing up blood. TB infection can cause weight loss, night sweats and fatigue. Left untreated, TB may spread to the spine, causing bone breakdown with deformity, to the lining of the brain, causing tuberculous meningitis, or, in fact, to any organ of the body (extrapulmonary TB).

People who are otherwise healthy, and who are infected with a strain of mycobacterium that is sensitive to standard drugs, can almost always be cured after 6-9 months of therapy. Persons infected with HIV, because of their lowered resistance to disease, have trouble clearing their TB infection, even if they use effective drugs faithfully. Therefore, they should be treated for one year. Regardless of length of treatment, during this time the germ may become resistant to the drug being used. Therefore treatment includes at least 2 drugs, so that a bacterium that develops resistance to one drug will still be killed by another one. Incomplete or interrupted treatment often leads to drug resistance. Germs that are resistant to multiple drugs may be passed to others, and are now a serious public health menace. Unfortunately, the HIV-infected patient is an ideal breeding ground for drug-resistant TB germs.

Persons with drug-sensitive TB who are otherwise healthy and will cooperate with treatment are generally treated by community physicians. Those with complicated medical status (HIV, drug-resistant organisms) or social difficulties (alcoholism, substance abuse, homelessness) generally require specialized public health clinics that can combine medical expertise with nursing and social outreach support.

Many persons who have been infected by TB keep it successfully contained by their own immune systems. There is some risk of the contained germ, however, even years later, overcoming the body's resistance and causing active disease. The tuberculin skin test (PPD) is used to widely screen certain high-risk populations, particularly those who have been exposed to an infectious individual. Prior, adequately treated infection may be diagnosed by a positive PPD, and is sometimes treated with antibiotics to reduce the risk of future disease.

National Agencies & Associations

9265 American Lung Association
1301 Pennsylvania Avenue NW
Washington, DC 20004
212-315-8700
800-LUN-GUSA
www.lungusa.org

The mission of the American Lung Association is to prevent lung disease and promote lung health. Founded in 1904 to fight tuberculosis the American Lung Association today fights disease in all its forms, with special emphasis on asthma and tobacco control.
H James Gooden, Secretary
Stephen J Nolan, Chair

9266 Centers for Disease Control and Prevention National Center for Prevention Services
National Center for Prevention Services
1600 Clifton Road
Atlanta, GA 30333
404-639-8135
800-CDC-INFO
TTY: 888-232-6348
e-mail: cdcinfo@cdc.gov
www.cdc.gov

CDC has been dedicated to protecting health and promoting quality of life through the prevention and control of disease, injury and disability.
Richard E Besser, Acting Director
Ileana Arias, Director Center Injury Prevention

9267 National Institute of Allergy and Infectious Diseases
6610 Rockledge Drive
Bethesda, MD 20892-6621
301-496-5717
866-284-4107
Fax: 301-402-3573
TTY: 800-877-8339
e-mail: afauci@niaid.nih.gov
www.niaid.nih.gov

Conducts and supports basic and applied research to better understand, treat and ultimately prevent infectious, immunologic and allergic diseases.
Anthony S Fauci MD, Director
H Clifford Lane MD, Acting Deputy Director

9268 New Jersey Medical School: National Tuberculosis Center
225 Warren Street
Newark, NJ 07101-1709
973-972-3270
800-482-3627
Fax: 973-972-3268
www.umdnj.edu/ntbcweb/tbsplash.html

Provides expert medical consultation, trains health care providers and other health related professionals, utilize innovative educational methodologies such as standardized patients, develop linkages with health care delivery systems and collaborate with health care professionals.
Lee B Reichman, Executive Director
Reynard J McDonald, Medical Director

9269 Occupational Safety & Health Administration
200 Constitution Avenue Northwest
Washington, DC 20210
800-321-6742
TTY: 877-889-5627
www.osha.gov

OSHA's mission is to assure the safety and health of America's workers by setting and enforcing standards, providing training, outreach and education, establishing partnerships and encouraging continual improvement in workplace safety and health.
Doug Kalinowski, Director

State Agencies & Associations

Alabama

9270 American Lung Association of Alabama
PO Box 3188
Bessemer, AL 35023
205-933-8821
800-LUN-GUSA
Fax: 205-930-1717
e-mail: kperry@alabamalung.org
www.alabamalung.org

Kim Perry, Director of Development

Alaska

9271 American Lung Association of Alaska
500 W International Airport Road   907-276-5864
Anchorage, AK 99518   800-LUN-GUSA
                                                    Fax: 907-565-5587
                                    e-mail: mlarson@aklung.org
                                                    www.aklung.org

Marge Larson, Director

Arizona

9272 American Lung Association of Arizona/New Mexico
102 W McDowell Road   602-258-7505
Phoenix, AZ 85003-1299   800-586-4872
                                                    Fax: 602-258-7507
                                                    www.lungusa.org

9273 Northern Arizona Branch:Phoenix Area
102 W McDowell Road   602-258-7505
Phoenix, AZ 85003-1299   800-LUN-GUSA
                                                    Fax: 602-258-7507
                                    e-mail: infophoenix@lungaz.org
                                                    www.lungarizona.org

Nancy Cohrs, Executive Director
Evelyn Frear, Office Manager

9274 Southern Arizona Branch: Tucson Area
2819 E Broadway   520-323-1812
Tuscon, AZ 85716   800-LUN-GUSA
                                                    Fax: 520-323-1816
                                    e-mail: infotucson@lungaz.org
                                                    www.lungarizona.org

Keith Kaback, Chairman
Heidi Miller, Vice Chairman

Arkansas

9275 American Lung Association of Arkansas
1 Castle Rock Cove   501-224-0773
Little Rock, AR 72212-1539   Fax: 866-571-9608
                                    e-mail: wdavenport@breethealthy.org
                                    www.lungusa2.org/arkansas/index.html

California

9276 American Lung Association of California
424 Pendleton Way   510-638-LUNG
Oakland, CA 94621-2189   800-LUN-GUSA
                                                    Fax: 510-638-8984
                                    e-mail: contact@californialung.org
                                                    www.californialung.org

Trisha Murakawa, Chairman
Laura Keegan Boudreau, Acting CEO

Colorado

9277 American Lung Association of Colorado
5600 Greenwood Plaza Boulevard   303-388-4327
Greenwood Village, CO 80111-2305   800-LUN-GUSA
                                                    Fax: 303-377-1102
                                    e-mail: cmichael@lungcolorado.org
                                                    www.lungcolorado.org

Curt Huber, Executive Director
Connor Michael, Communications Manager

Connecticut

9278 American Lung Association of Connecticut
45 Ash Street   860-289-5401
E Hartford, CT 06108-3272   800-992-2263
                                                    Fax: 860-289-5405
                                    e-mail: alaofct@alact.org
                                                    www.alact.org

Margaret LaCroix, Vice President Communications

Delaware

9279 American Lung Association of Delaware
1021 Gilpin Avenue   302-655-7258
Wilmington, DE 19806-3280   Fax: 302-655-8546
                                                    www.alade.org

Peter Shanley, Chairman

District of Columbia

9280 American Lung Association of the District of Columbia
530 7th Street SE   202-682-5864
Washington, DC 20003-2617   Fax: 202-682-5607
                                    e-mail: info@aladc.org
                                                    www.aladc.org

Jan Morgan, Special Events Director
Phoebe Robinson, Administrative Coordinator

Florida

9281 American Lung Association of Florida
6852 Belfort Oaks Place   904-743-2933
Jacksonville, FL 32216-5216   800-940-2933
                                                    Fax: 904-743-2916
                                    e-mail: alaf@lungfla.org
                                                    www.lungfla.org

Michael Diamond, President
Marilin K Glassberg, President-Elect

Georgia

9282 American Lung Association of Georgia
2452 Spring Road   770-434-5864
Smyrna, GA 30080   800-586-4872
                                                    Fax: 770-319-0349
                                    e-mail: mail@alaga.org
                                                    www.alase.org

Charles J White, Chief Executive Officer
June Deen, VP Public Affairs

Hawaii

9283 American Lung Association of Hawaii
680 Iwilei Road   808-537-5966
Honolulu, HI 96817   Fax: 808-537-5971
                                    e-mail: lung@ala-hawaii.org
                                                    www.ala-hawaii.org

Karen J Lee, President, Executive Director

Illinois

9284 American Lung Association of Illinois-Iowa
3000 Kelly Lane   217-787-5864
Springfield, IL 62707   800-586-4872
                                                    Fax: 217-787-5916
                                    e-mail: info@lungil.org
                                                    www.lungil.org

Harold Wimmer, CEO
Lori Younker, Manager

Indiana

**9285 American Lung Association of Indiana: State Office & Support
Office**
115 W Washington Street   317-819-1181
Indianapolis, IN 46204   800-LUN-GUSA
                                                    Fax: 317-819-1187
                                    e-mail: info@lungin.org
                                                    www.lungin.org

Dana Pitts, VP Communications/Marketing

Kansas

9286 American Lung Association of Kansas
PO Box 8630   785-246-0377
Topeka, KS 66618-2419   Fax: 866-575-1761
                                    e-mail: menisam@kylung.org
                                                    www.lungusa.org

Judy Keller, Executive Director

Kentucky

9287 American Lung Association of Kentucky
4100 Churchman Avenue
Louisville, KY 40209-0067

502-363-2652
800-LUN-GUSA
Fax: 502-363-0222
e-mail: info@kylung.org
www.kylung.org

Todd Adams, Development Director
Laura Collins, Executive Assistant

Louisiana

9288 American Lung Association of Louisiana
2325 Severn Avenue
Metairie, LA 70001-6918

504-828-5864
800-LUN-GUSA
Fax: 504-828-5867
e-mail: info@louisianalung.org
www.louisianalung.org

Aline Palmisano-Vita, Deputy Executive Director
Thomas P Lotz, Chief Executive Officer

Maine

9289 American Lung Association of Maine
122 State Street
Augusta, ME 04330

207-622-6394
800-LUN-GUSA
Fax: 639-426-2919
e-mail: info@lungme.org
www.mainelung.org

Lee Scott, President of Health Promotion
Edward Miller, Executive Director/SVP

Maryland

9290 American Lung Association of Maryland
11350 McCormick Road
Hunt Valley, MD 21031

410-560-2120
Fax: 410-560-0829
e-mail: info@marylandlung.org
www.marylandlung.org

Melina Davis-Martin, President and CEO
Krista Jennings, Chief Operations Officer

Massachusetts

9291 American Lung Association of Massachusetts
460 Totten Pond Road
Waltham, MA 02451

781-890-4262
Fax: 781-890-4280
e-mail: info@lungma.org
www.lungusa.org

Michigan

9292 American Lung Association of Michigan
25900 Greenfield Road
Oak Park, MI 48237

248-784-2000
800-543-5864
Fax: 248-784-2008
e-mail: alam@alam.org
www.alam.org

Colette Scholzen, President

Minnesota

9293 American Lung Association of Minnesota
490 Concordia Avenue
Saint Paul, MN 55103-2441

651-227-8014
800-LUN-GUSA
Fax: 651-227-5459
e-mail: info@alamn.org
www.alamn.org

Bill Westhoff, President

Mississippi

9294 American Lung Association of Mississippi
731 Pear Orchard Road
Ridgeland, MS 39158

601-206-5810
800-586-4872
Fax: 601-206-5813
www.alams.org

Greg Wynne, Chairman
Jennifer Cofer, Deputy Executive Director

Missouri

9295 American Lung Association of Missouri
1118 Hampton Avenue
Saint Louis, MO 63139

314-645-5505
Fax: 314-645-7128
e-mail: pickens@lungmo.org
www.lungusa2.org

Lori Pickens, Chief Executive Officer
Barry Freedman, VP Community Initiatives

Montana

**9296 American Lung Association of the Northern Rockies: Montana
and Wyoming**
825 Helena Avenue
Helene, MT 59601-3459

406-442-6556
Fax: 406-442-2346
e-mail: ala-nr@ala-nr.org
www.lungusa.org

Nebraska

9297 American Lung Association of Nebraska
7101 Newport Avenue
Omaha, NE 68152

402-502-4950
Fax: 402-502-3012
e-mail: jegerton@breathehealthy.org
www.lungusa.org

Nevada

9298 American Lung Association of Idaho/Nevada
10615 Double R Boulevard
Reno, NV 89521-7056

775-829-LUNG
800-LUN-GUSA
Fax: 775-829-5850
e-mail: lmartin@lungnevada.org
www.lungnevada.org/Reno

Louise Martin, Executive Director
Gwen Bourne, Development Manager - Events

New Hampshire

9299 American Lung Association of New Hampshire
20 Warren Street
Concord, NH 03301

603-369-3977
Fax: 603-369-3978
e-mail: info@nhlung.org
www.lungne.org

Jeff Seyler, President & CEO
David Ales, Senior Vice President

New Jersey

9300 American Lung Association of New Jersey
1600 Route 22 E
Union, NJ 07083-3407

908-687-9340
800-LUN-GUSA
Fax: 908-851-2625
e-mail: info@lunginfo.org
www.alanewjersey.org

John A Rutkowski, President

New Mexico

9301 New Mexico Branch
7001 Menaul Boulevard NE
Albuquerque, NM 87110

505-265-0732
800-LUN-GUSA
Fax: 505-260-1739
e-mail: ronh@alanm.org
www.lungusa.org

New York

9302   American Lung Association of Mid New York
155 Washington Avenue
Albany, NY 12210

518-465-2013
Fax: 518-465-2926
e-mail: info@alany.org
www.alany.org

The mission of the American Lung Association and the American Lung Association of New York State is to prevent lung disease and promote lung health. The American Lung Association is the oldest voluntary health organization in the United States.
Deborah Carioto, President
Michael Seilback, Vice President Public Policy

North Carolina

9303   American Lung Association of North Carolina
3801 Lake Boone Trail
Raleigh, NC 27607

919-832-8326
800-892-5650
Fax: 919-856-8530
e-mail: dbryan@lungnc.org
www.lungnc.org

Deborah C. Bryan, President

9304   American Lung Association of North Dakota
8300 Health Park
Raleigh, NC 27615

919-832-8326
Fax: 919-856-8530
e-mail: dbryan@lungnc.org
www.lungnc.org

Deborah C Bryan, VP Advocacy & Donor Value
Mendi Nieters, Regional VP Development

North Dakota

9305   American Lung Association of North Dakota
212 N 2nd Street
Bismarck, ND 58502-5004

701-223-5613
800-252-6325
Fax: 701-223-5727
e-mail: amerlungnd@gcentral.com
www.lungusa2.org/northdakota

Judy Mourhess, Office Manager

Ohio

9306   American Lung Association of Ohio
1950 Arlingate Lane
Columbus, OH 43228

614-279-1700
800-LUN-GUSA
Fax: 614-279-4940
e-mail: alao@ohiolung.org
www.ohiolung.org

Tracy Ross, President / CEO

Oklahoma

9307   American Lung Association of Oklahoma
1010 E 8th Street
Tulsa, OK 74120

918-747-3441
Fax: 918-747-4629
www.oklung.org

Sara Dreiling, Chief Executive Officer
Edward C Rosentel, Chief Financial and Operating Officer

Oregon

9308   American Lung Association of Oregon
7420 SW Bridgeport Road
Tigard, OR 97224

503-924-4094
Fax: 503-924-4120
e-mail: info@lungoregon.org
www.lungoregon.org

Jan Jensen, President
Dana Kaye, Executive Director

Pennsylvania

9309   American Lung Association of Pennsylvania
3001 Old Gettysburg Road
Camp Hill, PA 17011

717-541-5864
800-LUN-GUSA
Fax: 717-541-8828
e-mail: info@lunginfo.org
www.lunginfo.org

South Carolina

9310   American Lung Association of South Carolina
1817 Gadsen Street
Columbia, SC 29201-2392

803-779-5864
800-849-5864
Fax: 803-254-2711
e-mail: alasc@lungsc.org
www.lungsc.org

9311   American Lung Association of South Dakota
1817 Gadsen Street
Columbia, SC 29201

803-779-5864
Fax: 803-254-2711
e-mail: shelps@alase.org
www.alase.org

Amanda Strickland, Regional Manager Special Events
Sharon Helps, Regional Manager Programs

South Dakota

9312   American Lung Association of South Dakota
108 E 38th Street
Sioux Falls, SD 57105

605-336-7222
800-873-5864
Fax: 605-336-7227
e-mail: lung@americanlungsd.org
www.lungusa2.org/southdakota

Tennessee

9313   American Lung Association of Tennesse
One Vantage Way
Nashville, TN 37228

615-329-1151
800-LUN-GUSA
Fax: 615-329-1723
e-mail: alastaff@alatn.org
www.alatn.org

Texas

9314   American Lung Association of Texas
5926 Balcones Drive
Austin, TX 78731-0460

512-467-6753
800-252-5864
Fax: 512-467-7621
e-mail: info@texaslung.org
www.texaslung.org

Phillip J Hanson, Senior VP Resource Development
Margaret Crump, Senior VP Community Initiatives

Utah

9315   American Lung Association of Utah
1930 S 1100 E
Salt Lake City, UT 84106-2317

801-484-4456
Fax: 801-484-5461
e-mail: info@utahlung.org
www.lungusa2.org/utah

Vermont

9316   American Lung Association of Vermont
372 Hurricane Lane
Williston, VT 05495-6196

802-876-6500
Fax: 802-876-6505
e-mail: info@vtlung.org
www.lungne.org

Erin Hickey, Senior Manager Development
Margaret LaCroix, VP Marketing\Communications

Virginia

9317   American Lung Association of Virginia
9221 Forest Hill Avenue
Richmond, VA 23235

804-267-1900
Fax: 804-267-5634
e-mail: mdavismartin@lungva.org
www.lungva.org

Melina Davis-Martin, President and CEO
Krista Jennings, Chief Operating Officer

9318 American Lung Association of Washington
2625 Third Avenue   206-441-5100
Seattle, WA 98121   800-732-9339
                                          Fax: 206-441-3277
                                      e-mail: alaw@alaw.org
                                              www.alaw.org

Vivian Echavarria, Chair
Rick Weems, Secretary

West Virginia

9319 American Lung Association of West Virginia
415 Dickinson Street   304-342-6600
Charleston, WV 25301-3980   Fax: 304-342-6096
                                  e-mail: cfields@lunginfo.org
                                            www.lungusa.org

Sara Crickenberger, Executive Director

Wisconsin

9320 American Lung Association of Wisconsin
13100 W Lisbon Road   262-703-4200
Brookfield, WI 53005-2508   800-586-4872
                                          Fax: 262-781-5180
                                  e-mail: amlung@lungwi.org
                                             www.lungwi.org

Susan Gloede Swan, Executive Director
Dona Wininsky, Director of Public Policy

Research Centers

9321 University of Illinois at Chicago Lions
833 S Wood Street   312-355-1715
Chicago, IL 60612   Fax: 312-355-2693
                                www.uic.edu/pharmacy/research/itr
The Institute for Tuberculosis Research is comprised of approximately 30 individuals: biologists chemists pharmacologists and support staff -ÿ all working towards a single goal - the discovery of new drugs for tuberculosis.
Scott Franzblau, Director
Lorna Haubrich, ITR General Information

9322 University of Illinois at Chicago: Institute for Tuberculosis Research
833 S. Wood Street   312-355-1715
Chicago, IL 60612-7631   Fax: 312-355-2693
                                www.uic.edu/pharmacy/research/itr
Scott Franzblau, Director

Support Groups & Hotlines

9323 National Health Information Center
PO Box 1133   310-565-4167
Washington, DC 20013   800-336-4797
                                          Fax: 301-984-4256
                                       e-mail: info@nhic.org
                                          www.health.gov/nhic
Offers a nationwide information referral service, produces directories and resource guides.

Pamphlets

9324 Classification of Tuberculosis and Other Mycobacterial Diseases
American Lung Association
1740 Broadway   212-315-8700
New York, NY 10019-4315
Chart listing different classes of tuberculosis and other mycobacterial diseases.

9325 Facts About Tuberculosis
American Lung Association
1740 Broadway   212-315-8700
New York, NY 10019-4315

Primary public information leaflet on TB as well as on its impact and treatment.
8 pages

9326 TB Skin Test
American Lung Association
1740 Broadway   212-315-8700
New York, NY 10019-4315
Primary public information leaflet on the TB skin test.
8 pages

9327 TB: What You Should Know
American Lung Association of Connecticut
45 Ash Street   860-289-5401
East Hartford, CT 06108-3294   800-586-4872
                                          Fax: 860-289-5405
                                              www.alact.org
Offers a brief overview of tuberculosis, how transmission is possible, and TB skin testing.
John E Zinn, President/CEO

9328 This is Mr. TB Germ
American Lung Association
1740 Broadway   212-315-8700
New York, NY 10019-4315
Lively booklet of drawings and very brief text giving a basic description of TB and its treatments.
20 pages

Web Sites

9329 American Lung Association
                                  www.americanlungusa.org
Offers research, medical updates, fund-raising, educational materials and public awareness campaigns relating to lung disease and related disorders.

9330 Healing Well
                                        www.healingwell.org
An online health resource guide to medical news, chat, information and articles, newsgroups and message boards, disease-related web sites, medical directories, and more for patients, friends, and family coping with disabling diseases, disorders, or chronic illnesses.

9331 Health Finder
                                         www.healthfinder.gov
Searchable, carefully developed web site offering information on over 1000 topics. Developed by the US Department of Health and Human Services, the site can be used in both English and Spanish.

9332 Healthlink USA
                                       www.healthlinkusa.com
Health information concerning treatment, cures, prevention, diagnosis, risk factors, research, support groups, email lists, personal stories and much more. Updated regularly.

9333 Helios Health
                                        www.helioshealth.com
Online resource for your health information. Detailed information about specific health topics, access to expert advice from our Medical Advisory Board, and up-to-date health news.

9334 MedicineNet
                                         www.medicinenet.com
An online resource for consumers providing easy-to-read, authoritative medical and health information.

9335 Medscape
                                           www.medscape.com
Medscape offers specialists, primary care physicians, and other health professionals the Web's most robust and integrated medical information and educational tools.

9336 National Institute of Allergy & Inf. Dis.
                                           www.niaid.nih.gov
NAID is composed of four extramural divisions: the Division of AIDS; the Division of Allergy, Immunology and Transplantation; the Division of Microbology and Infectious Diseases; and the Division of Extramural Activities. In addition, NIAID scientists con-

duct intramural research in laboratories located in Bethesda, Rockville and Frederick, Maryland, and in Hamilton, Montana.

9337 WebMD

www.webmd.com

Information on Tuberculosis, including articles and resources.

Description

9338 Tuberous Sclerosis

Tuberous sclerosis is a genetic disorder that causes benign, (non-cancerous) tumors to form in different locations - primarily in the brain, skin, kidneys, heart, lungs and even eyes. The name is derived from tuber-like growths on the brain that become hard. It usually shows itself in infancy or early childhood, and may cause seizures and/or mental retardation. It is inherited through chromosome 9 or 16. Disease severity is highly variable, even within the same family. Those with tuberous sclerosis can have mental retardation as well as seizures.

There are various skin abnormalities that may provide a clue to the diagnosis when an infant or young child exhibits seizures or delayed development. The first is an area of decreased skin pigmentation, called an ash-leaf spot because of its shape. Multiple ash-leaf spots may appear on the trunk and limbs during infancy. At age 3 or 4, tiny red bumps, adenoma sebaceum, resembling acne may appear on the nose and cheeks. Finally, a roughened spot with the consistency of orange peel, shagren patch, may appear over the lower spine.

There is no cure so treatment is based on symptoms and can include anti-epileptic drugs for seizures, removal of skin lesions, treatment of high blood pressure caused by kidney problems, special education and, in some instances, surgery to remove growing tumors.

National Agencies & Associations

9339 National Tuberous Sclerosis Association
801 Roeder Road　　　　　　　　　　301-562-9890
Sliver Spring, MD 20910　　　　　　　800-225-6872
　　　　　　　　　　　　　　Fax: 301-562-9870
　　　　　　　　　e-mail: info@tsalliance.org
　　　　　　　　　　　　　　　www.ntsa.org
A voluntary nonprofit organization that is dedicated to fostering and supporting tuberous sclerosis research; to provide education of the public educators and health care professionals; and to providing support of individuals with tuberous sclerosis.
Kari Luther Carlson, President & Chief Executive Officer
Gail Alexander, Senior Manager of Operations

Support Groups & Hotlines

9340 National Health Information Center
PO Box 1133　　　　　　　　　　　310-565-4167
Washington, DC 20013　　　　　　　800-336-4797
　　　　　　　　　　　　　　Fax: 301-984-4256
　　　　　　　　　　e-mail: info@nhic.org
　　　　　　　　　　www.health.gov/nhic
Offers a nationwide information referral service, produces directories and resource guides.

Books

9341 Tuberous Sclerosis
Oxford University Press
2001 Evans Road
Cary, NC 27513
　　　　　　　　　　　　　　800-451-7556
　　　　　　　　　　　　Fax: 919-677-1303
　　　　　　　　　　　　www.oup-usa.org

A revision offering up-to-date medical information to families, researchers, and professionals on TS.

ISBN: 0-195122-10-0

Newsletters

9342 NTSA Perspective
National Tuberous Sclerosis Association
8181 Professional Place　　　　　　301-459-9888
Landover, MD 20785-2226　　　　　800-225-6872
　　　　　　　　　　　　　　Fax: 301-459-0394
　　　　　　　　　　　e-mail: ntsa@ntsa.org
　　　　　　　　　　　　　　　www.ntsa.org
Offers the latest research and medical information on tuberous sclerosis to physicians and health care professionals.
Quarterly

Web Sites

9343 Healing Well
　　　　　　　　　　　　　www.healingwell.com
An online health resource guide to medical news, chat, information and articles, newsgroups and message boards, books, disease-related web sites, medical directories, and more for patients, friends, and family coping with disabling diseases, disorders, or chronic illnesses.

9344 Health Finder
　　　　　　　　　　　　　www.healthfinder.gov
Searchable, carefully developed web site offering information on over 1000 topics. Developed by the US Department of Health and Human Services, the site can be used in both English and Spanish.

9345 Healthlink USA
　　　　　　　　　　　　　www.healthlinkusa.com
Health information concerning treatment, cures, prevention, diagnosis, risk factors, research, support groups, email lists, personal stories and much more. Updated regularly.

9346 Helios Health
　　　　　　　　　　　　　www.helioshealth.com
Online resource for your health information. Detailed information about specific health topics, access to expert advice from our Medical Advisory Board, and up-to-date health news.

9347 MedicineNet
　　　　　　　　　　　　　www.medicinenet.com
An online resource for consumers providing easy-to-read, authoritative medical and health information.

9348 Medscape
　　　　　　　　　　　　　www.medscape.com
Medscape offers specialists, primary care physicians, and other health professionals the Web's most robust and integrated medical information and educational tools.

9349 National Tuberous Sclerosis Association
　　　　　　　　　　　　　www.ntsa.org
NTSA provides information to individuals and families through its family support network, quarterly newsletters, brochures and other printed materials.

9350 WebMD
　　　　　　　　　　　　　www.webmd.com
Information on Tuberous Sclerosis, including articles and resources.

Description

9351 Turner Syndrome

Turner syndrome is a genetic disorder that occurs in 1 in 2,500 to 10,000 live female births. It only affects females because, rather than having two female sex (X) chromosomes, Turner syndrome patients have only one. The disease usually hinders sexual development and produces small stature and varying degrees of mental retardation. There may be associated anomalies such as webbed neck and defects of the heart or aorta, which may occur in up to 25 percent of individuals.

Turner syndrome cannot be cured, but hormonal treatment may give the patient a more normal life. Growth hormone injections can help the patient reach a taller adult height, and estrogen replacement can encourage breast development and other sex characteristics. A few patients will develop menstrual periods spontaneously, and a few have become pregnant; most, however, are infertile. Psychological support for the patient and her family is important.

National Agencies & Associations

9352 Human Growth Foundation: Turner Syndrome Division
997 Glen Cove Avenue
Glen Head, NY 11545-1554   800-451-6434
Fax: 516-671-4055
e-mail: hgf1@hgfound.org
www.hgfound.org
A nonprofit, national organization committed to expanding and accelerating research into growth and growth disorders, provides education and support to those affected by growth disorders and their families and fosters the exchange of information.
Frank Diamond, President
Emily Germain-Lee, Vice President

9353 MAGIC Foundation for Children's Growth: Turner's Syndrome Division
6645 W N Avenue   708-383-0808
Oak Park, IL 60302-1376   800-362-4423
Fax: 708-383-0899
e-mail: dianne@magicfoundation.org
www.magicfoundation.org
A national nonprofit organization created to provide support services for the families of children afflicted with a wide variety of chronic and/or critical disorders that affect a child's growth.
James Andrews, Director/Co-Founder
Mary Andrews, CEO

9354 Turner's Syndrome Society of Canada
323 Chapel Street   613-321-2267
Ottawa, K1N   800-465-6744
Fax: 613-321-2268
e-mail: tssincan@web.net
www.turnersyndrome.ca
International society providing support services, educational information and activities to persons with Turner's Syndrome, their families and the professionals who work with them.

9355 Turner's Syndrome Society of the United States
11250 W Road   832-249-9988
Houston, TX 77065   800-365-9944
Fax: 832-912-6446
e-mail: tssus@turnersyndrome.org
www.turnersyndrome.org
Through this society members have available a host of informational and support services including consultation services a resource center offering access to the most recently published articles on Turner's Syndrome conferences and advocacy.
Cindy Scurlock, Executive Director
Deborah Rios, Member Services Director

State Agencies & Associations

California

9356 Bay Area Turner Syndrome Society
Moraga, CA 94556   925-846-0608
e-mail: jenakiko@aol.com
www.turnersyndrome.org
Jennifer Saito, Contact

9357 Turner's Syndrome Society
11250 W Road   832-912-6006
Houston, TX 77065   800-365-9944
Fax: 832-912-6446
e-mail: tssus@turnersyndrome.org
www.turnersyndrome.org
Cindy Scurlock, Executive Director
Deborah Rios, Member Services Director

Colorado

9358 Turner's Syndrome Society of Rocky Mountain
Longmount, CO 80501   303-774-0720
e-mail: bpblick@earthlink.net
www.turnersyndrome.org
Brian Blick, President

Florida

9359 Florida Southwest Turner Syndrome Society
Orlando, FL 33919   407-859-3131
e-mail: cjubelt@affirmativemanagement.com
www.turnersyndrome.org
Lauren Jubelt, Leader

9360 Turner's Syndrome Society of South Florida
5215 N Dixie Highway   945-815-9100
Oakland Park, FL 33334   e-mail: tigger3927@aol.com
www.turnersyndrome.org
Rachel Nowak, Leader

Georgia

9361 Georgia Atlanta Turner Syndrome Society
10635 Jones Bridge Road   770-918-3120
Alpharetta, GA 30022   e-mail: jbrownlee@rockdale.org
www.turnersyndrome.org
Judy Brownlee, Contact

Illinois

9362 Metro Chicago Turner Syndrome Society
5467 S Ingleside #3E   773-667-1364
Chicago, IL 60615   e-mail: sgfhoff@sbcglobal.net
www.turnersyndrome.org
Susan Hoffman, President

9363 St. Louis Turner Syndrome Society
14450 TC Jester   832-689-3901
Houston, TX 77014   800-365-9944
Fax: 832-249-9987
e-mail: heatherandben@earthlink.net
www.turnersyndrome.org
Turner Syndrome is a chromosomal condition that describes girls and women with common features that are caused by complete or partial absence of the second sex chromosome.
Heather Derousse, Contact

Indiana

9364 Indiana Chapter Turner Syndrome Society
2030 S Odell Street   317-858-9398
Brownsburg, IN 46112   e-mail: candjgarland@yahoo.com
                                            www.turnersyndrome.org
Connie Garland, Contact

Iowa

9365 Turner's Syndrome Society of Iowa
2615 Meadow Glen Road   515-292-2757
Ames, IA 50014-8238   e-mail: mkepolashek@msn.com
                                            www.turnersyndrome.org
Mary Kay Polashek, Leader

Louisiana

9366 Southeast Louisiana Turner Syndrome Society
14450 TC Jester   832-249-9988
Houston, TX 77014   Fax: 832-249-9987
                          e-mail: cajungirl302003@yahoo.com
                                            www.turnersyndrome.org
The Turner Syndrome Society of the United States creates awareness promotes research and provides support for all persons
touched by Turner Syndrome.
Delaine Reed, Contact

Massachusetts

9367 Southern New England Turner Syndrome Society
1034 Maple Street   401-732-2136
Mansfield, MA 02048   e-mail: deb_pomerantz@hotmail.com
                                            www.turnersyndrome.org
Deborah Pomerantz, Leader

Michigan

9368 Michigan Chapter: Southeast
146 Meadow Lane Circle   248-608-6127
Rochester Hills, MI 48307   e-mail: ksemrau@aol.com
                                            www.turnersyndrome.org
Kim Semrau, President

9369 Michigan West Turner Syndrome Society
PO Box 307   517-852-9593
Nashville, MI 49073   e-mail: r-m-ohler4@triton.net
                                            www.turnersyndrome.org
Mary Ohler, Contact

Minnesota

9370 MN Chapter of the Turner Syndrome Society
1531 American Blvd E   952-854-1224
Bloomington, MN 55425   e-mail: jleon101@hotmail.com
                                            www.tssminnesota.org
Julie Leon, Contact

Missouri

9371 Kansas/Missouri- Turner Syndrome Society
Chapter Headquarters
6721 E 127th Street   816-763-9550
Grandview, MO 64030   Fax: 816-763-8884
                                    e-mail: tsskc@hotmail.com
                                            www.tsskc.com
Dennis McKenzie, Co-President
Carolyn McKenzie, Vice-President

9372 Missouri/St. Louis Turner Syndrome Society
8831 Madge   314-963-0565
Brentwood, MO 63144   e-mail: loch5@juno.com
                                            www.turnersyndrome.org
Mary Jo Lochmoeller, Co-President

9373 Turner's Syndrome Society of St. Louis/West Illinois
8831 Madge   314-963-0565
Brentwood, MO 63144   e-mail: loch5@juno.com
                                            www.turner-syndrome-us.org
Mary Jo Lochmoeller, President

New Hampshire

9374 Northern New England Turner Society
38 Beaman Street   603-524-6011
Laconia, NH 03246   e-mail: tssnnepa@hotmail.com
                                            www.turnersyndrome.org
Lori Ann Pawlowski, Leader

New Jersey

9375 New Jersey Metroplitan Turner Syndrome Society Association
107 Crabapple Lane   732-217-3021
Franklin Park, NJ 08823   e-mail: tssusnj@turnersyndromenj.com
                                            www.turnersyndrome.org
Laura Fasciano, Contact

New York

9376 Turner Syndrome Support Group of Central N Y
476 Ford Hill Road   607-223-4142
Berkshire, NY 13736   e-mail: tlkwwjd@frontiernet.net
                                            www.turnersyndrome.org
Tammy Kozak, President

9377 Turner's Syndrome Society New York - Metro
215 E 95th Street #24M   607-223-4142
New York, NY 10128   e-mail: tlkwwjd@frontiernet.net
                                            www.turnersyndrome.org
Tammy Kozak, Contact

North Carolina

9378 North Carolina Turner Syndrome Society
1223 Pine Springs Drive   828-699-1088
Hendersonville, NC 28739   e-mail: inmydna@charter.net
                                            www.turnersyndrome.org
Cheryl Tuttle, Contact

Ohio

9379 Turner Syndrome Chapter of Ohio
3333 Burnet Avenue ML 5006   513-697-0941
Cincinnati, OH 45229   e-mail: lwestcott@fuse.net
                                            www.turnersyndrome.org
Leslie Westcott, Contact

9380 Turner Syndrome Chapter of Oklahoma
5904 E Lattimer
Tulsa, OK 74115-6728   918-838-7355
                                            www.turnersyndrome.org
Jean Radtke, Contact

Pennsylvania

9381 Philadelphia Turner Syndrom Society
169 Trappe Lane   215-752-4405
Langhorne, PA 19047   e-mail: wolfepac5@comcast.net
                                            www.turnersyndrome.org
This society covers the 5 surrounding counties of Philadelphia,
along with Eastern Pennsylvania, Delaware and Southern New Jersey.
Eileen Wolfe, President

9382 SW Pennsylvania Turner Syndrome Support Gr oup
3110 Westchester   412-767-4321
Pittsburgh, PA 15238   e-mail: fay_larkin@pghcorning.com
                                            www.turnersyndrome.org
Fay Larkin, Contact

Rhode Island

9383 Rhode Island Turner Syndrome Society
24 Turner Street   401-732-2136
Warwick, RI 02886   e-mail: deb_pomerantz@hotmail.com
                                            www.turnersyndrome.org
Debbie Pomerantz, Contact

South Carolina

9384 South Carolina Palmetto Turner Syndrome So ciety
153 Gannet Point Road   843-521-4461
Beaufort, SC 29902   e-mail: auntrobin74@yahoo.com
                                      www.turnersyndrome.org

Robin Butler, Contact

9385 Turner's Syndrome Society: Palmetto Area
Drachman Hall 1295 N Martin   843-521-4461
Tucson, AZ 85721   888-285-3410
                          e-mail: auntrobin74@yahoo.com
                                      www.turnersyndrome.org
Teratology Information Services are comprehensive and
multidisciplinary resources for medical consultation on prenatal
exposures. TIS interpret information regarding known and poten-
tial reproductive risks into risk assessments.
Robin Butler, Leader

Texas

9386 Houston/South Texas Turner Syndrome Society
Houston, TX   832-689-3901
          e-mail: heatherandben@earthlink.net
                                      www.turnersyndrome.org

Heather Derousse, Contact

9387 Turner's Syndrome Society of North Texas
5633 Cork Lane   817-485-1684
N Richland Hills, TX 76180   e-mail: bright165@cs.com
                                      www.turnersyndrome.org

Hollye Bright, Leader

Utah

9388 Utah Turner Syndrome Society
American Fork, UT 84003
                                          801-754-1792
                       e-mail: abclaker@aol.com
                                      www.turnersyndrome.org

Angela Dawn Laker, Contact

Washington

9389 Washington Puget Sound Turner Syndrome Society
12321 22nd Street NE   206-417-6776
Seattle, WA 98125   e-mail: pugetsoundtss@gmail.com
                                      www.turnersyndrome.org

Larin Amos, President

Libraries & Resource Centers

9390 Turner Syndrome Society Resource Center
Turner Syndrome Society of the United States
14450 TC Jester   832-249-9988
Houston, TX 77014   800-365-9944
                                  Fax: 832-249-9987
               e-mail: tssus@tuRNersyndromeus.org
                                      www.turnersyndrome.org
The Turner Syndrome Society of the US creates awareness, pro-
motes research, and provides support for all persons touched by
Turner Syndrome.
Barbara Flink, President
Dr Catherine Ward, President Elect

Support Groups & Hotlines

9391 National Health Information Center
PO Box 1133
Washington, DC 20013   310-565-4167
                                          800-336-4797
                                     Fax: 301-984-4256
                             e-mail: info@nhic.org
                                     www.health.gov/nhic
Offers a nationwide information referral service, produces directo-
ries and resource guides.

Newsletters

9392 Turner's Syndrome News
Turner's Syndrome Society of the United States
1313 5th Street SE
Minneapolis, MN 55414-4509   800-365-9944
                                     Fax: 612-379-3619
                                     www.turner-syndrome.org
Includes articles addressing current issues in Turner's Syndrome,
updates on national and local activities and letters from girls and
women with Turner's syndrome and their families.
Quarterly

Pamphlets

9393 Answers to Some Commonly Asked Questions
Turner's Syndrome Society of the United States
1313 5th Street SE
Minneapolis, MN 55414-4509   800-365-9944
                                     Fax: 612-379-3619
                                     www.turner-syndrome-us.org
Offers information on the Society's activities and the role they play
in supporting people with Turner's syndrome.

9394 Facing the Challenges of Turner's Syndrome Together
Turner's Syndrome Society of the United States
1313 5th Street SE
Minneapolis, MN 55414-4509   800-365-9944
                                     Fax: 612-379-3619
                                     www.turner-syndrome-us.org
A brochure offering information on Turner's syndrome, statistics
on how widespread the disease is and the Society's role in conquering this disease and supporting their members.

9395 Facts About Turner's Syndrome
Turner's Syndrome Society of the United States
1313 5th Street SE
Minneapolis, MN 55414-4509   800-365-9944
                                     Fax: 612-379-3619
                                     www.turner-syndrome-us.org
Offers statistical and factual information on the disease of Turner's
syndrome, causes, symptoms, prevention and treatment.

9396 How to Start a Turner's Syndrome Support Group
Turner's Syndrome Society of the United States
1313 5th Street SE
Minneapolis, MN 55414-4509   800-365-9944
                                     Fax: 612-379-3619
                                     www.turner-syndrome-us.org
Offers information to the lay person on how to obtain material from
medical professionals, publicity aspects and funding aspects in
pertaining to starting a support group.

9397 Turner's Syndrome Society Resource Bibliographies
Turner's Syndrome Society of the United States
1313 5th Street SE
Minneapolis, MN 55414-4509   800-365-9944
                                     Fax: 612-379-3619
                                     www.turner-syndrome-us.org
These fact sheets offer information on books, videos and other re-
sources available on Turner's syndrome.

9398 Turner's Syndrome: A Guide for Families
Turner's Syndrome Society of the United States
1313 5th Street SE
Minneapolis, MN 55414-4509   800-365-9944
                                     Fax: 612-379-3619
                                     www.turner-syndrome-us.org
Offers information to parents on the causes, symptoms, diagnosis
and prognosis of Turner' syndrome, includes resources of where to
go for help and support.

9399 Turner's Syndrome: A Personal Perspective
Turner's Syndrome Society of the United States
1313 5th Street SE
Minneapolis, MN 55414-4509   800-365-9944
                                     Fax: 612-379-3619
                                     www.turner-syndrome-us.org

A reprint from the Adolescent and Pediatric Gynecology Journal offering a personal account of a woman with Turner's syndrome and her experiences.

9400 Turner's Syndrome: Hows and Whys of the Missing X Chromosome
Human Growth Foundation
977 Glen Cove Avenue   516-671-4041
Glen Head, NY 11545-1554   800-451-6434
                                               Fax: 516-671-4055
                                        e-mail: hgf1@hgfound.org
                                              www.hgfound.org
Provides a brief overview for parents about Turner's Syndrome.
Patricia D Costa, Executive Director

Web Sites

9401 Healing Well
                                          www.healingwell.com
An online health resource guide to medical news, chat, information and articles, newsgroups and message boards, books, disease-related web sites, medical directories, and more for patients, friends, and family coping with disabling diseases, disorders, or chronic illnesses.

9402 Health Finder
                                           www.healthfinder.gov
Searchable, carefully developed web site offering information on over 1000 topics. Developed by the US Department of Health and Human Services, the site can be used in both English and Spanish.

9403 Healthlink USA
                                          www.healthlinkusa.com
Health information concerning treatment, cures, prevention, diagnosis, risk factors, research, support groups, email lists, personal stories and much more. Updated regularly.

9404 Helios Health
                                            www.helioshealth.com
Online resource for your health information. Detailed information about specific health topics, access to expert advice from our Medical Advisory Board, and up-to-date health news.

9405 Human Growth Foundation
                                                www.genetic.org
National organization committed to expanding and accelerating research into growth and growth disorders, provides education and support to those affected by growth disorders and their families, and fosters the exchange of information with the medical community.

9406 MAGIC Foundation for Children's Growth: Turner's Syndrome Division
                                           www.magicfoundation.org
National organization created to provide support services for the families of children afflicted with a wide variety of chronic and/or critical disorders that affect a child's growth.

9407 MedicineNet
                                             www.medicinenet.com
An online resource for consumers providing easy-to-read, authoritative medical and health information.

9408 Medscape
                                               www.medscape.com
Medscape offers specialists, primary care physicians, and other health professionals the Web's most robust and integrated medical information and educational tools.

9409 Turner's Syndrome Society of the United States
                                          www.turner-syndrome-us.org
Through this society, members have available a host of informational and support services including consultation services, a resource center offering access to the most recently published articles on Turner's syndrome, conferences, advocacy, information and referral services and public relations activities.

9410 WebMD
                                                  www.webmd.com

Information on Turner's syndrome, including articles and resources.

Description

9411 Ulcerative Colitis

Ulcerative colitis is an inflammatory condition of the large bowel, or colon. The cause is unknown, but there is a strong genetic association. First degree relatives have a 3 to 9 percent lifetime risk of the disease, and the illness is much more common in certain racial groups.

Inflammation of the wall of the bowel leads to ulcerations of its surface. Symptoms include weight loss, fatigue, abdominal pain, and diarrhea, which may be bloody. Ulcerative colitis in patients who have a specific antibody in their system (HLA-B27) has a strong association with an arthritis called ankylosing spondylitis. Several kinds of liver and biliary tract disease, inflammation of the eye, and certain characteristic skin rashes may occur.

Treatment depends on the severity of symptoms. Mild cases may respond to simple anti-diarrheal medicines. More severe cases are treated with either rectal or oral forms of 5-ASA, marketed under several trade names. Corticosteroids are sometimes necessary. Disease confined to the rectum can generally be managed with steroid enemas. Extensive disease requires oral steroid medication. Immunosuppressive drugs like azathioprine and 6-mercaptopurine are sometimes given if the disease is resistant to steroids or if steroid side effects are unacceptable. Twenty percent of patients will eventually have their entire colon removed, which cures the disease.

After many years of active ulcerative there is an increased risk of colon cancer. It is usually preceded by warning signs visible on colonoscopy, so physicians generally begin an aggressive surveillance program after 8 to 10 years of disease.

National Agencies & Associations

9412 American Gastroenterological Association
4930 Del Ray Avenue
Bethesda, MD 20814

301-654-2055
Fax: 301-654-5920
e-mail: member@gastro.org
www.gastro.org

Dedicated to the mission of advancing the science and practice of gastroenterology. As the oldest specialty medical society in the United States the membership includes physicians and scientists who research diagnose and treat disorders.
Robert B Greenberg JD, Executive Vice President
Michael H Stolar PhD, Senior VP

9413 Crohn's & Colitis Foundation of America
386 Park Avenue S
New York, NY 10016-8804

212-685-3440
800-932-2423
Fax: 212-779-4098
e-mail: info@ccfa.org
www.ccfa.org

Supports basic and clinical research into a cure and prevent Crohn's disease and ulcerative colitis; conducts professional and patient education activities; produces public service programs and a wide variety of literature about inflammatory bowel disease.
Richard S Blumberg MD, Chairperson

9414 National Institute of Diabetes and Digestive Disorders
5 Information Way

31 Center Drive MSC 2560
Bethesda, MD 20892-3568

301-496-3583
800-860-8747
www2.niddk.nih.gov

Offers information and referrals to persons afflicted with ulcerative colitis.
Dora Abankwah, Staff
Adil Abdalla, Staff

9415 Reach Out for Youth with Ileitis and Colitis
84 Northgate Circle
Melville, NY 11747

631-293-3102
e-mail: info@reachourforyouth.org
www.reachoutforyouth.org

Provides educational seminars and individual and group support to patients and their families. Fundraising efforts support the Center's programs clinical and laboratory research and purchase of state-of-the-art equipment.
Irwin Maltz, President

9416 United Ostomy Association
PO Box 512
Northfield, MN 55057

800-826-0826
Fax: 507-645-5168
e-mail: info@uoaa.org
www.uoa.org

A national network for bowel and urinary diversion support groups in the United States. Its goal is to provide a nonprofit association that will serve to unify and strengthen its member support groups, which are organized for the benefit of people who have, or will have intestinal or urinary diversions and their caregivers.
David Rudzin, President

Support Groups & Hotlines

9417 National Health Information Center
PO Box 1133
Washington, DC 20013

310-565-4167
800-336-4797
Fax: 301-984-4256
e-mail: info@nhic.org
www.health.gov/nhic

Offers a nationwide information referral service, produces directories and resource guides.

Books

9418 Alive and Kicking
Rolf Benirschke Enterprises
PO Box 9922
Rancho Santa Fe, CA 92067-4922

800-571-4770

Football star writes of his struggle with ulcerative colitis.

9419 Ask Audrey
7466 Pebble Lane
West Bloomfield, MI 48322-3521

248-626-6960

A compilation of material and the personal story of a medical psychotherapist who has inflammatory bowel disease. Includes practical tips on issues such as handling diarrhea, sexuality, relationships, traveling, coping with hospital stays, ostomies, and TPN.

9420 IBD Nutrition Book
John Wiley & Sons
1 Wiley Drive
Somerset, NJ 08873-1222

800-225-5945

Clinical dietitian/nutritionist's overview of the role of diet in IBD, including recipes and meal plans.

9421 Inflammatory Bowel Disease
Williams & Wilkins
351 W Camden Street
Baltimore, MD 21201-7912

301-528-4000
800-638-0672

Detailed information on every aspect of IBD. Topics include medical and surgical management, epidemiology, fertility and pregnancy, psychosocial factors, and diagnostic techniques. Written for medical professionals and laypersons who are comfortable with medical terminology.

9422 **Treating IBD: A Patient's Guide to the Medical and Surgical Management**
Crohn's and Colitis Foundation of America
386 Park Avenue S
New York, NY 10016-8804
212-685-3440
800-932-2423
Fax: 212-779-4098
e-mail: info@ccfa.org
www.ccfa.org

Children's Books

9423 **You're Bigger Than it**
Hotel Dieu Hospital
613-544-3310
Ontario, Canada,
This cartoon book offers a lively, brief introduction to the basics of living with IBD. Contact can be reached at extension 2400.

Magazines

9424 **Phoenix Magazine**
United Ostomy Association of America
PO Box 512
Northfield, MN 55057
800-826-0826
Fax: 507-645-5168
e-mail: info@uoa.org
www.uoa.org
America's leading ostomy patient magazine providing colostomy, ileostomy, urostomy and continent diversion information, management techniques, new products and much more.
Quarterly
David Rudzin, President

Newsletters

9425 **Inner Circle**
Reach Out for Youth with Ileitis and Colitis
84 Northgate Circle
631-293-3102
Melville, NY 11747 e-mail: reachoutforyouth@reachoutforyouth.org
www.reachoutforyouth.org
Newsletter for youth with ileitis and colitis.
Irwin Maltz, President

Pamphlets

9426 **Bleeding in the Digestive Tract**
Nat'l Digestive Diseases Information Clearinghouse
9000 Rockville Pike
301-496-3583
Bethesda, MD 20892-0001
Informational fact sheet.

9427 **Inside Story**
Reach Out for Youth with Ileitis and Colitis
84 Northgate Circle
631-293-2102
Melville, NY 11747 e-mail: reachoutforyouth@reachoutforyouth.org
www.reachoutforyouth.org
Educational brochure for youth with illeitis and colitis.
Irwin Maltz, President

9428 **Ulcerative Colitis**
National Organization For Rare Disorders
PO Box 8923
203-746-6518
New Fairfield, CT 06812-8923
e-mail: orphan@rarediseases.org
www.rarediseases.org
Informational fact sheet.

Web Sites

9429 **Crohn's & Colitis Foundation of America**
www.ccfa.org
Supports basic and clinical research into a cure and prevent Crohn's disease and ulcerative colitis; conducts professional and patient education activities; produces public service programs and a wide variety of literature about inflammatory bowel disease for patients and their families, professionals and the public; and sponsors chapters nationwide.

9430 **Healing Well**
www.healingwell.com
An online health resource guide to medical news, chat, information and articles, newsgroups and message boards, books, disease-related web sites, medical directories, and more for patients, friends, and family coping with disabling diseases, disorders, or chronic illnesses.

9431 **Health Finder**
www.healthfinder.gov
Searchable, carefully developed web site offering information on over 1000 topics. Developed by the US Department of Health and Human Services, the site can be used in both English and Spanish.

9432 **Healthlink USA**
www.healthlinkusa.com
Health information concerning treatment, cures, prevention, diagnosis, risk factors, research, support groups, email lists, personal stories and much more. Updated regularly.

9433 **Helios Health**
www.helioshealth.com
Online resource for your health information. Detailed information about specific health topics, access to expert advice from our Medical Advisory Board, and up-to-date health news.

9434 **MedicineNet**
www.medicinenet.com
An online resource for consumers providing easy-to-read, authoritative medical and health information.

9435 **Medscape**
www.medscape.com
Medscape offers specialists, primary care physicians, and other health professionals the Web's most robust and integrated medical information and educational tools.

9436 **United Ostomy Association**
www.uoa.org
A national network for bowel and urinary diversion support groups in the United States. Its goal is to provide a nonprofit association that will serve to unify and strengthen its member support groups, which are organized for the benefit of people who have, or will have intestinal or urinary diversions and their caregivers.

9437 **WebMD**
www.webmd.com
Information on Ulcerative Colitis, including articles and resources.

Description

9438 **Visual Impairment**

Visual impairment encompasses a wide variety of disorders of the eye. It includes damage to the cornea or retina (macular degeneration or secondary to diabetes), cataracts, glaucoma, muscular imbalance, infections, congenital disorders and those associated with premature birth. Occasionally visual impairment reflects a disease behind the eye, involving some part of the brain that receives and processes images from the eyes.

Visual impairment covers a continuum from decreased visual acuity correctible by refractive means (glasses and contact lenses) to legal blindness, indicating less than 20/200 vision in the better eye, or an extremely limited field of vision. Totally blind represents the complete loss of sight.

Many health problems and eye injuries lead to visual impairment. Half a million Americans are visually impaired, and an additional 50,000 lose their sight each year. Cataracts account for one third of all visual impairments and cause 16 persons to lose their sight every day. Glaucoma causes vision impairment in 2 million persons. One thousand eye injuries resulting in some level of vision impairment occur in the workplace or home each day. Diabetic retinopathy is one of the leading causes of the new cases of blindness. Retinitis pigmentosa, a degeneration of the light-sensing tissue at the back of the eye, also causes vision (especially night vision) deterioration.

Depending on the cause of vision loss, the condition may be fully or partially correctible through surgery or visual aids. Sometimes treatment will not reverse prior losses, but will slow the progression of vision loss. When the visual loss cannot be reversed, a variety of supportive devices and services, improved over the past twenty years, can greatly enhance the person's functional status and quality of life.

Technology has played an increasing role in helping the visually impaired function in their daily lives. Recently, doctors implanted the first artificial retina, and relatively new laser technology allows eye specialists to surgically treat extreme degrees of nearsightedness and astigmatism (blurred vision caused by uneven curvature of the eye).

National Agencies & Associations

9439 **ACB Radio Amateurs**
2200 Wilson Boulevard   202-467-5081
Arlington, VA 22201   800-424-8666
                                       Fax: 703- 46- 508
                                       e-mail: info@acb.org
                                       www.acb.org
A radio amateur network of blind, visually impaired and sighted members who gather and share common problems and solutions to help members improve radio amateurs in getting started, provides

access to educational materials in special media and publishes a newsletter.
Mitch Pomerantz, President
Kim Charlson, First Vice President

9440 **Alliance for Aging Research**
2021 K Street NW   202-293-2856
Washington, DC 20006   Fax: 202-785-8574
                                       e-mail: info@agingresearch.org
                                       www.agingresearch.org
Alliance for Aging Research is the nation's leading citizen advocacy organization for improving the health and independence of Americans as they age. It was founded to promote medical and behavioral research into the aging process.
Daniel P Perry, Executive Director
Sarah Rhyne, Executive Coordinator

9441 **American Academy of Ophthalmology**
PO Box 7424   415-561-8500
San Francisco, CA 94120-7424   Fax: 415-561-8533
                                       e-mail: customer_service@aao.org
                                       www.aao.org
Sponsors National Eye Care Project that gives free eye care to the elderly.

9442 **American Association of the Deaf-Blind**
8630 Fenton Street   301-495-4403
Silver Spring, MD 20910-4500   Fax: 301-495-4404
                                       TTY: 301-495-4402
                                       e-mail: AADB-Info@aadb.org
                                       www.aadb.org
Promotes better opportunities and services for deaf-blind people. The mission of this organization is to assure that a comprehensive coordinated system of services is accessible to all deaf-blind people, enabling them to achieve their maximum potential.
35-50 pages 600 Members
Jamie McNama Pope, Executive Director
Elizabeth Spiers, Director of Information Services

9443 **American Coucnil of the Blind Impairment**
1155 15th Street NW Suite 1004   202-467-5081
Washington, DC 20005   800-424-8666
                                       Fax: 202-467-5085
                                       e-mail: cindybur@comcast.net
                                       www.acb.org
A network of blind or visually impaired people that offers support and outreach, shares experiences and exchanges information.
Cindy Burgett, President

9444 **American Council of Blind Lions**
148 Vernon Avenue   502-897-1472
Louisville, KY 40206   Fax: 502-721-9929
                                       e-mail: adam148@bellsouth.net
                                       www.acb.org/acbl
The American Council of Blind Lions (ACBL) is a specially chartered Lions club. The goal of this club is to assist other Lions clubs in understanding the issues surrounding people who are blind or visually impaired.
Adam Ruschival, President

9445 **American Council of the Blind**
2200 Wilson Boulevard   202-467-5081
Arlington, VA 22201-2706   800-424-8666
                                       Fax: 703-465-5085
                                       e-mail: info@acb.org
                                       www.acb.org
A national membership organization whose members are visually impaired and fully sighted individuals who are concerned about dignity and well-being of blind people throughout America. Formed in 1961, the Council has become the largest organization of blind individuals.
Mitch Pomerantz, President

9446 **American Foundation for the Blind**
11 Penn Plaza   212-502-7600
New York, NY 10001   800-232-5463
                                       Fax: 212-502-7777
                                       e-mail: afbinfo@afb.net
                                       www.afb.org

AFB is the cause and organization to which Helen Keller dedicated more than 40 years of her life. In addition to being a national information consultative and advocacy resource engaged in a wide variety of initiatives AFB is home to the Helen Keller Arch.
Carl R Augusto, President/CEO
Richard J O'Brien, Chair

9447 American Foundation for the Blind: National Employment Center
11 Penn Plaza   212-502-7600
New York, NY 10001   Fax: 212-502-7777
                                    e-mail: afbinfo@afb.net
                                              www.afb.org
Leads initiatives in the area of employment. Nationally offers consultation, technical assistance and support and undertakes local and national efforts such as training programs and public education in the area of employment. Responds to inquiries from blind and visually impaired people and thier families, service providers and the general public in the region and nationally.
Richard J O'Brien, Chair
John T Bourger, Vice Chair

9448 American Foundation for the Blind: SE National Literacy Center
100 Peachtree Street   404-525-2303
Atlanta, GA 30303   Fax: 404-659-6957
                                    e-mail: iteracy@afb.net
                                              www.afb.org
Leads initiatives in the area of literacy. Offers consultation technical assistance and support and undertakes local and national efforts such as training programs and public education in the area of literacy. Offers training and in-service opportunities.

9449 American Optometric Association
243 N Lindbergh Boulevard   314-991-4100
Saint Louis, MO 63141-7881   800-365-2219
                                         Fax: 314-991-4101
                                  e-mail: PHKehoe@aoa.org
                                            www.aoanet.org
The AOA and affiliates work to provide the public with quality vision and eye care. It sets professional standards helping its members conduct patient care efficiently and effectively. It also lobbies government and other organizations on behalf of the visually impaired population.
Peter H Kehoe, President
Joe E Ellis, Vice President

9450 American Printing House for the Blind
1839 Frankfort Avenue   502-895-2405
Louisville, KY 40206-0085   800-223-1839
                                         Fax: 502-899-2274
                                       e-mail: info@aph.org
                                               www.aph.org
The oldest nonprofit organization of its kind in the US that creates education, workplace and lifestyle products for visually impaired people. This organization promotes the independence of blind persons by providing special media, tools and materials.
Tuck Tinsley III, President
Bob Brasher, Vice President Advisory Services

9451 Assoc. for Education & Rehabilitation of the Blind & Visually Impaired
1703 N Beauregard Street   703-671-4500
Alexandria, VA 22311   877-492-2708
                                         Fax: 703-671-6391
                                e-mail: jkellyinom@msn.com
                                             www.aerbvi.org
The only professional membership organization dedicated to the advancement of education and rehabilitation of blind and visually impaired children and adults.
Jim Gandorf, Executive Director
Bette Anne Preston, Director of Affiliate Affairs

9452 Associated Services for the Blind
919 Walnut Street   215-627-0600
Philadelphia, PA 19107-5237   Fax: 215-922-0692
                                     e-mail: asbinfo@asb.org
                                               www.asb.org

Limited funding is available to assist aspiring visually impaired users in the purchase of helpful high tech equipment.
Patricia C Johnson, President/CEO
Victor Difelice, Director Strategic Analysis & Planning

9453 Association for Macular Diseases
210 E 64th Street   212-605-3719
New York, NY 10065-7480   Fax: 212-605-3795
                        e-mail: association@retinal-research.org
                                              www.macula.org
A nonprofit corporation to promote education and research in this scarcely-explored field. A nationwide support group for individuals and their families to adjust to the restrictions and changes brought about by macular disease.
Lawrence A Yannuzzi, President
Yale L Fisher, VP

9454 Blinded Veterans Association
477 H Street NW   202-371-8880
Washington, DC 20001-2694   800-669-7079
                                         Fax: 202-371-8258
                                       e-mail: bva@bva.org
                                               www.bva.org
The organization seeks and identifies legally blind veterans who need services linking them to appropriate benefits training and opportunities in both the public and the private sectors. It represents blinded veterans before congress.
Paperback
Thomas H Miller, Executive Director
Brigitte Jones, Administrative Director

9455 Braille Institute of America Library
741 North Vermont Avenue   323-663-1111
Los Angeles, CA 90029-3594   800-272-4553
                            e-mail: info@brailleinstitute.org
                                       www.brailleinstitute.org
Discs, cassettes, braille, Optacon, home visits, braille writer, reference materials on blindness and other handicaps. Closed-circuit TV, Optacon, braille writer, and large print copier also available. Home visits and cassette books are part of special services offered.
Adama Dyoniziak, Regional Program Director

9456 Canine Companions for Independence
2965 Dutton Ave   707-577-1000
Santa Rosa, CA 95407   800-572-2275
                                      TTY: 707-577-1756
                                       e-mail: info@cci.org
                                               www.cci.org
A non-profit organization that enhances the lives of people with disabilities by providing highly trained assistance dogs and ongoing support to ensure quality partnerships.
Corey Hudson, CEO
Kathy Pierson, Northwest Regional Executive Director

9457 Canine Helpers for the Disabled
5699 Ridge Road   716-433-4035
Lockport, NY 14094   e-mail: chhdogs@aol.com
                                        ww.caninehelpers.org
A non-profit organization devoted to training dogs to assist people with disabilities to lead more independent, secure lives.

9458 Catholic Guild for the Blind Catholic Charities of the Archdiocese of
Catholic Charities of the Archdiocese of New York
180 N Michigan Avenue   312-236-8569
Chicago, IL 60601-7463   Fax: 312-236-8128
                            e-mail: info@guildfortheblind.org
                                      www.guildfortheblind.org
A nonprofit organization under the sponsorship of the Catholic Charities of the Archdiocese of New York. Daily living skills, orientation and mobility training, communication skills and bilingual preparation for high school equivalency diplomas are among things covered.
Kathy Austin, Coordinator of Adult Rehabilitation
Lauri Dishman, Manager of Career Services

9459 Council for Exceptional Children
1110 N Glebe Road
Arlington, VA 22201

703-620-3660
888-232-7733
Fax: 703-264-9494
TTY: 866-915-5000
e-mail: service@cec.sped.org
www.cec.sped.org

Advocates appropriate policies standards and development for individuals with special needs. Provides professional development for special educators.
Bruce Ramirez, Executive Director
Joan Melner, Assistant Executive Director

9460 Council of Citizens with Low Vision International
1155 15th Street NW
Washington, DC 20005

714-630-8098
800-733-2258
www.cclvi.org

Affiliated with American Council of the Blind. Promotes the concept that persons with partial sight/low vision are not blind and should have every right to maximize the use of their residual vision.
John Horst, President
Richard Rueda, 1st Vice President

9461 Fidelco Guide Dog Foundation
103 Old Iron Ore Road
Bloomfield, CT 06002-0142

860-243-5200
Fax: 860-243-7215
e-mail: info@fidelco.org
www.fidelco.org

Fidelco breeds raises trains and places German shepherd guide dogs with men and women who are visually impaired primarily in the Northeast. The pioneer of in-community training in this country the visually impaired individual can remain independent.
Roberta C Kaman, Chairman
George J Salpietro, Executive Director

9462 Fight for Sight
381 Park Avenue S
New York, NY 10016

212-679-6060
Fax: 212-679-4466
e-mail: info@fightforsight.com
www.fightforsight.com

Voluntary health organization that works to conquer defective sight and blindness. Provides grants to accredited medical colleges and institutions to help supply equipment technical assistance and materials for research projects.
Mary Prudden, Executive Director
Kenneth R Barasch MD, President

9463 Foundation Fighting Blindness
7168 Columbia Gateway Drive
Columbia, MD 21046

410-423-0600
800-683-5555
Fax: 410-872-0438
TDD: 800-683-5551
e-mail: info@FightBlindness.org
www.blindness.org

Mission is to drive the research that will provide preventions, treatments, and cures for people affected by retinitis pigmentosa, macular degeneration, Usher syndrome and the entire spectrum of retinal degenerative diseases.
William T Schmidt, CEO

9464 Foundation for Glaucoma Research
251 Post Street
San Francisco, CA 94108

415-986-3162
800-826-6693
Fax: 415-986-3763
e-mail: question@glaucoma.org
www.glaucoma.org

A national organization dedicated to protecting the sight of people with glaucoma through research and education. The Foundation conducts and supports research that contributes to improved patient care and a better understanding of the disease process.
Andrew Jackson, Director of Communications
Thomas M Brunner, President and CEO

9465 Foundation for the Advancement of the Blind
4058 Moore Street
Los Angeles, CA 90066-5118

310-301-0344

Helps blind people attain and retain employment.

9466 Friends-In-Art
2331 Poincianna Street
Huntsville, AL 35801

202-467-5081
800-424-8666
Fax: 202-467-5085
e-mail: nansong@knology.net
www.friendsinart.com

Aims to enlarge the art experience of blind people encourages blind people to visit museums galleries concerts the theater etc. offers consultation to program planners in establishing accessible art and museum exhibits.
Nancy Pendegraph, President
Gordon Kent, Board Member

9467 Guide Dog Users
14311 Astrodome Drive
Silver Spring, MD 20906-2245

866-799-8436
e-mail: beckyb@cloud9.net
www.gdui.org

Promotes the acceptance of blind people and their dogs works for enforcement and expansion of laws admitting guide dogs into public places advocates for quality training and follow-up services.
Elizabeth Barnes, President
Rebecca Floyd-Collin, First Vice President

9468 Guide Dogs for the Blind
PO Box 151200
San Rafael, CA 94915

415-499-4000
800-298-4050
Fax: 415-499-4035
e-mail: information@guidedogs.com
www.guidedogs.com

Offers educational materials, transportation seminars, and newsletters for the blind providing 2 field offices.
Etta Allen, Board Chair
Morgan Watkins, Interim CEO

9469 Helen Keller National Center's National Parent Network
141 Middle Neck Road
Sands Point, NY 11050-1218

516-944-8900
Fax: 516-944-7302
TTY: 516-944-8637
e-mail: hkncinfo@hknc.org
www.hknc.org

Establishes a coalition of state parent organizations to promote the exchange of information among parents of deaf-blind youth. Provides training to parents to develop their legislative advocacy skills, empowers parents and their families to obtain needed services.
Kathy Mezack, Coordinator of Vocational Services

9470 Independent Visually Impaired Enterprises
230 Robinhood Lane
McMurray, PA 15317

e-mail: lengual@concentric.net
www.acb.org

Strives to broaden vocational opportunities in business for the visually impaired. Works to improve rehabilitation facilities for all types of business enterprises and publicizes the capabilities of blind and visually impaired business persons.
Carla Hayes, President

9471 International Agency for the Prevention of Blindness
National Eye Institute
2020 Vision Place
Bethesda, MD 20892-3655

301-496-5248
www.nei.nih.gov

Ophthalmic societies and committees for the prevention of blindness whose members include ophthalmologists public health officers nutritionists geneticists and other health workers. Coordinates international research into the causes of impaired vision.
Carl Kupfer, Volunteer
Paul A Sieving, Director

9472 Library Users of America
2200 Wilson Boulevard
Arlington, VA 22201

202-467-5081
800-424-8666
Fax: 703-465-5085
e-mail: info@acb.org
www.acb.org

Provides for chapters in states through the US to encourage the development acquisition and use of technology which enables blind

and visually impaired persons to use printed material independently in library settings and elsewhere.
Barry Levine, President

9473 Lighthouse International Headquarters
111 E 59th Street
New York, NY 10022-1202
212-821-9200
800-821-0500
Fax: 212-821-9707
TTY: 212-821-9713
e-mail: info@lighthouse.org
www.lighthouse.org
A leading resource worldwide on vision impairment and vision rehabilitation. Pioneer in vision rehabilitation services, education, research and advocacy enabling people of all ages who are blind or partially sighted to lead independent and productive lives.
Roger O Goldman, Chairman
Tara A Cortes, President/CEO

9474 Lions World Services for the Blind Lions Clubs International
Lions Clubs International
2811 Fair Park Boulevard
Little Rock, AR 72204
501-664-7100
800-248-0734
Fax: 501-664-2743
e-mail: training@lwsb.org
www.lwsb.org
Lions World Services for the Blind was founded in 1947 to serve people who are blind and visually impaired who needed to learn independent living skills or job training skills that considered the special requirements of their individual visual impairments.
Ramona Sangalli, President and Chief Executive Officer
Larry Morgan, Vice President for Development

9475 Macular Degeneration Foundation
PO Box 515
Northampton, MA 01061-0515
413-268-7660
888-622-8527
e-mail: amdf@macular.org
www.macular.org
The American Macular Degeneration Foundation is committed to the prevention and cure of macular degeneration and offers hope and support to those afflicted and their families.
Chip Goehring, President and Trustee
Mark E Torrey, Vice President and Trustee

9476 National Alliance of Blind Students
2200 Wilson Boulevard
Arlington, VA 22201
202-467-5081
800-424-8666
Fax: 703-465-5085
e-mail: info@acb.org
www.acb.org
Works to facilitate progress toward full accessibility of college programs and facilities provides opportunities for discussion of issues important to students and assists with National Student Seminars.
Rebecca Bridges, President

9477 National Association for Parents of the Visually Impaired
PO Box 317
Watertown, MA 02471-0317
617-972-7441
800-562-6265
Fax: 781-972-7444
e-mail: napvi@perkins.org
www.napvi.org
The only national organization that strives to serve families of children of all ages and ranges with visual loss. It is a community based organization whose members include parents parent organizations agencies and other persons with common objectives.
Susan LaVenture, Executive Director
Doug Halverson, President

9478 National Association for Visually Handicapped
22 West 21st Street
New York, NY 10010
212-889-3141
888-205-5951
Fax: 212-727-2931
e-mail: navh@navh.org
www.navh.org
NAVH ensures that those with limited vision do not lead limited lives. We offer emotional support; training in the use of and access to a wide variety of optical aids and lighting; a large print, nationwide, free-by-mail loan library; large print educational materials;

quarterly newsletter; referrals; self-help groups and educational outreach.
Cesar Gomez, Executive Director

9479 National Association for Visually Hand.
22 W 21st Street
New York, NY 10010
212-889-3141
Fax: 212-727-2931
e-mail: navh@navh.org
www.navh.org
NAVH ensures that those with limited vision do not lead limited lives. We offer emotional support; training in the use of and access to a wide variety of optical aids and lighting and a large print, nationwide, free-by-mail loan library.
Lorraine H Marchi, Founder & CEO
Miriam Rosen, Executive Director

9480 National Association of Blind Educators Sheila Koenig
Sheila Koenig
2214 Emerson Avenue S
Minneapolis, MN 55401
612-375-1625
e-mail: jsanders.nfb@comcast.net
www.nfb.org
Membership organization of blind teachers professors and instructors in all levels of education. Provides support and information regarding professional responsibilities classroom techniques national testing methods and career obstacles.
Judy Sanders, President

9481 National Association of Blind Lawyers Scott LaBarre
Scott LaBarre
1660 S Albion Street
Denver, CO 80222-4046
303-504-5979
Fax: 303-757-3640
e-mail: slabarre@labarrelaw.com
www.nfb.org
Membership organization of blind attorneys law students judges and others in the law field. Provides support and information regarding employment techniques used by the blind, advocacy, laws affecting the blind and current information about the American legal system.
Scott LaBarre, President

9482 National Association of Blind Musicians Linda Mentink
Linda Mentink
1865 42nd Avenue
Columbus, NE 68601-0952
402-563-8138
e-mail: mentink@frontiernet.net
www.nfb.org
Blind persons dedicated to advancing employment and entertainment opportunities in various music fields. Offers support and information regarding copyright publishing promotion and other career details.
Linda Mentik, Chairperson

9483 National Association of Blind Office Professionals
Lisa Hall
7001ÿHamilton Avenue
Cincinnati, OH 45231-6104
513-931-7070
e-mail: Lhall007@cinci.rr.com
www.nfb.org
Membership organization of blind secretaries and transcribers at all levels including medical and paralegal transcription office workers customer-service personnel and many other similar fields. Addresses issues such as technology, accommodation and caregivers.
Lisa Hall, President

9484 National Association of Blind Students Angela Wolf
Angela Wolf
3106 Barrett Place
Wichita Falls, TX 76308-1803
512-417-8190
e-mail: nabs.president@gmail.com
www.nfb.org
For over 30 years this national organization of blind students has provided support information and encouragement to blind college and university students. Leads the way in offering resources in issues such as national testing and accessible textbooks.
Terri Rupp, President

9485 National Association of Guide Dog Users Priscilla Ferris
Priscilla Ferris
1003 Papaya Drive
Tampa, FL 33619-3714
813-626-2789
800-558-8261
e-mail: president@nfb-nagdu.org
www.nfb-nagdu.org

Provides information and support for guide dog users and works to secure high standards in guide dog training. Addresses issues of discrimination of guide dog users and offers public education about guide dog use.
Marion Gwizdala, President

9486   National Association to Promote the Use of Braille
Nadine Jacobson
5805 Kellogg Avenue   952-927-7694
Edina, MN 55424-1819   e-mail: nadine.jacobson@visi.com
                                            www.nfb.org
Dedicated to securing improved Braille instruction increasing the number of Braille materials available to the blind and providing information about the importance of Braille in securing independence education and employment for the blind.
Nadine Jacobson, President

9487   National Braille Association
95 Allens Creek Road   585-427-8260
Rochester, NY 14618-2513   Fax: 585-427-0263
                      e-mail: nbaoffice@nationalbraille.org
                                   www.nationalbraille.org
Provides transcription service for and maintains a depository of braille books.
Diane Spence, President
Jan Carroll, Vice President

9488   National Braille Press
88 Saint Stephen Street   617-266-6160
Boston, MA 02115-4302   888-965-8965
                                        Fax: 617-437-0456
                                            www.nbp.org
The guiding purposes of National Braille Press are to promote the literacy of blind children through braille and to provide access to information that empowers blind people to actively engage in work family and community affairs.
Paul Parravano, Chair
Gayle L Yarnall, Clerk

9489   National Center for Vision and Aging Lighthouse
Lighthouse
111 E 59th Street   212-821-9200
New York, NY 10022-1202   800-829-0500
                                        Fax: 212-821-9707
                                        TTY: 212-821-9713
                                        TDD: 212-821-9713
                                   e-mail: info@lighthouse.org
                                        www.lighthouse.org
The National Center for Vision and Aging provides information on eye conditions and visual impairment of all ages resources education and professionally prepared multimedia and print material for community education lectures.
Roger O Goldman, Chairman
Tara A Cortes, President and Chief Executive Officer

9490   National Center for Vision and Child Development
Lighthouse
111 E 59th Street   212-821-9200
New York, NY 10022   800-829-0500
                                        Fax: 212-821-9707
                                        TTY: 212-821-9713
                                   e-mail: info@lighthouse.org
                                        www.lighthouse.org
Our mission is to overcome vision impairment for people of all ages through worldwide leadership in rehabilitation services education research prevention and advocacy.
Roger O Goldman, Chairman
Tara A Cortes PhD RN, President and Chief Executive Officer

9491   National Diabetes Action Network for the Blind
National Federation of the Blind
1800 Johnson Street   410-659-9314
Baltimore, MD 21230-7337   Fax: 410-685-5653
                                   e-mail: nfb@nfb.org
                                            www.nfb.org
Leading support and information organization of persons losing vision due to diabetes. Provides personal contact and resource information with other blind diabetics about non-visual techniques

of independently managing diabetes and monitoring glucose levels.
Marc Maurer, President
Fredric Schroeder, First Vice President

9492   National Eye Institute National Institutes of Health
National Institutes of Health
2020 Vision Place
Bethesda, MD 20892-3655   301-496-5248
                                            www.nei.nih.gov
Mission is to discover safe and effective methods to prevent diagnose and treat diseases and disorders of the visual system. In this way the Institute helps to prevent reduce and possibly eliminate blindness and visual impairment.
Paul A Sieving, Director
Carl Kupfer, Volunteer

9493   National Federation of the Blind
1800 Johnson Street   410-659-9314
Baltimore, MD 21230   Fax: 410-685-5653
                                   e-mail: pmaurer@nfb.org
                                            www.nfb.org
The largest consumer membership organization for the blind founded in 1940 it has 50 000 members nationwide in 52 affiliates and over 700 local chapters. Provides public education about blindness, support services to the newly blinded and scholarships.
50M Members
Marc Maurer, President
Fredric Schroeder, First Vice President

9494   National Federation of the Blind in Computer Science
Curtis Chong
3000 Grand Avenue   515-277-1288
Des Moines, IA 50312-4256   Fax: 515-281-1361
                                   e-mail: curtischong@earthlink.net
                                            www.nfb.org
National organization of blind persons knowledgeable in the computer science and technology fields. Works to develop new technologies, to secure access to current technology and to develop new ways of using current or new technologies by the blind.
Curtis Chong, President

9495   National Federation of the Blind: Blind/Deaf Division
Robert Eschbach
1186 North Verbena Place   520-836-3689
Casa Grande, AZ 85222-5440   e-mail: Resch@earthlink.net
                                            www.nfb-db.org
Deaf-blind persons working nationally to improve services, training and independence for the deaf-blind. Offers personal contact with other deaf-blind individuals knowledgeable in advocacy, education, employment, technology, discrimination and other issues surrounding deaf-blindness.
Robert Eschbach, President

9496   National Federation of the Blind: Blind Industrial Workers of America
National Federation of the Blind
1800 Johnson Street   410-659-9314
Baltimore, MD 21230-4998   Fax: 410-685-5653
                                   e-mail: nfb@nfb.org
                                            www.nfb.org
Membership organization of blind persons employed in industrial and manufacturing work or in government job programs for the blind. Dedicated to protecting the rights of blind workers in salary, job stability, advancement and labor issues.
Ken Staley, President

9497   National Federation of the Blind: Human Services Division
Melissa Riccobono
1026 E 36th Street   410-235-3073
Baltimore, MD 21218   e-mail: maricco@uwalumni.com
                                            www.nfb.org
Membership organization of blind persons working in counseling personnel psychology social work psychiatry rehabilitation and other social science and human resource fields. Dedicated to improving employment opportunities and advancement for blind persons.
Melissa Riccobono, President

9498   National Federation of the Blind: Masonic Square Club
Fred Flowers
46 Powderock Place
Baltimore, MD 21236-4766   410-598-0155
www.nfb.org
Blind individuals committed to sharing of Masonic experiences
goals and history.
Fred Flowers, President

9499   National Federation of the Blind: Public Employees Division
Ivan Weich
4301 Clogston Avenue NE   360-782-9575
Bremerton, WA 98310-3009   e-mail: IEWeich@comcast.net
www.nfb.org
Organization of blind persons holding local state or federal jobs.
Focuses on issues such as changes in governmental hiring and retention practices new job skills needed for the future, government
employment downsizing, new electronic means of finding employment and more.
Ivan Weich, President

**9500   National Federation of the Blind: Science and Engineering
Division**
John Miller
10955 Deering Street   858-527-1727
San Diego, CA 92126-1920   e-mail: j8miller@soe.ucsd.edu
www.nfb.org
Blind persons with expertise and experience in fields such as ge-
netics, telecommunications, biology, chemistry, physics and nu-
clear physics or mechanical electronic and chemical engineering.
This is a strong support group to encourage blind persons to excel
in science and engineering.
John Miller, President

9501   National Federation of the Blind: Writers Division
Tom Stevens
504 S 57th Street   402-556-3216
Omaha, NE 68106-0809   e-mail: newmanrl@cox.net
www.nfb-writers-division.org
Blind writers in all styles including poetry short story fiction
non-fiction magazine writing and theatrical work offer encouragement and support to blind writers and authors. Issues cover various
aspects of this business including selling your work.
Robert L Newman, President

9502   National Industries for the Blind
1310 Braddock Place
Alexandria, VA 22314-1727   703-310-0500
Fax: 703-998-8268
e-mail: communications@nib.org
www.nib.org
A nonprofit organization that represents over 100 associated industries serving people who are blind in thirty-six states. These
agencies serve people who are blind or visually impaired and help
them to reach their full potential.
Kevin Lynch, President/CEO
Steve Brice, Vice President/CFO

**9503   National Library Service for the Blind and Physically
Handicapped**
Library of Congress
1291 Taylor Street NW   202-707-5100
Washington, DC 20011   888-657-7323
TTY: 202-707-0744
TDD: 202-707-0744
e-mail: nls@loc.gov
www.loc.gov/nls
Administers a national library service that provides braille and re-
corded books and magazines on free loan to anyone who cannot
read standard print because of visual or physical disabilities who
are eligible residents of the United States.
12 pages Quarterly
Frank Kurt Cylke, Director
Michael M Moodie, Research and Development Officer

9504   National Organization of Parents of Blind Children
Barbara Cheadle
1152 106th Lane NE   763-784-8590
Minneapolis, MD 55434-4998   Fax: 410-685-5653
e-mail: carrie.gilmer@gmail.com
www.nfb.org/nfb/Parents_and_Teachers.asp

Support information and advocacy organization of parents of blind
or visually impaired children. Addresses issues ranging from help
to parents of a newborn blind infant, mobility and Braille instruction, education, social and community participation.
Carrie Gilmer, President

9505   New Eyes for the Needy
549 Milburn Avenue   973-376-4903
Short Hills, NJ 07078   Fax: 973-376-3807
e-mail: neweyesfortheneedy@yahoo.com
www.neweyesfortheneedy.org
Provides new glasses for those with low vision who may not be able
to afford them.

9506   Prevent Blindess America
211 W Wacker Drive
Chicago, IL 60606-5624   800-331-2020
e-mail: info@preventblindness.org
www.preventblindness.org
Information and referral services provided on specific eye disorders. Publishes literature and supports community screening and
testing programs.
Hugh R Parry, President/CEO

9507   Randolph-Sheppard Vendors of America
1808 Faith Place   504-368-7785
Terrytown, LA 70056-4104   800-467-5299
Fax: 504-368-7739
e-mail: rsva@juno.com
www.acb.org/rsva
Protects the interests of blind vendors seeks proper implementation of the Randolph-Sheppard Act and encourages facility locations in more visible and profitable areas.
Charles Glaser, President
John Gordon, First Vice President

9508   Recording for the Blind and Dyslexic
20 Roszel Road
Princeton, NJ 08540-6294   866-RFB-D585
www.rfbd.org
Provides materials for all people who cannot effectively read standard print because of a visual perceptual or other physical disability.

9509   Research to Prevent Blindness
645 Madison Avenue   212-752-4333
New York, NY 10022-1010   800-621-0026
Fax: 212-688-6231
e-mail: inforequest@rpbusa.org
www.rpbusa.org
National voluntary health foundation supported by foundations
corporations and voluntary gifts and bequests from individuals.
Established to stimulate basic and applied research into the causes
prevention and treatment of blinding eye diseases.
David Weeks, Chairman
Diane S Swift, President

9510   Seeing Eye
PO Box 375   973-539-4425
Morristown, NJ 07963-0375   Fax: 973-539-0922
e-mail: info@seeingeye.org
www.seeingeye.org
A training school for dogs to guide qualified blind persons.
James A Kutsch, President and Chief Executive Officer

9511   Smith-Kettlewell Eye Research Foundation
2318 Fillmore Street   415-345-2000
San Francisco, CA 94115   Fax: 415-345-8455
www.ski.org
Dedicated to research on human vision founded to encourage a productive collaboration between the medical clinic and the scientific
laboratories.

9512   Taping for the Blind
3935 Essex Lane   713-622-2767
Houston, TX 77027-5113   Fax: 713-622-2772
www.tapingfortheblind.org
Records reading material on audiotape copied onto cassettes for
use by blind and physically handicapped persons. Promotes in-

creased interest in and use of free audio materials. Books textbooks and technical manuals are recorded and sent to libraries.

Cynthia Franzetti, Executive Director
Ginger Gish, Volunteer Coordinator

9513 United States Association for Blind Athletes
33 N Institute Street   719-630-0422
Colorado Springs, CO 80903-3508   Fax: 719-630-0616
                               e-mail: mlucas@usaba.org
                                        www.usaba.org

Athletic association for blind athletes this association is the national governing body for the United States visually impaired athletes.

Mark Lucas, Executive Director
Nicole Jomantas, Communications Director

9514 Vision World Wide
5707 Brockton Drive   317-254-1332
Indianapolis, IN 46220-5481   800-431-1739
                                         Fax: 317-251-6588
                     e-mail: info@visionenhancement.org
                                        www.visionww.org

Believing there is hope when vision fails. It disseminates relevant information on a variety of topics through its information and referral helpline website e-mail announce list and journal Vision Enhancement all designed to encourage and support individuals with vision impairments.

Patricia Price, Editor-In-Chief
William Corbin, Board Chairman

9515 Washington Ear
12061 Tech Road   301-681-6636
Silver Spring, MD 20904-2437   Fax: 301-625-1986
                         e-mail: information@washear.org
                                        www.washear.org

A nonprofit organization providing reading and information services for the blind visually impaired and physically disabled persons who cannot effectively read print see plays watch television programs or view museum exhibits.

Margaret Pfanstiehl, President
George Long, Vice President

9516 National Federation of the Blind: Blind Merchants Division
Kevin Worley
1223 Lake Plaza Drive   719-527-0488
Colorado Springs, CO 80906-3591   866-543-6808
                                         Fax: 303-695-1828
                    e-mail: kevinworley@blindmerchants.org
                                        www.blindmerchants.org

Membership organization of blind persons employed in either self-employment work or the Randolph-Sheppard vending program. Provides information regarding rehabilitation social security tax and other issues which directly affect blind merchants.

Kevin Worley, President

State Agencies & Associations

Alabama

9517 Alabama Council of the Blind
1018 E Street S   256-362-5649
Talladega, AL 35160   e-mail: dart1018@charter.net
                                        www.acbalabama.org

David Trott, President

9518 National Federation of the Blind: Alabama
4905 Brooke Court   251-344-7960
Mobile, AL 36618-2708   e-mail: mwkoger21@bellsouth.net
                                        www.nfbofalabama.org

Minnie K Walker, President

Alaska

9519 National Federation of the Blind: Alaska
700 Hollywood   907-339-9578
Anchorage, AK 99501   e-mail: priddle@gci.net
                                        www.nfb.org

Steven Priddle, President

Arizona

9520 Arizona Center for the Blind and Visually Impaired
3100 E Roosevelt Street   602-273-7411
Phoenix, AZ 85008-5036   Fax: 602-273-7410
                                 e-mail: jlamay@acbvi.org
                                        www.acbvi.org

Provides services for individuals to enhance the quality of life of people who are blind or otherwise visually impaired. Services are available to adults who are either legally blind or visually impaired as well as those who have a degenerative eye condition.

Jim LaMay, Executive Director
Diana Miladin, Director of Communications/Development

9521 Arizona Industries for the Blind
515 N 51st Avenue   602-771-9100
Phoenix, AZ 85043   Fax: 602-353-5703
                             e-mail: LHudspeth@azdes.gov
                                        www.azdes.gov/aib

Arizona Industries for the Blind was established in 1952 to provide employment and training opportunities for Arizonans who are legally blind.

Lorraine Hudspeth, Controller
Letty Cerpa, Senior Accountant

9522 National Federation of the Blind: Arizona
9014 E Bellevue Street   520-733-5894
Tucson, AZ 85715-5652   e-mail: krezguy@cox.net
                                        www.nfbarizona.com

Bob Kresmer, President
Vicki Hodges, 1st Vice President

9523 Region 6 of the National Association for Parents of the Visually Impaired
Walnut Creek, CA 85282-5724   602-730-8282
                          e-mail: mebphillips@comcast.net
                                        www.spedex.com/napvi

Mary Beth Phillips, NAPVI Region 6 Representative

Arkansas

9524 Arkansas Lighthouse for the Blind
6818 Murray Street   510-562-2222
Little Rock, AR 72209-2666   Fax: 501-568-5275
                        e-mail: bjohnson@arkansaslighthouse.org
                                        www.arkansaslighthouse.org

Danny Novielli, COO
John McAtee, CFO

9525 National Federation of the Blind: Arkansas
608 Cedar Ridge   870-565-4484
Paragould, AR 72450-2304   e-mail: nfbofarkansas@yahoo.com
                                        www.nfb.org

Jerree Harris, President

California

9526 Helen Keller National Center: South Region
9939 Hibert Street   858-578-1600
San Diego, CA 92131   Fax: 858-578-3800
                                    TTY: 858-578-1600
                               e-mail: Ckirscher@att.net
                                        www.hknc.org

Cathy Kirscher, Regional Representative

9527 Lighthouse for the Blind and Visually Impaired
Lighthouse Industries
214 Van Ness Avenue   415-431-1481
San Francisco, CA 94102   Fax: 415-863-7568
                                    TTY: 415-431-4572
                             e-mail: info@lighthouse-sf.org
                                        www.lighthouse-sf.org

The LightHouse promotes the independence, equality and self-reliance of people who are blind or visually impaired through rehabilitation training and relevant services, such as access to employment, education, government, information, recreation and transportation.

Chuck Godwin, Executive Support
Anthony Fletcher, Associate Executive Director and COO

9528 National Federation of the Blind: California
5530 Corbin Avenue
Tarzana, CA 91356
818-342-6524
877-558-6524
Fax: 818-344-7930
e-mail: nfbcal@sbcglobal.net
http://www.nfbcal.org/
Robert Stigile, President

9529 Northwest Regional Training Center: Canine Companions for Independence
2965 Dutton Avenue
Santa Rosa, CA 95407-0446
707-577-1000
800-572-2275
TTY: 707-577-1756
e-mail: info@cci.org
www.cci.org
Canine Companions for Independence is a non-profit organization that enhances the lives of people with disabilities by providing highly trained assistance dogs and ongoing support to ensure quality partnerships.
Corey Hudson, CEO
Kathy Pierson, Northwest Regional Executive Director

9530 Southwest Regional Training Center: Canine Companions for Independence
124 Rancho del Oro Drive
Oceanside, CA 92057
760-901-4300
800-572-2275
Fax: 760-901-4350
TTY: 760-901-4326
TDD: 760-901-4350
www.cci.org
Canine Companions for Independence is a non-profit organization that enhances the lives of people with disabilities by providing highly trained assistance dogs and ongoing support to ensure quality partnerships.
Linda Valliant, Executive Director
Chuck Contreras, Director of Development

Colorado

9531 National Federation of the Blind: Colorado
2233 W Shepperd Avenue
Littleton, CO 80120
303-778-1130
800-401-4NFB
e-mail: slabarre@labarrelaw.com
www.nfbco.org
Scott LaBarre, President
Kevan Worley, 1st Vice President

9532 Rocky Mountain Region: Helen Keller National Center
1880 S Pierce Street
Lakewood, CO 80232
303-934-9037
Fax: 303-934-2939
TTY: 303-934-9037
e-mail: maureen.mcgowan@hknc.org
www.hknc.org
Maureen McGowan, Regional Representative

Connecticut

9533 BESB Industries
184 Windsor Avenue
Windsor, CT 06095-4536
860-602-4000
800-842-4510
Fax: 860-602-4220
TTY: 860-602-4221
e-mail: besb@ct.gov
www.ct.gov/besb
Brian S Sigman, Executive Director

9534 National Federation of the Blind: Connecticut
580 Burnside Avenue
East Hartford, CT 06108-3579
860-289-1971
e-mail: aldelucia@nfbct.org
http://www.nfbct.org/
Alfonse DeLucia, President

9535 Prevent Blindness Tri-State
101 Whitney Avenue
New Haven, CT 06510
800-850-2020
e-mail: info@preventblindnesstristate.org
www.preventblindness.org/tristate
Kathryn Garre-Ayars, President & CEO
Maria Giarratana, Grants Manager

9536 Region 1 of the National Association for Parents of the Visually Impaired
Hudson, MA 06016-9560
860-623-4129
e-mail: sue.rawley@verizon.net
www.spedex.com/napvi
Sue Rawley, NAPVI Region 1 Representative

Delaware

9537 Delaware Assocation for the Blind Department of Health & Social Services
Department of Health & Social Services
800 W Street
Wilmington, DE 19801-1526
302-655-2111
888-777-3925
Fax: 302-655-1442
e-mail: contact@dabdel.org
www.dabdel.org

9538 National Federation of the Blind: DC
627 Dahlia Street NW
Washington, DC 20012-1841
202-882-8090
e-mail: dnj.galloway@starpower.net
www.nfb.org
Don Galloway, President

District of Columbia

9539 American Foundation for the Blind: Governmental Relations
820 1st Street NE
Washington, DC 20002
202-408-0200
Fax: 202-289-7880
e-mail: afbgov@afb.net
www.afb.org
Advocates on behalf of people who are blind or visually impaired before Congress and Executive Branch offices, and participates in advocacy-related coalitions and initiatives nationwide.
Paul W Schroeder, Vice President, Governmental Relations
Barbara Jackson LeMoine, Legislative Assistant

9540 Columbia Lighthouse for the Blind
1825 K Street NW
Washington, DC 20006
202-454-6400
877-324-5252
Fax: 202-454-6401
e-mail: info@clb.org
www.clb.org
Columbia Lighthouse for the blind offers programs and services that enable individuals who are blind or visually impaired to obtain and maintain independence at home, school and in the community.
Anthony Cancelosi, President/CEO

9541 National Federation of the Blind: Delaware
3618 Kiamensi Street
Wilmington, DE 19808-2646
302-999-7242
e-mail: rhbennett.nfb@comcast.net
www.nfb.org
Richard Bennett, President

Florida

9542 Goodwill Industries-Suncoast
Goodwill Industries-Suncoast
10596 Gandy Boulevard
Saint Petersburg, FL 33702
727-523-1512
888-279-1988
Fax: 727-579-0850
TTY: 727-579-1068
e-mail: gw.marketing@goodwill-suncoast.com
www.goodwill-suncoast.org
A non-profit community based organization whose purpose is to improve the quality of life for people who are disabled, disadvantaged and/or aged. This mission is accomplished through a staff of over 1,200 employees providing independent living skills.
R Lee Waits, President/Chief Executive Officer
Chris Ward, Marketing and Media Relations Manager

9543 National Federation of the Blind: Florida
121 Deer Lake Circle
Ormond Beach, FL 32174-4266
386-677-6886
888-282-5972
e-mail: kdavisnfbf@cfl.rr.com
www.nfbflorida.org
Kathy Davis, President

9544 **Southeast Regional Center: Canine Companions for Independence**
Anheuser-Busch/SeaWorld Campus
8150 Clarcona Ocoee Road
Orlando, FL 32818-0388
407-522-3300
Fax: 407-522-3347
e-mail: mager@cci.org
www.cci.org
Canine Companions for Independence is a non-profit organization that enhances the lives of people with disabilities by providing highly trained assistance dogs and ongoing support to ensure quality partnerships.
Margaret S Ager, Executive Director
Nancy Baumann, President

9545 **Tampa Lighthouse for the Blind**
1106 W Platt Street
Tampa, FL 33606-2142
813-251-2407
866-251-2407
Fax: 813-254-4305
e-mail: TLH@tampalighthouse.org
www.tampalighthouse.org
Tampa Lighthouse for the Blind provides comprehensive rehabilitation programs for persons who are blind or visually impaired.
Cliff Olstrom, Executive Director

Georgia

9546 **Georgia Industries for the Blind**
700 Faceville Highway
Bainbridge, GA 39818-0218
229-248-2666
www.vocrehabga.org
The primary mission of the Georgia Industries for the Blind (GIB) is to provide employment opportunities for people who are visually impaired or blind.

9547 **National Federation of the Blind: Georgia**
315 Ponce de Leon Avenue
Decatur, GA 30030
404-371-1000
Fax: 404-371-1002
e-mail: alewis@nfbga.org
www.nfb.org

Anil Lewis, President

9548 **Southeastern Region: Helen Keller National Center**
1003 Virginia Avenue
Atlanta, GA 30354-1365
404-766-9625
Fax: 404-766-3447
TTY: 404-766-2820
e-mail: bc4hknc@aol.com
www.hknc.org

Barbara Chandler, Regional Representative

Hawaii

9549 **Division of Vocational Rehabilitation and Services for the Blind**
Department of Human Services
601 Kamokila Boulevard
Kapolei, HI 96707
808-692-7715
Fax: 808-692-7727
TTY: 808-692-7715
e-mail: info@hawaiivr.org
www.hawaiivr.org
The American Macular Degeneration Foundation is committed to the prevention and cure of macular degeneration and offers hope and support to those afflicted and their families. The Foundation is a major voice in establishing national research.
Joe Cordova, Administrator

9550 **Ho'opono Workshop for the Blind**
1901 Bachelor Street
Honolulu, HI 96817
808-586-5286
Fax: 808-586-5288
TTY: 808-586-5269
e-mail: hoopono@hawaiivr.org
www.hawaiivr.org

Dave Eveland, Administrator

9551 **National Federation of the Blind: Hawaii**
PO Box 4482
Honolulu, HI 96812
808-391-1214
e-mail: nanifife@aol.com
hawaii.nfb.org

Nani Fife, President
Charlene Ota, Vice-President

Idaho

9552 **National Federation of the Blind: Idaho**
300 Willard Avenue
Pocatello, ID 83201
208-377-9825
Fax: 208-232-5416
e-mail: ElsieLamp@yahoo.com
www.nfbidaho.org

Elsie H Lamp, President

Illinois

9553 **AFB Midwest: American Foundation for the Blind**
949 Third Avenue
Huntington, WV 25701
304-523-8651
e-mail: muslan@afb.net
www.afb.org

Leads initiatives in the area of technology. Nationally offers consultation technical assistance and support and undertakes local and national efforts such as training programs in the area of technology. Responds to inquiries from blind and visually impaired.
Mark Uslan, Director
Darren Burton, National Program Associate

9554 **Aid to the Aged, Blind or Disabled**
Department of Human Services
100 South Grand Avenue, East
Springfield, IL 62762
800-252-8635
TTY: 800-447-6404
www.macular.org/stagency/state_il.html
The American Macular Degeneration Foundation is committed to the prevention and cure of macular degeneration and offers hope and support to those afflicted and their families. The Foundation will be a major voice in establishing the national research agenda for macular degeneration through promoting an alliance among the scientific community, government, and victims of the disease and their families to ensure the prevention and cure of the disease.

9555 **Chicago Lighthouse for People Who are Blind and Visually Impaired**
1850 W Roosevelt Road
Chicago, IL 60608-1298
312-666-1331
Fax: 312-243-8539
TTY: 312-666-8874
TDD: 312-666-8874
e-mail: helpdesk@chicagolighthouse.org
www.thechicagolighthouse.org
The Chicago Lighthouse is a comprehensive private rehabilitation and educational facility dedicated exclusively to assisting children youth and adults who are blind visually impaired or multi-disabled.
Janet P Szlyk, Executive Director
William L Conaghan, Chairman

9556 **Helen Keller National Center Regional Representatives**
485 Avenue of the Cities
E Moline, IL 61244
309-755-0018
Fax: 309-755-0025
TTY: 309-755-0018
TDD: 309-755-0021
e-mail: HKNC5LJT@aol.com
www.hknc.org

Laura J Thomas, Regional Representative

9557 **National Federation of the Blind: Illinois**
6919 W Berwyn Avenue
Chicago, IL 60656-2040
773-307-6440
e-mail: president@nbfofillinois.org
www.nfbofillinois.org

Patti Gregory-Chang, President
Deborah Kent Stein, First Vice-President

9558 **Region 3 of the National Association for Parents of the Visually Impaired**
Highland Park, IL 60047-7711
847-438-0705
e-mail: wizoz4@aol.com
www.spedex.com/napvi

Pam Stern, NAPVI Region 3 Representative

Indiana

9559 Bosma Industries for the Blind
8020 Zionsville Road
Indianapolis, IN 46268-3876
317-684-0600
800-362-5463
Fax: 317-684-1946
e-mail: info@bosma.org
www.bosma.org

It is the mission of Bosma Industries for the Blind to enhance opportunities for individuals who are blind or visually impaired to achieve their potential in vocational, economic, social and personal independence.
Lou Moneymaker, CEO
Connie F Campbell, CFO/COO

9560 National Federation of the Blind: Indiana
6010 Winnpeny Lane
Indianapolis, IN 46220-5253
317-205-9226
e-mail: rb15@iquest.net
www.nfb.org

Ron Brown, President

Iowa

9561 National Federation of the Blind: Iowa
2721 34th Street
Des Moines, IA 50310
515-771-8348
e-mail: m.barber@mchsi.com
www.nfbi.org

Michael D Barber, President
April Enderton, First Vice-President

Kansas

9562 Great Plains Region: Helen Keller National Center
4330 Shawhee Mission Parkway
Shawnee Mission, KS 66205
913-677-4562
Fax: 913-677-1544
TTY: 913-677-4562
e-mail: hknc7bj@aol.com
www.helenkeller.org

Services are free and offer client advocacy consultation and technical assistance to schools and agencies; assistance in developing local services information and referral; public education and awareness; maintenance of the National Registry.
Beth Jordan, Regional Representative
Jody Searing, Administrative Assistant

9563 Kansas Industries for the Blind
425 MacVicar Street
Topeka, KS 66606
785-296-3211
Fax: 785-296-0728

9564 National Federation of the Blind: Kansas
11405 W Grant
Wichita, KS 67209-3621
913-339-9341
e-mail: donnajwood@cox.net
www.nfbks.org

Donna Wood, President
Susan L Stanzel, First Vice President

Kentucky

9565 Kentucky Industries for the Blind
1900 Brownsboro Road
Louisville, KY 40206-2102
502-893-0211
Fax: 502-893-3885

9566 National Federation of the Blind: Kentucky
210 Cambridge Drive
Louisville, KY 40214-2809
502-366-2317
e-mail: cathyj@iglou.com
www.nfbky.org

Cathy Jackson, President
Pamela Roark-Glisson, Vice President

Louisiana

9567 Industries for the Blind and Visually Impaired of Louisiana
PO Box 366
Delhi, LA 71232-0366
318-878-8171

9568 Louisiana Association for the Blind
1750 Claiborne Avenue
Shreveport, LA 71103
318-635-6471
877-913-6471
Fax: 318-635-8902
e-mail: labstore@lablind.com
www.lablind.com

LAB employs people who are blind in manufacturing administrative training and a variety of job positions that match an individual's goals and potential.
Shelly Taylor, President/CEO
William G Rogers, Vice President Administration

9569 National Federation of the Blind: Louisana
605 University Boulevard
Ruston, LA 71270-4862
318-251-1511
800-234-4166
e-mail: pallenp@lcb-ruston.com
www.nfbla.org

Pam Allen, President

Maine

9570 Maine Center for the Blind and Visually Impaired
189 Park Avenue
Portland, ME 04102-2909
207-774-6273
Fax: 207-774-0679
e-mail: info@theiris.org
www.theiris.org

Phipps, Executive Director
Retta Choate, Executive Assistant

9571 National Federation of the Blind: Maine
13 Whispering Pines Drive
Limington, ME 04049-9707
207-221-6710
e-mail: sallylaughlin@earthlink.net
www.nfb.org

Sally Laughlin, President

Maryland

9572 Blind Industries and Services of Maryland
3345 Washington Boulevard
Baltimore, MD 21227
410-737-2600
888-322-4567
Fax: 410-737-2665
www.bism.org

Blind Industries and Services of Maryland provides innovative rehabilitation services training and stable employment opportunities to our state's citizens who are blind or visually impaired.
Don Morris, Chairperson
Walter Brown, Vice-Chairperson

9573 East Central Region: Hellen Keller National Center
9320 Annapolis Road
Lanham, MD 20706
301-459-5474
Fax: 301-459-5070
TTY: 301-459-5433
TDD: 301-459-5433
e-mail: hkncreg3cl@aol.com
www.helenkeller.org

The Helen Keller National Center for Deaf- Blind Youths& Adu;ts offers intensive and comprehensive rehabilitation raining to individuals who are deaf- blind.
Cynthia L Ingraham, Regional Representative
Jackie Greenfield, Administrative Assistant

9574 National Federation of the Blind: Maryland
1026 E 36th Street
Baltimore, MD 21218
410-235-3073
e-mail: president@nfbmd.org
www.nfbmd.org/

Melissa Riccobono, President
Debbie Brown, First Vice President

Massachusetts

9575 Carroll Center for the Blind
770 Centre Street
Newton, MA 02458-2597
617-969-6200
800-852-3131
Fax: 617-969-6204
TTY: 617-969-6204
e-mail: info@carroll.org
www.carroll.org

Assists blind and visually impaired adults and adolescents to adjust to loss of vision. The goal of this dynamic program is to en-

courage independence, restore self-confidence, prepare for employment and improve the quality of life.
Dina Rosenbaum, Marketing Director

9576 Ferguson Industries for the Blind
One Highland Avenue   617-727-9840
Malden, MA 02148   Fax: 781-324-3111
www.state.ma.us/mcb/ferguson.html

9577 Massachusetts Commission for the Blind
48 Boylston Street   617-727-5550
Boston, MA 2116—4718   800-392-6450
                                         Fax: 617-626-7685
                                         TTY: 800-392-6556
                                         TDD: 800-392-6556
                         e-mail: cheryl.standley@state.ma.us
                                         www.state.ma.us/mcb
Provides services to blind citizens of Massachusetts, enabling them to lead more fulfilling and independent lives. Offers vocational rehabilitation, independent living, social services, home care and respite assistance, radio reading programs and print resources.
Cheryl Standley, Contact
Janet LaBreck, Commissioner

9578 National Federation of the Blind: Massachusetts
140 Wood Street   508-679-8543
Somerset, MA 02726-5225   e-mail: nfbmass@earthlink.net
                                  http://www.nfbmass.org/

Priscilla Ferris, President

9579 New England Region: Helen Keller National Center
152 Lincoln Road   781-259-7100
Lincoln, MA 01773   Fax: 781-259-4014
                             e-mail: hknc1meb@comcast.net
                                         www.hknc.org

Mary Ellen Barbiasz, Regional Representative
Peg Ouellette, Administrative Assistant

Michigan

9580 Association for the Blind & Visually Impaired
456 Cherry Southeast   616-458-1187
Grand Rapids, MI 49503   800-466-8084
                                         Fax: 616-458-7113
                           e-mail: blindser@abvimichigan.org
                                         www.abvimichigan.org
To advance the independence of people who are visually impaired and to promote the prevention of blindness.
Richard A Stevens, Executive Director
George Kremer, Director of Rehabilitation Services

9581 Greater Detroit Agency for the Blind and Visually Impaired
16625 Grand River Avenue   313-272-3900
Detroit, MI 48227-1419   Fax: 313-272-6893
                           e-mail: information@gdabvi.org
                                         www.gdabvi.org

We are a non-profit organization dedicated to preventing blindness reducing the impact of blindness and advocating for those with severe vision loss.
Gail L McEntee, President & CEO
Christina Schlitt, Administrative Manager

9582 National Federation of the Blind: Michigan
1212 N Foster Avenue   517-482-1800
Lansing, MI 48912-3309   e-mail: f.wurtzel@comcast.net
                                         www.nfbmi.org

Fred Wurtzel, President
Mary Ann Rojek, State Braille Coin Project Coordinator

Minnesota

9583 Duluth Lighthouse for the Blind
4505 W Superior Street   218-624-4828
Duluth, MN 55807-2728   800-422-0833
                                         Fax: 218-624-4479
                e-mail: info@lighthousefortheblind-duluth.org
                      www.lighthousefortheblind-duluth.org

The LightHouse for the blind is a teaching facility providing employment, training and rehab instruction for blind and visually-impaired individuals.
Mary Junnila, Executive Director
Julaine Netzel, Intervenor/Service Support Person

9584 National Federation of the Blind: Minnesota
5132 Queen Avenue South   612-872-9363
Minneapolis, MN 55410-2217 e-mail: joyce.scanlan@earthlink.net
                                   http://www.nfbmn.org/

Joyce Scanlan, President

Mississippi

9585 Mississippi Industries for the Blind
2501 N W Street   601-984-3200
Jackson, MS 39296-4417   866-859-4461
                                         Fax: 601-987-3892
                               e-mail: bcoy@msblind.org
                                         www.msblind.org
The Mississippi Industries for the Blind seeks to provide jobs for the blind and visually-impaired.
Michael Chew, Executive Director
Bob Coy, Sales Manager

9586 National Federation of the Blind: Mississippi
268 Lexington Avenue   601-969-3352
Jackson, MI 39209-5431   e-mail: samgleese@earthlink.net
Sam Gleese, President

Missouri

9587 Alphapointe Association for the Blind
7501 Prospect   816-421-5848
Kansas City, MO 64132   Fax: 816-237-2019
                          e-mail: sliptak@alphapointe.org.
                                         www.alphapointe.org
The Alphapointe Association for the Blind has a Braille library a Senior Adult Services Program and a dedication to finding employment for the blind and visually-impaired.
Reinhard Mabry, President/CEO
James E Van Winkle, VP Administration/CFO

9588 Kansas City Association for the Blind
1844 Broadway Street   816-333-2173
Kansas City, MO 64108-2007

9589 National Federation of the Blind: Missouri
3910 Tropical Lane   573-874-1774
Columbia, MO 65202-6205   e-mail: info@nfbmo.org
                                         www.nfbmo.org

Gary Wunder, President
Shelia Wright, First Vice President

Montana

9590 National Federation of the Blind: Montana
408 W Sussex Avenue   406-546-8546
Missoula, MT 59801   e-mail: burk.dall@gmail.com
                                         www.mt-blind.org

Daniel Burke, President
Dick Howse, 1st Vice President

Nebraska

9591 National Federation of the Blind: Nebraska
1033 O Street   402-477-7711
Lincoln, NE 68508-2468   866-254-6347
                            e-mail: amy.buresh@ncbvi.ne.gov
                                         nfbn.inebraska.com

Amy Buresh, President
Jeff Altman, First Vice President

Nevada

9592 National Federation of the Blind: Nevada
8455 W Sahara Avenue   702-639-9072
Las Vegas, NV 89117   e-mail: terri.rupp@gmail.com
                                         ww.nfb.org

Terri Rupp, President

9593 Southern Nevada Sightless
1001 N Bruce Street
Las Vegas, NV 89101-1247
702-642-6000
Fax: 702-649-6739
e-mail: info@blindcenter.org
www.blindcenter.org

Neal Marek, Chairman
Veronica Wilson, President/CEO

New Hampshire

9594 National Federation of the Blind: New Hampshire
11 Springfield Street
Concord, NH 03301
603-225-7917
e-mail: jomar2000@comcast.net
Marie Johnson, President

New Jersey

9595 Bestwork Industries for the Blind
801 E Clements Bridge Road
Runnemede, NJ 08078
856-939-5220
800-370-9560
Fax: 856-939-5022
e-mail: bestwork@bestworkindustries.org
www.bestworkindustries.org
Bestwork Industries for the Blind is dedicated to providing employment opportunities for those with visual impairments.
James Varsaci, Founder

9596 National Federation of the Blind: New Jersey
254 Spruce Street
Bloomfield, NJ 07003
973-743-0075
e-mail: nfbnj@yahoo.com
http://www.nfbnj.org/

Joe Ruffalo, President

New Mexico

9597 National Federation of the Blind: New Mexico
1331 Park Avenue Southwest
Albuquerque, NM 87102
505-243-6165
e-mail: blindart@myfreedombox.com
http://www.nfbnm.org/
Arthur Schreiber, President

9598 New Mexico Industries for the Blind
2200 Yale Boulevard SE
Albuquerque, NM 87106-4212
505-841-8844
888-513-7958
Fax: 505-841-8850
e-mail: Greg.Trapp@state.nm.us
www.state.nm.us/cftb

Greg Trapp, Executive Director
Dallas Allen, Commissioner

9599 Region 5 of the National Association for Parents of the Visually Impaired
PO Box 1337
Alamogordo, NM 88311-1337
505-682-2693
ww.spedex.com/napvi

9600 State of New Mexico Commission for the Blind
2905 Rodeo Park Drive E
Santa Fe, NM 87505
505-476-4479
888-513-7968
e-mail: Greg.Trapp@state.nm.us
www.state.nm.us/cftb
The mission of the New Mexico Commission for the Blind is to encourage and enable blind citizens to achieve vocational economic and social equality. It provides career preparation and training in the skills of blindness.
Greg Trapp, Executive Director
Arthur A Schreiber, Chairman

New York

9601 Association for the Blind & Visually Impaired of Greater Rochester
422 South Clinton Avenue
Rochester, NY 14620-1198
585-232-1111
www.raen.org
Our mission is to assist people who are blind or visually impaired to achieve their highest level of independence in all aspects of their lives.
A Gidget Hopf, EdD, President/CEO

9602 Blind Association of Western New York
1170 Main Street
Buffalo, NY 14209-2331
716-882-1025
e-mail: guildcarebuffalo@jgb.org
www.olmstedcenter.org

Ronald Maier, President
Milissa Acquard, Chief Operations Officer/CFO

9603 Blind Work Association
55 Washington Street
Binghamton, NY 13901-3770
607-724-2428
Fax: 607-771-8045
e-mail: bobh@clarityconnect.com
www.co.tompkins.ny.us

9604 Central Association for the Blind and Visually Impaired
507 Kent Street
Utica, NY 13501-2317
315-797-2233
877-719-9996
Fax: 315-797-2244
e-mail: info@cabui.org
www.cabvi.org

Paul Drejza, Chairman
Peter Emery Sr, Vice Chairman

9605 National Federation of the Blind: New York
PO Box 09-0363
Brooklyn, NY 11209-4617
718-567-7821
Fax: 718-765-1843
e-mail: office@nfbny.org
www.nfbny.org

Carl Jacobsen, President
Mindy Fliegelman, Vice President

9606 Northeast Regional Training Center: Canine Companions for Independence
SUNY Farmingdale
PO Box 205
Farmingdale, NY 11735-0205
631-694-6938
800-572-2275
TTY: 631-694-6938
e-mail: jdiamond@caninecompanions.org
www.caninecompanions.org
Canine Companions for Independence is a non-profit organization that enhances the lives of people with disabilities by providing highly trained assistance dogs and ongoing support to ensure quality partnerships.
Alan Feinne, CFO
Corey Hudson, CEO

9607 Northeastern Association of the Blind of Albany
301 Washington Avenue
Albany, NY 12206-3012
518-463-1211
Fax: 518-463-5883
e-mail: info@naba-vision.org
www.naba-vision.org
NABA offers a wide range of services to those with visual impairments from its free vision screening service for children to training and placing legally blind adults in professional employment. Also provides rehabilitation services to seniors with age-related conditions.
Christopher Burke, Interim Executive Director
Larry N Volk, Chair

9608 Southern Tier Association for the Visually Impaired
719 Lake Street
Elmira, NY 14901-2538
607-734-1554
Fax: 607-734-9467
e-mail: info@st-avi.org
www.st-avi.org

Timothy Hertlein, Executive Director
Cindy Young, Fiscal Administrator

North Carolina

9609 Lions Industries for the Blind
4126 Berkeley Avenue
Kinston, NC 28504-8321
252-523-1019
Fax: 252-523-7090
e-mail: ray_amyette@lionsindustries.org
www.lionsindustries.com
The Lions Industries for the Blind provides employment opportunities for the blind and visually-impaired.
Bob Smith, Executive Director
Danny Rice, Chairman

9610 National Federation of the Blind: North Carolina
128 Summerlea Drive
Charlotte, NC 28214-1324
704-491-1486
Fax: 704-391-3204
e-mail: tjnc2@carolina.rr.com
http://www.nfbofnc.org/
Tim Jones, President

9611 Winston-Salem Industries for the Blind
7730 N Point Drive
Winston-Salem, NC 27106-3310
336-759-0551
800-242-7726
Fax: 336-759-0990
e-mail: info@wsifb.com
www.wsifb.com
The Winston-Salem Industries for the Blind provides employment opportunities for the blind and visually-impaired.
Daniel J Boucher, Executive Chairman
Ann Johnston, Chairman

North Dakota

9612 National Federation of the Blind: North Dakota
2581 Villa Drive S
Fargo, ND 58103
701-298-2963
e-mail: jcbichler@msn.com
www.nfb.org
Jennelle Bichler, President

Ohio

9613 Cincinnati Association for the Blind
2045 Gilbert Avenue
Cincinnati, OH 45202-1490
513-221-8558
888-687-3935
Fax: 513-221-2995
e-mail: info@cincyblind.org
www.cincyblind.org
Persons who are blind visually impaired or print impaired may choose from a wide range of services to help them live more independently. Our services are provided by qualified certified instructors and staff with highly specialized skills.

9614 Cleveland Sight Center
1909 E 101st Street
Cleveland, OH 44106-8696
216-791-8118
Fax: 216-791-1101
e-mail: sfriedman@clevelandsightcenter.org
www.clevelandsightcenter.org
Mission is to enable people with vision impairment to reach their full potential and assure that adequate services are available to make a normal life possible.
Stanley E Wertheim, Chair
Steven M Friedman, President/CEO

9615 Cleveland Skilled Industries
2239 E 55th Street
Cleveland, OH 44103-4451
216-431-8085
Fax: 216-431-5123

9616 National Federation of the Blind: Ohio
237 Oak Street
Oberlin, OH 44074-1517
440-775-2216
e-mail: bbpierce@pobox.com
www.nfbohio.org
J Webster Smith, President
Barbara Pierce, President Emerita

9617 North Central Regional Training Center: Canine Companions for Independence
4989 State Route 37 E
Delaware, OH 43015-9682
740-548-4447
800-572-2275
Fax: 740-363-0555
TTY: 740-548-4447
www.caninecompanions.org
Canine Companions for Independence is a non-profit organization that enriches the lives of people with disabilities by providing highly trained assistance dogs and ongoing support to ensure quality partnerships.
Corey Hudson, CEO
Alan Feinne, CFO

9618 Region 2 of the National Association for Parents of the Visually Impaired
5786 Arlyne Lane
Medina, OH 44256-3825
330-722-6609
www.spedex.com/napvi
Victoria Gor Miller
Rachel Miller, President

9619 Society of the Blind: Akron Center
325 E Market Street
Akron, OH 44304-1340
330-253-2555
Fax: 330-996-4088

Oklahoma

9620 National Federation of the Blind: Oklahoma
242 E 35th Street
Tulsa, OK 74105
918-850-6751
e-mail: selena.j.sundling@irs.gov
www.nfb.org
Selena Sundling-Craw, President

9621 Oklahoma League for the Blind
501 N Douglas Avenue
Oklahoma City, OK 73106
405-232-4644
Fax: 405-236-5438
e-mail: info@olb.org
www.olb.org
The mission of the Oklahoma League for the Blind is to facilitate independence and improve the quality of life for people who are blind or vision impaired by providing employment opportunities and services.
Lauren White, President/CEO
Carol Campbell, Executive Assistant

Oregon

9622 Blind Enterprises of Oregon
6540 SE Foster Road
Portland, OR 97206
503-774-6387
Fax: 503-774-0585
e-mail: blindent@aol.com
www.blindenterprises.com
Jennifer Williams, Operations Manager
Tami Foss, Executive Director

9623 National Federation of the Blind: Oregon
1616 5th Street NE
Salem, OR 97301
503-585-4318
800-422-7093
e-mail: artds55@comcast.net
www.nfb.org
Art Stevenson, President

Pennsylvania

9624 Association for the Blind & Visually Impaired of Lehigh County
845 Wyoming Street
Allentown, PA 18103-2199
610-433-6018
Fax: 610-433-4856
e-mail: info@abvi.org
www.abvi.org
The ABVI mission is to strive to be our community's foremost provider and coordinator of preventative, educational, social and rehabilitative programs concerning vision loss. Our goal is to assist each individual and his/her family to achieve their greatest potential.
Kathleen Meckes, Executive Director

9625 Beaver County Association for the Blind
616 Fourth Street
Beaver Falls, PA 15010
724-843-1111
Fax: 724-843-8886
e-mail: bcab@forcomm.net
bcab2.tripoid.com
The Beaver County Association for the Blind conducts educational programs about blindness or vision problems by request and provides opportunities to learn experience share and celebrate in the lives of the blind and visually impaired in Beaver County.
Fay Lentz, Executive Director
Linda Borghi, Controller/Business Manager

9626 Cambria County Association for the Blind and Handicapped
211 Central Avenue
Johnstown, PA 15902
814-536-3531
Fax: 814-539-3270
e-mail: ccabh@ccabh.com
www.ccabh.com

The mission of the Cambria County Association for the Blind and Handicapped is to develop and support an environment for persons with disabilities which promotes vocational and employment training, independence and community involvement through rehabilitative programs.
Richard C Bosserman, President

9627 Chester County Association for the Blind
71 S First Avenue
Coatesville, PA 19320
610-384-2767
Fax: 610-384-8005
e-mail: info@chescoblind.org
www.chescoblind.org

Anita Cavuto, Executive Director
John W Esworthy, President

9628 Chester County Branch of the Pennsylvania Association for the Blind
71 S First Avenue
Coatesville, PA 19320-3461
610-384-2767
Fax: 610-384-8005
e-mail: info@chescoblind.org
www.chescoblind.org

John W Esworthy, President
Anita Cavuto, Executive Director

9629 DELCO Blind/Sight Center
100 W Fifteenth Street
Chester, PA 19013
610-874-1476
Fax: 610-874-6454
e-mail: info@delcoblind.org
www.delcoblind.org

This agency is dedicated to helping individuals in the greater Delaware Valley area to prevent, prepare for and adapt to vision loss in order to achieve independence. Our goal is to help those with blindness or vision loss to lead well adjusted, independent lives.
Robert M Nelson, Executive Director

9630 Delaware County Branch of the Pennsylvania Association for the Blind
100-106 W 15th Street
Chester, PA 19013
610-874-1476
Fax: 610-874-6454
e-mail: delcosce@liberty.org
www.libertynet.org

9631 Greater Wilkes-Barre Association for the Blind
1825 Wyoming Avenue
Exeter, PA 18643
570-693-3555
877-693-3555
Fax: 570-823-4841
e-mail: info@wilkesbarreblind.com
www.wilkesbarreblind.com

Our mission is to address the needs of those with limited vision and we also take an active role in the prevention of blindness.
Ronald V Petrilla, Executive Director
Denise Culver, Office Manager

9632 Indiana County Association for the Blind
31 S 10th Street
Indiana, PA 15701-2649
724-465-5549

9633 Keystone Blind Association
1230 Stambaugh Avenue
Sharon, PA 16146
724-347-5501
800-837-4122
Fax: 724-347-2204
e-mail: kba@keystoneblind.org
www.keystoneblind.org

The Keystone Blind Association is dedicated to maintaining and improving the quality of life for blind and/or visually impaired persons preventing blindness and providing employment opportunities and advocacy for persons who are disabled.
Jonathan G Fister, President/CEO
Perry Templeton, Vice President of Operations

9634 Lancaster County Association for the Blind
244 N Queen Street
Lancaster, PA 17603-3512
717-291-5951
www.sabvi.com

Dennis L Steiner, President/CEO
Kay L Macsi, VP Rehabilitation and Education

9635 Montgomery County Association for the Blind
212 N Main Street
North Wales, PA 19454-3117
215-661-9800
Fax: 215-661-9888
e-mail: mcab@mcab.org
www.mcab.org

MCAB's mission is to enhance the quality of life and independence of people coping with blindness and vision impairment through rehabilitation education support and advocacy.
Douglas Yingling, Executive Director
Sharon Zislis, Director of Development

9636 National Federation of the Blind: Pennsylvania
42 South 15th Street
Philadelphia, PA 19102-2206
215-988-0888
e-mail: nfbofpa@att.net
http://www.nfbp.org/

James Antonacci, President

9637 North Central Sight Services
2121 Reach Road
Williamsport, PA 17704-0292
570-323-9401
866-320-2580
Fax: 570-323-8194
e-mail: ncss@ncsight.org
www.ncsight.org

Our agency philosophy focuses on helping people help themselves and emphasizes the abilities and capabilities of the blind and visually impaired people we serve.
Robert B Garrett, President/CEO
Barbara Snauffer, Administrative Assistant

9638 Pennsylvania Association for the Blind
90 E Shady Lane
Enola, PA 17025
717-234-3261
Fax: 717-234-4733
e-mail: neal.carrigan@pablind.org
www.pablind.org

Neal J Carrigan, President/CEO
Willard D Brown, Vice-President for Finance

9639 Pittsburgh Branch for the Pennsylvania Association for the Blind
1800 W Street
Homestead, PA 15120-3707
412-368-4400
800-706-5050
Fax: 412-368-4090
TTY: 412-368-4095
e-mail: info&ref@pghvis.org
ww.pghvis.org

Stephen S Barrett, President
James Baumgartner, Vice President of Finance

9640 Pittsburgh Vision Services
1800 W Street
Homestead, PA 15120
412-368-4400
800-706-5050
Fax: 412-368-4090
TTY: 412-368-4095
e-mail: info&ref@pghvis.org
www.pghvis.org

Pittsburgh Vision Services is a private non-profit United Way agency whose mission is to reduce the limitations that may result from loss of vision.
Stephen S Barrett, President
James Baumgartner, Vice President of Finance

9641 Somerset County Blind Center
748 S Center Avenue
Somerset, PA 15501
814-445-1310
Fax: 814-445-3184
e-mail: rob@somersetblind.org
www.somersetblind.org

The Somerset Blind Center offers a number of services to those who are blind or visually impaired, including work opportunities, eyeglass prescription programs, free vision screenings, and training facilities.
Rob Stemple, Executive Director
Anna Hope, Finance Manager

9642 Tri-County Association for the Blind
1130 S 19th Street
Harrisburg, PA 17102-2200
717-238-2531
Fax: 717-238-0710
e-mail: info@tricountyblind.org
www.tricountyblind.org

The Tri-County Association for the Blind works to improve the quality of life for people who are visually-impaired in the

Tri-County region, by helping each person achieve his or her full potential and maximum independence.
Danette Blank, Executive Director
Laurie Thompson, Public Relations/Development Director

9643   VIABL Services of Northampton County
260 E Broad Street   610-866-8049
Bethlehem, PA 18018   Fax: 610-866-8730
e-mail: viabl@viablservices.org
www.viablservices.org
Our mission is to promote the social economic and physical self-sufficiency of blind deaf-blind and visually impaired individuals by providing them with the resources and skills needed to live rewarding productive and independent lives.
Jan Leon, Executive Director

9644   Washington-Greene County Branch for the Pennsylvania Association for Blind
566 E Maiden Street   412-228-0770
Washington, PA 15301-3720   Fax: 412-228-6617
e-mail: washgreene@verizon.net
www.pablind.org

Elaine R Welch, President/CEO
Willard D Brown, Vice-President for Finance

9645   York Industries for the Blind: Division of York County Blind Center
A Division of York County Blind Center
1380 Spahn Avenue   717-848-1690
York, PA 17403-5711   Fax: 717-845-3889
www.forsight.org

William H Rhinesmith, President

Rhode Island

9646   IN-SIGHT
43 Jefferson Boulevard   401-941-3322
Warwick, RI 02888   Fax: 401-941-3356
e-mail: insighttri@gmail.com
www.in-sight.org
IN-SIGHT is a private non-profit agency which has been serving the blind and visually impaired since 1925.
Gerard Goulet, President
Eleanor Acton, Director of Communications

9647   National Federation of the Blind: Rhode Island
PO Box 154564   401-433-2606
Riverside, RI 02915   Fax: 877-383-3682
e-mail: info@nfbri.org
www.nfbri.org

Richard Gaffney, President

South Carolina

9648   National Federation of the Blind: South Carolina
1293 Professional Drive   803-254-3777
Myrtle Beach, SC 29577   e-mail: parnell@sccoast.net
http://www.nfbsc.net/

Parnell Diggs, President

9649   Region 4 of the National Association for Parents of the Visually Impaired
1032 Trail Road
Belton, SC 29627-7926   864-338-9593
www.spedex.com/napvi

South Dakota

9650   National Federation of the Blind: South Dakota
903 Fulton Street   605-791-3939
Rapid City, SD 57701   e-mail: President@nfb-south-dakota.org
www.nfb-south-dakota.org
Kenneth Rollman, President

Tennessee

9651   Ed Lindsey Industries of the Blind
4110 Charlotte Avenue   615-741-2251
Nashville, TN 37209-3749   Fax: 615-741-5024

9652   National Federation of the Blind: Tennessee
1226 Goodman Circle West   901-452-6596
Memphis, TN 38111-6524   e-mail: michael.seay@ssa.gov
http://www.nfb-tennessee.org/

Michael Seay, President

9653   West Tennessee Lions Blind Industries
PO Box 2175   901-767-5466
Memphis, TN 38101-2175

Texas

9654   American Foundation for the Blind
11030 Ables Lane   214-352-7222
Dallas, TX 75229   Fax: 214-352-3214
e-mail: dallas@afb.net
www.afb.org
Leads initiatives in the areas of aging and education. Nationally offers consultation, technical assistance and support and undertakes local and national efforts such as training programs, public education and coalition building in the areas of aging and elder care.

9655   American Foundation for the Blind: National Aging Center
11030 Ables Lane   214-352-7222
Dallas, TX 75229   Fax: 214-352-3214
e-mail: dallas@afb.net
www.afb.org
Leads initiatives in the areas of aging and education. Nationally offers consultaion, technical assistance and support and undertakes local and national efforts such as training programs, public education and coalition building in the areas of aging and education. Responds to inquiries from blind and visually impaired people and their families, service providers and the general public in the region and nationally.

9656   Beacon Lighthouse
300 7th Street   940-767-0888
Wichita Falls, TX 76301-1699   800-262-6412
Fax: 817-767-0893
e-mail: jkoszarek@beaconwf.com
www.beaconwf.com

9657   Dallas Lighthouse for the Blind
4245 Office Parkway   214-821-2375
Dallas, TX 75204   Fax: 214-824-4612
www.dallaslighthouse.org
The Dallas Lighthouse for the Blind provides work opportunities for the blind and visually impaired.
Michael Orfinik, Chief Executive Officer
Nancy J Perkins, President

9658   East Texas Lighthouse for the Blind
500 N Bois D'Arc   903-595-3444
Tyler, TX 75702   888-595-3444
Fax: 903-595-3447
e-mail: customerservice@horizonind.com
www.horizonind.com

9659   El Paso Lighthouse for the Blind
200 Washington Street   915-532-4495
El Paso, TX 79905   Fax: 915-532-6338
e-mail: htyler@elp.rr.com
www.lighthouse-elpaso.com
Lighthouse is guided by the unwavering belief that its rehabilitative and employment services can help any person overcome his or her disability and enable them to reach their fullest potential for self-sufficiency and independence.
Harry Tyler, President/CEO
Rusty Hooten, CFO

9660   Lighthouse for the Blind of Houston
3602 W Dallas   713-527-9561
Houston, TX 77019-0435   Fax: 713-284-8451
e-mail: houstonlighthouse@houstonlighthouse.org
www.houstonlighthouse.org
Founded in 1839 the Lighthouse of Houston is a private nonprofit rehabilitation center dedicated to helping blind and visually impaired people live independently.
Gibson M DuTerroil, President

9661 Lighthouse of the Blind of Fort Worth
912 W Broadway Street 817-332-3341
Fort Worth, TX 76104 Fax: 817-332-3456
e-mail: plattallen@lighthousefw.org.
www.lighthousefw.org
The Lighthouse of the Blind of Fort Worth offers many services including skills assessment orientation and mobilty training assisted employment and senior services.
Platt Allen, President
Steve Peglar, Chairman

9662 National Federation of the Blind: Texas
314 E Highland Mall Boulevard 512-323-5444
Austin, TX 78752-3123 866-636-3289
Fax: 512-420-8160
e-mail: tecraig@earthlink.net
www.nfb-texas.org
Tommy Craig, President

9663 South Central Region: Helen Keller National Center
12160 Abrams Road 972-490-9677
Dallas, TX 75243-5903 Fax: 972-490-6042
TTY: 972-490-9677
e-mail: ccfutbol@aol.com
www.hknc.org
C C Davis, Regional Representative

9664 South Texas Lighthouse for the Blind
PO Box 9697 361-883-6553
Corpus Christi, TX 78469 888-255-8011
Fax: 361-883-1041
e-mail: Regisb@stlb.net
www.stlb.net
Regis Barber, President/CEO
Nicky Ooi, VP/COO

9665 Texas Association of Retinitis Pigmentosa
PO Box 8388 361-852-8515
Corpus Christi, TX 78468-8388 Fax: 361-852-8515
e-mail: tarpmail@homebiz101.com
www.geocities.com/HotSprings/7815
A nonprofit organization based in Texas serving as a national information-sharing center to provide human services to persons with progressive vision loss from retinitis pigmentosa and other retinal degenerative disorders.
Dorothy H Stiefel, Executive Director

9666 Travis Association for the Blind
2307 Business Center Drive 512-442-2329
Austin, TX 78764-3297 Fax: 512-442-5498
e-mail: info@austinlighthouse.org
www.austinlighthouse.org
Travis Association for the Blind (aka Austin Lighthouse) is a service oriented non-profit organization with the mission to assist people who are blind or vision impaired to attain the skills they need to become gainfully employed in the community.
Jerry A Mayfield, Executive Director
Benny Galloway, Chief Financial Officer

9667 West Texas Lighthouse for the Blind
2001 Austin Street 325-653-4231
San Angelo, TX 76903-8705 Fax: 325-657-9367
e-mail: d.wells@lighthousefortheblind.org
www.lighthousefortheblind.org
The West Texas Lighthouse for the Blind is a sheltered facility providing employment for blind and visually impaired individuals.
David Wells, Executive Director
Stephen Horton, Operations Manager

Utah

9668 National Federation of the Blind: Utah
161 W 600 S 801-292-3000
Salt Lake City, UT 84010-7634 888-292-3007
Fax: 801-294-6000
e-mail: president@nfbutah.org
www.nfbutah.org
Ron Gardner, President
Cheralyn Bra Creer, First Vice President

9669 Utah Industries for the Blind
PO Box 258 801-533-9689
Salt Lake Cty, UT 84110-1258

Vermont

9670 National Federation of the Blind: Vermont
1 Mechanic Street 802-229-0748
Montpelier, VT 5602 e-mail: fshiner@verizon.net
www.nfbvt.org
Franklin Shiner, President

Virginia

9671 National Federation of the Blind: Virginia
9522 Lagersfield Circle 703-319-9226
Vienna, VA 22181 e-mail: fschroeder@sks.com
www.nfbv.org
Fredric K Schroeder, President
Seville Allen, First Vice President

9672 Virginia Industries for the Blind
1102 Monticello Road 434-295-5168
Charlottesville, VA 22902 Fax: 434-977-0122
e-mail: Robert.Berrang@dbvi.virginia.gov
www.vdbvi.org/vib
Our mission is to be a self-sufficient and self-supporting industry enhance the quality of life for blind and visually impaired individuals through providing gainful employment; and provide opportunities in career development and employment related services.
Robert C Berrang, Deputy Commissioner
Richard C Bohrer, Plant Manager

Washington

9673 Lighthouse for the Blind of Washington
PO Box 14119 206-322-4200
Seattle, WA 98114 Fax: 206-329-3397

9674 National Federation of the Blind: Washington
101 NE 83rd Street 360-576-5965
Vancouver, WA 98665-7900 e-mail: k7uij@panix.com
Mike Freeman, President

9675 Northwestern Region: Helen Keller National Center
1620 18th Avenue 206-324-9120
Seattle, WA 98122-6501 Fax: 206-324-9159
TTY: 206-324-1133
e-mail: nwhknc@juno.com
www.hknc.org
Dorothy Walt, Regional Representative

9676 Washington State Department of Services for the Blind
402 Legion Way 360-725-3830
Olympia, WA 98504-0933 800-552-7103
Fax: 360-407-0679
e-mail: information@dsb.wa.gov
www.dsb.wa.gov
The Washington State Department of Services for the Blind (DSB) is a state rehabilitation agency that offers assistance to persons who are blind or visually impaired. We also provide various services for employers interested in accomodating or hiring workers with visual impairments.
Bill Palmer, Director

West Virginia

9677 AFB Technology & Employment Center
949 Third Avenue 304-523-8651
Huntington, WV 25701 800-824-2184
Fax: 304-523-8656
e-mail: AFBTECH@afb.net
www.afb.org
AFB Technology runs AFB's CareerConnect and the AFB TECH Product Evaluation Laboratory. Nationally offers consultation, technical assistance and support and undertakes local and national efforts in employment and technology.
Brad Hodges, National Technology Associate

9678 National Federation of the Blind: West Virginia
220 Buena Vista Avenue   304-622-0626
Clarksburg, WV 26301   e-mail: cs.nfbwv@verizon.net
                                          www.nfbwv.org
Charlene Smyth, President

Wisconsin

9679 National Federation of the Blind: Wisconsin
27824 Nuthatch Road   608-758-4800
Kendall, WI 54638   e-mail: johnfritz@centurytel.net
                                       http://www.nfbwis.org/
John Fritz, President

9680 National Federation of the Blind: Writers
27824 Nuthatch Road   608-758-4800
Kendall, WI 54638   e-mail: johnfritz@centurytel.net
                                          www.nfbwis.org
John Fritz, President

9681 Wiscraft: Wisconsin Enterprises for the Blind
5316 W State Street   414-778-5800
Milwaukee, WI 53208-2686   Fax: 414-778-5805
                               e-mail: sales@wiscraft.com
                                          www.wiscraft.com
Wiscraft provides long-term supportive employment for people who are blind. It is a manufacturing company that operates as a non-profit with the clear mission of employing people who are blind by sellng blind-made products and services.
Jim Kerlin, President
Ron Hutchinson, Chair

Wyoming

9682 National Federation of the Blind: Wyoming
PO Box 347
Sheridan, WY 82801-0347   307-672-1821
                                          www.nfb.org
Max Aguilar, President

Foundations

9683 Foundation Fighting Blindness
11435 Cronhill Drive   410-568-0150
Owings Mills, MD 21117-2220   800-683-5555
                                     TDD: 800-683-5551
                           e-mail: info@FightBlindness.org
                                       www.fightblindness.org
For a $25.00 annual membership fee, FFB offers information and referral services for affected individuals and their families as well as for doctors and eye care professionals. The Foundation also provides comprehensive information kits on retinitis pigmentosa, macular degeneration, and usher syndrome. Their newsletter, InFocus, and their e-newsletter, InSight, present articles on coping research updates, and Foundation news. A national conference is usually held every other year.
Gordon Gund, Chairman
Edward H. Gollob, President

9684 Glaucoma Research Foundation
251 Post Street   415-986-3162
San Francisco, CA 94108   800-826-6693
                                     Fax: 415-986-3763
                                e-mail: info@glaucoma.org
                                          www.glaucoma.org
The Glaucoma Research Foundation is a nationa nonprofit dedicated to curing glaucoma. We receive no government funding. Your contribution is tax-deductible as allowed by law.
Thomas M Brunner, President/CEO

Libraries & Resource Centers

9685 District of Columbia Public Library Librarian for the Deaf Community
901 G Street North West
Washington, DC 20001   202-727-1111
                                          www.dclibrary.org

Offers reference services through TDD, portable TDD for public use at pay phone, signers for library programs, sign language classes, information about deafness, print and non-print materials for persons who are deaf.
John W Hill, Jr, President
James W Lewis, Vice President

Alabama

9686 Alabama Radio Reading Service Network
WBHM
650 11th Street South   205-934-6576
Birmingham, AL 35294-4530   800-444-9246
                                     Fax: 205-934-5075
                                e-mail: philip@wbhm.org
                                          www.wbhm.org/ARRS
Services and readings are relayed over the radio to three-quarters of Alabama for the benefit of the visually impaired.
Philip Habeeb, Program Director

9687 Alabama Regional Library for the Blind and Physically Handicapped
Alabama Public Library Service
6030 Monticello Drive   334-213-3906
Montgomery, AL 36130-6000   800-392-5671
                                     Fax: 334-213-3993
                          e-mail: fzaleski@apls.state.al.us
                                 http://statelibrary.alabama.gov
To promote and support equitable access to library and information resources and services to enable all Alabamians to satisfy their educational, working, cultural, and leisure-time interests. These resources and services will be provided through APLS's statewide programs and through direct grants and assistance to libraries and library systems to meet user's needs.
Fara Zaleski, Regional Librarian
Rebecca Mitchell, Director (APLS)

9688 Houston Love Memorial Library
212 West Burdeshaw Street   334-793-9767
Dothan, AL 36303   e-mail: bforbus@yahoo.com
                                       www.houstonlovelibrary.org
Offers magnifiers, summer reading programs and more for the blind and physically handicapped. Scanner, software and jaws for windows.
Bettye Forbus, President

9689 Huntsville Subregional Library for the Blind and Physically Handicapped
P.O. Box 443   256-532-5980
Huntsville, AL 35804   Fax: 256-532-5994
                           e-mail: bphdept@hpl.lib.al.us
                               www.hpl.lib.al.us/departments/bph
The Subregional Library for the Blind and Physically Handicapped is located in the Main branch of the Huntsville-Madison County Public Library. It is also part of a Library of Congress administered nationwide network of libraries serving persons who cannot use conventional printed materials.
Joyce Welch, Librarian

9690 Library and Resource Center for the Blind and Physically Handicapped
Alabama Institute for Deaf and Blind
705 South Street   256-761-3237
Talladega, AL 35161   800-848-4722
                                     Fax: 256-761-3561
                        e-mail: lacy.teresa@aidb.state.al.us
                                          http://www.aidb.org
Using federal and state funds, the Resource Center purchases or produces braille textbooks and other necessary materials for students. The Resource Center also loans equipment, like braillewriters, to help students learn alternative methods of communication.
Teresa Lacy, Director

9691 Tuscaloosa Subregional Library for the Blind & Physically Handicapped
1801 Jack Warner Parkway   205-345-5820
Tuscaloosa, AL 35401   Fax: 205-752-8300
                        e-mail: bjordan@tuscaloosa-library.org
                                          www.tuscaloosa-library.org

Provide talking books to patrons who are unable to use standard print because of a visual or physical limitation. Deliver playback equipment to qualified patrons. Provides reference and referral service to this special population also.

Barbara Jordan, Librarian

Alaska

9692 Alaska State Library Talking Book Center
National Library Services
344 W 3rd Avenue   907-269-6575
Anchorage, AK 99501-2337   800-776-6566
                                      Fax: 907-269-6580
                                      TDD: 907-269-6575
                          e-mail: tbc@eed.state.ak.us
                              www.library.state.ak.us

The Alaska State Library Talking Book Center is a cooperative effort between the National Library Service and the Alaska State Library to provide print handicapped Alaskans with talking book and Braille service.

Bev Griffin, Library Assistant II
Stephanie Schott, Administrative Clerk I

Arizona

9693 Arizona State Braille and Talking Book Library
1030 N 32nd Street   602-255-5578
Phoenix, AZ 85008-5108   800-255-5578
                                      Fax: 602-255-4312
                               e-mail: btbl@lib.az.us
                                        www.lib.az.us

Closed-circuit TV, summer reading programs, volunteer-produced cassette books, braille writer, films, large-print photocopier and more.

Linda Montgomery, Division Director

9694 Flagstaff City Coconino County Public Library
300 W Aspen Avenue
Flagstaff, AZ 86001-5304   520-779-7670
                          www.flagstaffpubliclibrary.org

Reference materials on blindness and other handicaps, braille writer, magnifiers and large-print photocopier.

9695 Phoenix Public Library: Special Needs Section
Burton Barr Central Library
1221 North Central Avenue   602-262-4636
Phoenix, AZ 85004   TDD: 602-254-8205
                      e-mail: specialneeds@phxlib.org
                              www.phoenixpubliclibrary.org

The Special Needs Center is designed to make the services and resources of the Phoenix Public Library accessible to people with disabilities.

Toni Garvey, City Librarian

Arkansas

9696 Arkansas Regional Library for the Blind and Physically Handicapped
One Capitol Mall   501-682-1155
Little Rock, AR 72201-1049   866-660-0885
                                      Fax: 501-682-1529
                                      TDD: 501-682-1002
                        e-mail: nlsbooks@asl.lib.ar.us
                                    www.asl.lib.ar.us

Public library books in recorded or braille format. Popular fiction and nonfiction books for all ages, books and players are on free loan, sent to patrons by mail and may be returned postage free. Anyone who cannot see well enough to read regular print with glasses on or who has a disability that makes it difficult to hold a book or turn the pages is eligible.

John D Hall, Coordinator

9697 Library for the Blind and Handicapped, Southwest
Columbia County Library
220 East Main Street   870-234-0399
Magnolia, AR 71754   866-234-8273
                                      Fax: 870-234-5077
                          e-mail: lbph@hotmail.com
                          www.youseemore.com/columbia

The mission of the Columbia County Library is to help the people of our community in their pursuits of information and education , as well as vocational and recreational endeavors, by providing current materials, services, and programs. Our inviting public libraries are the cornerstone of our diverse communities where all people, regardless of age, race, or socio-economic circumstances can experience personal enrichment and literary growth.

Dana Thornton, Interim Director
Sandra Grissom, Librarian

California

9698 Blind Childrens Center
4120 Marathon Street   323-664-2153
Los Angeles, CA 90029-3584   Fax: 323-665-3828
                              www.blindchildrenscenter.org

The Blind Childrens Center is a family-centered agency which serves children with visual impairments from birth to school-age. The center-based and home-based programs and services help the children acquire skills and build their independence. The Center utilizes its expertise and experience to serve families and professionals worldwide through support services, education, and research.

Midge Horton, Executive Director
Muriel Scharf, Director Development

9699 Braille Institute Library Services
741 North Vermont Avenue   323-663-1111
Los Angeles, CA 90029-3594   800-808-2555
                                      Fax: 323-662-2440
                                      TDD: 323-660-3880
                     e-mail: dls@braillelibrary.org
                              www.braillelibrary.org

The Braille Institute is a non-profit organization whose mission is to eliminate barriers to a fulfilling life caused by blindness and severe sight loss. The Institute provides an environment of hope and encouragement for people who are blind and visually impaired through integrated educational, social and recreational services and programs.

Henry C. Chang, Librarian

9700 California State Library Braille and Talking Book Library
National Library Service
PO Box 942837   916-654-0640
Sacramento, CA 94237-0001   800-952-5666
                                      Fax: 916-654-1119
                        e-mail: btbl@library.ca.gov
                                      www.library.ca.gov

Library services in braille and recorded formats. Free to residents of Northern California who are unable to read ordinary print on hold a printed book.

Michael Marlin, Manager
Mary Jane Kayes, Outreach Coordinator

9701 Fresno County Public Library: Talking Book Library for the Blind
770 North San Pablo Avenue   559-488-3217
Fresno, CA 93728-3640   800-742-1011
                                      Fax: 559-488-1971
                                      TDD: 559-488-1642
           e-mail: wendy.eisenberg@fresnolibrary.org
                            www.fresnolibrary.org/tblb

We provide books and magazines on cassette tape and in Braille to people of all ages who are blind, visually impaired, or have physical disabilities preventing the reading of standard print.

Karen Bosch Cobb, County Librarian
Wendy Eisenberg, Librarian

9702 San Francisco Public Library for the Blind and Print Disabled
100 Larkin Street   415-557-4253
San Francisco, CA 94102-4733   TTY: 415-557-4433
                          e-mail: citylibrarian@sfpl.org
                                      www.sfpl.lib.ca.us

Foreign-language books on cassette, children's books on cassettes and more.

Luis Herrera, City Librarian
Marcia Schneider, Chief, Communications/Adult Services

9703 San Jose State University Library
1 Washington Square
San Jose, CA 95192-0001   408-924-1000
                                                www.library.sjsu.edu
Information on physical disabilities, accessibility and learning
disabilities.

Colorado

9704 Boulder Public Library
1000 Canyon Boulevard   303-441-3100
Boulder, CO 80302-1326   Fax: 303-442-1808
                                         e-mail: ask@boulder.lib.co.us
                                                www.boulder.lib.co.us
Offers braille books, cassettes, talking books, large print photo-
copier, large print books and more for the visually impaired.
Tony Tallent, Library & Arts Director

9705 Colorado Talking Book Library
180 Sheridan Boulevard   303-727-9277
Denver, CO 80226-8101   800-685-2136
                                                Fax: 303-727-9281
                                      e-mail: ctbl.info@cde.state.co.us
                                                 www.cde.state.co.us
Take advantage of the services offered by the Colorado Talking
Book Library (CTBL). CTBL provides postage-free recorded,
braille, and large print library materials to eligible residents in Col-
orado.
Debbi MacLeod, Director

Connecticut

**9706 Connecticut State Library for the Blind and Physically
Handicapped**
198 W Street   860-721-2020
Rocky Hill, CT 06067-3554   800-842-4516
                                                Fax: 860-721-2056
                                          e-mail: lbph@cslib.org
                                            www.cslib.org/lbph.htm
Free audio cassettes and braille books and magazines along with
reference materials on blindness and other handicaps. Necessary
playback equipment for eligible residents of Connecticut.
Carol Taylor, Director

Delaware

**9707 Delaware Division of Libraries: Library for the Blind and
Physically Handicapped**
43 South DuPont Highway   302-739-4748
Dover, DE 19901   800-282-8676
                                                Fax: 302-739-6787
                                              TDD: 302-739-4847
                                     e-mail: john.phillos@state.de.us
                                                www.state.lib.de.us
Since 1971, the Delaware Library for the Blind and Physically
Handicapped has provided books in Braille and audio books on re-
cord and cassette for the blind and physically handicapped resi-
dents of Delaware.
John Phillos, Librarian

District of Columbia

9708 Council of Families with Visual Impairment
American Council of the Blind
1155 15th Street NW   202-467-5081
Washington, DC 20005   800-424-8666
                                                Fax: 202-467-5085
                                             e-mail: info@acb.org
                                                    www.acb.org
Members are sighted parents of blind or visually impaired children. Offers a forum for support and outreach, sharing of experiences in parent-child relationships, and educational and cultural
information about child development. Monitors developments in
technical and legislative arenas.
Melanie Brunson, Executive Director

9709 DC Public Library Adaptive Services Division
901 G Street NW, Room 215   202-727-2142
Washington, DC 20001   Fax: 202-727-1129
                                                TTY: 202-727-2255
                                                TDD: 202-727-1129
                                          e-mail: lbph.dcpl@dc.gov
                                                www.dclibrary.org
The DC Public Library has a special Adaptive Technology Program to help older adults, the deaf, and those with visual and physi-
cal disabilities use library materials and resources.
Venetia V. Demson, Librarian

**9710 National Library Service for the Blind and Physically
Handicapped**
Library of Congress   202-707-9261
Washington, DC 20542   Fax: 202-707-0712
                                                TDD: 202-707-0744
                                             e-mail: raj@loc.gov
                                                www.loc.gov/nls
The NLS, Library of Congress, administers the free programs that
loans recorded and braille books and magazines, music scores in
braille and large print, and specially designed playback equipment
to residents of the United States who are unable to read or use standard print materials due to visual or physical impairment.
Yealuri Rathan Raj, Librarian

Florida

9711 Brevard County Libraries: Talking Books Library
308 Forrest Avenue   321-633-1810
Cocoa, FL 32922-7781   Fax: 321-633-1838
                                          e-mail: dmartin@brev.org
                                                    www.brev.org
The Talking Books/Homebound Services has many devices and
special materials to assist blind, physically handicapped and/or
homebound citizens to access library services.
Debra A. Martin, Librarian

9712 Broward County Talking Book Library
100 S Andrews Avenue   954-357-7555
Fort Lauderdale, FL 33301-1830   Fax: 954-577-20
                                    e-mail: talkingbooks@browardlibrary.org
                                       www.broward.org/library/talkingbooks
Reference materials on blindness and other handicaps, closed-circuit TV, Talking Book cassettes, print/Braille and descriptive videos.
William Forbes, Librarian

9713 Florida Bureau of Braille and Talking Book Library Services
421 Platt Street   386-239-6000
Daytona Beach, FL 32114-2803   800-226-6075
                                                Fax: 386-239-6069
                                     e-mail: mike.gunde@dbs.fldoe.org
                                        dbs.myflorida.com/library/index.php
The Florida Bureau of Braille and Talking Book Library Services
provides information and reading materials needed by Florida residents who are unable to use standard print as the result of visual,
physical, or reading disabilities.
Michael Gunde, Librarian

9714 Hillsborough County Talking Book Library
Jan Kaminis Platt Regional Library
3910 South Manahattan Avenue   813-272-6024
Tampa, FL 33611-1214   Fax: 813-272-6072
                                                TDD: 813-272-6305
                                  e-mail: talkingbooks@hillsboroughounty.org
                                           hcplc.org/hcplc/liblocales/tbl
This free program provides recorded and braille books and maga-
zines to people who are blind, visually impaired or physically
handicapped.
Ann Palmer, Librarian

9715 Jacksonville Public Library
303 North Laura Street
Jacksonville, FL 32202   904-630-2665
                                                  http//jpl.coj.net
Discs, cassettes, reference materials on blindness and other handi-
caps and children's books on cassettes.
Mark S. Wood, Chairperson
Bill E. Scheu, Vice Chair

9716 Lee County Talking Books Library
13240 North Cleveland Avenue, #5-6
North Ft. Myers, FL 33903-4855   239-995-2665
    800-854-8195
    Fax: 239-995-1681
    TDD: 2399952665
    e-mail: talkingbooks@leegov.com
    www.lee-county.com/library
Talking Books are books and magazines that are recorded for people who need to hear their reading. The books are played on special players provided free by the National Library Service for the Blind and Physically Handicapped.
Sheldon Kaye, Librarian

9717 Miami Dade Talking Book Library
Miami Dade Public Library System
2455 North West 183rd Street
Miami, FL 33056   305-751-8687
    800-451-9544
    Fax: 305-757-8401
    TDD: 305-474-7258
    e-mail: talkingbooks@mdpls.org
    www.mdpls.org
The Talking Books Library loans books and magazines on cassette tapes or in Braille FREE by mail to persons who have difficulty seeing or using standard small print.
Barbara Moyer, Librarian

9718 Orange County Library System: Orlando Public Library
101 E Central Boulevard   407-835-7323
Orlando, FL 32801-2462   Fax: 407-425-6779
    www.ocls.info
The library's collection consists of a wide variety of print materials, including fiction, nonfiction, world languages, genealogy, and special materials that comprise the Florida and Disney collections. The library also has audiovisual materials and electronic resources to meet customer needs.
Mary Anne Hodel, Library Director/CEO

9719 Palm Beach County Library Annex: Talking Books
Mil-Lake Plaza
4639 Lake Worth Road   561-649-5500
Lake Worth, FL 33463   888-780-5151
    Fax: 561-649-5402
    e-mail: talkingbooks@pbclibrary.org
    www.pbclibrary.org
The Talking Books Library is a special service of the Palm Beach County Library and a part of the Library of Congress National Library Service for the Blind and Physically Handicapped.
Pat Mistretta, Librarian

9720 Pinellas Talking Book Library for the Blind and Physically Handicapped
1330 Cleveland Street   727-441-9958
Clearwater, FL 33755-5103   Fax: 727-441-9068
    TDD: 727-441-3168
    www.pplc.us/tbl/
The Pinellas Talking Book Library's mission is to encourage and support reading by providing free library services to Pinellas County residents for whom conventional print is a barrier. The Pinellas Talking Book Library is part of a nationwide network of cooperating libraries serving people who have difficulty using or reading regular print.
Marilyn Stevenson, Access Services Librarian

9721 Sub Regional Talking Book Library
1755 Edgewood Avenue West
Jacksonville, FL 32208-7206   904-765-5588
    Fax: 904-768-7822
    TDD: 904-768-7822
    e-mail: jerryco@j.net
Susan V Arthur, Librarian
Laurie Baumgardner, Librarian

9722 West Florida Public Library: Talking Book Library
200 West Gregory Street   850-436-5065
Pensacola, FL 32502-4822   Fax: 850-436-5039
    e-mail: talkingbooks@ci.pensacola.fl.us
    www.cityofpensacola.com/library
As a subregional Talking Book Library, the Pensacola Public Library offers free service by mail to blind and physically handi-

capped adults and children who have difficulty reading ordinary print or holding or turning the pages of a book.
Susan C. Voss, Librarian

Georgia

9723 Albany Library for the Blind and Physically Handicapped
Dougherty County Public Library
300 Pine Avenue   229-420-3220
Albany, GA 31701   800-337-6251
    Fax: 229-420-3240
    e-mail: lbph@docolib.org
    www.docolib.org/libblind.html
The Library for the Blind and Physically Handicapped provides resources to individuals who are blind, visually impaired, physically handicapped or learning disabled in a thirteen-county area.
Kathryn Sinquefield, Librarian

9724 Atlanta Metro Subregional Library
1150 Murphy Avenue, SW   404-756-4619
Atlanta, GA 30310   800-248-6701
    Fax: 404-756-4618
    e-mail: glass@georgialibraries.org
    www.georgialibraries.org/public.glass
Through Georgia's Regional Library for the Blind and Physically Handicapped and cooperating local libraries, Georgians have access to a free national library program that offers books and magazines on cassette tape and in Braille.

9725 Augusta Regional Library Talking Book Center
425 James Brown Boulevard   706-821-2625
Augusta, GA 30901   Fax: 706-724-5403
    e-mail: talkbook@ecgrl.org
    www.ecgrl.public.lib.ga.ua/lbph.htm
Through the Georgia Library for Accessible Services, Georgians have access to a free national library program that offers books and magazines on cassette tape and in Braille.
Gary Swint, Librarian

9726 Bainbridge Subregional Library for the Blind and Physically Handicapped
Southwest Georgia Regional Library
301 South Monroe Street   229-248-2680
Bainbridge, GA 39819-4029   800-795-2680
    Fax: 229-248-2670
    TDD: 229-248-2665
    e-mail: lbph@swgrl.org
    www.swgrl.org
The library houses a large collection of recorded materials as well as reference materials.
Susan S. Whittle, Director

9727 Columbus Library for Accessible Services (CLASS)
The Columbus Public Library
3000 Macon Road   706-243-2686
Columbus, GA 31906-2201   800-652-0782
    Fax: 706-243-2710
    e-mail: sbarnes@cvrls.net
    www.thecolumbuslibrary.org
CLASS serves as one of the Georgia subregional distribution centers for books and magazines on audiocassettes published by the National Library Service for the Blind and Physically Handicapped.
Suzanne Barnes, Librarian

9728 Georgia Library for Accessible Services (GLASS)
1150 Murphy Avenue SW   404-756-4619
Atlanta, GA 30310-3803   800-248-6701
    Fax: 404-756-4618
    e-mail: glass@georgialibraries.org
    www.georgialibraries.org
Georgians have access to a free national library program that offers books and magazines on cassette tape and in Braille. These materials are provided by the Library of Congress, National Library Service for the Blind & Physically Handicapped (NLS),), to eligible persons with a visual or physical disability. All reading material and playback equipment is sent to borrowers and returned by postage-free mail.
Linda B Stetson, Director

9729 Hall County Library System: East Hall Branch and Special Needs Library
2434 Old Cornelia Highway
Gainesville, GA 30507
770-532-3311
Fax: 770-531-2502
TDD: 770-531-2530
e-mail: kevans@hallcountylibrary.org
www.hallcountylibrary.org/ehmap.htm
The East Hall Branch and Special Needs Library goal is to provide excellent service to those with disabilities including the blind, handicapped, mobility impaired and deaf.
Kathy Evans, Branch Manager

9730 Middle Georgia Subregional Library for the Blind and Physically Handicapped
Washington Memorial Library
1180 Washington Avenue
Macon, GA 31201-1790
478-744-0877
800-805-7613
Fax: 478-744-0840
e-mail: harringj@bibblib.org
www.co.bibb.ga.us/library/TBC.htm
Books, magazines, newspapers, radio programs and various publications are available. Assistive technology equipment is also available at the library.
Judy T. Harrington, Librarian

9731 Oconee Regional Library for the Blind and Physically Handicapped
801 Bellevue Avenue
Dublin, GA 31040
478-275-5382
800-453-5541
Fax: 478-275-3821
e-mail: wdaniel@ocrl.org
www.laurens.public.lib.ga.us
Through the Georgia Library for Accessible Services and cooperating local libraries, Georgians have access to a free national library program which offers braille and recorded materials.
Wanda Daniel, Librarian

9732 Rome Subregional Library for People with Disabilities
205 Riverside Parkway NE
Rome, GA 30161-2911
706-236-4618
888-263-0769
Fax: 706-236-4631
TDD: 706-236-4618
e-mail: dhickman@rome-lpd.org
www.rome-lpd.org
Provides free library service to the disabled in eleven counties of Northwest Georgia.
Delana Hickman, Coordinator

9733 Special Needs Library of Northeast Georgia
Athens-Clarke County Regional Library
2025 Baxter Street
Athens, GA 30606-6331
706-613-3655
800-531-2063
Fax: 706-613-3660
TDD: 706-613-3655
e-mail: specialneedslibrary@athenslibrary.org
www.clarke.public.lib.ga.us/specneeds
The Special Needs Library of Northeast Georgia provides free library services for patrons with visual, physical, and reading disabilities.
Claudia L. Markov, Librarian

9734 Subregional Library for the Blind and Physically Handicapped
Live Oak Public Libraries, Thunderbolt Branch
2708 Mechanics Avenue
Savannah, GA 31404
912-354-5864
800-342-4455
Fax: 912-354-5534
e-mail: stokesl@liveoakpl.org
www.liveoakpl.org
Library for the blind and physically handicapped.
LaTrelle Mobley, Manager

9735 Three Rivers Regional Library
Brunswick-Glynn County Regional Library
208 Gloucester Street
Brunswick, GA 31520-5324
912-267-1212
866-833-2878
Fax: 912-267-9597
e-mail: bransom@trrl.org
www.trrl.org

The Talking Book Center serves 12 counties with over 1200 patrons. The center provides talking books which are recorded at a slower speed which requires the use of a special player.
Betty D. Ransom, Librarian

9736 Valdosta Talking Book Library
South Georgia Regional Library
300 Woodrow Wilson Drive
Valdosta, GA 31602-2592
229-333-7658
800-246-6515
Fax: 229-333-0774
e-mail: djernigan@sgrl.org
www.sgrl.org
The Talking Book Center is available to blind persons with visual difficulty or physical handicaps which prevent them from using printed material.
Diane Jernigan, Librarian

Hawaii

9737 Hawaii State Library for the Blind and Physically Handicapped
402 Kapahulu Avenue
Honolulu, HI 96815
808-733-8444
800-559-4096
Fax: 808-733-8449
TDD: 808-733-8444
e-mail: olbcirc@librarieshawaii.org
www.librarieshawaii.org
The Library for the Blind and Physically Handicapped serves as the regional library and machine lending agency for the blind and physically disabled throughout the state and the outlying Pacific Islands in cooperation with the Library of Congress and the National Library Service for the Blind and Physically Handicapped.
Fusako Miyashiro, Librarian

Idaho

9738 Idaho Commission for Libraries Talking Book Service
325 West State Street
Boise, ID 83702-6072
208-334-2150
800-458-3271
Fax: 208-334-4016
TDD: 800-377-1363
e-mail: talkingbooks@libraries.idaho.gov
http://libraries.idaho.gov/tbs
The Idaho Talking Book Service provides books and magazines in cassette format for individuals who are unable to read standard print.
Sue Walker, Librarian

Illinois

9739 Catholic Guild for the Blind
180 N Michigan Avenue
Chicago, IL 60601
312-236-8569
Fax: 312-236-8128
e-mail: info@guildfortheblind.org
www.guildfortheblind.org
The Guild's adult rehabilitation services include a program geared towards seniors experiencing new vision loss called New Visions. This program promotes independence within the home and community by providing participants with the information, techniques, and tools they need to successfully adjust to their new lives with impaired sight. Two workshop series are available to beginners or to those ready for more advanced topics.
David J Tabak, Executive Director
Polly Abbott, Manager Adult Rehabilitation Services

9740 Illinois State Library Talking Book and Braille Service
401 East Washington
Springfield, IL 62701-1207
217-782-9435
800-665-5576
Fax: 217-558-4723
TDD: 888-261-7863
The Illinois State Library Talking Book and Braille Service plays a supporting rols for the Illinois Network of Libraries Serving the Blind and Physically Handicapped.

9741 Mid-Illinois Talking Book Center
600 Highpoint Lane
East Peoria, IL 61611
217-224-6619
800-426-0709
Fax: 217-224-9818
e-mail: info@mitbc.org
www.mitbc.org

We provide free library service for anyone unable to read regular print because of low vision, blindness, or a physical disability. We provide recorded and Braille books and popular magazines. There are over 60,000 titles available including popular fiction and non-fiction, bestsellers, classics, history, biographies, children's books and more.
Karen Bershe, Director
Valerie Brandon, PR/Outreach Coordinator

9742 Shawnee Library System: Southern Illinois Talking Book Center
607 South Greenbriar Road
Carterville, IL 62918
618-985-8375
800-445-2665
Fax: 618-985-4211
TDD: 618-985-8375
www.shawls.lib.il.us/talkingbooks
The Talking Book Program is a free library service for anyone who has difficulty reading print or holding books and turning pages due to any visual or physical limitation or medically diagnosed reading disability. Participants are loaned cassette players along with unabridged books and magazines on tape and in Braille.
Diana Brawley Sussman, Director/Librarian

9743 Skokie Accessible Library Services
Skokie Public Library
5215 Oakton Street
Skokie, IL 60077-3634
847-673-7774
Fax: 847-673-7797
e-mail: anthe@skokie.library.info
www.skokie.lib.il.us
Library services for people with disabilities, including electronic aids, materials in special formats, programs and special services, and access to the North Suburban Library System.
Carolyn A Anthony, Director

9744 Voices of Vision Talking Book Center
127 S First Street
Geneva, IL 60134
630-208-0398
800-227-0625
Fax: 630-208-0399
e-mail: kodean@dupagels.lib.il.us
www.vovtbc.org
Voices of Vision is part of a statewide and national network of libraries which provide the talking book and braille service. We provide free library service to persons unable to read or use conventional print material due to a visual or physical disability. There is no cost to eligible readers.
Karen Odean, Director

Indiana

9745 Bartholomew County Public Library
National Library Services
536 Fifth Street
Columbus, IN 47201
812-379-1277
800-685-0524
Fax: 812-791-75
e-mail: talkingbooks@barth.lib.in.us
www.barth.lib.in.us
Talking Books for the Blind and Physically Handicapped is a free library service for visually or physically challenged persons of all ages. Anyone who is unable to use regular printed materials as the result of a temporary or permanent visual or physical limitation is eligible.
Sharon Thompson, Librarian

9746 Evansville-Vanderburgh County Public Library
200 SE Martin Luther King Jr Blvd
Evansville, IN 47713
812-428-8200
Fax: 812-428-8397
www.evcpl.lib.in.us
The Evansville-Vanderburgh County Public Library, an essential provider of shared information and a core community service, promotes reading, lifelong learning, and economic vitality through its resources, services and programs to the residents of Vanderburgh County.
Mike Russ, President
Brenda Schiedler, Vice President

9747 Indiana Talking Book & Braille Library
140 North Senate Avenue
Indianapolis, IN 46204
317-232-3684
800-622-4970
e-mail: lbph@statelib.lib.in.us
www.in.gov/library/tbbl.htm

The TBBL provides large print books, braille books, and books on tape to Indiana residents who are unable to read regular print.
Roberta L Brooker, Interim Director

9748 Lake County Public Library
1919 W 81st Street
Merrillville, IN 46410
219-769-3541
Fax: 219-769-0690
www.lakeco.lib.in.us
Talking books provides cassette books, descriptive videos, magazines and large print books to people who are blind and physically handicapped. Materials are sent through the mail and the service is free to those who qualify.
Renee Lewis, Director

Iowa

9749 Iowa Department for the Blind
524 Fourth Street
Des Moines, IA 50309-2364
515-281-1333
800-362-2587
Fax: 515-281-1263
TTY: 515-281-1355
e-mail: information@blind.state.ia.us
www.blind.state.ia.us/Library/
Our program offers the specialized, integrated services that blind and severely visually impaired Iowans need to live independently and work competitively.
Allen Harris, Director

Kansas

9750 CKLS Headquarters
1409 Williams Street
Great Bend, KS 67530-4090
620-792-4865
800-362-2642
Fax: 620-793-7270
e-mail: jswan@ckls.org
www.ckls.org
Offers direct services to rural residents and those who need special services because of disability.
James Swan, Administrator
Joanita Doll-Masden, Department Head

9751 Manhattan Subregional Library of the Kansas Talking Books Service
629 Poyntz Avenue
Manhattan, KS 66502-6006
785-776-4741
800-432-2796
Fax: 785-776-1545
e-mail: annp@manhattan.lib.ks.us
www.manhattan.lib.ks.us
Books and magazines in braille and recorded format and playback equipment are provided to any Kansas citizen residing in the twelve county area of the North Central Kansas Libraries System who is unable to use standard print as a result of temporary or permanent visual or physical impairments.
Ann Pearce, Department Manager
Wandean Rivers, Assistive Technology Center Instructor

9752 Northwest Kansas Library System
Northwest Kansas Library System
2 Washington Square
Norton, KS 67654
785-877-5148
800-432-2858
Fax: 785-877-5697
www.skyways.lib.ks.us
The Kansas Library Network for the Blind and Physically Handicapped, in cooperation with the Library of Congress, National Library Service for the Blind and Physically Handicapped, provides library services and materials to Kansans unable to use conventional print.
Leslie Bell, Director
Clarice Howard, BPH Librarian

9753 South Central Kansas Library System
321A North Main Street
South Hutchinson, KS 67505
800-234-0529
Fax: 313-663-9797
e-mail: phawkins@sckls.info
www.sckls.info/
Summer reading programs, braille writer, magnifiers, closed-circuit TV, large-print photocopier, cassette books and magazines,

children's books on cassette, home visits and other reference materials on blindness and other handicaps.
Paul Hawkins, Director

9754 Talking Books Service
Topeka and Shawnee County Public Library
1515 SW 10th Avenue   785-580-4530
Topeka, KS 66604-1304   800-432-2925
Fax: 785-580-4530
e-mail: tbooks@tscpl.lib.ks.us
www.tscpl.org/services/talkingbooks
Summer reading programs, braille writer, magnifiers, closed-circuit TV, large-print photocopier, cassette books and magazines, children's books on cassette, home visits and other reference materials on blindness and other handicaps.
Suzanne Bundy, Librarian

9755 Wichita Public Library
223 S Main   316-261-8500
Wichita, KS 67202   Fax: 316-262-4540
TDD: 316-262-3972
www.wichita.lib.ks.us
Talking books provides cassette books, descriptive videos, magazines adn large print books to people who are blind and physically handicapped. Materials are sent through the mail and the service is free to those who qualify.
Brad Reha, Talking Books Manager

Kentucky

9756 Kentucky Talking Book Library
PO Box 537   502-564-8300
Frankfort, KY 40602-0537   800-372-2968
Fax: 502-564-5773
e-mail: Wendy.Hatfield@ky.gov
www.kdla.ky.gov
Our mission is to provide library service to individuals who have a visual or physical disability that prevents them from using standard print materials. We send books on tape and Braille books through the mail at no cost to our patrons.
Wendy Hatfield, Librarian, Talking Books

9757 Louisville Talking Book Library for the Blind and Physically Handicapped
301 York Street
Louisville, KY 40203-2205   502-574-1625
www.lfpl.org/tbl
The Louisville Talking Book Library offers recorded books and other materials to eligible visually and physically handicapped Jefferson County, KY residents. All recorded books & equipment may be sent to borrowers and returned by postage-free mail.
Linda Atzinger, Supervisor Accessibility Services

9758 Northern Kentucky Talking Book Library
502 Scott Boulevard   859-962-4095
Covington, KY 41011   866-491-7610
Fax: 859-962-4096
www.kenton.lib.ky.us
Our library provides books and magazines on specially recorded cassettes for people who are visually impaired and/or physically handicapped and live in Boone, Campbell, Carroll, Gallatin, Grant, Kenton, Owen and Pendleton counties.
Dave Schroeder, Director

Louisiana

9759 State Library of Louisiana
701 N 4th Street   225-342-4943
Baton Rouge, LA 70802   Fax: 225-219-4804
e-mail: admin@state.lib.la.us
www.state.lib.la.us
Talking books provides cassette books, descriptive videos, magazines and large print books to people who are blind and physically handicapped. Materials are sent through the mail and the service is free to those who qualify.

Maine

9760 Bangor Public Library
145 Harlow Street   207-947-8336
Bangor, ME 04401-4900   Fax: 207-945-6694
e-mail: bplill@bpl.lib.me.us
www.bpl.lib.me.us
Summer reading programs, braille writer, magnifiers, closed-circuit TV, large-print photocopier, cassette books and magazines, children's books on cassette, home visits and other reference materials on blindness and other handicaps.
Barbara McDade, Director

9761 Cary Library
107 Main Street   207-532-1302
Houlton, ME 04730-2196   Fax: 207-532-4350
www.cary.lib.me.us
Summer reading programs, braille writer, magnifiers, closed-circuit TV, large-print photocopier, cassette books and magazines, children's books on cassette, home visits and other reference materials on blindness and other handicaps.
Linda Faucher, Librarian

9762 Lewiston Public Library
200 Lisbon Street   207-784-0135
Lewiston, ME 04240-7203   Fax: 207-784-3011
TTY: 207-784-3123
e-mail: lplweb@lplonline.org
www.lplonline.org
Summer reading programs, braille writer, magnifiers, closed-circuit TV, large-print photocopier, cassette books and magazines, children's books on cassette, home visits and other reference materials on blindness and other handicaps.

9763 Maine State Library
64 State House Station   207-287-5650
Augusta, ME 04333-0064   800-452-8793
Fax: 207-287-5624
www.state.me.us/msl
Large Print Books is a service through Outreach Services for residents of Maine who are certified as visually impaired and public libraries who serve the visually impaired.
J Gary Nichols, Librarian

9764 Portland Public Library
5 Monument Square   207-871-1700
Portland, ME 04101-4072   Fax: 207-871-1715
e-mail: reference@portland.lib.me.us
www.portlandlibrary.com
Portland Public Library's Outreach Services brings library resources to those who are unable to visit the library in person. For people living in nursing homes or assisted living facilities, or for those confined to home due to illness or disability, the library will deliver print and audio books right to your doorstep.
Stephen J Podgajny, Director

9765 Waterville Public Library
73 Elm Street   207-872-5433
Waterville, ME 04901-6027   Fax: 207-873-4779
www.waterville.lib.me.us
Summer reading programs, braille writer, magnifiers, closed-circuit TV, large-print photocopier, cassette books and magazines, children's books on cassette, home visits and other reference materials on blindness and other handicaps.
Sarah Sugden, Director

Maryland

9766 American Action Fund for Blind Children and Adults
1800 Johnson Street, Suite 100   410-659-9315
Baltimore, MD 21230   e-mail: actionfund@actionfund.org
www.actionfund.org
Our mission is to assist blind persons in securing reading matter, to educate the public about blindness, to give aid to the deaf-blind, to provide specialized aids and appliances to the blind, to give consultation to governmental and private agencies serving the blind, to offer assistance to older blind persons, to offer services to blind

children and their parents, and to do any other lawful thing which it can to improve the quality of life for blind persons.
Barbara Loos, President
Ramona Walhof, First Vice President

9767   Disability Resource Center of Montgomery County Public Libraries
Rockville Library
21 Maryland Avenue   240-777-0140
Rockville, MD 20850   TTY: 240-777-0902
e-mail: drcinfo@montgomerycountymd.gov
www.montgomerycountymd.gov
The Disability Resource Center (DRC) is the focal point within the Montgomery County Public Libraries (MCPL) for library and literacy services to people with disabilities, their families, caretakers and professionals.
Kay Bowman, Agency Manager

9768   International Braille and Technology Center for the Blind
National Federation of the Blind
1800 Johnson Street
Baltimore, MD 21230-4998   410-659-9314
Fax: 410-685-5653
e-mail: ataylor@nfb.org
www.nfb.org
A comprehensive and complete evaluation and demonstration center for assistive technology used by the blind worldwide. Includes all Braille, synthetic speech, print-to-speech scanning, internet and portable devices and programs. Available for tours by appointment to blind persons, employers, technology manufacturers, teachers, parents and those working in the assistive technology field.
Ann Taylor, Director Technology

9769   Maryland State Library for the Blind and Physically Handicapped
415 Park Avenue   410-230-2424
Baltimore, MD 21201   800-964-9209
Fax: 410-333-2095
TTY: 800-934-2541
www.lbph.lib.md/us
The basic mission of the Maryland State Library for the Blind and Physically Handicapped is to provide comprehensive library services to the eligible blind and physically handicapped residents of the State of Maryland.
Jill Lewis, Director

9770   Prince George's County Memorial Library: Talking Book Center
6532 Adelphi Road
Hyattsville, MD 20782-2098   301-699-3500
www.prge.lib.md.us
Talking books provides cassette books, descriptive videos, magazines and large print books to people who are blind and physically handicapped. Materials are sent through the mail and the services are free to those who qualify.
Maralita Freeny, Director

Massachusetts

9771   Caption Center
125 Western Avenue   617-492-9225
Allston, MA 02134-1008   Fax: 617-562-0590
Provides closed captioning for videos, including training, safety, instructional and educational films. Maintains a consumer information service for overcoming communications barriers in the workplace.
Lori Kay, Co-Director
Tom Apone, Co-Director

9772   Laboure College Library
2120 Dorchester Avenue   617-296-8300
Boston, MA 02124-5617   e-mail: library@laboure.edu
www.laboure.edu
Offers information on physical disabilities, independent living, peer counseling and advocacy.
Maryann O'Toole, Director

9773   Perkins Braille and Talking Book Library
175 N Beacon Street   617-972-7240
Watertown, MA 02472-2751   800-852-3133
Fax: 617-972-7363
TTY: 617-972-7690
e-mail: library@perkins.org
www.perkins.org
The Perkins Braille & Talking Book Library, funded in part by the Massachusetts Board of Library Commissioners, provides free services to Massachusetts residents of any age who are unable to read traditional print materials due to a visual or physical disability.
Kim Charlson, Director

9774   Talking Book Library at Worcester Public Library
3 Salem Square   508-799-1730
Worcester, MA 1608-2074   800-762-0085
Fax: 508-799-1676
e-mail: talkbook@cwmars.org/talkingbook
www.cwmars.org/talkingbook
Adapted computers, braille embosser, magnifiers, closed circuit TV, large print books, cassette books and magazines, children's books on cassette, reference materials on blindness and other disabilities. Summer reading programs.
James L Izatt, Librarian

Michigan

9775   Detroit Subregional Library for the Blind and Physically Handicapped
Detroit Public Library
3666 Grand River Avenue   313-833-5494
Detroit, MI 48208   Fax: 313-325-97
TDD: 313-833-5492
e-mail: dmiddle@detroitpubliclibrary.org
www.detroit.lib.mi.us
Talking books along with talking book machines are available to eligible residents who live in a 14 ZIP code area of Detroit and Highland Park. Loans of the books and machines are made to individuals and to institutions such as schools, nursing homes and senior residences. Over 45,000 books are available. Magazines available in recorded format include Ebony, Good Housekeeping, and Sports Illustrated.
Dori V. Middleton, LBPH Specialist

9776   Grand Traverse Area Library for the Blind and Physically Handicapped
322 6th Street   616-935-6520
Traverse City, MI 49684-2414   Fax: 616-922-0904
TDD: 616-922-0901
Evelyn Welty

9777   Kent County Library for the Blind
775 Ball Avenue NE   616-336-3250
Grand Rapids, MI 49503-1397   Fax: 616-336-3256
e-mail: kdlem@lakeland.lib.mi.us
Summer reading programs, braille writer, magnifiers, closed-circuit TV, large-print photocopier, cassette books and magazines, children's books on cassette, home visits and other reference materials on blindness and other handicaps.
Claudya Muller, Librarian

9778   Library of Michigan Service for the Blind
PO Box 30007   517-373-5614
Lansing, MI 48909-7507   Fax: 517-735-65
e-mail: sbph@michigan.gov
www.michigan.gov/sbth
Braille writer, magnifiers, closed circuit TV, large print photocopier, cassette books and magazines, children's books on cassette, reference materials on blindness and other handicaps. Books on cassette and braille books and cassette players will be loaned and sent through the mail at no charge. For blind and those physically unable to read standard print or turn the pages.
Susan Thinault, Manager

9779   Macomb Library for the Blind and Physically Handicapped
16480 Hall Road   810-286-1580
Clinton Township, MI 48038-1132   Fax: 810-286-0634
                                         TDD: 8102869940
                          e-mail: macbld@libcoop.net
                          www.macomb.lib.mi.us/macspe
Summer reading programs, braille writer, closed-circuit TV, cassette books and magazines, children's books on cassette, reference materials on blindness and other handicaps.
Beverlee Babcock, Librarian

9780   Midwestern Michigan Library Cooperative
G4195 West Pasadena Avenue   810-732-1120
Flint, MI 48504   Fax: 810-321-15
                          www.mideasteRN.lib.mi.us

Roger Mendell, Director

9781   Muskegon County Library for the Blind
635 Ottawa Street   616-724-6248
Muskegon, MI 49442-1016   Fax: 616-724-6675
                                         TDD: 616-722-4103
Summer reading programs, braille typewriter, magnifiers, closed-circuit TV, large-print photocopier, cassette books and magazines, children's books on cassette, home visits and other reference materials on blindness and other handicaps, The Reading Edge, Perkins Brailler and large print books.
Linda Clapp, Librarian

9782   Northland Library Cooperative
316 E Chisholm Street   517-356-1622
Alpena, MI 49707-2892   Fax: 517-354-3939
                          e-mail: nlc.lib.mi.us/lbph.htm
Summer reading programs, braille writer, magnifiers, closed-circuit TV, large-print photocopier, cassette books and magazines, children's books on cassette, home visits and other reference materials on blindness and other handicaps.
Catherine Glomski, Librarian

9783   Oakland County Library for the Visually and Physically Impaired
1200 N Telegraph Road   248-858-5050
Pontiac, MI 48341-1032   800-774-4542
                                         Fax: 248-858-9313
                          e-mail: lVPi@co.oakland..mi.us
                          www.co.oakland.mi.us/lVPi
Free cassette book service to eligible visually or physically impaired Oakland County residents; demonstrations, CCTV and hand held magnifiers and a large print collection.
David Conklin, Head Librarian

9784   St. Clark County Library for the Blind and Physically Handicapped
210 McMorran Boulevard   810-987-7323
Port Huron, MI 48060-4014   Fax: 810-987-7327
Offers library services to the blind and visually impaired.
Jackie Skinner, Librarian

9785   Upper Peninsula Library for the Blind and Physically Handicapped
1615 Presque Isle Avenue   906-228-7697
Marquette, MI 49855-2811   Fax: 906-285-27
                          e-mail: uproc.lib.mi.us
                          www.michigan.gov/sbth
Summer reading programs, braille writer, magnifiers, closed-circuit TV, large-print photocopier, cassette books and magazines, children's books on cassette, home visits and other reference materials on blindness and other handicaps.
Susan Thinault, Manager

9786   Washtenaw County Library for the Blind and Physically Disabled
PO Box 8645   734-971-6059
Ann Arbor, MI 48107-8645   Fax: 734-971-3892
                          e-mail: lbpd@co.washtennaw.mi.us
                          comnet.org/cgi-bin/helpnet/viewitem?290+
Book lovers club.adaptive technology,cassette equipment, cassette books and magazines, described videos, low vision aids reference and referral services.
Margaret Wolfe, Cordinator

9787   Wayne County Regional Library for the Blind and Physically Handicapped
30555 Michigan Avenue   734-727-7300
Westland, MI 48186-5310   888-968-2737
                                         Fax: 734-727-7333
                                         TDD: 313-326-3008
                          e-mail: werlbph@tln.lib.mi.us
                          www.tln.lib.mi.us
Summer reading programs, braille writer, magnifiers, closed-circuit TV, large-print photocopier, cassette books and magazines, children's books on cassette, home visits and other reference materials on blindness and other handicaps.
Pat Klemans, Librarian

Minnesota

9788   Duluth Public Library
City of Duluth Department
520 W Superior Street   218-723-3800
Duluth, MN 55802-1578   Fax: 218-233-15
                          e-mail: webmail@duluth.li.mn.us
                          www.duluth.lib.mn.us
Adapted access to Apple computer, adapted toys and adapted library equipment.
Randall Deth Kelly, Director

9789   Minnesota Library for the Blind
388 South East 6 Avenue   507-333-4828
Faribault, MN 55021   800-722-0550
                                         Fax: 507-333-4832
                          e-mail: mn.lbph@state.mn.us
                          www.education.state.mn.us
Summer reading programs, braille writer, magnifiers, closed-circuit TV, large-print photocopier, cassette books and magazines, children's books on cassette, home visits and other reference materials on blindness and other handicaps.
Catherine Durivage, Director

Mississippi

9790   Mississippi Library Commission
1221 Ellis Avenue   601-961-4111
Jackson, MS 39209-7328   800-647-7542
                                         Fax: 601-961-4113
                                         TDD: 601-354-6411
                          e-mail: mslib@mic.lib.ms.us
                          www.mlc.lib.ms.us
Summer reading programs, braille writer, magnifiers, closed-circuit TV, large-print photocopier, cassette books and magazines, children's books on cassette, home visits and other reference materials on blindness and other handicaps.
Larry Mc Millan, Director

Missouri

9791   Adriene Resource Center for Blind Children
Assembly of God Center for Blind
1445 Boonville Avenue   417-831-1964
Springfield, MO 65802   Fax: 417-625-20
                          e-mail: blind@ag.org
                          www.blind.ag.org
Offers braille and cassette lending library, braille and cassette Sunday school materials for all ages, braille and cassette periodicals and resource assistance, and resources for blind children and children of blind parents.
Paul Weingariner, Director
Caryl Weingariner, Co-Director

9792   Assemblies of God National Center for the Blind
1445 Boonville Avenue   417-831-1964
Springfield, MO 65802   Fax: 417-627-66
                          e-mail: blind@ag.org
Offers braille and cassette lending library, braille and cassette Sunday school materials for all ages, braille and cassette periodicals and resource assistance, and resources for blind children and children of blind parents.
Paul Weingariner, Director

9793 Church of the Nazarene
Nazarene Publishing House
PO Box 419527 816-931-1900
Kansas City, MO 64141-6527 800-877-0700
e-mail: NPH@direct.nph.com
www.nph.com
Offers braille and large print books. Also offers a lending library
and cassettes for the blind.

9794 Lutheran Library for the Blind
Lutheran Church - Missouri Synod
1333 S Kirkwood Road 314-965-9000
Saint Louis, MO 63122-7295 800-843-5267
Fax: 314-996-1016
e-mail: infocenter@lems.org
www.lcms.org
Offers braille and large print books and cassettes for the blind and
visually impaired.

9795 Whitney Library for the Blind: Assemblies of God
1445 N Boonville Avenue 417-862-2781
Springfield, MO 65802-1894 Fax: 417-863-7566
www.gospelpublishing.com
Offers braille and cassette lending library, braille and cassette
Sunday school materials for all ages, braille and cassette periodi-
cals and resource assistance.
Paul Weingariner, Librarian

9796 Wolfner Memorial Library for the Blind
PO Box 387 573-751-8720
Jefferson City, MO 65102-387 800-392-2614
Fax: 573-526-2985
TDD: 800-347-1379
e-mail: wolfner@sos.mo.gov
www.sos.mo.gov/wolfner
Summer reading programs, braille writer, closed circuit TV, large
print photocopier, cassette books and magazines, children's books
on cassette, home visits and other reference materials on blindness
and other handicaps.
Richard J Smith, Director Wolfner Library
Debbie Musselman, Administrative Program Coordinator

Montana

9797 Montana State Library
1515 E 6th Avenue 406-444-3009
Helena, MT 59620-1800 Fax: 406-444-5612
Summer reading programs, braille writer, magnifiers, closed-circuit TV, large-print photocopier, cassette books and magazines,
children's books on cassette, home visits and other reference materials on blindness and other handicaps.
Darlene Staffeldt, Director

Nebraska

9798 Nebraska Library Commission Talking Book and Braille Services
1200 N Street, Suite 120 402-471-4038
Lincoln, NE 68508-2023 800-742-7691
e-mail: nlc.talkingbook@nebraska.gov
www.nlc.nebraska.gov/tbbs
Free loan of books and magazines on flash cartridge, cassette, and
in Braille, including children's materials, along with specially designed playback equipment. Summer reading program for children
and young adults, Braille embossing, closed circuit TV,large-print
copier. Reference materials on blindness and other disabilities.
David Oertli, Director
Kay Goehring, Reader Services Coordinator

9799 North Platte Public Library
120 W 4th Street 308-535-8036
North Platte, NE 69101-3901 Fax: 308-535-8296
e-mail: library@ci.north-platte.ne.us
www.ci.north-platte.ne.us/library
Summer reading programs, braille writer, magnifiers, closed-circuit TV, large-print photocopier, cassette books and magazines,
children's books on cassette, home visits and other reference materials on blindness and other handicaps.
Cecelia Lawrence, Library Director

Nevada

9800 Las Vegas Clark County Library District
833 Las Vegas Boulevard N
Las Vegas, NV 89101-5256 702-734-7323
www.lvccld.org
Summer reading programs, braille writer, magnifiers, closed circuit TV, large-print photocopier, cassette books and magazines,
children's books on cassette, home visits and other reference materials on blindness and other handicaps.
Daniel Walters, Executive Directors

9801 Nevada State Library and Archives
100 North Stewart Street 775-684-3360
Carson City, NV 89701-4285 800-922-2880
Fax: 775-684-3330
TDD: 775-687-8338
e-mail: nslref@clan.lib.nv.us
dmla.clan.lib.nv.us/
Summer reading programs, braille writer, magnifiers, closed-circuit TV, large-print photocopier, cassette books and magazines,
children's books on cassette, home visits and other reference materials on blindness and other handicaps.
Kevin E Putnam, Librarian

New Hampshire

9802 New Hampshire State Library
117 Pleasant Street 603-271-3429
Concord, NH 03301-3852 Fax: 603-271-8370
e-mail: talking@lilac.nhsh.lib.nh.us
www.state.nh.us
Summer reading programs, braille writer, magnifiers, closed-circuit TV, large-print photocopier, cassette books and magazines,
children's books on cassette, home visits and other reference materials on blindness and other handicaps.
Eileen Keim, Librarian

9803 Voices for the Blind
PO Box 781 603-332-9355
Barrington, NH 3825
Tape library and depository for people with visual and learning dis-
abilities. Recording services available by request.
Connie Hindman, Director

New Jersey

9804 New Jersey Library for the Blind and Handicapped
2300 Stuyvesant Avenue 609-530-4000
Trenton, NJ 08618-3226 800-792-8322
Fax: 609-530-6384
TDD: 877-882-5593
e-mail: nglbh@njstatelib.org
www2.njstatelib.org/lbh/index.htm
Summer reading programs, large print, cassette, braille books and
magazines, children's books on cassette and brailles and other reference materials on blindness and other handicaps.
Deborah Toomey, Director

New Mexico

9805 New Mexico State Library for the Blind and Physically Handicapped
National Library Services
1209 Camino Carlos Rey 505-476-9770
Santa Fe, NM 87507 800-456-5515
Fax: 505-476-9776
e-mail: lbph@stlib.state.nm.us
www.stlib.state.nm.us
Summer reading programs, braille writer, magnifiers, closed-circuit TV, large-print photocopier, cassette books and magazines,
children's books on cassette, home visits and other reference materials on blindness and other handicaps.
John Mugford, Library Manager

New York

9806 **Choice Magazine Listening**
85 Channel Drive   516-883-8280
Port Washington, NY 11050-2216   888-724-6423
Fax: 516-944-6849
e-mail: choicemag@aol.com
www.choicemagazinelistening.org
A free recorded spoken word magazine anthology for anyone college level and older unable to read large print because of visual or physical handicaps. Produced on special speed cassette format, playable on free library of congress player.
Sondra Mochson, Editor

9807 **JGB Cassette Library International**
Jewish Guild for the Blind
15 W 65th Street   212-769-6331
New York, NY 10023-6601   Fax: 212-769-6266
e-mail: bemass@aol.com
Summer reading programs, braille writer, magnifiers, closed-circuit TV, large-print photocopier, cassette books and magazines, children's books on cassette, home visits and other reference materials on blindness and other handicaps.
Bruce Massis

9808 **Nassau Library System**
900 Jerusalem Avenue   516-292-8920
Uniondale, NY 11553-3039   Fax: 516-481-4777
e-mail: nls@lilrc.org
Summer reading programs, braille writer, magnifiers, closed-circuit TV, large-print photocopier, cassette books and magazines, children's books on cassette, home visits and other reference materials on blindness and other handicaps.
Dorothy Pruyear, Librarian

9809 **New York State Talking Book & Braille Library, New York State Library, DOE**
Empire State Plaza, CEC   518-474-5935
Albany, NY 12230-0001   800-342-3688
Fax: 518-486-1957
e-mail: tbbl@mail.nysed.gov
www.nysl.nysed.gov/tbbl/
Books on audio cassette, cassette players, braille books, summer reading programs, braille writer, magnifiers, closed-circuit TV, large-print photocopier, cassette books and magazines, children's books on cassette, reference materials on blindness and other disabilities. Library is part of the National Service Network serving those with print disabilities. Available: audio and braille books sent post-free by mail, euipment loans, services to schools and institutions. Serves 55 New York counties.
Sharon B. Phillips, Program Director

9810 **Suffolk Cooperative Library System**
627 N Sunrise Service Road   631-286-1600
Bellport, NY 11713-9000   Fax: 631-286-1647
scls.suffolk.lib.ny.us
Talking books services.
Julie Klauber, Adjunct Professor

9811 **Xavier Society for the Blind**
154 E 23rd Street   212-473-7800
New York, NY 10010-4501   800-637-9193
Fax: 212-473-7801
e-mail: xaviersocietyfortheblind@yahoo.com
www.xaviersociety.com
Provides spiritual and inspirational reading material to visually impaired persons in suitable format: Braille, large print and cassette, throughout the USA and Canada. Services provided by way of regular periodicals which are non-returnable, and through our lending library where books are returned. All services are provided free of charge, and interested persons can write or phone.
Alfred Caruana, Executive Director
Margie Montenegro, Client Services Representative

North Carolina

9812 **North Carolina Library for the Blind**
1841 Capital Boulevard   919-733-4376
Raleigh, NC 27635   888-388-2460
Fax: 919-733-6910
TDD: 919-733-1462
e-mail: nclbph@ncdcr.gov
statelibrary.ncdcr.gov/lbph
A general interest library offering books and magazines at no cost in large print, in braille on audio cassette for anyone who cannot use regular print in North Carolina due to physical or visual disability. Summer reading programs, braille writer, magnifiers, closed circuit TV, large print photocopier, cassette books and magazines, children's books on cassette, digital, cartridges and large print and other reference materials.
Carl Keehn, Director

North Dakota

9813 **North Dakota State Library Services for the Disabled**
North Dakota State Library
604 E Boulevard Avenue   701-328-1408
Bismarck, ND 58505-800   800-843-9948
Fax: 701-328-2040
TDD: 800-892-8622
e-mail: tbooks@state.nd.us
ndsl.lib.state.nd.us

Stella Cone, Regional Librarian

9814 **North Dakota State Library Talking Book Services**
604 E Boulevard Avenue   701-328-1408
Bismarck, ND 58505-0800   800-843-9948
Fax: 701-328-2040
TDD: 800-892-8622
e-mail: twilhelm@state.nd.us
ndsl.lib.state.nd.us

Terria Wilhelm, Talking Book Manager

9815 **Services for the Visually Impaired**
8720 Georgia Avenue   301-589-0894
Silver, MD 20910   Fax: 301-589-7281
www.servicesvi.org
Eligible readers of North Dakota receive library service from the regional library in Pierre, South Dakota.
Betty Bender

Ohio

9816 **Case Western Reserve University**
10900 Euclid Avenue
Cleveland, OH 44117-2620   216-368-2000
www.cwru.edu
Research in electrical stimulation and rehabilitation technology.
Jeanne O'Malley Teeter, Manager

9817 **Ohio Regional Library for the Blind and Physically Handicapped**
800 Vine Street   513-369-6999
Cincinnati, OH 45202   800-528-0335
Fax: 513-369-3111
TDD: 513-369-6072
www.cincinatilibrary.org/main/lb.asp
Summer reading programs, braille writer, magnifiers, closed-circuit TV, large-print photocopier, cassette books and magazines, children's books on cassette, home visits and other reference materials on blindness and other handicaps.
Donna Foust, Librarian

9818 **State Library of Ohio Talking Book Program**
274 E First Avenue   614-644-6895
Columbus, OH 43201-3673   800-686-1531
Fax: 614-995-2186
winslo.state.oh.us/services
A machine-lending agency for the visually impaired.
Roger Verney, Head Supervisor

Oklahoma

9819 Oklahoma Library for the Blind and Physically Handicapped
300 NE 18th Street   405-521-3514
Oklahoma City, OK 73105-3212   Fax: 405-214-82
www.state.ok.us/~library
Summer reading programs, braille writer, magnifiers, closed-circuit TV, large-print photocopier, cassette books and magazines, children's books on cassette, home visits and other reference materials on blindness and other handicaps.
Geraldine Adams, Director

9820 Tulsa City: County Library System
400 Civic Center   918-596-7977
Tulsa, OK 74103-3830   Fax: 918-596-7990
www.tulsalibrary.org
Summer reading programs, braille writer, magnifiers, closed-circuit TV, large-print photocopier, cassette books and magazines, children's books on cassette, home visits and other reference materials on blindness and other handicaps.
Ellen Ontko, Librarian

Oregon

9821 Oregon State Library
250 Winter Street NE   503-378-4243
Salem, OR 97301-3950   800-452-0292
Fax: 503-588-7119
TDD: 503-378-4276
www.oregon.gov/osl
Summer reading programs, braille writer, magnifiers, closed-circuit TV, large-print photocopier, cassette books and magazines, children's books on cassette, home visits and other reference materials on blindness and other handicaps.
Jim Scheppke, Head Librarian

Pennsylvania

9822 Carnegie Library of Pittsburgh
4724 Baum Boulevard   412-687-2440
Pittsburgh, PA 15213-1321   800-242-0586
Fax: 412-687-2442
e-mail: lbph@carnegielibrary.org
www.clpgh.org/clp/LBPH
Provides on loan recorded books and magazines, large print books, and described videos to Western Pennsylvannia residents unable to use standard printed materials due to visual, physical, or physically-based reading disabilities. Also loans special cassette and disc machines; does not loan equipment to play described videos. Information about disabilities and related agencies is also available.
Sue Murdock, Director
Kathleen Kappel, Assistant Director

9823 Free Library of Philadelphia
919 Walnut Street   215-925-3213
Philadelphia, PA 19107-5237   Fax: 215-928-0856
e-mail: flpblind@library.phila.gov
Summer reading programs, braille writer, magnifiers, closed-circuit TV, large-print photocopier, cassette books and magazines, children's books on cassette, home visits and other reference materials on blindness and other handicaps.
Vickie Lange Collins, Librarian

Rhode Island

9824 Rhode Island Department of State Library for the Blind and Physically Handicapped
1 Capitol Hl   401-277-2726
Providence, RI 02908-5803   Fax: 401-277-4195
e-mail: richard@dsl.rhilinet.gov
Offers information and services for the visually impaired including reference materials, braille printers, braille writers, large-print books and more.
Richard Ledue, Librarian

South Carolina

9825 South Carolina State Library
PO Box 11469   803-734-8666
Columbia, SC 29202-0821   Fax: 803-734-8676
TDD: 803-734-7298
e-mail: guynell@leo.scsl.state.sc.us
www.state.sc.us/scsl
Summer reading programs, braille writer, magnifiers, closed-circuit TV, large-print photocopier, cassette books and magazines, children's books on cassette, home visits and other reference materials on blindness and other handicaps.
Guynell Williams, Librarian

South Dakota

9826 South Dakota State Library
800 Governors Drive   605-773-3131
Pierre, SD 57501-2235   Fax: 605-734-50
TDD: 605-773-4950
e-mail: daRN@stlib.state.sd.us
www.sdstatelibrary.com
Summer reading programs, braille writer, magnifiers, closed-circuit TV, large-print photocopier, cassette books and magazines, children's books on cassette, home visits and other reference materials on blindness and other handicaps.
Daniel Boyd, Librarian

Tennessee

9827 LRC for Students with Disabilities
MSU Library Reference Department
Memphis State University   901-678-2208
Memphis, TN 38152-0001   800-669-2267
Fax: 901-678-3070
www.memphis.edu
Information on physical disabilities, blindness and visual impairments.
Ross Johnson, Reference Librarian

9828 Tennessee Library for the Blind and Physically Handicapped
National Library Services
403 7th Avenue N   615-741-3915
Nashville, TN 37243-1409   800-342-3308
Fax: 615-532-8856
e-mail: tlbph@mail.state.tn/sos/statelib/LBPH/
www.state.tn.us
Offers free public library services to those unable to hold, read, or turn the pages of books and magazines due to physical or visual impairment. Collections include books and magazines in large print, braille and audio format. Players loaned for the audio books and magazines. All items are delivered and returned via the US Postal Service free matter mailing.
Ruth Hemphill, Director
Janie Murphee, Assistant Director

Texas

9829 Christian Resource for People Who Are Blind
Care Ministries Inc
PO Box 1830   662-323-4999
Starkville, MS 39760-1830   800-366-2232
e-mail: care@careministries.org
www.careministries.org
Offers braille and large print books and cassettes for the visually impaired.
B J LeJeune, Director

9830 Houston Public Library Access Center
500 McKinney Street   832-393-1313
Houston, TX 77002-2534   Fax: 832-931-83
e-mail: website@hpl.lib.tx.us
www.houstonlibrary.org
Offers Kurzweil Reading Machine 400, closed-circuit TV, braille writer, reference materials on visual impairments and other handicaps.
Heidi Miller, Supervisor

9831 **Texas State Library**
PO Box 12927
Austin, TX 78711-2927
512-463-5460
Fax: 512-635-36
TDD: 512-463-5449
e-mail: dale.propp@tsl.state.tx.us
Summer reading programs, braille writer, magnifiers, closed-circuit TV, large-print photocopier, cassette books and magazines, children's books on cassette, home visits and other reference materials on blindness and other handicaps.
Dale Propp, Librarian

9832 **Texas State Library: Talking Book Program**
1201 Brazos Street
Austin, TX 78711-2927
512-463-5458
800-252-9605
Fax: 512-936-0685
e-mail: tbp.services@tsl.state.tx.us
www.texastalkingbooks.org
Part of the free National Library Services. Provides equipment and books in alternate formats to qualified individuals who cannot read standard print. Certified applications required. Disabilities and information referral services available.
Ava Smith, Librarian
Dina Abramson, Disabilities/Information Referral

Utah

9833 **Utah State Library Division**
Program for the Blind and Disabled
250 North 1950 West, Suite A
Salt Lake City, UT 84116-7901
801-715-6789
800-662-5540
Fax: 801-715-6767
TDD: 801-715-6721
e-mail: blind@utah.gov
http://blindlibrary.utah.gov
Library providing services to individuals with visual impairments who cannot read standard print.
Bessie Y. Oakes, Director

Vermont

9834 **Vermont Department of Libraries Special Services Unit**
578 Paine Turnpike North
Berlin, VT 05602
802-828-3273
800-479-1711
Fax: 802-828-2199
e-mail: ssu@mail.dol.state.vt.us
dol.state.vt.us
Summer reading programs, braille writer, magnifiers, closed-circuit TV, large-print photocopier, cassette books and magazines, children's books on cassette, home visits and other reference materials on blindness and other handicaps.
Theresa Faust, Librarian

Virginia

9835 **Arlington County Department of Libraries**
1015 N Quincy Street
Arlington, VA 22201-4603
703-228-5959
Fax: 703-358-5962
TDD: 703-358-6320
Summer reading programs, braille writer, magnifiers, closed-circuit TV, large-print photocopier, cassette books and magazines, children's books on cassette, home visits and other reference materials on blindness and other handicaps.
Roxanne Barnes, Librarian

9836 **Central Rappahannock Regional Library**
1201 Caroline Street
Fredericksburg, VA 22401-3701
540-372-1144
Fax: 540-373-9411
TDD: 540-371-9165
e-mail: nschiff@hq.crrl.org
Offers reference materials on blindness and other disabilities.
Nancy Schiff, Librarian

9837 **Division for the Visually Handicapped**
1110 N Glebe Road
Arlington, VA 22201
703-620-3660
888-232-7733
Fax: 703-264-9494
e-mail: service@cec.sped.org
www.cec.sped.org

Members are teachers, college faculty members, administrators, supervisors and others concerned with the education and welfare of visually handicapped and blind children and youth. This is a division of the Council For Exceptional Children.

9838 **Fairfax County Public Library**
12000 Government Center Parkway
Fairfax, VA 22035-0012
703-660-6943
Fax: 703-765-5893
TDD: 703-660-8524
e-mail: sjapikse@leo.vsla.edu
www.co.fairfax.va.us
Summer reading programs, braille writer, magnifiers, closed-circuit TV, large-print photocopier, cassette books and magazines, children's books on cassette, home visits and other reference materials on blindness and other handicaps.
Jeanette Studley, Librarian

9839 **Hampton Subregional Library for the Blind**
1 South Malory Street
Hampton, VA 23663-4243
757-727-1900
800-552-7015
www.hamptonpubliclibrary.org
Summer reading programs, braille writer, magnifiers, closed-circuit TV, large-print photocopier, cassette books and magazines, children's books on cassette, home visits and other reference materials on blindness and other handicaps.
Douglas Perry, Director

9840 **Newport News Public Library System**
110 Main Street
Newport News, VA 23601-4105
757-591-4858
Fax: 757-591-7425
e-mail: shalswin@leo.vsla.edu
www.newport-news.va.us
Summer reading programs, braille writer, magnifiers, closed-circuit TV, large-print photocopier, cassette books and magazines, children's books on cassette, home visits and other reference materials on blindness and other handicaps.
Sue Balswin, Librarian

9841 **Roanoke City Public Library System**
2607 Salem Tpke NW
Roanoke, VA 24017-5333
540-853-2648
Fax: 540-853-1030
Summer reading programs, braille writer, magnifiers, closed-circuit TV, large-print photocopier, cassette books and magazines, children's books on cassette, home visits and other reference materials on blindness and other handicaps.
Rebecca Cooper, Librarian

9842 **Staunton Public Library: Talking Book Center**
1 Churchville Avenue
Staunton, VA 24401-3229
540-885-6215
800-995-6215
Fax: 540-332-3906
e-mail: talkingbook@ci.staunton.via.us
www.loc.gov/nls
Sub-regional library for those who are unable to use standard print materials due to visual, physical, or reading disability.
Oakley Pearson, Librarian

9843 **University Library Services**
Virginia Commonwealth University
901 Park Avenue
Richmond, VA 23284-2033
804-828-1105
Fax: 804-828-0150
www.ucu.edu
Library services for the visually disabled.
Sally Jacobs, Reference Librarian

9844 **Virginia Beach Public Library**
936 Independence Boulevard
Virginia Beach, VA 23455-6006
757-460-7518
Fax: 757-460-6741
vbgov.com/libraries
Summer reading programs, braille writer, magnifiers, closed-circuit TV, large-print photocopier, cassette books and magazines, children's books on cassette, home visits and other reference materials on blindness and other handicaps.
Susan Head, Librarian

9845 Washington Talking Book & Braille Library
2021 9th Avenue   206-615-0400
Seattle, WA 98121   Fax: 206-615-0437
                                      TTY: 206-615-0418
                          e-mail: wtbbl@spl.lib.wa.us
                                      www.wtbbl.org

Summer reading programs, braille writer, magnifiers, closed-circuit TV, large-print photocopier, cassette books and magazines, children's books on cassette, home visits and other reference materials on blindness and other handicaps.
Danielle Miller, Director

9846 Cabell County Public Library
455 9th Street   304-528-5700
Huntington, WV 25701-1417   Fax: 304-285-01
                          e-mail: tbooks@cabell.libwv.us
                                      www.cabell.lib.wv.us

Summer reading programs, braille writer, magnifiers, Arkenstone reader/scanner, cassette books and magazines, children's books on cassette, home visits and other reference materials on blindness and other handicaps.
Vicky Woods, Talking Books Coordinator
Kurle K Judy, Director

9847 Kanawha County Public Library
123 Capitol Street   304-343-4646
Charleston, WV 25301-2609   Fax: 304-348-6530
                                      kanawha.lib.wv.us

Summer reading programs, braille writer, magnifiers, closed-circuit TV, large-print photocopier, cassette books and magazines, children's books on cassette, home visits and other reference materials on blindness and other handicaps.
Dixie Smith, Librarian

9848 Ohio County Public Library Services for the Blind and Physically Handicapped
52 16th Street   304-232-0244
Wheeling, WV 26003-3671   Fax: 304-232-6848
                          e-mail: llnicholson@hotmail.com
Lori Nicholson, Subregional Librarian BIPH

9849 Parkersburg and Wood County Public Library
3100 Emerson Avenue   304-420-4587
Parkersburg, WV 26104-2414   800-642-8674
                                      Fax: 304-420-4589
                          e-mail: raitzb@hp9k.park.lib.wv.us
                                      parkersburg.lib.wv.us

Services for the bind and physically handicapped.
Michael Hickman

9850 West Virginia Library Commission
1900 Kanawha Boulevard E   304-558-2041
Charleston, WV 25305-0009   800-642-9021
                                      Fax: 304-558-2044
                          e-mail: web_one@wvlc.lib.wv.us
                                      librarycommission.lib.wv.us

Summer reading programs, braille writer, magnifiers, closed-circuit TV, large-print photocopier, cassette books and magazines, children's books on cassette, home visits and other reference materials on blindness and other handicaps.
Francis Fesenmainer, Librarian

9851 West Virginia School for the Blind
301 E Main Street   304-822-4800
Romney, WV 26757-1828   Fax: 304-822-3377
                          e-mail: cjohn@access.mountain.net

Summer reading programs, braille writer, magnifiers, closed-circuit TV, large-print photocopier, cassette books and magazines, children's books on cassette, home visits and other reference materials on blindness and other handicaps.
Cynthia Johnson, Librarian

9852 Brown County Library
515 Pine Street   920-448-4400
Green Bay, WI 54301-5194   Fax: 920-448-4376
                                      www.co.brown.wi.us

Summer reading programs, braille writer, magnifiers, closed-circuit TV, large-print photocopier, cassette books and magazines, children's books on cassette, home visits and other reference materials on blindness and other handicaps.
Lynn Stainbrook, Director

9853 Wisconsin Regional Library for the Blind Talking Book Program
813 W Wells Street   414-286-3045
Milwaukee, WI 53233-1436   800-242-8822
                                      Fax: 414-286-3102
                                      TDD: 414-286-3548
                          e-mail: mvalne@mpl.org
                                      www.regionallibrary.wi.gov

Circulates recorded materials, playback equipment and braille materials to print-handicapped Wisconsin residents.
Marsha Valance, Regional Librarian

9854 Wyoming Services for the Visually Disabled
State Department of Education
2300 Capitol Avenue Hathaway Buildi   307-777-7690
Cheyenne, WY 82002-50   Fax: 307-776-34
                                      http//www.k12.wy.us

Eligible readers of Wyoming receive library service from the regional library in Salt Lake City, Utah.
Duane Edmonds, Chairman
Ruby Calvert, Vice Chairman

Research Centers

9855 Baylor College of Medicine: Cullen Eye Institute
6565 Fannin   713-798-6100
Houston, TX 77030-2703   800-229-5676
                                      Fax: 713-798-4231
                          e-mail: ophthalmology@bcm.edu
                                      www.bcm.edu/eye

Research activities focus on restoring vision and preventing blindness through a better understanding of the disease.
Dan B Jones, Professor and Chair
Milton Boniuk, Professor

9856 BermanGund Laboratory for the Study of Retinal Degenerations
Massachusetts Eye & Eye Infirmary
243 Charles Street   617-523-7900
Boston, MA 02114-3002   Fax: 617-733-44
                          e-mail: directors@meei.harvard.edu
                                      www.meei.harvard.edu

We strive to offer you the highest quality care from our physicians nurses and clinical staff who are world-leaders in their specialties.ÿFrom the moment you arrive at Mass. Eye and Ear through the completion of your visit we hope that you will feel confident you are in the best hands for care of your eyes ears nose throat head and neck.ÿ
John Fernandez, President
Javier Balloffet, VP-Ophthalmology

9857 Braille Institute Desert Center
70251 Ramon Road   760-321-1111
Rancho Mirage, CA 92270-5203   800-212-4533
                                      Fax: 760-321-9715
                          e-mail: dc@brailleinstitute.org
                                      www.brailleinstitute.org

Dedicated to providing blind and visually impaired men women and children with the training programs and services they need to enjoy productive lives. Services offered include child development youth programs library services and adult education.
Leslie E Stocker Jr, President
Sally H Jameson, VP of Programs and Services

9858 Braille Institute Orange County Center
527 N Dale Avenue   714-821-5000
Anaheim, CA 92801-4899   Fax: 714-527-7621
                                          e-mail: oc@brailleinstitute.org
                                          www.brailleinstitute.org
Offers services publications information and programs to blind
and visually impaired persons.
Sheila F Daily, Orange County Regional Director
Gene Mathiowetz, Assistant Regional Director

**9859 Braille Institute Santa Barbara Center Braille Institute of Los
Angeles**
Braille Institute of Los Angeles
2031 De La Vina Street   805-682-6222
Santa Barbara, CA 93105-3895   800-272-4553
                                          Fax: 805-687-6141
                                          e-mail: sb@brailleinstitute.org
                                          www.brailleinstitute.org
Offers classes type library services and information for persons
with visual impairments.
Angela Nowlin, Assistant Regional Director
Michael Lazarovits, Santa Barbara Regional Director

9860 Braille Institute Sight Center
741 N Vermont Avenue   323-663-1111
Los Angeles, CA 90029   800-272-4553
                                          Fax: 323-663-0867
                                          e-mail: la@brailleinstitute.org
                                          www.brailleinstitute.org/los_angeles
Offers help programs services and information to the blind and vi-
sually impaired children and adults.
Dr Henry C Chang, Director of Library Services
Anita Wright, Los Angeles Regional Program Director

9861 Braille Institute Youth Center
3450 Cahuenga Boulevard W
Los Angeles, CA 90068-1381   800-272-4553
                                          Fax: 323-851-6961
                                          www.brailleinstitute.org
Offers various youth programs and services for the blind and visu-
ally impaired youngster.
Leslie E Stocker Jr, President
Sally H Jameson, Vice President of Programs and Services

9862 Braille Textbook Assignment Service National Braille Association
National Braille Association
95 Allens Creek Road   585-427-8260
Rochester, NY 14618-2537   Fax: 585-427-0263
                                          e-mail: nbaoffice@nationalbraille.org
                                          www.nationalbraille.org
Certified braillists provide readers with technical and nontechni-
cal materials by transcribing for this service.
Diane Spence, President
David W Shaffer, Executive Director

9863 Carroll Center for the Blind
770 Centre Street   617-969-6200
Newton, MA 02458-2597   800-852-3131
                                          Fax: 617-969-6204
                                          TTY: 617-969-6204
                                          e-mail: info@carroll.org
                                          www.carroll.org
Assists blind and visually impaired adults and adolescents to adjust to loss of vision. The goal of this dynamic program is to help
the person become more independent to restore self-confidence
prepare for employment and improve the quality of life. Programs
of individual counseling are offered as part of the program.
Dina Rosenbaum, Director of Marketing

9864 Clearinghouse for Specialized Media and Translation
California Department of Education/CSMT
1430 N Street   916-319-0800
Sacramento, CA 95814   Fax: 916-323-9732
                                          e-mail: jparissalb@cde.ca.gov
                                          www.cde.ca.gov/re/pn/sm
Assists schools and students in the identification and acquisition of
textbooks reference books and study materials in aural media,
braille, large print, and electronic media access technology.
Jonn Paris-Salb, Adminisrtator

9865 Clovernook Center for the Blind and Visually Impaired
7000 Hamilton Avenue   513-522-3860
Cincinnati, OH 45231-5240   888-234-7156
                                          Fax: 513-728-3946
                                          www.clovernook.org
Information and resources for the blind and visually impaired as
well as rehabilitation services for youth to mature adults braille
production and manufacturing of paper products.
Robin L Usalis, President
Jacqueline L Conner, VP of Multi-State Center East

9866 Dean A McGee Eye Institute
608 Stanton L Young Boulevard   405-271-6060
Oklahoma City, OK 73104-5065   800-787-9012
                                          Fax: 405-271-4442
                                          www.dmei.org
Basic and clinical investigations in visual sciences.
David W Parke II, President
Jean Ann Vickery, Director Contact Lens Services

9867 Department of Ophthalmology/Eye and Ear Infirmary
1855 W Taylor Street   312-996-6590
Chicago, IL 60612-7242   Fax: 312-996-7770
                                          e-mail: eyeweb@uic.edu
                                          www.uic.edu/com/eye
Offers help support information and research for persons with vi-
sion problems including Retinitis Pigmentosa.
Timothy McMahon, Director of Contact Lens Service
Elmer Tu, Director of Cornea Service

9868 Emory University: Laboratory for Ophthalmic Research
1365-B Clifton Road NE
Atlanta, GA 30322-1013   404-778-2020
                                          www.eyecenter.emory.edu
Various studies into the aspects of blindness.
Henry F Edelhauser, Director

9869 Eye Institute of New Jersey New Jersey Medical School
New Jersey Medical School
PO Box 1709   973-972-2036
Newark, NJ 07101-2425   Fax: 973-723-94
                                          njms.umdnj.edu
Ophthamology including research into cornea retina and
neuro-ophthamalogy.
Marco A Zarbin, Chair

9870 Florida Ophthalmic Institute
7106 NW 11th Pl   352-331-2020
Gainesville, FL 32605-3157   Fax: 352-331-2019
Nonprofit organization that understands and treats ocular diseases
including glaucoma.
Norman S Levy MD, Director

9871 Foundation for Glaucoma Research
251 Post Street   415-986-3162
San Francisco, CA 94108   800-826-6693
                                          Fax: 415-986-3763
                                          e-mail: info@glaucoma.org
                                          www.glaucoma.org
Clinical and laboratory studies of glaucoma.
Thomas M Brunner, Chief Executive Officer/President
Andrew Jackson, Director of Communications

9872 Glaucoma Laser Trabeculoplasty Study Sinai Hospital of Detroit
Sinai Hospital of Detroit
6767 W Outer Drive   313-966-3256
Detroit, MI 48235-2899   Fax: 313-966-4296
Examines the effectiveness and safety of the treatments of glau-
coma.
Hugh Beckman, Chairman

9873 Harvard University Howe Laboratory of Ophthalmology
Massachusetts Eye & Ear Infirmary
243 Charles Street
Boston, MA 02114-3002   617-523-7900
                                          www.masseyeandear.org
Development ophthalmology and eye research.
John Fernandez, President
Javier Balloffet, VP Ophthalmology

9874 Helen Keller International
352 Park Avenue S
New York, NY 10010

212-532-0544
877-535-5374
Fax: 212-532-6014
e-mail: info@hki.org
www.hki.org

Nonprofit organization for the blind.
Kathy Spahn, President/CEO
Shawn K Baker, VP/Regional Director-Africa

9875 Helen Keller National Center for Deaf/Blind Youths and Adults
141 Middle Neck Road
Sands Point, NY 11050-1299

516-944-8900
Fax: 516-944-7302
TTY: 516-944-8637
e-mail: hkncinfo@hknc.org
www.hknc.org

We enable all those who are deaf-blind to live and work in the community of their choice. We provide comprehensive vocational rehabilitation training at our headquarters in NY and assistance with job and residential placements when training is completed.
Joseph McNulty, Executive Director

9876 Institute for Visual Sciences
1 E 71st Street
New York, NY 10021-4102

212-305-2919

Ophthalmology with emphasis on the development of care for the eye.
Melissa Mount, Executive Director

9877 Jerusalem Center for Multi-Handicapped Blind Children
350 7th Avenue
New York, NY 10001-7903

212-279-4070
Fax: 212-279-4043
e-mail: info@keren-or.org
keren-or.org

Maintains the Keren-Or Center for the Multiply Handicapped Blind Child in Jerusalem for rehabilitation and training. Funds acquired through contributions bequests and legacies.
Madelyn Cohen, Executive Director
Tamara Silberberg, Director Keren-Or Center

9878 Johns Hopkins University: Dana Center for Preventive Ophthalmology
Wilmer Ophthalmology Institute
600 N Wolfe Street
Baltimore, MD 21287-0001

410-955-2777
www.hopkinsmedicine.org/wilmer/danacente

Research at the Dana Center focuses on national and international public health prevention of blinding eye disease.
Harry A Quigley, Director

9879 New Beginnings: The Blind Children's Center
4120 Marathon Street
Los Angeles, CA 90029-3505

213-664-2153
800-222-3566

The purpose of the Center is to turn initial fears into hope. Helps children and their families become independent by creating a climate of safety and trust. Children learn to develop self confidence and to master a wide range of skills. Services include an infant stimulation program, educational preschool, interdisciplinary assessment services, family services, correspondence program, toll free national hotline and a publication and research service.

9880 New Beginnings: The Blind Children's Cente
4120 Marathon Street
Los Angeles, CA 90029

323-664-2153
800-222-3566
Fax: 323-665-3828
www.blindchildrenscenter.org

The purpose of the Center is to turn initial fears into hope. Helps children and their families become independent by creating a climate of safety and trust. Children learn to develop self confidence and to master a wide range of skills. Services include an infant stimulation program educational preschool interdisciplinary assessment services family services correspondence program toll free national hotline and a publication and research service.

9881 Oregon Health Sciences University: Elk's Children's Eye Clinic
Casey Eye Institute
3375 SW Terwilliger Boulevard
Portland, OR 97239-4197

503-494-3000
Fax: 503-494-5347
www.ohsucasey.com

Our mission at the Casey Eye Institute is to provide excellent eye care in a quality cost-effective environment that combines education research clinical leadership and service to the community.
Earl Palmer, Director

9882 Reader-Transcriber Registry National Braille Association
National Braille Association
3 Townline Circle
Rochester, NY 14623-2537

716-427-8260

Certified braillists fill requests for college textbooks and other technical works through this service of the National Braille Association.

9883 Smith-Kettlewell Eye Research Institute
2318 Fillmore Street
San Francisco, CA 94115-1821

415-345-2000
Fax: 415-345-8455
www.ski.org

Dedicated to research on human vision. The Institute was founded to encourage a productive collaboration between the medical clinic and scientific laboratory. Research is conducted with clinical studies which relate directly to the diagnosis and treatment of eye diseases the development of devices and vocational programs to aid the partially sighted and basic research to understand how the eye and brain work for both the clinical and rehabilitation programs.
Arthur Jampolsky, Executive Director
Ruth S Poole, COO

9884 University of Illinois at Chicago Lions of Illinois Eye Research Institute
UIC Eye Center
1905 W Taylor Street
Chicago, IL 60612-7245

312-996-1466
Fax: 312-355-4248
www.uic.edu/com/eye/Lions

Visual impairments and blindness research including glaucoma studies.
Janet Szlyk, Presidentÿ
Julie Daraska, Secretaryÿ

9885 University of Miami: Bascom Palmer Eye Institute
Department of Ophthalmalogy
900 NW 17th Street
Miami, FL 33136-1015

305-326-6000
800-329-7000
Fax: 305-326-6306
www.bpei.med.miami.edu/site/default.asp

Clinical and basic research into blindness and visual impairments.
John G Clarkson, Dean Emeritus

9886 Visually Impaired Center
1422 W Court Street
Flint, MI 48503

810-767-4014
Fax: 810-767-0020
e-mail: info@vicflint.org
www.vicflint.org

A private non-profit agency which offers special programs and some very practical help to people who are blind or partially sighted. Offers rehabilitation low vision aids orientation and mobility vocational training reading and information recreation counseling services volunteer services and community awareness.
Fharon Reigle, Director

9887 Warren Grant Magnuson Clinical Center National Institute of Health
National Institute of Health
9000 Rockville Pike
Bethesda, MD 20892

301-496-4000
800-411-1222
Fax: 301-480-9793
TTY: 866-411-1010
e-mail: prpl@mail.cc.nih.gov
www.cc.nih.gov

Established in 1953 as the research hospital of the National Institutes of Health. Designed so that patient care facilities are close to research laboratories so new findings of basic and clinical scientists can be quickly applied to the treatment of patients. Upon referral by physicians patients are admitted to NIH clinical studies.
John I Gallin, Director
David Henderson, Deputy Director for Clinical Care

9888   Yale University: Vision Research Center
330 Cedar Street   203-785-5687
New Haven, CT 06510-3218   800-395-7949
                                                              Fax: 203-785-7401
                                          e-mail: sarah.gelo@yale.edu
                                          visionresearch.med.yale.edu
Vision including studies on growth and development.
Bruce Shields, Chair
Sarah Gelo, Administrator

Kansas

9889   Kansas Services for the Blind and Visually Impaired
Social Rehabilitation Services
915 SW Harrison   785-368-7471
Topeka, KS 66612-2445   800-547-5789
                                                              Fax: 785-368-7467
                                                              TTY: 785-368-7478
                                          e-mail: rehab@srs.ks.gov
                               www.srskansas.org/rehab/text/SBVI.htm
Instructional employment oriented services for blind adults.
Laura Howard, Deputy Secretary and Chief Financial Off
Theresa Addington, Accounting and Administrative Operations

Support Groups & Hotlines

9890   1-800-BRAILLE
Braille Institute
741 N Vermont Avenue   323-663-1111
Los Angeles, CA 90029-3594   800-272-4553
                                          www.brailleinstitute.org
A toll free information and referral service where callers can obtain information about community programs and referrals to organizations serving the blind in their local areas.
Carol Mora, Director

9891   AFB Toll-Free Hotline
American Foundation for the Blind
11 Penn Plaza   212-502-7600
New York, NY 10001-2018   800-232-5463
                                                              Fax: 212-502-7777
                                          e-mail: afbinfo@afb.net
                                                              www.afb.org
Supplies information on visual impairment and blindness, answers queries regarding AFB services, products, publications, technology, the Careers and Technology Information Bank (a national data bank) and much more.
Richard J. O'Brien, Chair

9892   American Foundation for the Blind Information Center
11 Penn Plaza   212-502-7600
New York, NY 10001   800-232-5463
                                                              Fax: 212-502-7777
                                          e-mail: afbinfo@afb.net
                                                              www.afb.org
Nationally recognized information clearinghouse on blindness and visual impairment. Serves people who are blind or visually impaired, professionals in the field of blindness and visual impairment — including the staff at AFB, business and government organizations and the general public. Provides a toll-free information line available 24 hours a day, online information and referral services, professional library and archival services.

9893   Aurora of Central New York
518 James Street   315-422-7263
Syracuse, NY 13203   Fax: 315-422-4792
                                                              TTY: 315-422-9746
                                                              TDD: 315-422-9746
                                    e-mail: auroracny@auroraofcny.org
                                          www.auroraofcny.org/
Professional counseling services to assist individuals and their families deal with the trauma of hearing or vision loss.
Earleen Foulk, President Board of Directors
Debra Chaiken, Executive Director

9894   Carroll Center for the Blind
770 Centre Street   617-969-6200
Newton, MA 2458-2597   800-852-3131
                                                              Fax: 617-969-6204
                                                              www.carroll.org
Rehabilition and educational facility for persons with vision loss.
Dina Rosenbaum, VP Marketing

9895   Department of Ophthalmology Information Line
Illinois Eye & Ear Infirmary
1855 W Taylor Street m/c 648   312-996-6500
Chicago, IL 60612-7242   Fax: 312-996-7770
                                          e-mail: eyeweb@uic.edu
                                          www.uic.edu/com/eye/
Offers eye clinic and physician referrals to persons suffering from vision disorders as well as offers emergency information.
Dimitri Azar, Director

9896   Glaucoma Support Network
490 Post Street   415-986-3162
San Francisco, CA 94102-1409   800-826-6693
                                                              Fax: 415-986-3763
                                          e-mail: info@glaucoma.org
                                                              www.glaucoma.org
A peer support service for glaucoma patients and their families. The Network provides meaningful, helpful answers to questions from individuals concerned about vision and glaucoma.
Thomas Brunner, President
Rita Loskill, Executive Director

9897   Job Opportunities for the Blind
National Federation of the Blind
1800 Johnson Street   410-659-9314
Baltimore, MD 21230-4998   Fax: 410-685-5653
                                          e-mail: nfb@nfb.org
                                                              www.nfb.org
A specialized service that provides free support, resources and information to blind persons seeking employment and to employers interested in hiring the blind. A partnership program with the US Department of Labor, this is the most successful program of it's kind in helping blind persons find competitive work.
Anthony Cobb, Dircetor

9898   National Association for Parents of the Visually Impaired
Watertown, MA 2471   617-972-7441
                                                              800-562-6265
                                                              Fax: 617-972-7444
                                          e-mail: napvi@perkins.org
                                                              www.napvi.org

Susan Laventure, Executive Director

9899   National Center for Sight
National Society to Prevent Blindness
211 Wacker Drive   312-363-6001
Chicago, IL 60606   800-331-2020
                                                              Fax: 312-363-6052
A toll-free line offering information on a broad range of vision, eye health and safety topics including sports eye safety, lazy eye, diabetic retinopathy, glaucoma, cataracts, children's eye disorders, and more.

9900   National Eye Health Education Program
1855 W Taylor Street   312-996-6590
Chicago, IL 60612-7242   800-786-3937
                                                              Fax: 312-996-9967
                                                              www.uic.edu
Offers information and support for persons with vision disorders, including Retinitis Pigmentosa.
Mary Go, Supervisor

9901   National Health Information Center
PO Box 1133   310-565-4167
Washington, DC 20013   800-336-4797
                                                              Fax: 301-984-4256
                                          e-mail: info@nhic.org
                                          www.health.gov/nhic
Offers a nationwide information referral service, produces directories and resource guides.

9902   National Service Dog Center
Delta society

875 124th Avenue, NE
Bellevue, WA 98005
425-226-7357
Fax: 425-235-1076
e-mail: info@deltasociety.org
www.deltasociety.org

A service of the Delta Society, provides information about the selection, training, stewardship, and roles of service dogs; referral to service dog training programs and related resources; education to businesses, health care professionals, and the general public regarding service dog issues; research assistance athrough a resource library and network of professional esperts; and advocacy on behalf of people with service dogs.
Linda M Hines, Director
Susan Duncan, Contact

9903 PXE International
4301 Connecticut Avenue NW
Washington, DC 20008-2369
202-362-9599
Fax: 202-966-8553
e-mail: info@pxe.org
www.pxe.org

Initiates, funds and conducts research; provides support for individuals and families affected by pseudoxanthoma elasticum; and provides resrouces for healthcare professionals.
Elizabeth Terry, Executive Director

9904 Recorded Periodicals
Associated Services for the Blind
919 Walnut Street
Philadelphia, PA 19107-5237
215-627-0600
Fax: 215-220-92
e-mail: asbinfo@asb.org
www.asb.org

A subscription service of Associated Services for the Blind, these periodicals provide 21 magazines through this subscription service. A magazine list can be sent, in both large print and on audio cassette.
Patricia C Johnson, President/Chief Executive Officer

9905 Recording for the Blind Helpline
20 Roszel Road
Princeton, NJ 08540-6294
609-452-0606
800-221-4792
e-mail: audioaccesssupport@rfbd.org
www.rfbd.org

An organization dedicated to helping people with print disabilities.
Jay Haggith, Director of Communications

9906 Vision Use in Employment
Carroll Center for the Blind
770 Centre Street
Newton, MA 02458-2597
617-969-6200
800-852-3131
Fax: 617-969-6204
www.carroll.org

VUE provides engineering solutions plus training to help people keep jobs despite their vision loss.
Dina Rosenbaum, Marketing Director

9907 Washington Connection
American Council of the Blind
1155 15th Street NW
Washington, DC 20005-2706
202-467-5081
800-424-8666
Fax: 202-467-5085
e-mail: info@acb.org
www.acb.org

Coverage of issues affecting blind people via legislative information, participates in law-making, legislative training seminars and networking of support resources across the US.
Melanie Brunson, Executive Director

Books

9908 AFB Directory of Services for Blind/Vis. Impaired Persons in the US & Canada
AFB Press: American Foundation for the Blind
11 Penn Plaza
New York, NY 10001
212-502-7600
800-232-3044
Fax: 212-502-7774
e-mail: afbdirectory@afb.net
www.afb.org/store

Provides the most comprehensive collection of information available on services for blind and visually impaired individuals. Over

800 pages of revised and updated information on more than 1,500 agencies and 45 new indexes. Includes complete descriptions of services offered by organizations and web sites and e-mail addresses. Available online on a subscription basis.

9909 APH Catalog of Accessible Books for People Who are Visually Impaired
American Printing House for the Blind
1839 Frankfort Avenue
Louisville, KY 40206-3148
502-895-2405
800-223-1839
Fax: 502-895-1509
e-mail: info@aph.org

Offers thousands of selections and publishers of large type and braille books for persons with visual impairments.

9910 Access to Mass Transit for Blind & Visually Impaired Travelers
AFB Press: American Foundation for the Blind
11 Penn Plaza
New York, NY 10001
212-502-7600
800-232-3044
Fax: 212-502-7774
www.afb.org/store

Addresses several travel issues vital to the independence of blind and visually impaired persons from serveral perspectives — those of the blind and visually impaired persons who use mass transit, orientation and mobility instructors and transportation professionals. Focusing on national and international issues, this information filled manual covers approaches to making mass transit available in several cities in the US and Canada, the United Kingdom and Japan.
192 pages Paperback
ISBN: 0-891281-66-5

9911 An Orientation and Mobility Primer for Families and Young Children
American Foundation for the Blind
11 Penn Plaza
New York, NY 10001-2018
212-502-7600
800-232-5463
Fax: 212-502-7777

Practical information for helping a child learn about his or her environment right from the start. Covers sensory training, concept development and orientation skills.
48 pages Papberback
ISBN: 0-891281-57-6

9912 Art Beyond Sight: Resource Guide to Art, Creativity and Visual Impairment
AFB Press: American Foundation for the Blind
11 Penn Plaza
New York, NY 10001
212-502-7600
800-232-3044
Fax: 212-502-7774
www.afb.org/store

AFB and Art Education for the Blind have joined together to co-publish this one-of-a-kind resource that provides vital information on all aspects of exploring art and creativity by people who are blind or visually impaired. Includes a section of reproducible pages for classroom or workshop activities.
504 pages Paperback
ISBN: 0-891288-50-3

9913 Art and Science of Teaching Orientation to the Visually Impaired
AFB Press: American Foundation for the Blind
11 Penn Plaza
New York, NY 10001
212-502-7600
800-232-3044
Fax: 212-502-7774
www.afb.org/store

Updated and comprehensive description of the techniques of teaching orientation and mobility, presented along with strategies for sensitive and effective teaching. Such factors as individual needs, environmental features and ethical issues are discussed in this important text.
200 pages Paperback
ISBN: 0-891282-59-9

9914 Beginning with Braille: Balanced Approach to Literacy
AFB Press: American Foundation for the Blind
11 Penn Plaza
New York, NY 10001
212-502-7600
800-232-3044
Fax: 212-502-7774
www.afb.org/store

Exciting resource from a skilled practitioner, this book provides a wealth of effective activitoes for promoting literacy at the early stages of braille instruction. The text includes creative and practical strategies for designing and delivering quality braille instruction and offers teacher-friendly suggestions for many areas, such as reading aloud to young children, selecting and making early tactile books and teaching tactile and hand movement skills. Tips on lessons and worksheets.

ISBN: 0-891283-23-4

9915 Behavioral Vision Approaches for Persons with Physical Disabilities
William V. Padula, author
Optometric Extension Program Foundation
1921 E. Carnegie Ave., Suite 3-L   949-250-8070
Santa Ana, CA 92705-5510   Fax: 949-250-8175
                                e-mail: smc.oep@worldnet.att.net
                                                www.oepf.org
A discussion of the behavioral vision/neuro-motor approach to providing directions for prescriptive and therapeutic services for the visually handicapped child or adult.
197 pages
ISBN: 0-943599-04-0
Beverly Roberts, President
Gregory Kitchener, O.D., Vice President

9916 Blindness and Early Childhood Development
AFB Press: American Foundation for the Blind
11 Penn Plaza   212-502-7600
New York, NY 10001   800-232-3044
                                           Fax: 212-502-7774
                                                www.afb.org/store
Reviews knowledge of motor and locomotor development, language and cognitive processes and social, emotional and personality development. It is a classic resource for teachers and those who work with children who are blind or visually impaired.
384 pages Paperback
ISBN: 0-891281-23-1

9917 Braille Book Bank: Music Catalog
National Braille Association
95 Allens Creek Road, 1-202   585-427-8260
Rochester, NY 14618   Fax: 585-427-0263
                                e-mail: NBAOffice@nationalbraille.org
                                                www.nationalbraille.org
Offers hundreds of musical titles in print form, braille and on cassette.
62 pages

9918 Building Blocks: Foundations for Learning for Young Blind & Vis. Impaired Children
AFB Press: American Foundation for the Blind
11 Penn Plaza   212-502-7600
New York, NY 10001   800-232-3044
                                           Fax: 212-502-7774
                                                www.afb.org/store
Available in English and Spanish, this work presents the essential components of a successful early intervention program, including collaboration with family members, positive relationships between parents and professionals, public education, and attention to important programming components such as space exploration, braille readiness, orientation and mobility, play, cooking and music. VHS video also available.
149 pages Paperback
ISBN: 0-891281-87-8

9919 Burns Braille Transcription Dictionary
AFB Press: American Foundation for the Blind
11 Penn Plaza   212-502-7600
New York, NY 10001   800-232-3044
                                           Fax: 212-502-7774
                                                www.afb.org/store
A handy, portable guide that is a quick reference for anyone who needs to check print-to-braille and braille-to-print meanings and symbols. This easy-to-use listing provides readers with the essential alphabet, contractions, punctuation and signs and symbols for braille, as well as brief descriptions of rules for thier use. Organized into four clear sections aimed at providing information at a glance, this valuable tool is an ideal reference for teachers, rehabilitation professionals and others.
96 pages Paperback
ISBN: 0-891292-32-7

9920 Business Owners Who Are Blind or Visually Impaired
AFB Press: American Foundation for the Blind
11 Penn Plaza   212-502-7600
New York, NY 10001   800-232-3044
                                           Fax: 212-502-7774
                                                www.afb.org/store
Demonstrates the wide range of careers and talents that can be pursued by persons with visual impairments. Each profile features a successful individual who has accomplised his or her dream of business ownership and who shares important insights. Available in paperback, audio cassette or ASCII disk.
148 pages
ISBN: 0-891283-24-2

9921 Career Perspectives: Interviews with Blind & Visually Impaired Professionals
AFB Press: American Foundation for the Blind
11 Penn Plaza   212-502-7600
New York, NY 10001   800-232-3044
                                           Fax: 212-502-7774
                                                www.afb.org/store
Profiles of 20 successful archivers who describe in their own words what it takes to pursue and attain professional success in a sighted world. From all around the country and representing a wide range of professions, including law, science, journalism, management and medicine, the blind and visually impaired individuals featured serve as role models for others who wnat to follow career paths.
96 pages Paperback
ISBN: 0-891281-70-3

9922 Childhood Glaucoma: A Reference Guide for Families
NAPVI
PO Box 317   617-972-7441
Watertown, MA 02471-0317   800-562-6265
                                           Fax: 617-972-7444
                                e-mail: napvi@perkins.org
                                                www.napvi.org

Susan LaVenture, Executive Director

9923 Communication Skills for Visually Impaired
Charles C Thomas Publisher
2600 S 1st Street   217-789-8980
Springfield, IL 62704-4730   Fax: 217-789-9130
                                e-mail: books@ccthomas.com
                                                www.ccthomas.com
322 pages
ISBN: 0-398066-92-2

9924 Concept Development for Visually Impaired Children: Resource Guide
AFB Press: American Foundation for the Blind
11 Penn Plaza   212-502-7600
New York, NY 10001   800-232-3044
                                           Fax: 212-502-7774
                                                www.afb.org/store
Program for integrating such concepts as body imagery, gross motor movement, posture and tactile discrimination into the curriculum from kindergarten on.
80 pages Paperback
ISBN: 0-891280-18-9

9925 Coping with Vision Loss
Bill Chapman, EdD, author
Hunter House Publishing
PO Box 2914   510-865-5282
Alameda, CA 94501   800-266-5592
                                           Fax: 510-865-4295
                                e-mail: ordering@hunterhouse.com
                                                www.hunterhouse.com
Maximizing what you can see and do. The Author explains the five leading causes of vision loss, and how to use new skills and vision aids.
2001 304 pages Paperback
Cristina Sverdrup, Customer Service Manager

9926 Development of Social Skills by Blind and Visually Impaired Students

AFB Press: American Foundation for the Blind

11 Penn Plaza 212-502-7600
New York, NY 10001 800-532-3044
Fax: 212-502-7774
www.afb.org/store

Examination of the social interactions of children with visual impairments, theory and research are combined to explore how these children can be helped to succeed socially. Innovative practical strategies are provided for educators, researchers and families on how to assist children in the development of social skills. Qualitative ethnographic approaches demonstrate how classroom teachers can work effectively with individual children and present valuable insights about children's interactions.

232 pages Paperback
ISBN: 0-891282-17-3

9927 Early Focus: Working with Young Children Who Are Blind or Visually Impaired

AFB Press: American Foundation for the Blind

11 Penn Plaza 212-502-7600
New York, NY 10001 Fax: 212-502-7777
www.afb.org/store

Early intervention has increasingly been recognized as critical in the development and growth of children with visual impairments and other disabilities. Federal regulations have mandated early indentifacation and assesment, underscoring its importance for children's well being. This revised and updated edition of Early Focus provides the important information you need to know including serving culturally diverse families with children who have multiple disabilities and practical tips.

376 pages Paperback
ISBN: 0-891282-15-7

9928 Encyclopedia of Blindness and Vision Impairment

Facts on File

11 Penn Plaza 212-967-8800
New York, NY 10001 800-322-8755
Fax: 800-678-3633

Designed to provide both laymen and professionals with concise, practical information on the second most common disability in the US.

340 pages Hardcover

9929 Equals in Partnership: Basic Rights for Families of Children with Blindness

NAPVI

PO Box 317 617-972-7441
Watertown, MA 02471-0317 800-562-6265
Fax: 617-972-7444
e-mail: napvi@perkins.org
www.napvi.org

Susan LaVenture, Executive Director

9930 Essential Elements in Early Intervention: Visual Impairment & Multiple Disability

AFB Press: American Foundation for the Blind

11 Penn Plaza 212-502-7600
New York, NY 10001 800-232-3044
Fax: 212-502-7774
www.afb.org/store

Latest comprehensive resource from an outstanding early childhood specialist, this guide provides a range of information on effective early intervention with young children who are visually impaired and have other disabilities.

503 pages Paperback
ISBN: 0-891283-05-6

9931 Eye and Your Vision

Dr Lorrain H Marchi, author

National Association for Visually Handicapped

22 W 21st Street 212-889-3141
New York, NY 10010-6904 Fax: 212-727-2931
e-mail: navh@navh.org
www.navh.org

A large booklet offering information, with illustrations, on the eye. Includes information on protection of eyesight, how the eye works and vision disorders.

19 pages $5.00 n/members
Lorraine Marchi LHD, Founder/CEO
Cesar Gomez, Executive Director

9932 First Steps

Blind Children's Center

4120 Marathon Street 213-664-2153
Los Angeles, CA 90029-3584 Fax: 213-665-3828
e-mail: info@blindcntr.org
www.blindcntr.org

A handbook for teaching young children who are visually impaired. Designed to assist students, professionals and parents working with children who are visually impaired.

203 pages

9933 Foundations of Education

AFB Press: American Foundation for the Blind

11 Penn Plaza 212-502-7600
New York, NY 10001 800-232-3044
Fax: 212-502-7774
www.afb.org/store

Complete revision of landmark text. Comprehensive compilation of state-of-the-art information is the essential resource on educating visually impaired students, the essential theory forming the knowledge base, and methodology of teaching visually impaired students in all areas.

2000
ISBN: 0-891283-49-8

9934 Foundations of Orientation and Mobility

AFB Press: American Foundation for the Blind

11 Penn Plaza 212-502-7600
New York, NY 10001 800-232-3044
Fax: 212-502-7774
www.afb.org

Updated and revised, this new edition of the field's founding classics includes current research fom a variety of disiplines, an international perspective, and expanded contents on low vision, aging, multiple disabilities, accessibility, program design and adaptive technology from more than 30 eminent subject experts. Divided into four main sections, the book explores every of Orientation and Mobility learning and instruction.

800 pages Hardcover
ISBN: 0-891289-46-1

9935 Foundations of Rehabilitation Counseling with Persons Who Are Blind/Visually Imp.

AFB Press: American Foundation for the Blind

11 Penn Plaza 212-502-7600
New York, NY 10001 800-232-3044
Fax: 212-502-7774
www.afb.org/store

Rehabilitation professionals have long recognized that the needs of people who are blind or visually impaired are unique and require a special knowledge and expertise for the provision and coordination of effective rehabilitation services. Contributions to this text from more than 25 experts provide essential information on subjects as functional, medical, vocational and phychological assessments, demographic and cultural issues, pacement and employment issues, and the rehabilitation team.

464 pages Hardcover
ISBN: 0-891289-45-3

9936 Get a Wiggle On

American Alliance For Health, Phys. Ed. & Dance

1900 Association Drive 703-476-3400
Reston, VA 20191-1598 800-213-7193
www.aahperd.org/

Gives teachers and parents practical suggestions for helping blind and visually impaired infants grow and learn like other children.

80 pages
ISBN: 0-883140-77-2

9937 Guide to Independence for the Visually Impaired and Their Families

Demos Medical Publishing

386 Park Avenue S
New York, NY 10016-8804
212-683-0072
800-532-8663
Fax: 212-683-0118
e-mail: orderdept@demopub.com
www.demosmedpub.com

This first comprehensive, hands-on book for the newly visually impaired and their families presents detailed instructions to deal with emotional reactions and fioght depression; contact organizations and get information; obtain federal and other types of financial aid; use the other senses more effectively; adapt their homes and do household chores; handle paperwork and become socially active.
248 pages Paperback
ISBN: 0-939957-61-2
Dr. Diana M Schneider, President

9938   Guidelines and Games for Teaching Efficient Braille Reading
AFB Press: American Foundation for the Blind
11 Penn Plaza
New York, NY 10001
212-502-7600
800-232-3044
Fax: 212-502-7774
www.afb.org/store

Based on research in the areas of rapid reading and precision teaching, these effective guidelines and games represent a unique adaptation of a general reading program to the needs of braille readers.
116 pages Paperback
ISBN: 0-891281-05-3

9939   Hammond Large Type World Atlas
American Map-Langensceidt Publishing Group
15 Tyger River Drive
Duncan, SC 29334
864-486-0214
800-432-6277
Fax: 888-773-7979
www.hammondmap.com

100 maps.

ISBN: 0-816159-11-4

9940   Handbook for Itinerant and Resource Teachers of Blind Students
National Federation of the Blind
1800 Johnson Street
Baltimore, MD 21230-4998
410-659-9314
Fax: 410-685-5653
e-mail: subscribe@diabetes.nfb.org
www.nfb.org

The Handbook provides help to teachers, school administrators or other school personnel that have experience with blind or visually impaired students. The Handbook devotes 45 pages to Braille and how to teach Braille for parents and teachers; other chapters iclude law, physical education, fitting in socially, testing and evaluation, home economics, daily living skills and more.
533 pages Softcover
Eileen Ley, Director of Publishing
Elizabeth Lunt, Editor

9941   Health Care Professionals Who are Blind or Visually Impaired
AFB Press: American Foundation for the Blind
11 Penn Plaza
New York, NY 10001
212-502-7600
800-232-3044
Fax: 212-502-7774
www.afb.org/store

Exciting career possibilities for people who are visually impaired as well as those who are sighted. Inspirational profiles of 15 sucessful role models. Written in an accesible, easy-to-read style, this book documents the stories and stategies of professionals ranging from a forensic psychiatrist to a radiology dark room technician. Information on technology and tactics that are used to perform demanding jobs are also included. Available in paperback, audio casette, or ASCII disk.
2001 166 pages
ISBN: 0-891283-88-9

9942   I Keep Five Pairs of Glasses in a Flower Pot
Henrietta Levner, author
National Association for Visually Handicapped
22 W 21st Street
New York, NY 10010-6904
212-889-3141
Fax: 212-727-2931
e-mail: navh@navh.org
www.navh.org

A short story, printed in 18 point type, is the saga of one womans struggle with low vision.
Lorraine Marchi LHD, Founder/CEO
Cesar Gomez, Executive Director

9943   If Blindness Comes
National Federation of the Blind
1800 Johnson Street
Baltimore, MD 21230-4998
410-659-9314
Fax: 410-685-5653
e-mail: subscribe@diabetes.nfb.org
www.nfb.org

An introduction to issues relating to vision loss and provides a positive, supportive philosophy about blindness. It is a general information book which includes answers to many common questions about blindness, information about services and programs for the blind and resource listings.
Eileen Ley, Director of Publishing
Elizabeth Lunt, Editor

9944   Independence Without Sight or Sound: Suggestions for Practitioners
AFB Press: American Foundation for the Blind
11 Penn Plaza
New York, NY 10001
212-502-7600
800-232-3044
Fax: 212-502-7774
www.afb.org/store

Written in a personal and informal style, this practical guidebook covers the essential aspects of communicating and working with deaf-blind persons. Full of valuable information on subjects such as how to talk with deaf-blind people, adapt orientation and mobility techniques for deaf-blind travelers, and interact with deaf-blind individuals socially, this useful manual also contains a substantial resource section detailing sources of information and adapted equipment. Also available in braille.
193 pages Paperback
ISBN: 0-891282-46-7

9945   Jewish Heritage for the Blind
1655 E 24th Street
Brooklyn, NY 11229-2401
718-338-4999
800-995-1888
Offers large print traditional prayer books for the High Holy days, festivals, fast days and daily rituals for those finding it difficult or impossible to read small print.

9946   Kernel Book Series
National Federation of the Blind
1800 Johnson Street
Baltimore, MD 21230-4998
410-659-9314
Fax: 410-685-5653
e-mail: subscribe@diabetes.nfb.org
www.nfb.org

A series of books written by the blind themselves. Each book is a collection of articles and stories about the real life experiences of blind persons. These books help educate the blind and the sighted alike about a positive philosophy regarding blindness.
Eileen Ley, Director of Publishing
Elizabeth Lunt, Editor

9947   King James Bible: Large Print
Science Products
PO Box 888
Southeastern, PA 19399-0888
800-888-7400
24 point type easily seen with 20/200 acuity. Makes bible reading for children easier too.

9948   Knotholes are for Seeing: Therapy Through Poetry, Prose & Other Writings
Business of Living Publications
PO Box 8388
Corpus Christi, TX 78468-8388
512-852-8515

ISBN: 1-879518-08-2

9949   Large Print American Heritage Dictionary
Houghton Mifflin Harcourt
222 Berkeley Street
Boston, MA 02116
617-351-5000
800-888-7400
www.hmco.com

More than 35,000 easy to read entries for those who prefer large type.

ISBN: 0-395929-32-6

9950 Legislative Handbook for Parents
NAPVI
PO Box 317   617-972-7441
Watertown, MA 02471-0317   800-562-6265
                                             Fax: 617-972-7444
                                      e-mail: napvi@perkins.org
                                              www.spedex.com
Written by parents for parents in dealing with legislative processes that ultimately affect their children's lives.
Susan LaVenture, Executive Director

9951 Library Resources for the Blind and Physically Handicapped
National Library Service for the Blind
1291 Taylor Street NW   202-707-5100
Washington, DC 20542-0002   Fax: 202-707-0712
                                                www.loc.gov/nls

9952 Low Vision: Reflections of the Past, Issues for the Future
AFB Press: American Foundation for the Blind
11 Penn Plaza   212-502-7600
New York, NY 10001   800-232-3044
                                             Fax: 212-502-7774
                                              www.afb.org/store
Research report based on a multiphase survey of professionals. Identifies important trends that will shape the field of low vision services into the next century. Designed for administrators, policy planners and university instructors, as well as for direct service providers, Low Vision includes overview papers by six eminent leaders in the low vision field.
181 pages Paperback
ISBN: 0-891282-18-1

9953 Madness of Usher's: Coping with Vision & Hearing Loss
Richard A. Lewis, Dorothy H. Stiefel, author
Business of Living Publications
PO Box 8388   512-852-8515
Corpus Christi, TX 78468-8388
Paperback
ISBN: 1-879518-06-6
Dorothy H Stiefel, Author

9954 Mainstreaming & the American Dream: Soc. Logical Perspectives on Parental Coping
AFB Press: American Foundation for the Blind
11 Penn Plaza   212-502-7600
New York, NY 10001   800-232-3044
                                             Fax: 212-502-7774
                                              www.afb.org/store
Based on in-depth interviews with parents and professionals, this research monograph presents a sociological framework for looking at the needs and aspirations of parents of blind and visually impaired children.
256 pages Paperback
ISBN: 0-891281-91-6

9955 Mainstreaming the Visually Impaired Child
NAPVI
PO Box 317   617-972-7441
Watertown, MA 02471-0317   800-562-6265
                                             Fax: 617-972-7444
                                      e-mail: napvi@perkins.org
                                               www.napvi.org
A unique, informative guide for teachers and educational professionals that work with the visually impaired.
Susan LaVenture, Executive Director

9956 Making Life More Livable: Adaptations for Living at Home After Vision Loss
AFB Press: American Foundation of the Blind
11 Penn Plaza   212-502-7600
New York, NY 10001   800-232-3044
                                             Fax: 212-502-7774
                                              www.afb.org/store
Essential guide for adults experiencing vision loss and an invaluable resource for their family and friends. Full of practical tips and

illustrated by numerous photographs, this easy-to-use resource shows how people who are visually impaired can continue living independent, productive lives at home on their own. Useful general guidelines and room-by-room specifics provide simple and effective solutions for making homes accessible and everyday activities doable for visually impaired individuals.
132 pages Cassette avail.
ISBN: 0-891281-15-0

9957 Occupational Therapy Practice Guidelines for Adults with Low Vision
American Occupational Therapy Association
4720 Montgomery Lane   301-652-2682
Bethesda, MD 20824-1220   Fax: 301-652-7711
                                             TDD: 800-377-8555
                                                 www.aota.org
25 pages
ISBN: 1-569001-50-2

9958 Perkins Activity and Resource Guide: A Handbook for Teachers
Perkins School for the Blind Publications
175 N Beacon Street   617-924-3434
Watertown, MA 02472-2790   Fax: 917-926-2027
This is a comprehensive, two volume guide with over 1,000 pages of activities, resources and instructional strategies for teachers and parents of students with visual and multiple disabilities.

9959 Preschool Learning Activities for the Visually Impaired Child
NAPVI
PO Box 317   617-972-7441
Watertown, MA 02471-0317   800-562-6265
                                             Fax: 617-972-7444
                                      e-mail: napvi@perkins.org
                                               www.napvi.org
This guide for parents offers games and activities to keep visually impaired children active during the preschool years.
Susan LaVenture, Executive Director

9960 Prescriptions for Independence: Working with Older People Who Are Visually Imp.
AFB Press: American Foundation for the Blind
11 Penn Plaza   212-502-7600
New York, NY 10001   800-232-3044
                                             Fax: 212-502-7774
                                              www.afb.org/store
Easy-to-read manual on how older persons with visual impairments can pursue their interests and activities in community residences, senior centers, long-term care facilities and other community settings. Topics covered include signs of vision loss, recreation, personal care, orientation and mobility and modifications in the environment.
87 pages Paperback
ISBN: 0-891282-44-0

9961 Providing Services for People with Vision Loss: Multidisciplinary Perspective
Resources For Rehabilitation
22 Bonad Road   781-368-9094
Winchester, MA 01890   Fax: 781-368-9096
                                          e-mail: info@rfr.org
                                                  www.rfr.org
A collection of articles by ophthalmologists and rehabilitation professionals, including chapters on operating a low vision service, starting self-help programs, mental health services, aids and techniques that help people with vision loss.
136 pages
ISBN: 0-929718-02-X

9962 Psychoeducational Assessment of Visually Impaired Students
Pro-Ed, Inc.
8700 Shoal Creek Boulevard   512-451-3246
Austin, TX 78757-6897   800-897-3202
                                             Fax: 800-397-7633
                                    e-mail: info@proedinc.com
                                              www.proedinc.com
Professional reference book that addresses the problems specific to assessment of visually impaired children. Of particular value to the practitioner are the extensive reviews of available tests, includ-

ing ways to adapt those not designed for use with the visually handicapped.
140 pages Paperback
Lindy Jordaan, Marketing Coordinator

9963 Resources Family Centered Intervention for Infants, Toddlers & Preschoolers
Hope
1856 N 1200 E   435-245-2888
North Logan, UT 84341   Fax: 435-245-2888
Describes children with vision impairment in terms of characteristics, needs, and parent concerns.
Hardcover

9964 Show Me How: Manual for Parents Preschool Visually Impaired & Blind Children
AFB Press: American Foundation for the Blind
11 Penn Plaza   212-502-7600
New York, NY 10001   800-232-3044
                                                   Fax: 212-502-7774
                                                   www.afb.org/store
Practical guide for parents, teachers and others who help preschool children attain age-related goals. Includes activities for growing and learning, building self-concept, moving around, playing, perfecting daily living skills and developing sensory awareness. It also covers such issues as observing safety precautions, choosing appropriate toys and facilitating relationships with playmates.
56 pages Paperback
ISBN: 0-891281-13-4

9965 Starting Points
Blind Children's Center
4120 Marathon Street   213-664-2153
Los Angeles, CA 90029-3584   Fax: 213-665-3828
Basic information for the classroom teacher of 3 to 8 year olds whose multiple disabilities include visual impairment.
160 pages

9966 Tactile Graphics
AFB Press: American Foundation for the Blind
11 Penn Plaza   212-502-7600
New York, NY 10001   800-232-3044
                                                   Fax: 212-502-7774
                                                   www.afb.org/store
Easy-to-read encyclopedia handbook on translating visual information into a three-dimensional form that the blind and visually impaired persons can understand. This heavily illustrated guide covers theory, techniques, materials and step-by-step instructions for educators, rehabilitators, graphic artists, museum and busines personnel, employers and anyone involved in producing tactile material for visually impaired persons.
544 pages Paperback
ISBN: 0-891281-94-0

9967 Teachers Who Are Blind or Visually Impaired
AFB Press: American Foundation for the Blind
11 Penn Plaza   212-502-7600
New York, NY 10001   800-232-3044
                                                   Fax: 212-502-7774
                                                   www.afb.org/store
First volume in the Jobs That Matter series, this book profiles 18 visually impaired individuals who have successfully fulfilled their dreams of becoming teachers. These engaging individuals demonstrate how visually impaired teachers can be effective in their jobs and achieve classroom success and satisfaction. Available in paperback, audio cassette or braille.
1998 176 pages
ISBN: 0-891283-06-4

9968 Textbook Catalog
National Braille Association
95 Allens Creek Road 1-202   585-427-8260
Rochester, NY 14618   Fax: 585-427-0263
                                                   www.nationalbraille.org
Lists hundreds of scholarly, college and professional textbooks offered in large print, braille or on cassette for visually impaired readers.
80 pages

9969 To Love This Life: Quotations by Helen Keller
AFB Press: American Foundation for the Blind
11 Penn Plaza   212-502-7600
New York, NY 10001   800-232-3044
                                                   Fax: 212-502-7774
                                                   www.afb.org/store
Beautiful and moving souvenir of one of the world's most admired women. This memorable collection of quotations from Helen Keller brings words of wisdom, courage and inspiration from a remarkable individual who above all wanted to make a difference in the lives of her fellow men and women. The thought captured here — many from unpublished letters and speeches — offer profound statements on the meaning of being human and on life in all its complexity. Available in hardcover and audio cassette.
2000 118 pages
ISBN: 0-891283-47-1

9970 Unseen Minority: Social History of Blindness in the US
Frances A. Koestler, author
David McKay Company/AFB Press, Distributor
11 Penn Plaza   412-741-1398
New York, NY 10001   800-232-3044
                                                   Fax: 412-741-0609
                                                   e-mail: afborder@abdintl.com
                                                   www.afb.org
Lively narrative, peppered with anecdotes, recounts how the blind overcame discrimination to gain full participation in the social, educational, economic and legislative spheres. Here are the gripping stories: Why it took a century for braille to become a universal medium in English, how america's first school for the blind began with a chance encounter on a Boston street, and how the talking book came into existence.
573 pages Hardcover
ISBN: 0-679505-39-3

9971 Vision and Aging: Crossroads for Service Delivery
AFB Press: American Foundation for the Blind
11 Penn Plaza   212-502-7600
New York, NY 10001   800-232-3044
                                                   Fax: 212-502-7774
                                                   www.afb.org/store
This overview of the service delivery systems in the aging and blindness fields covers the essential issues concerning vision loss among older persons in this country, the growth of visual impairment among the increasing number of elderly people in the US, and the policy and service questions that will demand national attention throughout this and the coming decades.
392 pages Paperback
ISBN: 0-891282-16-5

9972 Visual Aids and Informational Material
National Association for Visually Handicapped
22 W 21st Street   212-889-3141
New York, NY 10010-6904   Fax: 212-727-2931
                                                   e-mail: navh@navh.org
                                                   www.navh.org
A large reference guide offering a list of visual aids and resources for persons with visual impairments.
65 pages
Lorraine Marchi LHD, Founder/CEO
Cesar Gomez, Executive Director

9973 Visual Handicaps and Learning
Pro-Ed, Inc.
8700 Shoal Creek Boulevard   512-451-3246
Austin, TX 78757-6897   800-897-3202
                                                   Fax: 800-397-7633
                                                   e-mail: info@proedinc.com
                                                   www.proedinc.com
This text covers a range of topics associated with visual impairment, from past practices to up-to-date research, and from legal responsibilities to personal beliefs, without losing sight of the individual child.
180 pages
ISBN: 0-890795-15-0
Lindy Jordaan, Marketing Coordinator

9974 Visual Impairment: An Overview
AFB Press: American Foundation for the Blind

11 Penn Plaza
New York, NY 10001

212-502-7600
800-232-3044
Fax: 212-502-7774
www.afb.org/store

Down-to-earth look at the common forms of vision loss and their impact on the individual. Explains the different aspects of visual impairment, describes adaptive techniques and devices and provides information on available resources and services in a conscise and easy-to-understand manner for professionals and visually impaired people and their families.
56 pages Paperback
ISBN: 0-891281-74-6

9975 Walking Alone and Marching Together
Floyd Matson, author

National Federation of the Blind
1800 Johnson Street
Baltimore, MD 21230-4998

410-659-9314
Fax: 410-685-5653
e-mail: subscribe@diabetes.nfb.org
www.nfb.org

The history of the organized blind movement, this book spans more than 50 years of civil rights, social issues, attitudes and experiences of the blind. Published in 1990, it has been read by thousands of blind and sighted persons and is used in colleges, libraries and programs across the country as an important tool in understanding blindness and it's impact on both personal lives and the society at large.
1100 pages
Eileen Ley, Director of Publishing
Elizabeth Lunt, Editor

9976 Webster Large Print Dictionary
Random House
1745 Broadway, 15-3
New York, NY 10019

212-782-9000
800-888-7400
www.randomhouse.com

Ten point type, more than 60,000 word entries and illustrations.
880 pages
ISBN: 0-375722-32-7

9977 What Museum Guides Need to Know: Access for Blind & Visually Impaired Visitors
AFB Press: American Foundation for the Blind
11 Penn Plaza
New York, NY 10001

212-502-7600
800-232-3044
Fax: 212-502-7774
www.afb.org/store

Provides practical, easy-to-use guidelines on how to greet and help blind and visually impaired museum goers. With numerous photographs taken at the High School Museum of Art and the Atlanta Historical Society, this handbook also covers aesthetics and visual impairment, legal requirements for accessibility, resources, a training outline for museum requirements for accessibility, a bibliography on art and museum access for blind and visually impaired persons, and guidelines for preparing media.
64 pages Paperback
ISBN: 0-891281-58-4

Children's Books

9978 Belonging
Dial Books
375 Hudson Street
New York, NY 10014-3658

212-366-2000
www.penguingroup.com

Meg attended special schools for the blind until she was ready for high school. She decided that she wanted to go to a regular high school. She and her mother practiced her walks to school and studied the layout of the building prior to school starting, but Meg was unprepared for the trip when there were 1,500 students. She adjusted quickly to the crowds and the pace of the new school.
200 pages Hardcover
ISBN: 0-803705-30-1

9979 Beside Me
Leader Dogs For The Blind

1039 S. Rochester Road
Rochester Hills, MI 48307

248-651-9011
888-777-5332
Fax: 248-651-5812
TTY: 248-651-3713
e-mail: leaderdog@leaderdog.org
www.leaderdog.org

Marion became blind as an adult. She was totally dependent on her parents to move around and go places she wanted to be. Marion decided to go to the leader-dog program and learn to use a leader dog. Particularly she wanted the independence she would need to go to college. Marion enrolled at the Leader-Dog-For-The-Blind Program in Rochester, Michigan. After weeks of training she was given a German Shepherd named Heidi. Marion and Heidi trained together until they were a team and ready.
Films

9980 Guide Dog Goes to School
William Morrow and Company
105 Madison Avenue
New York, NY 10016-7418

212-889-3050
800-843-9389
william-morrow-co.1.searchbook.net

Cinderena is a golden retriever. As a puppy Cindy is outgoing and not afraid of things in her environment. This disposition is ideal for a guide dog to the blind, and Cindy is selected to be in a program for guide dogs. Follow Cindy as we focus on the guide dog training.
51 pages Hardcover
ISBN: 0-688068-44-8

9981 How Do You Kiss a Blind Girl?
Charles C Thomas Publisher
2600 S First Street
Springfield, IL 62704-4730

217-789-8980
Fax: 217-789-9130
e-mail: books@ccthomas.com
www.ccthomas.com

Focuses, in a humorous way, on the attitudes toward persons with visual impairments.
126 pages
ISBN: 0-398052-62-X

9982 Living with Blindness
Franklin Watts Grolier
90 Old Sherman Tpke
Danbury, CT 06816-0001

203-797-3500
800-621-1115
Fax: 203-797-3197
www.grolier.com

Shows how persons with visual impairments and blindness can overcome their disability and lead productive lives.
32 pages Grades 5-7
ISBN: 0-531108-43-0

9983 Man Who Sang in the Dark
Eth Clifford, author

Houghton, Mifflin & Company
1 Beacon Street
Boston, MA 02108-3107

617-725-5000

The story of a girl and a man who is blind and how they both come to an understanding about certain prejudices.
Grades 3-5

9984 Out of the Corner of My Eye
American Foundation for the Blind
15 W 16th Street
New York, NY 10011-6301

212-502-7600
Fax: 212-502-7777

A personal account of students' vision loss and subsequent adjustment that is full of practical advice and cheerful encouragement, told by an 87 year old retired college teacher who has maintained her independence and zest for life.

ISBN: 0-891281-93-2

9985 She'll Never Walk Alone
Leader Dog For The Blind
1964 Park Street
Regina, SK, S4P 3G4,

306-565-8211

Leader dogs for the blind require many weeks of training before they are ready to work with the blind individual. Two courses, basic and advanced, are provided for each dog.
Films

Magazines

9986 Access World: Technology and People with Visual Impairments
AFB Press: American Foundation for the Blind
11 Penn Plaza   212-502-7600
New York, NY 10001   800-232-3044
                            Fax: 212-502-7774
                    e-mail: afbdirectory@afb.net
                                www.afb.org/store
Comprehensive and reader friendly online magazine covering every aspect of assistive technology and visual impairment.
Bimonthly

9987 Blind Educator
National Federation of the Blind
1800 Johnson Street   410-659-9314
Baltimore, MD 21230-4998   Fax: 410-685-5653
                    e-mail: subscribe@diabetes.nfb.org
                                www.nfb.org
The articles in this newsletter are written by people who are blind. Blind people can teach. In fact, this newsletter captures a glimpse of the range of subjects and grade levels in which blind people are engaged.
Eileen Ley, Director of Publishing
Elizabeth Lunt, Editor

9988 Braille Forum
Penny Reeder, author
American Council of the Blind
1155 15th Street NW   202-467-5081
Washington, DC 20005-2706   800-424-8666
                            Fax: 202-467-5085
                        e-mail: info@acb.org
                                www.acb.org
Offered in large print, braille, half speed cassette, via email and on the website.
32 pages 10x/year
Sharon Lovering, Editor

9989 Braille Monitor
National Federation of the Blind
1800 Johnson Street   410-659-9314
Baltimore, MD 21230-4998   Fax: 410-685-5653
                    e-mail: subscribe@diabetes.nfb.org
                                www.nfb.org
The leading publication in the blindness field, with a circulation of 30,000, this publication addresses issues of concern to the blind and the philosophy and activities of the National Federation of the Blind.
100 pages Monthly
Eileen Leyrce, Director of Publishing
Elizabeth Lunt, Editor

9990 Dialogue Magazine
Blindskills
PO Box 5181   503-581-4224
Salem, OR 97304-0181   800-860-4224
                            Fax: 503-518-0178
                    e-mail: blindsici@teleport.com
                                www.teleport.com
Publishes quarterly magazine in braille, large-type, cassette and disk of news items, fiction and articles of special interest.
Quarterly

9991 Future Reflections
Barbara Cheadler, author
National Federation of the Blind
1800 Johnson Street   410-659-9314
Baltimore, MD 21230-4998   Fax: 410-685-5653
                    e-mail: subscribe@diabetes.nfb.org
                                www.nfb.org
National magazine written specifically for parents and educators of blind children. Each issue addresses various topics important to blind children, their families and to school personnel.
Quarterly
Eileen Ley, Director of Publishing
Elizabeth Lunt, Editor

9992 Illinois Braille Messenger
Illinois Council of the Blind
PO Box 1336   217-523-4967
Springfield, IL 62705-1336   888-698-1862
                            Fax: 217-523-4302
                        e-mail: icb@fgi.net
Quarterly
Laura Booker, Editor

9993 Journal of Vision Rehabilitation
Media Productions & Marketing
2440 O Street   402-474-2676
Lincoln, NE 68510-1125
Multidisciplinary journal containing articles and papers dealing with low vision, its evaluation, instrumentation and rehabilitation.

9994 Journal of Visual Impairment & Blindness
AFB Press: American Foundation for the Blind
11 Penn Plaza   212-502-7600
New York, NY 10001   800-232-3044
                            Fax: 212-502-7774
                                www.afb.org/store
Peer-reviewed journal reporting on the cutting-edge research, innovative practice and news on all aspects of visual impairment. Available online, on cassette and ASCII disk.
10 Issues

9995 Recorded Periodicals
Associated Services for the Blind
919 Walnut Street   215-627-0600
Philadelphia, PA 19107-5237 Fax: 215-922-0692
                        e-mail: asbinfo@asb.org
                                www.asb.org
A subscription service of Associated Services for the Blind, this service provides 26 recorded magazines for blind and visually impaired individuals.
Audio Cassette
Patricia C Johnson, President/CEO

9996 Review
AER
206 N Washington Street   703-823-9690
Alexandria, VA 22314-2528   Fax: 703-823-9695
The Association's practice-oriented journal.

9997 Tactic
Clovernook Ctr. for the Blind & Visually Impaired
7000 Hamilton Avenue   513-522-3860
Cincinnati, OH 45231-5240   888-224-7156
                            Fax: 513-728-3946
                                www.clovernook.org
Quarterly
Jeffrey D Brasie, President

9998 Vision Enhancement Journal
Vision World Wide
5707 Brockton Drive   317-254-1332
Indianapolis, IN 46220-5481   800-733-2258
                            Fax: 317-251-6588
                    e-mail: info@visionww.org
                                www.visionww.org
Leading International publication providing information and resources for people with vision loss. Journal is available in large print, audio cassette and computer disk.
68-78 pages Quarterly
Patricia Price, President/Managing Editor

9999 Vision World Wide
5707 Brockton Drive   317-254-1332
Indianapolis, IN 46220-5481   800-733-2258
                            Fax: 317-251-6588
                    e-mail: info@visionww.org
                                www.visionww.org
Believing there is hope when vision fails. It disseminates relevant information on a variety of topics through its information and referral helpline, website, e-mail announce list and journal Vision Enhancement, all designed to encourage and support individuals with vision loss, family memebers, professionals who serve them. Aims to enhance everyday living so as to maintain an independent

lifestyle. It also serves as a consumer protection against misrepresentation and fraud.
72-78 pages Quarterly
Patricia Price, President/Managing Editor

10000 Voice of the Diabetic
National Federation of the Blind
1800 Johnson Street   410-659-9314
Baltimore, MD 21230-4998   Fax: 410-685-5653
e-mail: subscribe@diabetes.nfb.org
www.nfb.org
The leading publication in the diabetes field. Each issue addresses the problems and concerns of diabetes, with a special emphasis for those who have lost vision due to diabetes. Available in print and on cassette.
30 pages Quarterly
Eileen Ley, Director of Publishing
Elizabeth Lunt, Editor

Newsletters

10001 ACB Reports
American Council of the Blind
1155 15th Street NW   202-467-5081
Washington, DC 20005-2706   800-424-8666
Fax: 202-467-5085
e-mail: info@acb.org
www.acb.org
Radio news feature program for radio information services.
Monthly
Melanie Brunson, Executive Director

10002 AER Report
AER
4600 Duke Street   703-823-9690
Alexandria, VA 22304   877-492-2708
Fax: 703-823-9695
www.aerbvi.org
Contains organizational news, conference dates and information concerning services to visually impaired people.
28 pages BiMonthly
Jackie Fairbarns, Assistant Director

10003 AFB News
American Foundation for the Blind
11 Penn Plaza   212-502-7600
New York, NY 10001-2018   800-232-5463
Fax: 212-502-7777
National newsletter for general readership about blindness and visual impairments featuring people, programs, services and activities.
12 pages Quarterly

10004 Aging and Vision News
National Center for Vision and Aging
800 2nd Avenue   212-808-0077
New York, NY 10017   800-334-5497
3x Year

10005 Awareness
NAPVI
PO Box 317   617-972-7441
Watertown, MA 02471-0317   800-562-6265
Fax: 617-972-7444
e-mail: napvi@perkins.org
www.napvi.org
Newsletter offering regional news, sports and activities, conferences, camps, legislative updates, book reviews, audio reviews, professional question and answer column and more for the visually impaired and their families.
Quarterly
Susan LaVenture, Executive Director

10006 Braille Book Review
National Library Service for the Blind
1291 Taylor Street NW   202-707-5100
Washington, DC 20542-0002   Fax: 202-707-0712
www.loc.gov/nls

New braille books and product news.
BiMonthly

10007 Bulletin
National Association for Visually Handicapped
22 W 21st Street   212-889-3141
New York, NY 10010-6904   Fax: 212-727-2931
e-mail: navh@navh.org
www.navh.org
Annual report offering information on association activities and events, conferences, vision aids and resources for the visually impaired.
Lorraine Marchi LHD, Founder/CEO
Cesar Gomez, Executive Director

10008 DVH Quarterly
University of Arkansas At Little Rock
2801 S University Avenue   501-296-1815
Little Rock, AR 72204-1000   Fax: 501-663-3536
Offers information on upcoming events, conferences and workshops on and for visual disabilities. Book reviews, information on the newest resources and technology, educational programs, want ads and more.
Quarterly
Bob Brasher, Editor

10009 Eye Research News
645 Madison Avenue   212-752-4333
New York, NY 10022-1010   800-621-0026
Fax: 212-688-6231
e-mail: inforequest@rpbusa.org
www.rpbusa.org
Newsletter on the latest development in eye research
Annual
David Weeks, Chairman
Diane S Swift, President

10010 Focus
Visually Impaired Center
1422 West Court Street   810-767-4014
Flint, MI 48503   Fax: 810-767-0020
e-mail: info@vicflint.org
www.vicflint.org
Newsletter offering information for the visually impaired person in the forms of legislative and law updates, ADA information, support groups, hotlines, and articles on the newest technology in the field.
Quarterly
Laurie MacArthur, Executive Director

10011 Gleams Newsletter
Glaucoma Research Foundation
251 Post Street   415-986-3162
San Francisco, CA 94108   800-826-6693
Fax: 415-986-3763
e-mail: question@glaucoma.org
www.glaucoma.org
It includes information about glaucoma, new treatments, updates on research findings, and more.
3x/year
Thomas M Brunner, President/CEO
Andrew Jackson, Director Communications

10012 Guide Dog Foundation for the Blind Newsletter
371 E Jericho Turnpike   631-265-2121
Smithtown, NY 11787-2976   800-548-4337
Fax: 631-361-5192
e-mail: info@guidedog.org
www.guidedog.org
This organization relies on voluntary public contributions to provide persons with blindness the gift of second sight through the eyes of a guide dog. This nonprofit organization furnishes guide dogs, free of charge, to qualified people who seek independence, mobility and companionship.
Wells B Jones CAE CFRE, CEO
Michelle Lavitt, Marketing Manager

10013 Guide Dog News
Guide Dogs for the Blind

PO Box 151200
San Rafael, CA 94915

415-499-4000
800-298-4050
Fax: 415-499-4035
e-mail: information@guidedogs.com
www.guidedogs.com

About graduates, volunteers and donors of Guide Dogs for the Blind.
Quarterly
Etta Allen, Board Chair
Morgan Watkins, Interim CEO

10014 Guideway
Guide Dog Foundation for the Blind
371 E Jericho Turnpike
Smithtown, NY 11787-2976

631-265-2121
800-548-4337
Fax: 631-361-5192
e-mail: info@guidedog.org
www.guidedog.org

Offers updates and information on the foundation's activities and guide dog programs. In print form but is also available on cassette.
6 pages Monthly
Wells B Jones CAE CFRE, CEO
Michelle Lavitt, Marketing Manager

10015 Hearsay
Radio Information Service
600 Forbes Avenue
Pittsburgh, PA 15282

412-488-3944
Fax: 412-488-3953
e-mail: info@readingservice.org
www.readingservice.org

Newsletter for persons interested in radio reading services.
Quarterly

10016 Hub
SPOKES Unlimited
415 Main Street
Klamath Falls, OR 97601

541-883-7547
Fax: 541-885-2469
www.spokesunlimited.org

Newsletter on rehabilitation, peer counseling, blindness, visual impairments, information and referral.
Meg Graf, Resource Librarian

10017 InSight
Foundation Fighting Blindness
11435 Cronhill Drive
Owings Mill, MD 21117-2220

410-568-0150
800-683-5555
Fax: 410-363-2393
TDD: 410-363-7139
e-mail: info@fightblindness.org
www.fightblindness.org

The Foundation Fighting Blindness newsletter, delivered to members monthly. The major emphasis is to report on research and science news, and FDA approved clinical trials around retinal degenerative dieseases.
20 pages 3 per year
William T. Schmidt, CEO

10018 Lion
Lions Clubs International
300 W 22nd Street
Oak Brook, IL 60523-8815

312-571-5466

Publication for the blind.

10019 Listen Up
Recording for the Blind & Dyslexic (RFB&D)
20 Roszel Road
Princeton, NJ 08540-6294

609-452-0606
800-221-4792
Fax: 609-987-8116
e-mail: custserv@rfbd.org
www.rfbd.org

RFB&D's bi-monthly newsletter for members.

10020 Long Cane News
American Foundation for the Blind
15 W 16th Street
New York, NY 10011-6301

212-502-7600
800-232-5463
Fax: 212-502-7777

Semiannual

10021 Musical Mainstream
National Library Service for the Blind
1291 Taylor Street NW
Washington, DC 20542-0002

202-707-5100
Fax: 202-707-0712

Articles selected from print music magazines.
Quarterly

10022 NAVH UPDATE
National Association for Visually Handicapped
22 W 21st Street
New York, NY 10010-6904

212-889-3141
Fax: 212-727-2931
e-mail: navh@navh.org
www.navh.org

This newsletter offers vision news, medical updates, assistive device information, resources and more for the visually impaired.
4 pages Quarterly
Lorraine Marchi LHD, Founder/CEO
Cesar Gomez, Executive Director

10023 NLS News
National Library Service for the Blind
1291 Taylor Street NW
Washington, DC 20542-0002

202-707-5100
Fax: 202-707-0712

Newsletter on current program developments.
Quarterly

10024 NLS Update
National Library Service for the Blind
1291 Taylor Street NW
Washington, DC 20542-0002

202-707-5100
Fax: 202-707-0712

Newsletter on the services volunteer activities.
Quarterly

10025 NOAH News
National Organization for Albinism
PO Box 959
E. Hampsted, NH 03826-0959

603-887-2310
800-473-2310
Fax: 603-887-2310
www.albinism.org

BiAnnually

10026 Newsline for the Blind
National Federation of the Blind
1800 Johnson Street
Baltimore, MD 21230-4998

410-659-9314
Fax: 410-685-5653
e-mail: subscribe@diabetes.nfb.org
www.nfb.org

Nation's only digital talking newspaper service for the blind. Allows the blind to read the full text of leading national and local newspapers by using a touch-tone telephone. Service is free of charge and available 24 hours a day, 7 days per week.
Eileen Ley, Director of Publishing
Elizabeth Lunt, Editor

10027 Open Windows
Sunday School Board of the Southern Baptists
127 9th Avenue N
Nashville, TN 37234-0001

800-458-2772

Guide for personal devotions on audio cassette tape, using Bible references, devotional readings, and prayer calendar of popular Open Windows devotional guide for visually handicapped adults.
Quarterly

10028 Personal Reader Update
Personal Reader Department
9 Centennial Drive
Peabody, MA 01960-7906

978-977-2000
800-343-0311
Fax: 978-977-2437

Offers information on new services, assistive devices and technology for the blind.

10029 Prevent Blindness America News
Prevent Blindness America
211 West Wacker Drive, Suite 1700
Chicago, IL 60606

847-843-2020
800-331-2020
www.preventblindness.org

Offers information and articles on eye safety, programs, and services of the Society.
Quarterly

10030 RP Messenger
Texas Association of Retinitis Pigmentosa
PO Box 8388
Corpus Christi, TX 78468-8388
361-852-8515
Fax: 361-852-8515
A bi-annual newsletter offering information on Retinitis Pigmentosa.
BiAnnual

10031 Raised Dot Computing Newsletter
Raised Dot Computing
211 S Paterson Street
Madison, WI 53703-3789
608-257-9595
Discusses braille computer techniques and devices for blind persons.

10032 SCENE
Braille Institute
741 N Vermont Avenue
Los Angeles, CA 90029-3594
213-663-1111
800-272-4553
www.brailleinstitute.org
Offers information on the organization, question and answer column, articles on the newest technology and more for visually impaired persons.
Paul J Porelli, Managing Editor

10033 Smith-Kettlewell Technical File
Smith-Kettlewell Eye Research Foundation
2232 Webster Street
San Francisco, CA 94115-1821
415-561-1619
Fax: 415-561-1610
Quarterly

10034 Student Advocate
National Alliance of Blind Students
1155 15th Street NW, Suite 1004
Washington, DC 20005
202-467-5081
800-424-8666
e-mail: president@acbstudents.org
www.acbstudents.org
A communication forum covering issues of concern to postsecondary students who are blind.

Cammie Vloedman, President
Olivia Norman, First Vice President

10035 Talking Book Topics
National Library Services For The Blind
1291 Taylor Street NW
Washington, DC 20542-0002
202-707-5100
Fax: 202-707-0712
Offers hundreds of listings of books, fiction and nonfiction, for adults and children on cassette. Also offers listings on foreign language books on cassette, talking magazines and reviews.
Bimonthly

10036 Tarheel Talk
North Carolina Library for the Blind
1841 Capital Boulevard
Raleigh, NC 27635
919-733-4376
888-388-2460
Fax: 919-733-6910
TDD: 919-733-1462
e-mail: nclbph@ncdcr.gov
statelibrary.ncdcr.gov/lbph
Quarterly
Carl Keehn, Director

10037 The Macula Foundation Manhattan Eye, Ear & Throat Hospital
American Macular Degeneration Foundation
8th Floor 210 East 64th St.
New York, NY 10021-0515
212-605-3777
Fax: 212-605-3795
e-mail: foundation@retinal-research.org
www.macular.org/spotlite.html
Newsletter of the American Macular Degeneration Foundation, a nationwide support group for individuals and their families to adjust to the restrictions and changes brought about by macular disease.
Quarterly
Nikolai Stevenson, President
Walter Ross, VP

10038 The Pioneer Projects and Programs Periodic al
TelecomPioneers

930 15th St. 12th Floor
Denver, CO 80202
303-571-1200
www.pioneersvolunteer.org
Monthly

10039 Viva Vital News
5016 Silk Oak Drive
Sarasota, FL 34232-5410
941-371-2153
Membership service organization offering information for veterans and is an affiliate of the American Council of the Blind.

10040 Voice of Vision
GW Micro
310 Racquet Drive
Fort Wayne, IN 46825-4229
219-483-3625
Fax: 219-489-2608
e-mail: webmaster@gwmicro.com
www.gwmicro.com
Offers product reviews, product announcements, tips for making systems or applications more accessible, or explanations of concepts of interest to any computer user or would-be computer user. This association newsletter is available in braille, in large print, on audio cassette and on 3.5 or 5.25 IBM format diskette.
Quarterly

10041 What's Line
Alabama Regional Library for the Blind
6030 Monticello Drive
Montgomery, AL 36130-6000
334-213-3906
800-392-5671
Fax: 334-213-3993
e-mail: fzaleski@apls.state.al.us
http://statelibrary.alabama.gov
Informational 4 page newsletter in large print. Also available in braille and e-text formats.
4 pages Quarterly
Fara Zaleski, Division
Rebecca Mitchell, Director

Pamphlets

10042 About Children's Vision: Guide for Parents
National Association for Visually Handicapped
22 W 21st Street
New York, NY 10010-6904
212-889-3141
Fax: 212-727-2931
e-mail: navh@navh.org
www.navh.org
Offers a better understanding of the normal and possible abnormal development of a childs eyesight.
Lorraine Marchi LHD, Founder/CEO
Cesar Gomez, Executive Director

10043 Age Related Macular Degeneration
National Association for Visually Handicapped
22 W 21st Street
New York, NY 10010-6904
212-889-3141
Fax: 212-727-2931
e-mail: navh@navh.org
www.navh.org
Describes various conditions which affect the macular area and how to best maximize the use of residual peripheral vision.
Lorraine Marchi LHD, Founder/CEO
Cesar Gomez, Executive Director

10044 Are You Looking for a Few Good Workers?
AFB Press: American Foundation for the Blind
11 Penn Plaza
New York, NY 10001
212-502-7600
800-232-3044
Fax: 212-502-7774
www.afb.org/store
Helpful pamphlet explores both the importance and the advantage of hiring workers who are blind or visually impaired. Designed for human resource and other professionals responsible for hiring, it answers critical questions about hiring blind or visually impaired applicants. This enlightening guide to employment practices relating to these individuals offers insights on interviewing, job performance, tax incentives for businesses, insurance issues and more.
7 pages Pack of 20
ISBN: 0-891283-60-9

10045 BVA Bulletin
Blinded Veterans Association

477 H Street NW
Washington, DC 20001-2694

202-371-8880
800-669-7079
Fax: 202-371-8258
e-mail: bva@bva.org
www.bva.org

The Bulletin informs blinded veterans, their families, and those of the general public with an interest in BVA issues, about the organization. The publication includes current information relating to technology for the blind, legislation affecting blinded veterans, and news about the people who have overcome the challenges of blindness and are doing amazing work in their lives.

32 pages Quarterly
Thomas Miller, Executive Director
Stuart Nelson, Coordinator Public Relations

10046 Books are Fun for Everyone
National Library Service for the Blind
1291 Taylor Street NW
Washington, DC 20542

202-707-5100
Fax: 202-707-0712

10047 Braille Alphabet and Numbers
AFB Press: American Foundation for the Blind
11 Penn Plaza
New York, NY 10001

212-502-7600
800-232-3044
Fax: 212-502-7774
www.afb.org/store

Embossed with the braille alphabet and numbers, this 9 x 4 inch display card includes an explanation of braille and a short history of its development.

Pack of 25
ISBN: 0-891281-98-3

10048 Braille Literacy: Blind Persons, Families, Prof. & Producers of Braille
AFB Press: American Foundation for the Blind
11 Penn Plaza
New York, NY 10001

212-502-7600
800-232-3044
Fax: 212-502-7774
www.afb.org/store

Vigorous defece of the use of braille and an explanation of the importance of positive attitudes toward it that states: Braille is an assertion of equality between blind and sighted persons with respect to written communication. For everyone who uses or teaches braille and is interested in its future.

12 pages Pack of 25
ISBN: 0-891289-28-3

10049 Braille: An Extraordinary Volunteer Opportunity
National Library Service for the Blind
1291 Taylor Street NW
Washington, DC 20542-0002

202-707-5100
Fax: 202-707-0712

10050 Cataracts
National Eye Institute, Information Office
31 Center Drive MSC 2510
Bethesda, MD 20892-2510

301-496-5248
e-mail: 2020@nei.nih.gov
www.nei.nih.gov

Provides information about this common condition and its treatment.

10051 Classification of Impaired Vision
National Association for Visually Handicapped
22 W 21st Street
New York, NY 10010-6904

212-889-3141
Fax: 212-727-2931
e-mail: navh@navh.org
www.navh.org

Describes various degrees of impaired vision.
Lorraine Marchi LHD, Founder/CEO
Cesar Gomez, Executive Director

10052 Communicating with People Who Have Trouble Hearing & Seeing: A Primer
National Association for Visually Handicapped
22 W 21st Street
New York, NY 10010-6904

212-889-3141
Fax: 212-727-2931
e-mail: navh@navh.org
www.navh.org

Line drawings that depict problems for those with both deficiencies.
Lorraine Marchi LHD, Founder/CEO
Cesar Gomez, Executive Director

10053 Dancing Cheek to Cheek
Blind Children's Center
4120 Marathon Street
Los Angeles, CA 90029-3584

213-664-2153
Fax: 213-665-3828

Discusses beginning social, play and language interactions.
33 pages

10054 Diabetes, Vision Impairment and Blindness
AFB Press: American Foundation for the Blind
11 Penn Plaza
New York, NY 10001

212-502-7600
800-232-3044
Fax: 212-502-7777
www.afb.org/store

Presentation of how chronic diabetes affects vision and how diabetes can be managed at home by blind and visually impaired individuals.
32 pages
ISBN: 0-891289-02-0

10055 Diabetic Retinopathy
National Association for Visually Handicapped
22 W 21st Street
New York, NY 10010-6904

212-889-3141
Fax: 212-727-2931
e-mail: navh@navh.org
www.navh.org

Describes types of this disease and methods of treatment.
Lorraine Marchi LHD, Founder/CEO
Cesar Gomez, Executive Director

10056 Directory of Radio Reading Services
Radio Information Service
600 Forbes Avenue
Pittsburgh, PA 15282

412-488-3944
Fax: 412-488-3953
e-mail: info@readingservice.org
www.readingservice.org

Annually

10057 Don't Lose Sight of Age-Related Macular Degeneration
National Eye Institute, Information Office
31 Center Drive MSC 2510
Bethesda, MD 20892-2510

301-496-5248
e-mail: 2020@nei.nih.gov
www.nei.nih.gov

10058 Don't Lose Sight of Cataracts
National Eye Institute, Information Office
31 Center Drive MSC 2510
Bethesda, MD 20892-2510

301-496-5248
e-mail: 2020@nei.nih.gov
www.nei.nih.gov

10059 Don't Lose Sight of Glaucoma
National Eye Institute, Information Office
31 Center Drive MSC 2510
Bethesda, MD 20892-2510

301-496-5248
e-mail: 2020@nei.nih.gov
www.nei.nih.gov

10060 Eye-Q Test
National Association for Visually Handicapped
22 W 21st Street
New York, NY 10010-6904

212-889-3141
Fax: 212-727-2931
e-mail: navh@navh.org
www.navh.org

Five questions and answers to assist in knowing more about vision.
Lorraine Marchi LHD, Founder/CEO
Cesar Gomez, Executive Director

10061 Facts: Books for Blind and Physically Handicapped Individuals
National Library Service for the Blind
1291 Taylor Street NW
Washington, DC 20542-0002

202-707-5100
Fax: 202-707-0712
www.loc.gov

Annual

10062 Facts: Music for Blind and Physically Handicapped Individuals
National Library Service for the Blind

1291 Taylor Street NW
Washington, DC 20542-0002

202-707-5100
Fax: 202-707-0712
www.loc.gov

Annual

10063 Facts: Playback Machines and Accessories Provided on Free Loan
National Library Service for the Blind
1291 Taylor Street NW
Washington, DC 20542-0002

202-707-5100
Fax: 202-707-0712
www.loc.gov

10064 Facts: Sources for Purchase of Cassette & Disc Players From NLS
National Library Service for the Blind
1291 Taylor Street NW
Washington, DC 20542-0002

202-707-5100
Fax: 202-707-0712
www.lov.gov

10065 Family Guide to Vision Care
American Optometric Association
243 N Lindbergh Boulevard
Saint Louis, MO 63141-7881

314-991-4100
Fax: 314-991-4101
www.aoanet.org

Offers information on the early developmental years of your vision, finding a family optometrist and how to take care of your eyesight through the learning years, the working years and the mature years.

10066 Family Guide: Growth & Development of the Partially Seeing Child
National Association for Visually Handicapped
22 W 21st Street
New York, NY 10010-6904

212-889-3141
Fax: 212-727-2931
e-mail: navh@navh.org
www.navh.org

Offers information for parents and guidelines in raising a partially seeing child.
Lorraine Marchi LHD, Founder/CEO
Cesar Gomez, Executive Director

10067 General Facts and Figures on Blindness
National Society to Prevent Blindness
500 Remington Road
Schaumburg, IL 60173-5624

800-331-2020

10068 General Interest Catalog
National Braille Association
3 Townline Circle
Rochester, NY 14623-2537

716-427-8260

Lists hundreds of titles of fiction and non-fiction books offered in large print, braille or on cassette to visually impaired readers.
19 pages

10069 Glaucoma
Foundation For Glaucoma Research
490 Post Street
San Francisco, CA 94102-1409

415-986-3162

Offers information on what glaucoma is, the causes, treatments, types of glaucoma, eye exams and prevention.

10070 Glaucoma: Sneak Thief of Sight
National Association for Visually Handicapped
22 W 21st Street
New York, NY 10010-6904

212-889-3141
Fax: 212-727-2931
e-mail: navh@navh.org
www.navh.org

A pamphlet describing the disease, treatment and medications.
Lorraine Marchi LHD, Founder/CEO
Cesar Gomez, Executive Director

10071 Guide Dog Foundation Flyer
Guide Dog Foundation for the Blind
371 E Jericho Turnpike
Smithtown, NY 11787-2976

631-265-2121
800-548-4337
Fax: 631-361-5192
e-mail: info@guidedog.org
www.guidedog.org

Offers information on the programs and services provided by the foundation.
Wells B Jones CAE CFRE, CEO
Michelle Lavitt, Marketing Manager

10072 Guidelines for Comprehensive Low Vision Care
National Association for Visually Handicapped
22 W 21st Street
New York, NY 10010-6904

212-889-3141
Fax: 212-727-2931
e-mail: navh@navh.org
www.navh.org

A description of the proper method to conduct a low vision evaluation.
Lorraine Marchi LHD, Founder/CEO
Cesar Gomez, Executive Director

10073 Guidelines for Helping Deaf/Blind Persons
Helen Keller National Center for Deaf/Blind
111 Middle Neck Road
Sands Point, NY 11050-1299

516-944-8900
Fax: 516-944-7302
TTY: 516-944-8637
e-mail: hkncinfo@rcn.com
www.hknc.org

Pamphlet offering information on how persons should interact with deaf/blind individuals. Includes drawings of the one hand manual alphabet.
Joseph McNulty, Executive Director

10074 Heart to Heart
Blind Children's Center
4120 Marathon Street
Los Angeles, CA 90029-3584

213-664-2153
Fax: 213-665-3828

Parents of blind and partially sighted children talk about their feelings.
12 pages

10075 Heartbreak of Being a Little Bit Blind
National Association for Visually Handicapped
22 W 21st Street
New York, NY 10010-6904

212-889-3141
Fax: 212-727-2931
e-mail: nvah@navh.org
www.navh.org

Summary of what it means to have impaired vision with illustrations. Free for members.
Lorraine Marchi LHD, Founder/CEO
Cesar Gomez, Executive Director

10076 Helen Keller
AFB Press: American Foundation for the Blind
11 Penn Plaza
New York, NY 10001

212-502-7600
800-232-3044
Fax: 212-502-7774
www.afb.org/store

Brief biography that focuses on the major events of Helen Keller's life, from her birth in Tuscumbia, Alabama on June 27, 1880 to her death in Connecticut on June 1, 1968.
6 pages Pack of 25
ISBN: 0-891282-03-3

10077 How Does a Blind Person Get Around?
AFB Press: American Foundation for the Blind
11 Penn Plaza
New York, NY 10001

212-502-7600
800-232-3044
Fax: 212-502-7774
www.afb.org/store

Offers information on daily living as a blind person.

10078 How to Develop a Self-Help Group for Elders Losing Eyesight
National Association for Visually Handicapped
22 W 21st Street
New York, NY 10010-6904

212-889-3141
Fax: 212-727-2931
e-mail: navh@navh.org
www.navh.org

The pioneer for development of self-help groups, using the NAVH model, this publication is designed to help start and facilitate self-help groups.
Lorraine Marchi LHD, Founder/CEO
Cesar Gomez, Executive Director

10079 How to Use Your Low Vision Glasses
National Association for Visually Handicapped

22 W 21st Street 212-889-3141
New York, NY 10010-6904 Fax: 212-727-2931
e-mail: navh@navh.org
www.navh.org

A line drawing showing the correct way to benefit from low vision glasses.
Lorraine Marchi LHD, Founder/CEO
Cesar Gomez, Executive Director

10080 Information on Glaucoma
Foundation for Glaucoma Research
490 Post Street 415-986-3162
San Francisco, CA 94102-1409

10081 Information on Macular Degeneration
American Council of the Blind
1155 15th Street NW
Washington, DC 20005-2706 202-467-5081
800-424-8666
Fax: 202-467-5085
e-mail: info@acb.org
www.acb.org

Melanie Brunson, Executive Director

10082 It's All Right to Be Angry
National Association for Visually Handicapped
22 W 21st Street 212-889-3141
New York, NY 10010-6904 Fax: 212-727-2931
e-mail: navh@navh.org
www.navh.org

A helpful pamphlet describing reactions to learning to live with vision impairment.
Lorraine Marchi LHD, Founder/CEO
Cesar Gomez, Executive Director

10083 Large Print Loan Library Catalog
National Association for Visually Handicapped
22 W 21st Street 212-889-3141
New York, NY 10010-6904 Fax: 212-727-2931
e-mail: navh@navh.org
www.navh.org

Listing of over 9,000 commercially published and NAVH large print books available through NAVH on a loan basis. Includes a limited selection of titles available for purchase.
Lorraine Marchi LHD, Founder/CEO
Cesar Gomez, Executive Director

10084 Learning to Play
Blind Children's Center
4120 Marathon Street 213-664-2153
Los Angeles, CA 90029-3584 Fax: 213-665-3828
Discusses how to present play activities to the visually impaired preschool child.
12 pages

10085 Let's Eat
Blind Children's Center
4120 Marathon Street 213-664-2153
Los Angeles, CA 90029-3584 Fax: 213-665-3828
Teaches competent feeding skills to children with visual impairments.
28 pages

10086 Low Vision Questions and Answers
AFB Press: American Foundation for the Blind
11 Penn Plaza 212-502-7600
New York, NY 10001 800-232-3044
Fax: 212-502-7774
www.afb.org/store
What does low vision mean? What do low vision services cost? What diseases cause low vision? Answers to these and other questions are presented in a straightforward yet comprehensive format. Photographs show how objects appear to people with low vision, what low vision devices look like, and how they are used.
21 pages Pack of 25
ISBN: 0-891281-96-7

10087 Magnifier
Macular Degeneration Foundation
PO Box 9752 408-260-1335
San Jose, CA 95157-0752 888-633-3937
www.eyesight.org

Large-font publication.

10088 Magnifier Highlights
Independent Living Aids
200 Robbins Lane
Jericho, NY 11753-2341 800-537-2118
Fax: 516-752-3135
e-mail: indlivaids@aol.com
www.independentliving.com
Full line of magnifiers, ranging from high-powered vision aids to instruments and accessories
Marvin Sandler, President

10089 Move with Me
Blind Children's Center
4120 Marathon Street 213-664-2153
Los Angeles, CA 90029-3584 Fax: 213-665-3828
A parent's guide to movement development for visually impaired babies.
12 pages

10090 Music Is for Everyone
National Library Service for the Blind
1291 Taylor Street NW 202-707-5100
Washington, DC 20542-0002 Fax: 202-707-0712

10091 Parenting Preschoolers: Raising Young Blind & Visually Impaired Child
AFB Press: American Foundation for the Blind
11 Penn Plaza 212-502-7600
New York, NY 10001 800-232-3044
Fax: 212-502-7774
www.afb.org/store
Why is my baby so quiet? Why does my child seem slower than other children? What will happen when my child goes to school? This primer provides practical answers to the questions most freqently asked by parents and gives advice on what to expect, how to adapt to the child's situation and needs, and what to look for in early education programs.
28 pages Pack of 25
ISBN: 0-891289-98-4

10092 Patient's Guide to Visual Aids and Illumination
National Association for Visually Handicapped
22 W 21st Street 212-889-3141
New York, NY 10010-6904 Fax: 212-727-2931
e-mail: navh@navh.org
www.navh.org
A reference booklet offering information on aids for the visually impaired.
Lorraine Marchi LHD, Founder/CEO
Cesar Gomez, Executive Director

10093 Puppy Walker Brochure
Guide Dog Foundation for the Blind
371 E Jericho Turnpike 631-265-2121
Smithtown, NY 11787-2976 800-548-4337
Fax: 631-361-5192
e-mail: info@guidedog.org
www.guidedog.org
Offers information on being a volunteer puppy walker family.
Wells B Jones CAE CFRE, CEO
Michelle Lavitt, Marketing Manager

10094 Reaching, Crawling, Walking-Let's Get Moving
Blind Children's Center
4120 Marathon Street 213-664-2153
Los Angeles, CA 90029-3584 Fax: 213-665-3828
Orientation and mobility for visually impaired preschool children.
24 pages

10095 Reading is for Everyone
National Library Service for the Blind
1291 Taylor Street NW 202-707-5100
Washington, DC 20542-0002 Fax: 202-707-0712

10096 Reading with Low Vision
National Library Service for the Blind
1291 Taylor Street NW 202-707-5100
Washington, DC 20542-0002 Fax: 202-707-0712

10097 Reference and Information Services from NLS
National Library Service for the Blind
1291 Taylor Street NW   202-707-5100
Washington, DC 20542-0002   Fax: 202-707-0712

10098 Resource List for Persons with Low Vision
American Council of the Blind
1155 15th Street NW   202-467-5081
Washington, DC 20005-2706   800-424-8666
                                 Fax: 202-467-5085
                                 e-mail: info@acb.org
                                 www.acb.org

Melanie Brunson, Executive Director

10099 Seeing Eye to Eye: An Administrator's Guide
AFB Press: American Foundation for the Blind
11 Penn Plaza   212-502-7600
New York, NY 10001   800-232-3044
                                 Fax: 212-502-7774
                                 www.afb.org/store
Visual impairment often has a profound impact on a child's ability to learn language and basic communication concepts. This easy-to-read booklet explains the student's needs and the practical services essential for helping them become literate and successful. An ideal tool for administrators and educators, it includes clear explanations of common terminology, the impact of visual impairment on learning, specialized services for visually impaired students, and in-service training for teachers.
72 pages Pack of 10
ISBN: 0-891283-59-5

10100 Selecting a Program
Blind Children's Center
4120 Marathon Street   213-664-2153
Los Angeles, CA 90029-3584   Fax: 213-665-3828
A guide for parents of infants and preschoolers with visual impairments.
28 pages

10101 Standing on My Own Two Feet
Blind Children's Center
4120 Marathon Street   213-664-2153
Los Angeles, CA 90029-3584   Fax: 213-665-3828
A step-by-step guide to designing and constructing simple, individually tailored adaptive mobility devices for preschool-age children who are visually impaired.
36 pages

10102 Talk to Me
Blind Children's Center
4120 Marathon Street   213-664-2153
Los Angeles, CA 90029-3584   Fax: 213-665-3828
A language guide for parents of deaf children.
11 pages

10103 Talk to Me II
Blind Children's Center
4120 Marathon Street   213-664-2153
Los Angeles, CA 90029-3584   Fax: 213-665-3828
A sequel to Talk To Me, available in English and Spanish.
15 pages

10104 Talking Books for Senior Adults
National Library Service for the Blind
1291 Taylor Street NW   202-707-5100
Washington, DC 20542-0002   Fax: 202-707-0712

10105 Touch the Baby: Blind & Visually Impaired Children as Patients
American Foundation for the Blind
11 Penn Plaza   212-502-7600
New York, NY 10001-2018   800-232-3044
                                 Fax: 212-502-7774
                                 www.afb.org/store
How-to manual for health care professionals working in hospitals, clinics and doctors' offices that teaches the special communication and touch-related techniques needed to prevent blind and visually impaired patients from withdrawing from healthcare staff and the outside world. includes how to talk to infants and how to signal to children that a procedure may cause discomfort.
13 pages Pack of 25
ISBN: 0-891281-97-5

10106 Volunteer at Your Braille and Talking Book Library
National Library Service for the Blind
1291 Taylor Street NW   202-707-5100
Washington, DC 20542-0002   Fax: 202-707-0712
Brochure

10107 What Do You Do When You See a Blind Person — and What Don't You Do?
AFB Press: American Foundation for the Blind
11 Penn Plaza   212-502-7600
New York, NY 10001   800-232-3044
                                 Fax: 212-502-7774
                                 www.afb.org/store
Examples of real-life situations that teach sighted persons how to interact effectively with blind persons. Topics covered include how to help someone across the street, how not to distract a guide dog and how to take leave of a blind person.
8 pages Pack of 25
ISBN: 0-891281-95-9

10108 Wings for the Future
American Printing House for the Blind
1839 Frankfort Avenue   502-895-2405
Louisville, KY 40206-3148   800-223-1839
                                 Fax: 502-895-1509
                                 e-mail: info@ahp.org
This booklet offers an introduction to the American Printing House For The Blind's programs, services, tools, aids and more.
13 pages

10109 Without Sight and Sound
Helen Keller National Center for Deaf/Blind
111 Middle Neck Road   516-944-8900
Sands Point, NY 11050-1299   Fax: 516-944-7302
                                 TTY: 516-944-8637
                                 e-mail: hkncinfo@rcn.com
                                 www.hknc.org
Pamphlet offering facts, causes, types and descriptions of deaf/blindness.
Joseph McNulty, Executive Director

10110 You Seem Like a Regular Kid to Me
AFB Press: American Foundation for the Blind
11 Penn Plaza   212-502-7600
New York, NY 10001   800-232-3044
                                 Fax: 212-502-7774
                                 www.afb.org/store
An interview with Jane, a blind child, allows other children to understand what it's like to be blind. Jane explains how she gets around, takes care of herself, does her school work, spends her leisure time and even pays for things when she can't see money. Photographs show Jane engaged in various activities.
16 pages Pack of 25
ISBN: 0-891289-21-6

Audio & Video

10111 Adult Bible Study
Sunday School Board of the Southern Baptists
127 9th Avenue N
Nashville, TN 37234-0001   800-458-2772
Unabridged Sunday School lessons recorded on audio cassette as printed in Adult Bible Study.
Quarterly

10112 Aging and Vision: Declarations of Independence
AFB Press: American Foundation for the Blind
11 Penn Plaza   212-502-7600
New York, NY 10001   800-232-3044
                                 Fax: 212-502-7774
                                 www.afb.org/store
Very personal look at five older people who have successfully coped with visual impairment and continue to lead active, satisfying lives. Their stories are not only inspirational, they also provide paractical, down-to-earth suggestions for adapting to vision loss later in life.
18 Minutes VHS
ISBN: 0-891282-20-3

10113 Bible Alliance
PO Box 621 941-748-3031
Bradenton, FL 34206-0621 e-mail: aurora@auroraministries.org
www.careministries.org
Offers the Christian bible on cassettes in over 52 languages for those finding it impossible to read small print.

10114 Blindness: A Family Matter
AFB Press: American Foundation for the Blind
11 Penn Plaza 212-502-7600
New York, NY 10001 800-232-3044
Fax: 212-502-7774
www.afb.org/store
Frank exploration of the effects of an individual's visual impairment on other members of the family and how family members can play a positive role in the rehablitation process. Features three families whose success stories provide advice and encouragement, as well as interviews with newly blinded adults currently involved in a rehabilitation program. Also available in PAL.
23 Minutes VHS
ISBN: 0-891282-22-X

10115 Braille Documents
Metrolina Sight Services
704 Louise Avenue 704-372-3870
Charlotte, NC 28204-2128 e-mail: braille@charlotte.infi.net
www.careministries.org
This production shop creates Braille and large-print documents.

10116 Brief Encounters of the Right Kind: How to Make Your Point in 10 Minutes or Less
AFB Press: American Foundation for the Blind
11 Penn Plaza 212-502-7600
New York, NY 10001 800-232-3044
Fax: 212-502-7774
www.afb.org/store
Humorous and instructional tour through the do's and don'ts of lobbying at the local, state and national levels. Three seasoned lobbyists discuss how professionals, families, consumers and volunteer advocates can use their expert knowledge to influence public policy. A Toolkit for Advocates, the accompanying manual, complements the video by providing a summary of the legislative process and key points on how to meet successfully with legislators.
VHS & PAL
ISBN: 0-891282-83-1

10117 Destination Unlimited
Leader Dog For The Blind
1964 Park Street 306-565-8211
Regina, SK, S4P 3G4,
This is a documentary about Leader-Dog-For-The-Blind Program. The needs of various people and how their dog fulfills their needs are shown. In addition, the overall leader-dog program is reviewed. This training program would be of interest to many teenagers.
Films

10118 Employed Ability: Blind Persons on the Job
AFB Press: American Foundation for the Blind
11 Penn Plaza 212-502-7600
New York, NY 10001 800-232-3044
Fax: 212-502-7774
www.afb.org/store
Blind and visually impaired people from a wide variety of occupations talk about career opportunities and their experiences in the workplace. Employers and coworkers are also interviewed and speak openly about supervising and working alongside visually impaired employees.
14 Minutes VHS
ISBN: 0-891282-24-6

10119 Focused On: Importance and Need for Skills
AFB Press: American Foundation for the Blind
11 Penn Plaza 212-502-7600
New York, NY 10001 800-232-3044
Fax: 212-502-7774
www.afb.org/store
Provides an overview of the importance of social competence and details the course of social skills development in children in general and in children who are blind or visually impaired in particu-

lar. This study guide examines both the development of social skills in general and how this process applies to children who are blind or who have visual impairments.
VHS & PAL
ISBN: 0-891283-25-0

10120 Hand in Hand: It Can Be Done
AFB Press: American Foundation for the Blind
11 Penn Plaza 212-502-7600
New York, NY 10001 800-232-3044
Fax: 212-502-7774
www.afb.org/store
One hour introduction to working effectively with individuals who are deaf-blind. Designed as both an overview and a reinforcer of the self-study text, this video can be used as a whole or in sections for parents and regular educators, as well as in the community. Includes a discussion guide. Available in audioscribed or open captioned VHS and PAL.
ISBN: 0-891283-25-0

10121 Heart to Heart
Blind Children's Center
4120 Marathon Street 213-664-2153
Los Angeles, CA 90029-3584 Fax: 213-665-3828
Parents of blind and partially sighted children talk about their feelings.
Videotape

10122 Helen Keller in Her Story
AFB Press: American Foundation for the Blind
11 Penn Plaza 212-502-7600
New York, NY 10001 800-232-3044
Fax: 212-502-7774
www.afb.org/store
Patty Duke, who portrayed the young Helen Keller on stage and on screen in The Miracle Worker, introduces this Oscar-winning documentary about the extraordinary lives of Ms. Keller, her teacher Anne Sullivan Macy and her friend and companion Polly Thompson. Includes vintage still photographs as well as early movie footage and newsreel footage.
VHS & PAL
ISBN: 0-891282-25-4

10123 Let's Eat
Blind Children's Center
4120 Marathon Street 213-664-2153
Los Angeles, CA 90029-3584 Fax: 213-665-3828
Teaches competent feeding skills to children with visual impairments.
Videotape

10124 Making the Most of Early Communication: Strategies for Supporting Communication
AFB Press: American Foundation for the Blind
11 Penn Plaza 212-502-7600
New York, NY 10001 800-232-3044
Fax: 212-502-7774
www.afb.org/store
Demonstrates selected interventions to assist infants and toddlers with multiple disabilities, including vision and hearing loss, in developing early communication and other skills. Emphasizing the critical importance of early intervention, this video is designed to help service providers and families create effective communication straegies that encourage cognitive development and funtional abilities in young children with multiple disabilities and those who are deaf-blind. 37 minutes.
VHS & PAL
ISBN: 0-891282-96-3

10125 New What Do You Do When You See a Blind Person?
AFB Press: American Foundation for the Blind
11 Penn Plaza 212-502-7600
New York, NY 10001 800-232-3044
Fax: 212-502-7774
www.afb.org/store
Engaging remake of the 1971 classic brings a fresh perspective on how to interact comfortably with someone who is visually impaired. The entertaining experiences of Mark Johnson, a computer programmer who is blind, and Dave Simon, a computer salesman

who is not, show the simple ways to provide assistance, if it is needed, to someone who is blind or visually impaired. 16 minutes.
VHS & PAL
ISBN: 0-891283-13-7

10126 Oh, I See
AFB Press: American Foundation for the Blind
11 Penn Plaza   212-502-7600
New York, NY 10001   800-232-3044
                                 Fax: 212-502-7774
                                 www.afb.org/store
Lively and entertaining video provides practical suggestions on helping students who are blind and visually impaired adapt to the mainstream classroom. The modifacations shown can easily be used by teachers, students, or anyone working with blind and visually impaired students. Seven minutes.
VHS & PAL
ISBN: 0-891282-52-1

10127 Out of Left Field
AFB Press: American Foundation for the Blind
11 Penn Plaza   212-502-7600
New York, NY 10001   800-232-3044
                                 Fax: 212-502-7774
                                 www.afb.org/store
Illustrates how youngsters who are blind or visually impaired are integrated with their sighted peers in a variety of recreational and athletic activites. 17 minutes.
VHS & PAL
ISBN: 0-891282-28-9

10128 Profiles in Aging and Vision
AFB Press: American Foundation for the Blind
11 Penn Plaza   212-502-7600
New York, NY 10001   800-232-3044
                                 Fax: 212-502-7774
                                 www.afb.org/store
Can be used on its own or in conjunction with the text, this is an informative overview of the common eye conditions that affect older people, with a detailed description of the vision-related services that help older people who are visually impaired continue to lead independent lives. Experienced professionals provide valuable information on crucial issues, and older visually impaired persons offering their own revealing perspectives. 33 minutes.
VHS
ISBN: 0-891289-48-8

10129 Reaching Out: A Creative Access Guide for Designing Exhibits & Cultural Programs
AFB Press: American Foundation for the Blind
11 Penn Plaza   212-502-7600
New York, NY 10001   800-232-3044
                                 Fax: 212-502-7774
                                 www.afb.org/store
Video and accompanying manual are a creative package for making information on cultural programs and facilities accessable to people who are blind or visually impaired. Created especially for libraries, museums, historical societies, outdoor cultural facilities, corporations and everyone whose mission involves providing information to the community, this video offers practical design and program solutions. 22 minutes.
VHS & PAL
ISBN: 0-891289-49-6

10130 Seven Minute Lesson
AFB Press: American Foundation for the Blind
11 Penn Plaza   212-502-7600
New York, NY 10001   800-232-3044
                                 Fax: 212-502-7774
                                 www.afb.org/store
Introduction to the basic techniques used when acting as a sighted guide for a person who is blind or visually impaired.
VHS & PAL
ISBN: 0-891282-29-7

10131 Solutions for Everyday Living for Older People with Visual Impairments
AFB Press: American Foundation for the Blind

11 Penn Plaza   212-502-7600
New York, NY 10001   800-232-3044
                                 Fax: 212-502-7774
                                 www.afb.org/store
Presents a positive and helpful view of how older people who have lost some or all of their vision can continue to lead satisfying lives within supportive environments. This engaing video shows how staff members in continuing care communities and other living settings for older people can help residents function as independently as possible.Different types of vision loss are explained, and simple solutions are offered for carrying out everyday activities. 34 minutes.
VHS & PAL
ISBN: 0-891288-52-X

10132 Strategies for Community Access: Braille & Raised Large Print Facility Signs
AFB Press: American Foundation for the Blind
11 Penn Plaza   212-502-7600
New York, NY 10001   800-232-3044
                                 Fax: 212-502-7774
                                 www.afb.org/store
Brief and effective advocacy tool that can be used to educate architects, planners, facility managers, sign makers and consumers about the value of accessible signs. Topics covered include ADA requirements for accessible signs, samples of signs designed to be compatible with an organization's interior design, demonstrations of how blind and print signs are a cost-effective way to provide access. Reproducible fact sheets on ADA signage guidelines are enclosed. Seven minutes.
VHS & PAL
ISBN: 0-891282-56-4

10133 Understanding Braille Literacy
AFB Press: American Foundation for the Blind
11 Penn Plaza   212-502-7600
New York, NY 10001   800-232-3044
                                 Fax: 212-502-7774
                                 www.afb.org/store
Motovational and intructional video covers all aspects of a successful braille education program. Teachers and students demonstate how braille is learned and used from preschool through high school and describes how braille skills contribute to literacy, independence, mastry of academic skills and successful education experiences in the regular classroom. Parents, classroom teachers and school administrators also speak out about the importance of braille. 25 minutes.
VHS & PAL
ISBN: 0-891282-61-0

10134 We Can Do it Together: Mobility for Students with Multiple Disabilities
AFB Press: American Foundation for the Blind
11 Penn Plaza   212-502-7600
New York, NY 10001   800-232-3044
                                 Fax: 212-502-7774
                                 www.afb.org/store
Illustrates a transdisiplinary team approach to teaching orientation and mobility to students with severe visual and multiple impairments, covering both adapted communication systems that are used to teach mobility skills and basic indoor mobility in the school. For mobility instructors, administrators, teachers of visually impaired and severely disabled students, occupational, physical and speech therapists and parents. Discussion guide included, 13 minutes.
VHS & PAL
ISBN: 0-891282-13-0

10135 What Can Baby See? Vision Tests & Intervention Strategies for Infants
AFB Press: American Foundation for the Blind
11 Penn Plaza   212-502-7600
New York, NY 10001   800-232-3044
                                 Fax: 212-502-7774
                                 www.afb.org/store
Presents common vision tests and methods of gathering information that can be used with infants and very young children to help indentify visual impairments that require early intervention services. Effective ways of working with families and early intervention strategies for encouraging infants with multiple disabilities to

use their vision in functional ways are demonstrated to help families and service providers contribute to children's growth and development.
VHS & PAL
ISBN: 0-891282-99-8

Web Sites

10136 ACB Government Employees

www.acb.org
Concerns of the organization include recruitment, placement and advancement of blind and visually impaired employees.

10137 ACB Radio Amateurs

www.acb.org
A radio amateur network of blind, visually impaired and sighted members who gather and share common problems and solutions to help members improve radio amateurs in getting started, provides access to educational materials in special media and publishes a directory for the visually impaired.

10138 ACB Social Service Providers

www.acb.org
Information on blind and visually impaired social workers, social service professionals, students pursuing careers in social work, and other interested persons.

10139 American Blind Lawyers Association

www.acb.org
Information on law school admission tests and bar exams, private sector and government employment relations and specialized work techniques for the blind and visually impaired.

10140 American Council of Blind Lions

www.acb.org
Information concerning Club activities in the field of work for the blind and encourages blind people to join Lions Clubs and other civic activities.

10141 American Council of the Blind

www.acb.org
Information for the visually impaired and fully sighted individuals who are concerned about the dignity and well-being of blind people throughout America.

10142 American Foundation for the Blind

www.afb.org
Our web site unique in that it combines state-of-the-art features, an attractive visual environment and an accessible design for people with all types of disabilities. Features include a searchable database of vision services nationwide, community message boards and the largest collection of Helen Keller memorbilia on the web. It meets the stringent AAA guidelines of the Web Accessibility Initiative of the World Wide Web Consortium, established to help organizations build accessible websites.

10143 American Printing House for the Blind

www.aph.org
This organization promotes the independence of blind persons by providing special media, tools and materials needed for education and life.

10144 Blinded Veterans Association

www.bva.org
Offers two main service programs without cost to blinded veterans. Field service program provides counseling to veterans and families, and information on benefits and rehabilitation.

10145 Braille Revival League

www.acb.org
Information for people to read and write in braille, advocates for mandatory braille instruction in educational facilities for the blind, strives to make available a supply of braille materials from libraries and printing houses and more.

10146 Council of Families with Visual Impairment

www.acb.org
Offers support and outreach, shares experiences in parent/child relationships, exchanges educational, cultural and medical information about child development and more.

10147 Fidelco Guide Dog Foundation

www.fidelco.org
Fidelco breeds, raises, trains, and places German shepherd guide dogs with men and women who are visually impaired, primarily in the Northeast.

10148 Friends-In-Art

www.acb.org
Offers consultation to program planners in establishing accessible art and museum exhibits and presents Performing Arts Showcases.

10149 Guide Dog Foundation for the Blind

www.guidedog.org
Furnishes guide dogs, free of charge, to qualified people who seek independence, mobility and companionship.

10150 Guide Dog Users

www.acb.org
Promotes the acceptance of blind people and their dogs, works for enforcement and expansion of laws admitting guide dogs into public places, advocates for quality training and follow-up services.

10151 Healing Well

www.healingwell.com
An online health resource guide to medical news, chat, information and articles, newsgroups and message boards, books, disease-related web sites, medical directories, and more for patients, friends, and family coping with disabling diseases, disorders, or chronic illnesses.

10152 Health Finder

www.healthfinder.gov
Searchable, carefully developed web site offering information on over 1000 topics. Developed by the US Department of Health and Human Services, the site can be used in both English and Spanish.

10153 Healthlink USA

www.healthlinkusa.com
Health information concerning treatment, cures, prevention, diagnosis, risk factors, research, support groups, email lists, personal stories and much more. Updated regularly.

10154 Helios Health

www.helioshealth.com
Online resource for your health information. Detailed information about specific health topics, access to expert advice from our Medical Advisory Board, and up-to-date health news.

10155 Independent Visually Impaired Enterprises

www.acb.org
Information on rehabilitation facilities for all types of business enterprises and publicizes the capabilities of blind and visually impaired business persons.

10156 Library Users of America

www.acb.org
Provides for chapters in states through the US to encourage the development, acquisition and use of technology which enables blind and visually impaired persons to use printed material independently in library settings and elsewhere.

10157 Lighthouse International

www.lighthouse .org
Offers information about vision impairment and vision rehabilitation, and provides referrals to services and support groups nationwide.

10158 MedicineNet

www.medicinenet.com
An online resource for consumers providing easy-to-read, authoritative medical and health information.

10159 Medscape

www.medscape.com
Medscape offers specialists, primary care physicians, and other health professionals the Web's most robust and integrated medical information and educational tools.

10160 National Alliance of Blind Students

www.acb.org
Works to facilitate progress toward full accessibility of college programs and facilities, provides opportunities for discussion of

issues important to students and assists with National Student Seminars.

10161 National Association for Visually Hand.

www.navh.org

NAVH ensures that those with limited vision do not lead limited lives. We offer emotional support; training in the use of and access to a wide variety of optical aids and lighting; a large print, nationwide, free-by-mail loan library; large print educational materials; quarterly newsletter; referrals; self-help groups and educational outreach.

10162 National Association of Blind Educators

www.nfb.org

Provides support and information regarding professional responsibilities, classroom techniques, national testing methods and career obstacles. Publishes The Blind Educator, national magazine specifically for blind educators.

10163 National Association of Blind Lawyers

www.nfb.org

Provides support and information regarding employment, techniques used by the blind, advocacy, laws affecting the blind, current information about the American Bar Association and other issues for blind lawyers.

10164 National Association of Blind Secretaries and Transcribers

www.nfb.org

Addresses issues such as technology, accomodation, career planning and job training.

10165 National Association of Blind Students

www.nfb.org

Provides support, information and encouragement to blind college and university students.

10166 National Association of Blind Teachers

www.acb.org

Works to advance the teaching profession for blind and visually impaired people, protects the interest of teachers, presents discussions and solutions for special problems encountered by blind teachers and publishes a directory of blind teachers in the US.

10167 National Association of Guide Dog Users

www.nfb.org

Provides information and support for guide dog users and works to secure high standards in guide dog training. Addresses issues of discrimination of guide dog users and offers public education about guide dog use.

10168 National Association to Promote the Use of Braille

www.nfb.org

Provides information about the importance of Braille in securing independence, education and employment for the blind.

10169 National Braille Association

www.nationalbraille.org/

Provides transciption service for, and maintains a depository of, braille books.

10170 National Federation of the Blind: Blind/Deaf Division

www.nfb.org

Offers personal contact with other deaf-blind individuals knowledgeable in advocacy, education, employment, technology, discrimination and other issues surrounding deaf-blindness.

10171 National Federation of the Blind

www.nfb.org

Provides public education about blindness, support services to the newly blinded, scholarships, publications about blindness, adaptive equipment for the blind, advocacy services, Newsline for the Blind, assistive technology information and Job Opportunities for the Blind.

10172 National Federation of the Blind in Computer Science

www.nfb.org

New technologies, to secure access to current technology and to develop new ways of using current or new technologies by the blind.

10173 National Federation of the Blind: Blind Merchants Division

www.nfb.org

Provides information regarding rehabilitation, social security, tax and other issues which directly affect blind merchants. Serves as advocacy and support group.

10174 National Federation of the Blind: Human Services Division

www.nfb.org

Organization of blind persons working in counseling, personnel, psychology, social work, psychiatry, rehabilitation and other social science and human resource fields. Provides resources regarding blindness-related techniques and methods used in these fields.

10175 National Federation of the Blind: Masonic Square Club

www.nfb.org

Blind individuals committed to sharing of Masonic experiences, goals and history.

10176 National Federation of the Blind: Music Division

www.nfb.org

Offers support and information regarding copyright, publishing, promotion and other career details.

10177 National Federation of the Blind: Public Employees Division

www.nfb.org

Focuses on issues such as changes in governmental hiring and retention practices, new job skills needed for the future, government employment downsizing, new electronic means of finding public sector jobs, self-advocacy and career planning strategies.

10178 National Federation of the Blind: Science and Engineering Division

www.nfb.org

This is a strong support group to encourage blind persons in pursuit of these careers, many of which have been considered not possible for the blind in the past.

10179 National Federation of the Blind: Writers Division

www.nfb.org

Covers various aspects of this business, including selling your work, publishing, technology, motivation and discovering writing and publishing resources.

10180 National Library Service for the Blind

www.loc.gov/nls

Administers a national library service that provides braille and recorded books and magazines on free loan to anyone who cannot read standard print because of visual or physical disabilities who are eligible residents of the United States or American citizens living abroad.

10181 National Organization of Parents of Blind Children

www.nfb.org

Addresses issues ranging from help to parents of a newborn blind infant, mobility and Braille instruction, education, social and community participation, development of self-confidence and other vital factors involved in the growth of a blind child.

10182 National Organization of the Senior Blind

www.nfb.org

Provides support and information to other blind seniors. Issues include concerns such as remaining active in community and social life, maintaining private homes or living in retirement communities or nursing homes, learning the techniques used by the blind, independently caring for oneself and maintaining a positive approach to vision loss.

10183 Randolph-Sheppard Vendors of America

www.acb.org

Protects the interests of blind vendors, seeks proper implementation of the Randolph-Sheppard Act and encourages facility locations in more visible and profitable areas.

10184 Vision World Wide

www.visionww.org

Aims is to enhance everyday living so as to maintain an independent lifestyle. It also serves as a consumer protection against misrepresentation and fraud.

10185 Visually Impaired Data Processors International

www.acb.org

Provides for the exchange of work technique ideas and works with agencies to increase the availability of braille and recorded materials.

10186 Visually Impaired Piano Tuners International

www.acb.org

Works to preserve, advance and enrich the skilled professional piano tuning for competent, well-trained blind and visually impaired persons.

10187 Visually Impaired Veterans of America

www.acb.org

Promotes the rights of visually impaired veterans to receive all benefits, encourages research and development of new products for blind people.

10188 WebMD

www.webmd.com

Information on Blindness and Visual Impairments, including articles and resources.

Description

10189 War Syndromes

War syndromes have plagued soldiers for centuries. Though symptoms may vary, soldiers may become affected by various postulated physiological diseases as well as psychological illnesses. Agent Orange and the Gulf War Syndrome are two of the conditions still prevalent today.

Agent Orange is the common name for a mix of chemicals developed by the military. It was first used during the Vietnam War to destroy vegetation that concealed the enemy. During the war, soldiers were exposed heavily to this chemical; years later, many of them contracted a variety of conditions. There has been an intense controversy about whether Agent Orange caused these conditions, with medical scientists, patients, politicians and advocacy groups all involved.

Among the conditions sometimes attributed to Agent Orange exposure are a variety of cancers, an acne-like skin condition called chloracne, neurological diseases, repeated infections, sterility, and birth defects in the children of exposed persons.

To further understand this condition, the Department of Veterans Affairs has been established a registry of Vietnam veterans concerned that they may have been exposed to Agent Orange. Veterans who suspect their symptoms are related to this exposure can contact the Department's Medical Administrative Services to request the Agent Orange Registry Examination, a complete health evaluation. The Department offers service-connected compensation for those veterans who develop a condition believed to be related to exposure to Agent Orange.

Gulf War Syndrome, GWS, or Persian Gulf War Syndrome is a constellation of illnesses experienced by 5,000 to 80,000 US veterans after returning from the Persian Gulf Wars in the 1990's and 2000's. Symptoms are predominately neurologic and consist of impaired cognition, with problems of attention, memory, reasoning, insomnia, depression and headaches. Complaints of muscle and joint pain, gastrointestinal difficulties, vertigo and weakness are also common. As veterans resumed family life, various birth defects were added to the list. The cause of GWS is unknown.

A 1997 study funded by the Centers for Disease Control shows that Gulf War personnel are more likely than others to report depression, syptoms similar to post-traumatic stress disorder, chronic fatigue, cognitive difficulties, bronchitis, asthma, fibromyalgia, alcohol abuse, anxiety and sexual dysfunction.

Many causes of GWS have been suggested, but none have been definitely identified or eliminated. These include: effects of chemical and/or biological weapons; exposure to pesticides; smoke from oil well fires; airborne contamination from munitions plants destroyed in Iraq, exposure to depleted uranium used as a material in some US munitions and exposure to volatile solvents used in the normal course of equipment maintenance. None of these exposures have been convincingly linked to a cause of the illness.

Given the range of reported GWS effects, treatment is highly individualized and symptomatic. A number of specialized support groups and websites have been established by members of the Persian Gulf War Community.

National Agencies & Associations

10190 Advocacy for the Gulf War Children
1692 6th Road
St Libory, NE 68872
308-795-2319
e-mail: Firefly@mail.hamilton.net
Gives listings of names and addresses of families with children with gulf war syndrome.

10191 Agent Orange Registry Department of Veterans Affairs
Department of Veterans Affairs
810 Vermont Avenue NW
Washington, DC 20420
202-233-4000
800-827-1000
www.va.gov
Offers a computerized index of examinations of Vietnam veterans who were worried that they may have been exposed to chemical herbicides which might be causing a variety of ill effects. Services available to any veteran, male or female, who had active military service.

10192 Centers for Disease Control
1600 Clifton Road
Atlanta, GA 30333
404-639-3311
800-232-4636
Fax: 404-639-3435
TTY: 888-232-6348
e-mail: cdcinfo@cdc.gov
www.cdc.gov
Offers reprints from the CDC Health Status of Vietnam veterans and the Journal of the American Medical Association. Also offers reports from the Centers for Disease Control Vietnam Experience Study, which was a multidimensional assessment of the health of Vietnam War veterans.
William H Gimson, Chief Operating Officer
John Tibbs, Director

10193 National Veterans Services Fund
PO Box 2465
Darien, CT 06820-0465
203-656-0003
800-521-0198
Fax: 203-656-1957
e-mail: philvet@NVSF.org
www.nvsf.org
Supports and informs those who were exposed to the defoliant Agent Orange or dioxin while serving the US in the conflict in Vietnam. The organization has developed a detailed exposure survey form to collect information on exposed veterans.
Phil Kraft, President Treasurer
Cathie Green Stansell, Vice President

10194 VA Data Processing Center
1615 E Woodward Street
Austin, TX 78772-0001
512-389-5380
Helps veterans register after receiving the Agent Orange examination.

State Agencies & Associations

Alabama

10195 Gulf War Veterans of Alabama
2344 Glendale Avenue
Montgomery, AL 36107
205-265-7723
e-mail: 76163 1323@compuserve.com
Don Reeves
Shannon Reeves

10196 Veterans Administration Medical Center: Alabama
3701 Loop Road E   205-554-2000
Tuscaloosa, AL 35404   Fax: 205-554-2034
www2.va.gov/directory

10197 Veterans Association Medical Center
700 S 19th Street   205-933-8101
Birmingham, AL 35233   866-487-4243
Fax: 205-933-4484
www2.va.gov/directory

Alaska

10198 Alaska Gulf War Syndrome Referral Coordinator
23740 Sunny Glen Drive   907-696-8688
Eagle River, AK 99577   Fax: 907-696-8688
e-mail: mcclure@alaska.net

Larry McClure

10199 Veterans Adm. Medical Center: Anchorage Outpatient Clinic
Outpatient Clinic
2925 DeBarr Road   907-257-4700
Anchorage, AK 99508   888-383-7574
Fax: 907-257-6774
www2.va.gov/directory

Arizona

10200 Veterans Adm. Medical Center: Arizona Carl T. Hayden VA Medical Center
Carl T. Hayden VA Medical Center
650 E Indian School Road   602-277-5551
Phoenix, AZ 85012   800-554-7174
www.phoenix.med.va.gov

Renee Stover, VA Employees Association President
Paula Pedene, Public Affairs Officer

10201 Veterans Adm. Medical Center: Tucson Southern Arizona VA Health Care System
Southern Arizona VA Health Care System
3601 S 6th Avenue   520-792-1450
Tucson, AZ 85723   800-470-8262
Fax: 520-629-1818
www2.va.gov/directory

Jonathan Gardner, Chief Executive Officer

Arkansas

10202 Central Arkansas Veterans Healthcare Syste Eugene J. Towbin Healthcare Center
Eugene J. Towbin Healthcare Center
2200 Fort Roots Drive
North Little Rock, AR 72114-1706   501-257-1000
www2.va.gov/directory

10203 Gulf War Veterans of Arkansas
11127 Eglia Valley Drive   501-225-9347
Little Rock, AR 72212
Lydia Pace

10204 Veterans Adm. Medical Center: Fayetville
1100 N College Avenue   479-443-4301
Fayetteville, AR 72703   800-691-8387
www2.va.gov/directory

10205 Veterans Adm. Medical Center: Little Rock
4300 W 7th Street
Little Rock, AR 72205-5484   501-257-1000
www2.va.gov/directory

California

10206 California Association of Persian Gulf Veterans
PO Box 3661   408-476-6684
Santa Cruz, CA 95063   Fax: 415-227-0848
e-mail: CAGulfVets@aol.com

Erika Lundholm

10207 Northern California Association of Persian Gulf Veterans
9141 East Stockton Boulevard   916-684-1693
Elk Grove, CA 95624   Fax: 916-684-1693
e-mail: NCAPGV@aol.com

Debbie Judd

10208 Sacramento Veterans Center
1111 Howe Avenue   916-566-7430
Sacramento, CA 95825   Fax: 916-566-7433
www2.va.gov/directory

Michael Miracle, Team Leader
Edna Gabaldon, Counselor

10209 Sepulveda Ambulatory Care Center
16111 Plummer Street   818-891-7711
North Hills, CA 91343   800-516-4567
Fax: 818-895-9559
www2.va.gov/directory

10210 VA Northern California Health Care System
10535 Hospital Way   916-843-7000
Mather, CA 95655   800-382-8387
Fax: 916-843-9001
www2.va.gov/directory

Lawrence Sandler, Disabilities Committee Chair

10211 Veterans Adm. Medical Center: Livermore
4951 Arroyo Road   925-373-4700
Livermore, CA 94550   800-455-0057
www2.va.gov/directory

10212 Veterans Adm. Medical Center: Long Beach
5901 E 7th Street   562-826-8000
Long Beach, CA 90822   Fax: 562-826-5972
www.long-beach.med.va.gov

10213 Veterans Adm. Medical Center: Los Angeles
11301 Willshire Boulevard   310-478-3711
Los Angeles, CA 90073   Fax: 310-268-3494
www.losangeles.va.gov

10214 Veterans Adm. Medical Center: Martinez
150 Muir Road   916-366-5366
Martinez, CA 94553   800-382-8387
Fax: 925-372-2020
www2.va.gov/directory

10215 Veterans Adm. Medical Center: Palo Alto
3801 Miranda Avenue   650-493-5000
Palo Alto, CA 94304   800-455-0057
Fax: 650-852-3228
www.palo-alto.med.va.gov/

John Didty, Director
Jeanette Hsu, Director of Training

10216 Veterans Adm. Medical Center: Salem
4150 Clement Street   415-221-4810
San Francisco, CA 94121   Fax: 415-750-2185
www.sanfrancisco.va.gov

Sheila M Cullen, Director
C Diana Nicoll, Chief of Staff

10217 Veterans Adm. Medical Center: San Francisco
4150 Clement Street   415-221-4810
San Francisco, CA 94121   Fax: 415-750-2185
Sheila M Cullen, Director
C Diana Nicoll, Chief of Staff

10218 Veterans Administration Medical Center: Fresno
3636 N 1st Street   559-487-5660
Fresno, CA 93726   Fax: 559-487-5399
www2.va.gov/directory

Herman Barretto, Counselor
Mary Jordan-Church, Counselor

10219 Veterans Affairs Medical Center: Loma Linda
11201 Benton Street   909-825-7084
Loma Linda, CA 92357   800-741-8387
Fax: 909-422-3106
www.lom.med.va.gov/

Annie Tuttle, Public Affairs Director

Colorado

10220 Persian Gulf Veterans of Colorado
405 Cody
Wheat Ridge, CO 80033
303-424-6235
Fax: 303-422-2962
e-mail: GJMF90B@prodigy.com

Denise Nichols

10221 Veterans Adm. Medical Center: Denver
300 S Jackson Street
Denver, CO 80206
303-331-7500
800-733-8387
Fax: 303-331-7800
e-mail: hac.inq@med.va.gov
www.va.gov/hac/

Ralph Charlip, Director

10222 Veterans Adm. Medical Center: Grand Junction
2121 N Avenue
Grand Junction, CO 81501
970-242-0731
866-206-6415
Fax: 970-244-1303
www1.va.gov/directory

Connecticut

10223 Gulf War Veterans of Connecticut: New England Chapter
8 Frances Lane
Windsor Locks, CT 6096
860-623-1456
Fax: 860-292-1849
e-mail: DIANEDULKA@aol.com

Diane Dulka

Delaware

10224 Veterans Adm. Medical Center: Wilmington VA Medical Center
Wilmington VA Medical Center
1601 Kirkwood Highway
Wilmington, DE 19805
302-994-2511
Fax: 302-633-5591
www2.va.gov/directory

District of Columbia

10225 Disabled American Veterans National Service Headquarters
807 Maine Avenue SW
Washington, DC 20024
202-554-3501
Fax: 202-554-3581
www.dav.org

Serves America's disabled veterans and their families. Direct services include legislative advocacy professional counseling about compensation pension educational and job training programs and VA health care. Also offers assistance in applying for those programs.
Arthur H Wilson, National Adjutant
David G Gorman, Executive Director

10226 US Veteran's Administration
810 Vermont Avenue NW
Washington, DC 20420
202-273-5400
Fax: 202-273-4877
www2.va.gov/directory

Provides a wide range of services for those who have been in the military and their dependents as well as offering information on driver assessment and education programs.
Louise R Van Diepen MS CGP, Chief of Staff
Patricia Van MHA BS, Assistant Deputy Policy/Planning

10227 Veterans Adm. Medical Center: Washington
50 Irving Street NW
Washington, DC 20422
202-745-8000
Fax: 202-754-8530
www.washington.med.va.gov

Sanford M Garfunkel, Medical Center Director
Ross D Fletcher, Chief of Staff

Florida

10228 Desert Storm Justice Foundation: Florida
10 Marlow Road
Frostproof, FL 33843-9321
813-635-3261
Fax: 813-635-3261
e-mail: BillCarpenter@cjewel.com

William Carpenter

10229 Desert Storm Veterans of Florida
PO Box 6081
Titusville, FL 32782
407-269-3453
e-mail: GulfVet@Metrolink.net

Kevin Knight

10230 Veterans Adm. Medical Center: Bay Pines
10000 Bay Pines Boulevard
Bay Pines, FL 33744
727-398-6661
Fax: 727-398-9442
www.va.gov/visn8/baypines

Wallace M Hopkins, Medical Center Director
George F Van Buskirk MD, Chief of Staff

10231 Veterans Adm. Medical Center: Gainesville
1601 SW Archer Road
Gainesville, FL 32608-1197
352-376-1611
Fax: 352-374-6113
www2.va.gov/directory

Frederick L Malphurs, Director
Bradley S Bender MD, Chief of Staff

10232 Veterans Adm. Medical Center: Lake City
Lake City Veterans Administration Medical Center
619 S Marion Avenue
Lake City, FL 32025-5808
386-755-3016
800-308-8387
Fax: 386-758-3209
www2.va.gov/directory

10233 Veterans Adm. Medical Center: Miami
1201 NW 16th Street
Miami, FL 33125
305-575-7000
888-276-1785
Fax: 305-575-5232
www.va.gov/visn8/miami

Stephen M Lucas, Director
John R Vara MD, Chief of Staff

10234 Veterans Adm. Medical Center: St. Petersburg
Bay Pines VA Medical Center
10000 Bay Pines Boulevard
Saint Petersburg, FL 33744
727-398-6661
888-820-0230
Fax: 727-322-1248
www2.va.gov/directory

10235 Veterans Adm. Medical Center: Tampa
Tampa Veterans Administration Medical Center
13000 Bruce B Downs Boulevard
Tampa, FL 33612
813-972-2000
Fax: 813-972-7673
www.va.gov/visn8/tampa

Richard A Silver, Medical Center Director
Thomas E Bowen, Chief of Staff

10236 Vietnam Veterans of Brevard The Vietnam And All Veterans Of Brevard
The Vietnam And All Veterans Of Brevard
1125 W King Street
Cocoa, FL 32922-0929
321-690-0805
Fax: 321-690-0106
e-mail: BVagianos@cfl.rr.com
www.vietnamandallveteransofbrevard.com

Bill Vagianos, President
Don Wassmer, Vice President

10237 West Palm Beach VA Medical Center
7305 N Military Trail
West Palm Beach, FL 33410-6400
561-422-8262
800-972-8262
Fax: 561-422-8613
www.westpalmbeach.va.gov

Edward H Seiler, Medical Center Director
Darin Rubin, Chief of Staff

Georgia

10238 Gulf War Veterans of Georgia
307 Adair Street
Decatur, GA 30030
404-373-3741
Fax: 404-377-3741
e-mail: 70711 3174@compuserve.com

Paul Sullivan

10239 VA Southeast Network: Georgia
3700 Crestwood Parkway NW
Duluth, GA 30096-5585
678-924-5700
Fax: 678-924-5757
www2.va.gov/directory

10240 Veterans Adm. Medical Center: Augusta
One Freedom Way 706-733-0188
Augusta, GA 30904 800-836-5561
Fax: 706-823-3934
www1.va.gov/augustaga

10241 Veterans Adm. Medical Center: Decatur Atlanta VA Medical Center
Atlanta VA Medical Center
1670 Clairmont Road 404-321-6111
Decatur, GA 30033 Fax: 404-728-7733
www.va.gov/atlanta

Thomas Cappello, Director
David J Bower, Chief of Staff

10242 Veterans Adm. Medical Center: Dublin Carl Vinson VA Medical Center
Carl Vinson VA Medical Center
1826 Veterans Boulevard 912-272-1210
Dublin, GA 31021 800-595-5229
Fax: 912-277-2717
www2.va.gov/directory

Hawaii

10243 Veterans Adm. Medical Centery: Honolulu VA Pacific Islands Health Care System
VA Pacific Islands Health Care System
459 Patterson Road 808-433-0600
Honolulu, HI 96819-1522 Fax: 808-433-0390
www.va.gov/hawaii

Idaho

10244 Idaho Persian Gulf Veterans
2055 Sotuh Colorado Street 208-344-3028
Boise, ID 83706
Vaughn Kidwell

10245 Veterans Adm. Medical Center: Boise Boise VA Medical Center
Boise VA Medical Center
500 W Fort Street 208-422-1000
Boise, ID 83702 866-437-5093
Fax: 208-422-1326
www2.va.gov/directory

Wayne Tippets, Director

Illinois

10246 Desert Storm Justice Foundation: Illinois
Rural Route 4 618-457-2621
Carbondale, IL 62901
Shan Now

10247 Edward J Hines Jr VA Hospital
5th & Roosevelt Road 708-202-8387
Hines, IL 60141 Fax: 708-202-7998
www2.va.gov/directory

10248 Great Lakes Health Care System
PO Box 5000 708-202-8400
Hines, IL 60141-5000 Fax: 708-202-8424
www.visn12.va.gov

10249 Jesse Brown VA Medical Center
820 S Damen Avenue
Chicago, IL 60612 312-569-8387
www.chicago.va.gov

10250 VA Illinois Health Care System
1900 E Main Street 217-554-3000
Danville, IL 61832-5198 Fax: 217-554-4552
www2.va.gov/directory

10251 Veterans Adm. Medical Center: Marion Marion VA Medical Center
Marion VA Medical Center
2401 W Main Street
Marion, IL 62959 618-997-5311
www2.va.gov/directory

10252 Veterans Adm. Medical Center: North Chicago
North Chicago VA Medical Center
3001 Green Bay Road 847-688-1900
North Chicago, IL 60064 Fax: 847-578-3806
www.vision12.med.va.gov/northchicag

10253 Veterans Adm. Medical Center: Northport North Chicago VA Medical Center
3001 Green Bay Road 847-688-1900
North Chicago, IL 60064 Fax: 847-578-3806
www.northchicago.va.gov

10254 Veterans Administration West Side Medical Center
820 S Damen Avenue 312-569-8387
Chicago, IL 60612 Fax: 312-569-6188
www2.va.gov/directory

Stan Johnson, Director
DeAnn Dietrich, Deputy Director

Indiana

10255 VA Northern Indiana Health Care System Marion Campus
1700 E 38th Street 765-674-3321
Marion, IN 46953-4589 800-360-8387
Fax: 765-677-3124
www2.va.gov/directory

10256 Veterans Adm. Medical Center: Fort Wayne
2121 Lake Avenue 260-426-5431
Fort Wayne, IN 46805 800-360-8387
Fax: 260-460-1336
www2.va.gov/directory

10257 Veterans Adm. Medical Center: Indianapolis
1481 W Tenth Street 317-554-0000
Indianapolis, IN 46202 888-878-6889
Fax: 317-554-0127
www2.va.gov/directory

Iowa

10258 Cedar Rapids Persian Gulf Veterans, Spouses and Children
909-28th Street Southeast 1 319-366-0756
Cedar Rapids, IA 52403
Mary Shears

10259 Des Moines Division: VA Central Iowa Health Care System
3600 30th Street 515-699-5999
Des Moines, IA 50310-5774 800-294-8387
Fax: 515-699-5862
www2.va.gov/directory

10260 Knoxville Division: VA Central Iowa Health Care System
1515 W Pleasant Street 641-842-3101
Knoxville, IA 50138 800-816-8878
Fax: 515-699-5862
www2.va.gov/directory

10261 Veterans Adm. Medical Center: Iowa City
601 Highway 6 W 319-338-0581
Iowa City, IA 52246-2208 800-637-0128
Fax: 319-339-7171
www2.va.gov/directory

Kansas

10262 Veterans Adm. Medical Center: Leavenwoth Dwight D. Eisenhower VA Medical Center
Dwight D. Eisenhower VA Medical Center
4101 S 4th Street 913-682-2000
Leavenworth, KS 66048-5055 800-952-8387
Fax: 913-758-4149
www2.va.gov/directory

10263 Veterans Adm. Medical Center: Topeka Colmery O'Neil VA Medical Center
Colmery O'Neil VA Medical Center
2200 SW Gage Boulevard
Topeka, KS 66622 785-350-3111
800-574-8387
Fax: 785-350-4336
www2.va.gov/directory

10264 Veterans Adm. Medical Center: Wichita Robert J. Dole Department Of VA Medical
Robert J. Dole Department Of VA Medical Center
5500 E Kellogg   316-685-2221
Wichita, KS 67218   888-878-6881
Fax: 316-651-3666
www2.va.gov/directory

Kentucky

10265 Carol and Dr. James W Stutts
108 Whispering Hills Drive   606-986-3267
Berea, KY 40403   e-mail: cstutts@kih.net

10266 National Association of State Directors of Veterans Affairs
Kentucky Department of Veteran Affairs
1111 Louisville Road   502-564-9203
Frankfort, KY 40601   Fax: 502-564-9240
e-mail: les.beavers@ky.gov
www.nasdva.net
Provides a medium for the exchange of ideas and information; facilitates reciprocal state services; fosters a better understanding of the national veterans' problems; and secures uniformity and equality of services in all states and territories.
Leslie Beavers, Commissioner
Terry Schow, Senior Vice President

10267 Veterans Adm. Medical Center: Lexington Lexington VA Medical Center
Lexington VA Medical Center
1101 Veterans Drive
Lexington, KY 40502   859-233-4511
www2.va.gov/directory

10268 Veterans Adm. Medical Center: Louisville Louisville VA Medical Center
Louisville VA Medical Center
800 Zorn Avenue   502-287-4000
Louisville, KY 40206   800-376-8387
Fax: 502-287-6225
www2.va.gov/directory

10269 Veterans Adm. Regional Office: Louisville Louisville Regional Office
Louisville Regional Office
1347 S 3rd Street   502-634-1916
Louisville, KY 40208   Fax: 502-625-7082
www2.va.gov/directory
Phillip Goudeau, Team Leader
Carolyn Beisler, Counselor

Louisiana

10270 Mission Project
PO Box 92574   318-236-3599
Lafayette, LA 70509-2574   e-mail: mission@linknet.net
Carol Picou
Tony Picou

10271 Veterans Adm. Medical Center: Alexandria Alexandria VA Medical Center
Alexandria VA Medical Center
PO Box 69004   318-473-0010
Alexandria, LA 71360   800-375-8387
Fax: 318-483-5029
www2.va.gov/directory
Barbara C Watkins, Medical Center Director
Hollis Reed MD, Chief of Staff

10272 Veterans Adm. Medical Center: New Orleans New Orleans VA Medical Center
New Orleans VA Medical Center
1601 Perdido Street   504-568-0811
New Orleans, LA 70146   Fax: 504-589-5210
www1.va.gov

10273 Veterans Adm. Medical Center: Shreveport Overton Brooks VA Medical Center
Overton Brooks VA Medical Center

510 E Stoner Avenue   318-221-8411
Shreveport, LA 7110   800-863-7441
Fax: 318-424-6156
www2.va.gov/directory

Maine

10274 Veterans Adm. Medical Center: Augusta Togus VA Medical Center
Togus VA Medical Center
1 VA Center   207-623-8411
Augusta, ME 4330   866-590-2976
Fax: 207-623-5792
TTY: 800-829-4833
TDD: 800-829-4833
e-mail: togus.query@vba.va.gov
www2.va.gov/directory
Dale Denners, Regional Office Director

Maryland

10275 Baltimore VA Rehabilitation and Extended Care Center (BRECC)
3900 Loch Raven Boulevard   410-605-7000
Baltimore, MD 21218   Fax: 410-605-7900
www2.va.gov/directory

10276 Fort Howard VA Outpatient Clinic
9600 N Point Road   410-477-1800
Fort Howard, MD 21052   800-351-8387
Fax: 410-477-7177
www.maryland.va.gov/facilities/Fort_Howa
Dennis H Smith, Director

10277 Maryland Group
8725 Fairhaven Place   301-725-4269
Jessup, MD 20794
Nancy Kaplan

10278 VA Capitol Health Care Network
849 International Drive   410-691-1131
Linthicum, MD 21090   Fax: 410-684-3189
www.va.gov/visn5
Sanford M Garfunkel, Network Director

10279 VA Maryland Health Care System Perry Point VA Medical Center
Perry Point VA Medical Center
Perry Point, MD 21902   410-642-2411
800-949-1003
Fax: 410-642-1161
www.maryland.va.gov/facilities/Perry_Poi
Dennis H Smith, Director
Dorothy M Snow, Chief of Staff

10280 Veterans Adm. Medical Center: Baltimore
10 N Greene Street   410-605-7000
Baltimore, MD 21201   800-463-6295
Fax: 410-605-7901
www.maryland.va.gov/facilities/Baltimore
Carol Nizzardini, Chief Nurse Executive
Dennis H Smith, Director

Massachusetts

10281 New England Health Care System
200 Springs Road   781-687-4821
Bedford, MA 01730   Fax: 781-687-3470
www.newengland.va.gov
Michael F Mayo-Smith, Network Director
Christine Croteau, Deputy Network Director

10282 Northhampton VA Medical Center
421 N Main Street   413-584-4040
Leeds, MA 01053-9764   800-893-1522
Fax: 413-582-3121
www.northampton.va.gov
Mary A Dowling, Director
George Fuller, Chief of Staff

10283 Persian Gulf Era Veterans
24 Beacon Street
Boston, MA 02133
617-329-8149
e-mail: jagmedic@pgev.org
www.pgev.org

VenusVal Hammack, Executive Director

10284 VA Boston Healthcare System: Jamaica Plain Jamaica Plain Campus
Jamaica Plain Campus
150 S Huntington Avenue
Jamiaca Plain, MA 02130
617-232-9500
Fax: 617-278-4508
www.boston.va.gov

Michael M Lawson, Director
Michael E Charness, Chief of Staff

10285 VA Boston Healthcare System: West Roxbury West Roxbury Campus
West Roxbury Campus
1400 VFW Parkway
W Roxbury, MA 02132
617-323-7700
www.boston.va.gov

Michael M Lawson, Director
Susan MacKenzie, Associate Director

10286 Veterans Adm. Medical Center: Bedford Edith Nourse Rogers Memorial Veterans
Edith Nourse Rogers Memorial Veterans Hospital
200 Springs Road
Bedford, MA 01730
781-687-2000
800-VET-MED1
Fax: 781-687-2101
www.bedford.va.gov

Tammy A Follensbee, Hospital Director
Gregory Binus, Chief Medical Officer

10287 Veterans Adm. Medical Center: Brockton Brockton Campus
Brockton Campus
940 Belmont Street
Brockton, MA 02301
508-583-4500
800-865-3384
Fax: 700-885-1000
www.boston.va.gov

Michael M Lawson, Director
Michael E Charness MD, Chief of Staff

Michigan

10288 Detroit VA Medical Center John D. Dingell VA Medical Center
John D. Dingell VA Medical Center
4646 John R
Detroit, MI 48201
313-576-1000
800-511-8056
Fax: 313-576-1025
www.detroit.va.gov

Pamela J Reeves, Director
Basim Dubaybo, Chief of Staff

10289 International Advocacy for Gulf War Syndrome
2297 Westfield Drive
Niles, MI 49102
616-684-5903
e-mail: DSVETERAN1@juno.com
Brian Martin

10290 Veterans Adm. Medical Center: Ann Arbor Ann Arbor Healthcare System
Ann Arbor Healthcare System
2215 Fuller Road
Ann Arbor, MI 48105
734-769-7100
800-361-8387
Fax: 734-845-3245
www.annarbor.va.gov

Eric W Young, Acting Director
Stacey Breedveld, Associate Director Patient Care

10291 Veterans Adm. Medical Center: Bath Battle Creek VA Medical Center
5500 Armostrong Road
Battle Creek, MI 49015
269-966-5600
Fax: 269-966-5483
www.battlecreek.va.gov

Denise Deitzen, Acting Director
Alan Sooho, Chief of Staff

10292 Veterans Adm. Medical Center: Battle Creek
Battle Creek VA Medical Center

5500 Armostrong Road
Battle Creek, MI 49016
269-966-5600
Fax: 269-966-5483
www.va.gov

10293 Veterans Adm. Medical Center: Iron Mountain
Iron Mountain VA Medical Center
325 E H Street
Iron Mountain, MI 49801
906-774-3300
800-215-8262
Fax: 906-779-3188
www.ironmountain.va.gov

Michael J Murphy, Director
Craig L Holmes, Chief of Staff

10294 Veterans Adm. Medical Center: Saginaw Aleda E. Lutz VA Medical Center
Aleda E. Lutz VA Medical Center
1500 Wiess Street
Saginaw, MI 48602
989-497-2500
800-406-5143
Fax: 989-321-4903
www.saginaw.va.gov

Gabriel Perez, Director
Gregory Movsesian, Acting Chief of Staff

10295 Veterans In Partnership
PO Box 134002
Ann Arbor, MI 48113-4002
734-222-4300
888-838-6446
Fax: 734-222-4340
www.visn11.va.gov

Minnesota

10296 Desert Storm Justice Foundation: Minnesota
PO Box 186
Buhl, MN 55713
218-258-3685
Jeff Zakula

10297 Desert Storm Justice Foundation: Virginia
PO Box 186
Buhl, MN 55713
218-258-3685
Jeff Zakula

10298 Veterans Adm. Medical Center: Minneapolis Minneapolis VA Medical Center
Minneapolis VA Medical Center
1 Veterans Drive
Minneapolis, MN 55417
612-725-2000
866-414-5058
Fax: 612-725-2049
www1.va.gov/minneapolis

Steven P Kleinglass, Director
John J Drucker, Chief of Staff

10299 Veterans Adm. Regional Office: St. Paul
1 Federal Drive Fort Snelling
Saint Paul, MN 55111
612-644-4022
800-827-1000
Fax: 612-970-5415
e-mail: VBCINQ@VBA.VA.GOV
www1.va.gov

Mississippi

10300 Gulf War Babies
PO Box 198
Clara, MS 39324
601-735-9206
Aimee West

10301 South Central VA Health Care Network
1600 E Woodrow Wilson
Jackson, MS 39216
601-364-7900
800-639-5137
Fax: 601-364-7996
www.visn16.med.va.gov

George Gray, Network Director
Gregg Parker, Chief Medical Officer

10302 VA Gulf Coast Veterans Health Care System
400 Veterans Avenue
Biloxi, MS 39531
228-523-5000
800-296-8872
Fax: 228-523-5719
www.biloxi.va.gov

Charles Sepich, Director
Ana Mello, Chief of Staff

10303 Veterans Adm. Medical Center: Jackson
1500 E Woodrow Wilson Drive
Jackson, MS 39216

601-362-4471
800-949-1009
Fax: 601-364-1359
www.jackson.va.gov

Linda F Watson, Director
Kent A Kirchner, Chief of Staff

10304 Veterans Adm. Regional Office: Jackson
1600 E Woodrow Wilson Avenue
Jackson, MS 32916

601-364-7000
800-827-1000
Fax: 601-364-7007
www.vba.va.gov/ro/south/jacks/JacksonInt

Missouri

10305 VA Heartland Network
1201 Walnut Street
Kansas City, MO 64106

816-701-3000
Fax: 816-221-0930
www.visn15.med.va.gov

10306 Veterans Adm. Medical Center: Columbia Harry S. Truman Memorial
Harry S. Truman Memorial
800 Hospital Drive
Columbia, MO 65202-5297

573-814-6000
800-349-8262
Fax: 573-814-6600
www.columbiamo.va.gov

10307 Veterans Adm. Medical Center: Kansas City Kansas City VA Medical Center
Kansas City VA Medical Center
4801 Linwood Boulevard
Kansas City, MO 64128

816-861-4700
800-525-1483
Fax: 816-922-3303
www.va.gov

10308 Veterans Adm. Medical Center: Poplar Bluff
John J. Pershing VA Medical Center
1500 N Westwood Boulevard
Poplar Bluff, MO 63901

573-686-4151
888-557-8262
Fax: 573-778-4559
www.poplarbluff.va.gov

Judy K McKee, Acting Director
Vijayachandr Nair, Chief of Staff

10309 Veterans Adm. Regional Office: St. Louis John Cochran Division
John Cochran Division
915 N Grand Boulevard
Saint Louis, MO 63125

314-652-4100
800-228-5459
Fax: 314-289-6557
www.stlouis.va.gov

Glen E Struchtemeyer, Director
Nathan Ravi, Chief of Staff

Montana

10310 Veterans Adm. Medical Center: Fort Harrison
VA Montana Health Care System
William Street
Fort Harrison, MT 59636

406-442-6410
800-827-1000
Fax: 406-477-7916
www.va.gov

10311 Veterans Adm. Medical Center: Miles City
210 S Winchester
Miles City, MT 59301

406-874-5600
877-468-8387
Fax: 406-232-8298
www1.va.gov

Nebraska

10312 Veterans Adm. Medical Center: Grand Island
2201 N Broadwell Avenue
Grand Island, NE 68803-2196

308-382-3660
866-580-1810
Fax: 308-389-5113
www.nebraska.va.gov

10313 Veterans Adm. Medical Center: Lincoln
600 S 70th Street
Lincoln, NE 68510

402-489-3802
866-851-6052
Fax: 402-486-7840
www.nebraska.va.gov

10314 Veterans Adm. Medical Center: Omaha Western Iowa Health Care System
Western Iowa Health Care System
4101 Woolworth Avenue
Omaha, NE 68105

402-346-8800
800-451-5796
Fax: 402-449-0684
www.nebraska.va.gov

Al Washko, Director
Thomas Lynch, Acting Chief of Staff

Nevada

10315 Veterans Adm. Medical Center: Las Vegas VA Southern Nevada Healthcare System
VA Southern Nevada Healthcare System (VASNHS)
901 Rancho Lane
Las Vegas, NV 89106

702-636-3000
877-252-4866
Fax: 702-636-3027
www.lasvegas.va.gov

John B Bright, Director
Ramu Komanduri, Chief of Staff

10316 Veterans Adm. Medical Center: Reno VA Sierra Nevada Health Care System
VA Sierra Nevada Health Care System
1000 Locust Street
Reno, NV 89502

775-786-7200
888-838-6256
Fax: 775-328-1464
www.reno.va.gov

Kurt W Schlegelmilch, Director
Steven E Brilliant, Chief of Staff

New Hampshire

10317 Veterans Adm. Medical Center: Manchester Manchester VA Medical Center
Manchester VA Medical Center
718 Smyth Road
Manchester, NH 03104

603-624-4366
800-892-8384
Fax: 603-626-6579
www.manchester.va.gov

Marc F Levenson MD, Director
Andrew Breuder, Chief of Staff

New Jersey

10318 Veterans Adm. Medical Center: East Orange East Orange Campus
East Orange Campus
385 Tremont Avenue
E Orange, NJ 07018

973-676-1000
Fax: 973-676-4226
www.eastorange.va.gov

Kenneth H Mizrach, Director
Steven L Lieberman, Chief of Staff

10319 Veterans Adm. Medical Center: Lyons Lyons Campus
Lyons Campus
151 Knollcroft Road
Lyons, NJ 07939

908-647-0180
Fax: 908-647-3452
www.lyons.va.gov

Kenneth H Mizrach, Director
Steven L Lieberman, Chief of Staff

New Mexico

10320 Veterans Adm. Medical Center: Albuquerque New Mexico VA Health Care System
New Mexico VA Health Care System
1501 San Pedro Drive SE
Albuquerque, NM 87108-5153

505-265-1711
800-465-8262
Fax: 505-256-2855
www.albuquerque.va.gov

George Marnell, Director
Meghan Gerety, Chief of Staff

New York

10321 Gulf War Veterans of Long Island, NY
100 Robinson
E Patchogue, NY 11772
516-289-1580
Fax: 516-447-5871
e-mail: DStormMom@aol.com

Jackie Olsen

10322 Persian Gulf Veterans
212 Garfield Avenue
E Rochester, NY 14445-1314
716-385-4097
Fax: 716-924-2161
Beverly Place

10323 VA Helathcare Network: Upstate New York
PO Box 8980
Albany, NY 12208-8980
518-626-7300
Fax: 518-626-7333
www.visn2.va.gov

Stephen L Lemons, Network Director
Lawrence H Flesh, Chief Medical Officer

10324 VA NY/NJ Veterans Healthcare Network
130 W Kingsbridge Road
Bronx, NY 10468
718-584-9000
Fax: 718-579-1671
www1.va.gov//visn03

Michael A Sabo, Network Director

10325 Veterans Adm. Medical Center: Albany Samuel S. Stratton: VA Medical Center
Samuel S. Stratton: VA Medical Center
113 Holland Avenue
Albany, NY 12208
518-626-5000
Fax: 518-626-5500
www.albany.va.gov

Mary-Ellen Pich,, Director
Lourdes Irizarry, Chief of Staff

10326 Veterans Adm. Medical Center: Batavia VA Western New York Healthcare System
VA Western New York Healthcare System at Batavia
222 Richmond Avenue
Batavia, NY 14020
585-297-1000
Fax: 716-344-3305
www.buffalo.va.gov/batavia.asp

David J West, Interim Director
Miguel Rainstein, Chief of Staff

10327 Veterans Adm. Medical Center: Bath Bath VA Medical Center
Bath VA Medical Center
76 Veterans Avenue
Bath, NY 14810
607-664-4000
877-845-3247
Fax: 607-664-4511
www.bath.va.gov

Thomas W Sharpe, Acting Medical Center Director
Steven Speroni, Acting Chief of Staff

10328 Veterans Adm. Medical Center: Brooklyn Brooklyn Campus
Brooklyn Campus
800 Poly Place
Brooklyn, NY 11209
718-836-6600
Fax: 718-630-2840
www.brooklyn.va.gov

John J Donnellan Jr, Director

10329 Veterans Adm. Medical Center: Buffalo
3495 Bailey Avenue
Buffalo, NY 14215
716-834-9200
800-532-8387
Fax: 716-862-8759
www.buffalo.va.gov

David J West, Interim Director
Miguel Rainstein, Chief of Staff

10330 Veterans Adm. Medical Center: Montrose Franklin Delano Roosevelt Campus
Franklin Delano Roosevelt Campus
2094 Albany Post Road
Montrose, NY 10548
914-737-4400
800-269-8749
Fax: 914-788-4244
www.hudsonvalley.va.gov

Gerald F Culliton, Director
Joanne Malina, Chief of Staff

10331 Veterans Adm. Medical Center: New York New York Campus
New York Campus

423 E 23rd Street
New York, NY 10010
212-686-7500
Fax: 718-567-4082
www.manhattan.va.gov

John J Donnellan Jr, Director

10332 Veterans Adm. Medical Center: Northport Northport VA Medical Center
Northport VA Medical Center
79 Middleville Road
Northport, NY 11768
516-261-4400
800-551-3996
Fax: 631-754-7933
www.northport.va.gov

Philip C Moschitta, Director
Edward Mack, Chief of Staff

10333 Veterans Adm. Medical Center: Syracuse Syracuse VA Medical Center
Syracuse VA Medical Center
800 Irving Avenue
Syracuse, NY 13210
315-425-4400
800-792-4334
Fax: 315-425-4375
www.syracuse.va.gov

James Cody, Director
William H Marx, Chief of Staff

10334 Veterans Affairs Medical Center Canandaigua
Canadaigua VA Medical Center
400 Fort Hill Avenue
Canandaigua, NY 14424
716-394-2000
Fax: 716-393-8328
www.va.gov/visns/visn02

Sally Martin, Geriatrics/Extended Care Line Co-Manager
Diane West, Geriatrics/Extended Care Line Co-Manager

North Carolina

10335 Charles George Veterans Affairs Medical Center
1100 Tunnel Road
Asheville, NC 28805
828-298-7911
800-932-6408
Fax: 828-299-2563
www.asheville.va.gov

Cynthia Breyfogle FACHE, Medical Center Director
David A Pattillo MHA FACHE, Associate Medical Center Director

10336 Desert Storm Veterans of North Carolina
739 E Haggard Avenue
Ellon College, NC 27224
910-584-5038
Kevin Treiber

10337 Veterans Adm. Medical Center: Durham Durham VA Medical Center
Durham VA Medical Center
508 Fulton Street
Durham, NC 27705
919-286-0411
888-878-6890
Fax: 919-286-6825
www.durham.va.gov

Ralph T Gigliotti, Director
John D Shelburne, Chief of Staff

10338 Veterans Adm. Medical Center: Fayetville Fayettville VA Medical Center
Fayettville VA Medical Center
2300 Ramsey Street
Fayetteville, NC 28301
910-488-2120
800-771-6106
Fax: 910-822-7093
www.fayettevillenc.va.gov

Bruce C Triplett, Director
Kanan Chatterjee, Interim Chief of Staff

10339 Veterans Adm. Medical Center: Salisbury W.G. Hefner VA Medical Center
W.G. Hefner VA Medical Center
1601 Brenner Avenue
Salisbury, NC 28144
704-683-9000
800-469-8262
Fax: 704-638-3395
www.salisbury.va.gov

Carolyn L Adams, Director
Miguel H LaPuz, Chief of Staff

North Dakota

10340 Veterans Adm. Regional Office: Fargo Regional Office Center
Fargo VA Medical.Regional Office Center
2101 N Elm Street 701-232-3241
Fargo, ND 58102 800-410-9723
Fax: 701-239-3705
www.fargo.va.gov

Robert P McDivitt, Director
Lavonne Liversage, Associate Medical Director

Ohio

10341 Persian Gulf War Veterans of Western Pennsylvania, W Virginia and NE Ohio
600 North Market Street 216-426-3203
East Palestine, OH 44413 Fax: 216-426-3309
Barry M Walker

10342 VA Healthcare System Of Ohio
11500 Northlake Drive 513-247-4621
Cincinnati, OH 45249 Fax: 513-247-4620
e-mail: visn10webmaster@med.va.gov
www.visn10.va.gov

10343 Veterans Adm. Medical Center: Chillicothe Chillicothe VA Medical Center
Chillicothe VA Medical Center
17273 State Route 104 740-773-1141
Chillicothe, OH 45601 800-358-8262
Fax: 740-773-1141
www.chillicothe.va.gov

Jeffrey T Gering, Director
Deborah M Meesig, Chief of Staff

10344 Veterans Adm. Medical Center: Cincinnati Cincinnati VA Medical Center
Cincinnati VA Medical Center
3200 Vine Street 513-861-3100
Cincinnati, OH 45220 888-267-7873
Fax: 513-475-6500
www.cincinnati.va.gov

Linda D Smith, Director
Sidney R Steinberg, Chief of Staff

10345 Veterans Adm. Medical Center: Cleveland Louis Stokes VA Medical Center
Louis Stokes VA Medical Center
10701 E Boulevard 216-791-3800
Cleveland, OH 44106 Fax: 216-421-3217
www.cleveland.va.gov

William Montague, Director
Murray D Altose, Chief of Staff

10346 Veterans Adm. Medical Center: Columbus Chalmers P. Wylie Outpatient Clinic
Chalmers P. Wylie Outpatient Clinic
420 N James Road 614-257-5200
Columbus, OH 43219-1278 888-615-9448
Fax: 614-257-5460
www.columbus.va.gov

Lilian T Thome, Director
Miguel LaPuz, Chief of Staff

10347 Veterans Adm. Medical Center: Dayton Dayton VA Medical Center
Dayton VA Medical Center
4100 W 3rd Street 937-268-6511
Dayton, OH 45428 800-368-8262
Fax: 937-262-2179
TTY: 800-829-4833
www.dayton.va.gov

Guy B Richardson, Medical Center Director
Terry E Taylor, Associate Director

10348 Veterans and Families Support Network Ohio
5488 State Route 7 216-457-0641
New Waterford, OH 44445 Fax: 216-457-1923
e-mail: VFSN@delphi.com
Gina Brown

Oklahoma

10349 American Veterans Justice Foundation
3908 NW Santa Fe 405-355-3811
Lawton, OK 73505 e-mail: dwolf@sirinet.net
Dannie Wolf

10350 Veterans Adm. Medical Center: Muskogee Dayton VA Medical Center
Dayton VA Medical Center
1011 Honor Heights Drive 918-577-3000
Muskogee, OK 74401 888-397-8387
Fax: 918-680-3648
www.muskogee.va.gov

Adam C Walmus, Director
A Rudy Klopfer, Associate Director

10351 Veterans Adm. Medical Center: Oklahoma City
Oklahoma City VA Medical Center
921 NE 13th Street 405-456-1000
Oklahoma City, OK 73104 866-835-5273
Fax: 405-270-1560
www.oklahoma.va.gov

David P Wood, Director
Anne Kreutzer, Associate Director

Oregon

10352 Northwest Network
PO Box 1035 360-619-5925
Portland, OR 97207 Fax: 360-737-1405
www.visn20.med.va.gov

10353 Northwest Vets for Peace
811 E Burnside Street 503-656-9785
Portland, OR 97214 e-mail: NWVP@teleport.com
Marvin Simmons

10354 Veterans Adm. Medical Center: Roseburg VA Roseburg Healthcare System
VA Roseburg Healthcare System
913 NW Garden Valley Boulevard 541-440-1000
Roseburg, OR 97470 800-549-8387
Fax: 541-440-1225
www.visn20.med.va.gov/roseburg

Susan Yeager, Acting Director
Stephen J Broskey, Associate Director

10355 Veterans Adm. Medical Center: White City VA S Oregon Rehabilitation Center
VA Southern Oregonrehabilitation Center & Clinics
8495 Crater Lake Highway 541-826-2111
White City, OR 97503 800-809-8725
Fax: 541-830-3500
www.visn20.med.va.gov/Southern-Oregon
Pam Harris, Human Resources Assistant

10356 Veterans Adm. Regional Office: Portland Portland VA Medical Center
Portland VA Medical Center
3710 SW US Veterans Hospital Road 503-220-8262
Portland, OR 97239 800-949-1004
Fax: 503-273-5319
www.visn20.med.va.gov

James Tuchschmidt, Director
John D Dryden, Chief of Staff

10357 Veterans Administration Domicillary
8495 Crater Lake Highway 541-826-2111
White City, OR 97503 Fax: 541-830-3519
e-mail: David.Schwing@med.va.gov
www1.va.gov/domiciliary

10358 Erie VA Medical Center
135 E 38th Street
Erie, PA 16504

814-868-8661
800-274-8387
Fax: 814-860-2120
www1.va.gov/erie

Michael D Adelman MD, Director
Melissa Sundin, Associate Director

10359 Pennsylvania Gulf War Veterans
RR 3
Clarion, PA 16214

814-226-4084
e-mail: kjsmith@penn.com

Kenneth J Smith, President
Daniel J Meck, VP

10360 VA Pittsburgh Healthcare System: University Drive Division
University Drive
Pittsburgh, PA 15240

866-482-7488
Fax: 412-688-6121
www.va.gov/pittsburgh

Terry Gerigk Wolf, Director
Rajiv Jain MD, Chief of Staff

10361 VA Stars & Stripes Healthcare Network
1010 Delafield Road
Pittsburgh, PA 15240

412-688-6000
866-482-7488
Fax: 412-784-3724
www.visn4.va.gov

Michael E Moreland FACHE, Network Director
Bradley P Shelton, Deputy Network Director

10362 Veterans Adm. Medical Center: Philadelphia
Philadelphia VA Medical Center
University & Woodland Avenues
Philadelphia, PA 19104

215-823-5800
877-626-2500
Fax: 215-823-6007
www.va.gov

10363 Veterans Adm. Medical Center: Altoona Coatesville VA Medical Center
James E. Van Zandt VA Medical Center
1400 Black Horse Hill Road
Coatesville, PA 19320-4377

610-384-7711
877-626-2500
Fax: 610-383-0207
e-mail: Coatesville.Query@med.va.gov
www.coatesville.med.va.gov

Gary W Devansky, Director
Donald R Means, Associate Director

10364 Veterans Adm. Medical Center: Coatesville
Coatesville VA Medical Center
1400 Black Horse Hill Road
Coatesville, PA 19320

610-384-7711
e-mail: coatesville.query@med.va.gov
www.coatesville.med.va.gov

10365 Veterans Adm. Medical Center: Lebanon Lebanon VA Medical Center
Lebanon VA Medical Center
1700 S Lincoln Avenue
Lebanon, PA 17042

717-272-6621
800-409-8771
Fax: 717-228-5907
e-mail: Norman.Faas@va.gov
www.lebanon.va.gov

Robert W Callahan Jr, Director
William H Mills, Associate Director

10366 Veterans Adm. Medical Center: Pittsburg VA Pittsburgh Healthcare System
VA Pittsburgh Healthcare System
7180 Highland Drive
Pittsburg, PA 15206

412-365-4900
866-482-7488
Fax: 412-365-4213
e-mail: VHAPTHwebteam@va.gov
www.pittsburgh.va.gov

Terry Gerigk Wolf, Director
Rajiv Jain MD, Chief of Staff

10367 Wilkes-Barre VA Medical Center
1111 E End Boulevard
Wilkes-Barre, PA 18711

570-824-3521
877-928-2621
Fax: 570-821-7278
www.wilkes-barre.va.gov

anice M Boss MS CHE, Director
C Gene Molino, Associate Director

10368 Veterans Adm. Medical Center: Providence Providence VA Medical Center
Providence VA Medical Center
830 Chalkstone Avenue
Providence, RI 02908-4799

401-273-7100
866-590-2976
Fax: 401-457-3370
www.providence.va.gov

Vincent Ng, Director
William J Burney, Associate Director

10369 Ralph H. Johnson VA Medical Center
109 Bee Street
Charleston, SC 29401-5799

843-577-5011
Fax: 843-937-6100
www2.va.gov

10370 William Jennings Bryan Dorn VA Medical Center
6439 Garners Ferry Road
Columbia, SC 29209

803-776-4000
800-293-8262
Fax: 803-695-6739
www.va.gov/columbiasc

Falea Maney, Program Manager

10371 Department of Veterans Affairs Medical Center: Sioux Falls
2501 W 22nd Street
Sioux Falls, SD 57117-5046

605-336-3230
800-316-8387
Fax: 605-333-6878
www.visn23.med.va.gov

Healthcare for eligible veterans.

10372 VA Black Hills Health Care System- Fort Meade Campus
113 Comanche Road
Fort Meade, SD 57741

605-347-2511
800-743-1070
Fax: 605-347-7171
e-mail: Jeffrey.Honeycutt@med.va.gov
www2.va.gov

Jeffrey Honeycutt

10373 VA Black Hills Health Care System- Hot Springs Campus
500 N 5th Street
Hot Springs, SD 57747

605-745-2000
800-764-5370
Fax: 605-745-2091
www2.va.gov

10374 Mountain Home VA Medical Center
PO Box 4000
Mountain Home, TN 37684

423-926-1171
877-573-3529
Fax: 423-979-3519
www2.va.gov

Carl J Gerber MD PhD, Director
John W McFadden, Associate Director

10375 Persian Gulf Information Network
PO Box 10160
Clarksville, TN 37042

931-674-1518
Fax: 615-431-5222
e-mail: pgin@knightwave.com
home.att.net/~vetcenter/vetgrps.htm

Paul Lyons

10376 Tennessee Valley Healthcare System- Nashville Campus
1310 24th Avenue, South
Nashville, TN 37212-2637

615-327-4751
Fax: 615-321-6350

10377 Tennessee Valley Healthcare System- Alvin C. York (Murfreesboro) Campus
3400 Lebanon Pike
Murfreesboro, TN 37129
615-867-6000
800-876-7093
Fax: 615-225-4901
www2.va.gov

10378 VISN 9: VA Mid South Healthcare Network
1801 W End Avenue
Nashville, TN 37203
615-695-2200
Fax: 615-695-2210
www.visn9.va.gov

10379 Veterans Adm. Medical Center: Murfreesboro
3400 Lebanon Road
Murfreesboro, TN 37130
615-893-1360
Fax: 615-898-4872

10380 Veterans Adm. Medical Center: Memphis
1030 Jefferson Avenue
Memphis, TN 38104
901-523-8990
800-636-8262
www.memphis.va.gov

10381 Veterans Adm. Medical Center: Muskogee
3400 Lebanon Pike
Murfreesboro, TN 37129
615-867-6000
Fax: 615-225-4901
www.tennesseevalley.va.gov

10382 Veterans Adm. Medical Center: Nashville
1310 24th Avenue S
Nashville, TN 37212
615-327-4751
800-228-4973
Fax: 901-577-7306
www.memphis.va.gov

10383 Veterans Affairs Medical Center
1030 Jefferson Avenue
Memphis, TN 38104
901-523-8990
800-636-8262
Fax: 901-577-7251
www.memphis.va.gov

10384 Veterans Affairs Medical Center, Memphis, Tennessee
1030 Jefferson Avenue
Memphis, TN 38104
901-523-8990
Fax: 901-577-7251

Texas

10385 Amarillo VA Health Care System
6010 Amarillo Boulevard W
Amarillo, TX 79106
806-355-9703
800-687-8262
Fax: 806-354-7860
www.amarillo.va.gov

10386 Austin Outpatient Clinic
2901 Montopolis Drive
Austin, TX 78741
512-389-1010
Fax: 512-389-6545
www2.va.gov

10387 Central Texas Veterans Health Care System
1901 Veterans Memorial Drive
Temple, TX 76504
254-778-4811
800-423-2111
www.centraltexas.va.gov

Bruce A Gordon, Director
Karen Spada MSN MPH MHA FN, Associate Director Nursing Services

10388 El Paso VA Health Care Center
5001 N Piedras
El Paso, TX 79930-4211
915-564-6100
800-672-3782
Fax: 915-564-7920
www.elpaso.va.gov

10389 Michael E. DeBakey VA Medical Center
2002 Holcombe Boulevard
Houston, TX 77030-4298
713-791-1414
800-639-5137
Fax: 713-794-7218
www.houston.med.va.gov

10390 Operation Desert Shield/Desert Storm
PO Box 1712
Odessa, TX 79760
915-368-4667
Fax: 915-580-7451
Vic Sylvester

10391 Persian Gulf Veterans of America
PO Box 190222
San Antonio, TX 78280
210-666-4409
e-mail: KathyPGVA@aol.com
Kathy Hughes

10392 South Texas Veterans Health Care System
7400 Merton Minter
San Antonio, TX 78229
210-617-5300
877-469-5300
www.south-texas.med.va.gov

10393 Thomas T. Connally Medical Center Marlin, T X

10394 VA Heart of Texas Health Care Network Dallas VA Medical Center, TX 76661
Dallas VA Medical Center
4500 S Lancaster Road
Dallas, TX 75216
214-742-8387
800-849-3597
Fax: 214-857-1171
www.northtexas.va.gov

10395 VISN 17: VA Heart of Texas Health Care Network
2301 E Lamar Boulevard
Arlington, TX 76006
817-652-1111
Fax: 817-385-3700
www.heartoftexas.va.gov

10396 Veterans Adm. Medical Center: Big Spring
300 Veterans Boulevard
Big Spring, TX 79720-5500
432-263-7361
800-472-1365
Fax: 432-264-4834
www2.va.gov

10397 Veterans Adm. Medical Center: Dallas
4500 S Lancaster Road
Dallas, TX 75216
214-742-8387
800-849-8387
Fax: 214-857-1171
www2.va.gov

10398 Veterans Adm. Medical Center: Kerrville
3600 Memorial Boulevard
Kerrville, TX 78028
830-896-2020
www2.va.gov

10399 Veterans Adm. Medical Center: Marlin
1016 Ward Street
Marlin, TX 76661
254-883-3511
Fax: 254-883-9240

10400 Veterans Adm. Medical Center: San Antonio
7400 Merton Minter Boulevard
San Antonio, TX 78284
210-617-5300
www.va.gov

10401 Veterans Adm. Medical Center: Temple
1901 Veterans Memorial Drive
Temple, TX 76504
254-778-4811
800-423-2111
Fax: 254-771-4588
www2.va.gov

10402 Waco VA Medical Center
4800 Memorial Drive
Waco, TX 76711
254-752-6581
800-423-2111
www2.va.gov

10403 West Texas VA Health Care System
300 Veterans Boulevard
Big Spring, TX 79720
432-263-7361
800-472-1365
Fax: 432-264-4834
www2.va.gov

Utah

10404 VA Salt Lake City Health Care System
500 Foothill Drive
Salt Lake City, UT 84148
801-582-1565
800-613-4012
Fax: 801-584-1289
www.va.gov

Vermont

10405 White River Junction VA Medical Center
215 N Main Street
White River Junction, VT 05009
802-295-9363
866-687-8387
Fax: 802-296-6354
www.va.gov

Virginia

10406 Desert Storm Justice Foundation: Virginia
PO Box 6812   703-550-1346
Alexandria, VA 22309   Fax: 703-550-1346
Diane St Julian

10407 Gulf War Veterans of Virginia
PO Box 3124   757-988-3PGW
Chesapeake, VA 23320
Ted Myers, President

10408 Veterans Adm. Medical Center: Hampton Hampton VA Medical Center
Hampton VA Medical Center
100 Emancipation Drive   757-722-9961
Hampton, VA 23667   888-869-6060
    Fax: 757-723-6620
www.hampton.va.gov

10409 Veterans Adm. Medical Center: Richmond Hunter Holmes McGuire VA Medical Center
Hunter Holmes McGuire VA Medical Center
1201 Broad Rock Boulevard   804-675-5000
Richmond, VA 23249   800-784-8381
    Fax: 804-675-5581
www.va.gov

10410 Veterans Adm. Medical Center: Roanoke Roanoke Vet Center
Roanoke Vet Center
350 Albemarle Avenue SW   540-342-9726
Roanoke, VA 24016   Fax: 540-857-2405
    www.va.gov

Lynn McGhee, Team Leader
John Whitlock, Counselor

10411 Veterans Adm. Medical Center: Salem Salem VA Medical Center
Salem VA Medical Center
1970 Roanoke Boulevard   540-982-2463
Salem, VA 24153   888-982-2463
    Fax: 540-983-1096
www.va.gov

Washington

10412 Persian Gulf Veterans of Washington
13523 202nd Street E   360-893-2480
Graham, WA 98338   Fax: 360-893-3998
    e-mail: amehl@ix.netcom.com
Alyssa Mehl

10413 VA Puget Sound Health Care System
1660 S Columbian Way   206-762-1010
Seattle, WA 98108-1597   800-329-8387
    Fax: 206-764-2224
www.va.gov/pugetsound

10414 Veterans Adm. Medical Center: Seattle
1660 S Columbian Way   206-762-1010
Seattle, WA 98108   800-329-8387
    Fax: 206-764-2224
www2.va.gov

10415 Veterans Adm. Medical Center: Spokane Spokane VA Medical Center
Spokane VA Medical Center
4815 N Assembly Street   509-434-7000
Spokane, WA 99205-6197   Fax: 509-434-7119
    www.va.gov

10416 Veterans Adm. Medical Center: Tacoma Tacoma Vet Center
Tacoma Vet Center
4916 Center Street   253-565-7038
Tacoma, WA 98409   Fax: 253-565-4981
    www.va.gov

Robert Ramsey, Team Leader
George Rippon, Counselor

10417 Veterans Adm. Medical Center: Walla Walla Johnathan M. Wainwright Memorial VA MC
Johnathan M. Wainwright Memorial VA Medical Center

77 Wainwright Drive   509-525-5200
Walla Walla, WA 99362   888-687-8863
    Fax: 509-527-3452
www.va.gov

West Virginia

10418 Veterans Adm. Medical Center: Beckley Beckley VA Medical Center
Beckley VA Medical Center
200 Veterans Avenue   304-255-2121
Beckley, WV 25801   877-902-5142
    Fax: 304-255-2431
www.va.gov

10419 Veterans Adm. Medical Center: Clarksburg Louis A. Johnson VA Medical Center
Louis A. Johnson VA Medical Center
One Medical Center Drive   304-623-3461
Clarksburg, WV 26301   800-733-0512
    Fax: 304-626-7026
www.va.gov

10420 Veterans Adm. Medical Center: Huntington
1540 Spring Valley Drive   304-429-6741
Huntington, WV 25704   800-827-8244
    Fax: 304-429-6713
www.va.gov

10421 Veterans Affairs Medical Center: Martinsburg
900 Winchester Avenue   304-263-6776
Martinsburg, WV 25401   800-817-3807
    Fax: 304-262-7448
www.va.gov

Robert Hogue, Counselor
Cindy Hughes, Counselor

Wisconsin

10422 Clement J. Zablocki Veterans Affairs Medical Center
5000 W National Avenue   414-382-5300
Milwaukee, WI 53295-1000   Fax: 414-382-5321
    www.va.gov

10423 Gulf War Veterans of Wisconsin
33 University Square   608-250-9645
Madison, WI 53715   e-mail: gulfwarwisc@geocities.com
Anthony Hardie

10424 MidWest Gulf War Veterans Association
PO Box 108   414-695-8694
Pewaukee, WI 53072   Fax: 414-695-8694
    e-mail: mrlbrty@execpc.com
Robert Schramm

10425 Veterans Adm. Medical Center: Tomah
500 E Veterans Street   608-372-3971
Tomah, WI 54660   800-872-8662
    www.va.gov

10426 William S. Middleton Memorial Veterans Hospital
2500 Overlook Terrace   608-256-1901
Madison, WI 53705-2286   Fax: 608-280-7096
    www.va.gov

Wyoming

10427 Veterans Adm. Medical Center: Cheyenne
2360 E Pershing Boulevard   307-778-7550
Cheyenne, WY 82001   888-483-9127
    Fax: 307-778-7336
www.va.gov

10428 Veterans Adm. Medical Center: Sheridan
1898 Fort Road   307-672-3473
Sheridan, WY 82801   866-822-6714
    Fax: 307-672-1900
www.va.gov

Libraries & Resource Centers

10429 ARCH Training Center
2427 Martin Luther King Jr Avenue
Washington, DC
202-889-6344

10430 American GI Forum NVOP
219 Tampico Street
San Antonio, TX 78207
210-212-4088

10431 COPIN Foundation
2644 North Avenue
Niagara Falls, NY 14305
716-283-5622
Fax: 716-283-5721

10432 Kennedy-Krieger Institute
707 N Broadway
Baltimore, MD 21205
443-923-9200
800-873-3377
Fax: 443-923-9405
www.kennedykrieger.org

10433 Shriver Center University Affiliated Program
Eunice Kennedy Shriver Center
200 Trapelo Road
781-642-0001
Waltham, MA 02452-6319   e-mail: shriver.center@umassmed.edu
www.shriver.org

10434 Veterans Benefits Clearinghouse
38 Dudley Street
Roxbury, MA 02119-1707
617-541-8846

Support Groups & Hotlines

10435 National Health Information Center
PO Box 1133
Washington, DC 20013
310-565-4167
800-336-4797
Fax: 301-984-4256
e-mail: info@nhic.org
www.health.gov/nhic

Offers a nationwide information referral service, produces directories and resource guides.

10436 National Veterans Services Fund
PO Box 2465
Darien, CT 06820-0465
203-656-0003
800-521-0198
Fax: 203-656-1957
e-mail: NatVetSvc@aol.com
www.nvsf.org

Agent Orange informational hotline.
Phil Kraft, President

Books

10437 An Assessment of Technical Issues Raised in RW Haley's Critique of Health Studies
Gus Haggstrom, author

Rand Corporation
1776 Main Street
Santa Monica, CA 90407-2138
310-393-0411
Fax: 310-393-4818

ISBN: 0-833027-52-2

10438 Gulf War and Health
National Academy Press
500 5th Street NW
Washington, DC 20055
202-334-3313
888-624-8373
Fax: 202-334-2793
e-mail: zjones@nas.edu

Lyla M Hernandez, Editor
Merwyn R Greenlick, Editor

10439 Natural Attenuation for Groundwater Remediation
National Academy Press
500 5th Street NW
Washington, DC 20055
202-334-3313
888-624-8373
Fax: 202-334-2793
e-mail: zjones@nas.edu

10440 Yes, You Can
Demos Medical Publishing
386 Park Avenue S
New York, NY 10016
212-683-0072
Fax: 212-683-0118
e-mail: orderdept@demospub.com
www.demosmedpub.com

112 pages
ISBN: 1-888799-48-x
Dr. Diana M Schneider

Newsletters

10441 Agent Orange Briefs
Department of Veterans Affairs
810 Vermont Avenue NW
Washington, DC 20420-0002
202-233-4000
Designed to answer questions regarding Agent Orange and related matters. This fact sheet series is prepared and updated annually.
Monthly

10442 Agent Orange Review
Department of Veterans Affairs
810 Vermont Avenue NW
Washington, DC 20420-0002
202-233-4000
Published periodically to provide information on Agent Orange to concerned veterans and their families. The most recent issues include updated information about Federal government studies and activities related to Agent Orange and the Vietnam experience.

Pamphlets

10443 Agent Orange Anxiety: The Human Response to Possable Oncogenicity and Mutagencity
National Veterans Services Fund
PO Box 2465
Darien, CT 06820-0465
203-656-0003
800-521-0198
Fax: 203-656-1957
e-mail: NatVetSvc@optonline.net
www.angelfire.com/ct2/natvetsvc

10444 Agent Orange Fact Sheet: A Historical Perspective
Veterans Of The Vietnam War
805 South Township Boulevard
Pittston, PA 18640-3327
570-603-9740
Fax: 570-603-9741
www.vvnw.org

Fact sheet designed to bring an awareness of Agent Orange and related herbicides to the American public, includes a bibliography for the professional.
10 pages

10445 Agent Orange and Birth Defects
Veterans Health Adminstration
810 Vermont Avenue Northwest
Washington, DC 20420-3517
202-273-8580
Fax: 202-273-9080
www.tpromo2.com/usvi/index2.htm
Letters to the editor, New England Journal of Medicine articles.

10446 Agent Orange and Chloracme
National Veterans Services Fund
PO Box 2465
Darien, CT 06820-0465
203-656-0003
800-521-0198
Fax: 203-656-1957
e-mail: NatVetSvc@optonline.net
www.angelfire.com/ct2/natvetsvc

10447 Agent Orange and Hodgkin's Disease
Veterans Health Administration
810 Vermont Avenue Northwest
Washington, DC 20420-3517
203-273-8580
Fax: 203-273-9080
www.tpromo2.com/usvi/index2.htm

10448 Agent Orange and Mutiple Myeloma
National Veterans Services Fund
PO Box 2465
Darien, CT 06820-0465
203-656-0003
800-521-0198
Fax: 203-656-1957
e-mail: NatVetSvc@optonline.net
www.angelfire.com/ct2/natvetsvc

10449 Agent Orange and Non-Hodgkin's Lymphoma
Veterans Health Administration
810 Vermont Avenue   203-273-8580
Washington, DC 20420-3517   Fax: 203-273-9080
www.tpromo2.com/usvi/index2.htm

10450 Agent Orange and Peripheral Neuropathy
Veterans Health Administration
810 Vermont Avenue   203-273-8580
Washington, DC 20420-3517   Fax: 203-273-9080
www.tpromo2.com/usvi/index2.htm

10451 Agent Orange and Porphyria Cutanea Tarda
National Veterans Services Fund
PO Box 2465   203-656-0003
Darien, CT 06820-0465   800-521-0198
Fax: 203-656-1957
e-mail: NatVetSvc@optonline.net
www.angelfire.com/ct2/natvetsvc

10452 Agent Orange and Prostate Cancer
National Veterans Services Fund
PO Box 2465   203-656-0003
Darien, CT 06820-0465   800-521-0198
Fax: 203-656-1957
e-mail: NatVetSvc@optonline.net
www.angelfire.com/ct2/natvetsvc

10453 Agent Orange and Respiratory Cancers
National Veterans Services Fund
PO Box 2465   203-656-0003
Darien, CT 06820-0465   800-521-0198
Fax: 203-656-1957
e-mail: NatVetSvc@optonline.net
www.angelfire.com/ct2/natvetsvc

10454 Agent Orange and Soft Tissue Sarcomas
National Veterans Services Fund
PO Box 2465   203-656-0003
Darien, CT 06820-0465   800-521-0198
Fax: 203-656-1957
e-mail: NatVetSvc@optonline.net
www.angelfire.com/ct2/natvetsvc

10455 Agent Orange and Spina Bifida
National Veterans Services Fund
PO Box 2465   203-656-0003
Darien, CT 06820-0465   800-521-0198
Fax: 203-656-1957
e-mail: NatVetSvc@optonline.net
www.angelfire.com/ct2/natvetsvc

10456 Agent Orange: It is Part of Your Life
National Veterans Services Fund
PO Box 2465   203-656-0003
Darien, CT 06820-0465   800-521-0198
Fax: 203-656-1957
e-mail: NatVetSvc@optonline.net
www.angelfire.com/ct2/natvetsvc

10457 Brief History of the Agent Orange Lawsuit
National Veterans Services Fund
PO Box 2465   203-656-0003
Darien, CT 06820-0465   800-521-0198
Fax: 203-656-1957
e-mail: NatVetSvc@optonline.net
www.angelfire.com/ct2/natvetsvc

10458 Case Control Study: Soft-Tissue Sarcomas and Exposure to Phenoxyacetic Acids
National Veterans Services Fund
PO Box 2465   203-656-0003
Darien, CT 06820-0465   800-521-0198
Fax: 203-656-1957
e-mail: NatVetSvc@optonline.net
www.angelfire.com/ct2/natvetsvc
Case control study: soft-tissue sarcoma and exposure to phenoxyacetic acids or chlorphenols.

10459 Children of Vietnam Veterans: Complex Concerns and Innovative Solutions
National Veterans Services Fund

PO Box 2465   203-656-0003
Darien, CT 06820-0465   800-521-0198
Fax: 203-656-1957
e-mail: NatVetSvc@optonline.net
www.angelfire.com/ct2/natvetsvc
7 pages

10460 Dioxin, A Case in Point
National Veterans Services Fund
PO Box 2465   203-656-0003
Darien, CT 06820-0465   800-521-0198
Fax: 203-656-1957
e-mail: NatVetSvc@optonline.net
www.angelfire.com/ct2/natvetsvc

10461 Enviromental Chloracne
National Veterans Services Fund
PO Box 2465   203-656-0003
Darien, CT 06820-0465   800-521-0198
Fax: 203-656-1957
e-mail: NatVetSvc@optonline.net
www.angelfire.com/ct2/natvetsvc

10462 History of the Agent Orange Litigation
National Veterans Services Fund
PO Box 2465   203-656-0003
Darien, CT 06820-0465   800-521-0198
Fax: 203-656-1957
e-mail: NatVetSvc@optonline.net
www.angelfire.com/ct2/natvetsvc

10463 List of Agent Orange-Related Illnesses Recognized By the VA
National Veterans Services Fund
PO Box 2465   203-656-0003
Darien, CT 06820-0465   800-521-0198
Fax: 203-656-1957
e-mail: NatVetSvc@optonline.net
www.angelfire.com/ct2/natvetsvc

10464 List of Diseases Accepted by the VA for Presumptive Service-Connection
National Veterans Services Fund
PO Box 2465   203-656-0003
Darien, CT 06820-0465   800-521-0198
Fax: 203-656-1957
e-mail: NatVetSvc@optonline.net
www.angelfire.com/ct2/natvetsvc
List of diseases accepted by the VA for presumptive service-connection that are associated with exposure to certain herbicide agents including Agent Orange.

10465 Relation of Soft-Tissue Sarcome, Malignant Lymphoma & Colon Cancer
National Veterans Services Fund
PO Box 2465   203-656-0003
Darien, CT 06820-0465   800-521-0198
Fax: 203-656-1957
e-mail: NatVetSvc@optonline.net
www.angelfire.com/ct2/natvetsvc
Relation to soft-tissue sarcomas, malignant lymphoma and colon cancer to phenoxy acids, chlorphenois and other agents.

10466 Spina Bifida Benefits Guide
National Veterans Services Fund
PO Box 2465   203-656-0003
Darien, CT 06820-0465   800-521-0198
Fax: 203-656-1957
e-mail: NatVetSvc@optonline.net
www.angelfire.com/ct2/natvetsvc
4 pages

Audio & Video

10467 Agent Orange Videotapes
Regional Learning Resources Service
915 N. Grand Boulevard   314-652-4100
St. Louis, MO 63106
Produces several Agent Orange videotape programs that explain what Agent Orange is, where, when and how it was used, why persons are concerned about exposure to it and what VA and other de-

partments and agencies are doing in response to these concerns. These videotapes are maintained at all VA medical centers across the country.

Web Sites

10468 Gulf War Syndrome Database

www.louisville.edu/library/ekstrom

This is a substantial database of relevant documents and studies kept by University of Louisville, Ekstrom Library.

10469 Gulf War Veteran Resource Pages

www.gulfweb.org

This page is administered by Gulf War veterans and provides a great range of information on a variety of Gulf War-related items, including GWS. The site includes many links to other groups interested in GWS and to GWS studies.

10470 Healing Well

www.healingwell.com

An online health resource guide to medical news, chat, information and articles, newsgroups and message boards, books, disease-related web sites, medical directories, and more for patients, friends, and family coping with disabling diseases, disorders, or chronic illnesses.

10471 Health Finder

www.healthfinder.gov

Searchable, carefully developed web site offering information on over 1000 topics. Developed by the US Department of Health and Human Services, the site can be used in both English and Spanish.

10472 Healthlink USA

www.healthlinkusa.com

Health information concerning treatment, cures, prevention, diagnosis, risk factors, research, support groups, email lists, personal stories and much more. Updated regularly.

10473 Heatlhcentral.com

www.healthcentral.com

The HealthCentral Network has a collection of owned and operated web sites and multimedia affiliate properties providing timely, in-depth, trusted medical information, personalized tools and resources for people seeking to manage and improve their health.

10474 Helios Health

www.helioshealth.com

Online resource for your health information. Detailed information about specific health topics, access to expert advice from our Medical Advisory Board, and up-to-date health news.

10475 InteliHealth

www.intelihealth.com

InteliHealth's mission is to empower people with treusted solutions for healthier lives. They accomplish this by providing credible information fromt he most trusted sources.
Brian Berkenstock, Writer/Editor

10476 MedicineNet

www.medicinenet.com

Medicine Net is an online healthcare media publishing company. It provides easy-to-read, in-depth, authoritative medical information for consumers via its robust, user-friendly, interactive web site.

10477 Medscape

www.medscape.com

Medscape offers specialists, primary care physicians, and other health professionals the Web's most robust and integrated medical information and educational tools.

10478 National Veterans Services Fund

www.nvsf.org

Supports and informs those who were exposed to the defoliant Agent Orange, or dioxin, while serving the US in the conflict in Vietnam.

10479 Office of the Special Assistant for Gulf War Illnesses

www.gulflink.osd.mil

This is a page sponsored by the Defense Department's Special Assistant for Gulf War Illnesses. It provides information on and linkes to Federal and State-funded studies of Gulf War Illnesses.

10480 WebMD

www.webmd.com

Information on Agent Orange related injuries, including articles and resources.

Description

10481 Wilson's Disease

Wilson's disease is a rare genetic disorder that results from an inability to adequately excrete copper. In the United States, approximately one person in 40,000 has this condition. The resulting accumulation of copper in the body's tissues and organs leads to disease of the brain and liver, and to a lesser extent, the kidney and red blood cells. The disease is genetic; if two carriers have children, the disease would have a 1 in 4 chance of being passed on.

Build-up of copper in the liver causes a hepatitis-like illness with loss of appetite, low grade fever, abdominal discomfort and jaundice. If not detected and treated, this process can lead to cirrhosis and fatal liver failure. In 40 to 50 percent of patients, the illness affects the brain and can include unsteadiness, tremors, slurred speech and intellectual deterioration. Copper rings may appear in the eye in up to 10 percent of patients. Although they do not cause any symptoms, their appearance may help establish the diagnosis.

In untreated Wilson's, the disease is fatal, generally before the age of 30. Continual, lifelong treatment is mandatory for any patient with confirmed Wilson's disease, whether symptomatic or not. The critical therapy is to administer a drug that helps the body release its copper stores. D-penicillamine is the most common such drug. Some patients have required liver transplantation.

National Agencies & Associations

10482 American Liver Foundation
75 Maiden Lane
New York, NY 00038
212-668-1000
800-465-4837
Fax: 212-483-8179
e-mail: info@liverfoundation.org
www.liverfoundation.org
The only national voluntary health group dedicated to fighting all liver diseases through research education and patient self-help groups.
Rick Smith, President/CEO
Newton Guerin, COO

10483 United Liver Foundation
11646 W Pico Boulevard
Los Angeles, CA 90064
213-445-4204
Foundation offering information public awareness materials support and medical research for persons suffering from liver diseases.

10484 Wilson's Disease Association
1802 Brookside Drive
Wooster, OH 44691
330-264-1450
888-264-1450
Fax: 330-264-0974
e-mail: info@wilsonsdisease.org
www.wilsonsdisease.org
Serves as a communications support network for individuals affected by Wilson's disease; distributes information to professionals and the public; makes referrals; and holds meetings.
8 pages
Kimberly Symonds, Executive Director

Foundations

10485 Hepatitis B Foundation
3805 Old Easton Road
Doylestown, PA 18902
215-489-4900
Fax: 215-489-4313
e-mail: info@hepb.org
www.hepb.org
We are dedicated to finding a cure and improving the quality of life for those affected by hepatitis B worldwide. Our commitment includes funding focused research, promoting disease awareness, supporting immunization and treatment initiatives, and serving as the primary source of information for patients and their families, the medical and scientific community, and the general public.

Molli Conti, Chair
Timothy Block, PhD, Founder/President

Support Groups & Hotlines

10486 National Health Information Center
PO Box 1133
Washington, DC 20013
310-565-4167
800-336-4797
Fax: 301-984-4256
e-mail: info@nhic.org
www.health.gov/nhic
Offers a nationwide information referral service, produces directories and resource guides.

Pamphlets

10487 Wilson's Disease
American Liver Foundation
1425 Pompton Avenue
Cedar Grove, NJ 07009
800-465-4837
Fax: 973-256-3214
e-mail: info@liverfoundation.org
www.liverfoundation.org
A brochure offering information on the causes, symptoms and treatments of Wilson's Disease.
Rick Smith, President & CEO

Web Sites

10488 Healing Well
e-mail: webmaster@healingwell.com
www.healingwell.com
An online health resource guide to medical news, chat, information and articles, newsgroups and message boards, books, disease-related web sites, medical directories, and more for patients, friends, and family coping with disabling diseases, disorders, or chronic illnesses.
Peter Waite, MS, MA, Founder/Editor

10489 Health Finder
PO Box 1133
Washington, DC 20013-1133
e-mail: healthfinder@nhic.org
www.healthfinder.gov
Searchable, carefully developed web site offering information on over 1000 topics. Developed by the US Department of Health and Human Services, the site can be used in both English and Spanish.

10490 Healthlink USA
www.healthlinkusa.com
Health information concerning treatment, cures, prevention, diagnosis, risk factors, research, support groups, email lists, personal stories and much more. Updated regularly.

10491 Helios Health
www.helioshealth.com
Online resource for your health information. Detailed information about specific health topics, access to expert advice from our Medical Advisory Board, and up-to-date health news.

10492 MedicineNet
www.medicinenet.com

An online resource for consumers providing easy-to-read, authoritative medical and health information.

10493 Medscape
Corporate Headquarters
111 8th Avenue
New York, NY 10011   212-624-3700
                                      www.medscape.com
Medscape offers specialists, primary care physicians, and other health professionals the Web's most robust and integrated medical information and educational tools.
Kate Hahn, Media Relations
Tony G Holcombe, President

10494 WebMD
                                      www.webmd.com
Information on Wilson's disease, including articles and resources.

National Agencies & Associations

10495 ABLEDATA
8630 Fenton Street 301-608-8998
Silver Spring, MD 20910 800-227-0216
Fax: 301-608-8958
TTY: 301-608-8912
e-mail: abledata@macrointernational.com
www.abledata.com

Provides objective information on assistive technology and rehabilitation equipment available from domestic and international sources to consumers, organizations, professionals, and caregivers within the United States.
Katherine Belknap, Project Director

10496 ABLEDATA-REHAB DATA Alliance for Technology Access (ATA)
8630 Fenton Street 301-608-8998
Silver Spring, MD 20910 800-227-0216
Fax: 301-608-8958
TTY: 301-608-8912
e-mail: abledata@macrointernational.com
www.abledata.com

National organization dedicated to providing access to technology for people with disabilities through its coalition of 45 community-based resource centers in 34 states and the Virgin Islands. Each center provides information, awareness and training.
Katherine Belknap, Project Director
Juanita Hardy, Information Specialist

10497 Access Unlimited
570 Hance Road
Binghamton, NY 13903 800-849-2143
Fax: 607-669-4595
e-mail: tom@accessunlimited.com
www.accessunlimited.com

Assists educators health care providers and parents in discovering lift and transfer aids help children and adults with disabilities compensate for some of the barriers imposed by their conditions. Access Unlimited markets and offers technical support.
Tom Cole, Owner

10498 American Academy of Pediatrics
141 NW Point Boulevard 847-434-4000
Elk Grove Village, IL 60007-1098 Fax: 847-434-8000
www.aap.org

To attain optimal physical, mental, and social health and well-being for all infants, children, adolescents, and young adults.
O Marion Burton MD FAAP, President
Errol T Alden MD FAAP, Executive Director

10499 American Association for the Advancement of Science
1200 New York Avenue NW 202-326-6640
Washington, DC 20005 Fax: 202-371-9526
e-mail: webmaster@aaas.org
www.aaas.org

Seeks to advance science, engineering, and innovation throughout the world for the benefit of all people.
Dr Alan I Leshner, AAAS CEO
Dr Peter C Agre, Chair

10500 American Association of People with Disabilities
1629 K Street NW 202-457-0046
Washington, DC 20006 800-840-8844
Fax: 202-457-0473
TTY: 202-457-0046
www.aapd-dc.org

A cross-disability membership organization, organizes the disability community to be a powerful voice for change-politically, economically, including their family, friends and supporters, and to be a national voice for change in implementing the goals of the Americans with Disabilities Act (ADA).
Helena Berger, Acting President/CEO/COO

10501 American Autoimmune Related Diseases Association
22100 Gratiot Avenue 586-776-3900
Eastpointe, MI 48021 Fax: 586-776-3903
e-mail: aarda@aarda.org
www.aarda.org

Dedicated to the eradication of autoimmune diseases and the alleviation of suffering and the socioeconomic impact of autoimmunity through fostering and facilitating collaboration in the areas of education, public awareness, research, and patient services in an effective, ethical and efficient manner.
Stanley M Finger PhD, Chairman
Virginia T Ladd, President/Executive Director

10502 American Bar Association Commission on Mental and Physical Disability Law
740 15th Street NW 202-662-1570
Washington, DC 20005 Fax: 202-442-3439
e-mail: campdl@americanbar.org
www.americanbar.org

The Commission's mission is to promote the ABA's commitment to justice and the rule of law for persons with mental, physical, and sensory disabilities and to promote their full and equal participation in the legal profession.
John W Parry, Director

10503 American Camp Association
5000 State Road 67 N 765-342-8456
Martinsville, IN 46151-7902 800-428-2267
Fax: 765-342-2065
www.acacamps.org

Formerly the American Camping Association, a community of camp professionals who have joined together to share the knowledge and experience and to ensure the quality of camp programs.
Peter Surgenor, President

10504 American Counseling Association
5999 Stevenson Avenue
Alexandria, VA 22304 800-347-6647
Fax: 703-823-0252
e-mail: ryep@counseling.org
www.counseling.org

A not-for-profit, professional and educational organization that is dedicated to the growth and enhancement of the counseling profession. Represents professional counselors in various practice settings.
Marcheta Evans, President
Richard Yep, Executive Director

10505 American Foundation for The Blind
2 Penn Plaza 212-502-7600
New York, NY 10121 800-232-5463
Fax: 888-545-8331
e-mail: afbinfo@afb.net
www.afb.org

AFB's priorities include broadening access to technology; elevating the quality of information and tools for the professionals who serve people with vision loss by providing them and their families with relevant and timely resources.
Carl R Augusto, President/CEO

10506 American Institute for Preventive Medicine
30445 NW Highway 248-539-1800
Farmington Hills, MI 48334 800-345-2476
Fax: 248-539-1808
e-mail: aipm@healthylife.com
www.healthylife.com

An award winning, internationally recognized authority on th development and implementation of health promotion, wellness, medical self-care, and disease management programs and publications.
Don R Powell PhD, President/CEO

10507 American Institute for Preventive Medicine
30445 NW Highway 248-539-1800
Farmington Hills, MI 48334 800-345-2476
Fax: 248-539-1808
e-mail: aipm@healthylife.com
www.healthylife.com

The institute provides health promotion programs disease management guides and self-care publications to hospitals HMOs corporations and government agencies. Programs are designed to lower health care costs, decrease absenteeism and improve productivity.
Don R Powell PhD, President and CEO
Larry Chapman, Senior Vice President

10508 American Organ Transplant Association
21175 Tomball Parkway
Houston, TX 77070
713-344-2402
Fax: 713-344-9422
www.aotaonline.org
Helps patients with free transportation to and from their transplant center, many times hundreds of miles away. Also provides transplant patients and their loved ones with resources regarding transplantation.
Pamela H Terry, Board President
David Hileman, Board VP

10509 American Red Cross National Headquarters
2025 E Street NW
Washington, DC 20006
202-303-5000
www.redcross.org
The nation's premier emergency response organization that aids victims of devastating natural disasters; community services that help the needy; support and comfort for military members and their families; the collection, processing and distribution of lifesaving blood and blood products; educational programs that promote health and safety; and international relief and development programs.
Gail J McGovern, President/CEO
Bonnie McElveen-Hunt, Chairman

10510 American Rehabilitation Counseling Association
5999 Stevenson Avenue
Alexandria, VA 22304-3300
800-347-6647
Fax: 800-473-2329
TTY: 703-823-6862
TDD: 7038236862
e-mail: webmaster@counseling.org
www.counseling.org
Mission of ARCA is to enhance the development of persons with disabilities throughout their life span and to promote excellence in the rehabilitation counseling professional.
Colleen Logan, President
Richard Yep, Executive Office

10511 American Society of Dermatology
PO Box 9013
Port St Lucie, FL 34984
561-873-8335
Fax: 561-344-8388
www.asd.org
The purpose of this organization is to make optimal care available to all citizens of this country by preserving, promoting and enhancing the practice of dermatology. It should represent its members in those scientific, educational, socio-economic and legislative areas that affect the practice of dermatology and shall endeavor to cooperate with other organizations of similar purpose.
W Gerald Klinger MD, President
M John Hanni Jr, Executive Director

10512 Americas Association for the Care of Children
PO Box 2154
Boulder, CO 80306-2154
303-527-2742
www.aaccchildren.net
To promote support for those who are involved in early childhood education through educational programs and projects, including among other things, citizen exchange programs, global communication networks, and resource assistance to participating communities.

Debbie Young, Executive Director

10513 Asbestos Information Association/North America
1745 Jefferson Davis Highway
Arlington, VA 22202
703-412-1150
Fax: 703-412-1586
e-mail: aiabjpigg@aol.com
Founded to represent the interests of the asbestos industry and to collect and disseminate information about asbestos and asbestos products with emphasis on safety health and environmental issues.

10514 Beach Center on Disability
University of Kansas
1200 Sunnyside Avenue
Lawrence, KS 66045
785-864-7600
Fax: 786-864-7605
e-mail: beachcenter@ku.edu
www.beachcenter.org
Through excellence in research, teaching and technical assistance, and service in Kansas, the United States of America, and globally, and through collaborations with those individuals and entities dedicated to the same ends, the Beach Center on Disability will make a significant and sustainable difference in the quality of life of families and individuals affected by disability and of those who are closely involved with them.
Wayne Sailor, Associate Director

10515 Breaking New Ground Resource Center
Purdue University, ABE Building
W Lafayette, IN 47907
765-494-5088
800-825-4264
Fax: 765-496-1356
e-mail: bng@enc.purdue.edu
www.ecn.purdue.edu
Has become internationally recoginzed as the primary source for information and resources on rehabilitation technology for persons working in agriculture.
Prof William Field, Project Leader

10516 Center for Children with Chronic Illness and Disability
University of Minnesota School of Public Health
2525 Chicago Avenue
Minneapolis, MN 55404
612-813-6000
www.childrensmn.org
Dr Joan Patterson, Director

10517 Center for Chronic Disease Prevention and Centers for Disease Control
1600 Clifton Road
Atlanta, GA 30333
404-639-3311
800-232-4636
TTY: 888-232-6348
e-mail: cdcinfo@cdc.gov
www.cdc.gov
Chronic diseases such as heart disease cancer and diabetes are the leading causes of death and disability in the United States. These diseases account for 7 of every 10 deaths and affect the quality of life of 90 million Americans.
Richard E Besser, Director

10518 Center for Developmental Disabilities University of South Carolina
8301 Farrow Road
Columbia, SC 29208
803-935-5231
Fax: 803-935-5059
uscm.med.sc.edu/cdrhome
The vision of The Center for Developmental Disabilities is to work as a team to create a quality environment in which the following values are embraced: Everyone is treated with dignity and respect. Individual strengths and abilities are recognized.

10519 Center for Disability Resources
University of South Carolina
8301 Farrow Road
Columbia, SC 29208
803-935-5231
Fax: 803-935-5059
e-mail: steve.wilson@uscmed.sc.edu
uscm.med.sc.edu/cdrhome
To enhance the well-being and quality of life of persons with disabilities and their families. Collaborates with persons with disabilities and their families to develop new knowledge and best practices, train leaders, and effect systems change.

10520 Center for Disease Control and Prevention
1600 Clifton Rd
Atlanta, GA 30333
800-232-4636
TTY: 800-232-6348
e-mail: cdcinfo@cdc.gov
www.cdc.gov
To collaborate to create the expertise, information, and tools that people and communities need to protect their health - through health promotion, prevention of disease, injury and disability, and preparedness for new health threats.
Thomas R Frieden MD MPH, Director

10521 Center for Health Research
Kaiser Permanente Northwest
3800 N Interstate Avenue
Portland, OR 97227-1098
503-335-2400
e-mail: information@kpchr.org
www.kpchr.org
Conducts professionally independent, public domain research and idsseminates its findings in the scholarly literature and scientific community.
Mary L Durham PhD, Director

10522 Center for Medical Consumers
239 Thompson Street
New York, NY 10012   212-674-7105
e-mail: centerformedicalconsumers@gmail.com
www.medicalconsumers.org
A non-profit advocacy organization that was founded with the philosophy: Whenever long-term drug therapy, elective surgery, or any other major treatment is prescribed, the question of whether the treatment has been proven safe and effective should come up.
Arthur Aaron Levin MPH, Director

10523 Center for Universal Design North Carolina State University
North Carolina State University
Campus Box 7701   919-513-2022
Raleigh, NC 27695-8613   800-647-6777
Fax: 919-515-8951
e-mail: nilda_cosco@ncsu.edu
www.design.ncsu.edu
National research information and technical assistance center that evaluates develops and promotes accessible and universal design in housing buildings outdoor and urban environments and related products.
Nilda Cosco PhD, Education Specialist
Leslie Young, Director of Design

10524 Child Center
3995 Marcola Road   541-726-1465
Springfield, OR 97477   Fax: 541-726-5085
e-mail: info@thechildcenter.org
www.thechildcenter.org
To provide individualized, diagnostic, therapeutic and educational services for the emotional and behavioral problems children exhibit in the home, school and community; provide integreated community based psychiatric and support services that are child centered, family driven and culturally competent
Scott Diehl, President
Dennis Konrady, Vice President

10525 Children's Hospice International
1101 King Street   703-684-0330
Alexandria, VA 22314   800-242-4453
e-mail: info@chionline.org
www.chionline.org
To ensure medical, psychological, social and spiritual support to all children with life-threatening conditions and their families by providing a network of resources and care.
Ann Armstrong-Dailey, Founding Director/CEO

10526 Children's National Medical Center
111 Michigan Avenue NW   202-476-3000
Washington, DC 20010   e-mail: webteam@cnmc.org
www.dcchildrens.com
The only exclusive provider of pediatric care in the metropolitan Washington area and is the only freestanding children's hospital between Philadelphia, Pittsburgh, Norfolk, and Atlanta; the leader in the development and application of innovative new treatments for childhood illness and injury.
Edwin K Zechman Jr, President/CEO

10527 Christian Horizons
PO Box 6646
Grand Rapids, MI 48608   989-493-4099
www.christian-horizons.org
Empowers individuals with exceptional needs, enabling them to embrace their God-given potential and enjoy hope and opportunity in everyday living.
Ed Sider, CEO
Beth Woof, Chair

10528 Clearinghouse on Disability Information Office of Special Education & Rehab Svcs
US Department of Education
550 12th Street SW   202-245-7307
Washington, DC 20202-2550   Fax: 202-245-7636
TTY: 202-205-5637
TDD: 2022055637
www.ed.gov
Provides information to people with disabilities or anyone requesting information by doing research and providing documents in response to inquiries. Information provided includes areas of federal funding for disability-related programs.
Carolyn Corlett, Contact

10529 Council for Learning Disabilities (CLD)
11184 Antioch Road   913-491-1011
Overland Park, KS 66210   Fax: 913-491-1012
e-mail: CLDInfo@ie-events.com
www.cldinternational.org
National professional organization dedicated solely to professionals working with individuals who have learning disabilities. Committed to enhancing the education and life span development of those individuals.
Caroline Dunn, President
Monica Lambert, President Elect

10530 Disabled & Alone: Life Services for the Handicapped
61 Broadway   212-532-6740
New York, NY 10006   800-995-0066
Fax: 212-532-3588
e-mail: info@disabledandalone.org
www.disabledandalone.org
A non-profit organization established to help families provide a secure future for their loved ones with a disability. Also believes that no person should have to live his life in loneliness and isolation because of a disability.
Leslie D Park, Chairman
Lee Alan Ackerman, Executive Director

10531 Distance Education and Training Council
1601 18th Street NW   202-234-5100
Washington, DC 20009   Fax: 202-332-1386
e-mail: brianna@detc.org
www.detc.org
A voluntary, non-governmental, educational organization that operates a nationally recognized accrediting association, the DETC Accrediting Commission.
Michael P Lambert, Executive Director

10532 Educational Equity Center at The Academy for Educational Development
100 Fifth Avenue   212-243-1110
New York, NY 10011   Fax: 212-627-0407
e-mail: lcolon@aed.org
www.edequity.org
A national non-profit organization promoting educational excellence for children.
Merle Froschl, Co-Director
Barbara Sprung, Co-Director

10533 Equal Opportunity Employment Commission
131 M Street NE
Washington, DC 20507   202-663-4900
www.eeoc.org
To promote equality of opportunity and enforce federal laws prohibiting employment discrimination.
Jacqueline A Berrien, Chair

10534 Estate Planning for the Disabled
2232 W Avenue 133   510-352-4127
San Leandro, CA 94577-1050   Fax: 510-352-4127
e-mail: EFM@EFMOODY.com
www.efmoody.com
Counsels and assists parents of children with special needs to develop viable estate plans, letters of intent, wills and special needs trusts. EPD will work with the appropriate professionals and agencies to help put together an effective comprehensive plan.

10535 Extensions for Independence
555 Saturn Boulevard   619-618-2154
San Diego, CA 92154   866-632-7149
Fax: 866-632-7149
e-mail: info@mouthstick.net
www.mouthstick.net
Designer and manufacturer of home and office related equipment for the functional independence of the most physically challenged.
Arthur Heyer, President

10536 Favarh
225 Commerce Drive
Canton, CT 06019-1099
860-693-6662
Fax: 860-693-8662
www.favarh.org

Provides a variety of programs and services to adults with developmental, physical or mental disabilities and their families, throughout the Farmington Valley communities of Avon, Burlington and more.
Stephen Morr MPA, Executive Director

10537 Federation for Children with Special Needs
1135 Tremont Street
Boston, MA 02120
617-236-7210
800-331-0688
Fax: 617-572-2094
e-mail: fcsninfo@fcsn.org
fcsn.org

Provides information, support, and assistance to parents of children with disabilities, their professional partners and their communities. Committed to listening to and learning from families, and encouraging full participation in community life by all people, especially those with disabilities.
Rich Robison, Executive Director
Sara Miranda, Associate Executive Director

10538 Florida Disabled Outdoor Association
2475 Apalachee Parkway
Tallahassee, FL 32301
850-201-2944
Fax: 850-201-2945
www.fdoa.org

Enriches lives through accessible inclusive recreation and active leisure for all.
David Jones, Director

10539 Goodwill Industries International
15810 Indianola Drive
Rockville, MD 20855
301-530-6500
800-741-0186
Fax: 301-530-1516
TTY: 301-530-9759
e-mail: contactus@goodwill.org
www.goodwill.org

Enhances the dignity and quality of life of individuals, families and communities by eliminating barriers to opportunity and helping people in need reach their fullest potential through the power of work.
Jim Gibbons, President/CEO
Bill J Kacal, Chair

10540 HEATH Resource Center
George Washington University
2134 G Street NW
Washington, DC 20052-0001
202-939-9329
800-544-3284
Fax: 202-994-3365
e-mail: AskHEATH@gwu.edu
www.heath.gwu.edu

Serves as a national clearinghouse on postsecondary education for individuals with disabilities.
Dr Lynda West, Principal Investigator
Dr Joel Gomez, Co-Principal Investigator

10541 Health Care For All
30 Winter Street
Boston, MA 02108
617-350-7279
Fax: 617-451-5838
TTY: 617-350-0974
e-mail: aslemmer@hcfama.org
www.hcfama.org

HCFA seeks to create a consumer-centered health care system that provides comprehensive, affordable, accessible, culturally competent, high quality care and consumer education for everyone, especially the most vulnerable.
Amy Whitcomb Slemmer, Executive Director

10542 International Association for the Study of Pain
111 Queen Anne Avenue N
Seattle, WA 98109-4955
206-283-0311
Fax: 206-283-9403
e-mail: iaspdesk@iasp-pain.org
www.iasp-pain.org

Brings together scientists, clinicians, health care providers, and policy makers to stimulate and support the study of pain and to translate that knowledge into improved pain relief worldwide.
Kathy Kreiter, Executive Director
Kathy Havers, Prorgam Coordinator

10543 International Council on Disability
1012 14th Street NW
Washington, DC 20005
202-347-0102
Fax: 202-347-0315
e-mail: info@usicd.org
www.usicd.org

To catalyze and help focus the energy, expertise and resources of the US disability community and the US government to optimize their impact on improving the lives of and circumstances of people with disabilities worldwide.
David Morrissey, Executive Director

10544 LAUNCH Department of Special Education
Department of Special Education
Commerce, TX 75428
903-886-5932

Provides resources for learning disabled individuals coordinates efforts of other local state and national LD organizations acts as a communication channel for people with learning disabilities through a monthly newsletter and provides programs.

10545 Learning Disabilities Association of America
4156 Library Road
Pittsburgh, PA 15234-1349
412-341-1515
888-300-6710
Fax: 412-344-0224
e-mail: info@ldaamerica.org
www.ldaamerica.org

To create opportunities for success for all individuals affected by learning disabilities and to reduce the incidence of learning disabilities in future generations.
Patricia Lillie, President
Andrea Turkheimer, Director Resource/Referral/Education

10546 Learning How
1583 Sulphur Spring Road
Baltimore, MD 21227
410-242-7100
Fax: 410-242-5246
e-mail: info@learninghow.com
www.learninghow.com

To provide educational materials for parents, teachers, and daycare providers that will encourage the learning process and help children reach their fullest potential.

10547 Life Development Institute
18001 N 79th Avenue
Glendale, AZ 85308
623-773-2774
Fax: 623-773-2788
e-mail: info@life-development-inst.org
www.lifedevelopmentinst.org

LDI's mission to inspire individuals to experience success while optimizing their potential for an enhanced quality of life in a challenging and supportive learning environment. LDI is a nonprofit private organization based in Glendale Arizona.
Rob Crawford, CEO
Veronica Crawford, Vice President

10548 Lions Quest
300 W 22nd Street
Oak Brook, IL 60523-8842
630-571-5466
Fax: 630-571-5735
e-mail: matthew.kiefer@lionsclub.org
www.lions-quest.org

To empower and support adults throughout the world to nuture caring and responsibility in young people.
Matthew Kiefer, Manager

10549 Lymphatic Research Foundation
40 Garvies Point Road
Glen Cove, NY 11542
516-625-9675
Fax: 516-625-9410
e-mail: lrf@lymphaticresearch.org
www.lymphaticresearch.org

A not-for-profit organization whose mission is to advance research of the lymphatic system and to find the cause of and cure for lymphatic diseases, lymphedema, and related disorders.
Jaqueline Reinhard, Executive Director
Wendy Chaite, Esq., Founder

10550 MedEscort International ABE International Airport
ABE International Airport
PO Box 8766
Allentown, PA 18105-8766
610-792-3111
800-255-7182
Fax: 610-791-9189
e-mail: medescort@fast.net
www.medescort.com

Offers specially trained escorts for individuals who cannot travel alone due to age or disability.
David M Stein DO, Medical Director
Sherry L Sefcik RN/BSN, Senior Flight Nurse

10551 MedicAlert Foundation International
2323 Colorado Avenue
Turlock, CA 95382-2018   800-432-5378
                                                    Fax: 800-863-3429
e-mail: customer_service@medicalert.org
www.medicalert.org
Organization offering persons with medical problems descriptive warning bracelets or neck chains to alert emergency personnel.
Andrew B Wigglesworth, President/CEO
Ramesh Srinivasan, SVP

10552 Mental Health Services Training Center
University of Maryland
3700 Koppers Street
Baltimore, MD 21227   410-646-7758
                                                    Fax: 410-646-7849
e-mail: ehansen@psych.umaryland.edu
trainingcenter.umaryland.edu
Formerly the Mental Health Services Training Collaborative, assists Mental Hygiene Administration in planning, organizing and implementing conference and training activities to support the continued growth and development of the public mental health system.
Eileen Hansen MSSW, Director
Wendy Baysmore MSHSA, Assistant Director

10553 National Association of Councils on Developmental Disabilities
1660 L Street NW   202-506-5813
Washington, DC 20036   Fax: 202-506-5846
e-mail: info@nacdd.org
www.nacdd.org
Serves as the national voice of State and Territorial Councils on Dvelopment Disabilities. Support Councils in implementing the Developmental Disabilities Assistance and Bill of Rights Act and promoting the interests and rights of people with developmental disabilities and their familes.
Michael Brogioli, CEO

10554 National Center for Family-Centered Care
695 Park Avenue   212-772-4000
New York, NY 10021   Fax: 212-452-7475
e-mail: gmallon@hunter.cuny.edu
www.hunter.cuny.edu/socwork/nrcfcpp//tra
Goals are to promote implementation of a family-centered care approach for children with special health care needs.
Karen Lawrence

10555 National Chronic Pain Outreach Association
PO Box 274   540-862-9437
Millboro, VA 24460   Fax: 540-862-9485
e-mail: ncpoa@cfw.com
www.chronicpain.org
Purpose is to lessen the suffering of people with chronic pain by educating pain sufferers, health care professionals, and the public about chronic pain and its management.

10556 National Clearinghouse of Rehabilitation Training Materials
Utah State University
6524 Old Main Hill
Logan, UT 84322-6524   866-821-5355
e-mail: jennifer.robinson@usu.edu
www.ncrtm.org
Offers reference materials on rehabilitation for professionals and the disabled.
Michael Millington, Ph.D, Director
Jennifer Robinson, Office Manager

10557 National Council on Disability
1331 F Street NW   202-272-2004
Washington, DC 20004   Fax: 202-272-2022
                                                    TTY: 202-272-2074
e-mail: ncd@ncd.gov
www.ncd.gov
The National Council on Disability is an independent federal agency that works with the President and Congress to increase the

inclusion independence and empowerment of Americans with disabilities. They are involved in policy making issues.
Jonathan Young, Ph.D., Chairman
Aaron Bishop, Executive Director

10558 National Council on Independent Living
1710 Rhode Island Avenue NW   202-207-0334
Washington, DC 20036   877-525-3400
                                                    Fax: 202-207-0341
                                                    TTY: 202-207-0340
e-mail: ncil@ncil.org
www.ncil.org
A membership organization that advanced independent living and the rights of people with disabilities through consumer-driven advocacy.
Kelly Buckland, Executive Director
Christine Boucher, Development Director

10559 National Digestive Diseases Information Clearinghouse
2 Information Way
Bethesda, MD 20892-3570   800-891-5389
                                                    Fax: 703-738-4929
                                                    TTY: 866-569-1162
e-mail: nddic@info.niddk.nih.gov
www.digestive.niddk.nih.gov
An information dissemination service of the National Institute of Diabetes and Digestive and Kidney Diseases that was established to increase knowledge and understanding about digestive diseases among people with these conditions and their families, health care professionals, and the general public.
Griffin P Rodgers MD MACP, Director

10560 National Dissemination Center for Children
1825 Connecticut Ave NW   202-884-8200
Washington, DC 20009   800-695-0285
                                                    Fax: 202-884-8441
                                                    TTY: 202-884-8200
e-mail: nichcy@aed.org
www.nichcy.org
Provides information to the nation on: disabilities in children and youth; programs and services for infants, children, and youth with disabilities; IDEA, the nation's special education law; No Child Left Behind, the nation's general education law; and research-based information on effective practices for children with disabilities.

10561 National Endowment for the Arts: Office for Accessability
1100 Pennsylvania Avenue NW   202-682-5400
Washington, DC 20506   TTY: 202-682-5496
e-mail: webmgr@arts.endow.gov
www.nea.gov
A public agency dedicated to supporting excellence in the arts, both new and established; bringing the arts to all Americans; and providing leadership in arts education.
Rocco Landesman, Chairman

10562 National Institute for People with Disabilities
460 W 34th Street
New York, NY 10001-2382   212-273-6100
www.yai.org
To create hope and opportunity for people with developmental and learning disabilities and their families.
Philip H Levy PhD, President/CEO

10563 National Institute of Child Health and Human Development
31 Center Drive   301-496-5133
Bethesda, MD 20892   800-370-2943
                                                    Fax: 301-496-7101
                                                    TTY: 888-320-6942
e-mail: guttmach@mail.nih.gov
www.nichd.nih.gov
NICHD conducts and supports research on topics related to the health of children, adults, families and populations. Some of these topics include: reducing infant deaths; improving the health of women, men and families; and understanding reproductive health and fertility/infertility; learning about growth and development; examining, preventing and treating problems of borth defects and intellectual and developmental disabilities.
Alan E Guttmacher, Director

10564 National Institute of Disability and Rehabilitation Research
US Department of Education
400 Maryland Avenue SW   202-245-7640
Washington, DC 20202   Fax: 202-245-7323
www2.ed.gov
provides leadership and support for a comprehensive program and research related to the rehabilitation of individuals with disabilities. All of the programmatic efforts are aimed at improving the lives of individuals with disabilities from birth through adulthood.

10565 National Job Accommodation Network
PO Box 6080   304-293-7186
Morgantown, WV 26506-6080   800-526-7234
Fax: 304-293-5407
TTY: 877-781-9403
e-mail: jan@askjan.org
askjan.org
The JAN is an international information service for people with disabilities and their employers. They have information about implementation of workplace accommodations as well as resources to promote an awareness of functional limitations.
Anne Hirsh, Co-Director
Louis Orslene, Co-Director

10566 National Legal Center for the Medically Dependent & Disabled
50 S Meridian Street   317-632-6245
Indianapolis, IN 46204-3537   Fax: 317-632-6542
Committed to defending the rights of vulnerable persons threatened by infanticide, euthanasia, assisted suicide, non-voluntary withdrawal/withholding of essential medical treatment and care and discrimination in health care financing.
Marilyn Bove, President

10567 National Network of Learning Disabled Adults
808 N 82nd Street   602-941-5112
Scottsdale, AZ 85257
Provides information and referral for LD adults involved with or in search of support groups and networking opportunities.

10568 National Organization for Rare Disorders
55 Kenosia Avenue   203-744-0100
Danbury, CT 06813-1968   800-999-6673
Fax: 203-798-2291
TDD: 203-797-9590
e-mail: orphan@rarediseases.org
www.rarediseases.org
The National Organization for Rare Disorders(NORD) a 501(c)3 organization is a unique federation of voluntary health organizations dedicated to helping people with rare orphan diseases and assisting the organizations that serve them.
Frank Sasinowski, Chair
Carolyn Asbury, PhD, Vice Chair

10569 National Organization on Disability
1625 K Street NW   202-293-5960
Washington, DC 20006   e-mail: ability@nod.org
www.nod.org
To expand the participation and contribution of America's 54 million men, women, and children with disabilities in all aspects of life.
Carol Glazer, President

10570 National Parent Network on Disabilities
1130 17th Street NW   202-434-8686
Washington, DC 20036   Fax: 202-638-7299
www.npnd.org
To provide a presence and national voice for all families of children, youth and adults with disabilities.
Linda Shepard, Executive Director
Jill Foss, Office Manager

10571 National Rehabilitation Information Center
8201 Corporate Drive   301-459-5900
Landover, MD 20785   800-346-2742
Fax: 301-459-4263
TTY: 301-459-5984
e-mail: naricinfo@heitechservices.com
www.naric.com
One of the three components of the office of Special Education and Rehabilitative Services. Mission is to generate, disseminate and promote new knowledge to improve the options available to disabled persons. The ultimate goal is to allow these individuals to perform their regular activities in the community and to bolster society's ability to provide full opportunities and appropriate supports for its disabled citizens.
Mark Odum, Director

10572 North American Society for Pediatric Gastroenterology, Hepatology & Nutrition
PO Box 6   215-233-0808
Flourtown, PA 19031   Fax: 215-233-3918
e-mail: naspghan@naspghan.org
www.naspghan.org
To advance understanding of normal development, physiology and pathophysiology of diseases of the gastrointestinal tract and liver in children, improve quality of care by fostering the dissemination of this knowledge through scientific meetings, professional and public education, and policy development, and serve as an effective voice for members and the profession.
Margaret K Stallings, Executive Director
Kate Ho, Associate Director

10573 Office of Civil Rights
US Department of Education
Lyndon B Johnson Dept of Ed Bldg
Washington, DC 20202-1100   800-421-3481
Fax: 202-453-6012
TTY: 877-521-2172
e-mail: ocr@ed.gov
www.ed.gov/about/offices/list/ocr
To ensure equal access to education and to promote educational excellence throughout the nation through vigorous enforcement of civil rights.
Russlynn Ali, Assistant Secretary

10574 Office of Policy Planning and Legislation
200 Independence Avenue SW   202-619-0257
Washington, DC 20201-0004   877-696-6775
www.hhs.gov/about/referlst.html
Administers grants to the states for social services under Title XX of the Social Security Act to welfare recipients and others likely to become welfare recipients.
G Barry Nielsen, Director

10575 Office of Special Education Programs
Department of Education
400 Maryland Avenue SW
Washington, DC 20202   202-245-7459
www2.ed.gov/about/offices/list/osers
Dedicated to improving results for infants, toddlers, children and youth with disabilities ages birth through 21 by providing leadership and financial support to assist states and local districts.
Melody Musgrove, Director
Bill Wolf, Acting Deputy Director

10576 Office on Smoking and Health
Centers for Disease Control and Prevention
4770 Buford Highway   404-639-3311
Atlanta, GA 30341-3717   800-232-4636
TTY: 888-232-6348
e-mail: tobaccoinfo@cdc.gov
www.cdc.gov/tobacco/osh/index.htm
The leading federal agency for comprehensive tobacco prevention and control, the Office develops, conducts, and supports strategic efforts to protect the public's health from the harmful effects of tobacco use.
Tim McAfee MD MPH, Director

10577 Option Institute International Learning & Training Center
2080 S Undermountain Road   413-229-2100
Sheffield, MA 01257   800-714-2779
Fax: 413-229-8931
e-mail: happiness@option.org
www.option.org
Offers self improvement and personal growth workshops and seminars that provide practical tools and strategies to help people worldwide to live happier, more confident, more empowered and

more fulfilling lives, and enjoy gratifying relationships and careers.
Barry Neil Kaufman, Co-Founder/Co-Director
Samahria Kaufman, Co-Founder/Co-Director

10578 Pediatric Neurology Georgetown University Hospital
Georgetown University Hospital
3800 Reservoir Road NW
Washington, DC 20007   202-444-8785
www.georgetownuniversityhospital.org
provides a wide range of consultative services, neurodiagnostic studies and therapies for children with neurodevelopmental disorders.
Cesar Santos MD, Chief

10579 People-to-People Committee for the Handicapped
PO Box 18131   301-774-7446
Washington, DC 20036-8131
Individuals concerned about the circumstances of handicapped people throughout the world. Disseminates information acts as a consultant in promoting exchange activities coordinates special assistance projects in developing countries and more.
David Brigham, Chairman

10580 President's Committee on the Employment of People with Disabilities
200 Constitution Avenue NW   202-693-6000
Washington, DC 20210   Fax: 202-693-7888
TTY: 877-889-5627
e-mail: webmaster@dol.gov
www.dol.gov
Independent federal agency to facilitate the communication coordination and promotion of public and private efforts to empower Americans with disabilities through employment.
John Davey, Deputy Assistant Secretary

10581 Rehabilitation International
25 E 21st Street   212-420-1500
New York, NY 10010   Fax: 212-505-0871
e-mail: ri@riglobal.org
www.riglobal.org
A global network with all important stakeholders, promoting the rights and inclusion of persons with disabilities and/or health problems, through means including advocacy, habilitation, rehabilitation to achieve an inclusive world where all people can enjoy active participation and full human rights.
Venus Ilagan, Secretary General
Megan Brinster, Development/Program Officer

10582 Rehabilitation Services Administration
US Department of Education
400 Maryland Avenue SW
Washington, DC 20202-2800   202-245-7488
www2.ed.gov/about/offices/list/osers/rsa
Oversees grant programs that help individuals with physical or mental disabilities to obtain employment and live more independently through the provision of such supports as counseling, medical and psychological services, job training and other individualized services.
Lynnae M Ruttledge, Commissioner

10583 Social Security Administration Office of Public Inquiries
Office of Public Inquiries
Windsor Park Building
Baltimore, MD 21235   800-772-1213
TTY: 800-325-0778
www.ssa.gov
Administers old age survivors and disability insurance programs under Title II of the Social Security Act. Also administers the federal income maintenance program under Title XVI of the Social Security Act. Maintains networks of local/regional offices.
Michael J Astrue, Commissioner
James A Winn, Chief of Staff

10584 US Department of Justice
950 Pennsylvania Avenue NW   202-514-2000
Washington, DC 20530-0001   e-mail: askdoj@usdoj.gov
www.usdoj.gov
To enforce the law and defend the interests of the United States according to the law; to ensure public safety against threats foreign

and domestic; to provide federal leadership in preventing and controlling crime; to seek just punishment for those guilty of unlawful behavior; and to ensure fair and impartial administration of justice for all Americans.
Eric Holder, Attorney General
James Cole, Deputy Attorney General

10585 US Department of Transportation
1200 New Jersey Avenue SE   202-366-4000
Washington, DC 20590   866-377-8642
TTY: 800-877-8339
e-mail: dot.comments@dot.gov
www.dot.gov
Serves the United States by ensuring a fast, safe, efficient, accessible and convenient transportation system that meets the vital national interests and enhances the quality of life of the American people, today and into the future.
Ray LaHood, Secretary of Transportation
Joan DeBoer, Chief of Staff

10586 US Office of Personnel Management
1900 E Street NW   202-606-1800
Washington, DC 20415   TTY: 202-606-2532
e-mail: General@opm.gov
www.opm.gov
Recruiting, retaining and honoring a world-class workforce to serve the American people.
John Berry, Director

10587 VSA Arts
818 Connecticut Avenue NW   202-628-2800
Washington, DC 20006   800-933-8721
Fax: 202-429-0868
TTY: 202-737-0645
e-mail: info@vsarts.org
www.vsarts.org
An international nonprofit organization founded by Ambassador Jean Kennedy Smith to create a society where people with disabilities learn through, participate in, and enjoy the arts.

10588 World Institute on Disability
510 16th Street   510-763-4100
Oakland, CA 94612-1520   Fax: 510-763-4109
TTY: 510-208-9493
e-mail: wid@wid.org
www.wid.org
A public policy center that is run by persons with disabilities. Conducts research, public education, training and advocacy campaigns.
Anita Shafer Aaron, Executive Director
Rebecca Palmer, Executive Assistant

State Agencies & Associations

Alabama

10589 Division of Rehabilitation: Montgomery
PO Box 11586   334-281-8780
Montgomery, AL 36111-0586
Marilyn Bove, President

Alaska

10590 Client Assistance Program: Anchorage
2900 Boniface Parkway   907-333-2211
Anchorage, AK 99504   800-478-0047
Fax: 907-333-1186
e-mail: akcap@alaska.com
home.gci.net/~alaskacap

Arizona

10591 HPV Support Groups: Arizona
7331 E Osborn Drive   602-994-8330
Scottsdale, AZ 85251-6422   800-223-2159
e-mail: sthf@home.com

Arkansas

10592 Disability Rights Center of Arkansas
1100 N University   501-296-1775
Little Rock, AR 72207   800-482-1174
                                         Fax: 501-296-1779
e-mail: panda@advocacyservices.org
www.advocacyservices.org
Protection and advocacy system for people with disabilities in Arkansas.
Traci Perrin, President

California

10593 Disability Rights California
100 Howe Avenue   916-488-9955
Sacramento, CA 95825   Fax: 916-488-9960
                                         TTY: 800-719-5798
e-mail: info@disabilityrightsca.org
www.disabilityrightsca.org
Mission is to advance the rights of Californians with disabilities.
Catherine Blakemore, Executive Director

Colorado

10594 Disability Careers
5760 E Evans Avenue   303-757-3070
Denver, CO 80222-5305   Fax: 303-757-3392
This is a non profit corporation that provides employee and employer services. Founder and Executive Director Ted Pavakis is a former commercial real estate broker with multiple sclerosis.

10595 Legal Center for People with Disabilities and Older People
455 Sherman Street   303-722-0300
Denver, CO 80203   800-288-1376
                                         Fax: 303-722-0720
                                         TTY: 303-722-3619
e-mail: tlcmail@thelegalcenter.org
www.thelegalcenter.org
An independent public interest non-profit specializing in civil rights and discrimination issues. We protect the human, civil and legal rights of people with mental and physical disabilities, people with HIV, and older people throughout Colorado.
Mary Anne Harvey, Executive Director

Connecticut

10596 Office of Protection and Advocacy for Persons with Disabilities
60B Weston Street   860-297-4300
Hartford, CT 06120-1551   800-842-7303
                                         TTY: 860-297-4380
                                         www.ct.gov
To advance the cause of equal rights for persons with disabilities and their families by: increasing the ability of individuals, groups and systems to safeguard rights; exposing instances and patterns of discrimination and abuse; seeking individual and systemic remediation when rights are violated; increasing public awareness of unjust situations and of means to address them; and empowering people with disabilities and their families to advocate effectively.

Delaware

10597 Client Assistance Program: Delaware
13 SW Front Street   302-422-6744
Milford, DE 19963-1900
Marilyn Bove, President

District of Columbia

10598 Client Assistance Program: District of Columbia
Rehabilitation Services Administration
605 G Street NW   202-727-0977
Washington, DC 20001-3705
Jim Tolbert, Director

10599 Information Protection & Advocacy Center for Handicapped Individuals
Center for Handicapped Individuals

4455 Connecticut Avenue NW   202-966-8081
Washington, DC 20008-2328
Marilyn Bove, President

Florida

10600 Disability Rights: Florida
2728 Centerview Drive   850-488-9071
Tallahassee, FL 32301   800-342-0823
                                         Fax: 850-488-8640
                                         TTY: 800-346-4127
e-mail: info@advocacycenter.org
www.advocacycenter.org
To advance the quality of life, dignity, equality, self-determination, and freedom of choice of persons with disabilities through collaboration, education, advocacy, as well, as legal and legislative issues.
Bob Whitney, Executive Director

10601 North Florida: HPV Support Group
126 Salem Court   850-877-3183
Tallahassee, FL 32301-2810

Georgia

10602 Division of Rehabilitation Service
148 Andrew Young Int'l Blvd NE   404-232-3910
Atlanta, GA 30303-1751   TTY: 404-232-3911
e-mail: rehab@dol.state.ga.us
www.vocrehabga.org
Operates five integrated and interdependent programs that share a primary goal — to help people with disabilities to become fully productive members of society by achieving independence and meaningful employment.

Hawaii

10603 Protection & Advocacy Agency
900 Fort Street Mall   808-949-2922
Honolulu, HI 96813-9607   800-882-1057
                                         Fax: 808-949-2928
                                         TTY: 808-949-2922
e-mail: info@hawaiidisabilityrights.org
www.hawaiidisabilityrights.org
Gary L Smith, Executive Director

Idaho

10604 Co-Ad
4477 Emerald   208-336-5353
900 Fort Street Mall, 90 900 F-2017   800-632-5125
                                         Fax: 208-336-5396
                                         TTY: 208-336-5353
e-mail: coadinc@cableone.net
users.moscow.com
Marilyn Bove, President

Illinois

10605 Illinois Client Assistance Program
Illinois Department of Human Services
100 N 1st Street
Springfield, IL 62702   800-641-3929
e-mail: dhs.cap@illinois.gov
www.dhs.state.il.us
Helps people with disabilities receive quality services by advocating for their interests and helping them identify resources, understand procedures, resolve problems, and protect their rights in the rehabilitation process, employment and home services.

Indiana

10606 Indiana Protection and Advocacy Services
4701 N Keystone Avenue
Indianapolis, IN 46205   800-622-4845
                                         TTY: 800-838-1131
e-mail: kpedevilla@ipas.in.gov
www.in.gov/ipas

To protect and promote the rights of individuals with disabilities, through empowerment and advocacy.
Karen Pedevilla, Education/Training Director

Iowa

10607 Client Assistance Program: Iowa Division o n Persons with Disabilities
Division on Persons with Disabilities
Lucas State Office Building   515-281-3656
Des Moines, IA 50310   800-652-4298
                                    Fax: 515-242-6119
                                    TTY: 800-652-4298
                                    e-mail: jackie.wipperman@iowa.gov
                                    www.icdri.org

Marilyn Bove, President

Kansas

10608 Disability Rights Center of Kansas
635 SW Harrison   785-273-9661
Topeka, KS 66603-3726   877-776-1541
                                    Fax: 785-273-9414
                                    TTY: 877-335-3725
                                    e-mail: rocky@drckansas.org
                                    www.icdri.org
A public interest legal advocacy agency empowered by federal law to advocate for the civil and legal rights of Kansans with disabilities.
Rocky Nichols MPA, Executive Director

Kentucky

10609 Client Assistance Program: Kentucky
275 E Main Street
Frankfort, KY 40621   800-633-6283
                                    e-mail: vanessa.denham@ky.gov
                                    http://ovr.ky.gov

Gerry Gordon Brown, Director

Louisiana

10610 Advocacy Center
1010 Common Street   504-522-2337
New Orleans, LA 70112   800-960-7705
                                    Fax: 504-522-5507
                                    TTY: 866-935-7348
                                    e-mail: advocacycenter@advocacyla.org
                                    www.advocacyla.org
Serves people with disabilities and senior citizens.
Lois Simpson, Executive Director

Maine

10611 Disability Rights Center: Maine
PO Box 2007   207-626-2774
Augusta, ME 04338-2007   800-452-1948
                                    Fax: 207-621-1419
                                    e-mail: advocate@drcme.org
                                    www.drcme.org
To enhance and promote the equality, self-determination, independence, productivity, integration, and inclusion of people with disabilities through education, strategic advocacy and legal intervention.
Kim Moody, Executive Director

Maryland

10612 Client Assistance Program: Maryland
Maryland State Department of Education
2301 Argonne Drive   410-554-9361
Baltimore, MD 21218   800-638-6243
                                    Fax: 410-554-9362
                                    TTY: 410-554-9360
                                    e-mail: cap@dors.state.md.us
                                    www.dors.state.md.us

Helps individuals who have concerns or difficulties when applying for or receiving rehabilitation services funded under the Rehabilitation Act.
Beth Lash, Director

Massachusetts

10613 Client Assistance Program: Massachusetts
250 Washington Street   617-727-7440
Boston, MA 02108-1518   800-322-2020
                                    e-mail: james.aprea@state.ma.us
                                    www.mass.gov
Provides advocacy and information services. CAP also works to ensure that consumers are placed in integrated settings and receive competitive wages. It helps people get services from the Massachusetts Rehabilitation Commission, the Massachusetts Commission for the Blind and the Independent Living Centers in Massachusetts, all of which receive Federal money under the Federal Vocational Rehabilitation Act.
Barbara E Lybarger Esq, Director

10614 Merrimack Valley HPV Support Group Holy Family Hospital
Holy Family Hospital
70 E Street   978-687-0156
Methuen, MA 01844-4597

10615 Neurosurgical Service
Massachusetts General Hospital
55 Fruit Street
Boston, MA 02114   617-726-2937
                                    neurosurgery.mgh.harvard.edu
Uses a multidisciplinary approach to provide a complete range of services for the diagnosis, treatment and rehabilitation of patients with neurological disorders.

Michigan

10616 Client Assistance Program: Michigan
Michigan Protection and Advocacy Service
4095 Legacy Parkway   517-487-1755
Lansing, MI 48911-7508   800-292-5896
                                    Fax: 517-487-0827
                                    e-mail: molson@mpas.org
                                    www.mpas.org
Assists people who are seeking or receiving services from Michigan Rehabilitation Services, Consumer Choice Programs, Michigan Commission for the Blind, Centers for Independent Living, and Supported Employment and Transition Programs.
Mark R Lezotte, President

10617 Commission for the Blind
201 N Washington 2nd Floor   517-373-2062
Lansing, MI 48909   800-292-4200
                                    Fax: 517-335-5140
                                    TDD: 517-373-4025
                                    e-mail: heibeckc@michigan.gov
                                    www.michigan.gov
To provide opportunity to individuals who are blind or visually impaired to achieve employability and/or function independently in society.
Patrick Cannon, Director

Minnesota

10618 Minnesota Disability Law Center
430 1st Avenue N   612-332-1441
Minneapolis, MN 55401-1780   Fax: 612-334-5755
                                    www.mndlc.org
Addresses the unique legal needs of Minnesotans with disabilities. Provides free civil legal assistance to individuals with disabilities statewide on legal issues related to their disabilities.
Jerry Lane, Executive Director

Mississippi

10619 Mississippi Client Assistance Program
Mississippi Society for Disabilities

PO Box 4958
Jackson, MS 39296

601-362-2585
800-962-2400
Fax: 601-982-1951
www.icdri.org

A federal grant to the State of Mississippi to provide advocacy services for clients and client applicants of the Office of Vocational Rehabilitation, Vocational Rehabilitation for the Blind, and the Independent Living programs.
Johnny McGinn, Director

Missouri

10620 Missouri Protection and Advocacy Services
925 S Country Club Drive
Jefferson City, MO 65109

573-893-3333
866-777-7199
Fax: 573-893-4231
TDD: 800-735-2966
e-mail: mopasjc@embarqmail.com
www.moadvocacy.org

To protect the rights of individuals with disabilities by providing advocacy and legal services.
Cathy Enfield, Chair

Montana

10621 Disability Rights Montana
1022 Chestnut Street
Helena, MT 59601

406-449-2344
800-245-4743
Fax: 406-449-2418
TDD: 406-449-2344
e-mail: advocate@disabilityrightsmt.org
www.disabilityrightsmt.org

Protects and advocates for the human, legal, and civil rights of Montanans with disabilities while advancing dignity, equality, and self-determination.
Bernadette Franks-Ongoy, Executive Director

Nebraska

10622 Client Assistance Program: Nebraska Division of Rehabilitative Services
Division of Rehabilitative Services
301 Centennial Mall S
Lincoln, NE 68509

402-471-3656
800-742-7594
e-mail: victoria.rasmussen@cap.ne.gov
www.cap.state.ne.us

The Nebraska Client Assistance Program is a free service to help you find solutions if you are having problems with any of the following programs: Vocational Rehabilitation, Nebraska Commission for the Blind and Visually Impaired or Centers for Independent Living.

10623 Omaha HPV Support Group: PP of Omaha
Planned Parenhood
4610 Dodge Street
Omaha, NE 68132-3234

402-397-2739
www.aad.org

Nevada

10624 Client Assistance Program: Nevada
2800 E Saint Louis Avenue
Las Vegas, NV 89104

775-684-3849
800-633-9879
Fax: 775-684-3850
e-mail: detradmn@nvdetr.org
http://detr.state.nv.us

Designed to assist individuals with disabilities resolve problems they may experience with any of Nevada's rehabilitation programs.
Maureen Cole, Rehabilitation Administrator

New Hampshire

10625 Client Assistance Program: New Hampshire
Governor's Commission for the Handicapped

57 Regional Drive
Concord, NH 03301-8518

603-271-2773
800-852-3405
Fax: 603-271-2837
e-mail: disability@nh.gov
www.nh.gov/disability/about/cap.htm

CAP provides information about vocational rehabilitation services; advises you of your rights and responsibilities; investigate your complaint; helps resolve problems with your vocational plan; and represents you at administratove reviews and fair hearings.
John Richards, Executive Director

New Jersey

10626 Disability Rights New Jersey
210 S Broad Street
Trenton, NJ 08608

609-292-9742
Fax: 609-777-0187
TTY: 609-633-7106
e-mail: adocate@drnj.org
www.drnj.org

To protect, advocate for and advance the rights of persons with disabilities in pursuit of a society in hich persons with disabilities exercise self-determination and choice, and are treated with dignity.
Joseph B Young, Executive Director

New Mexico

10627 Protection and Advocacy System of Alburque rque
1720 Louisiana Boulevard NE
Albuquerque, NM 87110-7070

505-256-3100
Fax: 505-256-3184
www.protectionandadvocacy.com

Marilyn Bove, President

New York

10628 Client Assistance Program: NY State Commission of Quality of Care
Advocacy Bureau
99 Washington Avenue
Albany, NY 12210-2810

518-473-4057
800-624-4143
Fax: 518-473-6296
e-mail: hn5344@handsnet.org

Marilyn Bove, President

10629 March of Dimes Foundation
1275 Mamaroneck Avenue
White Plains, NY 10605

914-997-4488
www.marchofdimes.com

Volunteers and professionals providing leadership in the treatment and prevention of birth defects and prematurity.
Jennifer L Howse, President/CEO

North Carolina

10630 North Carolina Client Assistance Program
2806 Mail Service Center
Raleigh, NC 27699-2806

919-855-3600
800-215-7227
Fax: 919-715-2456
e-mail: nccap@dhhs.nc.gov
cap.state.nc.us

Helping people understand and access rehabilitation services.
Kathy Brack, Director

North Dakota

10631 Client Assistance Program: North Dakota
1237 W Divide Avenue
Bismarck, ND 58501-1208

701-328-8947
800-207-6122
TDD: 707-328-8968
e-mail: cap@nd.gov
www.nd.gov/cap

Assists clients and client applicants of North Dakota Vocational Rehabilitation services, Tribal Vocational Rehabilitation, or Independent Living services.

Ohio

10632 Cincinnati HPV Support Group: PP of Cincin nati
Planned Parenthood

PO Box 12407
Cincinnati, OH 45212-0407
513-357-7300
www.dermconsultants.com

10633 Disability Rights Center at Ohio Legal Rights Service
50 W Broad Street
Columbus, OH 43215-5923
614-466-7264
800-282-9181
TTY: 614-728-2553
www.olrs.ohio.gov
To protect and advocate, in partnership with people with disabilities, for their human, civil and legal rights.
Kalpana Yalamanchili, Chair

10634 Richland County HPV Support Group
PO Box 3881
Mansfield, OH 44907-3881
419-525-3075
www.skinpatient.com

10635 Technology Resource Center
2140 Arbor Boulevard
Dayton, OH 45439
937-294-8086

Oklahoma

10636 Client Assistance Program: Oklahoma Office of Handicapped Concerns
Oklahoma Ofice of Handicapped Concerns
2401 NW 23rd
Oklahoma City, OK 73107-5106
405-521-3756
Fax: 405-522-6695
e-mail: Marilyn.Burr@ohc.state.ok.us
www.icdri.org

Marilyn Bove, President

10637 Oklahoma City HPV Support Group: PP of Cen tral Oklahoma
Planned Parenthood of Central Oklahoma
Oklahoma City, OK 73103-1415
405-528-0221
www.aad.org

Oregon

10638 Resources for Seniors and People with Disabilities
Department of Human Services
500 Summer Street NE
Salem, OR 97301-1097
503-947-5110
Fax: 503-378-2897
TTY: 503-947-5080
e-mail: dhs.directorsoffice@state.or.us
www.oregon.gov
To secure economic, social, legal and political justice for individuals with disabilities through systems change
Dr Bruce Goldberg, Director
Margaret Carter, Deputy Director Human Services Program

Pennsylvania

10639 Client Assistance Program: Medical Center East
Medical Center East
4200 Forbes Boulevard
Lanham, MD 20706
301-459-2742
Fax: 215-557-7602
TTY: 301-459-5984
The Advocacy Center for Persons with Disabilities is a non-profit organization providing protection and advocacy services. Its mission is to advance the dignity, equality, self-determination and expressed choices of individuals with disabilities.
Marilyn Bove, President

10640 Client Assistance Program: Philadelphia
1515 Market Street
Philadelphia, PA 19102
215-557-7112
888-745-2357
Fax: 215-557-7602
TDD: 215-557-7112
e-mail: info@equalemployment.org
www.equalemployment.org
Ensuring that vocation rehabilitation is open and responsive to your needs. Provides information and advice about rehabilitation programs; to advise you of your legal rights and responsibilities; to help resolve probelms that may arise while you are seeking services from rehabilitation programs; to help you pursue administrative and legal remedies to protect your rights.
Stephen S Pennington, Executive Director
Jamie C Ray- Leonetti, Assistant Director

Rhode Island

10641 Rhode Island Disability Law Center
275 Westminster Street
Providence, RI 02903-3434
401-831-3150
Fax: 401-274-5568
TTY: 401-831-5335
e-mail: info@ridlc.org
www.ridlc.org
Provides free legal assistance to persons with disabilities. Services include individual representation to protect rights or to secure benefits and services; self-help information; educational programs; and administrative and legislative advocacy.

South Carolina

10642 South Carolina Protection & Advocacy System for the Handicapped
3710 Landmark Drive
Columbia, SC 29204-4034
803-782-0639
800-922-5225
Marilyn Bove, President

10643 Tri County HPV Support Group
PO Box 1997
Mt Pleasant, SC 29465-1997
843-884-7333
www.aad.org

South Dakota

10644 South Dakota Advocacy Services
221 S Central Avenue
Pierre, SD 57501
605-224-8294
800-658-4782
Fax: 605-224-5125
TTY: 800-658-4782
e-mail: sdas@sdadvocacy.com
www.sdadvocacy.com
To protect and advocate the rights of South Dakotans with disabilities through legal, administrative, and other remedies.

Tennessee

10645 Disability Law & Advocacy Center of Tennessee
2416 21st Avenue S
Nashville, TN 37212
615-298-1080
Fax: 615-298-2046
e-mail: gethelp@dlactn.org
www.dlactn.org
Advocates for the rights of Tennesseans with disabilities to ensure they have an equal opportunity to be productive and respected members of the society.
Jerry Gonzalez, Chair

Texas

10646 Dallas/Ft.Worth Metroplex HPV Support Group
8215 Westchester Drive
Dallas, TX 75225-6116
214-363-6733

10647 Disability Rights Texas
Advocacy Inc
7800 Shoal Creek Boulevard
Austin, TX 78757-1024
512-454-4816
Fax: 512-323-0902
www.advocacyinc.org
Protecting and advocating the rights of Texans with disabilities - because all people have dignity and worth.
Mary Faithfull, Executive Director

Utah

10648 Legal Center for People with Disabilities
455 E 400 S
Salt Lake City, UT 84111-3076
801-363-1347
800-662-9080
Marilyn Bove, President

Vermont

10649 Citizen Advocacy of Burlington
Chase Mill 1 Mill Street   802-655-0329
Burlington, VT 05401
Marilyn Bove, President

10650 Client Assistance Program: Vermont Ladd Hall
Ladd Hall
57 N Main Street   802-775-0021
Rutland, VT 05701-8409   800-769-7459
          Fax: 802-775-0022
          e-mail: nbreiden@vtlegalaid.org
          www.icdri.org

Marilyn Bove, President

Virginia

10651 Richmond HPV Support Group: Fan Free Clini c
Fan Free Clinic
PO Box 5669
Richmond, VA 23220-0669
          804-358-6343
          www.ashastd.org

10652 Virginia Office for Protection and Advocacy
1910 Byrd Avenue   804-225-2042
Richmond, VA 23230   800-552-3962
          Fax: 804-662-7057
          e-mail: general.vopa@vopa.virginia.gov
          www.vopa.state.va.us
Helps with disability-related problems like abuse, neglect, and discrimination. Also help people with disabilities obtain services and treatment.
Coleen Miller, Executive Director

Washington

10653 Seattle HPV Support Group
PO Box 31171
Seattle, WA 98103-1171   425-619-7190
          www.aad.org

10654 Washington State Client Assistance Program
2531 Rainer Avenue S   206-721-5999
Seattle, WA 98144-9510   800-544-2121
          Fax: 206-721-5980
          TTY: 206-721-6072
          e-mail: caprogram@qwestoffice.net
          http://washingtoncap.org

Marilyn Bove, President

West Virginia

10655 Northcentral West Virginia HPV Support Group
Monongalia County Health Department
453 Van Voorhis Road
Morgantown, WV 26505-3408   304-598-5100

10656 West Virginia Advocates
1207 Quarrier Street   304-346-0847
Charleston, WV 25301   800-950-5250
          Fax: 304-346-0867
          e-mail: contact@wvadvocates.org
          www.wvadvocates.org
Protects and advocates for the human and legal rights of persons with disabilities.
Clarice Hausch, Executive Director
Barbara Criner, Administrative Director

Wisconsin

10657 Governor's Committee for People with Disabilities
Wisconsin Department of Health Services
1 W Wilson Street   608-261-7816
Madison, WI 53703   Fax: 608-266-3386
          e-mail: sarah.lincoln@wisconsin.gov
          www.dhs.wisconsin.gov

Sarah Lincoln, Director

Wyoming

10658 Wyoming Protection & Advocacy System
7344 Stockman Street   307-632-3496
Cheyenne, WY 82009   Fax: 307-638-0815
          e-mail: wypanda@wypanda.com
          www.wypanda.com
To establish, expand, protect and enforce the human and civil rights of persons with disabilities through administrative, legal, and other appropriate remedies.
Mary Carson Barks, President
Jeanne A Thobro, CEO

Libraries & Resource Centers

Alabama

10659 Horizons Schools
2018 15th Avenue South   205-322-6606
Birmingham, AL 35205   800-822-6242
          Fax: 205-322-6605
          www.horizonsschool.org
Offers our young adults a college-like experience as they live away from home, develop a group of lifelong friends, prepare for careers and establish and practice setting, planning and evaluating personal goals. We offer individuals and their families an inclusive, holistic life preparatory program as we try to consider all aspects of a student and families learning and living needs.
Jade K Carter EdD, Director
Marie McElheny MAE, Assistant Director

Arizona

10660 Life Development Institute
18001 N 79th Avenue   623-773-2774
Glendale, AZ 85308   Fax: 623-773-2788
          e-mail: info@life-development-inst.org
          www.lifedevelopmentinst.org
LDI'S mission is to inspire individuals to experience success while optimizing their potential for an enhanced quality of life in a challenging and supportive learning environment. LDI is a non-profit, private organization based in Glendale, Arizona, and provides a supportive residential community that gives individuals the education, skills and training they need to live independently.
Rob Crawford, CEO
Veronica Crawford, Vice President

California

10661 Center for Adaptive Learning
3227 Clayton Road   925-827-3863
Concord, CA 94519   Fax: 925-827-4080
          e-mail: info@centerforadaptivelearning.org
          www.centerforadaptivelearning.org
Committed to creating and maintaining a living and working environment for neurologically impaired individuals, which will promote dignity and support a sense of community. The CAL program provides each participant with an individual program for growth. CAL is committed to maintaining the highest quality of living possible, which will allow each client to develop a sense of pride, to augment self-esteem and to foster a sense of self-worth.
Genevieve Stolarz, Executive Director
Don Bone, President

10662 Independence Center
3640 S Sepulveda Boulevard   310-202-7102
Los Angeles, CA 90034   Fax: 310-202-7180
          e-mail: judym@independencecenter.com
          www.independencecenter.com
A mainstreamed transitional residential program for young adults (18-30) with learning disabilities. Program highlights include training in independent living, social and vocational skills, counseling and more.
Judith Maizlish, Executive Director
Gloria Ogletree, Administrative Director

Connecticut

10663 Chapel Haven
1040 Whalley Avenue
New Haven, CT 06515
203-397-1714
Fax: 203-392-3698
e-mail: admissions@chapelhaven.org
www.chapelhaven.org
Providing an array of lifelong individualized support services for adults (18+) on the autism spectrum and those with developmental and social disabilities, enabling them to lead independent and productive lives.
Betsey Parlato, CEO/Executive Director

Georgia

10664 Creative Community Services (CCS)
4487 Park Drive
Norcross, GA 30093
770-469-6226
866-618-2823
Fax: 770-469-6210
e-mail: info@ccsgeorgia.org
www.ccsgeorgia.org
Provides therapeutic foster care services for children and home-based support for adults with developmental disabilities. CCS improves the quality of life for children, adults and families through its community-based support and services. CCS gives both kids and adults hope by encouraging independent living resulting in involved, engaged citizens and community members.
Sally Buchanan, Executive Director

Massachusetts

10665 Berkshire Center
18 Park Street
Lee, MA 01238
413-243-2576
Fax: 413-243-3351
www.berkshirecenter.org
The College Internship Program at the Berkshire Center provides individualized, post-secondary academic, internship and independent living experiences for young adults with Asperger's Syndrome and other Learning Differences.
Lucy Gosselin MSBM, Program Director

Minnesota

10666 National Resource Library on Youth with Disabilities
University of Minnesota
Box 721-UMHC
Minneapolis, MN 55455
612-626-3087
800-276-8642
Fax: 612-626-2134
TTY: 612-624-3939
e-mail: kdwb-var@umn.edu
www.peds.umn.edu
Offers comprehensive sources of information related to adolescents, disability and transition. The database contains bibliographic, programs, training/education and technical assistance files for the medical community, families, parents and children with chronic illnesses.
Peggy Mann Reinhart, Director
Elizabeth Latts, Resource Coordinator

New Hampshire

10667 Camp Allen
56 Camp Road
Bedford, NH 03110-6606
603-622-8471
Fax: 603-626-4295
e-mail: mary@campallennh.orgg
www.campallennh.org
Camp Allen welcomes about 600 campers each summer. They are persons of all ages with special needs and extraordinary challenges, including cerebral palsy, autism, muscular dystrophy, Down syndrome, and other developmental disabilities.
Mary Constance, Executive Director

New Jersey

10668 HealthyWomen
157 Broad Street
Red Bank, NJ 07701
877-986-9472
Fax: 732-530-3347
e-mail: info@healthywomen.org
www.healthywomen.org
Independent health information source for women whose mission is to educate, inform and empower women to make smart health choices for themselves and their families.
Elizabeth Battaglino Cahill, RN, Executive Director
Marisa Bushee, Director of Marketing & Communications

New York

10669 Center for Medical Consumers
239 Thompson Street
New York, NY 10012
212-674-7105
Fax: 212-674-7100
e-mail: centersformedicalconsumers@gmail.com
www.medicalconsumers.org
A non-profit advocacy organization that was founded with the philosophy of: Whenever long-term drug therapy, elective surgery, or any other major treatment is prescribed, the question of whether the treatment has been proven safe and effective should come up. And the prescribing physician should be expected to cite the relevant studies.
Arthur Aaron Levin MPH, Director
Maryann Napoli, Associate Director

Virginia

10670 ERIC Clearinghouse on Disabilities and Gifted Education
ERIC Project
C/O Computer Sciences Corporation
Washington, DC 20008
800-538-3742
Fax: 703-620-4334
TTY: 703-264-9449
www.eric.ed.gov
The ERIC mission is to provide a comprehensive, easy-to-use, searchable, Internet-based bibliographic and full-text database of education research and information. The simple version of that is that it provides an enormous amount of print materials online, for easy access to important research and journal materials.
Cheryl Racey, Director

Support Groups & Hotlines

10671 Behavioral Pediatrics Program
KDWP Variety Family Center
200 Oak Street SE
Minneapolis, MN 55455-2002
612-626-4260
800-276-8642
Fax: 612-624-0997
TTY: 612-624-3939
www.peds.umn.edu/pedsadol
Behavioral Pediatrics Staff help children, teen and their families with a wide variety of behavioral concerns including adjustment to coping with chronic illness. Treatments vary depending on the age, developmental state and needs of each child and family. Often, children are taught to self-regulate their behavior.
Daniel Kohen MD, Director

10672 Childrens Hospice International
1101 King Street
Alexandria, VA 22314
703-684-0330
800-242-4453
Fax: 703-684-0226
e-mail: info@chionline.org
www.chionline.org
To ensure medical, psychological, social and spiritual support to all children with like-threatening conditions and their families by providing a network of resources and care.
Ann Armstrong Dailey, Founding Director/CEO

10673 Fetal Alcohol Network
KDWP Variety Family Center

200 Oak Street SE
Minneapolis, MN 55455-2002

612-626-4260
800-276-8642
Fax: 612-624-0997
TTY: 612-624-3939
e-mail: kdwb-var@umn.edu
www.peds.umn.edu/peds-adol

Staff provide assessment, intervention and consultation regarding the physical, developmental learning, behavioral and emotional well-being of children and individuals affected by prenatal exposure to alcohol and drugs.
Daniel Kohen MD, Director

10674 Foundation for Hospice and Homecare
3801 Vanesta Drive
Manhattan, KS 66503

785-537-0688
800-748-7474
Fax: 785-537-1309
e-mail: business@homecareandhospice.org
www.homecarehospice.org

A charitable organization to support the mission of Homecare & Hospice, Inc.
Lowell Kohlmeier, Chair

10675 Friends Health Connection
PO Box 114
New Brunswick, NJ 08903

732-418-1811
800-483-7436
Fax: 732-249-9897
e-mail: info@friendshealthconnection.org
www.friendshealthconnection.org

Enhances mind, body and soul through our personalized support network and dynamic educational and motivational programs. Works with hospitals and other nonprofit organizations to complement their program offerings and connect people with resources and support that can enrich their lives.

10676 Genetic Alliance
4301 Connecticut Avenue NW
Washington, DC 20008

202-966-5557
Fax: 202-966-8553
e-mail: info@geneticalliance.org
www.geneticalliance.org

Improves health through the authentic engagement of communities and individuals. The goal is to build capacity within the genetics community. Transform health through genetics and promote an environment of openness centered on the health of individuals, families, and communities.
Sharon F Terry, President/CEO

10677 KDWB Family Resource Center
200 Oak Street SE
Minneapolis, MN 55455-2002

612-626-3087
800-276-8642
Fax: 612-624-0997
TTY: 612-624-3939
e-mail: kdwb-var@umn.edu
www.peds.umn.edu/peds-adol

A place families can visit to learn about their child's chronic illness or disability, identify psychological and developmental issues, and link-up with program and community resources. Information will be available by telephone and via the web site.
Elizabeth Latts, Resource Coordinator

10678 KDWB Variety Family Canter
200 Oak Street SE
Minneapolis, MN 55455-2002

612-626-3087
800-276-8642
Fax: 612-624-0997
TTY: 612-624-3939
e-mail: kdwbvar@umn.edu
www.peds.umn.edu/pedsadol/

University-Community pertnership that provides family-centered services that promote physical, emotional, psychological and social health and well being for children and youth at risk, including children and youth with disabilities. The Center is dedicated to teaching, research, outreach, and community services.
Peggy Mann Reinhart, Director
Elizabeth Latts, Resource Coordinator

10679 National Association for Home Care
228 Seventh Street SE
Washington, DC 20003

202-547-7424
Fax: 202-547-3540
e-mail: exec@nahc.org
www.nahc.org

Trade association representing the interests and concerns of home care agencies, hospices, and home care aide organizations.
Val J Halamandaris, President

10680 National Family Caregivers Association
10400 Connecticut Avenue
Kensington, MD 20895-3944

301-942-6430
800-896-3650
Fax: 301-942-2302
e-mail: info@thefamilycaregiver.org
www.thefamilycaregiver.org

Educates, supports, empowers and speaks up for the more than 65 million Americans who care for loved ones with a chronic illness or disability or the frailties of old age. Reaches across the boundaries of diagnosis, relationships and life stages to help transform family caregivers' lives by removing barriers to health and well being
Suzanne Mintz, President/CEO

10681 National Health Information Center
PO Box 1133
Washington, DC 20013

310-565-4167
800-336-4797
Fax: 301-984-4256
e-mail: info@nhic.org
www.health.gov/nhic

Offers a nationwide information referral service, produces directories and resource guides.

10682 National Parent to Parent Support and Information System
3805 Presidential Parkway
Atlanta, GA 30340

770-451-5484
Fax: 770-458-4091
e-mail: info@p2pga.org
www.p2pusa.org

NPPSIS is a nonprofit organization established to support, strengthen, and empower families through one-on-one parent contacts. They link families nationally whose children have special health care needs and rare disorders. They provide parents with heath care information, resources and referrals to allow them to identify appropriate services.
Nancy DiVenere, President
Debra S. Tucker, Executive Director

10683 Okizu Foundation Camps
16 Digital Drive
Novato, CA 94949-6115

415-382-9083
Fax: 415-382-8384
e-mail: info@okizu.org
www.okizu.org

This foundation runs family camp programs for children who have cancer and their families, and for children who have or had a parent with cancer.
Suzie Randall, Executive Director
Heather Ferrier, Asst. Executive Director

10684 Parent to Parent of New York State
500 Balltown Road
Schenectady, NY 12304-2247

518-381-4350
800-305-8817
Fax: 518-393-9607
e-mail: staciap2p@verizon.net
www.parenttoparentnys.org

Parent to Parent programs provide informational and emotional support to parents who have a child, adolescent or adult family member with special needs. Offers an important connection for a parent who is seeking support for special disability issues, by matching him or her with a trained veteran parent who has already been there. Because the two parents share so many common concerns and interests, the support given and received is often uniquely meaningful. Also helps families locate information
Stacia Kooney, Regional Coordinator
Jim Swart, Regional Coordinator

10685 Pediatric Psychology
KDWP Variety Family Center
200 Oak Street SE
Minneapolis, MN 55455-2002

612-626-4260
800-276-8642
Fax: 612-624-0997
TTY: 612-624-3939
e-mail: kdwbvar@umn.edu
www.peds.umn.edu/pedsadol

Staff provide assessment, intervention and consultation regarding the physical, developmental, learning, behavioral and emotional

well-being of children and individuals affected by prenatal exposure to alcohol and drugs.
Daniel Kohen MD, Director

10686 STAR Center for Family Health
KDWB University Pediatrics Family Center
200 Oak St, SE, Suite 160   612-626-4260
Minneapolis, MN 55455-2002   Fax: 612-624-0997
                                                          TTY: 6126243939
                                          e-mail: kdwb-var@umn.edu
                                          www.peds.umn.edu/peds-adol/
Helps children, youth and families develop new and enhanced ways of coping with stress, learn strategies for adjusting to living with a chronic illness, and discover new ways of finding health, balance and well-being.
Lavon Anderson, M.A., Administrator
Linda Boche, Executive Secretary to Division Director

10687 U Special Kids
KDWB Variety Family Center
200 Oak Street SE   612-626-3081
Minneapolis, MN 55455-2002   800-276-8642
                                                          Fax: 612-624-0997
                                                          TTY: 6126243939
                                          e-mail: uspclkid@umn.edu
                                          www.peds.umn.edu/peds-adol/
A program that provides care coordinators for children with complex medical conditions. A team of health care providers advocates for children and their families within the health care system.
Anne Kelly MD, Director

10688 Visiting Nurse Association of America
900 19th Street, NW   202-384-1420
Washington, DC 20006   Fax: 202-384-1444
                                          e-mail: vnaa@vnaa.org
                                          www.vnaa.org
This agency represents independent VNA units across the United States. Each VNA unit may vary in their services, but most provide skilled nursing, physical therapy, occupational therapy, speech therapy, and home health aid services.
Andy Carter, President/CEO

10689 Well Spouse Association
63 W Main Street
Freehold, NJ 07728   800-838-0879
                                          e-mail: info@wellspouse.org
                                          www.wellspouse.org
This association is a nonprofit national self-help organization serving the well spouse of the chronically ill. Members help each other develop coping and survival skills through local support groups (including bereavement), letter and telephone networks, and personal outreach and a quarterly newsletter.
Lawrence Bocchiere, President
Gerald Bishop, Board Chair

Books

10690 A History of Childhood and Disability
Philip Safford and Elizabeth Safford, author

Teachers College Press
1234 Amsterdam Avenue   212-678-3929
New York, NY 10027   Fax: 212-678-4149
                                          e-mail: tcpress@tc.columbia.edu
                                          www.teacherscollegepress.com
This book presents an interdisciplinary perspective on children considered exceptional and how services have evolved in reponse to their diverse neeeds.
1996 352 pages
ISBN: 0-807734-85-3

10691 Art of Getting Well
David Spero, RN, author

Hunter House Publishing
1515 1/2 Park Street   510-865-5282
Alameda, CA 94501   800-266-5592
                                                          Fax: 510-865-4295
                                          e-mail: ordering@hunterhouse.com
                                          www.hunterhouse.com

A five step plan for maximazing health when you have a chronic illness.
224 pages Paperback

10692 Assisstive Technology for Young Children: A Guide to Family-Centered Services
Sharon Lesar Judge and Howard P Parette, author

Brookline Books
PO Box 1209   617-734-6772
Brookline, MA 02445   800-666-2665
                                                          Fax: 617-734-3952
                                          www.brooklinebooks.com
Explores the wide range of considerations involved in evaluating children's needs, selecting and prescribing devices, and training children, families, and teachers to use the technology.
1998 Softcover
ISBN: 1-571290-51-6

10693 Awaking to Disability
Volcano Press
PO Box 270   209-296-3445
Volcano, CA 95689-0270   800-879-9636
                                                          Fax: 209-296-4995
                                          e-mail: sales@volcanopress.com
                                          www.volcanopress.com
From the disability activist whose columns have been avidly followed by readers of the Albuquerque Journal and Miami Herald comes this revealing compedium of her thoughts. It offers a perspective for parents of children with disabilites, or for newly disabled people.
1997 288 pages
ISBN: 1-884244-14-9

10694 Blood Pressure Book: How to Get it Down & Keep it Down
Bull Publishing
PO Box 1377   303-545-6350
Boulder, CO 80306   800-676-2855
                                                          Fax: 303-545-6354
                                          www.bullpub.com
Provides basic information on the causes and treatment of high blood pressure includes check up charts and illustrations that will help readers find out where they stand and lead them to practical advice tailored to their own needs.
1996
ISBN: 0-923521-97-6

10695 Building Partnerships in Hospital Care
Bull Publishing
PO Box 1377
Boulder, CO 80306   800-676-2855
                                                          Fax: 303-545-6354
                                          www.bullpub.com
Aims to desensetize patients and families to their fears of illness, hospital machinery and authority figures at the same time resensitize institution weary professionals to the feelings, instincts and emotions that brought them into the field in the first place.
304 pages
ISBN: 0-923521-07-0

10696 Child of Mine: Feeding with Love and Good Sense
Bull Publishing
PO Box 1377
Boulder, CO 80306   800-676-2855
                                          www.bullpub.com
Parents need to learn how to provide a nutritionally wholesome diet, but they also need to know how to feed in a way that nurtures a child's senses of autonomy and trust in themselves and their bodies.
470 pages
ISBN: 0-923521-51-8

10697 Childhood Emergencies: What to Do A Quick Refrence Guide
Bull Publishing
PO Box 1377
Boulder, CO 80306   800-676-2855
                                          www.bullpub.com
Handy book contains clear and quick referance for most common injuries including cuts and wounds, broken bones, abdominal pain, burns, toothaches, convulsion, eye and ear injuries, abrasions,

bites insect and animal, bleeding, choking, seizures, freezing and frostbite, CPR, etc.
44 pages
ISBN: 0-923521-62-3

10698 Chiropractor's Self-Help Back and Body Book
Samuel Homola, DC, author
Hunter House Publishers
1515 1/2 Park Street
Alameda, CA 94501
510-865-5282
800-266-5592
e-mail: ordering@hunterhouse.com
www.hunterhouse.com
How to relieve common aches and pains at home and on the job.
2002 320 pages Paperback
ISBN: 0-897933-76-6

10699 Choose the Right Long Term Care
NOLO
950 Parker Street
Berkeley, CA 94710-2524
800-728-3555
Fax: 800-645-0895
e-mail: cs@nolo.com
www.nolo.com
You can use this book to figure out how to choose a nursing home, or find a viable alternative. Covers how to get the most out of Medicare and other benefit programs.
336 pages
ISBN: 0-873375-15-7
Ralph Warner, Executive Chairman & Co-Founder
Bob Dubow, CEO

10700 Chronic Physical Illness
S. Newman, E. Steed, K. Mulligan, author
McGraw-Hill Companies
Returns Department
Dubuque, IA 52002
877-833-5524
Fax: 609-308-4484
e-mail: pbg.ecommerce_custserv@mcgraw-hill.com
www.mcgraw-hill.com
Provides an overview of self-management in chronic physical illness, theoretical and conceptual background, and examines issues related to the delivery of self-management. Discussion of a range of chronic conditions including: asthma, coronary artery disease, heart failure, COPD, hypertension, diabetes and rheumatoid arthritis. Authored by a number of leading international experts in the diseases they discuss. Hardcover also available for $136.95.
2008 240 pages
ISBN: 0-335217-86-9

10701 Directory of Health Grants
Research Grant Guides
PO Box 1214
Loxahatchee, FL 33470-1214
561-795-6129
Fax: 561-795-7794
1000 foundation profiles.
Second edition
ISBN: 0-945078-19-6

10702 Directory of Social Service Grants
Research Grant Guides
PO Box 1214
Loxahatchee, FL 33470-1214
561-795-6129
Fax: 561-795-7794
1100 foundation profiles.
Second edition
ISBN: 0-945078-18-8

10703 Disabled Woman's Guide to Pregnancy and Birth
Judith Rogers OTR, author
Demos Medical Publishing
11 W 42nd Street
New York, NY 10036
212-683-0072
800-532-8663
Fax: 212-683-0118
e-mail: info@demosmedpub.com
www.demosmedpub.com
Based on the experiences of ninety women with disabilities who chose to have children. Contains in-depth interviews with women

with 22 different types of disabilities and with a total of 143 pregnancies.
528 pages
ISBN: 1-932603-08-8
Dr. Diana M Schneider, President

10704 Family Interventions Throughout Chronic Illness and Disability
Springer Publishing Company
536 Broadway
New York, NY 10012-3955
212-431-4370
Fax: 212-941-7842
e-mail: marketing@springerpub.com
www.springerpub.com
This book provides usable methods for professionals to help families deal with the reality of chronic illness of disability of a family member. Included at the end of each section are study questions and suggested activities for those working with the disabled, as well as for students.
336 pages Hardcover
ISBN: 0-826155-80-1
Annette Imperati, Marketing Director

10705 Get Fit While You Sit: Easy Workouts From Your Chair
Charlene Torkelson, author
Hunter House Publishing
1515 1/2 Park Street
Alameda, CA 94501
510-865-5282
800-266-5592
e-mail: ordering@hunterhouse.com
www.hunterhouse.com
A total body workout that can be done right from your chair, anywhere. Perfect for office workers, travelers, and those with age-related movement limitations or special conditions.
Paperback
ISBN: 0-897932-53-0

10706 Good Bones: Complete Guide to Building and Maintaining the Healthiest Bones
Barbara Luke, author
Bull Publishing
PO Box 1377
Boulder, CO 80306
800-676-2855
Fax: 303-545-6354
www.bullpub.com
Examines 17 major risks in bone health with women. Author offers nutrional advice and preventative nutritional advice and prevenative measures in this comprehensive and scientifically sound guide for woman of all ages.
192 pages
ISBN: 0-923521-44-5

10707 Grants for Organizations Serving People with Disabilities
Research Grant Guides
PO Box 1214
Loxahatchee, FL 33470-1214
Fax: 561-795-7794
800 foundation profiles, including funding for all types of nonprofits. Also two key articles on winning grant strategies.
Tenth edition
ISBN: 0-945078-17-X

10708 Habits Not Diets: Secret to Lifetime Weight Control
James M Ferguson MD, Cassandra Ferguson, author
Bull Publishing
PO Box 1377
Boulder, CO 80306
303-545-6350
800-676-2855
Fax: 303-545-6354
www.bullpub.com
This sensible approach puts the emphasis on how to eat rather than what. Uses the cognitive aspects of weight management including thinking skills, stress management and problem solving to help analyze individual eating habits , break undesirable patterns and establish new ones.
352 pages
ISBN: 0-923521-70-7

10709 Health
Sage Publications

2455 Teller Road
Thousand Oaks, CA 91320

805-499-9774
800-818-7243
Fax: 805-499-0871
e-mail: journals@sagepub.com
www.sagepublications.com

A interdisciplinary and international journal committed to the social and cultural study of health, illness and medicine with a particular focus on the changing place of health matters in modern society and in public onsciousness.
Quarterly

10710 I Can't Chew Cookbook

J Randy Wilson, author

Hunter House Publishing
1515 1/2 Park Street
Alameda, CA 94501

510-865-5282
800-266-5592
Fax: 510-865-4295
e-mail: ordering@hunterhouse.com
www.hunterhouse.com

Delicious soft-diet recipes for people with chewing, swallowing and dry-mouth disorders.
224 pages Paperback
ISBN: 0-897934-00-8

10711 Informed Woman's Guide to Breast Health

Kerry McGinn RN, author

Bull Publishing
PO Box 1377
Boulder, CO 80306

303-545-6350
800-676-2855
Fax: 303-545-6354
www.bullpub.com

Covers all elements of self-examination, mammography, medical exams and tests; includes new information about the genes BRCA 1 and BRCA 2, possible early predictors of cancer

ISBN: 0-923521-61-5

10712 Insider's Guide to HMOs

Penguin Putnam
PO Box 999
Bergenfield, NJ 07621-0903

800-526-0275
Fax: 800-227-9604

ISBN: 0-452276-91-8

10713 Journel to Pain Relief

Phyllis Berger, author

Hunter House Publishing
PO Box 2194
Alameda, CA 94501

510-865-5282
800-266-5592
Fax: 510-865-4295
e-mail: ordering@hunterhouse.com
www.hunterhouse.com

Hands-on guide to breakthroughs in pain treatment.
2007 288 pages Paperback
Cristina Sverdrup, Customer Service Manager

10714 Joy of Laziness

Peter Axt, PhD, Michaela Axt-Gardermann, author

Hunter House Publishing
1515 1/2 Park Street
Alameda, CA 94501

510-865-5282
800-266-5592
Fax: 510-865-4295
e-mail: ordering@hunterhouse.com
www.hunterhouse.com

Explains that every human being has a limited amount of energy at his or her disposal.
160 pages Paperback
ISBN: 0-897934-01-5
Cristina Sverdrup, Customer Service Manager

10715 Just Like Everyone Else

World Institute on Disability
510 16th Street, Suite 100
Oakland, CA 94612-1520

510-763-4100
Fax: 510-763-4109
TTY: 510-208-9493
e-mail: wid@wid.org
www.wid.org

Provides perspective, inspiration and information about the Independent Living Movement and the Americans with Disabilities Act.
16 pages
Kathy Martinez, Executive Director

10716 Laurel's Kitchen Caring: Recipes for Everyday Home Caregiving
Ten Speed Press
PO Box 7123
Berkeley, CA 94707-0123

510-559-1600
800-841-2665
Fax: 510-524-4588
e-mail: order@tenspeed.com
www.tenspeed.com

A cookbook tailored to the nutritional needs of recovering patients as well as morale booster, caregiving primer, and resource book.
1997 158 pages
ISBN: 0-898159-51-2

10717 Living a Healthy Life with Chronic Conditions

Kate Lorig, Halsted Holman, David Sobel, author

Bull Publishing
PO Box 1377
Boulder, CO 80306

303-545-6350
800-676-2855
Fax: 303-545-6354
www.bullpub.com

Full of tips, suggestions, and strategies to deal with chronic illness and common symptoms, such as fatigue, pain, shortness of breath, disability, and depression. Encourages readers to develop individual approaches to setting goals, making decisions, and finding resources and support so they are able to do the things they want, and need, to accomplish.
292 pages
ISBN: 1-933503-01-1

10718 Maximize Your Body Potential

Joyce D Nash PhD, author

Bull Publishing
PO Box 1377
Boulder, CO 80306

303-545-6350
800-676-2855
Fax: 303-545-6354
www.bullpub.com

Using selftests, checklists, and fill-in forms, shows readers how to make a committment, how to set realistic goals, and how to design an individualized exercise and eating program.
640 pages
ISBN: 0-923521-71-4

10719 Menopause Without Medicine

Linda Ojeda, author

Hunter House Publishing
1515 1/2 Park Street
Alameda, CA 94501

510-865-5282
800-266-5592
Fax: 510-865-4295
e-mail: ordering@hunterhouse.com
www.hunterhouse.com

Provides complete information on the symptoms of menopause - hot flashes, sexual changes, deperssion and osteoporosis - and how to alleviate them.
400 pages Paperback
ISBN: 0-897934-05-3

10720 Nolo's Guide to Soc. Security Disability: Getting and Keeping Your Benefits

David Morton MD, author

NOLO
950 Parker Street
Berkeley, CA 94710-2524

800-728-3555
Fax: 800-645-0895
e-mail: cs@nolo.com
www.nolo.com

The essential book for anyone dealing with a long-term or permanent disability. Written both for first-time applicants and existing recipients of Social Security disability, this guide demystifies the program and tells you everything you need to know about qualifying and applying for benefits, maintaining your benefits, and appealing the denial of a claim.
512 pages
ISBN: 1-413311-04-4

10721 Ostomy Book: Living Comfortably with Colostomies, Ileostomies and Urostomies

Barbara Dorr Mullen, Kerry Anne McGinn, author

Bull Publishing
PO Box 1377
Boulder, CO 80306

303-545-6350
800-676-2855
Fax: 303-545-6354
www.bullpub.com

For people who have a colostomy, ileostomy or urinary diversion (utostomy), either permanent or temporary, as well as for family, friends and health professionals.

ISBN: 0-933503-13-4

10722 Psychological Management of Chronic Pain: A Treatment Manual

Springer Publishing Company
536 Broadway
New York, NY 10012-3955

212-431-4370
Fax: 212-941-7842

This volume provides the clinician with a practical guide to help clients manage and alleviate problems associated with chronic pain and places an emphasis on the cognitive components of treatment. The manual illustrates a time-limited, therapist-guide/self-management program.

1996 80 pages Softcover
ISBN: 0-826161-12-X

10723 Self Help: Your Strategy for Living with COPD

Bull Publishing
PO Box 1377
Boulder, CO 80306

800-676-2855
Fax: 303-545-6354
www.bullpub.com

Contains vital information for patients suffering from asthma, emphysema, or chronic bronchitis. Colorful charts, graphs and illustrations highlight major concepts and help make the booklet user friendly.

1997 32 pages
ISBN: 0-923521-40-2

10724 ShapeWalking

Marilyn Bach, PhD, Lorie Schleck, author

Hunter House Publishing
1515 1/2 Park Street
Alameda, CA 94501

510-865-5282
800-266-5592
Fax: 510-865-4295
e-mail: ordering@hunterhouse.com
www.hunterhouse.com

An easy low cost total fitness program that is suited for exercisers of all levels.

144 pages Paperback
ISBN: 0-897933-73-5

10725 Social Security, Medicare and Government Pensions

Dorothy Matthews Berman, author

NOLO
950 Parker Street
Berkeley, CA 94710-2524

800-728-3555
Fax: 800-645-0895
e-mail: cs@nolo.com
www.nolo.com

Gets you the most out of your retirement benefits

496 pages
ISBN: 1-413310-97-9

10726 Strength Training for Seniors

Michael Fekete, CSCS; ACE, author

Hunter House Publishing
PO Box 2194
Alameda, CA 94501

510-865-5282
800-266-5592
Fax: 510-865-4295
e-mail: ordering@hunterhouse.com
www.hunterhouse.com

How to rewind your biological clock. Reduce a person's biological age by 10-20 years.

2006 160 pages Paperback
Cristina Sverdrup, Customer Service Manager

10727 Succeeding Against the Odds: Strategies and Insights from the Learning Disabled

Jeremy P Tarcher
5858 Wilshire Boulevard
Los Angeles, CA 90036-4521

213-935-9980

Filled with information on adults with learning disabilities, including the hidden handicaps, the definition of learning disabilities, and characteristics of individuals with learning disabilities. The book also looks at the responsibility of preparing for adulthood, and includes information for parents and teachers.

Lex Frieden, Program Director

10728 Taking Care of Caregivers

D Jeanne Roberts MA, author

Bull Publishing
PO Box 1377
Boulder, CO 80306

303-545-6350
800-676-2855
Fax: 303-545-6354
www.bullpub.com

Covers the needs of caregivers; their feelings; stress management techniques; communication; grief; sharing and support

ISBN: 0-923521-09-7

10729 Tax Options and Strategies for People with Disabilities

Demos Vermande
386 Park Avenue S
New York, NY 10016-8804

212-683-0072
800-532-8663
Fax: 212-683-0118
e-mail: info@demospub.com

1996 288 pages
ISBN: 0-939957-85-

10730 Teens Face to Face with Chronic Illness

Asthma and Allergy Foundation of America
1233 20th Street NW
Washington, DC 20036-2330

202-466-7643
800-727-8462
Fax: 202-466-8940
www.aafa.org

Young people easily relate to this book, which uses anecdotes from teens dealing with chronic illness. Teens address issues such as peer pressure and feeling different.

129 pages Paperback

10731 The Personal Care Attendant Guide: The Art of Finding, Keeping, or Being One

Katie Rodriguez Banister, author

Program Development Associates
5620 Business Avenue
Cicero, NY 13039-9576

315-452-0643
800-543-2119
Fax: 315-452-0710
e-mail: info@disabilitytraining.com
www.disabilitytraining.com/pcgb.html

To live independently, many people with chronic illness and/or disabilitiy hire a personal attendant to assist with day-to-day tasks. Finding a qualified caregiver can be challenging, but not impossible. The Guide teaches readers how to find a competent caregiver, and gives prospective attendants vital information and real-life examples to help them succeed. Includes easy-to-use forms and worksheets to make the search easy and organized, anecdotes, and resources.

2007 160 pages

10732 Time for Healing: Relaxation for Mind and Body

Bull Publishing
PO Box 1377
Boulder, CO 80306

800-676-2855
Fax: 303-545-6354
www.bullpub.com

Helps and guides listeners release tension and acheive deep muscular relaxation, heightened self-awareness and total relaxation.

10733 Understanding Addiction

Elizabeth Connell Henderson MD, author

University Press of Mississippi
3825 Ridgewood Road
Jackson, MS 39211

601-432-6205
800-737-7788
www.upress.state.ms.us

A concise overview of this complex affliction for all those affected by addiction — addicts, family members, and even employers
224 pages Paperback
ISBN: 1-578062-40-9

10734 Understanding Anemia
Ed Uthman, MD, author

University Press of Mississippi
3825 Ridgewood Road
Jackson, MS 39211   601-432-6205
                                     www.upress.state.ms.us
Gently builds upon elementary knowledge of biology to provide the general reader with a fairly sophisticated understanding of the various causes of anemia, of the methods used to make diagnoses, and of the principles of treatment.
160 pages Paperback
ISBN: 1-578060-39-9

10735 Understanding Child Sexual Abuse
Edward L Rowan, MD, author

University Press of Mississippi
3825 Ridgewood Road
Jackson, MS 39211   601-432-6205
                                 Fax: 601-432-6217
                                     www.upress.state.ms.us
For those looking to comrephend and to prevent child sexual abuse, a succinct guidebook of advice and resources.
96 pages Paperback
ISBN: 1-578068-07-X

10736 Understanding Cosmetic Laser Surgery
Robert Langdon, MD, author

University Press of Mississippi
3825 Ridgewood Road
Jackson, MS 39211   601-432-6205
                                 Fax: 601-432-6217
                                     www.upress.state.ms.us
A description of the processes and procedures available in cosmetic laser surgery.
112 pages
ISBN: 1-578065-87-9

10737 Understanding Dental Health
Francis G Serio, DMD; MS, author

University Press of Mississippi
3825 Ridgewood Road
Jackson, MS 39211   601-432-6205
                                 Fax: 601-432-6217
                                     www.upress.state.ms.us
A user-friendly manual on the basics of dental health.
128 pages Paperback
ISBN: 1-578060-10-9

10738 Understanding Dietary Supplements
Jenna Hollenstein, author

University Press of Mississippi
3825 Ridgewood Road
Jackson, MS 39211   601-432-6205
                                 Fax: 601-432-6217
                                     www.upress.state.ms.us
A handy guide to the evaluation and use of vitamins, minerals, herbs, botanicals, and more.
96 pages Paperback
ISBN: 1-578069-81-5

10739 Understanding Stuttering
Nathan Lavid, MD, author

University Press of Mississippi
3825 Ridgewood Road
Jackson, MS 39211   601-432-6205
                                 Fax: 601-432-6217
                                     www.upress.state.ms.us
Insight into an ailment that impairs more than sixty million in the world population.
112 pages Paperback
ISBN: 1-578065-73-9

10740 Understanding Your Learning Disability
Cheri Warner, author

Ohio State University at Newark

1179 University Drive
Newark, OH 43055   740-366-3321
                                     newark.osu.edu
Provides tips for students based on the author's experience as a Learning Disability Specialist. Offers definitions, characteristics, and suggestions related to reading, math, note taking, test taking, social interactions, and organizational strategies.

10741 Writing from Within
Bernard Selling, author

Hunter House Publishers
1515 1/2 Park Street   510-865-5282
Alameda, CA 94501   800-266-5592
                                 Fax: 510-865-4295
                        e-mail: ordering@hunterhouse.com
                                     www.hunterhouse.com
A guide to creativity and life story writing
320 pages Paperback
ISBN: 0-897932-17-2

10742 Yes, You Can!: Go Beyond Physical Adversity and Live Life to Its Fullest
Janis Dietz PhD, author

Demos Medical Publishing
11 W 42nd Street   212-683-0072
New York, NY 10036   800-532-8663
                        e-mail: info@demosmedpub.com
                                     www.demosmedpub.com
Based on the premise that life should be lived to the fullest extent possible, disability or no disability.
102 pages Paperback
ISBN: 1-888799-48-x

Children's Books

10743 Are You Tired Again?...I Understand: An Activities Workbook for Children
Marilyn W Deutsch PhD, author

Western Psychological Services
12031 Wilshire Boulevard   310-478-2061
Los Angeles, CA 90025-1251   800-648-8857
                                 Fax: 310-478-7838
                    e-mail: customerservice@wpspublish.com
                                     www.wpspublish.com
This reassuring activity and coloring book is for children with a chronically ill parent—children who often feel guilty, neglected, lonely, helpless, and afraid. It gives these youngsters the tools they need to work through their feelings, while gently explaining why Mom isn't getting better, why she's always tired, and how the family can still enjoy life and function as a family. It can be used with individuals or with support groups.

10744 In the Hospital
Peter Alsop, Bill Harley, author

Compassion Books
7036 State Highway 80 S   828-675-5909
Burnsville, NC 28714-7569   800-970-4220
                                 Fax: 828-675-9687
                         e-mail: heal2grow@aol.com
                                     www.compassionbooks.com
Wonderful songs and entertaining stories dealing with being sick, being different, being scared and finding strength and hope.
Audiotape/Book
Bruce Greene, Director

10745 Zink the Zebra
Gareth Stevens, Inc
330 West Olive Street   414-332-3520
Milwaukee, WI 53212-3952   800-542-2595
                                 Fax: 414-336-0156
                           e-mail: info@gspub.com
                                     www.garethstevens.com
Zink is a zebra with spots instead of stripes. Here is an inspiring and touching tale about being different in ways that don't matter and shouldn't get in the way when it comes to making friends and enjoying companionship and respect. Written by 11-year-old

Kelly Weil in the last year of a battle she bravely fought, but ultimately lost, against cancer.
1997
ISBN: 0-836816-26-9

Magazines

10746 Advance: for Directors in Rehabilitation
Merion Publications
2900 Horizon Drive   215-265-7812
King of Prussia, PA 19406-2651   800-355-5627
rehabilitation-director.advanceweb.com
An informational magazine designed to provide a balance of material concerning all aspects of a rehabilitation manager's job.
Scott Huelskamp, Editor
Johnathan Bassett, Senior Associate Editor

10747 Closing the Gap
526 Main Street   507-248-3294
Henderson, MN 56044   Fax: 507-248-3810
e-mail: info@closingthegap.com
www.closingthegap.com
Strives to provide parents and educators alike, the information and training necessary to locate, compare, and implement assistive technology.
BiMonthly
Budd Hagen, Co-Founder
Connie Kneip, VP/General Manager

10748 Exceptional Parent Magazine
209 Harvard Street   617-730-5800
Brookline, MA 02446-5005   800-852-2884
Fax: 617-730-8742

Lex Frieden, Program Director

Newsletters

10749 Asbestos Watch
PO Box 1483   301-243-5864
Baltimore, MD 21203-1483   Fax: 301-243-5234
A national nonprofit organization dedicated to the education of the public to the hazards of asbestos exposure. The association developed programs of public education and consults with victims of asbestos exposure, school boards, building owners, government agencies, and others interested in identifying asbestos hazards and developing control programs.
Annual

10750 Chronic Pain Letter
Dolak
Old Chelsea Station   718-797-0015
New York, NY 10011
Brings current information on the management of chronic pain to the sufferer and the health professional.

Dorothy Fabian, Circulation Manager

10751 Health Facts
Center for Medical Consumers
237 Thompson Street   212-674-7105
New York, NY 10012-1017   Fax: 212-674-7100
www.medicalconsumers.org
Analyses of topics such as cancer, nutrition, depression, exercise, prescription drugs and nonmedical therapies.
6 pages Monthly

10752 In Confidence
American Health Information Management Association
233 N Michigan Avenue, 21st Floor   312-233-1100
Chicago, IL 60601   800-621-6828
Fax: 312-233-1090
e-mail: info@ahima.org
www.ahima.org

Provides medical, legal and other professionals with a forum to exchange ideas and share knowledge about the confidentiality of health information and people's rights to privacy.
12 pages BiMonthly
Linda Kloss, Chief Executive Officer
Becky Perry, Executive Vice President & CFO

10753 Johns Hopkins Health Insider
Intelihealth
960C Harvest Drive
Blue Bell, PA 19422   800-988-1127
Fax: 800-676-3299
e-mail: service@jhinsider.com
www.jhinsider.com
Expert advice and information from America's leading health institution. The most authoritative, cutting-edge health information available today, straight from the leading specialists and experts.
David B Hellmann MD, Associate Editor
Linda A Lewandowski PhD, RN, Associate Editor

10754 Learning Disability Quarterly
Council for Learning Disabilities
11184 Antioch Road   913-491-1011
Overland Park, KS 66210   Fax: 913-491-1012
e-mail: CLDInfo@ie-events.com
www.cldinternational.org
Caroline Dunn, President
Monica Lambert, President Elect

10755 Lifelines
Disabled & Alone/Life Services for the Handicapped
61 Broadway   212-532-6740
New York, NY 10006   800-995-0066
Fax: 212-532-3588
e-mail: info@disabledandalone.org
www.disabledandalone.org
8 pages Quarterly
Leslie D Park, Chairman
Lee Alan Ackerman BA, Executive Director

10756 Lymphatic Research Matters
Lymphatic Research Foundation
40 Garvies Point Road   516-625-9675
Glen Cove, NY 11542   Fax: 516-625-9410
e-mail: lrf@lymphaticresearch.org
www.lymphaticresearch.org
Reporting information about LRF activities and current research. The newsletters are sent to registrants in our data base: patients, their families, the scientific community and health care providers.
Bi-Annual
Jacqueline Reinhard, Executive Director
Wendy Chaite, Esq., Founder

10757 Mainstay
Well Spouse Association
63 W Main Street   732-577-8899
Freehold, NJ 7728   800-838-0879
Fax: 732-577-8644
e-mail: info@wellspouse.org
www.wellspouse.org
The Well Spouse Association quarterly newsletter featuring articles written by WSA members.

10758 NHF Head Lines
National Headache Foundation
820 N Orleans   312-274-2650
Chicago, IL 60610   888-643-5552
Fax: 312-640-9049
e-mail: info@headaches.org
www.headaches.org
Up-to-date information on the latest developments in headache treatment; breaking news about newly-approved drugs; reviews of topical books; reader's mail feature, where the nation's leading medical experts answer questions about headaches; and a list of support group meetings where you can learn how to make a positive change in your life.
Bimonthly
Robert R Dalton, Executive Director

10759 National Networker
National Network of Learning Disabled Adults
808 N 82nd Street   602-941-5112
Scottsdale, AZ 85257-3850
For adults with learning disabilities.
Quarterly
Lex Frieden, Program Director

10760 Orphan Disease Update
National Organization for Rare Disorders
PO Box 8923   203-746-6518
New Fairfield, CT 06812-8923   800-999-6673
                                          Fax: 203-756-6481
                                   e-mail: orphan@rarediseases.org
                                          www.rarediseases.org
Information about rare disorders for families with similar disorders.

10761 VSA Arts
JFK Center for the Performing Arts
1300 Connecticut Avenue NW   202-628-2600
Washington, DC 20036-1715   800-933-8721
                                          Fax: 202-737-0725
                                          TDD: 202-737-0645
                                     e-mail: info@vsarts.org
                                              www.vsarts.org
VSA arts is an international, nonprofit organization dedicated to promoting artistic excellence and providing educational opportunities through the arts for children and adults with disabilities. The Creative Spirit is a quarterly newsletter that features VSA arts special events throughout the world, interviews with artistd and articles relating to disability and the arts.
8 pages
D Dixon, CEO
S Datton-Kumins, Writer/Research Coordinator

10762 Wheel Life News
University of Virginia, Rehab Engineering Centers
3363 University Station   804-924-0311
Charlottesville, VA 22903
Features tie downs and other adaptive technology for persons with disabilities.

10763 Worklife: A Publication of Employment and People with Disabilities
Office of Disability Employment Policy
200 Constitution Avenue NW   202-693-7880
Washington, DC 20210   Fax: 202-693-7888
                                          TDD: 202-376-6205

Quarterly

Pamphlets

10764 Campus Opportunities for Students with Learning Differences
Judith & Stephen Crooker, author

Octameron Associates
PO Box 2748   703-836-5480
Alexandria, VA 22301   Fax: 703-836-5650
                                     e-mail: octameron@aol.com
                                              www.octameron.com
Tells learning disabled students what questions to ask when selecting a school, how to prepare for the more rigorous academic schedule and when to get special assistance.
36 pages
ISBN: 1-575090-52-x

10765 Issues in Independent Living
Independent Living Research Utilization
2323 S Shepherd Drive   713-520-0232
Houston, TX 77019-7024   Fax: 713-520-5785
This booklet is a report of the National Study Group on the Implications of Health Care Reform for Americans with Disabilities and Chronic Health Conditions.
30 pages
Lex Frieden, Program Director

10766 OSERS News in Print: Office of Special Education & Rehabilitative Services
US Department of Education
400 Maryland Avenue SW   202-205-8241
Washington, DC 20202-0001   800-872-5327
                                              www.ed.gov
Provides information, research, and resources in the area of special learning needs.
Quarterly
Lex Frieden, Program Director

Audio & Video

10767 Assisting Parents Through the Mourning Process
Hope
55 E 100 N   435-752-9533
Logan, UT 84321-4648   Fax: 435-752-9533
Describes the mourning process experienced by some parents of children with disabilities and ways in which the professional can help them through the process.
20 minutes

10768 No Fears, No Tears
Leora Kuttner, PhD, author

Fanlight Productions
4196 Washington Street   617-469-4999
Boston, MA 02131-1731   800-937-4113
                                          Fax: 617-469-3379
                                   e-mail: fanlight@fanlight.com
                                              www.fanlight.com
Dr. Leora Kuttner explores the effects of childrens pain management.
1985 28 Minutes

10769 No Fears, No Tears: 13 Years Later
Leora Kuttner, PhD, author

Fanlight Productions
4196 Washington Street   617-469-4999
Boston, MA 02131-1731   800-937-4113
                                          Fax: 617-469-3379
                                   e-mail: fanlight@fanlight.com
                                              www.fanlight.com
Dr. Leora Kutner explores the effects of childrens pain management therapies 13 years after their use.
1998 47 Minutes
ISBN: 1-572952-77-6

Web Sites

10770 Access Unlimited
                                  www.accessunlimited.com
Assists educators, health care providers and parents in discovering how personal computers help children and adults with disabilities compensate for some of the barriers imposed by their conditions.

10771 American Academy of Pediatrics
                                              www.aap.org
Committed to the attainment of optimal physical, mental and social health and well-being for all infants, children, adolescents and yound adults.

10772 American Association for the Advancement of Science
                                              www.aaas.org
An international non-profit organization dedicated to advancing science around the world by serving as an educators, leader, spokesperson and professional association.

10773 American Bar Association Commission
                                  www.abanet.org/disability

10774 American Camp Association
                                          www.acacamps.org
Enriching the lives of children, youth and adults through the camp experience.

10775 American Counseling Association
                                          www.counseling.org

Dedicated to the growth and development of the counseling profession and those who are served.

10776 American Institute for Preventive Medicine

www.healthylife.com

An award winning, internationally recognized authority on the development and implementation of health promotion, wellness, medical self-care and disease management programs and publications.

10777 American Organ Transplant Association

www.aotaonline.org

To help transplant patients lead happy, productinve lives by helping them obtain and sustain transplantation.

10778 American Red Cross

www.redcross.org

In addition to domestic disaster relief, the American Red Cross offers compassionate services in five other areas: community services that help the needy; support and comfort for military members and their families; the collection, processing and distribution of lifesaving blood and blood products; educational programs that promote health and safety; and international relief and development programs.

10779 American Self-Help Group Clearinghouse

www.selfhelpgroups.org

A keyword-searchable database of over 1,100 national, international, model and online self-help support groups for addictions, bereavement, health, mental health, disabilities, abuse, parenting, caregiver concerns and many other stressful life situations.

10780 American Society of Dermatology

www.asd.org

A non-partisan professional association of dematologists across the country whose mission is to facilitate optimal dermatologic care being available to all citizens of this country by preserving, promoting and enhancing the private practice of dermatology.

10781 Americas Association for the Care of the Children

www.aaccchildren.net

To promote support for those who are involved in early childhood care and education through educational programs and projects, including among other things, citizen exchange programs, global communication networks, and resource assistance to participating communities.

10782 Beach Center on Families and Disability

www.beachcenter.org

Makes a significant and sustainable difference in the quality of life of families and individuals affected by disability and of those who are closely involved with them.

10783 Center for Chronic Disease Prevention and Health Promotion

www.cdc.gov/nccdphp

The forefront of the nation's efforts to prevent and control chronic diseases. Leads efforts that promote health and well-being through prevention and control of chronic diseases.

10784 Center for Developmental Disabilities

www.centerfor.com

Committed to its mission of helping children and adults with differing abilities achieve their dreams by overcoming barriers to living, working, learning and enjoying recreational opportunities in the community of their choice.

10785 ChiroWeb.com

www.chiroweb.com

Chiropractic news source for chiropractors, students, patients and health care professionals. Over 7,000 articles are available.

10786 Commission on Accreditation of Rehabilitation Services

www.carf.org

An independent, nonprofit accreditor of health and human services that promotes the quality, value and optimal outcomes of services through a consultative accreditation process that centers on enhancing the lives of the persons served.

10787 Disabled & Alone/Life Services for the Handicapped

www.disabledandalone.org

A non-profit organization established to help families provide a secure future for their loved ones with a disability. Believes that no person should have to live his life in loneliness and isolation because of a disability.

10788 Discovery Health

www.health.discovery.com

A large website covering various health topics; such as male and female health, senior health, children's health, mental health, alternative medicine, nutrition, fitness, and more.

10789 Educational Equity Center at AED

www.edequity.org

EEC at AED is an outgrowth of Educational Equity Concepts, a national not-for-profit organization with a 22-year history of promoting educational excellence for all children.

10790 Federation for Children with Special Needs

www.fcsn.org

Provides information, support, and assistance to parents with children with disabilities, their professional partners, and their communities.

10791 Healing Well

www.healingwell.com

A social network and support community for patients, caregivers, and families coping with the daily struggles of diseases, disorders and chronic illness.

10792 Health Care For All

www.hcfa.org

HCFA seeks to create a consumer-centered health care system that provides comprehensive, affordable, accessible, culturally competent, high quality care and consumer education for everyone, especially the most vulnerable.

10793 Health Finder

www.healthfinder.gov

A government website that contains information and tools to help you and those you care about stay healthy.

10794 Health on the Net Foundation

www.hon.ch

Promotes and guides the deployment of useful and reliable online health information, and its appropriate and efficient use.

10795 Healthcentral.com

www.healthcentral.com

Empower millions of people to improve and take control of their health and well-being.

10796 Healthlink USA

www.healthlinkusa.com

Discussion forum for treatments, symptoms and causes of 700 health conditions, diseases and topics.

10797 Helios Health

www.helioshealth.com

Online resource for your health information. Detailed information about specific health topics, access to expert advice from our Medical Advisory Board, and up-to-date health news.

10798 Life Development Institute

www.lifedevelopmentinst.org

Serving men and women between the ages of 18-30 who have Asperger's Syndrome, ADHD, learning disabilities, anxiety, depression and other disorders

10799 MedicineNet

www.medicinenet.com

An online resource for consumers providing easy-to-read, authoritative medical and health information.

10800 Medscape

www.medscape.com

Medscape offers specialists, primary care physicians, and other health professionals the Web's most robust and integrated medical information and educational tools.

10801 Medtronic

www.medtronic.com

Medtronic is changing the face of chronic disease. By working closely with physicians around the world, they create therapies to help patients do things they never thought were possible.

10802 **National Clearinghouse of Rehabilitation Training Materials**

www.ncrtm.org

The mission of the NCRTM is to advocate for the advancement of best practice in rehabilitation counseling through the development, collection, dissemination, and utilization of professional knowledge, information and skill.

10803 **National Council on Disability**

www.ncd.gov

The National Council on Disability is an independent federal agency that works with the President and Congress to increase the inclusion, independence and empowerment of Americans with disabilities.

10804 **National Organization for Rare Disorders (NORD)**

www.rarediseases.org

Serves as a clearinghouse for information about rare disorders and brings together families with similar disorders for mutual support; fosters communication among rare disease voluntary agencies, Government agencies, industry, scientific researchers, academic institutions, and concerned individuals; and encourages and promotes research and education on rare disorders and orphan drugs.

10805 **Office of Special Education and Rehabilitative Services**

www2.ed.gov/osers

The Office of Special Education and Rehabilitative Servics (OSERS) is committed to improving the results and outcomes for people with disabilities of all ages.

10806 **WebMD**

www.webmd.com

General information, including articles.

10807 **World Institute on Disability**

www.wid.org

A public policy center that is run by persons with disabilities. Conducts research, public education, and advocacy campaigns.

National Agencies & Associations

10808 A Kid Again
777-G Dearborn Park Lane   614-797-9735
Columbus, OH 43085   800-543-9735
Fax: 614-797-9600
e-mail: customerservice@akidagain.org
www.akidagain.org
Enriches the lives of children with life threatening illnesses and their families by providing year round fun-filled group activities and destination events by fostering joy, laughter, normalcy and supportive networking opportunities. Includes regional chapters.
Jeffrey Damron, CFRE, CEO
Kathy Derr, Director of Programs and Volunteers

10809 A Wish with Wings, Inc.
917 W Sanford   817-469-9474
Arlington, TX 76012   Fax: 817-275-6005
e-mail: wish@awishwithwings.org
www.awishwithwings.org
Grants the wishes of Texas children with life-threatening diseases.
Pat Skaggs, Founder
Judy Youngs, Executive Director

10810 BASE Camp Children's Cancer Foundation
140 N Orlando Avenue   407-673-5060
Winter Park, FL 32789-3679   Fax: 407-673-5095
e-mail: email@basecamp.org
www.basecamp.org
Supports children and their families who are facing the challenge of living with cancer or other life-threatening hematological illnesses. Offers year round programs, monthly overnight camps, support groups, and weekly events.
Terri Jones, President/Founder
Jackie Ellis, Executive Director

10811 Believe In Tomorrow Children's Foundation
6601 Frederick Road   410-744-1984
Baltimore, MD 21228   800-933-5470
Fax: 410-744-1984
e-mail: info@believeintomorrow.org
www.believeintomorrow.org
Formerly Grant-A-Wish Foundation, this Foundation provides exceptional hospital and retreat housing services to critically ill children and their families. The Foundation also believes that keeping families together during a child's medical crisis, and that the gentle caring environment is crucial.
Brian R Morrison, Founder
Richard E McCready, Chairman

10812 Camp Good Days
1332 Pittsford-Mendon Road   585-624-5555
Mendon, NY 14506   800-785-2135
Fax: 585-624-5799
www.campgooddays.org
A non-profit organization that provides a camping experience and more for children and adults facing the toughest challenges of life. Accepts the wishes of terminal ill children through age eighteen.
Gary Mervis, Founder/Chairman
Wendy Bleier-Mervis, Executive Director

10813 Children's Wish Foundation International
8615 Roswell Road   770-393-9474
Atlanta, GA 30350-7526   800-323-9474
Fax: 770-393-0683
e-mail: arthurs@childrenswish.org
www.childrenswish.org
Committed to bringing joy and happiness to seriously ill children throughout the world and this dedication has created special experiences for children around the globe. Our commitment is also developing hospital enrichment programs.
Linda Dozoretz, Executive Director
Jacque Niles, Director of Program Services

10814 Cure Our Children Foundation
711 S Carson Street   310-355-6046
Carson City, NV 89701   Fax: 310-454-9592
e-mail: barry@cureourchildren.org
www.cureourchildren.org
Support medical approaches to treatment of Ewings Sarcoma. Alternate and complimentary treatment information is provided only for use in conjunction with traditional approaches.
Barry Sugarman, President

10815 Dream Come True
PO Box 21167   610-865-3475
Lehigh Valley, PA 18002   Fax: 610-865-4710
e-mail: RVasko@aol.com
www.dreamcometrue.org
Seeks to fulfill the dreams of children ages 4 - 17 who are seriously, chronically and terminally ill and whom live in the Lehigh Valley area. Includes regional offices.
Rayann Vasko, Director
Jeane Hockenbury, President

10816 Dream Factory, Inc.
National Headquarters
120 W Broadway   502-561-3001
Louisville, KY 40202   800-456-7556
Fax: 502-561-3004
e-mail: dfinfo@dreamfactoryinc.org
www.dreamfactoryinc.org
Grants wishes to children and young adults ages 3 - 18 with a critical or chronic illness.
Janice Harris, President
Ralph Coldiron, Vice President

10817 Dream Foundation
1528 Chapala Street   805-564-2131
Santa Barbara, CA 93101   Fax: 805-564-7002
www.dreamfoundation.org
Enhances the quality of life for individuals and families battling terminal illnesses ages 18 and over.
Thomas Rollerson, Founder/President
Carol Brown, Chief Operating Officer

10818 Fairygodmother Foundation
550 W Webster Avenue   773-388-1160
Chicago, IL 60614   Fax: 773-883-3656
e-mail: info@fairygodmother.org
www.fairygodmother.org
Our wish granting program brings joy to the lives of adults (18 and older) and loved ones in their time of greatest need by turning dreams into reality. In the process of fulfilling wishes, we create an opportunity for peace, closure and a sense of belonging.
Lena Clement, Program Director

10819 Friends of Karen
118 Titicus Road   914-277-4547
Purdys, NY 10578   e-mail: info@friendsofkaren.org
www.friendsofkaren.org
Provides financial, emotional and advocacy support to children with life-threatening illnesses and their families.
Judith Factor, Executive Director
Nancy Mariano, Regional Director

10820 Give Kids the World Village
210 S Bass Road   407-396-1114
Kissimmee, FL 34746   800-995-KIDS
Fax: 407-396-1207
e-mail: dream@gktw.org
www.gktw.org
A 70-acre non-profit resort in Central Florida that creates magical memories for children with life-threatening illnesses and their families. GKTW provides accommodations at its whimsical resort, donated attractions, tickets, meals and more for a week-long stay.
Pamela Landwirth, President

10821 High Hopes Foundation of New Hampshire, Inc.
301 Daniel Webster Highway   603-429-1010
Merrimack, NH 03054   800-639-6804
Fax: 603-429-0037
e-mail: info@highhopesnh.net
www.highhopesnh.org
Grants wishes for severely and chronically ill children and young adults ages 3-18 who live in New Hampshire.
Jacque Yinger, Founder
Dawn Cavanaugh, Founder

10822 Hopes & Dreams Foundation, Inc.
517 Cedarbrook Road   215-264-2859
Southampton, PA 18966-mail: info@hopesanddreamsfoundation.org
                   www.hopesanddreamsfoundation.org
For children and young adults with disabilities such as down syndrome and other specific challenges. Helps to promote education and community involvement through social activities.
Vick Franklin, President

10823 Kidd's Kids
220 E Las Colinas Boulevard   972-432-8595
Irving, TX 75039   866-541-5437
                   Fax: 214-853-5212
                   e-mail: derrick@kiddlive.com
                   www.kiddskids.com
Founded by nationally syndicated morning show personality Kidd Kraddick. Provides chronically ill and/or physically challenged children between the ages of 5 to 12 with an unforgettable adventure.
Toby Wilson, President
Dr. Kevin Wylie, Vice President

10824 Kids Incorporated
9300 Old Keene Mill Road   703-455-5437
Burke, VA 22015-4277   Fax: 703-440-9208
                   www.jcambellinc.com
Grants wishes to gravely ill children 16 years and younger. Children older than 16 are sometimes eligible depending on child's situation and the availability of resources.
John Campbell, President

10825 Kids Wish Network
4060 Louis Avenue   727-937-3600
Holiday, FL 34691   888-918-9004
                   Fax: 727-937-3688
                   e-mail: info@kidswishnetwork.org
                   www.kidswishnetwork.org
A nationally recognized charitable organization dedicated to infusing hope creating happy memories and improving the quality of life for children. The Network also fulfills the wishes of children ages 3 to 18 with life threatening medical conditions.
Shelley Breiner, Founder

10826 Magic Moments
1600 7th Avenue South   205-939-9372
Birmingham, AL 35233   Fax: 205-939-6717
                   e-mail: info@magicmoments.org
                   www.magicmoments.org
Grants wishes to children 4 to 19 living or being treated in Alabama who have chronic life-threatening diseases or who have severe trauma (burn, spinal cord or head trauma).
Pam Jones, Executive Director
Courtney Austin, Project Manager

10827 Make-A-Wish Foundation of America
4742 N. 24th Street   602-279-9474
Phoenix, AZ 85016-4862   800-722-9474
                   Fax: 602-279-0855
                   e-mail: mawfa@wish.org
                   www.wish.org
A national organization that grants wishes for children with terminally or life threatening diseases and who are 18 years of age or younger. Includes regional chapters.
David Williams, President/CEO

10828 Marty Lyons Foundation, Inc.
326 W 48th Street   212-977-9474
New York, NY 10036   Fax: 212-977-1752
                   e-mail: mac@martylyonsfoundation.org
                   www.martylyonsfoundation.org
A national organization that grants wishes of children between the ages of three and seventeen who have life-threatening diseases or terminal illnesses. Those interested can submit applications for their wish fulfillment.
Mary Ann Canapi, Executive Director
Marty Lyons, Sr. Vice President, Operations

10829 New Hope for Kids Wish Program
205 E. SR 436   407-331-3059
Fern Park, FL 32730   Fax: 407-331-3063
                   e-mail: information@newhopeforkids.org
                   www.newhopeforkids.org
Grants wishes to children ages 3-18 who have been diagnosed with a life-threatening illness.
Dave Joswick, Executive Director
Dana Duffie, Office Manager

10830 Rainbow Connection
621 W University   248-601-9474
Rochester, MI 48307   877-649-4743
                   Fax: 248-601-0086
                   e-mail: info@rainbowconnection.org
                   www.rainbowwishconnection.org
Make the special wishes of children with life-threatening or terminal illnesses come true.
L. Brooks Patterson, Founder
Janet Dobson Vernier, 2nd Vice President

10831 Special Wish Foundation
1250 Memory Lane   614-258-3186
Columbus, OH 43209   800-486-9474
                   Fax: 614-258-3518
                   e-mail: info@spwish.org
                   www.spwish.org
A Special Wish Foundation Inc. is a non-profit charitable organization dedicated to granting the wishes of children under the age of 21 who have been diagnosed with a life-threatening disorder.
Laura Marchetta, Contact/Chicago Chapter
Patti Piening, Contact/Cincinnati

10832 Starlight Foundation
5757 Wilshire Boulevard   310-479-1212
Los Angeles, CA 90036-1035   800-274-7827
                   e-mail: info@starlight.org
                   www.starlight.org
A non-profit organization dedicated to brightening the lives of seriously ill children and their families.
Jacqueline Hart-Ibrahim, CEO
Jane Van Stedum, VP, Operations

10833 Sunshine Foundation National Headquarters
1041 Mill Creek Drive   215-396-4770
Feasterville, PA 19053   Fax: 215-396-4774
                   e-mail: philly@sunshinefoundation.org
                   www.sunshinefoundation.org
Answers the dreams of seriously ill physically challenged and abused children aged three to eighteen whose families cannot fulfill their requests due to financial strain that the child's illness may cause.
Kate Sample, President
Sandra Carr, Director of Development

10834 Vision Foundation
8901 Strafford Circle   865-357-4603
Knoxville, TN 37923-1567   Fax: 865-690-9322
                   e-mail: gordon@visionfoundation.net
                   www.visionfoundation.net
Offers counseling support groups seminars and transportation for the blind providing 600 members.
Gordon Adams, Executive Director/President
Hank Brink, Vice President

10835 Wish Upon A Star
PO Box 4000   559-733-7753
Visalia, CA 93278   800-821-6805
                   Fax: 559-733-0962
                   e-mail: info@wishuponastar.org
                   www.wishuponastar.org
A non-profit law enforcement effort designed to grant the wishes of children afflicted with high-risk and life threatening illnesses.
Wally Nelson, President
Carmen Perez, Executive Director

10836 Wishing Star Foundation
139 S Sherman
Spokane, WA 99202
509-744-3411
Fax: 509-744-3414
e-mail: paulan@wishingstar.org
www.wishingstar.org
Grants wishes to children with life threatening illnesses. Ages 3-21 in Eastern Washington and all of Idaho.
Paula Nordgaarden, M.Ed. MSW, Executive Director
Sarah Carpenter, Program Director

10837 Wishing Well Foundation USA, Inc.
3000 W Esplanade Avenue
Metairie, LA 70002
504-841-0001
888-663-9474
e-mail: wellfoundation@bellsouth.net
www.wishingwellusa.org
To bring joy to children with life threatening illnesses by providing them with their fondest wish in life.
Elwin Lebeau, President

Foundations

10838 Angelwish, Inc.
PO Box 186
Rutherford, NJ 07070
201-672-0722
Fax: 201-672-0733
e-mail: info@angelwish.org
www.angelwish.org
Provides the public with an easy way to grant wishes to the millions of children that are living with HIV/AIDS around the world. Infected or affected by the disease, their opportunities for a normal childhood are virtually impossible. By harnessing the power of the Internet, Angelwish helps donors add a ray of hope to their lives.
Shimmy Mehta, Founder/CEO
Tom Fuller, Director

10839 Chef David's Kids
1100 E Oakland Park Boulevard
Fort Lauderdale, FL 33334   e-mail: chefdavidmitchell@gmail.com
954-594-1024
www.chefdavidskids.com
Helps children afflicted with any form of terminal illness such as cancer, leukemia, and pediatric HIV. Also helps neglected and abused children.
Chef David Mitchell, Founder/Director of Operations
Laurie Amber, National Hospital Events Director

10840 Children's Wish Foundation of Canada
7-725 Westney Road South
Ajax, Ontario, L1S-7J7
905-427-5353
Fax: 905-427-0536
e-mail: on@childrenswish.ca
www.childrenswish.ca
Works with the community to provide children living with high risk life threatening illnesses the opportunity to realize their most heartfelt wish.
Chris Kotsopoulos, Director
Linda Marco, Communications/Development Nat'l Manager

10841 Dreams Come True
6803 Southpoint Parkway
Jacksonville, FL 32216
904-296-3030
Fax: 904-296-4244
www.dreamscometrue.org
Grants the dreams of children with life-threatening illnesses.
Jeffrey Conn, President
Eddie Allen, Managing Director

10842 Dreams for Seniors Charity Inc
512 Court Street
Pekin, IL 61554
309-353-7306
Fax: 309-353-7311
e-mail: ddavison@grics.net
www.dreamsforseniorscharity.net
Grant dreams to chronically/critically ill children between ages of 3-18 years in a 30 mile radiu of Pekin, Illinois
Debbie Davison, President/Founder

10843 Jason's Dreams for Kids Foundation, Inc.
20 Monmouth Street
Red Bank, NJ 07701
732-758-0060
Fax: 732-758-0070
e-mail: jasonsdreams@comcast.net
www.jasonsdreamsforkids.com

Devoted to granting wishes to children diagnosed with life-threatening illnesses. Holds a variety of fundraising events to meet the cost of fulfilling these childrens' wishes.

10844 Little Star Foundation
256 Rancho Milagro Way
Hesperus, CO 81326
800-543-6565
e-mail: info@littlestar.org
www.littlestar.org
Provides lifetime opportunities for children with cancer to enhance the quality of their lives.
Andrea Jaeger, Co-Founder & President

10845 Starlight Children's Foundation
5757 Wilshire Boulevard
Los Angeles, CA 90036
310-479-1212
e-mail: info@starlight.org
www.starlight.org
Helps seriously ill children and their families cope with their pain, fear and isolation through entertainment, education and family activities.
Jacqueline Hart-Ibrahim, CEO
Jane Van Stedum, VP, Operations

10846 Sunshine Dreams for Kids
495 Richmond Street
London, Ontario, N6A-5A9
519-642-0990
800-461-7475
Fax: 519-642-1201
e-mail: info@sunshine.ca
www.sunshine.ca
Grants dreams to children who are between the ages of 3 and 19 who are challenged by severe physical disabilities or life threatening illnesses.
Patrick DeMeester, MBA, President
Shawn Melito, MBA, Vice-President

10847 United Special Sportsman Alliance
7864 Shotwell Road
Pittsville, WI 54466
715-884-2256
800-518-8019
Fax: 715-884-7388
www.childswish.com
A dream wish granting charity that specializes in sending critically ill and disabled youth on the outdoor adventure of their dreams.
Brigid O'Donoghue, CEO/Founder
Ron Johnson, President

National Agencies & Associations

10848 Children's Hospice International
1101 King Street
Alexandria, VA 22314
703-684-0330
800-24C-HILD
e-mail: info@chionline.org
www.chionline.org
This organization was founded to provide a network of support and care for children with life threatening conditions and their families. The hospice is a team effort which provides medical, psychological, social and spiritual expertise in the US and abroad.
Ann Armstrong-Dailey, Founding Director/CEO
Rebecca Brant, Director

10849 Compassionate Friends
PO Box 3696
Oak Brook, IL 60522-3696
630-990-0010
877-969-0010
Fax: 630-990-0246
e-mail: nationaloffice@compassionatefriends.org
www.compassionatefriends.org
A national organization that gives support to people who have experienced the death of a child. Offers monthly support meetings to get through the difficult times and learn how to cope.
Patricia Loder, Executive Director

10850 HOSPICELINK Hospice Education Institute
Hospice Education Institute
3 Unity Square
Machiasport, MA 04655-0098
207-255-8800
800-331-1620
Fax: 207-255-8008
e-mail: info@hospiceworld.org
www.hospiceworld.org
Provides educational and informational services to health professionals and the public on subjects such as hospice care, death and dying and bereavement counseling.

10851 Helping Other Parents in Normal Grief
Underwood Memorial Hospital
509 N Broad Street
Woodbury, NJ 08096
856-845-0100
www.umhospital.org
Offers support to newly bereaved parents through trained parents who have suffered a similar loss and resolved their grief.
Eileen K. Cardile, RN, MS, CNA, President/CEO
John Graham, FACHE, Executive Vice President/COO

10852 National Association for Home Care and Hospice
228 7th Street SE
Washington, DC 20003-4306
202-547-7424
Fax: 202-547-3540
e-mail: hospice@nahc.org
www.nahc.org
Promotes the concepts of hospice, a philosophy of health care which is expressed through the provision of a variety of medical and nonmedical services to terminally ill patients and their families.
Val J. Halamandaris, President
Andrea Devoti, Chair

10853 National Hospice & Palliative Care Organization
1731 King Street
Alexandria, VA 22314
703-837-1500
800-658-8898
Fax: 703-837-1233
e-mail: nhpco_info@nhpco.org
www.nhpco.org
The nation's only advocate for terminally ill patients and their families. Founded in 1978, the NHPCO is the only organization devoted to hospice in the United States. Support is included from state hospice organizations, patients, families, communities, provider program members and professional/volunteer members. Represents hospice care interests to Congress, regulatory agencies, courts, voluntary organizations and the public.
J. Donald Schumacher, PsyD, President/CEO
Galen Miller, PhD, Executive Vice President

10854 National Hospice & Palliative Care Organization
1731 King Street
Alexandria, VA 22314
703-837-1500
800-658-8898
Fax: 703-837-1233
e-mail: nhpco_info@nhpco.org
www.nhpco.org
The nation's only advocate for terminally ill patients and their families. Founded in 1978, the NHPCO is the only organization devoted to hospice in the United States. Support is included from state hospice organizations, patients, families and communities.
J. Donald Schumacher, President/CEO
Galen Miller, Executive Vice President

10855 National Institute for Jewish Hospice
732 University Street
North Woodmere, NY 11581
516-791-9888
800-446-4448
Fax: 516-791-6999
e-mail: mlamm@nijh.org
www.nijh.org
Serves as a resource center that seeks to help terminal patients and their families deal with their grief by providing information on traditional Jewish views on death, dying and managing the loss of a loved one.
Shirley Lamm, Executive Director
Maurice Lamm, Founder/President

10856 Share Pregnancy and Infant Loss Support, Inc.
The National Share Office
402 Jackson Street
St. Charles, MO 63301
636-947-6164
800-821-6819
Fax: 636-947-7486
www.nationalshare.org
Serving those whose lives have been touched by the tragic death of a baby through pregnancy loss, stillbirth or the first few months of life.
Cathie Lammert, Executive Director
Rose Carlson, Program Director

10857 Wrap Myself in a Rainbow Compassion Books
Compassion Books
7036 State Highway 80 S
Burnsville, NC 28714-7569
828-675-5909
800-970-4220
Fax: 828-675-9687
e-mail: bruce@compassionbooks.com
www.compassionbooks.com
This is a collection of poignant songs and sensitive guided images that validates and transforms loss with hope. Side I is guided meditation Side II delivers powerful performances of Over The Rainbow, Rainbow Connection and Bring Rainbows to Children.
Audio Cassette
Bruce Greene, Director
Karen Walker, Staff

Support Groups & Hotlines

10858 Bereavement Group for Children
Corstone Center
33 Buchanan Drive
Sausalito, CA 94965-2535
415-331-6161
Fax: 415-331-4545
e-mail: info@corstone.org
www.corstone.org
For children who have suffered the loss of a close loved one. Parent group meets separately at the same time.
Steve Leventhal, Executive Director
Richard Cuadra, MS, Program Director

10859 Grief & Loss Support Group
First Love Outreach Ministries
PO Box 06204
Milwaukee, WI 53206
414-263-1323
Fax: 414-263-1148
e-mail: zelodius@aol.com
www.firstlovelifecoaching.com
Pr Zelodius Morton, CEO

10860 National Hospice Helpline
1700 Diaganal Road
Alexandria, VA 22314
703-837-1500
800-658-8898
Fax: 703-525-5762
e-mail: nhpcoinfo@nhpco.org
www.nhpco.org
Offers more information on hospice in general and offers referrals to a hospice program in your area.
Scott Vickers, Manager Consumer Resources
John Radulovic, Vice President of Communications

10861 Rainbows for All God's Children
1360 Hamilton Parkway
Itasca, IL 60143
847-952-1770
800-266-3206
Fax: 847-952-1774
e-mail: info@rainbows.org
www.rainbows.org
A support program for children who have suffered a significant loss in their lives due to death, divorce or any other painful transition.
Suzy Yehl Marta, Founder & President

Books

10862 A Good Death: Conversations with East Londoners
Lesley Cullen and Michael Young, author
Routledge
270 Madison Avenue
New York, NY 10016
212-216-7800
800-634-7064
Fax: 212-563-2269
e-mail: orders@taylorandfrancis.com
www.routledge.com
Based on a survey in East London and provides a wide range of fascinating and helpful insights into all aspects of experiencing death and surviving grief. The voices in the book are those of people who have managed to cope despite being under the shadow of impending death. Their experience could be a comfort to anybody in a similar situation. A Good Death is intended for people who are dying, and for student doctors, nurses, and social workers.
272 pages
ISBN: 0-415137-97-3

10863 Anatomy of Bereavement
Beverly Raphael, author
Rowman & Littlefield Publishers, Inc.
15200 NBN Way
Blue Ridge Summit, PA 17214
717-794-3800
800-462-6420
Fax: 717-794-3803
e-mail: orders@rowman.com
customercare@rowman.com
In this comprehensive book, Dr. Raphael describes all the stages of mourning and healing.
454 pages Softcover
ISBN: 1-568212-70-4

10864 Bereaved Children: A Support Guide for for Parents And Professionals
Earl A. Grollman, author
Beacon Press
25 Beacon Street
Boston, MA 02108-2824
617-742-2110
Fax: 617-723-3097
www.beacon.org
Comprehensive guide that helps children and teens cope with the loss of a loved one.
256 pages
ISBN: 0-807023-07-5

10865 Bereaved Parent
Harriet Sarnoff Schiff, author
Penguin USA
375 Hudson Street
New York, NY 10014
212-366-2372
800-847-5515
Fax: 212-366-2933
e-mail: insidesales@us.penguingroup.com
www.penguingroup.com
Supportive advice for bereaved parents and professionals who work with them.
146 pages
ISBN: 0-140050-43-4

10866 Concerning Death: A Practical Guide for the Living
Earl A. Grollman, author
Beacon Press
25 Beacon Street
Boston, MA 02108-2824
617-742-2110
Fax: 617-723-3097
www.beacon.org

A guide for people to learn how to cope with death and dying, and the many decisions involved in the process.
265 pages
ISBN: 0-807027-65-0

10867 Conversations At Midnight
William Morrow & Company/Order Department
39 Plymouth Street
Fairfield, NJ 07004-1633
973-227-7200
800-821-1513
Herbert Kramer is dying of cancer. For him, as for everyone someday, death is now an unavoidable companion. This book tells how Herb learns to acknowledge this presence and come to terms with human mortality. This book is a powerful way to look at death and to deal with losing a loved one.
256 pages Hardcover
ISBN: 0-688120-84-9

10868 Death and the Quest for Meaning
Stephen Strack & Herman Feifel, author
Rowman & Littlefield Publishers, Inc.
4501 Forbes Blvd., Suite 200
Lanham, MD 20706
800-462-6420
www.rowmanlittlefield.com
This work covers all aspects of the study of death and dying and the care of the bereaved.
Hardcover
ISBN: 0-765700-14-x

10869 Death: The Final Stage of Growth
Elisabeth Kubler-Ross, author
Simon & Schuster
1230 Avenue of the Americas
New York, NY 10020
212-698-7000
www.simonandschuster.com
This books shows readers how to come to terms with death as a part of human development, and how death can provide us with a key meaning of human existence.
208 pages

10870 Difference in the Family
Penguin Putnam
PO Box 999
Bergenfield, NJ 07621-0903
201-387-0600
800-526-0275
Fax: 800-227-9604
A frank chronicle of the grief, rage and guilt everyone in a family suffers after a death, and the adjustments each make to cope.
Helen Featherstone, Editor

10871 Dying and Disabled Children
Haworth Press
10 Alice Street
Binghamton, NY 13904-1580
607-722-5857
800-429-6784
Fax: 607-722-0012
www.haworthpress.com
In this sensitive and compassionate look at terminally ill and disabled children, professionals from the medical community examine the stresses faced by their parents and siblings. They address crucial element of communication in dealing with a child's serious illness. Ethical decision making, learning to recognize the child's suffering, and talking to children about death are honestly and clearly discussed.
153 pages Hardcover
ISBN: 0-866567-59-0

10872 For Those Who Live: Helping Children Cope with Death of a Brother or Sister
Centering Corporation
7230 Maple Street
Omaha, NE 68134
402-553-1200
866-218-0101
Fax: 402-553-0507
e-mail: danni@centeringcorp.com
www.centering.org
Deals with the grieving family as a whole and offers references for further help.
122 pages
Kathy LaTour, Editor

10873 Grief, Dying and Death: Clinical Intervention for Caregivers
Research Press

2612 N Mattis Avenue
Champaign, IL 61822-1053

217-352-3273
800-519-2707
Fax: 217-352-1221
e-mail: rp@researchpress.com
www.researchpress.com

In this comprehensive manual, the author provides both the theoretical background and the practical treatment interventions necessary for working with those who are bereaved or dying. Important topics such as anticipatory grief, postdeath mourning and the stress of grief are described in detail. Grief reactions, both normal and abnormal, as well as their causes are analyzed. Special attention is given to grief caused by death of a child or spouse, death by suicide, and children's grief.
488 pages Softcover
ISBN: 0-878222-32-4

10874 Helper's Journey
Dr. Dale G. Larson, author

Research Press
Dept. 11W
Champaign, IL 61826

217-352-3273
800-519-2707
Fax: 217-352-1221
e-mail: orders@researchpress.com
www.researchpress.com

This groundbreaking work, written for both professional and volunteer caregivers, provides exercises, activities and specific strategies for more successful caregiving, increased personal growth and effective stress management. In this thoughtfully written book, Dr. Larson explores the theory and practice of helping. He includes numerous case examples and verbatim disclosures of fellow caregivers that powerfully convey the joys and sorrows of the helpers journey.
292 pages Softcover
ISBN: 0-878223-44-4

10875 On Death & Dying
Dr. Elizabeth Kubler-Ross, author

MacMillan Publishing Company
175 Fifth Avenue
New York, NY 10010   e-mail: customerservice@mpsvirginia.com

646-307-5151
www.macmillan.com

Offers a new perspective on the terminally ill by refocusing on the patient as a human being and teacher, in hopes of learning from him or her about the final stages of life.
277 pages Paperback

10876 On Death and Dying
MacMillan Publishing Company
175 Fifth Avenue
New York, NY 10010

646-307-5151

A wonderful book offering information on how to deal and cope with death and dying.
Paperback

10877 Recovery from Bereavement
Rowman & Littlefield Publishers, Inc.
4501 Forbes Blvd.
Lanham, MD 20706

717-794-3800
800-462-6420
Fax: 717-794-3803
e-mail: orders@rowman.com
www.rowmanlittlefield.com

Outstanding authorities on loss and bereavement discuss the factors that play a role in successful recovery.
344 pages Softcover
ISBN: 1-568213-61-1

10878 Talking About Death - A Dialog Between Parent and Child
Earl A. Grollman, author

Beacon Press
25 Beacon Street
Boston, MA 02108-2824

617-742-2110
Fax: 617-723-3097
e-mail: bp_information@beacon.org
www.beacon.org

A compassionate guide for children and adults. Also includes listings of resources and organizations.
128 pages

10879 Treatment of Complicated Mourning
Dr. Therese A. Rando, author

Research Press
Dept. 11W
Champaign, IL 61826

217-352-3273
800-519-2707
Fax: 217-352-1221
e-mail: orders@researchpress.com
www.researchpress.com

This is the first book to focus specifically on complicated mourning, often referred to as pathological, unresolved, or abnormal grief. It provides caregivers with practical therapeutic strategies with and specific interventions that are necessary when traditional grief counseling is insufficient. The author provides critically important information on the prediction, identification, assessment, classification and treatment of complicated mourning.
768 pages Hardcover
ISBN: 0-878223-29-0

10880 What Helped Me When My Loved One Died
Beacon Press
25 Beacon Street
Boston, MA 02108-2824

617-742-2110
Fax: 617-723-3097
www.beacon.org

Children's Books

10881 Aarvy Aardvark Finds Hope
Donna O'Toole, author

Centering Corporation
7230 Maple Street
Omaha, NE 68134

402-553-1200
866-218-0101
www.centering.org

A best selling, illustrated, read-aloud story of the pain and sadness of loss and the hope of grief recovery.
80 pages Paperback
Janet Sieff, Executive Director

10882 Badger's Parting Gifts
Susan Varley, author

Compassion Books, Inc.
7036 State Highway 80 South
Burnsville, NC 28714-7569

828-675-5909
800-970-4220
Fax: 828-675-9687
e-mail: orders@compassionbooks.com
www.compassionbooks.com

A story of the death of old Badger. As the animals talk about Badger they remember the gift of skills and kindnesses he taught them.
23 pages Paperback
Bruce Greene, Director

10883 Compassion Books, Inc.
7036 State Highway 80 South
Burnsville, NC 28714-7569

828-675-5909
800-970-4220
Fax: 828-675-9687
e-mail: orders@compassionbooks.com
www.compassionbooks.com

Hand picked resources to help people through loss, grief and changes of all kinds. Carry over 400 books and videos on death and dying, bereavement and change, comfort and healing, hope and much more.
Bruce Greene, VP

10884 Fire in My Heart: Ice in My Veins
Enid Samuel Traisman, author

Compassion Books, Inc.
7036 State Highway 80 South
Burnsville, NC 28714-7569

828-675-5909
800-970-4220
Fax: 828-675-9687
e-mail: orders@compassionbooks.com
www.compassionbooks.com

A fill in scrapbook/journal to help teenagers experiencing a loss express feelings, sort out their thoughts and gather memories.
70 pages Paperback
Bruce Greene, Director

10885 Gentle Willow: A Story for Children About Dying
Joyce C. Mills, PhD, author

Magination Press (American Psychological Assoc.)
750 First Street NE
Washington, DC 20002-4242   202-336-5500
                                   800-374-2721
                                   TDD: 202-336-6123
                                   e-mail: order@apa.org
                                   www.apa.org

This book is written for children who may not survive their own illness or for children who know them. This tender and touching tale helps address feelings of disbelief, anger, and sadness, along with love and compassion.
2003 32 pages Hardcover
ISBN: 1-591470-71-7
Melba Vasquez, PhD, President

10886 Great Change
Compassion Books, Inc.
7036 State Highway 80 S   828-675-5909
Burnsville, NC 28714-7569   800-970-4220
                                 Fax: 828-675-9687
                                 e-mail: orders@compassionbooks.com
                                 www.compassionbooks.com

In this deeply moving Native American story, grandmother uses nature to explain death, the great change, to a grieving granddaughter.
32 pages Hardcover
Bruce Greene, Director

10887 Let's Talk About When A Parent Dies
Rosen Publishing Group's PowerKids Press
29 E 21st Street   212-777-3017
New York, NY 10010   800-237-9932
                                 Fax: 888-436-4643
                                 e-mail: customerservice@rosenpub.com
                                 www.rosenpublishing.com

This book guides children through the grieving process in a language they can understand. Recommended for grades K-4.

ISBN: 0-823923-09-6
Elizabeth Weitzman, Author

10888 Nana Upstairs and Nana Downstairs
Compassion Books
7036 State Highway 80 S   828-675-5909
Burnsville, NC 28714-7569   800-970-4220
                                 Fax: 828-675-9687
                                 e-mail: heal2grow@aol.com
                                 www.compassionbooks.com

This charming picture book recognizes that even after a family member dies the love connections continue in heart and home.
32 pages Paperback
Bruce Greene, Director

Magazines

10889 Compassion Books Catalog
Compassion Books
7036 State Highway 80 South   828-675-5909
Burnsville, NC 28714-7569   800-970-4220
                                 Fax: 828-675-9687
                                 e-mail: orders@compassionbooks.com
                                 www.compassionbooks.com

More than 400 books and videos to help with serious illness, death and dying, and losses of all kinds.
32 pages
Bruce Greene, VP

Pamphlets

10890 Approaching Grief
Richard Deitrick/Ann Armstrong Dailey, author

Children's Hospice International

1101 King Street   703-684-0330
Alexandria, VA 22314   800-242-4453
                                 e-mail: info@chionline.org
                                 www.chionline.org

Delves into the different stages of grief, guilt, depression, fear and anger. Also tells how children approach grief and ways in which to help your children get past the sorrow.
Ann Armstrong-Dailey, Founding Director/CEO
Rebecca Brant, Director

10891 Pregnancy After a Loss
Abbott Northwestern Hospital Parent Education
800 E 28th Street-Chicago Avenue   612-863-4000
Minneapolis, MN 55407

This booklet is written by a group of parents that have experienced a pregnancy after a loss, sensitively written with suggestions for coping with the fears and anxieties of the new pregnancy.

10892 Pregnancy Heartbreak: Unfulfilled Promises
Abbott Northwestern Hospital Parent Education
800 E 28th Street-Chicago Avenue   612-863-4000
Minneapolis, MN 55407

This handbook is written for parents who had to face the reality of the diagnosis and birth of a baby with life-threatening conditions.

Audio & Video

10893 Encounters with Grief
Fanlight Productions
C/O Icarus Films   718-488-8642
Brooklyn, NY 11201   800-876-1710
                                 Fax: 718-488-8642
                                 e-mail: info@fanlight.com
                                 www.fanlight.com

A mother who lost her teenage son, a woman widowed in her sixties and a man whose wife died at fifty-two discuss the emotional upheaval that followed and their moving perspectives on the process of recovery.
1992 13 Minutes
ISBN: 1-572950-91-9

10894 Grave Words: Tools for Discussing End of Life Choices
Maren Monson, MD, author

Fanlight Productions
C/O Icarus Films   718-488-8900
Brooklyn, NY 11201   800-876-1710
                                 Fax: 718-488-8642
                                 e-mail: info@fanlight.com
                                 www.fanlight.com

Blends humor, music and insightful interviews to confront the issues that arise in discussions between physicians and healthcare providers and patients about end-of-life care decisions.
1996 25 Minutes
ISBN: 1-572952-24-5

10895 Pitch of Grief
Eric Strange, author

Fanlight Productions
C/O Icarus Films   718-488-8900
Brooklyn, NY 11201   Fax: 718-488-8642
                                 e-mail: info@fanlight.com
                                 www.fanlight.com

Explores the process of grieving through interviews with four bereaved men and women, and is helpful to not only the grieving person, but for others within the family who have faced the loss of a loved one.
1985 28 Minutes
ISBN: 1-572950-18-8

10896 There Was a Child
Fred Simon, author

Fanlight Productions
C/O Icarus Film   718-488-8642
Brooklyn, NY 11201   800-876-1710
                                 Fax: 718-488-8642
                                 e-mail: orders@fanlight.com
                                 www.fanlight.com

Demonstrates the impact that losing a pregnancy, or the birth of a stillborn child, has had on three mothers and a father. Validates the emotions of parents who feel alone with their loss, while helping health care workers and families to give appropriate, meaningful support.

1991 32 Minutes
ISBN: 1-572950-48-X

10897 We Will Remember
Compassion Books, Inc.
7036 State Highway 80 South   828-675-5909
Burnsville, NC 28714-7569   800-970-4220
                                     Fax: 828-675-9687
                   e-mail: orders@compassionbooks.com
                              www.compassionbooks.com

A video meditation that uses the beauty of natural photography, soothing music and gentle words to give permission and encouragement in using the memories of the past for healing in the present.

11 minutes
Bruce Greene, Director

10898 When the Bough Breaks
Fanlight Productions
4196 Washington Street   617-469-4999
Boston, MA 02131-1731   800-937-4113
                                     Fax: 617-469-3379
                        e-mail: fanlight@fanlight.com
                                     www.fanlight.com

Based on the real story of a patient who experienced a stillbirth, these ten vignettes dramatically recreate her interactions with health care providers during the final weeks of pregnancy. Study guide included.

1992 71 Minutes
ISBN: 1-572951-08-7

Web Sites

10899 Compassionate Friends
                              www.compassionatefriends.org
Gives support to people who have experienced the death of a child.

10900 Hospice Association of America
                                            www.nahc.org
Promotes the concepts of hospice, a philosophy of health care which is expressed through the provision of a variety of medical and nonmedical services to terminally ill patients and their families.

10901 National Hospice & Palliative Care Organization
                                           www.nhpco.org
The nation's only advocate for terminally ill patients and their families. Founded in 1978, the NHPCO is the only organization devoted to hospice in the United States. Support is included from state hospice organizations, patients, families, communities, provider program members and professional/volunteer members. Represents hospice care interests to Congress, regulatory agencies, courts, voluntary organizations and the public.

10902 Share Pregnancy and Infant Loss Support, Inc.
                                     www.nationalshare.org
Offers studies, information, statistics, help and support to parents who have suffered the loss of a child.

B

C

D

DC Department of Health Maternal and Family Health Administration, 8823
DC Public Library Adaptive Services Division, 9709
DC Threshold Alliance for the Mentally Ill, 6076
DELCO Blind/Sight Center, 9629
DVH Quarterly, 10008
Daddy's Girl, 3580
Dads and Daughters, 3605
Daily Reflections: A Book of Reflections by AA Members for AA Members, 8381
Dallas Lighthouse for the Blind, 9657
Dallas/Ft.Worth Metroplex HPV Support Group, 10646
Dana Alliance for Brain Initiatives, 4064
Dana Farber Cancer Institute National Drug Discovery Group for AIDS Treatment, 345
Dana-Farber Institute: Department of Biostatistics and Computational Biology, 2242
Dancing Against the Darkness: A Journey Through America in the Age of AIDS, 406, 435
Dancing Cheek to Cheek, 10053
Dancing Without Music, 4404
Dano Cerebral: Guia Para Familias y Cuidadores, 4134
Darker Side of Tanning, 7759
Dartmouth Medical School: Microbiology Department, 3721
Dartmouth-Hitchcock Medical Center - Genetics and Development, 3511
David T Siegel Institute for Communicative Disorders, 4311
A Day At A Time, 2741
Day We Met Cindy, 4591
Day at a Time: Daily Reflections for Recovering People, 8382
Day by Day, 8383
A Day in the Life of a Child, 3914
Days of Healing, Days of Joy, 8384
Deadly Diet: Recovering from Anorexia & Bulimia, 3655
Deaf AIDS Project Family Service Foundation, 201
Deaf Artists of America, 4245, 4673
Deaf Association of Wyoming, 4298
Deaf Children Signers, 4732
Deaf Children in Public Schools Placement, Context, and Consequences, 4405
Deaf Culture Autobiographies, 4733
Deaf Culture Series, 4734
Deaf Culture Videotapes, 4700
Deaf Culture, Our Way, 4406
Deaf Culture: Suggested Readings, 4701
Deaf Empowerment, Emergence, Struggle and Rhetoric, 4407
Deaf Episcopalian, 4674
Deaf Heritage: A Narrative History of Deaf America, 4408
Deaf Heritage: Student Text and Workbook, 4409
Deaf History Unveiled: Interpretations from the New Scholarship, 4410
Deaf Life, 4646
Deaf Like Me, 4411
Deaf Mosaic Series, 4735
Deaf President Now! The 1988 Revolution at Gallaudet University, 4412
Deaf REACH, 4246
Deaf Sport: The Impact of Sports Within the Deaf Community, 4413
Deaf Sports Review, 4647
Deaf Students and the School-to-Work Transition, 4414
Deaf Studies Curriculum Guide, 4415
Deaf USA, 4648
Deaf Women: A Parade Through the Decades, 4416
Deaf Work, 4675
Deaf and Hard of Hearing Individuals, 4417
Deaf in America: Voices from a Culture, 4418
Deaf-Blind American, 4649
Deafness Research Foundation, 4247, 4781
Deafness and Child Development, 4419
Deafness and Communicative Disorders Branch, 4248
Deafness: 1993-2013, 4420
Deafness: A Fact Sheet, 4702
Deafness: A Personal Account, 4421

Deafness: An Autobiography, 4422
Deafness: Historical Perspectives, 4423
Deafness: Life and Culture II, 4424
Deafpride Advocate, 4676
Dealing with Mental Incapacity, 6255
Dean A McGee Eye Institute, 9866
Death Be Not Proud: A Memoir, 1948
Death and the Quest for Meaning, 10868
Death: The Final Stage of Growth, 10869
Deenie, 7464
Deep Brain Stimulation for Parkinson's Disease, 7131
Delaware Assocation for the Blind Department of Health & Social Services, 9537
Delaware County Branch of the Pennsylvania Association for the Blind, 9630
Delaware Department of Health and Social Services, 252
Delaware Division of Alcoholism, Drug Abuse and Mental Health, 8242
Delaware Division of Libraries: Library for the Blind and Physically Handicapped, 9707
Delaware FFMCH, 6074
Delaware SIDS Alliance, 8821
Delaware Valley Chapter of the National Hemophilia Foundation, 4947
Delicate Balance: Living Successfully with Chronic Illness, 3794
Delware Valley Brain Tumor Support Group at Jefferson, 1923
Dementia Care Practice Recommendations Phases 1 and 2, 945
Denial, 8623
Dental Care for the Patient with Parkinson's Disease, 7132
Dental Tips for Diabetics, 3445
Dental Treatment of Patients with Gilles de la Tourette Syndrome, 9100
Dentists Concerned for Dentists, 8261, 8779
Denver Childrens Hospital, 3031
Denver Support Group: National Ataxia Foundation, 1436
Department of Alcohol and Drug Programs, 8239
Department of Alcoholism and Substance Abuse, 8248
Department of Epidemiology and Health Policy Research: University of Florida, 327
Department of Health, 8270
Department of Health and Human Services, 8885
Department of Health and Welfare Department Of Health And Welfare, 8247
Department of Human Services, 8848
Department of Institutions, Alcohol and Drug Abuse Division, 8265
Department of Mental Health and Mental Retardation, Alcohol & Drug Service, 8284
Department of Ophthalmology Information Line, 9895
Department of Ophthalmology/Eye and Ear Infirmary, 9867
Department of Pediatrics Medical College of Georgia, 3038
Department of Pediatrics, Division of Rheumatology, 1145
Department of Public Health and Human Services, 8867
Department of Public Health: Adult and Child Health Division, 8844
Department of Public Health: Division of Substance Abuse and Health, 8252
Department of Public Instruction: Division of Alcoholism and Drug Abuse, 8266
Department of Reproductive Genetics: Magee Women's Hospital, 1744
Department of Social Services: Division of Substance Abuse, 8286
Department of State Health Offices, 8903
Department of Veterans Affairs Medical Center: Sioux Falls, 10371
Departments of Neurology & Neurosurgery: University of California, San Francisco, 8138
Depression Sourcebook, 6371
Depression and Bipolar Support Alliance, 6367
Depression and Dementia in Parkinson's Disease, 7133

Depression and Recovery from Chemical Dependency, 8624
Depression and its Treatment, 6372
Depression is a Treatable Illness: A Patients Guide, 6393
Depressive Illnesses: Treatments Bring New Hope, 6373
Derma Doctor, 7803
Dermatitis Herpetiformis, 2575
Dermatology Focus, 7749
Dermatology Foundation, 2182, 7718, 7804
Dermatology World, 7750
Des Moines Division: VA Central Iowa Health Care System, 10259
Desert Southwest Chapter 1 National Multiple Sclerosis Society, 6514
Desert Southwest Chapter 2 National Multiple Sclerosis Society, 6515
Desert Southwest Chapter 3 National Multiple Sclerosis Society, 6556
Desert Storm Justice Foundation: Florida, 10228
Desert Storm Justice Foundation: Illinois, 10246
Desert Storm Justice Foundation: Minnesota, 10296
Desert Storm Justice Foundation: Virginia, 10297, 10406
Desert Storm Veterans of Florida, 10229
Desert Storm Veterans of North Carolina, 10336
Desferal Q&A, 2909
Design of Rehabilitation Services in Psychiatric Hospital Settings, 6256
Designs on Life, 5424
Destination Unlimited, 10117
Detaching with Love, 8625
Detachment, 8626
Detroit Subregional Library for the Blind and Physically Handicapped, 9775
Detroit Support Group: National Ataxia Foundation, 1448
Detroit VA Medical Center John D. Dingell VA Medical Center, 10288
Developing Chemical Dependency Services for Black People, 8385
Developing Cognition in Young Children Who are Deaf, 4703
Developing IEPs Under the New Idea Regulations, 1704
Developing Support Groups for Individuals with Early-Stage Alzheimer's Disease, 906
Developing a Functional and Longitudinal Individual Plan, 1693
Development of Behavioral and Emotional Problems in TS, 9101
Development of Social Skills by Blind and Visually Impaired Students, 9926
Developmental Delays and Developmental Disorders, 8938
Developmental Evaluation Clinic, 3512
Developmental Medicine Center (DMC), 3513
Developmental Medicine Center Children's Hospital Boston, 346
Diabetes, 3424, 3434
Diabetes & Exercise Video, 3463
Diabetes & Pregnancy: What to Expect, 3366
Diabetes A to Z, 3367
Diabetes Advisor, 3441
Diabetes Care, 3435
Diabetes Care Made Easy, 3368
Diabetes Control Program, 3314
Diabetes Dateline, 3442, 3446
Diabetes Dictionary, 3472
Diabetes Education Goals, 3369
Diabetes Education and Research Center The Franklin House, 3325
Diabetes Educator, 3443
Diabetes Exercise and Sports Association, 3149, 3473
Diabetes Forecast, 3436
Diabetes Low-Fat & No-Fat Meals in Minutes, 3370
Diabetes Medical Nutrition Therapy, 3371
Diabetes Mellitus: A Practical Handbook, 3372
Diabetes Research and Training Center: University of Alabama at Birmingham, 3326
Diabetes Self-Management, 3373
Diabetes Society, 3353
Diabetes Society of Santa Clara Valley, 3165
Diabetes Sourcebook, 3374

E

H

I

K

L

M

N

National Treatment Consortium for Alcohol and Other Drugs, 8314

National Tuberous Sclerosis Association, 9339, 9349

National Veterans Services Fund, 10193, 10436, 10478

National Volunteer Training Center for Sub CSAP Division of Communications Programs, 8316

National Volunteer Training Center for Substance Abuse Prevention, 8315

National Women's Health Information Center, 3616

National Women's Health Network, 3718

National Women's Health Resource Center, 5402, 9002, 9020

National Womens Health Resource Center, 3720

Nationwide Survey of Sudden Infant Death Syndrome (SIDS) Service, 8942

Natural Attenuation for Groundwater Remediation, 10439

Navaho Nation K'E Project Children and Families Advocacy Corp, 6123

Navaho Nation K'E Project: Tuba City Children & Families Advocacy Corp, 6061

Navaho Nation K'E Project: Winslow Children & Families Advocacy Corp, 6062

Navajo Nation K'E Project: Shiprock Children & Families Advocacy Corp, 6124

Navajo Nation Office Special Education & R ehabilitation Services, 6185

Navajo Nation Office of Special Education & Rehabilitation Services (OSERS), 6186

Navigating the Social World: A Curriculum for Individuals with Asperger's Syndrome, 1665

Nebraska Chapter of the National Hemophilia Foundation, 4934

Nebraska Department of Health Perinatal Child and Adolescent Health, 8869

Nebraska Information Service, 1762

Nebraska Kidney Association, 5599

Nebraska Library Commission Talking Book and Braille Services, 9798

Nebraska Organ Retrieval System, 9204

Nebraska SIDS Foundation University of Nebraska Medical Center, 8870

Need to Know, 9113

Negotiating the Special Education Maze: A Guide for Parents and Teachers, 7988

Nemours Childrens Clinic, 3037

Neuro-Oncology Information and Support Group, 1843

Neurobiology of Autism, 1666

Neurocognitive Aspects of CFS, 2826

Neurofibromatosis, 6823, 6859, 6864, 6870

Neurofibromatosis Association of Arizona, 6827

Neurofibromatosis Foundation: Colorado, 6860

Neurofibromatosis Kansas and Central Plains, 6843

Neurofibromatosis Society of Ontario, 6824

Neurofibromatosis Support Network, 6861

Neurofibromatosis Type 2: Information for Patients and Families, 6871

Neurofibromatosis: Mid-Atlantic, 6845

Neurofibromatosis: Minnesota, 6847

Neurofibromatosis: New England, 6846

Neurological Center of Iowa, 1875

Neurological Science Federation, 6825

Neurological Support Group of St. Luke's Hospital, 1891

Neurology Channel, 987, 1080, 2555, 2751, 3837, 4218, 5207, 6503, 6682, 6816, 6880, 7184, 7612, 7921, 8186, 9071

Neurology Institute, 8132

Neurology Research Center Helen Hayes Hospital, 7537

Neurology of Down Syndrome, 3571

Neuromuscular Dis. of Infancy, Childhood & Adolesece: A Clinician's Approach, 6705

Neuromuscular Treatment Center: Univ. of Texas Southwestern Medical Center, 6607

Neuromuscular and ALS Center The Clinical Academic Building, 1040

Neuropsychological Assessment: What it Does & Does Not Do, 4203

Neuropsychological Performance in Adults with TS, 9114

Neuropsychological Rehabilitation Suggestions/Techniques, 2812

Neuropsychology and Parkinson's Disease, 7147

Neuropsychology of Attention and Memory, 4184

Neurosarcoidosis, 7325

Neurosarcoidosis or Multiple Sclerosis?, 7326

Neuroscience Institute Brain Tumor Hotline, 1844

Neuroscience Institute at Mercy Hospital, 6862

Neurosciences Institute of the Neurosciences Research Program, 872

Neurosurgical Service, 10615

Neurotrophic Factors in Parkinson's Disease, 7148

Nevada Alliance for the Mentally Ill, 6116

Nevada Department of Human Resources: Health Program Section, 275

Nevada Donor Network, 9205

Nevada PEP, 6224

Nevada State Health Division Bureau of Family Health Services, 8871

Nevada State Library and Archives, 9801

Never the Twain Shall Meet: The Communications Debate, 4503

Never to Be a Mother, 5452

The New ADD in Adults Workbook, 1532

New Beginnings: The Blind Children's Cente, 9880

New Beginnings: The Blind Children's Center, 9879

New Brunswick Innovation Foundation, 2029

New Challenge: Responding to Families, 6327

A New Civil Right: Telecommunications Equality for Deaf and Hard of Hearing, 4358

New England AIDS Education & Training Center (NEHEC), 269

New England AIDS Education & Training Ctr., 552

New England AIDS Education and Training Center, 225

New England Area Support Group: National Ataxia Foundation, 1447

New England Health Care System, 10281

New England Hemophilia Association, 4929

New England Hemophilia Association Newsletter, 5045

New England Medical Center: ALS Laboratory, 1041

New England Organ Bank Connecticut, 9181

New England Organ Bank Maine, 9195

New England Organ Bank Massachusetts, 9198

New England Organ Bank New Hampshire, 9206

New England Organ Bank Rhode Island, 9223

New England Organ Bank Vermont, 9228

New England Region: Helen Keller National Center, 9579

New England Regional Genetics Group, 1748

New Expectations, 3584

New Eyes for the Needy, 9505

New Food Labels, 608

New Hampshire Cancer Pain Initiative, 2119

New Hampshire Chapter NSCIA, 8052

New Hampshire Cystic Fibrosis Care Teaching and Research Center, 3075

New Hampshire Department of Health and Human Services, 276

New Hampshire Lupus Foundation, 5941

New Hampshire SIDS Alliance, 8872

New Hampshire SIDS Program, 8873

New Hampshire State Library, 9802

New Hope for Kids Wish Program, 10829

New Jersey Alliance for the Mentally Ill, 6122

New Jersey Department of Health: Child Health Program, 8874

New Jersey Department of Health: Division of AIDS Prevention & Control, 277

New Jersey Institute of Technology Center for Biomedical Engineering, 3980

New Jersey Library for the Blind and Handicapped, 9804

New Jersey Medical School, 3078

New Jersey Medical School: National Tuberculosis Center, 9268

New Jersey Metroplitan Turner Syndrome Society Association, 9375

New Jersey Parkinson's Disease Information Center, 7099

New Jersey Pregnancy Risk Information Service, 1763

New Jersey SIDS Alliance, 8875

New Jersey Woman AIDS Network, 278

New Language of Toys: Teaching Communication Skills to Children..., 7989

New Mexico Alliance for the Mentally Ill, 6125

New Mexico Branch, 9301

New Mexico Chapter of the Myasthenia Gravis Foundation of America, 6772

New Mexico Donor Services, 9209

New Mexico Health Department: Public Health Division, 279

New Mexico Industries for the Blind, 9598

New Mexico SIDS Information and Counseling Program, 8878

New Mexico State Library for the Blind and Physically Handicapped, 9805

New Parents, 3572

New Set of Fears, a New Set of Hopes, 3585

New Sjogren's Syndrome Handbook, 7698

New Start News, 9249

New What Do You Do When You See a Blind Person?, 10125

New York Alliance for the Mentally Ill, 6128

New York Ambassador National Ataxia Foundation, 1455

New York Brain Tumor Support Group, 1910

New York Chapter of the American Association of Kidney Patients, 5612

New York Chapter of the Arthritis Foundation, 1138

New York City Center for SIDS, 8881

New York College of Osteopathic Medicine, 7101

New York Department of Health, Office of Public Health: AIDS Institute, 280

New York Male Reproductive Center: Sexual Dysfunction Unit, 5269

New York Obesity/Nutrition Research Center, 6892

New York Obesity/Nutrition Research Center (ONRC), 6943

New York Organ Donor Network, Inc, 9212

New York State Center for SIDS: School of Social Welfare, 8882

New York State Talking Book & Braille Library, New York State Library, DOE, 9809

New York University Cancer Institute New York University Medical Center, 2272

New York University General Clinical Research Center, 5220

New York University Medical Center Auxiliary of Tisch Hospital, 5177

New York University Medical Center Head Trauma Program, 4066

Newcomer Asks, 8698

Newport News Public Library System, 9840

News & Notes, 6318

News & Review, 7121

News Across Our Horizons, 1194

News Report, 5238

News from the Border: A Mother's Memoir of Her Autistic Son, 1667

NewsLine, 1780

Newsletter of American Hearing Research, 4683

Newsletter of the Central Pennsylvania Chapter, 1195

Newsletter: SIDS, 8935

Newsline, 4684

Newsline for the Blind, 10026

Next Step, 4504

Niagara Cerebral Palsy, 2679

Nick Joins In, 7990

Nick's Mission, 4617

Nicotine Addiction and Cigarettes, 8699

Night Kites, 417, 438

Night Light: A Book of Nighttime Meditations, 8441

Night-Side: CFS and the Illness Experience, 2784

No Fears, No Tears, 10768

No Fears, No Tears: 13 Years Later, 10769

No Less a Woman, 2376

No Longer Immune: A Counselor's Guide to AIDS, 418

No Smoking Coloring Book, 8700

No Smoking: Lungs At Work, 8701

No Sound, 4505

No Walls of Stone: An Anthology of Literature by Deaf Writers, 4506

No-Hysterectomy Option, 5453

No. Colorado FFCMH, 6070

Nobody Knows!, 2738

Nocturnal Asthma, 1371

Noise Can Be Harmful to Your Health, 4716

O

U

W

X

Y

Z

Alabama

AIDS Alabama, 372
Alabama Ambassador: National Ataxia Foundation, 1427
Alabama Association of the Deaf, 4276
Alabama Chapter of the American Association of Kidney Patients, 5554
Alabama Chapter of the Arthritis Foundation, 1090
Alabama Chapter of the Myasthenia Gravis Foundation of America, 6750
Alabama Chapter of the National Hemaphilia Foundation, 4912
Alabama Council of the Blind, 9517
Alabama Department of Public Health, 238
Alabama Education of Homeless Children and Youth Program, 6183
Alabama Head Injury Foundation, 4010
Alabama Head Injury Foundation Helpline, 4079
Alabama Organ Center, 9173
Alabama Radio Reading Service Network, 9686
Alabama Regional Library for the Blind and Physically Handicapped, 9687
Alabama Support Group: National Ataxia Foundation, 1428
Alzheimer's Association: North Alabama Chapter, 654
Alzheimer's Association: Southeast Alabama Chapter, 655
Alzheimer's Association: Southwest Alabama Chapter, 656
Alzheimer's Disease Center: University of Alabama at Birmingham, 856
American Cancer Society: Alabama, 2034
American Diabetes Association: Alabama, 3154
American Lung Association of Alabama, 5798
American Lung Association of Alabama, 9270
American Society for Reproductive Medicine, 3713
American Society for Reproductive Medicine, 5344
Arthritis and Musculoskeletal Center: UAB Shelby Interdisciplinary Biomedical Rese, 1140
Autism Society of Alabama, 1573
Autism Society of North Alabama, 1574
Birmingham VA Medical Center: Research and Development, 2188
Breast Cancer Resource Foundation of Alabama, 2189
Bureau of Family Health Services: Alabama Department of Public Health, 8807
CCFA Alabama Chapter, 2931
Cardiovascular Research and Training Center University of Alabama, 4815
Center for Neuroimmunology: University of Alabama at Birmingham, 6605
Centers for AIDS Research: University of Alabama at Birmingham, 305
Civitan International Research Center, 4309
Diabetes Research and Training Center: University of Alabama at Birmingham, 3326
Division of Mental Illness and Substance Abuse Community Programs, 8234
Division of Rehabilitation: Montgomery, 10589
Friends-In-Art, 9466
General Clinical Research Center: UAB, 306
Gulf War Veterans of Alabama, 10195
Hemophilia Clinic: Childrens' Rehabilitation Service, 4985
Horizons Schools, 10659
Houston Love Memorial Library, 9688
Huntsville Subregional Library for the Blind and Physically Handicapped, 9689
Juvenile Diabetes Research Foundation: Birmingham, 3155
Knollwoodpark Hospital Sleep Disorders Cen, 7835
Knollwoodpark Hospital Sleep Disorders Center, 7834
Leukemia and Lymphoma Society: Alabama Chapter, 2035
Library and Resource Center for the Blind and Physically Handicapped, 9690
Lupus Foundation of America: Alabama Chapter, 5892
Lyme Disease Network Support Group of Alabama: Mobile Chapter, 9032
Magic Moments, 10826

NNFF Alabama Affiliate, 6826
National Alliance on Mental Illness of Alabama: NAMI Alabama, 6056
National Federation of the Blind: Alabama, 9518
National Kidney Foundation of Alabama, 5555
National Multiple Sclerosis Society: Alabama Chapter, 6511
National Mutiple Sclerosis Society: Alabama Chapter, 6512
National Society for MVP and Dysautonomia, 4866
National Spinal Cord Injury Statistical Center, 8033
National Spinal Cord Injury Support Groups, 8073
Pediatric Brain Tumor Support Group, 1822
Pull-thru Network, 3877
Pushin On: RRTC on Secondary Conditions of Spinal, 8062
Sickle Cell Foundation of Greater Montgomery, 7665
Specialized Center of Research in Ischemic Heart Disease, 4841
Spina Bifida Association of Alabama, 7930
Stroke Research and Treatment Center UAB Medical Center, 8141
Tuscaloosa Subregional Library for the Blind & Physically Handicapped, 9691
United Cerebral Palsy of Alabama, 2599
United Cerebral Palsy of East Central Alabama, 2600
United Cerebral Palsy of Greater Birmingha m, 2601
United Cerebral Palsy of Huntsville & Tennessee Valley, 2602
United Cerebral Palsy of Mobile, 2603
United Cerebral Palsy of Northwest Alabama, 2604
United Cerebral Palsy of West Alabama, 2605
University Alzheimer Center University of Alabama at Birmingham, 878
University of Alabama At Birmingham Comprehensive Cancer Center, 2190
University of Alabama Birmingham, 7420
University of Alabama Speech and Hearing Center, 4335
University of Alabama at Birmingham Parkinsons Disease Center, 7087
University of Alabama at Birmingham: Congenital Heart Disease Center, 4843
University of Alabama at Birmingham: National Cooperative Drug/AIDS, 307
Veterans Administration Medical Center: Alabama, 10196
Veterans Association Medical Center, 10197

Alaska

AARP Alaska State Office, 29
Alaska Department of Health and Social Services: AIDS/STD Program, 239
Alaska Gulf War Syndrome Referral Coordinator, 10198
Alaska State Library Talking Book Center, 9692
Alaskan Statewide AIDS Helpline, 376
Alzheimer's Disease Resource Agency of Alaska, 657
American Cancer Society: Alaska, 2036
American Diabetes Association: Alaska, 3156
American Lung Association of Alaska, 5799
American Lung Association of Alaska, 9271
Asthma and Allergy Foundation of America: Alaska Chapter, 1278
Client Assistance Program: Anchorage, 10590
Lupus Foundation of America: Alaska Chapter, 5893
National Alliance for the Mentally Ill (NA MI) Alaska, 6184
National Alliance on Mental Illness of Alaska, 6057
National Federation of the Blind: Alaska, 9519
National Multiple Sclerosis Society: Alaska Chapter, 6513
Office of Alcohol and Substance Abuse Department of Health and Social Services, 8235
SIDS Information and Counseling Program: Alaska Department of Health, 8808
United Cerebral Palsy of Alaska/PARENTS, 2606
Veterans Adm. Medical Center: Anchorage Outpatient Clinic, 10199

Arizona

AARP Arizona: Phoenix Collier Center, 30
Alcoholism and Drug Abuse: Office of Community Behavioral Health, 8236
Alzheimer's Association: Desert Southwest Chapter, 658
Alzheimer's Association: Northern Arizona, 659
Alzheimer's Association: Northern Nevada, 660
Alzheimer's Association: Southern Arizona, 661
Alzheimer's Association: Southern Arizona Region, 662
American Cancer Society: Arizona, 2037
American Council on Alcohol Problems, 8195
American Diabetes Association: Arizona, 3157
American Diabetes Association: Arizona, Border Area, 3158
American Diabetes Association: Atlanta Met, 3159
American Diabetes Association: Northern Arizona, 3160
American Fibromyalgia Syndrome Association, 3779
American Liver Foundation Arizona Chapter, 5718
American Lung Association of Arizona, 5800
American Lung Association of Arizona/New Mexico, 9272
Arizona Association of the Deaf, 4277
Arizona Brain Tumor Support Group, 1823
Arizona Center for the Blind and Visually Impaired, 9520
Arizona Chapter of the ALS Association, 991
Arizona Chapter of the National Parkinson Foundation, 7047
Arizona Department of Health Services, 240
Arizona Heart Institute, 4808
Arizona Industries for the Blind, 9521
Arizona Kidney Foundation, 5556
Arizona SIDS Founation, 8809
Arizona State Braille and Talking Book Library, 9693
Arizona Telemedicine Program, 7273
Arizona United Spinal Cord Association Samaritan Rehab Institute R-2, 8039
Arthritis Foundation: Central Arizona Chapter, 1091
Arthritis Foundation: Greater Southwest Chapter, 1092
Arthritis Foundation: New Mexico Chapter, 1117
Autism Society of Pima County, 1575
Body Positive HIV and AIDS Research and Re Southwest Center for HIV/AIDS, 254
Brain Injury Association of Arizona, 4012
Brain Injury Association of Arizona, 4080
CCFA Southwest Chapter: Arizona, 2932
Center for Neurodevelopmental Studies, 1624
Center for Neurology & Stroke Baptist Hospital Office, 2542
Central Arizona Chapter of the American Association of Kidney Patients, 5557
Commission on Accreditation of Rehabilitation Services, 21
Cystic Fibrosis Center: Phoenix Childrens Hospital, 3021
Desert Southwest Chapter 1 National Multiple Sclerosis Society, 6514
Desert Southwest Chapter 2 National Multiple Sclerosis Society, 6515
Do it Now Foundation, 8300
Eating Disorders Anonymous, 3607
Fibromyalgia Network, 3792
Flagstaff City Coconino County Public Library, 9694
HPV Support Groups: Arizona, 10591
International Holistic Center, 2038
Jim L Walker: Arizona Chapter of the Myasthenia Gravis Foundation of America, 6751
Juvenile Diabetes Research Foundation: Phoenix Chapter, 3161
Leukemia and Lymphoma Society: Mountain States Chapter, 2039
Life Development Institute, 10547
Life Development Institute, 10660
Lupus Foundation of America: Greater Arizona Chapter, 5894
Lupus Foundation of America: Southern Arizona Chapter, 5895
Make-A-Wish Foundation of America, 10827
Mayo Clinic Scottsdale Center for Scleroderma Care & Research, 7415

Mentally Ill Kids In Distress, 6058
Mentally Ill Kids in Distress Sue Gilbertson, 6059
Mountain State Regional Hemophilia Center
  University of Arizona Health Sciences Ce, 4993
Muscular Dystrophy Association, 6685
Muscular Dystrophy Association, 6694
National Alliance on Mental Illness of Arizona, 6060
National Federation of the Blind: Arizona, 9522
National Federation of the Blind: Blind/Deaf
  Division, 9495
National Network of Learning Disabled Adults,
  10567
National Sjogren's Syndrome Foundation NSSA,
  7695
Navaho Nation K'E Project: Tuba City Children &
  Families Advocacy Corp, 6061
Navaho Nation K'E Project: Winslow Children &
  Families Advocacy Corp, 6062
Navajo Nation Office of Special Education &
  Rehabilitation Services (OSERS), 6186
Neurofibromatosis Association of Arizona, 6827
New Mexico Chapter of the Myasthenia Gravis
  Foundation of America, 6772
Northern Arizona Branch:Phoenix Area, 9273
Office of Chronic Disease Prevention and Nutrition
  Services, 6895
Office of Womens And Childrens Health: Alabama
  Department of Health, 8810
Phoenix Area Support Group: National Ataxi
  Foundation, 1429
Phoenix Public Library: Special Needs Section, 9695
Prader-Willi Syndrome Arizona Association
  Prader-Willi Syndrome Association, 7207
Prader-Willi Syndrome Arizona Association: Phoenix
  Area, 7206
RESOLVE of Valley of the Sun, 5349
Ruth E Golding Clinical Pharmacokinetics
  Laboratory, 8324
Scleroderma Foundation: Arizona Chapter, 7376
Southern Arizona Brain Tumor Support Group, 1824
Southern Arizona Branch: Tucson Area, 9274
Southwest Association for Education in Biomedical
  Research, 2191
Spina Bifida Association of Arizona, 7931
St. Joseph's Hemophilia Center, 5009
Teratology OTIS, 1749
Tucson Interfaith HIV/AIDS Network (TIHAN), 241
Tucson Support Group: National Ataxia Foundation,
  1430
Turner's Syndrome Society: Palmetto Area, 9385
United Cerebral Palsy of Central Arizona, 2607
United Cerebral Palsy of Southern Arizona, 2608
University of Arizona Cancer Center, 2192
Veterans Adm. Medical Center: Arizona Carl T.
  Hayden VA Medical Center, 10200
Veterans Adm. Medical Center: Tucson Southern
  Arizona VA Health Care System, 10201

Arkansas

AARP Arkansas State Office: Little Rock, 31
Alzheimer's Arkansas Programs and Services, 663
Alzheimer's Association: Western Arkansas Chapter,
  664
American Cancer Society: Arkansas, 2040
American Diabetes Association: Arkansas, 3162
American Lung Association of Arkansas, 5801
American Lung Association of Arkansas, 9275
Arkansas Association of the Deaf, 4278
Arkansas Chapter of the Myasthenia Gravis
  Foundation of America, 6752
Arkansas Cystic Fibrosis Center Arkansas Children's
  Hospital, 3022
Arkansas Department of Health AIDS Prevention
  Program, 242
Arkansas Department of Health: SIDS Information &
  Counseling Program, 8811
Arkansas FFCMH Jane Burgan, 6063
Arkansas Lighthouse for the Blind, 9524
Arkansas Regional Library for the Blind and
  Physically Handicapped, 9696
Arkansas Regional Organ Recovery Agency, 9175
Arthritis Foundation: Arkansas Chapter, 1093
Brain Injury Association of Arkansas, 4013

Brain Injury Association of Arkansas Helpl ine, 4081
Central Arkansas Veterans Healthcare Syste Eugene J.
  Towbin Healthcare Center, 10202
Disability Rights Center of Arkansas, 10592
Donor Network of Arizona, 9174
Gulf War Veterans of Arkansas, 10203
Health Resource, 2041
Hemophilia Foundation of Arkansas, 4913
John L McClellan Memorial Veterans' Hospital
  Research Office, 4830
Juvenile Diabetes Research Foundation: Northwest
  Arkansas Branch, 3163
Library for the Blind and Handicapped, Southwest,
  9697
Lions World Services for the Blind Lions Clubs
  International, 9474
Lupus Foundation of America: Arkansas Chapter,
  5896
NAMI Arkansas, 6064
NNFF Arkansas Affilaite, 6828
National Federation of the Blind: Arkansas, 9525
National Kidney Foundation of Arkansas, 5558
National Multiple Sclerosis Society: Arkansas
  Chapter, 6516
Office of Alcohol and Drug Abuse Prevention, 8237
Prader-Willi Arkansas Association Prader-Willi
  Syndrome Association, 7208
RESOLVE Affiliate of Northwest Arkansas, 5350
Research and Training Center for Persons Who are
  Deaf or Hard of Hearing, 4325
Spina Bifida Association of Arkansas, 7932
United Cerebral Palsy of Central Arkansas, 2609
United Cerebral Palsy of South Arkansas, 2610
Veterans Adm. Medical Center: Fayetville, 10204
Veterans Adm. Medical Center: Little Rock, 10205

California

1-800-BRAILLE, 9890
AARP California State Office: Pasadena, 32
AARP California State Office: Sacramento, 33
AEGIS AIDS Education Global Information System,
  371
AIDS Clinical Trials Unit CARES Clinic, 308
AIDS.ORG, 179
ALS Association Free Standing Support Groups, 1045
ALS Association: Bay Area Chapter, 992
ALS Association: Greater Los Angeles Chapter, 993
ALS Association: Greater Sacramento Chapter, 994
ALS Association: Greater San Diego CIO, 995
ALS Center at UCSF, 1032
Adopt-A-Special-Kid America, 5342
Adult Research Opportunities, 309
Advocates 4 Health: Tick-borne Disease Self-Help
  Group, 9028
Aids, Medicine and Miracles, 243
Alcohol Drug Treatment Referral, 8339
Alcohol Research Group Public Health Institute, 8296
Alta Bates Summit Medical Center, 6161
Alzheimer's Association San Diego/Imperial
  Chapter, 665
Alzheimer's Association: California Central Chapter:
  Ventura County Office, 666
Alzheimer's Association: Greater North Valley
  Chapter, 668
Alzheimer's Association: Greater Sacramento, 667
Alzheimer's Association: Los Angeles Chapter, 669
Alzheimer's Association: Monterey County Chapter,
  670
Alzheimer's Association: North Bay Chapter, 671
Alzheimer's Association: Orange County Chapter,
  672
Alzheimer's Association: Riverside/San Bernardino
  Counties Chapter, 673
Alzheimer's Association: San Francisco Bay Area
  Chapter, 674
Alzheimer's Association: Santa Barbara Central Coast
  Chapter, 675
Alzheimer's Association: Santa Cruz County Chapter,
  676
Alzheimer's Disease Center: University of California,
  Davis, 855
American Academy of Ophthalmology, 9441

American Association of Gynecologic Laproscopists,
  3712
American Cancer Society Santa Clara County /
  Silicon Valley / Central Coast Region, 2042
American Cancer Society: Central Los Angeles, 2043
American Cancer Society: East Bay/Metro Region,
  2044
American Cancer Society: Fresno/Madera Counties,
  2045
American Cancer Society: Inland Empire, 2046
American Cancer Society: Orange County, 2047
American Cancer Society: Sacramento County, 2048
American Cancer Society: San Diego County, 2049
American Cancer Society: San Francisco County,
  2050
American Cancer Society: San Jose Prostate Cancer
  Support Group, 2318
American Cancer Society: Santa Maria Valley, 2051
American Cancer Society: Sonoma County, 2052
American Chronic Pain Association, 2538
American Chronic Pain Association, 2841
American Diabetes Association: California, 3164
American Liver Foundation Greater Los Angeles
  Chapter, 5719
American Liver Foundation Northern CA Chapter,
  5720
American Liver Foundation San Diego Chapte r, 5721
American Lung Association of California, 5802
American Lung Association of California, 9276
American Narcolepsy Association, 7817
Amyotrophic Lateral Sclerosis Toll Free Hotline,
  1047
Arthritis Foundation: Northern California Chapter,
  1094
Arthritis Foundation: San Diego Area Chapter, 1095
Arthritis Foundation: Southern California Chapter,
  1096
Asian & Pacific Islander Wellness Center Community
  HIV/AIDS Services, 188
Asian and Pacific Island Wellness Center, 189
Association for the Cure of Cancer of the Prostate,
  2001
Asthma and Allergy Foundation of America:
  Southern California Chapter, 572
Asthma and Allergy Foundation of America:
  Southern California Chapter, 1279
Autism Research Institute, 1566
Autism Society of California, 1576
Bay Area LE Foundation, 5897
Bay Area Turner Syndrome Society, 9356
Bees-Stealy Research Foundation, 4811
Bereavement Group for Children, 1825
Bereavement Group for Children, 10858
Blind Childrens Center, 9698
Braille Institute Desert Center, 9857
Braille Institute Library Services, 9699
Braille Institute Orange County Center, 9858
Braille Institute Santa Barbara Center Braille Institute
  of Los Angeles, 9859
Braille Institute Sight Center, 9860
Braille Institute Youth Center, 9861
Braille Institute of America Library, 9455
Brain Injury Association of California Hel pline, 4082
Brain Tumor Society, 1826
Brain Tumor Support Group: Duarte, 1827
Brain Tumor Support Group: Fresno, 1828
Brain Tumor Support Group: Fullerton, 1829
Brain Tumor Support Group: Newport Beach, 1830
Brain Tumor Support Group: Orange, 1831
Brain Tumor Support Group: Redding, 1832
Brain Tumor Support Group: Sacramento, 1833
Brain Tumor Support Group: San Diego, 1834
Brain Tumor Support Group: San Francisco, 1835
Brain Tumor Support Group: Santa Barbara, 1836
Brain Tumor Support Group: Stanford, 1837
Brain Tumor Support Group: Westlake Village, 1838
Brain Tumor/Pituitary Patient Support Group, 1839
Breast Cancer Action, 2003
Burnham Institute Cancer Center The Burnham
  Institute for Medical Resear, 2193
CCFA California: Greater Los Angeles Chapter, 2934
California Ambassador: National Ataxia Foundation,
  1431
California Association of Persian Gulf Veterans,
  10206

California Collaborative Treatment Group CCTG Data Center, 244

California Department of Health Services Office of Aids, 245

California Institute for Medical Research, 7085

California Lyme Disease Association, 9025

California SIDS Program, 8812

California State Library Braille and Talking Book Library, 9700

California Teratogen Information Service UC San Diego School of Medicine Dept of, 1743

California Transplant Donor Network, 9176

California Women's Commission on Alcohol and Drug Dependencies, 8238

Cancer Control Society and Cancer Book House, 2053

Cancer Federation, 2184

Cancer Support Community, 2322

Cancervive, 2323

Canine Companions for Independence, 9456

Celiac Disease Foundation, 2563

Center for AIDS Prevention Studies AIDS Research Institute University of C, 310

Center for Adaptive Learning, 10661

Center for Cancer Survival, 2324

Center for Interdisciplinary Research in Immunology and Diseases at UCLA, 311

Centers for AIDS Research: North-Central California, 312

Centers for AIDS Research: USCD Center for AIDS Research, 313

Centers for AIDS Research: University of California, Los Angeles, 314

Central California Chapter National Multiple Sclerosis Society, 6517

Central California Chapter of the National Hemophilia Foundation, 4914

Cerebrospinal Fluid Shunt Systems for the Management of Hydrocephalus, 5166

Children Affected by AIDS Foundation, 196

Children Living with Illness, 1840

Children of Deaf Adults, 4350

Children's Gaucher Research Fund, 3952

Children's Hospital of Los Angeles, 3023

Children's Hospital of Orange County, 3019

Children's Liver Association for Support S ervices, 5747

Childrens Hospital at Oakland, 3024

City of Hope Comprehensive Cancer Research Center, 2194

City of Hope National Medical Center Beckman Research Institute, 2054

City of Hope National Medical Center Drug Discover/AIDS Group, 315

Clearinghouse for Specialized Media and Translation, 9864

Coalition for Pulmonary Fibrosis, 5789

Cocaine Anonymous: World Service Office, 8203

Collaborative Medicine Center, 2325

Commonwealth Cancer Help Program, 2326

Comprehensive Gaucher Treatment Center at Tower Hermatology Oncology, 3953

Continuum, 200

Cooley's Anemia Foundation (CAF): California, 2888

Cystic Fibrosis Center: Cedars-Sinai Medic Cedars-Sinai Medical Center, 3026

Cystic Fibrosis Center: Cedars-Sinai Medical Center, 3025

Cystic Fibrosis Center: University of California at San Francisco, 3027

Cystic Fibrosis Research, 3028

Department of Alcohol and Drug Programs, 8239

Departments of Neurology & Neurosurgery: University of California, San Francisco, 8138

Diabetes Control Program, 3314

Diabetes Society, 3353

Diabetes Society of Santa Clara Valley, 3165

Disability Rights California, 10593

Down Syndrome Association of Los Angeles, 3491

Dream Foundation, 10817

Drug Abuse Resistance Education of America, 8204

Dwarf Athletic Association of America, 3970

Eczema Association for Science and Education, 568

Eczema Association for Science and Education, 7719

Enzymology Research Laboratory Dept. of Veterans Affairs Medical Center, 5852

Epilepsy Foundation of Northern California, 7522

Ernest Gallo Clinic and Research Center, 8302

Estate Planning for the Disabled, 10534

Extensions for Independence, 10535

Families Anonymous, 8206

Family Caregiver Alliance/National Center on Caregiving, 4006

Foundation for Glaucoma Research, 9464

Foundation for Glaucoma Research, 9871

Foundation for the Advancement of the Blind, 9465

Fresno County Public Library: Talking Book Library for the Blind, 9701

Friday Night Live, 8342

Friends Medical Science Research Center, 8304

General Clinical Research Center: University of California at LA, 4823

Geraldine Brush Cancer Research Institute California Pacific Medical Center, 2195

Glaucoma Research Foundation, 9684

Glaucoma Support Network, 9896

Glendale Adventist Medical Center Brain Tumor Support Group, 1841

Golden State Donor Services, 9177

Guide Dogs for the Blind, 9468

HIV/Hepatitis C in Prison (HIP) Committee, 206

HIV/Hepatitis C in Prison (HIP) Committee, 5091

Harbor-South Bay Orange County Chapter of the American Assoc. of Kidney Patients, 5559

Heads Up!, 1842

Hear Center, 4315

Hearing Education and Awareness for Rocker s, 4253

Heart Research Foundation of Sacramento, 4828

Heart Touch™ Project, 209

Helen Keller National Center: South Region, 9526

Hemophilia Association of San Diego County, 4915

Hemophilia Center of the Huntington Hospital, 4983

Hemophilia Foundation of Northern California, 4916

Hemophilia Foundation of Southern California, 4917

House Ear Institute, 4255

Hydrocephalus Association Hydrocephalus Association, 5152

Hydrocephalus Support Group of Southern California, 5159

Ida and Joseph Friend Cancer Resource Center, 2196

Independence Center, 10662

International Association of Cancer Victors and Friends, 2334

International Association of Laryngectomees, 2014

International Skeletal Dysplasia Registry Medical Genetics Institute, 3979

International Spinal Cord Regeneration Center, 8030

Jodi House, 4083

John Douglas French Alzheimer's Foundation, 653

John Tracy Clinic, 4258

John Tracy Clinic on Deafness, 4354

Jonsson Comprehensive Cancer Center University of California At Los Angeles, 2197

Juvenile Diabetes Research Foundation: Bakersfield Chapter, 3166

Juvenile Diabetes Research Foundation: Gre ater Bay Area Chapter, 3167

Juvenile Diabetes Research Foundation: Inl and Empire Chapter, 3168

Juvenile Diabetes Research Foundation: Los Angeles Chapter, 3169

Juvenile Diabetes Research Foundation: Nor thern California Inland Chapter, 3170

Juvenile Diabetes Research Foundation: Ora nge County Chapter, 3171

Juvenile Diabetes Research Foundation: San Diego Chapter, 3172

Juvenile Scleroderma Network, 7410

Kaiser Foundation Research Institute, 316

LAC/USC Imaging Science Center, 3954

LINK Program, 5165

Langley Porter Psychiatric Institute University of California, 6167

Leukemia & Lymphoma Society: Orange, Riverside, And San Bernadino Counties, 2055

Leukemia and Lymphoma Society: Greater Los Angeles Chapter, 2058

Leukemia and Lymphoma Society: Greater Sacramento Area Chapter, 2057

Leukemia and Lymphoma Society: Northern California Chapter, 2059

Leukemia and Lymphoma Society: Orange, Riverside, And San Bernadino Counties, 2060

Leukemia and Lymphoma Society: San Diego/Hawaii Chapter, 2056

Leukemia and Lymphoma Society: Tri-County Chapter, 2061

LifeSharing Community Organ & Tissue Donation, 9178

Lighthouse for the Blind and Visually Impaired, 9527

Little People of America, 3972

Loma Linda University Sleep Disorders Clinic, 7836

Los Angeles Alliance Against Parkinson's Disease, 7048

Los Angeles Chapter of the American Association of Kidney Patients, 5560

Los Angeles County Department of Health Services, 246

Los Angeles Support Group: National Ataxia Foundation, 1432

Lupus Foundation of America: Northern California Chapter, 5899

Lupus Foundation of America: Sacramento Chapter, 5900

Lupus Foundation of America: San Diego/Imperial County Chapter, 5898

Lupus Foundation of America: Southern California Chapter, 5901

Marijuana Anonymous: World Services, 8211

Marin Institute, 8310

MedicAlert Foundation International, 10551

Memorial Miller Children's Hospital Cystic Fibrosis Center, 3029

NAMI California, 6065

Narcotics Anonymous World Service Office, 8213

National Association to Advance Fat Acceptance, 6886

National Brain Tumor Foundation, 1809

National Brain Tumor Society, 1810

National Federation of the Blind: California, 9528

National Federation of the Blind: Science and Engineering Division, 9500

National Fibromyalgia Association, 3783

National Health Federation, 2062

National Hepatitis C Coalition, 5096

National Hydrocephalus Foundation, 5155

National Kidney Foundation of Northern California, 5561

National Kidney Foundation of Southern California, 5562

National Multiple Sclerosis Society Channel Islands Chapter, 6519

National Multiple Sclerosis Society: Silicon Valley Chapter, 6520

National Multiple Sclerosis Society: Southern California Chapter, 6518

National Parkinson Foundation: California Office, 7049

National Parkinson Foundation: Orange County Chapter, 7050

National Spinal Cord Injury Association: Los Angeles Chapter, 8041

National Spinal Cord Injury Association: San Diego County Chapter, 8040

Neuro-Oncology Information and Support Group, 1843

Neurofibromatosis Support Network, 6861

Neuroscience Institute Brain Tumor Hotline, 1844

Neurosciences Institute of the Neurosciences Research Program, 872

New Beginnings: The Blind Children's Cente, 9880

New Beginnings: The Blind Children's Center, 9879

Northern California Association of Persian Gulf Veterans, 10207

Northern California Cancer Center, 2199

Northern California Chapter National Multiple Sclerosis Society, 6521

Northern California Support Group: National Ataxia Foundation, 1433

Northstate Parkinson's Chapter, 7051

Northwest Regional Training Center: Canine Companions for Independence, 9529

Okizu Foundation Camps, 10683

One Legacy Transplant Donor Network, 9179

Canada

National Network for Mental Health (NNMH) s, 6051
Post Polio Awareness and Support Society o f British Columbia, 7187
Rick Hansen Foundation, 8036
Scleroderma Society of Ontario, 7375
Sickle Cell Association of Ontario, 7659
Society for Muscular Dystrophy Information International, 6688
Spina Bifida and Hydrocephalus Association of Canada, 7929
Stroke Recovery Canada, 8133
Sunshine Dreams for Kids, 10846
Thyroid Federation International, 9003
Thyroid Foundation of Canada, 9004
Tourette Syndrome Foundation of Canada, 9079
Turner's Syndrome Society of Canada, 9354
World Federation of Hemophilia, 4911

Colorado

AARP Colorado State Office: Denver, 34
ALS Association: Rocky Mountain Chapter, 997
AMC Cancer Research Center, 2209
Aging Support Group, 85
Alcohol and Drug Abuse Division Department of Human Services, 8240
Alzheimer's Association: Greater Grand Junction Area Chapter, 677
Alzheimer's Association: Rocky Mountain Chapter, 678
American Cancer Society: Colorado, 2064
American Diabetes Association: Denver, 3173
American Homes for the Aging: Western, 679
American Liver Foundation Rocky Mountain Division, 5722
American Lung Association of Colorado, 5803
American Lung Association of Colorado, 9277
Americas Association for the Care of Children, 10512
Americas Association for the Care of the Children, 1999
Arthritis Foundation: Rocky Mountain Chapter, 1097
Autism Society of Colorado, 1577
BACCHUS of the US, 8199
Barbara Davis Center for Childhood Diabetes, 3322
Boulder Public Library, 9704
Brain Injury Association of Colorado, 4014
Brain Injury Association of Colorado Helpline, 4084
Brain Tumor Resource and Vital Encouragement, 1853
CCFA Rocky Mountain Chapter: Colorado, 2935
CO Center for AIDS Research: University Colorado Health Sciences Center/CFAR, 249
Centers for AIDS Research: University of Colorado Health Sciences Center, 324
Centers for Disease Control Division of Vector Borne Infectious Diseases, 9027
Colorado Brain Tumor Support Group, 1854
Colorado Cancer Research Program, 2210
Colorado Chapter of the American Association of Kidney Patients, 5565
Colorado FFCMH, 6067
Colorado SIDS Program, 8816
Colorado Talking Book Library, 9705
Colordao Department of Health and Environment, 8817
Denver Childrens Hospital, 3031
Denver Support Group: National Ataxia Foundation, 1436
Disability Careers, 10594
Donor Alliance, 9180
Donor Alliance, 9233
FFCMH: Denver/Aurora Chapter, 6068
Hemophilia Society of Colorado, 4918
International Hearing Dog, 4256
Jimmie Heuga Center, 6606
Juvenile Diabetes Research Foundation: Colorado Springs Chapter, 3174
Juvenile Diabetes Research Foundation: Roc ky Mountain Chapter, 3175
Laradon Services for Children and Adults w ith Developmental Disabilities, 6187
Legal Center for People with Disabilities and Older People, 10595
Little Star Foundation, 10844

Lung Facts, 5857
Lupus Foundation of Colorado, 5902
Mile High Down Syndrome Association, 3492
Mountain-Plains AIDS Education and Training Center (MPAETC), 573
Myasthenia Gravis Association of Colorado, 6790
NNFF Colorado Chapter, 6829
National Alliance for the Mentally Ill of Colorado, 6069
National Association of Blind Lawyers Scott LaBarre, 9481
National Federation of the Blind: Blind Merchants Division, 9516
National Federation of the Blind: Colorado, 9531
National Jewish Center for Immunology, 586
National Jewish Center for Immunology, 5853
National Jewish Center for Immunology and Respiratory Medicine, 587
National Jewish Division of Immunology National Jewish Medical and Research Cen, 1296
National Jewish Medical and Research Center, 5791
National Kidney Foundation of Colorado,, 5598
National Kidney Foundation of Colorado,, 5646
National Kidney Foundation of Colorado, Idaho, Montana, and Wyoming, 5580
National Kidney Foundation of Colorado/Idaho/Montana/Wyoming, 5597
National Kidney Foundation of Colorado/Idaho/Montana/Wyoming, 5645
National MS Society: Colorado Chapter, 6524
National Native American AIDS Prevention Center, 222
National Stroke Association, 5214
National Stroke Association, 8131
Neurofibromatosis Foundation: Colorado, 6860
No. Colorado FFCMH, 6070
Persian Gulf Veterans of Colorado, 10220
Prader-Willi Colorado Association Prader-Willi Syndrome Association, 7211
RESOLVE of Colorado, 5355
Region VIII Office Program Consultants for Maternal and Child Health, 8818
Rocky Mountain CFIDS/FMS Association, 3791
Rocky Mountain Region: Helen Keller National Center, 9532
Scleroderma Foundation: Colorado Chapter, 7380
Spina Bifida Association of Colorado, 7934
Turner's Syndrome Society of Rocky Mountain, 9358
United Cerebral Palsy of Colorado, 2624
United States Association for Blind Athletes, 9513
University of Colorado Cancer Center, 2211
University of Colorado: General Clinical Research Center, Pediatric, 3337
Veterans Adm. Medical Center: Denver, 10221
Veterans Adm. Medical Center: Grand Junction, 10222
Western Slope Chapter of the American Association of Kidney Patients, 5567

Connecticut

Alzheimer's Association: Connecticut Chapter, 680
Alzheimer's Association: South Central Connecticut Chapter, 681
American Cancer Society: Connecticut, 2065
American Diabetes Association: Connecticut, 3176
American Epilepsy Society, 7518
American Liver Foundation: Connecticut Chapter, 5723
American Lung Association of Connecticut, 5804
American Lung Association of Connecticut, 9278
American Lyme Disease Foundation, 9029
Arthritis Foundation: Southern New England Chapter, 1098
Arthritis Foundation: Southern New England Chapter, 1130
Autism Society of Connecticut, 1578
BESB Industries, 9533
Brain Injury Association of Connecticut, 4015
Brain Injury Association of Connecticut Helpline, 4085
CCFA Central Connecticut Chapter, 2936
CCFA Northern Connecticut Affiliate Chapter, 2937
Chapel Haven, 10663

Connecticut Alcohol and Drug Abuse Commission, 8241
Connecticut Brain Tumor Support Group, 1855
Connecticut Chapter of the ALS Association, 998
Connecticut Chapter of the Myasthenia Gravis Foundation of America, 6753
Connecticut Department of Health Services AIDS Programs, 250
Connecticut Down Syndrome Congress, 3493
Connecticut Pregnancy Exposure Information Service, 1757
Connecticut SIDS Alliance, 8819
Connecticut State Library for the Blind and Physically Handicapped, 9706
Cornelia de Lange Syndrome Foundation, 1735
Exceptional Cancer Patients/ECaP, 2328
Families United For CMH, Inc., 6071
Favarh, 10536
Fidelco Guide Dog Foundation, 9461
Gulf War Veterans of Connecticut: New England Chapter, 10223
International Lawyers in Alcoholics Anonymous, 8344
Juvenile Diabetes Research Foundation: Fai rfield County Chapter, 3178
Juvenile Diabetes Research Foundation: Greater New Haven Chapter, 3177
Juvenile Diabetes Research Foundation: Nor th Central CT and Western MA, 3179
Leukemia and Lymphoma Society: Central Connecticut Chapter, 2067
Leukemia and Lymphoma Society: Connecticut Chapter, 2066
Leukemia and Lymphoma Society: Fairfield County Chapter, 2068
Lupus Foundation of America: Connecticut Chapter, 5903
Lupus Network, 5891
Lyme Disease Foundation, 9024
Massachusetts Chapter of SIDS Alliance Boston Medical Center, 8852
Motor Neuron Disease Clinic University of Connecticut Health Center, 1038
NNFF Connecticut Chapter, 6830
National Alliance for the Mentally Ill of Connecticut, 6072
National Federation of the Blind: Connecticut, 9534
National Kidney Foundation of Connecticut, 5568
National MS Society: Greater Connecticut Chapter, 6525
National MS Society: Western Connecticut Chapter, 6526
National Organization for Rare Disorders, 8967
National Organization for Rare Disorders, 10568
National Organization for Rare Disorders (NORD), 3759
National Organization for Rare Disorders (NORD), 3951
National Organization for Rare Disorders (NORD), 8802
National Spinal Cord Injury Association: Connecticut Chapter, 8042
National Veterans Services Fund, 10193
National Veterans Services Fund, 10436
NorthEast Organ Procurement Organization, 9199
Northwestern Connecticut AIDS Project, 251
Office of Protection and Advocacy for Persons with Disabilities, 10596
Prader-Willi Connecticut Association Prader-Willi Syndrome Association, 7212
Prevent Blindness Tri-State, 9535
RESOLVE of Fairfield County, 5356
RESOLVE of Greater Hartford, 5357
Reflex Sympathetic Dystrophy Syndrome Association (RSDSA), 2845
Renfrew Center of Connecticut, 3618
Rhode Island 'Hope' Chapter, 6782
SIDS Program: Connecticut Department of Health, 8820
Spina Bifida Association of Connecticut, 7935
Sudden Infant Death Syndrome (SIDS) Network, 8805
TBI Support Group, 4086
Terri Gotthelf Lupus Research Institute, 5991

National Health Information Center, 2545
National Health Information Center, 2564
National Health Information Center, 2727
National Health Information Center, 2767
National Health Information Center, 2846
National Health Information Center, 2902
National Health Information Center, 2975
National Health Information Center, 3120
National Health Information Center, 3355
National Health Information Center, 3645
National Health Information Center, 3728
National Health Information Center, 3790
National Health Information Center, 3876
National Health Information Center, 3956
National Health Information Center, 3982
National Health Information Center, 4078
National Health Information Center, 4355
National Health Information Center, 4865
National Health Information Center, 5022
National Health Information Center, 5101
National Health Information Center, 5168
National Health Information Center, 5226
National Health Information Center, 5272
National Health Information Center, 5305
National Health Information Center, 5413
National Health Information Center, 5659
National Health Information Center, 5749
National Health Information Center, 5858
National Health Information Center, 5992
National Health Information Center, 6182
National Health Information Center, 6368
National Health Information Center, 6427
National Health Information Center, 6459
National Health Information Center, 6612
National Health Information Center, 6697
National Health Information Center, 6795
National Health Information Center, 6858
National Health Information Center, 6957
National Health Information Center, 6988
National Health Information Center, 7027
National Health Information Center, 7089
National Health Information Center, 7247
National Health Information Center, 7274
National Health Information Center, 7290
National Health Information Center, 7426
National Health Information Center, 7457
National Health Information Center, 7542
National Health Information Center, 7625
National Health Information Center, 7681
National Health Information Center, 7697
National Health Information Center, 7737
National Health Information Center, 7882
National Health Information Center, 7980
National Health Information Center, 8067
National Health Information Center, 8147
National Health Information Center, 8345
National Health Information Center, 8927
National Health Information Center, 8970
National Health Information Center, 9035
National Health Information Center, 9081
National Health Information Center, 9323
National Health Information Center, 9340
National Health Information Center, 9391
National Health Information Center, 9417
National Health Information Center, 9901
National Health Information Center, 10435
National Health Information Center, 10486
National Health Information Center, 10681
National Hispanic Coalition of Health and Human
    Service Organizations, 6048
National Institute of Disability and Rehabilitation
    Research, 10564
National Kidney Foundation of the National Capital
    Area, 5570
National Kidney Foundation of the Texas, 5571
National Library Service for the Blind and Physically
    Handicapped, 9503
National Library Service for the Blind and Physically
    Handicapped, 9710
National MS Society: National Capital Chapter, 6528
National Mental Health Information Center, 6360
National Mental Health Services Knowledge
    Exchange Network, 6050
National Minority AIDS Education Training Center,
    221

National Organization on Disability, 10569
National Organization on Fetal Alcohol Syndrome,
    8222
National Osteoporosis Foundation, 6980
National Osteoporosis Foundation (NOF), 6989
National Parent Network on Disabilities, 10570
National Sleep Foundation, 7824
National Treatment Consortium for Alcohol and
    Other Drugs, 8314
National Women's Health Network, 3718
Occupational Safety & Health Administration, 9269
Office of Civil Rights, 10573
Office of Policy Planning and Legislation, 10574
Office of Special Education Programs, 10575
PXE International, 9903
Paralysis Society of America, 8034
Paralyzed Veterans of America, 8035
Parkinson's Action Network (PAN), 7044
Parkinson's Action Network (PAN) Parkinson's
    Action Network, 7054
Pediatric Neurology Georgetown University Hospital,
    10578
People-to-People Committee for the Handicapped,
    10579
President's Committee on the Employment of People
    with Disabilities, 10580
Problems of the Elderly Committee, 26
Project Eyes and Ears, 4356
Public Information Center US Environmental
    Protection Agency, 5792
Region III Office Program: Consultants for Maternal
    and Child Health, 8895
Rehabilitation Engineering Center for Technological
    Aids for the Deaf, 4324
Rehabilitation Services Administration, 10582
Sarcoidosis Support Group: Washington DC, 7298
Scottish Rite Center for Childhood Language
    Disorders, 4327
Shiloh Senior Center for the Hearing Impaired, 4279
Spina Bifida Association of America, 7928
US Administration on Aging, 28
US Department of Justice, 10584
US Department of Transportation, 10585
US Environmental Protection Agency: Indoor
    Environments Division, 5796
US Office of Personnel Management, 10586
US Veteran's Administration, 10226
United Cerebral Palsy Associations, 2598
United Cerebral Palsy of Washington DC, 2718
United Cerebral Palsy of Washington DC & Northern
    Virginia, 2629
VSA Arts, 10587
Veterans Adm. Medical Center: Washington, 10227
Visiting Nurse Association of America, 10688
Washington Connection, 9907
Washington DC Department of Health HIV/AIDS
    Administration, 253
Washington DC Metropolitan Area Support Group,
    1857
Whitman Walker Clinic AIDS/Medical Services
    Programs, 326
Ysthma and Allergy Foundation of America:
    Washington Chapter, 1289

Florida

AARP Florida State Office: St. Petersburg, 35
ALS Association: Florida Chapter, 1000
ALS Association: Florida Chapter East Coast
    Regional Office, 1001
Alcohol and Drug Abuse Program Department Of
    Children And Families, 8244
Alzheimer's Association: Broward County Chapter,
    683
Alzheimer's Association: East Central Florida
    Chapter, 684
Alzheimer's Association: Florida Gulf Coast Chapter,
    685
Alzheimer's Association: Greater Miami Chapter, 686

Alzheimer's Association: Greater Orlando Area
    Chapter, 687
Alzheimer's Association: Greater Palm Beach Area
    Chapter, 688
Alzheimer's Association: Northeast Florida, 689
Alzheimer's Association: Northern Central Florida
    Chapter, 690
Alzheimer's Association: Northwest Florida Chapter,
    691
Alzheimer's Association: Southwest Florida Chapter,
    692
Alzheimer's Association: Tampa Bay Chapter, 693
Alzheimer's Association: Volusia/Flagler Branch, 694
Alzheimer's Association: West Central Florida
    Chapter, 695
Alzheimer/Parkinson Association of Indian River
    County, 7056
American Association of Kidney Patients, 5549
American Cancer Society: Florida, 2075
American Diabetes Association: Northeast F
    lorida/Southeast Georgia, 3184
American Diabetes Association: Seattle, 3185
American Diabetes Association: South Coast
    Regional/Central Florida, 3186
American Hemochromatosis Society, 3844
American Liver Foundation Gulf Coast Chapter, 5724
American Lung Association of Florida, 5808
American Lung Association of Florida, 9281
American Society of Dermatology, 10511
Angels in the Sun Brain Tumor Support Group, 1858
Arthritis Foundation: Florida Chapter, Gulf Coast
    Branch, 1100
Association of Birth Defect Children Birth Defect
    Research for Children, 565
Association of Birth Defect Children Birth Defect
    Research for Children, 1274
Asthma and Allergy Foundation of America: Florida
    Chapter, 574
Autism Society of Greater Orlando, 1581
BASE Camp Children's Cancer Foundation, 10810
Birth Defect Research for Children, 1732
Brain Injury Association of Florida, 4017
Brain Injury Association of Florida, 4088
Brain Tumor Support Group, 1859
Brave Kids, 3955
Brevard County Libraries: Talking Books Library,
    9711
Broward County Talking Book Library, 9712
CCFA Florida Chapter, 2938
Career Assessment & Planning Services Goodwill
    Industries-Suncoast, 6078
Central Florida Chapter, 6529
Chef David's Kids, 10839
Children's Medical Services Program: Florida SIDS
    Program, 8824
Choices for Work Program Goodwill
    Industries-Suncoast, 4018
Coconut Creek Eating Disorders Support Group, 3640
Colorado Parkinson Foundation, 7055
Comprehensive Pediatric Hemophilia Center
    University of South Florida, 4968
Cystic Fibrosis Center: All Children's Hospital, 3035
Department of Epidemiology and Health Policy
    Research: University of Florida, 327
Desert Storm Justice Foundation: Florida, 10228
Desert Storm Veterans of Florida, 10229
Disability Rights: Florida, 10600
Dreams Come True, 10841
East Central Florida Chapter of the Myasthenia
    Gravis Foundation of America, 6756
Endometriosis Association, 3714
Endometriosis Reseach Center and Women's H The
    Endometriosis Research Center, 3724
Endometriosis Reseach Center and Women's
    Hospital, 3723
Endometriosis Research Center 0, 3725
Endometriosis Research Center 0, 3726
Epilepsy Association of Big Bend, 7523
Epilepsy Foundation of South Florida, 7524
Epilepsy Services Foundation, 7525
Epilepsy Services of North Central Florida, 7526
Epilepsy Services of Northeast Florida, 7527
Epilepsy Services of Southwest Florida, 7528
Florida Alliance for the Mentally Ill, 6079

Florida Ambassador: National Ataxia Foundation, 1437

Florida Association of the Deaf, 4280

Florida Brain Tumor Association, 1860

Florida Brain Tumor Support Group, 1861

Florida Brain Tumor Support Group: Deerfield Beach, 1862

Florida Bureau of Braille and Talking Book Library Services, 9713

Florida Chapter of the National Hemophilia Foundation, 4919

Florida Department of Health, 8825

Florida Department of Health Bureau of HIV/AIDS, 255

Florida Disabled Outdoor Association, 10538

Florida FFCMH: Tampa Chapter, 6080

Florida Gulf Coast Chapter National Multiple Sclerosis Society, 6530

Florida Institute for Family Involvement (FIFI), 6188

Florida Ophthalmic Institute, 9870

Florida SIDS Alliance, 8826

Florida Southwest Turner Syndrome Society, 9359

Gilda's Club: South Florida, 2332

Give Kids the World Village, 10820

Gold Coast Down Syndrome Organization, 3494

Goodwill Industries-Suncoast, 36

Goodwill Industries-Suncoast, 3495

Goodwill Industries-Suncoast, 4019

Goodwill Industries-Suncoast, 4281

Goodwill Industries-Suncoast, 5809

Goodwill Industries-Suncoast, 6531

Goodwill Industries-Suncoast, 7057

Goodwill Industries-Suncoast, 8043

Goodwill Industries-Suncoast, 9542

Greater Daytona Area Parkinson Support Group, 7091

HEALTHSOUTH Capital Rehabilitation Hospital, 8065

Hillsborough County Talking Book Library, 9714

Hollywood Area Brain Tumor Support Group, 1863

International Society of Dermatology, 7720

Iron Overload Diseases Association, 3856

Jacksonville Public Library, 9715

Juvenile Diabetes Research Foundation: Cen tral Florida Chapter, 3187

Juvenile Diabetes Research Foundation: Flo rida Sun Coast Chapter, 3188

Juvenile Diabetes Research Foundation: Gre ater Palm Beach County Chapter, 3189

Juvenile Diabetes Research Foundation: Nor th Florida Chapter, 3190

Juvenile Diabetes Research Foundation: Sou th Florida Chapter, 3191

Juvenile Diabetes Research Foundation: Tam pa Bay Chapter, 3192

Kids Wish Network, 10825

Lee County Talking Books Library, 9716

Leukemia & Lymphoma Society: Suncoast Chapter, 2076

Leukemia and Lymphoma Society: Southern Florida Chapter, 2077

Leukemia and Lymphoma Society: Central Florida Chapter, 2078

Leukemia and Lymphoma Society: Northern Florida Chapter, 2079

Leukemia and Lymphoma Society: Palm Beach Area Chapter, 2080

Leukemia and Lymphoma Society: Suncoast Chapter, 2081

LifeLink of Florida, 9184

LifeLink of Southwest Florida, 9185

Lupus Foundation of America: Northeast Florida Chapter, 5905

Lupus Foundation of America: Northwest Florida Chapter, 5906

Lupus Foundation of America: Southeast Florida Chapter, 5907

Lupus Foundation of America: Suncoast Chapter, 5908

Lupus Foundation of America: Tampa Area Chapter, 5909

Lupus Foundation of Florida, 5910

MSWorld, 6610

Manattee County Office Epilepsy Services of Southwest Florida, 7529

Metabolic Research Institute, 3334

Miami Childrens Hospital Division of Pulmonology, 3036

Miami Comprehensive Hemophilia Center Jackson Medical Towers, 4990

Miami Dade Talking Book Library, 9717

Miami Heart Institute, 4833

Miami Heart Research Institute, 4834

Miami Project to Cure Paralysis, 8060

Multiple Sclerosis Foundation, 6507

NF Center: North Broward Medical Center Neurofibromatosis, 6831

NNFF Florida Chapter, 6832

National Association of Guide Dog Users Priscilla Ferris, 9485

National Federation of the Blind: Florida, 9543

National Kidney Foundation of Florida, 5572

National Multiple Sclerosis Society: North Florida Chapter, 6533

National Parkinson Foundation, 7042

National Parkinson Foundation Hotline, 7092

National Spinal Cord Injury Support Goups, 8069

National Spinal Cord Injury Support Groups, 8072

Nemours Childrens Clinic, 3037

New Hope for Kids Wish Program, 10829

North Florida: HPV Support Group, 10601

Northwest Florida Support Group: National Ataxia Foundation, 1438

Orange County Library System: Orlando Public Library, 9718

Palm Beach Chapter of the American Association of Kidney Patients, 5573

Palm Beach County Library Annex: Talking Books, 9719

Parent Education Network (PEN) Project Health, 6189

Parkinson Association of Greater Daytona Beach, 7058

Parkinson Association of Greater Kansas, 7059

Parkinson Association of Southwest Florida, 7060

Parkinson Educational Society of Puget Sound, 7081

Pembroke Pines Parkinson Support Group, 7093

Pensacola Brain Injury TBI/ABI Support Group, 4020

Pinellas Talking Book Library for the Blind and Physically Handicapped, 9720

Positive Voices, 256

Prader-Willi Florida Assoction Prader-Willi Syndrome Association, 7214

Prader-Willi Syndrome Association (USA) Prader-Willi Syndrome Association, 7205

PraderWilli Syndrome Association, 7248

RESOLVE Affiliate of Central Florida, 5359

RESOLVE of North Florida, 5360

RESOLVE of South Florida, 5361

Rambaugh-Goodwin Institute for Cancer Research, 2215

Renfrew Center of Miami, 3619

Renfrew Center of South Florida, 3620

Sarasota Area Brain Tumor Support Group, 1864

Scleroderma Foundation: Southeast Florida Chapter, 7384

Scoliosis Association, 7453

South Florida Chapter National Multiple Sclerosis Society, 6534

South Florida Chapter of the American Association of Kidney Patients, 5574

South Florida Gold Coast Chapter of the Myasthenia Gravis Foundation of America, 6757

South Palm Beach County Chapter of NFP, 7061

Southeast Parkinson Disease Association, 7062

Southeast Regional Center: Canine Companions for Independence, 9544

Spina Bifida Association of Florida Space Coast, 7937

Spina Bifida Association of Jacksonville, 7938

Spina Bifida Association of Tampa, 7939

Sub Regional Talking Book Library, 9721

Suncoast Residential Training Center/Developmental Services Program, 6081

Sunshine Chapter of the American Association of Kidney Patients, 5575

TBAN, 257

TPN: The Perspective Network, 4009

Tallahassee Memorial Diabetes Center, 3321

Tampa Bay Research Institute, 328

Tampa Lighthouse for the Blind, 9545

Teratogen Information Services, 1768

TransLife/Florida Hospital, 9186

Turner's Syndrome Society of South Florida, 9360

UM/Sylvester Comprehensive Cancer Center, 2216

United Cerebral Palsy of Central Florida, 2630

United Cerebral Palsy of East Central Florida, 2631

United Cerebral Palsy of Florida, 2632

United Cerebral Palsy of North Florida: Tender Loving Care, 2633

United Cerebral Palsy of Northeast Florida, 2634

United Cerebral Palsy of Northwest Florida, 2635

United Cerebral Palsy of Sarasota-Manatee, 2636

United Cerebral Palsy of South Florida, 2637

United Cerebral Palsy of Tallahassee, 2638

United Cerebral Palsy of Tampa Bay, 2639

University of Florida: General Clinical Research Center, 591

University of Miami School of Medicine Department of Neurology, 8144

University of Miami: Bascom Palmer Eye Institute, 9885

University of Miami: Center on Aging Center on Aging, 883

University of Miami: Diabetes Research Institute, 3341

University of Miami: Mailman Center for Child Development, 1753

University of South Florida Center for HIV Education and Research, 329

Veterans Adm. Medical Center: Bay Pines, 10230

Veterans Adm. Medical Center: Gainesville, 10231

Veterans Adm. Medical Center: Lake City, 10232

Veterans Adm. Medical Center: Miami, 10233

Veterans Adm. Medical Center: St. Petersburg, 10234

Veterans Adm. Medical Center: Tampa, 10235

Vietnam Veterans of Brevard The Vietnam And All Veterans Of Brevard, 10236

West Central FL Support Group: National Ataxia Foundation, 1439

West Central Florida Chapter of the Myasthenia Gravis Foundation of America, 6758

West Florida Public Library: Talking Book Library, 9722

West Palm Beach Area Brain Tumor Support Group, 1865

West Palm Beach VA Medical Center, 10237

Georgia

AARP Georgia: Atlanta, 37

AIDS School Health Education Database Centers for Disease Control, 330

ALS Association of Georgia, 1002

Albany Library for the Blind and Physically Handicapped, 9723

Alcohol and Drug Services Addictive Diseases Program, 8245

All Ages Support Group, 1866

Alzheimer's Association: Atlanta Chapter, 696

Alzheimer's Association: Augusta Chapter, 697

Alzheimer's Association: Central Georgia Chapter, 698

Alzheimer's Association: Greater Columbus Chapter, 699

Alzheimer's Association: Greater Georgia Chapter, 700

Alzheimer's Association: Southeast Georgia Chapter, 701

Alzheimer's Association: Southwest Georgia Chapter, 702

Alzheimer's Disease Center Emory University/VA Medical Center, 849

American Cancer Society, 1996

American Cancer Society: Georgia, 2082

American Diabetes Association: Atlanta Met ro, 3193

American Diabetes Association: Savannah, 3194

American Foundation for the Blind: SE National Literacy Center, 9448

American Juvenile Arthritis Organization, 5888

American Juvenile Arthritis Organization (AJAO), 5887

American Juvenile Arthritis Organization Arthritis Foundation, 1083

American Lung Association of Georgia, 5810
American Lung Association of Georgia, 9282
American SIDS Institute, 8798
American Spinal Cord Injury Association, 8023
American Spinal Injury Association (ASIA), 8024
Arthritis Foundation, 1085
Arthritis Foundation, 7025
Arthritis Foundation, 7270
Arthritis Foundation Information Hotline, 1155
Arthritis Foundation: Georgia Chapter, 1101
Atlanta Georgia Chapter of the American Association
of Kidney Patients, 5576
Atlanta Metro Subregional Library, 9724
Augusta Regional Library Talking Book Center, 9725
Autism Society of Greater Georgia, 1582
Bainbridge Subregional Library for the Blind and
Physically Handicapped, 9726
Brain Tumor Foundation for Children, 1812
CCFA Georgia Chapter, 2939
Center for AIDS Research: Emory University Rollins
School of Public Health, 331
Center for Chronic Disease Prevention and Centers
for Disease Control, 10517
Center for Disease Control and Prevention, 10520
Centers for Disease Control, 10192
Centers for Disease Control and Prevention, 2764
Centers for Disease Control and Prevention, 7618
Centers for Disease Control and Prevention Hepatitis
Branch, 5090
Centers for Disease Control and Prevention National
Center for Prevention Services, 9266
Children's Wish Foundation International, 10813
Columbus Library for Accessible Services (CLASS),
9727
Comprehensive Sickle Cell Center, 7657
Creative Community Services (CCS), 10664
Department of Pediatrics Medical College of Georgia,
3038
Division of Diabetes Translation, 3315
Division of Rehabilitation Service, 10602
Down Syndrome Association of Atlanta, 3496
Educational Materials Database Centers for Disease
Control, 332
Emory Autism Resource Center, 1622
Emory Brain Tumor Support Group, 1867
Emory University: Cystic Fibrosis Center, 3039
Emory University: Georgia Center for Cancer
Statistics, 2217
Emory University: Laboratory for Ophthalmic
Research, 9868
Emory University: National Cooperative Drug
Discovery for AIDS Treatment, 333
Emory University: Winship Cancer Institute, 2218
Families in Action National Drug Information Center,
8207
Fertility Clinic at the Shepherd Spinal Center, 5403
Funding Database Centers for Disease Control, 334
Georgia Alliance for the Mentally Ill, 6082
Georgia Association of the Deaf, 4282
Georgia Atlanta Turner Syndrome Society, 9361
Georgia Chapter of the Myasthenia Gravis
Foundation of America, 6759
Georgia Department of Human Resources: Center for
Family Resource Planning, 8827
Georgia Department of Human Resources: Division
of Public Health, 258
Georgia Department of Human Resources: Infant and
Child Health, 8828
Georgia Industries for the Blind, 9546
Georgia Library for Accessible Services (GLASS),
9728
Georgia National Spinal Cord Injury Association
Support Group Network, 8064
Georgia Parent Support Network (GPSN), 6190
Georgia SIDS Project, 8829
Georgia Support Group: National Ataxia Foundation,
1440
Gulf War Veterans of Georgia, 10238
HIV/AIDS Prevention Program, 382
Hall County Library System: East Hall Branch and
Special Needs Library, 9729
Hearts and Minds, 1868
Hemophilia Foundation of Georgia, 4920
I Can Cope, 2333

Immunization Division Centers for Disease Control,
383
Impotence Resource Center of the Geddings Osbon Sr
Foundation, 5264
Juvenile Diabetes Research Foundation: Georgia
Chapter, 3195
Kids on the Block Arthritis Programs, 1156
Kidscope, 2083
Leukemia and Lymphoma Society: Georgia Chapter,
2084
LifeLink of Georgia, 9187
Look Good... Feel Better, 2336
Lupus Foundation of America: Columbus Chapter,
5911
Lupus Foundation of America: Greater Atlanta
Chapter, 5912
Marcus Institute for Development and Learning, 3519
Medical College of Georgia Alzheimers Research
Center, 869
Medical College of Georgia: Sickle Cell Center, 7670
Middle Georgia Subregional Library for the Blind and
Physically Handicapped, 9730
NAMES Project Foundation AIDS Memorial Quilt,
216
NNFF Georgia Affiliate, 6833
National Down Syndrome Congress, 3488
National Down Syndrome Congress, 3534
National Families in Action, 8221
National Federation of the Blind: Georgia, 9547
National Gaucher Disease Foundation, 3762
National Gaucher Foundation, 3950
National Gaucher Foundation (NGF), 5748
National Kidney Foundation of Georgia, 5577
National MS Society: Georgia Chapter, 6535
National Parent to Parent Support and Information
System, 10682
National Spinal Cord Injury Support Groups, 8071
Northwest Georgia Parkinson Disease Association,
7063
Oconee Regional Library for the Blind and Physically
Handicapped, 9731
Office on Smoking and Health, 10576
Office on Smoking and Health: CDCP, 8227
PWSA of Georgia Prader-Willi Syndrome
Association, 7215
RESOLVE of Georgia, 5362
Reach to Recovery, 2342
Region IV Office Program Consultants for Maternal
and Child Health, 8830
Rome Georgia Chapter of the American Association
of Kidney Patients, 5578
Rome Subregional Library for People with
Disabilities, 9732
SBTF Brain Tumor Support Group, 1869
Shepherd Spinal Center, 8044
Sickle Cell Foundation of Georgia, 7664
Sickle Cell Information Center Grady Memorial
Hospital, 7661
Southeastern Region: Helen Keller National Center,
9548
Special Needs Library of Northeast Georgia, 9733
Spina Bifida Association of Georgia, 7940
Subregional Library for the Blind and Physically
Handicapped, 9734
Three Rivers Regional Library, 9735
United Cerebral Palsy of Georgia, 2640
VA Southeast Network: Georgia, 10239
Valdosta Talking Book Library, 9736
Veterans Adm. Medical Center: Augusta, 10240
Veterans Adm. Medical Center: Decatur Atlanta VA
Medical Center, 10241
Veterans Adm. Medical Center: Dublin Carl Vinson
VA Medical Center, 10242
Well Project, 235

Hawaii

AARP Hawaii State Office: Honolulu, 38
Alcohol and Drug Abuse Division Department of
Health, 8246
Alzheimer's Association: Honolulu Chapter, 703
Alzheimer's Association: West Hawaii Chapter, 704
American Cancer Society: Hawaii, 2085
American Diabetes Association: Hawaii, 3196

American Liver Foundation Hawaii Chapter, 5725
American Lung Association of Hawaii, 5811
American Lung Association of Hawaii, 9283
Autism Society of Hawaii, 1583
Brain Injury Association of Hawaii, 4021
Brain Injury Association of Hawaii, 4089
Division of Vocational Rehabilitation and Services for
the Blind, 9549
Hawaii Department of Health: Communicable
Disease Division, 259
Hawaii Department of Health: Family Health
Division, 8831
Hawaii Down Syndrome Congress, 3497
Hawaii Families As Allies (HFAA), 6191
Hawaii Lupus Foundation, 5913
Hawaii Parkinson Association Gwendolyn A
Montibon President, 7064
Hawaii State Library for the Blind and Physically
Handicapped, 9737
Hemophilia Foundation of Hawaii Kapiolani Medical
Center, 4921
Ho'opono Workshop for the Blind, 9550
Juvenile Diabetes Research Foundation: Hawaii
Chapter, 3197
Kuakini Parkinson Disease (PD) Information &
Referral, 7094
NAMI: The Local Affiliate of the National Alliance
for the Mentally Ill, 6083
National Federation of the Blind: Hawaii, 9551
National Kidney Foundation of Hawaii, 5579
National MS Society: Hawaii Chapter, 6536
Organ Donor Center of Hawaii, 9188
Pacific Health Research Institute, 2219
Prader-Willi Northwest Association, 7216
Protection & Advocacy Agency, 10603
RESOLVE of Hawaii, 5363
United Cerebral Palsy of Hawaii, 2641
University of Hawaii: Cancer Research Center, 2220
Veterans Adm. Medical Centery: Honolulu VA
Pacific Islands Health Care System, 10243

Idaho

AARP Idaho State Office: Meridian, 39
Alzheimer's Association: Greater Idaho Chapter, 705
Alzheimer's Association: Northern Idaho Chapter,
706
American Cancer Society: Idaho, 2086
American Lung Association of Idaho, 5812
Autism Society of Treasure Valley, 1584
Brain Injury Association of Idaho, 4022
Child Health Improvement Program: Idaho
Department of Health, 8832
Department of Health and Welfare Department Of
Health And Welfare, 8247
FFCMH: Idaho Chapter, 6084
Hemophilia Foundation of Idaho, 4922
Idaho Alliance for the Mentally Ill, 6085
Idaho Commission for Libraries Talking Book
Service, 9738
Idaho Department of Health and Welfare, 8833
Idaho Department of Health and Welfare The
STD/AIDS Program, 260
Idaho Persian Gulf Veterans, 10244
Lupus Foundation of America: Idaho Chapter, 5914
NNFF Idaho Chapter, 6834
National Federation of the Blind: Idaho, 9552
National MS Society: Idaho Division, 6537
Prader-Willi Northwest Association, 7217
United Cerebral Palsy of Idaho, 2642
Veterans Adm. Medical Center: Boise Boise VA
Medical Center, 10245

Illinois

AARP Illinois State Office: Chicago, 40
AIDS Legal Council of Chicago, 261
ARRISE, 1565
Academy for Eating Disorders, 3601
Academy for Eating Disorders, 3633
Adult Down Syndrome Center of Lutheran General
Hospital, 3508
Aid to the Aged, Blind or Disabled, 9554

Alzheimer's Association: Central Illinois Chapter, 707

Alzheimer's Association: East Central Illinois Chapter, 708

Alzheimer's Association: Four Rivers Chapter, 709

Alzheimer's Association: Greater Illinois Chapter, 710

Alzheimer's Association: Greater Illinois Chapter: Carbondale Office, 711

Alzheimer's Association: Land of Lincoln Chapter, 712

Alzheimer's Disease and Related Disorders Association, 650

American Academy of Dermatology, 7713

American Academy of Orthopaedic Surgeons, 2537

American Academy of Orthopaedic Surgeons, 7450

American Academy of Pediatrics, 10498

American Academy of Sleep Medicine, 2755

American Association of Diabetes Educators, 3147

American Board of Dermatology American Society for Dermatologic Surger, 7714

American Brain Tumor Association, 1807

American Brain Tumor Association, 4002

American Brain Tumor Association Patient Line, 4090

American Cancer Society: Illinois, 2087

American College of Allergy, Asthma & Immunology, 563

American Dental Association Department of Library Services, 8196

American Diabetes Association: Greater Ill inois, 3198

American Diabetes Association: Northern Il linois, 3199

American Dietetic Association, 564

American Dietetic Association, 3602

American Dietetic Association, 3842

American Hearing Research Foundation, 4232

American Homes for the Aging: Midwest Regional Office, 713

American Liver Foundation Illinois Chapter, 5726

American Lung Association Help Line, 5856

American Lung Association of Illinois, 5813

American Lung Association of Illinois-Iowa, 9284

American Pain Society, 2842

American Society for Dermatologic Surgery, 7716

American Society for Gastrointestinal Endoscopy, 3848

American Society for Surgery of the Hand, 2539

American Society of Colon and Rectal Surgeons, 1998

American Society of Plastic and Reconstructive Surgeons, 7717

Arthritis Foundation: Greater Chicago Chapter, 1102

Arthritis Foundation: Greater Illinois Chapter, 1103

Arthritis Foundation: Northwestern Ohio Chapter, 1125

Associates in Nephrology, 5647

Association of Halfway House Alcoholism Programs of North America, 8198

Association of Late-Deafened Adults, 4236

Association of Professional Sleep Societies, 7819

Autism Society of Illinois, 1585

Baxter Hyland Division, 4906

Benjamin B Greenfield National Alzheimer's Center, 651

Better Existence with HIV, 190

Brain Injury Association of Illinois, 4023

Brain Injury Association of Illinois Helpline, 4091

Brain Research Foundation, 1816

Brain Tumor Support Group, 1870

CANDU Parent Group, 6192

CCFA Illinois: Carol Fisher Chapter, 2940

Cancer and Leukemia Group B, 2255

Catholic Guild for the Blind, 9739

Catholic Guild for the Blind Catholic Charities of the Archdiocese of, 9458

Center for Digestive Disorders: Central, 3851

Center for Narcolepsy Research at the University of Illinois at Chicago, 7828

Central Brain Tumor Registry of the US, 1818

Chicago Area Support Group: National Ataxia Foundation, 1441

Chicago Department of Health, 262

Chicago Lighthouse for People Who are Blind and Visually Impaired, 9555

Chicago Metro Support Group: National Ataxia Foundation, 1442

Chicagoland Chapter of the American Association of Kidney Patients, 5581

Citizens Alliance for VD Awareness, 7619

Clinical Research Center Northwestern Center for Clinical Researc, 335

Cognitive Neurology and Alzheimer's Disease Center, 860

Comer Children's Hospital at the Universit, 3041

Comer Children's Hospital at the University of Chicago, 3040

Compassionate Friends, 8800

Compassionate Friends, 10849

Cooley's Anemia Foundation (CAF): Illinois Oakbrook Towers, 2889

Cystic Fibrosis Center: Childrens Memorial Hospital, 3042

Cystic Fibrosis Center: Park Ridge Lutheran General Children's Hospital, 3043

David T Siegel Institute for Communicative Disorders, 4311

Department of Alcoholism and Substance Abuse, 8248

Department of Ophthalmology Information Line, 9895

Department of Ophthalmology/Eye and Ear Infirmary, 9867

Depression and Bipolar Support Alliance, 6367

Dermatology Foundation, 2182

Dermatology Foundation, 7718

Desert Storm Justice Foundation: Illinois, 10246

Division on Endocrinology Northwestern University Feinberg School, 3327

Dreams for Seniors Charity Inc, 10842

Easter Seals, 1736

Easter Seals, 2595

Easter Seals, 7926

Edward J Hines Jr VA Hospital, 10247

Fairygodmother Foundation, 10818

Gastro-Intestinal Research Foundation, 3867

Gastrointestinal Research Foundation, 3871

Great Lakes Health Care System, 10248

Hands Organization: Advocacy Network for the Deaf and Hearing Impaired, 4251

Helen Keller National Center Regional Representatives, 9556

Hemophilia Foundation of Illinois, 4923

Ileitis and Colitis Educational Foundation, 2924

Illinois Alliance for the Mentally Ill, 6086

Illinois Association of the Deaf, 4283

Illinois Church Action on Alcohol Problems, 8249

Illinois Client Assistance Program, 10605

Illinois Department of Public Health: Division of Infectious Diseases, 263

Illinois Federation of Families, 6087

Illinois Midwest Neurofibromatosis, 6835

Illinois Spina Bifida Association, 7941

Illinois State Library Talking Book and Braille Service, 9740

Illinois Teratogen Information Service (IT IS), 1758

International Association for Chronic Fatigue, 2756

International Association of Eating Disorders Professionals, 3610

International Pelvic Pain Society Women's Medical Plaza, 2844

International Pelvic Pain Society Women's Medical Plaza, 3717

Jesse Brown VA Medical Center, 10249

Juvenile Diabetes Research Foundation: Gre ater Chicago Chapter, 3200

KALEIDOSCOPE, 6193

Kellogg Cancer Care Center Evanston Hospital, 2221

LaRabida Children's Hospital: Developmental Disabilities & Delays, 3525

Les Turner Amyotrophic Lateral Sclerosis Foundation, 1048

Les Turner Research Laboratory Northwestern University Medical School, 1036

Let's Breathe Sarcoidosis Support Group, 7287

Leukemia Research Foundation, 2222

Leukemia and Lymphoma Society: Illinois Chapter, 2088

Lions Quest, 10548

Lois Insolia ALS Center at Northwestern Memorial Hospital, 1003

Loyola University Medical Center: Departme, 3045

Loyola University Medical Center: Department of Pediatrics, 3044

Loyola University of Chicago Cardiac Transplant Program, 4832

Loyola University of Children: Parmly Hearing Institute, 4317

Lupus Foundation of America: Illinois Chapter, 5915

MAGIC Foundation for Children's Growth, 3976

MAGIC Foundation for Children's Growth: Turner's Syndrome Division, 9353

Male Sexual Dysfunction Clinic, 5268

Medical Library Association, 214

Metro Chicago Turner Syndrome Society, 9362

Mid-Illinois Talking Book Center, 9741

Myasthenia Gravis Support Group East Central Illinois, 6792

NNFF Illinois Chapter: Chicago Area, 6836

NNFF Illinois Chapter: Silvis Area, 6837

NNFF Illinois Chapter: Springfield Area, 6838

NNFF Illinois Chapter:Peoria Region, 6839

National Association for Down Syndrome, 3486

National Association of Anorexia Nervosa and Associated Disorders, 3612

National Center for Sight, 9899

National Certification Board for Diabetes Educators, 3151

National Eye Health Education Program, 9900

National Federation of the Blind: Illinois, 9557

National Fraternal Society of the Deaf, 4265

National Headache Foundation, 6456

National Kidney Foundation of Illinois, 5582

National MS Society: Chicago, Greater Illinois Chapter, 6538

Northern Illinois University Research and Training Center, 4319

Northwestern University: Division of Allergy and Immunology, 1297

Oncology Hematology Associates of Central Illinois, 2223

PWSA Illinois Prader-Willi Syndrome Association, 7218

Parents Information Network FFCMH, 6194

Parents of Children with Brain Tumors PCBT, 1871

Parkside Medical Services Corporation, 8250

Prevent Blindess America, 9506

Pulmonary Fibrosis Association, 5793

Pulmonary Fibrosis Foundation, 5794

RESOLVE of Illinois, 5364

Rainbow House, 4008

Rainbows for All God's Children, 10861

Raynaud's Foundation, 7271

Region 3 of the National Association for Parents of the Visually Impaired, 9558

Regional Organ Bank of Illinois, Inc., 9189

Rehabilitation Institute of Chicago, 1151

Robert H Lurie Comprehensive Cancer Center of Northwestern University, 2224

Rockford Parkinson's Support Group, 7095

Rush University Multiple Sclerosis Center, 6608

SIDS of Illinois, 8834

Saint Francis Medical Center Peoria Pulmon, 3047

Saint Francis Medical Center Peoria Pulmonary Association, 3046

Scleroderma Foundation: Greater Chicago Chapter, 7386

Shawnee Library System: Southern Illinois Talking Book Center, 9742

Shriners Hospital for Crippled Children Chicago Unit, 7456

Simon Foundation Helpline for Incontinence Information, 5306

Simon Foundation for Continence, 5303

Skokie Accessible Library Services, 9743

Sleep Research Society American Academy of Sleep Medicine, 7825

Society of Gastroenterology Nurses and Associates, 3864

Society of Mitral Valve Prolapse Syndrome, 4868

Spinal Cord Injury Association of Illinois, 8045

Statewide SIDS Program: Illinois Department of Public Health, 8835

Sulzberger Institute for Dermatologic Educ, 7734
Sulzberger Institute for Dermatologic Education, 7733
Test Positive Aware Network (TPAN), 264
Thresholds Psychiatric Rehabilitation, 6172
United Cerebral Palsy Land of Lincoln, 2643
United Cerebral Palsy of East Central Illinois, 2644
United Cerebral Palsy of Greater Chicago, 2645
United Cerebral Palsy of Illinois, 2646
United Cerebral Palsy of Southern Illinois, 2647
United Cerebral Palsy of Will County, 2648
United Cerebral Palsy of the Blackhawk Region, 2649
United Cerebral Palsy: Eastern Seals, 2650
University of Chicago Cancer Research Center, 2225
University of Chicago Center for Advanced Medicine Duchossis Center, 7421
University of Chicago Committee on Virology, 7624
University of Chicago Dept of Neurology University of Chicago Hospital, 880
University of Chicago: Clinical Nutrition Research Unit, 2226
University of Chicago: Comprehensive Diabetes Center, 3336
University of Chicago: Temporal Bone Laboratory for Ear Research, 4336
University of Illinois Health Services Research, 881
University of Illinois at Chicago Consultation Clinic for Epilepsy, 7538
University of Illinois at Chicago Craniofacial Center, 1751
University of Illinois at Chicago Lions, 9321
University of Illinois at Chicago Lions of Illinois Eye Research Institute, 9884
University of Illinois at Chicago Medical Center Outpatient Clinical Center, 7422
University of Illinois at Chicago: Institute for Tuberculosis Research, 9322
VA Illinois Health Care System, 10250
Veterans Adm. Medical Center: Marion Marion VA Medical Center, 10251
Veterans Adm. Medical Center: North Chicago, 10252
Veterans Adm. Medical Center: Northport North Chicago VA Medical Center, 10253
Veterans Administration West Side Medical Center, 10254
Voices of Vision Talking Book Center, 9744
Y-ME National Breast Cancer Organization, 2033

Indiana

AARP Indiana State Office: Indianapolis, 41
ALS Association: Indiana Chapter, 1004
Alzheimer's Association: Central Indiana, 714
Alzheimer's Association: Central Indiana Chapter-Columbus Office, 715
Alzheimer's Association: Central Virginia, 716
Alzheimer's Association: Northern Indiana Chapter, 717
Alzheimer's Support Group, 886
American Camp Association, 10503
American Cancer Society: Indiana, 2089
American Diabetes Association: Northern Indiana/Northern Ohio, 3201
American Liver Foundation Indiana Chapter, 5727
American Lung Association of Indiana, 5814
American Lung Association of Indiana: State Office & Support Office, 9285
Ann Whitehill Down Syndrome Program, 3509
Arthritis Foundation: Indiana Chapter, 1104
Autism Society of Indiana, 1586
Ball State University Public Health Entomology Laboratory, 9026
Bartholomew County Public Library, 9745
Bloomington: NAMI Bloomington, 6195
Bosma Industries for the Blind, 9559
Brain Injury Association of Indiana, 4024
Brain Injury Association of Indiana Helpli ne, 4092
Brain Tumor Support Group, 1872
Breaking New Ground Resource Center, 10515
CCFA Indiana Chapter, 2941
Children's Organ Transplant Association (COTA), 9163

Chronic Fatigue Syndrome & Fibromyalgia Support, 2765
Diabetes Youth Foundation of Indiana, 3202
Division of Addiction Services Department of Mental Health, 8251
Elkhart: NAMI Elkhart County, 6196
Evansville NAMI Evansville, 6197
Evansville-Vanderburgh County Public Library, 9746
FFCMH: Indiana Chapter, 6088
Family Action Network, 6089
Fort Wayne: NAMI Fort Wayne, 6198
Greater Indianapolis Chapter of the Myasthenia Gravis Foundation of America, 6760
Hemophilia Foundation of Indiana, 4924
Indiana Chapter Turner Syndrome Society, 9364
Indiana Down Syndrome Foundation, 3498
Indiana Organ Procurement Organization,, 9190
Indiana Protection and Advocacy Services, 10606
Indiana Resource Center for Autism (IRCA), 1623
Indiana State Board of Health: SIDS Project, 8836
Indiana State Department of Health Maternal And Child Health Services, 8837
Indiana Talking Book & Braille Library, 9747
Indiana Teratogen Information Service, 1759
Indiana University Center for Aging Research, 864
Indiana University: Area Health Education Center, 3329
Indiana University: Center for Diabetes Research, 3330
Indiana University: Human Genetics Center of Medical & Molecular Genetics, 865
Indiana University: Hypertension Research Center, 5219
Indiana University: Pharmacology Research Laboratory, 3331
Indianapolis: NAMI Indianapolis, 6199
International Academy of Proctology, 3854
Jeffersonville: NAMI Sunnyside, 6200
Juvenile Diabetes Research Foundation: Ind iana State Chapter, 3203
Juvenile Diabetes Research Foundation: Nor thern Indiana Chapter, 3204
Kendallville NAMI Northeast, 6201
Kokomo NAMI Kokomo, 6202
Krannert Institute of Cardiology, 4831
Lafayette: NAMI West Central, 6203
Lake County Public Library, 9748
Lake County: NAMI Lake County, 6204
Lawrenceburg: NAMI Southeast, 6205
Leukemia and Lymphoma Society: Indiana Chapter, 2090
Logansport: NAMI Cass County, 6206
Lupus Foundation of America: Northeast Indiana Chapter, 5916
Lupus Foundation of America: Northwest Indiana Lupus Chapter, 5917
Lupus Foundation of Indiana, 5918
Marion NAMI Grant Blackford Counties, 6207
Mary Margaret Walther Program Walther Cancer Institute, 2227
Methodist Hospital Sleep Center Winona Memorial Hospital, 7837
MidWest Medical Center: Sleep Disorders Center, 7838
Multipurpose Arthritis and Musculoskeletal Disease Center, 1149
Muncie: NAMI Delaware County, 6208
NAMI Highland, 6209
NAMI Indiana, 6090
NAMI Indiana - National Alliance on Mental Illness, 6210
NAMI South Central Indiana, 6211
NNFF Indiana Chapter, 6840
National Federation of the Blind: Indiana, 9560
National Kidney Foundation of Indiana, 5583
National Legal Center for the Medically Dependent & Disabled, 10566
National MS Society: Indiana State Chapter, 6539
National Spinal Cord Injury Association: Central Indiana Chapter, 8046
PWSA of Indiana Prader-Willi Syndrome Association, 7219
Parent Care, 8803
Primary Brain Cancer Support Group, 1873
Purdue Cancer Center Purdue University, 2187

Purdue University Center for AIDS Research, 336
Purdue University William A Hillenbrand Biomedical Engineering Center, 4838
Purdue University: Center for Research on Aging, 82
RESOLVE of Indiana, 5365
Richmond: NAMI East Central, 6212
Riley Hemophilia & Hemophilia Center Riley Hospital for Children, 5006
SIDS Center of Indiana, 8838
Sleep Alertness Center: Lafayette Home Hospital, 7844
Sleep/Wake Disorders Center: Community Hospitals of Indianapolis, 7875
South Bend: NAMI St. Joseph County, 6213
Southern Indiana Support Group: National Ataxia Foundation, 1443
Spina Bifida Association of Central Indiana, 7942
Terre Haute: NAMI Wabash Valley, 6214
The Riley Cystic Fibrosis Center, 3048
United Cerebral Palsy Association of Indiana, 2651
United Cerebral Palsy Associations, 2652
United Cerebral Palsy of the Wabash Valley, 2653
VA Northern Indiana Health Care System Marion Campus, 10255
Veterans Adm. Medical Center: Fort Wayne, 10256
Veterans Adm. Medical Center: Indianapolis, 10257
Vision World Wide, 9514
Warsaw NAMI Warsaw, 6215

Iowa

AARP Iowa State Office: Des Moines, 42
Alzheimer's Association: Big Sioux Chapter, 718
Alzheimer's Association: East Central Iowa Chapter, 719
Alzheimer's Association: Greater Iowa Chapter, 720
Alzheimer's Association: Heart of Iowa Chapter, 721
American Cancer Society: Iowa, 2091
American Dermatological Association University of Iowa Hospital and Clinics, 7715
American Diabetes Association: Cedar Rapid s District, 3205
American Lung Association of Iowa, 5815
Arthritis Foundation: Iowa Chapter, 1105
Autism Society of Iowa, 1587
Blank Childrens Hospital Pediatric Pulmonology Clinic, 3049
Brain Injury Association of Iowa, 4025
Brain Injury Association of Iowa Helpline, 4093
CCFA Iowa Chapter, 2942
Cedar Rapids Persian Gulf Veterans, Spouses and Children, 10258
Center for Disabilities and Development, 3526
Client Assistance Program: Iowa Division o n Persons with Disabilities, 10607
Department of Public Health: Division of Substance Abuse and Health, 8252
Des Moines Division: VA Central Iowa Health Care System, 10259
FFCMH: Iowa Chapter, 6091
Gilda's Club: Quad Cities, 2331
Great Plains Regional Hemophilia Center University of Iowa Hospitals, 4972
Greater Iowa Chapter Alzheimer's Association Quadcity Office, 722
Iowa Brain Tumor Support Group, 1874
Iowa Department for the Blind, 9749
Iowa Department of Public Health Center for Congenital and Inherited Disorders, 8839
Iowa Donor Network, 9191
Iowa Federaion of Families for Children's Mental Health (FFCMH), 6216
Iowa Oncology Research Association, 2228
Iowa SIDS Alliance, 8840
Iowa SIDS Program Iowa Department of Public Health, 8841
Juvenile Diabetes Research Foundation: Eas tern Iowa Chapter, 3206
Juvenile Diabetes Research Foundation: Gre ater Iowa Chapter, 3207
Kidneeds, 5658
Knoxville Division: VA Central Iowa Health Care System, 10260
Lupus Foundation of America: Iowa Chapter, 5919

Kansas

Kentucky

Louisiana

Juvenile Diabetes Research Foundation: Bat on Rouge Chapter, 3212
Juvenile Diabetes Research Foundation: Lou isiana Chapter, 3213
Juvenile Diabetes Research Foundation: Shr eveport Chapter, 3214
Louisiana Alliance for the Mentally Ill, 6097
Louisiana Association for the Blind, 9568
Louisiana Association of the Deaf, 4286
Louisiana Chapter of the National Hemophilia Foundation, 4926
Louisiana Comprehensive Hemophilia Care Center, 4987
Louisiana Department of Health & Hospitals : Office of Public Health, 266
Louisiana Lupus Foundation, 5923
Louisiana Organ Procurement Agency, 9194
Louisiana State University Genetics Section of Pediatrics, 1747
Louisiana Support Group: National Ataxia Foundation, 1444
Lupus Foundation of America: Cenla Chapter, 5924
Lupus Foundation of America: Northeast Louisiana, 5925
Lupus Foundation of America: Shreveport Chapter, 5926
Mission Project, 10270
NNFF Louisiana Chapter, 6844
National Federation of the Blind: Louisana, 9569
National Kidney Foundation of Louisiana, 5589
National Multiple Sclerosis Society, 6544
National Multiple Sclerosis Society: Louisiana Chapter 3, 6545
National Spinal Cord Injury Association: Louisiana Chapter, 8048
Northeast Louisiana Sickle Cell Anemia Foundation, 7663
Office of Human Services: Division of Alcohol and Drug Abuse, 8255
Office of Public Health, 8846
Public Health Services of Louisiana, 8847
RESOLVE of Louisiana, 5368
Randolph-Sheppard Vendors of America, 9507
Sickle Cell Anemia Research Foundation, 7673
Spina Bifida Association of Greater New Orleans, 7945
State Library of Louisiana, 9759
Tulane University Pulmonary Diseases Critical Care and Enviromental Medicine, 2236
Tulane University: US-Japan Biomedical Research Laboratories, 4071
United Cerebral Palsy of Baton Rouge McMains Children's Developmental Center, 2655
United Cerebral Palsy of Greater New Orleans, 2656
Veterans Adm. Medical Center: Alexandria Alexandria VA Medical Center, 10271
Veterans Adm. Medical Center: New Orleans New Orleans VA Medical Center, 10272
Veterans Adm. Medical Center: Shreveport Overton Brooks VA Medical Center, 10273
Wishing Well Foundation USA, Inc., 10837

Maine

AARP Maine State Office: Portland, 46
Alzheimer's Association: Maine Chapter, 731
American Cancer Society: Maine, 2099
American Diabetes Association: Maine, 3215
American Lung Association of Maine, 5819
American Lung Association of Maine, 9289
Autism Society of Maine, 1592
Bangor Public Library, 9760
Brain Injury Association of Maine, 4028
Brain Injury Association of Maine Helpline, 4096
Brain Tumor Support Group of Maine, 1882
Cary Library, 9761
Central Maine Cystic Fibrosis Center, 3056
Department of Human Services, 8848
Disability Rights Center: Maine, 10611

Juvenile Diabetes Research Foundation: New England/Maine Chapter, 3216
Lewiston Public Library, 9762
Lupus Group of Maine, 5927
Maine Alliance for the Mentally Ill, 6098
Maine Alzheimer's Care Center, 732
Maine Bureau of Health: Division of Disease Control, 267
Maine Center for the Blind and Visually Impaired, 9570
Maine Hemophilia Treatment Center, 4988
Maine Medical Center: Cystic Fibrosis Clin, 3058
Maine Medical Center: Cystic Fibrosis Clinical Center, 3057
Maine SIDS Foundation, 8849
Maine SIDS Program Department Of Human Services, 8850
Maine State Library, 9763
Maine Support Group: National Ataxia Foundation, 1445
National Federation of the Blind: Maine, 9571
National Kidney Foundation of Maine, 5590
National MS Society: Maine Chapter, 6546
Office of Alcohol and Drug Abuse Prevention, 8256
Portland Public Library, 9764
Sleep Laboratory, Maine Medical Center, 7869
United Cerebral Palsy of Northeastern Maine, 2657
United Families for Children's Mental Health, 6099
University of Maine: Conley Speech and Hearing Center, 4337
Veterans Adm. Medical Center: Augusta Togus VA Medical Center, 10274
Waterville Public Library, 9765

Maryland

ABLEDATA, 4223
ABLEDATA, 10495
ABLEDATA-REHAB DATA Alliance for Technology Access (ATA), 10496
ADARA, 4224
AIDSinfo, 180
AIDSinfo, 375
ALS Association: National Capital Area Chapter, 999
Alzheimer's Association: Central Maryland Chapter, 733
Alzheimer's Association: Eastern Shore Chapter, 734
Alzheimer's Association: Western Maryland Chapter, 736
Alzheimer's Disease Center: Johns Hopkins University School of Medicine, 854
Alzheimer's Disease Education and Referral Center, 649
American Action Fund for Blind Children and Adults, 9766
American Association of the Deaf-Blind, 4230
American Association of the Deaf-Blind, 9442
American Cancer Society: Maryland, 2100
American College of Gastroenterology, 3841
American Diabetes Association: Maryland, 3217
American Foundation for Urologic Disease: Us Too Line, 2319
American Gastroenterological Association, 9412
American Gastroenterological Association National Office, 3843
American Kidney Fund, 5550
American Lung Association of Maryland, 5820
American Lung Association of Maryland, 9290
American Prostate Society, 1997
American Society for Parenteral and Enteral Nutrition (ASPEN), 3849
American Society of Human Genetics, 1046
American Speech-Language-Hearing Association, 4234
American Urological Association, 5298
American Venereal Disease Association, 7617
Anxiety Disorders Association of America, 6354
Arthritis Foundation: Maryland Chapter, 1108
Asthma and Allergy Foundation of America, 566
Asthma and Allergy Foundation of America: Maryland/Greater Washington, DC, 575
Asthma and Allergy Information Association, 1276
Autism Society of America, 1568
Autism Society of America, 1631

Autism Society of Baltimore-Chesapeake, 1593
Baltimore Headache Institute, 6457
Baltimore VA Rehabilitation and Extended Care Center (BRECC), 10275
Believe In Tomorrow Children's Foundation, 10811
Blind Industries and Services of Maryland, 9572
Brain Injury Association of Maryland, 4029
Brain Injury Association of Maryland Helpl ine, 4097
Brain Tumor Networking Group, 1883
Brain Tumor Support Group: Maryland, 1884
Brainiacs, 1885
CCFA Maryland Chapter, 2946
CDC National Prevention Information Network (NPIN), 193
CDC National Prevention Information Network (NPIN), 304
CSAP State Liason Program CSAP Division of Communications Programs, 8200
Cancer Information Service, 2185
Candlelighters Childhood Cancer Foundation, 2009
Captioned Films/Videos, 4300
Center for AIDS Research: Johns Hopkins University School of Medicine, 337
Center for Research for Mothers & Children, 8799
Center for Substance Abuse Prevention, 8201
Chesapeake Area Support Group: National Ataxia Foundation, 1446
Children & Adults with Attention Deficit Disorders, 1506
Client Assistance Program: Maryland, 10612
Client Assistance Program: Medical Center East, 10639
Clinical Focus on Primary Immune Deficiency Diseases, 198
Community Services for Autistic Adults & Children, 1571
Cooley's Anemia Foundation (CAF): Capital Area, 2890
Cystic Fibrosis Center: National Institute of Health NIDDK, 3059
Cystic Fibrosis Foundation, 3018
Cystic Fibrosis Foundation, 3020
Deaf AIDS Project Family Service Foundation, 201
Digestive Disorders Associates Ridgely Oaks Professional Center, 3870
Disability Resource Center of Montgomery County Public Libraries, 9767
Drug Free Workplace Hotline, 8341
East Central Region: Hellen Keller National Center, 9573
Endocrine Society, 2
Epilepsy Foundation, 7519
Epilepsy Foundation of America Helpline, 7541
Fort Howard VA Outpatient Clinic, 10276
Foundation Fighting Blindness, 9463
Foundation Fighting Blindness, 9683
Frederick Cancer Research Center, 2237
Friends of Libraries for Deaf Action USA, 4302
Genetic and Rare Diseases Information Center, 3756
Goodwill Industries International, 10539
Guide Dog Users, 9467
Health Resources and Services Administration (HRSA), 9165
Hemophilia Foundation of Maryland, 4927
Hepatitis Foundation International, 5093
Immune Deficiency Foundation, 210
Immune Deficiency Foundation, 570
Impotents Anonymous, 5271
Indian Health Service, 8209
Institute of Psychiatry and Human Behavior: University of Maryland, 6166
International Agency for the Prevention of Blindness, 9471
International Braille and Technology Center for the Blind, 9768
Job Opportunities for the Blind, 9897
Johns Hopkins Brain Tumor Education Group, 1886
Johns Hopkins University: Asthma and Allergy Center, 1295
Johns Hopkins University: Behavioral Pharmacology Research Unit, 8308
Johns Hopkins University: Center for Communication Programs, 338
Johns Hopkins University: Dana Center for Preventive Ophthalmology, 9878

University of Maryland: Department of Pediatrics, 3523

University of Maryland: Division of Infectious Diseases, 882

University of Maryland: Medical Biotechnology Center, 341

Urban Cardiology Research Center, 4859

VA Capitol Health Care Network, 10278

VA Maryland Health Care System Perry Point VA Medical Center, 10279

Veterans Adm. Medical Center: Baltimore, 10280

Warren Grant Magnuson Clinical Center, 595

Warren Grant Magnuson Clinical Center, 1154

Warren Grant Magnuson Clinical Center, 2240

Warren Grant Magnuson Clinical Center, 3350

Warren Grant Magnuson Clinical Center, 4860

Warren Grant Magnuson Clinical Center, 5656

Warren Grant Magnuson Clinical Center, 5855

Warren Grant Magnuson Clinical Center National Institute of Health, 6180

Warren Grant Magnuson Clinical Center National Institute of Health, 9887

Washington DC Metropolitan Area Brain Tumor Support Group, 1887

Washington Ear, 9515

Weight-control Information Network, 6889

Weight-control Information Network National Institutes of Health, 3617

White Lung Association, 5797

Workplace Program CSAP Division of Communication Programs, 8233

Massachusetts

AARP Massachusetts State Office: Boston, 47

AIDS Support Group of Cape Cod, 374

ALS Association: Massachusetts Chapter, Wakefield Office, 1008

Affiliated Children's Arthritis Centers of New England, 1139

Alzheimer's Association, 737

Alzheimer's Association: Massachusetts Chapter, 738

Alzheimer's Association: Western Regional Office: Massachusetts Chapter, 739

Alzheimer's Disease Center: Boston University, 853

American Cancer Society: Boston, 2103

American Cancer Society: Central New England Region-Weston MA, 2104

American Diabetes Association: Boston, 3219

American Liver Foundation New England Chapter, 5728

American Lung Association of Massachusetts, 5821

American Lung Association of Massachusetts, 9291

American Society of Adults with Pseudo-Obstruction, 3850

Arthritis Foundation: Massachusetts Chapter, 1109

Association of Gastrointestinal Motility D isorders, 3639

Asthma and Allergy Foundation of America: New England Chapter, 576

Asthma and Allergy Foundation of America: New England Chapter, 1280

Attention Deficit Information Network, 1513

Autism Society of Massachusetts, 1594

Autism Treatment Center of America, 1569

Autism Treatment Center of America: Son-Rise Program, 1570

Baystate Medical Center Wesson Memorial Unit, 3060

Berkshire Center, 10665

BermanGund Laboratory for the Study of Retinal Degenerations, 9856

Boston Hemophilia Center Fegan 5 Children's Hospital, 4963

Boston Sickle Cell Center Boston Medical Center, 7666

Boston University Arthritis Center, 1141

Boston University Cancer Research Center, 2241

Boston University Center for Human Genetics, 1742

Boston University Laboratory of Neuropsychology, 8297

Boston University Medical Campus General Clinical Research Center, 1142

Boston University University Medical Center, 7411

Boston University, Whitaker Cardiovascular Institute, 4813

Brain Injury Association of Massachusetts, 4030

Brain Injury Association of Massachusetts Helpline, 4098

Brain Tissue Resource Center McLean Hospital, 1817

Brain Tumor Patient and Caregiver Support Group, 1888

Brain Tumor Society, 1808

Brain Tumor Support Group: Lahey, 1889

Brain Tumor Support Group: Worcester, 1890

Brigham and Women's Hospital: Center for Neurologic Diseases, 6604

Brigham and Women's Hospital: Rheumatology Immunology, and Allergy Division, 1291

Brigham and Women's Orthopedica and Arthritis Center, 1143

CAPP National Parent Resource Center, 1733

CCFA New England Chapter: Massachusetts, 2947

Cape Cod Chapter National Parkinson Foundation, 7068

Caption Center, 9771

Carroll Center for the Blind, 9575

Carroll Center for the Blind, 9863

Carroll Center for the Blind, 9894

Center for AIDS Research: Harvard Medical School, Division of AIDS, 342

Center for Blood Research Harvard Medical School/CBR, 343

Centers for AIDS Research: University of Massachusetts Medical School, 344

Childrens Hospital Immunology Division Children's Hospital, 1292

Childrens Hospital Medical Center Cystic Fibrosis Center, 3061

Client Assistance Program: Massachusetts, 10613

Cooley's Anemia Foundation (CAF): Massachusetts Chapter, 2891

Cystic Fibrosis Worldwide, 3017

Cystic Firbrosis Center: Tufts New England Medical Center, 3062

Dana Farber Cancer Institute National Drug Discovery Group for AIDS Treatment, 345

Dana-Farber Institute: Department of Biostatistics and Computational Biology, 2242

Developmental Medicine Center (DMC), 3513

Developmental Medicine Center Children's Hospital Boston, 346

Division of Substance Abuse, 8258

Eaton-Peabody Laboratory of Auditory Physiology, 4312

Facioscapulohumeral Muscular Dystrophy Soc iety (FSH Society), 6696

Federation for Children with Special Needs, 1737

Federation for Children with Special Needs, 10537

Ferguson Industries for the Blind, 9576

Fertility and Women's Health Care Center, 5404

Framingham Heart Study, 4821

General Clinical Research Center at Beth Israel Hospital, 4822

HOSPICELINK Hospice Education Institute, 10850

Harris Center for Education and Advocacy in Eating Disorders, 3636

Harvard Clinical Nutrition Research Center, 6890

Harvard Cocaine Recovery Project, 8306

Harvard Throndike Laboratory Harvard Medical Center, 4826

Harvard University Howe Laboratory of Ophthalmology, 9873

Health Care For All, 10541

Hemophilia Center of the New England Medical Center, 4984

Hydrocephalus Foundation, 5153

Joslin Diabetes Center, 3333

Juvenile Diabetes Research Foundation: New England/Bay State Chapter, 3220

Laboure College Library, 9772

Lupus Foundation of America: Massachusetts Chapter, 5929

Macular Degeneration Foundation, 9475

Mass./New Hampshire Chapter of the Myasthenia Gravis Foundation of America, 6763

Mass./New Hampshire Chapter of the Myasthenia Gravis Foundation of America, 6770

Massachusetts Alliance for the Mentally Ill, 6102

Massachusetts Alzheimers Disease Research Center, 868

Massachusetts Chapter of the MG Foundation, 6764

Massachusetts Commission for the Blind, 9577

Massachusetts Department of Health HIV/AIDS Bureau, 268

Massachusetts Down Syndrome Congress, 3499

Massachusetts Eating Disorder Association, 3622

Massachusetts General Departments of Neurology and Neurosurgery, 8140

Massachusetts General Hospital, 3063

Massachusetts General Hospital: Harvard Cutaneous Biology Research Center, 7727

Massachusetts Institute of Technology Center for Cancer Research, 2243

Massachusetts Institute of Technology: Center for Cancer Research, 2244

Massachusetts State Association of the Deaf, 4287

Massachusetts Sudden Infant Death Syndrome Boston City Hospital, 8922

Merrimack Valley HPV Support Group Holy Family Hospital, 10614

Myasthenia Gravis: Massachusetts Chapter, 6765

NNFF Northern New England Chapter, 6849

National Association for Parents of the Visually Impaired, 9477

National Association for Parents of the Visually Impaired, 9898

National Braille Press, 9488

National CFIDS Foundation, 2762

National Eating Disorders Screening Program, 3615

National Federation of the Blind: Massachusetts, 9578

National Kidney Foundation of MA/RI/NH/VT, 5592

National Kidney Foundation of MA/RI/NH/VT, 5601

National Kidney Foundation of MA/RI/NH/VT, 5624

National Kidney Foundation of MA/RI/NH/VT, 5641

National MS Society: Central New England Chapter, 6548

National MS Society: Central New England Chapter, 6558

National MS Society: Massachusetts Chapter, 6549

National Parkinson Foundation:Cape Cod Chapter, 7069

National Scoliosis Foundation, 7452

National Spinal Cord Injury Association, 8050

National Spinal Cord Injury Association: Greater Boston Chapter, 8051

National Tay-Sachs and Allied Disease Association, 3760

National Tay-Sachs and Allied Diseases Association (NTSAD), 8968

National Tay-Sachs and Allied Diseases Association (NTSAD), 8969

National TaySachs & Allied Diseases, 8972

Neurofibromatosis: New England, 6846

Neurological Support Group of St. Luke's Hospital, 1891

Neurosurgical Service, 10615

New England AIDS Education & Training Center (NEHEC), 269

New England AIDS Education and Training Center, 225

New England Area Support Group: National Ataxia Foundation, 1447

New England Health Care System, 10281

New England Hemophilia Association, 4929

New England Medical Center: ALS Laboratory, 1041

New England Organ Bank Connecticut, 9181

New England Organ Bank Maine, 9195

New England Organ Bank Massachusetts, 9198

New England Organ Bank New Hampshire, 9206

New England Organ Bank Rhode Island, 9223

New England Organ Bank Vermont, 9228

New England Region: Helen Keller National Center, 9579

New England Regional Genetics Group, 1748

Northeast Parkinson's and Caregivers, 7070

Northhampton VA Medical Center, 10282

Option Institute, 2761

Option Institute, 3787

Option Institute, 6361

Option Institute International Learning & Training Center, 10577

Option Istitute Learning and Training Center, 6053

PALS Support Groups, 1764
Parent Education/Support Group, 1892
Parent Professional Advocacy League, 1741
Parent Professional Advocacy League, 6218
Pediatric Crohn's and Colitis Association, 2927
Pediatric Pulmonary Unit Massachusetts General Hospital, 8923
Perkins Braille and Talking Book Library, 9773
Persian Gulf Era Veterans, 10283
Prader-Willi New England Association, 7223
Prader-Willi New England Association Prader-Willi Syndrome Association, 7224
Prader-Willi Syndrome of Western Massachusetts, 7225
RESOLVE of the Bay State, 5371
Region 1 of the National Association for Parents of the Visually Impaired, 9536
Region I Office Program: Consultants for Maternal and Child Health, 8853
SIDS Support Group, 8930
Safe Homes, 8230
Scleroderma Foundation, 7374
Scleroderma Foundation: New England Chapter, 7387
Scleroderma Foundation: New England Chapter, 7389
Scleroderma Foundation: New England Chapter, 7394
Scleroderma Foundation: New England Chapter, 7403
Scleroderma Foundation: New England Chapter, 7407
Scleroderma Support Groups, 7428
Screening For Mental Health, 6362
Shriver Center University Affiliated Program, 10433
Sleep Disorders Unit Beth Israel Deaconess Medical Center, 7867
Sleep Research Foundation, 7871
Society for Surgery of the Alimentary Tract, 3862
Southern New England Turner Syndrome Society, 9367
Spina Bifida Association of Massachusetts, 7948
Spinal Connection National Scoliosis Foundation, 7454
Students Against Destructive Decisions, 8231
Talking Book Library at Worcester Public Library, 9774
Traditional Tibetan Healing, 6613
Tufts University: Baystate Medical Center, 5406
United Cerebral Palsy of Berkshire County, 2661
United Cerebral Palsy of MetroBoston, 2662
United Scleroderma Foundation, 7272
University of Massachusetts Memorial Medical Center, 3064
University of Massachusetts: Diabetes and Endocrinology Research Center, 3340
VA Boston Healthcare System: Jamaica Plain Jamaica Plain Campus, 10284
VA Boston Healthcare System: West Roxbury West Roxbury Campus, 10285
VALT Support Group (Vital Active Life After Trauma), 4099
Veterans Adm. Medical Center: Bedford Edith Nourse Rogers Memorial Veterans, 10286
Veterans Adm. Medical Center: Brockton Brockton Campus, 10287
Veterans Benefits Clearinghouse, 10434
Vision Use in Employment, 9906
Windhorse Associates, 6219

Michigan

AARP Michigan State Office: Lansing, 48
ALS Association: Michigan Chapter, 1009
ALS Association: West Michigan Chapter, 1010
Alzheimer's Association: East Central Michigan Chapter, 740
Alzheimer's Association: Greater Michigan Chapter, 741
Alzheimer's Association: Greater Michigan Chapter: Upper Peninsula Region, 742
Alzheimer's Association: Michigan Great Lakes Chapter: West Shore Region, 743
Alzheimer's Association: Mid-Michigan Chapter, 744
Alzheimer's Association: Northeast Michigan Chapter, 745
Alzheimer's Association: Northwest Michigan Chapter, 746

American Autoimmune Related Diseases Association, 184
American Autoimmune Related Diseases Association, 4862
American Autoimmune Related Diseases Association, 10501
American Diabetes Association: Michigan, 3221
American Institute for Preventive Medicine, 10506
American Institute for Preventive Medicine, 10507
American Liver Foundation Michigan Chapter, 5729
American Lung Association of Michigan, 5822
American Lung Association of Michigan, 9292
American Motility Society, 3845
Apnea Identification Program Children's Ho spital of Michigan, 8854
Arthritis Foundation: Michigan Chapter Chapter and Metro Detroit, 1110
Association for Children's Mental Health, 6103
Association for the Blind & Visually Impaired, 9580
Asthma and Allergy Foundation of America: Michigan Chapter, 577
Asthma and Allergy Foundation of America: Michigan Chapter, 1281
Autism Society of Michigan, 1595
Autoimmune Diseases Association, 5889
Brain Injury Association of Michigan, 4031
Brain Injury Association of Michigan Helpline, 4100
Brain Tumor Networking Club, 1893
Brain Tumor Support Group for Patients & Families, 1894
Brain Tumor Support Group: Ann Arbor, 1895
Brain Tumor Support Group: West Bloomfield, 1896
CCFA Michigan Chapter: Farmington Hills, 2948
Christian Horizons, 10527
Client Assistance Program: Michigan, 10616
Commission for the Blind, 10617
Detroit Subregional Library for the Blind and Physically Handicapped, 9775
Detroit Support Group: National Ataxia Foundation, 1448
Detroit VA Medical Center John D. Dingell VA Medical Center, 10288
Dynamic Rehab, 4004
East Lansing Cystic Fibrosis Center Michigan State University, 3065
Eastern Michigan Hemophilia Center St. Joseph Hospital, 4969
Genesee County Health Department, 8855
Gershenson Radiation Oncology Center Barbara Ann Karmanos Cancer Institute, 2245
Gilda's Club: Grand Rapids, 2329
Glaucoma Laser Trabeculoplasty Study Sinai Hospital of Detroit, 9872
Grand Traverse Area Library for the Blind and Physically Handicapped, 9776
Great Lakes Chapter of the Myasthenia Gravis Foundation of America, 6766
Greater Detroit Agency for the Blind and Visually Impaired, 9581
Greater Grand Rapids Pediatric Hemophilia Program, 4973
Hearing Aid Helpline, 4353
Hemophilia Foundation of Michigan, 4930
Henry Ford Hospital: Hypertension and Vascular Research Division, 5218
Hydrocephalus Support Group of Michigan Children's Hospital of Michigan, 5160
International Advocacy for Gulf War Syndrome, 10289
International Hearing Society, 4257
JIMHO Affiliated Centers (Justice in Mental Health Organization), 6104
Juvenile Diabetes Research Foundation: Metropolitan Detroit/SE Michigan, 3222
Juvenile Diabetes Research Foundation: Wes t Michigan Chapter, 3223
Kalamazoo Center for Medical Studies Michigan State University, 3066
Kent County Health Department, 8856
Kent County Library for the Blind, 9777
Leukemia and Lymphoma Society: Michigan Chapter, 2105
Library of Michigan Service for the Blind, 9778
Lupus Foundation of America: Michigan Lupus Foundation, 5930

Lyme Alliance, 9030
Macomb Library for the Blind and Physically Handicapped, 9779
Meyer L Prentis Comprehensive Cancer Cente Barbara Ann Karmanos Cancer Institute, 2247
Meyer L Prentis Comprehensive Cancer Center of Metropolitan Detroit, 2246
Michigan Alliance for the Mentally Ill, 6105
Michigan Alzheimer's Disease Research Center, 870
Michigan Chapter: Southeast, 9368
Michigan Deaf Association, 4288
Michigan Department of Community Health, 8857
Michigan Department of Community Health HIV/AIDS Prevention & Intervention Secti, 270
Michigan Hand Center, 2543
Michigan State University Hemophilia Comprehensive Care Clinic, 4991
Michigan West Turner Syndrome Society, 9369
Midwestern Michigan Library Cooperative, 9780
Motor Neuron Disease Program University of Michigan Health System, 1039
Muskegon County Library for the Blind, 9781
Myasthenia Gravis Association, 6767
NF Support Group of West Michigan, 6857
National Federation of the Blind: Michigan, 9582
National Federation of the Blind: Mississippi, 9586
National Kidney Foundation of Michigan, 5593
National MS Society: Michigan Chapter, 6550
National Parents Resources Institute for Drug Education, 8223
Northland Library Cooperative, 9782
Oakland County Health Division: SIDS Project, 8858
Oakland County Library for the Visually and Physically Impaired, 9783
Office of Substance Abuse Services Department of Public Health, 8259
Patient Advocates for Advanced Cancer Treatments (PAACT), 2186
Prader-Willi Syndrome Association of Michigan, 7226
RESOLVE of Michigan, 5372
Rainbow Connection, 10830
Regional Hemophilia Treatment Center Children's Hospital of Michigan, 5004
Rehabilitation Institute of Michigan, 4068
SIDS LEAD: Children's Special Health Care Services, 8859
Scleroderma Foundation: Michigan Chapter, 7390
Spina Bifida Association of Grand Rapids, 7949
Spina Bifida Association of Upper Peninsula Michigan, 7950
Spina Bifida and Hydrocephalus Association, 7952
Spina Bifida and Hydrocephalus Association of Southwestern Michigan, 7951
St. Clark County Library for the Blind and Physically Handicapped, 9784
Transplantation Society of Michigan, 9200
United Cerebral Palsy of Metropolitan Detroit, 2663
United Cerebral Palsy of Michigan, 2664
University of Michigan Communicative Disorders Clinic, 4338
University of Michigan Hemophilia Center, 5017
University of Michigan Michigan Gastrointestinal Peptide Research Ctr., 3874
University of Michigan Montgomery: John M. Sheldon Allergy Society, 593
University of Michigan Nephrology Division, 5654
University of Michigan Pulmonary and Critical Care Division, 4848
University of Michigan Reproductive Sciences Program, 5408
University of Michigan: Alcohol Research Center, 8329
University of Michigan: Cancer Center Cancer Research Committee, 2248
University of Michigan: Cystic Fibrosis Center, 3067
University of Michigan: Division of Cardiology, 4849
University of Michigan: Division of Hypertension, 5221
University of Michigan: Kresge Hearing Research Institute, 4339
University of Michigan: Mental Health Research Institute, 6174

University of Michigan: National Cooperative Drug/AIDS Group, 347
University of Michigan: Orthopaedic Research Laboratories, 1153
University of Michigan: Psychiatric Center, 8330
Upper Peninsula Library for the Blind and Physically Handicapped, 9785
Veterans Adm. Medical Center: Ann Arbor Ann Arbor Healthcare System, 10290
Veterans Adm. Medical Center: Bath Battle Creek VA Medical Center, 10291
Veterans Adm. Medical Center: Battle Creek, 10292
Veterans Adm. Medical Center: Iron Mountain, 10293
Veterans Adm. Medical Center: Saginaw Aleda E. Lutz VA Medical Center, 10294
Veterans In Partnership, 10295
Visually Impaired Center, 9886
Washtenaw County Library for the Blind and Physically Disabled, 9786
Wayne County Regional Library for the Blind and Physically Handicapped, 9787
Wayne State University, 5411
Wayne State University Center for Health Research, 348
Wayne State University Center for Molecular Medicine and Genetics, 2249
Wayne State University: CS Mott Center for Human Growth and Development, 1754
Wayne State University: Comprehensive Sickle Cell Center, 7678
Wayne State University: Gurdjian-Lissner Biomechanics Laboratory, 4077
Wayne State University: University Women's Care, 5412
William T Gossett Parkinson's Disease Center, 7088

Minnesota

AARP Minnesota State Office: Saint Paul, 49
ALS Association: Minnesota Chapter, 1011
African American Family Services, 8190
Alzheimer's Association: Minnesota/Dakotas, 747
Alzheimer's Disease Center Mayo Clinic Mayo Medical School, 851
American Academy of Neurology, 6450
American Academy of Neurology: Tourette Syndrome, 9076
American Cancer Society: Duluth, 2106
American Cancer Society: Mendota Heights Mendota Heights, 2107
American Cancer Society: Rochester, 2108
American Cancer Society: Saint Cloud, 2109
American Diabetes Association: Minnesota, 3224
American Liver Foundation Minnesota Chapte r, 5730
American Lung Association of Minnesota, 5823
American Lung Association of Minnesota, 9293
American Pancreatic Association, 3846
Anna Westin Foundation, 3603
Arthritis Foundation: North Central Chapter, 1111
Autism Society of Minnesota, 1596
Behavioral Pediatrics Program, 10671
Brain Injury Association of Minnesota, 4032
Brain Injury Association of Minnesota Helpline, 4101
CCFA Minnesota Chapter, 2949
Center for Children with Chronic Illness and Disability, 10516
Chemical Dependency Program Division Department of Human Services, 8260
Dads and Daughters, 3605
Dentists Concerned for Dentists, 8261
Desert Storm Justice Foundation: Minnesota, 10296
Desert Storm Justice Foundation: Virginia, 10297
Down Syndrome Association of Minnesota, 3500
Duluth Lighthouse for the Blind, 9583
Duluth Public Library, 9788
Emotional Health Anonymous, 6220
Fairview-University Hemophilia & Thrombosis Center, 4971
Fetal Alcohol Network, 10673
Hazelden, 8208
Hear Now: Starkey Hearin Foundation, 4252
Hemophilia Foundation of Minnesota and the Dakotas, 4931

Hepatitis B Coalition, 5092
Immunization Action Coalition, 5094
Impotence Information Center, 5270
International Diabetes Center at Nicollet, 3332
Juvenile Diabetes Research Foundation: Min nesota Chapter, 3225
KDWB Family Resource Center, 10677
KDWB Variety Family Canter, 10678
Lawyers Concerned for Lawyers, 8210
Leukemia and Lymphoma Society: Minnesota Chapter, 2110
LifeSource, Upper Midwest Organ Procurement Organization, Inc., 9201
Lupus Foundation of America: Minnesota Chapter, 5931
Lyme Disease Network, 9031
MN Chapter of the Turner Syndrome Society, 9370
Mayo Clinic and Foundation Mayo Foundation, 6693
Mayo Clinic and Foundation: Division of Allergic Diseases, 585
Mayo Clinic: Department of Neurology, 1037
Mayo Comprehensive Cancer Center, 2250
Mayo Comprehensive Hemophilia Center Mayo Clinic, 4989
Melpomene Institute for Women's Health Research, 5405
Minnesota AIDS Project AIDSLine, 385
Minnesota Alliance for the Mentally Ill, 6106
Minnesota Ambassador: National Ataxia Foundation, 1449
Minnesota Association for Children's Mental Health, 6107
Minnesota Department of Health: AIDS/STD Prevention Service, 271
Minnesota Disability Law Center, 10618
Minnesota Library for the Blind, 9789
Minnesota Obesity Center, 6891
Minnesota State Chapter of the Myasthenia Gravis Foundation of America, 6768
Minnesota Sudden Infant Death Center Minneapolis Children's Medical Center, 8860
Myasthenia Gravis Foundation, 6748
Myasthenia Gravis Foundation of America, 6749
National Association of Blind Educators Sheila Koenig, 9480
National Association of Epilepsy Centers, 7520
National Association to Promote the Use of Braille, 9486
National Ataxia Foundation, 1425
National Federation of the Blind: Minnesota, 9584
National Kidney Foundation of Minnesota, 5594
National MS Society: Minnesota Chapter, 6551
National Marrow Donor Program, 2027
National Resource Library on Youth with Disabilities, 10666
Neurofibromatosis, 6823
Neurofibromatosis: Minnesota, 6847
PACER Center, 6221
PWSA of Minnesota Prader-Willi Syndrome Association, 7227
Parkinson Association of Minnesota, 7071
Pediatric Psychology, 10685
RESOLVE: Minnesota Chapter, 5373
STAR Center for Family Health, 10686
STOP-SIDS Minnesota, 8861
Schulze Diabetes Institute, 3320
Scleroderma Foundation: Minnesota Chapter, 7391
Spina Bifida Association of Minnesota, 7953
Spinal Cord Society, 8038
Twin Cities Area Support Group: National Ataxia Foundation, 1450
U Special Kids, 10687
United Cerebral Palsy of Central Minnesota, 2665
United Cerebral Palsy of Central Ohio, 2666
United Cerebral Palsy of Minnesota, 2667
United Ostomy Association, 2929
United Ostomy Association, 3865
United Ostomy Association, 9416
United Ostomy Associations of America Advocacy Hotline, 2343
University of Minnesota Department of Psychiatry, 6175
University of Minnesota Masonic Cancer Center, 2251
University of Minnesota: Cystic Fibrosis Center, 3068

University of Minnesota: Hypertensive Research Group, 5222
University of Minnesota: Program on Alcohol/Drug Control, 8331
Veterans Adm. Medical Center: Minneapolis Minneapolis VA Medical Center, 10298
Veterans Adm. Regional Office: St. Paul, 10299

Mississippi

Alzheimer's Association: Mississippi Chapter, 748
Alzheimer's Foundation of the South: Mississippi Division, 749
American Cancer Society: Jackson, 2111
American Diabetes Association: Mississippi, 3226
American Lung Association of Mississippi, 5824
American Lung Association of Mississippi, 9294
American Lung Association of Missouri, 5825
Arthritis Foundation: Mississippi Chapter, 1112
Brain Injury Association of Mississippi, 4033
Brain Injury Association of Mississippi Helpline, 4102
Christian Resource for People Who Are Blind, 9829
Division of Alcohol & Drug Abuse: Mississippi, 8262
Division of Alcohol & Drug Abuse: South Department of Mental Health, 8263
Gulf War Babies, 10300
Leukemia and Lymphoma Society: Mississippi Chapter, 2112
Lupus Foundation of America: Mississippi Chapter, 5932
Mississippi Alliance for the Mentally Ill, 6108
Mississippi Area Support Group: National Ataxia Foundation, 1451
Mississippi Client Assistance Program, 10619
Mississippi Department of Public Health: STD/HIV Prevention Program, 272
Mississippi Families as Allies, 6109
Mississippi Hemophilia Foundation, 4932
Mississippi Industries for the Blind, 9585
Mississippi Library Commission, 9790
Mississippi Organ Recovery, 9202
Mississippi SIDS Alliance, 8862
Mississippi State Department of Health and Child Health Services, 8863
National Kidney Foundation of Mississippi, 5595
National Multiple Sclerosis Society: Alaba ma-Mississippi Chapter, 6552
South Central VA Health Care Network, 10301
University of Mississippi Medical Center, 3069
VA Gulf Coast Veterans Health Care System, 10302
Veterans Adm. Medical Center: Jackson, 10303
Veterans Adm. Regional Office: Jackson, 10304

Missouri

AARP Missouri State Office: Kansas City, 50
ALS Association: Keith Worthington Chapter Central Missouri Branch Office, 1012
ALS Association: St. Louis Regional Chapter, 1013
APDA Center for Advanced Parkinson Disease Research, 7097
Adriene Resource Center for Blind Children, 9791
Alphapointe Association for the Blind, 9587
Alzheimer's Association: Mid-Missouri Chapter, 750
Alzheimer's Association: Northwest Missouri-Chapter, 751
Alzheimer's Association: Southwest Missouri Chapter, 752
Alzheimer's Association: St. Louis Chapter, 753
Alzheimer's Disease Research Center Washington University School of Medicine, 858
American Cancer Society: Saint Louis, 2113
American Diabetes Association: Missouri, 3227
American Liver Foundation Greater Kansas Greater kC Chapter, 5731
American Lung Association of Eastern Missouri, 5826
American Lung Association of Missouri, 9295

American Lung Association: Kansas City Office, 5827
American Optometric Association, 9449
Arthritis Foundation: Eastern Missouri Chapter, 1113
Assemblies of God National Center for the Blind, 9792
Asthma and Allergy Foundation of America: Greater Kansas City Chapter, 1282
Asthma and Allergy Foundation of America: St. Louis Chapter, 578
Asthma and Allergy Foundation of America: St. Louis Chapter, 1283
Autism Society of Gateway Chapter, 1597
Brain Cancer Support Group, 1897
Brain Injury Association of Kansas and Greater Kansas City Helpline, 4103
Brain Injury Association of Missouri, 4034
Brain Injury Association of Missouri Helpline, 4104
Brain Tumor Support Group: Kansas City, 1898
Brain Tumor Support and Networking Group, 1899
CCFA Mid-America Chapter: Kansas, 2943
CCFA Mid-America Chapter: Missouri, 2951
Cancer Research Center, 2252
Canine Assistance for the Disabled CADI, 4240
Central Institute for the Deaf, 4307
Central Missouri Regional Arthritis Center Stephen's College Campus, 1144
Children's Mercy Hospital Children's Mercy Hospitals & Clinics, 3070
Church of the Nazarene, 9793
Fabry Support & Information Group, 3763
Gateway Hemophilia Association, 4933
Juvenile Diabetes Research Foundation: St. Louis Chapter, 3228
Kansas City Association for the Blind, 9588
Kansas City Support Group: National Ataxia Foundation, 1452
Kansas/Missouri- Turner Syndrome Society, 9371
Lupus Foundation of America: Kansas City Chapter, 5933
Lupus Foundation of America: Missouri Chapter, 5934
Lupus Foundation of America: Ozarks Chapter, 5935
Lutheran Library for the Blind, 9794
MO-SPAN, 6110
MO-SPAN Southwest Region, 6222
MOSPAN Northwest Region, 6223
Make Today Count, 2017
Mid Missouri Support Group: National Ataxia Foundation, 1453
Mid-America Transplant Services, 9203
Missouri Coalition Alliance for the Mentally Ill, 6111
Missouri Department of Health: Bureau of AIDS Prevention, 273
Missouri Division of Alcohol and Drug Abuse, 8264
Missouri Illinois Regional Hemophilia Comprehensive Treatment Center, 4992
Missouri Protection and Advocacy Services, 10620
Missouri Teratogen Information Service, 1760
Missouri/St. Louis Turner Syndrome Society, 9372
NAMI of Missouri, 6112
NNFF Kansas Affiliate, 6842
National CFS Association, 2757
National Children's Cancer Society, 2183
National Chronic Fatigue Syndrome and Fibr, 2759
National Chronic Fatigue Syndrome and Fibr, 3782
National Chronic Fatigue Syndrome and Fibr omyalgia Association Support Group, 3789
National Chronic Fatigue Syndrome and Fibromyalgia Association, 2758
National Chronic Fatigue Syndrome and Fibromyalgia Association, 2766
National Chronic Fatigue Syndrome and Fibromyalgia Association, 3781
National Federation of the Blind: Missouri, 9589
National Kidney Foundation of Eastern Missouri and Metro East, 5596
National MS Society: Gateway Area Chapter, 6553
Ozarks Parkinson Support Group, 7098
PKD Foundation Polycystic Kidney Disease Foundation, 5652
PWSA Missouri Chapter Prader-Willi Syndrome Association, 7228
PWSA of Kansas Prader-Willi Syndrome Association, 7221

PostPolio Health International, 7188
RESOLVE of St. Louis, Missouri, 5374
SIDS Resources, 8865
Scleroderma Foundation: Missouri Chapter, 7392
Share Pregnancy and Infant Loss Support, Inc., 8804
Share Pregnancy and Infant Loss Support, Inc., 10856
Spina Bifida Association of Greater St. Louis, 7954
Turner's Syndrome Society of St. Louis/West Illinois, 9373
United Cerebral Palsy of Greater Kansas City, 2668
United Cerebral Palsy of Greater St. Louis, 2669
United Cerebral Palsy of Northwest Missouri, 2670
United Cerebral Palsy of Northwestern, 2671
University of Missouri Columbia Cystic Fibrosis Center, 3071
University of Missouri Columbia Division of Cardiothoracic Surgery, 4850
University of Missouri: Columbia Missouri Institute of Mental Health, 6176
University of Missouri: Kansas City Drug Information Service, 8332
VA Heartland Network, 10305
Veterans Adm. Medical Center: Columbia Harry S. Truman Memorial, 10306
Veterans Adm. Medical Center: Kansas City Kansas City VA Medical Center, 10307
Veterans Adm. Medical Center: Poplar Bluff, 10308
Veterans Adm. Regional Office: St. Louis John Cochran Division, 10309
Washington University Chromalloy American Kidney Center, 5657
Washington University School of Medicine, 8146
Washington University: Cystic Fibrosis Center, 3072
Washington University: Diabetes Research and Training Center, 3351
Western Region SIDS Resources, 8866
Whitney Library for the Blind: Assemblies of God, 9795
Wolfner Memorial Library for the Blind, 9796

Montana

AARP Montana State Office: Helena, 51
Alzheimer's Association: Greater Billings Area Chapter, 754
American Cancer Society: Montana, 2114
American Diabetes Association: Montana, 3229
American Lung Association of Northern Rockies, 5828
American Lung Association of the Northern Rockies: Montana and Wyoming, 9296
Brain Injury Association of Montana, 4035
Brain Injury Association of Montana Helpline, 4105
Cancer Patient/Caregiver Support Group, 1900
Department of Institutions, Alcohol and Drug Abuse Division, 8265
Department of Public Health and Human Services, 8867
Disability Rights Montana, 10621
Family Support Network, 6113
Lupus Foundation of America: Montana Chapter, 5936
Montana Alliance for the Mentally Ill Mihelish's Residence, 6114
Montana Department of Health & Environmental Sciences, 8868
Montana Deptartment of Health And Human Services, 274
Montana State Library, 9797
National Federation of the Blind: Montana, 9590
National MS Society: Montana Division, 6554
Veterans Adm. Medical Center: Fort Harrison, 10310
Veterans Adm. Medical Center: Miles City, 10311

Nebraska

AARP Nebraska State Office: Lincoln, 52
ALS Association: Keith Worthington Chapter Nebraska Branch Office, 1014
Advocacy for the Gulf War Children, 10190
Alzheimer's Association: Lincoln/Greater Nebraska Chapter, 755

Alzheimer's Association: Omaha/Eastern Nebraska Chapter, 756
Alzheimer's Association: Wyoming Chapter, 845
American Cancer Society: Nebraska, 2115
American Diabetes Association: Nebraska, 3230
American Lung Association of Nebraska, 5829
American Lung Association of Nebraska, 9297
Arthritis Foundation: Nebraska Chapter, 1115
Autism Society of Nebraska, 1598
Boys Town National Research Hospital, 4305
Celiac Sprue Association: USA, 2560
Center for Hearing Loss in Children Boystown National Research Hospital, 4306
Client Assistance Program: Nebraska Division of Rehabilitative Services, 10622
Creighton University Allergic Disease Center, 584
Creighton University Cardiac Center, 4819
Creighton University Center for Healthy Aging, 80
Creighton University Midwest Hypertension Research Center, 5216
Department of Public Instruction: Division of Alcoholism and Drug Abuse, 8266
Family Support Network, 2726
Juvenile Diabetes Research Foundation: Lin coln Chapter, 3231
Juvenile Diabetes Research Foundation: Oma ha Council Bluffs Chapter, 3232
Leukemia and Lymphoma Society: Nebraska Chapter, 2116
Lincoln Cancer Center, 2253
Lupus Foundation of America: Omaha Chapter, 5937
Lupus Foundation of America: Western Nebraska Chapter, 5938
National Alliance for the Mentally Ill: Nebraska (NAMI), 6115
National Association of Blind Musicians Linda Mentink, 9482
National Federation of the Blind: Nebraska, 9591
National Federation of the Blind: Writers Division, 9501
National MS Society: Midlands Chapter Community Health Plaza, 6555
Nebraska Chapter of the National Hemophilia Foundation, 4934
Nebraska Department of Health Perinatal Child and Adolescent Health, 8869
Nebraska Information Service, 1762
Nebraska Kidney Association, 5599
Nebraska Library Commission Talking Book and Braille Services, 9798
Nebraska Organ Retrieval System, 9204
Nebraska SIDS Foundation University of Nebraska Medical Center, 8870
North Platte Public Library, 9799
Omaha HPV Support Group: PP of Omaha, 10623
PWSA Nebraska Chapter Prader-Willi Syndrome Association, 7230
Spina Bifida Association of Nebraska, 7955
United Cerebral Palsy of Nebraska, 2672
University of Nebraska Medical Center Cystic Fibrosis Center, 3073
University of Nebraska Medical Center Tera Togen Project, 1771
University of Nebraska at Omaha Eppley Institute for Research in Cancer, 2254
University of Nebraska: Lincoln Barkley Memorial Center, 4340
Veterans Adm. Medical Center: Grand Island, 10312
Veterans Adm. Medical Center: Lincoln, 10313
Veterans Adm. Medical Center: Omaha Western Iowa Health Care System, 10314

Nevada

AARP Nevada State Office: Las Vegas, 53
Alcohol and Drug Abuse Bureau: Department of Human Resources, 8267
Alzheimer's Association: Northern Nevada Chapter, 757
Alzheimer's Association: Southern Nevada Chapter, 758
American Cancer Society: Nevada, 2117
American Diabetes Association: Nevada, 3233
American Lung Association of Idaho/Nevada, 9298

American Lung Association of Nevada, 5830
Autism Society of Northern Nevada, 1599
Children's Lung Specialists, 3074
Client Assistance Program: Nevada, 10624
Cure Our Children Foundation, 10814
Desert Southwest Chapter 3 National Multiple
  Sclerosis Society, 6556
Hemophilia Foundation of Nevada, 4935
Juvenile Diabetes Research Foundation: Nevada
  Chapter, 3234
Juvenile Diabetes Research Foundation: Nor thern
  Nevada Branch, 3235
Kantor Nephrology Consultants, 5648
Las Vegas Clark County Library District, 9800
Lupus Foundation of America: Las Vegas Chapter,
  5939
Lupus Foundation of America: Northern Nevada
  Chapter, 5940
NNFF Nevada Affiliate: Reno Area, 6848
National Federation of the Blind: Nevada, 9592
National Kidney Foundation of Nevada, 5600
National MS Society: Great Basin Sierra Chapter,
  6557
Nevada Alliance for the Mentally Ill, 6116
Nevada Department of Human Resources: Health
  Program Section, 275
Nevada Donor Network, 9205
Nevada PEP, 6224
Nevada State Health Division Bureau of Family
  Health Services, 8871
Nevada State Library and Archives, 9801
RESOLVE of Nevada Barbara Greenspun Women's
  Care Center, 5375
Scleroderma Foundation: Nevada Chapter, 7393
Southern Nevada Sightless, 9593
United Cerebral Palsy of Northern Nevada, 2673
University Medical Center Hemophilia Program,
  5014
Veterans Adm. Medical Center: Las Vegas VA
  Southern Nevada Healthcare System, 10315
Veterans Adm. Medical Center: Reno VA Sierra
  Nevada Health Care System, 10316

New Hampshire

AARP New Hampshire State Office-Manchester, 54
ALS Association: Northern New England Chapter,
  1028
Alzheimer's Association of Vermont and New
  Hampshire, 759
American Cancer Society: New Hampshire Gail
  Singer Memorial Building, 2118
American Diabetes Association: New Hampshire,
  3236
American Lung Association of New Hampshire, 5831
American Lung Association of New Hampshire, 9299
Arthritis Foundation: Northern New England Chapter,
  1134
Autism Society of New Hampshire, 1600
Brain Injury Association of New Hampshire, 4036
Brain Injury Association of New Hampshire, 4107
Brain Injury/Brain Tumor Support Group, 1901
Camp Allen, 10667
Client Assistance Program: New Hampshire, 10625
Dartmouth Medical School: Microbiology
  Department, 3721
Dartmouth-Hitchcock Medical Center - Genetics and
  Development, 3511
Granite State FFCMH, 6117
High Hopes Foundation of New Hampshire, Inc.,
  10821
Juvenile Diabetes Research Foundation: New
  England/New Hampshire Chapter, 3237
National Alliance for the Mentally Ill, 6118
National Alliance for the Mentally Ill: New
  Hampshire, 6119
National Alliance for the Mentally Ill: New
  Hampshire, 6225
National Federation of the Blind: New Hampshire,
  9594
New Hampshire Cancer Pain Initiative, 2119
New Hampshire Chapter NSCIA, 8052
New Hampshire Cystic Fibrosis Care Teaching and
  Research Center, 3075

New Hampshire Department of Health and Human
  Services, 276
New Hampshire Lupus Foundation, 5941
New Hampshire SIDS Alliance, 8872
New Hampshire SIDS Program, 8873
New Hampshire State Library, 9802
Norris Cotton Cancer Center Dartmouth-Hitchcock
  Medical Center, 2256
Northern New England Turner Society, 9374
Office of Alcohol and Drug Abuse Prevention, 8268
Office of Alcohol and Drug Abuse Programs State
  Office Park South, 8269
RESOLVE of New Hampshire, 5376
Sleep Disorders Center Dartmouth Hitchcock Medical
  Center, 7848
Sleep/Wake Disorders Center: Hampstead Hospital,
  7876
Veterans Adm. Medical Center: Manchester
  Manchester VA Medical Center, 10317
Voices for the Blind, 9803

New Jersey

AARP New Jersey State Office: Princeton, 55
Alcohol Disease Foundation, 8295
Alzheimer's Association: Greater New Jersey
  Chapter, 760
Alzheimer's Association: South Jersey Chapter, 761
American Anorexia Bulimia Association: New Jersey
  Chapter, 3623
American Auditory Society, 4231
American Cancer Society: New Jersey, 2120
American Council for Headache Education, 6451
American Diabetes Association: New Jersey, 3238
American Headache Society, 6452
American Lung Association of New Jersey, 5832
American Lung Association of New Jersey, 9300
American Society of Transplantation (AST), 9161
Angelwish, Inc., 10838
Arthritis Foundation: New Jersey Chapter, 1116
Association for Advancement of Mental Health, 6120
Asthma and Allergy Foundation of America:
  Southeast Pennsylvania Chapter, 1284
Asthma and Allergy Foundation of America:
  Southern Pennsylvania Chapter, 580
Autism Society of Southwest New Jersey, 1601
Bestwork Industries for the Blind, 9595
Brain Injury Association of New Jersey, 4037
Brain Injury Association of New Jersey Helpline,
  4108
Brain Tumor Support Group: New Jersey, 1902
Brain Tumor Support Group: Toms River, 1903
CCFA New Jersey Chapter, 2952
CanHelp, 2175
Central New Jersey Brain Tumor Support Group,
  1904
Christ Hospital Hepatitis C Support Group, 5099
Christopher & Dana Reeve Foundation Paralysis
  Resource Center, 8026
Community Mental Health Foundation, 6121
Congenital Heart Information Network, 2878
Cooley's Anemia Foundation (CAF): New Jersey
  Chapter, 2892
Department of Health, 8270
Disability Rights New Jersey, 10626
Division of Narcotic and Drug Abuse Control, 8271
Eating Disorders Association of New Jersey, 3642
Epilepsy Foundation of New Jersey, 7530
Eye Institute of New Jersey New Jersey Medical
  School, 9869
Friends Health Connection, 10675
Garden State Chapter of the Myasthenia Gravis
  Foundation of America, 6771
Garrett Mountain Chapter of the American
  Association of Kidney Patients, 5602
Greater New York Pull-Thru Network, 5304
HealthyWomen, 10668
Helping Other Parents in Normal Grief, 10851
Huxley Insititute-American Schizophrenic
  Association, 6420

Hydrocephalus Parents Support Group, 5167
Jason's Dreams for Kids Foundation, Inc., 10843
Juvenile Diabetes Research Foundation: Cen tral
  Jersey Chapter, 3240
Juvenile Diabetes Research Foundation: Mid -Jersey
  Chapter, 3241
Juvenile Diabetes Research Foundation: Roc kland
  County/Northern New Jersey, 3242
Juvenile Diabetes Research Foundation: South Jersey
  Chapter, 3239
Leukemia and Lymphoma Society: Northern New
  Jersey Chapter, 2121
Leukemia and Lymphoma Society: Southern New
  Jersey Chapter, 2122
Lupus Foundation of America: New Jersey Chapter,
  5942
Lupus Foundation of America: South Jersey Chapter,
  5943
Lyme Disease Network of New Jersey, 9033
Meadowlands Chapter of the American Association
  of Kidney Patients, 5603
Monmouth Medical Center: Cystic Fibrosis &
  Monmouth Medical Center, 3077
Monmouth Medical Center: Cystic Fibrosis &
  Pediatric Pulmonary Center, 3076
Multiple Sclerosis Association of America, 6506
Musculoskeletal Transplant Foundation, 9235
Nadeene Brunini Comprehensive Hemophilia Care
  Center, 4994
National Federation of the Blind: New Jersey, 9596
National MS Society: Greater North Jersey Chapter,
  6559
National MS Society: Mid-Jersey Chapter, 6560
National Sarcoidosis Family Aid and Research
  Foundation, 7281
National Sarcoidosis Resource Center, 7282
National Women's Health Resource Center, 5402
National Women's Health Resource Center, 9002
National Womens Health Resource Center, 3720
Neuromuscular and ALS Center The Clinical
  Academic Building, 1040
New Eyes for the Needy, 9505
New Jersey Alliance for the Mentally Ill, 6122
New Jersey Department of Health: Child Health
  Program, 8874
New Jersey Department of Health: Division of AIDS
  Prevention & Control, 277
New Jersey Institute of Technology Center for
  Biomedical Engineering, 3980
New Jersey Library for the Blind and Handicapped,
  9804
New Jersey Medical School, 3078
New Jersey Medical School: National Tuberculosis
  Center, 9268
New Jersey Metroplitan Turner Syndrome Society
  Association, 9375
New Jersey Parkinson's Disease Information Center,
  7099
New Jersey Pregnancy Risk Information Service,
  1763
New Jersey SIDS Alliance, 8875
New Jersey Woman AIDS Network, 278
Northern New Jersey Chapter of the American
  Association of Kidney Patients, 5604
Parkinson Alliance, 7072
Prader-Willi New Jersey Association Prader-Willi
  Syndrome Association, 7231
RESOLVE of New Jersey, 5377
Recording for the Blind Helpline, 9905
Recording for the Blind and Dyslexic, 9508
Renfrew Center of Northern New Jersey, 3624
Rutgers University Center of Alcohol Studies, 8322
Rutgers University: Controlled Drug- Delivery
  Research Center, 8323
SIDS Center of New Jersey, 8876
SIDS Center of New Jersey: Northern Site, 8877
Sarcoidosis Networking Program National
  Sarcoidosis Resource Center, 7283
Sarcoidosis Support Group: New Jersey, 7297
Scleroderma Foundation: Delaware Valley Chapter,
  7382
Scleroderma Foundation: Delaware Valley Chapter,
  7401
Seeing Eye, 9510

Columbia University Comprehensive Cancer Center, 2269

Columbia University Irving Center for Clinical Research Adult Unit, 4818

Columbia University: Comprehensive Sickle Cell Center, 7667

Community Access, 6040

Cooley's Anemia Foundation (CAF): Buffalo, 2894

Cooley's Anemia Foundation (CAF): Long Island, 2895

Cooley's Anemia Foundation (CAF): Queens, 2896

Cooley's Anemia Foundation (CAF): Staten Island, 2897

Cooley's Anemia Foundation (CAF): Suffolk Chapter Office, 2898

Cooley's Anemia Foundation (CAF): Westches ter/Rockland Chapter, 2899

Cooleys Anemia Foundation, 2901

Cornell University: Winifred Masterson Burke Medical Research-Dementia, 861

Cornerstone Medical Arts Center Hospital, 8299

Corporate Angel Network, 2327

Crohn's & Colitis Foundation of America, 2923

Crohn's & Colitis Foundation of America, 9413

Crohn's & Colitis Foundation of America Hotline, 2974

Cystic Fibrosis Center St. Vincent's Hospital & Medical Center, 3083

Dana Alliance for Brain Initiatives, 4064

Deaf Artists of America, 4245

Deafness Research Foundation, 4247

Developmental Evaluation Clinic, 3512

Disabled & Alone: Life Services for the Handicapped, 10530

Division of Digestive & Liver Diseases of Cloumbia University, 3635

Division of Substance Abuse Services Substance Abuse Services, 8273

Drugs Anonymous, 8205

ENCORE YWCA-National Board, 2012

Eastern Paralyzed Veterans Association of America, 8027

Eating Disorder Resource Center, 3641

Educational Equity Center at The Academy for Educational Development, 10532

Endocrinology Research Laboratory Cabrini Medical Center, 3328

Epilepsy Foundation of Long Island, 7531

Families Together in New York State, 6127

Family Ties of Orange County, 6226

Feingold Association of the US, 1508

Fertility Research Foundation, 3719

Fertility Research Foundation, 5401

Fibromyalgia Resources Group, 3788

Fight for Sight, 9462

Finger Lakes Donor Recovery Network, 9211

First Presbyterian Church in the City of New York Support Groups, 3643

Foundation for Advancement in Cancer Therapy, 2130

Friends of Karen, 10819

General Clinical Research Center Mount Sinai School of Medicine, 353

Gilda's Club: New York City, 2330

Greater New York Metro Intergroup of Overeaters Anonymous, 6894

Greater Rochester Area Chapter NSCIA, 8053

Guardians of Hydrocephalus Research Foundation, 5151

Gulf War Veterans of Long Island, NY, 10321

HEAL, 381

HIV Center for Clinical and Behavioral Studies, 354

Heart Disease Research Foundation, 4827

Helen Keller International, 9874

Helen Keller National Center for Deaf/Blind Youth and Adults, 4254

Helen Keller National Center for Deaf/Blind Youths and Adults, 9875

Helen Keller National Center's National Parent Network, 9469

Hemophilia Center of Western New York, 4937

Hemophilia Center of Western New York Erie County Medical Center, 4982

Holliswood Hospital Psychiatric Care, Serv ices and Self-Help/Support Groups, 3644

Human Growth Foundation, 3975

Human Growth Foundation: Turner Syndrome Division, 9352

Hy Feinstein Clubhouse, 4112

Images Within: A Child's View of Parental Alcoholism, 8343

Information Resource Center and Library, 6602

Institute for Basic Research in Developmental Disabilities, 866

Institute for Basic Research in Developmental Disabilities, 1626

Institute for Basic Research in Developmental Disabilities, 3530

Institute for Clinical Research Weill Cornell Medical College, 355

Institute for Visual Sciences, 9876

Institute on Communication and Inclusion at Syracuse University, 1627

International Center for Fabry Disease Mt. Sinai School of Medicine, 3757

International Union Against Venereal Diseases, 7623

JGB Cassette Library International, 9807

Jerusalem Center for Multi-Handicapped Blind Children, 9877

Juvenile Diabetes Foundation: International, 3150

Juvenile Diabetes International Hotline, 3354

Juvenile Diabetes Research Foundation Executive Office/Corporate Headquarters, 3246

Juvenile Diabetes Research Foundation: Buf falo/Western New York Chapter, 3248

Juvenile Diabetes Research Foundation: Hud son Valley Chapter, 3249

Juvenile Diabetes Research Foundation: Long Island/South Shore Chapter, 3247

Juvenile Diabetes Research Foundation: New York Chapter, 3250

Juvenile Diabetes Research Foundation: Nor theastern New York, 3251

Juvenile Diabetes Research Foundation: Roc hester Branch/Western New York Chapter, 3252

Juvenile Diabetes Research Foundation: Wes tchester County Chapter, 3253

Kidney & Urology Foundation of America, 5606

Kidney Disease Institute Wadsworth Center for Laboratories and Re, 5649

Laboratory of Dermatology Research Memorial Sloane-Kettering Cancer Center, 7726

League for the Hard of Hearing, 4289

Leukemia & Lymphoma Society Chapter: New York City, 2131

Leukemia & Lymphoma Society: Westchester/ Hudson Valley Chapter, 2132

Leukemia and Lymphoma Society, 2016

Leukemia and Lymphoma Society Chapter: New York City, 2133

Leukemia and Lymphoma Society: Central New York Chapter, 2134

Leukemia and Lymphoma Society: Long Island Chapter, 2135

Leukemia and Lymphoma Society: Upstate New York Chapter, 2136

Leukemia and Lymphoma Society: Western New York & Finger Lakes Chapter, 2137

Life Force: Women Fighting AIDS, 212

Lighthouse International Headquarters, 9473

Long Island Alzheimers Foundation, 847

Long Island Alzheimers Foundation, 867

Long Island Brain Tumor Support Group, 1908

Long Island Chapter of the American Association of Kidney Patients, 5607

Lupus Alliance of America LIQ Affiliate, 5945

Lupus Foundation of America: Bronx Chapter, 5946

Lupus Foundation of America: Central New York Chapter, 5947

Lupus Foundation of America: Genessee Valley Chapter, 5948

Lupus Foundation of America: Marguerite Curri Chapter, 5949

Lupus Foundation of America: New York Southern Tier Chapter, 5950

Lupus Foundation of America: Westchester, 5952

Lupus Foundation of America: Western New York Chapter, 5953

Lymphatic Research Foundation, 10549

MS Toll-Free Information Line, 6609

March of Dimes Birth Defects Foundation, 1738

March of Dimes Birth Defects Foundation, 3977

March of Dimes Birth Defects Foundation, 7927

March of Dimes Foundation, 10629

Marty Lyons Foundation, Inc., 10828

Mary M Gooley Hemophilia Center: A Chapter of the NHF, 4938

Medical Foundation of Buffalo Hauptman-Woodward Medical Research Insti, 2270

Memorial Sloan-Kettering Cancer Center, 2271

Mental Health Association in Dutchess Coun ty, 6227

Metro New York Chapter of Myasthenia Gravis Foundation of America, 6773

Michael J. Fox Foundation for Parkinson's Research, 7040

Mid Florida Chapter National Multiple Sclerosis Society, 6532

Mount Sinai Medical Center Brain Tumor Support Group, 1909

Mount Sinai Sarcoidosis Support Group, 7289

Mount Sinai School of Medicine: Alzheimers Disease Research Center, 871

Multiple Sclerosis Action Group, 6611

Myasthenia Gravis Support Group: Long Island, 6774

NARSAD: Mental Health Research Association, 6355

NARSAD: Mental Health Research Association, 6418

NYS Center for SIDS, 8879

NYS Center for Sudden Infant Death: Eastern Satellite Office, 8880

Naomi Berrie Diabetes Center at Columbia University Medical Center, 3318

Narcolepsy Institute/Montefiore Medical Center, 7822

Narcolepsy Institute/Montefiore Medical Center, 7880

Narcolepsy Network, 7823

Narcotic and Drug Research, 8311

Nassau Library System, 9808

National AIDS Treatment Advocacy Project, 218

National Adrenal Diseases Foundation, 3

National Alliance for Autism Research, 1628

National Alliance for Research on Schizophrenia and Depression, 6422

National Alliance of Breast Cancer Organizations, 2018

National Association for Visually Hand., 9479

National Association for Visually Handicapped, 9478

National Association on Drug Abuse Problems, 8217

National Braille Association, 9487

National Center for Family-Centered Care, 10554

National Center for Learning Disabilities, 1510

National Center for Vision and Aging Lighthouse, 9489

National Center for Vision and Child Development, 9490

National Center on Addiction and Substance Abuse, 8312

National Council on Alcoholism and Drug Dependence, 8219

National Down Syndrome Society, 3489

National Down Syndrome Society Hotline, 3535

National Family Association for Deaf-Blind, 4264

National Federation of the Blind: New York, 9605

National Foundation for Depressive Illness, 6358

National Foundation for Facial Reconstruction, 1740

National Foundation for Jewish Genetic Diseases, 3949

National Foundation for Jewish Genetic Diseases, 8964

National Hemophilia Foundation, 301

National Hemophilia Foundation, 4909

National Hemophilia Foundation, 4960

National Hemophilia Foundation's Information Center, 4910

National Hemophilia Foundation/Hemophilia and AIDS/HIV Network (HANDI), 3785

National Hypertension Association, 5213

National Infertility Network Exchange, 5414

National Institute for Jewish Hospice, 10855

National Institute for People with Disabil ities, 10562

National Kidney Foundation, 5552

National Kidney Foundation of Central New York, 5608

National Kidney Foundation of Colorado: Idaho, Montana, and Wyoming, 5566

National Kidney Foundation of Northeast New York, 5609

North Carolina

Alzheimer's Association: Eastern North Carolina Chapter, 774

Alzheimer's Association: Western Carolina Chapter, 775

Alzheimer's Association: Western North Carolina Chapter, 776

Alzheimer's Disease Research Center Duke University, 859

American Cancer Society: North Carolina, 2138

American Diabetes Association: North Carolina, 3255

American Lung Association of North Carolina, 5835

American Lung Association of North Carolina, 9303

American Lung Association of North Dakota, 9304

American Social Health Association, 7616

Arthritis Foundation: Carolinas Chapter, 1122

Autism Society of North Carolina, 1604

Beginnings for Parents of Children Who are Deaf or Hard of Hearing, 4349

Bowman Gray School of Medicine, 8135

Bowman Grey School of Medicine: Hemophilia Diagnostic Center, 4964

Brain Injury Association of North Carolina, 4042

Brain Injury Association of North Carolina Helpline, 4113

Brain Injury Association of North Dakota H, 4043

Brain Tumor Support Group: Raleigh Area, 1911

CCFA Carolinas Chapter, 2958

CCFA South Carolina Chapter, 2965

Cancer Center of Wake Forest University at Bowman Gray School of Medicine, 2276

Carolinas Chapter of the Myasthenia Gravis Foundation of America, 6776

Carolinas Chapter of the Myasthenia Gravis Foundation of America, 6783

Center for Universal Design North Carolina State University, 10523

Centers for AIDS Research: Univeristy of North Carolina at Chapel Hill, 359

Charles George Veterans Affairs Medical Center, 10335

Cleft Palate Foundation, 1734

Comprehensive Hemophilia Diagnostic and Treatment Center, 4967

Department of Pediatrics, Division of Rheumatology, 1145

Desert Storm Veterans of North Carolina, 10336

Division TEACCH University of North Carolina at Chapel H, 1625

Dorothea Dix Hospital Clinical Research Unit, 8301

Duke Asthma, Allergy and Airway Center, 1294

Duke Comprehensive Cancer Center, 2277

Duke Pediatric Brain Tumor Family Support Program, 1912

Duke University Center for the Advanced Study of Epilepsy, 7535

Duke University Center for the Study of Aging and Human Development, 862

Duke University Clinical Research Institute, 863

Duke University Epilepsy Research Center, 7536

Duke University Medical Center: Division of Pulmonary and Critical Care Medicine, 3087

Duke University Pediatric Cardiac Catheterization Laboratory, 4820

Duke University Plastic Surgery Research Laboratories, 7725

Easter Seals UCP North Carolina & Virginia, 2692

Families in Action National Drug Abuse Center, 8303

Hemophilia Foundation of North Carolina, 4939

Herpes Resource Center, 7620

Herpes Resource Center, 7622

International Federation of Spine Associations, 7451

Juvenile Diabetes Research Foundation: Cha rlotte Chapter, 3257

Juvenile Diabetes Research Foundation: Pie dmont Triad Chapter, 3258

Juvenile Diabetes Research Foundation: Triangle/Eastern North Carolina Chapter, 3256

Leukemia and Lymphoma Society: Eastern North Carolina Chapter, 2139

Leukemia and Lymphoma Society: North Carolina Chapter, 2140

Leukemia and Lymphoma Society: North Texas, 2141

Life Share of the Carolinas, 9214

Lions Industries for the Blind, 9609

Lupus Foundation of America: Charlotte Chapter, 5956

Lupus Foundation of America: Raleigh Chapter, 5957

Lupus Foundation of America: Winston-Triad Lupus Chapter NCLF, 5955

National Early Childhood Technical Assistance Center, 1739

National Early Childhood Technical Assistance System, 3490

National Federation of the Blind: North Carolina, 9610

National Kidney Foundation of North Carolina, 5613

National Kidney Foundation of North Texas, 5614

National MS Society: Central North Carolina Chapter, 6569

National MS Society: Eastern North Carolina Chapter, 6570

National Multiple Sclerosis Society, 6571

North Carolina Association of the Deaf, 4290

North Carolina Client Assistance Program, 10630

North Carolina Department of Health & Natural Resources, 281

North Carolina Library for the Blind, 9812

North Carolina Turner Syndrome Society, 9378

Pediatric Brain Tumor Foundation, 1814

Prader-Willi Syndrome Association of North Carolina, 7233

Preston Robert Tisch Brain Tumor Center at Duke, 1913

RESOLVE of North Carolina, 5382

SIDS Alliance of the Carolinas, 8886

Sickle Cell Anemia Foundation, 7658

Spina Bifida Association of North Carolina, 7961

Triangle Area Sarcoidosis Support Group, 7299

UNC Cystic Fibrosis Center Department of Pediatrics, 3088

University of North Carolina Sarcoidosis Support Group, 7301

University of North Carolina UNC Lineberger Comprehensive Cancer Center, 2278

University of North Carolina at Chapel Hill Division of Speech & Hearing, 4341

Veterans Adm. Medical Center: Durham Durham VA Medical Center, 10337

Veterans Adm. Medical Center: Fayetville Fayetville VA Medical Center, 10338

Veterans Adm. Medical Center: Salisbury W.G. Hefner VA Medical Center, 10339

Wake Forest University: Arteriosclerosis Research Center, 5225

Wake Forest University: Cerebrovascular Research Center, 8145

Winston-Salem Industries for the Blind, 9611

Wrap Myself in a Rainbow Compassion Books, 10857

North Dakota

AARP North Dakota State Office: Bismarck, 60

Alzheimer's Association: Fargo/Moorhead Regional Center, 777

American Cancer Society: North Dakota, 2142

American Diabetes Association: Nashville, 3259

American Diabetes Association: North Dakota, 3260

American Lung Association of North Dakota, 5836

American Lung Association of North Dakota, 9305

Autism Society of North Dakota, 1605

Brain Injury Association of North Dakota H elpline, 4114

Client Assistance Program: North Dakota, 10631

Division of Alcoholism & Drug Abuse: Department of Human Services, 8275

Healthy Weight Network, 3609

MeritCare Children's Hospital Down Syndrome Outpatient Service, 3520

ND FFCMH Region II, 6228

ND Region V FFCMH Chapter-Federation of Fa milies for Children's Mental Health, 6229

ND Region VII FFCMH-Federation of Families for Children's Mental Health, 6230

National Federation of the Blind: North Dakota, 9612

National MS Society: Dakota Chapter, 6572

North Dakota Alliance for the Mentally Ill, 6130

North Dakota Association of the Deaf, 4291

North Dakota Comprehensive Hemophilia Center, 4995

North Dakota FFCMH, 6131

North Dakota Hemostasis and Thrombosis Treatment Center, 4996

North Dakota SIDS Alliance, 8887

North Dakota SIDS Management Program, 8888

North Dakota State Library Services for the Disabled, 9813

North Dakota State Library Talking Book Services, 9814

PWSA Fargo Chapter Prader-Willi Syndrome Association, 7234

St. Alexius Medical Heart and Lung Clinic, 3089

Veterans Adm. Regional Office: Fargo Regional Office Center, 10340

ON

Ontario HIV Treatment Network, 227

Ohio

1st Capital FFCMH, 6132

A Kid Again, 10808

AARP Ohio State Office: Columbus, 61

ALS Association: Northeast Ohio Chapter, 1018

ALS Association: Western Ohio Chapter, 1019

Alzheimer's Association: Canton Chapter, 778

Alzheimer's Association: Central Ohio Chapter, 779

Alzheimer's Association: Clark/Champaign, Miami Valley Chapter, 780

Alzheimer's Association: Cleveland Area Chapter, 781

Alzheimer's Association: Greater Cincinnati Chapter, 782

Alzheimer's Association: Greater East Ohio Chapter: Greater Youngstown Office, 783

Alzheimer's Association: Miami Valley Chapter, 784

Alzheimer's Association: Northwest Ohio Chapter, 785

Alzheimer's Association: West Central Ohio Chapter, 786

American Cancer Society: Ohio, 2143

American Diabetes Association: Ohio, 3261

American Liver Foundation Ohio Chapter, 5734

American Lung Association of Ohio, 5837

American Lung Association of Ohio, 9306

American Sickle Cell Anemia, 7656

Arthritis Foundation: Central Ohio Chapter, 1123

Arthritis Foundation: Northeastern Ohio Chapter, 1124

Arthritis Foundation: Ohio River Valley Chapter, 1126

Arthritis Foundation; Great Lakes Region, Northeastern Ohio, 1127

Autism Society of Greater Cincinnati, 1606

Autism Society of Ohio Tri-County Chapter, 1607

Blick Clinic for Developmental Disabilities, 3510

Brain Injury Association of Ohio, 4044

Brain Injury Association of Ohio, 4115

Brain Tumor Support Group: Cincinnati, 1914

Bureau on Alcohol Abuse and Recovery Ohio Department of Health, 8276

Bureau on Drug Abuse: Ohio Department of Health, 8277

CCFA Central Ohio Chapter, 2959

CCFA Northeast Ohio Chapter, 2960

CCFA Southwest Ohio Chapter, 2961

CHASER Congenital Heart Disease Anomalies Anomalies Support, Education & Resources, 4814

Case Western Reserve University, 9816

Case Western Reserve University: Bolton Brush Growth Study Center, 3978

Case Western Reserve University: Center on Aging and Health, 77

Case Western Reserve University: Cystic Fi, 3091

Case Western Reserve University: Cystic Fibrosis Center, 3090

Case Western Reserve University: Ireland C University Hospitals of Cleveland, 2280

Case Western Reserve University: Ireland Cancer Center, 2279

Center for ALS and Related Diorders The Cleveland Clinic DepartmentOf Neurol, 1035

Center for Research in Sleep Disorders Affiliated with Mercy Hospital, 7829

Center for Sleep & Wake Disorders: Miami Valley Hospital, 7830

Centers for AIDS Research: Case Western University, 360

Central Ohio Chapter of the National Hemophilia Foundation, 4940

Central Ohio Support Group: National Ataxia Foundation, 1457

Child & Adolescent Service Center (CASC), 6231

Children's Hospital Hemophilia Treatment Center, 4965

Children's Hospital Research Foundation, 2281

Cincinnati Association for the Blind, 9613

Cincinnati HPV Support Group: PP of Cincin nati, 10632

Cleveland Clinic Foundation Research Institute, 4817

Cleveland Hearing and Speech Center, 4310

Cleveland Sight Center, 9614

Cleveland Skilled Industries, 9615

Clinical Research Center: Pediatrics Children's Hospital Research Foundation, 5742

Clovernook Center for the Blind and Visually Impaired, 9865

Columbus Center of the National Multiple Sclerosis Society, 6573

Columbus Children's Hospital: Cystic Fibrosis Center, 3092

Columbus Children's Research Institute, 583

Comprehensive Sickle Cell Center Children's Hospital Research Foundation, 7668

Disability Rights Center at Ohio Legal Rights Service, 10633

District Board of Health: Mahoning County, 8889

Division Of Developmental and Behavioral Pediatrics, 1745

Down Syndrome Association of Greater Cinci nnati, 3502

Down Syndrome Association of Greater Cinci nnati, 3533

FES Information Center WO Walker Industrial Rehabilitation Cent, 8028

First Ohio Chapter: FFCMH, 6232

Greater Cincinnati/Northern Kentucky Chapter of the NHF, 4941

JamesCare For Life Support Groups & Services, 2335

Jane and Richard Thomas Center for Down Syndrome, 3517

Juvenile Diabetes Research Foundation/JDRF, 3262

Juvenile Diabetes Research Foundation: Akr on/Canton Chapter, 3264

Juvenile Diabetes Research Foundation: Gre ater Cincinnati Chapter, 3265

Juvenile Diabetes Research Foundation: Mid-Ohio Chapter, 3263

Juvenile Diabetes Research Foundation: Tol edo/Northwest Ohio Chapter, 3266

Kettering-Scott Magnetic Resonance Laboratory, 8309

Leukemia and Lymphoma Society: Central Ohio Chapter, 2144

Leukemia and Lymphoma Society: Northern Ohio Chapter, 2145

Leukemia and Lymphoma Society: Southern Ohio Chapter, 2146

Lewis H Walker MD: Cystic Fibrosis Center Children's Hospital Medical Center of Ak, 3093

Life Connection of Ohio, 9215

LifeBanc, 9216

Lifeline of Ohio Organ Procurement Agency, Inc., 9217

Lupus Foundation of America: Akron Area Chapter, 5958

Lupus Foundation of America: Columbus, 5959

Lupus Foundation of America: Columbus, Marcy Zitron Chapter, 5960

Lupus Foundation of America: Greater Cleveland Chapter, 5961

Lupus Foundation of America: North Texas, 5962

Lupus Foundation of America: Northwest Ohio Lupus Chapter, 5963

Mahoning-Shenango Chapter of the Myasthenia Gravis Foundation of America, 6777

Medical College of Toledo: Cancer Research Division, 2282

Miami Valley Ohio Chapter of the American Association of Kidney Patients, 5615

Mitral Valve Prolapse Program of Cincinnati Support Group, 4864

National Association of Blind Office Professionals, 9483

National Federation of the Blind: Ohio, 9616

National Kidney Foundation of Ohio, 5616

National MS Soceity: Western Ohio Chapter The Woolpert Building, 6574

National MS Society: Northeast Ohio Chapter, 6576

National MS Society: Northwest Ohio Chapter, 6577

National MS Society: Southwestern Ohio/Northern Kentucky, 6575

National Reye's Syndrome Foundation, 5750

North Central Regional Training Center: Canine Companions for Independence, 9617

North East Ohio Support Group National Ataxia Foundation, 1458

Northern Ohio Chapter of the National Hemophilia Foundation, 4942

Northwest Ohio Hemophilia Association, 4943

Northwest Ohio Hemophilia Treatment Center, 4999

Northwest Ohio Sleep Disorders Center Toledo Hospital, 7839

Ohio Alliance for the Mentally Ill, 6133

Ohio Ambassador: National Ataxia Foundation, 1459

Ohio Chapter of the Myasthenia Gravis Foundation of America, 6778

Ohio Department of Health, 8890

Ohio Department of Health: Division of Preventive Medicine, 282

Ohio Regional Library for the Blind and Physically Handicapped, 9817

Ohio Sleep Medicine Institute, 7840

Ohio State University Clinical Pharmacolog College of Medicine, 8318

Ohio State University Clinical Pharmacology Division, 8317

Ohio State University Comprehensive Cancer Center, 2283

Ohio State University General Clinical Research Center, 2284

Ohio State University Laboratory of Psychobiology, 4067

Ohio State University Neuroscience Program, 873

Ohio State University Otological Research Laboratories, 4320

Ohio University Therapy Associates: Hearing, Speech and Language Clinic, 4321

Ohio Valley LifeCenter, 9218

PWSA Ohio Chapter Prader-Willi Syndrome Association, 7235

Parent Project: Muscular Dystrophy, 6687

Pediatric Pulmonary Center The Children's Medical Center of Dayton, 3094

Persian Gulf War Veterans of Western Pennsylvania, W Virginia and NE Ohio, 10341

RESOLVE of Ohio, 5383

Rainbow Alliance of the Deaf, 4269

Region 2 of the National Association for Parents of the Visually Impaired, 9618

Richland County HPV Support Group, 10634

SIDS Network of Ohio, 8891

Scleroderma Foundation: Ohio Chapter, 7399

Sleep Disorders Center Bethesda Oak Hospital, 7846

Sleep Disorders Center Ohio State University Medical Center, 7850

Sleep Disorders Center: Cleveland Clinic Foundation, 7856

Sleep Disorders Center: Kettering Medical Center, 7860

Sleep Disorders Center: St. Vincent Medical Center, 7864

Society of the Blind: Akron Center, 9619

Southwest Ohio Brain Tumor Support Group, 1915

Southwestern Ohio Chapter of the National Hemophilia Foundation, 4944

Special Wish Foundation, 10831

Spina Bifida Association of Canton, 7962

Spina Bifida Association of Central Ohio, 7963

Spina Bifida Association of Cincinnati, 7964

Spina Bifida Association of Greater Dayton, 7965

Spina Bifida Association of Northwest Ohio, 7966

State Library of Ohio Talking Book Program, 9818

Support Group for Parents of Children with Brain Tumors, 1916

Technology Resource Center, 10635

The Cancer Prevention Institute, 2285

Turner Syndrome Chapter of Ohio, 9379

United Cerebral Palsy of Central Ohio, 2693

United Cerebral Palsy of Cincinnati, 2694

United Cerebral Palsy of Greater Cleveland, 2695

United Cerebral Palsy of Greater Dane, 2696

University Alzheimer Center UHC: Case Western Reserve University, 879

University Treatment Center of University Hospitals of Cleveland, 5015

University of Cincinnati Adult Hemophilia Treatment Program, 5016

University of Cincinnati College of Medicine Division of Pediatrics, 3095

University of Cincinnati Department of Pathology & Laboratory Medicine, 4846

VA Healthcare System Of Ohio, 10342

Veterans Adm. Medical Center: Chillicothe Chillicothe VA Medical Center, 10343

Veterans Adm. Medical Center: Cincinnati Cincinnati VA Medical Center, 10344

Veterans Adm. Medical Center: Cleveland Louis Stokes VA Medical Center, 10345

Veterans Adm. Medical Center: Columbus Chalmers P. Wylie Outpatient Clinic, 10346

Veterans Adm. Medical Center: Dayton Dayton VA Medical Center, 10347

Veterans and Families Support Network Ohio, 10348

West Central Ohio Hemophilia Center Childens Medical Center, 5021

Wilson's Disease Association, 5751

Wilson's Disease Association, 10484

World Hypertension League, 5158

Oklahoma

AARP Oklahoma State Office: Edmond, 62

Alzheimer's Association: Oklahoma Chapter, 787

American Association of Kidney Patients, 5617

American Association of Kidney Patients: Tulsa Chapter, 5618

American Cancer Society: Oklahoma, 2147

American Diabetes Association: Oklahoma, 3267

American Lung Association of Oklahoma, 5838

American Lung Association of Oklahoma, 9307

American Veterans Justice Foundation, 10349

Arthritis Foundation: Oklahoma Chapter, 1128

Autism Society of Central Oklahoma, 1608

Brain Injury Association of Oklahoma, 4045

Brain Injury Association of Oklahoma Helpl ine, 4116

CCFA Oklahoma Chapter, 2962

Client Assistance Program: Oklahoma Office of Handicapped Concerns, 10636

Dean A McGee Eye Institute, 9866

Juvenile Diabetes Research Foundation: Cen tral Oklahoma Chapter, 3268

Juvenile Diabetes Research Foundation: Tul sa Green County Chapter, 3269

Leukemia and Lymphoma Society: Oklahoma Chapter, 2148

Myasthenia Gravis Support Group, 6791

Natalie Warren Bryant Cancer Center St. Francis Hospital, 2286

National Federation of the Blind: Oklahoma, 9620

National Kidney Foundation of Oklahoma, 5619

National MS Society: Oklahoma Chapter, 6578

Neuroscience Institute at Mercy Hospital, 6862

Oklahoma Alliance for the Mentally Ill, 6134

Oklahoma Ambassador: National Ataxia Foundation, 1460

Oklahoma Association of the Deaf, 4292

Oklahoma Chapter of the Myasthenia Gravis Foundation of America, 6779

Oklahoma Chapter of the National Hemophilia Foundation, 4945

Oklahoma City HPV Support Group: PP of Cen tral Oklahoma, 10637

Rhode Island

Alzheimer's Association: Rhode Island Chapter, 799
American Cancer Society: Rhode Island, 2157
American Diabetes Association: Central Virginia Office, 3279
American Diabetes Association: Rhode Island, 3280
American Diabetes Association: Richmond, 3281
American Lung Association of Rhode Island, 5842
Autism Society of Rhode Island, 1611
Brain Injury Association of Rhode Island, 4048
Brain Injury Association of Rhode Island H, 4049
Brain Injury Association of Rhode Island H elpline, 4118
Brain Tumor Support Group: Providence, 1925
Brown University Division of Biology and Medicine, 2295
Center for Alcohol & Addiction Studies Brown University, 8298
Centers for AIDS Research: Brown University, 364
Children's Neurodevelopment Center, 3529
Division of Substance Abuse: Department of Mental Health and Hospitals, 8281
Hemophilia Center of Rhode Island Rhode Island Hospital, 4980
Hydrocephalus Association of Rhode Island, 5162
IN-SIGHT, 9646
Leukemia and Lymphoma Society: Rhode Island Chapter, 2158
Lupus Foundation of America: Rhode Island Chapter, 5972
Narcolepsy Network, 7881
National Alliance for the Mentally Ill, 6140
National Alliance for the Mentally Ill of Rhode Island (NAMI), 6141
National Federation of the Blind: Rhode Island, 9647
National MS Society: Rhode Island Chapter, 6582
Parent Support Network, 6233
Parent Support Network of Rhode Island, 6234
RESOLVE of the Ocean State, 5389
Rhode Island Association of the Deaf, 4294
Rhode Island Brain & Spine Tumor Foundation, 1926
Rhode Island Department of Health, 8897
Rhode Island Department of Health: Division of Disease Prevention & Control, 287
Rhode Island Department of Health: National SIDS Foundation, 8898
Rhode Island Department of State Library for the Blind and Physically Handicapped, 9824
Rhode Island Disability Law Center, 10641
Rhode Island Hemophilia Foundation, 4949
Rhode Island Hospital: Cystic Fibrosis Center, 3102
Rhode Island Scleroderma Support Group, 7427
Rhode Island Turner Syndrome Society, 9383
Roger Williams Clinical Cancer Research Ce Roger Williams General Hospital, 2297
Roger Williams Clinical Cancer Research Center, 2296
Sleep Disorders Center: Rhode Island Hospital, 7863
Spina Bifida Association of Rhode Island, 7970
United Cerebral Palsy of Rhode Island, 2709
Veterans Adm. Medical Center: Providence Providence VA Medical Center, 10368

South Carolina

AARP South Carolina Office: Columbia, 65
Agromedicine Program Medical University of South Carolina, 7724
Alzheimer's Association: Low Country Chapter, 800
Alzheimer's Association: Mid-State South Carolina Chapter, 801
Alzheimer's Association: Upstate South Carolina Chapter, 802
American Cancer Society: South Carolina, 2159
American Diabetes Association: South Carolina, 3282
American Diabetes Association: South Coast, 3283
American Lung Association of South Carolina, 5843
American Lung Association of South Carolina, 9310
American Lung Association of South Dakota, 9311
Autism Society of South Carolina, 1612
Brain Injury Association of South Carolina, 4050
Brain Tumor Support Group: Charleston, 1927

Brain Tumor Support Group: Florence, 1928
Captioned Media Program, 4301
Carolinas Support Group: National Ataxia National Ataxia Foundation, 1463
Center for Developmental Disabilities University of South Carolina, 10518
Center for Disability Resources, 10519
Children's Center for Cancer and Blood Dis University of South Carolina School of M, 2299
Children's Center for Cancer and Blood Disorders, 2298
Division of Perinatal Systems Mills Jarret Complex, 8899
FFCMH: South Carolina Chapter, 6235
Family Support Network/SC AMI, 6236
Federation of Families of South Carolina, 6237
Hemophilia Association of South Carolina, 4950
Interdisciplinary Program in Cell and Molecular Pharmacology, 8307
James R Clark Memorial Sickle Cell Foundation, 7662
Juvenile Diabetes Research Foundation: Low Country Chapter, 3285
Juvenile Diabetes Research Foundation: Palmetto Chapter, 3284
Leukemia and Lymphoma Society: South Carolina Chapter, 2160
Leukemia and Lymphoma Society: South/West, 2161
LifePoint, 9224
Lupus Foundation of America: South Carolina Chapter, 5973
Lyme Disease Network of South Carolina, 9034
Medical University of South Carolina, 1147
Medical University of South Carolina Health Services Administration, 365
Medical University of South Carolina Medical University of South Carolina, 7416
Medical University of South Carolina: Cyst Department of Pediatrics, 3104
Medical University of South Carolina: Cystic Fibrosis Center, 3103
Medical University of South Carolina: Division of Rheumatology & Immunology, 1148
NAMI-SC: National Alliance on Mental Illness: South Carolina, 6142
NNFF South Carolina Chapter, 6853
National Association for Continence, 5301
National Federation of the Blind: South Carolina, 9648
National Kidney Foundation of South Carolina, 5625
National MS Society: South Carolina Branch, 6583
PWSA South Carolina Chapter Prader-Willi Syndrome Association, 7240
RESOLVE of South Carolina, 5390
Ralph H. Johnson VA Medical Center, 10369
Region 4 of the National Association for Parents of the Visually Impaired, 9649
Richland Memorial Comprehensive Pediatric Hemophilia Center, 5005
Scleroderma Foundation: South Carolina Chapter, 7404
South Carolina Commission on Alcohol and Drug Abuse, 8282
South Carolina Department of Health & Environmental Control, 288
South Carolina Palmetto Turner Syndrome So ciety, 9384
South Carolina Protection & Advocacy System for the Handicapped, 10642
South Carolina State Library, 9825
Tri County HPV Support Group, 10643
William Jennings Bryan Dorn VA Medical Center, 10370

South Dakota

American Cancer Society: South Dakota, 2162
American Lung Association of South Dakota, 5844
American Lung Association of South Dakota, 9312
Autism Society of Black Hills, 1613
Cancer Support Group, 1929
Department of Veterans Affairs Medical Center: Sioux Falls, 10371

Division of Alcohol & Drug Abuse: South Dakota, 8283
Juvenile Diabetes Research Foundation: Sio ux Falls Chapter, 3286
NAMI South Dakota, 6143
National Federation of the Blind: South Dakota, 9650
National Kidney Foundation of South Dakota, 5626
National Kidney Foundation of South Dakota, 5627
Parkinson Association of South Dakota, 7079
South Dakota Advocacy Services, 10644
South Dakota Department of Health, 8900
South Dakota State Library, 9826
Teratogen and Birth Defects Information Project, 1769
VA Black Hills Health Care System- Fort Meade Campus, 10372
VA Black Hills Health Care System- Hot Springs Campus, 10373

Tennessee

AARP Tennessee State Office: Nashville, 66
ALS Association: Middle Tennessee Chapter, 1024
Alzheimer's Association: Eastern Tennessee Chapter, 803
Alzheimer's Association: Highland Rim Chapter, 804
Alzheimer's Association: Memphis Area Office, 805
Alzheimer's Association: Middle Tennessee Chapter, 806
Alzheimer's Association: Northeast Tennessee Chapter, 807
Alzheimer's Association: Southeast Tennessee Chapter, 808
American Cancer Society: Tennessee, 2163
American Diabetes Association: Nashville, 3287
American Diabetes Association: Tennessee, 3288
American Liver Foundation Midsouth Chapter, 5737
American Lung Association of Tennessee, 9313
American Lung Association of Tennessee, 5845
Arthritis Foundation: Southeast Region, 1131
Arthritis Trust of America, 2540
Autism Society of East Tennessee, 1614
Brain Injury Association of Tennessee, 4051
Brain Injury Association of Tennessee Help, 4052
Brain Injury Association of Tennessee Help line, 4119
CCFA Kentucky Chapter c/o CCFA Indiana Chapter, 2944
CCFA Tennessee Chapter, 2966
Cancer Support Group: Knoxville, 1930
Cancer Support Group: Nashville, 1931
Centers for AIDS Research: Vanderbilt University Medical Center, 366
Department of Mental Health and Mental Retardation, Alcohol & Drug Service, 8284
Disability Law & Advocacy Center of Tennessee, 10645
Down Syndrome Association of Middle Tennessee, 3503
EAR Foundation, 4250
Ed Lindsey Industries of the Blind, 9651
Endometriosis Association Research Program : Vanderbuilt University, 3722
Hemophilia Health Services, 4908
Impotence Institute of America, 5263
Juvenile Diabetes Research Foundation: East Tennessee Chapter, 3289
Juvenile Diabetes Research Foundation: Mid dle Tennessee Chapter, 3290
LRC for Students with Disabilities, 9827
Leukemia & Lymphoma Society: Tennessee Chapter, 2164
Lupus Foundation of America Memphis Area Chapter, 5974
Lupus Foundation of America: East Tennessee Chapter, 5975
Lupus Foundation of America: Mid-South Area Chapter, 5976
Memphis Cystic Fibrosis Center LeBonheur Children's Medical Center, 3105
Memphis Regional Brain Tumor Survivors Group, 1932
Memphis State University Center for the Communicatively Impaired, 4318

Mid-South Transplant Foundation, Inc. Tennessee, 9225

Middle Tennessee Sarcoidosis Support Group, 7288

Mountain Home VA Medical Center, 10374

National Federation of the Blind: Tennessee, 9652

National Foundation for Transplants, 9167

National Kidney Foundation of East Tennessee, 5628

National Kidney Foundation of West Tennessee, 5629

National Kidney Foundation of West Texas, 5630

National MS Society: Mid-South Chapter, 6585

National MS Society: Mid-South Chapter, Nashville Office, 6586

National MS Society: Sutheast Tennessee/North Georgia Chapter, 6584

PWSA Tennessee Chapter Prader-Willi Syndrome Association, 7241

Persian Gulf Information Network, 10375

RESOLVE of Tennessee, 5391

Sarcoidosis Center, 7284

Sarcoidosis Research Institute (SRI), 7293

Scleroderma Foundation: Tennessee Chapter, 7405

Spina Bifida Association of Tennessee, 7971

St. Jude Children's Research Hospital, 2300

TN Hemo & Bleeding Disorders Foundation, 4951

Tenessee Department of Health, 8901

Tennessee Alliance for the Mentally Ill, 6144

Tennessee Department of Health: AIDS Program, 289

Tennessee Donor Services, 9226

Tennessee Kidney Foundation, 5631

Tennessee Library for the Blind and Physically Handicapped, 9828

Tennessee Neuropsychiatric Institute Middle Tennessee Mental Health Institute, 6425

Tennessee SIDS Alliance, 8902

Tennessee Valley Healthcare System- Alvin C. York (Murfreesboro) Campus, 10377

Tennessee Valley Healthcare System- Nashville Campus, 10376

Tennessee Voices for Children, 6238

United Cerebral Palsy of Middle Tennessee, 2710

United Cerebral Palsy of the Mid-South, 2711

University of Tennessee Drug Information Center, 8333

University of Tennessee Hemophilia Clinic, 5018

University of Tennessee Medical Group, 7424

University of Tennessee Memphis: Cancer Center, 2301

University of Tennessee: Center for Neuroscience, 7539

University of Tennessee: Division of Cardiovascular Diseases, 4855

University of Tennessee: Division of Reproductive Endocrinology, 3727

University of Tennessee: General Clinical Research Center, 3345

University of Tennessee: Memphis State University of Neuropsychology Lab, 4075

VISN 9: VA Mid South Healthcare Network, 10378

Vand erbilt University: Center for Fertili, 5409

Vanderbilt Children's Hospital, 3106

Vanderbilt Comprehensive Hemophilia Center, 5019

Vanderbilt University Diabetes Center, 3348

Vanderbilt University John F Kennedy Center for Research/Human Development, 6178

Vanderbilt University: Center for Fertility and Reproductive Research, 5410

Veterans Adm. Medical Center: Murfreesboro, 10379

Veterans Adm. Medical Center: Memphis, 10380

Veterans Adm. Medical Center: Muskogee, 10381

Veterans Adm. Medical Center: Nashville, 10382

Veterans Affairs Medical Center, 10383

Veterans Affairs Medical Center, Memphis, Tennessee, 10384

Vision Foundation, 10834

West Tennessee Lions Blind Industries, 9653

West Tennessee Sarcoidosis Support Group, 7302

Texas

A Wish with Wings, Inc., 10809

AARP Texas State Office: Austin, 67

AIDS Outreach Center (AOC), 290

ALS Association: Greater Houston CIO, 1025

ALS Association: North Texas Chapter, 1026

ALS Association: South Texas Chapter, 1027

Academy of Rehabilitative Audiology, 4226

Alzheimer's Alliance of Smith County, 809

Alzheimer's Alliance: Texarkana Area, 810

Alzheimer's Association: Capital of Texas Chapter, 811

Alzheimer's Association: El Paso Chapter, 812

Alzheimer's Association: Greater Beaumont Area Chapter, 813

Alzheimer's Association: Greater Dallas Chapter, 814

Alzheimer's Association: Greater East Texas Chapter, 815

Alzheimer's Association: Greater Wichita Falls Chapter, 816

Alzheimer's Association: Houston and Southeast Texas Chapter, 817

Alzheimer's Association: Northeast Texas Chapter, 818

Alzheimer's Association: Rio Grande Valley Region, 819

Alzheimer's Association: STAR Chapter, Midland Region, 820

Alzheimer's Association: South Central Texas, 821

Alzheimer's Association: Tarrant County Chapter, 822

Amarillo VA Health Care System, 10385

American Association for Respiratory Care, 5787

American Association of Kidney Patients, 5632

American Association of Kidney Patients: Piney Woods Chapter, 5633

American Cancer Society: Texas, 2165

American Diabetes Association: Texas, 3291

American Foundation for the Blind, 9654

American Foundation for the Blind: National Aging Center, 9655

American GI Forum NVOP, 10430

American Heart Association, 4803

American Heart Association, 8126

American Liver Foundation South Texas Chap ter, 5738

American Lung Association of Texas, 5846

American Lung Association of Texas, 9314

American Organ Transplant Association, 10508

American Porphyria Foundation, 3866

American Stroke Association, 8127

Arthritis Foundation: North Texas Chapter, 1132

Asthma and Allergy Foundation of America, 1287

Asthma and Allergy Foundation of America: North Texas Chapter, 581

Asthma and Allergy Foundation of America: North Texas Chapter, 1288

Austin Outpatient Clinic, 10386

Autism Society of Dallas, 1615

Baylor College of Medicine: Children's General Clinical Research Center, 3323

Baylor College of Medicine: Cullen Eye Institute, 9855

Baylor College of Medicine: Debakey Heart Center, 4809

Baylor College of Medicine: Epilepsy Research Center, 7534

Baylor College of Medicine: General Clinical Research Center for Adults, 3869

Baylor College of Medicine: General Clinical Research Center Adults, 4810

Baylor College of Medicine: Jerry Lewis Neuromuscular Disease Research, 6689

Baylor College of Medicine: Sleep Disorder and Research Center, 7826

Baylor University Bone Marrow Transplantat Baylor Research Institute, 2303

Baylor University Bone Marrow Transplantation Research Center, 2302

Beacon Lighthouse, 9656

Brain Injury Association of Texas, 4053

Brain Tumor Support Group: El Paso, 1933

CCFA Houston Gulf Coast/South Texas Chapter, 2967

CCFA North Texas Chapter, 2968

Cancer Therapy and Research Center, 2304

Centers for AIDS Research: Baylor College of Medicine, 367

Central Texas Brain Tumor Support Group, 1934

Central Texas FFCMH, 6145

Central Texas Veterans Health Care System, 10387

Cerebral Blood Flow Laboratories Veterans Administration Medical Center, 8136

Children's Heart Institute of Texas, 4816

Convention of American Instructors of the Deaf, 4243

Cook Children's Medical Center: Cystic Fibrosis Clinic, 3107

Cooley's Anemia Foundation (CAF): Texas, 2900

Cystic Fibrosis Care and Teaching Center Children's Medical Center, 3108

Cystic Fibrosis-Lung Disease Center: Santa Rosa Children's Hospital, 3109

Dallas Lighthouse for the Blind, 9657

Dallas/Ft.Worth Metroplex HPV Support Group, 10646

Department of State Health Offices, 8903

Disability Rights Texas, 10647

Down Syndrome Clinic of Houston, 3515

Down Syndrome Guild of Dallas, 3504

East Texas Lighthouse for the Blind, 9658

El Paso Lighthouse for the Blind, 9659

El Paso VA Health Care Center, 10388

Greater Houston Chapter SIDS Alliance, 8904

Greater South Texas Chapter of the Myasthenia Gravis Foundation of America, 6784

Gulf States Hemophilia Diagnostic and Treatment Center, 4974

Harris County FFCMH, 6239

Harris County Public Health and Environmental Services, 8905

Houston Area Brain Tumor Network, 1935

Houston Department of Health and Human Services: Bureau of HIV Prevention, 291

Houston Ear Research Foundation, 4316

Houston Public Library Access Center, 9830

Houston Support Group: National Ataxia Foundation, 1464

Houston/South Texas Turner Syndrome Society, 9386

Hydrocephalus Association of North Texas, 5163

Independent Living Research Utilization Project, 2596

Institute for Rehabilitation and Research, 4065

International Medical Society of Paralegia: US Office, 8029

Juvenile Diabetes Research Foundation: Dal las Chapter, 3293

Juvenile Diabetes Research Foundation: Gre ater Fort Worth/ Arlington Chapter, 3294

Juvenile Diabetes Research Foundation: Hou ston/Gulf Coast Chapter, 3295

Juvenile Diabetes Research Foundation: South Central Texas Chapter, 3292

Juvenile Diabetes Research Foundation: Wes t Texas Chapter, 3296

Kent Waldrep National Paralysis Foundation Main Office, 8031

Kidd's Kids, 10823

LAUNCH Department of Special Education, 10544

Leukemia and Lymphoma Society: North Texas Chapter, 2166

Leukemia and Lymphoma Society: South/West Texas Chapter, 2167

Leukemia and Lymphoma Society: Texas Gulf Coast Chapter, 2168

Lighthouse for the Blind of Houston, 9660

Lighthouse of the Blind of Fort Worth, 9661

Lone Star Chapter of the American Association of Kidney Patients, 5634

Lone Star Chapter of the National Hemophilia Foundation, 4952

Lupus Foundation of America: North Texas Chapter, 5977

Lupus Foundation of America: South Central Texas Chapter, 5978

Lupus Foundation of America: Texas Gulf Coast Chapter, 5979

Lupus Foundation of America: West Texas Chapter, 5980

Mended Hearts, 4863

Michael E. DeBakey VA Medical Center, 10389

Mothers Against Drunk Driving (MADD), 8212

National Association of Blind Students Angela Wolf, 9484

National Federation of the Blind: Texas, 9662

National Kidney Foundation of North Texas, 5635

National Kidney Foundation of South Texas, 5636

National Kidney Foundation of Southeast Texas, 5637
National Kidney Foundation of West Texas, 5638
National Kidney Foundation of the Texas Coastal Bend, 5639
National MS Society: North Central Texas Chapter, 6587
National MS Society: Panhandle Chapter, 6588
National MS Society: Southern Texas, 6589
National MS Society: West Texas Division, 6590
National MS Socisty: Southeast Texas Chapter, 6591
National Ovarian Cancer Coalition, 2028
Neuromuscular Treatment Center: Univ. of Texas Southwestern Medical Center, 6607
North Texas Comprehensive Adult Hemophilia Center, 4997
North Texas Comprehensive Pediatric Hemophilia Center, 4998
North Texas FFCMH, 6146
North Texas Support Group: National Ataxia Foundation, 1465
Northwest Texas Chapter of the Myasthenia Gravis Foundation of America, 6785
Operation Desert Shield/Desert Storm, 10390
PWSA Texas Chapter Prader-Willi Syndrome Association, 7242
Persian Gulf Veterans of America, 10391
Presbyterian Hospital of Dallas, 7107
RESOLVE of Central Texas, 5392
RESOLVE of Dallas/Fort Worth, 5393
RESOLVE of Houston, 5394
RESOLVE of South Texas, 5395
RRTC on Community Integration of Persons with TBI, 4041
Region VI Office Program Consultants for Maternal and Child Health, 8906
Rio Grande Chapter: NSCIA Rio Vista Rehabilitation Hospital, 8056
Roy M and Phyllis Gough Huffington Center on Aging, 83
San Antonio Bexar County FFCMH, 6147
San Antonio Cancer Institute, 2305
Santa Rosa Medical Center, 3521
Scleroderma Foundation: Bluebonnet Chapter, 7406
Sickle Cell Anemia Association of Austin: Marc Thomas Chapter, 7682
Sickle Cell Association of the Texas Gulf Coast, 7674
Sleep Medicine Associates of Texas, 7870
South Central Region: Helen Keller National Center, 9663
South Texas Brain Tumor Foundation Support Group, 1936
South Texas Comprehensive Hemophilia Center: Santa Rosa Health Corporation, 5007
South Texas Lighthouse for the Blind, 9664
South Texas Veterans Health Care System, 10392
Southeast Louisiana Turner Syndrome Society, 9366
Southwest Foundation for Biomedical Research, 2306
Southwest SIDS Research Institute, 8907
Spina Bifida Association of Austin, 7972
Spina Bifida Association of Dallas, 7973
Spina Bifida Association of Texas, Gulf Coast, 7974
St. Louis Turner Syndrome Society, 9363
Stroke Clubs International, 8148
Taping for the Blind, 9512
Texas Alliance for the Mentally Ill, 6148
Texas Ambassador: National Ataxia Foundation, 1466
Texas Association of Retinitis Pigmentosa, 9665
Texas Association of the Deaf, 4295
Texas Association on Mental Retardation, 3505
Texas Central Chapter of the National Hemophilia Foundation, 4953
Texas Children's Allergy and Immunology Clinic, 590
Texas Childrens Cystic Fibrosis Care Center, 3110
Texas Commission on Alcohol and Drug Abuse Department Of State Health, 8285
Texas Department of Health: Bureau of HIV and STD Prevention, 292
Texas FFCMH, 6149
Texas Heart Institute St Lukes Episcopal Hospital, 4842
Texas Mining and Reclamation Association, 6054
Texas Neurofibromatosis Foundation, 6863
Texas State Library, 9831
Texas State Library: Talking Book Program, 9832

Texas Tech University Tarbox Parkinson's Disease Institute, 7086
The Alzheimer's Disease & Memory Disorders Center, 876
Thomas T. Connally Medical Center Marlin,T X, 10393
Travis Association for the Blind, 9666
Tri-Services Military Cystic Fibrosis Center, 3111
Turner Syndrome Society Resource Center, 9390
Turner's Syndrome Society, 9357
Turner's Syndrome Society of North Texas, 9387
Turner's Syndrome Society of the United States, 9355
United Cerebral Palsy of Greater Houston, 2712
United Cerebral Palsy of Metropolitan Dallas, 2713
United Cerebral Palsy of Tarrant County, 2714
United Cerebral Palsy of Texas, 2715
University of Texas General Clinical Research Center, 3346
University of Texas HSC at San Antonio, 7108
University of Texas Health Science Center, 7425
University of Texas Health Science Center Neurophysiology Research Center, 8334
University of Texas Mental Health Clinical Research Center, 6364
University of Texas Sleep/Wake Disorders Center, 7879
University of Texas Southwestern Medical, 5745
University of Texas Southwestern Medical Center, 5744
University of Texas Southwestern Medical Center at Dallas, 594
University of Texas Southwestern Medical Center at Dallas, 4856
University of Texas Southwestern Medical Center/Sickle Cell Management, 7677
University of Texas at Austin: Drug Synamics Institute, 8335
University of Texas at Dallas Callier Center for Communication Disorders, 4343
University of Texas: MD Anderson Cancer Center, 2307
University of Texas: Medical Branch at Galveston Cancer Center, 2308
University of Texas: Southwestern Medical Center at Dallas, Immunodermatology, 7736
VA Data Processing Center, 10194
VA Heart of Texas Health Care Network Dallas VA Medical Center, 10394
VISN 17: VA Heart of Texas Health Care Network, 10395
VIVA!, 8070
Veterans Adm. Medical Center: Big Spring, 10396
Veterans Adm. Medical Center: Dallas, 10397
Veterans Adm. Medical Center: Kerrville, 10398
Veterans Adm. Medical Center: Marlin, 10399
Veterans Adm. Medical Center: San Antonio, 10400
Veterans Adm. Medical Center: Temple, 10401
Waco VA Medical Center, 10402
West Texas Lighthouse for the Blind, 9667
West Texas VA Health Care System, 10403

Utah

AARP Utah State Office: Midvale, 68
Allies with Families, 6240
Alzheimer's Association: Utah Chapter, 823
American Cancer Society: Utah, 2169
American Diabetes Association: Utah, 3297
American Lung Association of Utah, 5847
American Lung Association of Utah, 9315
Arthritis Foundation: Utah/Idaho Chapter, 1133
Brain Injury Association of Utah, 4054
Brain Injury Association of Utah Helpline, 4120
Brigham Young University Cancer Research Center, 2309
Cancer Wellness House, 1937
Department of Social Services: Division of Substance Abuse, 8286
Huntsman Cancer Institute University of Utah School of Medicine, 2310

Intermountain Donor Services, 9227
Legal Center for People with Disabilities, 10648
Lupus Foundation of America Utah Chapter, 5981
National Clearinghouse of Rehabilitation Training Materials, 10556
National Federation of the Blind: Utah, 9668
National Kidney Foundation of Utah, 5640
National MS Society: Utah State Chapter, 6592
Prader-Willi Utah Association Prader-Willi Syndrome Association, 7243
Pregnancy Risk Line, 1766
RESOLVE of Utah, 5396
United Cerebral Palsy of Utah, 2716
University of Utah Intermountain Cystic Fibrosis Center, 3112
University of Utah Rocky Mountain Center for Occupational & Environmental Health, 5854
University of Utah Utah Genome Depot University of Utah, 6695
University of Utah: Artificial Heart Research Laboratory, 4857
University of Utah: Cardiovascular Genetic Research Clinic, 4858
University of Utah: Center for Human Toxicology, 8336
Utah Alliance for the Mentally Ill, 6150
Utah Chapter of the National Hemophilia Foundation, 4954
Utah Department of Health, 8908
Utah Department of Health: Bureau of Communicable Disease Control, 293
Utah Industries for the Blind, 9669
Utah SIDS Alliance, 8909
Utah State Intermountain Chapter of the Myasthenia Gravis Foundation of America, 6786
Utah State Library Division, 9833
Utah Support Group: National Ataxia Foundation, 1467
Utah Turner Syndrome Society, 9388
VA Salt Lake City Health Care System, 10404
Veterans Affairs Medical Center: Research Service, 3349

VI

AARP Virgin Islands State Office: St Croix, 75

Vermont

AARP Vermont State Office: Montpelier, 69
ALS Clinical Department of Neurology College of Medicine of the University of, 1034
Alcohol and Drug Abuse Programs of Vermont Department Of Health, 8287
Alzheimer's Association: Vermont Chapter, 824
American Cancer Society: Vermont, 2170
American Diabetes Association: Vermont, 3298
American Lung Association of Vermont, 9316
Autism Society of Vermont Autism Society of America, 1616
Brain Injury Association of Vermont, 4055
Brain Injury Association of Vermont Helpli ne, 4121
Citizen Advocacy of Burlington, 10649
Client Assistance Program: Vermont Ladd Hall, 10650
Lupus Foundation of America: Vermont Chapter, 5982
Medical Center Hospital of Vermont Cystic Fibrosis Center, 3113
National Federation of the Blind: Vermont, 9670
National MS Society: Vermont Division, 6593
RESOLVE of Vermont, 5397
University of Vermont Cancer Center University of Vermont, 2311
University of Vermont: Office of Health Promotion Research, 368
Vermont Alliance for the Mentally Ill, 6151
Vermont Department of Health: Health Surveillance HIV/AIDS/STD/TB Program, 294
Vermont Department of Health: SIDS Information and Counseling Program, 8910
Vermont Department of Libraries Special Services Unit, 9834

Autism Society of Washington, 1618
BABES Network-YWCA, 377
Benaroya Research Institute Virginia Mason Medical Center, 3324
Brain Cancer Support Group: Port Orchard, 1940
Brain Cancer Support Group: Seattle, 1941
Brain Injury Association of Washington, 4057
Brain Injury Association of Washington Hel, 4058
Brain Injury Association of Washington Hel pline, 4124
CCFA Washington State Chapter, 2970
Cancer Information Service, 2321
Centers for AIDS Research: University of Washington, Harborview Medical Center, 369
Common Voice for Pierce County Parents, 6244
Dunshee House, 380
Epilepsy Foundation of North West Washington, 7533
Fred Hutchinson Cancer Research Center, 2314
Gluten Intolerance Group: GIG, 2561
HIV Prevention Trials Unit University of Washington/Seattle HPTU Si, 370
Head Injury Hotline, 4125
Health Information Network, 207
Health Information Network for Women and AIDS, 208
Hemophilia Foundation of Washington, 4957
Hepatitis Education Project, 5098
Hepatitis Education Project, 5100
Hope Heart Institute, 4829
Hydrocephalus Support Group of Seattle, 5164
Inland Empire Bleeding Disorders, 4958
International Association for the Study of Pain, 2843
International Association for the Study of Pain, 10542
Juvenile Diabetes Research Foundation: Sea ttle Chapter, 3305
Juvenile Diabetes Research Foundation: Seattle Guild, 3304
Juvenile Diabetes Research Foundation: Spo kane County Area Chapter, 3306
LifeCenter Northwest, 9230
Lighthouse for the Blind of Washington, 9673
Lupus Foundation of America: Pacific Northwest Chapter, 5986
Mental Illness Research and Education Institute, 6170
Multifaith Works, 215
Myasthenia Gravis Foundation: Greater St. Louis Chapter, 6769
NAMI Washington (National Alliance for the Mentally Ill of Washington), 6154
National Association for Native American Children of Alcoholics, 8215
National Eating Disorders Association, 3614
National Eating Disorders Association Long Island, 3625
National Federation of the Blind: Public Employees Division, 9499
National Federation of the Blind: Washington, 9674
National MS Society: Greater Washington Chapter, 6597
National MS Society: Inland Northwest Chapter, 6598
National Service Dog Center, 9902
Northwest AIDS Education and Training Center (AETC), 296
Northwestern Region: Helen Keller National Center, 9675
Pacific NW Support Group, 7291
Pacific Northwest Chapter of the Myasthenia Gravis Foundation of America, 6788
Persian Gulf Veterans of Washington, 10412
Prader-Willi Northwest Association, 7229
Prader-Willi Northwest Association Prader-Willi Syndrome Association, 7245
Puget Sound Blood Center, 5002
Region X Office Program Consultants for Maternal and Child Health, 8914
SIDS Foundation of Washington, 8915
SIDS Northwest Regional Center, 8916
Scleroderma Foundation: Evergreen Chapter, 7409
Seattle HPV Support Group, 10653
Seattle Support Group: National Ataxia Foundation, 1468
Solomon Park Research Institute, 1042
Spina Bifida Association of Evergreen, 7975
United Cerebral Palsy of Pierce County, 2719
University of Washington, 7109

University of Washington Department of Speech & Hearing Sciences, 4344
University of Washington Diabetes: Endocrinology Research Center, 3347
University of Washington Speech and Hearing Clinic, 4345
University of Washington: Cystic Fibrosis Center, 3116
University of Washington: Experimental Education Unit, 3524
VA Puget Sound Health Care System, 10413
Veterans Adm. Medical Center: Seattle, 10414
Veterans Adm. Medical Center: Spokane Spokane VA Medical Center, 10415
Veterans Adm. Medical Center: Tacoma Tacoma Vet Center, 10416
Veterans Adm. Medical Center: Walla Walla Johnathan M. Wainwright Memorial VA MC, 10417
Virginia Mason Brain Tumor Support Group, 1942
Virginia Mason Medical Center Neuroscience Institute, 1044
Washington Ambassador National Ataxia Foundation, 1469
Washington Department of Health: Division of HIV/AIDS Prevention Services, 297
Washington Department of Social and Health Services, Alcohol and Drug Prog., 8289
Washington FFCMH, 6155
Washington Leukemia and Lymphoma Society: Alaska Chapter, 2176
Washington Puget Sound Turner Syndrome Society, 9389
Washington State Client Assistance Program, 10654
Washington State Department of Health Maternal & Child Health Office, 8917
Washington State Department of Services for the Blind, 9676
Washington Talking Book & Braille Library, 9845
Wenatchee Valley Brain Tumor Support Group, 1943
Wishing Star Foundation, 10836

West Virginia

AARP West Virginia Office: Charleston, 72
AFB Midwest: American Foundation for the Blind, 9553
AFB Technology & Employment Center, 9677
Alzheimer's Association: Greater Mid-Ohio Valley Chapter, 834
Alzheimer's Association: N Central West Virginia Chapter, 835
Alzheimer's Association: South West Virginia Chapter, 836
American Cancer Society: West Virginia, 2177
American Diabetes Association: West Virginia, 3307
American Diabetes Association: Wisconsin, 3308
American Lung Association of West Virginia, 5850
American Lung Association of West Virginia, 9319
Autism Services Center, 1567
Autism Services Center, 1621
Autism Socity of West Virginia, 1619
Brain Injury Association of West Virginia, 4059
Brain Injury Association of West Virginia Helpline, 4126
Brain Tumor Support Group: Southern West Virginia, 1944
Cabell County Public Library, 9846
Health Science Library, 3316
Hemophilia Association of the Huntington A Marshall University School of Medicine, 4978
Hemophilia Association of the Huntington Area, 4977
Hemophilia Center of West Virginia University Health Sciences Center, 4981
Juvenile Diabetes Research Foundation: Hun tington Chapter, 3309
Kanawha County Public Library, 9847
Mountain State/Parents/Children/ Adolescents Network, 6156
NAMI West Virginia, 6157
National Association of Therapeutic Wilderness Camps, 6046
National Autism Hotline Autism Services Center, 1633

National Federation of the Blind: West Virginia, 9678
National Job Accommodation Network, 10565
Northcentral West Virginia HPV Support Group, 10655
Office of Maternal, Child & Family Health, 8918
Ohio County Public Library Services for the Blind and Physically Handicapped, 9848
Parkersburg and Wood County Public Library, 9849
The West Virginia Autism Training Center Marshall University, 1630
Veterans Adm. Medical Center: Beckley Beckley VA Medical Center, 10418
Veterans Adm. Medical Center: Clarksburg Louis A. Johnson VA Medical Center, 10419
Veterans Adm. Medical Center: Huntington, 10420
Veterans Affairs Medical Center: Martinsburg, 10421
West Virginia Advocates, 10656
West Virginia Department of Health & Human Resources, 298
West Virginia Division of Alcohol & Drug Abuse, 8290
West Virginia Library Commission, 9850
West Virginia Mountaineer Chapter: NSCIA, 8058
West Virginia School for the Blind, 9851
West Virginia University Cystic Fibrosis Center, 3117
West Virginia University: Mary Babb Randolph Cancer Center, 2315

Wisconsin

AARP Wisconsin State Office: Madison, 73
AIDS Network, 173
ALS Association: Southeast Wisconsin Chapter, 1031
ASTHMA Hotline, 596
About Kids GI Disorders, 3638
Alzheimer's Association: Greater Wisconsin Chapter, 837
Alzheimer's Association: Indianhead Chapter, 838
Alzheimer's Association: Lake Superior Chapter, 839
Alzheimer's Association: Midstate Wisconsin Chapter, 840
Alzheimer's Association: North Central Wisconsin Chapter, 841
Alzheimer's Association: Northeast Wisconsin Chapter, 842
Alzheimer's Association: South Central Wisconsin Chapter, 843
Alzheimer's Association: Southeast Wisconsin Chapter, 844
American Academy for Cerebral Palsy and Developmental Medicine, 2593
American Academy of Allergy, Asthma & Immunology, 561
American Academy of Allergy, Asthma & Immunology, 1272
American Association of Children's Residential Centers, 6031
American Cancer Society: Wisconsin, 2178
American Diabetes Association: Wisconsin, 3310
American Liver Foundation Wisconsin Chapter, 5741
American Lung Association of Wisconsin, 5851
American Lung Association of Wisconsin, 9320
American Red Cross Hemophilia Center, 4962
Anxiety Disorders Center University of Wisconsin, 6165
Arthritis Foundation: Wisconsin Chapter Foundation, 1137
Autism Society of Wisconsin, 1620
Brain Injury Association of Wisconsin, 4060
Brain Injury Association of Wisconsin Help line, 4127
Brain Tumor Support Group: John Sierzant Lutheran Hospital, Gunderson Clinic, 1945
Brown County Library, 9852
CCFA Wisconsin Chapter, 2971
Children's Brittle Bone Foundation, 6956
Clement J. Zablocki Veterans Affairs Medical Center, 10422
Counseling and Research Center for SIDS, 8919
Cyclic Vomiting Syndrome Association, 3852
Down Syndrome Association of Wisconsin, 3507
Eau Claire Hemophilia Center, 4970
Endometriosis Association International, 3715
FASST, Friends & Survivors Standing Together, 4005

Governor's Committee for People with Disabilities, 10657
Great Lakes Hemophilia Foundation, 4959
Greater Milwaukee Area Chapter: NSCIA Sacred Heart Rehabilitation Hospital, 8059
Grief & Loss Support Group, 10859
Gulf War Veterans of Wisconsin, 10423
Gundersen Clinic Comprehensive Hemophilia Treatment Center, 4975
Hematology Treatment Center of the Great Lakes Hemophilia Foundation, 4976
Infant Death Center of Wisconsin Childrens Hospital Of Wisconsin, 8920
International Foundation for Functional Gastrointestinal Disorders (IFFGD), 2925
International Foundation for Functional Gastrointestinal Disorders, 3855
International Foundation for Functional Gastrointestinal Disorders (IFFGD), 5299
Juvenile Diabetes Research Foundation: Gre ater Madison Chapter, 3312
Juvenile Diabetes Research Foundation: Nor theast Wisconsin Chapter, 3313
Juvenile Diabetes Research Foundation: Southeastern Chapter, 3311
Kids with Heart National Association for Children's Heart Disorders, 2879
LODAT: Brain Tumor Support Group, 1946
Leukemia and Lymphoma Society: Wisconsin Chapter, 2179
Lupus Foundation of America: Wisconsin Chapter, 5987
Medical College of Wisconsin: Cystic Fibrosis Clinic, 3118
MidWest Gulf War Veterans Association, 10424
Myasthenia Gravis Support Group of Wiscons in, 6793
NNFF Wisconsin Chapter, 6855
National Federation of the Blind: Wisconsin, 9679
National Federation of the Blind: Writers, 9680
National Kidney Foundation of Wisconsin, 5644
National MS Society: Wisconsin Chapter, 6600
Obsessive Compulsive Information Center Dean Foundation, 6052
Office of Alcohol and Other Drug Abuse, 8291
PWSA of Wisconsin Prader-Willi Syndrome Association, 7246
Physician Referral and Information Line, 1303
RESOLVE of Wisconsin, 5399
Scoliosis Research Society, 7455
Society for the Study of Reproduction, 5400
Spina Bifida Association of Northern Wisconsin, 7976
Spina Bifida Association of Northwest Ohio, 7977
Spina Bifida Association of Southeastern Wisconsin, 7978
Spina Bifida Association of the Greater Fox Valley, 7979
Stem Cell Research Program University of Wisconsin-Madison, 1043
Trace Center University of Wisconsin: Madison, 4334
United Cerebral Palsy of Greater Dane County, 2720
United Cerebral Palsy of North Central Wisconsin, 2721
United Cerebral Palsy of Southeastern Wisconsin, 2722
United Cerebral Palsy of West Central Wisconsin, 2723
United Cerebral Palsy of Wisconsin, 2724
United Special Sportsman Alliance, 10847
University of Wisconsin Madison Neurophysiology Laboratory, 7540
University of Wisconsin Milwaukee Medicinal Chemistry Group, 8337
University of Wisconsin Organ Procurement Organization, 9231
University of Wisconsin Paul P Carbone Comprehensive Cancer Center, 2317
University of Wisconsin-Madison: Cystic Fibrosis/Pulmonary Center, 3119
University of Wisconsin: Asthma, Allergy and Pulmonary Research Center, 1299
University of Wisconsin: Auditory Physiology Center, 4346
Veterans Adm. Medical Center: Tomah, 10425

We Are the Children's Hope/Support Group, 6245
William S. Middleton Memorial Veterans Hospital, 10426
Wisconsin Alliance for the Mentally Ill, 6158
Wisconsin Association of the Deaf, 4297
Wisconsin Chapter of the Myasthenia Gravis Foundation of America, 6789
Wisconsin Department of Health and Social Services: Division of Health, 299
Wisconsin Family Ties, 6159
Wisconsin Parkinson Association, 7082
Wisconsin Regional Library for the Blind Talking Book Program, 9853
Wiscraft: Wisconsin Enterprises for the Blind, 9681
Wisonsin Donor Network, 9232

Wyoming

AARP Wyoming State Office: Cheyenne, 74
Alcohol & Drug Abuse Programs of Wyoming Department Of Health, 8292
Alzheimer's Wyoming, 846
American Cancer Society: Wyoming, 2180
Brain Injury Association of Wyoming, 4061
Brain Injury Association of Wyoming, 4128
Concerned Parent Coalition, 6246
Deaf Association of Wyoming, 4298
National Federation of the Blind: Wyoming, 9682
National MS Society: Wyoming Chapter, 6601
Uplift, 6247
Veterans Adm. Medical Center: Cheyenne, 10427
Veterans Adm. Medical Center: Sheridan, 10428
Wyoming Alliance for the Mentally Ill, 6160
Wyoming Department of Health, 8921
Wyoming Department of Health HIV/AIDS/Hepatitis Program, 300
Wyoming Protection & Advocacy System, 10658
Wyoming Services for the Visually Disabled, 9854

General Reference

American Environmental Leaders: From Colonial Times to the Present
An African Biographical Dictionary
Encyclopedia of African-American Writing
Encyclopedia of American Industries
Encyclopedia of Emerging Industries
Encyclopedia of Global Industries
Encyclopedia of Gun Control & Gun Rights
Encyclopedia of Invasions & Conquests
Encyclopedia of Prisoners of War & Internment
Encyclopedia of Religion & Law in America
Encyclopedia of Rural America
Encyclopedia of the United States Cabinet, 1789-2010
Encyclopedia of Warrior Peoples & Fighting Groups
Environmental Resource Handbook
From Suffrage to the Senate: America's Political Women
Global Terror & Political Risk Assessment
Historical Dictionary of War Journalism
Human Rights in the United States
Nations of the World
Political Corruption in America
Speakers of the House of Representatives, 1789-2009
The Environmental Debate: A Documentary History
The Evolution Wars: A Guide to the Debates
The Religious Right: A Reference Handbook
The Value of a Dollar: 1860-2009
The Value of a Dollar: Colonial Era
University & College Museums, Galleries & Related Facilities
Weather America
World Cultural Leaders of the 20th & 21st Centuries
Working Americans 1880-1999 Vol. I: The Working Class
Working Americans 1880-1999 Vol. II: The Middle Class
Working Americans 1880-1999 Vol. III: The Upper Class
Working Americans 1880-1999 Vol. IV: Their Children
Working Americans 1880-2003 Vol. V: At War
Working Americans 1880-2005 Vol. VI: Women at Work
Working Americans 1880-2006 Vol. VII: Social Movements
Working Americans 1880-2007 Vol. VIII: Immigrants
Working Americans 1770-1869 Vol. IX: Revol. War to the Civil War
Working Americans 1880-2009 Vol. X: Sports & Recreation
Working Americans 1880-2010 Vol. XI: Entrepreneurs & Inventors

Bowker's Books In Print®Titles

Books In Print®
Books In Print® Supplement
American Book Publishing Record® Annual
American Book Publishing Record® Monthly
Books Out Loud™
Bowker's Complete Video Directory™
Children's Books In Print®
Complete Directory of Large Print Books & Serials™
El-Hi Textbooks & Serials In Print®
Forthcoming Books®
Law Books & Serials In Print™
Medical & Health Care Books In Print™
Publishers, Distributors & Wholesalers of the US™
Subject Guide to Books In Print®
Subject Guide to Children's Books In Print®

Business Information

Directory of Business Information Resources
Directory of Mail Order Catalogs
Directory of Venture Capital & Private Equity Firms
Food & Beverage Market Place
Grey House Homeland Security Directory
Grey House Performing Arts Directory
Hudson's Washington News Media Contacts Directory
New York State Directory
Sports Market Place Directory
The Rauch Guides – Industry Market Research Reports

Statistics & Demographics

America's Top-Rated Cities
America's Top-Rated Small Towns & Cities
America's Top-Rated Smaller Cities
Comparative Guide to American Suburbs
Comparative Guide to Health in America
Profiles of... Series – State Handbooks

Health Information

Comparative Guide to American Hospitals
Comparative Guide to Health in America
Complete Directory for Pediatric Disorders
Complete Directory for People with Chronic Illness
Complete Directory for People with Disabilities
Complete Mental Health Directory
Directory of Health Care Group Purchasing Organizations
Directory of Hospital Personnel
HMO/PPO Directory
Medical Device Register
Older Americans Information Directory

Education Information

Charter School Movement
Comparative Guide to American Elementary & Secondary Schools
Complete Learning Disabilities Directory
Educators Resource Directory
Special Education

TheStreet.com Ratings Guides

TheStreet.com Ratings Consumer Box Set
TheStreet.com Ratings Guide to Bank Fees & Service Charges
TheStreet.com Ratings Guide to Banks & Thrifts
TheStreet.com Ratings Guide to Bond & Money Market Mutual Funds
TheStreet.com Ratings Guide to Common Stocks
TheStreet.com Ratings Guide to Credit Unions
TheStreet.com Ratings Guide to Exchange-Traded Funds
TheStreet.com Ratings Guide to Health Insurers
TheStreet.com Ratings Guide to Life & Annuity Insurers
TheStreet.com Ratings Guide to Property & Casualty Insurers
TheStreet.com Ratings Guide to Stock Mutual Funds
TheStreet.com Ratings Ultimate Guided Tour of Stock Investing

Canadian General Reference

Associations Canada
Canadian Almanac & Directory
Canadian Environmental Resource Guide
Canadian Parliamentary Guide
Financial Services Canada
History of Canada
Libraries Canada

Grey House Publishing
4919 Route 22, PO Box 56, Amenia NY 12501-0056 | (800) 562-2139 | www.greyhouse.com | books@greyhouse.com